PEARSON'S

Comprehensive
Medical Assisting

Administrative and Clinical Competencies

Nina Beaman, MS, RNC, CMA
Bryant and Stratton College
Richmond, VA

Lorraine Fleming-McPhillips, MS, MT, CMA
Medical Assisting Program Coordinator (retired)
Quinebaug Valley Community College
Danielson, Connecticut

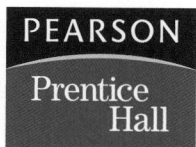

PEARSON
Prentice
Hall

Upper Saddle River, New Jersey 07458

Library of Congress Cataloging-in-Publication Data

Pearson's administrative medical assisting.
   p. ; cm.
   Includes index.
   ISBN 0-13-220904-7 (v. 1)—ISBN 0-13-199042-X (v. 2)—
ISBN 0-13-174206-X (v. 3)—ISBN 0-13-171577-1 (v. 4)
1. Medical assistants.   2. Medical secretaries.   3. Medical
offices—Management.
   [DNLM: 1. Physician Assistants.   2. Medical Secretaries.
3. Practice Management, Medical. W 21.5 P362 2006]
I. Title: Administrative medical assisting.   II. Pearson/
Prentice Hall.
R728.8.P43 2006
610.73'7—dc22
                                                          2005036391

Publisher: Julie Levin Alexander
Publisher's Assistant: Regina Bruno
Executive Editor: Joan Gill
Assistant Editor: Bronwen Glowacki
Development Editor: Teri Zak
Associate Development Editor: Triple SSS Press Media
   Development
Senior Marketing Manager: Harper Coles
Director of Marketing: Karen Allman
Marketing Coordinator: Michael Sirinides
Marketing Assistant: Wayne Celia, Jr.
Director of Production and Manufacturing: Bruce Johnson
Media Product Manager: John Jordan
Manager of Media Production: Amy Peltier
New Media Project Manager: Tina Rudowski
Manufacturing Manager: Ilene Sanford
Managing Editor: Patrick Walsh

Production Liaison: Julie Li
Project Manager: Shelley L. Creager
Senior Design Coordinator: Christopher Weigand
Interior Designer: Brigid Kavanagh and Pearson Education
   Development Group
Cover Designer: Yin Wong, Pearson Education
   Development Group
Director, Image Resource Center: Melinda Reo
Manager, Rights and Permissions: Zina Arabia
Manager, Visual Research: Beth Brenzel
Manager, Cover Visual Research & Permissions:
   Karen Sanatar
Image Permission Coordinator: Frances Toepfer
Composition: Techbooks
Printing and Binding: Courier Kendallville
Cover Printer: Phoenix Color Corporation

Pearson Education Ltd., *London*
Pearson Education Australia Pty. Limited, *Sydney*
Pearson Education Singapore, Pte. Ltd.
Pearson Education North Asia Ltd., *Hong Kong*
Pearson Education Canada, Ltd., *Toronto*
Pearson Educación de Mexico, S.A. de C.V.
Pearson Education—Japan, *Tokyo*
Pearson Education Malaysia, Pte. Ltd.
Pearson Education, Upper Saddle River, New Jersey

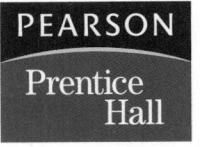

10 9 8 7 6 5 4 3 2 1
ISBN 0-13-171577-1

Brief Contents

Unit One   Introduction to Health Care   1

Chapter 1   Medical Assisting: The Profession . 2
Chapter 2   Medical Science: History and Practice 14
Chapter 3   Medical Law and Ethics 42
Chapter 4   Communications: Verbal and Nonverbal 64

Unit Two   Administrative Medical Assisting   93

Chapter 5   The Office Environment 94
Chapter 6   Telephone Techniques 112
Chapter 7   Patient Reception 128
Chapter 8   Appointment Scheduling 142
Chapter 9   Office Facilities, Equipment, and Supplies 158
Chapter 10 Written Communication 170
Chapter 11 Computers in the Medical Office 192
Chapter 12 Managing Medical Records 206
Chapter 13 Fees, Billing, Collections, and Credit. 226
Chapter 14 Financial Management 246
Chapter 15 Medical Insurance. 268
Chapter 16 Medical Insurance Claims 284
Chapter 17 Medical Coding 298
Chapter 18 Medical Office Management. . . . 316

Unit Three   Anatomy and Physiology   339

Chapter 19 Body Structure and Function . . . 340
Chapter 20 The Integumentary System 360
Chapter 21 The Skeletal System 376
Chapter 22 The Muscular System 392
Chapter 23 The Nervous System 404
Chapter 24 The Senses 422
Chapter 25 The Circulatory System. 434
Chapter 26 The Immune System 460
Chapter 27 The Respiratory System 472
Chapter 28 The Digestive System 488

Chapter 29 The Urinary System 508
Chapter 30 The Endocrine System. 520
Chapter 31 The Reproductive System 536

Unit Four   Clinical Medical Assisting   559

Chapter 32 Infection Control 560
Chapter 33 Vital Signs. 588
Chapter 34 Assisting with Physical Examinations 630
Chapter 35 Assisting with Medical Specialties 658
Chapter 36 Assisting in Eye and Ear Care . . . 706
Chapter 37 Assisting in Life Span Specialties 730
Chapter 38 Assisting with Minor Surgery . . . 762
Chapter 39 Assisting with Medical Emergencies 800
Chapter 40 The Clinical Laboratory 834
Chapter 41 Microbiology 850
Chapter 42 Urinalysis 878
Chapter 43 Hematology 900
Chapter 44 Radiology 928
Chapter 45 Electrocardiography and Pulmonary Function 954
Chapter 46 Physical Therapy and Rehabilitation 978
Chapter 47 Math for Pharmacology 1010
Chapter 48 Pharmacology. 1022
Chapter 49 Administering Medications 1046
Chapter 50 Patient Education 1080
Chapter 51 Nutrition 1096
Chapter 52 Psychology 1120

Unit Five   Career Assistance   1139

Chapter 53 Externship and Career Opportunities 1140

Appendices. A-1
Glossary G-1
Index I-1

Contents

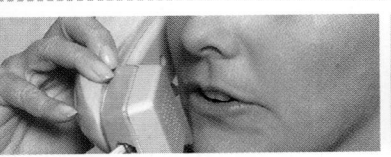
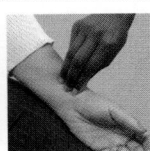

Unit One   Introduction to Health Care   1

Chapter 1

Medical Assisting: The Profession   2

History of Medical Assisting 4
Education and Training for the
     Medical Assistant 4
Role of the Medical Assistant 5
Characteristics of a Good Medical Assistant 7
Professional Organizations 9
Career Opportunities 10

Chapter 2

Medical Science: History and Practice   14

History of Medicine 16
Medical Practitioners 23
Medical Practice Acts 24
Health Care Costs and Payments 25
Types of Medical Practices 26
Medical and Surgical Specialties. 27
Health Care Institutions. 30
Allied Health Professionals 33
Centers for Disease Control 38

Chapter 3

Medical Law and Ethics   42

Classification of Law 44
Professional Liability 46
Patient/Physician Relationship 49
Documentation 52
Public Duties of Physicians 53

Drug Regulations 53
Role of the Medical Assistant 54
Code of Ethics 56
Medical Ethics 56
AMA Principles of Medical Ethics 57
Medical Assistant's Principles of
     Medical Ethics 57
Medical Assistant's Standard of Care 58
The Patient's Bill of Rights 58
Confidentiality 59
Ethical Issues and Personal Choice 60

Chapter 4

Communications:
Verbal and Nonverbal   64

Interpersonal Dynamics 66
The Communication Process 68
Communication Techniques 72
Procedure 4-1: Effective Listening Skills 73
Assertive versus Aggressive Behavior 75
Barriers to Communication 76
Communication in Special Circumstances 80
Procedure 4-2: Assisting the Hearing
     Impaired Patient 81
Intraoffice Communication 84
Staff Arrangements 85
Communication and Patients' Rights 87
Advising Patients 89
Communication and Patient Education 89

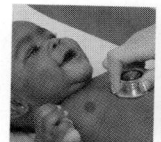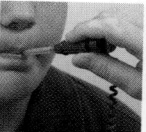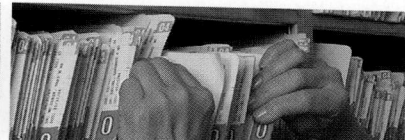

Unit Two

Administrative Medical Assisting

93

Chapter 5

The Office Environment 94

General Safety Measures 96
Guidelines 5-1: General Safety Measures 96
Guidelines 5-2: Handling a Disaster 97
Employee Safety. 98
Hazardous Medical Waste 99
OSHA Bloodborne Pathogens
    Standards/Universal Precautions 100
Housekeeping Safety 101
Guidelines 5-3: Using Personal Protective
    Equipment and Clothing from OSHA 101
Proper Body Mechanics 102
Office Security 102
Guidelines 5-4: Housekeeping Procedures
    from OSHA. 103
Ergonomics in the Medical Office 105
Quality Medical Care. 105
What Is Quality Assurance? 106

Chapter 6

Telephone Techniques 112

Telephone Techniques 114
Procedure 6-1: Taking a
    Telephone Message 117
Typical Incoming Calls. 119
Prescription Refill Requests 121
Telephone Triage 121
Handling Difficult Calls. 122
Using a Telephone Directory 122
Procedure 6-2: Taking a Prescription
    Refill Message 122
Long Distance Calls 123
Using an Answering Service 124
Procedure 6-3: Placing a Conference
    Call 124
Handling an Emergency Telephone
    Call 125

Chapter 7

Patient Reception 128

Duties of a Receptionist 130
Personal Characteristics and
    Physical Appearance 131
Opening the Office. 132
Collating Records. 132
Procedure 7-1: Opening the Office 133
Procedure 7-2: Collating Records. 133
Greeting the Patient Upon Arrival 134
Registering New Patients 135
Charge Slips. 135
Consideration for the Patient's Time 135
Escorting the Patient into the
    Examination Room 136
Managing Disturbances 137
No-Shows 138
Closing the Office 138
Procedure 7-3: Closing the Office. 139

Chapter 8

Appointment Scheduling 142

Appointment Schedules 144
Scheduling Systems 146
Patient Scheduling Process 148
Procedure 8-1: Scheduling Patients. 150
Patient Referrals 151
Hospital Admission Scheduling 151
Scheduling Surgery 151
Appointment Exceptions 151
Procedure 8-2: Scheduling Inpatient
    Surgical Procedures 152
Procedure 8-3: Scheduling an Outpatient
    Procedure. 153
Telephone and E-mail Scheduling. 154
New Patient Appointments 154
Established Patient Appointments 155
Scheduling Other Types of Appointments 155

Contents *continued*

Chapter 9

Office Facilities, Equipment, and Supplies   158

Medical Office Facility 160
Office Layout 160
Office Equipment 163
Procedure 9-1: Operating a Transcriber 165
Supplies 166

Chapter 10

Written Communication   170

Letter Writing 172
Word Choice 172
Composing Letters 174
Guidelines 10-1: Using Courtesy Titles 179
Letter Styles 180
Procedure 10-1: Composing a Business Letter . . 180
Interoffice Memoranda 181
Proofreading 181
Editing 181
Guidelines 10-2: Proofreading 181
Abbreviations 183
Reference Materials 183
Preparing Outgoing Mail 183
Classifications of Mail 185
Size Requirements for Mail 187
Mail Handling Tips 187
Electronic Mail (E-mail) 187
Procedure 10-2: Opening the Daily Mail 188
Reflection on the Medical Practice 189

Chapter 11

Computers in the Medical Office   192

Use of Computers in Medicine 194
Types of Computers 194
Basic Computer Components 194
Security for the Computer System 198
Selecting a Computer System 199
The Internet 199
Electronic Signatures 201
Computers and Ergonomics 202

Chapter 12

Managing Medical Records   206

The Medical Record 208
Procedure 12-1: Adding or Changing Items
    on a Patient's Record 210
Filing 212
Procedure 12-2: Organize a Patient's
    Medical Record 213
Procedure 12-3: Filing a Record
    Alphabetically 216
Procedure 12-4: Filing a Record
    Numerically Using the Terminal Digit
    Filing System 217
Guidelines 12-1: Locating Missing
    Files 219
Quality Assurance for Quality
    Medical Care 219
Releasing Medical Records 221
Storing Medical Records 221
Medical Transcription 222
Ownership of the Medical Record 222
Retention and Destruction of
    Medical Records 223

Chapter 13

Fees, Billing, Collections, and Credit   226

Professional Fees 228
Billing 229
Credit Policy 231
Collections 232
Guidelines 13-1: Collections 232
Guidelines 13-2: Making Collections 233
Accounting Systems 235
Guidelines 13-3: Manual Bookkeeping 235
Bookkeeping Systems 237
Procedure 13-1: Perform Accounts
    Receivable 237
Procedure 13-2: Pegboard System 241
Computerized Systems 243
Professional Courtesy 244

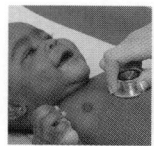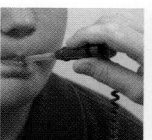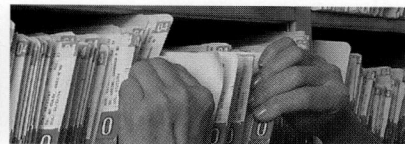

Chapter 14
Financial Management 246

Function of Banking. 248
Checks 249
Procedure 14-1: Prepare a Check 250
Paying Bills 254
Procedure 14-2: Post Non-sufficient
   Funds Checks 255
Deposits. 256
Procedure 14-3: Prepare a Deposit Slip 256
Accepting Cash 257
Cash Disbursement 258
Bank Hold on Accounts. 258
Bank Statement 258
Saving Documentation. 259
Procedure 14-4: Reconciling a Bank
   Statement 259
Petty Cash 260
Payroll 260
Procedure 14-5: Generating Payroll
   in a Medical Office 262

Chapter 15
Medical Insurance 268

Purpose of Health Insurance 270
Health Insurance and Availability of
   Health Insurance 270
Managed Care Organizations (MCOs). 270
Commercial Plans 273
Government Programs 274
Types of Health Insurance Benefits. 276
Payment of Benefits 276
Procedure 15-1: Perform Billing and
   Collection Procedures 278
Verification of Insurance Benefits. 279
Procedure 15-2: Apply Third Party
   Guidelines 279
Fee Schedules 280
Procedure 15-3: Apply Managed Care
   Policies and Procedures 280
Health Care Cost Containment 280
The Federal Register 281

Chapter 16
Medical Insurance Claims 284

Types of Health Insurance Claim Forms 286
Type of Claims. 288
The Claim Form 290
Claims Processing 290
Procedure 16-1: Completing
   the CMS-1500 Form 291
Claim Security 295
Tracking Claim Forms 295

Chapter 17
Medical Coding 298

Insurance Coding. 300
Understanding the ICD-9-CM 300
Procedure Coding 303
Procedure 17-1: ICD-9-CM Coding 305
Getting to Know the CPT. 305
Insurance Fraud 308
Procedure 17-2: Assigning a CPT Code 310
Compliance Plan 311

Chapter 18
Medical Office Management 316

Systems Approach to Office Management 318
The Office Manager. 319
Procedure 18-1: Staff Meeting Procedures 321
Leadership Styles 322
Creating a Team Atmosphere. 323
Hiring Procedures: Selecting the Right
   Staff Members 324
Orientation and Training 326
Using Performance Evaluation Effectively 328
Time Management 330
Personnel Policy Manual 331
Office Procedures Manual 332
Medical Meetings and Speaking Engagements . . 332
Patient Information Booklet. 333
Medical Practice Marketing and
   Customer Service 333
Procedure 18-2: Developing a Patient
   Information Booklet 334

Contents *continued*

Unit Three — Anatomy and Physiology

339

Chapter 19
Body Structure and Function 340

The Human Body: Levels of Organization 342
Anatomical Locations and Positions. 350
Chemistry. 354
Genetics and Heredity 355

Chapter 20
The Integumentary System 360

Overview of the Integumentary System 362
Functions of the Integumentary System 362
Layers of the Skin. 362
Accessory Structures of the Skin. 363
Common Disorders Associated with the
    Integumentary System 364

Chapter 21
The Skeletal System 376

Bones and Their Classification. 378
Joints and Movement. 380
The Axial Skeleton. 381
The Appendicular Skeleton 383
Common Disorders Associated with the
    Skeletal System 383

Chapter 22
The Muscular System 392

Functions of Muscle. 394
Types of Muscle Tissue. 395
Energy Production for Muscle 396
Structure of Skeletal Muscles 396
Major Skeletal Muscles 397
Common Disorders Associated
    with the Muscular System 398

Chapter 23
The Nervous System 404

Functions of the Nervous System 407
Neurons. 407
Nerve Fiber, Nerves, and Tracts 407
Nerve Impulses and Synapses. 408
Central Nervous System. 408
Peripheral Nervous System. 411
Autonomic Nervous System. 414
Common Disorders Associated
    with the Nervous System 415

Chapter 24
The Special Senses 422

The Eye and the Sense of Vision. 424
The Ear and the Sense of Hearing 428
The Senses of Taste and Smell 430
The Sense of Touch 431

Chapter 25
The Circulatory System 434

Overview of the Circulatory System. 436
The Heart. 436
Blood Vessels 439
Blood Pressure 440
Pulmonary and Systemic Circulation 442
Blood. 442
Hemostasis and Bleeding Control. 446
Blood Types 446
The Lymphatic System 448
Common Disorders Associated
    with the Circulatory System. 450

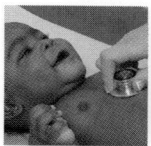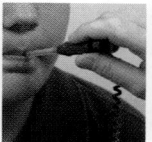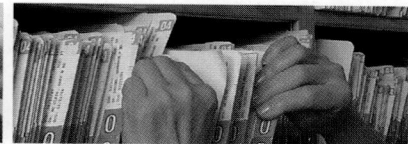

Chapter 26

The Immune System 460

Anatomy of the Immune System. 462

The Immune System and the
Body's Defense. 464

Common Disorders Associated
with the Immune System 465

Chapter 27

The Respiratory System 472

Organs of the Respiratory System 474

Mechanism of Breathing 478

Respiratory Volumes and Capacities 479

Common Disorders Associated
with the Respiratory System 480

Chapter 28

The Digestive System 488

Organs of the Digestive System 491

Common Disorders Associated
with the Digestive System 495

Chapter 29

The Urinary System 508

Organs of the Urinary System 511

Urine 512

Common Disorders Associated
with the Urinary System. 513

Chapter 30

The Endocrine System 520

Pituitary Gland. 523

Pineal Gland. 524

Thyroid Gland 524

Parathyroid Glands 524

Pancreas (Islets of Langerhans). 525

Adrenal Glands 525

Ovaries. 527

Testes 527

Placenta 527

Gastrointestinal Mucosa 527

Thymus Gland 527

Common Disorders Associated
with the Endocrine System. 527

Chapter 31

The Reproductive System 536

Female Reproductive System 538

The Menstrual Cycle 542

Male Reproductive System. 542

Common Disorders Associated
with the Female Reproductive System 544

Common Disorders Associated
with the Male Reproductive System. 554

Contents *continued*

Unit Four — Clinical Medical Assisting — 559

Chapter 32

Infection Control 560

History of Asepsis 562
Microorganisms 562
The Infection Control System. 564
Universal Precautions. 565
Procedure 32-1: Disposal of Infectious
Waste and Substances 570
Procedure 32-2: Hand Hygiene 572
Procedure 32-3: Sanitizing Instruments 578
Procedure 32-4: Wrapping Instruments
for Autoclaving 581
Hepatitis and AIDS 582
Bioterrorism 585

Chapter 33

Vital Signs 588

Interviewing the Patient 590
Patient History 591
Correct Documentation 593
Measuring Weight and Height 593
Procedure 33-1: Measuring Adult
Weight and Height 595
Vital Signs 595
Temperature 596
Procedure 33-2: Measuring Oral Temperatures
Using a Glass Non-Mercury Thermometer . . 602
Procedure 33-3: Measuring a Rectal
Temperature Using a Glass
Non-Mercury Thermometer 604
Procedure 33-4: Cleaning and Storing
Glass Non-Mercury Thermometers 605
Pulse 606
Procedure 33-5: Measuring Oral Temperature
Using an Electronic or Digital Thermometer . . . 607
Procedure 33-6: Measuring Temperature
Using an Aural (Tympanic Membrane)
Thermometer 608

Procedure 33-7: Measuring Axillary
Temperature 609
Procedure 33-8: Measuring Radial
Pulse Rate 612
Respiration 612
Procedure 33-9: Measuring Apical-Radial
Pulse (Two-Person) 614
Procedure 33-10: Measuring Respirations 615
Blood Pressure 616
Procedure 33-11: Measuring Oxygen
Saturation Using a Pulse Oximeter. 617
Pain 623
Procedure 33-12: Measuring Systolic
Blood Pressure Using Palpatory Method 624
Procedure 33-13: Measuring Blood Pressure . . 625
Body Fat Measurement 626

Chapter 34

Assisting with Physical Examinations 630

Preparing the Exam Room 632
Procedure 34-1: Cleaning the Examination
Room 633
Equipment and Supplies Used
for Physical Examinations 634
Examination Methods Used
by the Physician 635
Adult Examination 639
Assisting the Physician with a Physical Exam . . . 640
Sequence of Examination Procedures 645
Procedure 34-2: Assisting with a Complete
Physical Examination 648
Documentation of Patient Medical
Information 651
Procedure 34-3: Interview New Patient
to Obtain Medical History Information
and Prepare for Physical Examination 652
Guidelines 34-1: Charting 655

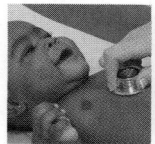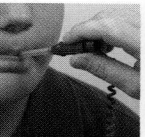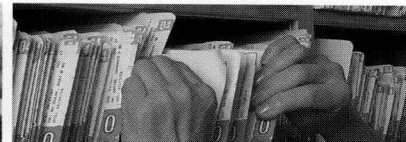

Chapter 35
Assisting with Medical Specialties   658
Allergy 660
Dermatology 662
Cardiovascular System 663
Procedure 35-1: Taking a Wound Culture 666
Endocrinology 669
Gastrointestinal System 672
Procedure 35-2: Assisting
    with a Sigmoidoscopy 676
Lymphatic System 677
Musculoskeletal System 678
Nervous System 679
Reproductive Systems 684
Female Reproductive System 684
Procedure 35-3: Instructing a Patient
    on Breast Self-Examination 686
Procedure 35-4: Assisting with a Pelvic
    Examination and Pap Test 691
Male Reproductive System 695
Sexually Transmitted Diseases (STDs) 696
Urinary System 699

Chapter 36
Assisting in Eye and Ear Care   706
The Study of the Eye 708
Procedure 36-1: Testing Visual Acuity
    Using a Snellen Eye Chart 710
Procedure 36-2: Screening for Near
    Vision Acuity 711
Procedure 36-3: Screening for Color
    Vision Acuity 712
Procedure 36-4: Irrigation of the Eye 714
Procedure 36-5: Instilling Eye Medication 715
Irrigation of the Eye 715
Instillation of Eye Medications 715
Patient Safety Guidelines 715

Assisting the Blind Patient 716
The Study of the Ear 717
Guidelines 36-1: Assisting the
    Vision-Impaired Patient to Prepare
    for Physical Examination 717
Hearing Acuity and Assessment 719
Examination of the Nose and Throat 722
Procedure 36-6: Irrigation of the Ear 723
Procedure 36-7: Instilling Ear Medication 724
Procedure 36-8: Assisting with Audiometry . . . 725

Chapter 37
Assisting in Life Span Specialties   730
Assisting in Pediatrics 732
The Pediatric Office 732
The Pediatric Patient 733
Pediatric Office Visits and Procedures 733
Procedure 37-1: Measuring Pediatric
    Vital Signs 736
Procedure 37-2: Measuring the Weight
    and Height of Infants 739
Procedure 37-3: Measuring Infant
    Head Circumference 740
Procedure 37-4: Perform a Snellen Eye
    Exam on a Child 741
Procedure 37-5: Applying Pediatric
    Urine Collection Device 742
Pediatric Diseases and Disorders 743
Assisting the Elderly 747
Aging Population 747
Facts about the Elderly 749
The Aging Process 750
The Aging Body 750
Legal and Medical Decisions 756
Procedure 37-6: Communicating
    Effectively with the Elderly 757
Elder Abuse 758
Safety Guidelines for Children and Elders 758

Contents *continued*

Chapter 38
Assisting with Minor Surgery   762

Ambulatory Surgery 764
Principles of Surgical Asepsis 764
Guidelines 38-1: Surgical Asepsis 765
Procedure 38-1: Surgical Hand
    Hygiene/Sterile Scrub 766
Handling Sterile Instruments 769
Procedure 38-2: Surgical Gloving 770
Procedure 38-3: Opening a Sterile Packet 772
Procedure 38-4: Dropping Sterile
    Packet onto a Sterile Field 773
Procedure 38-5: Transferring Sterile
    Objects Using Transfer Forceps 774
Surgical Assisting 779
Guidelines 38-2: Handling Instruments 779
Guidelines 38-3: Sterile Techniques
    for Scrub Assistants 780
Procedure 38-6: Transferring Sterile
    Solutions onto a Sterile Field 781
Procedure 38-7: Assisting with Minor Surgery . . 782
Guidelines 38-4: Floating Assistants
    during Surgery 783
Preparing the Patient for Minor Surgery 783
Procedure 38-8: Preparing the
    Patient's Skin for Surgical Procedure 786
Postoperative Patient Care 786
Procedure 38-9: Assisting with Suturing 790
Surgical Procedures Performed
    in the Medical Office 791
Procedure 38-10: Removing Sutures 792
Procedure 38-11: Changing a Sterile Dressing . . 793
Procedure 38-12: Applying a Bandage
    over a Sterile Dressing 795

Chapter 39
Assisting with Medical Emergencies   800

The Emergency Medical Services System 802
Guidelines for Providing Emergency Care 802
The Office Emergency Crash Kit 806
Medical Emergencies 806
Procedure 39-1: Responding to an Obstructed
    Airway (Conscious Adult, Child, or Infant) . . 808
Procedure 39-2: Administering Adult CPR 818

Procedure 39-3: Applying an Arm Sling 824
Procedure 39-4: Controlling Bleeding 829

Chapter 40
The Clinical Laboratory   834

Role of Clinical Laboratory in Patient Care 836
Laboratory Safety Regulations 837
Laboratory Hazards 838
Quality Assurance 839
Guidelines 40-1: Laboratory Safety 840
Laboratory Equipment 841
Laboratory Measurements and Equipment 842
Procedure 40-1: Using the Microscope 843
Guidelines 40-2: Care and Maintenance
    of Microscope 843
Clinical Laboratory and
    Patient Communication 845

Chapter 41
Microbiology   850

Role of the Medical Assistant in Microbiology . . 852
Classifications of Microorganisms 853
Types of Microorganisms 854
Specimen Collection and Transportation 860
Guidelines 41-1: Specimen Collection 861
Overview of the Process of Diagnosing
    Infection 862
Microbiology Equipment and Procedures 863
Procedure 41-1: Preparing a Smear 866
Procedure 41-2: Preparing a
    Wet Mount Slide 867
Types of Specimens 867
Procedure 41-3: Performing a Gram Stain 868
Procedure 41-4: Obtaining a Throat Culture . . 870
Procedure 41-5: Obtaining a Sputum
    Specimen for Culture 871
Procedure 41-6: Performing a Urine Culture . . . 872
Procedure 41-7: Obtaining Stool
    Specimen for Culture and Sensitivity 873
Procedure 41-8: Obtaining a Stool
    Specimen for Ova and Parasites 874
Procedure 41-9: Obtaining a Stool
    Specimen for Examination for Pinworms 875
Serology Testing 875

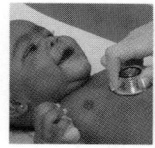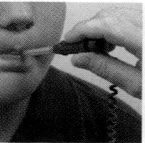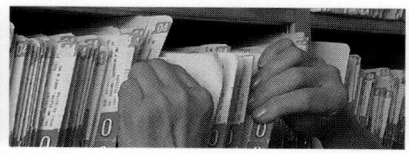

Chapter 42

Urinalysis 878

Asepsis................................. 880
Collecting the Specimen 880
Guidelines 42-1: Collecting a Routine
Urine Specimen 881
Guidelines 42-2: Collecting a 24-Hour
Specimen 882
Procedure 42-1: Collecting a Clean-Catch
Midstream Urine Specimen 883
Routine Urinalysis 884
Procedure 42-2: Evaluating the Physical
Characteristics of Urine 885
Procedure 42-3: Measuring Specific
Gravity (SG) with a Refractometer 887
Procedure 42-4: Testing Urine with
Reagent Strips 888
Procedure 42-5: Testing for Sugar
in the Urine Using Tablets 890
Procedure 42-6: Preparing a Specimen for a
Microscopic Urine Specimen Examination... 893
Urine Pregnancy Testing.................. 894
Procedure 42-7: Performing a Urine Pregnancy
Test Using the Enzyme Immunoassay Method.. 896
Quality Control 896

Chapter 43

Hematology 900

The Medical Assistant's Role 902
Blood Formation and Components 902
Function of Blood 903
Blood Specimen Collection................ 904
Procedure 43-1: Quality Control
for Collecting a Blood Specimen 904
Procedure 43-2: Obtaining Venous
Blood with a Sterile Syringe and Needle..... 906
Routine Blood Tests..................... 909
Procedure 43-3: Performing a Venipuncture
Using the Vacutainer Method............ 910
Procedure 43-4: Performing a Capillary
Puncture (Manual)..................... 915
Procedure 43-5: Screening for Glucose
(Blood Sugar) Level 917
Procedure 43-6: Performing a Microhematocrit.. 918
Procedure 43-7: Determining Hemoglobin
Using the Hemoglobinometer 920
Erythrocyte Sedimentation Rate............ 921

Phenylketonuria 921
Mono Testing........................... 921
Procedure 43-8: Preparing Slides 922
Procedure 43-9: Performing an Erythrocyte
Sedimentation Rate Test Using
the Wintrobe Method 924
Procedure 43-10: Performing a PKU Test 925
Procedure 43-11: Performing a Mono Test.... 925

Chapter 44

Radiology 928

Radiology............................... 930
Diagnostic Imaging Overview 931
Preparing and Positioning the Patient........ 932
Procedure 44-1: Procedure for General
X-ray Examination 935
Guidelines 44-1: Sequencing Multiple
Radiographic Procedures................ 936
Diagnostic Imaging Procedures 936
Guidelines 44-2: Upper GI Series 939
Guidelines 44-3: Lower GI Series 939
Radiation Therapy....................... 945
Nuclear Medicine........................ 946
Safety Precautions 947
Radiographic Equipment 949
Guidelines 44-4: Maintaining Personnel Safety.. 950
Guidelines 44-5: Maintaining Patient Safety... 950
Processing X-ray Film 950
Storage and Records...................... 951
Ownership of Film....................... 951

Chapter 45

Electrocardiography and
Pulmonary Function 954

Heart Structure and Function.............. 956
The Electrocardiogram.................... 957
Procedure 45-1: Recording a 12-Lead
Electrocardiograph 965
Special Tests............................ 967
Procedure 45-2: Treadmill Stress Test........ 969
Pulmonary Function...................... 970
Pulmonary Function Tests 970
Procedure 45-3: Applying a Holter Monitor .. 971
Procedure 45-4: Performing a Spirometer
Test to Measure Forced Vital Capacity...... 974
Treatments............................. 975
Pulmonary Diseases 975

Contents *continued*

Chapter 46

Physical Therapy and Rehabilitation   978

Therapeutic Team 980
Rehabilitation 982
Patient Assessment...................... 983
Conditions Requiring Physical Therapy 983
Physical Therapy Methods.................. 983
Guidelines 46-1: Performing Range of
Motion (ROM) Exercises................ 986
Procedure 46-1: Applying a Hot Compress ... 990
Procedure 46-2: Application of Hot Soak..... 991
Procedure 46-3: Application of a Heating Pad . 992
Procedure 46-4: Application of Cold Compress . 993
Procedure 46-5: Application of Ice Bag 994
Procedure 46-6: Application of
Cold Chemical Pack.................... 995
Adaptive Equipment and Devices............ 996
Procedure 46-7: Instructing a Patient
to Use Crutches Correctly 1001
Procedure 46-8: Instructing a Patient
to Use a Cane or Single Crutch Correctly... 1003
Procedure 46-9: Teaching a Patient
to Correctly Use a Walker 1005
Procedure 46-10: Wheelchair Transfer
to Chair or Examination Table 1006
Diagnostic Testing 1007

Chapter 47

Math for Pharmacology   1010

Weights and Measures 1012
Drug Calculations 1013
Guidelines 47-1: Conversion
within the Metric System 1014
Calculating Dosages..................... 1017
Rules for Conversion 1017
Calculating Pediatric Dosages 1018
Guidelines 47-2: Conversion 1018

Chapter 48

Pharmacology   1022

Drug Names........................... 1024
Regulation and Standards 1024
References 1024
Legal Classification of Drugs 1025
Drug Abuse 1028

General Classes of Drugs 1029
Routes and Methods of Drug Administration .. 1033
Frequently Administered Drugs 1036
Side Effects of Medications 1037
Drug Interactions....................... 1037
Drug Use During Pregnancy.............. 1038
Reading and Writing a Prescription 1038
Guidelines 48-1: Administration of Medication . 1040
Abbreviations Used in Pharmacology........ 1041

Chapter 49

Administering Medications   1046

Administration Procedures: OSHA Standards .. 1048
Medication Administration 1048
Procedure 49-1: Administering (Inserting)
a Rectal or Vaginal Suppository.......... 1050
Procedure 49-2: Administering Sublingual
or Buccal Medication.................. 1051
Procedure 49-3: Administering Oral
Medications.......................... 1052
Equipment Used for Medication Administration.. 1053
Procedure 49-4: Using an Ampule 1055
Procedure 49-5: Withdrawing Medication
from a Single-Dose or Multiple-Dose Vial .. 1056
Sites for Intramuscular Injection............ 1057
Sites for Subcutaneous Injection............ 1061
Procedure 49-6: Administering Parenteral
Subcutaneous (SC) or Intramuscular
(IM) Injections 1063
Procedure 49-7: Administering a Z-Track
Injection............................ 1066
Intradermal Injection 1066
Tuberculin Skin Test..................... 1067
Procedure 49-8: Administering
an Intradermal Injection 1068
Procedure 49-9: Performing a Tuberculin
Skin Test 1070
Intravenous Therapy 1071
Procedure 49-10: Preparing
an Intravenous (IV) Tray 1072
Immunizations 1072
Reconstituting a Powdered Medication
for Administration.................... 1076
Procedure 49-11: Reconstituting a Powdered
Medication for Administration 1076
Charting Medications.................... 1077

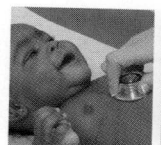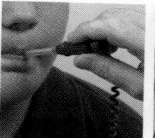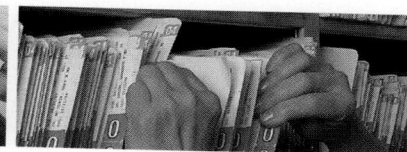

Chapter 50
Patient Education 1080
Patient Education 1082
Procedure 50-1: Creating a Community
   Resource Brochure 1082
Procedure 50-2: Creating a Public
   Relations Brochure 1083
Guidelines 50-1: Effective Health Instructions . . 1084
Procedure 50-3: Instructing Patients
   According to Their Needs
   for Health Maintenance
   and Promotion 1089
Developing a Teaching Plan 1089
Teaching Patients with Disabilities 1089
Handling Noncompliance 1091
Teaching about Cast Care 1091

Chapter 51
Nutrition 1096
Nutrition 1098
Stress Management 1116
Time Management 1116

Chapter 52
Psychology 1120
Psychology 1122
Psychological Disorders 1122
Treatments 1124
Developmental Stages of the Life Cycle 1125
The Mind–Body Connection 1126
Maslow's Hierarchy of Needs 1126
Heredity and Environmental and Cultural
   Influences on Behavior 1127
Procedure 52-1: Role-Playing a Situation
   in Which a Patient Is from Another Culture . . 1128
Interpersonal Skills and Human Behavior 1128
Emotions 1129
Motivation 1130
Stress 1130
Procedure 52-2: Role-Playing a Situation
   When a Patient Is Frightened, Angry,
   and Depressed 1131
Procedure 52-3: Develop a Patient
   Teaching Handout about Stress 1135
Assisting the Patient with Terminal Illness 1135

Unit Five
Career Assistance
1139

Chapter 53
Externship and Career Opportunities 1140
What Is an Externship? 1142
Preparing for the Certification Examination . . . 1145
The Job Search 1146
Procedure 53-1: Conducting a Job Search . . . 1148
The Résumé 1148
Procedure 53-2: Preparing Your Résumé 1150
The Cover Letter 1151
The Interview 1151
Procedure 53-3: Preparing a Cover Letter . . . 1153
Guidelines 53-1: Successful Interviewing 1154
Procedure 53-4: Role-Playing an Interview . . . 1155

Follow-Up after the Interview 1156
What Does the Employer Want? 1156
Procedure 53-5: Preparing
   a Follow-Up Letter 1157

Appendix I
Abbreviations and Symbols A-1

Appendix II
Glossary of Word Parts A-7

Glossary G-1

Index I-1

Preface

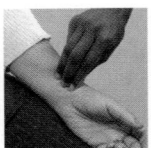

Pearson's Comprehensive Medical Assisting

Pearson's Comprehensive Medical Assisting is a brand new approach to learning the profession of Medical Assisting. It is all about Successful Skill Building so that you will be successful in the classroom and in the physician's office. To help ensure that success, Professionalism and Cultural Considerations are also explored. These are skills that will help you, the Medical Assistant, relate to your whole workplace: your administrative responsibilities, your patients, and your physicians. It's about making the connection between your skills and your whole profession.

Medical Assisting is, after all, a "people helping people" profession. What could be more important than the connections that make the Medical Assistant the vital link between people and their personal health and well-being? This comprehensive textbook helps the student learn the right skills for becoming the very best and most effective Medical Assistant through a step-by-step, competency based approach that covers virtually all the facets of the medical assisting profession. Through up to the minute content and careful planning, *Pearson's Comprehensive Medical Assisting* prepares students to make successful connections in class, in their externships, and in their professional placements.

How does *Pearson's Comprehensive Medical Assisting* accomplish these goals? A thorough table of contents that covers all the material necessary for student success, a curriculum that follows the AAMA and AMT competencies, a fully developed instructional package that contains everything an instructor needs to successfully connect with the student and challenge their skills, and the latest in interactive technology that will engage students and instructors alike. The entire package is comprehensive, easily implemented, simple to follow, and completely up to date.

Each chapter in *Pearson's Comprehensive Medical Assisting* begins with a Role Delineation Chart highlighted with the concepts covered in that chapter. Both students and their instructors easily see which AAMA or AMT competencies will be covered in the chapter. Learning Objectives underscore the chart, listing the skills and procedures the student will be able to demonstrate after completing the chapter. Terms to Learn are also included so that the student can immediately see the new vocabulary that she will experience. A case study vignette introduces the reader to central concepts and is followed up on later in the chapter with critical thinking questions. Other learning aids in the book include hundreds of color photos and photo sequences; hundreds of full color, detailed drawings; easy to understand charts and tables; step-by-step procedures; and clear, informative guidelines.

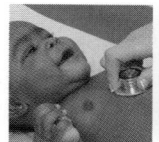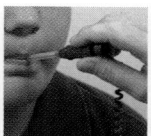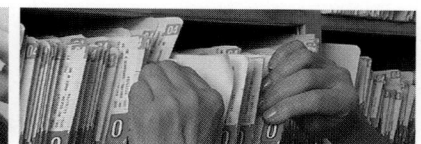

A helpful chapter review allows the student to check her knowledge in several ways:

- Chapter review questions test the student's understanding of key chapter concepts.
- Critical Thinking questions relate back to the case study vignette that opens each chapter.
- "On the Job" presents the student with a new scenario with more critical thinking opportunities.
- Certification Exam-style questions help prepare the student for the CMA and RMA exams and review the chapter material.
- An Internet Activity and a MediaLink is also included in each chapter review.

Developed by Pearson Education and Legacy Interactive, Inc., the Medical Assisting Interactive CD-ROM found in the back of the book provides a fascinating journey through the responsibilities, the technical skills, and the "people skills" of the Medical Assistant. The CD-ROM opens to the waiting room of a typical Doctor's office. The player can move from room to room in the medical office or, for the more sequentially-minded student, from chapter to chapter. There are medical assisting terminology memory games to play, interactive animations and simulations, tips from professionals, decision-making and critical thinking scenarios, an audio glossary, a resource library, and many other wonderful things to do.

Special features throughout the book include segments on *Patient Education*; important *Legal and Ethical* concerns: and *LifeSpan Considerations* which focus on the pediatric patient and the geriatric patient. *Preparing for Externship* deals with topics and issues relating to students' participation in an externship program as a capstone to their training. It addresses pertinent issues including student responsibilities, caring attitudes, enthusiasm, grooming/dress, interpersonal skills with patients and colleagues, language skills, poise under pressure and other issues.

Cultural Considerations addresses the Medical Assistant's encounters with people of different cultural backgrounds, a brief tip, advice, or general guideline on how to deal with a specific cultural or communication issue. Many different cultural issues arise in any physician's office. There may be taboos against certain procedures, removal of clothing, discussion of birth control, showing emotions or feelings, eating certain foods, or taking certain kinds of medication. In our multi-cultural world today, every Medical Assistant will deal with all kinds of people from many different backgrounds. This feature will help the Medical Assistant react with grace, graciousness, and a professional manner.

In the medical office today, the Medical Assistant must go a step further than mastering a myriad of challenging, detailed, and precise Administrative and Clinical skills. The Medical Assistant must show complete *Professionalism* in the office. This element of each chapter provides a focus on grooming and dress, interpersonal skills, ethical standards, language skills, punctuality, dependability, and a caring attitude. These highly important qualities help the Medical Assistant maintain a completely professional demeanor at all times. Coupled with mastery of technical skills, these "soft" skills will guarantee the professional status of the new Medical Assistant.

All care has been taken to ensure that *Pearson's Comprehensive Medical Assisting* covers all the current content and competencies of both the American Association of Medical Assistants (AAMA) and the American Medical Technologists (AMT). This text is aimed at preparing you for either the AAMA or the AMT certification examinations.

Use this book in any of a variety of learning environments and situations including the traditional classroom; the self-paced or individualized course; as a review for those seeking certification and preparing for a certification examination; or in an on-the-job training program in a doctor's office.

The Learning Package:

The Student Package:
- Textbook
- Interactive CD-ROM with exercises, learning games, skills review, medical office simulation for real-life application, skills videos, simulations, animations, resources, audio glossary.
- Student Workbook that contains chapter-specific assignments: step by step procedures and guidelines with Procedure checklists for instructor review; review questions; terminology review; skill exercise; vocabulary exercises; forms; other activities designed to reinforce the content of the text. This workbook has perforated pages so that assignments can be submitted for grading.
- Vango Notes are chapter highlights and in-depth summaries that are downloaded to an MP3

The Instructional Package:
- Instructor's Resource Guide with detailed CAAHEP Competency Correlation guide
- CD-ROM with Test Gen and over 5000 test questions and Classroom Management software.
- Lesson Plans
- Hundreds of PowerPoint slides for daily lessons
- Syllabus, teaching tips, notes, additional exercises, instructional strategies, answers to all text questions and workbook questions.
- Administrative and Clinical Medical Assisting videos in VHS or DVD format
- Pearson Solutions Medical Assisting Curriculum and Pearson Training Master Instructional Training
- *"Klickerz"* Classroom Response System for interactive classroom PowerPoint presentations; chapter review and test preparation; and classroom games.
- Transition Guides to help make text implementation easy

Reviewers

The invaluable editorial advice and direction provided by the following educators and health care professionals is deeply appreciated:

Cindy Abel, BS, CMA, Pbt
Program Chair
Ivy Tech Community College
Lafayette, IN

Kendra Allen, LPN
Program Manager Healthcare Office
    Technologies
Ohio Institute of Health Careers
Columbus, OH

James Baird, MBA, CAHI
Medical Program Director
Computer Career Center
El Paso, TX

Jennifer Barr, MT, M.Ed., CMA
Chairperson, Medical Assisting
    Technology
Sinclair Community College
Dayton, OH

Sue Beaman, RN
Wayne Community College
Goldsboro, NC

**Suzanne Bitters, RMA, NCPT,
    NCICS**
Former Instructor
CHI Institute
Southampton, PA

Lou Brown, MT (ASCP), CMA
Medical Assisting Program Director
Wayne Community College
Goldsboro, NC

Minda Brown, RMA
Pima Medical Institute
Colorado Springs, CO

Beth Anne Buchholz, BS, CMA
Medical Assisting Department Chair
Wichita Area Technical College
Wichita, KS

Cara Carreon, BS, RRT, CMA, CPC
Faculty
Ivy Tech Community College
Lafayette, IN

**Denise Carsillo, MS, BS, AS, RMA,
    BXMO**
Director of Academic Services
New England Tech
West Palm Beach, FL

Lisa Cook, CMA
Medical Assisting Education
    Program Chair
Bryman College
Port Orchard, WA

Janie Corbitt, RN, BSL
Central Georgia Technical College
Milledgeville, GA

Anita Denson, CMA
Director of Health Care Education
National College of Business
    & Technology
Danville, KY

George Fakhoury, MD, DORCP, CMA
Academic Program Manager
  Healthcare
Head College's Central Administrative
  Office
San Francisco, CA

Suzanne Feathers, CMA, EMT
Medical Program Coordinator
Computer Learning Network
Altoona, PA

Pamela Fleming, RN, CMA, MPA
Professor
Quinsigamond Community College
Worcester, MA

Beverley Giteles, CPC, CMM
Instructor
Gibbs College
Livingston, NJ

Robyn Gohsman, RMA, CMAS
Medical Assisting Department Head
Medical Careers Institute
Newport News, VA

Wendy Hall-Campbell, ADN
Medical Assisting Program Director
Concorde Career Institute
Portland, OR

Carrie Hammond, CMA
Medical Assisting Program Director
Utah Career College
West Jordan, UT

Jessica Hart, CMA
Director of Healthcare Education
National College of Business &
  Technology
Lexington, KY

Marsha Perkins Hemby, RN, CMA
Medical Assisting Department
  Chair
Pitt Community College
Greenville, NC

Elizabeth Henisse, BAS, MA
Allied Health Program Director
Florida Metropolitan University
Orlando, FL

Jessica Holtsberry
HIT Program Instructor
Ohio Institute of Health Careers
Columbus, OH

Marsha M. Holtsberry, CMA
HOT Program Director
Ohio Institute of Health Careers
Columbus, OH

Demetria Jackson
Former Program Director
Virginia College
Birmingham, AL

Shirley Jelmo, CMA
Faculty Coordinator
Pima Medical Institute
Colorado Springs, CO

Amy Knight, CMA
Allied Health Instructor
Remington College
Largo, FL

Holly A. Lincoln, BA
Academic Coordinator
St. Louis College of Health
  Careers
Fenton, MO

Marta Lopez, LM, CPM
Medical Assisting Program
   Coordinator
Miami Dade College
Miami, FL

Mary M. Marks, MSN, RN-BC,
   Pbt (ASCP)
Program Coordinator
Mitchell Community College
Mooresville, NC

Natalie McBride, CMA
Instructor
ICM School of Business &
   Medical Careers
Pittsburgh, PA

DeLeesa G. Meashintubby, BS,
   CMA, RMA
MOA/HRT Program Coordinator
Lane Community College
Eugene, OR

Tanya Mercer, BS, RN, RMA
Curriculum Specialist
KAPLAN Higher Education
Rowell, GA

Lisa Nagle, BS.Ed., CMA
Medical Assisting Program Director
Augusta Technical College
Augusta, GA

Kay Nave, CMA, MRT
Medical Assisting Program Director
Hagerstown Business College
Hagerstown, MD

Everlee O'Nan, RMA
Director of Health Care Education
National College of Business &
   Technology
Florence, KY

Karen Patrick, NCMA, CPI
Director
CAPPS College
Dothan, AL

Diane Peavy, RN, ASN, AHI
Director of Educational Services
Capps College
Foley, AL

Christina Rauberts-Conklin,
   AA, RMA
Medical Department Chair
Florida Metropolitan University
Tampa, FL

Deanna T. Rieke, BSRN, MSHA
Program Director
Montana State University—
Billings College of Technology
Billings, MT

Jim Rocco, MS, CAHI, CHI, CPI,
   CEI, CPCI, CMPCI, CCMA
Medical Assisting Instructor
Illinois School of Health Careers
Chicago, IL

Susan Saullo, RN, MS, MT (ASCP)
Medical Assisting Program
   Coordinator
Webster College
Ocala, FL

Lory Lee Serrato, CCS-P
Everest College
Springfield, MO

Janet Sesser, RMA, CMA, BS Ed.Admin.
Corporate Director of Education
Chubb Institute
Phoenix, AZ

Gary Shandrew, MSIA
Campus Director
Certified Careers Institute
Clearfield, UT

Maria L. Simard, LVN
Director of Allied Health Programs
Maric College
San Diego, CA

Lynn Slack, CMA
Medical Programs Director
ICM School of Business and
    Medical Careers
Pittsburgh, PA

Richard Snyder-Flohr, EdD, RN, CMA
Director of Medical Assisting
    Program
Hagerstown Business College
Hagerstown, MD

Sherry Stanfield, RN, BSN, MS
Medical Assisting Assistant Program
    Director
Miller-Motte Technical College
North Charleston, SC

Pollyanna Strunk, RN, BSN
Lead Medical Instructor
Daymar College
Louisville, KY

Deborah Sulkowski, CMA
Medical Department Chair
Pittsburgh Technical Institute
Oakdale, PA

Dr, Ruth Torres, MD, MA
Medical Instructor
Indiana Business College
Terre Haute, IN

Roberta C. Weiss, Ed.D.
Allied Health Curriculum Specialist
    and Instructional Designer

Nancy Wright, RN, BS, CNOR
Virginia College
Birmingham, AL

Authors & Contributors

It is with the greatest appreciation and admiration that we acknowledge the following Health Professions Educators for their contributions to the content of this text. Their dedication to the Medical Assisting profession and to the education of successful Medical Assistants has made this text the premier learning tool.

Authors

Nina Beaman, MS, RNC, CMA
Bryant and Stratton College
Richmond, VA

Lorraine Fleming-McPhillips, MS, MT, CMA
Medical Assisting Program
Coordinator (retired)
Quinebaug Valley Community College
Danielson, Connecticut

Contributors

Cindy Abel, BS, CMA, Pbt
Program Chair
Ivy Tech Community College
Lafayette, IN

Kendra Allen, LPN
Program Manager Healthcare Office
Technologies
Ohio Institute of Health Careers
Columbus, OH

Michelle Buchman, BSN, RN, BC
Everest College
Springfield, MO

Janie Corbitt, RN, BSL
Central Georgia Technical College
Milledgeville, GA

Jessica Holtsberry
HIT Program Instructor
Ohio Institute of Health Careers
Columbus, OH

Susie Huyer, MSN, RN
University of Phoenix Online Affiliate
Faculty
Heartland Hospice, Administrator

Demetria Jackson
Former Program Director
Virginia College
Birmingham, AL

Cathy Kelley-Arney, CMA, MLTC, BSHS
Institutional Director of Health Care
Education
National College of Business and
Technology
Bluefield, VA

Christine Malone, BS
Everett Community College
Everett, WA

Karen Minchella, Ph.D., CMA
Consulting Management Associates,
LLC
Warren, MI

Shelly Rainer, LPN
Vatterott College
Springfield, MO

Authors & Contributors, *continued*

Melanie Sheffield, LPN, AHI
Allied Medical Instructor
Remington College
Mobile, AL

Lynn Slack, CMA
Medical Programs Director
ICM School of Business and Medical
  Careers
Pittsburgh, PA

Lori Tyler, MS
President
Innova Inc.
Littleton, Colorado

Mary Warren-Oliver, BA
Clinical Coordinator, Medical Assisting
Gibbs College
Vienna, VA

Roberta C. Weiss, Ed.D.
Allied Health Curriculum Specialist
  and Instructional Designer

Nancy Wright, RN, BS, CNOR
Virginia College
Birmingham, AL

Special Acknowledgments

The Editor wishes to give special acknowledgments to Teri Zak, the Development Editor of Pearson's Comprehensive Medical Assisting. She worked tirelessly to ensure that this text is the very epitome and most current of Medical Assisting textbooks.

The Editor further gives special thanks to Assistant Editor Bronwen Glowacki. Bronwen's many hours analyzing reviews, monitoring ancillary contributors, and responding to every request—small and large—have helped to ensure this project's success.

Acknowledgments

Cover Photo Credits

Photodisc (background); Adam Smith/SuperStock (center); Thinkstock/Age Fotostock (bottom left); Arthur Tilley/Taxi/Getty Images (top left)

Interior Photo Credits

Dr. Klaus Boller/Photo Researchers, Inc. 858(BL); Matthew Brady/National Archives and Records Administration 22; R. Calentine/Visuals Unlimited 859(BR); Patrick Clark/Getty Images, Inc./Photodisc 171(BR); Stewart Cohen/Getty Images, Inc./Stone Allstock 29(TR); Corbis/Stock Market 37; Jim Cummins/Getty Images, Inc./Taxi 1126; Tomas del Amo/Pacific Stock 1081(BR); Custom Medical Stock Photography, Inc. 567(CR); Antonia Deutsch/ Dorling Kindersley Media Library 1097; Al Dodge/Pearson Education/PH College 801(BR); George Dodson/Pearson Education/PH College 1124; Dorling Kindersley Media Library 361, 363, 444, 445, 473, 489, 842, 859, 931, 1047, 1097; Laimute E. Druskis/Pearson Education/PH College 1121(BR); Laura Dwight/Laura Dwight Photography 1125(BR); Paul Ekman, Ph.D./David Matsumoto and Paul Ekman, www.PaulEkman.com 1129; Laura Elliott/Comstock Images 1125(TR); EyeWire Collection/Getty Images/Photodisc 341(BR); Denis Finnin and Jackie Beckett/ Dorling Kindersley Media Library 856, 858(BR); Futura Medical Corporation 102; Mike Gallitelli/Pearson Education/PH College 350, 405; Getty Images, Inc./Photodisc 159 (BR), 247, 1093; Getty Images, Inc./Stone Allstock 1132; Eric Grave/Phototake NYC 858(TL); Gary Hansen/Phototake NYC 561(BR); Adrienne Hart-Davis/Photo Researchers, Inc. 608(BR); Will Hart 1130(BL); Michal Heron/Pearson Education/Prentice Hall College 1, 2, 3, 4, 6, 7, 8, 15(BR), 31, 32, 33, 43, 48, 50, 57, 61, 64, 65(TL), 70, 71, 72, 76, 80, 84, 93, 94, 95, 103, 107, 108, 112, 113, 114, 115, 118, 119, 128, 129, 130, 131, 134, 137, 138, 142, 143, 144, 145, 146, 151, 158, 159(TL), 160, 162, 163, 164, 170, 171(TL), 178, 185, 186, 192, 193, 195, 202, 206, 207, 208, 211, 217, 219, 226, 227(TL), 228, 229, 231, 232, 236, 240, 268, 274, 278, 285, 299, 314, 315, 320, 324, 328, 377, 537(BR), 567(TR), 589(BR), 722, 901, 1092; Michal Heron Photography 29(BR), 70(CL); Ingenix, Inc. 304, 305; Dave King/ Dorling Kindersley Media Library 393, 423; Library of Congress 21; Michael Littlejohn/Pearson Education/PH College 1142(BR); Richard Logan/Pearson Education/PH College 351; Richard Lord/The Image Works 1130(BR); Dr. P. Marazzi/Photo Researchers, Inc. 453(TL); Matt Meadows/Science Photo Library/Photo Researchers, Inc. 194; Moredun Animal Health Ltd./Photo Researchers, Inc. 857(BR); Multimed Media 567(BR); Anthony Neste 627; Michael Newman/PhotoEdit, Inc. 269; Nova Biomedical 197; Omni-Photo Communications, Inc. 227(BR); Tom Pantages 600(BL); Pearson Education/PH College 452(CL/BL), 509, 1121(TL), 853; Barbara Penoyar/Getty Images, Inc./Photodisc 461(BR); R. Spencer Phippen/Phototake NYC 453(TR); Photo Researchers, Inc. 18, 938; Phototake NYC 857(TR); Roy Ramsey/Pearson Education/PH College 955(BR); A.M. Siegelman/Visuals Unlimited 853(BR); Justin Slide/ Dorling Kindersley Media Library 1130; Simon Smith/ Dorling Kindersley Media Library 521; Southern Illinois University/Photo Researchers, Inc. 28(BL); Paul Steel/ Corbis/Stock Market 42, 43; Tom Stewart/Corbis/Stock Market 28(TL); Stockbyte 3(BR), 65(BR); SuperStock, Inc. 452(TL); William Taufic/Corbis/Stock Market 196, 248; The Stock Photo Shop, Inc. 30(TL); US Healthcare 273; Brian Warling/American Association of Medical Assistants 9; Brian Warling/International Museum of Surgical Science; Chicago, IL 14, 15(TL), 16, 19, 22, 30(BL), 56; Brian Warling/Japan Airlines 218; Brian Warling/Pearson Education/Prentice Hall College 302, 879(TL); James Wilson/Woodfin Camp & Associates 1097(TL); John Woodcock/ Dorling Kindersley Media Library 431

Illustration Credits

All illustration created by Imagineering Inc. for Prentice Hall.

Additional Acknowledgments

Employment Forms Courtesy of Bibbero Systems, Inc., Petaluma, CA, (800) 242-2374, www.bibbero.com, 330 RMA Duty Pin Courtesy of the American Medical Technologists, 9

Successful Connections

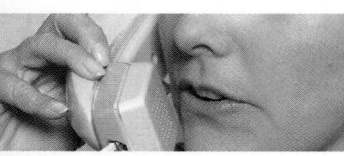

Pearson's Comprehensive Medical Assisting

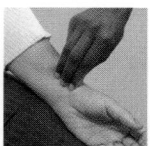

This is the first book to connect skills in the classroom and skills on the job, by helping medical assistant students achieve success in school and in their careers.

With *Pearson's Comprehensive Medical Assisting*, students learn what to do and how to do it. Strong integration of tips, hints, and guidelines help students avoid common performance problems, including timeliness, presentation, and interpersonal relations.

Skills in the Classroom

- Preparing for the Certification Exam
- Applied learning activities
- Open design makes using the text easy and clear to the student
- Role Delineation Chart shows student and instructor which skills and competencies will be covered in the chapter

Skills on the Job

- Case Study
- Legal and Ethical Issues
- Cultural Considerations
- Lifespan Considerations
- Professionalism
- Patient Education
- Preparing for Externship

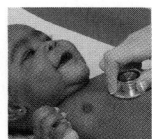
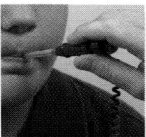
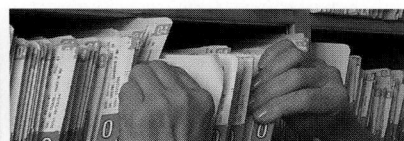

Chapter Opener Features...

Role Delineation Chart

Role Delineation Chart sets the stage and directly links the material that students need to master for passing the Certification Exam.

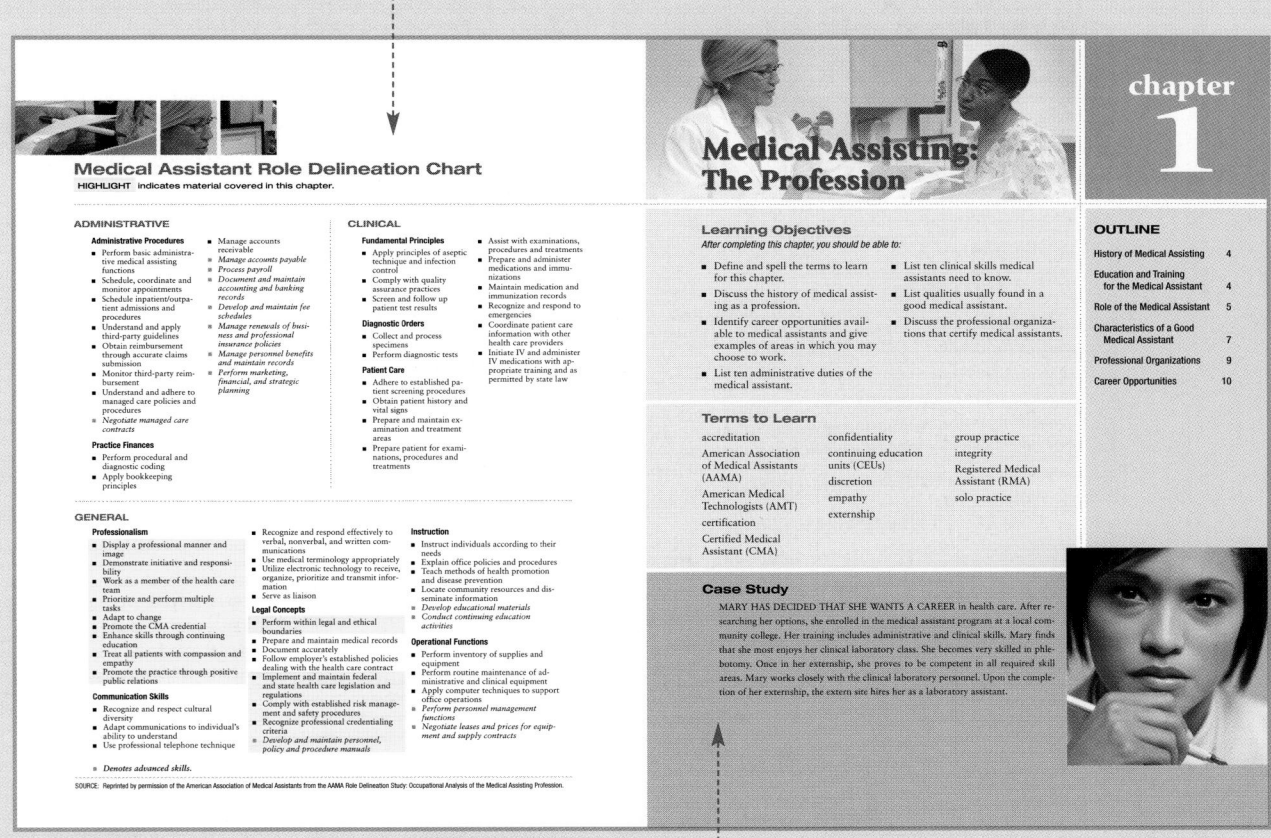

Medical Assistant Role Delineation Chart

HIGHLIGHT indicates material covered in this chapter.

ADMINISTRATIVE

Administrative Procedures
- Perform basic administrative medical assisting functions
- Schedule, coordinate and monitor appointments
- Schedule inpatient/outpatient admissions and procedures
- Understand and apply third-party guidelines
- Obtain reimbursement through accurate claims submission
- Monitor third-party reimbursement
- Understand and adhere to managed care policies and procedures
- *Negotiate managed care contracts*

- Manage accounts receivable
- *Manage accounts payable*
- *Process payroll*
- *Document and maintain accounting and banking records*
- *Develop and maintain fee schedules*
- *Manage renewals of business and professional insurance policies*
- *Manage personnel benefits and maintain records*
- *Perform marketing, financial, and strategic planning*

Practice Finances
- Perform procedural and diagnostic coding
- Apply bookkeeping principles

CLINICAL

Fundamental Principles
- Apply principles of aseptic technique and infection control
- Comply with quality assurance practices
- Screen and follow up patient test results

Diagnostic Orders
- Collect and process specimens
- Perform diagnostic tests

Patient Care
- Adhere to established patient screening procedures
- Obtain patient history and vital signs
- Prepare and maintain examination and treatment areas
- Prepare patient for examinations, procedures and treatments

- Assist with examinations, procedures and treatments
- Prepare and administer medications and immunizations
- Maintain medication and immunization records
- Recognize and respond to emergencies
- Coordinate patient care information with other health care providers
- Initiate IV and administer IV medications with appropriate training and as permitted by state law

GENERAL

Professionalism
- Display a professional manner and image
- Demonstrate initiative and responsibility
- Work as a member of the health care team
- Prioritize and perform multiple tasks
- Adapt to change
- Promote the CMA credential
- Enhance skills through continuing education
- Treat all patients with compassion and empathy
- Promote the practice through positive public relations

Communication Skills
- Recognize and respect cultural diversity
- Adapt communications to individual's ability to understand
- Use professional telephone technique

- Recognize and respond effectively to verbal, nonverbal, and written communications
- Use medical terminology appropriately
- Utilize electronic technology to receive, organize, prioritize and transmit information
- Serve as liaison

Legal Concepts
- Perform within legal and ethical boundaries
- Prepare and maintain medical records
- Document accurately
- Follow employer's established policies dealing with the health care contract
- Implement and maintain federal and state health care legislation and regulations
- Comply with established risk management and safety procedures
- Recognize professional credentialing criteria
- *Develop and maintain personnel, policy and procedure manuals*

Instruction
- Instruct individuals according to their needs
- Explain office policies and procedures
- Teach methods of health promotion and disease prevention
- Locate community resources and disseminate information
- *Develop educational materials*
- *Conduct continuing education activities*

Operational Functions
- Perform inventory of supplies and equipment
- Perform routine maintenance of administrative and clinical equipment
- Apply computer techniques to support office operations
- *Perform personnel management functions*
- *Negotiate leases and prices for equipment and supply contracts*

- *Denotes advanced skills.*

SOURCE: Reprinted by permission of the American Association of Medical Assistants from the AAMA Role Delineation Study: Occupational Analysis of the Medical Assisting Profession.

Medical Assisting: The Profession

chapter 1

Learning Objectives

After completing this chapter, you should be able to:

- Define and spell the terms to learn for this chapter.
- Discuss the history of medical assisting as a profession.
- Identify career opportunities available to medical assistants and give examples of areas in which you may choose to work.
- List ten administrative duties of the medical assistant.
- List ten clinical skills medical assistants need to know.
- List qualities usually found in a good medical assistant.
- Discuss the professional organizations that certify medical assistants.

Terms to Learn

accreditation
American Association of Medical Assistants (AAMA)
American Medical Technologists (AMT)
certification
Certified Medical Assistant (CMA)

confidentiality
continuing education units (CEUs)
discretion
empathy
externship

group practice
integrity
Registered Medical Assistant (RMA)
solo practice

OUTLINE

History of Medical Assisting 4

Education and Training for the Medical Assistant 4

Role of the Medical Assistant 5

Characteristics of a Good Medical Assistant 7

Professional Organizations 9

Career Opportunities 10

Case Study

MARY HAS DECIDED THAT SHE WANTS A CAREER in health care. After researching her options, she enrolled in the medical assistant program at a local community college. Her training includes administrative and clinical skills. Mary finds that she most enjoys her clinical laboratory class. She becomes very skilled in phlebotomy. Once in her externship, she proves to be competent in all required skill areas. Mary works closely with the clinical laboratory personnel. Upon the completion of her externship, the extern site hires her as a laboratory assistant.

Case Study

Case Study provides brief vignettes that help students understand how the chapter information relates to their careers. It increases retention of chapter material because students have a context for the topics.

Additional Features...

Open design is ideal for visual learners. Material is presented in smaller chunks with relevant applications to provide context.

Legal
and Ethical Issues

Licensure and continuing medical education (CME) are two areas in which you can assist the physician. The renewal of licenses is usually dependent on the completion of re-registration forms and filing these forms on time with the necessary fees. Always take care to maintain accurate records of continuing medical education units earned by the physician since CME is an important part of the licensing process. Be alert to this legal obligation and remind your employing physician in advance of such renewals.

Medical assistants dedicate themselves to the care and well-being of all patients, according to the American Association of Medical Assistants code of ethics. In addition, medical assistants should take the Oath of Hippocrates, Òdo no harm to the patient" as seriously as the physicians who state it at the time of their graduation from medical school. As a medical assistant, you will act as a representative of the physician and must be well versed on all legal issues that affect the physician's practice.

Legal and Ethical Issues

Legal and Ethical Issues address the complex topics in a practical and relevant manner, making it easier for students to apply.

Professionalism

The professional medical assistant will occasionally have days on which the physician is seeing patients later than their appointments. This can create discomfort for both the patients and the medical assistant. Explain to patients that the physician is running behind, and give them the option to reschedule their appointment. If they choose to wait, be sure to move them to an exam room as quickly as possible, and plan ahead as much as possible to help the physician be as efficient as possible. Explaining to patients that the physician is providing the same care to other patients that he or she will provide to them will help to alleviate their frustrations with the delays. Always remember that if patients verbalize their frustrations about the delay, their attack is never personal; instead, they are just venting their frustration.

Professionalism

Professionalism is one of the most important keys to career success. These featured highlights help students understand the importance of adopting and maintaining a professional demeanor.

Cultural Considerations

Cultural Considerations give students the skills to connect with both patients and other health professionals from diverse backgrounds.

Cultural Considerations

Family in some populations is extremely important to the patient. Family members provide not only emotional and physical support but are an essential part of the medical decision-making process. Do not be surprised if your patient brings along the entire family, including parents, grandparents, siblings, aunts, and uncles to discuss an important medical condition. Be prepared for a large crowd and do not get annoyed. Make them as comfortable as possible and consider them part of the healing process.

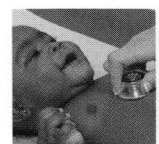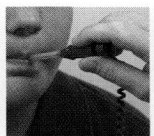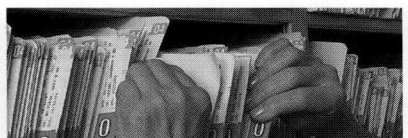

Lifespan
Considerations

Drawing blood from an older individual can sometimes be challenging due to the condition of their veins. Patients do not want to have any more needle sticks than necessary. To ensure that a successful needle stick occurs requires both experience and patience. If patients will be returning to the office for blood work at a later time, inform the patient to drink a lot of fluids prior to arrival at the office. Being well hydrated is helpful for finding veins. Use of items such as a small ball placed in the patient's hand to squeeze in order to pump up the veins is also helpful. If the hand must be used for the draw site, place a warm cloth over the area to allow for the vein to rise up. All of these techniques can help in making the first try a success.

Lifespan Considerations

Lifespan Considerations help students develop the skills to relate to patients of all ages.

Patient Education

Skin care is a very important part of hygiene. Patients should be taught that they should moisturize their skin on a daily basis, or more often as necessary. Sunscreen is one of the easiest ways to avoid skin cancer, and teaching patients about using adequate sun protection may be one duty of the medical assistant. Write down the correct sun protection factor prescribed by the physician so that the patient can easily locate the appropriate lotion in the store. Patients should be taught to avoid sunburn as much as possible. Some medications can increase the risk of sunburn, and education for patients who take these medications is extremely important.

Patient Education

Patient Education provides hints and important tips on how to share information with patients in a professional and complete manner.

Preparing for Externship

Preparing for Externship discusses topics and issues students may encounter during participation in an externship program.

Preparing for
Externship

When preparing for a procedure, *carefully plan the steps you will take. Make sure that you not only do exactly what you have been asked to do or prepare for, but be ready to take the next step. Always think ahead. Ask yourself what the physician might need next, whether it is having paperwork for labs ready to go or a prescription pad or being ready for a follow-up procedure. If the physician will be performing a minor surgical procedure, be sure that all the necessary supplies, including dressings, are ready for use.*

Certification

Certification Exam Success end-of-the-chapter self-assessment and practice help students build exam confidence.

PREPARING FOR THE CERTIFICATION EXAM

1. Which of the following is the amount of air that can be forcibly inspired after a normal inhalation?
   A. tidal volume
   B. expiratory reserve
   C. inspiratory reserve
   D. total lung capacity
   E. residual volume

2. When performing an ECG on a patient with a right lower leg cast, the leg sensors are placed:
   A. on the left leg
   B. on both upper legs
   C. on both upper arms
   D. on the bottom of the feet
   E. they are eliminated.

3. An electrocardiogram is a:
   A. recording of the voltage with respect to time
   B. recording of the mechanical action of the heart
   C. technique for making recordings of heart activity
   D. machine used to make cardiac tracings.
   E. recording of the size

4. Normally, a complete ECG consists of _____ sensors and _____ leads.
   A. 10, 10
   B. 8, 10
   C. 6, 12
   D. 12, 10
   E. 10, 12

5. The Purkinje fibers are located on or in the:
   A. right atrium
   B. left atrium
   C. apex
   D. ventricles
   E. septum between the atria

6. The portion of the ECG that relates to ventricular depolarization is the:
   A. P wave
   B. QRS complex
   C. T wave
   D. U wave
   E. P-R interval

CRITICAL THINKING

1. Did Betsy greet Stacy appropriately?
2. What was the benefit of sending Stacy the paperwork in the mail before her visit?
3. Why did Betsy give Stacy the Notice of Privacy Practice?
4. Did Betsy handle the phone call appropriately? If not, how should she have handled it?

ON THE JOB

Dr. Morrison, a child psychiatrist, who is in solo practice, employs one medical assistant in her office. This medical assistant is multiskilled, like all medical assistants, and, essentially, handles all of the administrative and clinical tasks in the office.

It is 3:00 P.M. and a parent has just arrived for a 3:30 P.M. appointment with her 10-year old daughter. The child is a new patient of Dr. Morrison and was referred by her attending physician. She has a relatively long history of combative and destructive behavior and the referring pediatrician is seeking a psychological evaluation from Dr. Morrison. Psychotropic medication of some sort may be a viable treatment option. The medical assistant has asked the mother and daughter to please be seated and to fill out some registration forms. The child is acting out—pulling cushions off of the reception room couch, wildly ripping the pages of the magazines, whining and kicking at her mother. The behavior seems to be escalating as the mother tries to frantically control her child while, at the same time, follow the instructions of the medical assistant and fill out the registration forms.

What is your response?

1. What if anything, should the medical assistant do?
2. Would it be appropriate, for example, for the medical assistant to interrupt Dr. Morrison's current session?
3. Might this be considered a medical emergency?

INTERNET ACTIVITY

1. Find out how HIPAA has changed the way the medical office handles patient reception.
2. Look for companies that produce forms that can be used by a medical receptionist.

MediaLink More on patient reception in the medical office environment, including interactive resources, can be found on the Student CD-ROM accompanying this textbook.

applied learning activities

Applied learning activities like "On the Job" scenarios help students increase retention and success by linking concepts to their job functions.

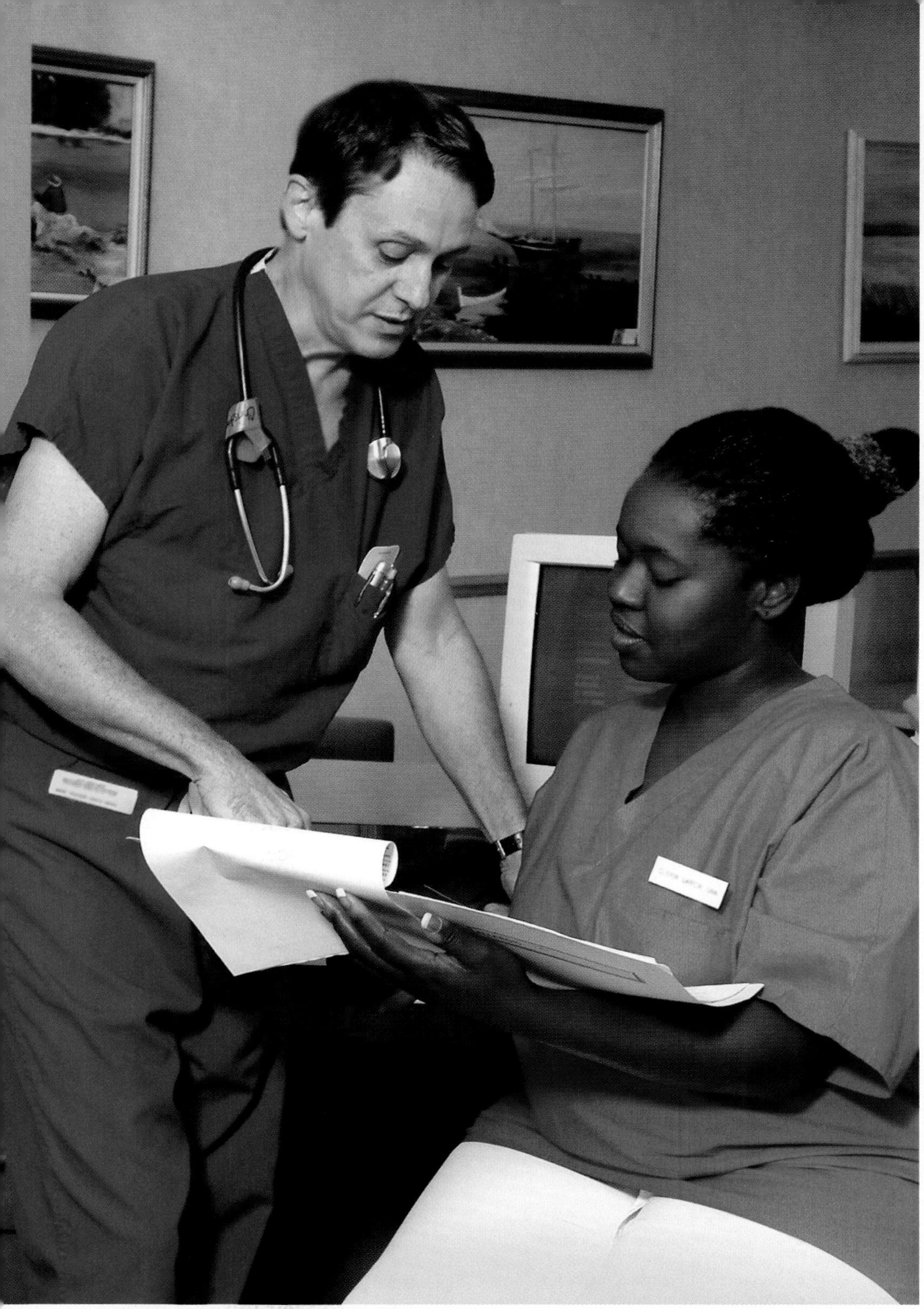

Unit One

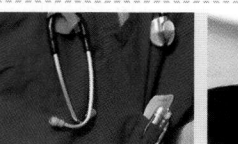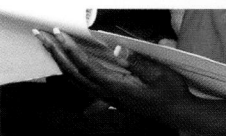

Introduction to Health Care

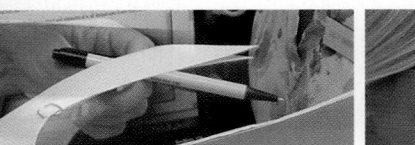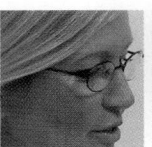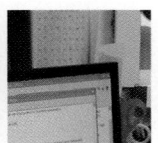

Medical Assistant Role Delineation Chart

HIGHLIGHT indicates material covered in this chapter.

ADMINISTRATIVE

Administrative Procedures

- Perform basic administrative medical assisting functions
- Schedule, coordinate and monitor appointments
- Schedule inpatient/outpatient admissions and procedures
- Understand and apply third-party guidelines
- Obtain reimbursement through accurate claims submission
- Monitor third-party reimbursement
- Understand and adhere to managed care policies and procedures
- *Negotiate managed care contracts*

Practice Finances

- Perform procedural and diagnostic coding
- Apply bookkeeping principles

- Manage accounts receivable
- *Manage accounts payable*
- *Process payroll*
- *Document and maintain accounting and banking records*
- *Develop and maintain fee schedules*
- *Manage renewals of business and professional insurance policies*
- *Manage personnel benefits and maintain records*
- *Perform marketing, financial, and strategic planning*

CLINICAL

Fundamental Principles

- Apply principles of aseptic technique and infection control
- Comply with quality assurance practices
- Screen and follow up patient test results

Diagnostic Orders

- Collect and process specimens
- Perform diagnostic tests

Patient Care

- Adhere to established patient screening procedures
- Obtain patient history and vital signs
- Prepare and maintain examination and treatment areas
- Prepare patient for examinations, procedures and treatments

- Assist with examinations, procedures and treatments
- Prepare and administer medications and immunizations
- Maintain medication and immunization records
- Recognize and respond to emergencies
- Coordinate patient care information with other health care providers
- Initiate IV and administer IV medications with appropriate training and as permitted by state law

GENERAL

Professionalism

- Display a professional manner and image
- Demonstrate initiative and responsibility
- Work as a member of the health care team
- Prioritize and perform multiple tasks
- Adapt to change
- Promote the CMA credential
- Enhance skills through continuing education
- Treat all patients with compassion and empathy
- Promote the practice through positive public relations

Communication Skills

- Recognize and respect cultural diversity
- Adapt communications to individual's ability to understand
- Use professional telephone technique

- Recognize and respond effectively to verbal, nonverbal, and written communications
- Use medical terminology appropriately
- Utilize electronic technology to receive, organize, prioritize and transmit information
- Serve as liaison

Legal Concepts

- Perform within legal and ethical boundaries
- Prepare and maintain medical records
- Document accurately
- Follow employer's established policies dealing with the health care contract
- Implement and maintain federal and state health care legislation and regulations
- Comply with established risk management and safety procedures
- Recognize professional credentialing criteria
- *Develop and maintain personnel, policy and procedure manuals*

Instruction

- Instruct individuals according to their needs
- Explain office policies and procedures
- Teach methods of health promotion and disease prevention
- Locate community resources and disseminate information
- *Develop educational materials*
- *Conduct continuing education activities*

Operational Functions

- Perform inventory of supplies and equipment
- Perform routine maintenance of administrative and clinical equipment
- Apply computer techniques to support office operations
- *Perform personnel management functions*
- *Negotiate leases and prices for equipment and supply contracts*

■ *Denotes advanced skills.*

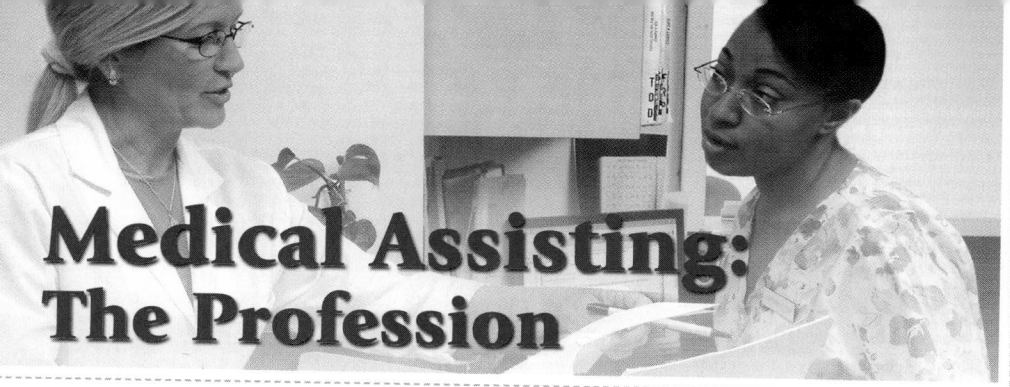

Medical Assisting: The Profession

Learning Objectives

After completing this chapter, you should be able to:

- Define and spell the terms to learn for this chapter.
- Discuss the history of medical assisting as a profession.
- Identify career opportunities available to medical assistants and give examples of areas in which you may choose to work.
- List ten administrative duties of the medical assistant.

- List ten clinical skills medical assistants need to know.
- List qualities usually found in a good medical assistant.
- Discuss the professional organizations that certify medical assistants.

OUTLINE

History of Medical Assisting 4

Education and Training
  for the Medical Assistant 4

Role of the Medical Assistant 5

Characteristics of a Good
  Medical Assistant 7

Professional Organizations 9

Career Opportunities 10

Terms to Learn

accreditation	confidentiality	group practice
American Association of Medical Assistants (AAMA)	continuing education units (CEUs)	integrity
	discretion	Registered Medical Assistant (RMA)
American Medical Technologists (AMT)	empathy	solo practice
certification	externship	
Certified Medical Assistant (CMA)		

Case Study

MARY HAS DECIDED THAT SHE WANTS A CAREER in health care. After researching her options, she enrolled in the medical assistant program at a local community college. Her training includes administrative and clinical skills. Mary finds that she most enjoys her clinical laboratory class. She becomes very skilled in phlebotomy. Once in her externship, she proves to be competent in all required skill areas. Mary works closely with the clinical laboratory personnel. Upon the completion of her externship, the extern site hires her as a laboratory assistant.

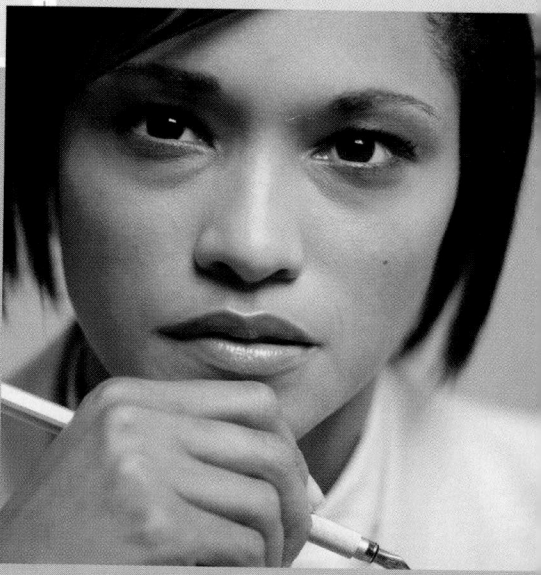

The rapidly changing health care environment has caused health care providers to rely more heavily on assistive personnel. As a result, medical assistants have become an important part the health care team. No matter the setting, these multifunctional team members provide valuable services and support. Medical assistants can be found in a variety of settings from pediatric to chiropractic offices. No matter how varied the roles or duties of the medical assistant (MA), the essential skills and personal qualities needed in all good medical assistants are quite similar.

As a well-trained, multiskilled health care professional, the medical assistant fulfills many roles in the allied health field where the challenges of everyday are balanced by opportunities for advancement, personal growth, and satisfaction. Professional organizations that oversee or regulate the education, training, and certification of medical assistants are also discussed in this chapter along with current career opportunities and the future of the medical assisting field.

History of Medical Assisting

Historically, medical assistants were trained on the job by a physician. They became skilled through the day-to-day education and training provided in the medical office. Due to the increasing responsibilities, most clinics staff their offices with individuals who have received some form of formal training. Many physicians had become familiar with the clinical skills of nurses while working closely with nurses in the hospital setting, so they chose to hire registered nurses to work in their offices. When a shortage of nursing personnel occurred, physicians had to look elsewhere for professionally trained office personnel who could handle both the administrative and clinical responsibilities of a medical office practice (Figure 1-1). Patient Education addresses the need to distinguish nurses and medical assistants.

The American Association of Medical Assistants (AAMA), organized in 1956, offers the following definition of medical assisting:

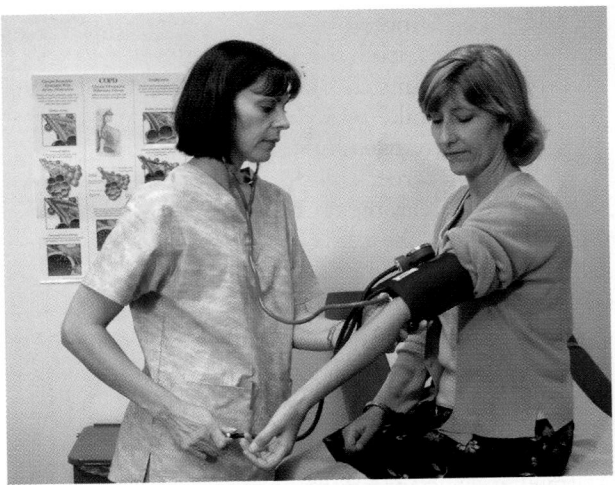

FIGURE 1-1 Medical assistants perform many functions in a physician's office or a clinic.

Medical assisting is a multiskilled allied health profession whose practitioners work primarily in ambulatory settings such as medical offices and clinics. Medical assistants function as members of the health care delivery team and perform administrative and clinical procedures.

(From Essentials and Guidelines for an Accredited Educational Program for the Medical Assistant, adopted by the AAMA's Endowment and the American Medical Association in 1969, revised 1971, 1977, 1984, 1991, 1999, and 2003. Copyright by the American Association of Medical Assistants, Inc. Reprinted by permission.)

Education and Training for the Medical Assistant

Over the years, the education and training of medical assistants has undergone many changes and today, medical assistants are well-trained and respected practitioners in the allied health field. Students may obtain a certificate, diploma, or associate degree in the field of medical assisting.

Patient Education

Patients do not always clearly understand the distinctions among the professions of medical assistant, physician's assistant, and nurse. It is your responsibility to clarify for the patients what you are permitted to do. Do not accept being addressed as "nurse," since the nursing license carries different responsibilities and standards than does the medical assistant's certificate.

- Certificate programs: The length of the course of study varies from one institution to the next. Some programs are six weeks in length, while others may take up to a year to complete. These programs are usually offered in either vocational schools or career colleges. The focus tends to be on the development of clinical skills. Students may choose the traditional classroom setting or may opt for distance learning (online). Most certificate programs require a hands-on externship to complete the program. Depending on the accreditation, graduates of certificate programs may be eligible to sit for a national certification examination. Students who choose this training option may be supplementing prior training or may want an introduction to the health care field.

- Diploma program: These programs tend to be similar to the certificate programs. Most diploma programs are nine months to a year in length. Career and community colleges most often offer this course of study. Training focuses on developing clinical skills, as well as limited administrative skills. Completion of an externship is required and most students qualify to sit for a national certification examination. Students selecting this option may be interested in a career as a medical assistant. Others may want to use this as a stepping stone to other health care careers.

- Degree program: This course of study is approximately two years in length. It is usually offered in a traditional classroom setting at a career or community college. Along with clinical and administrative courses, courses to assist in professional development are offered as part of the curriculum. This option is usually chosen by those who know that they want a career as a medical assistant.

Accreditation

Accreditation is the process in which an institution voluntarily completes an extensive self-study after which an accrediting association visits the school to verify the self-study statements. Accreditation ensures that a school meets an established list of criteria.

Schools may also seek programmatic accreditation for their medical assisting programs. The learning outcomes for these programs are competency based. The U.S. Department of Education recognizes two agencies to accredit programs in medical assisting:

- The Commission on Accreditation of Allied Health Education Programs (CAAHEP)

- The Accrediting Bureau of Health Education Schools (ABHES)

The Joint Review Committee for Ophthalmic Medical Personnel accredits programs in ophthalmic medical assisting.

The CAAHEP Essentials state that to provide for student attainment of "*Entry-Level Competencies for the Medical Assistant*," the curriculum—"shall include, but is not limited to the following units, modules, and/or courses of instruction:"

- Anatomy and Physiology
- Medical Terminology
- Medical Law and Ethics
- Psychology
- Communication (oral and written)
- Medical Assistant Administrative Procedures
- Medical Assisting Clinical Procedures
- Professional Components
- Externship

An externship experience is required in which students work without payment in a physician's office, clinic, or hospital setting for a specified number of hours over several weeks during the final stage of their training.

Role of the Medical Assistant

The medical assistant's main responsibility is to assist the physician in providing patient care. Central to a medical assistant's responsibilities are sound clinical skills. He or she must be able to obtain vital signs, collect specimens, administer medication, and run basic laboratory tests. It is not unusual to find medical assistants who take x-rays, conduct cardiac stress tests, and assist with minor office surgeries. Administrative duties may be part of the job description. In small clinics or physicians' offices, the medical assistant may function as the receptionist or insurance clerk.

The field of medical assisting is open to both men and women in a variety of work settings such as physicians' offices, ambulatory care clinics, government agencies, extended-care centers, hospitals, urgent care facilities, and free-standing facilities (Figure 1-2).

Responsibilities of the Medical Assistant

The list of responsibilities that medical assistants perform is extensive. For this reason, the education and training for this field is carefully designed and must involve both theory and hands-on experience. The actual duties of the medical assistant vary from office to office. However, a good medical assistant, who has received a well-rounded education, will be able to adjust to different work environments. Never perform

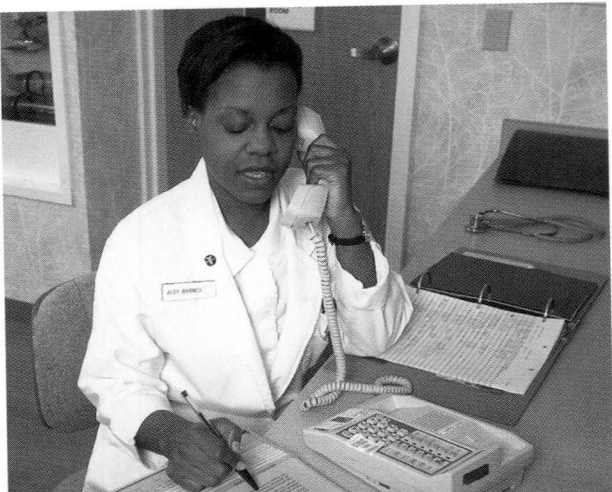

FIGURE 1-2 The medical assisting profession offers many settings in which to pursue your career. Good communication and social skills are required in each of them.

duties that are beyond your level of responsibility—education and training (Legal and Ethical Issues).

Medical assistants' responsibilities will also vary according to the size and type of setting and state laws that apply. Always familiarize yourself with federal and state regulations and guidelines governing the procedures that medical assistants are allowed to perform in whatever environment you work. Generally, the medical assistants' duties are grouped into two categories: administrative and clinical and include the following competencies.

Administrative Competencies—Business and Front Office

- Scheduling patients, including referrals to specialists
- Greeting and receiving patients
- Screening nonpatients and visitors
- Making arrangements for patient admissions to hospitals, patient tests, and procedures such as x-rays and laboratory tests
- Providing patient instruction regarding procedures and tests performed in the physician's office and hospitals
- Updating and filing patient medical records
- Coding diagnoses and procedures for insurance purposes
- Computer skills (Figure 1-3)
- Handling financial arrangements with patients
- Introduction to, or transcribing medical dictation
- Handling the telephone, reports, correspondence, and filing
- Handling mail, billing, insurance claims, credit, and collections
- Operating office equipment
- Preparing and maintaining employee records
- Handling petty cash
- Reconciling bank statements
- Maintaining records for license renewals, membership fees, and insurance premiums

Legal and Ethical Issues

It is important to fully understand what your credentials allow you to do. The medical assistant is uniquely qualified to perform the administrative and clinical procedures associated with responsibilities assigned in the particular setting by the physician. In fulfilling these responsibilities, however, you must always be aware that the potential for psychological, financial, and physical injury to the patient exists. It is your ethical responsibility to patients and your employer that you do your utmost to maintain a high level of skill performance in all that you do. The medical assistant always works as an agent of the physician.

Many of the jobs and careers discussed in this chapter require additional education, including passing a written certification examination. Be mindful that patients understand what your title—Certified Medical Assistant (CMA) or Registered Medical Assistant (RMA)—means. Never be afraid to say, "I am not qualified to do that."

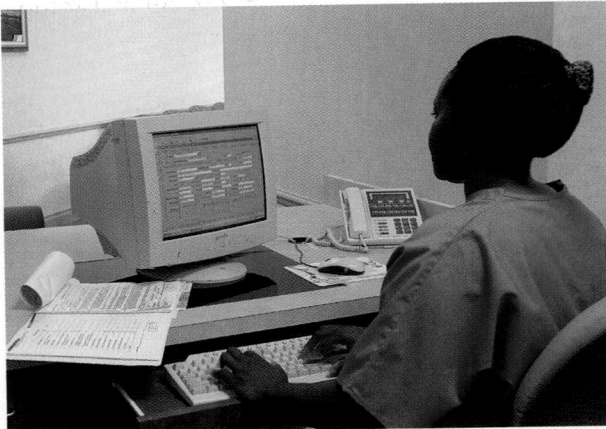

FIGURE 1-3 Good computer skills are now required to be a successful member of an office staff.

- Handling the office in the physician's absence
- Assisting the physician with articles, lectures, and manuscripts
- Utilization review of necessary procedures and referrals
- Coordinating managed-care coverage for patients and physicians
- Ensure compliance with HIPAA guidelines

Clinical Competencies—Care and Treatment of Patients

- Assisting patients in preparation for physical examinations and procedures
- Obtaining a medical history (Figure 1-4)
- Performing routine clinical and laboratory procedures under the supervision of a physician
- Collecting, preparing, and transporting laboratory specimens
- Venipuncture, where permitted
- Assisting the physician with procedures
- Instructing and educating patients on treatments and procedures
- Cleaning and sterilizing equipment
- Obtaining patient's height, weight, and vital signs
- Preparing and maintaining examination and treatment rooms
- Inventory control—ordering and storing of supplies
- Disposing of hazardous waste and other materials
- Administering medications under the supervision and orders of the physician, where permitted
- Changing bandages and dressings, and suture removal, where permitted
- Handling drug refills as directed by the physician
- Performing ECGs
- Occupational Safety and Health Administration (OSHA) guidelines compliance and employee instruction
- Performing skills relevant to a particular practice (for example: audiometry, spirometry, halter monitor)
- Disposing of contaminated supplies
- Sterilizing medical instruments
- Preparing patients for x-rays

Medical assistants who specialize will have additional duties. Some of these specialties include pediatric medical assistants, ophthalmic medical assistants, and surgical medical assistants.

Medical assistants must also meet technical standards such as bending requirements, correct bending

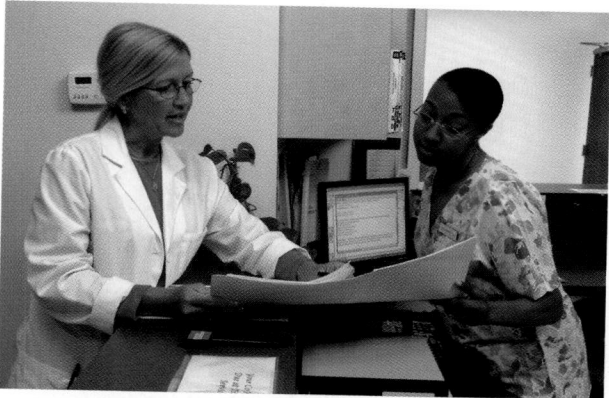

FIGURE 1-4 Helping maintain accurate patient records is a critical part of the medical assistant's work.

procedures, being able to stand for long periods of time, being able to reach overhead, and being able to lift 30 pounds.

Role Delineation

The AAMA analyzed the medical assisting field in 1979 to determine the responsibilities of the medical assistant. As a result of this survey and analysis, the AAMA used a process for developing a curriculum called DACUM (Developing A Curriculum) based on the skills performed daily by medical assistants. The DACUM philosophy is based on the belief that expert workers can describe and define their job more accurately than anyone else. In 1984 and 1990, the DACUM list was revised to reflect the major changes in medicine and the health care delivery system.

The Role Delineation Study released in 1997 and updated in 2003 by the AAMA updates and replaces DACUM. This study is the result of a composite of current competencies essential for medical assistants based upon the practice experience of an expert panel. A Role Delineation Chart, which outlines the study, identifies three major categories of competence—administrative, clinical, and general, or interdisciplinary—for entry-level medical assistants. These areas are further expanded to include competencies that should be taught in medical assisting programs. See the Role Delineation Chart included with each chapter.

Characteristics of a Good Medical Assistant

In addition to having a general medical knowledge, including medical terminology, and being able to perform administrative and clinical responsibilities, medical assistants must genuinely care about others. Cultural Considerations discusses how cultural background and personal beliefs may impact your relationship with patients.

The nature of the patient and health care worker relationship demands medical assistants be able to communicate effectively and get along with others. Qualities or characteristic regularly found in good medical assistants are integrity, discretion, empathy, and the ability to safeguard the patient's right to confidentiality (Figure 1-5).

- Integrity—A medical assistant with integrity will do what is expected, when it is expected, for the simple reason that it is expected. Someone with integrity is usually honest, dependable, punctual, and dedicated to high standards.

- Empathy—The ability to work with the sick and the infirm depend on one's ability and willingness to show empathy. A medical assistant with empathy has the ability to be sensitive to or understand the feelings of another individual. An empathic person is able to stand in the shoes of another and identify with what he or she is experiencing. For example, when a medical assistant has some insight or understanding of the pain or distress a patient is feeling, he or she acts in a kindly way that expresses sensitivity to the patient's feelings.

- Discretion—A medical assistant who uses discretion is able to make decisions responsibly. Someone who uses discretion is tactful in communicating with others. It is important to be able to be fair and be familiar with policies and regulations. Discretion is important in patient interaction, as well as interaction with coworkers.

- Confidentiality—The ability to safeguard patient confidences, particularly information in the medical record regarding family history, past or current diseases or illnesses, test results, and medications is vital to the patient and health care professional relationship. No information about the patient is to be disclosed without the written permission of the patient. This is a legal and ethical issue with penalties for violating patient confidentiality. Without this trust, there can be no relationship. As the person with most frequent access to patient records and verbal confidences, the medical assistant has a serious professional responsibility to safeguard the patient's right to confidentiality.

In many cases, the medical assistant will be the first health professional with whom the patient interacts and on whom the patient bases his or her opinion of the physician (Professionalism). It is important to present a confident, professional image that helps put the patient at ease. A calm, pleasant speaking voice conveys a professional attitude. Remember, eating, drinking, or chewing gum while working are not appropriate in areas open to the public. Along with a basic understanding of human behavior and good communication skills—written, spoken, and nonverbal—the medical assistant must be able to handle tasks requiring basic mathematics, grammar, and spelling skills.

Daily habits of good personal hygiene and grooming are expected from the medical assistant. The use of strong perfumes and showy jewelry is not professional and may

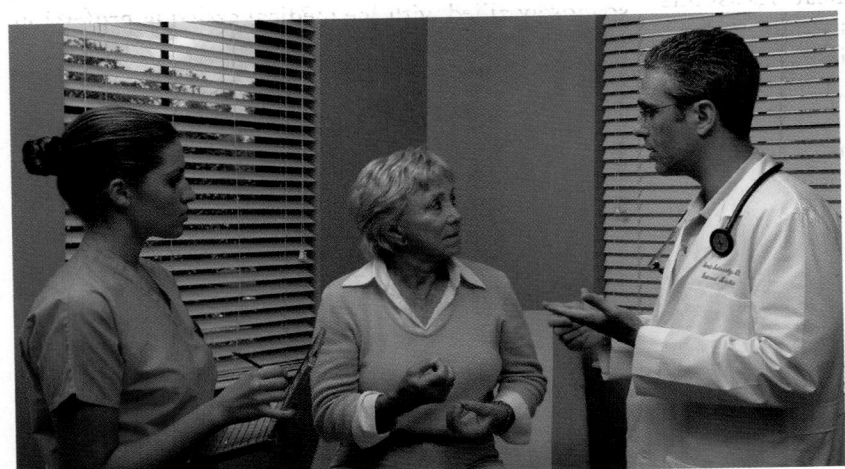

FIGURE 1-5 Medical assistants are often involved in confidential conversations between the physician and the patient.

Professionalism

Lifespan
Considerations

even be harmful. For example, strong perfume may actually trigger headaches in some individuals and loose dangling jewelry may get in the way while treating a patient. Loose, long hair and extended nails should be avoided.

Medical assistants provide the quality of care that they would wish to have given to themselves or to members of their own families. The medical assistant must have the ability to see beyond the gruff or complaining manner of the patient who is not feeling well and project a professional, pleasant, and caring attitude. Lifespan Considerations discusses patients at various life stages that medical assistants will encounter.

Professional Organizations

The American Association of Medical Assistants (AAMA), founded in 1959, is a key association in the field of medical assisting. Chicago, Illinois is national headquarters for the AAMA. This organization is responsible for the Certified Medical Assistant (CMA) certification process and offers the certification examination in January, June and in October. Certification indicates that a candidate has met the standards of the AAMA by achieving a satisfactory test result. A certificate, or legal document, is issued to such a person. The first examination given to certify medical assistants was administered in 1963.

The certification examination is offered to graduates of programs accredited by the Commission of Accreditation of Allied Health Education Program (CAAHEP) or by the Accrediting Bureau of Health Education Schools (ABHES). Upon successful completion of the certification examination, candidates will

receive a certificate, confirming them as certified medical assistants (Figure 1-6).

Membership in the AAMA is not necessary to take the certification examination. For the credential to remain current, it must be revalidated every five years, either by earning a designated number of continuing education units (CEUs) or through reexamination. The AAMA sponsors workshops, seminars, and county, state, and national conferences for medical assistants to remain current in their field.

The AAMA accredits medical assisting education/training programs and has set the minimum standards for the entry-level in this profession. Since the AAMA is so closely allied with the medical assisting profession,

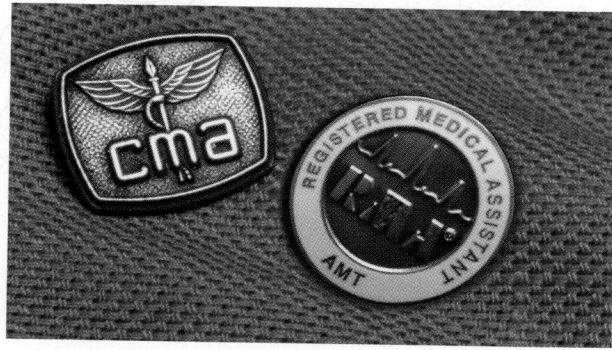

FIGURE 1-6 Becoming a Certified Medical Assistant may demonstrate your commitment to the profession and the continuing education required to maintain the CMA credential.

it is able to monitor the needs and skill education/ training of the students. Education programs are periodically reevaluated by the AAMA to assure that the curriculum is adequate and maintained. Recommendations for re-accreditation are then made by the AAMA to the new accrediting agency, Commission on Accreditation of Allied Health Education Program (CAAHEP).

The American Medical Technologists (AMT) association provides oversight for the registration and testing of medical assistants, medical technologists and phlebotomists. This association, in cooperation with the AMT Institute for Education (AMTIE) has developed a continuing education (CE) program and recording system.

The AMT, a nonprofit certifying body, provides a Registered Medical Assistant (RMA) certification examination for medical assistants who meet the eligibility requirements and who can prove their competency to perform entry-level skills through written examination. The RMA is awarded to candidates who pass the AMT certification examination. The RMA certification examination is formed around the following parameters:

I. General Medical Assisting Knowledge
   a. Anatomy and Physiology
   b. Medical Terminology
   c. Medical Law
   d. Medical Ethics
   e. Human Rights
   f. Patient Education

II. Administrative Medical Assisting
   a. Insurance
   b. Financial Bookkeeping
   c. Medical Secretarial—Receptionist

III. Clinical Medical Assisting
   a. Asepsis
   b. Sterilization
   c. Instruments
   d. Vital Signs
   e. Physical Examinations
   f. Clinical Pharmacology
   g. Minor Surgery
   h. Therapeutic Modalities
   i. Laboratory Procedures
   j. Electrocardiography
   k. First Aid

Career Opportunities

According to US Department of Labor Statistics (2003–2004 edition), medical assistants held about 365,000 jobs in 2002. Nearly 60 percent were employed by physicians' offices; 14 percent held positions in public and private hospitals; and almost 10 percent worked in the offices of other health care practitioners.

The medical assistant is the most frequently employed allied health professional in the physician's office and most physicians have more than one medical assistant working in their office. The US Bureau of Labor Statistics projects medical assisting to be the fastest growing occupation over the 2002–2012 period. (Bureau of Labor Statistics, US Department of Labor: Employment by Occupation and Industry, 2004, Washington, DC, US Government Printing Office.)

The anticipated need for more health professionals is based on the expected increase in the number of older adults who will require the care of a physician and the tremendous growth in the number of outpatient facilities. The wide range of health care settings presents many opportunities for the medical assistant who is trained in both clinical and administrative duties. Table 1-1 lists several inpatient and ambulatory care (outpatient) facilities or settings with descriptions of some possible job opportunities for medical assistants in each setting. Table 1-2 lists departments or specialties in which medical assistants may seek employment in either inpatient or ambulatory care settings. In some states and settings, additional education and training may be required for medical assistants to fulfill certain responsibilities. While the general category, "medical assistant," may be used in some career ads, some of the jobs title opportunities may include:

- Clinic aide
- Data processing clerk
- Billing or collection assistant
- Insurance claims coder
- Medical records clerk
- Clinical assistant
- Medical receptionist
- Multifunctional technician

With Additional Education and Credentials, You May Even Respond to Ads For:

- A medical laboratory assistant
- An electrocardiography (ECG) technician
- A phlebotomist

Experienced medical assistants may find work as office managers, medical records managers, hospital ward clerks, and teachers of medical assistants. With additional schooling, medical assistants can enter other health care occupations such as nursing, occupational therapy, physical therapy, medical and x-ray technologists.

Since your education and training includes general, administrative, and clinical skills, you can seek employment in many different types of work. Then, too, you may work for a physician who practices alone in a solo practice or one who participates in a group practice with other physicians. If you choose to work for a

TABLE 1-1 Job Opportunities for Medical Assistants in Inpatient and Ambulatory Care Settings

Inpatient Setting	Description of Job
Rehabilitation facility	Perform both clinical and administrative tasks in medical setting focused on rehabilitation and physical therapy.
Extended care center	Work with patients who require a protective environment.
Hospital	Perform both clinical and administrative tasks as a member of the health care team.
Nursing home	Perform clinical and administrative tasks working with older adult patients.

Ambulatory Care Setting	Description of Job
Clinic	Use clinical and administrative skills to schedule and assist with patients who require special medical attention (for example, eye clinic, orthopedic clinic, mental health clinic).
Free-standing facility	Care for patients who require immediate medical treatment.
Physician's office	Use clinical and administrative skills in the private office setting for physicians of all specialties.
Rehabilitation center	Provide care for patients recovering from illness or injury.

physician, he or she may specialize in an area of medicine such as family practice, internal medicine, pediatrics, surgery, gerontology, psychiatry, obstetrics and gynecology, sports medicine, or dermatology, just to name a few. According to the US Department of Labor Statistics (2003–2004 edition), "job prospects should be best for medical assistants with formal training or experience, particularly those with certification."

TABLE 1-2 Job Opportunities for Medical Assistants in Healthcare Departments and Specialties

Department/Specialty	Description of Job
Admissions	Handle pre-admission interviews, schedule laboratory testing, and document insurance coverage.
Billing and Insurance	Work with patients, third-party payers, insurance companies to process insurance forms, claims forms, and DRG, ICD9, CPT, and HCPC coding.
EKG/ECG Tech	Perform electrocardiogram studies on patients.
Medical Records	Use administrative skills of transcription, medical terminology, and insurance coding. Requires use of the computer.
Phlebotomy	Use clinical skills to draw blood samples for testing and blood bank use.
Surgery	Use clinical skills to sterilize surgical instruments and set up surgical trays, and assist when needed.
Treatment/Procedure/ Emergency Room (ER)	Assist with minor surgeries and procedures performed in physicians' offices, hospitals, rehabilitation centers, and emergency rooms (ER).

SUMMARY

The field of medical assisting is growing in response to increasing health care needs of consumers. The profession of medical assistant offers many opportunities—roles, responsibilities, and settings for employment. Most medical assistants work in ambulatory settings such as physicians' offices where they fulfill the administrative and clinical responsibilities associated with running medical offices. The size and nature of the medical office practice will determine the number of medical assistants and the actual work they will do.

Caring individuals, who are dedicated professionals with a commitment to maintain their skills through continuing education, make the best medical assistants. The important thing to remember is the opportunities presented are many and the future of medical assisting looks attractive. A career in medical assisting is emotionally and professionally challenging.

Chapter Review

COMPETENCY REVIEW

1. Define and spell the terms to learn for this chapter.
2. List several health care facilities or specialties to work at as a medical assistant.
3. Explain the difference between administrative and clinical functions of medical assisting.
4. Name a medical assistant's professional organization.
5. What qualities are regularly found in good medical assistants?
6. Explain what the curriculum in medical assisting should include.
7. List the job titles for which a medical assistant may qualify.
8. List the educational options available to one who is interested in medical assisting.

PREPARING FOR THE CERTIFICATION EXAM

1. What is the AAMA?
   A. All American Medical Association
   B. Allied American Medical Association
   C. Administrative (division) of the American Medical Association
   D. American Association of Medical Assistants
   E. American Association of Medical Assistance

2. What are two general categories that BEST describe the responsibilities of a medical assistant?
   A. administrative and laboratory
   B. secretarial and direct patient care
   C. assisting the physician and secretarial
   D. clinical and secretarial
   E. administrative and clinical

3. Which of following is NOT a category of the AAMA Role Delineation Chart?
   A. administrative
   B. clinical
   C. professional
   D. transdisciplinary
   E. instruction

4. Which administrative tasks falls beyond the scope of practice for a medical assistant?
   A. coordinating managed care coverage
   B. handling petty cash
   C. assisting the physician with a journal article
   D. utilization review of necessary procedures
   E. posting patient information on the Internet

5. Which of the following clinical tasks falls beyond the scope of practice for a medical assistant?
   A. vital signs
   B. patient education
   C. phlebotomy
   D. handling drug refills
   E. prescribing medications

6. How many total CEUs over what period of time must a CMA obtain to remain certified?
   A. 15 CEUs over 2 years
   B. 30 CEUs over 5 years
   C. 60 CEUs over 5 years
   D. 45 CEUs over 3 years
   E. 50 CEUs over 5 years

continued on next page

7. Which of the following statements is TRUE?
   A. a MA is equivalent to a nurse
   B. a MA is equivalent to a physician assistant
   C. it is acceptable for patients to refer to a medical assistant as a "nurse"
   D. an advertisement for a medical assistant might include "medical records clerk"
   E. an advertisement for a medical assistant might include "x-ray technician"

8. As per the CAAHEP Essentials, at a minimum, the curriculum of a medical assisting school does NOT include
   A. medical assistant administrative procedures
   B. medical assistant clinical procedures
   C. medical law and ethics
   D. externship of 160 to 190 hours
   E. medical nurse training

9. Necessary characteristics of a good medical assistant should include all EXCEPT
   A. confidentiality
   B. discretion
   C. empathy
   D. integrity
   E. physical attractiveness

10. Which of the following statements is TRUE?
    A. MAs work only in physicians' offices
    B. all MA programs are diploma programs
    C. medical assistants may work as ECG technicians, with additional training
    D. MAs do not work in hospitals
    E. MAs do not need good communication skills

CRITICAL THINKING

1. Mary decides to further her health care career. What additional training will fit her interests?
2. Because Mary wants a career and not just a job as a medical assistant, what level of education might best support her goals?
3. Mary sits for the AAMA Certification Examination. What are the benefits of certification?

ON THE JOB

Darlene Smith, a CMA, has been employed six years by a Cardiology practice of three physicians. She is a graduate of a CAAHEP accredited school. Furthermore, Darlene received extensive hands-on training performing ECGs while doing her required externship.

Darlene has completed an ECG ordered by Dr. Patel for Mrs. Warner, a 76-year old patient. Dr. Patel, Darlene's boss, has telephoned her explaining that he was behind schedule doing rounds at the hospital. He asked her to do him a favor and interpret Mrs. Warner's ECG, sign his name and fax the report to Mrs. Warner's referring internist who is expecting the results.

1. Given the scope of Darlene's education, training, and years of experience as a CMA, would this "favor" fall within the AAMA guidelines of her responsibilities?
2. Would any portion of Dr. Patel's request fall within the guidelines, if so, which portion(s)? Is there ever a case for an exception to these guidelines?
3. What, if anything, should Darlene say to Dr. Patel?

INTERNET ACTIVITY

Conduct an Internet search for local medical assistant positions. How many positions require certification? What are other job titles a medical assistant would be qualified to take?

MediaLink  More on the profession of medical assisting, including interactive resources, can be found on the Student CD-ROM accompanying this textbook.

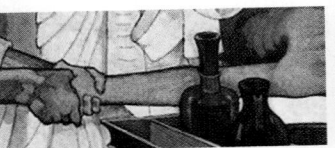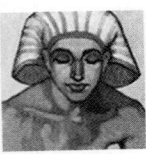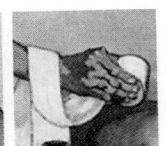

Medical Assistant Role Delineation Chart

HIGHLIGHT indicates material covered in this chapter.

ADMINISTRATIVE

Administrative Procedures

- Perform basic administrative medical assisting functions
- Schedule, coordinate and monitor appointments
- Schedule inpatient/outpatient admissions and procedures
- Understand and apply third-party guidelines
- Obtain reimbursement through accurate claims submission
- Monitor third-party reimbursement
- Understand and adhere to managed care policies and procedures
- *Negotiate managed care contracts*

Practice Finances

- Perform procedural and diagnostic coding
- Apply bookkeeping principles

- Manage accounts receivable
- *Manage accounts payable*
- *Process payroll*
- *Document and maintain accounting and banking records*
- *Develop and maintain fee schedules*
- *Manage renewals of business and professional insurance policies*
- *Manage personnel benefits and maintain records*
- *Perform marketing, financial, and strategic planning*

CLINICAL

Fundamental Principles

- Apply principles of aseptic technique and infection control
- Comply with quality assurance practices
- Screen and follow up patient test results

Diagnostic Orders

- Collect and process specimens
- Perform diagnostic tests

Patient Care

- Adhere to established patient screening procedures
- Obtain patient history and vital signs
- Prepare and maintain examination and treatment areas
- Prepare patient for examinations, procedures and treatments

- Assist with examinations, procedures and treatments
- Prepare and administer medications and immunizations
- Maintain medication and immunization records
- Recognize and respond to emergencies
- Coordinate patient care information with other health care providers
- Initiate IV and administer IV medications with appropriate training and as permitted by state law

GENERAL

Professionalism

- Display a professional manner and image
- Demonstrate initiative and responsibility
- Work as a member of the health care team
- Prioritize and perform multiple tasks
- Adapt to change
- Promote the CMA credential
- Enhance skills through continuing education
- Treat all patients with compassion and empathy
- Promote the practice through positive public relations

Communication Skills

- Recognize and respect cultural diversity
- Adapt communications to individual's ability to understand
- Use professional telephone technique

- Recognize and respond effectively to verbal, nonverbal, and written communications
- Use medical terminology appropriately
- Utilize electronic technology to receive, organize, prioritize and transmit information
- Serve as liaison

Legal Concepts

- Perform within legal and ethical boundaries
- Prepare and maintain medical records
- Document accurately
- Follow employer's established policies dealing with the health care contract
- Implement and maintain federal and state health care legislation and regulations
- Comply with established risk management and safety procedures
- Recognize professional credentialing criteria
- *Develop and maintain personnel, policy and procedure manuals*

Instruction

- Instruct individuals according to their needs
- Explain office policies and procedures
- Teach methods of health promotion and disease prevention
- Locate community resources and disseminate information
- *Develop educational materials*
- *Conduct continuing education activities*

Operational Functions

- Perform inventory of supplies and equipment
- Perform routine maintenance of administrative and clinical equipment
- Apply computer techniques to support office operations
- *Perform personnel management functions*
- *Negotiate leases and prices for equipment and supply contracts*

- *Denotes advanced skills.*

SOURCE: Reprinted by permission of the American Association of Medical Assistants from the AAMA Role Delineation Study: Occupational Analysis of the Medical Assisting Profession.

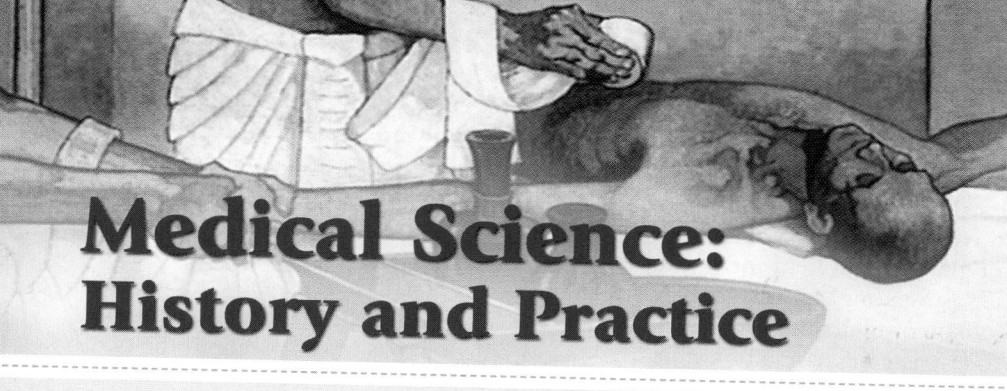

Medical Science: History and Practice

Learning Objectives

After completing this chapter, you should be able to:

- Define and spell the terms to learn for this chapter.
- Identify the major achievements during each of these periods: early medicine, 18th century, 19th century, 20th century, and modern medicine.
- Name three women and explain the contributions they made to medicine.
- Describe the difference between an internship and a residency in the training of physicians.

- State which type of medical practice is addressed under the medical and surgical specialties.
- Discuss ten allied health fields and the educational requirements for each of them.
- Discuss the current trends in health care that are driving changes in medical practice.

OUTLINE

History of Medicine	16
Medical Practitioners	23
Medical Practice Acts	24
Health Care Costs and Payments	25
Types of Medical Practices	26
Medical and Surgical Specialties	27
Health Care Institutions	30
Allied Health Professionals	33
Center for Disease Control	38

Terms to Learn

acquired immune deficiency syndrome (AIDS)

anesthesia

anthrax

bacteria

cadaver

caduceus

Diagnostic Related Groups (DRGs)

hospice

immunology

licensure

medical privilege

microbe

microorganism

morbidity rate

osteopath

pandemic

pasteurization

registration

stem cell

Case Study

ELIZABETH IS A MEDICAL ASSISTANT WHO HAS WORKED in a HMO in California for 6 years. One of her duties is to facilitate the provision of care as HMO subscribers transition from one type of patient care environment to another.

Elizabeth has been working with the family of a 22-year old man who is to be discharged from the hospital following acute care for depression and drug and alcohol abuse. The patient has a history of progressively worsening reactive violence and depression. He is unable to live on his own and care for himself at this time.

In addition, the family is afraid of him and do not want to assume responsibility for his care. The primary physician, medical social worker, and clinical psychologist assigned to his case recommended that he be placed in a suitable long-term care facility.

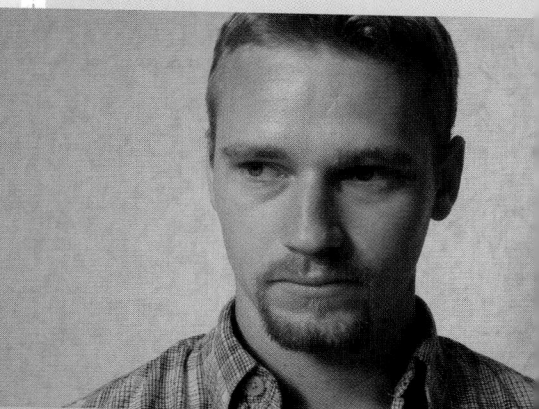

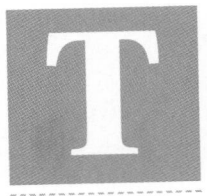

T he healing art of medicine was taught and practiced before humans kept written records. This chapter describes the science and practice of medicine from the earliest evidence of healing when disease was considered to be of supernatural origin or the field of demons to the present—a time of astounding research, discovery, and healing. Contributions of many ancient peoples still influence medicine today. The discussion of present day medical codes of ethics, rules about sanitation, personal hygiene, herbal cures, acupuncture, and other medical and surgical practices highlights the specific contributions of ancient peoples and the men and women whose accomplishments catapulted the science of medicine along in leaps and bounds.

This chapter provides a picture of today's medical practitioners—issues of licensure, including evaluations, credentials, reciprocity, renewals, suspensions, and doctor's titles. In addition, current trends in health care, health care costs, types of practices, medical and surgical specialties, and roles and educational requirements of a variety of health care team members are covered.

History of Medicine

Drawings, bony remains, and some surgical tools are evidence of early human attempts to practice medicine. Folk medicine, using plants, adopted a trial-and-error method to determine which plants were poisonous and which had medicinal value. Early humans attributed supernatural origins to some ailments. In early medicine,

some diseases were considered the work of a demon, evil spirit, or an offended god who had placed some object, such as a worm, into the body of the patient. Treatment consisted of trying to remove the evil intruder.

The first doctors, "medicine men," were shaman, witch doctors, or sorcerers (Figure 2-1). In 3000 BC, Babylonian physicians practiced using the written "Code of Hammurabi." This code, named after Hammurabi, an early king of Babylon, has laws relating to the practice of medicine, which included severe penalties for errors. For example, according to the Code, a doctor who killed a patient while opening an abscess, would have his hands cut off.

Contributions of Ancient Civilizations

A study of medical practice in early Egypt offers greater insight into the basis of modern medicine. The Egyptians left behind lists of remedies, surgical treatments of wounds and injuries, and records for rules of sanitation. Personal hygiene, the sanitary preparation of food, and other matters of public health were pioneered by the practices of the Jewish religion. Other cultures contributed to moving the practice forward.

The early Greeks have records of using nonpoisonous snakes to treat the wounds of patients. The caduceus (Figure 2-2), which has become the recognized symbol for medicine, depicts a healing staff with two snakes coiled around the staff.

Herbal medical remedies from ancient India are recorded from 800 BC. The Chinese culture wrote about human blood pulses around the time of 250 BC. Early Japanese and Chinese cultures practiced acupuncture successfully.

Ancient Cures Are Today's Legacy

Early medicine, while often based on superstition, actually provided medicinal remedies that are still used today. The effect of opium produced by the poppy plant was known in ancient times and even now is used in the medication morphine to relieve severe pain. Other remedies include using:

- Nitroglycerin to treat heart patients
- Digitalis from the foxglove plant to regulate and strengthen the heartbeat
- Sulfur and cayenne pepper to stop bleeding
- Chamomile and licorice to aid digestion
- Cranberry to treat urinary tract infections

Early Medicine

Early medicine began with Hippocrates and the shift from the belief in magical sources of illness and disease to more scientific study, which looked to physical causes of disease. The medieval period from the 5th century to the 16th century was a time of little or no progress in

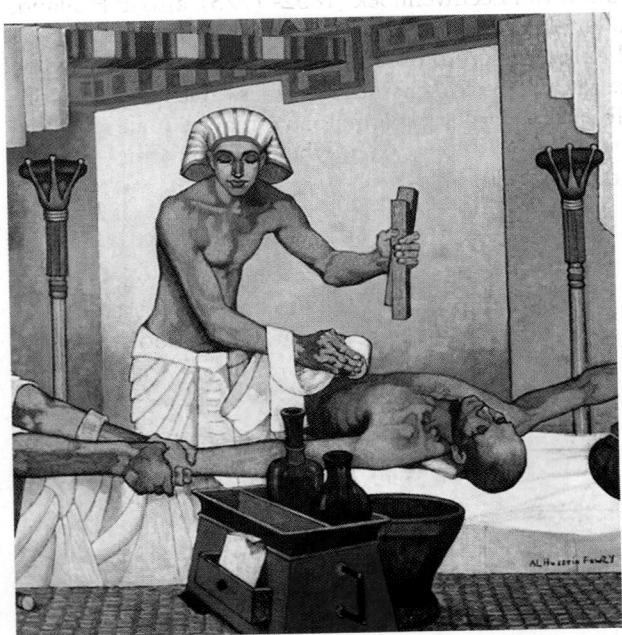

FIGURE 2-1 An early physician.

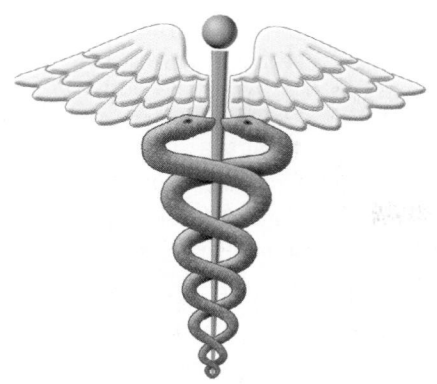

FIGURE 2-2 Caduceus, the emblem of the medical profession.

medical practices. The lack of sanitation, poor personal hygiene, and poor nutrition led to many epidemics. An epidemic is a disease, which infects a large part of a population in one region or location at the same time. The bubonic plague was a pandemic because it affected many people in different countries at the same time. It was known as the "black plague" or "black death" because the corpses appeared dark due to hemorrhage under the skin. Death was extensive in China, India, Europe, Russia, Egypt, and North Africa. The cause of bubonic plague was not discovered until 1905. It was determined then that it was bacteria which grew in the fleas of infected rats. Bacteria are microorganisms, some of which are capable of causing disease. Microorganisms are minute living organisms.

During the medieval period, medical teaching was mostly oral. Surgeons, at the time, only treated the wealthy. Other patients had to rely on the local barber to perform surgical procedures. The red and white stripe pole we are familiar with today was the sign that barbers used—a white pole wrapped with bloody bandages to solicit business. This period concludes with the introduction of the microscope and the ability to see and measure bacteria previously not observed with the naked eye.

Hippocrates (Father of Medicine)

Historically, the first scientific system of medicine is of Greek origin and is usually associated with Hippocrates (460–377 BC) who has become known as the "Father of Medicine." Hippocrates shifted medicine from the realm of mysticism and into the area of scientific practice. He stressed the body's healing nature, clinical descriptions of diseases, and the ability to discover some diseases by listening to the chest. He practiced medicine at a time in history when little was known about anatomy and physiology. Nevertheless, his writings and descriptions of symptoms remain accurate today.

The Hippocratic Oath (Box 2-1) is part of the writings of this fifth century BC physician. The oath serves as a widely used ethical guide for physicians who pledge to work for the good of the patient, to do him or her no harm, to prescribe no deadly drugs, to give no advice that could cause death, and to keep confidential medical information regarding the patient. The oath is still often administered as part of graduation ceremonies in medical schools.

Galen

Galen (130–201 AD), a Greek physician who practiced in Rome, initially followed the Hippocratic method. He stressed the value of anatomy and founded experimental physiology. He stated that arteries contained blood and not air as previously believed. Since the dissection of humans was illegal during Galen's time, he based his theories on the examination of pigs and apes. While some of his work is inaccurate due to the lack of human cadavers, or dead bodies from which to study the human anatomy, he is still known as the "Prince of Physicians."

William Harvey

In England during the 17th century, William Harvey (1578–1657) began writing on the topic of blood circulation and using the experimental method in medicine. Unfortunately for Harvey, the microscope had not yet been invented and he was never able to view capillaries.

Galileo

Galileo (1564–1642) was the first to use a telescope to study the skies. Applications of the telescope lens led to the invention of the microscope. Zacharias Janssen in Holland was an eyeglass maker who invented the microscope.

Anton van Leeuwenhoek

Anton van Leeuwenhoek (1632–1723), also in Holland, devoted his life to microscopic studies. He is known as the first person to observe and describe bacteria, which he referred to as "tiny little beasties." He is also responsible for describing spermatozoa (mature male sex cells) and protozoa. Protozoa are the simplest forms—usually one cell—of animals.

Medicine During the 18th Century

In England, formal medical training began when it was required that anyone wishing to become a doctor must first become an apprentice. Medical schools in Edinburgh and Glasgow, Scotland were developed during this era.

John Hunter

John Hunter (1728–1793) developed surgery and surgical pathology into a science. He is noted as the "Founder of Scientific Surgery." Some of his contributions to medical science include the introduction of a flexible feeding tube into the stomach. The term "surgeon" comes from the Greek word "cheir," which means hand, and "ergeon," which means work.

BOX 2-1
The Hippocratic Oath

I swear by Apollo Physician, by Asclepias, by Health, by Heal All, and by all the gods and goddesses, that according to my ability and judgment, I will keep this oath and stipulation; to reckon him who taught me this art equally dear to me as my parents, and share my substance with him and relieve his necessities if required. To regard his offspring as on the same footing with my own brothers and to teach them this art if they should wish to learn it, without fee or stipulation; and that by precept, lecture, and every other mode of instruction I will impart a knowledge of my art to my own sons and to those of my teachers and to disciples bound by a stipulation and oath according to the law of medicine, but to none others.

I will follow that method of treatment which according to my ability and judgment, I consider for the benefit of my patients, and abstain from whatever is deleterious and mischievous. I will give not deadly medicine to anyone if asked, nor suggest any counsel.

Furthermore, I will not give to a woman an instrument to produce an abortion.

With Purity and with Holiness, I will pass my life and practice my art. I will not cut a person who is suffering with a stone, but will leave this to the practitioners of this work. Into whatever houses I enter I will go into them for the benefit of the sick and will abstain from every voluntary act of mischief and corruption; and further from the seduction of females or males, bond or free.

Whatever, in connection with my professional practice, or not in connection with it, I may see or hear in the lives of men which ought not to be spoken abroad, I will not divulge, as reckoning that all such should be kept secret.

While I continue to keep this oath inviolated, may it be granted to me to enjoy life and practice the art respected by all men, at all times, but should I trespass and violate this oath, may the reverse be my lot.

Edward Jenner

Public health and hygiene began to attract attention during the 18th century. A country doctor, Edward Jenner (1749–1823), a pupil of John Hunter, observed that dairy maids who had become infected with the disease cowpox would not become infected with the deadly disease smallpox. Jenner overcame ridicule from the medical community and went on to perform the first vaccination using the smallpox vaccine.

The term vaccination comes from the Latin term "vacca" meaning cow. Cowpox was referred to as "vaccinia." Today the term vaccine means to give live or attenuated material to a person to establish resistance to disease. Vaccines come from animals other than cows today and from synthetic sources.

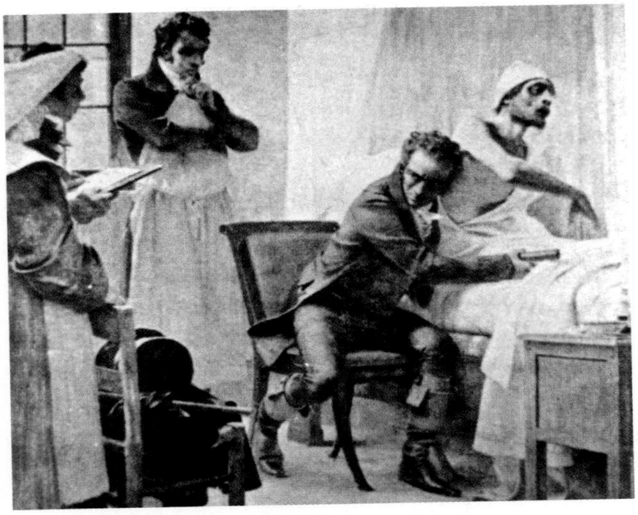

Rene Laennec

Another major advancement in medicine was made by Rene Laennec (1781–1826), who invented the stethoscope. His invention (Figure 2-3) was based on the use of paper wrapped into a cone shape, which was then placed over the patient's chest to listen to the heart.

Benjamin Franklin

The American statesman, Benjamin Franklin (1706–1790), was an inventor and, in addition to inventing bifocals, one of his important contributions to medical science was the discovery that colds could be passed from one person to another.

FIGURE 2-3 Rene Laennec and the stethoscope.

Medicine During the 19th Century

During the 19th century, the practice of medicine advanced rapidly. The documentation of accurate anatomy and physiology allowed physicians to better understand the human body. The use of sophisticated microscopes, injection materials, and instruments such as the ophthalmoscope all moved the practice of medicine forward.

The discovery of the cell was one of the most enlightening discoveries of this era. Many believe that the greatest achievement of the 19th century was the knowledge that certain diseases, as well as surgical wound infections, were directly caused by microorganisms. The practice of surgery changed as a result of this knowledge along with advances in the use of anesthetics.

Louis Pasteur

Louis Pasteur (1822–1895) is credited for establishing the science of bacteriology (Figure 2-4). His experiments proved that putrefaction or decay was caused by living organisms known as bacteria. His work solved many medical problems during his day including rabies, anthrax in sheep and cattle, and chicken cholera. Anthrax is a deadly infectious disease caused by *Bacillus anthracisis*. Humans can contract the disease from infected animal hair, hides, or waste. Cholera, an acute infection of the small bowel causing severe diarrhea, was determined to be a bacillus transmitted through water, milk, or food contaminated with excreta of carriers. The process of pasteurization is named after Pasteur. Pasteurization is the process during which substances, such as milk and cheese, are heated to a certain temperature to eliminate bacteria.

Joseph Lister

Joseph Lister (1827–1912) borrowed Pasteur's theories and eventually introduced the antiseptic system in surgery (Figure 2-4). Until that time, surgeons and obstetricians did not wash their hands between patients. Disease was being spread from one patient to another. Lister advised placing an antiseptic barrier between the wound and the germ-containing atmosphere. Present day aseptic techniques can be attributed to Lister's work.

Ignaz Semmelweiss

Ignaz Semmelweiss (1818–1865), an obstetrician in Vienna, advised medical students to disinfect the hands and clothing of anyone who attended a birth. During the early practice of obstetrics, a physician would wear the same "butcher's coat" for all deliveries in the hospital. Figure 2-5 shows a Cesarean section. There was a high death rate from puerperal sepsis or childbed fever. Women avoided having a baby in the hospital because of the high mortality rate or death rate. Eventually, the use of contaminated clothing and contaminated hands were traced to the spread of puerperal sepsis thanks to Dr. Semmelweiss. The term puerperal comes from the Latin word "puer" meaning child and "pario" meaning to bring forth. The term puerperium is now used to denote a period of time after a delivery.

Semmelweiss noted that the medical students would attend a mother in childbirth immediately after having

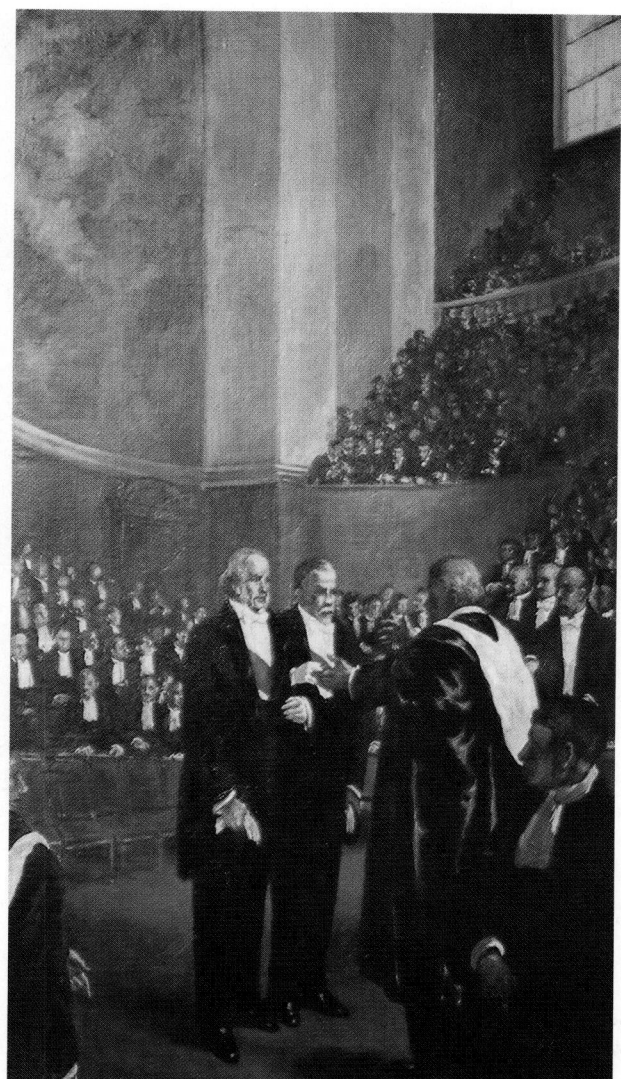

FIGURE 2-4 Louis Pasteur and Joseph Lister.

participated in an autopsy. An autopsy is an examination of the organs and tissues of a deceased body to determine the cause of death. After he advised students to disinfect their hands before attending childbirth, the incidence of disease went down dramatically. In the 1800s, the men who advocated disinfection were ridiculed and in Semmelweiss' case considered insane.

Robert Koch

Robert Koch (1843–1910) showed how bacteria could be cultivated and stained. He discovered the tubercle bacillus, the cause of tuberculosis. His investigation into the cause of cholera led to knowledge that contaminated food and water can cause disease.

Paul Ehrlich

Paul Ehrlich (1854–1915) was a pioneer in the study of microbiology. He was a pioneer in the fields of immunology, bacteriology, and the use of chemotherapy.

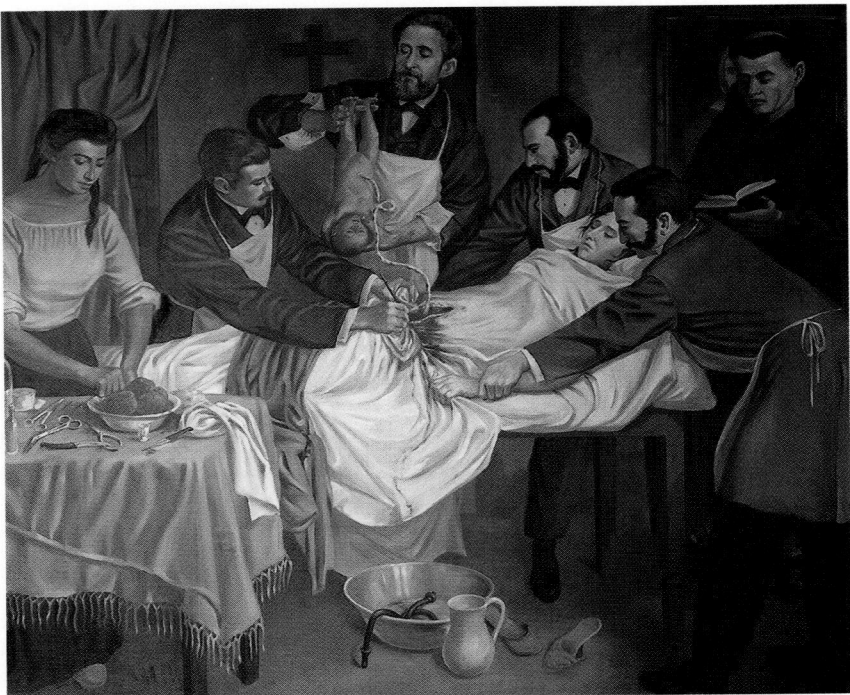

FIGURE 2-5 A cesarean section from an old medicine text book.

partial or complete sensation. An anesthetic is a substance used to produce anesthesia. These two men worked independently of each other and made possible life-saving operations that previously could not be performed without anesthetics.

WALTER REED Walter Reed (1851–1902) and others helped to conquer yellow fever, which allowed for completion of the Panama Canal by reducing the death rate for the workers. Dr. Reed gathered volunteers who allowed him to inject them with yellow fever in order to find a cure.

Medicine During the 20th Century

The first half of the 20th century resulted in major medical advances. Death rates from diseases such as tuberculosis and diphtheria dropped dramatically. The overall mortality rates decreased due to improved medical care and new emphasis was placed on morbidity rates (rates of disease and illness). Four major developments dominate this period:

- The development of chemotherapy and the specialty of oncology
- The development of immunology
- Progress in endocrinology
- Progress in nutrition

Alexander Fleming

One of the most dramatic episodes of the modern era was the discovery of antibiotics. Sir Alexander Fleming (1881–1955) accidentally discovered that a stray mold on his culture plate of staphylococci would cause the bacteria to stop growing. He called this mold Penicillium and it has became known throughout the world as penicillin. Fleming's discovery took place in 1928. He, along with two other scientists, won the Nobel Prize for their work with penicillin. The use of penicillin was one of the first examples of using chemicals to treat infections. Today, the term chemotherapy generally refers to drugs used to treat forms of cancer.

Jonas Salk and Albert Sabin

The study of immunology advanced with the discovery of vaccines against typhoid, tetanus, diphtheria, tuberculosis, yellow fever, influenza, and measles. During the 1950s, Doctors Jonas Salk (1914–1996) and

Immunology is the study of immunity, the resistance to or protection from disease. Chemotherapy is the use of chemicals including drugs to treat or control infections and disease. He developed a method for staining bacteria and cells, which eventually, led to a means for providing a differential diagnosis based on classifying organisms. He was one of the original "microbe hunters." Microbes are one-celled forms of life such as bacteria. His greatest achievement was the discovery, on his 606th attempt, of the "magic bullet" to treat syphilis. Syphilis is an infectious chronic venereal disease.

Other Major Advances During This Period

William Roentgen (1845–1923) discovered x-rays, Pierre (1859–1906) and Marie (1867–1934) Curie discovered radium, and Sigmund Freud (1856–1939) worked in the field of psychiatry.

American Medicine During This Period

Significant contributions were made to medicine through the work of William Norton, Crawford Long, and Walter Reed. The specific work of each of these individuals is highlighted here.

WILLIAM MORTON AND CRAWFORD LONG An important American contribution to the practice of medicine during this period was the discovery of anesthesia. William Morton (1819–1868), a dentist at Massachusetts General Hospital, and Crawford Long (1815–1878), a Georgia physician, are generally credited with having first demonstrated the use of ether as a general anesthetic. Anesthesia refers to the absence of

Albert Sabin (1906–1993) developed vaccines, which eradicated the crippling disease polio.

Women in Medicine

Few women were allowed to practice medicine in the early years. In part, this was due to social constraints on women appearing in public. However, many women did practice as midwives and became skilled at delivering babies. There are also some remarkable female physicians and nurses who overcame great odds to practice in their profession.

Elizabeth Blackwell

Elizabeth Blackwell (1821–1910) was the first female physician in the United States. After being turned down by several medical schools, she was finally awarded a degree in 1849 in New York. She went on to open a medical college for women and her own dispensary.

Florence Nightingale

Florence Nightingale (1820–1910) is considered the founder of modern nursing (Figure 2-6). She studied nursing in Europe and cared for wounded soldiers during the Crimean War (1850–1853). Nightingale and her fellow nurses were treated poorly by the doctors at that time.

Nightingale's attention to detail, record keeping, and compassionate nursing care changed the way nursing was practiced. She advocated the use of the nursing process and elevated nursing to an honored profession. She is referred to as "The Lady with the Lamp" due to her tireless work night and day to supervise the nursing care of wounded soldiers. She started the first school of nursing in 1860 at St. Thomas Hospital in London.

Clara Barton

Clara Barton (1821–1912) was a contemporary of Florence Nightingale, but nursed soldiers in a different war, the Civil War in the United States. She established the American Red Cross when she became aware of the need for support services for the soldiers (Figures 2-7 and 2-8). She also established the Federal Bureau of Records to help track injured and dead soldiers.

Modern Medicine and the Future

In the last 25 years, technological discoveries have permitted medical science to advance faster than in the previous one hundred years. There is the potential for greater advances in the 21st century. The average life span of ancient humans was 30 years. According to the U.S. Census Bureau (2001), a person born in 1900 had the life expectancy of 47 years and someone born in 1991 had the life expectancy of 76 years. With rapid

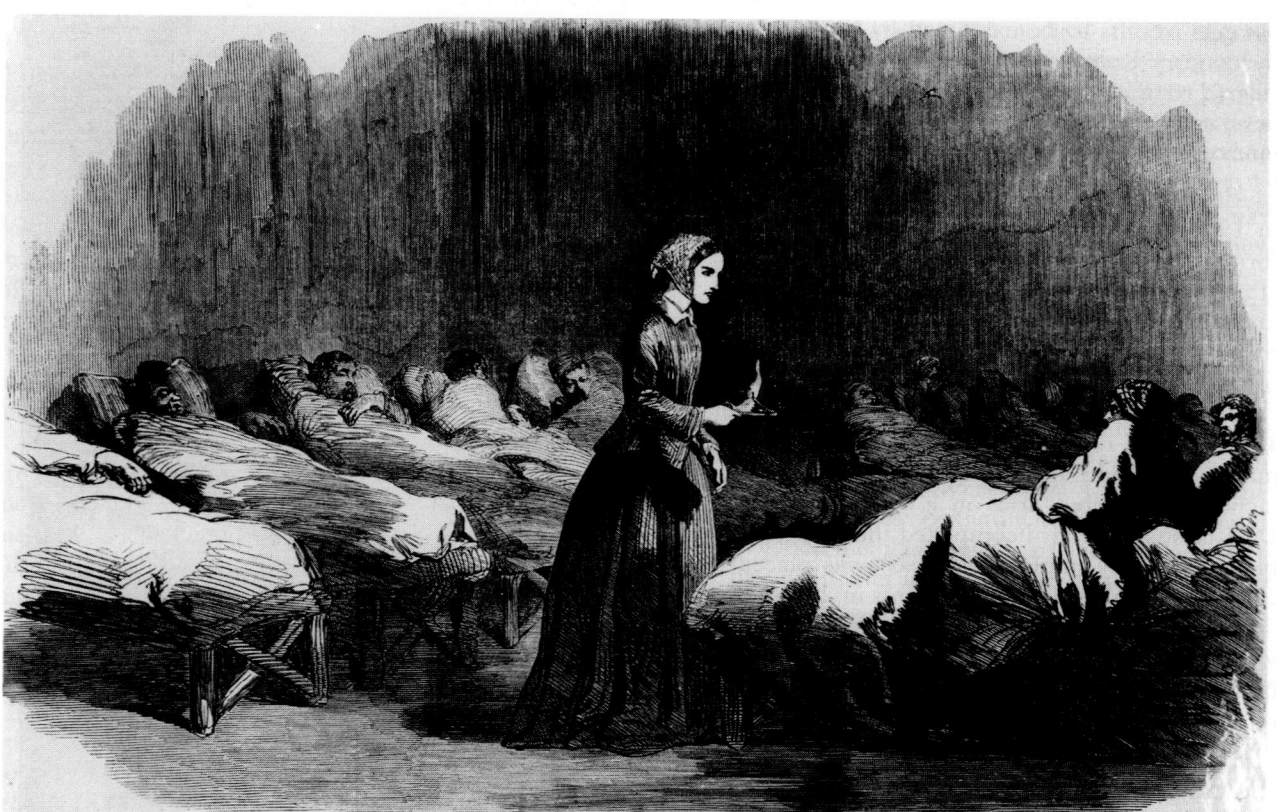

FIGURE 2-6 Florence Nightingale, the founder of modern nursing.

TABLE 2-1 Designations and Initials for Doctors

Term	Initials
Doctor of Chiropractic	DC
Doctor Of Dental Medicine	DMD
Doctor of Dental Surgery	DDS
Doctor of Education	EdD
Doctor of Medicine	MD
Doctor of Optometry	OD
Doctor of Osteopathy	DO
Doctor of Philosophy	PhD
Doctor of Podiatric Medicine	DPM

degree in his or her field. Several designations for doctor are listed in Table 2-1 with the corresponding initials. Patient Education stresses how knowing the physician's credentials is helpful.

Doctor of Osteopathy or DO has similar educational requirements to the medical doctor. Both MDs and DOs are licensed physicians. Both categories of physicians use similar approaches to medicine, including the use of drugs, therapy, and radiation. Both groups must pass state board examinations to become licensed in their states. Doctors of Osteopathy learn the skill of manipulation therapy in schools of osteopathy. The osteopath places great emphasis on the relationship between the musculoskeletal systems and the organs of the body. In most states, the osteopath is able to perform the same procedures as a medical doctor.

A chiropractor (DC) is trained in manipulation of the spinal cord and other areas of the body. This field requires two years of premedical studies and four years of training in a licensed chiropractic school. Most states license chiropractors.

Medical Practice Acts

Each state has regulations that direct the practice of medicine in that state. While there are some slight differences from state to state, in general, these medical practice acts uphold who must be licensed to perform certain procedures. These acts also maintain the requirements for licensure (granting of a license), duties of that license, grounds on which the license can be revoked or taken away, and reports that must be made to the government. Medical practice acts also cover the penalties for practicing without a valid license.

If a physician moves to another state, he or she must obtain a license to practice in that state. It may mean taking and passing another state medical examination. See the section on reciprocity later in this chapter.

Generally, physicians in different states may consult with each other without being licensed in each other's states. Physicians who practice in governmental institutions, such as Veteran's Administration hospitals or in military service, may practice medicine without the local licensure.

Licensure

The Board of Medical Examiners in each state grants a license to practice medicine. Licensure may be granted through one of three ways: examination, endorsement, or through reciprocity.

Examination

Each state will offer its examination for licensure. This examination is usually taken before the end of medical school. Within the United States, the official medical licensing examination is called the Federation Licensing

Patient Education

Some patients require information about the physician's specialty and credentials. A patient often has questions regarding the skill level of the physician or the amount of the bill. The medical assistant can discuss these concerns with the patient. Explaining the physician's credentials, including the years of education and training required to become a doctor, particularly if the doctor specializes, often increases the patient's level of confidence in the physician.

A patient welcomes an explanation of reasons for being referred to a specialist by his or her physician. In many cases, you will provide the patient with a list of referral specialists approved by your employer. You may be required to schedule an appointment for the patient and to follow up with the patient to see that he or she visited the specialist.

Examination (FLEX). The license is then issued after an internship is completed. Successful performance on this examination entitles one to set up private practice as a general practitioner. The United States Medical Licensing Examination (USMLE), which began in 1992, provides a single licensing examination for graduates from accredited medical schools.

Endorsement

Endorsement, meaning an approval or sanction, is granted to applicants who have successfully passed the National Board Medical Examination (NBME). In fact, most physicians in the United States are licensed by endorsement. Any medical school graduate who is not licensed by endorsement is required to pass the state board examination (FLEX). Graduates of foreign medical schools must pass the same requirements as American graduates.

Reciprocity

In some cases, the state to which the physician is applying for a license will accept the state license, which the physician already holds so that the physician will not have to take another examination. This practice is known as reciprocity.

Registration

It is necessary for physicians to maintain their license by periodic re-registration either annually or bi-annually. The physician is notified by mail when to re-register and must submit the re-registration fee within a designated time period. In addition to payment of a fee to re-register, 75 hours in a three-year period of continuing medical education (CME) units are required to assure that the physician is remaining current in the field of practice. Legal and Ethical Issues discusses how a medical assistant can oversee re-registrations and renewals for the physician.

Suspension or Revoking a Medical License

A physician's license may be revoked in cases of severe misconduct, which include unprofessional conduct, commission of a crime, or personal incapacity to perform one's duties. Unprofessional conduct relates to behavior that fails to meet the ethical standards of the profession, such as inappropriate use of drugs or alcohol. Crimes include rape, murder, larceny, and narcotics convictions. Personal incapacity relates to the physician's inability to perform due to physical or mental incapacities.

Health Care Costs and Payments

Before discussing medical specialties, types of medical practices, health care facilities, and the role and education of allied health professions, it is important to look

Legal and Ethical Issues

Licensure and continuing medical education (CME) are two areas in which you can assist the physician. The renewal of licenses is usually dependent on the completion of re-registration forms and filing these forms on time with the necessary fees. Always take care to maintain accurate records of continuing medical education units earned by the physician since CME is an important part of the licensing process. Be alert to this legal obligation and remind your employing physician in advance of such renewals.

Medical assistants dedicate themselves to the care and well-being of all patients, according to the American Association of Medical Assistants code of ethics. In addition, medical assistants should take the Oath of Hippocrates, "do no harm to the patient" as seriously as the physicians who state it at the time of their graduation from medical school. As a medical assistant, you will act as a representative of the physician and must be well versed on all legal issues that affect the physician's practice.

at some health care costs and trends. Comprehending these trends and their impact on health care make you a more informed professional and will lead to a better understanding of problems that patients may have obtaining and paying for health care.

Health care has changed dramatically in the past 25 years. It has become the largest industry in the nation providing 12.9 million jobs according to the Bureau of Labor Statistics. The costs of health care are increasing faster than the cost of living. It is estimated that more than 14% of our gross national product (GNP) is spent on health care totaling about $1.5 trillion dollars per year. According to CNN Money, in 2003, 15.6% of the population or over 45 million Americans were uninsured. The costs of employer-sponsored health care increased by 13.9% between 2002 and 2003 according to Kaiser Family Foundation. The number of working Americans without health care is increasing because they cannot afford the premiums. According to Kaiser, the annual premium for a family would be more than $9,000 a year for health care coverage. The United States is the only industrialized nation that does not provide some sort of basic health care for all citizens.

What are some of the factors that are driving the skyrocketing costs of health care delivery today?

- Technological advances are expensive
- Knowledge growth and technology has led to physician specialization
- Specialization has damaged the long term doctor-patient relationship; patients do not feel close to the specialists and are more inclined to sue these doctors
- Drug costs are skyrocketing
- The population is aging and the older segment of the population uses the most health care services
- Longer life expectancy means greater need for care for a longer time
- Patients are not passive; they are active, informed consumers who demand more tests and options
- The uninsured rely on emergency room visits for primary care and do not seek medical care until absolutely necessary
- The uninsured have less or no access to preventive care and often require treatment for more advanced illness or ailments
- Social conditions, such as homelessness, substance abuse, poverty, child abuse, break up of the family unit, and increased number of people living alone, impact individual health, health care delivery systems, and health care costs

These trends need to be considered as we continue with our discussion of the types of practices, governmental regulations, and steps utilized to control the costs of health care. Insurance companies, managed care plans, such as health maintenance organizations (HMOs), Diagnostic Related Groups (DRGs), and government legislation have attempted to control costs and have had significant impact on the way health care services are delivered.

In 1983, Medicare instituted a hospital payment system called DRGS, which classifies each Medicare patient according to his or her illness. There are 467 illness categories. Under this system, hospitals receive a preset sum for treatment, regardless of the actual number of "bed days" of care used by a patient. This method of payment provides further incentive to keep costs down. However, it has also led to early discharge of patients, increased number of re-admissions, and discouraged treatment of severely ill patients. Cultural Considerations explains that community resources can be helpful to a diverse client population.

Types of Medical Practices

In the early part of the 20th century, the main form of medical practice was the solo practice. In this type of practice, a family practitioner set up a medical practice within a designated town and geographic area. Over the years, the practice of medicine and the legal environment have changed. Other forms of medical practice have become popular to meet patients' needs for around-the-clock medical coverage. Alternative forms of practice also provide the opportunity for a group of physicians to share insurance premium costs, staff, and facilities investments.

Solo Practice

In a solo practice, a physician practices alone. This is a common type of practice for dentists. However, physicians generally enter into agreements with other

Cultural Considerations

The diversity of the client population will present many challenges to you as a medical assistant. Non-English speaking patients will need brochures and handouts in their own languages if possible. Many brochures are available in Spanish for example. Often these patients are unaware of the community resources available to help them in emergency situations. In some cultures, it is considered unthinkable to ask strangers for help. Understanding how some ethnic groups dread not being self-reliant will help you treat them with more tolerance.

Names, addresses, and telephone numbers of service agencies, such as the American Red Cross, abuse hotlines, homeless shelters, soup kitchens, and poison control centers, all are available from a number of sources such as the phone book, local library, Chamber of Commerce, and the Internet. As a medical assistant, having a typed list of all facilities and information at your fingertips will enable you to be prepared for any contingency. After completing this chapter, you will have a greater understanding of the difficulties that patients face obtaining and paying for medical care. You must be ready to help them regardless of their income levels, cultural origin, race, or attitude.

physicians to provide coverage for each other's patients and to share office expenses.

Sole Proprietorship

In a sole proprietorship, one physician is still responsible for making all the administrative decisions. However, this physician may employ other physicians and pay them a salary. The physician-owner will pay all expenses and retain all assets. In the sole proprietorship form of practice, the owner is responsible and liable for the actions of all the employees.

Partnership

A partnership is a legal agreement to share in the business operation of a medical practice. A partnership is between two or more physicians. In this legal arrangement, each of the partners becomes responsible for the actions of all the partners. This refers to debts and all legal actions, unless otherwise stipulated in the legal partnership agreement.

Associate Practice

The associate practice is a legal arrangement in which physicians agree to share a facility and staff. They do not, as a general rule, share responsibility for the legal actions of each other as in the partnership. The legal contract of agreement stipulates the responsibilities of each party. The physicians act as if their practice is a sole proprietorship.

The legal arrangement must be carefully described and discussed with patients. In some cases, patients have mistakenly believed that there was a shared responsibility by all the physicians in the practice.

Group Practice

A group practice consists of three or more physicians who share the same facility (office or clinic) and practice medicine together. This is a legal form of practice in which the physicians share all expenses, income, personnel, equipment, and records. Some areas of medicine frequently found in group practice are anesthesiology, rehabilitative or obstetrical services, radiology, and pathology.

A group practice can also be designated as a health maintenance organization (HMO) or as an independent practice association (IPA). Group practices have grown rapidly during the last decade. Large groups with over 100 doctors are not uncommon. A large group practice will often form a legal corporation.

Professional Corporation

During the 1960s, state legislatures passed laws (statutes) allowing professionals, for example physicians, lawyers, and accountants, to incorporate. A corporation is managed by a board of directors and there are legal and financial benefits from incorporating.

Professional corporation members are known as shareholders. Therefore, the physician-members become the shareholders in the corporation. Some of the benefits that can be offered to employees of a corporation include medical expense reimbursement, profit sharing, pension plans, and disability insurance. These fringe benefits would not be taxable to the employee and are generally tax deductible to the employer. While a corporation can be sued, the individual assets of the members cannot be touched as in a solo practice. A corporation will remain after a member leaves or dies. Other forms of practice, such as the sole proprietorship, may die with the death of the owner.

Medical and Surgical Specialties

Due to the dramatic advances in medicine over the past two decades, there continues to be an interest in specialization among physicians. Transplant surgery, including the liver, kidneys, lungs, and pancreas, has expanded the need for medical and surgical specialties.

Medical Specialties

A description of some more common medical specialties follows.

Allergy and Immunology

An allergist treats abnormal responses or acquired hypersensitivity to substances with medical methods including testing and desensitization. Pediatricians and internists may sit for the board examination in allergy and immunology after taking several years of additional training.

Anesthesiology

An anesthesiologist is trained to administer both local and general drugs to induce a complete or partial loss of feeling (anesthesia) during a surgical procedure (Figure 2-9). This physician also provides respiratory and cardiovascular support during surgery. The anesthesiologist meets with the patient before the surgical procedure to explain the type of anesthetic that will be used. Certified registered nurse anesthesiologists (CRNA) also may administer anesthetics.

Cardiology

A cardiologist is trained to treat cardiovascular disease. This physician has received special training in the diseases and disorders of the heart and blood vessels. A cardiologist specializing in the treatment of children's heart disease would receive special training as a pediatric cardiologist.

Dermatology

A dermatologist treats injuries, growths, and infections relating to the skin, hair, and nails. This physician may treat patients either medically or surgically.

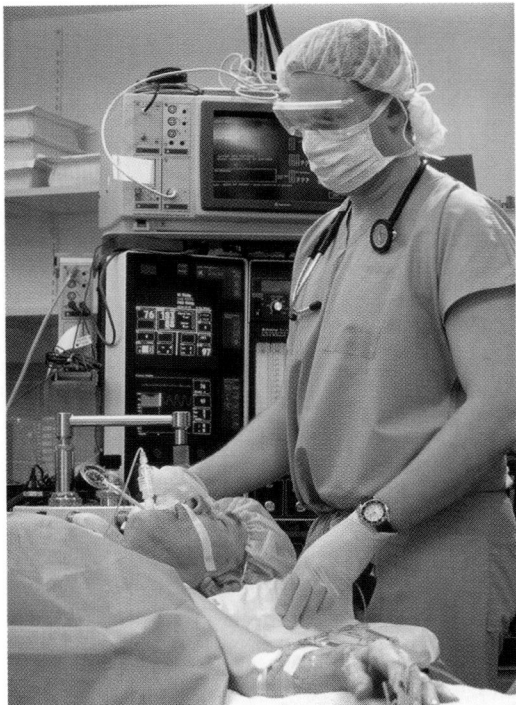

FIGURE 2-9 Anesthesiologist.

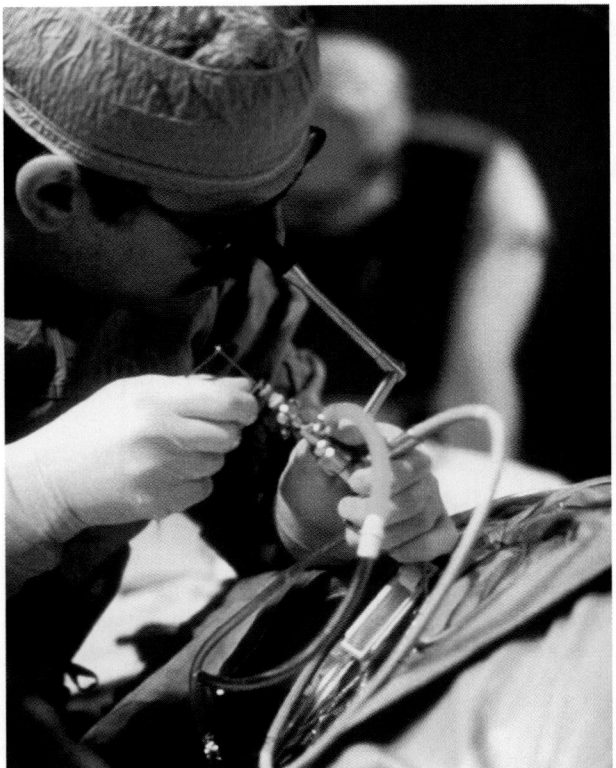

FIGURE 2-10 Nephrologist.

A dermatologist may remove growths such as warts, moles, benign cysts, birthmarks, and skin cancers.

Emergency Medicine
The physician who specializes in emergency medicine has received additional training as an emergency medical resident. Emergency medicine specialists typically work in hospital emergency rooms and freestanding, walk-in emergency centers. They acquire the ability and skills to quickly recognize and prioritize (triage) acute injuries, trauma, and illnesses. They also supervise paramedic pre-hospital care.

Family Practice (Primary Care Medicine)
The family practitioner physician will treat the entire family regardless of age and sex. In some cases, they will refer patients with specific medical conditions to specialists, such as nephrologists for the treatment of renal (kidney) diseases.

Geriatric Medicine
The practice of geriatrics is focused on the care of diseases and disorders of the elderly. Gerontology is a relatively new field of medicine and is the direct result of the larger aging population.

Hematology
Hematology is the study of blood and blood-forming tissues.

Oncology
Oncology is the study of cancer and cancer-related tumors.

Internal Medicine (Primary Medicine)
The internist is a physician who treats adult patients. This physician is skilled in diagnosis and treatment of non-surgical problems. There are subspecialties within the area of internal medicine including: cardiology, endocrinology, gastroenterology, hematology, immunology, nephrology, oncology, and pulmonary medicine.

Neurology
The neurologist treats the non-surgical patient who has a disorder or disease of the nervous system.

Nephrology
A nephrologist specializes in pathology of the kidney including disorders and diseases. A nephrologist is skilled in both medical and surgical treatments including kidney dialysis (Figure 2-10).

Nuclear Medicine
The physician specializing in this field uses radioactive substances for the diagnosis and treatment of diseases such as cancer.

Obstetrics and Gynecology

An obstetrician treats the female as she begins prenatal care and continues through labor, delivery, and the postpartum period (Figure 2-11). A gynecologist provides both medical and surgical treatment of diseases and disorders of the female reproductive system. This is a sub-specialty, which also deals with infertility, the study of a diminished capacity or inability to produce offspring.

Ophthalmology

An ophthalmologist treats disorders of the eye. The study of ophthalmology includes the diagnosis and treatment of vision problems using both medical and surgical procedures.

Orthopedics

An orthopedist or orthopod specializes in the branch of medicine that deals with the prevention and correction of disorders of the musculoskeletal system (Figure 2-12). An orthopedic surgeon specializes in surgical procedures relating to this specialty.

Otorhinolaryngology

The otorhinolaryngologist (ENT) specializes in the medical and surgical treatment of ear, nose, and throat disorders. This includes the study of otology (ear), rhinology (nose), and laryngology (throat), and is also known as otorhinolaryngology.

Pathology

A pathologist specializes in diagnosing abnormal changes in tissues that are removed during a surgical operation and in postmortem examinations. A forensic pathologist is an expert in determining the identity of a person based on such evidence as body parts, dental records, and tissue samples.

Pediatrics

The pediatrician specializes in the development and care of children from birth to maturity (Figure 2-13).

Physical Medicine and Rehabilitative Medicine

Physical medicine and/or rehabilitative medicine specialists treat patients after they have suffered an injury or disability. The purpose of treatment is to return patients to their former state of physical health if possible. This rapidly growing field is closely associated with sports medicine in which the physician treats athletes using preventive and diagnostic medicine.

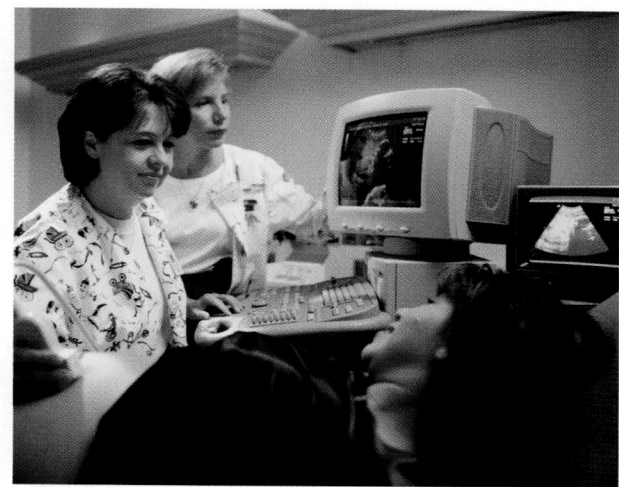

FIGURE 2-11   An obstetrician.

Psychiatry

The psychiatrist specializes in the diagnosis and treatment of patients with mental, behavioral, or emotional disorders. A psychiatrist is qualified to prescribe and administer medications. This specialist may also practice psychotherapy.

Radiology

A radiologist specializes in the study of tissue and organs that is based on x-ray visualization. This physician has been tested and approved by the American Board of Radiology.

Rheumatology

A rheumatologist treats disorders and diseases characterized by inflammation of the joints such as arthritis.

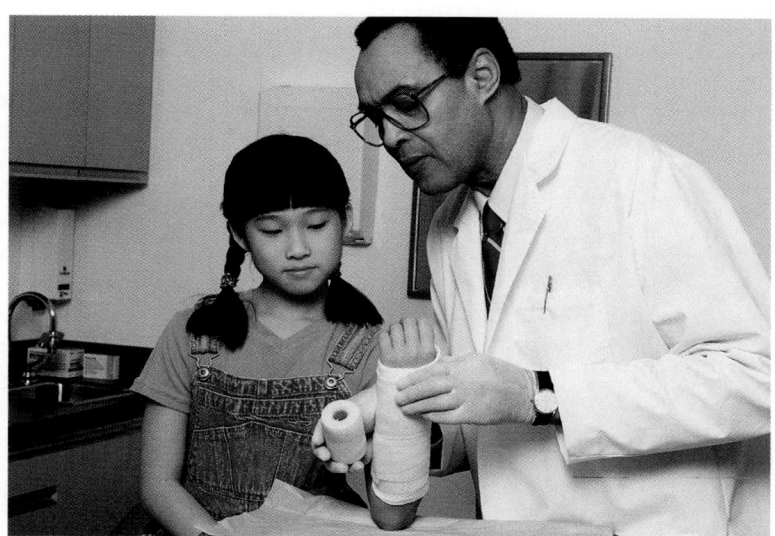

FIGURE 2-12   An orthopedist putting a cast on a young girl.

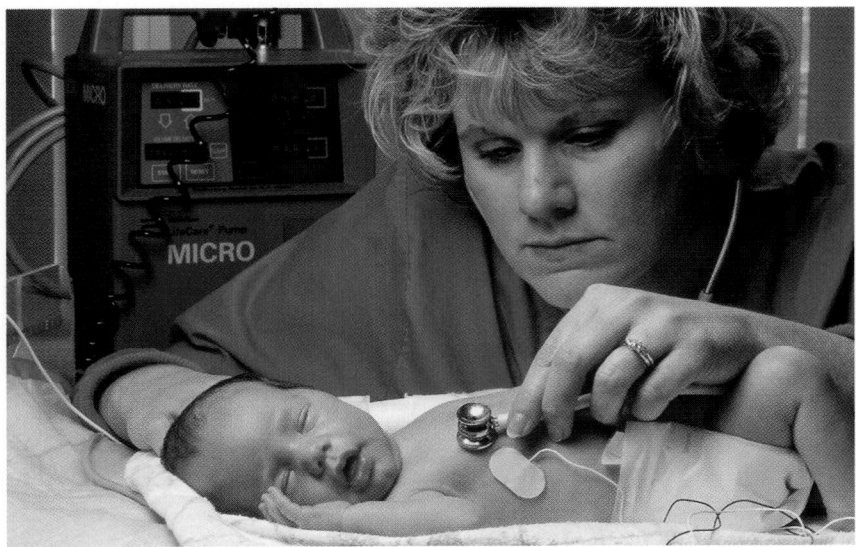

FIGURE 2-13 A pediatrician with a baby.

Surgery

A surgeon corrects illness, trauma, and deformities using an operative procedure (Figure 2-14). Surgery is any invasive procedure that requires entering the body by making an incision or passing instruments through the skin and organs.

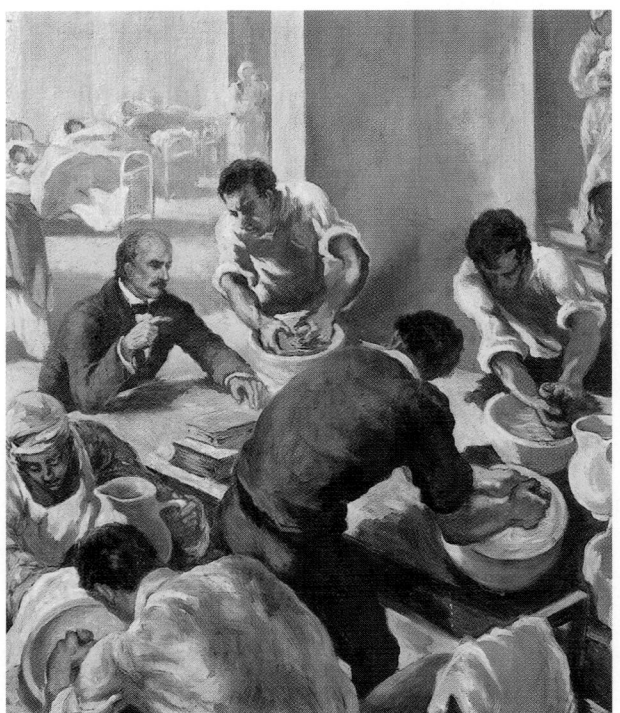

FIGURE 2-14 Surgical procedures are safer today because of hand hygiene and disinfection techniques introduced by Dr. Semmelweiss.

Surgical Specialties

General surgery includes all areas of surgery. General surgeons may restrict their practices to abdominal surgical procedures. However, many surgeons specialize in areas such as neurosurgery, cardiovascular surgery, and orthopedic surgery. Some of the more common surgical specialties are described in Table 2-2.

Health Care Institutions

Hospitals are the largest employers in the nation. According to the Bureau of Labor Statistics, in 2004, hospitals employed 41% of health care workers. In recent years, there has been increased demand from the public, government, and insurance companies to curb hospital expenses. The length of stay in the hospital has been decreasing steadily over the past decade as a result of the DRGs system of payment and better medical and surgical procedures. The result has been an increased emphasis on outpatient rather than inpatient care, especially in the area of minor surgery. Outpatient care refers to services provided to patients on a walk-in basis where no overnight stay is required; inpatient care refers to services provided to patients who are in a facility overnight or on a long-term basis.

Same-day surgery sites, home health agencies, and physical therapy/rehabilitative and sports medicine are all growing rapidly. Also, care that can be provided to older adults in their own homes is encouraged.

Hospitals

The hospital is still considered the key resource for health care in America. While the patient's primary care is delivered in the physician's office, hospitals deliver care for acute illnesses, are sites for major surgical procedures, train and educate health care professionals, conduct research, and provide educational resources to the public. Hospital sizes vary depending on the needs within the community where the hospital was built. The size is based on the number of patient beds.

As hospitals try to curb costs but maintain a rate of bed occupancy, new models are developing. Some services will be eliminated from one hospital if they are available at other nearby hospitals. Many hospitals will merge to share expenses and services or may be purchased by large national corporations.

To ensure quality health care, many hospitals seek accreditation by an association such as Joint Commission

TABLE 2-2 Surgical Specialties and Their Descriptions

Surgical Specialty	Description
Cardiovascular	Cardiovascular surgery is the surgical treatment of the heart and blood vessels.
Colorectal	Colorectal surgery involves the surgical treatment of the lower intestinal tract (colon and rectum).
Cosmetic Surgery/Plastic	Cosmetic surgery involves the reconstruction of underlying tissues. This surgical intervention is used to correct structural defects or remove scars and signs of aging.
Hand	Hand surgery is orthopedic surgery that involves surgical treatment of defects, traumas, and disorders of the hand. Hand surgeons may employ a physical therapy staff and have x-ray equipment at their disposal.
Neurosurgery	Neurosurgery involves surgical intervention for diseases and disorders of the central nervous system.
Orthopedic	Orthopedic surgery treats musculoskeletal injuries and disorders, congenital deformities, and spinal curvatures through surgical means.
Oral (Periodontics, Orthodontics)	Oral surgery involves treatment of disorders of the jaws and teeth by means of incision and surgery as well as extraction of teeth.
Thoracic	Thoracic surgery involves treatment of disorders and diseases of the chest with surgical intervention.

on the Accreditation of Health Care Organizations (JCAHO). JCAHO is a private nonprofit organization that encourages high standards of medical care. Strict guidelines must be met by the institution seeking accreditation.

There are four categories of hospitals:

- General hospital—(Figure 2-15) provides both routine care and special care such as intensive-care units and emergency rooms. They range in size from fifty beds to several hundred beds and are usually found in most towns and communities.

- Teaching hospital—provides the same type of care as in a general hospital. Teaching hospitals are generally located near a university medical school and have medical students, interns, and residents who treat patients under the supervision of staff physicians. Teaching hospitals may have more specialists on staff in order to educate and train interns and residents.

- Research hospital—provides patient care and conducts research to combat disease. Veteran's Administration hospitals throughout the nation and Shriner's hospitals for crippled children are examples of research hospitals.

- Specialty hospital—provides specialized care for certain types of patients such as children, psychiatric patients, or burn victims.

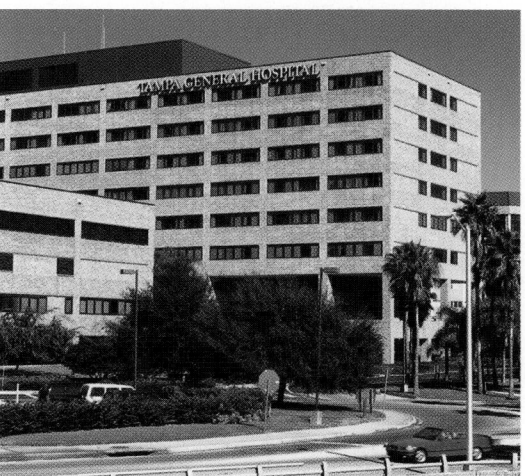

FIGURE 2-15 A general hospital.

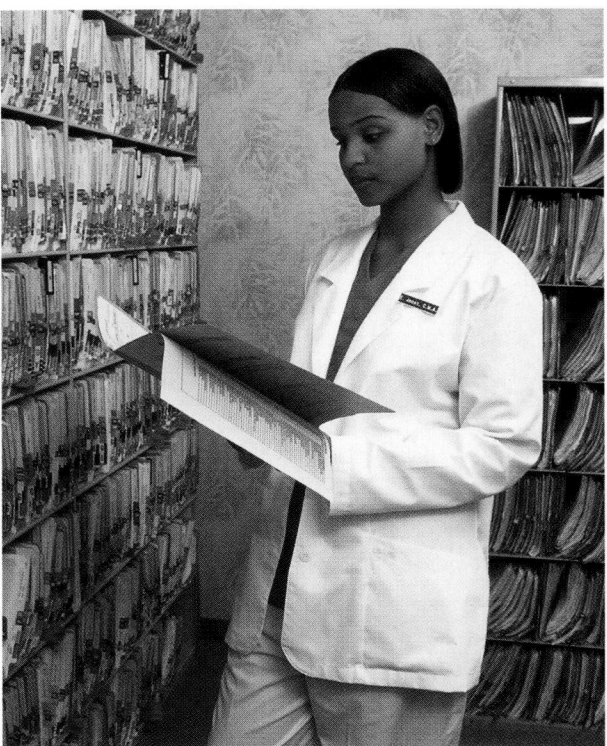

FIGURE 2-16 The medical records department.

Many larger hospitals provide all three services: general patient care, teaching, and research. The hospital organization contains many departments that interact to provide comprehensive health care for the patient. Hospital departments include emergency services, laboratory, radiology, oncology, nuclear medicine, psychiatry, pathology, immunology, respiratory, physical

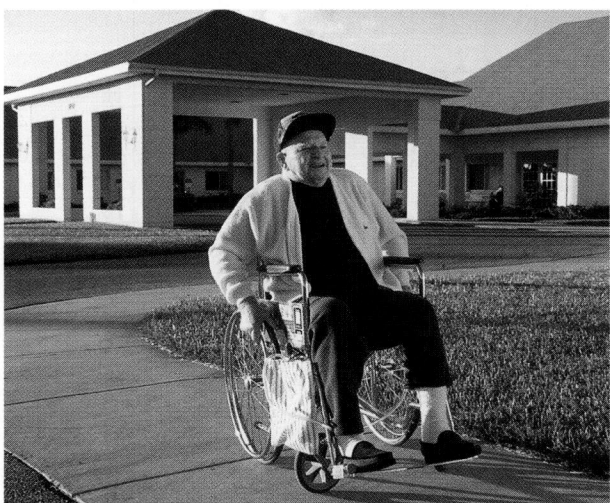

FIGURE 2-17 Skilled nursing facilities provide care for patients requiring longer stays than hospitals allow.

and occupational therapy, nursing, dietary, pharmacy, central supply, housekeeping, engineering, and health information. See Figure 2-16 for an example of a medical records department. The social services department will assist in locating medical care, treatment and/ or placement for the patient after discharge from the hospital.

Physicians generally serve on the staff of more than one hospital, but seldom more than three. Physicians will then refer their patients to one of these hospitals in which they have medical privileges. Medical privileges refer to the physician's right to practice medicine in a particular hospital or other health care facility. A physician may also have "courtesy" or "visiting privileges" at a hospital where he or she may be called to see a patient on a referral basis, but in which the physician does not have admitting privileges.

Nursing Homes

Nursing homes were established in the 19th century to provide food, clothing, and shelter for the poor. Over the past century, the quality of care has improved in nursing homes and most homes care for the elderly. Many homes are owned and operated by church groups, but the majority of homes are for-profit run by nursing home corporations. There is much tighter control over the quality of care because of stricter regulations by state public health departments and Medicare. Due to the increased costs of nursing home care, some patients have to convert to Medicaid, the national health insurance for the poor, when their funds are depleted. The present day nursing home is a long-term facility that cares for elderly persons who are sick, too feeble to care for themselves, and have no other source of care. According to the U.S. Medicare Web site, approximately nine million men and women over the age of 65 needed long-term care in 2005. Seventy percent are being cared for by family and friends. The remaining thirty percent or three million needed care in long-term care facilities.

Types of Long-Term-Care Institutions

Long-term-care institutions are classified by federal regulations either as skilled nursing facilities (SNF), intermediate-care facilities (ICF), and extended-care facilities (ECF). A description of these facilities and of assisted living follows.

- Skilled nursing facility (SNF)— intended for patients who require skilled nursing care round the clock (Figure 2-17). Patients must be re-certified every 100 days to allow them to remain in a skilled-care facility.

- Intermediate-care facility (ICF)—intended for patients who are no longer able to live alone and care for themselves, but who do not require skilled nursing care on a 24-hour basis. Many ICFs also have occupational and rehabilitative therapists on their staff. Intermediate-care facilities must meet federal guidelines in order to receive federal funds for services provided to Medicare patients.

- Extended-care facility (ECF)—provides services to patients who no longer need the skilled nursing care of a hospital, but are still too ill or incapacitated to return home. Many hospitals have opened extended-care facilities for such patients (Figure 2-18). An extended-care facility provides custodial care and thus does not employ skilled personnel.

- Assisted-living facility—offers living arrangements for the older adult in which each resident or couple has a separate apartment and pays a fixed fee to have some meals and services provided. Older adults who are able to care for themselves and require a minimum of supervision are living in this relatively new environment.

Hospice

Through the hospice movement, which began in medieval England, the wounded, sick, and dying were cared for by religious communities of sisters. Today's modern hospice movement emphasizes improved quality of care for the dying. Most hospice care is provided at home, but some programs also provide care in centers. This interdisciplinary program of care and supportive services facilitates the care of the patient by family members or significant others in the privacy of the patient's home or in a hospice facility.

On home visits, hospice personnel provide nursing care for the special needs of the dying patient, including pain management, but not necessarily treatment for the disease. These visits often provide great emotional support to the patient and the patient's family. Often the visiting health care worker can offer suggestions that might make the patient more comfortable. Most patients in a hospice facility are suffering from terminal illnesses, such as cancer, and Medicare currently covers part of this care in a hospice setting. Medicare (Part B) will cover a part of home care if there is a qualifying diagnosis.

Allied Health Professionals

There are many health care professions and it would be impossible to cover them all in this chapter. As a member of the health care team, it is important that you understand the role and educational require-

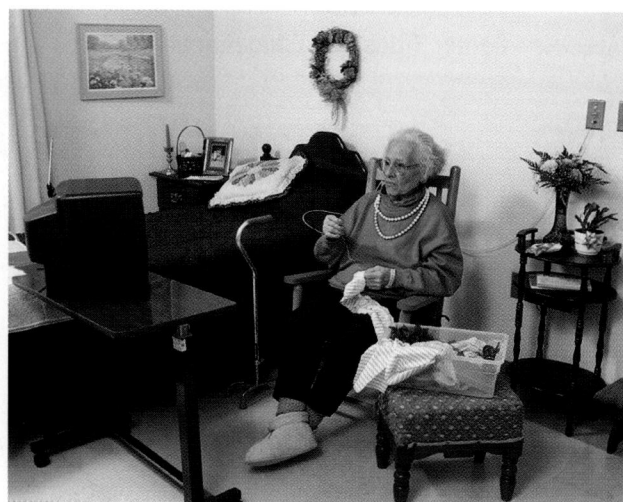

FIGURE 2-18 An extended care facility.

ments of others. Before we consider some of the specific professions, you will need an understanding of the terms certification, licensure, and registration as they relates to allied health professionals. A discussion of levels of education and degree titles will be covered as well.

Certification involves the issuing of a certificate and credentials by a professional organization to one who has met the educational/experience standards of that organization. An example would be certification as a medical assistant or CMA by the AAMA, or RMA certification by the American Medical Technologists after a candidate has passed the national examination. Registration means that a professional organization in a specific health care field administers examinations and/or maintains a list of qualified individuals. Licensure means a government agency authorizes individuals to work in a given occupation, such as registered nurses (RN), licensed practical nurses (LPN), and physical therapists (PT).

Educational requirements for health careers vary from state to state. In all cases, a high school diploma or equivalency is necessary. Post secondary education in a vocational/technical school, community college, or university may be required. Table 2-3 illustrates a career ladder in health care, educational requirements, degree designations, and some examples of professions in each category. Health care institutions may require the applicant to pass a national registration or certification examination in his or her field of study as a condition of hire. See Professionalism for continuing education requirements.

Careers in the health care field involve many types of duties or responsibilities. An extensive list of possible career choices follows and are categorized into

TABLE 2-3 Career Titles and Educational Levels

Professional	Educational Requirement	Diploma/ Degree	Examples
Professional	4-year degree, advanced degree and clinical training	Bachelor (BA, BS), Master or Doctorate	Medical Doctor (MD) Patholgist
Technologist	4-year college program	Bachelor (BA, BS)	Medical Technologist (MT)
Technician	2-year community college or vocational program	Associate's degree (AS)	Medical Laboratory Technician (MLT)
Assistant	Up to 1-year classroom and clinical preparation	Diploma	Laboratory Assistant
Aide	On-the-job training	High school diploma or GED	Laboratory Aide

Professionalism

Physicians must obtain continuing education to retain their license. Medical assistants also need to keep abreast of new medical information. AAMA requires Certified Medical Assistants (CMA) to earn 60 continuing education credits (CEUs) in five years to maintain their certification. Registered Medical Assistants (RMAs) who earn certification by passing the American Medical Technologists' examination are also encouraged to earn CEUs. Being a life-long learner should be the goal of every medical assistant. The body of knowledge in health care is growing tremendously each year and you will need to be vigilant about keeping up with new information. The following are a few ideas to help you become a well-informed, life-long learner.

- Read *CMA Today*, the AAMA medical assisting journal or AMT Events, the RMA professional publications and complete the continuing education article and test in each edition if provided.
- Select an interesting condition or disease each month to research on the Internet or local library; Keep this research information in a binder for future reference.
- Subscribe to other medical publications or ask your physician if you may read some periodicals that she/he receives.
- Attend seminars provided by the local hospital, HMO, and state or local chapters of medical assisting groups.

National Heath Care Skills Standards (NHCSS) career clusters. The National Health Care Skill Standards were developed to define the body of knowledge and specific skills health care workers are expected to possess for entry-level and technical-level positions. These core standards are used by schools, colleges, and health care facilities to establish curriculum and competencies for a wide variety of fields. The health care careers discussed will be broken down according to National Health Care Skill Standards career clusters and a few examples from each category will be examined.

Therapeutic Cluster Careers

Careers in this cluster include those that involve the health care status of the patient including treatment, evaluation, collection of patient data, and evaluation of patient status.

Nurse

The term nurse refers to a diversified group of health care professionals with a range of qualifications. A description follows of a certified nursing assistant (CNA), licensed practical nurse (LPN), registered nurse (RN), and nurse practitioner (NP).

CERTIFIED NURSING ASSISTANT (CNA) A certified nursing assistant is a member of the health care team who has completed a training program and taken a state examination to qualify to assist nurses in nursing homes, hospitals, and other health care facilities. The CNA provides such patient care as bed baths, vital signs, feeding, and ambulation. Cross training of employees has led to positions such as patient care technician (PCT). The PCT may have a CNA or medical assisting background and perform more technical tasks such as drawing blood and performing EKGs. The nursing assistant may also be referred to as a nurses' aid or orderly.

LICENSED PRACTICAL NURSE (LPN) A licensed practical nurse performs some of the same, but not all, clinical nursing tasks as a registered nurse. The LPN must have graduated from a recognized one-year program and become licensed by the National Federation of Licensed Practical Nurses. In some states, the LPN is known as a licensed vocational nurse (LVN).

REGISTERED NURSE (RN) A nursing career is ideal for the person who wishes to provide hands-on patient care. Nurses work in hospitals, physicians' offices, industry, governmental agencies, ambulatory care units, emergency services, and schools. Their work ranges from managed care organizations providing direct patient care, to teaching and supervising other staff, performing research, and managing agencies. Nurses receive their education and training in either a two-year or four-year program. To become licensed as a registered nurse requires successful completion of a national licensure examination known as the National Council Licensure Examination (NCLEX). A nurse practitioner (NP) is a registered nurse who has received additional training to provide basic patient care including diagnosing and prescribing medications and treatments for common illnesses. This nurse is a masters-degree, trained individual.

Occupational Therapist (OT)

Occupational therapy provides treatment to people who are physically, mentally, developmentally, or emotionally disabled. Occupational therapists evaluate the patient's ability for self-care, work, and leisure skills. The goal of the occupational therapist is to develop programs that will help to restore the patient's ability to manage activities of daily living (ADL). Occupational therapists require a bachelor's degree from an approved program in occupational therapy. In addition, certification by the American Occupational Therapy Association (AOTA) and six months of on-the-job training are needed.

An occupational therapy assistant must complete a two-year vocational training program and be certified by AOTA. This individual works under the supervision of an OT and implements patient treatments designated by the OT.

Physical Therapist (PT)

Physical therapy is the treatment of diseases or disabilities of the joints, bones, and nerves by massage, therapeutic exercises, and heat and cold treatments. Conditions treated by means of physical therapy include: multiple sclerosis, cerebral palsy, arthritis, fractures, spinal cord injuries, and heart disease.

Practitioners work in a variety of facilities including hospitals, ambulatory care, rehabilitation centers, private practice, and schools for the physically challenged. A physical therapist is required to hold a four-year degree in physical therapy, participate in a four-month clinical internship, and successfully pass the state licensure examination. After obtaining a master's degree, some physical therapists set up private practices and provide services on a contract basis.

A physical therapy assistant may be required to have a degree from an accredited two-year college and pass a written licensure examination in some states. He or she works under the supervision of a physical therapist and implement treatments designated by the PT.

Physician's Assistant (PA)

The field of physician's assistant is relatively new, emerging since the 1970s. The goal of this profession is to assist the physician in the primary care of patients. The job description for a physician's assistant includes evaluation, monitoring, diagnostics, therapeutics, counseling, and referral skills. In nearly all states, the PA can prescribe medications. The profession has expanded to include surgeon's, pathologist's, anesthesiologist's, and radiologist's assistant, among others. The general educational program is similar to a master's level program with two years education after a bachelor's degree. In most programs, the student must have work and/or internship experience and pass an accreditation examination.

Respiratory Therapist (RT)

A respiratory therapist evaluates, treats, and cares for patients with breathing problems. A respiratory therapist tests lung capacity, administers breathing treatments, teaches self-care to patients, and provides emergency care. An RT can be employed in hospitals, cardiopulmonary laboratories, nursing homes, health maintenance organizations (HMOs), and ambulatory care facilities. To become a certified respiratory therapy technician (CRTT), the candidate must complete a one-year internship and pass a written examination given by the National Board of Respiratory Therapy.

To become a registered respiratory therapist (RRT) requires completion of a college program, an approved training program, one year's experience in the field, and the successful completion of a written examination given by the National Board of Respiratory Therapy.

Dietician

Dietitians are skilled in applying the principles of good nutrition to food selection and meal preparation. They will work closely with a patient's physician to coordinate the patient's diet with other treatments such as medications. Dietitians also provide consulting services, offer seminars, author books, counsel patients, plan food service systems, and design nutrition plans within fitness programs for athletes. A dietitian must have a bachelor's degree with a major in foods and nutrition. In addition, an internship in a dietary department is required. To become registered requires successful completion of an examination. Dietitians work in a variety of settings including hospitals, long-term-care facilities, schools, and prisons. The employment opportunities for dietitians are currently excellent.

Dental Hygienist

A dental hygienist works directly with the patient to clean teeth, take oral x-rays, teach oral health, and discusses results of dental examinations with the dentist. The dental hygienist must graduate from a two-year community college program or a four-year bachelor's program and pass both a state written and clinical examination.

Emergency Medical Technicians (EMTs)/Paramedics

Emergency medical technicians/paramedics (EMTs/paramedics) are trained in providing emergency care and transporting injured patients to a medical facility. They are skilled in recognizing emergency conditions such as cardiac arrhythmias, airway obstruction, and psychological crisis. Emergency medical technicians and paramedics always work under the direct supervision of a physician and follow a physician's orders. There are different levels of EMTs:

- Basic—the beginner EMT performs basic life support.
- Advanced—an advanced EMT has more training and advanced skills beyond the basic level.
- Paramedic—as the highest level of EMT, a paramedic is able to treat cardiac arrest, perform defibrillation, and administer certain drugs.

EMTs receive certification after completion of an approved EMT program. They must be recertified every two years and receive ongoing education and training in their field.

Diagnostic Career Cluster

The careers in this cluster are involved with procedures that create a picture of the patient's health status at a specific point in time. These careers involve measuring, evaluating, and reporting patient information.

Ultrasound Technologist (AART)

An ultrasound technologist receives training in the use of ultrasound equipment, which uses inaudible sound waves to outline shapes of tissues and organs. Ultrasound equipment produces an image of the shapes. Ultrasound images of fetal development in the uterus are commonly used to assist with fetal monitoring.

X-ray Technologist (Radiologic Technologist)

An x-ray or radiologic technologist must hold a bachelor's degree in radiologic technology, have experience in two or more radiologic disciplines such as nuclear medicine and radiation therapy, and be a registered radiologic technologist (ARRT).

Electroencephalograph Technician

Electroencephalography (EEG) is the field devoted to recording and studying the electrical activity of the brain. An EEG technician operates an electroencephalograph, which records the activity of the brain with a written tracing of the brain's electrical impulses. EEG technologists work primarily in hospitals.

Pharmacist

The field of pharmacy deals with the ordering, maintaining, preparing, and distributing prescription medications. Several pharmacy roles are described here along with the educational requirements.

A pharmacist must complete five years of education in an accredited pharmacy program. In addition, a pharmacy student must serve a one-year internship and become licensed in the state where he or she is employed. A registered pharmacist can work in a variety of institutions including hospitals, drug stores, or may open a pharmacy.

Pharmacy technicians attend a community college or private vocational program. They are able to assist the pharmacist in preparing medications. In some states, they are issued a Pharmacy Technician Certificate upon completion of an examination. A pharmacy clerk assists the pharmacist with typing prescription labels, assigning prescription numbers, and maintaining supplies and records. A high school degree is necessary for this position.

Medical Social Worker

Social work involves programs and services that are developed to meet the special needs of the ill, physically and mentally challenged, and the elderly. A medical social worker cares for the total person, including the emotional, cultural, social, and physical needs of the patient.

Medical social workers assist patients and their families in handling problems associated with a long-term illness or disability. Social workers need a thorough understanding of a community's resources for the disabled. A medical social worker requires a bachelor's degree. Many states require licensing or registration for social workers and a master's degree.

Diagnostic Imaging Technician

Diagnostic Imaging Technicians are trained in the operation of x-ray equipment such as ultrasound, computerized tomography (CT) scan, and magnetic resonance imaging (MRI). Radiology practitioners include: darkroom attendants with a minimum of education or training; radiologic technicians who are graduates of an accredited program; radiologists, who are graduates of an accredited medical school; and licensed physicians with specialized training in radiology.

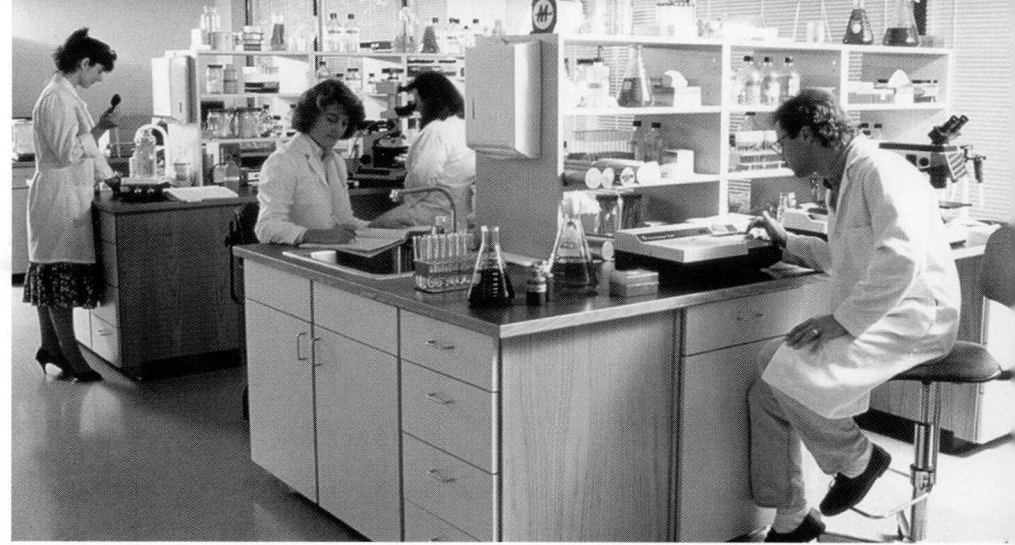

FIGURE 2-19 Hospital laboratory.

Employment opportunities are available in physicians' offices, hospitals, trauma centers, and other ambulatory care facilities.

Medical Laboratory

A medical laboratory is a facility that is equipped for testing, research, scientific experimentation, or clinical studies of materials, fluids, or tissues taken from patients. Independent laboratories provide routine analysis of patient's blood, urine, tissue, and other materials. Hospital laboratories perform tests for both inpatients and outpatients (Figure 2-19). In some instances, a physician's office (POL) will contain a small laboratory where routine tests can be conducted.

PHLEBOTOMIST OR VENIPUNCTURE TECHNICIAN   A phlebotomist is skilled in drawing blood from patients. This requires the ability to maintain standard precautions, aseptic technique, excellent venipuncture technique, and good communication skills. Training in a vocational education program is required. In some cases, certification as a phlebotomist is required.

LABORATORY TECHNICIAN (MLT AND CLT)   The medical laboratory technician (MLT) and the clinical laboratory technician (CLT) are laboratory technicians skilled in testing blood, urine, lymph, and body tissues. This career requires two years of training in a vocational education program and certification by the National Certification Agency for Medical Laboratory Personnel.

MEDICAL TECHNOLOGIST (MT) OR CLINICAL LABORATORY SCIENTIST (CLS).   A laboratory or medical technologist must complete a four-year medical technology program in a college or university to become a certified medical technologist (CMT) or certified laboratory scientist (CLS). This person directs the work of other laboratory staff, is responsible for maintaining quality assurance standards for all equipment, and performs laboratory analysis. The examination for this profession is prepared by the Board of Registry of the American Society of Clinical Pathologists (ASCP) or American Association of Medical Technologists.

The American Medical Technologists (AMT) certifies phlebotomists, medical laboratory technicians, and medical technologists.

Information Services Career Clusters

Careers in this cluster are involved with documenting client information, including managing, coding, analyzing, maintaining, and retrieving information.

Health Information Technology (Medical Records Technician)

Health information technology refers to the massive database known as medical records. Every person seen by a health care professional has a medical record. Medical records technicians, now more commonly referred to as health information technologists, maintain the permanent records relating to a patient's condition and treatment. The medical record is a legal document that can be used in a court of law.

A medical records technician (ART) must graduate from an accredited medical records program, have a two-year associates degree, have several years experience as a medical records clerk, and have 30 credit hours from an accredited college. Successful completion of the accredited record technical examination allows the technician to use the initials ART after his or her name.

A registered medical records administrator (RRA) requires a bachelor's degree in health information technology and the successful completion of an examination.

Medical Transcription

A medical transcriptionist types or enters into the computer dictation that is taken from a recording machine or tape. This dictation consists of medical reports from physicians and surgeons. Skills required for this profession include typing ability, good spelling understanding of medical terminology, and data processing equipment.

Office Management

The role of office manager is a choice open to some allied health professionals, including medical assistants and nurses. Office managers supervise the entire support staff. The position requires someone with a sound knowledge of the type of work performed in the office or institution, strong supervisory skills, and the ability to work closely with top management. Excellent time-management and communication skills are a must for office managers.

Unit Clerk/Communications Clerk

The unit clerk, or ward secretary, is responsible for clerical duties, reception work, and other communication duties in hospitals, long-term-care facilities, and clinics. The unit clerk in a hospital performs varied tasks, for example, taking physicians' orders from the charts and assisting the nursing staff. A knowledge of medical terminology is required.

Environmental Services Career Cluster

This career cluster includes careers involved with the patient's health care environment such as aseptic procedures, resource management, maintaining equipment, and providing sterile supplies.

Biomedical Equipment Technician

A biomedical equipment technician maintains and repairs medical testing equipment either in a health care facility or for a private company. Educational requirements vary from an associate's to a bachelor's degree.

Other health care workers in this career cluster, which do not require postsecondary education, include central supply/sterile supply workers, housekeeping staff, and food-service aides.

Centers for Disease Control (CDC)

The Centers for Disease Control (CDC), a division of Department of Health and Human Services (DHHS), was established in 1946. The CDC's main headquarters and laboratories are in Atlanta, Georgia. This is a governmental agency that employs over 8,600 people.

The purpose of the CDC is to safeguard public health by preventing and controlling disease, and act as a resource for the medical profession. The CDC seeks information about causes of disease to find cures, alerts the medical profession to potential outbreaks of diseases such as influenza, describes the group who will be at highest risk during an outbreak of disease such as the elderly, and recommends the proper treatment. In addition, the CDC conducts disease research, prevention, control, and education programs nationally and in several other countries. These programs help to train doctors, provide public health information, develop immunization services with state and local agencies, and establish standards for healthful working conditions.

SUMMARY

The medical profession contains a rich history of achievement and progress. The history of medicine can be broken into four categories: early medicine going back to 3000 BC, the 18th century, 19th century, and 20th century. Major advancements include the eradication of many deadly diseases with the advent of vaccines, the decrease of infections due to the discovery of aseptic technique and antibiotics, the harnessing of radium to treat disease, the inventions of the microscope and surgical instruments, the discovery of anesthesia, and a better understanding of anatomy and physiology.

Contemporary licensed physicians must maintain their knowledge base by completing 75 continuing

medical education (CME) units over a period of three years. There are 24 medical specialty boards for the purpose of improving the quality of care by encouraging physicians to seek further education and training. The medical assistant will have the opportunity to pursue a career working for physicians in all areas of specialization.

The health care environment can be confusing and intimidating to the patient. It is important to have an understanding of the health care system and the diversity of institutions that deliver health care services. The descriptions provided in this chapter of inpatient facilities including hospitals, nursing homes, hospices, as well as ambulatory care settings and services provide a basic explanation of a rather complex structure. Patients need to know the options that are available as they seek out services and follow up on the referrals made by their primary physician for treatment, procedures, or further diagnosis. The medical assistant's understanding of the system is key to providing clear explanations to the patient. Understanding managed care plans and using the proper insurance codes (see CPT and ICD-9 in Chapter 17) for services provided to patients are necessary to assure insurance claims reimbursement.

Chapter Review

COMPETENCY REVIEW

1. Define and spell the terms to learn for this chapter.
2. State some of the major achievements in medicine during each of these periods: early medicine, 18th century, 19th century, and 20th century or modern medicine.
3. List the three methods by which a physician can become licensed.
4. Explain three circumstances that would justify the suspension or revocation of a physician's license.
5. Describe four types of medical practices.
6. Identify and explain issues in this chapter that might require patient education.
7. Find examples of four board certified physicians in your local telephone directory.
8. Describe the role of the medical assistant as it relates to patient education concerning the physician's credentials.
9. Using the local telephone directory, find examples of names and addresses of three hospitals, a hospice, an extended-care facility, and a medical laboratory.
10. Discuss the role of the medical assistant in relationship to other health care providers.

PREPARING FOR THE CERTIFICATION EXAMINATION

1. What is the symbol for healing that incorporates a staff with two coiled snakes?
   A. colliculus
   B. caisson
   C. cachination
   D. choleretic
   E. caduceus

2. The number of individual cases of a disease within a defined population is known as the
   A. morbidity rate
   B. mortality rate
   C. illness factor
   D. disease factor
   E. illness rate

3. The first written source of medical ethics for the first doctors in history is called the
   A. Code of Medical Conduct
   B. Code of Hammurabi
   C. Hippocratic Oath
   D. Code of Caduceus
   E. Oath of Medical Healing

4. One source of medicine to treat pain in early human history was
   A. the poppy plant
   B. cayenne pepper
   C. chamomile tea
   D. licorice
   E. the foxglove plant

continued on next page

5. The "father of medicine" is
   A. Caduceus
   B. Galen
   C. Hippocrates
   D. Vesalius
   E. Galileo

6. Who discovered penicillin?
   A. Sabin
   B. Salk
   C. Fleming
   D. Banting
   E. Nightingale

7. The state law which governs the licensure of physicians is the
   A. Medical Licensure Act
   B. Code of Medical Conduct and Licensure
   C. Medical Practice Act
   D. Physicians' Practice Act
   E. Physicians' Conduct Oath

8. Which physician in the late 1800s helped find a cure for yellow fever?
   A. Morton
   B. Reed
   C. Long
   D. Hahnemann
   E. Beaumont

9. Which government agency was established to safeguard public health by preventing and controlling disease through research?
   A. ICF
   B. ECF
   C. FDA
   D. HMO
   E. CDC

10. DRGs stands for
   A. Diagnostic Related Groups
   B. Diagnostic Research Groups
   C. Delivery Related Groups
   D. Drug Related Groups
   E. Drug Reactive Groups

CRITICAL THINKING

1. Is it beyond the scope of her training for Elizabeth to arrange for such care and the physical transition for this patient?

2. If yes, how could Elizabeth handle this situation with the physician and other providers that are involved in this case?

3. If no, what options could Elizabeth investigate in order to help facilitate the placement of this patient?

4. Are patient and family education merited in this particular situation or is some sort of intervention applicable?

5. Does the fact that alcohol and drug abuses are involved alter potential treatment options?

6. Because the patient has a history of violent behavior, should this fact limit the placement options?

ON THE JOB

One of the important characteristics of a medical assistant is to have a concrete foundation in the practice of medicine. This would include a complete understanding of the many medical and surgical specialties and subspecialties in which a physician can be board certified.

An important responsibility for the medical assistant is to have the ability to convey this information about the treating physician to the anxious patient and the patient's family. This is part of patient education.

Mary is employed as a medical assistant for a physician who is a pediatric cardiovascular surgeon. She is taking a history on the patient, a newborn, by interviewing the parents, Mr. and Mrs. Appleby. They are extremely anxious and upset over the condition of their newborn who was diagnosed shortly after birth with a serious, yet quite treatable, heart defect. The prognosis, should the parents agree to the corrective surgery, is quite good. However, the parents are having a difficult time understanding how the physician could help their newborn. They are not even quite sure why they were referred to this specialist and why their pediatrician could not treat the infant.

1. How could Mary comfort and reassure these parents?
2. What could she possibly say about the physician that might help the parents to understand why they were referred and how their newborn could be helped?

INTERNET ACTIVITY

Research ethical arguments for and against the use of fetal stem cells for medical treatment.

MediaLink More on medical practices and health care environment, including interactive resources, can be found on the Student CD-ROM accompanying this textbook.

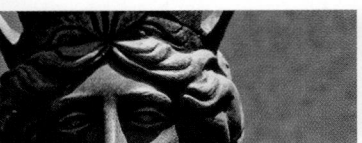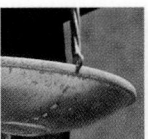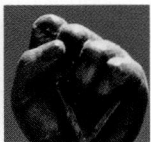

Medical Assistant Role Delineation Chart

HIGHLIGHT indicates material covered in this chapter.

ADMINISTRATIVE

Administrative Procedures

- Perform basic administrative medical assisting functions
- Schedule, coordinate and monitor appointments
- Schedule inpatient/outpatient admissions and procedures
- Understand and apply third-party guidelines
- Obtain reimbursement through accurate claims submission
- Monitor third-party reimbursement
- Understand and adhere to managed care policies and procedures
- *Negotiate managed care contracts*

Practice Finances

- Perform procedural and diagnostic coding
- Apply bookkeeping principles

- Manage accounts receivable
- *Manage accounts payable*
- *Process payroll*
- *Document and maintain accounting and banking records*
- *Develop and maintain fee schedules*
- *Manage renewals of business and professional insurance policies*
- *Manage personnel benefits and maintain records*
- *Perform marketing, financial, and strategic planning*

CLINICAL

Fundamental Principles

- Apply principles of aseptic technique and infection control
- Comply with quality assurance practices
- Screen and follow up patient test results

Diagnostic Orders

- Collect and process specimens
- Perform diagnostic tests

Patient Care

- Adhere to established patient screening procedures
- Obtain patient history and vital signs
- Prepare and maintain examination and treatment areas
- Prepare patient for examinations, procedures and treatments

- Assist with examinations, procedures and treatments
- Prepare and administer medications and immunizations
- Maintain medication and immunization records
- Recognize and respond to emergencies
- Coordinate patient care information with other health care providers
- Initiate IV and administer IV medications with appropriate training and as permitted by state law

GENERAL

Professionalism

- Display a professional manner and image
- Demonstrate initiative and responsibility
- Work as a member of the health care team
- Prioritize and perform multiple tasks
- Adapt to change
- Promote the CMA credential
- Enhance skills through continuing education
- Treat all patients with compassion and empathy
- Promote the practice through positive public relations

Communication Skills

- Recognize and respect cultural diversity
- Adapt communications to individual's ability to understand
- Use professional telephone technique

- Recognize and respond effectively to verbal, nonverbal, and written communications
- Use medical terminology appropriately
- Utilize electronic technology to receive, organize, prioritize and transmit information
- Serve as liaison

Legal Concepts

- Perform within legal and ethical boundaries
- Prepare and maintain medical records
- Document accurately
- Follow employer's established policies dealing with the health care contract
- Implement and maintain federal and state health care legislation and regulations
- Comply with established risk management and safety procedures
- Recognize professional credentialing criteria
- *Develop and maintain personnel, policy and procedure manuals*

Instruction

- Instruct individuals according to their needs
- Explain office policies and procedures
- Teach methods of health promotion and disease prevention
- Locate community resources and disseminate information
- *Develop educational materials*
- *Conduct continuing education activities*

Operational Functions

- Perform inventory of supplies and equipment
- Perform routine maintenance of administrative and clinical equipment
- Apply computer techniques to support office operations
- *Perform personnel management functions*
- *Negotiate leases and prices for equipment and supply contracts*

- *Denotes advanced skills.*

SOURCE: Reprinted by permission of the American Association of Medical Assistants from the AAMA Role Delineation Study: Occupational Analysis of the Medical Assisting Profession.

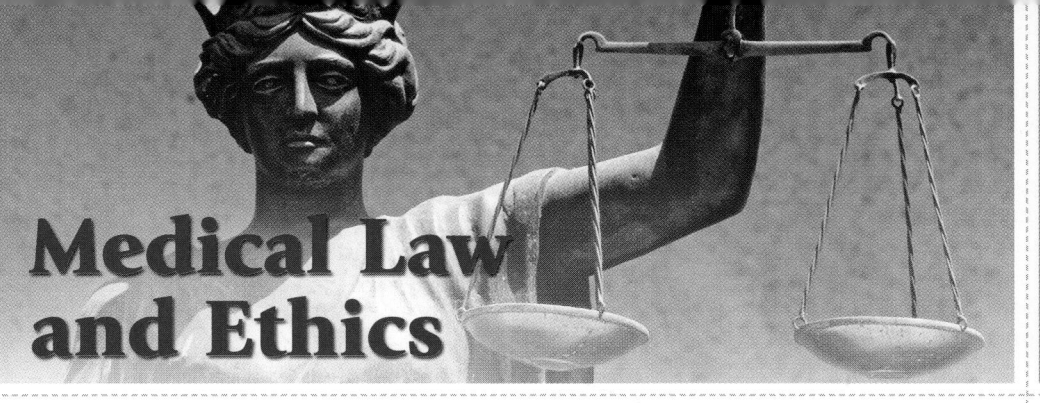

Medical Law and Ethics

Learning Objectives

After completing this chapter, you should be able to:

- Define and spell the terms to learn for this chapter.
- Differentiate between criminal and civil law.
- Discuss the four Ds of negligence.
- Discuss what can be done to avoid a claim of abandonment.
- Discuss informed consent.
- Discuss the role of the medical assistant relating to legal issues in the medical office.
- Explain the importance of the Hippocratic oath today.

- List the seven main points of the AMA Principles of Medical Ethics.
- List and discuss the main points of the AAMA Principles of Medical Ethics.
- Discuss what is meant by the medical assistant's standards of care.
- Describe the Patient's Bill of Rights.
- Explain the HIPAA guidelines concerning the patient's right to privacy and confidentiality in the medical office.

OUTLINE

Classification of the Law	44
Professional Liability	46
Patient/Physician Relationship	49
Documentation	52
Public Duties of Physicians	53
Drug Regulations	53
Role of the Medical Assistant	54
Code of Ethics	56
Medical Ethics	56
AMA Principles of Medical Ethics	57
Medical Assistant's Principles of Medical Ethics	57
Medical Assistant's Standard of Care	58
The Patient's Bill of Rights	58
Confidentiality	59
Ethical Issues and Personal Choice	60

Terms to Learn

breach of contract
contributory negligence
defamation of character
guardian ad litem
informed consent

living will
practice of medicine
proximate cause
reasonable person standard

res ipsa loquitur
respondeat superior
standard of care
statute of limitations

Case Study

DR. BARNS IS A BOARD CERTIFIED ONCOLOGIST. Although in a solo practice, she employs a staff of five—an office manager, insurance administrator, receptionist, registered nurse, and medical assistant. They have worked in the practice together for more than three years.

Dr. Barnes has asked the medical assistant, Sue Halt, to take over the insurance administrator's duties in her absence. Since the medical assistant is multiskilled, she is the best choice on staff.

Sue was surprised to discover that insurance companies were being billed for medication that is, according to the FDA, experimental. She also was troubled by the fact that insurance companies were being billed as if the patients were being treated on an outpatient basis. In reality, many of the patients resided out of the state and had been shipped the experimental medication for self-administration.

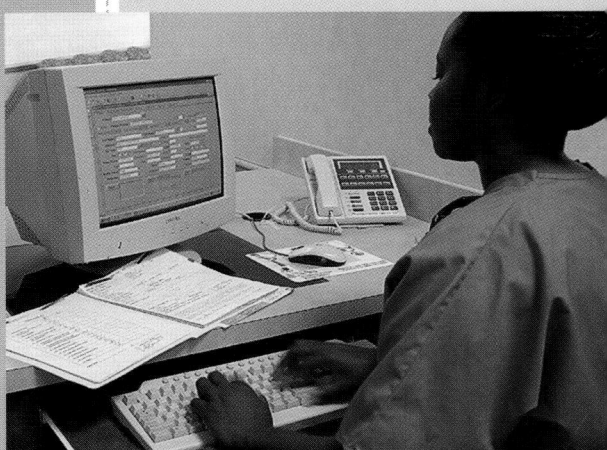

oday's health care consumer demands more of a partnership with the physician and the rest of the health care team. Patients should be part of the decision-making process regarding their care and treatment. This chapter discusses issues such as malpractice, abandonment, and litigation, as well as specific regulations and documents protecting the patient, the patient's family, physicians, and medical staff involved in care and treatment. Some examples are the Uniform Anatomical Gift Act and the Patient Self-Determination Act. Other topics presented include the public duties of the physician, documentation of medical records, regulations relating to controlled substances and the medical assistant's role in preventing liability suits.

Classification of the Law

Laws are classified into four types:

- Criminal
- Civil
- International
- Military

Only criminal and civil law are discussed here.

Criminal Law

Criminal laws are made to protect the public as a whole from the harmful acts of others.

Criminal acts fall into two categories: felony and misdemeanor. A felony carries a punishment of imprisonment in a state or federal prison or death. These crimes include murder, rape, robbery, and practicing medicine without a license. Misdemeanors are less serious offenses and carry a punishment of fines or imprisonment in jail for up to a year. They include traffic violations, disturbing the peace, and theft.

A physician's license may be revoked or taken away if he or she is convicted of a crime. Criminal cases have included revocation of a license for sexual misconduct, murder, violating narcotics laws, and practicing medicine without a license. The practice of medicine is defined as diagnosing and prescribing treatment or medication. The medical assistant must make sure that he or she always assists the physician, and does not try to treat or diagnose a patient's condition.

Civil Law

Civil law concerns relationships between individuals or between individuals and the government. Civil law includes contract law, tort law, and administrative law. Contract law includes enforceable promises and agreements between two or more persons to do or not do a particular action. Tort law covers acts that result in

TABLE 3-1 Intentional Torts

Tort	Description	Example
Assault	The threat of bodily harm to another. There does not have to be actual touching (battery) or injury for assault to take place.	Threatening to harm a patient or to perform a procedure for which he or she does not consent.
Battery	Actual bodily harm to another person without permission. This is also referred to as unlawful touching or touching without consent.	Performing surgery or a procedure without the informed consent (permission) of the patient.
False imprisonment	A violation of the personal liberty of another person through unlawful restraint.	Refusing to allow a patient to leave an office, hospital, or medical facility, when he or she requests.
Defamation of character	Damage caused to a person's reputation through spoken or written word.	Making a negative statement about another physician's ability.
Fraud	Deceitful practice.	Promising a miracle cure.
Invasion of privacy	The unauthorized publicity of information about a patient.	Allowing personal information, such as test results for HIV, to become public without the patient's permission.

harm to another. Administrative law covers regulations that are set by governmental agencies. Health care employees are most frequently involved in cases of civil law, in particular, tort and contract law.

Tort Law

A tort is a wrongful act that is committed against another person or property that results in harm. In order to meet the definition of a tort, there must be damage or injury to the patient that was caused by the physician or the physician's employee.

Intentional torts include assault, battery, false imprisonment, defamation of character, fraud, and invasion of privacy. Table 3-1 provides a description and example of these torts.

Unintentional torts, such as negligence, occur when the patient is injured as a result of the health care professional not exercising the ordinary standard of care. The health care professional must exercise the type of care that a "reasonable" person would use in a similar circumstance. This is known as the reasonable person standard.

Negligence and malpractice are the same thing. It is easier to prevent negligence than it is to defend it. Physicians can take steps to avoid negligence suits by:

- Protecting the physician-client relationship.
- Being above any reproach in the performance of their medical duties.

In order to obtain a judgment for negligence against a physician, the patient must be able to show what is referred to as the "four Ds": Duty, Dereliction or neglect of duty, Direct cause, and Damages (Box 3-1).

In legal terms, a plaintiff is a person or group of people who file a lawsuit. The defendant is the person, or group of people, who are accused of wrongdoing in a court of law.

In a case of negligence, the plaintiff must prove proximate cause. This means that the plaintiff must prove that the defendant's acts (or failure to act) directly caused the injury. For example, if a patient returns to his room after having prostate surgery and experiences severe headaches that were not present before having the surgery, the patient must prove that the physician's performance of the prostate surgery was the cause of the headaches. Contributory negligence relates to the patient's contribution to the injury, which if proven, would release the physician as the direct cause. For example, the patient did not keep an appointment causing an undetected infection to advance.

Contract Law

The branch of law known as contract law is generally concerned with a breach or neglect of an understanding between two parties.

BOX 3-1
The Four Ds of Negligence

- **Duty** refers to the physician-client relationship. The patient must prove that this relationship has been established. When the patient has made an appointment and been seen by the physician, a relationship has been established. Further office visits and treatment will establish that the physician had a duty or obligation to the patient. (Contract)
- **Dereliction or neglect of duty** refers to a physician's failure to act as any ordinary and prudent physician (a peer) within the same community would act in a similar circumstance when treating a patient. To prove dereliction or neglect of duty, a patient would have to prove that the physician's performance or treatment did not comply with the acceptable standard of care based on the norm of the ordinary and prudent physician described above. (Standard of Care)
- **Direct cause** requires the patient to prove that the physician's derelict or breach of duty was the direct cause for the injury that resulted.
- **Damages** refers to any injuries that were received by the patient. The court may award compensatory damages to pay for the patient's injuries.

A contract is a voluntary agreement that two parties enter into with the intent of mutual benefit for both parties. Something of value, which is termed *consideration*, is part of the agreement. In the medical profession, the consideration might be the performance of a hysterectomy in exchange for a specific fee. An agreement would take place between the two parties, which would include the offer ("I will perform the hysterectomy") and the acceptance of the offer ("I will allow you to perform a hysterectomy") and the consideration (performance of the hysterectomy in exchange for the fee).

In order for a contract to be legal, there are several considerations. For one thing, the concerned party (the patient) must be mentally competent at the time the contract is made. For example, the patient must not be under the influence of drugs or alcohol at the time the contract is entered.

A breach of contract occurs when either party fails to comply with the terms of the agreement. In the previous example, a breach of contract would occur if the

BOX 3-2
Premature Termination of the Physician-Patient Contract

A medical office should document any of the incidents below with a certified letter.

- Failure to pay for service.
- Missed appointments.
- Failure to follow instructions.
- The patient states (orally or in writing) that he or she is seeking the care of another physician. Reasons for seeking another physician are many. For example, the patient's insurance may have changed and the patient's physician may not be covered by the new insurance, or the patient may move.

physician removed the appendix along with the uterus during a hysterectomy without the expressed consent of the patient, or if the patient failed to pay the agreed-upon fee.

Abandonment

Once a physician has agreed to take care of a patient that contract may not be terminated improperly. The physician may be charged with abandonment of the patient if he or she does not give formal notice of withdrawal from the case. In addition, the physician must allow the patient enough time to seek the services of another physician. The best method to protect the physician from a charge of abandonment is to send a letter by certified mail.

An example of abandonment is the patient who is under treatment for a heart ailment but has not kept appointments for periodic checkups to assess his or her condition. The physician may decide that he or she can no longer accept responsibility for the medical treatment of this patient without periodic physical examinations to assess medication dosage and other factors. In this case, the physician makes a decision to no longer treat this patient. Abandonment would occur if the physician did not provide enough notice to the patient of withdrawal from the case. This notice must be sufficient for the patient to find another physician who will provide treatment. The time varies from state to state.

Termination of Contract

The termination of the contract between a physician and a patient generally occurs when the treatment has ended and the fee has been paid. However, there are serious issues that arise causing premature termination of a contract between the physician and the patient. It should be noted that both physicians and patients have the right to terminate the contractual relationship. Letters from the physician should indicate the date the physician's services will be terminated. The medical assistant needs to understand these situations and handle them correctly (Box 3-2).

Collections

Several laws have been enacted to provide protection against unscrupulous collection practices that harm individuals. The medical assistant needs to be familiar with these laws since he or she is responsible for following the administrative procedures these laws require. The laws relating to the collection process are discussed in Table 3-2.

Professional Liability

Lawsuits related to health care have greatly increased during the past decade and the average liability award granted to plaintiffs in medical malpractice cases is now over one million dollars. Professional liability is determined by the federal, state, and local laws governing the patient/physician relationship and relates to the standard of care, legal contracts, and informed consent. An important issue in the question of liability is the physician/employee relationship. Some factors impacting on this relationship are discussed here. They include respondeat superior, standard of care, malpractice, res ipsa loquitur, statute of limitations, Good Samaritan laws, and defamation of character.

Respondeat Superior

Physician/employers are especially concerned that their employees have a complete understanding of the law. The Latin term respondeat superior literally means, "Let the master answer." What this means to your employer, the physician, is that he or she is liable for the negligent actions of anyone working for him or her. In some cases and in some states, both the physician and the employee may be liable.

In effect, under respondeat superior, the physician delegates certain duties to you and if you perform them incorrectly, then the ultimate liability rests with the physician/employer. However, medical assistants and other health care workers can also be named in malpractice suits.

TABLE 3-2 Laws Governing Collection

Law	Description
Equal Credit Opportunity Act of 1975	Prohibits discrimination—unfair treatment—in the granting of credit. This law mandates that women and minorities must be issued credit if they qualify for it, based on the premise that if credit is given to one patient it should be given to all patients that request it.
Fair Debt Collection Practices Act of 1978	Provides a guide for determining what are considered the fair collections practices for creditors.
Fair Credit Reporting Act of 1971	Provides guidelines for collecting an individual's credit information. Individuals are able to learn what credit information is available about them. Consumers can correct and update this credit information.
Notice on "Use of Telephone for Debt Collection" from the Federal Communications Commission	Provides guidelines for the specific times that credit collection phone calls can be made. It prohibits using the telephone for harassment and threats. Telephone calls for the purposes of collections must be made between the hours of 8 A.M. and 9 P.M.
Truth in Lending Act of 1969	Requires a full, written disclosure concerning the payment of any fee that will be collected in more than 4 installments. Also referred to as Regulation Z of the Consumer Protection Act.

For example, if you are authorized by your employer to draw a sample of blood from a patient and you inadvertently enter a nerve causing permanent damage to the patient's arm, then you may also be liable for that patient's injury. Since the physician's medical license is in jeopardy when errors are made, it is vital that you understand the law.

Standard of Care

While a physician is under no obligation to treat everyone, once he or she does accept a patient for treatment, the physician has then entered into the physician/patient relationship and must provide a certain standard of care. This standard of care asserts that the physician must then provide the *same* knowledge, care, and skill that a similarly trained physician would provide under the same circumstances in the same locality. The law requires only reasonable, ordinary care and skill.

The physician is expected to perform the same acts that a "reasonable and prudent" physician would. This standard also states that a physician will not perform any acts that a "reasonable and prudent" physician would not. Physicians are expected to exhaust all the resources available to them when they are treating a patient. This would include:

- Taking a thorough medical history.
- Giving a complete physical examination.

- Conducting the necessary laboratory tests and x-rays.

Physicians are not expected to expose their patients to undue risk. If the physician violates this standard of care, he or she is liable for negligence.

The medical assistant must also adhere to a standard of care. This standard will depend on training, skills, experience, education, and the responsibility assigned. Employees going outside of their competency risk being sued for negligence. Preparing for Externship advises reviewing applicable laws in your state and region.

Preparing for
Externship

Be sure that you have reviewed the local laws regarding the standards of care for medical assistants in your state. If you happen to move to, or work in another state, then be sure, prior to beginning working in the new state, that you are aware of applicable laws so that you can follow the regulations.

Malpractice

Professional misconduct or demonstration of an unreasonable lack of skill with the result of injury, loss, or damage to the patient is considered malpractice. It means the physician was negligent. Every mistake or error, however, is not considered malpractice. Therefore, when a treatment or diagnosis does not turn out well, the physician is not necessarily liable. The physician/employer and all staff must each act within the "standard of care" appropriate for the particular practice of medicine. All health care providers are held to this same standard.

Malpractice Insurance

In most cases, employers carry insurance to cover acts of their employees during the course of carrying out their duties. This is general liability coverage. Employees should request to see your employer's "certificate of insurance" to determine policy coverage.

Some physicians carry a rider, or addition, to their professional liability or malpractice policy to cover any negligence on the part of their clinical assistants. An example of this is the patient who slips and falls while getting off the examination table, even though you had warned the patient to sit up slowly and use the foot stool. If this type of fall were to result in a broken bone, the insurance company might settle the case even though negligence was not found.

The time taken away from the job to hire and meet with a lawyer, in order to discuss a case prior to appearing in court, as well as the court appearance itself, could become quite costly. So, if you are not covered by your employer's malpractice policy, then you must purchase your own professional liability coverage from an insurance carrier who specializes in this type of coverage.

Res Ipsa Loquitur

The doctrine of res ipsa loquitur, which means "the thing speaks for itself," applies to the law of negligence. This doctrine tells us that the breach (neglect) of duty is so obvious that it does not need further explanation or "it speaks for itself." For instance, leaving a sponge in the patient during abdominal surgery, dropping a surgical instrument causing injury to the patient, and operating on the wrong body part are all examples of res ipsa loquitur. None of these examples would have occurred without the negligence of someone involved in the procedure.

Statute of Limitations

The statute of limitations refers to the period of time during which a patient has to file a lawsuit. The court will not hear a case that is filed after the time limit has run out. This varies from state to state. In some states, the time period is one or two years.

The statute of limitations does not always start "running" when the treatment is administered. It may begin when the problem is discovered, which may be some time after the actual treatment. This is known as *the rule of discovery*. For instance, there is a case in which a physician accidentally left a surgical sponge in a patient's body during an abdominal operation. After sixteen years of abdominal discomfort, the patient required more surgery but the physician who had performed the original operation had died. So, another surgeon, who found the sponge and removed it, performed the second surgery. The patient then sued the estate of the original surgeon for malpractice and won because the statute of limitations, which was two years in that state, started running when the sponge was discovered.

The reverse of a statute "running" is a situation in which the statute is prevented from coming into play. This occurs when the injury is to a minor child. Generally, the court will appoint a guardian ad litem, an adult who will act in the court on behalf of the child. However, the child does not have to sue through a guardian ad litem as a minor, but may wait until he or she reaches adulthood. In such a case, an obstetrician and his or her assistants can be sued twenty-one years and nine months (plus the statute of limitations period in that state) after a birth injury has occurred.

Good Samaritan Laws

Good Samaritan laws are state laws that help to protect a health care professional from liability while giving emergency care to an accident victim. Such laws are in effect in all states to encourage physicians and other health care professionals to offer aid.

No one is required to provide aid in the event of an emergency, except in the state of Vermont (Figure 3-1). Someone responding in an emergency situation is only required to act within the limits of his or her skill and training. A medical assistant would not be expected, nor advised, to perform emergency treatment that is within the area practiced by physicians and nurses.

Defamation of Character

Defamation of character is a scandalous statement about someone that can injure the person's reputation. Defamation can result even when the statement is true.

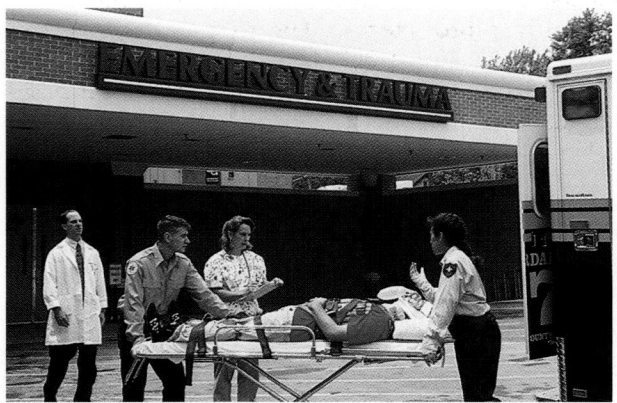

FIGURE 3-1 An accident victim gets emergency care.

Slander occurs when the defaming statement is spoken. *Libel* refers to written defamation.

As a medical assistant, you will have access to privileged information about patients that may seem harmless, but, in reality, the information could be very damaging to their reputations. For instance, a patient who has a test for an infectious disease, such as hepatitis or AIDS, may not wish an employer to know the test took place even if the test result is negative. If you call the patient's place of employment and leave a message regarding a test result of this nature, the action could be considered a breach of confidentiality and defamation.

The fact that a physician saw a patient must be kept confidential. The medical assistant should not fax information or leave messages on answering machines unless specifically instructed to do so in writing by the patient. Such instructions should be documented.

In order to protect yourself and avoid involvement in lawsuits, you must practice your skills with care, be concerned about maintaining good public relations with patients and other staff members, and understand the law.

Patient/Physician Relationship

Both physician and patient must agree to form a relationship if there is to be a contract for service and treatment. In order to receive proper treatment, the patient must confide truthfully in the physician. Failure to state all the facts may result in serious consequences for the patient. The physician is not liable if the patient has withheld critical information. Patients can expect to be treated as long as necessary.

Physician Rights

Physicians have the right to select the patients they wish to treat. They also have the right to refuse service to patients. From an ethical standpoint, most physicians do treat patients who need their skills. This is particularly true in cases of emergency.

Physicians may also state the type of services they will provide, the hours their offices will be open, and where they are located. The physician has the right to expect payment for treatment given.

Physicians have a right to take vacations and time off from their practices. Care must be taken to inform patients if their physician will be unavailable. In most cases, another physician will cover or take care of a colleague's patients while he or she is away.

Patient Rights

The patient has the right to approve or give consent or permission for all treatment. In giving consent for treatment, the patient reasonably expects that his or her physician will use the appropriate "standard of care" in providing care and treatment. That is, that the physician will use the same skill that is used by other physicians in treating patients with the same ailments. Patients also expect that all information and records about their cases will be kept confidential by the physician and staff. The patient's right to privacy prohibits the presence of unauthorized persons during physical examinations or treatments.

In addition to these rights, the patient also has certain obligations. For example, the patient is expected to follow the instructions given by the physician. And finally, the patient is expected to pay the physician for medical services.

Informed Consent

The patient can expect to receive information concerning the advantages and potential risks of all treatments. Informed consent means that the patient is informed about the possible consequences of both having and not having certain procedures and treatment. The physician must carefully explain that in some cases, the treatment may even make the patient's condition worse.

The Doctrine of Informed Consent (Figure 3-2) includes the following:

- Explanation of advantages and risks to the treatment.
- Alternatives available to the patient.
- Potential outcomes to the treatment.
- What might occur if there is no treatment.
- The use of understandable language.

Touching someone without the person's consent is referred to as battery. Since consent means to give permission or approval for something, for example, when a patient is seen for a routine examination for medical treatment, there is implied consent that the physician will touch the person during the examination. Therefore, the "touching" required for the examination would not be considered a crime of battery.

It is very difficult to "fully" inform a patient about all the things that can go wrong with a treatment. In an emergency situation in which the patient is not able to understand the explanation, nor sign a consent form, a physician is protected by law to provide care. The process of obtaining consent cannot be delegated by the physician to someone else, except in emergency situations (Figure 3-3).

Does the signed informed consent protect the physician and staff? If after the physician has carefully explained the treatment, the patient acknowledges understanding the explanation and risks involved and signs the consent form, then, generally speaking, there is some protection from lawsuits. However, patients have sued and won cases in which they were presented the risks of a procedure, signed the form, and then proceeded to sue the physician when the treatment failed.

MEMORIAL HEALTH

COMPLETE ORIGINAL IN INK FOR HOSPITAL CHART
PATIENT MUST BE AWAKE, ALERT AND ORIENTED WHEN SIGNING
DATE: _____ TIME: _____ ☐ AM ☐ PM

I AUTHORIZE THE PERFORMANCE UPON _____
OF THE FOLLOWING OPERATION (state nature and extent): _____
_____
_____

TO BE PERFORMED UNDER THE DIRECTION OF DR. _____

1. I HAVE BEEN ADVISED THAT THERE IS A FAVORABLE LIKELIHOOD OF SUCCESS, BUT I UNDERSTAND THAT A COMPLETELY SUCCESSFUL OUTCOME MAY NOT BE ACHIEVABLE, AND THERE ARE NO GUARANTEES REGARDING THE OUTCOME. I ALSO UNDERSTAND THAT CERTAIN ADVERSE EVENTS COULD OCCUR AS A RESULT OF THE PERFORMANCE OF THE PROCEDURE OR TREATMENT, INCLUDING PAIN, INFECTION, LACERATION OR PUNCTURE OF INTERNAL ORGANS, BLEEDING, NERVE DAMAGE OR EVEN IN RARE CASES, DEATH. I UNDERSTAND THAT HOSPITALIZATION OR OTHER INSTITUTIONAL CARE, HOME CARE OR CARE BY HEALTH PROFESSIONALS MAY BE NEEDED FOLLOWING THE PROCEDURE OR TREATMENT, RELATED TO FULL RECOVERY, RECUPERATION OR CONVALESCENCE. I UNDERSTAND THE ALTERNATIVES TO THIS PROCEDURE, INCLUDING MY RIGHT TO REFUSE TO CONSENT TO IT, AND I NEVERTHELESS HAVE DECIDED TO CONSENT TO PERFORMANCE OF THE PROCEDURE OR TREATMENT.

2. I CONSENT TO THE PERFORMANCE OF OPERATIONS AND PROCEDURES IN ADDITION TO OR DIFFERENT FROM THOSE NOW CONTEMPLATED, WHETHER OR NOT ARISING FROM PRESENTLY UNFORESEEN CONDITIONS WHICH THE ABOVE NAMED DOCTOR OR HIS/HER ASSOCIATES OR ASSISTANTS MAY CONSIDER NECESSARY OR ADVISABLE IN THE COURSE OF THE OPERATION.

3. I CONSENT TO THE DISPOSAL BY HOSPITAL AUTHORITIES OF ANY TISSUES OR PARTS WHICH MAY BE REMOVED.

4. THE NATURE AND PURPOSE OF THE OPERATION/PROCEDURE, POSSIBLE ALTERNATIVE METHODS OF TREATMENT, THE RISK AND BENEFITS INVOLVED, AND THE COURSE OF RECUPERATION HAVE BEEN FULLY EXPLAINED TO ME. NO GUARANTEE OR ASSURANCE HAS BEEN GIVEN BY ANYONE AS TO THE RESULTS THAT MAY BE OBTAINED.

5. I UNDERSTAND AND AGREE WITH THE ABOVE INFORMATION. I HAVE NO QUESTIONS WHICH HAVE NOT BEEN ANSWERED TO MY FULL SATISFACTION. I UNDERSTAND THAT I HAVE THE RIGHT TO ASK FOR FURTHER INFORMATION BEFORE SIGNING THIS CONSENT.

I have crossed out any paragraph above which does not apply or to which I do not give consent.

PATIENT SIGNATURE: _____   WITNESS SIGNATURE: _____
(OR PARENT OR GUARDIAN IF PATIENT IS UNDER 18 YEARS OF AGE)   *(OF PATIENT, PARENT OR GUARDIAN SIGNATURE)*

RELATIONSHIP: _____   WITNESS SIGNATURE: _____
☐ **TELEPHONE CONSENT** *(2ND WITNESS NEEDED FOR TELEPHONE CONSENT)*

FIGURE 3-2   Sample of an informed consent document to perform an operation, sedation, anesthetics, and other medical services.

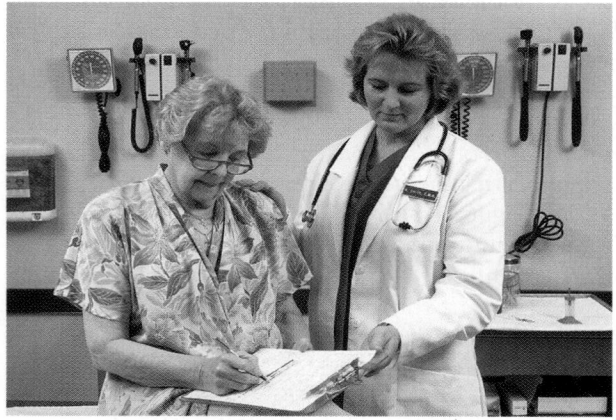

FIGURE 3-3   The patient's signature on the informed consent form indicates that the patient understands the limits and risks involved in the treatment or surgical procedure as explained by the physician.

Outpatient surgical forms or procedure forms used in clinic settings may be shorter in content. There are exceptions to the informed consent doctrine that are unique to each state. Some of the more general exceptions follow.

- A physician does not have to inform a patient about risks that are commonly known. For example, a patient could choke swallowing a pill.

- If the physician feels the disclosure of risks may be detrimental to the patient, then he or she is not responsible for disclosing them. This might occur if a patient has a severe heart condition that may be worsened by an announcement of risks.

- If the patient requests the physician not to disclose the risks, then the physician is not responsible for failing to do so.

Cultural Considerations

Patients have the right to refuse treatment. Cultural Considerations looks at accommodating different cultural groups. Some members of religious groups, such as Jehovah's Witnesses and Christian Scientists, do not wish to receive blood transfusions or certain types of medical treatment. The adults would not receive the treatment against their wishes. In the case of a minor child, the court may appoint a guardian who can then give consent for the procedure.

Rights of Minors

A minor is considered a person who has not reached the age of majority, which varies from state to state, but usually, is 18. In most states, minors are unable to give consent for treatment. Exceptions are special cases involving pregnancy, request for birth control information, abortion, testing and treatment for sexually transmitted diseases, problems with substance abuse, and a need for psychiatric care. There are two types of minors who can give consent for treatment:

- Mature minors
- Emancipated minors

A mature minor is a young person, generally under the age of 18, who possesses a maturity to understand the nature and consequences of the treatment in spite of his or her young age. Emancipated minors actually have the same legal capacity as an adult under any of the following five conditions:

- They live on their own.
- They are married.
- They are self-supporting.
- They are in the armed forces.
- Any combination of the above conditions.

Since not all states recognize the categories of mature and emancipated minors, it is wise to handle consent on a case-by-case basis. Following are some legal implications to consider when treating a minor.

- Right to confidentiality—a 16-year old who is seeking birth control information has a right to have her records remain confidential.
- Financial responsibility—the 16-year old girl seeking birth control information may not be able to pay for the office visit. Contacting her parents for payment may breach confidentiality.
- Minor's legal guardian—this is sometimes difficult to determine if the child lives with the mother but the father is financially responsible for care and treatment.

Patient Self-Determination Act

Several documents executed by the patient provide protection for the patient and physician. Such documents also provide direction for the patient's caregiver or proxy to make health-care-related decisions according to the patient's wishes at a point in time when the patient is unable to do so. These documents include the following:

Living Will

The living will allows patients to request that life-sustaining treatments and nutritional support not be used to prolong their life. This document gives patients the legal right to direct the type of care they wish to receive when their death is imminent. The document provides protection for physicians and hospitals when they follow the patient's wishes. This process is often discussed in the office with patients when they are capable of making the decision. Other family members or significant others can also be part of the discussion and decision. One copy of the living will should be kept with the patient's record.

Durable Power of Attorney

The durable power of attorney, when signed by the patient, allows an agent or representative to act on behalf of the patient. If the durable power of attorney is for health care only, then the agent may only make health-care-related decisions on behalf of the patient. The agent may be a spouse, grown child, friend, or, in some cases, an attorney.

The durable power of attorney (DPOA) is a safeguard that someone will be able to act on the patient's behalf if he or she becomes physically or mentally incapacitated. This document is in effect until the patient cancels it. A copy of the durable power of attorney should be kept with the patient's record. The person who is the patient's DPOA acts on behalf of the patient until the patient is again capable of making his or her own decisions.

Uniform Anatomical Gift Act

The Uniform Anatomical Gift Act allows persons 18 years or older and of sound mind to make a gift of any or all parts of their body for purposes of organ transplantation or medical research. One of the regulations of the act is that a physician who is not involved in the transplant will determine the time of death. No money is allowed to change hands for organ donations.

The donor will carry a card that has been signed in the presence of two witnesses. In some states, the back of the driver's license has a space to indicate the desire to be an organ donor with space for a signature.

In some cases, the family will make the decision for the donor if this was not done while the donor was alive. It is generally agreed that if a member of the family opposes the donation of organs, then the physician and hospital do not insist upon it.

Documentation

Carefully document all calls, visits, treatments, no-shows, appointment cancellations, medications, prescription refills, vital signs, and other pertinent information in the patient's chart. If an action is not recorded on the medical chart, then it is considered by most courts not to have been performed.

Use of Records in Litigation

Litigation refers to a lawsuit tried in court. For this purpose, a court of law may subpoena a medical record. When this is done, only the parts of the record that are requested should be copied and sent to the requesting attorney. Unless the original record is subpoenaed, a certified photocopy may be sent. If the original record is subpoenaed, then make a copy and return the copy to the locked file. A receipt for the subpoenaed record should then be placed in the patient's file. The patient should also be notified that his or her record has been subpoenaed. Both the subpoenaed record and the notification to the patient should be sent by certified mail.

Be especially careful when using a fax transmission for medical records. The person receiving the fax should assure you that the machine is located in a restricted area. Confidential material is not generally sent over a fax transmission. Of course, a fax is not usable when an original record is requested. A disclaimer should be placed on the fax cover sheet explaining that the records are confidential.

Should you or your employing physician receive a *subpoena duces tecum*, meaning an order to appear in court and to bring certain records or other materials to a trial or deposition, remember only the records specifically stated in the subpoena are required.

Court Testimony

Not everyone who has information relating to a case will be called into court to testify. An attorney may interrogate, or ask questions, of a witness. Another means of obtaining information from a witness to be used during a court case is to submit a deposition. In this case, a written statement is taken of oral testimony given in front of a court officer. The person who gives the oral testimony and then signs a deposition does not have to actually appear in court. An attorney submits the deposition during the court case. Arraignment occurs when a defendant is called before the court to answer a charge.

An expert witness is a person called upon to testify in court regarding what standard of care for a patient is in a similar community. An expert witness in a medical malpractice suit is generally a physician.

In the event that you are called upon to appear in court, you will want to be as comfortable as you can when giving testimony. It will be well to remember a few pointers.

- *Be professional.* You will be judged by your appearance and behavior as well as by what you say. Your attorney can advise you on this more fully.
- *Remain calm, dignified, and serious at all times.* The opposing attorney may try to make you nervous.
- *Do not answer questions you do not understand.* Simply ask the attorney to repeat the question or state, "I don't know."
- *Just present the facts surrounding the case.* Do not give any information for what is not asked. Do not insert your opinion. "The patient was shouting" is stating a fact. Stating, "He was angry," is your opinion.
- *Do not memorize your testimony ahead of time.* You will generally be allowed to take some notes with you to refresh your memory concerning dates.
- *Always tell the truth.*

Giving testimony in court is a crucial and sensitive matter. It is best to consult an attorney if you have any questions.

Public Duties of Physicians

There are responsibilities the physician has to the public. Some of these duties include reports of births, still-births and deaths, communicable illnesses or diseases, drug abuse, certain injuries such as rape, abuse of children, spouses, and older adults, gunshot and knife wounds, and animal bites.

Exact reporting requirements vary from state to state, so the medical assistant should be familiar with the requirements of his or her state. Office personnel, including the medical assistant, carry out many of the duties that relate to these responsibilities (Table 3-3).

Drug Regulations

The Food and Drug Administration (FDA) is the agency within the federal government that has jurisdiction over testing and approving drugs for public use. The Drug Enforcement Administration (DEA), a branch of the Justice Department, regulates the sale and use of schedule drugs.

TABLE 3-3 **Public Duties of the Physician**

Duty	Description
Births	Issuing of a legal certificate, which will be maintained during a person's life as proof of age. Many benefits and documents, including social security, passport, and driver's license, depend on having a valid birth certificate.
Deaths	Physicians sign a certificate indicating the cause of a natural death. Check with your state public health department to determine specific requirements. For example, in the case of a stillbirth before the 20th week of gestation, you will have to determine if both a birth and death certificate are required. A coroner or health official will have to sign a certificate in the following cases: ■ No physician present at the time of death ■ Violent death, unlawful death ■ Death as a result of criminal action ■ Death from an undetermined cause
Reportable communicable diseases	Physicians must report all diseases that can be transmitted from one person to another and are considered a general threat to the public. The list of reportable diseases differs from state to state. The report can be either by mail or phone. The following childhood vaccines and toxoids are required by law (The National Childhood Vaccine Injury Act of 1986): ■ Diphtheria, tetanus toxoids, pertussis vaccine (DTP) ■ Pertussis vaccine (whooping cough) ■ Measles, mumps, rubella (MMR) ■ Poliovirus vaccine, live ■ Poliovirus vaccine, inactivated ■ Hepatitis B vaccine ■ Tuberculosis test
Reportable injuries	Certain injuries are reportable according to state requirements. These injuries include gun or knife wounds, rape and battered persons injuries, and spousal, child, and elder abuse.
Child abuse	Questionable injuries of children, including bruises, fractured bones, and burns, must be reported. Signs of neglect, such as malnutrition, poor growth, and lack of hygiene, are reportable in some states.
Elder abuse	Physical abuse, neglect, and abandonment of older adults is reportable in most states. The reporting agency varies by state but generally includes social service agencies.
Drug abuse	Abuse of prescription drugs is reportable according to the law. Such abuse can be difficult to determine since the abuser may seek prescriptions for the same drug from several different physicians. A physician will want to see a patient before prescribing a medication.

Both the physician and the medical assistant are responsible for understanding patient education relating to legal issues. The medical assistant can assist the physician by providing good patient care and avoiding litigation by following practical recommendations. Patients must understand all papers they sign, including permission for treatment, insurance payments, and other billing materials. You may have to read and explain this material to patients if you have any doubts about their comprehension of the written materials.

The Controlled Substances Act of 1970 requires physicians to handle controlled drugs that are highly addictive in very specific ways. The physician who dispenses, purchases, administers, prescribes, or handles drugs is required to register with the Drug Enforcement Administration. The physician then receives a DEA registration number that must appear on all prescriptions for controlled substances. A DEA number is required for every location in which controlled drugs are stored. If a physician practices in two states, then two DEA numbers must be obtained. DEA registration numbers are generally printed on physician's prescription blanks. See Chapter 48 for a sample prescription form.

Controlled drugs must be kept in a locked or even double-locked cabinet and any theft must be immediately reported to both the regional DEA office and the local police. In addition, the physician's black bag and prescription blanks should always be stored in a secure locked location.

Records must be kept to document the administering and dispensing of controlled drugs. In addition, federal regulations require a written inventory in triplicate of drug supplies, based on daily use, be made every two years and kept for two more years.

Controlled drugs are classified into five schedules, or categories that indicate levels of potential abuse. Schedule I drugs have the highest potential for addiction and abuse while Schedule V drugs have the least. In Chapter 48, a Schedule for Controlled Substances shows the meaning of each classification and examples of drugs for each category.

The physician's medical assistant may not dispense controlled substances; however, he or she must be knowledgeable about the regulations governing the documentation and control of drugs. Only licensed personnel are permitted to dispense drugs. Be sure to report to the physician any unusual patient behavior indicating addictive drug use.

Role of the Medical Assistant

The role of the medical assistant in preventing liability suits is of paramount importance to both you and your employer. Remember that in many cases, you are the only one in the office who will hear a patient's complaint. Your ability to handle the complaint professionally and efficiently may eliminate a potential lawsuit for the physician. Patient Education discusses how providing good patient care can help to prevent litigation.

Acting under a code of ethics that compels you to safeguard any patient whose care and safety are affected by the negligent action of someone else, you must follow the chain of command, the authority structure within your office, and report to your immediate supervisor any negligent action you observe. It goes without saying that if you accidentally make an error, you will bring this to your supervisor's attention so that it can be corrected immediately (Professionalism).

You can help your employer and protect yourself, by remembering the recommendations and cautions that follow. These recommendations and cautions are clustered around major areas of responsibility you address daily in your role as a medical assistant.

Professionalism

Telling the truth is one of the most important parts of being a medical professional. Every human will make mistakes; it is part of being human. However, the most important thing any professional can do is admit that he or she made a mistake and seek to correct the mistake. However, do not offer extra information to the patient. Just state that there is a correction to be made. Be sure to speak with the supervising physician, and document clearly in the chart the mistake that was made and how it was corrected. Honesty goes a very long way in preventing litigation and providing good, quality care to all patients.

Confidentiality/Privacy

- Never make any statements about your employing physician that could be interpreted as an admission of fault. On the other hand, as a medical assistant, you cannot remain silent if you are aware that your employing physician is doing something illegal. You can be held liable for remaining silent.

- Do not participate in negative or critical discussions of the physician(s) or other practitioners in your office with your patients. Do not comment on a patient's negative criticism of a current or former physician.

- Never discuss anything about the patient outside of the office.

- Make sure that a female medical assistant is present when the physician (male or female) examines a female patient.

- Treat all patients with dignity and respect.

Office Management

- Treat all patients with the same courtesy and dignity you would expect to receive. Log and return telephone calls promptly. Explain any delays to patients who are waiting to see the physician. Offer to set up another appointment if the delay will be very long.

- Never make promises regarding what the physician can do for the patient.

- Carefully explain all fees and responsibilities for bills to the patient, relating any concerns the patient may have to the physician.

- Relay any dissatisfied patient's comments to the physician.

- If the physician will be out of town or absent from the office, post these dates. Include this announcement in the monthly billing envelopes. Also provide the name and telephone number of the physician available for patients who need care when their own physician is absent.

- If a physician is withdrawing from a case, then a certified letter must be sent to the patient declaring this. Send the letter certified mail with return receipt requested and keep a copy of the letter and receipt with the patient's record. The physician can be brought up on charges of abandonment if there is no documentation or evidence that there was a formal withdrawal.

Documentation

- Carefully sign or initial every note. Remember: medical documents are considered legal documents and may be used in a court of law.

- If the patient did not keep an appointment, be sure to document the fact as a no-show. Document canceled appointments and follow-up to determine why the patient missed the appointment.

- Document when a patient is referred to another physician and follow up to make sure the patient did see the referral physician.

- Document all patient contacts, including telephone prescription refills and tests and procedures that have been ordered. Call all patients the day after surgery to check on their progress. Document this telephone call.

- Record all care and treatment given as soon as possible after the patient's visit. This will keep patient records current and ensure appropriate follow-up treatment if it is required.

- Be sure the physician sees and initials all diagnostic reports in a timely fashion before they are filed.

- Provide all instructions to patients in writing.

Drug Regulations

- A medical assistant may administer medication only under the direct supervision of a physician. Follow the Controlled Substances Act by careful procedure and documentation. This may vary from state to state.

- Secure the supply of prescription pads from theft at all times.

- When preparing medications for administration, check the medication three times. Remember the "three befores." Check the medication **before removing it from the shelf**; check the name and dosage **again before preparing the dosage**; and check the label again **before returning the medication** to the shelf.

Certification and Licensing

- Have a thorough understanding of the limits of certification and standards of care for the medical assisting profession. Never perform any procedure for which you are not trained or qualified.

- Do not diagnose or prescribe over the telephone. This applies to all drugs even those that can be obtained over the counter. You could be charged with practicing medicine without a license.

- Do not call yourself a "nurse" or allow anyone else to refer to you as the nurse. You must be held to your own standard of care and not that of a nurse.

- Participate in continuing education and training programs to maintain your skill levels.

Informed Consent

- The physician must thoroughly explain all procedures to the patient. The medical assistant is responsible for making sure there is a signed consent form. Never have the patient sign a document that he or she does not understand.

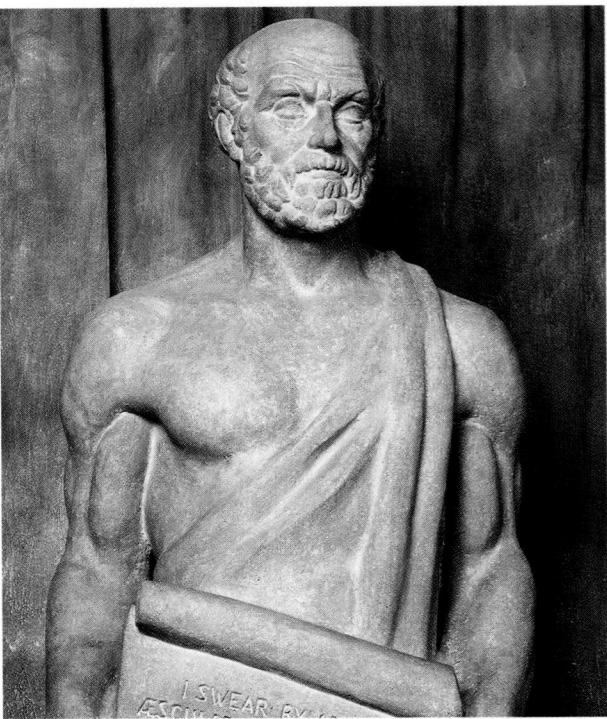
FIGURE 3-4 An artist's interpretation of Hippocrates.

- Obtain a parent or guardian's signature before any procedure is performed on a minor. The only exception is in a case of emergency, when the parent or guardian cannot be reached. File the signed consent form immediately.

Safety
- Maintain a safe environment in the office or work site for the patients and staff. Handle requests for maintenance repairs. Report any safety

hazards at once. If you knowingly overlook a hazard that a "reasonable person" would report and eliminate, you can be guilty of negligence.

- Carefully check and document medical waste disposal. Be concerned about the safety of maintenance personnel who must handle the waste containers. Always dispose of syringes and needles correctly in designated hazardous waste containers.

- Maintain and document careful quality checks on laboratory testing equipment.

Code of Ethics

Ethics is the branch of philosophy relating to morals or moral principles. It involves the examination of human character and conduct, the distinction between right and wrong, and a person's moral duty and obligations to the community. Ethics has been part of the medical profession since the early beginning of the profession.

The earliest code of ethics, or principles to govern conduct for those in medicine, dates back to around 1800 BC, to the Code of Hammurabi. In 400 BC, Hippocrates, a Greek physician referred to as the "father of medicine," wrote a statement of principles for his medical students to follow (Figure 3-4). This statement of principles is known as the Hippocratic oath, and is still important today. This oath reminds medical students of the importance of their profession, the need to teach others, and the obligation they have to act in such a way as to never knowingly harm a patient or divulge a confidence. The Hippocratic oath is still recited at medical school graduation ceremonies, and has been for centuries, as it carries an important ethical message for physicians. Modern codes of ethics have been developed as medical science has continued to advance.

Medical Ethics

Medical ethics refers to the moral conduct of people in medical professions. This moral conduct of medical professionals is governed by the high principles and standards that these professionals set for themselves and willingly choose to follow through personal dedication. Every medical profession has a "Code of Ethics" that sets moral standards that are expected to be adhered to by the members of that profession (Legal and Ethical Issues).

Ethical Standards and Behavior

Ethical standards are generally more severe than those standards that are required by law. In many cases, ethical standards are more demanding than the law. A violation of an ethical standard could mean the loss of the physician's reputation.

Ethical behavior, according to the American Medical Association (AMA), refers to moral principles or practices, the customs of the medical profession, and matters of medical policy. Unethical behavior would be any actions that did not follow these ethical standards. When a physician is accused of unethical behavior or conduct in violation of these standards, he or she can be issued a warning or censure (criticism) by the AMA. The AMA Board of Examiners may recommend the expulsion or suspension of a physician from membership in the association. Expulsion, or being put out of the association, is a severe penalty for physicians since it limits the physician's ability to practice medicine. Not all physicians are members of the AMA, and the AMA does not have authority to bring legal action against nonmembers for unethical conduct. However, the State Medical Board that issued the physician his or her license may limit the physician's practice or revoke the license altogether for ethical misconduct. If it is alleged that a physician has committed a criminal act, the medical society is required to report it to the state board or governmental agency. Allege means assert or declare without proof. Violation of the law, which is followed by a conviction for the crime, may result in a fine, imprisonment, or both. The State Medical Board can then revoke the physician's license. Revocation means that the physician no longer has a license to practice medicine.

AMA Principles of Medical Ethics

In the United States, the AMA has taken a leadership role in setting standards for the ethical behavior of physicians. The AMA was organized in New York City in 1846 and the first Code of Ethics was formed shortly after that in 1847. Figure 3-5 shows a patient with a physician being assisted by a medical assistant.

The AMA Principles of Medical Ethics discusses human dignity, honesty, responsibility to society, confidentiality, the need for continued study, freedom of choice, and a responsibility of the physician to improve the community. Box 3-3 presents this statement of principles in its entirety.

Medical Assistant's Princples of Medical Ethics

Medical assistants may not be involved with the life and death ethical decisions that face the physician; however, they do face many dilemmas regarding right or wrong behavior on an almost daily basis. Examples include when a coworker violates patient confidentiality, uses foul language in front of a client, or how the team treats a patient whose body may smell of urine or alcohol. Ethical issues involve doing the right thing at the right time.

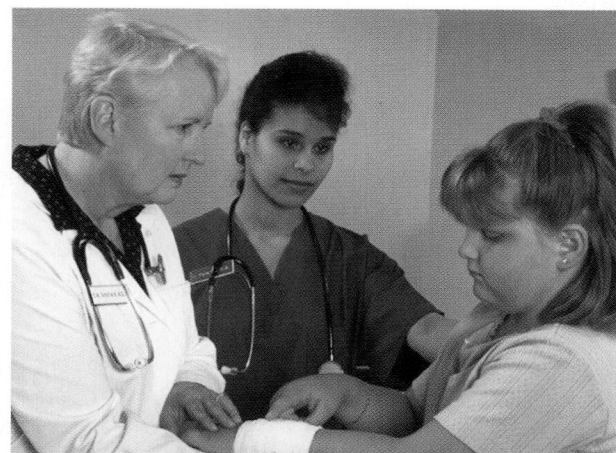

FIGURE 3-5 Medical assistant helps the physician with a patient.

Code of Ethics of the AAMA

The Code of Ethics of the American Association of Medical Assistants (AAMA) is a standard that medical assistants are expected to follow. The Code, which describes ethical and moral conduct for the medical assistant, is similar to the AMA's Principles of Medical Ethics. Box 3-4 lists the code of ethics of the AAMA. Medical assistants assume a position of trust and must try to live up to the standards of the profession as stated in the Code.

Creed of the AAMA

The Creed of the American Association of Medical Assistants can be best followed by the medical assistant who spends time reading about and discussing ethical problems, such as transplants, artificial insemination, the right to die with dignity, and abortion. To be true to this Creed, the medical assistant must know about the ethical issues the patient faces and be committed to treat the patient with respectful care regardless of the patient's religious beliefs or cultural practices.

Creed of the American Association of Medical Assistants:

I believe in the principles and purposes of the profession of medical assisting.

I endeavor to be more effective.

I aspire to render greater service.

I protect the confidence entrusted to me.

I am dedicated to the care and well-being of all people.

I am loyal to my employer.

I am true to the ethics of my profession.

I am strengthened by compassion, courage, and faith.

Copyright by the American Association of Medical Assistants, Inc. Reprinted by permission.

Medical Assistant's Standard of Care

As a medical assistant, you must remember that your actions can have legal consequences for the physician who employs you. You are not held to the same standard of care as a physician due to differing credentials, licensure, and education. However, you will carry out your duties under the direction of a physician and, therefore, you must use the same approved methods that a physician would use. For example, you must have the same quality standard, as any physician would use when taking an electrocardiogram, drawing blood, and collecting specimens.

A medical assistant is not expected to diagnose medical conditions, interpret electrocardiograms, or prescribe medications since these are all within the area of the physician's standard of care. In fact, a medical assistant must continually use caution and not take on any tasks or duties for which he or she is not trained within the scope of his or her practice.

The actions of medical assistants reflect upon their physician employers. Many duties performed by medical assistants could result in harm to the patient if not done properly. There have been lawsuits in which the physician has been found guilty of negligence due to improper performance of his or her medical assistant.

The Patient's Bill of Rights

The American Hospital Association developed a statement called "The Patient's Bill of Rights," which describes the patient-physician relationship. Medical assistants also follow these guidelines when working with the physician's patients. Box 3-5 states these rights. Most offices have these rights printed for their patients.

BOX 3-4
Code of Ethics of the American Association of Medical Assistants

Preamble

The Code of Ethics of AAMA shall set forth principles of ethical and moral conduct as they relate to the medical profession and the particular practice of medical assisting.

Members of the AAMA dedicated to the conscientious pursuit of their profession, and thus desiring to merit the high regard of the entire medical profession and the respect of the general public which they serve, do hereby pledge themselves to strive always to:

Human Dignity

I. Render service with full respect for the dignity of humanity;

Confidentiality

II. Respect confidential information obtained through employment unless legally authorized or required by responsible performance of duty to divulge such information;

Honor

III. Uphold the honor and high principles of the profession and accept its disciplines;

Continued Study

IV. Seek to continually improve the knowledge and skills of medical assistants for the benefit of patients and professional colleagues;

Responsibility for Improved Community

V. Participate in additional service activities aimed toward improving the health and well-being of the community.

Copyright by the American Association of Medical Assistants, Inc. Reprinted by permission.

Confidentiality

According to the Medical Patients Rights Act, all patients have the right to have their personal privacy respected and their medical records handled with confidentiality. Any information, such as test results, patient histories, and even the fact that the patient is a patient, cannot be told to another person. No information can be given over the telephone without the patient's permission. No patient records can be given to another person or physician without the patient's written permission or unless the court has subpoenaed it. A subpoena is a court order for a person to appear in court or for documents to be presented to the court.

A further set of rules towards maintaining confidentiality is called the Health Insurance Portability and Accountability Act (HIPAA). All medical office employees must undergo HIPAA training during their orientation. HIPAA rules ensure that private patient information remains private. Without written authorization, patient information may not be shared with other entities. HIPAA extends to making sure that computers with confidential patient information cannot be seen or accessed by individuals who are not authorized to see the information. All faxes and e-mails that contain private patient information must have a note stating that the information is confidential, and if the information is accidentally transmitted to someone without clearance to read the information, they must immediately notify the office, and destroy the information.

The medical assistant's treatment and concern for the patient reflects the physician's high standards of care. The human dignity of each patient must be preserved regardless of the patient's socioeconomic background, race, age, nationality, sexual orientation, or gender (Figure 3-6). Any promise or commitment that the medical assistant makes to a patient can be legally binding to his or her physician and employer. This means that the physician can be held responsible for something the staff has said or implied with regard to the physician improving the patient's condition. Keep all matters relating to patients in confidence. If you believe that any health professional is acting in an unethical or unprofessional manner, you should discuss this with your employer or another physician.

Any information that is given to a physician by a patient is considered confidential and it may not be given to an unauthorized person. The physician's medical

The Patient's Bill of Rights

1. The patient has the right to considerate and respectful care.
2. The patient has the right to and is encouraged to obtain from physicians and other direct caregivers relevant, current, understandable information concerning diagnosis, treatment, and prognosis.
3. The patient has the right to make decisions about the plan of care prior to and during the course of treatment and to refuse a recommended treatment or plan of care to the extent permitted by law and hospital policy and to be informed of the consequences of this action.
4. The patient has the right to have an advance directive (such as a living will, health care proxy, or durable power of attorney for health care) concerning treatment or designating a surrogate decision maker with the expectation that the hospital will honor the intent of that directive to the extent permitted by law and hospital policy.
5. The patient has the right to every consideration of privacy.
6. The patient has the right to expect that all communications and records pertaining to his or her care will be treated as confidential by the hospital, except in cases such as suspected abuse and public health hazards when reporting is permitted or required by law.
7. The patient has the right to review the records pertaining to his or her medical care and to have the information explained or interpreted as necessary, except when restricted by law.
8. The patient has the right to expect that, within its capacity and policies, a hospital will make reasonable responses to the request of a patient for appropriate and medically indicated care and service.
9. The patient has the right to ask and be informed of the existence of business relationships among the hospital, educational institutions, other health care providers, or payers that may influence the patient's treatment or care.
10. The patient has the right to consent to or decline to participate in proposed research studies or human experimentation affecting care and treatment or requiring direct patient involvement, and to have those studies fully explained prior to consent.
11. The patient has the right to expect reasonable continuity of care when appropriate and to be informed by physicians and other caregivers of available and realistic patient care options when hospital care is no longer appropriate.
12. The patient has the right to be informed of hospital policies and practices that relate to patient care, treatment, and responsibilities.

assistant is considered to be an authorized person with access to the patient's file and information. This information may not be divulged without permission of the doctor or patient. The physician must be notified of any information the patient gives the medical assistant, such as the patient is not taking prescribed medications or complying with treatment (Figure 3-7).

Ethical Issues and Personal Choice

In some cases, the medical assistant may have a personal, religious, or ethical reason for wishing not to be involved in particular procedures, such as abortions or artificial insemination. This preference should be stated to the employer prior to employment, allowing for this information to be considered when making a hiring decision. In the event that the situation arises after employment begins, all concerns should be communicated to the employer immediately. It is very important not to judge what the physician is doing since he or she is acting within ethical guidelines. An individual should request to refrain from participating in the procedures in question if he or she has ethical doubts. If the medical assistant's choice to not assist the physician in a specific procedure jeopardizes the health and safety of a patient, or interferes with the physician's ability to do the procedures, it may be necessary to seek other employment.

Scientific Discovery and Ethical Issues

There are still many areas of medical ethics for which there are no conclusive answers. For instance, when should life support be withdrawn; when does a life begin; is euthanasia ever permissible; and should the

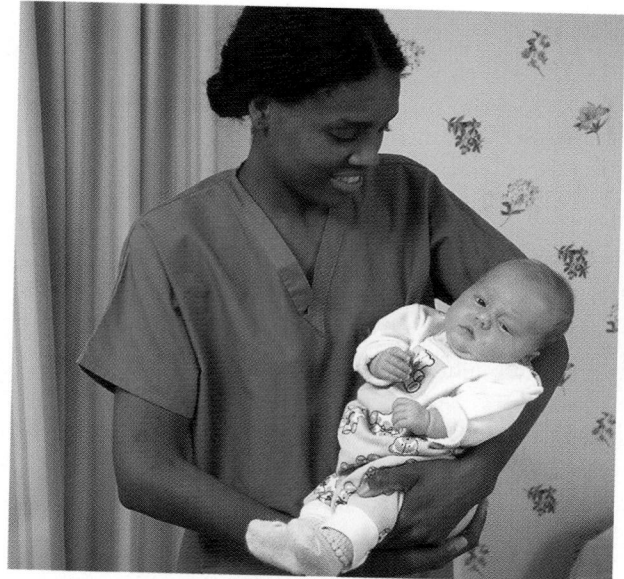

FIGURE 3-6 Patients of all socioeconomic backgrounds should be given equal care.

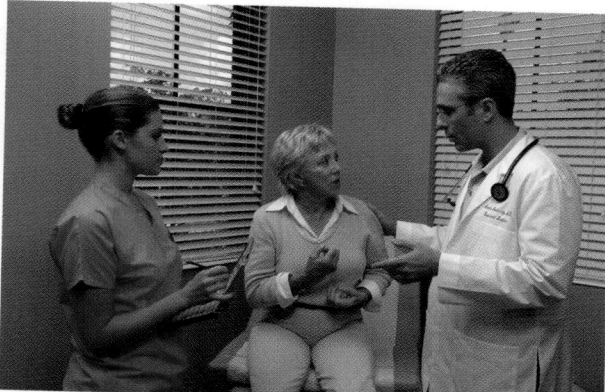

FIGURE 3-7 A medical assistant listening to the patient and physician discussing the patient's care.

unborn baby's life be sacrificed to save the mother? Scientific discoveries present new medical possibilities and choices every day. With these possibilities, there are often more complicated ethical issues to be addressed before choices can be made. The medical assistant has a responsibility to keep current on medical advances and form opinions based on sound medical ethics and practice.

SUMMARY

Medical law is based on the Hippocratic oath. Patients must be treated equally, using the best possible standards of care.

The medical and legal issues governing the medical profession and medical assistants are multifaceted. The medical assistant must be knowledgeable in many areas of the law. Laws governing medicine are different than those governing criminal behavior. Medicine is covered by civil law, often referred to as torts. It is both the physician's and the medical assistant's responsibility to be aware of these guidelines.

Chapter Review

COMPETENCY REVIEW

1. What are the elements of a contract?
2. Why is the Oath of Hippocrates still valid today?
3. Compare the principles of the AAMA or RMA with the AMA Principles of Medical Ethics.
4. What is informed consent?
5. Describe the medical assistant's responsibilities concerning medical ethics.
6. What is the difference between criminal and civil law?
7. List and describe the four Ds of negligence.
8. What are Good Samaritan laws, and how do they apply to you?
9. Why do you need thorough understanding of the law as it impacts your employer's practice?
10. State ten steps that can be taken to help protect the physician and staff from liability.

1. The earliest principles of ethical conduct, established to govern the practice of medicine, were known as
   A. Code of Hammurabi
   B. Code of Ethical Medical Practice
   C. Hippocratic oath
   D. AMA Principles of Medical Ethics
   E. Code of Medical Practice and Conduct

2. Medical ethics, by definition, refers to the
   A. regulations and standards established by the government
   B. moral conduct of medical professionals
   C. standards by which medical practice is deemed illegal
   D. ethical standards that are less severe than those required by law
   E. revocation of a physician's license to practice medicine

3. The Code of Ethics of the AAMA describes all of the following EXCEPT
   A. ethical conduct for the medical assistant
   B. moral conduct for the medical assistant
   C. a commitment to the patients to maintain their dignity and confidentiality
   D. a responsibility to improve the health and well-being of the community
   E. the legal responsibilities of the medical assistant

4. Which of the following falls INSIDE the medical assistant's standard of care?
   A. all medical assisting duties should always be under the direction of the treating physician
   B. the same standard of quality that is applicable to a physician in performing a procedure, for example, an ECG, is applicable to the medical assistant
   C. the medical assistant is allowed to, for example, prescribe over the counter medications
   D. the medical assistant is not responsible for giving physical exams
   E. the medical assistant must take a thorough medical history

5. What are the four types of written laws?
   A. misdemeanor, felony, civil, tort
   B. felony, tort, negligence, contract
   C. civil, tort, multi-national, governmental
   D. criminal, civil, tort, military
   E. civil, criminal, international, military

6. Performing surgery on a patient without the proper informed consent of the patient is an example of
   A. intentional tort
   B. abandonment
   C. breach of contract
   D. contribution negligence
   E. res ipsa loquitur

7. What might a physician be guilty of when, for example, a treatment that was below an acceptable standard of care was the direct cause of an injury?
   A. negligence
   B. malpractice
   C. abandonment
   D. A and B
   E. respondent superior

8. All actions must be carefully documented in a patient's medical chart. This would include all of the following EXCEPT
   A. calls and office visits
   B. office visits and treatments
   C. appointments and appointment cancellations
   D. personal opinions
   E. prescribed medications and their refills

9. Which, when signed by a patient, allows a representative to act on behalf of the patient in regards to medical treatment and care?
   A. durable power of attorney
   B. living will
   C. advanced directives
   D. the Uniform Anatomical Gift accord
   E. the Good Samaritan accord

10. Which statement(s) regarding patient/physician relationships is NOT true?
    A. Physicians have the right to select the patients they wish to treat.
    B. Patients expect that their physicians will use the appropriate "standard of care" in providing treatment.
    C. Consent refers to giving permission to treat.
    D. Patients can expect to receive information concerning both the advantages and potential risks of a given treatment.
    E. Patients can expect to have expensive treatment options withheld from them by their physician.

CRITICAL THINKING

1. What should Sue report to the physician?
2. Who should Sue report this to beside the physician?
3. Would Sue be legally responsible if she chooses to continue the billing practice?

ON THE JOB

Dr. Spring, a board certified obstetrician and gynecologist, has been in practice for more than ten years. He is licensed to practice medicine in both New York and Pennsylvania. Dr. Spring employs a staff that includes two medical assistants.

On Monday one of the medical assistants, Nancy Watts, took a history on a new patient that was referred to Dr. Spring by her internist. The 40-year old, married patient has had vaginal spotting for more than six weeks.

As part of the history, Nancy learned that the patient has been under the care and supervision of a fertility specialist for more than two years. In fact, although not always compliant, the patient has been on a medication treatment regime for fertility problems.

After examining the patient, Dr. Spring ordered a uterine biopsy to be performed in the office. The patient returns the following week, undergoes the biopsy and is sent home. Soon after, the patient's husband had telephoned the office, requesting to speak to Dr. Spring immediately. His wife had just been admitted to the hospital because of intense vaginal bleeding.

1. Was there anything in the patient's history that should have caused Nancy to alert the physician about performing a uterine biopsy?
2. Should Nancy have given this patient special instructions prior to the biopsy because of her history?
3. How should Nancy have handled the husband's telephone call?
4. Would it violate patient confidentiality to fax the patient's records to the emergency room physician, if requested?
5. Is this a potential case of medical negligence and malpractice? Could Nancy, as the medical assistant, have complicity in this particular case?

INTERNET ACTIVITY

Do an Internet search to explore the AAMA and AMA Web sites, especially concerning the code of ethics.

MediaLink More on medical law and ethics, including interactive resources, can be found on the Student CD-ROM accompanying this textbook.

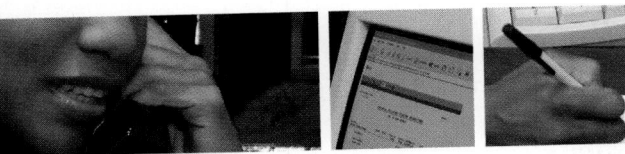

Medical Assistant Role Delineation Chart

HIGHLIGHT indicates material covered in this chapter.

ADMINISTRATIVE

Administrative Procedures

- Perform basic administrative medical assisting functions
- Schedule, coordinate and monitor appointments
- Schedule inpatient/outpatient admissions and procedures
- Understand and apply third-party guidelines
- Obtain reimbursement through accurate claims submission
- Monitor third-party reimbursement
- Understand and adhere to managed care policies and procedures
- *Negotiate managed care contracts*

Practice Finances

- Perform procedural and diagnostic coding
- Apply bookkeeping principles

- Manage accounts receivable
- *Manage accounts payable*
- *Process payroll*
- *Document and maintain accounting and banking records*
- *Develop and maintain fee schedules*
- *Manage renewals of business and professional insurance policies*
- *Manage personnel benefits and maintain records*
- *Perform marketing, financial, and strategic planning*

CLINICAL

Fundamental Principles

- Apply principles of aseptic technique and infection control
- Comply with quality assurance practices
- Screen and follow up patient test results

Diagnostic Orders

- Collect and process specimens
- Perform diagnostic tests

Patient Care

- Adhere to established patient screening procedures
- Obtain patient history and vital signs
- Prepare and maintain examination and treatment areas
- Prepare patient for examinations, procedures and treatments

- Assist with examinations, procedures and treatments
- Prepare and administer medications and immunizations
- Maintain medication and immunization records
- Recognize and respond to emergencies
- Coordinate patient care information with other health care providers
- Initiate IV and administer IV medications with appropriate training and as permitted by state law

GENERAL

Professionalism

- Display a professional manner and image
- Demonstrate initiative and responsibility
- Work as a member of the health care team
- Prioritize and perform multiple tasks
- Adapt to change
- Promote the CMA credential
- Enhance skills through continuing education
- Treat all patients with compassion and empathy
- Promote the practice through positive public relations

Communication Skills

- Recognize and respect cultural diversity
- Adapt communications to individual's ability to understand
- Use professional telephone technique

- Recognize and respond effectively to verbal, nonverbal, and written communications
- Use medical terminology appropriately
- Utilize electronic technology to receive, organize, prioritize and transmit information
- Serve as liaison

Legal Concepts

- Perform within legal and ethical boundaries
- Prepare and maintain medical records
- Document accurately
- Follow employer's established policies dealing with the health care contract
- Implement and maintain federal and state health care legislation and regulations
- Comply with established risk management and safety procedures
- Recognize professional credentialing criteria
- *Develop and maintain personnel, policy and procedure manuals*

Instruction

- Instruct individuals according to their needs
- Explain office policies and procedures
- Teach methods of health promotion and disease prevention
- Locate community resources and disseminate information
- *Develop educational materials*
- *Conduct continuing education activities*

Operational Functions

- Perform inventory of supplies and equipment
- Perform routine maintenance of administrative and clinical equipment
- Apply computer techniques to support office operations
- *Perform personnel management functions*
- *Negotiate leases and prices for equipment and supply contracts*

- *Denotes advanced skills.*

SOURCE: Reprinted by permission of the American Association of Medical Assistants from the AAMA Role Delineation Study: Occupational Analysis of the Medical Assisting Profession.

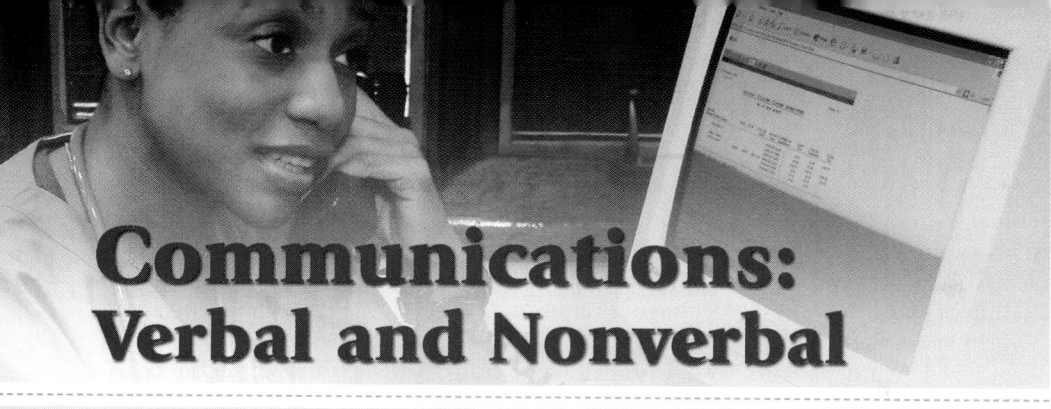

Communications: Verbal and Nonverbal

Learning Objectives

After reading this chapter, you should be able to:

- Define and spell the terms to learn for this chapter.
- Explain the importance of communication in health care today.
- Define the terms *values*, *attitudes*, and *behavior*, and explain their roles in self-awareness.
- Describe the communication process.
- Explain verbal and nonverbal communication.

- List several examples of nonverbal communication conveying impatience.
- List six guidelines for effective listening.
- Describe the difference between assertive and aggressive behavior.
- Describe two types of listening.
- List six types of defensive behavior, giving an example of each.
- Explain the importance of feedback in patient care.

OUTLINE

Interpersonal Dynamics	66
The Communication Process	68
Communication Techniques	72
Assertive versus Aggressive Behavior	75
Barriers to Communication	76
Communication in Special Circumstances	80
Intraoffice Communication	84
Staff Arrangements	85
Communication and Patients' Rights	87
Advising Patients	89
Communication and Patient Education	89

Terms to Learn

active listening
aggressive
assertive
assessment
attitudes
auditory
behavior
bias
character
close-ended questions
condescending
culture

defensive behaviors
empathy
ethnicity
ethnocentric
feedback
hierarchy
Health Insurance Portability and Accountability Act (HIPAA)
holistic
kinesthetic
nonverbal communication

open-ended questions
passive listening
prejudice
rapport
risk management
stereotyping
sympathy
values
verbal communication
visual

Case Study

MARY BROWN IS A 78-YEAR-OLD NEW PATIENT in Dr. Barry's office. She is very anxious in any new situation. When she arrived a few minutes early for her appointment, she was unsure what to do. She approached the glass window, which was closed, and waited for several minutes; no one acknowledged her. Susan and the other medical assistants were all busy talking to one another and laughing at a comment someone had made.

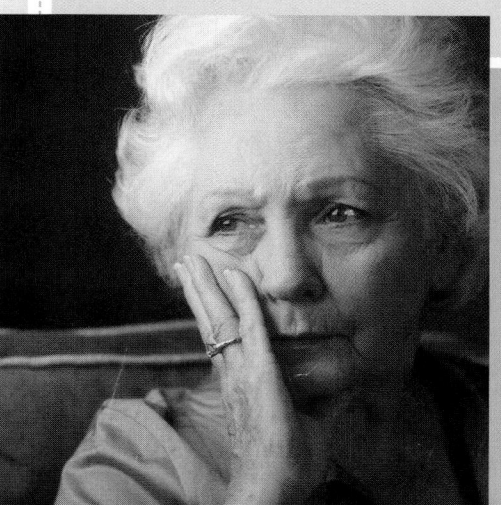

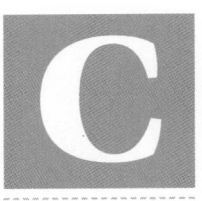

ommunication is a necessary requirement in any field, but is particularly essential in the health care field. As a medical assistant, you will relate to a variety of people, including sick and worried patients, your physician/employer, fellow staff members, vendors, and even some personal acquaintances of the physician. Some individuals you will interact with will be angry, frustrated, or simply ill and tired. Many patients who come into the physician's office or clinic will have physical or emotional problems that are not the main reason for their appointment. In addition, given the widely diverse population in the United States, you will be encountering people from a variety of countries and cultures. The medical assistant must be able to care for the entire patient in a holistic (viewing the overall situation) fashion and treat everyone with respect and courtesy.

It is not enough for the medical assistant to have excellent technical skills. Good interpersonal skills as well as good oral and written communication skills are needed to relate well to patients and fellow staff. In this chapter, you will learn about self-awareness and interpersonal dynamics. You will study the communication process, including directive techniques to improve effective communication, barriers to good communication, and defensive behaviors. Examining multicultural issues, communicating in special circumstances, and communicating with special needs patients will help you to be prepared for various situations you may encounter. Communication in the workplace, working as a member of a team, and understanding some conflict resolution strategies will help in your day-to-day work environment as well.

Interpersonal Dynamics

For the medical assistant to be able to provide effective communication in the delivery of health care, he or she must have a basic understanding of self. Why do you have the personality you exhibit? How do you communicate in everyday situations? Where do the impressions of others you hold originate? In other words, how did you get to be the person you are today? We will examine some concepts related to individuality and relationships with others.

Self-awareness

Understanding oneself and understanding the differences among others helps the medical assistant communicate more effectively. Personality is a sum of the traits, characteristics, and behaviors that makes us individuals. We all recognize different personalities, even among close family members.

Character is the sum of the values, attitudes, and behaviors a person exhibits. Psychologists tell us that values are a set of standards a person uses to measure the worth or importance of someone or something. Attitudes are opinions that develop from our value system. Values are acquired at home, in our family unit, and in the culture we live in and often are difficult to change. Prejudice, an opinion formed based on incorrect or irrational facts, is learned from experience and environment and colors our actions with others. An example of prejudice is viewing individuals with different skin color as inferior. Behavior, the actions others see, is based on our attitudes. To sum up, values form attitudes. Attitudes are reflected in behavior or actions that can be seen by others. Society prefers some behaviors and disapproves of others. For example, in the United States we are not permitted to have more than one spouse. In other cultures this is perfectly acceptable.

To be an effective communicator in all areas of our lives, it is important to look at our attitudes and our prejudices. How do others see us? How do we see ourselves? Examining ourselves leads to greater self-awareness and can lead to better communication skills. Patients and coworkers expect certain attitudes and professional behavior in the health care setting.

Life Stages

Understanding the stages of life through which we all pass will help the medical assistant be more sensitive to patients and their problems. Human growth and development refers not only to physical growth but also to emotional and psychological growth. Criteria, or norms, have been determined by professionals as guidelines to be used to ascertain development. The pace of development may differ widely and be irregular at times. Table 4-1 lists nine categories that make up the stages of life. Notice some corresponding characteristics listed along each stage.

Hierarchy of Needs

Along with recognizing the stages of development, it is important to understand Maslow's hierarchy, a ranked order of human needs. Psychologist Abraham Maslow established a ranking of human needs that is still widely used to help comprehend human behavior. Maslow maintained that people had needs and moved through various levels in achieving satisfaction in life. The hierarchy of needs is based on five elements or levels. These levels are:

Level I   Physiological needs such as food, water, and shelter.

Level II   Safety needs, which include physical safety as well as security—one's employment is associated with this level.

TABLE 4-1   The Nine Stages of Life

Infant (birth to 1 year)	Rapid physical growth, uncoordinated movements, may develop separation anxiety.
Toddler (1 to 2 years)	Less rapid growth, more coordination especially hands, begins walking speaking, quick mood changes.
Early childhood (3 to 5 years)	Grows taller, develops fine motor skills, becomes social, develops sense of self and body image.
Middle childhood (6 to 8 years)	Primary teeth lost, grows more slowly, begin cursive writing, begins to reason, friends are important.
Late childhood (9 to 12 years)	Muscles increase, secondary sexual signs begin, learns to communicate and compromise.
Adolescent (13 to 18 years)	Rapid physical growth, sexual maturation occurs, forms own identity, may rebel against authority.
Young adult (19 to 45 years)	Little physical growth, develops place in society, establishes family, life goals.
Middle age adult (46 to 65 years)	Aging changes occur, metabolism slows, earns most money, may question goals.
Older adult (66 years plus)	Declines in strength, slower neurological responses, hearing loss, less able to respond to stress, endures loss of family members, faces own death.

Level III   Social needs, which include having a sense of belonging to a group and the need for social interaction.

Level IV   Self-esteem, which includes having a sense of self-worth and pride.

Level V   Self-actualization, which occurs when the individual achieves all he or she is capable of achieving and derives a sense of accomplishment.

Maslow said that he believed a person could not move to a higher level until the basic needs at a lower level were met. An understanding of Maslow's hierarchy of needs is important for the medical assistant since patients he or she will encounter daily are at different stages or levels of fulfillment of their needs.

For example, one patient may be at Level I and be concerned about how he or she will pay a medical bill. Another patient, whose Level II and Level III needs are met, may wish to see the physician about cosmetic surgery as the patient attempts to have his or her self-esteem (Level V) needs met. Patients who have life-threatening illness require that their Level II needs for future security be met. For an illustration of Maslow's hierarchy of needs, see Figure 4-1.

Health and the Mind-Body Connection

Psychologists have discovered that there is a link between stress and illness. There are predisposing factors that

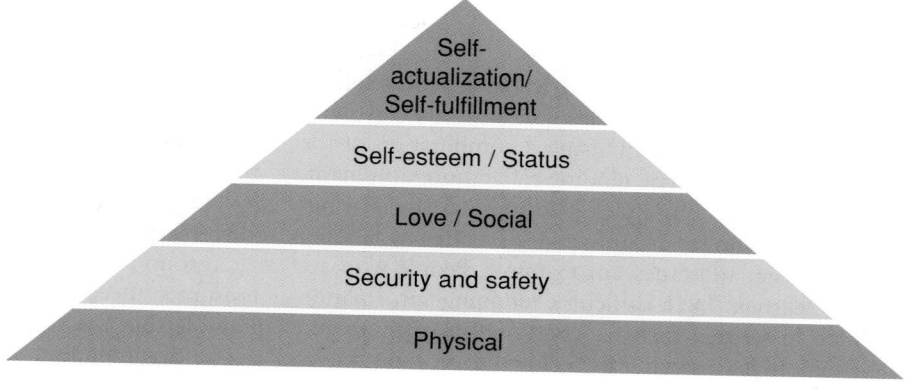

FIGURE 4-1 Maslow's hierarchy of needs.

create a tendency or susceptibility to becoming stresses. These include attitudes and feelings (emotions such as optimism or pessimism); health habits (smoking, exercise, drug use, and diet); the individual patient's methods for coping; economic and social resources; kind of job; sense of security; and the state of the patient's immune system.

The factors mentioned above also affect health care workers who have stress causing issues in their own lives and are dealing with patients who have many stress causing issues. Understanding stress factors and how to deal with them will make the medical assistant able to communicate more effectively and avoid burnout. *Burnout* is the result of experiencing prolonged periods of stress with no relief and can affect your health and career. For instance, a family member who cares for a patient with Alzheimer's disease and has no outside help may feel overwhelmed. Such a person may experience burnout and may also become ill.

Major life events, such as death of a loved one, divorce, an unexpected move away from family and friends, unemployment, or illness, can trigger stress. Some people who experience these life events may turn to unhealthy habits such as increased smoking or drinking. Others may exhibit negative behaviors such as anger outbursts, hostility, irritability, or depression. The following is a brief list of some ways to manage stress. They may be utilized by patients and caregivers alike.

- Develop a strong support system, including family and friends.
- Find a balance between striving for perfection and fear of failure.
- Eat nutritious meals.
- Avoid harmful habits such as smoking, drinking, and recreational drug use.
- Exercise regularly—walking, jogging, dancing, biking, and swimming.
- Look outward to develop social interests by understanding other people's problems and needs.
- Try to see the humor in situations.
- Limit the number of activities you engage in to a manageable few.
- Learn to budget time realistically.

Learning Styles

Examining the various styles of learning will help our self-awareness. Learning styles fall into several categories. Most of us learn by using a combination of the three styles with one style tending to be more dominant. There are three learning styles. The auditory (by hearing) learner is one who retains information better by hearing lectures, music, and tapes, for example. People who are auditory learners have difficulty retaining information presented in written format. The visual learner, as you would expect, learns better by seeing the information, by

means of reading, drawings, diagrams, and films. Visual learners find it more difficult to follow lectures unless visual aids are used with the presentation. The kinesthetic (involving movement) learner learns better by hands-on activities such as experiments, games, lab exercises, and movement. Such people have difficulty grasping a procedure until they have performed it themselves. Understanding these learning styles will help prepare the medical assistant for his or her role as patient educator.

The Communication Process

The basic units of the communication process are the source, message, channel, and receiver. Think of this as the acronym S-M-C-R:

S stands for the communication—who is sending the message?

M represents the actual message or the actual words that are placed on paper if the message is in writing.

C indicates the channel or channels through which the message moves from the source to the receiver. These channels include the senses: sight, smell, taste, hearing, and touch. Another set of channels consists of pathways like the telephone or interoffice mail.

R stands for the receiver of the message.

For example, a physician (S) writes a prescription (M) that the medical assistant then reads over the telephone (C) to the pharmacist (R). If any link in this chain is broken, an incorrect message is relayed. The same holds true if you relay a message to a patient. If the medical assistant (S) explains a procedure (M) to a patient who has a hearing loss (C), then the patient (R) will not hear the message as it was intended.

The communication process, then, is a chain effect that requires a source (S) and a receiver (R). The source (S) acts upon a stimulus to encode or transmit a message (M) in a particular form. The actual message can be transmitted in a variety of ways (C), including face-to-face, over the telephone, or in written form. The receiver (R) decodes or translates the message, based on his or her emotional state, perceptions, education, socioeconomic background, and many other factors.

Add to this process, the ever-present background noises that are part of the daily functioning of a medical office, and keeping the channels of communication open is as much a daily task for the medical assistant as any other. Some examples of background noises are conversations between patients or patients and staff, background music, ringing telephones, or requests for assistance. Because of this background buzz, it is very possible that the receiver may not receive the message the sender intended.

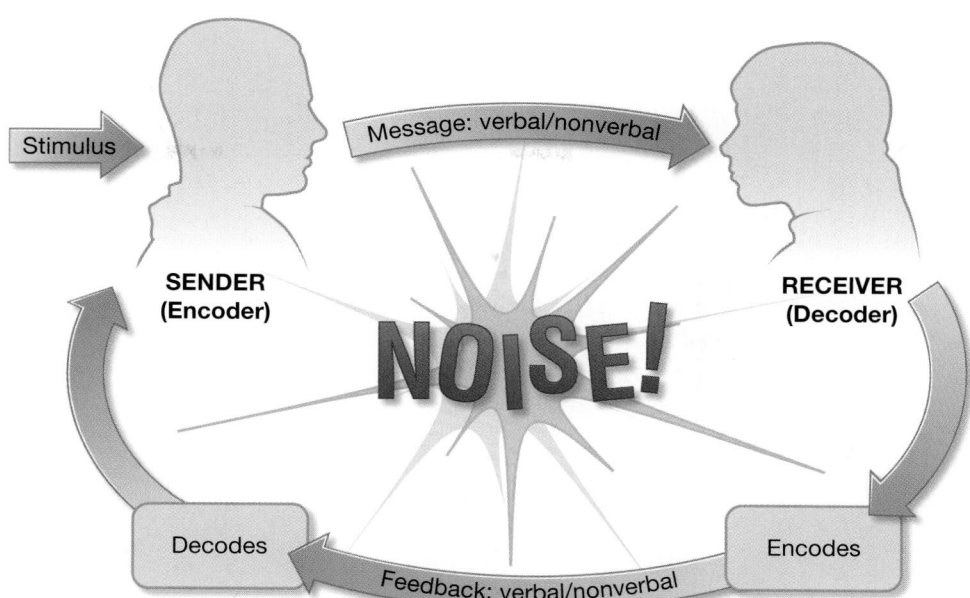

Channels of Communication

Channels of communication include the various means by which the spoken or written word is communicated from one person to another. Information is said to be "rich" if it conveys to the listener or reader the intent of the speaker. The greatest amount of information richness is gained from face-to-face discussion (Figure 4-2). The least amount of information is generally gained from formal numeric documents such as budget reports. When you wish to convey an important message to someone, it is better to do it face-to-face than to put the information into writing. This becomes important to remember when determining how to adequately educate patients regarding their medications. If you place all the important facts into a pamphlet, patients may never read it or might not understand your meaning. You need to consider the learning styles discussed previously and the fact that using a variety of styles better reinforces the message. However, it is important to give written instructions in addition to any verbal explanation you give the patient. Table 4-2 illustrates the varying degrees of "richness" of various information channels.

TABLE 4-2 **Information Richness Channels**

Information Channel	Level of Richness
Face-to-face discussion	Highest
Telephone conversations	High
Written letter/memos (individually addressed)	Moderate
Formal written documents (general bulletins or reports)	Low
Fax (facsimile)	Low
E-mail	Low
Internet	Low
Formal numeric document (printouts, budget reports)	Lowest

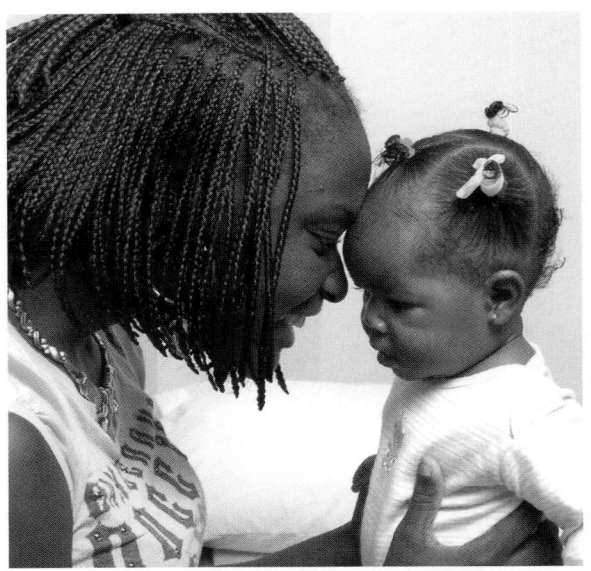
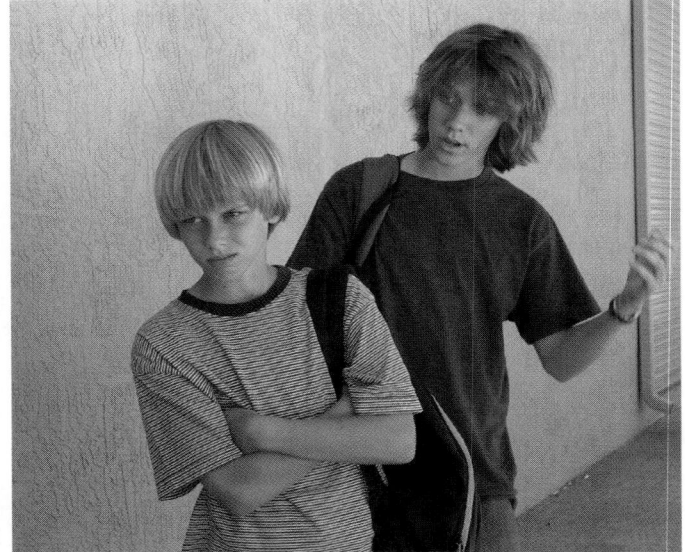
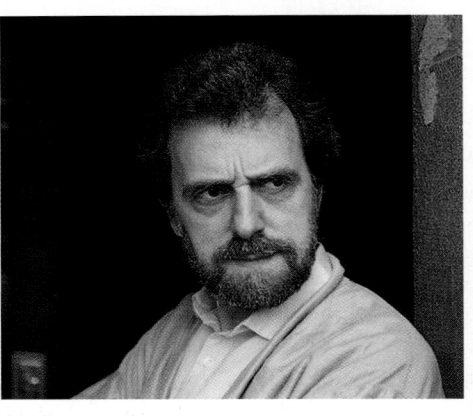
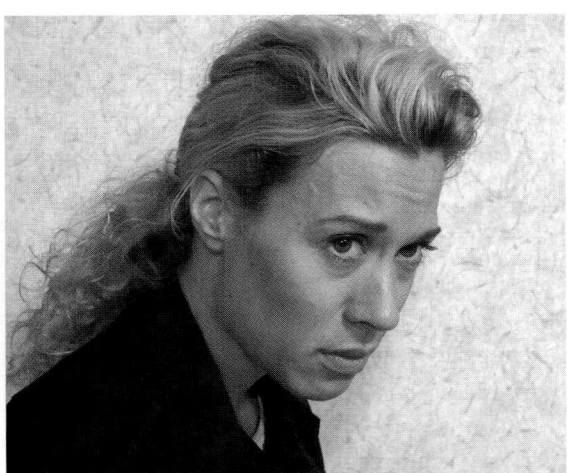

FIGURE 4-3 Nonverbal communications convey strong, powerful messages that may be negative or positive.

Verbal and Nonverbal Communication

Virtually everything a person does from birth to death is a form of communication. Smiling is a form of nonverbal communication, while talking "with a smile in your voice" is verbal communication. Nonverbal communication is the language of gesture and actions, including body language. In many cases, people are not even aware of the image they project with their bodies. The way a person holds his or her arms, makes eye contact, gestures, frowns, or turns toward or away from the speaker frequently conveys more than just words could convey (Figure 4-3). Box 4-1 offers some examples of messages that convey impatience.

Verbal Communication

Verbal communication depends on words and sounds or tone of voice. The sounds a person makes when

BOX 4-1
Communication Messages Conveying Impatience

- Interrupting people when they are speaking
- Answering telephone calls curtly
- Finishing another person's sentence
- Rushing the patient
- Eating lunch at your desk
- Looking at your watch or the clock
- Doing two things at once
- Not looking up from your work when someone approaches
- Rushing around the office

speaking cover a wide range and can convey vastly different meanings. The tone in which you speak to a patient is vitally important in making a positive impression on the patient and his or her family. Generally when someone is speaking, that person will raise his or her tone at the end of a statement when asking a question and drop the tone of voice when completing a sentence. When the speaker's tone drops it is appropriate to begin your part of the conversation. Interrupting speakers is a negative behavior that creates a barrier to good communication.

The medical assistant should speak loudly enough to be heard but not so loudly that a patient's confidentiality is compromised. Speaking clearly and properly pronouncing your words is important in conveying the message.

WORD SELECTION Choosing the right words to present a message is critical. We can all think of instances when we called a medical facility only to have been spoken to as though we were an annoyance to the person at the front desk. Other times, telephoning the medical assistant was a very pleasant experience and when the conversation was completed, we had a positive feeling. Sarcasm and ridicule have no place in the professional setting. The goal of the medical assistant is to promote an open, comfortable environment for the patient while keeping in mind that the patient is the customer. Choose your words carefully and take care not to be rude or impatient in your interpersonal relationships. See Lifespan Considerations for more on communicating with patients.

POSITIVE ATTITUDE The ability to convey a positive attitude is so important in working with people. Smiling immediately reassures the patient that he or she is welcome. When in the presence of a patient, always involve the patient in your conversation. Excluding the patient and talking "over his or her head" is disrespectful (Figure 4-4). If the conversation is of a business or confidential nature, it should be held elsewhere.

Effective medical assistants are able to demonstrate empathy but should be cautious about using sympathy for their patients. Empathy is the willingness or the ability to understand what the patient is feeling without necessarily experiencing the same thing. Sympathy, on the other hand, is feeling sorry for or pitying the patient. Patients react much better to an empathetic listener than to a sympathetic one. You can acquire the skill of empathetic listening using these simple nonverbal techniques: nodding, leaning toward the patient, or positioning yourself so you are at the patient's eye level, and indicating by your facial expression that you understand what he or she is saying (Figure 4-5).

Since we all share the same human emotions, there will be instances when you become distressed over a patient's situation. It is not possible to be a concerned health care provider and remain totally unemotional at all times. If you become upset, you can excuse yourself for a few moments. Realize that your emotions and concerns are another indication that you have chosen the correct field.

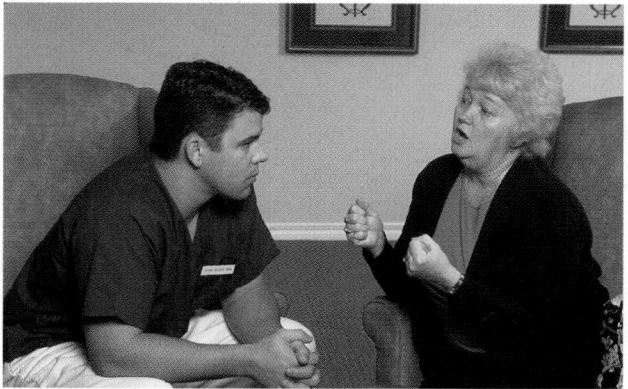

FIGURE 4-4 It is important to be concerned when a patient is upset.

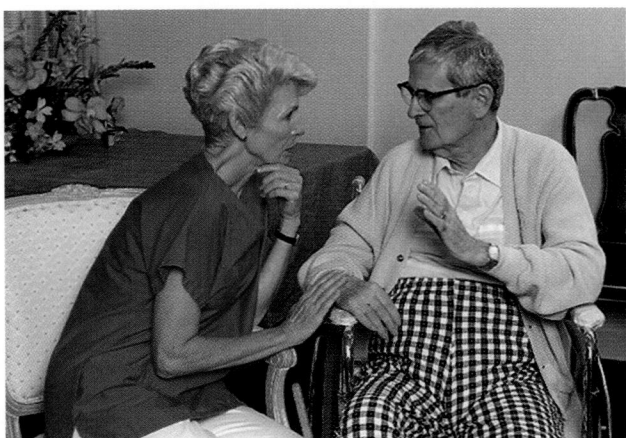

FIGURE 4-5 Empathy draws a more positive response from the patient since it is based on the willingness of the medical assistant to understand what the patient is experiencing.

Nonverbal Communication

Nonverbal communication involves facial expressions, gestures, body language, eye contact, good grooming, and mannerisms. It is important that verbal and nonverbal messages agree. Body language is learned by imitation, by being taught, and by instinct. For example, consider the hand gestures that are a normal part of communication among individuals from Italy and other Mediterranean countries. Appearance is a nonverbal form of communication. Patients expect certain types of behaviors, attitudes, and appearance in the health care setting. Unprofessional attire, visible tattoos, and overpowering perfume send a negative message. See Professionalism for more on maintaining a professional appearance.

The gesture of touch is considered a form of nonverbal communication and a form of body language. Gently touching a distraught patient's arm can reassure and comfort the patient. However, one must be cautious that the receiver does not misinterpret a

Professionalism

As a health care representative, the medical assistant should set a good example. The medical assistant sets the first impression of the office and is in many ways, the marketing representative of the practice. The medical assistant must always present a professional appearance. Good personal hygiene and grooming is a must. Nails should be kept short and unpolished, and jewelry should be kept to a minimum.

touch. In some cultures, for instance, it is considered rude to touch a child's head without permission. At times, abused children can be fearful of even innocent touching. Use caution when touching a patient unless you know him or her well.

Communication Techniques

The ability to encourage a patient to communicate effectively is critical when you wish to perform a patient assessment or evaluation to determine the patient's problems. For example, how are you to stop a patient who is talking about seemingly irrelevant issues? First of all, it is important to understand that the patient is nervous. Before we discuss specific techniques, there are several questions we need to consider as we examine the overall communication process. Each communication experience has unique qualities and must be considered carefully.

- What is the goal of your communication?
- What message do you want to give?
- What channel are you going to deliver (face-to-face, written, etc.)?
- How are you going to listen to the response (listening and observational skills)?
- How are you going to get clarification/feedback?
- Was your goal met or do you need to revise the message (assess or evaluate)?

Listening Skills

Listening involves verbal and nonverbal cues. The medical assistant must pay attention to both. Listening is either active or passive. Active listening involves paying attention to the speaker completely, concentrating on the verbal message, observing for nonverbal cues, and offering a response. It is difficult in a medical office to actively listen at times when so many things are happening at once. One skill you will gain with experience is the ability to prioritize simultaneous events. Passive listening is simply listening to someone without having to reply, such as when you are listening as a member of an audience. How we hear a message is often colored by the message being delivered. If it is criticism of your work and you disagree, you hear it one way. If it is praise for your work, you hear it another way. Sometimes we are formulating a response before the speaker is finished with his or her message. In either circumstance, the listener's mind or thoughts may wander and the message may not be delivered effectively or may be distorted. Part of effective listening is to know when it is your turn to speak and allowing enough time for the message to be completed. With

PROCEDURE

Effective Listening Skills

OBJECTIVE: Use effective listening skills to obtain chief complaint from a patient.

Equipment and Supplies
patient history form

Method
1. Identify patient.
2. Ask patient the reason for current appointment.
3. Smile and establish eye contact.
4. Seat the patient in appropriate area.
5. Focus full attention on patient.
6. Ask open-ended questions.
7. Do not interrupt patient.
8. Provide feedback by paraphrasing what the patient said.
9. Observe patient for signs of needing to give more information.
10. Restate the chief complaint before leaving patient.
11. Conclude patient interview in appropriate manner.
12. Document the chief complaint with 100% accuracy.

---

practice we can become good listeners. Procedure 4-1 provides steps to practice with fellow students and to employ with patients. The following are some guidelines for good listening:

- Avoid distractions.
- Face the speaker.
- Give the person your full attention.
- Maintain eye contact as suitable for culture.
- Do not be judgmental about what is said.
- Be aware of nonverbal cues.
- Note anything that seems unclear.
- Do not interrupt.
- Maintain personal space.
- Ask questions if you do not understand.

Directive Communication Techniques

The medical assistant can often assist the communication process by directing the patient's comments, using specific communication techniques so that the sharing between the patient and the medical assistant is productive.

Types of Questions

Asking questions to deliver a message and to obtain information is a directive technique. The medical assistant will be asking many questions of the patient. It is helpful to keep in mind the goal of your question before you choose the type of question to ask. Four types of questions will be discussed.

CLOSE-ENDED QUESTIONS Close-ended questions can be answered with a yes or a no. Often these types of questions are appropriate to obtain background information, such as "Is your mother still living?" However, there may be times when you ask a patient, "Do you understand what I mean," and the patient will answer, "yes" even if he or she does not comprehend what you are saying. Usually this happens because the patient does not want to be a "bother" or appear stupid. You need to consider the situation carefully when you use close-ended questions.

OPEN-ENDED QUESTIONS Open-ended questions, those that require more than yes or no responses, can be useful in gaining feedback or drawing out patient information. Using such questions or directive methods, you will be able to obtain information the physician will require to treat the patient. See Table 4-3 for a list of other directive communication techniques, including a description and an example of each technique.

PROBING QUESTIONS Probing questions are used to ask the patient for further information to more fully discuss the subject. For example, if a patient says, "My head hurts" a probing question would ask, "Where does it hurt?" or "How long have you had this pain?" In this example, other probing questions would seek information about type of pain, when it started, and when it occurs. The medical assistant is often the person the patient feels more comfortable speaking to and questioning. It is important to be empathetic and try to put the patient at ease.

TABLE 4-3 **Directive Communication Techniques**

Technique	Description	Example
Open-ended statement	Encourage the patient to discuss freely.	"Please describe your pain for me."
Closed-ended statement	Direct the patient to make a yes/no or simple response.	"Are you having pain?"
Reflecting	Direct the conversation back to the patient by repeating the patient's words.	Patient: "I'm afraid of what the doctor will find." MA: "You're afraid of what the doctor will find?"
Acknowledgment	Indicate understanding.	"I understand what you are saying."
Restating	State what the patient has said but in different terms.	Patient: "I can't sleep." MA: "You say you're having trouble getting to sleep at night?"
Add to an implied statement	Verbalize implied information.	Patient: "I'm usually relaxed." MA: "And today you're not relaxed?"
Seek clarification	Request more information in order to better understand.	Patient: "I don't feel good." MA: "Tell me what your symptoms are."
Silence	Remain silent or make no gesture in response to a statement.	Patient: I don't know what's wrong but something is."

LEADING QUESTIONS Leading questions are those questions in which part of the answer is in the question. For example, when asked, "Do you have to urinate two, three, or four times a night?" the patient then has to select one answer from your choices. This may be helpful in dealing with patients who do not understand English. However, the medical assistant must be careful not to ask the specific type of leading question in order to get the exact answer he or she desires.

Feedback

Feedback, any response to a communication, is critically important when working with patients since you must determine if they really understand what they have heard. Feedback can be either verbal or nonverbal. Sometimes the verbal message and the nonverbal message that patients send do not agree. For instance, as a medical assistant you may ask, "How are you feeling?" and the patient might state, "Fine." Since the patient is walking with a painful limp, you doubt the verbal statement. Always try to ask specific questions such as, "Do you have pain?" "Tell me about your medication," or "Tell me what you need to see the doctor about." When documenting the information

that the patient provides, use the patient's words, not yours.

REFLECTING Reflecting is a directive technique in which you mirror the patient's message back to the individual to ensure that you have understood him or her correctly. For example, you may say in response to a patient who needs an appointment, "You say you can't come in on Wednesdays?" The reflecting technique is also helpful in resolving conflicts, clearing up confusing statements, and requires more detail from the other person.

RESTATING Restating or paraphrasing is repeating the patient's message to him or her in your own words. For example, "I heard you say that you will not be able to pay your bill this month. Is that correct?" This technique helps to confirm that both parties understand the message clearly.

CLARIFICATION The ultimate goal in effective communication is to deliver the message so it is understood clearly. Clarification is a directive technique in which the medical assistant requests more information in order to better understand what the patient has stated. Many times patients use words such as "a lot" or "much worse" in explaining their symptoms. It is important to ask them to be more specific in order to accurately diagnose or treat them. For example, the patient says, "My right arm hurts a lot." The medical assistant should employ the directive techniques mentioned to clarify this information

The following questions are examples of follow-up questions and statements useful in this situation: "You say that your right arm hurts. Is that correct? Where on your arm do you feel the pain? What kind of pain is it? When did it start? Does it hurt all the time? Are you able to sleep? Are you taking any medications for the pain?"

Assertive versus Aggressive Behavior

Most instances of communication within the work setting involve convincing someone else to cooperate with you. Whether patient or staff communication is your goal, the methods to achieve cooperation are the same. As a medical assistant there are occasions when you will have to convince both patients and staff to listen to you. Using assertive behavior techniques can make this easier.

Being assertive means that you make a point in a positive manner by standing firm, making decisions based on your principles or values, and trusting you own ideas or instincts in the situation. Being aggressive, on the other hand, is trying to impose your point of view on others or trying to manipulate others. Aggressiveness is considered a negative behavior and indicates a type of pushiness when trying to convince others. In fact, it has been compared to making a

verbal attack against another. Many people resort to aggressive behavior in order to impose their ideas on others or when they are angry or fearful. Aggressive people are bossy and inconsiderate of the feelings of others. See Table 4-4 for a comparison of assertive and aggressive behavior.

Assertive Behavior Techniques

Acquiring the ability to use assertive behavior means that you will learn to offer new ideas or even unwanted ideas to people in such a manner that they will not feel threatened. Some assertive behaviors include being direct and honest, using positive body language, and using "I" statements such as "I feel." For instance, when calling a patient regarding nonpayment of a bill you will need to gain the patient's acceptance. The patient may become angry at the beginning of the conversation in response to an aggressive comment, such as "Are you aware that your bill is now two months overdue? When are you going to pay it?" He or she could become defensive and hang up. Since most patients know when they have not paid a bill, it is not necessary to use threatening language. A better approach would be to identify yourself and indicate that you are helping Dr. Thompson with his billings. In a calm but assertive manner, you would ask questions that would prompt a positive response from the patient. These questions might include, "How can I help you in clearing up these payments? Perhaps we can discuss your making a small payment on your account twice a month. What would be an amount that you could afford?"

Assertive Behavior Guidelines

Assertiveness is a learned skill that helps one to maintain self-confidence under stressful conditions. The basis for assertiveness is that everyone has the

TABLE 4-4 Comparison of Assertive and Aggressive Behavior	
Assertive Behavior	**Aggressive Behavior**
"This medication works best when it is taken on a regular daily basis."	"You know you can't expect this medication to work when you're not taking it every day."
"Let me find someone who can answer that question for you."	"That's not my job."
"Your behavior is inappropriate."	"Why did you do that? It was stupid."
Knocking on door and then coming into an exam to say: "Excuse me, Dr. Thompson, you are needed on the telephone."	Rushing into an exam room to say: "Doctor, you've got a telephone call."

right to express opinions or beliefs in an appropriate, respectful manner without fear of being humiliated or made to feel guilty. Aggressiveness results in violation of a person's right during communication. The results of aggressive behavior are resentment and loss of respect. To practice assertive behavior use the following steps:

- Take a few deep breaths to calm yourself.
- Describe the behavior that you would like the other person to change in unemotional tones.
- Describe how you feel when the behavior occurs.
- State the positive behavior you would like to see.
- Describe the consequences that will result if the person does not change his or her behavior.
- Consequences must be appropriate, reasonable, and enforceable.
- Follow through with consequences if the behavior does not change.
- Commend the individual for the behavioral change.
- Evaluate your confrontation.

Discussing Sensitive Issues

Discussing issues involving money, such as the patient's bill and personal financial responsibility, can be very sensitive. Patients should be advised before the first visit of physician's charges for specific services or treatment. Inquiries regarding patient's medical insurance and procedure for payment of fees should also be reviewed prior to the first visit. Complying with the federal regulations regarding the patient's right to privacy of all health related information should be addressed at the first visit. The Health Insurance Portability and Accountability Act (HIPAA), is a federal act designed to improve portability and continuity of health insurance coverage; to combat waste, fraud, and abuse in health insurance and health care delivery; to promote the use of medical savings accounts; to improve access to long-term care services and coverage; to simplify the administration of health insurance and ensure the privacy of personal health information and appropriate release of that information. The medical assistant should have each patient sign a release of information form on his or her first visit.

Always consider a patient's feelings when asking questions within hearing distance of others. If questions involve personal patient health care information, HIPAA requires that the medical assistant inquire about these issues in private, where others will not overhear it. When telephoning a patient you must keep in mind that all conversation about personal health care information must be private.

The Customer-Friendly Environment

Using good interpersonal skills to set a positive environment in the health care setting generates a customer-friendly atmosphere and comfortable workplace. A warm, friendly greeting, showing respect to the patient, being sincere and sensitive, and demonstrating empathy can help set a positive tone.

Greeting Patients

A patient should be greeted within one minute of entering the office. If you are speaking on the telephone when the patient comes in, be sure to acknowledge the patient's presence with a smile and nod. Give your full attention to the patient as soon as you complete the telephone conversation.

Barriers to Communication

There are many barriers to communication. Identifying and overcoming these barriers is essential for effective communication. Some are obvious barriers, such as the distraction of loud background noise, and can be eliminated by the medical assistant. However, there are other barriers that we are not even aware of that result in either no communication or a distorted message being received. In order to understand the patient, you must overcome the barriers to effective communication (Figure 4-6).

Giving the patient false reassurance that "everything will be all right" can result in the patient's reluctance to talk to you about personal or health related fears. Such comments can also lead to liability issues for the physician if the patient believes that a promise for recovery has been made. See Legal and Ethical Issues.

The medical assistant may also put up barriers to communication without meaning to. These include not looking at the patient when he or she is speaking, interrupting the patient, abruptly changing the subject,

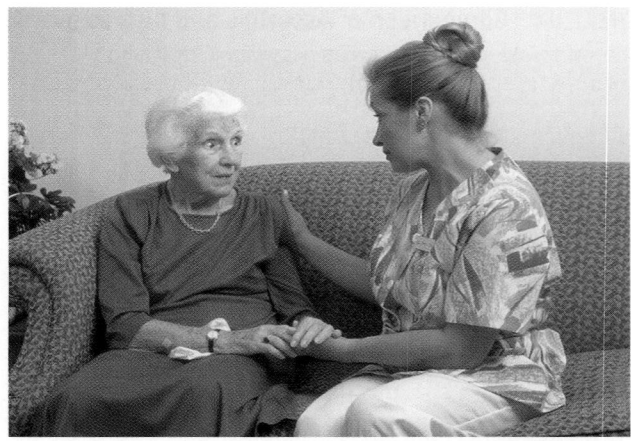

FIGURE 4-6 Effective listening skills demonstrates empathy to the patient and breaks down barriers to communication.

and using meaningless statements to soothe the patient, just to name a few. Medical assistants must remember that the patient is coming to see the physician because he or she has a problem. Patients should never be treated in a condescending manner.

Defensive Behaviors

Patients will also put up barriers to effective communication when they are under the stress of illness. These barriers are called defensive behaviors. A defensive behavior is a reaction to a perceived threat that is usually unconscious. Defensive behaviors are also referred to as coping behaviors. Not all coping behaviors are defensive or have a negative impact. For example, when trying to meet a deadline, you may have learned that using good time management skills and prioritizing tasks permits you to reach the deadline. Coping mechanisms are learned either consciously or unconsciously. As a member of the health care team, you need to be aware of your defensive behaviors in the professional setting at home. Some defensive behaviors are discussed in Table 4-5.

Use of Medical Language

You will become adept at understanding the language of medicine. The abbreviations that are used in medicine are a form of communication for people working in the health care field. However, your patients have little understanding of medical terminology. You may wish to teach patients a few simple terms so that they can better understand the physician's instructions on prescriptions. Otherwise, you must make an effort to avoid using medical terminology or abbreviations when speaking with patients. For example, abbreviations such as "NPO," meaning nothing by mouth, are not readily recognized or understood by patients. Always write out or state clear instructions regarding preparations for tests and taking medications. Patients may be reluctant to admit they do not understand. You will then assume that they have been properly instructed which is not the case. Failure to inform patients in terms they are able to understand could be construed as negligence on the part of the health care provider and increase the risk of a lawsuit.

Multicultural Issues

As a medical assistant, you will come in contact with people from many different cultures. A culture consists of the values, beliefs, attitudes, and customs shared by a group of people and passed on through the generations. Behaviors exhibited by the members of a culture are based on their beliefs and values. Health care beliefs may differ widely from those which we are accustomed. The medical assistant must be tolerant in attitude, not condescending, and treat each patient with empathy and respect. The medical assistant will encounter cultural diversity when interacting with individuals

Legal and Ethical Issues

Medical assistants must use caution when communicating with patients. Providing false hopes for recovery or implying that the physician may be able to cure a patient is not only unethical but can also result in liability for the physician and the medical assistant.

Putting incidents in writing also involves careful thought and caution. It is important to chart exactly what occurred and what the patient stated rather than the medical assistant's feelings about the situation. Recording the patient's comment, "I have an overwhelming feeling of hopelessness," is a better indication of the patient's emotional state than the comment, "I think the patient is depressed." This last comment reflects the medical assistant's judgment of the patient's appearance or what the patient said, not what the patient has said about himself or herself. As with everything that transpires in the medical environment, the HIPAA regulations must be kept in mind.

from other cultures. Cultural diversity presents its own set of barriers to effective communication. See Cultural Considerations for more on dealing with individuals from different cultures.

Language

A non-English speaking patient is at a disadvantage when trying to obtain health care. Imagine for a minute how you would feel if you were traveling in a foreign country and had an accident that required you to go to the hospital. Not only would you not understand anyone in the hospital, but also, their health care practices might be very different. The feelings of fear, frustration, and confusion you would feel would be augmented if you had no one with you to act as an interpreter.

You will encounter patients and other health care workers who speak a wide variety of languages. However, Hispanics make up the largest non-English speaking group in the United States today. It would be helpful for you to learn a few phrases and some simple words in the patient's language to help communicate with the patient and coworkers. If at all possible, you should try to get someone to interpret for the patient. Perhaps a fellow worker or family member would be able to help. If a patient has a limited ability to understand English, speak slowly and clearly, using simple

TABLE 4-5 Defensive Behaviors

Behavior	Description	Example
Compensation	Substitution of an attitude, feeling, or behavior with its opposite.	Mrs. Matthews believes the lump in her breast is cancer. However, she smiles and laughs whenever you talk to her about it.
Denial	Unconsciously avoiding an unwanted feeling or situation.	Mr. Morgan cancels an appointment to have a PSA (blood) test for prostate cancer in spite of having symptoms associated with prostate trouble.
Displaced anger	Expressing angry feelings toward persons or objects that are unrelated to the problem.	Mrs. Matthews is angry at being diagnosed with cancer. She takes this anger out on her family members.
Disassociation	Not connecting one event with another.	Mary Sims is a nurse who works with alcoholic patients. In her free time she drinks to excess.
Introjection	Adopting the feeling of someone else.	Mr. Morgan's friends have said that the PSA test is reliable and could relieve his anxiety about having prostate cancer. He believes them and has the test.
Projection	Placing your own feelings onto another person.	Mr. Morgan becomes irritated when the medical assistant calls to remind him of his appointment. He wrongly decides that she is irritated with him or dislikes him. In reality, he is upset with himself.
Rationalization	Justifying thoughts or behavior to avoid the truth.	Mary Sims believes that the appetite suppressant benefit of smoking offsets the risk of developing cancer.
Regression	Turning back to former behavior patterns in times of stress.	Jimmy, who is toilet trained, reverts to bed-wetting during hospitalization.
Repression	Keeping unpleasant thoughts or feelings out or one's mind.	Mr. Morgan denies any urinary frequency when questioned by the physician.
Sublimation	Directing or changing unacceptable drives for security, affection or power into socially or culturally acceptable channels.	Mrs. Matthews is worried about having cancer and uses up energy cleaning her house.

words or phrases. Smiling and other positive nonverbal cues are helpful. Use pictures if they are available. It will help you be more tolerant if you put yourself in the patient's position for a moment.

Culture

People from other cultures have different views and customs relating to health care delivery. Our views and customs are not better than theirs, just different. They may have different views about the causes of illness, treatments, and the expected behavior of the health care provider. In some cultures, illness is thought to be caused by winds or forces, blood being too thick or thin, or the ill will of others.

Encouraging patients from a different culture to relate their symptoms and signs to you may be another problem. They may feel that to talk about pain is a sign of weakness or to mention psychological problems is

Cultural Considerations

Medical assistants must work with and provide care for individuals from a wide variety of racial, ethnic, cultural, religious, and socioeconomic backgrounds. In every instance, it is important to respect the individuality of everyone. Patients from other cultures may be completely unfamiliar with the Western model of medical treatment. When communicating with others who are different from ourselves we must avoid prejudging or generalizing about them. The following are just a few examples of cultural concepts or traditions you as a medical assistant may encounter: nodding the head up and down means yes to us, but it means no in some other cultures; touching someone in certain areas of the body is not permissible in some cultures; shaving body hair to prepare the patient for a procedure is not permitted in some cultures; eye contact is not acceptable in some cultures.

not permitted. One of the duties of the medical assistant is to help ensure that the patient complies with the treatment physicians prescribe whether it is in the form of medication or therapy or diagnostic examinations. It may be necessary to ask for assistance from a family member who understands the issues and can communicate more easily. See Table 4-6 for a list of some diverse cultural traditions.

Bias, Prejudice, and Stereotyping

Bias, prejudice, and stereotyping are barriers to effective communication that directly relate to cultural diversity. In order to understand these barriers, a few more definitions are in order. We defined culture as the values, attitudes, and behaviors peculiar to a group of people. Ethnicity is a classification of people based on national origin. People from the same ethnic background share similar traditions, beliefs, and language. We have all heard street names that are negative in connotation being used to describe people of specific national origin. Stereotyping results when negative generalities concerning specific characteristics of a group are applied unfairly to an entire population. Race is a classification of people based on their physical or

TABLE 4-6 **Cultural Traditions in Health Care**

Country	Sick Care Practices	Health Care Beliefs	Family Role in Care
China	Holistic and traditional includes acupuncture, herbal medicine.	Upset in body energy causes disease. Stigma attached to mental illness. Health promotion important.	Family takes care of sick even in hospital.
Former Soviet Union	Holistic, folk, and Western medical practices.	Health promotion is important. Acute sick care practiced, rehabilitation not stressed.	Family members provide care in hospital: bathing, feeding, linen change.
Philippines	Health promotion important. Mental illness a disgrace. Evil can cause illness through eyes on another.	Family may give hospital care.	Children feel obligated to care for elderly.
Vietnam	Magical and religious health care practices. Eastern, herbal medicine important. Self-care and self-medication used to treat illness.	Acute sick care only. Believe health is restoration of yin/yang and hot/cold balance.	Patient care is a family responsibility.

biological characteristics such as skin color, shape of eyes, hair, bone structure, or facial features. Race is often used to classify people unfairly and unjustly in a negative way. Bias is an unfair preference or dislike of something. A bias prevents an impartial opinion of someone or something. People who are ethnocentric believe that their cultural background is better than any other. This leads to prejudice or prejudging and stereotyping, which impact negatively on communication and acceptance of others in all relationships. To avoid these negative behaviors the medical assistant should:

- Be aware of his or her beliefs.

- Learn as much as possible about other cultures, races, and nationalities.

- Be sensitive to the feelings of others.

- Evaluate information before accepting it as a belief.

- Avoid ethnic jokes.

- Be open to differences.

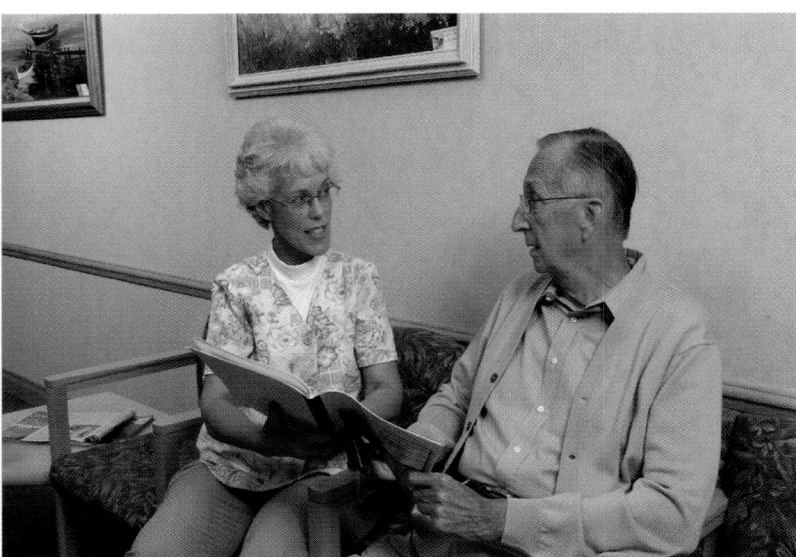

FIGURE 4-7 The medical assistant often has to reassure and comfort the patient before effective communication can take place.

Communication in Special Circumstances

The medical assistant will encounter special circumstances in the office when dealing with patients. At times, you will meet an angry patient, a patient who is terminally ill, one who is anxious, who is visually or hearing impaired, or who is mentally or emotionally impaired. Each of these types of patients must be treated with respect, empathy, and professionalism.

The Angry Patient

One of the most difficult communication problems involves the angry patient. It can be a difficult task for the medical assistant to refrain from taking the patient's comments personally. People have different styles and coping behaviors when they are frightened (Figure 4-7). Many patients who enter the physician's office are fearful of the diagnosis they may hear. Some patients become frightened of the equipment in the office or have an unwarranted fear of pain. In addition to fear, another cause of anger is loss of control. Many of us have had this feeling when we were hospitalized as a patient.

The job of the medical assistant is to remain calm and use positive communication and professional techniques to direct the patient's anger into a positive channel. Try to defuse the patient's anger. For instance, many patients will gain control over their anger when the medical assistant offers a comment such as, "I'm really sorry you feel this way. Let's see if we can solve the problem." You may have to take the patient into a private office if you cannot calm the patient immediately. Disruptive patients can upset others waiting to see the physician. While it is not necessary to give in to the unreasonable demands of a patient, realize that an upset patient is often expressing the need for you to listen carefully, without judging, and assist in solving the problem. Whenever possible, try to direct the patient's comments to the solution of the problem.

In the case of an angry caller, you must remember that no matter how angry a patient becomes, you cannot respond in anger. The role of the medical assistant is to assess or evaluate the situation. Remain calm and speak to the patient in a quiet, calm tone of voice, projecting your concern for the patient in the present situation. Often this will be enough to calm the patient down. If it does not work, however, ask your supervisor or office manager for assistance. Otherwise, ask the patient if you may return the call after you have been able to gather more information that will enable you to be of help.

In the case of a patient who becomes abusive or violent, you need to obtain assistance to protect yourself, other staff, and patients. Once the incident has been resolved, be sure to document it appropriately according to office policies.

The Anxious Patient

Many patients exhibit what is known as "white coat" syndrome. Whenever they have to encounter anyone in a white uniform, they become extremely anxious. Some signs of anxiety are trembling, flushing, perspiring, fidgeting, talking excessively, and remaining unusually quiet. Hypertensive patients who suffer from "white coat" syndrome should have their blood pressure measured at the beginning and the end of the visit to get a more representative value. To deal with anxious patients, use the communication skills you have learned in this chapter: speak calmly, reassure patients, smile, touch them respectfully on the hand, and be empathetic.

Patients with Special Needs

Meeting the needs of these patients requires some extra sensitivity, patience, and empathy on the part of the medical assistant. We will consider several types of patients individually along with some procedural guidelines.

The Hearing Impaired Patient

Hearing loss can vary from a slight loss to total deafness. Total hearing impairment is considered by many to be the most difficult of all handicaps since it keeps people isolated from communication and social interaction. If a child cannot hear, he or she will have difficulty speaking since learning speech involves imitating speech of others. Many such people communicate by means of sign language. Basic sign language is not difficult to learn. Simple phrases in sign language should be a part of every medical professional's knowledge base.

The manner in which you try to communicate will differ depending on whether the patient has a hearing aid, can lip-read, or has a family member or aid with him or her. Loss of hearing is a normal but frustrating sign of aging. The following are some guidelines to help the hearing impaired.

- Select a quiet environment to communicate with the patient.
- Reduce outside noise as much as possible.
- Never shout. Speak slowly and clearly.
- If the patient does not understand you the first time, rephrase the statement.
- Explain everything carefully before performing a procedure.
- Face the patient when speaking.
- Have a paper and pen available so that the patient can communicate in writing.

Basic hearing tests or screening tests are often performed by the medical assistant in the physician's office. An audiogram may be ordered by the physician when there is a suspicion of moderate to severe hearing loss. This test will determine the faintest sounds a patient can hear during audiometric testing. Audiometric testing, conducted by an audiologist, tests hearing ability by determining the lowest and highest intensity and frequencies that a person can distinguish. The patient may sit in a soundproof booth and receive sounds through earphones as the technician decreases the sounds or tones. Procedure 4-2 provides the steps for you to employ with the hearing impaired patient.

4-2 **PROCEDURE**

Assisting the Hearing Impaired Patient

OBJECTIVE: Use effective communication skills to assist a hearing impaired patient prepare for a physical examination.

Equipment and Supplies
none

Method
1. Identify patient.
2. Reduce external noise as much as possible.
3. Smile and establish eye contact and face patient.
4. Speak slowly and do not shout.
5. Provide careful explanation of procedure.
6. Provide paper and pencil for patient to use if desired.
7. Use written information for the patient to reinforce message.
8. Have patient repeat your response to ensure accuracy of message, if possible.
9. Give directions using actions as well as words.
10. Be sensitive to patient's needs.
11. Employ an empathetic, professional attitude.
12. Notify physician of patient's concerns.

The Visually Impaired Patient

Blindness can be present at birth or may develop as a result of a disease such as diabetes mellitus. Patients who are blind can remain independent. The visually impaired patient cannot rely on nonverbal cues that make up much of the communication process for those with sight. The medical assistant can communicate and help the vision impaired patient by remembering to follow the guidelines suggested.

- Always speak to announce your presence when you are near a blind person.
- Offer to guide the patient into the examination room by offering your arm. Do not grab the patient without offering your arm first.
- Face the patient and speak clearly.
- Describe the patient's surroundings.
- Explain all procedures in detail before beginning.
- Try not to leave the patient alone for any length of time.
- Have available large print educational materials for patients who might benefit from them.
- Do not be condescending toward the patient.

The Terminally Ill Patient

The medical assistant will come into contact with patients who have a terminal illness. A terminal illness is one that is expected to end in death. This includes conditions and diseases such as cancer, acquired immune deficiency syndrome (AIDS), progressive heart disease, amyotrophic lateral sclerosis (Lou Gehrig's disease), cystic fibrosis, and multiple sclerosis. In such cases in which the dying process is slow for the patient, the medical assistant may encounter the patient on several office visits. While there is always hope for recovery or finding a cure through research for a disease such as AIDS, it is wise to listen to a patient express his or her fears and concerns rather than to offer false hope for a recovery. Death is a natural process that everyone must face. People have different ways of coping with death based on a variety of influences including culture, religion, personal experience, and age.

Religious, Cultural, and Personal Experience

People learn what their own culture expects of them at a very early age by observing family and friends as they handle life events such as births and deaths. In some cultures, death is considered a normal end to the life process and accepted with peace. In others, death may be feared. The terminally ill patient and family may have already established a very personal approach or method for handling death and dying. The medical assistant may also have a strong cultural attitude toward death.

Religious beliefs play an important role in the manner patients handle death and dying. Some patients will have a strong belief in an afterlife. Other patients will follow no particular religious belief. In both cases, the patient's death and dying process can be meaningful and peaceful. It is considered unacceptable for the medical assistant to attempt to convert the patient to the medical assistant's religious faith. Professionalism mandates that the medical assistant and other staff members recognize and support the patient's right to embrace his or her own religious beliefs. Table 4-7 provides a comparison of religious beliefs about birth, death, and health care practices.

The past experiences of the patient and the medical assistant will mold how they approach the topic of death. If the patient has been closely involved with the care of someone who has died a painful death, the patient may fear the same type of death for himself or herself. These patients will need to be able to discuss their fears. In the same manner, if the medical assistant has had past experiences with the death of friends or relatives, it may be easier for him or her to assist the patient.

The Stages of Grief

Dr. Elizabeth Kübler-Ross devoted much of her life to the study of the dying process and to working with dying patients. She divided the dying process into five stages that she believed all persons go through. It is helpful to understand these stages when attempting to help the dying patient. According to Kübler-Ross, all those involved with the dying process may go through five stages. This would include the patient, family members, and caregivers (such as the medical assistant).

The five stages are denial, anger, bargaining, depression, and acceptance. The stages may overlap and may not be experienced by everyone in the stated order but are all present in the dying patient according to Kübler-Ross. The five stages are discussed in Table 4-8.

As the time of death approaches, some of the earlier stages may be repeated. For example, patients may become angry when they are not able to care for themselves. The critical point to remember when assisting a patient who is dying is that the grieving period is a normal part of the dying process. At no time should the medical assistant try to tell the patient, "Don't feel that way." A patient has a right to have his or her feelings accepted unconditionally.

Hospice care, which is physical and emotional care provided to the dying person and his or her family, is a growing movement throughout the United States. The medical assistant should be acquainted with this option of care for the terminally ill.

The Mentally/Emotionally Impaired Patient

Psychology is the science of behavior and the human thought process. This behavioral science is primarily concerned with human beings acting alone or in groups.

TABLE 4-7 Religious Beliefs about Birth, Death, and Health Care

Religion	Beliefs about Birth	Beliefs about Death	Health Care Beliefs
Christian, Roman Catholic	Infant baptism is mandatory. Baptism necessary for salvation. Any Christian may perform emergency baptism.	Sacrament of anointing the sick (last rites) performed by priest. Autopsy, organ donation, and cremation permitted.	Life is sacred. Abortion and contraception prohibited. Rite of communion important.
Hinduism	No ritual at birth.	Believe in reincarnation as humans, animals, or plants. Priest ties thread around neck or wrist of deceased, pour water in mouth. Only family or friends may wash the body. Autopsy, organ donation up to individual. Cremation preferred.	Illness as punishment for sins is a belief held by some. Faith healing important to some. Will accept most medical treatments, advice.
Islam (Muslim)	No ritual at birth. Circumcision at 7 days.	Family must be present at death. Dying person must ask forgiveness of sins. Body turned toward Mecca after death. Autopsy only if required by law. Organ donation permitted. Cremation not allowed.	Illness is atonement for sins. May pray facing toward Mecca five times a day (southeastern direction in United States). Ritual washing before and after prayer. Must take medications with right hand only, left hand considered dirty.
Jehovah's Witness (Christian)	No infant baptism.	No last rites. Autopsy only when required by law and body parts must not be removed. Organ donation discouraged. Cremation permitted.	May not receive blood or blood products. Church elders pray for healing. Medications permitted if not derived from blood products.
Judaism (Orthodox)	No infant baptism, circumcision by mohel (circumcisor), child's father, or Jewish physician.	Person should never die alone. Body is ritually cleaned and dead must be buried within 24 hours. Organ donation only by permission of rabbi. Cremation forbidden.	May refuse treatments on Sabbath or holy days. Family may want to bury body parts surgically removed. Ritual hand washing on rising and before eating.

There is a distinction between normal and abnormal behavior when studying psychology. All social interactions such as those that occur during the communication process may pose a problem for some people. The medical assistant will encounter patients, family members, staff, and caregivers who exhibit a wide scope of behavior patterns. These behavior patterns may be due to diseases, mental disorders, anxiety, drug abuse, trauma, the aging process, cultural customs, or a combination of several of these causes. The medical assistant must be tolerant and respectful of others in all circumstances.

When dealing with an emotionally or mentally impaired patient, it is important to determine, if possible, what level of communication the patient can understand. Often by observing the patient with a caregiver, if there is one, you will get clues on how to communicate with the patient. Speak slowly and clearly, stay calm, and keep your messages short. If you have to touch the patient for a procedure be sure to explain

TABLE 4-8 Five Stages of Grief

Stage	Description
Denial	A refusal to believe that dying is taking place. This may be a time when the patient (or family member) needs time to adjust to the reality of approaching death. This stage cannot be hurried.
Anger	At this stage, the patient may be angry at everyone and may express this intense anger at God, family, and even health care professionals. The patient may take this anger out on the closest person to him or her. Usually this is a family member. In reality the patient is angry about dying.
Bargaining	The third stage of grief involves attempting to gain time by making promises in return. Bargaining may be done between the patient and God. The patient may indicate a need to talk at this stage.
Depression	This stage is marked with a deep sadness over the loss of health, independence, and eventually life. There is an additional sadness of leaving loved ones behind. The grieving patient may become withdrawn at this time.
Acceptance	The acceptance stage is reached when there is a sense of peace and calm. The patient may make comments such as, "I have no regrets. I'm ready to die." It is better to let the patient talk and not make denial statements such as, "Don't talk like that. You're not going to die."

what you are doing first. Ask the caregiver for assistance in calming the patient, if possible.

The Non-English Speaking Patient

As mentioned in the previous discussion of cultural diversity, the non-English speaking patient is at a disadvantage in the medical environment. You should employ the communication skills discussed previously and consider the following guidelines: smile at the patient, determine if he or she has any ability to speak or understand English, speak in normal tones, use pantomime or pictures to demonstrate, and ask assistance of a family member.

Intraoffice Communication

The goal in the medical office should be to establish a sense of rapport—an environment of cooperation—with patients, coworkers, supervisors, and vendors. To create this cooperative environment, all of the communication skills we have examined in this chapter will need to be utilized.

Establishing Trust

In order to communicate effectively in the health care environment and in everyday life, we must establish trust in our relationships. Being open, honest, and firm in our convictions, presenting a professional image, and using positive body language, help create a positive environment. Some of the most difficult communication problems occur with other staff members (Figure 4-8). Good staff communication depends on positive respectful

interactions. When thoughtless or condescending comments are made, permanent damage to relationships can occur. To be condescending is to adopt a superior attitude and act as though you are better than someone else. Withdrawing from the group, feeling angry and hurt, and discussing other staff members behind their backs causes office morale to suffer. Using assertive behavior with fellow staff means that you assert your own needs without threatening theirs. For instance, if it is your turn to have a holiday off and you have been scheduled to work, it is better to state, "I'm sorry I can't work that day. Since I worked overtime on the last holiday, I have made plans for this one." An aggressive statement, such as, "It's not fair. I always have to work on holidays and the others don't," would imply that favoritism or special

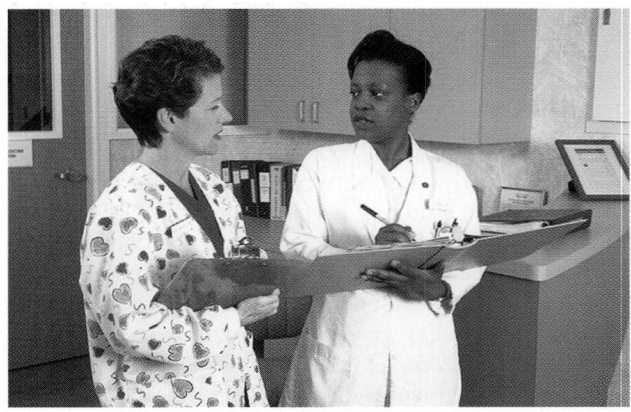

FIGURE 4-8 Staff members often find it difficult to communicate with other coworkers.

treatment has been shown to some staff members and might cause the supervisor to become defensive.

Rapport and Team Building

A positive attitude can make the difference between keeping and losing a job. A positive attitude is easier to project if you are happy in your work. The work group you are a part of is an important factor in your attitude. Work groups need to become a cohesive team. In order to do this, some degree of socializing is beneficial. Discussions about hobbies, travel, sports, family, and friends with other staff members help to establish an atmosphere of trust and understanding. However, the social aspect of staff communication should not interfere with work productivity.

Gossip is unnecessary, often negative conversation usually about someone who is not present. The medical assistant needs to learn to recognize gossip and not participate in it. Gossip can be extremely hurtful and is destructive to the atmosphere of cooperation needed in the medical facility.

Research has found that patients who have established a good relationship with their physicians and office staff are less willing to bring a lawsuit against them. It goes without saying that patients must always be provided quality medical care. However, courteous treatment of patients does pay extra dividends.

Patient as a Consumer

The patient today needs to be viewed as a consumer of health care. Patients and family members are more knowledgeable about health care options because of the Internet and other media. They no longer place the physician on a pedestal as older patients may have done when physicians made house calls. In fact, many patients can experience a certain amount of alienation from their health care providers because most physicians are specialists. Specialization can lead to viewing the patient as the sum of his or her injury or procedure—"a broken leg" or "appendectomy"—a viewpoint that is degrading. Instead, the patient should be treated holistically, and with dignity and respect. Medical assistants are the first to encounter the patient in many instances. Therefore, they are responsible for the initial impression the patient has of the practice or facility. The concept of "the customer comes first" should be a primary goal for all health care providers and needs to be considered to sustain a satisfied client base. Communication with other physicians, hospitals, and clinics is vitally important to the economic stability of practices and facilities.

Staff Arrangements

Staffing arrangements are as varied as the types of medical practices. The solo practice with its staff of one, the multi-physician practice with a variety of staff, including an office manager, the clinic with many registered nurses (RNs), and other types of allied health care workers are only a few of the types of practices in which the medical assistant may work. Regardless of the type of practice, communication is vitally important to keep conflict at a minimum, establish a positive environment, and provide quality health care.

Whatever the staffing arrangements, the physician/office manager must be clear about the chain of command and convey that information to the employees. In the solo office with one medical assistant, there is usually no problem. However, in larger practices, the health care professional with most seniority is often the unofficial office manager. This person may not be the most qualified, the most multiskilled, or an accomplished manager. Friction among coworkers is often a common problem in many of these larger practices. To avoid this problem, clearly defined areas of responsibility and authority should be established. The office policy and procedure manual can help resolve conflict about authority and responsibility.

Conflict Resolution

Inevitably there will be strife and conflict among coworkers. The procedure and policy manual is a valuable tool to begin to resolve issues. It should state clearly what standards are acceptable in all areas of the facility. Conflicts occur when there is miscommunication or misunderstanding of the message. Conflict also can occur when there are prejudices or preconceived ideas. Conflict interferes with establishing rapport and cooperation, which are essential in the workplace. To avoid conflict on a personal level, it would be helpful for you not to engage in gossip and to avoid the "downer," the negative person in the office who will try to bring you down to his or her level of pessimism. Conflict can be positive if it resolves issues of disagreement in an appropriate manner.

Critical Thinking and Problem Solving

Problem solving and critical thinking are necessary skills for health care workers. Problem solving is a way of looking at a problem and ultimately arriving at a decision. Box 4-2 lists the steps to evaluate the factors and risks involved in solving problems. Most problems have more than one solution. Weighing all the factors involved and evaluating the results will help later with other problems.

Critical thinking (Box 4-3) includes the ability to think imaginatively, solve problems, visualize situations, learn new information, and think logically. Both problem solving and critical thinking skills are important concepts to employ before trying to resolve any conflict. Box 4-4 illustrates the steps in conflict resolution.

BOX 4-2
Steps for Problem Solving

- Recognize that a problem exists. Recognition may result from a feeling, observation, or conversation with others.
- Describe the problem and clarify what the basic issue or question is and the factors that affect it.
- Identify alternative methods of resolving the problem. Any alternative can be considered even if is not immediately seen as practical.
- Choose the best method for resolving the problem and implement it.
- As the plan is being put into affect, evaluate the results and adjust the method if necessary.

BOX 4-3
Elements of Critical Thinking

- Ask questions
- Define a problem
- Examine evidence
- Avoid emotional reasoning
- Analyze assumptions and bias
- Avoid oversimplification
- Consider other interpretations
- Tolerate ambiguity
- Think about one's own thinking

BOX 4-4
Steps in Conflict Resolution

- Communicate your needs in simple terms.
- Know when to express your feelings.
- Do not assume you know the other person's feelings.
- Look at the issue from the other person's perspective.

Office Procedure and Policy Manual

A policy and procedure manual is a collection of policies and procedures for carrying out day-to-day operations in an office or facility and a vital instrument of communication in the medical office. The manual should be available to every employee, full time or part time, and must be updated on a regular basis. Every clinical procedure performed in the office should be included. For example, the procedure manual should include, but not be limited by, the following: step-by-step procedures for every test performed in the office including all reagents and calculations; quality control policies, normal values, and location and maintenance of instrumentation used. All policies related to hiring, firing, employee evaluation, personal records, job descriptions, dress code, supplies, maintenance of equipment, and rules and regulations should be included in the policy manual. The availability of policy and procedure manual to all personnel contributes to a more smoothly run office.

The Difficult Employee

A difficult or problem employee may disrupt the flow of work in an office. Negativity becomes contagious if there are no policies in place to deal with the difficult employee. Consulting the policy manual, meeting individually with the employee to obtain her side of the problem, setting goals for the employee, all may reduce the conflict. All meetings should be documented in case the positive steps recommended to the employee are not effective and termination is necessary.

Staff Meetings

Establishing a regularly scheduled staff meeting is an important step in having a smoothly functioning office. One of the most frequent complaints office managers receive is from employees who want to meet with physician/physicians and have some consistent way to address questions and concerns. The frequency of staff meetings is directly related to the type of practice, the number of staff, the office schedule, and the willingness of the practice managers/physicians.

There are many types of staff meetings. Some practices use lunch/coffee break time to gather staff. Others schedule them before or after working hours. A staff meeting may be held to offer in-service training on new equipment, updates on new procedures, to celebrate a holiday or special occasion, or any other reason office management deem appropriate. To have a successful staff meeting, you should have an agenda available ahead of time, stick to the agenda, and not let the meeting end in a gripe session. Chapter 18 will cover office management in detail.

Scope of Practice Issues

As a medical assistant, you are truly a multiskilled health care provider and are capable of functioning throughout a facility in many different areas. From the clinical

TABLE 4-9 Responses that Communicate Loyalty

Question/Comment	Sample Response
"I guess Dr. Thompson can't see me on Wednesday because he's playing golf."	"Dr. Thompson's day off is Wednesday, but he could see you on Saturday."
"I hear Dr. Thompson and his wife are divorcing?"	"I really have no information about Dr. Thompson's personal life."
"I've been waiting one hour to see Dr. Thompson. Why is he so slow?"	"I'm sorry you've had a long wait. Dr. Thompson has had many very ill patients today. May I reschedule your appointment?"

area where you have direct patient contact, to working in the front office, and including your handling of administrative procedures, you are cross-trained to effectively perform all of these duties. Other employees, like registered nurses (RNs) and licensed practical nurses (LPNs) who are working in the facility, may only be able to handle the clinical areas. Medical secretaries, coding, and billing employees usually can only perform the administrative functions. Because of your multifunctional training, you may encounter some jealousy or resentment from other staff members. It is important to work within your own scope of practice and job description. In other words, do not perform skills that are beyond your training. On the other hand, don't be afraid to promote your profession and all that it stands for.

Communicating with Superiors

In dealing with your superiors as with your coworkers, communication should be kept positive. If conflicts do arise and you need to speak with your superior, choose an appropriate time or ask for an appointment to speak with him or her. Be direct and to the point and do not promote any gossip you may have heard. If you have been given an order to do something and you need clarification on how to complete it, be sure to ask for help. Most supervisors would rather be asked a question than to have you perform a function about which you are not clear. Show initiative in your daily work. If a task needs to be done, volunteer to do it without being asked as long as it falls within your job description. Too often staff members are too busy keeping score of which employees do more or less work as compared to others.

Loyalty to Your Employer

You represent your employer or physician every time you speak to a patient or caller. You must support the physician and his or her reputation in every instance. In your position, you may become privileged to personal information about your employer. Under no circumstances, whether inside or outside of the office,

should that personal information be discussed. It is perfectly acceptable to state, "I really can't answer that," or "I'm sorry, but I don't know," in response to a patient's or other staff member's questions.

A loyal employee protects and defends an employer when other employees engage in negative conversation. See Table 4-9 for examples of loyal responses to questions or comments about your employer's personal life.

Communication and Patients' Rights

Every patient has the right to privacy and confidentiality. Any information dealing with a patient is considered privileged information. The American Hospital Association developed a statement called "The Patient's Bill of Rights," which describes the patient-physician relationship. Table 4-10 lists these rights. A copy of the "Patient's Bill of Rights" should be in every health care facility.

Confidentiality

All patients have the right to have their personal privacy respected and their medical records handled with confidentiality. Any information such as test results, patient histories, and even the fact that the patient is a patient, cannot be told to another person. No information can be given over the telephone without the patient's permission or unless a court has subpoenaed it. Your treatment and concern for the patient reflects the physician's high standards of care. The human dignity of each patient must be preserved regardless of the patient's socioeconomic background, race, age, nationality, sexual orientation, or gender.

Health Insurance Portability and Accountability Act (HIPAA)

The Health Insurance Portability and Accountability Act (HIPAA), previously mentioned, was passed in 1996 by Congress. The HIPAA Privacy Rule, which is

TABLE 4-10 Patient's Bill of Rights

1. The patient has the right to considerate and respectful care.

2. The patient has the right to and is encouraged to obtain from physicians and other direct caregivers relevant, current, understandable information concerning diagnosis, treatment, and prognosis.

3. The patient has the right to make decisions about the plan of care prior to and during the course of treatment and to refuse a recommended treatment or plan of care to the extent permitted by law and hospital policy and to be informed of the consequences of this action.

4. The patient has the right to have an advance directive (such as a living will, health care proxy, or durable power of attorney for health care) concerning treatment or designating a surrogate decision maker with the expectation that the hospital will honor the intent of that directive to the extent permitted by law and hospital policy.

5. The patient has the right to every consideration of privacy.

6. The patient has the right to expect that all communications and records pertaining to his or her care will be treated as confidential by the hospital, except in cases such as suspected abuse and public health hazards when reporting is permitted or required by law.

7. The patient has the right to review the records pertaining to his or her medical care and to have the information explained or interpreted as necessary, except when restricted by law.

8. The patient has the right to expect that, within its capacity and policies, a hospital will make reasonable response to the request of a patient for appropriate and medically indicated care and service.

9. The patient has the right to ask and be informed of the existence of business relationships among the hospital, educational institutions, other health care providers, or players that may influence the patient's treatment or care.

10. The patient has the right to consent to or decline to participate in proposed research studies or human experimentation affecting care and treatment or requiring direct patient involvement, and to have those studies fully explained prior to consent.

11. The patient has the right to expect reasonable continuity of care when appropriate and to be informed by physicians and other caregivers of available and realistic patient care options when hospital care is no longer appropriate.

12. The patient has the right to be informed of hospital policies and practices that relate to patient care, treatment, and responsibilities.

---

a part of HIPAA, provides for the federal protection of health information. This rule, while protecting patients' privacy, also allows for patients to have better access to their medical records and to have more control about how and to whom the information can be released. HIPAA designates the following information as protected health information or PHI:

- Name
- Address
- Phone numbers
- Fax numbers
- Dates (birth, death, admission, discharge, etc.)
- Social Security number
- E-mail address
- Medical record numbers

- Health plan beneficiary numbers
- Account numbers
- Certificate or license numbers
- Vehicle identifiers, serial numbers, and license plate numbers
- Device identifiers and serial numbers
- Web Universal Resource Locators (URLs)
- Internet Protocol (IP) address numbers

This means that any or all of this information cannot be given out by any means (electronic, paper, or orally) for any reason without the written authorization of the patient. The written authorization covers any information necessary for treatment, payment, and operations (TPO). If you are in doubt whether to release personal patient information, do not do it.

Check and make sure that you have obtained the appropriate authorization.

Appropriate Documentation

One way to reduce the risk of lawsuits is to document appropriately. The patient's record is a source of communication both within and outside the office necessary to provide the best quality of care. Keep in mind these steps to better documentation:

- Use the patient's own words.
- Use precise descriptions, incorporating acceptable terminology and abbreviations, and write clearly.
- Provide complete information on all forms.
- Be brief and clear when documenting and spell correctly.
- Date all entries.
- Sign all entries.
- Use ink.
- Correct and sign all charting errors appropriately.
- Maintain confidentiality.

Advising Patients

As a medical assistant, you are the physician's representative. Because you are part of the staff, wear a uniform, and assist with treatments, patients may view you as an authority figure. The physician advises the patient on a course of treatment or procedure based on his or her examination and diagnostic test results. You are not permitted to offer your opinion about the physician's diagnosis, the course of action the physician has set forth, or tell the patient what you would do in his or her position. Those opinions are beyond your scope of practice and could put you and the physician at risk of being sued. If asked by a patient, "What would you do if you were me?" you must not offer advice. Explain to the patient that the physician will be pleased to review the course of action, answer any questions, and that you will be happy to arrange for that meeting. A medical assistant giving advice to a patient could be construed as "practicing medicine without a license" and is an offense in most states.

Patient Decision Making

Patients who have received bad news from the physician or are faced with difficult choices do need help to come to a decision. Your role is to listen empathetically to the patient, ask him or her reflecting or clarifying questions, and make clear the information the physician has related to the patient to help him or her come to a decision on a course of treatment. For example, Mrs. Santos has been told by the physician that her breast biopsy was positive and mastectomy is recom-

mended as soon as possible. When the physician leaves the room, she asks you what she should do. Your response should be, "Mrs. Santos, you seem upset about having to have a mastectomy. What is concerning you about the procedure?" If she asks what you would do in her circumstances, suggest that she get a second opinion or offer to explain again in simple terms what the doctor has said. Sometimes patients are so nervous in the presence of a physician that they do not hear information correctly. It would be permissible to give her written information about the procedure, offer to bring her concerns to the physician, and encourage her to call back once she is home if she has more questions.

Risk Management

The term risk management refers to reducing the physician's risk of lawsuit in the medical setting. As a medical assistant, dealing so closely with patients, you are in a position to help reduce those risks. Communicating effectively with the patient is certainly one of primary ways to reduce the risk of being sued. On the other hand, any promise or commitment that you make to a patient can be legally binding to the physician who employs you. This means that the physician can be held responsible for something you have said or implied to the patient with regard to how the physician might improve the patient's condition. Keep all matters relating to patients' personal health information confidential. If you believe that any health professional is acting in an unethical or unprofessional manner, you should discuss this with your employer or another physician. For example, a comment such as "Did Miss Jones come in for her pregnancy test?" can result in a breach of confidentiality lawsuit against the physician if it is overheard by others.

Communication and Patient Education

The medical assistant is in a position to promote patient education. You are the staff person who interacts with the patient and spends more time with him or her than many of the other staff members. Effective communication is the goal in all interpersonal dealings. Often it falls to the medical assistant to have to explain again what the physician has already said to the patient. Many times the patient is too anxious when the physician is speaking to him or her to fully comprehend what is being said. The medical assistant should be careful not to promise outcomes. Your job is to reinforce what the physician has said, not change it. See Patient Education for additional ways to educate your patients.

Setting Goals

At times the medical assistant has to assume the role of patient educator to ensure that the patient is following through with the recommended treatments or

Patient education must be presented in a manner suited to the patient. In most cases, direct contact between the learner (patient) and the instructor (medical assistant) provides the best atmosphere for learning. As a medical assistant, it will be a great advantage if you are able to use the communication techniques discussed in this chapter effectively.

Life style changes can greatly affect the ability to acquire new information and some patients may use several barriers to block communication such as rationalization and denial. A patient concerned over a life-threatening diagnosis may not be in a receptive mood for education or

instruction. If you sense that a patient's uncooperativeness comes from defensive or anxious behavior, you may be able to draw the person out using open-ended questions. With a mutual trust established, it is more likely that needed instruction can be given.

Brochures and pamphlets can also be helpful for explaining health care issues. Material should be clearly and simply written. The patient with a language barrier will need an interpreter when an explanation regarding treatment or medications is given. Free brochures are available to physicians through organizations, such as American Diabetes Association.

instructions. To this end your role may become that of "cheerleader" to encourage the compliance of the patient. Before a patient can follow through with a plan, the goals of the plan must be set. The physician sets the goal and you will reinforce it with the patient. Keep the goals simple and small. If the patient needs to lose weight to lower his or her blood pressure, it is not realistic to expect the patient to lose 5 pounds every week.

Compliance and Wellness

Health care today is frequently more wellness care than illness care. Much of the time the physician is trying to encourage healthy life styles that lead to better health overall. Often times it has been said, "if I could only give patients a pill for motivation," it would be

easy. Unfortunately, this isn't possible. Positive communication—the rapport and comfort level you establish with the patient—has a direct bearing on patients' compliance with the goals that have been set. The tools already learned in this chapter can play a big role in compliance. Positive feedback—a smile, a word of praise, or a pat on the back—can help to further compliance. Be sure that you follow up on the patient's progress to encourage his or her new wellness behaviors. Written information is a powerful tool in educating the patient. However, the medical assistant should review the information with the patient to ensure that he or she understands what is written. The medical assistant should be a role model for the patient in behavior, dress, and promoting wellness.

SUMMARY

Communication is a necessary requirement for everyday living. In the health care field, the ability to communicate effectively is essential for success—for example, to call and request a prescription be renewed, to document the patient's symptoms and help the patient be diagnosed properly, to provide patient education, to arrange travel plans for the physician. The concern you have for patients will come through

in your words, actions, gestures, and your tone of voice. The special needs of some patients may not be the presenting problems when they arrive in the physician's office. However, these special needs must be dealt with to accommodate the patients as much as possible. The medical assistant must remain flexible and learn to be able to handle all unusual situations professionally.

Chapter Review

COMPETENCY REVIEW

1. Define and spell the terms to learn for this chapter.
2. Explain what you would say to a patient who says that the medication Dr. Thompson gave her last week have made her sick.
3. Explain what you would say to the patient who is angry at the delay in the waiting room.
4. Explain what you would say to the patient who complains to you about Dr. Thompson.

5. What are Kübler-Ross's five stages of dying and why are they important to know?
6. Describe how to communicate to a profoundly deaf patient that or she must remove all clothing and put on a gown.
7. Describe some cultural problems that can arise when treating patients from other cultures.
8. List five impressions you believe non-Americans have of U.S. citizens.
9. Discuss several defense mechanisms that you feel you sometimes exhibit. How do they impact negatively on your relationships with others?
10. Mary Brown's neighbor calls to see if she kept her appointment because she says Mary is sometimes forgetful. What would you say?

PREPARING FOR THE CERTIFICATION EXAM

1. The basic units of the communication process are
   A. source, message, receiver, patient
   B. message, receiver
   C. channel, message, receiver, patient
   D. receiver, message, source
   E. source, message, channel, receiver

2. A nonverbal form of communication would include
   A. doing one thing at a time
   B. smiling and saying, "Hi"
   C. finishing a sentence for a patient
   D. interrupting a patient
   E. folding one's arms across one's chest

3. Consider the statement a medical assistant might make to a patient: "You say you are still in pain from your hysterectomy. On a scale of 1 to 10, with 1 being very little pain and 10 being the worst you could imagine, how would you rank your pain level at this moment?" What directive communication technique is this statement?
   A. open-ended statement
   B. closed-ended statement
   C. reflective statement
   D. acknowledgment
   E. seeking clarification

4. Which of the following statements regarding assertive versus aggressive behavior is FALSE?
   A. assertiveness is generally considered a very positive form of communication
   B. aggressiveness is generally considered a very negative form of communication
   C. assertiveness can be compared to a verbal attack against another person
   D. aggressiveness can be compared to a verbal attack against another person

E. assertiveness is trying to impose ones point of view on others

5. Placing your own feelings onto another person is an example of which of the following defensive behaviors?
   A. rationalization
   B. projection
   C. compensation
   D. displaced anger
   E. disassociation

6. When dealing with a very angry patient, which of the following statements would be BEST to defuse the situation?
   A. "I am very sorry there was an error on your billing statement. Let me see if our billing clerk can fix it while you are here."
   B. "Please come back when you are less angry. It will be easier to talk to you then."
   C. "I will not listen to you while you are expressing your anger, but I will listen soon as soon as you calm down."
   D. "I think you are feeling angry because, without a medical background like mine, you simply do not understand the situation."
   E. "I am going to refer you to my supervisor."

7. What is the best way to help a blind patient?
   A. Take the patient by the arm and lead him or her into an examination room.
   B. Speak loudly to the patient so he or she can hear you since the patient cannot read your lips.
   C. Offer your arm for the patient to take.
   D. Allow the patient to remain independent by doing as little as possible to help.
   E. Tell the patient not to go outside without assistance.

continued on next page

8. When assisting patients who have a terminal disease, the BEST method is to
   A. allow them to talk about it
   B. do not allow them to dwell on the depressing subject of death
   C. encourage them by telling them they look wonderful
   D. avoid them
   E. speak loudly and clearly

9. Defensive behavior
   A. is conscious or unconscious
   B. can alienate the patient
   C. is a natural but unacceptable response
   D. is encouraged at times
   E. is on office policy

CRITICAL THINKING

1. What should Susan do to make Mrs. Brown feel more at ease once Susan has acknowledged her presence?

2. How could the staff at Dr. Barry's office avoid making the same mistake with other patients? What would have made Mrs. Brown feel more comfortable on her first visit?

3. Have you ever experienced the same problem in a physician's office and how did it make you feel? What did you do? What would have made you feel more comfortable?

4. If you were the office manager of Dr. Barry's office, what steps would you take to correct this problem?

5. What issues discussed in this chapter are illustrated in this case study?

ON THE JOB

Amy Freeman is a new medical assistant who has recently passed the CMA examination. She has studied Dr. Kübler-Ross's five stages of dying and believes they make sense. Renee Baker, a young mother of two small children, has an appointment to see Dr. Williams for follow-up care after having been diagnosed with terminal ovarian cancer. Renee bitterly tells Amy that she is angry at the doctors for not diagnosing her condition sooner; angry at God for allowing this to happen; angry at her husband for not being more supportive; and angry at herself for not demanding better health care.

Since Renee has opened up to Amy about her feelings, Amy wants to try to help her. What should Amy do?

1. Keeping in mind Dr. Kübler-Ross's five stages of dying, what exactly should Amy say to Renee?

2. Does Amy have a responsibility to inform the physician?

INTERNET ACTIVITY

Perform a search for information on hospice care. What information can you discover that will help you communicate with Renee, the terminal ovarian cancer patient, in the above On the Job exercise?

MediaLink  More on communication in the medical office environment, including interactive resources, can be found on the Student CD-ROM accompanying this textbook.

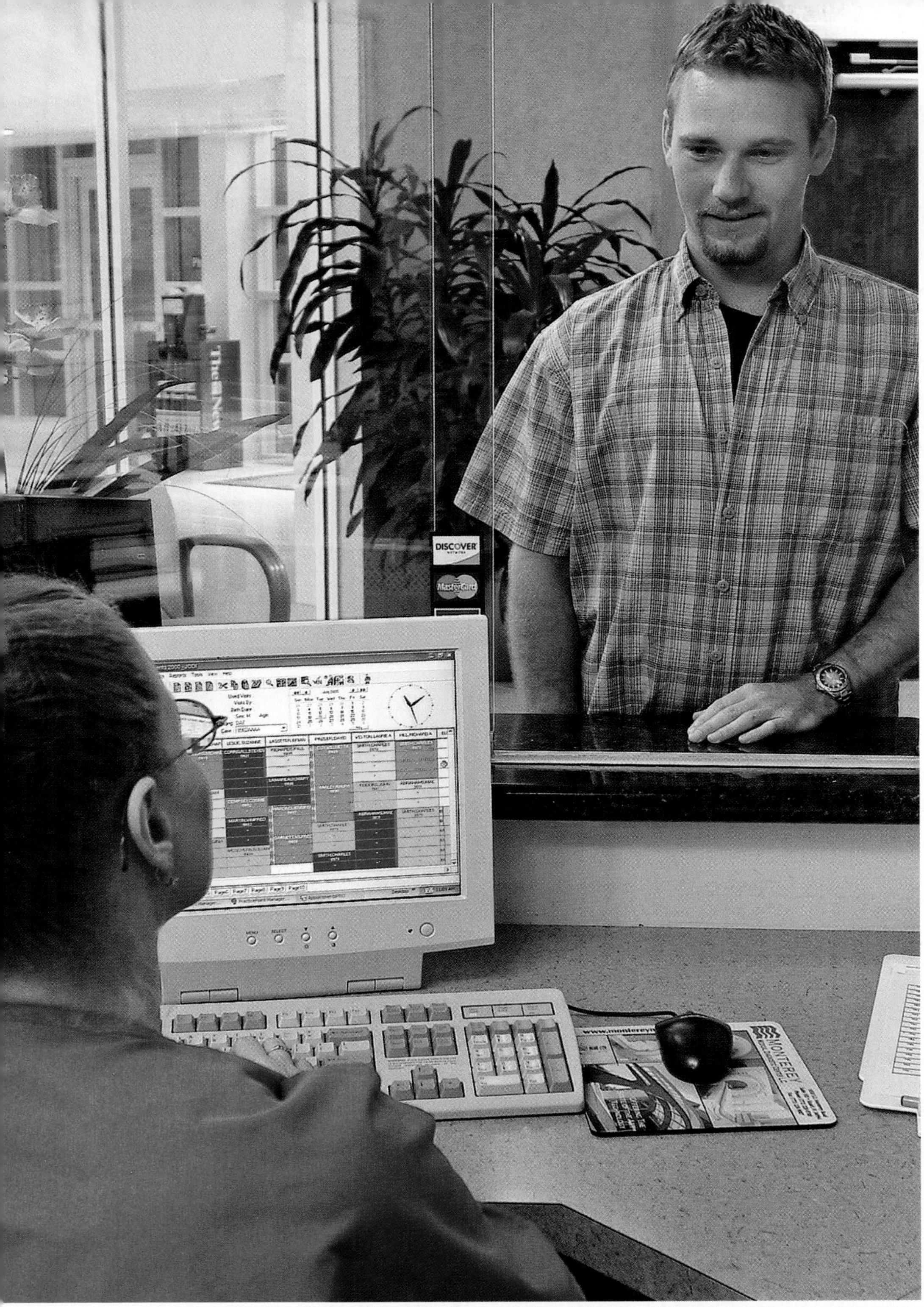

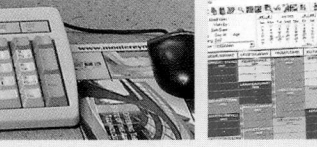

Unit Two

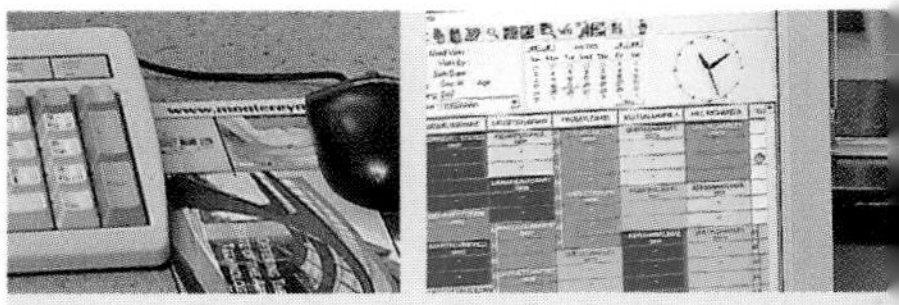

Administrative Medical Assisting

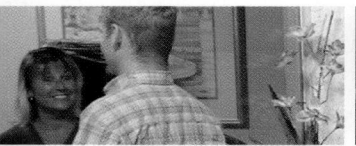 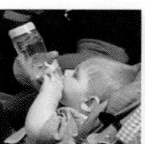 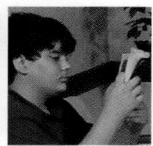

Medical Assistant Role Delineation Chart

HIGHLIGHT indicates material covered in this chapter.

ADMINISTRATIVE

Administrative Procedures

- Perform basic administrative medical assisting functions
- Schedule, coordinate and monitor appointments
- Schedule inpatient/outpatient admissions and procedures
- Understand and apply third-party guidelines
- Obtain reimbursement through accurate claims submission
- Monitor third-party reimbursement
- Understand and adhere to managed care policies and procedures
- *Negotiate managed care contracts*

Practice Finances

- Perform procedural and diagnostic coding
- Apply bookkeeping principles

- Manage accounts receivable
- *Manage accounts payable*
- *Process payroll*
- *Document and maintain accounting and banking records*
- *Develop and maintain fee schedules*
- *Manage renewals of business and professional insurance policies*
- *Manage personnel benefits and maintain records*
- *Perform marketing, financial, and strategic planning*

CLINICAL

Fundamental Principles

- Apply principles of aseptic technique and infection control
- Comply with quality assurance practices
- Screen and follow up patient test results

Diagnostic Orders

- Collect and process specimens
- Perform diagnostic tests

Patient Care

- Adhere to established patient screening procedures
- Obtain patient history and vital signs
- Prepare and maintain examination and treatment areas
- Prepare patient for examinations, procedures and treatments

- Assist with examinations, procedures and treatments
- Prepare and administer medications and immunizations
- Maintain medication and immunization records
- Recognize and respond to emergencies
- Coordinate patient care information with other health care providers
- Initiate IV and administer IV medications with appropriate training and as permitted by state law

GENERAL

Professionalism

- Display a professional manner and image
- Demonstrate initiative and responsibility
- Work as a member of the health care team
- Prioritize and perform multiple tasks
- Adapt to change
- Promote the CMA credential
- Enhance skills through continuing education
- Treat all patients with compassion and empathy
- Promote the practice through positive public relations

Communication Skills

- Recognize and respect cultural diversity
- Adapt communications to individual's ability to understand
- Use professional telephone technique

- Recognize and respond effectively to verbal, nonverbal, and written communications
- Use medical terminology appropriately
- Utilize electronic technology to receive, organize, prioritize and transmit information
- Serve as liaison

Legal Concepts

- Perform within legal and ethical boundaries
- Prepare and maintain medical records
- Document accurately
- Follow employer's established policies dealing with the health care contract
- Implement and maintain federal and state health care legislation and regulations
- Comply with established risk management and safety procedures
- Recognize professional credentialing criteria
- *Develop and maintain personnel, policy and procedure manuals*

Instruction

- Instruct individuals according to their needs
- Explain office policies and procedures
- Teach methods of health promotion and disease prevention
- Locate community resources and disseminate information
- *Develop educational materials*
- *Conduct continuing education activities*

Operational Functions

- Perform inventory of supplies and equipment
- Perform routine maintenance of administrative and clinical equipment
- Apply computer techniques to support office operations
- *Perform personnel management functions*
- *Negotiate leases and prices for equipment and supply contracts*

- *Denotes advanced skills.*

SOURCE: Reprinted by permission of the American Association of Medical Assistants from the AAMA Role Delineation Study: Occupational Analysis of the Medical Assisting Profession.

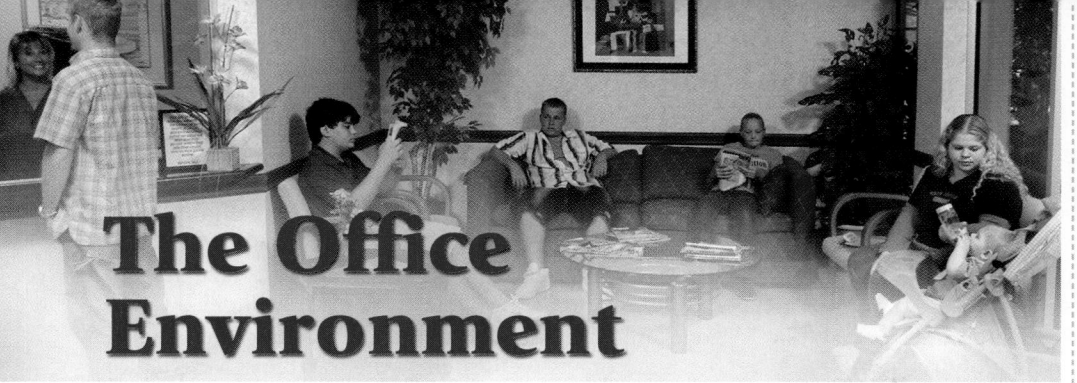

The Office Environment

Learning Objectives

After reading this chapter, you should be able to:

- Define and spell the terms to learn for this chapter.
- Identify six general safety measures.
- Discuss six disaster rules.
- Describe electrical, radiation, mechanical, and chemical safety hazards.
- List and describe four types of medical waste.
- Define OSHA Bloodborne Pathogens Standards.
- Describe the three points that must be included in an exposure plan.
- List and discuss five guidelines for using protective measures as indicated by OSHA.
- Discuss the importance of Universal Precautions for the medical assistant.
- List and describe six rules for proper body mechanics.

OUTLINE

General Safety Measures	96
Employee Safety	98
Hazardous Medical Waste	99
OSHA Bloodborne Pathogens Standards/Universal Precautions	100
Housekeeping Safety	101
Proper Body Mechanics	102
Office Security	102
Ergonomics in the Medical Office	105
Quality Medical Care	105
What is Quality Assurance?	106

Terms to Learn

biohazard

body mechanics

ergonomics

Ground Fault Circuit Interrupter (GFCI)

incident report

Material Safety Data Sheet (MSDS)

National Committee for Quality Assurance (NCQA)

Occupational Safety and Hazard Administration (OSHA)

quality assurance (QA)

Case Study

GLORIA, A MEDICAL ASSISTANT, PREPARES A MEDICATION for Mrs. Garner that is to be given by an intramuscular injection technique. She has both safety needles and non-safety needles at hand for use in this procedure. Since she has not been told to use only the safety needles, and she feels more comfortable with the old-style, she chooses to use the non-safety needle. After giving the injection, Gloria proceeds to dispose of the needle and syringe in the sharps container. As she places the non-safety needle on the flip-lid, it begins to slide off. Gloria catches it, receiving a needle stick in the process. She continues to put the needle and syringe into the sharps container and finishes up with the patient.

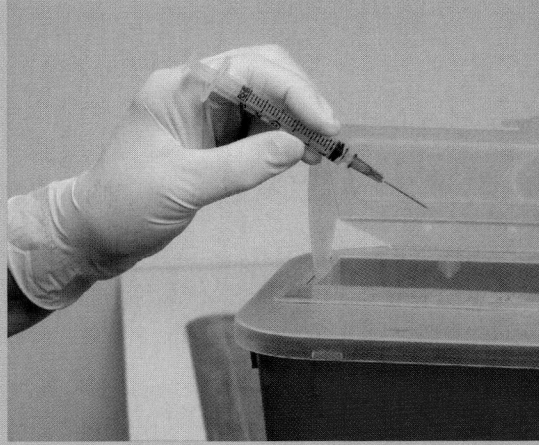

After dismissing the patient, Gloria reports the needle stick to her supervisor, Linda, who then asks Gloria why she chose not to use a safety needle. Gloria explains that she didn't think she needed to and wasn't really trained to use them. Linda tells Gloria to fill out an incident report, explaining the situation in full. Then all steps are taken to provide for testing of both the patient and Gloria.

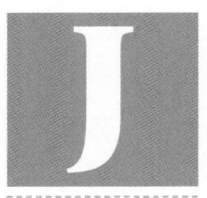

Just as in any workplace, general safety measures, employee safety, housekeeping, proper body mechanics, office security, and measures to ensure a clean, pleasant environment are critical to maintaining the safety and comfort of the medical assistant and the patient in the medical office. Additional safety issues may arise in a medical workplace, including biological hazards, bloodborne pathogens, and the handling of drug samples.

General Safety Measures

The Occupational Safety and Hazard Administration (OSHA) is a governmental agency responsible for the safety of all employees of companies operating in the United States. OSHA assures the safety and health of America's workers by setting and enforcing standards; providing training, outreach, and education; establishing partnerships; and encouraging continual improvement in workplace safety and health. They have the authority to inspect a workplace without notification and to levy fines on any deficiencies they find relating to the health and safety of employees.

Many offices make the mistake of believing the only OSHA issues they need to be concerned with are the Bloodborne Pathogens Standards. While these regulations are important and will be covered later, many other safety factors fall under the regulations of OSHA.

OSHA is concerned with any workplace hazard that may impact the safety of an employee. Other governmental agencies may have standards regarding these factors as well, such as the local Fire Marshal or local law enforcement agencies. In addition, insurance companies that your office may contract might have rules and regulations above and beyond these other agencies.

A workplace hazard could be defined as any issue that could affect the health or safety of an employee—either upon immediate exposure or in the long-term. Matters surrounding workplace hazards will be discussed in the material that follows. See Guidelines 5-1 for some general safety measures to adhere to in the office.

Disaster Plan

A disaster is anything that can cause injury or damage to a group of people. Disasters in a medical office include:

5-1 GUIDELINES **General Safety Measures**

- Walk never run in a medical office. If an emergency situation occurs, move quickly without running.
- Always walk on the right-hand side of the hallway. Wheelchairs and carts bearing patients use the same hallways as do employees and visitors. Some medical facilities have a mirror on the wall or ceiling at hallway junctions so that people do not collide.
- Use handrails when using stairways.
- Never carry uncapped syringes or sharp instruments in hallways or between examination rooms.
- Keep floors clear. Immediately wipe up spills or call housekeeping to assist. Never pick up broken glass with bare hands. Use OSHA standards when cleaning up glass, spilled specimens, and liquids.
- Open doors carefully to avoid injuring someone on the other side.
- Replace burned out light bulbs immediately, especially over exit signs.
- Report all unsafe conditions immediately.
- Wear long hair pulled back and tied to prevent it from coming into contact with hazardous materials.

- Shoes should cover the entire foot. Open toe, open heel, or high heel shoes are not recommended in the medical office due to the danger of slipping and other injuries.
- Do not ever place food in the same refrigerator with laboratory specimens or refrigerated drugs.
- There should be no eating, drinking, or smoking in the medical office, except in designated areas.
- File cabinets should be mounted against the walls to avoid accidental tipping when a heavy top drawer is open.
- Floors should be clean but not so highly polished that they cause slipping. All spills must be cleaned immediately. A hazard sign should always be placed near a wet floor.
- All controlled substances (narcotics) must be stored in a locked cabinet. A record of all narcotic administration must be maintained according to the Drug Enforcement Administration (DEA) regulations. Any loss of drugs must be reported to the regional office of the DEA immediately. The local police should also be notified.

---

fire, flood, tornado, earthquake, or explosions. Recent events have also given rise to the need for security from terrorist attacks. Every office should have a written disaster plan in place and all employees should be familiar with the steps to be taken in any emergency. All new hires should be trained in these emergency steps within the first day of employment. This training should be documented in writing to assure compliance with OSHA regulations. If a particular medical facility has radiation equipment on site, further regulations may be required to be instituted. See Guidelines 5-2 for basic rules for handling a disaster.

Fire Safety

Floor plans showing all exits, fire extinguishers, and stairwells should be placed in conspicuous areas all around the facility. These should include arrows showing the most direct route out of the building. They should be large enough to be easily read in dim light. For each area of the facility, a person should be designated to make sure that all employees are out of that area safely.

Portable fire extinguishers should be attached to walls in areas that are no more that 75 feet away from any employee area. Appropriate types of extinguishers for medical offices are ABC types. They are capable of putting out many types of fires. Each employee should be instructed on the proper use of fire equipment.

Most medical offices are now in buildings with smoke detectors and sprinkler systems. Smoke detectors and alarms should be tested regularly. Nothing should be placed within 18 inches of a sprinkler head.

Fire drills should be held at least once a year and with all employees present. During a mandatory staff meeting would be an ideal time to hold a fire drill. The drill should reinforce the location of fire exits, how to direct people to the fire exits, and how to act in a calm manner during such an emergency.

Because of the widespread "No Smoking" policies now in place in medical facilities, cigarettes are not as much of a fire hazard as before. However, safe disposal systems should be placed in designated areas to prevent people from throwing cigarettes into wastebaskets or other trash receptacles.

The following items should be in place in the event of a fire:

- Telephone numbers of fire and police departments attached to all telephones, including extensions
- Fire extinguishers that have been properly maintained through monthly maintenance checks, the date and initials of the person responsible for testing the equipment should be legible

---

5-2 GUIDELINES

Handling a Disaster

- Remain calm. Count to 10 and assess the situation.
- Make sure that you are not in danger.
- Remove all others (patients and employees) who are in immediate danger, if it is safe for you to do so.
- Make sure that the fire department has been called in the event of a fire.
- Notify others of the emergency according to the policy of the facility.
- Use stairs, never the elevator.

- Exits and stairways that are clearly marked and free of debris, a diagram of all exits should be posted near the fire extinguishers
- Fireproof file cabinets to protect vital records

After notifying the fire department, the most important function during a fire is to see that all patients and employees are safely out of danger. All patients should be told to immediately leave the building. Any patients who need assistance should be helped. Examination rooms and bathrooms need to be inspected in the event a patient is still in the building. Use the stairs, never the elevators. See Figure 5-1 for the basic steps of a fire safety plan.

Electrical Safety

Electrical shock is a hazard in the medical office. All equipment should be grounded according to the manufacturer's instructions. Never use extension cords. They are both an electrical and a trip/fall hazard. No circuit should be overloaded. Surge protectors should be used for all electronic equipment. A power surge can short circuit or "fry" the sensitive components of electronics. You should never plug a surge protector into another surge protector to double up the number of outlets.

All electric cords to equipment should be checked regularly for any cracks, loss of insulation, or other problems. In "wet" areas, such as near sinks, a Ground Fault Circuit Interrupter (GFCI) outlet must be used. GFCIs are designed to protect people from severe or fatal electric shocks. Because a GFCI detects ground faults, it can also prevent some electrical fires and reduce the severity of others by interrupting the flow of electric current. These outlets will break the circuit if water gets into them, protecting both the user and any plugged-in equipment.

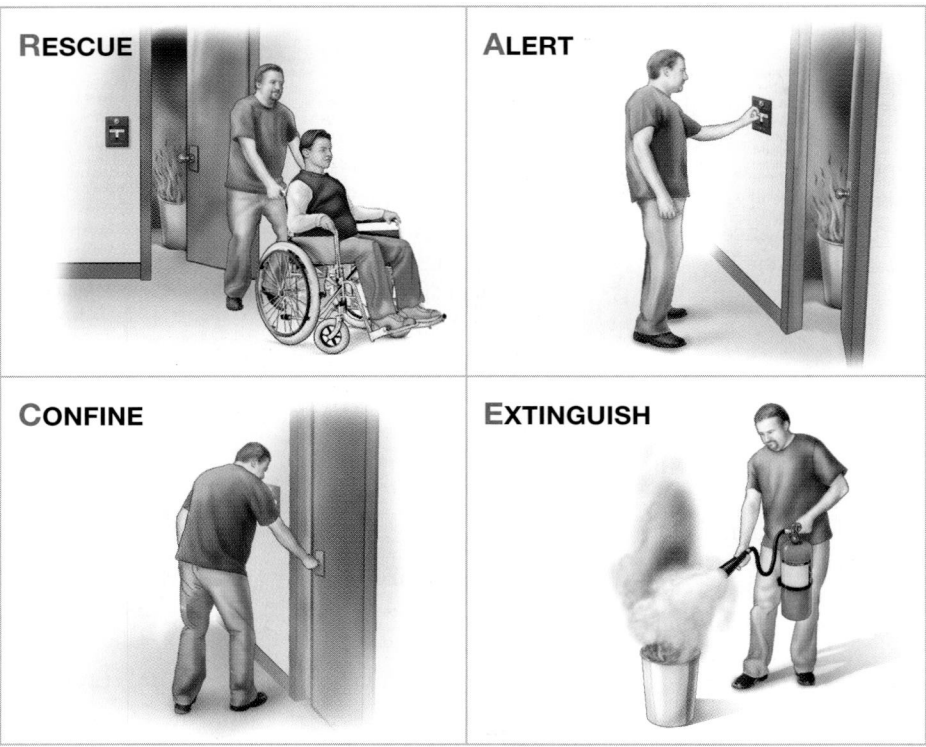

FIGURE 5-1 A fire safety plan like RACE saves lives.

Mechanical Safety

Many pieces of equipment in the medical office can cause harm if they are not used properly. Some of these include the centrifuge, autoclave, sterilizers, and oxygen equipment. You should always read the entire instruction manual before installing or using any type of equipment.

Chemical Hazards (OSHA Hazardous Communications)

Medical offices may contain chemicals that are hazardous to the human body. Materials may be considered harmful in several ways. Biohazards are biological substances, such as medical waste and samples of a virus or bacterium, that pose a threat to human beings and are potentially infectious. Corrosive materials cause burns, and flammable materials can burst into flame. Toxic materials can cause serious illness or death by exposure through skin contact, ingestion, or inhalation.

OSHA has very specific regulations regarding chemical hazards. These are covered under the Hazardous Communications sections. Each office should have an OSHA compliance officer who is trained and aware of all the required controls for the use and storage of such materials. All employees must have annual training for Hazardous Communications.

Each manufacturer of a product is required to provide the consumer with a Material Safety Data Sheet (MSDS), which contains written or printed material concerning a hazardous chemical. MSDSs offer basic information needed to ensure the safety and health of the user at all stages of manufacture, storage, use, and disposal of a hazardous chemical product.

MSDSs give information regarding the hazards of using the product and how to protect oneself from injury by using the appropriate Personal Protection Equipment (PPE). PPE consists of protective gloves, fluid resistant lab coats, safety glasses and a surgical mask, shield, or respirator. All MSDSs must be filed into a HAZCOM binder that is available to all employees at any time. Figure 5-2 is an example of an MSDS label that should be attached to any product that does not include a label.

Employee Safety

Safety is the responsibility of every member of the staff. While it is imperative that the practice provides a safe working environment, the staff needs to be constantly aware of their surroundings and any possible hazards. Employees must be willing to implement all safeguards to keep themselves and their patients safe.

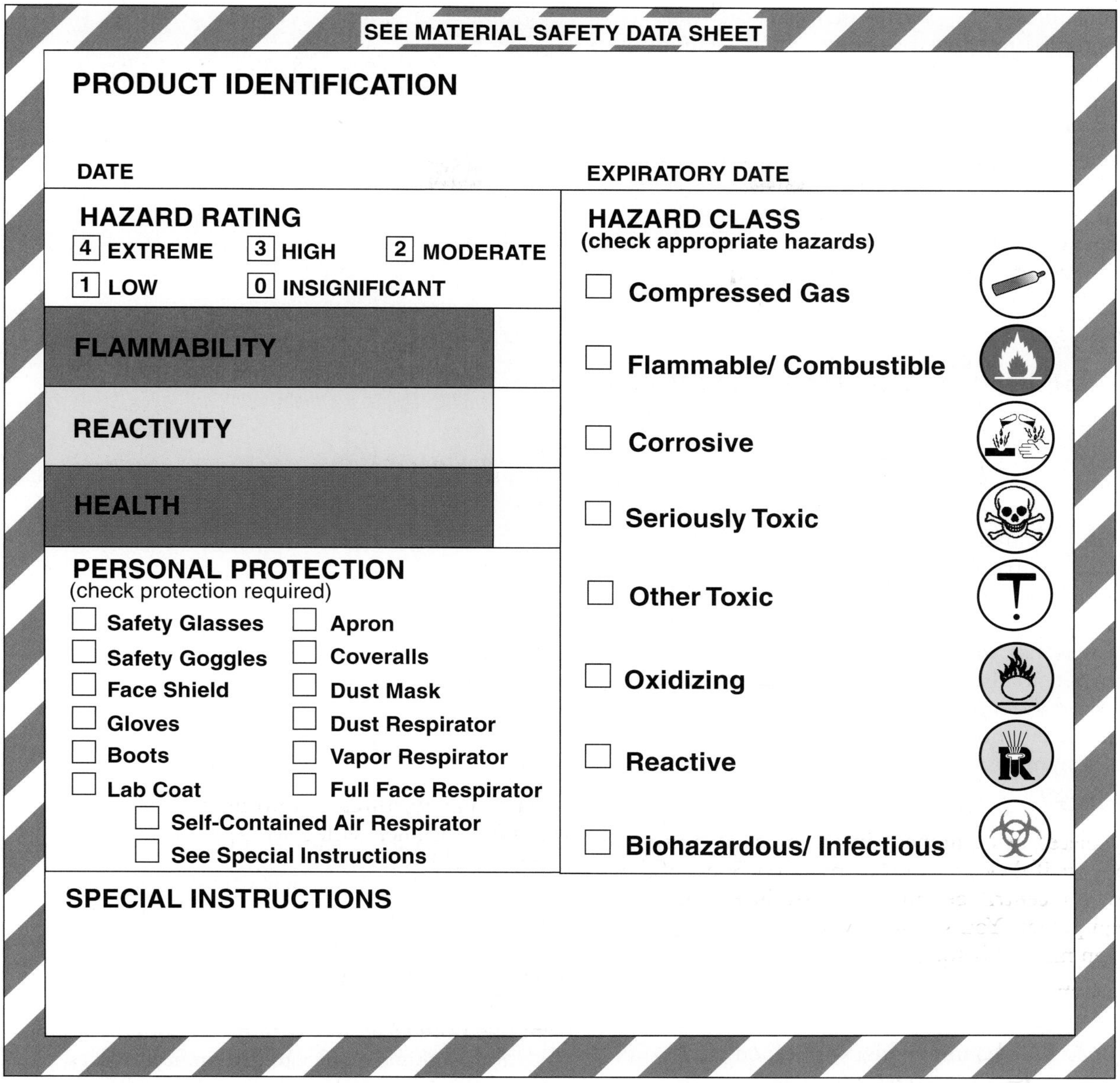

PRODUCT IDENTIFICATION

DATE   **EXPIRATORY DATE**

HAZARD RATING

| 4 | EXTREME | | 3 | HIGH | | 2 | MODERATE |
| 1 | LOW | | 0 | INSIGNIFICANT |

FLAMMABILITY

REACTIVITY

HEALTH

PERSONAL PROTECTION
(check protection required)

☐ Safety Glasses   ☐ Apron
☐ Safety Goggles   ☐ Coveralls
☐ Face Shield   ☐ Dust Mask
☐ Gloves   ☐ Dust Respirator
☐ Boots   ☐ Vapor Respirator
☐ Lab Coat   ☐ Full Face Respirator
        ☐ Self-Contained Air Respirator
        ☐ See Special Instructions

HAZARD CLASS
(check appropriate hazards)

☐ Compressed Gas

☐ Flammable/ Combustible

☐ Corrosive

☐ Seriously Toxic

☐ Other Toxic

☐ Oxidizing

☐ Reactive

☐ Biohazardous/ Infectious

SPECIAL INSTRUCTIONS

FIGURE 5-2   An example of a Material Safety Data Sheet (MSDS).

Hazardous Medical Waste

Hospitals, dental practices, veterinary clinics, laboratories, nursing homes, medical offices, and other health care facilities generate 3.2 million tons of hazardous medical waste each year. Much of this waste is potentially infectious or radioactive. There are four major types of medical waste.

- Solid—generated in every aspect of medicine, including administration, cafeterias, patient rooms, and medical offices. It includes trash such as paper, bottles, cardboard, and cans. Solid waste is not considered hazardous but can cause pollution of the environment. Mandatory recycling can reduce the amount of solid waste produced.

- Chemical—includes substances like germicides, cleaning solvents, and pharmaceuticals. This waste can create a hazardous situation like a fire or explosion. The safe manner in which to handle and dispose of chemicals is included in the MSDS.

- Radioactive—any waste that contains or is contaminated with liquid or solid radioactive material, such as Iodine 123, Iodine 131, and Thallium 201. Radioactive waste must be clearly labeled as "radioactive" and must be removed by a licensed facility.

- Infectious—any waste material that has the potential to carry disease. It includes laboratory cultures, blood and blood products from blood banks, operating rooms, emergency rooms, doctor and dentist offices, autopsy suites, and patient rooms. Infectious waste must be separated from other solid and chemical waste at the point of origin. A licensed medical waste removal agency must dispose of these materials. This is covered in more detail under the Bloodborne Pathogens Standards section.

OSHA Bloodborne Pathogens Standards/Universal Precautions

Medical office laboratories must follow the OSHA guidelines for handling contaminated materials. These guidelines are available from the U.S. Department of Labor in Washington, DC. Most offices contract with a private company to provide assistance in meeting OSHA guidelines.

OSHA standards must be adhered to by every employee who has the possibility of occupational exposure to potentially infectious materials (Preparing for Externship). Occupational exposure is defined as a reasonable anticipation that the employee's duties will result in skin, mucous membrane, eye, or parenteral (for example, assisting with blood work) contact with infectious material. Examples of employees at risk are physicians, nurses, laboratory workers, medical assistants, dental assistants, and, in some cases, housekeeping personnel. The OSHA standards mandate that each at-risk employee must be offered the Hepatitis B vaccine series at the expense of the employer. If an employee refuses the vaccine, he or she must sign a waiver. Potential infectious materials include:

- Body fluid contaminated with blood
- Saliva in dental procedures

Legal and Ethical Issues

The employer has the *responsibility, according to OSHA guidelines, to protect each employee's health from infectious disease. The medical assistant has a responsibility to correctly follow OSHA guidelines for self-protection and to protect other employees and patients.*

The medical assistant has a duty to report any incident such as the accidental administration of medication to a patient, a patient fall or injury, or theft.

- Amniotic fluid
- Cerebrospinal fluid
- Human biopsy tissue or cells
- Microbiological waste (kits or inoculated culture media)
- Any unidentified body fluid
- Urine, stool, sputum, nasal secretions; vomitus and sweat are considered contaminated only if there is visible evidence of blood present

OSHA requires that each medical office have a written Exposure Control Plan to assist in minimizing employee exposure to infectious materials. This plan must be reviewed by all office staff and updated annually. An Exposure Control Plan must include:

- Exposure Determination—listing of job classifications within the office to determine at-risk employees (those with potential exposure to infectious materials).
- Method of Compliance—specific measures to reduce the risk of exposure.
- Post-Exposure—evaluation and follow-up, which specify the steps followed when an exposure incident occurs.

A record for each employee must be kept on file for 30 years after the termination of employment. This includes documentation of the employee's annual review of the Exposure Control Plan for the facility. In addition, these records must contain information regarding the administration of Hepatitis B vaccine series or waiver signed by the employee within three days of initial employment, and a copy of any exposure incident reports. These records must be confidential and kept

TABLE 5-1   Personal Protective Equipment (PPE) and Clothing

Clothing/Equipment	When Used
Gloves	Anticipate contact with blood, infectious material, open wounds or broken skin on hands. Examples: venipuncture, capillary stick, wound care, injections, minor surgery, cleaning contaminated equipment, such as contaminated surfaces of thermometers.
Mask	Anticipate spray with blood or infectious materials. Often used with eye shields.
Eye/Face Shield	Anticipate spray with infectious materials, droplets of blood, or other infectious matter. Example: performing blood smear.
Gowns, Lab Coats	Anticipate gross contamination of clothing during a procedure. Examples: minor surgery, laboratory procedures.

under lock and key. Legal and Ethical Issues touches on more about this issue.

Universal Precautions

The U.S. Centers for Disease Control (CDC) in Atlanta issued recommendations for protection of health care workers. These became known as the Universal Precautions. According to Universal Precautions, all blood and body fluids should be treated as if it were contaminated with any bloodborne pathogen. The most commonly noted diseases related to bloodborne exposure are HIV and HBV. Personal protective equipment (PPE) used to fulfill the recommendations includes gloves, protective eyewear, masks, and fluid resistant lab coats. Table 5-1 describes what protective clothing is appropriate, and Guidelines 5-3 lists details in the use of personal protective equipment and clothing. In addition, the MSDS will contain information regarding PPE. In 1996, the CDC issued more complete guidelines known as Standard Precautions. These guidelines are discussed more fully in Chapter 32.

If there is a situation where infectious material has been spilled, proper procedures must be followed in the cleanup. A spill kit should be used. Commercial kits are available but a simple kit can be assembled with the following equipment:

- Plain clay kitty litter
- A small dust pan
- A biohazard bag

The kitty litter is used as a drying agent to allow sweep-up of the material without spreading it. The material is then placed in a biohazard bag to be disposed of with other biohazardous waste. Patient Education emphasizes more about safety precautions.

Housekeeping Safety

All members of the housekeeping department must receive careful instruction regarding OSHA standards. Housekeeping personnel should not empty biohazard waste and sharps containers. They only empty office trash containers. However, since housekeeping personnel are around potentially infectious materials, they

---

5-3   GUIDELINES

Using Personal Protective Equipment and Clothing from OSHA

- The employer must supply the protective clothing and provide cleaning or disposal of it.
- The clothing or other equipment must be of strength to act as a barrier to infectious materials reaching the employee's street clothing, work clothing, eyes, mouth, or skin.
- Disposable gloves may not be reused.
- Protective eye equipment must have solid sides to prevent infectious material from entering the area.
- All equipment and clothing must be removed and placed in a designated container before leaving the medical office.

Safety precautions are the responsibility of all medical office personnel. The medical assistant's thorough understanding of medical office policy regarding fire safety, infectious waste, and office security results in better patient education, understanding, and protection.

Some patients are insulted when the person caring for them applies gloves before touching them. The medical assistant may need to explain to patients the rationale for wearing protective clothing by medical personnel.

must receive training. If the office contracts with an outside agency for housekeeping duties, the contract should state that all of the agency's employees should be trained in Bloodborne Pathogen Standards and Universal Precautions. The medical office is then not required to train the personnel.

If a contracted agency brings in cleaning products and does not leave them on the premises, the practice is not responsible for maintaining MSDS for those products. However, if the supplies are left in the office, MSDS must be kept in the HAZCOM (hazard communication) book and made available at all times.

Proper storage of all chemical products is essential for the safety of employees and the patients. Guidelines 5-4 presents some rules for the storage and use of cleaning products. Figures 5-3 and 5-4 show some products.

Proper Body Mechanics

Ergonomics applies scientific information and data regarding human body mechanics to the design of objects and overall environments for human use. While OSHA abandoned the ergonomic portion of the regulations, proper body mechanics—coordination of body alignment, balance, and movement—should still be a part of the medical assistant's training.

Medical assistants move, lift, and carry many things, including equipment, supplies, and even patients. Correct methods of standing and lifting objects will help prevent pain and injury. Table 5-2 describes the principles of proper body mechanics and provides a demonstration of proper lifting techniques.

Office Security

There are unique security issues in a physician's office. Medical offices make an attractive target for a thief or addict looking for drugs. Doors and windows need to have secure locks. Only a few authorized personnel should have keys for opening and closing the office. If a key is missing all locks should be changed. Many offices have electronic security systems that are activated when the last person leaves the office. In order to

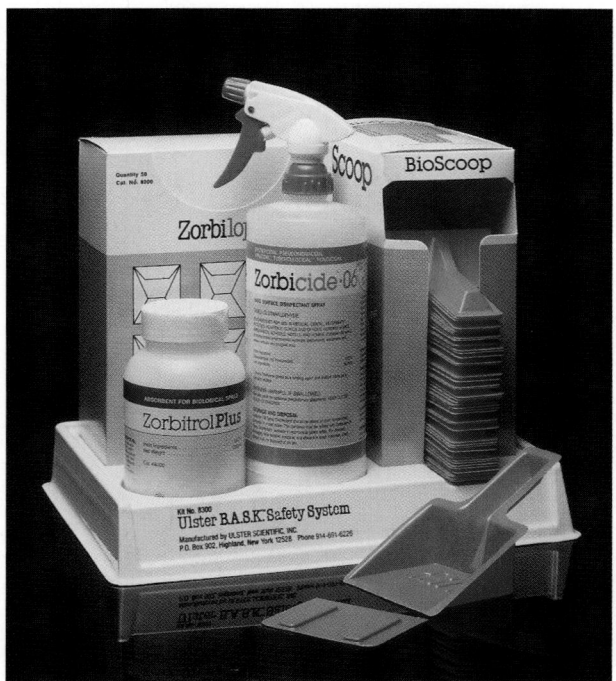

FIGURE 5-3 One type of single-use cleanup kit.

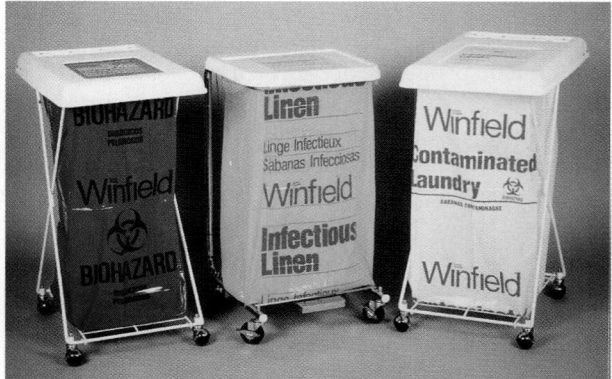

FIGURE 5-4 Examples of waste and hazard containers.

- Immediately clean and disinfect contaminated surfaces after exposure to infectious materials. Figure 5-3 shows one type of single-use cleanup kit. All surfaces must be decontaminated on a regular schedule that is posted, signed, and kept with OSHA records.
- Never pick up broken glass with hands. Use a dustpan or other mechanical device.
- Properly bag contaminated clothing and laundry in leak-proof labeled bags. Contaminated laundry should not be handled or washed at the medical office or with other noncontaminated clothing.
- Handle regulated waste (highly infectious material such as contaminated needles and surgical waste) by placing in clearly labeled biohazards waste containers (Figure 5-4). Waste must be removed by a licensed waste disposal service and incinerated or autoclaved before placing in a designated landfill area.

- Replace a damaged biohazard bag by placing a second bag around the first. Do not remove infectious material from the damaged bag.
- Use puncture-proof, sealable, biohazard sharps containers for all needles and sharps, such as razors and glass pipettes.
  - Place the container close to the work area.
  - Keep sharp container upright.
  - Never reach into the sharps container or push sharps further into the container.
  - Replace sharps container when 2/3 full.
  - Seal and label sharps containers before placing with biohazard waste for removal by disposal service.
- Perform hand hygiene both before and after using gloves.
- Personal protective equipment (PPE) may not be worn out of the laboratory areas. Failure to observe this precaution may result in an OSHA citation.

TABLE 5-2 **Principles of Proper Body Mechanics**

Movement	Description
Stoop	<ul><li>Do not bend from your back.</li><li>Stand close to the object you are moving.</li><li>Keep your feet 6–8 inches apart to create a base of support.</li><li>Place one foot slightly ahead of the other.</li><li>Bend at the hips and knees, keeping the back straight, and lower the body and hands down to the object (Figure 5-5).</li><li>Use the large leg muscles to assist in returning to a standing position (Figure 5-6).</li></ul> 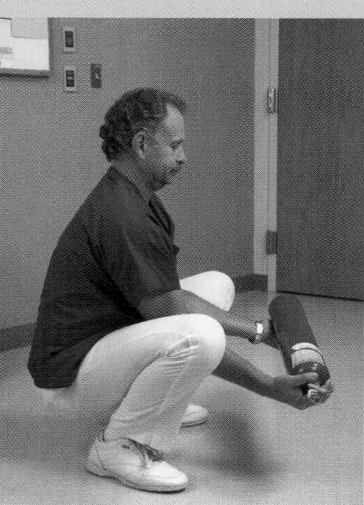 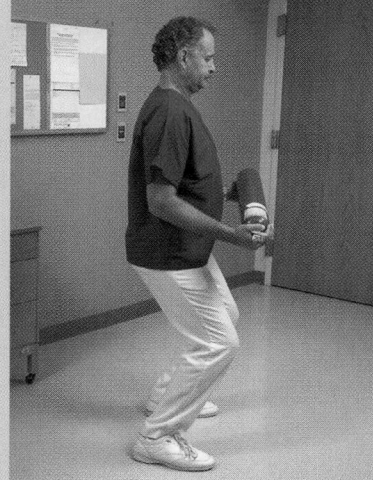 **FIGURE 5-5** Correct position when lifting a heavy object off the floor. **FIGURE 5-6** Use strong leg muscles, keeping back straight, when lifting.

(continued)

TABLE 5-2 Principles of Proper Body Mechanics, (*continued*)

Movement	Description
Lift firmly and smoothly	■ If you think you cannot move a heavy or awkward load, get help. ■ Grasp the load by using the large leg muscles. ■ Keep the load close to the body.
Use the center of gravity for carrying a load	■ Keep your back as straight as possible. (Hint: You should not be able to feel your clothing touch your back if you are standing straight.) ■ Keep the weight of the load close to your body and centered over the hips. ■ Put the load down by bending at the hips and knees. ■ When two or more people carry the load, have one person give the commands to lift or move the object.
Pull or push rather than lift or load	■ Remain close to the object you are moving. ■ Keep feet apart with one slightly forward. ■ Have a firm grasp on the object. ■ Crouch down with feet apart if the object is on the floor. ■ Bend your elbows and place hands on the load at chest level. ■ Keep your back straight. ■ Push up with your legs in order to stand up with the load.
Avoid reaching	■ Evaluate the distance before reaching too far for an object. ■ Stand close to the object. ■ Do not reach to the point of straining. ■ To change direction, point your feet in the direction you wish to go. ■ Keep the object close to your body as you lower it.
Avoid twisting	■ Do not twist your body.

enter the building a predetermined code has to be entered into the system. If the code is not entered within a specified number of seconds an alarm will be activated at the security system company's office. They will then alert the appropriate agency (fire, police, etc.).

Security doesn't just need to be in place when the office is closed. Procedures should take into account the need to secure patients and staff, patient medical records, computer stations, medical supplies, and, particularly, prescription pads from intruders and disorderly persons. HIPAA has raised awareness of many security issues regarding the privacy of each patient's personal medical history.

Incident Reports

Any unusual occurrence or accident is referred to as an incident in the medical setting. Following are some examples of incidents:

- A patient falls on a wet floor
- A housekeeping employee is stuck by a needle while emptying the trash
- A patient receives the wrong medication
- A patient misplaces or loses personal property, such as a hearing aid or glasses, while in the office
- Syringes or needles missing from the supply cupboard
- A medical assistant receives a needle stick from a contaminated needle
- An employee's purse is missing
- An abusive patient uses vulgar language
- A prescription pad is missing

Whenever any accident, injury, or unusual occurrence takes place, a written report must be made. This is called the incident report and can protect both the employer and the medical assistant against possible lawsuits. Some incidents should also be reported to the police or to the liability insurance carrier. For example, stolen property should be reported to the police, and a slip and fall should be reported to the insurance carrier.

Incident reports should be completed immediately in black ink. The incident should be described as simply as possible. Only objective information should be included, such as "Patient fell while getting onto exam table." Do not include subjective comment, such as "Patient was not paying attention to what he was doing." Your medical office should have its own customized form. However, most incident forms include the following information.

- Names of all persons involved
- Date and time of the incident
- Exact location of the incident (including the address of the medical facility and the location of the incident within the facility)
- Name of the person to whom the incident is reported and the time of the report
- Brief description of what happened
- Names of all witnesses
- Name and description of any equipment involved in the incident
- Action taken at the time of the incident
- Action taken to prevent a recurrence
- Signature and title of person completing the report

The incident report, like all other information relating to the patient, is subject to subpoena in litigation (lawsuits). A copy of the incident report should be placed in a master incident report file, the patient's file, and the employee's record. Figure 5-7 is an example of an incident report form. Professionalism addresses some information that can prevent incidents from occurring.

Ergonomics in the Medical Office

OSHA eliminated the ergonomics section of the regulations for medical facilities, but that doesn't mean they aren't important to the well-being and productivity of employees. If well designed, systems of work, sports and leisure, and health and safety all incorporate ergonomic principles.

In the medical setting, ergonomics applies to all aspects of the facility. The most common area for problems is the computer workstation. The keyboard should be at elbow height, the monitor at eye level, and the chair should be adjustable, with a lumbar support. The operator's feet should be able to rest on the floor comfortably, with no strain. A wrist rest and mouse wrist support should be used.

Lighting should be appropriate for the task. Overhead fluorescent lights should not reflect on the computer monitor screens, causing a glare. This can be prevented by adding an anti-glare shield to the monitor or tilting the screen so that the light does not hit it directly. Clinical areas should be well lit. Repetitive motions should be limited, and the proper tools should be available for any procedure.

Professionalism

Maintaining a professional demeanor in the medical office can prevent many incidents from occurring. Wearing the appropriate apparel, avoiding excessive jewelry, and pulling back long hair can eliminate hazards that might result in injuries.

Quality Medical Care

Quality medical care is an expectation of all patients and requires that the health care team use procedures and techniques that result in the best possible outcome for the patient. In addition, the patient must be satisfied with the care (Lifespan Considerations).

INCIDENT REPORT

Name of injured party _____ Date _____

Address _____ Telephone _____

_____

The injured party was: ☐ Employee   ☐ Patient   ☐ Other _____

Date of accident/incident _____   Time of incident _____

Where did incident occur? _____

Names of witnesses (include titles):

_____   _____

_____   _____

What first aid/treatment was given at the time of the incident?

_____

_____

Who administered first aid? _____

Briefly describe the incident. _____

_____

_____

_____

_____

Names of employees present at time of incident/injury:

_____

What, in your opinion, caused the accident? _____

_____

Follow-up: What steps have been taken to prevent a similar accident? _____

_____

_____

Date _____   Employee's signature _____

Date _____   Supervisor's signature _____

FIGURE 5-7   An example of a typical incident report.

Remember that when dealing with elderly patients, they may have balance problems or gait disabilities that make them more prone to falls. Consider this when preparing the waiting room and the examination rooms. Avoid throw rugs, extension cords, or anything that may be a trip/fall hazard.

The major parameters or attributes of health care that are regularly examined include treatment, benefit of treatment, cost/benefit, accessibility to health care, and delivery location. The outcome factor actually requires a measurable change in the health status of the

BOX 5-1
The AMA's Eight Essentials of Quality Care

- Bring about the optimal in the patient's condition within the earliest time frame possible based on the patient's comfort and physical condition.
- Have an emphasis on early detection and treatment as well as health promotion and disease prevention.
- Receive treatment in a timely fashion without unnecessary delay, termination, interruption, or prolongation.
- Encourage the patient's participation in the decision process regarding his or her treatment.
- Base the treatment on skillful use of technology and the health professional's use of accepted principles of medical science.
- Demonstrate concern for the patient and patient's family, with sensitivity to the stress caused by illness.
- Achieve the treatment goal through the wise use of technology and other resources.
- Provide adequate documentation in the patient's medical record to facilitate peer evaluation and continuity of care.

patient that is a direct result of the care received. Cost/benefit refers to the expenditure or cost in terms of time, money, and effort, and the relationship of this cost to the actual benefit the patient receives. Accessibility to health care refers to the effort a patient must make to receive health care. The American Medical Association (AMA) has defined quality care by listing eight essential elements (Box 5-1).

What is Quality Assurance?

In the early 1960s, the health care industry began to feel an increasing demand from the public for accountable quality care. From that initial swell of public pressure developed a continuing effort on the part of health care providers to deliver satisfactory, achievable excellence in care. Quality assurance (QA) is gathering and evaluating information about the services provided (as well as the results achieved) and comparing this information with an accepted standard.

Quality assessment measures consist of formal, systematic evaluations of overall patterns of care. The goal of the actual programs and activities of quality assurance have a desired degree of care in a health care setting. The results of the evaluations are then compared to standard results. As deficiencies are identified, recommendations for improvement in care are made. Quality Improvement Programs (QIPs) utilize the data gathered by quality assurance/assessment to make quality improvements in health care.

Quality Assurance Program

A quality assurance program (QAP) in a hospital, ambulatory health care setting, long-term-care facility, or health maintenance organization (HMO) consists of a system for reviewing records maintained by staff. These records may consist of medical or nursing records, data regarding days of hospitalization or treatment, progress reports, and other statistics that provide a firm indication of the care received by patients. A quality assurance program must include evaluation and educational components to identify and correct problems. Quality assurance programs such as these are required in order for the facility to receive funding by the Public Health Service Act, (which defines the requirements) as well as to achieve and maintain accreditation. The basic components of a quality assurance program include the following:

- Establish a QA Committee—representatives from the entire patient care team (such as physician, nurse, and medical assistant) should be part of a QA committee (Figure 5-8).
- Review all clinical and administrative services and procedures—committee members or an

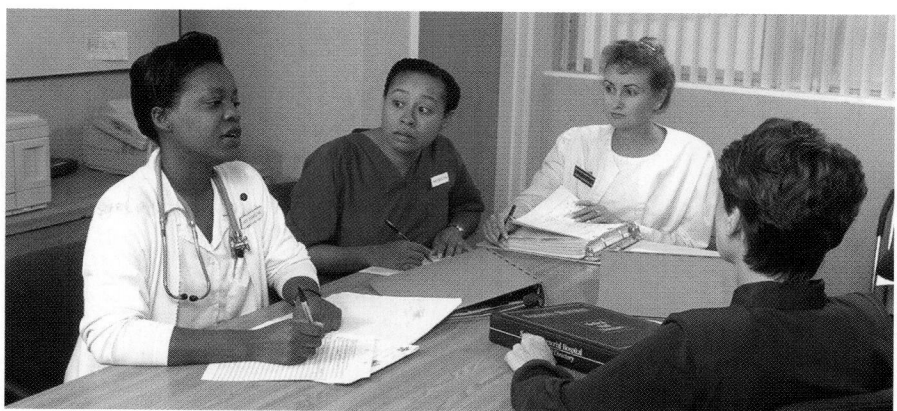

FIGURE 5-8 A quality assurance (QA) committee meeting.

assigned individual can conduct the review. All team members should have a role in the QA process, from designing the QA forms to selecting issues for review. Procedure and policy manuals are also subject to review during this process.

• Set up a structure for identifying items to review; pay particular attention to problem issues.

• Quantify all issues. For example:

 –average length of waiting time in minutes to see physician

 –number of errors in writing items on patient records

–number of insurance claims disallowed per 100 filed

–number of failed "needle sticks" per 50 attempts

• Limit the number of issues—set a limit to the number of issues or problems reviewed at any one session. Emphasis should be placed on taking corrective measures.

• Maintain careful records—review all records, such as incident reports and committee records, and progress or improvement with the entire medical team.

Box 5-2 lists examples of issues that a QA committee might review in a physician's office.

BOX 5-2

Issues Reviewed by a QA Committee in a Physician's Office

- Disallowed insurance claims
- Errors in dispensing medications (use incident reports)
- Errors in labeling of laboratory specimens
- Incorrect coding of diagnosis for insurance claims
- Long waiting time for patients
- Adverse reactions to treatments and/or medications (use incident reports)
- Inability to obtain venous blood on the first attempt
- Patient satisfaction (from survey/questionnaire results)
- Patients who leave the office without seeing the physician

- Patient complaints relating to confidentiality
- Appearance of office
- Handicapped parking availability
- Safety
- Provider availability
- Emergency preparations
- 16 Treatment areas
- Safety/monitoring practices for radiology and laboratory
- Medications
- Infection control
- Patient education/rights
- Medical records
- Collection procedures
- Telephone and reception behaviors

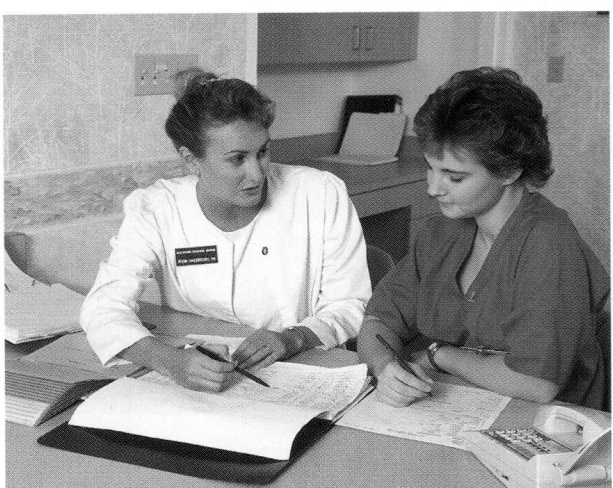

FIGURE 5-9 A medical assistant at a QA meeting.

Implementing a Quality Assurance Program (QAP)

The ultimate goal of a formal quality assurance program is to improve the quality of care so that there is no difference between what should be done and what is actually being done. Professionals in the field who are expert in a particular health care area develop these norms or standards.

To put a QAP into place, requires the development of patient-centered criteria based on acceptable stan-

dards of care. Criteria are standards used to compare something in order to make a decision. For example, years ago some patients were discharged from a hospital without being given any formal information or education about what to do when they returned home. Now all hospitalized patients should receive instructions at discharge regarding medications, diet, activity, and follow-up appointments with the physician. This discharge plan is explained to the patient, who then signs the plan and keeps a copy. A copy of the signed plan is also put in the patient's chart, indicating this instruction took place. A quality assurance program would monitor the discharge planning process.

The Medical Assistant's Role in a QAP

The medical assistant is trained in clinical and administrative skills with the expectation for the highest level of performance. To assist the physician/employer, pay rigorous attention to the quality of care given to patients. Patient satisfaction is a key element in quality of care. The medical assistant may be the first person to respond to a patient's complaint or discomfort. Medical assistants have the opportunity to present patients' concerns or complaints at a team QA meeting so that corrective measures can be taken (Figure 5-9). Some of the areas in which to assist the physician with quality assurance are noted in Box 5-3.

Health Plan Employer Data and Information Set (HEDIS)

Under HEDIS, managed care plans that serve Medicare patients must collect data relating to eight categories of performance:

- Effectiveness of care
- Access to/availability of care
- Member satisfaction
- Informed health care choices
- Health plan descriptive information
- Cost of care
- Health plan stability
- Use of service

Medicare, HMOs, and other plans seeking accreditation from the National Committee for Quality Assurance (NCQA), must also report data. The NCQA evaluates the quality of health plans in order to help consumers and employers make more informed decisions about their health care. Eventually, most of the health plans (HMOs and PPOs) a physician contracts with will be collecting data for the medical practice.

Box 5-3
The Medical Assistant's Role in QA

- Resolve patient complaints about items such as billing questions and long waiting times in the reception room.
- Perform patient education regarding diet, laboratory and procedure instructions, and personal care.
- Perform telephone follow-up regarding a patient's condition and progress.
- Double-check laboratory tests performed in the office.
- Verify the results of laboratory tests given over the telephone. Always ask the laboratory to repeat any results that are abnormal or unclear. Request to have a written report sent by mail or fax.
- Bring patient complaints to the attention of the physician.

TABLE 5-3 Clinical Laboratory Improvement Amendment (CLIA)

Category	Explanation
Simple Testing	Incorrect test results pose little risk for the patient. Laboratory is subject to random inspectors only. Some physician's laboratories fall in this category.
Intermediate-Level Testing (Level II)	Poses risk to patient if there is an incorrect test result. Must be certified by approved accrediting agency. Must be staffed by credentialed personnel. Must meet quality assurance standards.
Complex Testing (Level III)	Poses high risk to patient if there is an incorrect test result. Must be certified by approved accrediting agency. Must be staffed by credentialed personnel. Must meet quality assurance standards.

Clinical Laboratory Improvement Amendment (CLIA)

The federal government now requires that all clinical laboratories that test human specimens must be controlled. The Clinical Laboratories Improvement Amendment of 1988 (CLIA88) divides laboratories into three categories. These are described in Table 5-3. Refer to Chapter 40 for further discussion of the Clinical Laboratory Improvement Act (CLIA), which mandates quality control of laboratory tests by categories and documentation.

SUMMARY

Safety measures including general safety, employee safety, emergency plans, such as fire, the handling of biological hazards and bloodborne pathogens, housekeeping procedures, proper body mechanics, security, and environment are essential to maintaining a safe and pleasant workplace. The efforts of a medical assistant can be critical in ensuring that all of these components are carefully regarded.

Chapter Review

COMPETENCY REVIEW

1. Define and spell the terms to learn for this chapter.
2. List six safety rules to follow in medical offices.
3. You have been asked to draft the OSHA Exposure Plan for your office. What three points must you include in this plan?

PREPARING FOR THE CERTIFICATION EXAM

1. A formal written description of an accident that has occurred in a medical setting is a/an
   A. quality assurance report
   B. incident report
   C. evaluation
   D. policy manual
   E. procedure manual

2. A material safety data sheet (MSDS) contains information about
   A. OSHA guidelines
   B. hazardous chemicals and other substances
   C. office policy
   D. vendor information
   E. medical surgical devices

continued on next page

3. OSHA guidelines are available from
   A. U.S. Department of Labor
   B. AAMA
   C. AMA
   D. FDA
   E. BNDD

4. The law regulating laboratory safety precautions is
   A. OSHA
   B. FUTA
   C. CLIA
   D. FICA
   E. A and C

5. Universal precautions mandate that
   A. all blood and bodily fluid contact is to be treated as if it contains HIV, HBV, or other bloodborne pathogens
   B. precautions must be taken only when there is visible blood present
   C. precautions are not necessary if the health care professional uses proper hand hygiene
   D. only medical assistants and nurses must follow the guidelines
   E. all employees have the Hepatitis B vaccine series

6. An OSHA citation may be issued as a result of failure to
   A. use proper telephone and reception behavior
   B. affix hazardous waste container to the wall
   C. remove street clothing before coming to and leaving from work
   D. remove PPE before leaving from work
   E. bend when lifting a heavy object

7. Medical waste consists of the following, EXCEPT
   A. radioactive waste
   B. occupational waste
   C. infectious waste
   D. chemical waste
   E. solid waste

8. Proper body mechanics involves the following muscles, EXCEPT
   A. arm
   B. back
   C. leg
   D. neck
   E. eye lid

9. OSHA reports for employee Hepatitis B vaccine records must be maintained for at least
   A. 30 years
   B. 3 years
   C. 1 year
   D. 30 months
   E. 3 months

10. The following include potential infectious materials, EXCEPT
    A. amniotic fluids
    B. body fluid with blood
    C. saliva
    D. sweat
    E. bloody vomitus

CRITICAL THINKING

1. What errors did Gloria make in preparing the injection?
2. What tests must be performed as a result of this needlestick?
3. Does Linda hold any responsibility in this situation?
4. How would this pertain to OSHA's Bloodborne Pathogens Standards?

ON THE JOB

Bonnie feels that the office is always too cold, so she keeps a heater under her desk. In order to use the heater, she needs to run an extension cord across to another electrical outlet. Several times, the safety officer in the practice asks her to discontinue using the heater. Bonnie will put the heater away for a couple of days, then bring it back out when she feels it won't be noticed. The safety officer comes by one day and confiscates the heater and extension cord. Bonnie feels that this is unfair because she is cold during the day and thinks she should be allowed to use the heater which allows her to perform her duties in comfort and more efficently.

1. What OSHA violations are of concern in this situation?
2. Did the safety officer handle the situation correctly the first few times?
3. Did the safety officer have the right to confiscate the heater and extension cord?
4. How might the situation be rectified to make Bonnie comfortable?

INTERNET ACTIVITY

Search the Internet to find private companies that are in business to provide services to prepare an office for OSHA requirements.

MediaLink More on the medical office environment, including interactive resources, can be found on the Student CD-ROM accompanying this textbook.

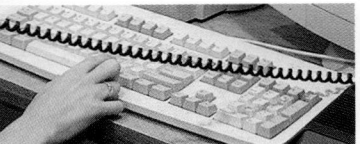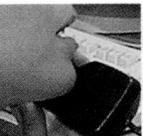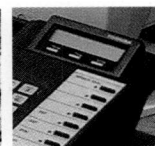

Medical Assistant Role Delineation Chart

HIGHLIGHT indicates material covered in this chapter.

ADMINISTRATIVE

Administrative Procedures

- Perform basic administrative medical assisting functions
- Schedule, coordinate and monitor appointments
- Schedule inpatient/outpatient admissions and procedures
- Understand and apply third-party guidelines
- Obtain reimbursement through accurate claims submission
- Monitor third-party reimbursement
- Understand and adhere to managed care policies and procedures
- *Negotiate managed care contracts*

- Manage accounts receivable
- *Manage accounts payable*
- *Process payroll*
- *Document and maintain accounting and banking records*
- *Develop and maintain fee schedules*
- *Manage renewals of business and professional insurance policies*
- *Manage personnel benefits and maintain records*
- *Perform marketing, financial, and strategic planning*

Practice Finances

- Perform procedural and diagnostic coding
- Apply bookkeeping principles

CLINICAL

Fundamental Principles

- Apply principles of aseptic technique and infection control
- Comply with quality assurance practices
- Screen and follow up patient test results

Diagnostic Orders

- Collect and process specimens
- Perform diagnostic tests

Patient Care

- Adhere to established patient screening procedures
- Obtain patient history and vital signs
- Prepare and maintain examination and treatment areas
- Prepare patient for examinations, procedures and treatments

- Assist with examinations, procedures and treatments
- Prepare and administer medications and immunizations
- Maintain medication and immunization records
- Recognize and respond to emergencies
- Coordinate patient care information with other health care providers
- Initiate IV and administer IV medications with appropriate training and as permitted by state law

GENERAL

Professionalism

- Display a professional manner and image
- Demonstrate initiative and responsibility
- Work as a member of the health care team
- Prioritize and perform multiple tasks
- Adapt to change
- Promote the CMA credential
- Enhance skills through continuing education
- Treat all patients with compassion and empathy
- Promote the practice through positive public relations

Communication Skills

- Recognize and respect cultural diversity
- Adapt communications to individual's ability to understand
- Use professional telephone technique

- Recognize and respond effectively to verbal, nonverbal, and written communications
- Use medical terminology appropriately
- Utilize electronic technology to receive, organize, prioritize and transmit information
- Serve as liaison

Legal Concepts

- Perform within legal and ethical boundaries
- Prepare and maintain medical records
- Document accurately
- Follow employer's established policies dealing with the health care contract
- Implement and maintain federal and state health care legislation and regulations
- Comply with established risk management and safety procedures
- Recognize professional credentialing criteria
- *Develop and maintain personnel, policy and procedure manuals*

Instruction

- Instruct individuals according to their needs
- Explain office policies and procedures
- Teach methods of health promotion and disease prevention
- Locate community resources and disseminate information
- *Develop educational materials*
- *Conduct continuing education activities*

Operational Functions

- Perform inventory of supplies and equipment
- Perform routine maintenance of administrative and clinical equipment
- Apply computer techniques to support office operations
- *Perform personnel management functions*
- *Negotiate leases and prices for equipment and supply contracts*

- *Denotes advanced skills.*

SOURCE: Reprinted by permission of the American Association of Medical Assistants from the AAMA Role Delineation Study: Occupational Analysis of the Medical Assisting Profession.

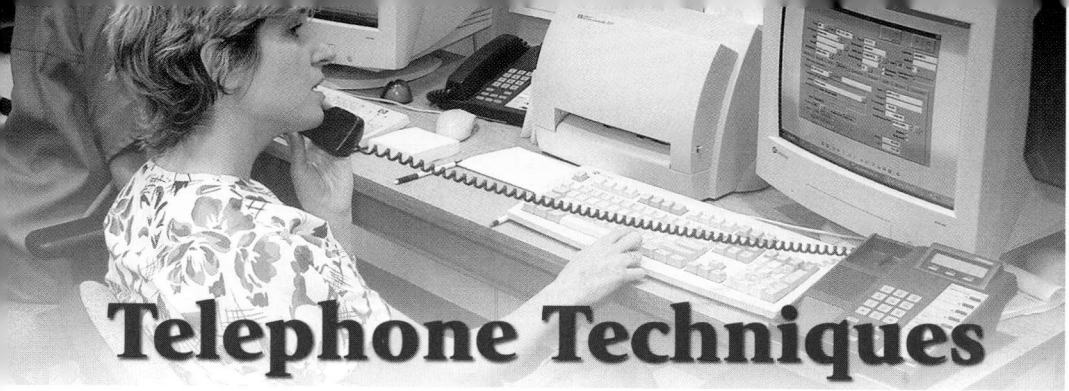

Telephone Techniques

Learning Objectives

After completing this chapter, you should be able to:

- Define and spell the terms to learn for this chapter.
- Take detailed and efficient telephone messages.
- Use the hold function effectively and professionally.
- Answer the telephone with a proper greeting and pleasant tone.

- Handle difficult callers.
- Understand what telephone triage is and how it is used in the medical office.
- Place long distance calls and conference calls.
- Handle emergency phone calls.

OUTLINE

Telephone Techniques	114
Typical Incoming Calls	119
Prescription Refill Requests	121
Telephone Triage	121
Handling Difficult Calls	122
Using a Telephone Directory	122
Long Distance Calls	123
Using an Answering Service	124
Handling an Emergency Telephone Call	125

Terms to Learn

answering service	conference call	queue
automated assistance program	enunciation	referrals
caller ID	inflection	telephone triage
clarity	pitch	voice messaging system

Case Study

CINDY HAS BEEN LOOKING FOR A NEW PHYSICIAN. She has decided to try Dr. Brown since the office is near her place of work. When Cindy calls the office to set up an appointment, she is first greeted by a machine, which tells her she is calling Dr. Brown's office. She receives many options and dials "2" to schedule an appointment. Cindy then waits as the system transfers her to the appropriate person. When the transfer is done, she is greeted by Tonya, a new medical assistant in Dr. Brown's office. Tonya greets her with "Good Afternoon, this is Dr. Brown's office. This is Tonya, how may I help you?" Although Cindy is left with a cold feeling because she detects an insincere tone in Tonya's voice, she decides to ignore this and tells Tonya that she would like to make a new patient appointment. Tonya then tells Cindy to hold, and Cindy finds herself waiting and listening to rather distracting music. She has been on hold for two minutes when Tonya returns to the phone. Tonya gives no reason for the wait. At this point, Cindy is rather frustrated and informs Tonya that she will seek another physician.

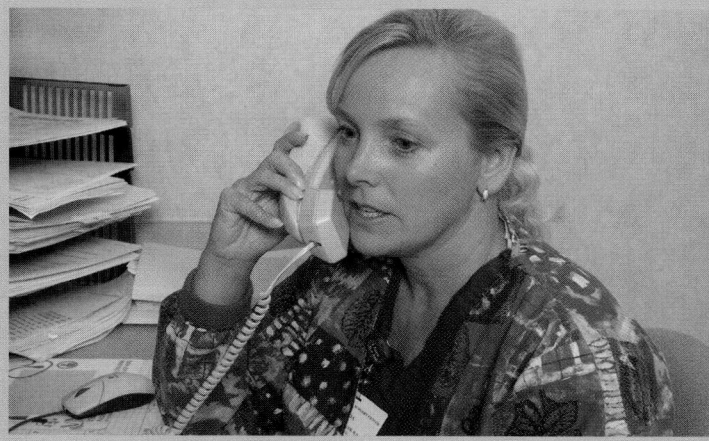

The telephone is the backbone of the medical office. It provides a key communication pathway between the physician, the staff, and the patient. As such, there are keys to using this pathway effectively. Every member of the health care team is responsible for communicating with patients and other callers and should know how to do so in the most professional way possible.

Telephone Techniques

If you work in the "front office" area, much of your day will be spent on the telephone. A fundamental rule to remember when answering your medical office's telephone is that you are not answering a home telephone. The telephone techniques used when speaking on home telephones are generally more informal and chatty than the style of conversation that is expected in a medical office. It is inappropriate to answer the office line with personal greetings, such as "Hello" or "Hi." A professional manner must always be presented to your callers.

Answering the Telephone

Your manner of answering the telephone frequently determines how the conversation will flow. It is also the first impression that callers, including potential new patients, receive of your office. Following are some important techniques that will assist you in answering your medical office's telephone in the most professional manner.

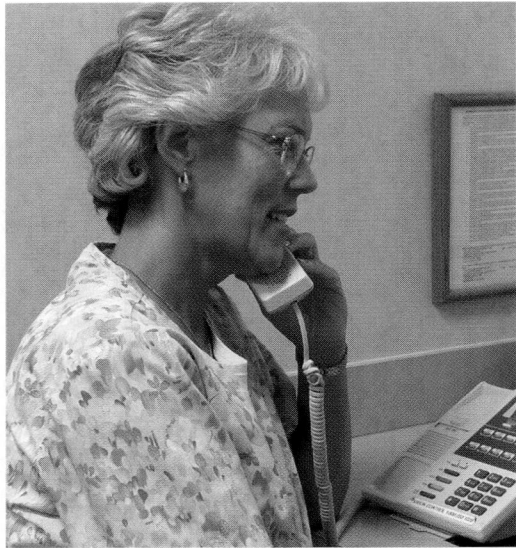

FIGURE 6-1 A pleasant smile can go a long way, even through telephone lines.

Smiling
Always answer the telephone with a smile. A human voice has so many nuances to it that most callers will be able to "hear" the warmth or indifference in your voice (Figure 6-1).

Greetings
When the medical office telephone rings, it is important that you answer the telephone quickly, usually by the third ring, and with a friendly, professional greeting. Your medical office supervisor will teach you the office's preferred method of answering the telephone. It is important that the greeting include the name of the office/physician and that all members of the staff use the same greeting. This will make the patient more comfortable in contacting your office. An example of a typical office greeting might be, "Good morning, Main Street Physicians. This is Jessica, how may I help you?"

Speech
We do not often think about how important it is to speak clearly on the telephone, but it is vital to good office management. There are four words used in reference to your speaking voice: clarity, enunciation, inflection, and pitch.

Clarity refers to the quality or state of being understandable. How clear is your voice to the caller? Are you holding the telephone receiver close to your mouth so that the best sound gets through to the caller? Many people tend to drop the receiver so that it sits just below the chin. This does not produce clear sound for the person on the other end of the telephone. You also need to make sure that there is nothing in your mouth that could garble your words. There should never be any gum, candy, or food in your mouth when addressing a caller.

Enunciation refers to the clear articulation and pronouncement of your words. Be careful not to speak too rapidly. Because you use the same greeting and phrase over and over again, it is easy to fall into the habit of speaking hurriedly. Remember to slow down, and pronounce your words slowly and properly. Avoid using regional pronunciations in the office setting. Remember that your patients come from many different cultures and may not understand your particular pronunciation. The sound of your voice ranges from high to low, depending on the context of your phrase. Have you ever noticed that when you ask a question your voice tends to rise at the end of the phrase? This is an example of the use of pitch or loudness of your voice. You will need to be aware of your voice pitch when speaking with patients. Inflection refers to the pitch and tone of your voice and the way you utter your words and phrases. Remember that speaking on the telephone is an opportunity to display excellent customer service. Try to avoid using a monotone voice (one single tone). The caller may feel you are bored and that you are not interested in helping.

Identify the Caller

Protection of a patient's information is vital in every medical office and health care facility. It is important to remember that some individuals may seek confidential information by dubious means, such as claiming to be the patient or even a specialist treating a patient. Therefore, steps must be taken to protect patient records. For example, each time a person calls in and claims to be a patient, it is a good idea to ask for some identifying information, especially his or her first and last names, social security number, and date of birth. You can check this information against the patient's computer record. You may also pull the patient's paper chart and check against that record. This will help to ensure that the person speaking is the patient.

The Business Telephone System

There are many types of business telephone systems in use today (Figure 6-2). Most medical offices will use some form of a multi-line telephone. Some may have all of the lines separate, where you must press that particular line's button to answer it, or a system that will feed calls to you from a queue or waiting line. More and more offices have systems that will answer the initial call with a recording and then feed the calls to the appropriate people.

Whether you are answering initially (without an automated system) or an automated system answers (calls are queued), remember to follow the rules of greeting callers discussed earlier.

Making Calls

Just as often as you answer calls in a medical office, you will have to make them. On most business telephones, you will be required to dial "9" to get an outside line. Some telephones may just have an outside line button that you will need to hit before you dial. Depending on the office's location, you may also need to dial the area code with all calls. Large cities have begun to make this a common practice because of the need for multiple area codes within a local calling zone. The telephone calls that you make in the office should be limited to business calls. All offices have different policies on the use of the office telephone for personal calls. Some may prohibit them all together, while others may allow them in limited number. It is important to keep in mind that the office telephone is for patients and emergencies, so you need to keep the lines open.

Using the Hold Function

One of the most sensitive issues relating to telephone courtesy is the use of the "hold" function. The hold function refers to the ability to keep more than one call on the line at a time. Holding the call is permissible when the person being called will come on the line

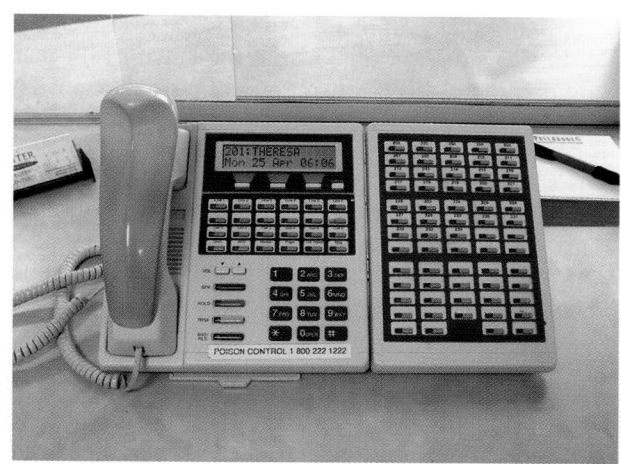

FIGURE 6-2 Choose the telephone unit that offers the features needed in your office.

within a short period of time or when you are already speaking to a caller on another line. However, the hold function is abused when callers are left "on hold" for indefinite periods of time.

If you are already speaking with a caller when a second call comes in, it is proper to ask the first caller if you may place him or her on hold for a moment in order to answer the second call. It is discourteous to handle the second caller before returning to the first call. An example of a typical conversation is as follows:

First caller: "Mrs. Brown, may I place you on hold for a moment? I have another call."

Second caller: "Good afternoon, Drs. Garcia and Jensen. Would you please hold?"

It is important to allow the second caller time to respond. If the second call is an emergency, you will need to take care of it before returning to the original call. If it is not an emergency, finish the original call before moving onto the second call. With all calls that you place on hold, try to keep the wait time to a minimum. Nobody likes to be on hold.

There are other situations where you may need to place a caller on hold. For example, you may need to pull a chart to answer a patient's question. When this happens, explain to the patient what you need to do to get the appropriate information, and then ask if you may place him or her on hold. Again, always wait for a response and then retrieve the information in the timeliest manner possible. If you have trouble getting the information and need more time, let the caller know. Do not leave callers on hold without checking back with them. To avoid forgetting that you have a caller on hold, be wary of distractions and do not do tasks that are unrelated to helping that caller.

Another situation that will require you to put a caller on hold is when a patient needs to speak with the doctor or another staff member who is not readily available. In this situation, make sure the person calling is aware that there will be a wait and offer to take a message and a number for a return call. As much as possible, it is best to keep the telephone lines open. If the caller chooses to wait, you will need to check on him or her approximately every 30 seconds. Let the caller know that the person he or she is waiting on is still unavailable. Then check to see if the caller would like to leave a name and number so as to have the call returned. See Box 6-1 for a list of things to avoid when using the hold function.

Transferring Calls

As you field calls in the medical office, you will find that it is often necessary to transfer or send them from one office telephone extension to another extension in the same office. Most business telephones will have the ability to transfer the call from your desk. There are a few steps that you should follow to make this a smooth transition for the caller.

First, once you have identified the person to whom you will be transferring the call, tell the caller the name of this person. This lets the caller know who to expect on the other end of the line as well as who to call back in case of disconnection during the transfer. If you have an extension number available, it is also helpful to provide that number to the patient before transferring him or her. When you start the transfer, make sure that the caller is aware of your actions. Do not transfer a patient without his or her prior knowledge and consent. Also, avoid transferring the call and hanging up without knowledge of whether the person was available to help the caller. Most telephones systems allow you to announce a call that you are transferring. Let the person to whom you

are transferring the call know the caller's name and the reason for the call. That person may tell you that he or she is unavailable to take the call. You may get a busy signal when you try to transfer the call. In these situations, take a message, or let the caller leave a recorded message.

Taking a Message

Medical offices are busy by nature. Medical assistants will often take messages from patients, other physicians, health care facilities, businesses, etc. Be prepared by keeping a notebook on hand to take notes while speaking with the caller. This will ensure that you have the information correct, such as the caller's name and the reason for the call. It is best not to trust your memory.

All messages should include the first and last name of the caller, a telephone number at which he or she can be reached for a callback, the reason for the call, and the name of the person he or she is trying to reach. If at any time you do not understand what a caller has stated, you will need to clarify the message with that caller. You may repeat to the caller what you believe you heard, or you may ask the caller to repeat back what was said to you. Always repeat the telephone number for a call back to the caller. The caller may interpret the lack of a return call due to an incorrect number, as lack of concern or disrespect. All telephone messages regarding a patient should be placed in the patient's chart.

It is very important to remember not to throw anything away that contains patient information. If a sheet of paper from the notepad you use to take proper messages has patient information, it must be shredded. It is a violation of the HIPAA privacy rule to throw patient information into the trash.

See Procedure 6-1 for instructions on how to take telephone messages. Legal and Ethical Issues discusses more about following office protocol.

The Voice Messaging System

In the medical office, you will deal with a voice messaging system for both incoming and outgoing calls. A voice messaging system allows for messages (voice mail) to be left or recorded when the medical assistant is unavailable to answer the telephone.

For incoming calls, your office may have a voice messaging system to record messages for you when you are away from your desk. If you are using a voice message system, remember to include your name and number in your recorded greeting. Your voice messaging system should also allow for the caller to dial "0" for immediate assistance.

When calling patients, you will find that most of them will have some form of voice messaging system, whether with a land line or cell phone. This does present a problem in the context of patient privacy. It is important to know your office's policy as to what kind of message should be left on a patient's voice messaging system.

BOX 6-1
Placing a Caller on Hold: Things to Avoid

When placing a caller on hold always avoid:
- Switching the caller to "hold" before he or she states the reason for the call
- Placing several callers on hold at the same time
- Going back to the "hold" call and asking, "Who are you waiting for?"
- Cutting off calls by careless use of the hold button
- Leaving a caller "on hold" for several minutes without checking back on the caller
- Playing loud music on the telephone line while the patient is "on hold"
- Stating rudely "Hold" or "hold please" without giving any explanation

Call Forwarding

The call forwarding feature allows for a telephone user to forward calls to another telephone. For example, a physician may wish to forward his or her cell phone calls to a home telephone. You will often use this feature if your office uses an answering service. Your office calls will be forwarded to the answering services lines.

Caller ID

Caller ID is an increasingly popular telephone option. This function allows for telephone owners to know who is calling each time the telephone rings. In the office, it is unlikely that you will have caller ID, but many of your patients may have this telephone feature. It is important to understand that a medical office may need to block the office number from showing up on the patient's caller ID. This is because most offices often have multiple telephone lines, some designated for incoming calls and others for outgoing calls. Each of these lines may have a different telephone number. "Backlines"—lines meant only for incoming calls from patients—should be left open at all times. If a patient has caller ID, he or she may get the number to one of your "backlines." This can become very confusing to both the patient and the staff.

Privacy Manager

Privacy manager is a fairly recent addition to the variety of telephone options. This option allows patients to block access to their home telephones. When you call a telephone number that has privacy manager attached, you will be asked to state from where you are calling. Once you have given this information, unless you are cleared, you'll be directed to a voice mail system, where you will leave a message.

Speakerphone and Headsets

There are times when you will feel the need to free up your hands for administrative duties, while still being available to answer the telephone. There are two options that can be utilized: the speakerphone and the headset.

Most telephones have a built in speakerphone or a microphone and speaker. The speakerphone allows you

---

6-1 PROCEDURE

Taking a Telephone Message

OBJECTIVE: Ensure that correct and relevant information is retrieved when taking a telephone message.

Equipment and Supplies
message form or pad with carbon or carbonless for duplicates; pen

1. Give the correct greeting.
2. Use a message form or pad with a carbon copy to keep a record of the message.
3. Print the date and time of the call.
4. Print the caller's full name and telephone number. (Always ask the caller to spell his or her name.)
5. Write the name of the person being called.
6. Write down the complete message. Avoid using abbreviations other than accepted medical abbreviations. Include symptoms such as temperature, rash, emesis, and duration of symptoms.
7. Write your initials to indicate that you took the message.

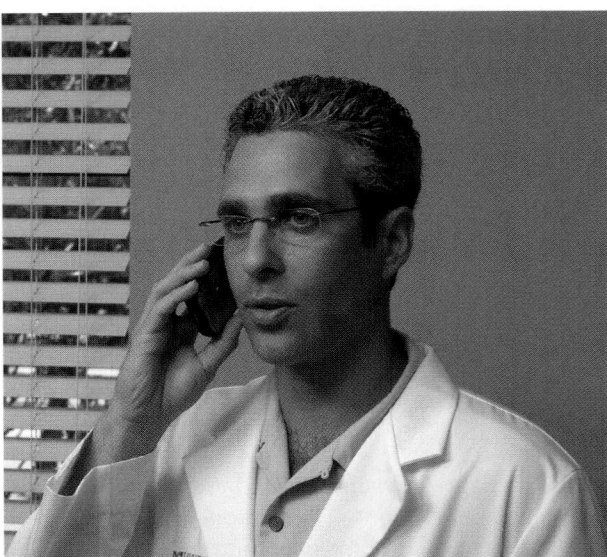

FIGURE 6-3 Many physicians use cell phones to stay in touch with their offices.

to hear and speak without having to pick up the handset of the telephone. There are a few drawbacks, however, to the speakerphone. Others nearby may overhear your conversation; also, the caller on the other end will be able to hear any background noise. Patient confidentiality should be a foremost concern when using the speakerphone.

Another hands-free feature is a headset. This is a microphone and earpiece that is worn on your head like a headband, an ergonomically safe feature. Headsets are either connected to the telephone with a cord, or they are cordless. When using a headset, you will need to remember to keep the microphone close to your mouth for the clearest delivery.

Pagers and Cell Phones

Many physicians carry pagers with them on a regular basis. It will be important for you to know if the physician(s) in your office carries a pager. This will be one of the most important methods for getting in touch with him or her in emergency situations. You will find that most pager systems are user-friendly. One simply has to call the pager number and when instructed, enter in the callback telephone number. Some offices may use a coded message system. For example, certain numbers may be designated for different types of emergencies or situations. Using a specific number will give the physician a heads up as to what the call is referencing. You will need to find out how your particular office uses the pager system.

Cell phones have become fundamental to business and social life. Most physicians and office managers now use cell phones to conduct day-to-day business

(Figure 6-3). Some have even replaced their conventional pagers with cell phones because most cell phones also have a pager function. However, cell phones do have a disadvantage in that certain parts of the hospitals do not allow them because they interfere with electronic monitors. Usually, hospital buildings are clearly marked as to where cell phones are allowed and where they are not allowed. In most of these cell-phone-free zones, pagers will still be allowed. It is important to check with the hospitals your office frequently deals with to understand their rules regarding cell phones and pagers.

Screening Telephone Calls

One of the most important ways to keep the office running smoothly and one of your key functions in the front office is to screen telephone calls effectively. When answering the telephone, you will need to determine quickly what type of call you have received and the proper way to handle it. Whenever you answer the telephone, you should ask the person the reason for the call. From there, you will either transfer the call to the appropriate person, or you will handle the call yourself. The different types of telephone calls you may receive will be discussed later in the chapter.

Making Reminder Calls and Doing Callbacks

Most offices will require medical assistants to make calls to patients to remind them of upcoming appointments. Offices might do this a week before the appointment and then again the day before the appointment.

As a medical assistant, you will also be required to make "callbacks"—return calls to patients or other callers. For instance, messages left by patients usually contain a question for the physician or deal with prescription refill requests. Your callback will relay the physician's response. Sometimes the physician may have you call a patient to check on his or her status.

When making any of these calls to a patient's house or place of business, you will need to take care in protecting the patient's privacy. Remember that this is one of the most important issues concerning a medical facility. The first thing that you should do when calling any patient is to make sure that it is the patient that you are speaking with on the telephone. Start every callback to the patient by identifying yourself, and then ask to speak to the patient. You should not indicate why you are calling until you have the patient on the telephone line. If the person who answers asks you why you are calling, explain that confidentiality laws prevent you from revealing that information.

Typical Incoming Calls

You will receive many different types of calls in the medical office. Most are from patients, but many are not. The following are some types of telephone calls you will handle on a daily basis.

Patient Calls

Most calls coming into the medical office will be from patients (Figure 6-4). We will discuss a few of the reasons why patients call.

Appointment Requests

One of the most common types of calls you receive in the office will be appointment requests. These calls will often involve patients with health problems, so you need to follow telephone triage procedures (discussed later in the chapter) to schedule them appropriately. The caller may be a current patient or a new patient. For patients who need routine appointments, give an appointment time that is convenient for both the patient and the medical office. You will learn more about scheduling appointments in Chapter 8.

Insurance and Billing Questions

It is a fact that most patients will not understand the way medical insurance works. You should anticipate receiving calls on a daily basis from patients with questions about their accounts and medical insurance. You may be able to answer some of these questions, but most will be directed to the billing department.

PROBLEMS WITH BILLS Patients will often call with the question, "Why did I receive a bill?" Many patients have the misconception that their insurance company will pay the entire bill. You may have to explain to the patient the details of what was billed. In your explanation, you will need to include what steps the insurance company has taken in regards to covering the charges. This could include discussing deductibles, co-payments, and coinsurance. You may also need to explain reasons for denial of certain charges. If you are unable to help the patient with questions concerning insurance coverage, you may refer him or her to the insurance company or to the human resources department of your employer.

ARE YOU A PARTICIPATING PROVIDER? The medical assistant should have a list of the most common insurance providers with whom the practice is affiliated. Specific questions patients have regarding provider participation should be directed to the insurance company.

Fees

Specific questions regarding fees should always be referred to the billing department. You should keep in mind that more often than not, you will be unable to give any exact figures until the patient has been seen by the physician.

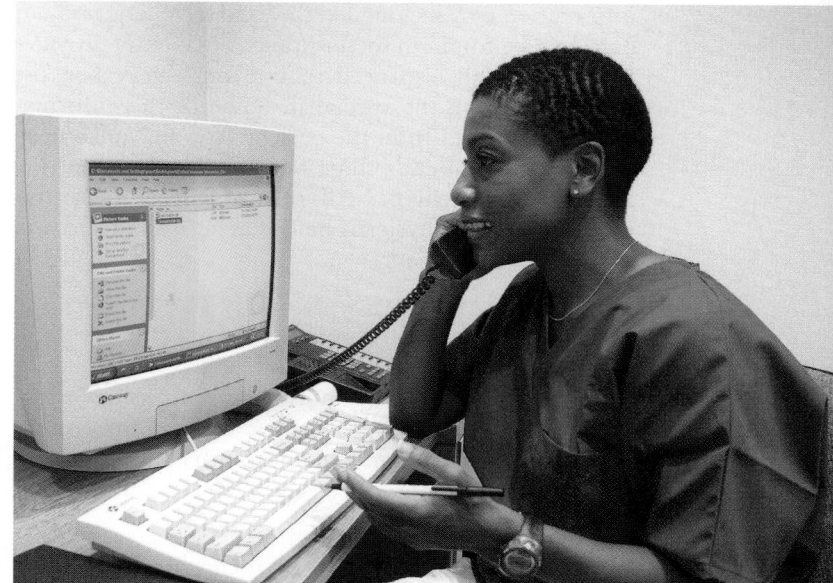

FIGURE 6-4 The medical assistant spends many hours on the telephone assisting patients.

Office Hours and Directions

Most offices now include the office hours and directions in the office's automated assistance systems. However, you may have to handle some of the calls yourself. You should have your office address and hours posted near your telephone. It is also a good idea to have directions posted near the telephone. The directions should include routes to the office from all directions—north, south, east, and west—when applicable.

Laboratory Test Results

Many patients will call the office, to get the results from recent procedures and tests. Follow your office policy regarding disseminating results to patients. Certain tests may require follow up testing or procedures. In that case, follow up is necessary to ensure that the patient performed as instructed.

Follow-Up Calls From Patients

It is common for a physician to have a patient call the office as a follow-up to certain procedures and to relate the status of certain problems. When these calls come into the office, you will need to take a message to convey this information to the physician.

Referral Requests

Many insurance companies require that patients get referrals (special paperwork) from primary care physicians when patients see a specialist. So it will often happen that a patient may call asking for the referral to be done. Referrals are done before the patient is to see the specialist and may be done over the telephone or by fax. You will need to get all of the information necessary to place the referral, including the name, address, and telephone number of the specialist's office. This information may be found in the local telephone book. It may also be found in the insurance company's provider book. You will also need to find out the reason the patient is seeing the specialist. Some of this information you may get from the patient. You may also need to check the patient's chart for the diagnosis that the referral is referencing. All referrals need to be approved by your physician before being completed and released to the patient.

Patients Who Refuse to Identify Themselves

Occasionally you will run into patients who refuse to identify themselves to you. You will need to let the caller know that you will not be of assistance without his or her name and reason for calling. Inform the caller that the physician will not return calls to patients who refuse to identify themselves.

The Persistent Talker

Every medical office has those patients who call in and draw the staff into long conversations. Unfortunately, your time is valuable and limited. You will need to end these conversations kindly, but promptly. You may simply state to the patient that you are busy helping another patient and apologize for the inconvenience.

Nonpatient Calls

Not all telephone calls to the office will be from patients. You will find that a large number of calls will come from sales people, hospitals, other physicians, and other health care facilities.

Sales Calls

Answering calls from sales representatives is part of the medical assistant's telephone responsibilities. You may have to become the wall between the sales calls and your physician and office manager. Most physicians will not take any type of sales calls while seeing patients. They may wish you to take messages or ask the sales representative to fax or email the information to them. The same will probably hold true with office managers. They will ask you to take messages from most sales calls to return the calls at a more convenient time.

Reports From Hospitals and Other Patient Care Facilities

If your physician has patients in a hospital or nursing facility, it will be common to receive calls from those facilities. The facilities will often call with status checks on patients or changes in patients' conditions. In many cases, you will need to interrupt the physician for these calls. You should knock on the examination room door and let the physician know that there is an important call.

There will also be times when you will just need to take a message for the physician. The message may just be information to relay or the physician may need to return the call. It is important that you find out whether or not the call should be returned.

BOX 6-2

Information to Request From the Patient

- Patient's name
- The caller's name, if different from the patient
- Telephone number
- Date of the call
- Time of the call
- The patient's physician, if a multi-physician practice
- Any medications that the patient is taking
- Any allergies the patient may have
- The patient's insurance
- The manner of the patient's problem

General Office Matters

Some calls received in the office deal with general office business, including telephone calls from accountants or calls regarding rented office equipment and suppliers. These calls should be handled on a case-by-case basis. It is important to screen calls from your suppliers carefully. Make sure the supplier gives you his or her name, the business' name, address, and telephone number.

Physician's Personal Calls

The physician will also receive personal calls in the office. Physicians work long hours and often encourage family members to call them at the office. Most physicians will instruct you on how they wish their personal calls to be handled. In some cases, they will want you to knock on the examination room door and simply state, "Doctor, you are wanted on the telephone." In other cases, physicians may ask you to give them telephone messages as soon as they come out of the examination room. Generally, family members do not wish to interrupt the physician during a patient examination.

Calls From Another Physician

Personal calls from other physicians are handled in a similar manner. Physicians may wish to talk to other physicians as soon as the call comes into the office. These calls may relate to a patient consultation question that needs to be answered immediately. Again, you may take a message to be delivered to the physician as he or she exits the examination room, or you may interrupt the physician with the call. You will need to follow the wishes of your employer.

Obscene or Prank Calls

It is a fact that if you have a telephone, you are at risk for receiving prank calls. You should hang up immediately if you receive obscene or prank calls. You may also report the call to the telephone operator, especially if it is an ongoing problem involving the same caller. Usually, the telephone company can trace the call.

Prescription Refill Requests

One of the most common telephone calls received in the office are requests for prescription refills. Because of the high volume of calls, many offices will have a voice mail system answer most of these calls. The medical assistant is often responsible for taking these messages off the voice mail system and responding to them. This will need to be done more than just once a day. The messages should be checked a minimum of twice a day and in larger offices, even more frequently. All of the prescription refill requests will need to be signed-off by the physician. Some physicians will request to have the patient's chart with the message before giving it an okay. It is advisable to be prepared and attach the message to the chart ahead of time. See Procedure 6-2 for important information on taking a prescription refill message.

Telephone Triage

Triage is a process used to determine the order in which patients should be treated. The patient's severity of illness or injury determines the order of treatment. Telephone triage—determining the order to take patient calls—is an issue for the telephone screening process. By asking specific questions, the medical assistant can determine how to handle a patient's problem. Each office should have a procedure manual that will outline the office's preferred method of screening telephone calls.

Most of your patients will be calling because they feel they need to see the physician. It will be one of your responsibilities to see that the patient is helped in the most appropriate manner. You will need to gather information from the patient. As with all telephone calls, the first thing you'll need to find out is

Lifespan
Considerations

When handling pediatric cases, the information received about the patient will most likely be from a parent or guardian. You will find that first-time parents may call often. As these parents' primary contact in the medical office, you will need to always treat them with respect and patience. Remember, what may be perceived as a minor health situation for most people, can be perceived as a major health situation for first-time parents.

the patient's name and telephone number, in case you become disconnected. Remember to have the patient spell out his or her name to avoid mistakes. During the course of your conversation, you should ask for some basic demographic information as well as for medical information. Box 6-2 lists information that you should request from the patient. When scheduling the patient, make sure to include the information that you received from the patient. Then place the information in the patient's chart. This will help you or another medical assistant know how to prepare for the appointment. Cultural Considerations discusses more about obtaining information from patients.

The medical assistant must be careful when screening patients on the telephone. You will be assessing a patient's symptoms. This, however, is very close to going outside of the medical assistant's scope of practice. Make sure that you are closely following the established telephone protocols that were agreed upon by the physician. If ever a situation arises that is not covered in the procedure manual, the medical assistant will need to ask the physician how to handle that

Cultural Considerations

You will encounter an array cultural differences when fielding calls in a medical office. When dealing with a patient, it is always best to speak directly with him or her to get the best information. However, there are some cultures that may not allow direct contact with certain members of the family. Even though it is often difficult to obtain vital information by proxy (a third person), it is sometimes necessary so as to avoid cultural clashes.

You may also deal with patients with very poor English skills. Sometimes a translator is necessary. Your main goal when taking calls is to make the patient as comfortable as possible while providing the appropriate assistance.

particular problem. Physicians will often purchase one of many triage manuals that are available on the market. Again, remember to follow only the protocols that the physician has approved. Lifespan Considerations addresses more on assessing symptoms.

If a patient refuses to tell you the reason for the call, you should explain the need for specific information so as to assist him or her. Try to make the caller comfortable in sharing the information with you.

Handling Difficult Calls

The most important thing to remember when dealing with a difficult patient is not to lose your temper. There are many types of problematic calls that you may receive. They can vary from patients who are angry and yelling, to people attempting to get confidential information. With any difficult caller, you must try and keep the situation as calm as possible. It is best to keep in mind that the patient, more often than not, is displacing anger and is probably frustrated with some other situation. It could be anything from worry over an illness, to having had a bad day, to suffering from pain.

When you have a difficult patient on the telephone line, the best approach is to be empathetic while remaining in control of the situation. Take the time to listen and find out the exact problem. Once you determine where the problem lies, then you can begin to help.

Using a Telephone Directory

When calling most insurance companies and hospitals, you will find that they have an automated telephone directory or automated assistance program—telephone systems that direct callers to the appropriate people through a series of questions.

After the call is answered, the caller is presented with options so that the telephone system can direct him or her to the proper person or department to handle the call. Be aware that many large business systems will also provide additional options. When using one of these systems, it is important to pay close attention to the options that are being offered. It can be easy to miss your cue. When you hear an option, the system will instruct you either to press the appropriate button or to state the option verbally. Keep in mind that in most systems, if you cannot find an option to fit your needs, you can dial "0" to have the operator of the system direct you manually. Patient Education highlights more uses of an automatic assistance program.

The term telephone directory can also pertain to the telephone book. These books are provided to you by your local telephone company. They come in two main forms, white pages and yellow pages. The white pages list the name, address, and telephone number of the telephone customers; the yellow pages are used to list the name, address, and telephone number of local businesses. It does cost to have your business listed. Some resources that are provided in the telephone book

---

| 6-2 | **PROCEDURE** |

Taking a Prescription Refill Message

OBJECTIVE: Ensure that correct information is acquired when refilling a patient's prescription.

Equipment and Supplies
message pad or paper; pen

1. Print the name of the patient. (This name may be different from the name of the caller.)
2. Write down the patient's telephone number.
3. Write down the name of the medication. Ask the caller to spell the medication if you are unclear about what the caller is saying.
4. Write down how long the patient has been on the medication.
5. Write down the patient's symptoms and why the prescription is still needed.
6. Take the patient's age and weight (if a child).
7. Ask for the name and telephone number of the pharmacy and the prescription number.
8. Tell the caller you will give the message to the physician.
9. Tell the caller that you will call back if the prescription cannot be refilled.
10. Pull out the patient's chart for the physician to review and attach the telephone message to it.

---

include emergency numbers, local government numbers, national area codes, and zip codes from your region. The telephone book is also where you will find directions on making long distance calls, including international calls.

Long Distance Calls

Occasionally, you will be asked to make long distance telephone calls for office business. For a time, a long distance call would be any call outside of your area code. This is no longer true. Many of the larger cities have had to add area codes within local calling regions. It will be necessary for you to learn what is considered long distance in your area. Long distance calls can be very costly, so your office may limit how many are made.

Telephone Logs

You will find that many offices maintain a telephone log to keep track of the long distance calls being made. When the telephone bill arrives, then the log and the bill can be compared. This can help to identify any abuses of the business telephone with personal calls. Many logs will have you list the name of the person, the facility or company being called, the number being called, the name of the person placing the call, the date and time of the call, the city and state where the call is being placed, the duration of the call, and the reason for it.

Making a Long Distance Call

Direct Distance Dialing (DDD) is the most common way of making a long distance call. To place a long distance call using DDD, dial "1," then the area code followed by the number you are calling. If you need to find an area code, you will find the listing of area codes at the front of the telephone book. The telephone book will also give you instructions for making international calls, if you are required to make them.

Another way of calling long distance is to make a collect call—reversing the call charges to the person

recieving the call. When collect calls are placed, the person being called is asked by the operator whether or not he or she will accept the charges. Your office should have a policy in place regarding accepting or denying collect calls.

Conference Calls

When several people from different locations wish to have a telephone discussion, you would place a conference call. This means, for example, two physicians at a distance from each other may speak with a patient at a third location at the same time. While these calls are more expensive than regular long distance calls, they can save money in the long run, since you do not have to make several long distance calls to relay the same information.

Most business telephone systems allow you to make conference calls without using the telephone operator. You will need to look into your telephone system to see if it allows you to set up a conference call. If your system is not set up to do conference calls, you may use the operator to place the calls. See Procedure 6-3 for placing a conference call.

Time Zones

You must be aware of time zones within the United States and foreign countries when placing long distance telephone calls. The continental United States and parts of Canada are divided into four time zones based on their location in the country: eastern, central, mountain, and pacific. As you move from east to west across the United States, there is a one-hour difference (earlier) in each time zone. For example, if it is 9:00 A.M. in Ohio (eastern time zone), then it will be 8:00 A.M. in Illinois (central time zone).

It is a good idea to have a time zone map posted near your office telephone (Figure 6-5). This way you can plan long distance calls based on "office hours" in each time zone. A call placed at 3:00 P.M. in California will be received in New York at 6:00 P.M., which is usually after office closing hours.

Placing a Conference Call

OBJECTIVE: Allow for a discussion via the telephone between three or more parties from various locations.

Equipment and Supplies
Telephone numbers of participating parties

1. Gather the telephone numbers of all participants before beginning the call.
2. Determine the time that everyone will be available for the conference call. You may have to call people in advance to determine a convenient time. Be aware of time zone differences when arranging conference calls.
3. Dial "0" for operator and give the operator the name and telephone number (area code first) for each person to be called.

4. The operator will then place a call to each of the parties. When all the participants are on the line, the operator will come back to the original caller (you) and the conversation can then begin. If you are placing this call for your physician, he or she will then pick up on your line.
5. If you are setting the conference call up ahead of time, tell the operator when you wish the conference call to begin.

Using an Answering Service

Many offices use an answering service for times when no one is available in the office. This service can be in effect 24-hours a day or just at designated times, for example: during the night, during lunch, or during peak hours of the day to relieve office staff.

The system works by forwarding your office calls to the service, which is at an off-site location. The answering service personnel answer the calls that come in and inform the patients that the office is closed. They will also take some non-emergency messages, which will be delivered to the staff when you return your telephone calls back to your care. When emergency calls come in, the answering service will contact the physician by pager or telephone.

This service does have a fee attached, but many offices will consider this a necessary service. You do have the option of using an answering machine or voice messaging system while the office is closed. This option is less expensive, but the patients' problems may not be addressed as quickly. If you do use an answering machine or voice messaging system, you will need to make sure that the messages are retrieved in a timely manner and that the recorded office greeting provides a number to call in case of an emergency.

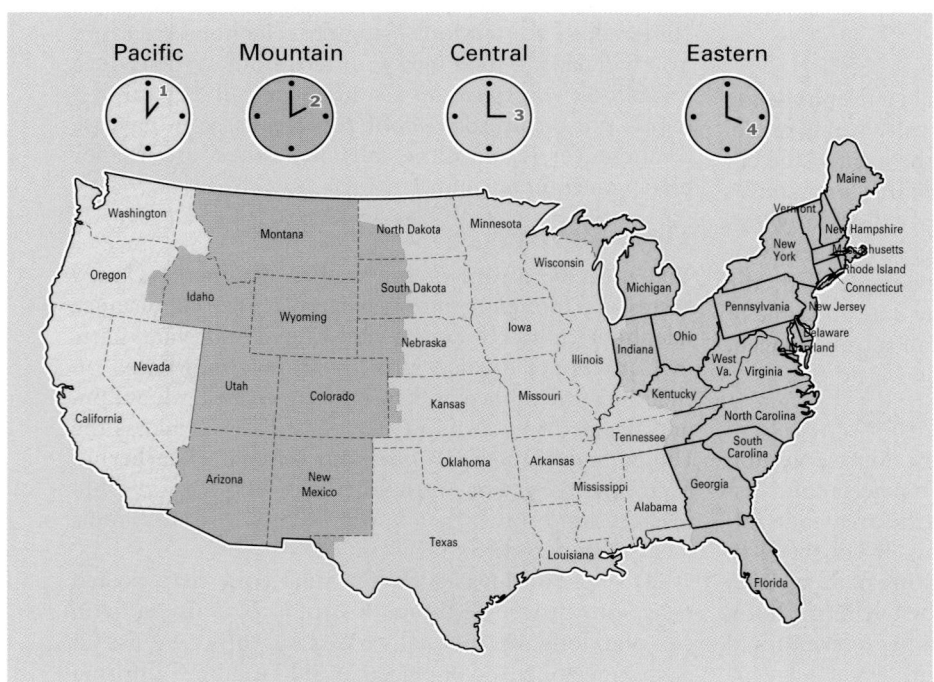

FIGURE 6-5 Having a time zone map located near the telephone will assist you with long distance calls outside your time zone.

Handling an Emergency Telephone Call

Every office should have a written protocol for handling emergency calls. Since you cannot see the telephone caller, it can be difficult to determine a true emergency by talking to someone over the telephone. It is critical to get the caller's name and telephone number immediately in case you are disconnected. You will then proceed by asking the patient specific questions. Examples of questions that you may ask, depending upon your office's procedure, are listed in Box 6-3. If an emergency is taking place during the telephone call, then alert the physician immediately.

In some cases, the patient may be hysterical or crying. Your job, in a situation such as this, is to calm the patient. If your voice remains calm and reassuring, you may be able to soothe the patient. If the caller is extremely upset, ask if there is someone else who can come to the telephone. Your role is to gain as much information from the caller as possible so that the emergency can be handled quickly. Following are some types of emergencies you may face.

- allergic reactions (anaphylactic shock)
- asthma
- broken bone
- drug overdose
- eye injury/foreign body
- gunshot/stabbing wound
- heart attack
- inability to breathe (or difficulty breathing)
- loss of consciousness
- premature labor
- profuse bleeding
- severe pain, including chest pain
- severe vomiting and/or diarrhea
- suicide attempt or suicide threats
- high temperature

BOX 6-3

Questions to Ask When Handling a Telephone Emergency

- What is your name?
- What is your telephone number?
- What is your relationship to the caller? (if a parent, spouse, friend, or passer-by is calling).
- What is the emergency?
- When did the emergency occur?
- How severe is the emergency?
- What are the patient's symptoms? (Problems breathing? Bleeding? Extreme pain? Other symptoms?)
- What has been done for the patient?
- Has anyone called an ambulance?
- Who is the patient's primary physician?
- Where is the emergency?

Note: Some specialists, such as obstetricians and cardiologists, may have additional questions they wish to have you ask the caller.

If your physician is not present, your office should have a policy in place for how to handle emergency calls. You may be required to call 911 while the patient is on the line, or you may need to instruct the patient to hang up and dial 911 directly from his or her home telephone.

Never take an emergency call lightly. Emergencies can become life-threatening if no treatment is provided. Even if you have questions as to whether the call is actually an emergency, you must always assume it is and alert the physician. Malpractice suits have been brought against medical assistants who have failed to correctly handle an emergency.

SUMMARY

A medical assistant who is working in a front desk position will find that the majority of his or her time is spent on the telephone. It is important to remember that when you are on the telephone, you are representing the medical office. Always greet the caller warmly and professionally. On a typical day, you will field many different types of calls. Take each call one at a time, and use the techniques and procedures from the chapter to work more efficiently.

Chapter Review

COMPETENCY REVIEW

1. When it is 9:00 A.M. in New York, what time is it in Pittsburgh, PA; St. Paul, MN; Los Angeles, CA; and Denver, CO?
2. Write a telephone message for a patient who calls for a refill of *Estrace* 1 mg. daily.
3. How might you handle receiving a prank telephone call?
4. Why should you smile when answering the telephone?
5. What do you do when you are helping a patient on one line and another line begins to ring?

PREPARING FOR THE CERTIFICATION EXAM

1. When taking a prescription refill message from a patient you should include writing down the following, EXCEPT
   A. patient's name and telephone number
   B. medication and length of time the patient has been taking it
   C. patient's symptoms
   D. pharmacy's prescription number, name, and telephone number
   E. patient's social security number

2. The type of long distance call that might be used to facilitate the consultation of one physician with another is called a/an
   A. operator-assisted call
   B. DDD
   C. conference call
   D. collect call
   E. station-to-station call

3. When handling an emergency telephone call from a patient, the FIRST thing a medical assistant should do is
   A. get the caller's name and telephone number
   B. ascertain whether or not it is, in fact, an emergency
   C. gather as much information about the emergency in the shortest amount of time
   D. ask to speak with someone other than the patient/caller, who is too hysterical to communicate the details of the situation
   E. ask if an ambulance has been summoned

4. A proper initial greeting upon answering the telephone would be
   A. "Gynecology Associates."
   B. "Please hold."
   C. "Good afternoon."
   D. "This is Mary King, may I help you?"
   E. "Gynecology Associates, Ms. King speaking, may I help you?"

5. After a patient is placed on hold, it is proper to check back every
   A. 10 seconds
   B. 20 seconds
   C. 30 seconds
   D. 1 minute
   E. 2 minutes

6. When handling a request for a prescription refill, a medical assistant
   A. may call in the request, but only for a non-controlled substance
   B. should ask the patient to come into the office to obtain a written prescription
   C. may never call in a refill without the physician's direct order
   D. is certified to call in all prescription refills
   E. should call in the prescription if directed to do so by a nurse

7. A ringing telephone should be answered by the
   A. first ring
   B. second ring
   C. third ring
   D. fourth ring
   E. fifth ring

8. If a medical assistant is already speaking to a patient when another phone line rings, it is best to
   A. call to another medical assistant to answer the other line
   B. let the other line be picked up by the voice mail
   C. let the patient finish his or her question and then say, "Would you please hold?"
   D. ask the patient if you may place him or her on hold
   E. answer the second caller and handle the problem right away

continued on next page

9. A system of prioritizing patient calls according to the most ill or injured is known as
   A. classifying
   B. telephone triage
   C. insurance pre-approval
   D. mortality rate
   E. morbidity rate

10. If an emergency is taking place to the person making the telephone call, the first action the medical assistant should take is to
    A. alert the physician immediately
    B. call 911
    C. put the caller on the speaker phone
    D. record the call for liability purposes
    E. tell the person to go to the hospital immediately

CRITICAL THINKING

1. What do you think was wrong with Tonya's greeting?

2. How could Tonya improve the impressions that Cindy received so as to prevent Cindy from seeking another physician?

3. What was wrong with the way Cindy was put on hold? How could this have been improved?

4. What else in Cindy's phone call could have increased her frustration, and how could it have been helped?

ON THE JOB

For over two years, medical assistant Linda Lewis has been employed by Drs. Norek and Klein, who are gerontologists. Also on staff are two registered nurses, a medical laboratory technician, and a medical social worker. The daughter of one of the doctor's patients has just called the office. She is very distraught at the seemingly diminished capacity of her mother and insists on speaking to the doctor.

Linda explains that both of the physicians only take emergency calls during patient appointment hours, but that she will take a detailed message. The caller, however, suggests that not only should her call be considered an emergency, but that she will sue the doctor if the call is not handled accordingly.

1. What should Linda do immediately to diffuse the situation?
2. Is this clearly a case where the call should be passed on to one of the registered nurses or even the medical social worker?
3. Is this a case where, because of the threat of an impending suit, the physician should be called to the telephone?
4. How could Linda ascertain whether or not this, indeed, is an emergency? Is it even up to her as a medical assistant to make such a determination?
5. Since this is the patient's daughter, rather than the patient herself, does Linda have any reason to even enter into a conversation with the caller? Could Linda be ethically bound by confidentiality to not even admit the woman's mother is a patient?

INTERNET ACTIVITY

Use the Internet and research the ways HIPAA has affected the use of the telephone in the medical office.

 MediaLink More on telephone techniques in the medical office environment, including interactive resources, can be found on the Student CD-ROM accompanying this textbook.

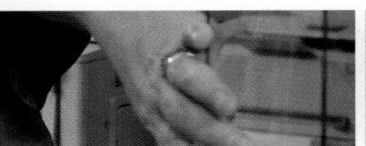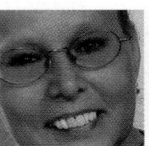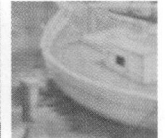

Medical Assistant Role Delineation Chart

HIGHLIGHT indicates material covered in this chapter.

ADMINISTRATIVE

Administrative Procedures

- Perform basic administrative medical assisting functions
- Schedule, coordinate and monitor appointments
- Schedule inpatient/outpatient admissions and procedures
- Understand and apply third-party guidelines
- Obtain reimbursement through accurate claims submission
- Monitor third-party reimbursement
- Understand and adhere to managed care policies and procedures
- *Negotiate managed care contracts*

- Manage accounts receivable
- *Manage accounts payable*
- *Process payroll*
- *Document and maintain accounting and banking records*
- *Develop and maintain fee schedules*
- *Manage renewals of business and professional insurance policies*
- *Manage personnel benefits and maintain records*
- *Perform marketing, financial, and strategic planning*

Practice Finances

- Perform procedural and diagnostic coding
- Apply bookkeeping principles

CLINICAL

Fundamental Principles

- Apply principles of aseptic technique and infection control
- Comply with quality assurance practices
- Screen and follow up patient test results

Diagnostic Orders

- Collect and process specimens
- Perform diagnostic tests

Patient Care

- Adhere to established patient screening procedures
- Obtain patient history and vital signs
- Prepare and maintain examination and treatment areas
- Prepare patient for examinations, procedures and treatments

- Assist with examinations, procedures and treatments
- Prepare and administer medications and immunizations
- Maintain medication and immunization records
- Recognize and respond to emergencies
- Coordinate patient care information with other health care providers
- Initiate IV and administer IV medications with appropriate training and as permitted by state law

GENERAL

Professionalism

- Display a professional manner and image
- Demonstrate initiative and responsibility
- Work as a member of the health care team
- Prioritize and perform multiple tasks
- Adapt to change
- Promote the CMA credential
- Enhance skills through continuing education
- Treat all patients with compassion and empathy
- Promote the practice through positive public relations

Communication Skills

- Recognize and respect cultural diversity
- Adapt communications to individual's ability to understand
- Use professional telephone technique

- Recognize and respond effectively to verbal, nonverbal, and written communications
- Use medical terminology appropriately
- Utilize electronic technology to receive, organize, prioritize and transmit information
- Serve as liaison

Legal Concepts

- Perform within legal and ethical boundaries
- Prepare and maintain medical records
- Document accurately
- Follow employer's established policies dealing with the health care contract
- Implement and maintain federal and state health care legislation and regulations
- Comply with established risk management and safety procedures
- Recognize professional credentialing criteria
- *Develop and maintain personnel, policy and procedure manuals*

Instruction

- Instruct individuals according to their needs
- Explain office policies and procedures
- Teach methods of health promotion and disease prevention
- Locate community resources and disseminate information
- *Develop educational materials*
- *Conduct continuing education activities*

Operational Functions

- Perform inventory of supplies and equipment
- Perform routine maintenance of administrative and clinical equipment
- Apply computer techniques to support office operations
- *Perform personnel management functions*
- *Negotiate leases and prices for equipment and supply contracts*

- *Denotes advanced skills.*

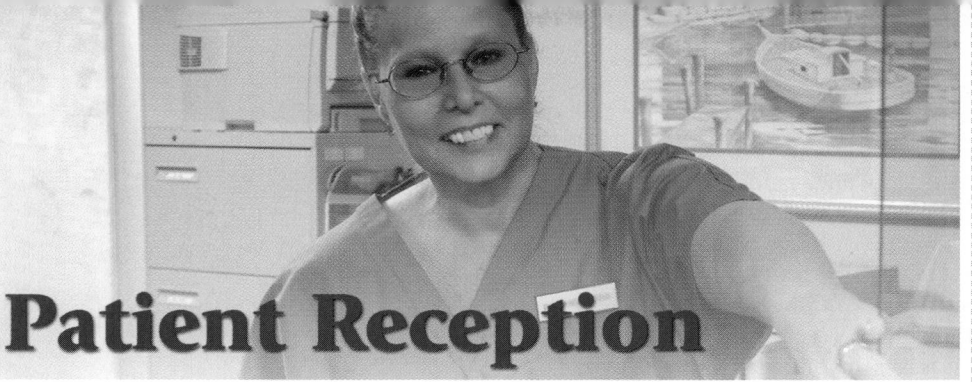

Patient Reception

Learning Objectives

After completing this chapter, you should be able to:

- Define and spell the terms to learn for this chapter.
- List the receptionist's responsibilities.
- Explain the procedure for opening the office.
- List the information to be obtained from the new patient.
- Describe how to handle the angry patient.
- Describe how to handle a waiting room emergency.
- Explain the procedure for closing the office.
- Explain the legal and ethical issues related to the duties of the receptionist.
- Describe the look of a professional medical assistant.

Terms to Learn

collating

co-payment

demographic

facsimile (fax)

medical emergency

no-show

overbooking

receptionist

OUTLINE

Duties of a Receptionist   130

Personal Characteristics and
  Physical Appearance   131

Opening the Office   132

Collating Records   132

Greeting the Patient Upon
  Arrival   134

Registering New Patients   135

Charge Slips   135

Consideration for the
  Patient's Time   136

Escorting the Patient into
  the Examination Room   136

Managing Disturbances   137

No-Shows   138

Closing the Office   138

Case Study

STACY IS A NEW PATIENT COMING INTO DR. MATHIAS' OFFICE. She was sent her new patient paperwork in the mail when she made her appointment. She has the papers already completed as she goes up to the receptionist. Betsy has been the receptionist for Dr. Mathias for only three months. When Stacy comes to the window, Betsy greets her with a smile and welcomes her to the office. She then asks for Stacy's paperwork. Betsy goes through the papers to make sure that everything was signed and completed. She then asks for Stacy's insurance cards and ID to make copies. Betsy gives Stacy the HIPAA notice of privacy practice to read over and has her sign an acknowledgement of receipt. Betsy makes front and back copies of Stacy's insurance card and ID. She notes that Stacy has a $15.00 co-payment. She collects it before Stacy goes back for her appointment. During this time the phone rings, and the only person available to answer is Betsy. She answers it by the third ring, places the patient on hold, and returns to helping Stacy. Once Betsy has completed checking in Stacy, she returns to the phone call. About two minutes has elapsed and the patient on the line has hung up.

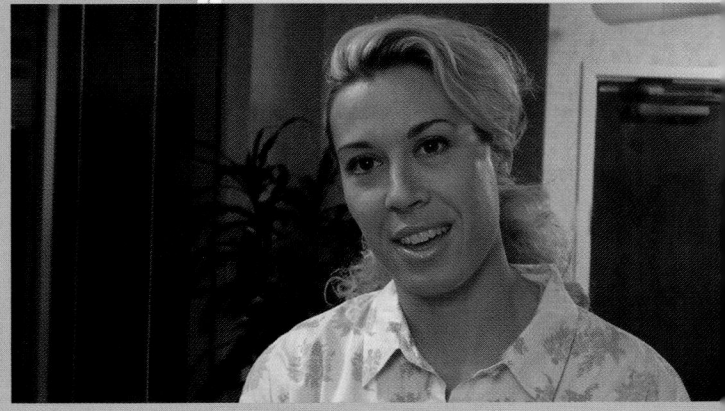

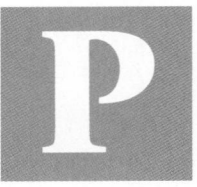

Patient reception requires a multiskilled individual whose manner, physical appearance, and tone of voice projects a professional, confident, and caring manner. A small office will have fewer employees than one with several physicians; therefore, the medical assistant in a small office will perform many of the tasks described in this chapter. In the role of receptionist, the medical assistant greets and assists incoming patients and performs many important duties, which make the office run smoothly and efficiently. Some of these duties are quiet and behind the scenes; others require constant interaction with patients. The medical assistant who functions as a receptionist must do everything possible to ensure patient safety and confidentiality at all times during the office visit.

Duties of a Receptionist

The number of patients as well as the nature of the medical practice—for example, whether it is a solo practice or a corporation of several physicians—will determine what duties or tasks the medical assistant performs in the role of receptionist (Figure 7-1).

The duties of a receptionist may include opening the office, greeting patients upon arrival, assisting a new patient with completion of the proper forms, maintaining a clean and safe environment in the reception area, managing any disturbance in the reception area, and handling a medical emergency or patient condition, which may be life threatening if left untreated. In addition, the receptionist may also handle

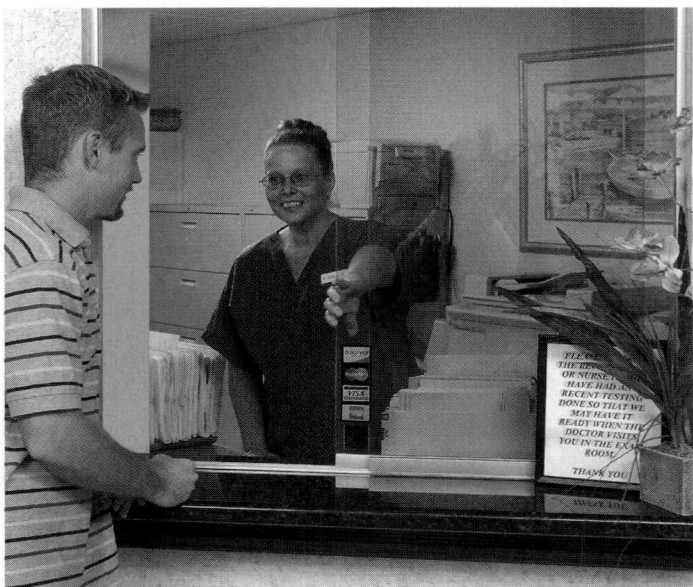

FIGURE 7-1 The medical assistant as receptionist in a medical office.

BOX 7-1
Duties of a Medical Receptionist

- Opening the office
- Pulling charts for the next day's appointments
- Collating patient records
- Checking in patients
- Greeting patients as they arrive
- Getting updated patient demographics
- Helping new patients fill out new paperwork
- Keeping the reception area clean and safe
- Managing any reception area disturbances
- Handling any reception area emergencies
- Handling some incoming calls
- Scheduling return appointments
- Possibly escorting patients to the exam rooms
- Keeping in mind the patient's time
- Documenting patient no-shows
- Closing the office

incoming telephone calls for the office, schedule returning appointments, and make reminder calls for upcoming appointments. Many of these jobs will be discussed in more detail throughout the chapter. See Box 7-1 for a list of reception duties.

The Reception Room

One of the most forgotten roles of the medical assistant will be taking care of the reception area. Many offices still refer to this area as the waiting room. However, many now call it the reception area to avoid the negative term *waiting*. This area must be kept clean and free from any hazards that may injure the patient. It is the first impression of the office that the patient gets. The receptionist will need to monitor the cleanliness of the room. If the room begins to get messy, the receptionist may need to take the time to straighten it up. Magazines, brochures, patient education documents, and toys should be arranged neatly. Any papers that may lie around need either to be thrown away or destroyed, depending upon the information they may contain. See Figure 7-2 and Professionalism for more on the reception room.

Lost and Found

It may also be the responsibility of the receptionist to take care of items left by patients in the reception area. The office may have a lost and found box in which these items may be kept. Many offices will try to contact a patient if it is known to whom the item belongs. The office may have a policy as to how long unclaimed items are kept before being thrown away or donated to a local charity.

Handling Incoming Money

The receptionist is often the person in charge of accepting office payments. They will often be responsible for collecting balances on accounts and co-payments. Co-payments are designated amounts that some medical insurance plans require patients to pay for medical services or medication, usually at the time of service. It is important to keep excellent records of all incoming money so that balancing at the end of the day is easier. See Chapter 13 for more on the handling of money in the medical office.

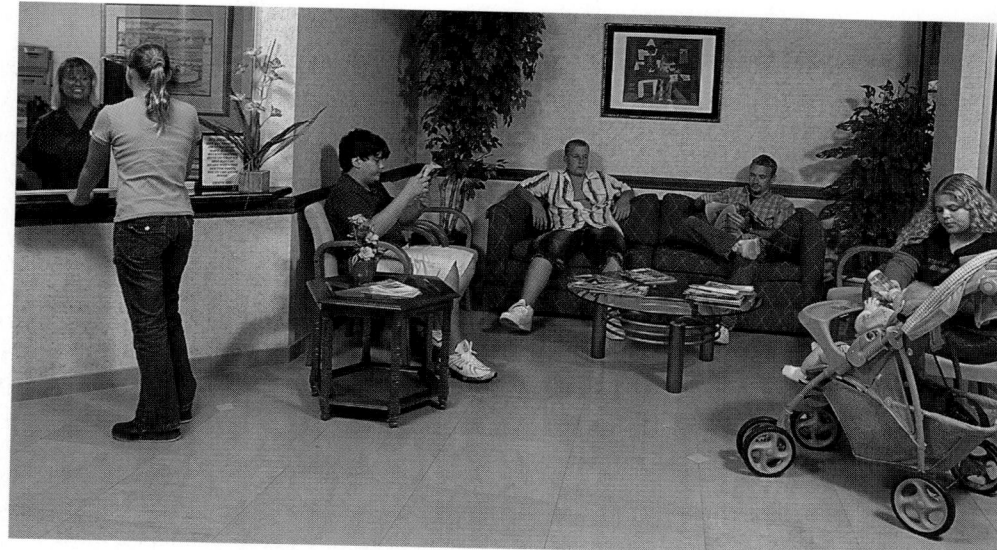

FIGURE 7-2 A typical reception area in a medical office.

Care and Maintenance of Office Equipment

The receptionist is often responsible for taking care of certain equipment such as the copiers, computers, printers, and facsimile or fax machines. It is important to learn the many functions of these machines. Knowledge of how to repair small problems, such as paper jams, is also helpful. If you are unable to fix something, it is important to know what numbers to call for service. The receptionist may also need to know how to replace certain things such as toner and ink cartridges. It is very important to make sure that these machines are filled with paper. See Chapter 11 for more information regarding the use of computers and troubleshooting.

Personal Characteristics and Physical Appearance

The receptionist is the first person a patient will see upon entering the office. Presenting a positive public image is important since your appearance reflects upon the entire staff. Careful grooming, good hygiene, and appropriate dress need to be observed. Office policy will dictate the preferred clothing. In most offices, the clinical staff wear uniforms of the same type. This can consist of scrub type pants and top with a lab coat. The advantage of this type of uniform is that it can be worn by both male and female staff and is relatively inexpensive. Colors and patterns of uniforms are usually determined by the management of the practice. Receptionists frequently wear the same style uniform as the clinical staff but without a lab coat, or they may be allowed to dress in business casual dress.

Hygiene, at a minimum, consists of daily bathing, use of a deodorant without a strong scent, good oral care, and clean, well-pressed clothing. Make-up, hairstyles, and jewelry worn by male and female medical assistants should reflect professionalism. Accessories should be conservative and minimal—generally limited to one finger ring, a watch with a second hand, name tag and a professional association pin. Long hair should be worn tied back and off the shoulders. Nails should be well trimmed and only clear polish should be used. No perfumes should be worn as patients can be allergic to certain scents. Lifespan Considerations discusses more about personal hygiene.

Name pins/tags should be visible at all times. More offices are requiring a picture ID for security reasons. These tags can serve dual purposes. With a magnetic strip, they can allow entrance into a secure area and can also be used to clock in and out the hours worked.

Professionalism

The receptionist is the first representative of the medical office that the patient is exposed to either by phone or in person. It is important that the first impression inspire confidence in the patient to the office's ability to meet his or her needs. This means that receptionists need to take great care in their appearance. Their clothes should be clean and pressed. The receptionist's hygiene influences the patient's perception of the cleanliness of the office. Receptionists need to keep their area of the office neat and organized. If patients see a messy, disorganized area, then they may wonder about the way their information will be handled.

Opening the Office

The medical assistant whose responsibility it is to open the office should arrive 15–30 minutes prior to the start of office hours. In addition to the receptionist's welcoming greeting, a well-lighted, clean, and inviting environment does much to cheer patients. The receptionist should begin checking the security alarm and disengaging it. Turn on all lights and check the general status of the reception room. It should be tidy and clean. Any area used for children's toys should be neat and safe. Magazines and books should be stacked or placed in wall racks.

Next, the medical assistant should check to see that the charts are pulled and prepared for that day's patients. Charge slips should be printed in advance for the day. The previous day's receipts should have been taken to the bank and the receptionist may have the responsibility of checking the cash box to see that the correct amount of change has been given. This will provide a way to double check the balance at the end of the day.

All office machines should be turned on and ready for use. Many copiers take several minutes to warm up in order to make copies. Be sure to add paper to the copier, fax machine, and any printers in the office. Nothing is more frustrating and time consuming than to find a fax machine with no paper and a queue of faxes waiting to be printed. Having the office machines turned on and ready can make the start of the day more efficient.

A master list of patient appointments should be printed out and copies placed on the desks of the clinical medical assistants and each of the doctors.

The final task prior to opening the office is to check the answering service and/or machine. If, additional appointments were made, pull the charts and make up a charge slip. It may be the responsibility of the opening medical assistant to make sure that all examination rooms are prepared for use. See Procedure 7-1 for more about opening the office.

Collating Records

Collating records refers to collecting all records, test results, and information pertaining to the patient, who is scheduled to be seen by the physician. Collating also refers to organizing the sub-group information (for example, laboratory and x-ray results) in records for the day's appointments as well as when filing. This should be part of pulling records, which may also be referred to as pulling charts. A record or chart refers to a medical record containing information such as laboratory and x-ray results. This is different from the patient's file. The file will refer to the financial record. It may contain billing, payment, and insurance information. The patient's file will most likely be contained on a computer, rather than on paper.

Collating records is usually done the day before patients are seen. The records of patients scheduled for a Monday are pulled and collated on the previous Friday. In some medical offices with several physicians, the number of patients seen may require collating records earlier than the day before the patient's visit. Always follow the policy of your office.

The physician's orders and notations from the previous visit must be reviewed to make sure that all necessary information has been received and is in the record. If laboratory tests or x-ray results are not present in the record, then you will have to call the laboratory or radiology department to obtain an oral report. This telephone report is written into the patient's record; however, when the originating report is received, it is placed in the patient's record also. This is quite often done by the clinical medical assistant. In some offices and laboratories, the facsimile (fax) machine can be used to send reports between facilities. A facsimile, or fax, is an electronically transmitted document containing print and/or graphic information.

In some offices, the records are to be placed in the order in which the patients will be seen. A printed appointment list is placed on top of the collated records. This list serves as a checklist to keep track of patients who have been seen by the physician. As a patient is seen, his or her name is checked off the list. A copy of this same list is placed on the physician's desk on the morning of the patient's visit. A list may also be given to the medical assistant that will be rooming patients that day, if different from the receptionist. Procedure 7-2 is provided for the process of collating records.

PROCEDURE

Opening the Office

OBJECTIVE: Prepare and set up the office to receive patients and operate efficiently.

Equipment and Supplies

checklist of opening office procedures; office keys for rooms and files; message forms or pads; master lists of scheduled patients

1. Turn on the lights in the patient reception area before the first patient arrives.
2. Check that the heating or air conditioning and computers are working properly.
3. Observe overall reception room for safety hazards such as frayed electrical cords, slippery floor, or torn carpeting. Place a warning sign near any safety hazard and report it immediately to the office manager.
4. Check magazines and recycle or discard any that are torn, damaged, or outdated.
5. Check for level of cleanliness per housekeeping services and report inadequate services.
6. Unlock file rooms or cabinets where records are kept.
7. Take calls from the answering machine or answering service. Handle any that need immediate attention.

8. Unlock any money that may be used for the day. Count and balance the money to make sure that the amount is the same as it was the day before when closing the office.
9. Unlock the outer office door.
10. Compare the master list of all patients who will be seen during the day against the patient records that were pulled during previous office hours. A patient may have been added to the schedule after the records were pulled. This patient's record must be pulled, reviewed, and added to the other records. Make phone calls to gather any laboratory test information that is missing from the record. Provide the physician(s) and nurse(s) with a copy of the list of any laboratory test information that you have called for, but has not yet been received.
11. Type and place a list of all patients who will be seen that day on the physician's desk.

PROCEDURE

Collating Records

OBJECTIVE: Prepare medical records of scheduled patients for review by the physician.

Equipment and Supplies

master list of scheduled patients; charts and records of scheduled patients

1. Print or copy the day's appointment schedule.
2. Pull all of the medical records of patients that are scheduled to be seen.
3. In each record, review the patient's last appointment and make note of any results that should have been received, including laboratory tests, x-rays results, consultation notes, and other tests.

4. If any of the results are not in the patient's chart, call the appropriate places to retrieve the results. You may take oral results, but request that the results be faxed to the office as soon as possible.
5. Make a list of all results that have been called to retrieve and any that are outstanding. Let the physician know what is still outstanding.
6. Put all information that is received onto the chart for the physician to review.

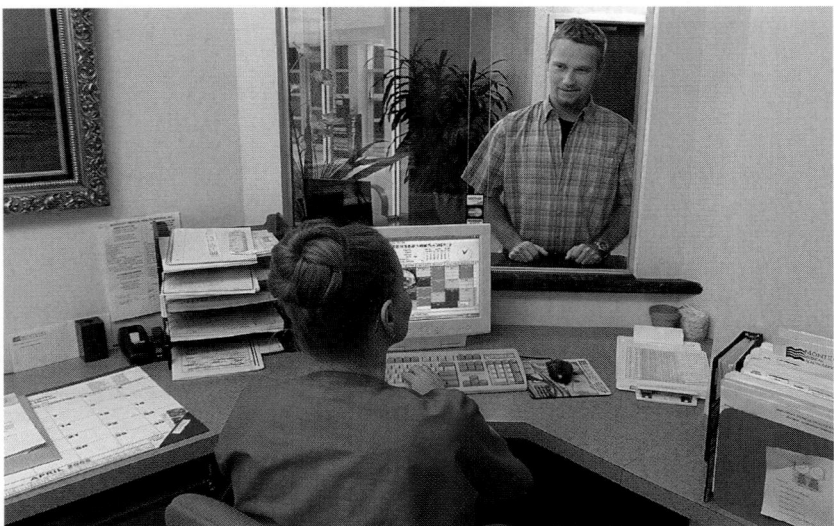

FIGURE 7-3 Each patient is greeted by the receptionist.

Patients must always take precedence over other visitors to the office (for example, a medical supplier or pharmaceutical representative). Scheduling such a visit when there are few or no patients in the office might be a better solution. Non-emergency conversations with other staff persons should always be interrupted to respond to a patient.

Use caution and speak in a low voice when mentioning another patient's name over the telephone or to another staff member within hearing distance of any patients in the reception room. A violation of confidentiality can be grounds for a lawsuit. The reason for the glass enclosure is to protect the confidentiality of patients. Always close the partition when you are speaking on the telephone.

Quickly pick up ringing phones by the second ring if possible, and always take a message if you are busy with another call or a patient in the office. It is better to call the patient back if you are unable to answer a question or have to look up information rather than to leave the patient on hold. Callers should not be left on hold for longer than one minute. See Chapter 6 for more information regarding the use of the telephone. Also see Patient Education for more on patient interaction.

Greeting the Patient Upon Arrival

In the role of receptionist, the impression the medical assistant makes on the patient is often the patient's first impression of the physician and the medical office staff. The impression you make—good or bad—tends to flavor the patient's opinion of everyone related to the office. Therefore, that first impression is very, very important.

Emergency patients or those with a contagious disease should enter the office through a private office entrance (if there is one) and be escorted directly into an examination room. This is done to limit exposure to contagious germs and not to alarm the other patients.

In some offices, the receptionist sits behind a glass window, which slides open easily, allowing the receptionist to personally greet each patient entering the office (Figure 7-3). If the receptionist is on the telephone when a patient enters, then looking up and smiling is a good way to acknowledge the patient's presence. Cultural Considerations addresses more about interacting with patients.

Signing-in

A sign-in sheet or patient register is maintained at the reception desk. The sign-in sheet, which will differ from office to office, usually has space for the patient's name, time of arrival, and the name of the physician the patient will see. The sign-in sheet allows the receptionist to maintain a continuous record of all patients who come into the office.

It is important to have every patient sign the register. The receptionist should verbally relate address and telephone information to the patient outside the hearing range of other patients, for example, "Mrs. Jones, do

Cultural Considerations

It is important to remember that different cultures have different ways of working with people. In your culture, you may feel that it is good manners to look someone in the eye when speaking with them. However, there are cultures that may be uncomfortable with looking a person in the eye because in that culture it is disrespectful. You will need to be aware of some of these cultural differences, especially if your office is located in an area in which you will deal with many people of different cultures.

Patient education often begins when the patient's call for an appointment. Two other important sites for patient education are at the reception desk and in the waiting room. For example, education regarding office hours, policies, insurance form submissions, and emergency telephone numbers can be handled at the reception desk. The receptionist may give instructions regarding tests and procedures such as fasting before a particular blood test. In smaller offices where the receptionist handles insurance processing, education can take place regarding the patient's responsibility in the process.

Patient education is supported through the use of descriptive informational office practice brochures, literature from the American Cancer Society, American Diabetic Association, and American Heart Association, and bulletin displays on various aspects of health. Some offices provide a brief video presentation about selected procedures or health concerns.

you still live at 43 Home Avenue? Is your telephone number still . . . ?" The sheet should be checked for accuracy and completeness. This can be critical for billing purposes. As each patient is taken into the examination room, a check mark is placed next to the patient's name. This is only one way of patients signing in; each office develops a system that works for its flow of patients.

In some offices, the sign-in sheet is filed in a designated folder at the end of the day to provide another record of the patients seen during that day. If the office policy is to destroy the sign-in sheet to maintain confidentiality, make sure these papers are shredded. Note: Some offices are starting to move away from sign-in sheets due to confidentiality concerns. HIPAA does allow for the use of sign-in sheets, but you may not include the reason for the visit on the sign-in sheet. Only the patient's name, time of arrival, and the physicians name should be used.

Registering New Patients

New patients will need to fill out a complete patient registration form containing demographic information, which is data relating to descriptive information such as age, gender, ethnic background, education, and Social Security number (Figure 7-4). Place the registration form on a clipboard with a pen attached and have the patient complete the form while he or she is waiting to be seen by the physician. Some offices send forms to patients to be completed at home and submitted at the time of the first visit; others request new patients arrive 15–30 minutes early to complete the necessary forms. Give precise instructions. Indicate what portion of the form the patient must complete, if there are two sides to be completed, and where the patient's signature is required. Assist patients who are unable to read and write either because they are illiterate or have a physical disability. Realize that many patients who cannot read or write may be embarrassed by this. You may want to help them to fill out the form in a private area of the office.

You will need to explain to the patient your office's policies on billing and payment. Along with verbally telling him or her the policies, you may give each new patient informational brochures. Then have the patient sign an assignment of benefits form so that the insurance company may send payments directly to the physician.

Make sure that all forms are completed correctly in their entirety and that all signatures have been received. With computer-assisted registration, you can input dictation directly onto the computer terminal. Refer to Chapter 11 for more information on computer-assisted office functions.

Request to see the patient's insurance card(s). It is a good rule to ask the patient politely if any insurance information has changed. This can decrease the chances of lapsed coverage. Photocopy both sides of the card(s) and be sure that the copy is legible. Insurance billing cannot be processed without complete information. Check on the insurance card to see if there is a patient co-payment, which requires the patient pay a certain amount of the total bill. Indicate the co-payment in the appropriate place on the patient's file. The amount may be collected before or after the visit, depending upon your office's procedure.

Charge Slips

The charge slip (also referred to as encounter form or superbill) used in most medical offices is a part of the billing process. Some offices use a charge plate system or computer program that will imprint the patient's name and identification number on all forms used including the charge slip. The appropriate charge slip is attached to the medical record of each patient who is to be seen by the physician on that day. At the end of the visit, the physician indicates what treatment was given and what the charge is. The charge slip is then given to the

PATIENT REGISTRATION FORM
(Please Print)

Date: _____

Patient's
Name: _____
       First   Middle   Last

DOB: _____ / _____ / _____
     Month   Day   Year

Address: _____
         Street   City   State   Zip

Phone: _____
       (Area code)

Patient's SS#: _____-_____-_____   Driver's License #: _____   Occupation: _____

Method of payment (circle):   cash   check   credit card   insurance co-payment

Primary Insurance Co.: _____   Policy/Group #: _____

Medicare #: _____   Medicaid #: _____

Person
Responsible
For Payment: _____
             First   Middle   Last   Relationship

Address: _____   Phone: _____ / _____-_____
         Street   City   State   Zip   (Area code)

Employer Name: _____   Dept: _____
               First   Middle   Last

Address: _____   Phone: _____ / _____-_____
         Street   City   State   Zip   (Area code)

Spouse or
Nearest Relative: _____
                  First   Middle   Last   Relationship

Address: _____   Phone: _____ / _____-_____
         Street   City   State   Zip   (Area code)

How were you referred to this office?_____

_____

Statement of Financial Responsibility: I, _____
do hereby agree to pay all medical charges incurred by the above listed patient. I further understand
that these charges are my responsibility, regardless of insurance coverage.

Responsible Person's Signature: _____

FIGURE 7-4 Patient Registration Form.

receptionist or the cashier. Payment or arrangements for payment are made before the patient leaves the office.

All patients must be issued a charge slip before they leave the office. When there is no charge for the visit, as in a follow-up visit after surgery, the physician will write "no charge" or N/C on the slip. For accounting purposes there should be a charge slip number for each patient. The patient is entitled to and should receive a copy of the charges. The charge slip will contain a list of the most common current procedural terminology (CPT) and International Classification of Diseases (ICD-9). These codes identifying diagnosis-related charges used by the office.

Consideration for the Patient's Time

One of the most common complaints heard from patients is the excessive amount of time they have to spend in the reception room before being seen by a physician. Patients generally understand when they are told the physician has an emergency that has resulted in a schedule delay. However, in many cases, the physician is running behind schedule because of errors with the scheduling system, such as overbooking, when more than one patient is scheduled in the same time slot. Delays are also caused by not allowing enough time on the schedule for patient visits. This usually occurs because inaccurate information is obtained concerning the reason a patient wishes to see the doctor.

In general, a 20-minute wait is accepted by most patients. If the wait is going to be longer, then you should approach each patient and ask if the patient prefers to wait or wishes to reschedule the appointment. Patients generally respond well to a quiet explanation from the receptionist regarding how long the wait will be. Unfortunately patients after they sign in are sometimes forgotten by the receptionist. Since the patient's only contact in the office is the receptionist, it is critical that a concerned approach be used. Periodically check on your waiting patients. Know the office policy regarding which type of complaint is seen to immediately by the physician.

When a patient complains of a long delay in seeing the physician, never become angry in return or tell the patient, "It's not my fault." An empathetic medical assistant can imagine how nervous and ill the patient must feel. Make every effort to calm an angry patient so that he or she is no longer angry when going in to see the physician.

Escorting the Patient into the Examination Room

All patients should be personally escorted into the examination room (Figure 7-5). In most instances, this is done by a medical assistant assigned to patient care rather than by the receptionist. Select the correct record and clearly call the patient's name. If there is doubt that you have the correct patient, ask the patient to give you his or her name. Verify the name with the record you have requesting additional information, such as senior (Sr.) or junior (Jr.), if necessary. Make sure to also ask the patient how his or her would like to be addressed. Never call a patient by his or her first name unless the patient has asked you to do so. Walk at the patient's rate of speed and offer special assistance to patients using a wheelchair, crutches, walker, or cane. You may wish to make pleasant conversation to make the patient feel at ease.

Place the patient's record in the proper location. Do not leave the chart in the room with the patient. Often there is a slot on the outside of the examination room door for the record. Enter the room with the patient. Clearly explain exactly what articles of clothing the patient should remove. It is important to be specific because it can extend a patient's appointment time if the physician is unable to perform an examination because the patient has not been correctly prepared. Point out the gown or sheet to be used after the patient has undressed. Assist any patient who is unable to remove his or her clothing. Always protect the patient's modesty as you help the patient undress. Efforts made by medical staff to protect a patient's modesty are important to the patient.

After the examination has been completed, return to the examination room and knock before entering. Give the patient instructions about what to do next. For example, you might say to the patient, "You may dress now. The doctor will come back to talk to you shortly," or "Stop at the reception desk (or other designated area) after you have dressed, and I'll explain the test the doctor has ordered."

Make it a point to speak with each patient before he or she leaves. In some cases, the patient may need to make a payment, talk to the cashier, make another appointment, or have a specific test or procedure explained. A simple "good-bye" brings closure to each patient's office visit.

If discussion is needed, it should be done in a private area out of the hearing range and view of the other patients. Remember that HIPAA regulations prohibit discussions with patients to take place in any area where another patient may overhear.

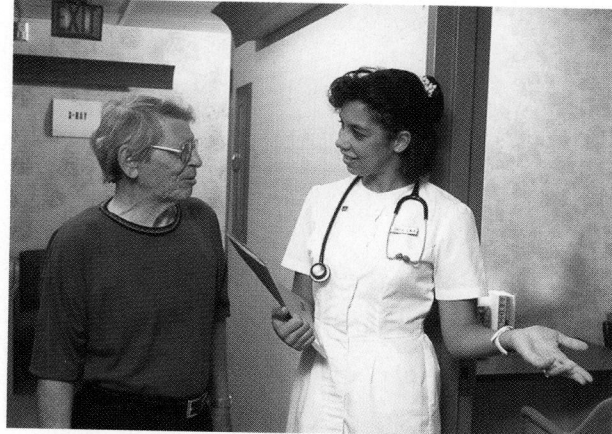

FIGURE 7-5 The medical assistant escorts the patient into the examination room.

Managing Disturbances

If a patient becomes angry or starts speaking in a loud voice, try to handle the situation immediately. It is always advisable to ask the patient to come into a quiet office where the problem can be discussed and handled.

If a private office is not available, the problem must be handled quickly and quietly in another area. Generally, people will respond to a sincere statement such as, "I'm sorry there's a problem. Let's see how we can solve it." Ask the patient to identify what he or she perceives the problem to be and then discuss the possible solutions. Frequently, the angry patient will respond well if the medical assistant uses a very quiet,

calm manner. Keep your voice low to help calm the patient. With practice, a medical assistant can become adept at calming the angry patient. If the patient is drunk or disorderly, follow the office policy regarding when to call the police.

Children

Children pose a special challenge. Usually, children go into the examination room with the adult patient and are removed only if private areas are to be examined on the parent. If a child is left alone in the office while the parent is seen by the physician, then the medical assistant must observe that the child remains safe at all times. It is advisable to explain to the parent before he or she leaves the office that children cannot be left unattended.

On rare occasions, a physician treats a child without the parent being present. In such a case, a medical assistant or other staff person will stay with the child during the examination or procedure. Teenagers often have things to ask the doctor that they may not want their parents to hear.

Medical Emergencies in the Reception Room

There will be occasions when a medical emergency occurs in the physician's office (Figure 7-6). Ill patients may come directly to the physician's office instead of first calling the physician or 911. In this case, you must stop whatever you are doing to give assistance immediately. Ask another staff member to alert the physician. Tell available staff to give you assistance or to call 911 if emergency transport to a hospital is necessary. If all the rooms are full, you can ask the other waiting patients to step into the hall to prevent these patients becoming anxious during the emergency.

In certain emergency situations, the medical assistant may be required to start first aid procedures. It may be necessary to begin cardiopulmonary resuscitation

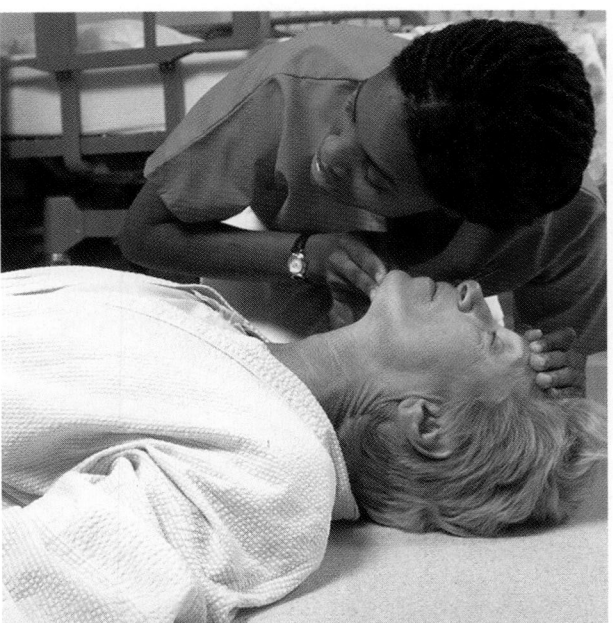

FIGURE 7-6 The medical assistant handles an emergency.

(CPR) on the patient. Your office should have guidelines set as to the proper procedure for handling this form of in-office emergency. See Legal and Ethical Issues for more about dealing with medical emergencies in the office.

If a patient's condition requires emergency treatment and equipment, which your physician is able to provide in the office setting, then immediately take the patient into an examination room. Assist the patient onto an examination table if possible. This patient should not be left unattended. Another staff member should alert the physician that the patient requires immediate attention. Many offices have an intercom system that allows communication from the reception area to all rooms in the office to quickly summon medical personnel.

If a family member who is present wishes to accompany the patient into the examination room, allow the person to do so unless prohibited by office policy. When treatment begins, a staff member should ask the family member to step out of the room.

No-Shows

No-show patients are any patients who do not keep their appointment and do not call to cancel their appointment. At the end of each day, one of the responsibilities of the receptionist is to account for these patients. Some offices have a standard practice to call the patient to determine why the appointment was not kept and to reschedule another appointment. There is sometimes a policy to charge for no-show appointments. It is important that the receptionist learn and use the procedure for "no-shows" as stated in the office's policy manual.

One person, usually the office manager, is responsible for alerting the physician to the patient "no-shows." Calling patients the day before their visits to remind them of the appointments may lower the number of no-shows.

After the patient has been rescheduled, place a notation on the patient's record about the failed appointment, the date, action taken, the result, and initials of the person performing the documentation. This documentation is important in protecting the physician should there ever be a lawsuit.

If the patient fails to keep two or more appointments, the physician should be informed. The physician may wish to send a letter declining to continue treating the patient or dismissing the patient from the practice. The letter should be sent both certified and regular mail.

Closing the Office

Closing the office at the end of the day and opening the office in the morning are two major functions of the medical assistant. These functions are key to operating a well-run office. A procedure for closing the office at the end of the day is presented in Procedure 7-3.

PROCEDURE

Closing the Office

OBJECTIVE: Secure the office properly during nonoperating hours.

Equipment and Supplies
checklist of office closing procedures; bank deposit forms and envelope/pouch; office keys for rooms and files

1. Leave at least 15 to 30 minutes at the end of the day to close the office.
2. Check all records used during the day for any orders that may have been missed. In addition, make sure that every visit is posted to be billed.
3. Records for patients who will be seen during the next day should be pulled, reviewed, and collated during the day. Place the collated records with the charge slips attached and the master list of the next day's scheduled patients together in the appropriate place. Also, make a copy of this master list of patients for each physician.
4. All money received from patient payments must either be deposited in a bank or locked in the office safe. It is wise to have the person designated to make the daily bank deposit vary the time of deposit. Many offices now use a courier for this task. For purposes of quality control, the person completing the bank deposit and the person making the deposit should not be the same. Both people should be bonded. Completing a bank deposit is discussed in Chapter 14.
5. Turn off electrical equipment and appliances. Note: Some equipment such as an incubator, fax machine, and computers, may require 24-hour operation. Check with your supervisor regarding the special requirements of your office.
6. Check all examination rooms to make sure they are clean and supplied for the next day. Note: This step may be done by the medical assistant who was in charge of rooming patients that day.
7. Straighten the reception room. Put away all magazines and pick up any toys.
8. The answering service must be activated before leaving. Know the name of the physician who is accepting emergency calls, or on call, until morning. Remind the physician who is on call.
9. Activate the security system if there is one.
10. Always double-check to make sure the door is locked.

SUMMARY

The receptionist's role can be one of the most demanding and most interesting positions in the medical office. While attending to the general running of the office, the medical assistant, as receptionist must greet all patients, assist new patients in registering while being sure to get necessary health and insurance information, answer calls, schedule patients, open and close the office, contact and document "no-shows," and more. All this requires a calm, caring, and organized individual who can keep patient information confidential and protect the safety of the patient during the office visit. The patient is most important.

Chapter Review

COMPETENCY REVIEW

1. Define and spell the terms to learn for this chapter.
2. Explain the steps you would take if you are the first person to arrive and must open the medical office.
3. Describe how a professionally groomed receptionist would appear.
4. Explain what you would do if a patient suddenly collapsed in the reception room.
5. Discuss steps a medical assistant would take to assist in preventing a claim of abandonment against a physician.
6. Describe the important characteristics of a typical waiting area.

1. At Mrs. Mendez' first appointment to see Dr. Williams, you would have the following forms for her to read and/or sign EXCEPT
   A. patient information sheet
   B. physician's emergency phone numbers
   C. authorization to pay physician form
   D. sign-in sheet
   E. bank deposit slip

2. When a patient enters the office and you are on the telephone, what is the correct procedure?
   A. continue speaking on the telephone, and after you have completed the conversation, look up and handle the walk-in patient
   B. place the telephone patient "on-hold" and tell the walk-in patient to sign in
   C. smile at the walk-in patient to indicate that you see him or her and finish talking with the patient on the telephone
   D. tell the patient on the telephone you will call back later, then handle the walk-in patient
   E. smile to answer the telephone

3. When handling the angry patient, it is best to
   A. ask the patient to have a seat
   B. calmly tell the patient you are sorry he or she is angry and take the patient to an empty examination room
   C. tell the patient that you have to cancel his appointment since you cannot have loud, angry patients in the office
   D. let the patient continue to talk until the patient's anger is gone
   E. answer the ringing telephone

4. "No-Show" appointments are documented
   A. when the staff person assigned to document "no-shows" comes in for work
   B. at the beginning of the next day
   C. at the end of the day of the failed appointment
   D. only on the sign-in sheet
   E. but do not have to be documented

5. Mr. James has walked into the office and collapsed. Dr. Williams is not there. Which of the following would a medical assistant do?
   A. alert a staff member to help Mr. James
   B. assist Mr. James and call out or ask another staff member to call 911 for help
   C. call 911 immediately and wait by the door to direct the emergency team
   D. if Mr. James is alert, advise him to go to the hospital to meet Dr. Williams, then call Dr. Williams to alert her that an emergency patient is on his way to the hospital
   E. answer the ringing telephone

6. Which of the following statements, regarding the collation of patient records is TRUE?
   A. patient records for the day's appointments are usually pulled and collated 2 days before the appointment
   B. patient records are usually pulled and collated for an appointment immediately after the reminder call
   C. only a written report of test results is entered into a patient's records not the actual laboratory report
   D. records for patients scheduled on Tuesday are pulled on Monday
   E. patient records include billing and insurance information

7. What is the name of the billing document used in most medical offices where the physician indicates a patient's treatment and charges?
   A. assignment of benefits form
   B. authorization to pay form
   C. charge slip
   D. insurance slip
   E. billing slip

8. What, in general, is the maximum acceptable amount of time for a patient to wait on the day of a scheduled appointment?
   A. 10 minutes
   B. 15 minutes
   C. 20 minutes
   D. 25 minutes
   E. 30 minutes

9. Which of the following should be considered a medical emergency in an office waiting room?
   A. a potentially contagious patient's incessant coughing
   B. a crying child with a very upset stomach
   C. a patient, whose chief complaint is nausea over the past several days, who has just vomited
   D. a disgruntled patient
   E. a patient requiring CPR

10. It is proper, when addressing patients, to
    A. call them by their surname only
    B. address them by their first name, in order to sound friendly
    C. ask them how they prefer to be addressed
    D. avoid all use of name to keep from offending the patient
    E. use a familiar nickname

CRITICAL THINKING

1. Did Betsy greet Stacy appropriately?
2. What was the benefit of sending Stacy the paperwork in the mail before her visit?
3. Why did Betsy give Stacy the Notice of Privacy Practice?
4. Did Betsy handle the phone call appropriately? If not, how should she have handled it?

ON THE JOB

Dr. Morrison, a child psychiatrist, who is in solo practice, employs one medical assistant in her office. This medical assistant is multiskilled, like all medical assistants, and, essentially, handles all of the administrative and clinical tasks in the office.

It is 3:00 P.M. and a parent has just arrived for a 3:30 P.M. appointment with her 10-year old daughter. The child is a new patient of Dr. Morrison and was referred by her attending physician. She has a relatively long history of combative and destructive behavior and the referring pediatrician is seeking a psychological evaluation from Dr. Morrison. Psychotropic medication of some sort may be a viable treatment option. The medical assistant has asked the mother and daughter to please be seated and to fill out some registration forms. The child is acting out—pulling cushions off of the reception room couch, wildly ripping the pages of the magazines, whining and kicking at her mother. The behavior seems to be escalating as the mother tries to frantically control her child while, at the same time, follow the instructions of the medical assistant and fill out the registration forms.

What is your response?

1. What if anything, should the medical assistant do?
2. Would it be appropriate, for example, for the medical assistant to interrupt Dr. Morrison's current session?
3. Might this be considered a medical emergency?

INTERNET ACTIVITY

1. Find out how HIPAA has changed the way the medical office handles patient reception.
2. Look for companies that produce forms that can be used by a medical receptionist.

MediaLink More on patient reception in the medical office environment, including interactive resources, can be found on the Student CD-ROM accompanying this textbook.

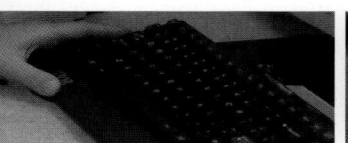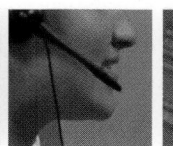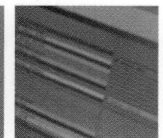

Medical Assistant Role Delineation Chart

HIGHLIGHT indicates material covered in this chapter.

ADMINISTRATIVE

Administrative Procedures

- Perform basic administrative medical assisting functions
- Schedule, coordinate and monitor appointments
- Schedule inpatient/outpatient admissions and procedures
- Understand and apply third-party guidelines
- Obtain reimbursement through accurate claims submission
- Monitor third-party reimbursement
- Understand and adhere to managed care policies and procedures
- *Negotiate managed care contracts*

- Manage accounts receivable
- *Manage accounts payable*
- *Process payroll*
- *Document and maintain accounting and banking records*
- *Develop and maintain fee schedules*
- *Manage renewals of business and professional insurance policies*
- *Manage personnel benefits and maintain records*
- *Perform marketing, financial, and strategic planning*

Practice Finances

- Perform procedural and diagnostic coding
- Apply bookkeeping principles

CLINICAL

Fundamental Principles

- Apply principles of aseptic technique and infection control
- Comply with quality assurance practices
- Screen and follow up patient test results

Diagnostic Orders

- Collect and process specimens
- Perform diagnostic tests

Patient Care

- Adhere to established patient screening procedures
- Obtain patient history and vital signs
- Prepare and maintain examination and treatment areas
- Prepare patient for examinations, procedures and treatments

- Assist with examinations, procedures and treatments
- Prepare and administer medications and immunizations
- Maintain medication and immunization records
- Recognize and respond to emergencies
- Coordinate patient care information with other health care providers
- Initiate IV and administer IV medications with appropriate training and as permitted by state law

GENERAL

Professionalism

- Display a professional manner and image
- Demonstrate initiative and responsibility
- Work as a member of the health care team
- Prioritize and perform multiple tasks
- Adapt to change
- Promote the CMA credential
- Enhance skills through continuing education
- Treat all patients with compassion and empathy
- Promote the practice through positive public relations

Communication Skills

- Recognize and respect cultural diversity
- Adapt communications to individual's ability to understand
- Use professional telephone technique

- Recognize and respond effectively to verbal, nonverbal, and written communications
- Use medical terminology appropriately
- Utilize electronic technology to receive, organize, prioritize and transmit information
- Serve as liaison

Legal Concepts

- Perform within legal and ethical boundaries
- Prepare and maintain medical records
- Document accurately
- Follow employer's established policies dealing with the health care contract
- Implement and maintain federal and state health care legislation and regulations
- Comply with established risk management and safety procedures
- Recognize professional credentialing criteria
- *Develop and maintain personnel, policy and procedure manuals*

Instruction

- Instruct individuals according to their needs
- Explain office policies and procedures
- Teach methods of health promotion and disease prevention
- Locate community resources and disseminate information
- *Develop educational materials*
- *Conduct continuing education activities*

Operational Functions

- Perform inventory of supplies and equipment
- Perform routine maintenance of administrative and clinical equipment
- Apply computer techniques to support office operations
- *Perform personnel management functions*
- *Negotiate leases and prices for equipment and supply contracts*

- *Denotes advanced skills.*

SOURCE: Reprinted by permission of the American Association of Medical Assistants from the AAMA Role Delineation Study: Occupational Analysis of the Medical Assisting Profession.

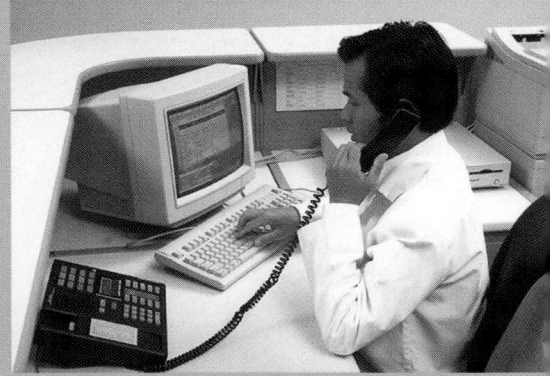

Appointment Scheduling

Learning Objectives

After completing this chapter, you should be able to:

- Define and spell the terms to learn for this chapter.
- Name and describe four scheduling systems.
- List and describe four pieces of equipment used in the scheduling process.
- Identify ten conditions that qualify as emergencies.

- Explain the importance of correct documentation when a patient does not keep an appointment.
- Describe the appointment scheduling process.
- Describe and arrange the process for scheduling a hospital admission and surgery.
- Summarize the ethical implications related to scheduling.

OUTLINE

Appointment Schedules	144
Scheduling Systems	146
Patient Scheduling Process	148
Patient Referrals	151
Hospital Admission Scheduling	151
Scheduling Surgery	151
Appointment Exceptions	151
Telephone and E-mail Scheduling	153
New Patient Appointments	154
Established Patient Appointments	154
Scheduling Other Types of Appointments	155

Terms to Learn

acute conditions	matrix	surgical scheduler
archived	modified wave scheduling	tickler file
cycle time	real time	time patterns
double booking	scheduling system	triage
established patient	specific time	wave scheduling

Case Study

MARC, CMA, IS WORKING THE FRONT DESK TODAY. He is looking ahead to tomorrow's (Friday) schedule. Fridays are Dr. Miller's short day for seeing established patients. The office usually closes from noon until 1:00 P.M. for lunch. Marc sees that Dr. Miller has the following appointments:

11:00	Laura White	2:00	Rinna Brown
	Joe Tanner		Monica Floyd
	Lucy Smith		Peter Conner
1:00	Justin Ivy		
	Ramona Pierce		
	Lucas Abrams		

Ramona Pierce calls to cancel her appointment. Shannon Reece wants to know if she can schedule a new patient appointment for tomorrow. Marcus Fowler, a familiar drug representative, wants to know if he can drop in briefly tomorrow.

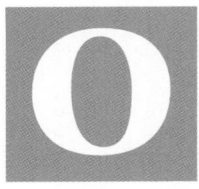**O**ffice hours are usually determined by the physician or group of physicians in a practice. The scheduling system used in each office is dependent on a variety of factors, including the physician's preference, type and size of practice, equipment availability, staff availability, amount of flexibility required by the physician(s), insurance coverage issues, and patient needs (Figure 8-1). The two basic types of appointment scheduling systems are (1) scheduled appointments, and (2) open office hours.

There are some medical facilities, such as independent ambulatory urgent care clinics, that offer extended evening hours and may be open 24-hours a day. Independent ambulatory urgent care clinics are facilities that are prepared to handle situations requiring immediate but not life-threatening medical care. These facilities are not always attached to a hospital or other large treatment center. The patients arrive without an appointment and are generally seen in the order of arrival. A medical office or facility using such a system is said to have "open" office hours.

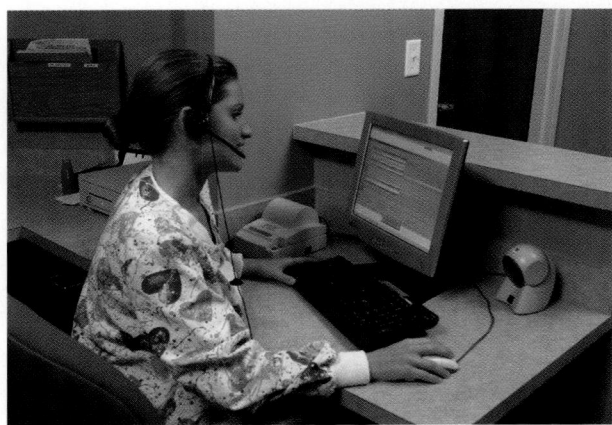
FIGURE 8-1 Scheduling patient appointments by telephone.

Appointment Schedules

Some physicians prefer to see patients according to a set schedule, depending on the specialty. As soon as a day's schedule of time slots is filled, then that day is closed to any new appointments. In this way, the physician is better able to spend an appropriate amount of time with each patient. There are several variations used for scheduling, including specified time, wave and modified wave, procedure grouping, double booking, and open hours system (Figure 8-2). All of these scheduling variations are described here along with the benefits and limitations of each type. Applying these scheduling variations in an office environment is discussed in Preparing for Externship.

Specified Time Scheduling

With specified time scheduling, each patient is given a specific time slot, which means the time allocated to each patient will depend upon the reason for the office visit or the type of examination or testing that is to be done. For example, a complete physical examination may require one and one-half hours. In an office based on 15-minute increments, or time slots, this patient would be given six time slots in a row equaling the one and one-half hours needed. This method prevents a large backlog of waiting patients or cycle time—the length of time the average patient spends in the medical office. Each staff member has a chance to maintain the office flow by reducing patient cycle time.

The drawback to specified time scheduling is that some patients may not provide enough information about their medical problems at the time the appointment is scheduled, in spite of careful questioning by the medical assistant. For instance, consider the case of a patient who is given a thirty-minute appointment but who really needs to have one or one and one-half hours for a thorough physical examination. Since not enough time was allocated for the visits, the schedule will back up. Some ways to deal with patients when the schedule backs up are discussed in Professionalism.

Some patients will discuss topics that are unrelated to the complaint that brought them into the office. This can be time consuming, frustrating for the physician, and not beneficial to the patient. It is the medical assistant's responsibility to get accurate information when scheduling patients so that the correct amount of time on the schedule is reserved for them. If the patient requires more time than was originally scheduled, the physician might have to ask the patient to make another appointment. In an attempt to prevent this from happening, many offices will build in time—known as "catch up" time—in either the morning or afternoon for emergencies.

Preparing for
Externship

Appointment scheduling is an administrative task or front office procedure. Be aware that the scheduling variation you learned in class may not be the one used at your externship site. Do not be afraid to ask questions. It is to your advantage to learn different variations. Because there is always more than one way of performing a task, you may be able to show what you learned in your office procedures class. Shared ideas sometimes lead to more effective ways of performing tasks.

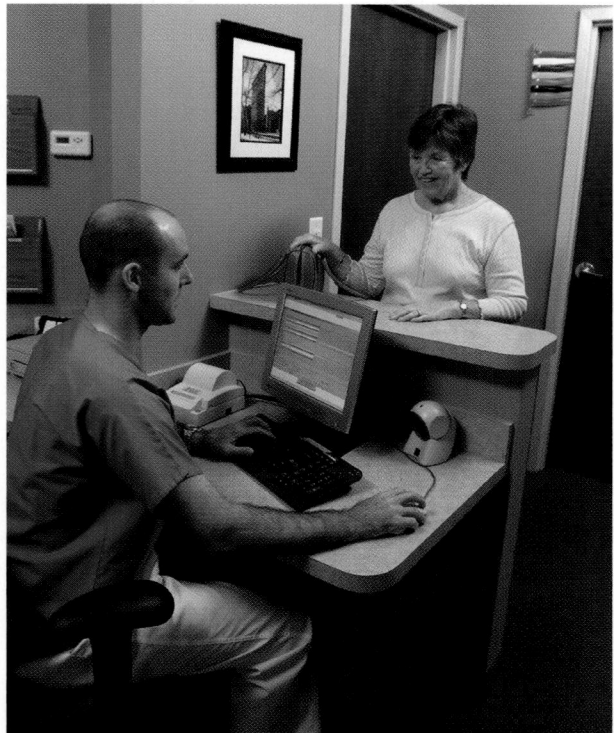

FIGURE 8-2 Scheduling appointments in a physician's office.

Wave Scheduling

Wave scheduling provides built-in flexibility to accommodate unforeseen situations, such as patients who require more time with the physician, a late arriving patient, or the patient who fails to keep an appointment (no-show). The purpose of wave scheduling is to begin and end each hour on time. Each hour is divided into equal segments of time, depending on how many patients can be seen within an hour.

For appointments averaging 20 minutes, three 20-minute appointments would be scheduled within each hour period of time, and for appointments averaging 15 minutes each, four appointments would be scheduled during the entire hour.

Using wave scheduling, all the patients are told to come in at the beginning of the hour in which they are to be seen. These patients are then seen in the order in which they arrive. Since some of the patients require more time, and others may be late, or some may not come in at all, wave scheduling allows for the actual time used by patient appointments to average out over the hour.

Modified Wave Scheduling

Wave scheduling can be modified to avoid the possibility that any patient would have to wait 40 minutes to be seen by the physician. Modified wave scheduling is also built on the hour as the base of each block of time. There are many variations of this type of scheduling.

One example would be to have three patients scheduled at intervals during the first half hour with none scheduled for the second half hour. All three patients would be seen during the entire hour period, but the physician would not be waiting for a late arriving patient. With this system the physician can still spend 20 minutes with each patient without having to wait for any patients to arrive. Table 8-1 is a comparison chart providing examples of specified time, wave, and modified wave scheduling.

Scheduling by Grouping Procedures

Many physicians prefer to have similar procedures and examinations scheduled during a particular block of time. For example, an obstetrician may prefer to have all new patients scheduled together on two mornings a week since they will require a longer physical examination. An allergist may group all skin testing together on three afternoons a week. A pediatrician may do well-baby checkups during particular hours each day.

Double Booking Patients

Double booking, which is the practice of scheduling two patients to be seen during the same time slot without allowing for any additional time in the schedule, is considered to be an ineffective method. If each patient will need a 20-minute appointment, and both are scheduled from 1:00 P.M. to 1:20 P.M., then the entire afternoon's schedule will be late by 20 minutes, at least. Using a modified form of wave scheduling will eliminate this problem since enough time is actually allowed in the schedule for all the patients.

Open Office Hours System

An open office hours system is the least structured of all the systems. The hours in which the office is open are posted, and patients may arrive at any time during those hours. The patients are seen in the order of their arrival.

Some physicians prefer this method because the schedule is not disrupted by patients who miss appointments. The disadvantages to this method include having too many patients arrive at the same time, which frequently

Professionalism

No matter how well a scheduling system may work, there may be times when the physician gets behind schedule. It is important to communicate to patients immediately that the wait may be a little longer than anticipated. Provide updates as often as possible. Some patients may get tired of waiting and become rude and demanding. Remain courteous and assure the patient that the staff is working as quickly and safely as possible and that he or she will be seen. If the wait time is much longer, ask patients with non-urgent, less serious problems if they want to reschedule (if office policy allows).

TABLE 8-1 Comparison of Scheduling Methods

Specified Time		Wave		Modified Wave		
1:00	Ed Trombley—ear irrigation	1:00	Ed Trombley Jerry Richard Janet Orlando	1:00	Ed Trombley	
1:20	Jerry Richard—well-baby checkup with vaccines			1:10	Jerry Richard	
1:40	Janet Orlando—PAP smear			1:20	Janet Orlando	
2:00	Lena Mezza—well-baby checkup with vaccines	2:00	Lena Mezza David Ingiolo Christina Soave	1:30	↓	↓
2:20	David Ingiolo—BP check			1:40	↓	↓
2:40	Christina Soave—skin rash (poss. contagious)			2:00	Lena Mezza	
3:00		3:00		2:10	David Ingiolo	
3:20				2:20	Christina Soave	
3:40				2:30	↓	↓
4:00		4:00		2:40	↓	↓

results in longer patient cycle time than necessary. The physician and staff can be overworked during peak times of the day and may have no patients during other times.

Scheduling Systems

Appointment scheduling is key to the business aspects of the office process flow (Chapter 9), time management, increased efficiency, and quality patient care. A scheduling system facilitates the coordination of appropriate time segments for staff, patients, and the practice's available equipment. In order for a medical practice to coordinate time, an appointment scheduling system is applied, no matter what the practice size, specialty, and patient load. Scheduling systems establish the appropriate office process flow and coordination of time with the ability for flexibility as necessary. Appointment systems include computerized and manual. Either system can accomplish scheduling coordination of time when managed appropriately for the medical practice while adhering to HIPAA compliance guidelines.

Computerized Systems

Many medical practices of various sizes and specialties are utilizing computers to schedule appointments (Figure 8-3). Computerized systems may be purchased based on the medical practice's specific needs. Some practices will purchase a commercial software product while others will contract a commercial appointment scheduling service. The responsibility of the medical assistant is to understand, demonstrate, and follow the computerized appointment system while adhering to HIPAA guidelines. There is no official government body or standards agency that will certify a commercial computerized product or service as a "HIPAA compliant." It is up to the health care providers to make sure

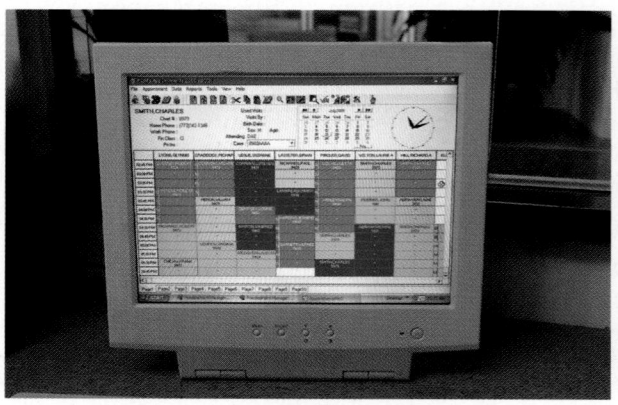

FIGURE 8-3 An example of computerized scheduling format.

the computerized product purchased for the medical practice will address the specific needs of the practice and their own HIPAA compliance issues, which will include patient safety, confidentiality, and security.

Computerized appointment systems are completed in a real time environment. Real time refers to automatically placing the appointment, patient needs, and information within the appropriate areas of the computer program versus the manual systems. The medical professional can key in the information to maximize the efficiency of the workflow. In addition, a computerized system provides the medical assistant with the ability to view times, dates, and open appointments with ease and consideration for the appointment criteria. Another advantage to computerized appointments is the ability to view and access patient appointments with a click or touch of a button. Whether a patient has a future appointment or a series of appointments, the computerized system can produce the information without the need of flipping the multiple pages in a manual schedule book.

While computerized systems maximize office process flow and patient cycle time (Chapter 9), there are some disadvantages and concerns the medical practice will need to consider. Some obvious concerns include privacy and technological factors, such as power outages, glitches within the software, and security. Computerized systems must be secured in a private space in accordance with HIPAA compliance. This can be accomplished by placing the computer in an area of the office where there is limited public walk-through traffic and visitors' ability to overhear a conversation. The computer screen should be set to a screen saver after a few short minutes to block others from viewing the screen when the medical assistant is away from the desk.

For technological concerns, in accordance with HIPAA, each medical practice should have an emergency action plan devised for such events. The medical assistant will need to back up the computerized schedule frequently to prevent loss of important information. If there were a power outage, the emergency action plan should provide information that will ensure that the medical office can operate and function for 48 to 72 hours without power. Office policies would dictate how the scheduling would be handled during the power outages, such as printing a hardcopy of the appointment schedule for the week versus one day at a time.

Another advantage of computerized appointment scheduling includes the ability to track regular patterns within the medical practice. For example, the office could track how many no-shows, or how many patients were scheduled for the same type of appointment, i.e. flu, or even how often the physician was late within a specific period of time. These tracking features provide the medical practice with an additional tool and analytical report for audit and review of the best methods within the office. Time management could be modified as needed based on the reports.

Security concerns should be outlined in accordance with the office policies and HIPAA compliance issues. Specified security guidelines are usually dictated by the medical office functions and flow. Security includes some of the following but are not limited to them: positioning and location of the computer monitor for visibility and confidentiality, employee computer authorization and accessibility requirements, the changing of employee passwords every 30 days, proper computer firewalls for patient confidentiality, and proper computer encryption.

Manual Systems

Some medical practices have not converted to computerized systems and instead use manual appointment systems. Utilizing computers to schedule appointments often depends on the size of practices and specialties. Manual systems are comprised of a hardcopy schedule book and a pencil or pen. Appointment books are purchased from various commercial office supply companies and offer a variety of styles, sizes, and features. Each office will determine the type of book needed based on the practice needs and preferences. Refer to Figure 8-4 for a sample of an appointment book. In accordance with HIPAA compliance, the appointment book and schedule must maintain patient confidentiality at all times. The appointment book should never be left in an

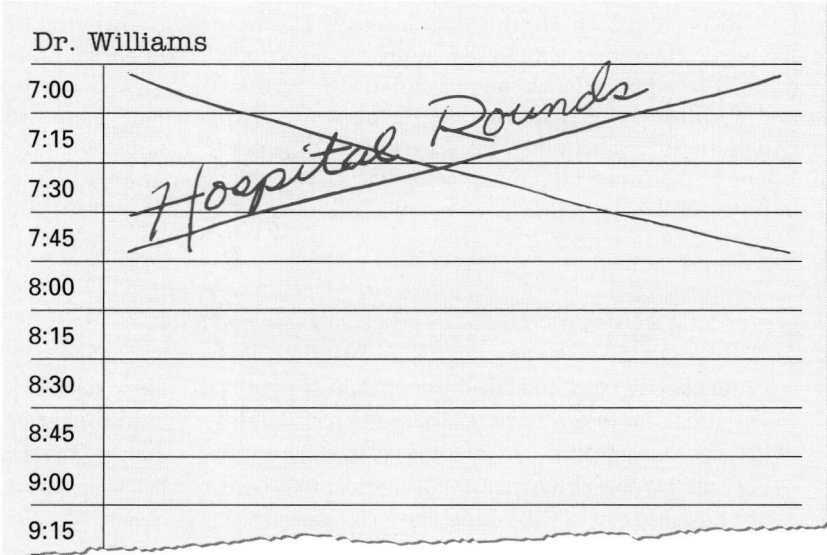

FIGURE 8-4 An example of manual appointment book.

area that is visible to visitors at the reception desk. The appointment schedule for the day should not be taped on the wall for all to view. Instead, secure a private location for required staff to reference.

The similarities and responsibilities of computerized and manual systems should be noted. The appointment book is a legal document that can be subpoenaed by the court (Legal and Ethical Issues). It is a record of the physician's day and time spent in contact with patients. Appointment books should be archived for future reference for several years in case of a court case. If there are any changes from the scheduled patients in the appointment book, such as a cancellation or no-show, these should be noted both in the appointment book and in the patient medical record. If the appointment has been rescheduled, then this should be appropriately documented. The appointment book should be archived (stored) for future reference with a hard copy or back up tape for computer scheduling. Files are archived by placing them in a storage container or facility and keeping them for several years as backup documentation.

Patient Scheduling Process

Every office will utilize its own method for appointment scheduling in accordance with the needs of the practice. However, the scheduling process remains the same for actually scheduling the appointment. The process includes either the computerized or manual system. The appointment is either entered into a manual appointment book or into the computer program.

The first step in the patient scheduling process is to be organized and efficient. Gather all required equipment, including the patient chart, computer scheduling system, pencil, manual schedule book, and office criteria requirement checklist. The medical assistant should be sure the schedule depicts all unavailable times, which is known as forming a matrix—periods of time blocked out on the daily schedule when an appointment is unavailable. Some of these blocked-out segments include times when the physician is seeing patients in the hospital, in surgery, out to lunch, on break, returning telephone calls, in meetings, and out of town. Several weeks of the schedule are blocked out or prepared at one time. It is not good practice to block out the entire schedule for the year since there may be unexpected changes in the physician's schedule. All blocking out and scheduling in the manual system is done in pencil. The medical assistant should cross out the blocks of time when the physician is unavailable, and write the reason across the line.

The next step in the process is to utilize effective communication skills. Listening to the patient's information and requests will help determine the type of appointment that is actually needed. When scheduling a patient appointment, always project a professional, caring, and willing demeanor with the patient. This can be accomplished by demonstrating effective listening and speaking skills so that the patient can understand and interpret the dialogue conveyed. Begin by asking for the patient's name, telephone contact, and purpose for the visit. Once the patient has described the purpose of his or her visit, the medical assistant should use the office criteria requirements checklist to help determine the type of and time needed for the appointment. Next, the medical assistant will need to determine the facility, equipment, and staff availability to meet the patient's needs. Based on the determination steps, the medical assistant can then discuss available dates and times with the patient. Refer to Table 8-2 for estimates of the amount of time to be allotted for specific office procedures. For more information that may need to be conveyed to patients before their appointment date, see Patient Education.

The medical assistant should offer one or two choices of dates, days and times for the patient to determine his or her availability. Be sure to always state the date, day, and time for reassurance that the patient has correctly understood when the appointment is scheduled. Once the patient and the medical assistant have mutually determined the time, either key in the information into the computer or use a pencil to enter the patient name and telephone number into the scheduled time slot in the schedule book. If the patient is making the appointment in person, write the date, day, and time on an appointment card for the patient. If the patient is on the telephone, have the patient repeat the day, date, and time. Procedure 8-1 provides information on how to schedule patients.

Missed Appointments and Delays

Appointments are cancelled for any number of reasons. Sometimes the patient experiences an unforeseen emergency, is too ill or too fatigued to get to the office, or actually forgets the appointment. Some medical practices charge patients for no-show appointments as well as rescheduled appointments. If the medical practice has a cancellation charge, the patients must be made aware of the policy prior to cancellation.

TABLE 8-2 **Time Estimates for Specific Office Procedures**

Procedure	Time in Minutes
Allergy testing	30–60
Cast check	10
Cast change	30
Complete physical with EKG	60
Blood pressure check	15
Dressing change	15
Minor surgery procedure	30–45
Office visit: Established patient	
Low complexity	5–10
Medium complexity	15–20
High complexity	20–30
Office visit: New Patient	
Low complexity	10–15
Medium complexity	15–30
Complete physical	30–45
Pelvic examination with PAP test	30
Patient education	30–45
Post-operative checkup	15–20
Prenatal examination (first visit)	30–60
Prenatal checkup	15
Prostate examination	30
School physical	15–30
Suture removal	10
Well-baby checkup	15

On the other hand, the physician may have a delay or the need to cancel appointments due to an emergency at the hospital or even a patient emergency in the office. Also, the medical office may not have all the necessary physical equipment for certain procedures, or building issues may arise as well as other unforeseen

Scheduling Patients

OBJECTIVE: Use an appointment scheduling system to schedule patients with efficiency.

Equipment and Supplies

pencil or pen (if preferred by office management); appointment schedule book

Method

1. Understand the scheduling system used in your office.

2. Use a pencil so that appointments can be erased to make changes as needed. Please note, some offices prefer the use of black or blue ink instead of pencil.

3. Set up a matrix by blocking out all time periods when the physician is not available (hospital rounds, vacation) for appointments before scheduling patients. Ideally, setting up a matrix or appointment blocking on the computer is done three months ahead of time.

4. Schedule appointments by beginning with the first empty appointment in the morning or early in the afternoon, and then fill in the day. Do not schedule appointments at the end of the day with large open gaps in between.

5. Print the patient's full first and last name next to the appropriate time on the schedule. Add Jr. for *junior* and Sr. for *senior* if there are two patients with the same name in a family.

6. Ask the patient for a current work and home telephone number, including the area code. Write these numbers next to the patient's name.

7. Write the reason for the visit on the schedule using accepted medical abbreviations.

8. Allow the correct amount of time for the appointment. If an appointment will take more than the minimum time allotted on the schedule, then use an arrow to indicate that the patient will be using 2 or 3 blocks of time. In some offices, a line is drawn across the time blocks.

NOTE: In offices where scheduling is done by computer, enter the patient information as directed by the on-screen prompts.

---

circumstances. In all cases, the medical assistant should provide patients with an explanation and reschedule appointments. Missed appointments happen with no warning, so the medical assistant has less opportunity to make satisfactory adjustments. No matter what the reason for a missed appointment, the medical assistant must contact the patient, reschedule the appointment, and document it as a missed and rescheduled appointment in the patient medical record. Careful legible documentation is necessary for HIPAA compliance as well as to legally protect the physician from a claim of patient abandonment.

Patient No-Shows

No-shows or failed appointments occur when a patient does not show up to keep an appointment. If a patient misses an appointment, write no-show (NS), or cancellation (xll) on the appointment schedule sheet and in the patient chart. Make every attempt to fill up a void in the schedule caused by a patient cancellation. One method is to call the patient who has the last appointment for the day and ask the patient if it is possible to come in earlier. In the event that a long appointment, such as a one and one-half hour appointment for a complete physical, has been canceled, you will have to attempt to move up an entire group of patients. Many offices maintain a list of patients who wish to be called if there is an appointment open at the last minute. This approach is beneficial to maintaining good customer service as well as being an effective use of time for the office schedule.

Advance Booking

Ideally, before leaving the office, the patient will schedule his or her next appointment. This routine is known as advance booking. It is possible to book patients far in advance because most medical offices prepare the schedule books from three to six months ahead of time. Advance booking is done for regularly scheduled checkups or required follow-up appointments, such as after physical therapy treatments, or blood pressure checks. Appointment cards with the name, address, and telephone number of the physician's practice have space to write in the date and time of the next appointment and should be given to each patient at the time the next appointment is made (Figure 8-5).

Follow-up

Some offices have the patient complete a self-addressed postcard reminder to use in an appointment reminder system known as a tickler file. The tickler card is filed in a small file box (tickler file) under the date the postcard should be mailed. Such reminders are used for annual PAP tests. The tickler file is very handy for the follow-up appointments. When possible, the follow-up should be scheduled before the patient leaves the office. Follow-ups can be made in writing, by telephone, or e-mail. All follow-up methods should include the day, date, and time of the next appointment. Some offices make personal telephone calls one to two days prior to the actual appointment. Either follow-up method is considered a good approach for maintaining customer service and smart office management to decrease the no-show rate.

Patient Referrals

The physician will often refer patients to another facility or physician for further testing and treatment. Ideally, the appointment is scheduled as soon as possible. Whether referring a patient to another location or receiving a referral, the medical assistant must exchange pertinent information regarding the patient's name, contact number, insurance, and referral needs as well as the referral physician's name, address, and contact number. In some cases, depending on the insurance, pre-certification (approval) is necessary before scheduling the appointment.

Hospital Admission Scheduling

The medical assistant is responsible for scheduling all patient admissions to the hospital. Patients do not schedule their own hospital admissions (admits). When scheduling a direct admit to the hospital, be sure to contact the patient's insurance company for pre-admissions approval. Table 8-3 provides a description of the patient information supplied when scheduling hospital admissions.

Provide the patient with a detailed explanation of the day, date, time, and preparation needed for the admission. It is always better to place details in writing. Many offices have preprinted information to distribute to the patient. This should, however, be personalized with the patient's name. Even when preprinted materials are used, a complete, concise, verbal explanation of the important points should be given by the medical assistant.

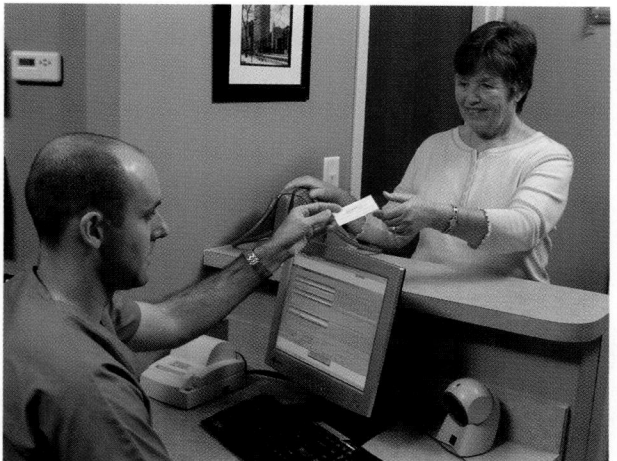

FIGURE 8-5   The medical assistant gives a patient an appointment card.

Scheduling Surgery and Outpatient Procedures

Scheduling a surgical procedure is determined on the patient's need and diagnosis, type of surgery, insurance carrier, physician, anesthesia, and facility availability. The medical assistant will contact the surgical boarding department and arrange with the surgical boarder the necessary pre-surgical appointments (i.e. blood work, chest x-ray, etc.), the actual surgery, and postoperative appointments, if necessary. The surgical boarder may request all patient information, including legal name, telephone contacts, insurance information (prior authorization for some elective surgeries), advanced directives, or other pre-admittance information.

Sometimes the medical assistant will be asked to assist a patient in scheduling an outpatient procedure with the surgical scheduler—the person in the surgery department who schedules the procedures. Procedure 8-2 provides instructions on how to schedule inpatient surgical procedures. Procedure 8-3 reviews the steps for scheduling outpatient procedures.

Appointment Exceptions

On occasion, nonscheduled patients will contact the office with a need for an immediate appointment. These include patient emergencies and patients with acute conditions. Acute conditions are illnesses or injuries that patients suddenly experience and require treatment but may not be life threatening.

The medical assistant must listen carefully to all the patient's complaints and assess the seriousness of the patient's condition. The medical assistant will ask questions regarding where the pain is located, when it first appeared, the duration of strength or measure of the pain, and if the patient has experienced the same pain

TABLE 8-3 **Patient Information Supplied when Scheduling Hospital Admissions**

■ Patient's full name	Verify spelling of first and last name.
■ Address	Ask the patient to state current address.
■ Social Security number	May be taken from the patient record. (Note: This is not in compliance with HIPAA, however, medical institutions still ask for this information.)
■ Age/Date of birth	Verify birth date in patient record.
■ Telephone number	Ask patient for current number and area code.
■ Requirement	Type of room or special requirement.
■ Admitting diagnosis	Give the physician's statement from the patient record.
■ Recent prior admission	Ask the patient for last admission date in any hospital.
■ Physician's name	Give physician's name.
■ Insurance information	May fax copy of insurance card.
■ Person's name at insurance company who gave pre-approval.	Forms are also available from insurance company.

8-2 PROCEDURE

Scheduling Inpatient Surgical Procedures

OBJECTIVE: Perform proper procedure to schedule inpatient surgical procedures.

Equipment and Supplies
patient's chart; written instructions for patients (if required)

Method

1. Review the patient's chart for the most current information. Make sure the chart contains the physician's notes and orders regarding the surgical procedure.
2. Verify with the physician the type of procedure for which you are to schedule the patient. Then you should:
   - determine which category the surgical procedure falls under (routine, elective, urgent).
   - find out the name of the surgeon to perform the procedure.
   - obtain the surgeon's scheduling preference for this type of procedure.
   - get an estimated length of time for the procedure.
3. Gather the following information from the patient and patient's chart:
   - patient's full name, age, sex, and any other pertinent identification or information.
   - physician's current diagnosis.
   - special pre-op orders and patient instructions.
   - patient's insurance information.
4. Obtain pre-authorization from the patient's insurance company, if required.
5. Contact the surgery scheduler.
6. Follow office procedure and surgeon's request for contacting other members of the surgical team.
7. Instruct patient on special preparation and admission procedures. Provide written instructions, if available.

Scheduling an Outpatient Procedure

OBJECTIVE: To demonstrate the ability to schedule outpatient procedures in the health care setting.

Equipment and Supplies

telephone; patient's insurance card; notepad; pen

Method

1. Access the appointment system (manual or computer).
2. According to the facility policy, contact the outpatient scheduler at the local hospital or clinic and identify yourself and your office.
3. Instruct the facility about the type of procedure and amount of time the physician expects to need the operating room.
4. Determine available days at the facility.
5. Offer options to patient and have patient choose the best option.
6. Notify the facility of the date and time chosen.
7. Create patient instruction sheet to include date and time of procedure and necessary preoperative information.
8. Document conversation in the patient chart.

Charting Example

Patient has cervical conization scheduled for 12:30 p.m. on November 9, 2005. Patient was given instruction sheet and stated she understood that she would have to go for preoperative testing on November 3 and is not to eat after midnight on the night prior to surgery.

---

before. Also ask the patient for a telephone number from where he or she is calling and determine if the patient is alone. It is best for the medical assistant to use the office policy and emergency criteria list to assess the situation. The physician should always be informed immediately regarding a potential emergency.

The medical assistant will need to apply his on her triage skills. Triage is the process of sorting or grouping patients according to the seriousness of their condition. Triage becomes necessary when there is more than one seriously ill patient waiting to see the physician. In general, sudden onset of pain must be considered an emergency until otherwise determined.

If an emergency exists, such as in the case of severe chest pain, then the physician is informed of the call immediately. If a physician is not available, then the medical assistant refers the patient to the nearest emergency center. If the patient is not able to make his or her own arrangements for transportation, then the medical assistant will arrange for taxi or med-van service. Table 8-4 lists acute illnesses that will require that the patient be seen by a physician as soon a possible, while Table 8-5 lists emergency (life-threatening) conditions, which will require immediate physician assistance.

In order to eliminate the need to "squeeze in" an emergency or nonscheduled appointments and disrupt the time management office flow, the medical assistant should set time patterns. Time patterns are similar to matrixing off time within the schedule for catch-up time or nonscheduled appointments. Ideally, there should be a few minutes built into the schedule between the end of one patient visit and the beginning of another patient's visit. However, most schedule systems do not allow for time between patients. Therefore, it is important to build small blocks of

TABLE 8-4 **Examples of Acute Conditions**

Earache	Eye infection
Fever lasting more than 24 hours	Infection that is visible to patient (for example, a red, swollen area after an injury)
Pain or burning upon urination	Pain in abdomen that is not severe
Skin rash	Stabbing chest pain
Unusual discharge (for example, blood in urine)	Sore throat and/or swollen glands

TABLE 8-5	Examples of Emergency Conditions
Acute allergic reaction	Head injury
Allergic reaction with respiratory distress	Laceration
Chest pain	Loss of consciousness
Coma	Pain and/or numbness after the application of a cast for fracture
Convulsions	Poisoning
Diabetic reaction	Severe bleeding
Difficulty breathing	Severe dizziness
Drowning/near-drowning	Severe nausea, vomiting, and diarrhea lasting more than 24 hours
Drug overdose	Severe pain
Foreign object in the eye	Sudden acute illness
Fracture	Sudden paralysis of part or all of the body
Gunshot wounds	Temperature over 104° F

time into the schedule during the day when the physician can return telephone calls, catch up on charting, read mail and journals, or just rest. The best time for this is at the end of the morning's schedule and again, at the end of the day. Some physicians prefer to return all morning telephone calls when they return from lunch.

Building this free time block into the office daily schedule at the same time each day is very important. Every effort should be made not to schedule last minute appointments during this time. These "buffer" periods are excellent backup times for emergencies that may have to be seen that day.

Telephone and E-mail Scheduling

Many offices use the telephone and e-mail (electronic mail) to schedule appointments. The medical assistant will need to apply professional, legal, and effective communication skills when using these forms of technology.

Following are some professional considerations to include while communicating with the patient:

- Determine if you are speaking directly with the patient.
- Use the patient's name while addressing him or her on the telephone and in the e-mail.
- On the telephone, confirm the appointment by having the patient repeat the day, date, time, and location of the appointment.
- In an e-mail, request that the patient provide a return communication for verification of received information.
- Communicate with the patient the desire to meet his or her requested appointment time; however, an explanation may be necessary when offering an alternative time.
- Be specific and inform the patient of the office policies for cancellations and missed appointments.
- Be sure to gather all pertinent information from the patient, i.e. name, telephone contacts, e-mail address, reason for visit, insurance carrier, and whether the patient needs directions to the office.

New Patient Appointments

Scheduling a new patient's appointment requires additional time, patience, and effective organizational skills. Always project a professional and positive image with the patient. Using effective communication skills will be most beneficial from a customer service perspective, since managing this appointment will set the stage for the patient's actual in-office visit. The following steps are guidelines for scheduling a new patient:

- Assemble necessary appointment scheduling equipment.
- Obtain the patient's full legal name and correct spelling, birth date, full address, telephone contacts (home, office, cell), and e-mail address.
- Record the patient's chief complaint and symptoms.
- Request the name of the patient's insurance carrier and policy number.
- Ask how the patient was referred to the medical office (physician referral, friend, colleague, insurance company, etc.).
- Ask the patient for a preferred appointment time.
- Attempt to accommodate the new patient's request for his or her preferred appointment time.
- Confirm the day, date, and time of the appointment and have the new patient repeat the information for verification and mutual understanding.

- Provide the new patient with directions to the office.
- Inform the new patient of all materials to bring with him or her for the first visit, i.e. insurance verification, photo identification, list of current medications, past medical records (if available), current lab, x-ray, and other medical reports, as available.
- Welcome and thank the new patient by name for selecting your medical office.
- Provide all information as discussed to the new patient via mail.
- Document new patient information in a new medical record.

When scheduling pediatric and elderly patients, it is important to note that they may need specific times and may have other special needs. Lifespan Considerations discusses some ways to make the office environment more welcoming for these patients.

Lifespan Considerations

Young children often find it hard to wait patiently for extended periods of time. Try to be sensitive to this when scheduling pediatric patients. Some adult patients may have to bring their children with them. In the waiting area, have some quiet activities and magazines geared toward children. Animated and children's videos may help children wait more patiently.

Also remember that the elderly may have difficulty waiting for long periods of time. Take measures to help make them as comfortable as possible. Comfortable seating, large print reading materials, and light refreshments may be ways to make their wait easier.

Established Patient Appointments

Any patient who has been previously seen by the physician is considered an established patient. Established patients will have an existing medical record/chart that will need to be accessed each time the patient contacts the physician for an appointment. It is a good approach to verify the established patient's telephone contact, address, and insurance information prior to scheduling an appointment. Maintaining good customer service with established patients includes appointment reminders and observing patient cycle time.

SUMMARY

An efficiently managed medical office requires careful attention to the scheduling function. The medical assistant is responsible for carefully assessing the patient's need for an appointment. Providing the correct amount of time on the schedule for the patient visit works to ensure that the needs of patient and physician are met. However, the medical assistant must remain flexible in scheduling since patients with emergencies and acute illnesses must be seen immediately.

Scheduling Other Types of Appointments

Medical practices may have non-patient appointments to schedule. These appointments may include, sales representatives from various companies, including office equipment, pharmaceuticals, insurance, or community service leaders. Each visitor will need an appointment to update the staff and physician on the newest product, drug(s), equipment, or community issue(s). Most offices have a policy for working with the non-patient visitors and vendor representatives.

A professional and ethical manner is the best approach to handling a schedule that has fallen behind. Quick thinking and planning by rescheduling patients can alleviate stress for the physician who falls behind. Careful documentation and HIPAA compliance of all patients who fail to keep appointments, either through cancellation or no-show, can assist the physician in avoiding a lawsuit for abandonment of the patient.

Chapter Review

COMPETENCY REVIEW

1. Define and spell the terms to learn for this chapter.
2. Write an office policy for scheduling emergency appointments.

3. Role-play instructing a patient on admission to the hospital for a surgical procedure. Use another student as the patient.
4. Correctly document a patient appointment cancellation.
5. Use a computerized scheduling system to integrate patient information and appointment scheduling.

PREPARING FOR THE CERTIFICATION EXAM

1. David is scheduled to have a post-operative checkup. He has been given a 15-minute appointment at 1:00 P.M. His wife, Christina, has an appointment on the same day at 1:15 P.M. What type of scheduling system is the physician using?
   A. wave scheduling
   B. specified time scheduling
   C. modified wave scheduling
   C. double booking
   E. open office hours

2. How far ahead of time should a medical office appointment schedule be "blocked out?"
   A. one year
   B. six months
   C. three months
   D. to be done when you make an appointment
   E. one week

3. What is the best method to use when a patient cancels an early afternoon one-hour appointment?
   A. move up the last appointment (15-minute exam) for the day into that slot
   B. leave the time free for the physician to get caught up with paper work
   C. do nothing since the physician is always running late
   D. call several patients who have asked to be placed on a waiting list and try to fill the entire hour
   E. try to change all of the rest of the afternoon appointments to one hour earlier

4. When the patient requires surgery, the medical assistant will
   A. give all the information to the patient so that the patient can schedule the surgery at a convenient time
   B. ask the surgeon who will be performing the surgery to schedule it
   C. call the surgery scheduler where the surgery will be performed and schedule the time
   D. place the surgery request in writing and send it to the surgical center
   E. tell the physician/employer to schedule it

5. All the following are either medical emergencies or acute conditions that require an appointment as soon as possible EXCEPT
   A. earache
   B. severe pain
   C. eye infection
   D. pain with urination
   E. fever of 99.8° F for the past two weeks

6. After a no-show and to assist the physician in avoiding a claim by a patient for abandonment, the medical assistant would
   A. tell the patient that he or she will have to find another physician for treatment
   B. screen out all patients who really do not need to be seen by the physician
   C. call the patient to attempt to re-schedule the appointment and document the telephone call
   D. nothing special needs to be done
   E. refer the patient to a specialist

7. Double booking patients
   A. is one of the most acceptable ways of patient scheduling in terms of practice time management
   B. is generally considered poor practice
   C. involves scheduling two members of the same family at the same time
   D. always forces the physician to utilize less time per patient
   E. does not cause daily scheduling problems

8. What procedure for appointment scheduling refers to crossing out periods of time when the physician is unavailable?
   A. double booking
   B. wave scheduling
   C. forming a matrix
   D. modified wave scheduling
   E. archiving

continued on next page

9. When a patient does not show up for an appointment, the medical assistant should do all of the following EXCEPT
   A. write "N/S" above the scheduled appointment
   B. record the missed appointment in the patient's record
   C. record the reason for the missed appointment in the patient's record
   D. notify the physician
   E. track down the patient

10. Which of the following is applicable to appointment cards?
    A. include the name, address and telephone number of the practice
    B. should be given to each patient whether the patient wants one or not
    C. includes all of the same information as the follow-up reminder card
    D. are generally only used for past no-shows
    E. are preprinted with the patient's name prior to the day's appointment

CRITICAL THINKING

1. What scheduling variation is in use?
2. Using a modified wave format, recreate the original schedule for Dr. Miller's Friday appointments.
3. On the new schedule, indicate Ramona Pierce's cancelled appointment.
4. The office is usually closed from 12 P.M. to 1 P.M. for lunch. New patient visits usually last about one hour. Can Shannon Reece see Dr. Miller tomorrow?
5. How should Marc handle scheduling Marcus Fowler?

ON THE JOB

A pharmaceutical representative has just arrived at the office of Dr. Joseph Henderson, a board certified orthopedic surgeon. The waiting room is literally swarming with patients waiting to see Dr. Henderson because he was delayed with an unexpectedly complicated lumbar spinal fusion and laminectomy.

The representative is very insistent, almost belligerent about seeing the physician immediately, even though she did not have an appointment to see him. In fact, the visit was totally unexpected as the representative had just been in two weeks prior to today. Last time the representative was in, she gave Dr. Henderson a variety of readily usable and dispensable medication. She has more of the same today—injectable cortisone with Novocain, muscle relaxants, NSAIDS, and even some Tylenol with codeine. Usually, Dr. Henderson is quite receptive to receiving these samples as they help ease the financial burden of his patients on whom he uses or to whom he dispenses the samples. The office is, in fact, running quite low on these particular medications because of Dr. Henderson's heavy patient load.

1. What is your response to the sales representative?
2. Should a representative ever take precedence over scheduled appointments?
3. Does the fact that Dr. Joseph is usually quite anxious to receive any and all samples for his patients enter in as a factor?
4. Does the diminished supply of these samples alter the situation?
5. Can the medical assistant ever accept delivery of any or all of these samples?

INTERNET ACTIVITY

Locate three different medical appointment scheduling software programs on the Internet. Compare and contrast the products, services, features, and costs to fit the needs of a general practitioner's medical practice. Then, locate the HIPAA compliance guidelines for appointment scheduling and develop a useful list for future reference.

MediaLink More on scheduling appointments, including interactive resources, can be found on the Student CD-ROM accompanying this textbook.

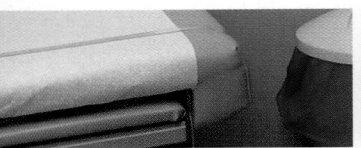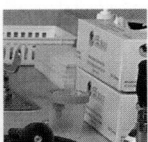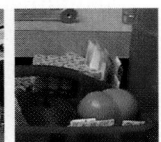

Medical Assistant Role Delineation Chart

HIGHLIGHT indicates material covered in this chapter.

ADMINISTRATIVE

Administrative Procedures

- Perform basic administrative medical assisting functions
- Schedule, coordinate and monitor appointments
- Schedule inpatient/outpatient admissions and procedures
- Understand and apply third-party guidelines
- Obtain reimbursement through accurate claims submission
- Monitor third-party reimbursement
- Understand and adhere to managed care policies and procedures
- *Negotiate managed care contracts*

Practice Finances

- Perform procedural and diagnostic coding
- Apply bookkeeping principles

- Manage accounts receivable
- *Manage accounts payable*
- *Process payroll*
- *Document and maintain accounting and banking records*
- *Develop and maintain fee schedules*
- *Manage renewals of business and professional insurance policies*
- *Manage personnel benefits and maintain records*
- *Perform marketing, financial, and strategic planning*

CLINICAL

Fundamental Principles

- Apply principles of aseptic technique and infection control
- Comply with quality assurance practices
- Screen and follow up patient test results

Diagnostic Orders

- Collect and process specimens
- Perform diagnostic tests

Patient Care

- Adhere to established patient screening procedures
- Obtain patient history and vital signs
- Prepare and maintain examination and treatment areas
- Prepare patient for examinations, procedures and treatments

- Assist with examinations, procedures and treatments
- Prepare and administer medications and immunizations
- Maintain medication and immunization records
- Recognize and respond to emergencies
- Coordinate patient care information with other health care providers
- Initiate IV and administer IV medications with appropriate training and as permitted by state law

GENERAL

Professionalism

- Display a professional manner and image
- Demonstrate initiative and responsibility
- Work as a member of the health care team
- Prioritize and perform multiple tasks
- Adapt to change
- Promote the CMA credential
- Enhance skills through continuing education
- Treat all patients with compassion and empathy
- Promote the practice through positive public relations

Communication Skills

- Recognize and respect cultural diversity
- Adapt communications to individual's ability to understand
- Use professional telephone technique

- *Denotes advanced skills.*

- Recognize and respond effectively to verbal, nonverbal, and written communications
- Use medical terminology appropriately
- Utilize electronic technology to receive, organize, prioritize and transmit information
- Serve as liaison

Legal Concepts

- Perform within legal and ethical boundaries
- Prepare and maintain medical records
- Document accurately
- Follow employer's established policies dealing with the health care contract
- Implement and maintain federal and state health care legislation and regulations
- Comply with established risk management and safety procedures
- Recognize professional credentialing criteria
- *Develop and maintain personnel, policy and procedure manuals*

Instruction

- Instruct individuals according to their needs
- Explain office policies and procedures
- Teach methods of health promotion and disease prevention
- Locate community resources and disseminate information
- *Develop educational materials*
- *Conduct continuing education activities*

Operational Functions

- Perform inventory of supplies and equipment
- Perform routine maintenance of administrative and clinical equipment
- Apply computer techniques to support office operations
- *Perform personnel management functions*
- *Negotiate leases and prices for equipment and supply contracts*

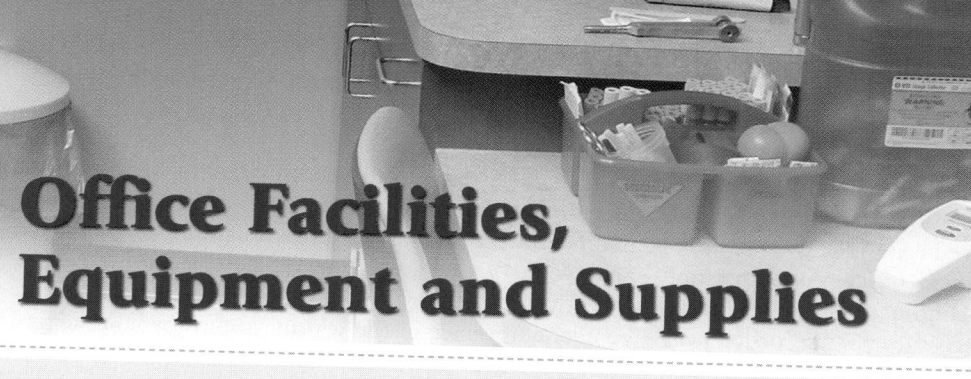

Office Facilities, Equipment and Supplies

Learning Objectives

After completing this chapter, you should be able to:

- Define and spell the terms to learn for this chapter.
- Discuss the elements of office flow.
- State the difference between capital equipment and expendable equipment.

- Discuss basic office equipment and their functions.
- Discuss HIPAA regulations as related to basic office equipment.
- State the proper procedure for handling drug samples.

OUTLINE

Medical Office Facility	160
Office Layout	160
Office Equipment	163
Supplies	166

Terms to Learn

Americans with Disabilities Act (ADA)

capital equipment

cycle time

inventory

morale

office flow

vendor

warranty

Case Study

YOU ARRIVE AT WORK TO FIND THE OFFICE CARPETS have just been cleaned and all the patient waiting room furniture is stacked in the hallway. Several patients are starting to walk in the front door. The cleaning crew cleaned the office administration area and most of the office equipment, including computers and the fax machine have been moved or unplugged. You find an entire shelf of patient records on the floor and in your work area, and you also noticed a few boxes out in the hallway that contain patient supplies.

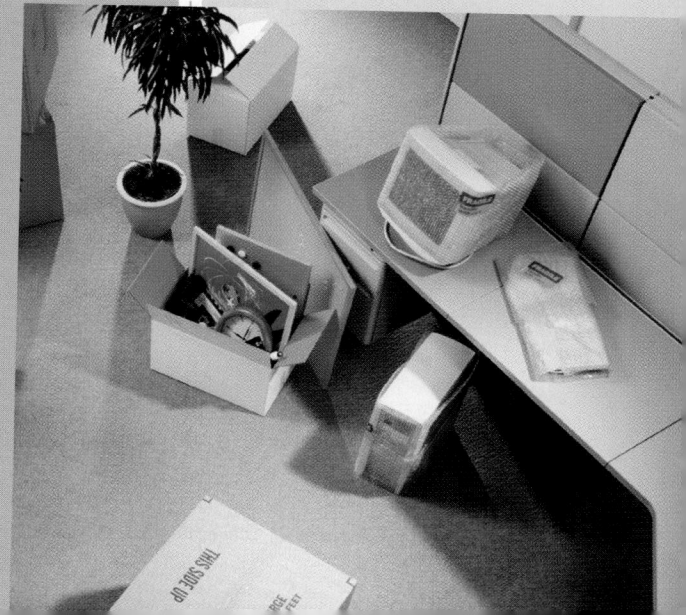

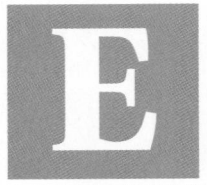

Every medical workplace should be clean to ensure employee and patient safety and health, the traffic should flow smoothly, and it should adhere to Federal, State, and local safety and health regulations. In recent years, changes have been made to many regulations that affect the medical office. As communication processes and technology become more sophisticated, it becomes necessary for the office personnel to both stay informed, and to adhere to the rules that make the medical office safe and protect everyone's right to privacy.

Medical Office Facility

The pleasant physical atmosphere created by a cheerful, clean office makes an immediate impression upon patients. It also adds to the general positive morale of the employees. Morale refers to the positive or negative state of mind of employees (regarding a feeling of well-being) with relationship to their work or work environment. Things to be considered in setting up and maintaining a medical office include the office layout and design that set the tone, attitude, climate, and culture of the office. Elements of the layout include the design of traffic flow, the color of the walls, room temperature, lighting, ventilation, furniture and placement of the furniture, equipment, supplies, and overall organization.

Facilities Planning

The medical assistant will need to view the medical office through the eyes of the patient. What does the patient see when he or she enters the doors and beyond?

One of the first considerations in planning a medical office facility is the Americans with Disabilities Act (ADA), legislation to protect the rights of the disabled regarding access to employment, public buildings, transportation, housing, schools, and health care facilities. The Americans with Disabilities Act allows for every public facility to be easily accessible to the handicapped, including unrestricted hallways, elevators or ramps, and handicapped restroom facilities. Furnishings should be arranged to create an easy traffic pattern for patients to follow as they enter and leave the office. There should be adequate space in the waiting room for wheelchairs to be maneuvered with ease.

All patients should walk into a medical office environment that is comfortable and bright. Some medical offices have patients walk into a reception room with a window that allows patients to look outside during their wait time. External light shines into the office making the room well lit and comfortable. Reception rooms generally should be painted with bright colors and have pleasing and tasteful art on the walls (Figure 9-1). If your office has a fish tank, it is important to regularly maintain the tank for patient safety and general cleanliness. Fish tanks are very inviting for children and adults to watch. It is important to position the tank up high enough so children cannot disturb the fish or push over the tank.

Office Layout

Medical offices are generally divided into two areas: administrative and clinical. The administrative area may contain the reception area to perform patient processing and scheduling, office equipment, file storage, payment collections, insurance, billing, and mail processing. The administrative area usually includes office equipment such as computers, printers, scanners, fax machines, postage meters, calculators, telephone system, paper shredder, dictation and transcribing equipment as well as all office supplies. The area may also include a children's play area and staff area. Child safety in the office is discussed in Lifespan Considerations.

The clinical area contains the examination rooms, physician's office and consultation room, treatment room for office surgical procedures, supply room, clean and contaminated utility areas, rest rooms, a laboratory that can house blood drawing, specimen analyzing, and electrocardiogram (ECG) equipment, and in some offices, a radiology room. Some medical facilities also have a small recovery room with a bed or cot for patients recovering from minor surgical procedures. Of course, not every

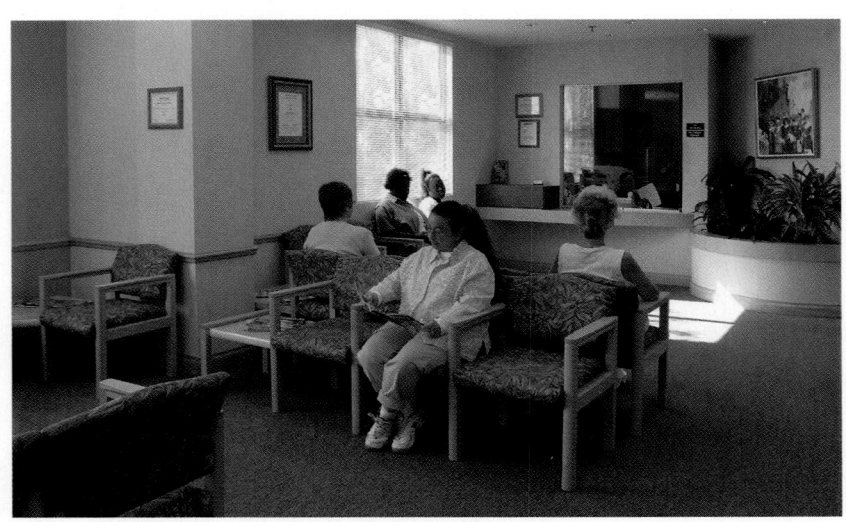

FIGURE 9-1 A reception area should be comfortable and bright.

office will have all of these areas. Specialty practices may have other departments and equipment specific to the type of procedures done.

Office Flow

The medical facility generally has a flow that lends itself easily to teamwork, time management, organized and efficient office equipment usage, and patient flow. This is known as office flow. The more organized the office area, the more effective the office flow will be managed by staff and patients (Professionalism). All staff members will be involved in the office flow process from the time the patients arrive to their departure time. Each staff member has a chance to maintain the office flow by reducing patient cycle time. Cycle time is the length of time the average patient spends in the medical office. With proper office layout, the cycle time can be managed more effectively for a smoother office flow. Let's take a closer look at how these elements impact the office flow (Figure 9-2).

The first element of the office flow is the patient entrance. The first impression the patient receives begins at the medical facility door. Getting patients into the office presents the opportunity to accommodate any type of patient. The office entranceways should include handrails, elevators, ramps, wheelchair-accessible door frames, patient lifts if necessary, and well lit walkways. High steps should be marked with reflector tape and should include slip protection sheets. Doors and door handles should be marked with a push or pull indicator. Keeping doors clean and clear is vital to office aesthetics and patient safety.

Reception Area

The reception area consists of the waiting room and the reception desk. The desk should be enclosed with a glass partition that can be closed for privacy so that personal medical information cannot be overheard in the waiting room. The desk surface should be neat and not

contain confidential patient information such as records, an open appointment book, and billing information.

The medical records area should be close to the receptionist's area for quick accessibility to charts for telephone calls. The Health Insurance Portability and Accountability Act (HIPAA) states that the medical records area should not be accessible to patients and that they should not be able to read the labels of the charts. Figure 9-3 shows a typical file room.

Seating that provides good support and can be easily cleaned is most suitable for the patient reception area. Over-stuffed chairs and couches should be avoided. Housekeeping staff cannot move such furniture easily. In addition, deep chairs are difficult to get in and out of for the elderly and the infirm.

Almost every office has magazines for patients to read. All materials placed for patient reading must be screened to make sure they meet the standards of your

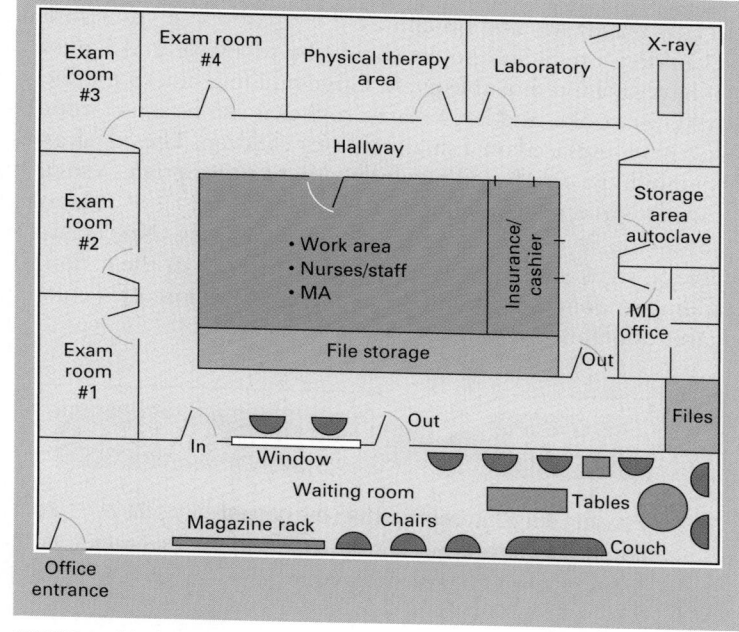

FIGURE 9-2 A typical office layout.

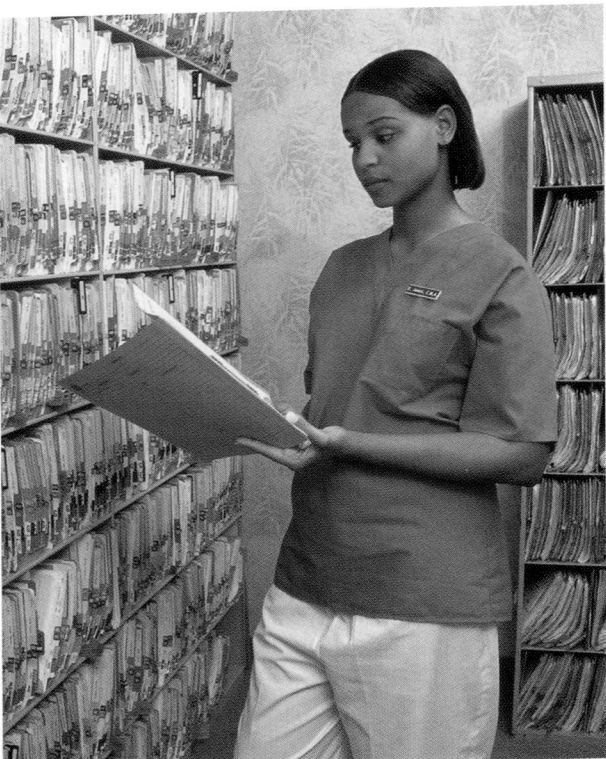

FIGURE 9-3 A typical office file room.

office and would not upset the patients. Patient Education discusses types of materials used to educate patients. It is important to organize the magazines and materials neatly in order to show that the office is clean and well maintained. Periodically, the receptionist or another staff member assigned may need to straighten up the reception area and waiting room, especially magazines and brochures.

Children's toys and books should be washable and not have small, removable parts. Large building blocks, hardcover books, and large plastic toys that can be sanitized may be placed on a small table for children. These toys should be disinfected regularly with an appropriate cleaner to prevent cross contamination.

Smoking is not allowed in medical facilities. No smoking signs should be placed at the entrance of the building. A container should be available to dispose of cigarettes before entering the building.

If a person with a communicable disease visits the office, he or she should be placed in a designated area to minimize spreading the disease. After the visit is over, the office should be disinfected immediately.

Patient orientation begins when the patient arrives in the reception area. Many medical offices prefer that a medical professional escort the patient through the office. However, this is not always possible and patients may need to get around by themselves. For patients to navigate for themselves requires clear markings that indicate the location of the registration and check-in desk, office entrance and exits, where patients should sit if there is more than one doctor in the office, and restroom locations. Hallways and walkways should be clear of any obstructions. In some offices, color-coded indicators on the floor or wall help to facilitate patient flow. It is important to have signs that show patients where they need to go.

Clearly marked areas will assist patient exits as well. When a patient is ready to leave the office, it is important to confirm the route a patient needs to take to exit the office. For example, if a patient has just been seen by a physician and you are showing the patient out, it is best to lead the way. This should prevent patients from accidentally walking into another examination room or into private areas of the office. Patients should have a direct route to the checkout desk and there should be markings on the walls to help patients to direct themselves toward the exit.

Examination Rooms

Examination rooms should only contain furnishings and equipment needed to examine a patient. Most examination rooms have only enough space for the necessities and little else. Figure 9-4 illustrates a typical patient examination room. All instruments and supplies, such as disposable gowns, towels, tissues, and sheets are kept in a sufficient number in examination room supply cabinets. Most examination tables have drawers for the convenient storage of these items. A small sink for hand hygiene, an adjustable gooseneck lamp, telephone, chair, examination table, and physician's stool are the only furnishings necessary. Examination rooms should be painted in a pleasant, comforting color. Paintings or pictures can also enhance the serenity of the room. The temperature throughout the reception

Patient Education

Patient Education begins when the patient enters the office. Many offices now offer videotapes on various health care topics that the patients may view while waiting to be seen by the physician. Become involved in keeping all patient education pamphlets up to date and displayed on tables in the reception area or in a rack designed for literature.

area and examination rooms should be maintained at around 74° F. Patients in the examination rooms must frequently disrobe and may be chilled in just a disposable gown.

At least one examination room should be configured for a wheelchair-bound patient. It should be larger than a normal sized examination room to allow both the patient and physician to maneuver comfortably.

Examination rooms should be soundproof so that conversations cannot be heard from one room to another. The examination table should be arranged so that the patient is not exposed when the door is opened. "White noise," such as pleasant, soothing background music, can also filter sounds.

Bathrooms

Bathrooms should be kept clean and odor-free. Every bathroom should have hot and cold water, soap, paper towels or other drying system, a trashcan, and toilet tissue. Since bathrooms in the medical office are multifunctional, they should also be large enough to accommodate a wheelchair, and at least one of the bathrooms should meet ADA guidelines for a handicapped restroom facility such as handrails around the toilet. Bathrooms are used by both staff and patients. They are also used by patients who are collecting urine specimens and should have a place to set the specimen while the patient washes his or her hands after collecting the sample.

Housekeeping

Housekeeping or medical office cleaning services can be contracted to clean the front office area and the examination room every night. Regular housekeeping services are usually not responsible for handling hazardous waste containers. Instead, hazardous waste, including sharps, should be disposed of in designated containers and removed from the office or facility properly.

Office Equipment

In order for a medical office to maintain effective office flow, certain office machines and equipment are most beneficial. As mentioned above, a copier, computers, printers, scanners, fax machines (Figure 9-5), postage meters, calculators, telephone system, dictation and transcribing equipment, and paper shredder would be considered essentials for the office. This equipment and other equipment, such as examination tables, refrigerators, x-ray and EKG machines, office furnishings, and carpeting, are categorized as capital equipment.

Capital equipment refers to items that require a large dollar amount to purchase (generally over $500) and have a relatively long life. The distinguishing factor between capital equipment and general office

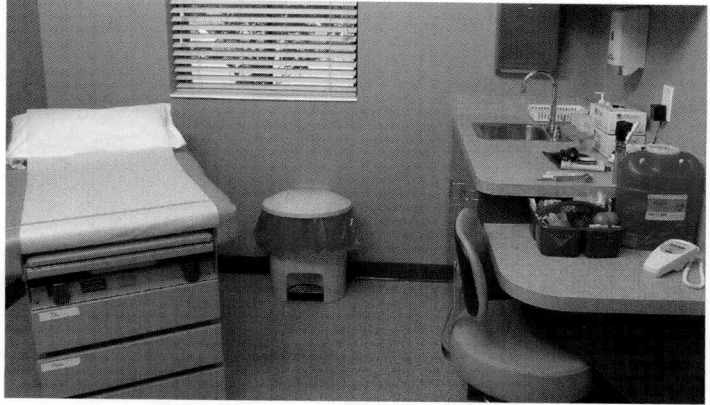

FIGURE 9-4 A patient examination room should be simple and efficiently designed.

supplies is the life expectancy (functional life period) of the product.

Capital equipment also has a financial life, which is referred to as depreciation. Depreciation is a loss in value of the product resulting from normal aging, use, or deterioration. An allowance is made for this type of loss of value for tax purposes. Therefore, the office accountant will credit capital items differently than for general office supplies. A master inventory, or list, should be detailed and maintained of all the physical assets, or capital equipment, in an office.

Determining what equipment to have begins with the office need. Obtaining the equipment requires research to gather equipment information, the actual purchase, delivery, setup, proper training, safe use, and general maintenance. Most medical offices will have the following administrative equipment.

- Calculator—used for mathematical calculation for billing and determining medication dosages.

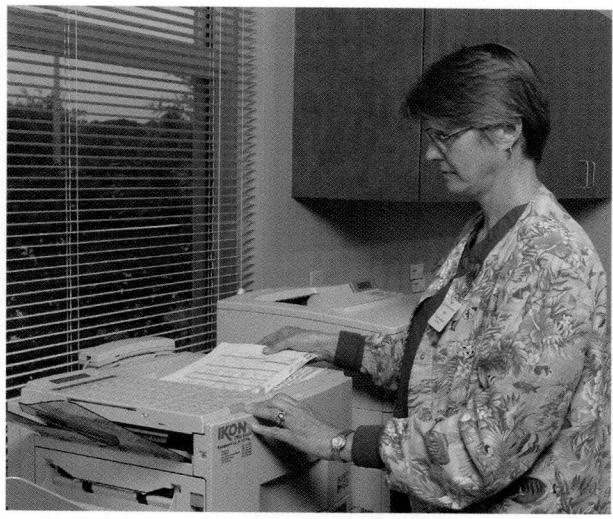

FIGURE 9-5 Fax machines are necessary in all medical offices.

- Computer—discussed in Chapter 11.
- Laser printer—used in conjunction with a computer for letter quality printing. Creates images with a laser beam and then transfers the image to paper with pressure and heat.
- Facsimile (fax) machine—used to send and receive copies to and from the office via the telephone system.
- Transcription equipment (dictation/transcription machine)—used to dictate and then transcribe information for documents and letters.
- Telephone system—discussed in Chapter 6.
- Scanners—used to "read" text and graphic files.
- Copy machine—used to copy, reduce, enlarge, and collate documents in the medical office (Figure 9-6).
- Electronic paper shredder—used to shred paper documents into thin strips so that the information on the documents cannot be retrieved.
- Postage meter—used to stamp envelopes and packages for offices with large mailings.

Transcription Equipment

The dictation equipment required for medical transcription includes transcribers, typewriters, word processing equipment, and reference materials. Newer methods of transcription include computerized voice recognition technology (VRT). Explanations of each follow.

Transcription Equipment for the Physically Challenged

There are many adaptations for persons with a physical impairment, such as lower limb paralysis, blindness, and deafness. For example, foot pedals can be replaced with hand or voice-activated equipment for a person in a wheelchair or with lower limb impairment.

The blind and visually impaired can use video magnifiers that use high-powered lenses to enlarge copy. A device called a tactile converter allows the blind person to read printed material by placing one hand inside the converter holding a printed document and "reading" the material with the index finger resting on the transmitter plate.

Blind transcriptionists are able to proofread their material through the use of a voice synthesizer. A Braille-Edit program allows blind and sighted persons to work together using a microcomputer.

The deaf or hearing-impaired are able to use a telecommunication device for the deaf (TDD) that will place sound onto paper. They can then type it into the correct format for a medical record.

Transcribers

Medical transcribers are machines that allow the transcriptionist to take oral dictation and turn this into written material and documents. These typically have an audiocassette tape (onto which the physician or other health care worker has dictated information); headphones for private listening, a speed, volume, and tone control; and a foot pedal to free the hands for typing.

The cassette mechanism of transcription equipment has the ability to play, stop, rewind, and fast-forward the tape. However, the foot pedal is used for most playing and rewinding since it is faster (Procedure 9-1).

Word Processing

Word processing has made medical transcription more efficient. The word processor has the ability to create and maneuver text without having to cut and paste a paper document. The word processor also is able to save the document. This allows the typist to work on a document, save it, retrieve it at a later time, and work on it again. Corrections during the typing process can easily be made. For example, if a dictated word or phrase is not clear on the tape, the transcriptionist can leave a blank with a question mark, speak to the dictator (physician) about the word or phrase, and add the correct word or phrase before finishing the document.

Another advantage of the word processor over the typewriter is the ability to make multiple original copies of the document.

Voice Recognition Technology (VRT)

This new technology allows the physician to speak into a microphone connected to a computer program that translates the dictation into a typed report. VRT requires the physician to provide several samples of his or her speech by reading manufacturer-provided scripts to activate the program. Since this is a time consuming process, not too many physicians have adopted this system in their offices. However, it is used in some

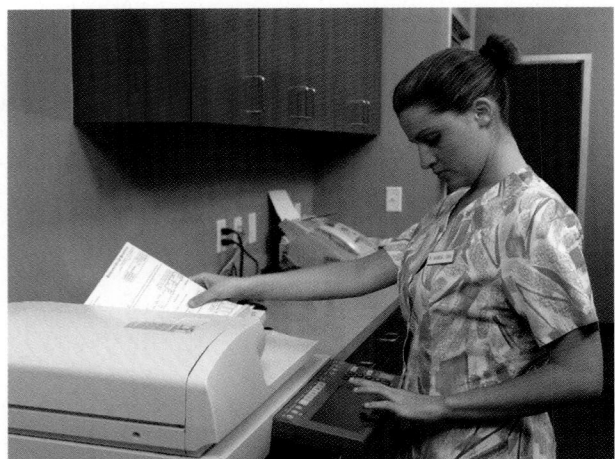

FIGURE 9-6 Copiers should meet the particular needs of the medical office.

PROCEDURE

Operating a Transcriber

OBJECTIVE: Understand basic information on how to operate a transcriber, which can produce a printed document of voice-recorded material.

Equipment and Supplies
transcriber; headset; computer; paper; printer; possibly a foot pedal

Method
1. Assure the transcriber and all ancillary equipment is turned on and is working.
2. Be sure to adjust the volume, tone, and speed controls to avoid any interruptions in the communication and transcription.

3. Listen for physician's instructions. The physician's instructions will guide the order of priority of reports and format.
4. Set all computer software formatting, such as margins, font, line spacing and indentation, and alignment.
5. Listen to the physician's recording and enter the information.
6. Complete, archive, and save all information according to the physician's procedures.

---

hospital medical records departments and as the equipment becomes more user-friendly, it will become more accessible.

Using a Postage Meter

Many offices use a postage meter that will automatically stamp large mailings. The postage can be printed directly onto an envelope with a meter. Postage can also be printed onto an adhesive backed strip that is placed directly onto a package. Metered mail does not have to be stamped when it arrives at the post office. The meter is taken into the post office for calibrating.

Purchasing Equipment

When a business determines the need for specific equipment, the purchase process begins. The medical assistant may be asked to research and compare equipment based on the manufacturer, quality, size, service, price, and other determining factors. The medical assistant can search the Internet, contact local vendors and other offices as part of the fact-gathering quest. Collecting information, printed materials, and resources will enable the physician to make the right choice when actually purchasing the equipment.

Warranties

A warranty is a guarantee in writing from the manufacturer that the product will perform correctly under normal conditions of use. The warranty provides for a replacement of defective parts at no charge within a certain period of time. An extended warranty can be purchased to cover the period of time after the warranty has expired. For example, a copier may have a one-year warranty, but an extended warranty can be purchased to cover parts replacement after that year has expired.

Some office equipment that is heavily used, such as a copy machine, has a service contract for preventive maintenance. A service contract provides maintenance and cleaning of equipment even when it is working properly to avoid a breakdown. A maintenance contract will state in detail what is actually covered by the contract. The dates and frequency of service should be noted carefully. Literature relating to warranties and preventative maintenance contracts should be kept in a designated file. Since office equipment is expensive these contracts are important.

Equipment Records

Records relating to office equipment need to be maintained. Receipts for major purchases, operating manuals, instructions, warranties, and repair and maintenance instructions need to be filed. Lists of service people with contact information should be maintained. Many offices maintain a current file of business cards representing the companies from which equipment has been purchased. Ideally, the registration and ID number of each item is maintained in a separate file from the warranty.

Remember to record any unusual occurrences of equipment in writing. Memory of what actually happened may fail over time. A written record of exactly what happened and the corrective action that was

TABLE 9-1 **Equipment Inventory Record**

Item	Serial #	Purchase Date	Location
Laptop	XX 12345	2/14/05	Reception
IBM Selectric II Typewriter	XC54321	2/14/05	Laboratory
IBM G40 Computer	4-190-L1001	9/19/05	Reception
Hewlett-Packard Color LaserJet Printer	JPHAC15531	9/19/05	Reception
Ricoh Copier	RC39C452	6/2/04	Billing

taken can assist in determining if something was an accident or negligence.

A list of inventory items should be kept in the procedure manual. Many inventory records are now maintained on the computer. Table 9-1 provides an example of an office inventory record.

Equipment Life and Safety

All equipment is purchased with the accompanying manufacturer's training manual to maintain the life of the machine and the safety of the user. The medical assistant should read all manuals prior to use and have the vendor provide training for the office staff. Usually, the retailer's training and manual will suggest using the equipment defaults and turning the equipment off when not in use. Training and manuals provide cleaning, maintenance and operation directions, and other important information. The suggestions usually place safety of the user first, longevity of the equipment second, and reordering or service information third. Either way, the staff should be familiar with and able to apply the general equipment features, defaults, and safety guidelines.

Legal and Ethical Issues

The medical assistant has a duty to report any incident such as equipment defects that may harm the employee. Working with inventory requires integrity. Office and medical supplies must not leave the medical office unless the physician orders them. Vendors and suppliers must be dealt with in an honest manner.

Supplies

Vendors, or suppliers, are selected based on several factors including: the quality, price, service, and availability that they provide. In general, it takes multiple vendors to provide all supplies for a medical practice. Catalog or online services can provide ease of availability, competitive pricing, and fast delivery. A wise purchaser will develop a good working relationship with vendors either in person, on the telephone, in writing, or online in preparation for negotiating a contract. Contracts or purchase agreements may include payment schedules, shipment times, product discounts, extended warranty, training sessions, and other incentives. Legal and Ethical Issues has more on equipment and supplies.

Many vendors will provide a discount on supplies when they are ordered in large quantities. This results in a unit cost savings. The drawback to this method is that many offices do not have enough storage space to handle a large inventory of supplies. Some suppliers will store excess inventory for you.

Supplies should be rotated on the shelves so that the newer supplies are in the back of the shelf and the older supplies are used first.

Expendable supplies and equipment include items that are used up in a short period of time and have a relatively inexpensive unit cost. Examples of expendable office supplies are found in Table 9-2.

Supply Inventory

Supply inventory control requires constant supervision since a medical office cannot afford to run out of supplies. Many supplies are purchased in large quantities at lower cost. It can be costly to run out and have to suddenly purchase supplies at full price with additional shipping costs for faster service.

Most offices maintain an ongoing inventory system that helps to determine when to reorder supplies. Whenever an item is removed from the supply cabinet

TABLE 9-2 Expendable Office Supplies

Paper supplies	Examination table paper, disposable gowns, drapes, paper towels, sterilization bags and tapes, stationery, photocopy paper, insurance and chart forms, laboratory order forms, appointment books, ECG paper, receipt book, appointment cards, current CPT and ICD-9 coding books.
Clinical equipment	Disposable speculums, ear and nose speculum covers, catheters, tongue blades, thermometers, cotton-tipped applicators, lubricant, needles, syringes, suture material, dressings, tape, elastic bandages, gloves, goggles.
Office Supplies	Pens, pencils, highlighters, copy paper, stapler(s), stapler removers, printer cartridge, CD-ROMs.

it is marked on the inventory sheet. A staff member is assigned the responsibility of reordering all supplies when items get to a certain level so that the supply is never totally depleted. The amount of time necessary to have the order processed and delivered should be factored in when reordering supplies. See Figure 9-7 for a sample inventory order form.

Order System

It takes experience to be able to calculate how long inventory items will last. However, records can be reviewed to determine when half the supply has been used. Then, by calculating the amount of time it takes to receive a new order, an estimate can be made when to place and how much to reorder. For example, if one printer cartridge is used in one month and there is a three-week reorder period, then a new order must be placed when half the supply has been used. Since print cartridges may be used more during a certain part of the billing periods, or when the office is busier, it would be advisable to reorder cartridges in advance to prevent running out of the supply.

Many offices use color-coded reorder reminder cards that are inserted into the stack of inventory items. As the color card comes to the top of the stack it is time to reorder. Inventory reminder cards can be maintained with a date for reorder.

Some suppliers maintain their own records and will notify the medical office when it is time to reorder. Remember to keep a list of inventory items in the procedure manual and maintain the inventory records on computer files. Some offices use an automated scanning system for inventory control and ordering system.

Drug Samples

Pharmaceutical representatives from the drug companies will often supply medical offices with samples of medications. Drug samples are small packages of a medication for distribution by the physician to the patients. An inventory list of all sample drugs should be maintained to adhere to HIPAA and in some cases, state regulations (check your local state).

Even though these drug samples are small and "free," the medical office must secure and organize the samples in a supply cupboard or drawer that is locked. It is advisable to keep all drugs together by category (for example, sedatives, antibiotics, hypertensive drugs). The expiration dates on drug samples have to be carefully monitored. All samples should be discarded in accordance with HIPAA and federal regulations when they have reached the manufactures expiration date.

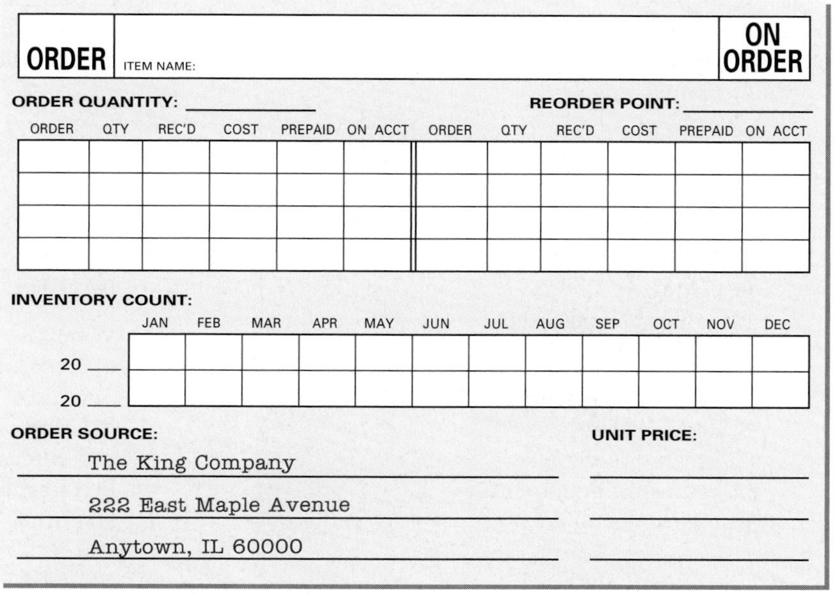
ORDER | ITEM NAME: | ON ORDER

ORDER QUANTITY: ______ REORDER POINT: ______

ORDER	QTY	REC'D	COST	PREPAID	ON ACCT	ORDER	QTY	REC'D	COST	PREPAID	ON ACCT

INVENTORY COUNT:

	JAN	FEB	MAR	APR	MAY	JUN	JUL	AUG	SEP	OCT	NOV	DEC
20 __												
20 __												

ORDER SOURCE: UNIT PRICE:

The King Company

222 East Maple Avenue

Anytown, IL 60000

FIGURE 9-7 Sample inventory order form.

SUMMARY

The office layout contributes to the physical atmosphere, organization and impression that patients and employees will encounter. An organized office layout can affect the office flow, and decrease patient cycle time, and positively impact employee morale and patients' attitudes.

The medical assistant will maintain an inventory list for all office equipment purchased, supplies, and drug samples. All staff members should be trained on the use and operation functions of the equipment.

Chapter Review

COMPETENCY REVIEW

1. Define and spell the terms to learn for this chapter.
2. Discuss how following the manufacturer's suggestions enhances equipment longevity.
3. Discuss the importance of patient flow.
4. Discuss how inventory control methods contribute to efficient office management.
5. Discuss the handling of pharmaceutical samples in the medical office.

PREPARING FOR THE CERTIFICATION EXAM

1. Expendable medical office equipment includes the following, EXCEPT
   A. paper supplies
   B. typewriter
   C. word processor
   D. computer printer
   E. fax machine

2. Which supplies are NOT expendable clinical equipment supplies?
   A. catheters
   B. syringes
   C. gloves
   D. gloves and goggles
   E. paper towels

3. Drug samples should be kept in a locked cabinet and organized by
   A. expiration date
   B. shipment date
   C. bottle color
   D. category
   E. alphabetical order

4. A fax machine is used primarily to
   A. copy documents
   B. transcribe
   C. scan documents
   D. transmit documents
   E. store documents

5. Equipment purchase agreements may include the following, EXCEPT
   A. training
   B. warranty
   C. service
   D. price
   E. office flow

6. Office flow includes
   A. furniture placement and current periodicals
   B. traffic flow and general eye appeal
   C. temperature and lighting
   D. ventilation and clearly marked hallways
   E. purchase agreements and warranties

7. At which temperature setting should a medical office be kept?
   A. 80° F
   B. 72° F
   C. 75° F
   D. 73° F
   E. 74° F

8. What two distinct areas are set up in a medical office facility?
   A. staff room and administration offices
   B. physicians office and clinical area
   C. clinical and administrative offices
   D. staff room and reception area
   E. office and traffic flow areas

continued on next page

9. Capital equipment includes the following, EXCEPT
   A. carpeting
   B. EKG machine
   C. refrigerator
   D. files
   E. typewriter

10. When working with vendors you should expect the following, EXCEPT
    A. unit pricing
    B. inventory count
    C. competitive pricing
    D. fast delivery
    E. quality assurance

CRITICAL THINKING

1. What is the first thing you would do to fix the situation after the office carpets were cleaned?

2. How do you function in the office? Based on your knowledge about physical hazards and office safety, what precautions should you take to resolve the problem?

3. What happens to patient flow in this situation?

ON THE JOB

Develop an inventory using an electronic spreadsheet of all equipment, machines, and supplies for the clinical and administrative areas. Include purchase date, maintenance schedule, and purchase price.

INTERNET ACTIVITY

Go to the Americans with Disabilities Act Web site (www.ada.gov) and research the standards for bathrooms in public places that accommodate wheelchairs.

MediaLink More on medical office facilities, equipment, and supplies, including interactive resources, can be found in the Student CD-ROM accompanying this textbook.

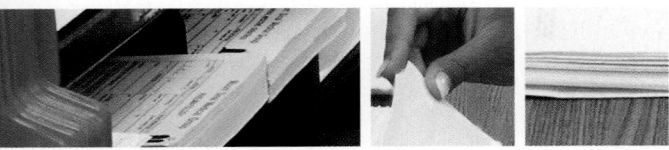

Medical Assistant Role Delineation Chart

HIGHLIGHT indicates material covered in this chapter.

ADMINISTRATIVE

Administrative Procedures

- Perform basic administrative medical assisting functions
- Schedule, coordinate and monitor appointments
- Schedule inpatient/outpatient admissions and procedures
- Understand and apply third-party guidelines
- Obtain reimbursement through accurate claims submission
- Monitor third-party reimbursement
- Understand and adhere to managed care policies and procedures
- *Negotiate managed care contracts*

Practice Finances

- Perform procedural and diagnostic coding
- Apply bookkeeping principles

- Manage accounts receivable
- *Manage accounts payable*
- *Process payroll*
- *Document and maintain accounting and banking records*
- *Develop and maintain fee schedules*
- *Manage renewals of business and professional insurance policies*
- *Manage personnel benefits and maintain records*
- *Perform marketing, financial, and strategic planning*

CLINICAL

Fundamental Principles

- Apply principles of aseptic technique and infection control
- Comply with quality assurance practices
- Screen and follow up patient test results

Diagnostic Orders

- Collect and process specimens
- Perform diagnostic tests

Patient Care

- Adhere to established patient screening procedures
- Obtain patient history and vital signs
- Prepare and maintain examination and treatment areas
- Prepare patient for examinations, procedures and treatments

- Assist with examinations, procedures and treatments
- Prepare and administer medications and immunizations
- Maintain medication and immunization records
- Recognize and respond to emergencies
- Coordinate patient care information with other health care providers
- Initiate IV and administer IV medications with appropriate training and as permitted by state law

GENERAL

Professionalism

- Display a professional manner and image
- Demonstrate initiative and responsibility
- Work as a member of the health care team
- Prioritize and perform multiple tasks
- Adapt to change
- Promote the CMA credential
- Enhance skills through continuing education
- Treat all patients with compassion and empathy
- Promote the practice through positive public relations

Communication Skills

- Recognize and respect cultural diversity
- Adapt communications to individual's ability to understand
- Use professional telephone technique

- Recognize and respond effectively to verbal, nonverbal, and written communications
- Use medical terminology appropriately
- Utilize electronic technology to receive, organize, prioritize and transmit information
- Serve as liaison

Legal Concepts

- Perform within legal and ethical boundaries
- Prepare and maintain medical records
- Document accurately
- Follow employer's established policies dealing with the health care contract
- Implement and maintain federal and state health care legislation and regulations
- Comply with established risk management and safety procedures
- Recognize professional credentialing criteria
- *Develop and maintain personnel, policy and procedure manuals*

Instruction

- Instruct individuals according to their needs
- Explain office policies and procedures
- Teach methods of health promotion and disease prevention
- Locate community resources and disseminate information
- *Develop educational materials*
- *Conduct continuing education activities*

Operational Functions

- Perform inventory of supplies and equipment
- Perform routine maintenance of administrative and clinical equipment
- Apply computer techniques to support office operations
- *Perform personnel management functions*
- *Negotiate leases and prices for equipment and supply contracts*

- *Denotes advanced skills.*

SOURCE: Reprinted by permission of the American Association of Medical Assistants from the AAMA Role Delineation Study: Occupational Analysis of the Medical Assisting Profession.

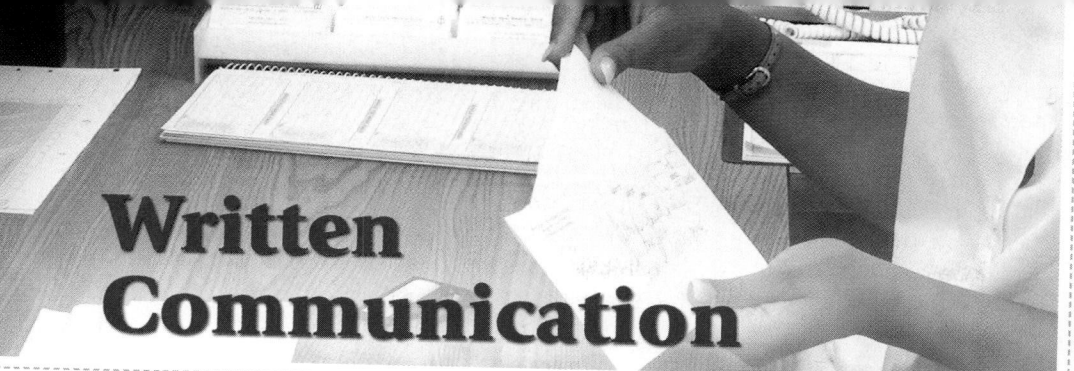

Written Communication

Learning Objectives

After completing this chapter, you should be able to:

- Define and spell the terms to learn for this chapter.
- Name and describe eight areas to consider when letter writing.
- Identify the eight parts of speech and use them correctly.
- Explain the process of proofreading and editing.
- Describe the process of drafting correspondence, using the four methods of letter styles.

- List and describe how to prepare an envelope to meet the standards of the U.S. Postal Service.
- State the four classifications of mail service.
- List and describe six special services offered by the U.S. Postal Service.
- Summarize the ethical implications related to written correspondence.
- Define an instant message and identify its purpose.

OUTLINE

Letter Writing	172
Word Choice	172
Composing Letters	174
Letter Styles	180
Interoffice Memoranda	181
Proofreading	181
Editing	181
Abbreviations	183
Reference Materials	183
Preparing Outgoing Mail	183
Classifications of Mail	185
Size Requirements for Mail	187
Mail Handling Tips	187
Electronic Mail (E-mail)	187
Reflection on the Medical Practice	189

Terms to Learn

active voice	homophones	proofreading
block	modified block	redundant
gender bias	passive voice	thesaurus

Case Study

THE STUDENT IN YOUR EXTERNSHIP PROGRAM has been asked by the physician to write a letter to refer a patient to another physician for a second opinion. The student writes the letter and asks you, the medical assistant, to review it. You find many spelling and grammatical errors and address these issues with the student. Following is the letter written by the extern:

Dear Dr Johnson

I am referring a patient to your office for further evaluation. I have been seeing this patient for several years now for right metatarsal injury. It is in my opinion that this patient should seek additional information on having the right metatarsal removed. This patient has been in my office on several occasions unable to walk with much swelling.

I trust your medical opinion and would appreciate you advising the proper action to take for this patient. For your review I have enclosed past x-rays, please feel free to contact my office as soon as possible.

Sincerely,
Dr. J. Ancella

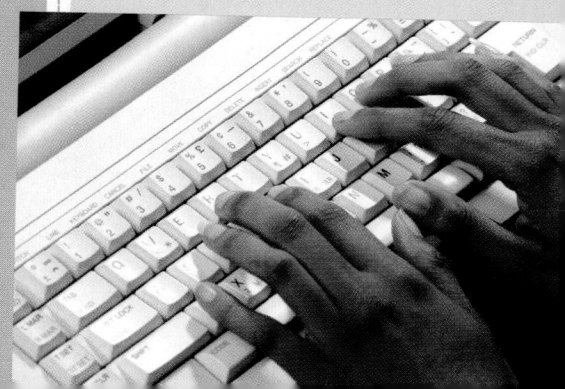

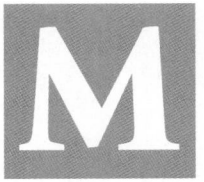

Medical assistants draft many types of correspondence to be signed by the physician/employer. These letters must reflect the professionalism of the medical practice. The physical appearance of letters depends on the quality of paper, letterhead design, and the choice of formats for the letters. However, even the most professional-looking correspondence is quickly and harshly judged when the letter is written in a negative or condescending tone, or is filled with grammatical errors. Correspondence should be positive in tone and well written.

Handling incoming mail requires efficiency in sorting, dating, and reading all correspondence. Correct handling of the mail can save money and time for the medical practice. Initiative in handling mail quickly and accurately is paramount.

Letter Writing

Letters from a medical office must be professional, courteous, business like, project a positive tone, and protect the confidentiality of the physician and the patient. This requires some diplomacy. For example, when drafting a sensitive letter requesting payment for a long overdue bill or to advise a patient to seek the services of another physician, such letters should be clear and to the point. The situation should be explained and the expected outcome presented—"Please send a check for (amount due)" or "Please call to make payment arrangements." Threats or derogatory comments are never acceptable in professional correspondence and may have legal consequences for the sender (Legal and Ethical Issues). The following letters are examples of positive and negative tones in writing.

Negative Example:

Dear Mrs. Murray:
You have repeatedly failed to take medications as prescribed and follow my recommended treatment. Since you have again failed to keep an appointment, I am forced to withdraw as your physician, and I request that you find another physician immediately.

Positive Example:

Dear Mrs. Murray:
During your last visit, we discussed the necessity of continuing medical treatment for you to recover fully from your recent medical problems. Therefore, I am concerned that you failed to keep your appointment this week and have not called the office to schedule a new appointment. Your health continues to be important to me, so I am requesting that you call me as soon as possible to discuss future treatment.

Legal and Ethical Issues

The medical assistant must carefully monitor all dated material to assure that replies are made on a timely basis. Confidential mail and correspondence including checks and payments are handled on a regular basis. This is a grave responsibility. Since the U.S. Postal Services is regulated by the federal government, any tampering or deliberate mishandling of mail is a federal offense.

A non-threatening tone of correspondence can promote the medical profession to the reader. Any attempts to threaten a patient in writing can lead to charges of harassment. Courteous language, presented in a diplomatic manner, can result in compliance and prevent a lawsuit.

An error in correspondence may not be caught by the physician before he or she signs the document. The medical assistant must carefully proofread all correspondence before it leaves the office to protect the physician from legal problems.

If we are unable to reach a mutual understanding about your medical treatment and appointment schedule, I regret that I will not be able to continue as your physician. In that event, you will receive a letter indicating that you have a month's notice in which to secure the services of another physician.

Word Choice

The use of correct words when writing office correspondence includes avoidance of the use of technical terms, gender bias (indicating either male or female by type of language used), long sentences and paragraphs, excessive use of the personal pronoun *I*, repetition, and the passive voice.

Technical Terminology

When writing a letter to medical professionals or institutions that employ medically trained staff, the use of correct medical terminology is essential. This terminology is specialized and is easily understood by medically trained professionals. Many patients are not familiar with medical terminology and, in fact, may not understand or may be intimidated by this style of writing. Table 10-1 lists selected medical terms with corresponding synonyms. The medical terms in the left-hand column are appropriate for medically trained personnel

TABLE 10-1 Medical Terms and Corresponding Synonyms

Medical Term	Synonym
Carcinoma	Cancer
Cardiac	Heart
Dermatitis	Skin irritation
Diabetes mellitus	Diabetes
Gastric	Stomach
Gynecology	Study of female diseases
Hepatic disease	Liver disease
Hyperglycemic	Excessive blood sugar
Hypertension	High blood pressure
Larynx	Voice box
Leukocytes	White blood cells
MI	Myocardial infarction
Nephroses	Kidney disease
NPO	Nothing by mouth
Otolaryngology	Study of ear and throat
Para I	First delivery
Pc	After meals
Thrombus	Blood clot

correspondence (physician to physician, physician to the medical record, medical assistant to hospital); the terms in the right-hand column are more easily understood by patients. The use and explanation of terminology in correspondence and other medical office printed matter as well as the facilitating of patient understanding with these materials is discussed in Patient Education.

Removing Gender Bias

Unfortunately it is quite common in the medical field to assume that every nurse is female and all physicians are male since this was the case many generations ago. Because this is no longer the case, gender-neutral terms are preferred. This means that any reference to a particular gender (male or female) should be eliminated. For example, a male orderly should be referred to as a medical attendant, and cleaning ladies are called housekeepers or cleaning personnel.

Written correspondence must also reflect this same neutral bias toward the genders. When writing about physicians, do not refer to them as males or nurses and medical assistants as females. For example, "The patient was referred to a hospital dietitian for diabetic diet instruction. The patient was told to ask her about a food exchange list." This wording assumes the dietitian is a female. A better statement would be, "The patient was instructed to ask the dietitian about a food exchange list." In order to write in a gender-neutral style, you may have to rewrite the sentence and choose alternate words or phrases.

Sentence and Paragraph Length

Short, concise sentences and paragraphs are preferred in medical writing. Sentence length should never exceed twenty words. Eliminate all words that are unnecessary. The paragraph should only cover one point. A good paragraph contains from two to six sentences. Your reader may stop reading if the paragraph is too long.

Patient Education

Many patient education materials used in the medical office are prepared and distributed in printed form. They include pamphlets, brochures, and letters of instructions. In many cases, the information will have to be interpreted for the patients who have language barriers, difficulty with vision, reading, or understanding medical information. This is an excellent opportunity to provide additional patient teaching. By asking the patient to repeat some of the material that has been explained, you can test the patient's understanding and comprehension.

When advising patients about correspondence, they should be cautioned about sending cash in the mail. Payments should always be made by check or money order when using the mail.

Personal Pronoun

Whenever possible, it is preferable to avoid the use of the personal pronoun *I* in professional writing. It is better to use *you* since this involves the reader. For example, a message such as, "I am asking that any overdue balance be cleared up immediately. I will have to take steps to send this account to a collection agency if it is not paid immediately," is negative. When requesting a patient to pay an overdue bill, it is better to write, "We know that you will want to clear up any overdue account. This overdue balance may have been an oversight on your part. If that is the case, would you kindly remit your payment in the enclosed envelope."

Repetition, Redundancy, and Inflated Phrases

The reader of your correspondence wants to know in concise terms what you are telling them. Avoid being redundant—repeating the same statement over again. Redundant expressions include such terms as *each and every*, *first and foremost*, and *physician's patient*. The above examples can be simplified by stating *each*, *first*, or *the patient*.

Inflated phrases can usually be eliminated without any loss of meaning. Common examples are introductory word groups such as *in my opinion*, *I think that*, *it seems that*, *one must*, and so on. Table 10-2 contains examples of inflated patterns of writing versus concise terms.

Active Versus Passive Voice

The active verbs can make writing more interesting. In the active voice, the subject of the sentence does the action; in the passive voice, the subject receives the action. Although both voices are grammatically correct, the active voice is considered more effective because it is simpler, more direct, and less wordy.

To transform a sentence from the passive to active voice, make the actor the subject of the sentence. Table 10-3 contains examples of statements in both active and passive voice.

Composing Letters

Composing letters can be a simple process when an organized approach is used. Use the guidelines presented in this chapter. The most import element in an organized letter writing approach is to get to the point quickly.

TABLE 10-2 Inflated Phrases Versus Concise Terms

Inflated	Concise
Along the lines of	Like
As a matter of fact	In fact
At all times	Always
At the present time	Now, currently
At this point in time	Now, currently
Because of the fact that	Because
By means of	By
By virtue of the fact that	Because
Due to the fact that	Because
For the purpose of	For
For the reason that	Because
Have the ability to	Be able to
In light of the fact that	Because
In the nature of	Like
In order to	To
In spite of the fact that	Although, though
In the event that	If
In the final analysis	Finally
In the neighborhood of	About
Until such time as	Until

TABLE 10-3 Active Versus Passive Voice

Active	Passive
The medical assistant took the patient's blood pressure measurement	The patient's blood pressure measurement was taken by the medical assistant.
The surgeon performed an appendectomy on the patient.	An appendectomy was performed on the patient by the surgeon.
The medical committee reached a decision.	A decision was reached by the medical committee.

TABLE 10-4 Common Homophones

Word	Meaning	Word	Meaning
accept	to receive	lose	to be deprived of
except	to take or leave out	pair	set of two
advice	opinion about what to do for a problem	pare	to trim
advise	to offer advice	pear	fruit
affect	to exert an influence	patience	calm endurance
effect	result; accomplishment	patients	a doctor's clients
all ready	prepared	personal	private; intimate
already	by this time	personnel	a group of employees
altar	a structure on which religious ceremonies are held	precede	to come before
alter	to change	proceed	to go forward
always	every time; forever	quiet	silent; calm
all ways	every way	quite	very
bare	naked	right	proper or just; correct
bear	to carry; to put up with	rite	a ritual
brake	something used to stop movement, to stop	write	to put words on paper
break	to split or smash	stationary	standing still
buy	to purchase	stationery	writing paper
by	near	taught	past tense of *teach*
choose	to select	taut	tight
chose	past tense of *choose*	than	besides
cite	to quote	then	at that time; next
sight	vision	their	belonging to them
site	position, place	they're	contraction of *they are*
complement	to complete	there	that place or position
compliment	praise	through	by means of; finished
conscience	sense of right and wrong	threw	past tense of *throw*
conscious	awake; aware	thorough	careful; complete
elicit	to draw or bring out	to	toward
illicit	illegal	too	also
fair	lovely; light-colored	two	one or more in number
fare	money for transportation, food or drink	waist	midsection
hear	to sense by the ear	waste	to squander
here	this place	weak	feeble
hole	hollow place	week	seven days
whole	entire; unhurt	weather	state of the atmosphere
its	of or belonging to it	whether	indicating a choice between alternatives
it's	contraction for *it is*	who's	contraction of *who is*
know	to be aware of	whose	possessive of *who*
no	opposite of yes	your	possessive of *you*
lessen	to make less	you're	contraction of *you are*
lesson	something learned		
loose	free; not secured		

Spelling

There are several words in the English language that have similar pronunciations but very different meanings and spellings. These words are called homophones. They pose problems unless the writer is careful about their usage. Table 10-4 contains some of the most common homophones.

Computer software programs cannot be depended upon to correct word use since they do not "understand" the data input or content of the correspondence. For example, use of the word *effect* or *affect* depends on the content and cannot be determined by the software program. Both spellings are correct and only the individual using the word in the sentence would be able to determine if the word is the correct choice. See Table 10-5 for examples of the most commonly misspelled medical terms. General rules for capitalization are given in Box 10-1.

Plurals

Following are some basic rules for forming plurals of words:

- Abbreviations are formed into plurals by adding an *s* (ECGs, DRGs).

TABLE 10-5 Commonly Misspelled Medical Terms

abscess	epistaxis	neuron	pneumonia
additive	eustachian	occlusion	polyp
aerosol	fissure	oscilloscope	prophylaxis
agglutination	glaucoma	osseous	prostate
albumin	gonorrhea	palliative	prosthesis
anastomosis	hemorrhage	parasite	pruritis
aneurysm	hemorrhoids	parenteral	psoriasis
anteflexion	homeostasis	parietal	pyrexia
arrhythmia	humerus	paroxysmal	respiratory
bilirubin	idiosyncrasy	pemphigus	roentgenology
bronchial	ileum	percussion	sagittal
calcaneus	ilium	perforation	sciatica
capillary	infarction	pericardium	serous
cervical	intussusception	perineum	sphincter
chromosome	ischemia	peristalsis	sphygmomanometer
cirrhosis	ischium	peritoneum	squamous
clavicle	larynx	petit mal	staphylococcus
curettage	leukemia	pharynx	suppuration
cyanosis	malaise	pituitary	trochanter
defibrillator	malleus	plantar	venous
ecchymosis	mellitus	pleura	wheal
effusion	menstruation	pleurisy	xiphoid
epididymis	metastasis		

BOX 10-1
Rules for Capitalization

First word of
- Sentences
- Expressions used as sentences
- Each item in a list or outline
- Salutation and closing of a letter

Proper name of person, place, or thing
- John F. Kennedy
- New York City
- Sears Tower

Noun that is part of a proper name
- Professor Mary King
- Dr. Beth Williams
- Michigan Avenue

- Plurals of nouns are formed by adding an *s* or an *es* (physicians, suffixes).

Basic rules for forming plurals of medical terms with specific endings are listed in Table 10-6 along with examples for each.

Numbers

In general, the numbers 1 to 10 are spelled out —one to ten— in correspondence. For numbers greater than ten, it is acceptable to use the number designation, as in

TABLE 10-6 Rules for Forming Plurals of Medical Terms (nouns)

Ending	Rule	Example
a	ae	vertebra to vertebrae
ax	aces	thorax to thoraces
ex, ix	ices	apex to apices
is	es	metastasis to metastases
on	a	ganglion to ganglia
um	a	ovum to ova
us	i	nucleus to nuclei
y	ies	biopsy to biopsies
nx	ges	phalanx to phalanges

TABLE 10-7 Use of Numbers in Correspondence

Type	Explanation of When to Use
Decimals	Write using figure without commas (23.04).
Figures	Only numbers (including 1–10) are used in tables, statistical data, dates, money, percentages, and time.
Measurements	Write out in figures (23 inches).
Percentages	Write out in figures and spell out percent (20 percent).
Tables	When typing numbers or placing them in columns align as follows: - Arabic numerals (1, 2, 3) aligned on the right. - Decimals (1.33) are aligned on the decimal. - Roman numerals (I, II, III) are aligned on the left.
Time	Do not use zeros when writing on-the-hour time. Use A.M. and P.M. with the time designation (10 A.M., not 10:00 A.M.).

128, 1020, 32. The only exception to this rule is when the number is at the beginning of a sentence. It should then be spelled out. See Table 10-7 for a further description of the use of numbers in correspondence.

Parts of Speech

Traditional grammar recognizes eight parts of speech: noun, pronoun, verb, adjective, adverb, preposition, conjunction, and interjection. Many words are able to function as more than one part of speech. For example, depending on its use in a sentence, the word *cut* can be a noun, as in "The cut is fresh," or a verb, as in "The surgeon cut into the organ." Table 10-8 provides a quick reference to parts of speech.

Error Correction in Office Correspondence

Word processing has made correspondence correction much easier. Word processing allows the writer to display the document on the computer screen, enter the

TABLE 10-8 **Eight Parts of Speech**

Part of Speech	Definition
Noun	Names a person, place, or thing. Example: medical assistant, office
Pronoun	Substitutes for a noun. Example: I, me, you, he, him, she, her, it, we, us, they, them
Verb	Helping verb: comes before main verb. Main verb: asserts action, being, or state of being. Example: operate, write, speak, obtain, is, are, am
Adjective	Modifies a noun or pronoun, usually answering the questions: Which one? What kind of? How many? Example: responsible medical assistant
Adverb	Modifies a verb, adjective, or adverb usually answering the questions: When? Where? Why? How? Under what conditions? To what degree? Example: gently, extremely, nicely, quietly
Preposition	Indicates the relationship between the noun and pronoun that follows it and another word in the sentence. Example: about, above, after, for, in, on, over, through
Conjunction	Connects words or word groups. Example: and, but, nor, or
Interjection	Word used to express strong feeling. Example: oh, hurrah, ouch

FIGURE 10-1 Different letterhead stationery and envelopes.

document, and make changes. This new document is then saved and printed.

Corrections made to letters typed on a typewriter require the use of correction ribbons, tapes, or fluids. Any corrections on correspondence should be inconspicuous. If more than a few words need correction, then the entire document needs to be retyped. It is considered unprofessional for a document to have correction fluid apparent on the document.

Standard Components of the Business Letter

All letters contain the same basic parts, starting at the top of a letter and moving down to the end. These include the heading, date, inside address, salutation, body, closing, and reference initials. In some specialized cases, such as with insurance correspondence, there may be special components added for clarification, such as the insurer's identification number.

Heading

Medical office letters are usually typed on letterhead stationery bearing the name of the physician (Beth Williams, MD) or practice (Windy City Clinic), address, telephone number, and fax number. See Figure 10-1 for an illustration of letterhead stationery. If the physician does not use letterhead stationery, the letter should be typed or printed on good quality bond paper with the return address typed above the date on the upper left side of the paper.

Date

Every correspondence must have a current date. The month must not be abbreviated, and is followed by the day and year (January 1, 2005). The date is usually placed three lines (spaces) below the letterhead or on line 15 if there is no letterhead. Four to six lines (spaces) are left after the date before the inside address.

Inside Address

The inside address contains the name, title, company name (if applicable), and address of the person who is to receive the correspondence. This is typed at the left margin and single-spaced. If there is a company name (for example, medical practice, clinic, hospital) it must be typed exactly as shown on the company's own letterhead.

All words in the inside address (such as the street name) are spelled out fully. The name of the city is followed by a comma; the two-letter state abbreviation is followed by two spaces; then the ZIP code is added. If the inside address contains a long line, it may be divided into two lines so that the inside address is in balance. The second of these two lines would be indented two spaces. See the example below.

Marvin Hammer, MD
123 Bonneymeadow
  Plaza in the Park
Chicago, IL 60610

Business courtesy recommends always including a title with the receiver's name on the inside address.

Salutation

The salutation, a courteous greeting, is typed at the left margin and spaced two lines below the inside address. The name in the salutation must agree with the name in the inside address. If the letter is going to a physician named Williams, the salutation would read, "Dear Dr. Williams:" with a colon placed after this type of salutation. If the person is well known to the writer, the first name is often used, for example "Dear Beth," followed by a comma. Guidelines 10-1 provides information on using courtesy titles in correspondence.

Body

The body contains the purpose of the letter. The body begins two spaces below the salutation and is single spaced, with a double space between each paragraph. The paragraphs of the body are either blocked or indented, depending on the style (format) of the letter. A letter may be any length, however, most letters bearing a single message are usually two to three paragraphs in length and confined to a single page.

Closing

The letter closing consists of a complimentary close containing a courtesy word(s), such as "Sincerely," "Sincerely yours," or "Yours truly." This appears two spaces below the end of the body of the letter.

The signature line is typed four spaces below the complimentary close and contains the name and title of the writer. The signature of the writer must be placed on the letter directly above the typed signature line before it is sent. If the name and title are on the same line, they are divided with a comma. The personal title of the writer (such as Mr. and Ms.) is not included in the signature line. The exception to this is when the writer may wish to indicate his or her gender to prevent the reader from being confused (for example, Ms. Leslie Lapointe or Mr. Pat Timmons).

Reference Initials

The medical professional uses reference initials to indicate who keyed the letter. Reference initials, when used, are placed at the lower left margin in lowercase, for example *bff*.

Enclosure Notation

When other documents are included along with the letter a notation is made on the letter indicating the enclosure. Examples of enclosures are x-ray films, medical records, and brochures. The abbreviation ENC. is used or the word "Enclosures" can be written out.

For example:

Enclosures (2)
x-ray lumbar spine
surgical report 12/10/20xx

10-1 GUIDELINES

Using Courtesy Titles

- *Mr.* is always an appropriate title for men.
- If there is a professional title, such as *MD* or *PhD,* this is used instead of the courtesy title.
- *Ms.* is used when the marital status of a woman is unknown.
- *Mrs.* is appropriate for a married woman if she prefers that title. However it is always safe to use *Ms.*
- *Miss* is appropriate for unmarried women who prefer that title. It is also used for young girls.
- Two people at the same address with different last names should be addressed individually. For example: Dr. Beth Williams and Mr. Allan Radde.
- A professional title, such as *owner, president, manager,* may be placed next to the name or below it depending on which is a better balance.

Allan Radde, President   Dinesh Shey, PhD
Radde and Associates   Department Chair

- If there is no record of the correct spelling of a receiver's name, then call the company or office and ask for the correct spelling.

Copy Notation

A copy of all correspondence is always filed in the office. In some cases, a copy of the letter is sent to someone other than the addressee. This is noted at the bottom left of the letter by typing the initial "c:" before the recipient's name. The title of the recipient is often added.

For example:

c: Jane Paulson, Office Manager

Procedure 10-1 lists important guidelines for composing business letters.

Two-Page Letter

When the letter is too long to fit on one page, a second sheet of plain stationery is used. Letterhead stationery is used only for the top sheet. The plain, bond second sheet should be of the same quality and color as the top letterhead stationery. A margin of one inch is left at the bottom of the first page.

Form Letters

Form letters can save time for the medical assistant. A form letter is developed when the same letter is sent to several different people. Figure 10-2 illustrates an example of a form letter that can be used as a base when constructing a letter of withdrawal. The letter would be personalized with the patient's name and the signature of the physician.

Composing a Business Letter

OBJECTIVE: Compose a business letter using proper guidelines.

Equipment and Supplies
computer or typewriter; office stationery

Method

1. Gather all necessary information and supplies.
2. Determine the reason for the correspondence. Write down the main purpose of the letter.
3. Make a list of all the points you will cover in the letter. Prepare a rough draft.
4. Arrange the ideas in a logical manner. Make sure the letter has a beginning, middle, and end.
   - The beginning or introduction should be appropriate for the intended reader. Use appropriate greetings and titles.
   - The middle should contain all the supporting facts and details. Make sure the content relates to the purpose of the letter.
   - The end should be brief, pleasant, and indicate any action that is to be taken by the reader or writer.
5. Use a natural style of writing; avoid pretentious language. Avoid medical terms when writing to the layperson. Also avoid inflated phrases (refer to Table 10-2).
6. Use a positive tone—negative writing should always be avoided.
7. Pay particular attention to spelling, punctuation, and grammar.
8. Once the rough draft is satisfactory, compose the final draft of the letter. Proofread for mistakes.
9. Obtain any necessary signatures. Include any enclosures as indicated.

WINDY CITY CLINIC
Beth Williams, M.D.
123 Michigan Avenue
Chicago, IL 60610
(312) 123-1234

Date

Dear (Patient):

I find it necessary to inform you that I am withdrawing from providing you medical care for the following reason(s): _____

_____

_____

Since your condition requires medical attention, I suggest that you place yourself under the care of another physician. If you do not know of other physicians, you may wish to contact the county medical society for a referral.

I shall be available to attend to you for a reasonable time after you have received this letter, but in no event for more than 15 days.

When you have selected a new physician, I would be pleased to make available to him or her a copy of your medical chart or a summary of your treatment.

Sincerely yours,

Beth Williams, M.D.

FIGURE 10-2 A form letter is a type of letter that is sent repeatedly to many patients.

The use of a computer or a word processor with memory individualizes the form letter. The body of the letter, called the constant information, is retained in the computer's memory or on a computer disk or CD. The areas of the letter that require personalization, such as the date, inside address, and salutation, are called the *variables*. The variables can be stored on a separate CD or database and then merged into the disk or main drive of the computer, which stores the constant information. In this manner, a set of data, such as names and addresses of patients for billing purposes, can be used with a form letter enclosed with the monthly bill. Chapter 11 contains more information regarding the use of computers in the medical office.

Letter Styles

Letter styles vary depending on the purpose. Letter styles include block, modified block (standard), modified block with indented paragraphs, and a simplified letter style. Block and modified block are the most commonly used in the medical office.

The block letter style format is spaced with all lines, from the date through the signature line, flush with the left margin. There is a space separating each paragraph and between inside address, salutation, body, and close. Since there are no indentations for paragraphs, this format saves typing time.

The modified block (standard) style letter has the date, complimentary closing, and the signature line beginning at the center and moving toward the right margin. All other lines are flush with the left margin. This is often preferred since it has a professional, neat appearance. This format requires more time to type since the typist must set and use tabs. The modified block style letter with indented paragraphs is identical to the modified block except that the paragraphs are indented five spaces.

A simplified letter style format is spaced with all lines flush with the left margin. The salutation line is omitted. In its place is a subject line, which appears on the third line below the inside address. This subject line is in capital letters and draws the reader's attention to the purpose of the letter. A complimentary closing is also omitted. The signature is also typed in all capital letters on the fifth line below the body. This format is an abbreviated style of writing letters relating to patients. Figure 10-3 shows sample letter formats: block, modified block (standard), modified block with indented paragraphs, and simplified letter style.

A semi-simplified letter style format is spaced with all lines flush with the left margin except for the first line of each paragraph. The first line of each paragraph is indented five spaces. All other aspects of the simplified letter style format apply to this format.

Interoffice Memoranda

Interoffice memoranda, also called *memos*, are correspondence sent to people within the office or organization. They are used to inform personnel about meetings, general changes that affect everyone, special projects, or news items. The memo is an inexpensive means to communicate with others in the office setting. They do not require postage and are delivered through the interoffice mail route.

Memos are generally written on a short form developed for that purpose. Memos may contain a heading much like the letterhead stationery to indicate the office where they originated. They contain the word MEMORANDUM at the top of the form. Also included are the typed words DATE:, TO:, FROM:, and RE: or SUBJECT:. The memo form is meant to be used within the office setting and should never be used to send information outside of the office. Figure 10-4 illustrates an example of a memo form.

Proofreading

Proofreading or checking for errors in content and typing is critical. The professionalism of the office is judged, in part, by the appearance of correspondence

---

| 10-2 | **GUIDELINES** |

Proofreading

- Proofread and correct errors before printing the document, whenever possible.
- Use a ruler, pencil, or edge of a piece of paper to follow each line as you proofread.
- Check the content to see if it flows in a logical order.
- Check for missing and repeated words.
- Check grammar, spelling, and punctuation.
- Check where the word breaks occur.
- Verify the spelling of proper names and titles.
- Verify numbers in dates, figures, and time (hours of the day).
- Read the opening and closing carefully.
- Proofread at least twice.
- Check the general appearance of the letter for spacing and format.

---

and documents that come out of that office. Proofreading cannot be overemphasized. Even small omissions, such as commas, are noticed by readers. Most computer programs contain spelling and grammar check components. These should always be used before printing the document. You may have to add frequently used medical terms to the program. After printing out the document, there should be a careful reading of all correspondence to catch any content or typing errors. Pay close attention to the spelling of names and procedures. When typing figures always double-check to make sure all decimal points are placed in the correct position. Look for sound-alike terms, such as *right* and *write* or *anti-* and *ante-*. Important points to remember when proofreading letters and other documents are listed in Guidelines 10-2.

Proofreader's Marks

There are marks that are generally accepted for use when proofreading large documents. These are especially helpful when a second person is proofing the document, such as the physician. See Figure 10-5 for a list of proofreader's marks.

Editing

Editing is similar to proofreading in that you must read the final material to check for accuracy. Editing also involves reading the printed material to determine if it is clear. When editing medical reports, you cannot change the content of the report or alter the meaning in

(A)

WINDY CITY CLINIC
Beth Williams, M.D.
123 Michigan Avenue, Chicago, IL 60610
(312) 123-1234

August 1, 20xx

Thomas Moore
123 Lee Street
Louisville, KY 40223

Dear Mr. Moore:

With the season for colds and flu fast approaching, it is time once again for flu shots. Supplies have arrived and flu shots will be administered starting October 3. Please call the office to schedule a visit for your flu shot at your earliest convenience.

If you wish to wait to get your flu shot at the time of your next appointment, it is not necessary to call the office. An appointment card with the date and time of your next appointment is enclosed.

Sincerely,

Beth Williams, MD

ENC: Appointment card
c: B. Reed, Office Manager

(B)

WINDY CITY CLINIC
Beth Williams, M.D.
123 Michigan Avenue, Chicago, IL 60610
(312) 123-1234

August 1, 20xx

Thomas Moore
123 Lee Street
Louisville, KY 40223

Dear Mr. Moore:

With the season for colds and flu fast approaching, it is time once again for flu shots. Supplies have arrived and flu shots will be administered starting October 3. Please call the office to schedule a visit for your flu shot at your earliest convenience.

If you wish to wait to get your flu shot at the time of your next appointment, it is not necessary to call the office. An appointment card with the date and time of your next appointment is enclosed.

Sincerely,

Beth Williams, MD

ENC: Appointment card
c: B. Reed, Office Manager

(C)

WINDY CITY CLINIC
Beth Williams, M.D.
123 Michigan Avenue, Chicago, IL 60610
(312) 123-1234

August 1, 20xx

Thomas Moore
123 Lee Street
Louisville, KY 40223

Dear Mr. Moore:

With the season for colds and flu fast approaching, it is time once again for flu shots. Supplies have arrived and flu shots will be administered starting October 3. Please call the office to schedule a visit for your flu shot at your earliest convenience.

If you wish to wait to get your flu shot at the time of your next appointment, it is not necessary to call the office. An appointment card with the date and time of your next appointment is enclosed.

Sincerely,

Beth Williams, MD

ENC: Appointment card
c: B. Reed, Office Manager

(D)

WINDY CITY CLINIC
Beth Williams, M.D.
123 Michigan Avenue, Chicago, IL 60610
(312) 123-1234

August 1, 20xx

Thomas Moore
123 Lee Street
Louisville, KY 40223

RE: FLU SHOT

With the season for colds and flu fast approaching, it is time once again for flu shots. Supplies have arrived and flu shots will be administered starting October 3. Please call the office to schedule a visit for your flu shot at your earliest convenience.

If you wish to wait to get your flu shot at the time of your next appointment, it is not necessary to call the office. An appointment card with the date and time of your next appointment is enclosed.

BETH WILLIAMS, M.D.

ENC: Appointment card
c: B. Reed, Office Manager

FIGURE 10-3 Examples of four letter formats: (A) block style; (B) modified block style; (C) modified block style with indented paragraphs; and (D) simplified letter style.

```
            WINDY CITY MEDICAL CENTER
                  MEMORANDUM
      DATE:

         TO:

      FROM:

   SUBJECT:


      c:
```

FIGURE 10-4 An example of a memo form.

any way. If you believe the meaning is unclear, you must check with the writer of the report before making any editorial changes.

When editing material you have composed, such as an informational form letter to be sent to all patients, changes can be made to increase clarity.

Abbreviations

Only accepted medical abbreviations can be used in medical reports and when filing insurance documents. A list of accepted medical abbreviations is included in the appendix of this textbook.

Individual physician offices may use an abbreviation on progress notes that is related to that practice. For example, a urologist may write "L," meaning leaking urine when coughing, on his or her progress notes. While this is not an acceptable abbreviation, it can be used to conserve space and simplify documentation within that particular office. It is important that a list of those abbreviations is shared with each employee and physically posted so that all employees are clear on the meaning of each abbreviation and are using the same abbreviation for the same term.

Reference Materials

Every physician's office contains general reference books and medical dictionaries as well as textbooks related to the physician's specialization. A complete office library should include the following:

- A desk dictionary, and access to an online dictionary.
- A medical dictionary, as well as access to an online medical dictionary, assists with the correct spelling, pronunciation, acronyms, abbreviations and meaning of medical terms and diagnoses.
- A Physician's Desk Reference (PDR) to verify the correct spelling and meaning of drugs.
- Current coding books including CPT (Current Procedural Terminology), ICD-9-CM.
- A thesaurus (which provides synonyms or similar meanings for words) such as Roget's International Thesaurus and access to an online thesaurus.

Preparing Outgoing Mail

Letterhead stationery, which contains the name and address of the sender, comes in three commonly used sizes. These sizes are standard, monarch or executive, and baronial. The more common letter sizes with their matching envelope sizes are shown in Table 10-9.

The standard letterhead is used for most office correspondence. A smaller version of the standard letterhead—the monarch or executive style—is used by some physicians for their social correspondence. The baronial letterhead is a half-sheet of the standard size and is used for brief letters and memoranda. Each size of letterhead stationery has an appropriate size envelope. See Figure 10-6 for an illustration of different letter sizes.

Folding Letters and Inserting into Envelopes

Following are recommended methods for folding and inserting letters into envelopes so the contents can

TABLE 10-9 Stationery and Envelopes

Stationery	Dimensions	Envelope	Dimensions
Standard	8 1/2″ × 11″	No. 10	9 1/2″ × 4 1/8″
Monarch	7 1/4″ × 10 1/2″	No. 7	7 1/2″ × 3 7/8″
Baronial	5 1/2″ × 8 1/2	No. 6 3/4	6 1/2″ × 3 5/8″

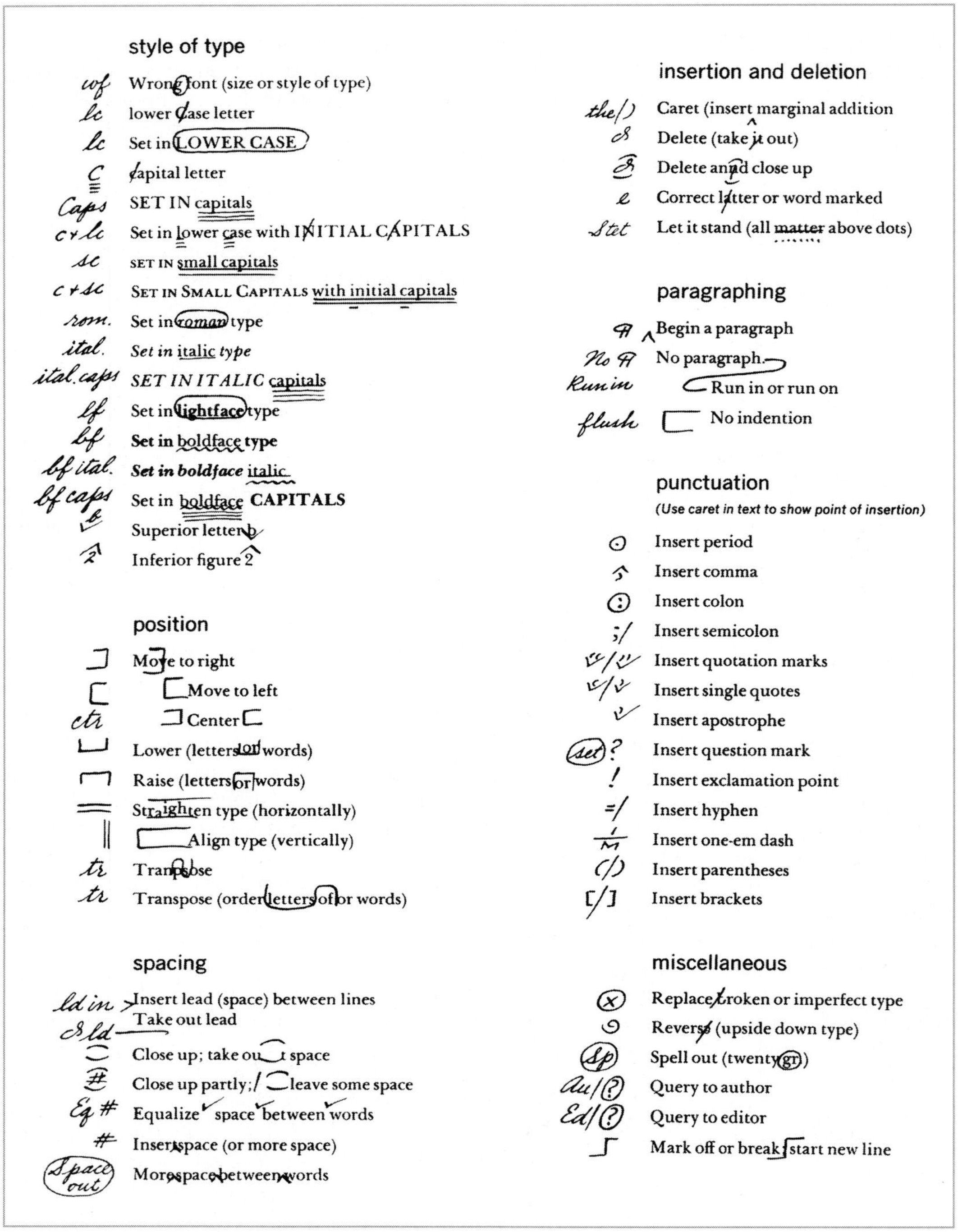

style of type

wf — Wrong font (size or style of type)

lc — lower case letter

lc — Set in LOWER CASE

C — capital letter

Caps — SET IN capitals

c+lc — Set in lower case with INITIAL CAPITALS

sc — SET IN small capitals

c+sc — SET IN SMALL CAPITALS with initial capitals

rom. — Set in roman type

ital. — Set in italic type

ital.caps — SET IN ITALIC capitals

lf — Set in lightface type

bf — Set in boldface type

bf ital. — Set in boldface italic

bf caps — Set in boldface CAPITALS

— Superior letter

— Inferior figure 2

position

— Move to right

— Move to left

ctr — Center

— Lower (letters or words)

— Raise (letters or words)

— Straighten type (horizontally)

— Align type (vertically)

tr — Transpose

tr — Transpose (order letters of or words)

spacing

ld in — Insert lead (space) between lines

— Take out lead

— Close up; take out space

— Close up partly; leave some space

Eq # — Equalize space between words

— Insert space (or more space)

Space out — More space between words

insertion and deletion

the/ — Caret (insert marginal addition)

— Delete (take it out)

— Delete and close up

e — Correct letter or word marked

Stet — Let it stand (all matter above dots)

paragraphing

— Begin a paragraph

No — No paragraph.

Run in — Run in or run on

flush — No indention

punctuation

(Use caret in text to show point of insertion)

— Insert period

— Insert comma

— Insert colon

— Insert semicolon

— Insert quotation marks

— Insert single quotes

— Insert apostrophe

(set)? — Insert question mark

! — Insert exclamation point

— Insert hyphen

— Insert one-em dash

— Insert parentheses

— Insert brackets

miscellaneous

— Replace broken or imperfect type

— Reverse (upside down type)

sp — Spell out (twenty gr)

Au/(?) — Query to author

Ed/(?) — Query to editor

— Mark off or break start new line

FIGURE 10-5 Proofreader's marks.

remain confidential and be easily removed. See Figure 10-7 for an illustration of folding a letter.

Number 10 Envelope

1. Bring up the bottom third of the letter and fold with a crease.
2. Fold the top of the letter down to 3/8 inch from the first creased edge.
3. Make a second crease at the fold and place this edge into the envelope first.

Number 6 3/4 Envelope

1. Bring the bottom edge up to 3/8 inch from the top edge.
2. Make a crease at the fold.
3. Fold the right edge one third of the width of the paper, and press a crease at this fold.
4. Fold the left edge to 3/8 inch from the previous crease and insert this edge into the envelope first.

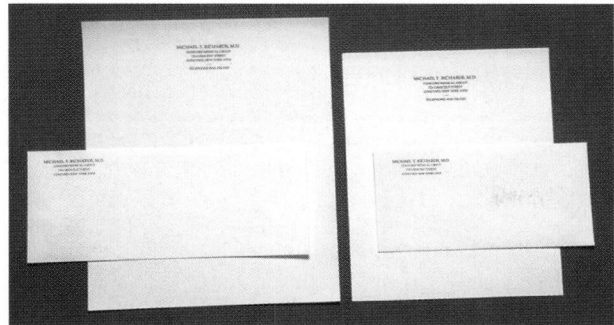

FIGURE 10-6 Letterhead stationery sizes are varied to suit the needs of the sender. Envelopes are sized to match different letter sizes.

Envelope Formats

The United States Postal Service (USPS) has recommended guidelines when typing envelopes. This is meant to improve the handling and delivery of the mail. Optical Character Recognition (OCR) equipment used by the postal service scans, reads, and sorts the envelope. For optimal efficiency of OCR scanning, the address must be typed on the envelope, using single spacing and all capital letters with no punctuation.

The last line in the address must include the city, state two-digit code, and the ZIP code. It cannot exceed 27 characters in length. See Figure 10-8 for a listing of the two digit letter abbreviations for states.

A more traditional style of typing envelopes with the initial letter in capital letters and small letters for the rest of the address is still accepted by the post office.

The bottom margin of the No. 10 envelope (business size) should be 5/8 inch with one-inch margins on the left and right sides. The No. 6 3/4 envelope should have a two-inch margin on the left side with the address 12 lines from the top of the envelope.

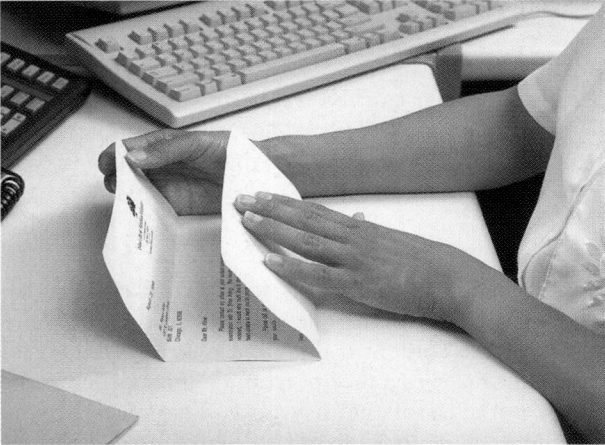

FIGURE 10-7 A well-folded letter fits easily into the envelope and is easily removed by the person who receives it.

A return address for the sender should always be placed in the upper left hand corner in the event the letter must be returned to the sender. Envelopes can be printed with the address of the sender in this position.

ZIP Codes

The five-digit ZIP code was introduced in the 1960s to increase the post office's efficiency in mail handling. ZIP codes begin on the East Coast with the number "0" eventually increasing to the number "9" on the West Coast and Hawaii. The first three numbers of the ZIP code identify the city and all five digits combine to identify the individual post office and zone within the city. Four more digits have been added to the ZIP code by the USPS. These four digits follow a hyphen behind the first five and represent the addressee's street location. The 9-digit ZIP code has eliminated many handling steps at the postal service and improved service.

Classifications of Mail

The classifications of mail vary according to weight, type, and destination. Mail is weighed in ounces and pounds. The most common types of mail are: first class, priority, second class, third class, fourth class, and express mail. Table 10-10 describes these classifications of mail.

TWO-LETTER ABBREVIATIONS
UNITED STATES and TERRITORIES

Alabama	AL	Montana	MT
Alaska	AK	Nebraska	NE
Arizona	AZ	Nevada	NV
Arkansas	AR	New Hampshire	NH
California	CA	New Jersey	NJ
Canal Zone	CZ	New Mexico	NM
Colorado	CO	New York	NY
Connecticut	CT	North Carolina	NC
Delaware	DE	North Dakota	ND
District of Columbia	DC	Ohio	OH
Florida	FL	Oklahoma	OK
Georgia	GA	Oregon	OR
Guam	GU	Pennsylvania	PA
Hawaii	HI	Puerto Rico	PR
Idaho	ID	Rhode Island	RI
Illinois	IL	South Carolina	SC
Indiana	IN	South Dakota	SD
Iowa	IA	Tennessee	TN
Kansas	KS	Texas	TX
Kentucky	KY	Utah	UT
Louisiana	LA	Vermont	VT
Maine	ME	Virgin Islands	VI
Maryland	MD	Virginia	VA
Massachusetts	MA	Washington	WA
Michigan	MI	West Virginia	WV
Minnesota	MN	Wisconsin	WI
Mississippi	MS	Wyoming	WY
Missouri	MO		

FIGURE 10-8 Every state has a two digit letter abbreviation.

TABLE 10-10 Classifications of Mail

Type	Description
First Class	Letters, postcards, business reply cards; letters weighing less than 11 ounces; sealed and unsealed, handwritten or typed material.
Priority	First class mail weighing more than 11 ounces; maximum weight of 70 pounds; postage calculated based on weight and destination.
Second Class	Newspapers and periodicals that have received second class mail authorization; copies of newspapers and periodicals mailed by the general public are not able to receive the second-class rate.
Third Class	Catalogs, books, photographs, flyers, and other printed materials (also called "bulk mail"); must be marked "Third Class;" must be sealed.
Fourth Class	Printed material, books, and merchandise not included in First and Second Class; must weigh between 16 ounces and 70 pounds; there are size limitations also.
Express Mail/Next Day Service	Available seven days a week; up to 70 pounds in weight and 108 inches around; expected delivery by noon; shipping containers are supplied; pickup service in some area.

Special Postal Services

Specialized services include certified mail, certificate of mailing, special delivery, registered mail and special handling.

Certified Mail

Mail that includes contracts, mortgages, birth certificates, deeds and checks, which are not valuable themselves but would be difficult to replace if lost, can be mailed as certified mail (Figure 10-9). They would need to be mailed at the first class rate with a special fee added for certified mail. Certified mail assists in tracking and collecting this mail. A receipt verifying delivery can be requested for a fee. Certified mail can also be sent by special delivery if the extra fee is paid. Certified mail records are maintained at the post office for two years.

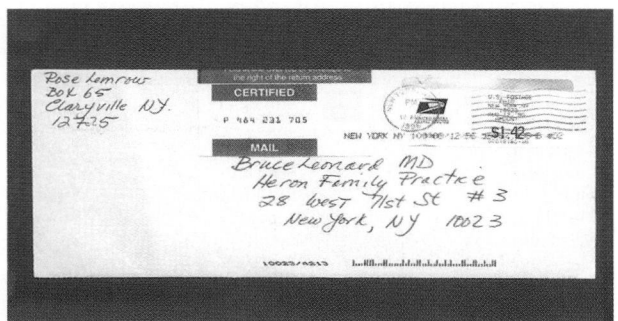

FIGURE 10-9 Items that would be difficult to replace bearing legal significance are sent by certified mail.

Certificate of Mailing

For a small fee, a certificate of mailing can be obtained at the post office. This document will demonstrate proof that mail was posted. This is useful for mailing items such as tax returns, which need to be received by a certain date.

Special Delivery

When fast delivery of an item is needed, special delivery service can be requested from the postal service. Special delivery is useful for shipping perishables, such as specimens, since the post office will deliver these items beyond the regular delivery service hours (for example, on Sundays and holidays). There is a fee for this service.

Special Handling

Special handling can be requested for third- and fourth-class items. "Special handling" is stamped across the package. The fee for this service is based on the weight of the item.

Insurance

Insurance can be purchased for third-class, fourth-class, and priority mail. The sender will then be reimbursed for the content if this mail is lost or damaged. The sender receives a receipt from the post office at the time of purchase of the insurance. This receipt along with the damaged goods must be presented when reimbursement is necessary.

Registered Mail

Registered mail is the safest way to send first-class or priority mail. A fee is paid for this service and a signed record is kept for each piece of registered mail. Registered mail is tracked as it moves throughout the mail system, which helps to reduce loss. Registered mail is insured for the value declared at the time of registration. For an additional fee the sender can request a return receipt indicating the time, place of delivery, and the receiver's signature.

Postal Money Orders

A postal money order can be purchased at the post office. The money order is replaceable if lost or stolen and can be mailed instead of the actual cash. It is available in several denominations and the fee varies according to the amount of the postal money order.

Forwarding Mail

First class is the only type of mail that can be forwarded to another address without paying an additional fee. Cross out the incorrect address and insert the new address and return to the mail carrier or post office. The post office will forward mail for up to six months.

Mail Recall

If mail has been placed into the mailbox or given to a postal carrier by mistake, it can be recalled by the sender. The sender can call the post office and request the item be held for them. When the sender goes to the post office to reclaim the mail, he or she will be asked to complete a "Sender's Application for Recall of Mail." If the mail is still at the post office, it will be returned to the sender upon completion of this form. If the mail has already left the post office, the postal clerk will call the post office where that mail has been sent and ask that the mail be returned. The sender must pay all the expenses incurred in an attempt to recall the mail, including the telephone calls placed by the postal service. If the mail has already been delivered to the addressee, the sender will be notified.

Tracing Lost Mail

All receipts for mailed goods should be retained until receipt of the mail has been acknowledged. If the mail has not arrived after a reasonable period of time, the post office will attempt to trace it for you. First class mail is not easy to trace since there is no receipt for it. The postal service requires a special form to be completed before they will trace mail.

Returned Mail

When mail has been returned and marked "undeliverable," it cannot be re-mailed until new postage is added. It is advisable to place the contents into a new envelope with the correct address, place the proper postage according to weight on the envelope, and re-mail.

Size Requirements for Mail

The USPS standardized envelope sizes in order to machine sort mail. Minimum mail sizes have been established. Domestic mail must be at least 0.0007 inch thick. A further restriction on size requires that mail 1/4 inch or less in thickness must be 3 1/2 inches in height and at least 5 inches long. All mail not meeting this requirement is considered nonstandard.

While postage is generally based on a package's weight, items that are bulky and lightweight are charged a 15-pound balloon rate surcharge. This balloon rate is applied to all Priority Mail® and Parcel Post® items that weigh less than 15 pounds and measure over 84 inches—but not more than 108 inches—in length and girth combined. Following are some general requirement guidelines for preparing mail to be metered.

- Separate all international mail from domestic mail. Separate all Canada and Mexico mail from the rest of the international mail.

- Face all letter size envelopes in the same direction. Make sure none are upside down. When mailing letter size envelopes, flaps must be sealed, tucked in, or nested (overlapped).

- Try not to overstuff letter-size envelopes. If this is not possible, you must seal the envelopes with tape.

- All envelopes larger than a No. 10 size letter envelope must be sealed before being sent.

- Keep the top right corner of each mailing piece clear of all markings. This is where the postmark will appear.

The medical assistant should always consult the USPS for specific mailing, size, weight, and pricing requirements to ensure the outgoing mail is properly prepared. This may include either a visit to the nearest postal office or browsing the USPS Web site.

Mail Handling Tips

To facilitate time management within the medical office, all mail should be handled only once. For ease and efficiency in handling large amounts of mail, follow the steps in Procedure 10-2.

Electronic Mail (E-mail)

All written materials that are transmitted electronically are referred to as electronic mail (e-mail). The documents may include letters, reports, and pictures. These e-mails may be sent over telephone lines, cables, computers, and satellites. Electronic mail allows the medical assistant to edit, correct, and transmit documents very quickly to another location. Electronic mail cannot be used if the original signature on the document

Opening the Daily Mail

OBJECTIVE: Sort and distribute the medical office's daily mail.

Equipment and Supplies
office stamps (one with date and one with name of medical office); ink pad; paper clips; pencil

Method
1. Have all supplies in one place when processing the mail.
2. Sort the mail before opening into first-class, personal/confidential, second-, third- and fourth class.
3. Discard and recycle all unwanted third-class mail.
4. Place a current date and time of arrival on each piece of mail. Purchase rubber stamp and pad from an office supply store so that the date can be changed each day.
5. Stamp the name of the medical office across all periodicals and newspapers.
6. Lay all of the envelopes flap down to reduce the motions involved in opening a large amount of mail.
7. Do not open mail marked "personal" or "confidential." Place it in the physician's box unopened unless otherwise instructed.
8. Attach all enclosures in each envelope with a paper clip. Avoid stapling since these will have to be removed later and may damage sensitive materials, such as x-rays. If an enclosure is noted within the correspondence but is not included in the envelope, write "no" next to enclosure with your initials to indicate it was not included. Clip the opened envelope to the mail until the mail is completely processed. In some cases, a return address is only on the envelope and not on the inside correspondence.
9. Open all the mail and clip together the inside contents before handling the individual correspondence.
10. Annotate the mail as soon as possible after it is opened. An annotation consists of writing a short comment in pencil to indicate the purpose of the letter, and underline the critical portions of the letter. If another document is referred to in the letter, then take initiative by pulling it from the file and attaching it to this correspondence.
11. Route the mail immediately after opening. Another department or physician may be waiting for the document.

needs to be sent. When creating e-mail, remember that e-mail is considered part of the patient's record or part of the office management, therefore all standard proofreading and confidentiality guidelines apply.

E-mail can take different forms. Just like a written letter, e-mail can take the form of a composed letter, form letter, or interoffice memorandum. Some offices use e-mail to confirm office visits. Every office has a particular format to utilize for this purpose.

Another form of e-mail is the instant message format. Instant mail can be defined as a way to communicate with another person in real-time. There are several offices that allow users to instant message each other both internally (within the office) or externally. The internal instant message format is usually connected to the office server and allows for messages to be sent quickly to each person. The external type of instant messages is generally linked to an account that is purchased from an Internet company. You would need to establish your own screen name and passwords to access and communicate with users by instant mail messages. It is important to remember that instant messages are not permanent documents and cannot be attached to a person's medical records or be used in a court of law.

If e-mail is offered to patients as a mode of communication, it is imperative to check it frequently in order to avoid liability. E-mail is not efficient to use for emergencies.

Facsimile (Fax)

Another electronic means of sending a written communication is by using a fax machine. The fax is an exact duplication of a document that is then transmitted to another location via a facsimile (fax) machine. The telephone lines are used to transmit fax documents. The original document is inserted into the fax machine, the receiver's fax phone number is dialed and when the connection is made, the document is transmitted over the telephone lines, resulting in a printed document at the receiver's fax machine. A cover sheet should be sent first, which includes information about the sender (company, name, and telephone and fax numbers) telephone number of the receiver, date, and number of pages. The cover sheet should contain verbiage to encourage the recipient to notify the sender if they have received the fax in error, and asking the recipient to destroy the document after notification.

Reflection on the Medical Practice

Medical assistants are often responsible for preparing interoffice memos and letters to patients. The letter you send is a direct reflection on the physician and the medical office as a whole. If the letter is filled with errors, incorrect diagnosis, or sent to the wrong patient, it reflects poorly on the medical office and can harm the physician's business. If your responsibilities as a medical assistant include letter writing, it is always a good idea to have someone in the office review your correspondence. To facilitate time management within the medical office, remember that you can utilize a form letter that you or the physician has created. Remember to proofread each letter and check for any inappropriate content, misspellings, grammatical or punctuation errors, and margin restrictions.

SUMMARY

The responsibilities of the medical assistant relating to office correspondence are multifaceted. These include being able to draft correspondence using correct grammar and style and efficiently handling mail. Effective mail handling includes using the most efficient and cost-saving form of mail service. These responsibilities must be handled in a professional, courteous, and diplomatic manner. Correct handling of written communication allows the medical assistant to demonstrate competence.

Chapter Review

COMPETENCY REVIEW

1. Define and spell the terms to learn for this chapter.
2. How would you track a missing piece of mail?
3. Address an envelope using the method recommended by the USPS for use with Optical Character Recognition Equipment (OCR).
4. Describe what types of material you would send by certified mail.
5. Type a short letter using both block and modified block with indented paragraph styles.
6. Why do you think companies (and medical offices) use letterhead stationery?

PREPARING FOR THE CERTIFICATION EXAM

1. Which of the following is NOT a method used for classifying mail?
   A. weight
   B. date
   C. destination
   D. type
   E. sender

2. What is the maximum weight (in pounds) for priority mail?
   A. 100
   B. 150
   C. 17
   D. 70
   E. 50

3. What is the term that means "to note the important points or items in a letter or document?"
   A. annotate
   B. announce
   C. notify
   D. proofread
   E. classify

4. Which term means "to indicate the presence of an error or correction needed on a letter or document?"
   A. annotate
   B. sort
   C. notify
   D. proofread
   E. classify

continued on next page

5. What type of mail is used to send laboratory specimens?
   A. special handling
   B. priority mail
   C. registered mail
   D. special delivery
   E. ground shipping

6. The following categories of mail can be insured EXCEPT
   A. first class
   B. second class
   C. third class
   D. fourth class
   E. first class e-mail

7. The two-letter abbreviation for Michigan is
   A. MH
   B. MN
   C. MI
   D. MG
   E. MA

8. Which of the following would NOT be used on a memorandum?
   A. writer's name
   B. subject
   C. complimentary close
   D. date
   E. receiving office

9. Which of the following is NOT found in a thesaurus?
   A. alphabetical listing
   B. index
   C. synonyms
   D. medical terminology
   E. Greek or Latin roots

10. The proofreader's mark that means "insert a space" is
    A. #
    B. //
    C. [
    D. sp
    E. tr

CRITICAL THINKING

1. According to the standard practices of written communication, what is incorrect about the student's letter?

2. What can be done to correct the problems seen in this letter?

3. In what voice is this letter written?

4. Since you have to rewrite the letter, what would you change about the letter? Why?

5. Once you have rewritten the letter, does the letter reflect the physician in a positive or negative manner? Why?

ON THE JOB

Diane Webb, a medical assistant in Dr. Williams' office, has been asked to proofread a letter that was prepared by a temporary assistant. Follow the rules for proofreading, grammar, capitalization, and spelling found in this chapter to correct the errors in this letter. Type this letter using the modified block style and prepare it for Dr. Beth Williams' signature.

Dear Docter Stacey:

I right this letter to inform you that I am pleased that you would chose me to present at your conference. Its a great complement.

Their are several cases which I can site. I would like you're recommendation since I no you will be frank with me. We must all ways be discrete and conscience of patience's rights when presenting cases relating to there conditions. We must remain mindful that patients have there legal rites.

I have the following x-ray studies which I can include: xyphoid process, greater trocanter, peretoneal abcess, left calcanus, fracture of right clavical, and a fractured ileum and ischeum. Let me know which of these rentgeneology studies you would prefer.

Please advise me on how to procede.

Sincerely yours,
Dr. Beth Williams

INTERNET ACTIVITY

Access the Internet and locate information on how to write professional medical letters and other information you may need, such as your extended ZIP code, online proofreader's marks to use as a reference tool, an online dictionary, medical dictionary, and thesaurus, and e-mail etiquette guidelines.

MediaLink  More on written communication, including interactive resources, can be found on the Student CD-ROM accompanying this textbook.

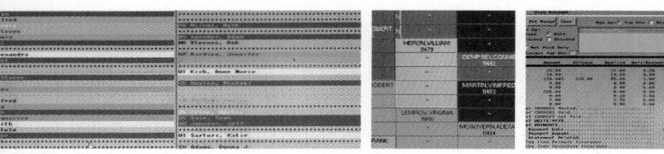

Medical Assistant Role Delineation Chart

HIGHLIGHT indicates material covered in this chapter.

ADMINISTRATIVE

Administrative Procedures
- Perform basic administrative medical assisting functions
- Schedule, coordinate and monitor appointments
- Schedule inpatient/outpatient admissions and procedures
- Understand and apply third-party guidelines
- Obtain reimbursement through accurate claims submission
- Monitor third-party reimbursement
- Understand and adhere to managed care policies and procedures
- *Negotiate managed care contracts*

Practice Finances
- Perform procedural and diagnostic coding
- Apply bookkeeping principles

- Manage accounts receivable
- *Manage accounts payable*
- *Process payroll*
- *Document and maintain accounting and banking records*
- *Develop and maintain fee schedules*
- *Manage renewals of business and professional insurance policies*
- *Manage personnel benefits and maintain records*
- *Perform marketing, financial, and strategic planning*

CLINICAL

Fundamental Principles
- Apply principles of aseptic technique and infection control
- Comply with quality assurance practices
- Screen and follow up patient test results

Diagnostic Orders
- Collect and process specimens
- Perform diagnostic tests

Patient Care
- Adhere to established patient screening procedures
- Obtain patient history and vital signs
- Prepare and maintain examination and treatment areas
- Prepare patient for examinations, procedures and treatments

- Assist with examinations, procedures and treatments
- Prepare and administer medications and immunizations
- Maintain medication and immunization records
- Recognize and respond to emergencies
- Coordinate patient care information with other health care providers
- Initiate IV and administer IV medications with appropriate training and as permitted by state law

GENERAL

Professionalism
- Display a professional manner and image
- Demonstrate initiative and responsibility
- Work as a member of the health care team
- Prioritize and perform multiple tasks
- Adapt to change
- Promote the CMA credential
- Enhance skills through continuing education
- Treat all patients with compassion and empathy
- Promote the practice through positive public relations

Communication Skills
- Recognize and respect cultural diversity
- Adapt communications to individual's ability to understand
- Use professional telephone technique

- *Denotes advanced skills.*

- Recognize and respond effectively to verbal, nonverbal, and written communications
- Use medical terminology appropriately
- Utilize electronic technology to receive, organize, prioritize and transmit information
- Serve as liaison

Legal Concepts
- Perform within legal and ethical boundaries
- Prepare and maintain medical records
- Document accurately
- Follow employer's established policies dealing with the health care contract
- Implement and maintain federal and state health care legislation and regulations
- Comply with established risk management and safety procedures
- Recognize professional credentialing criteria
- *Develop and maintain personnel, policy and procedure manuals*

Instruction
- Instruct individuals according to their needs
- Explain office policies and procedures
- Teach methods of health promotion and disease prevention
- Locate community resources and disseminate information
- *Develop educational materials*
- *Conduct continuing education activities*

Operational Functions
- Perform inventory of supplies and equipment
- Perform routine maintenance of administrative and clinical equipment
- Apply computer techniques to support office operations
- *Perform personnel management functions*
- *Negotiate leases and prices for equipment and supply contracts*
- *Denotes advanced skills.*

SOURCE: Reprinted by permission of the American Association of Medical Assistants from the AAMA Role Delineation Study: Occupational Analysis of the Medical Assisting Profession.

Computers in the Medical Office

Learning Objectives

After completing this chapter, you should be able to:

- Define and spell the terms to learn for this chapter.
- Discuss the functions and applications of the computer.
- Explain the difference between hardware and software.
- List three methods to ensure confidentiality of medical records when using a computer.
- List four methods to be ergonomically correct at your workstation.
- Describe computer maintenance and security.
- Distinguish the difference between the Internet and World Wide Web.

OUTLINE

Use of Computers in Medicine   194

Types of Computers   194

Basic Computer Components   194

Security for the Computer System   198

Selecting a Computer System   199

The Internet   199

Electronic Signatures   201

Computers and Ergonomics   202

Terms to Learn

bandwidth

clock speed

computer

central processing unit (CPU)

floppy disk

Internet

Internet service provider (ISP)

kilobyte (K or Kb)

main memory

mass storage device

megahertz (MHz)

memory

microprocessor

monitor

mouse

printer

random-access memory (RAM)

read-only memory (ROM)

software

Telnet

universal serial bus (USB)

Usenet

World Wide Web (WWW)

Case Study

HELDA KRENZ IS A MEDICAL ASSISTANT WHO WORKS for a family practice physician. She has been asked to develop some continuing education materials for a community service project her office will conduct at the local shopping mall. She will need to locate the most current information, design and develop the materials for distribution, and include marketing materials for the event as well as her office.

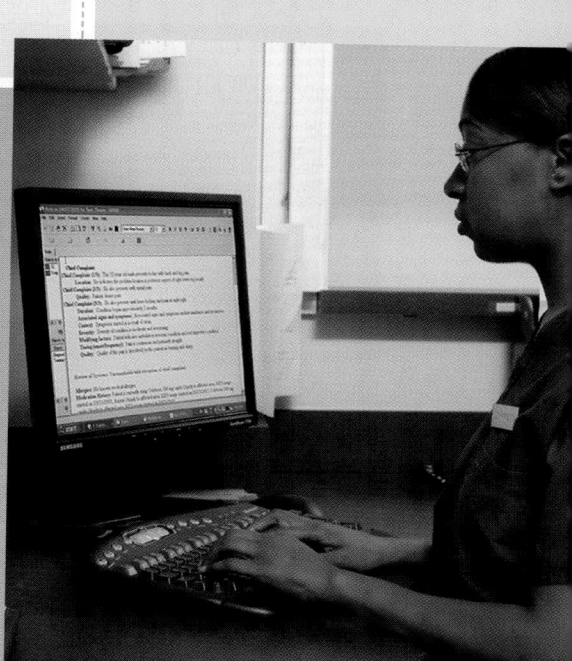

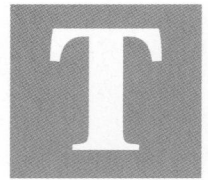

The uses of computers in medicine are many and varied. Depending on the size of the medical practice, some or all of the functions normally performed in the front office may be done with computers and specialized programs. In order to be successful in the administrative, clinical, and lab areas, the medical assistant must be familiar with computers and how they can be used.

Use of Computers in Medicine

Technology advancements have enabled medical offices to function with increased efficiency and speed using computers. Computers are considered a fundamental piece of operating equipment to perform and enhance quality patient care through data collection, eliminate duplication of work, and decrease errors. Figures 11-1 and 11-2 illustrate ways that computers have become invaluable in diagnosing, monitoring, and reporting the patient's progress. Medical assistants will be responsible for computer entries, electronic medical records, electronic bookkeeping, billing, insurance processing, appointment scheduling, inventory data, and many other functions. These responsibilities dictate the medical assistant's knowledge and application of computer literacy. Medical assistants must have competent computer skills and stay current as technology continues to advance.

Types of Computers

The types of computers used in medical offices today are microcomputers. This means that a small piece of electronic hardware, called a chip, allows the processing of information in a very small amount of space. The microchip revolutionized computers and today they

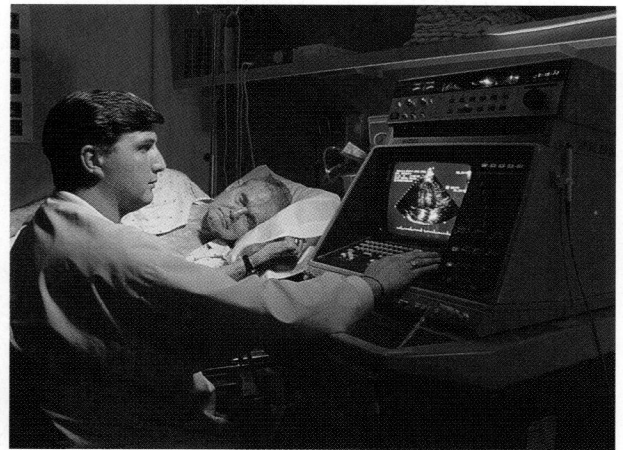

FIGURE 11-1 Echocardiography examination.

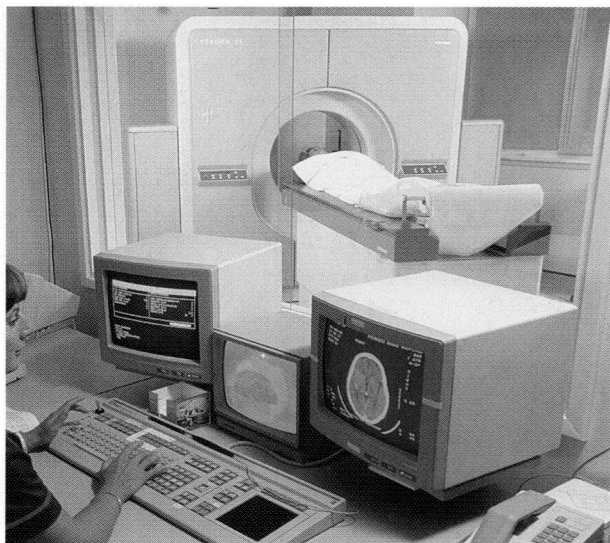

FIGURE 11-2 CT brain scanning.

can fit on a desk, in your lap, or even in a device the size of a hand-held calculator. Before the microchip was developed, computers took up a great deal of room and used a vastly different technology. In the early days, a computer that took up an entire room had the same amount of memory as what now fits on top of your desk.

As computers evolve, two characteristics have changed: size and portability. It has become more important to have computer access anywhere including in transit. Laptop computers allow users to carry their work with them (Figure 11-3). A laptop computer can fit in a case about the size of a small briefcase. Laptop computers offer the same functionality as desktop computers, only in a smaller package. Palm pilots and personal digital assistants (PDAs) are other portable devices used in the medical field. These devices store data that can be recalled as needed. Palm pilots and PDAs are so small that they can easily fit in the pocket of a lab jacket.

Basic Computer Components

A computer is a programmable machine, or system of hardware (Figure 11-4), which responds to a specific set of instructions and performs a list of instructions in programmed language called software. Table 11-1 lists the different types of hardware, software, and storage components. Generally, computers require the following components to function:

- memory makes it possible for a computer to temporarily store data and programs.
- mass storage device makes it possible for a computer to permanently retain large amounts of data. Common mass storage devices include disk drives or zip drives.

- **input** device, such as the keyboard and mouse, is a conduit through which data and instructions enter a computer.

- **output** device, such as a display screen, printer, and other devices, permits the visual capability to see what the computer has accomplished.

- central processing unit (CPU) is the brain of the computer that executes the specific set of instructions.

The CPU, or main memory of a computer, acts as a traffic controller, directing the computer's activities and sending electronic signals to the right place at the right time. The time it takes for the electronic signals to come and go is measured in megahertz (MHz). The higher the megahertz, the faster the computer can move information from one place to another. At the heart of the CPU is the microprocessor, which has a number indicating its size. Microprocessors have three differentiated characteristics: instruction set; bandwidth (the number of bits processed at one time to represent and address); and clock speed (represented in MHz for how many instructions per second the processor can execute). The higher the numbers, the more power the CPU will function.

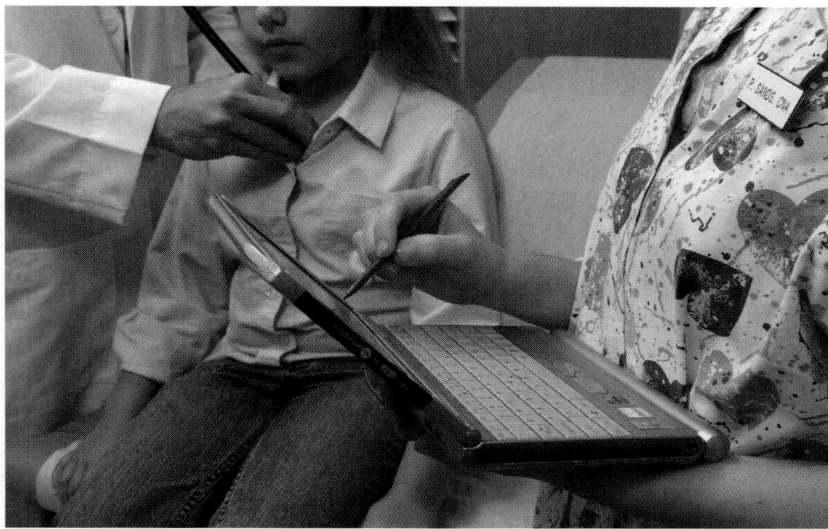

FIGURE 11-3   Medical assistant uses a laptop computer for bedside charting.

Memory

A computer's memory is measured and stored in kilobytes (Kb or K). Each kilobyte is 1,000 bytes (or characters) of information. This memory is further divided into RAM and ROM. RAM, or random-access memory, is the highest number of kilobytes a computer can hold all at once. The ROM, or read-only memory, is used to store information that is not actively being used by the computer at that moment. RAM, however, is only good as long as the computer is not turned off.

Once the computer is turned off, or powered down, all information stored in RAM is lost. The higher the number of kilobytes, the more information a particular storage media can hold.

Monitor

In order to communicate with a computer, the user needs to see what is happening. The monitor is the display screen that allows the user to observe that the computer does what it is directed to do. Monitors are categorized as monochrome, gray scale, or color. Monochrome monitors display two colors: one for the background and one for the foreground. The colors can be black and white, green and black, or amber and black. A gray scale monitor is a special type of monochrome monitor capable of displaying different shades of gray. Color or RGB (red, green, and blue) monitors display anywhere from 16 to over one million different colors (Figure 11-5). In addition to these monitor categories, monitors are available in a variety of sizes and styles similar to television screens. The screen size is measured in diagonal inches, the distance from one corner to the opposite diagonal corner.

TABLE 11-1   Hardware, Software, and Storage Components

Hardware	Software	Storage
Central processing unit (CPU)	Systems	Diskettes/floppy disks
Peripherals: monitor, printer, CD-ROM, modem, scanner, cables, and other equipment	Applications	Hard disks Magnetic tapes

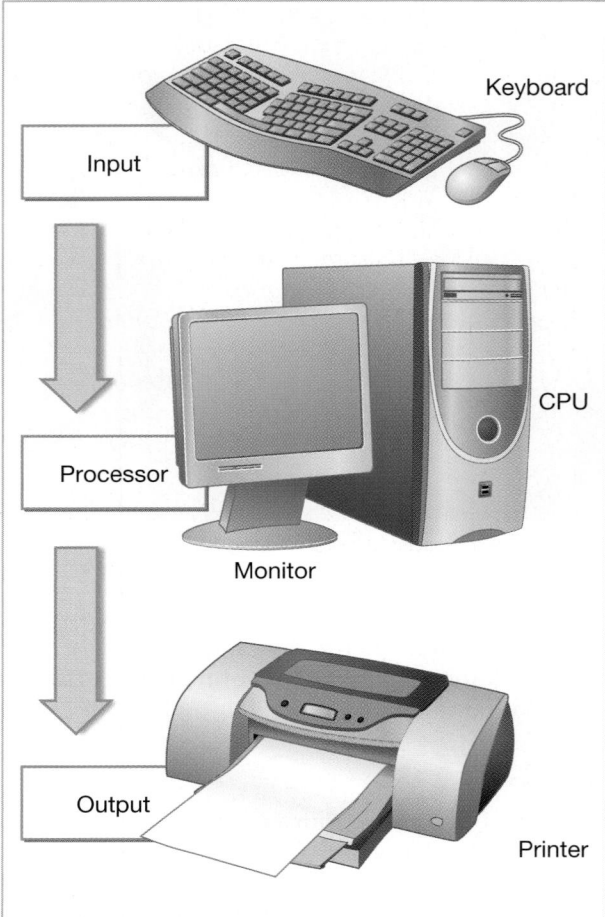

FIGURE 11-4 Components of a computer system.

Drives

Computers are based on hard-disk drive technology. By programming convention, the hard-disk drive, a magnetic storage media contained inside the computer, is usually called the "C drive." This storage area is controlled by the CPU, and information written to this magnetic media is accessed by the CPU when needed to make the computer run. Both programs and information can be stored on a hard-disk drive. The more visual the software, the larger the amount of storage space required. Disk drives can be either internal or external and there are different types of disk drives: hard-disk drive (HDD), floppy-drive (FDD), magnetic disk, and optical drive.

CD-ROM

CD-ROM stands for "Compact Disc Read-Only Memory." It is a data storage system for computers using internal or external CD-ROM players with CD-ROM. Computer programs, databases, and other large amounts of information on CD-ROM are digitally encoded and may not be changed by the user. Stored data may include simple text programs, entire encyclopedia pro-

grams, photo and sound libraries, and complex motion pictures or animations. The data is randomly accessed in the same manner as a floppy disk, which is a small flexible, magnetic disk in a rigid plastic case that stores data on and retrieves data by a computer. A CD-ROM is capable of holding or storing more information than 1,000 floppy disks.

Some computers have multimedia capabilities that allow the user to record and access a variety of sounds and music, photos, animations, and videos. Multimedia functions require the large storage capacity that a CD-ROM offers.

DVD stands for digital videodisc or digital versatile disc. DVDs use the same size disc as CD-ROMs; however they can hold much more information and can be recorded on both sides.

Removable Disk Drive

A removable disk drive uses disks mounted in cartridges. They are generally small and can fit on your key ring or in your pocket. Removable disks come in a variety of sizes ranging from 125 megabytes (MB) to 4 gigabytes (Gs). Their advantage is that multiple disks can be used to increase the amount of stored material, and that once removed, the disk can be stored away to prevent unauthorized use.

A portable universal serial bus (USB) drive, also known as jump drive, thumb drive, or flash drive, is a small portable storage device that can hold up to 4Gs of data. USB hard-disk devices can be purchased in a variety of sizes, styles, and shapes depending on the overall need.

Keyboard

Usually the keyboard is a set of keys utilized to input data. The keyboard is designed with function keys, alphanumeric keys, punctuation keys, arrow keys, and conjunction keys. Function keys serve as dual purpose

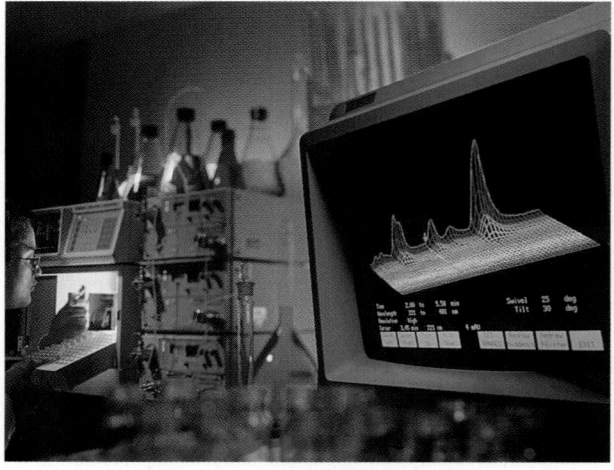

FIGURE 11-5 Color monitor for a computer system.

keys depending on the program that is running. The F1-key and the F12-key execute specific word processing operations. Conjunction keys execute directions in conjunction with the program running and at least two other keys at the same time, for example the control key+alt key+delete key = Windows task manager.

Mouse

In addition to the computer keyboard, a device that gives the user control of the computer is known as a mouse. As the mouse rolls along a hard, flat surface, it controls the movement of the cursor, or pointer on the monitor. The mouse contains at least one button, and up to three, each performing different functions depending on the program in use.

Printers

To output information from the computer monitor onto paper or hardcopy, printers are used. Popular printer options include dot matrix printers, ink-jet printers, and laser printers.

An ink-jet printer works on the dot matrix principle, so that the characters are made up of dots when the ink is blown onto the paper. Ink-jet printers are usually quieter and faster than dot matrix printers, and they can print graphics and in color if the proper ink cartridge and software have been installed. Ink-jet printers are also more costly than the dot matrix printers.

Laser printers use lasers to burn the ink onto the paper. While they are the most expensive of the three printer options, these non-impact printers are the most versatile printers available today. Laser printers are faster and quieter than either dot matrix or ink-jet printers, they can produce typewritten quality work, and they are able to add color to documents with available color print options.

Software

Software or program is the name given to the set or sets of instructions that allow the computer to perform its functions. Every computer starts with an operating system. Computer programs that work with the operating system are called "overlays." These overlay programs allow the user to choose from a menu instead of typing a command at the opening prompt. Each prompt (a symbol or message informing the user that some input is needed) directs the user what action to take. By using arrow keys, function keys, or a mouse, the user can choose the desired program from words or pictures (icons), allowing even an inexperienced user to choose a task more easily. The overlay programs that most users know are from Microsoft Windows, which lets the user choose a function from pictures or icons. Using a mouse, the user moves the cursor to the icon of the program and clicks the proper button on the mouse. The Windows program translates this command for the CPU, and the program is called to the screen.

Another layer of computer programs are called application programs. These programs can perform a special function such as spreadsheets, word processing, or data management. Spreadsheet application programs allow the user to manipulate data in table values by rows and columns. Values are input into specific cells on the spreadsheet and can be assigned a relationship between cells with formulas and labels electronically. Word processing applications provide the user the ability to create, edit, store, and print written documents such as letters, manuscripts, transmittals, and many other professional documents. Word processing programs can visually enhance the content's appearance on documents with numerous features such as bold, italics, color fonts, etc. Data management applications are similar to an electronic filing system (Figure 11-6). Data is stored in collections of information that are organized within the software application and can be sorted for quick data selection of specific desired information pieces. For example, the user would select the field for a directory of patient telephones numbers, diagnoses, or other information needed.

Advantages of medical management programs are many. After entering patient information into the program only once, the practice is able to schedule an appointment, record charges and payments, generate an insurance form, print a statement (including

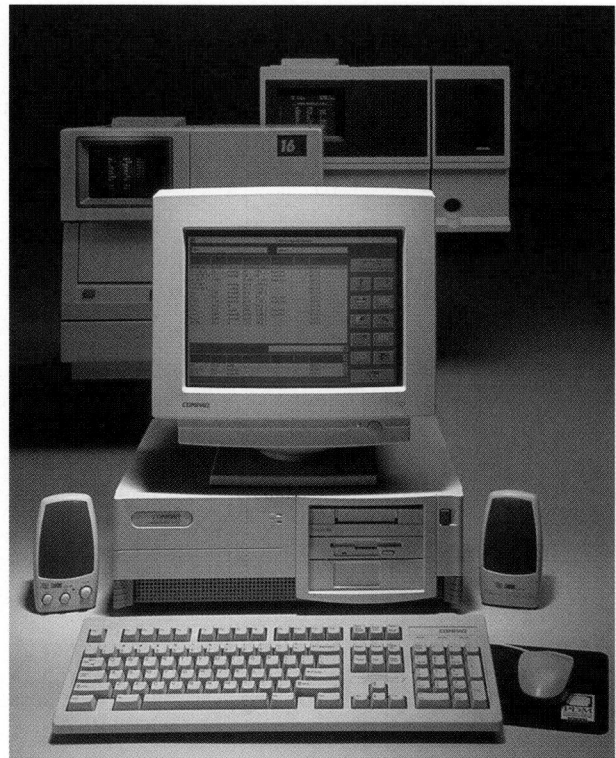

FIGURE 11-6 Patient data management system.

notices of delinquency accounts or aged accounts), track the number of days before payment is received from the insurance company, and write a reminder letter or postcard to the patient about an upcoming appointment.

Security for the Computer System

The same legal standards of confidentiality and the Health Insurance Portability and Accountability Act (HIPAA) compliance apply to all patient records, whether on paper or on the computer. Patient Education discusses reassuring patients about confidentiality in the medical office. It is absolutely essential for the successful medical assistant to understand that other patients should not be able to see computerized records any more easily than paper records. This may require some thought and planning when a computer system is used for record keeping in the front office.

The computer screen should be positioned so that it cannot be easily seen by patients. A privacy screen

around the computer workstation may be necessary, depending on the office layout. Another safeguard available is a screen saver that uses an image or texture to cover up the screen without removing any data allowing no one but the user to see it.

It is imperative that the records are accessible only to those who are authorized to use them. Keeping patient records safe may require using a password. Medical management programs often have several tiers of security, allowing one system administrator (the person in charge of the computer program) to limit access for patient records to those who need to see them. For example, the person who does appointment scheduling in a particular practice may not need to see a patient's financial records. The system administrator can "lock" the appointment scheduler out of financial records altogether, or assign limited access to the data.

Without a proper password, the user has no access to the data and must "log in" or type in his or her password, followed by an acceptance key (ENTER or RETURN) in order to use the program. It is important to guard a password carefully as discussed in Preparing for Externship. It should not be shared with coworkers or written where someone else will see it. When choosing a password, avoid using the names of children or significant others (these would be too easy for someone else to guess). Use a word or a set of numbers that has significance to you, but is also easily remembered. If you must write your password down, write it in a secure place and do not identify it as a system password. Passwords should be changed on a regular basis. Many medical offices change passwords monthly for added security and HIPAA compliance measures.

In addition to in-office security, a medical office needs to protect the computer from outside invaders (Legal and Ethical Issues). Outside invaders include hackers, crackers, viruses, or cyberbullies that access confidential information and commit identity theft. Computer security begins with regular maintenance of the computer systems such as firewalls, antivirus programs, defragmentation, deleting temporary Internet files, cookies, and the Internet history. Maintenance programs can be scheduled automatically or manually and should be run often. In addition to the internal maintenance, the external equipment should be cleaned regularly with appropriate cleaning solution to protect the user from spreading contact germs.

In order to avoid losing all data in the event of a system failure, fire, or equipment theft, it is also recommended that all data be backed up (copied onto disks or CD-ROMs) at regular intervals and that those back-ups be stored in a secure location outside the office. Again, confidentiality is of the utmost importance, and access to backup files should be carefully guarded.

Selecting a Computer System

Before beginning the search for a new computer system, it is important to establish the following:

- How will the computer be used?
- How many people will be using the computer system?
- How much storage space is needed now and for several years into the future?

Remember, the more visual the computer program, the more space will be required to run it. The more patients added to a particular database, the more storage space will be needed to keep pace with the size of the practice.

The second phase of the computer search should focus on the software currently being used.

- Is it meeting the needs of the practice?
- Does everyone who uses it understand how to use it?
- Will the current programs transfer to a new system?

The third critical element of a computer search is the budget and costs related to the budget, such as monthly billing and insurance claim mailings. Changing programs adds to the cost of a new computer system and must be considered carefully in any system change.

Once the hardware and software analysis has been completed, it is time to look at the products on the market.

- Are there manufacturers who have a better service record than others?
- What happens if the computer system breaks down?
- Who pays to have it fixed? Is there a warranty?

Identify a support system of computer experts who can provide ongoing technical assistance and quick on-site service for computer software and hardware problems. Purchasing a service contract to take effect when the warranty covering parts, repair,

Legal and Ethical Issues

The same standards of patient confidentiality apply to data stored on computers that apply to any and all patient records. The medical office must guard against unethical and illegal accessing and use of computer equipment for illegal purposes. Information contained within the computer must be protected, as must the computer hardware and software.

Employees of the practice must be educated and trained to understand the importance of security methods and to prevent loss or damage to valuable equipment and programs. Informed employees can follow the proper procedures to report suspicious occurrences within the workplace. The medical assistant must have an understanding of his or her own liability and the physician's liability in the processing of medical records.

and service expires is an option that you may wish to consider. Training contracts are available with firms that will provide employee training on new software and hardware.

Computer system selection is a large responsibility and while the final decision usually rests with a financial manager, the system's users can make or break the success of any given installation. Users who are unhappy with the selection are not as apt to use the system to its fullest capability, and this will, in the end, cost the practice money. Therefore, it is imperative that as many users as possible be involved in the selection process in order to make sure that the money being spent on a system is well spent. Table 11-2 lists commonly used computer terms.

The Internet

The Internet is a computer network made up of thousands of interfacing networks worldwide. Millions of computers are connected to the Internet. There are organizations that develop technical aspects of this network and set standards for creating applications on it, but no governing body is in control. Access to the Internet is through a commercial Internet service provider (ISP). Using the ISP and modem connection, you can browse the Internet for a wide variety of services: electronic mail, file transfer, vast information

TABLE 11-2 List of Frequently Used Computer Terms

Term	Definition
backup	A copy of work or software batch data stored for processing at periodic intervals.
batch	Data stored for processing at periodic intervals.
boot	To start up the computer.
catalog	List of all files stored on a storage device.
characters per second	Speed measurement for printers.
cursor	Flashing bar, arrow, or symbol that indicates where the next character will be placed.
daisy wheel printer	An impact printer that "strikes" characters onto a page, much like a typewriter; unable to produce graphic images; but does produce letter quality output.
database	Computer application that contains records or files.
data debugging	Process of eliminating errors from input data.
disk drive	A container that holds a read/write head, an access arm, and a magnetic disk for storage.
DOS	Disk operating system.
downtime	Time a computer cannot be used because of maintenance or mechanical failure.
electronic mail (e-mail)	Use of a telephone, modem, and appropriate hardware and software to allow transmission of data electronically from computer to computer.
file	A collection of related records.
file maintenance	Data entry operations including additions, deletions, and modifications.
format	Methods for setting margins, tabs, line spacing, and other layout features.
GIGO	"Garbage in, garbage out," which means if you input incorrect information you will receive incorrect output.
hard copy	A printed copy of data in a file.
hardware	The actual physical equipment that is used by a computer to process data.
input	Entering data into the computer system.
interface	Technology that allows two or more non-connected computers to exchange programs and data. Also referred to as a network.
keyboard	An input device, similar to a typewriter keyboard.
menu	A list of options available to the user.
modem	Hardware device which converts digital signals to analog signals for transfer over communication lines or links.
output	Processed data translated into final form or information to be used.
peripheral	Device required for the input, output, processing, and storage of data; Includes mouse, disk drive, keyboards, printers, and joysticks.
scrolling	Feature that allows the computer operator to control the location of the cursor within a document.
security code	A group of characters that allows an authorized computer operator access to certain programs or features. Password.
write protect	Feature of storage devices that allows the data to be seen, but not changed.

resources, interest group membership, interactive collaboration, multimedia displays, real-time broadcasting, shopping opportunities, breaking news, and much more.

With the advent of remote communications through electronic mail (e-mail) and modems, computers in one location can "talk" to computers across the street, across the state, across the country, and across the world (Professionalism).

Internet technology has allowed many medical insurance companies to offer electronic claims services or ECT (electronic claims transmission). ECT service speeds up the insurance claim process and puts the payment for services rendered into the practice's bank account in as few as three working days. Such access can be obtained through a "clearinghouse" or remote computer with transfer to multiple insurance carriers.

The World Wide Web (WWW or the Web) is a system of Internet servers. The initial purpose of the Web was to facilitate communication among its members, who were located in several countries. Rapid growth in the number of both developers and users ensued. In addition to hypertext (computer-based text), the Web began to incorporate graphics, video, and sound. The use of the Web has reached global proportions and has become a defining aspect of human culture in an amazingly short period of time.

Almost every protocol type available on the Internet is accessible on the Web. Internet protocols are sets of rules that allow for inter-machine communication on the Internet. The following is a sample of major protocols accessible on the Web:

- **E-mail** (Simple Mail Transport Protocol or SMTP)
  Distributes electronic messages and files to one or more electronic mailboxes.

- Telnet (Telnet Protocol)
  Facilitates login to a computer host to execute commands.

- **FTP** (File Transfer Protocol)
  Transfers text or binary files between an FTP server and client.

- Usenet (Network News Transfer Protocol or NNTP)
  Distributes Usenet news articles derived from topical discussions on newsgroups.

- **HTTP** (HyperText Transfer Protocol)
  Transmits hypertext over networks.

Many other protocols are available such as, the Voice over Internet Protocol (VoIP) that allows users to place a telephone call over the Web.

The World Wide Web provides almost instant access to information. The convenient and user-friendly environment of the Web makes it easy for patients to research information about a new medication, physi-

cians to share test results with specialists assisting in diagnosing patients, or as a tool to further educate members of the health care team. Lifespan Considerations encourages you to assist older patients with making use of computers to help in their patient care. Because of the Web's ability to work with multimedia and advanced programming languages, the Web is by far the most popular component of the Internet.

Electronic Signatures

The traditional "signature" on documents is becoming a thing of the past. The traditional signature can now be converted into a mathematical process (or a set of numbers) to create an electronic signature. This set of numbers, in computing terminology a "file," will be recorded temporarily in a computer's working memory or permanently on some storage medium such as a disk. The file that constitutes the electronic document can be copied from place to place via telecommunication devices. An increasing proportion of both commercial and private communications takes place in purely electronic form. Some of those communications will need to be signed to achieve their intended legal effects, and even where this is not strictly necessary, the parties to a transaction are likely to wish the transaction document or communication to be signed.

HIPAA requires health care organizations to protect the privacy and security of confidential health information and calls for standard formats of electronic transactions. These standardized national requirements apply to the electronic transmission of patient history and health records such as health insurance enrollment detail and claims. The need to maintain confidentiality and privacy of medical information and rules for medical document security, including standards related to electronic signatures, is also outlined in HIPAA.

Computers and Ergonomics

If you are a long time computer user, you might have noticed the occasional discomforts that accompany spending lengthy periods of time in front of the computer. After staring at a monitor for extended amounts of time, year after year, you may start to notice the discomfort increase in frequency and severity. As use and hours on the computer continues over the years, the discomfort could become part of the daily routine when you sit down to work or game at a computer. In order to safely incorporate computer use in your daily routine and to work effectively, you should be aware of some ergonomic tips, such as appropriately positioning computer equipment (Figure 11-7).

Your Chair

When sitting in your chair, make sure that you push your hips as far back as they can go in the chair. Adjust

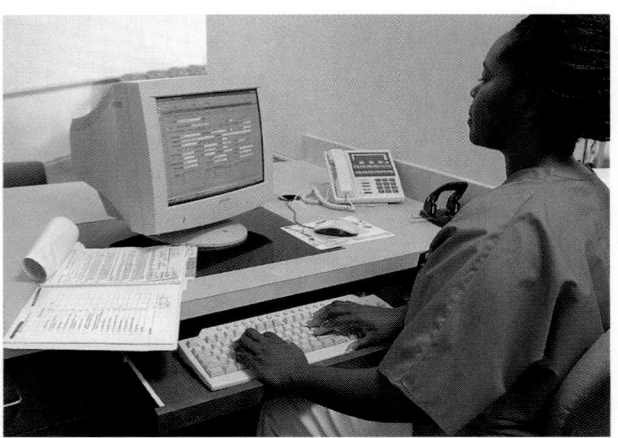

FIGURE 11-7 Ergonomically correct desk, chair and keyboard.

the seat height so your feet are flat on the floor and your knees are equal to, or slightly lower than, your hips. Adjust the back of the chair to a 100° to 110° reclined angle. Make sure your upper and lower back are supported. It may be necessary to use inflatable cushions or small pillows. If you have an active back mechanism on your chair, use it to make frequent position changes. For chairs with armrests, adjust them so that your shoulders are relaxed. If necessary, remove the armrests if they are in the way.

Your Keyboard

An articulating keyboard tray can provide optimal positioning of input devices. However, it should accommodate the mouse, enable leg clearance, and have an adjustable height and tilt mechanism. The tray should not push you too far away from other work materials such as your telephone. It is helpful if you pull up close to your keyboard and position it directly in front of your body. If possible, adjust the keyboard height so that your shoulders are relaxed, your elbows are in a slightly open position, and your wrists and hands are straight. Wrist rests can help to maintain neutral postures and pad hard surfaces. However, the wrist rest should only be used to rest the palms of the hands between keystrokes. Resting on the wrist rest while typing is not recommended.

Your Monitor

Incorrect positioning of the screen and source documents can result in awkward postures. Adjust the monitor and source documents so that your neck is in a neutral, relaxed position. Your monitor should be centered directly in front of you, above your keyboard. Position the top of the monitor approximately two to three inches above seated eye level. To reduce glare, it may be helpful to place the screen at right angles to windows and adjust curtains or blinds. Optical glass glare filters, light filters, or secondary task lights can also help reduce glare.

Your Body

Once you have correctly set up your computer workstation, use good work habits. No matter how perfect the environment, prolonged, static postures will inhibit blood circulation and take a toll on your body. Take short one to two minute stretch breaks every 20 to 30 minutes. After each hour of work, take a break or change tasks for at least five to ten minutes. Always try to get away from your computer during lunch breaks. Avoid eye fatigue by resting and refocusing your eyes periodically. Look away from the monitor and focus on something in the distance. Rest your eyes by covering them with your palms for 10 to 15 seconds. Use correct posture when working. Shift you position as much as possible.

SUMMARY

The use of computers is essential for medical offices to meet the process flow of business today. Computers enhance quality patient care through data collection, eliminate duplication of work, and decrease errors. Computers execute input, processing, output, and storage of medical data. In medical offices, computer use is especially useful in eliminating some of the more time-consuming tasks associated with appointment scheduling, charting, billing, and insurance processing.

Computers are composed of many parts including the microprocessor, CPU, monitor, keyboard, and printer. Safety on the computer includes regular maintenance, passwords, antivirus protection, HIPAA compliance, and general cleaning. The successful medical assistant is a computer literate professional who deals easily with the challenge of finding new and efficient ways to use available technology.

Chapter Review

COMPETENCY REVIEW

1. Define and spell the terms to learn for this chapter.
2. Using a microcomputer, boot up the computer. Notice what information is displayed on the screen before the computer is "ready" to work. What disk operating system is being used? Does a menu or sub-menu appear when the computer has been booted or is the computer using a version of Windows? Are any security codes required to use the programs listed? If so, what are they?
3. What type of printer is used by the computer system? Is it an impact or a non-impact printer?
4. Print a list of all the files on the hard drive.
5. Select a word processing program and type a simple letter reminding a patient that he or she is due for a blood pressure check. Use the spell-checking feature before printing the letter.
6. Enter a patient into a medical management software database. Use yourself and your own information as the data.

PREPARING FOR THE CERTIFICATION EXAM

1. Which is considered a software element of computers?
   A. hard disk
   B. central processing unit
   C. diskette
   D. kilobyte
   E. program

2. Which is NOT considered hardware?
   A. printer
   B. Windows
   C. monitor
   D. keyboard
   E. central processing unit

3. What type of printer is considered the most versatile?
   A. laser
   B. dot matrix
   C. ink jet
   D. word processor
   E. color printer

4. Which is NOT an advantage of a medical data base management program?
   A. enter patient information only once
   B. can print statements
   C. can track days before payment is received from insurer
   D. can print delinquency notices
   E. can measure storage capacity

continued on next page

5. Which is NOT recommended to establish computer security?
   A. position screen away from patients
   B. use a password that is unknown to the patient but that you can remember easily
   C. have tiers of security that limit access to patient information to authorized employees
   D. use screen savers to cover up the screen
   E. change password frequently

6. Electronic mail is
   A. entering data into the computer system
   B. a backup copy of work or software
   C. a process of eliminating errors from input data
   D. use of a telephone, modem, or hardware with software to transmit data from one computer to another
   E. physical equipment used by a computer to process data

7. A prompt is
   A. a set of instructions that tells the computer hardware what to do
   B. a reminder or hint to the user that some action must be taken
   C. processed data translated into final form
   D. methods for setting margins, tabs, and layout features
   E. a measure of storage capacity

8. The computer program that contains all records and files is known as
   A. software
   B. catalog
   C. database
   D. batch
   E. format

9. Which office function CANNOT be performed by word processing?
   A. user can input information using a typewriter-like keyboard
   B. user can see the copy that will be printed
   C. user can correct errors on the screen before printing takes place
   D. user can generate form letters
   E. user can print x-ray films

10. To protect against a loss of data and information processed by the computer, a medical assistant should
   A. change the password frequently
   B. use electronic mail
   C. use word-processing whenever possible
   D. make backup copies on a diskette
   E. handwrite a backup copy for the file

CRITICAL THINKING

1. Where should Helda begin?
2. Which software programs should she use to design and develop the educational materials and the marketing materials?
3. What should she do to become more familiar with the software features to design the materials?

ON THE JOB

Elizabeth Maxwell, a medical assistant for Dr. Casey, often works at the front desk. One of Dr. Casey's patients, Stephanie Cross, has arrived for a scheduled appointment. One her way in, Stephanie saw a neighbor leaving the office. She asks Elizabeth to look on the office system and tell her why her neighbor was in to see Dr. Casey.

Later the same day, Diana Mulderr, who sits at the desk next to Elizabeth, has forgotten her computer password. She asks to use Elizabeth's password "just for today."

1. What should Elizabeth tell Stephanie Cross?
2. Is it ever permissible to use the computer to look up information on patients for personal reasons?
3. What should Elizabeth tell Diana Mulderr?

INTERNET ACTIVITY

When researching information on the Internet, it is important that the Web sites used are reputable and provide accurate information. Perform a search using any of the search engines (a Web site that allows you to search the entire Web for related Web sites) available to you. Search for popular health-related Web sites. Make a list of ten Web sites and comment on each: ease of use, relevant information, easy to understand, etc.

MediaLink  More on computers in the medical office, including interactive resources, can be found on the Student CD-ROM accompanying this textbook.

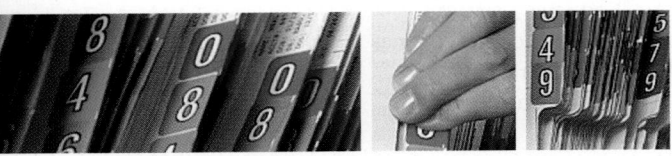

Medical Assistant Role Delineation Chart

HIGHLIGHT indicates material covered in this chapter.

ADMINISTRATIVE

Administrative Procedures

- Perform basic administrative medical assisting functions
- Schedule, coordinate and monitor appointments
- Schedule inpatient/outpatient admissions and procedures
- Understand and apply third-party guidelines
- Obtain reimbursement through accurate claims submission
- Monitor third-party reimbursement
- Understand and adhere to managed care policies and procedures
- *Negotiate managed care contracts*

Practice Finances

- Perform procedural and diagnostic coding
- Apply bookkeeping principles

- Manage accounts receivable
- *Manage accounts payable*
- *Process payroll*
- *Document and maintain accounting and banking records*
- *Develop and maintain fee schedules*
- *Manage renewals of business and professional insurance policies*
- *Manage personnel benefits and maintain records*
- *Perform marketing, financial, and strategic planning*

CLINICAL

Fundamental Principles

- Apply principles of aseptic technique and infection control
- Comply with quality assurance practices
- Screen and follow up patient test results

Diagnostic Orders

- Collect and process specimens
- Perform diagnostic tests

Patient Care

- Adhere to established patient screening procedures
- Obtain patient history and vital signs
- Prepare and maintain examination and treatment areas
- Prepare patient for examinations, procedures and treatments

- Assist with examinations, procedures and treatments
- Prepare and administer medications and immunizations
- Maintain medication and immunization records
- Recognize and respond to emergencies
- Coordinate patient care information with other health care providers
- Initiate IV and administer IV medications with appropriate training and as permitted by state law

GENERAL

Professionalism

- Display a professional manner and image
- Demonstrate initiative and responsibility
- Work as a member of the health care team
- Prioritize and perform multiple tasks
- Adapt to change
- Promote the CMA credential
- Enhance skills through continuing education
- Treat all patients with compassion and empathy
- Promote the practice through positive public relations

Communication Skills

- Recognize and respect cultural diversity
- Adapt communications to individual's ability to understand
- Use professional telephone technique

- Recognize and respond effectively to verbal, nonverbal, and written communications
- Use medical terminology appropriately
- Utilize electronic technology to receive, organize, prioritize and transmit information
- Serve as liaison

Legal Concepts

- Perform within legal and ethical boundaries
- Prepare and maintain medical records
- Document accurately
- Follow employer's established policies dealing with the health care contract
- Implement and maintain federal and state health care legislation and regulations
- Comply with established risk management and safety procedures
- Recognize professional credentialing criteria
- *Develop and maintain personnel, policy and procedure manuals*

Instruction

- Instruct individuals according to their needs
- Explain office policies and procedures
- Teach methods of health promotion and disease prevention
- Locate community resources and disseminate information
- *Develop educational materials*
- *Conduct continuing education activities*

Operational Functions

- Perform inventory of supplies and equipment
- Perform routine maintenance of administrative and clinical equipment
- Apply computer techniques to support office operations
- *Perform personnel management functions*
- *Negotiate leases and prices for equipment and supply contracts*

- *Denotes advanced skills.*

SOURCE: Reprinted by permission of the American Association of Medical Assistants from the AAMA Role Delineation Study: Occupational Analysis of the Medical Assisting Profession.

Managing Medical Records

Learning Objectives

After completing this chapter, you should be able to:

- Define and spell the terms to learn for this chapter.
- Describe three types of file storage units.
- State the "Rules for Filing."
- List and discuss five types of numerical filing systems.
- Describe color-coded, alphabetic, and numerical filing systems.
- State an effective system used for cross-referencing.

- Describe how to find a missing file.
- Describe a tickler file.
- Describe the process for medical transcribing and a variety of medical reports.
- Discuss quality assurance.
- Discuss ownership of the medical record.
- Discuss the medical record's statute of limitations.

OUTLINE

The Medical Record	208
Filing	212
Quality Assurance for Quality Medical Care	219
Releasing Medical Records	221
Storing Medical Records	221
Medical Transcription	222
Ownership of the Medical Record	222
Retention and Destruction of Medical Records	223

Terms to Learn

active record

alphabetic filling

closed record

electronic medical record (EMR)

inactive record

medical record

microfiche

microfilm

numerical filing

problem oriented medical record (POMR)

source oriented medical record

subjective, objective, assessment, and plan (SOAP)

terminal digit filing

Case Study

YOU ARE EMPLOYED AS A MEDICAL ASSISTANT in Dr. Salpega's office. A patient, Terry Dewey, has been diagnosed with a lung cancer with metastasis to the brain. Dr. Salpega has told him that his cancer is inoperable. Mr. Dewey wants the opinion of another physician and requests that his medical records, including all test results, be released to another physician in the same city. In preparing Mr. Dewey's record, you discover that there are no x-ray results in his chart, although you know he had x-rays done. In addition, you discover that Mr. Dewey has an unpaid balance of $742.21 for services previously rendered.

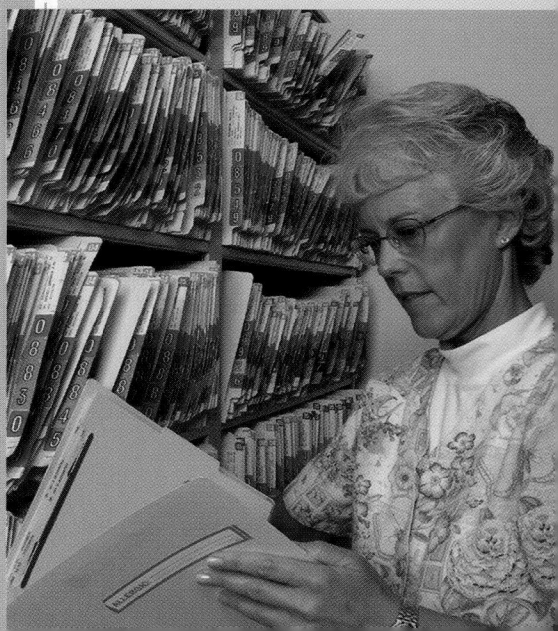

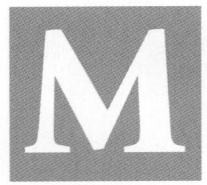

edical records are the sources of all documentation relating to the patient. The medical record contains past patient history information, current diagnosis and treatment, and correspondence relating to the patient. Billing materials are often maintained in a separate accounting record. Medical records can be maintained in a variety of methods, which include paper (hard copy files), computer database files on location or off with an online separate backup system, electronic medical records (EMR), microfilm (miniaturized photographs of records) and microfiche (sheets of microfilm) and other electronic medium. Medical records management requires careful attention to accuracy, confidentiality, and proper filing and storage.

The Medical Record

The medical record contains all the written documentation that relates to the patient's health care. Each patient's medical record will contain essentially the same categories of material but information unique to each patient. Information contained in a source-oriented medical record is filed within a section with tabs. Each medical record may or may not include all standard categories based on the patient's individual health care needs. For example, not every patient will have a consultation report from another physician, or a surgical report. See Box 12-1 for a summary list of standard

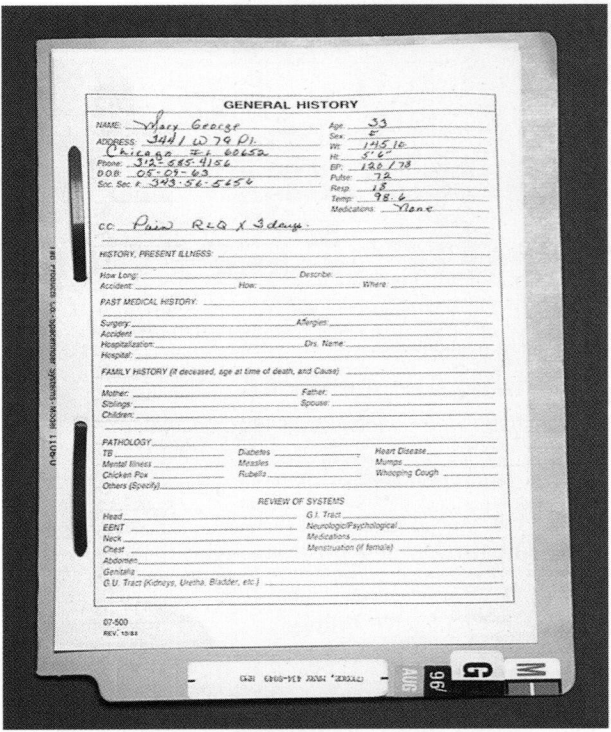

FIGURE 12-1 Handwritten documentation.

categories and reports that are covered in more detail in this chapter. Figure 12-1 is an example of handwritten documentation in a medical chart. This demonstrates just one part of what is in the standard patient's chart.

Types of Medical Records

Various medical reports are filed in the medical records with tabs that label the source, such as lab, x-ray, consultations, and special studies. These medical records are referred to as source oriented medical records.

Most medical offices and hospitals use subjective, objective, assessment, and plan (SOAP) charting and the problem oriented medical record (POMR). See Figure 12-2 for an example of SOAP charting. Chapter 34 contains a detailed description of the SOAP method.

For a physician to easily track the progress of a patient, the POMR system can be used. There are four sections to the POMR approach:

- Database—this section contains information about present illness, chief complaint, review of systems, laboratory reports, and physical examinations.

- Problem list—in this section each problem the patient has experienced is separately listed and numbered.

- Treatment plan—each treatment plan is numbered and corresponds to the numbered problem.

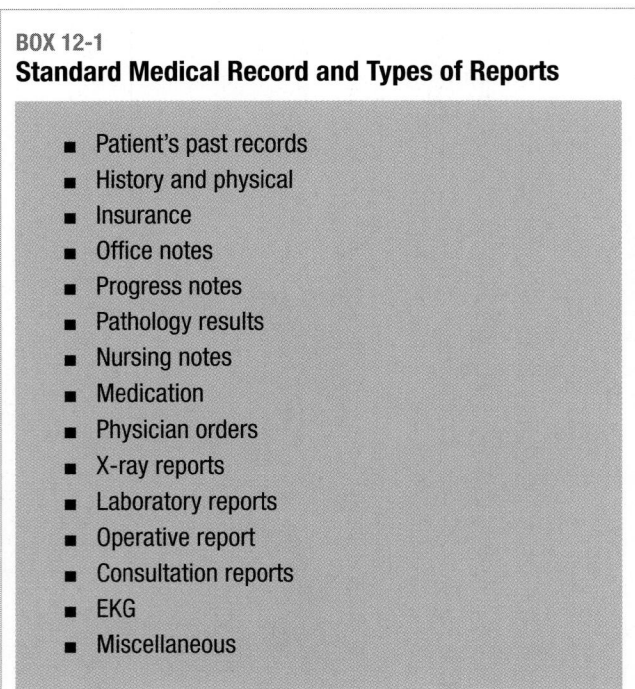

BOX 12-1
Standard Medical Record and Types of Reports

- Patient's past records
- History and physical
- Insurance
- Office notes
- Progress notes
- Pathology results
- Nursing notes
- Medication
- Physician orders
- X-ray reports
- Laboratory reports
- Operative report
- Consultation reports
- EKG
- Miscellaneous

PROGRESS NOTES

| Patient's name: Jessica Lopez | | | | | | | | Page: 1 |

Date	Problem Number	**S**	**O**	**A**	**P**	**S** = Subjective **O** = Objective **A** = Assessment **P** = Plan
3/12/05	1	"I'm having dizzy spells and have not been taking my BP med."				
			BP 170/110 both arms, lying down, sitting & standing; WT. 202#			
				Hypertension		
					Rx for Norvasc 5mg daily; to monitor BP and return in 1 week	
					for BP check; placed on 1200 calorie diet to lose 20#	

FIGURE 12-2   An example of SOAP charting.

- Progress notes—every progress note entered in the chart must correspond to one of the numbered problems. Each progress note will follow the structured format of SOAP charting.

Always keep in mind that the medical record is a legal document, permanent record, and a tool used to communicate between staff members to deliver services to the patient. The patient's chart is not the place to document your opinion or internal office problems. Statements such as, "Patient not administered injection due to lack of staffing" or "Patient very angry with physician" are opinions, or subjective. All documentation should be objective, not subjective.

Everything that is done during a patient's medical visit, ordered over the telephone, or discussed with a patient over the telephone or e-mail, must be docu-mented in the medical record. Write legibly in black ink. If you make an error, do not erase or totally oblit-erate the original error with commercial products like correcting fluid. If the error is made during the typing process, then it should be corrected as any other errors are corrected. However, if the error is noted later, then you must draw a line through the error, enter your ini-tials, the date, and write in the correction. Handwrit-ten errors on the medical chart are handled in the same manner. Procedure 12-1 lists steps the medical assis-tant should follow when changing or adding items to a patient's chart. Figure 12-3 is an example of a cor-rected chart notation.

The following items cannot be overemphasized as part of the medical assistant's responsibility to ensure an efficiently run medical office.

Date	Time	Order	Doctor	Administered by
9/9/05	3 pm	Erythromycin ~~500 mg~~ 250 mg BT 9/9	Williams	B. Tremgen RN.

FIGURE 12-3   An example of a corrected chart notation.

PROCEDURE

Adding or Changing Items on a Patient's Record

OBJECTIVE: Add an item to a patient record and correctly change an error in documentation.

Equipment and Supplies
medical record to be added to or changed; black pen; correct information or documentation to be added or changed

Method
Adding items to a record:

1. An item is added to a patient record as soon as it is discovered that the item was omitted.
2. Locate the last entry in the medical record.
3. Using a pen with black ink, on the next line of the record, immediately after the last entry, place the current date.
4. On the same line, after the date, place the statement, "Late entry."
5. Note the date on which the information to be added was gathered.
6. Enter the information that was originally omitted.

7. Sign the entry with your full name and credentials.

Changing items in a record:

1. If an entry was made in a record that was incorrect, or made in the wrong record, it must be corrected.
2. Locate the incorrect information.
3. Using a pen with black ink, draw one single line through the incorrect information, so that the incorrect information is not obscured, but can still be read.
4. NEVER erase in a medical record. NEVER use correction fluid in a medical record. NEVER mark through information so that it cannot be read.
5. Place the date of the correction, your initials, and the letters "m.e." (for mistaken entry) above the incorrect information.
6. Enter the correct information.

- Clear handwriting—the medical records that are handwritten should be easily read by anyone. Pay particular attention to numbers and spelling.

- Accurate records—keeping in mind that records are legal documents and can be used in a court of law, the physician must be able to trust the accuracy of the data. As simple as it sounds, never guessing about information and double-checking your work each time will help ensure this is the case.

- Records that are up to date and available—do not wait to update records; make it an office habit to update records either as they occur or daily. This updating should include telephone calls, lab reports, and office visits. Make sure that the files are easily accessible. If there is a patient emergency, for example, the medical history will be needed immediately.

Electronic and Computerized Medical Records
Many health care professionals remain wary of computerizing patient records because of confidentiality

worries. Electronic medical records, however, are becoming more common. Here are some advantages to electronic records:

- All office workers can have immediate access to the same files; a procedure for updating files needs to be in place.

- A physician may have offsite access to records on the network.

- Records can be sent via e-mail attachments to relevant and valid heath care inquiries or to satellite offices in different cities.

- Reminders for updating files can be set for staff members when updated information is due.

Types of Forms and Reports
A standard medical record is one of the most important items in an office setting. It is imperative that you are familiar with all components of it, such as medical forms and reports, in order to maintain the integrity and accuracy of patient records.

Patient Registration

The patient registration form usually includes the patient's name, the date of the visit, as well as the patient's age, date of birth (DOB), Social Security number, driver's license number (if applicable), address, and medical insurance information. The medical assistant should also note the patient's occupation, marital status, number of children (if applicable), emergency contact information, family medical history and current medical problems, as well as the chief complaint (CC). Figure 12-4 shows an example of a chief complaint. Other information the medical assistant may wish to note is mentioned in Cultural Considerations.

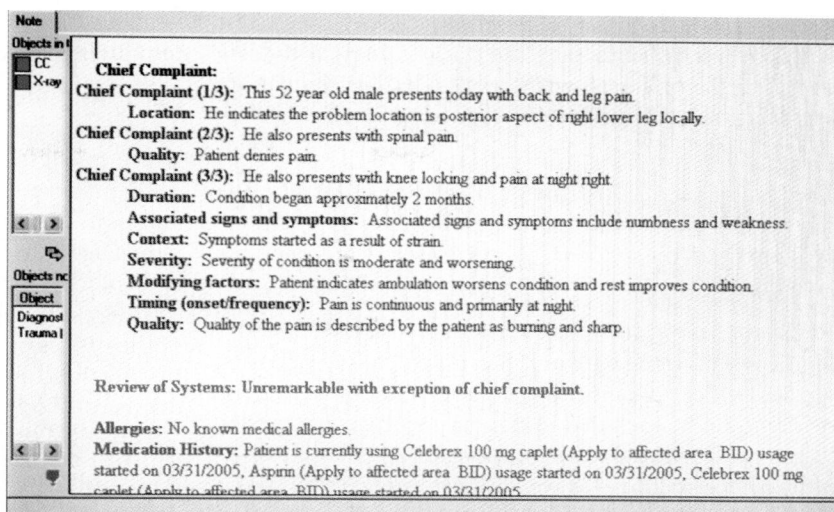

FIGURE 12-4 An example of a chief complaint chart notation in computerized patient records.

Family and Medical History

Sometimes the patient's family and medical history is listed on a separate form. This information should include the patient's past medical history of illness, surgery, allergies, current prescriptions, medications, and over-the-counter medications. It should also include herbal medications, and recreational drugs used by the patient. It should contain the patient's social and occupational history, including the amount of exercise done by the patient, whether the patient uses tobacco and the type of tobacco product, as well as alcohol use. Also, the medical assistant should note the current complaint and details of the present illness. Managed care insurances often require that the patient's current chief complaint be entered into the medical record as a history against the diagnosis. Use of the patient's own words is often requested. Relevant past family and social history is also vital, as well as the patient's medication history. Inventory of body systems is usually included as part of the patient's history.

Physical Examination Results

Not all patients receive general physical examinations. Some offices have a separate form to chart the outcome of a physical examination. The comprehensive physical examination form charts the results included in the examination, such as the patient's general appearance, nutrition, blood pressure (B/P), and head—an ear, eyes, nose, and throat examination (EENT), mouth, and scalp. Results from neck and thyroid examinations are also charted, as well as those of the thorax and breasts. Lymphadenothapy, and examinations done on the heart and lungs, the abdomen, the pelvic, genital and rectal areas, the skin, and overall impression and treatment plan also appear on the chart.

Results of All Tests

All results from tests performed on patients, such as office tests, laboratory tests, and hospital tests, should be tracked and filed in patients' records for easy accessibility should the physician need to consult them.

Records from Referred Physicians or Hospital Visits

New patients require incoming records from past offices to be placed in their records. Include a copy of the patient's written request and release for transferring records from past offices. Also, include information and relevant diagnoses from specialty physicians to whom the patient was referred for specific follow-ups.

Informed Consent Forms

A signed informed consent form documents that a patient has understood and consents to a treatment offered and has knowledge of the potential outcome and side effects of that treatment. The form must have

Cultural Considerations

Take note of the patient's cultural and ethnic background as well as that of friends or family accompanying the patient on his or her visit. It may be beneficial to make specific notes in that patient's chart regarding language spoken or other cultural considerations that the patient has mentioned in conversation.

a signature with the corresponding date. Moreover, it is important to note that the patient may withdraw consent if he or she so wishes. See Chapter 3 for more information on informed consent forms.

Diagnosis and Treatment Plan

The diagnosis and treatment plan should include the physician's diagnosis, the treatment plan, and options presented to the patient, as well as any instructions given to the patient.

Patient Correspondence and Follow-up Care

Invoices sent to the patient, procedures, follow-up visits, medical office care, and any notations involving the patient should be included in patient records. Also added to the records are documentations of telephone calls— often a separate log—as well as correspondence with or about the patient from all sources, such as laboratories, health care agencies, and referred consultations.

Consultation Report

There are many situations in which a physician will ask another physician to provide a second opinion on a patient's case. The second physician generally examines the patient, and then a report is dictated. The report is then sent to the attending physician (the requesting physician). The consultation report will include:

- Patient's name and medical record number
- Date of consultation
- Medical transcriptionist's name
- Referring physician
- Reason for the consultation
- Physical and laboratory evaluations
- Consulting physician's impression and recommendations

It is appropriate to close this report, which is supplied in letter format, with a complimentary close such as, "Thank you for allowing me to participate in the care of this patient."

Operative Note

The operative report describes a surgical procedure. The surgeon is expected to dictate this report as soon as possible, preferably immediately after the procedure is completed. The surgeon's name, date of procedure, preoperative and postoperative diagnosis, and the actual findings during the procedure are contained in this report.

This report is comprised of a description for the actual procedure, which will include location and length of the incision, the layers of skin and tissue that were incised, types of instruments used (in some cases), which organs and tissues were removed, all materials that were used in closing the wound, the estimated amount of blood loss, and a sponge count. The condition of the patient at the end of the procedure is stated, such as

"Patient tolerated procedure well," "Patient awake and responding," or "Patient taken to recovery room."

Pathology Report

The pathology report is generated by the pathologist as the result of examining tissue and organs removed during a surgical procedure (such as a biopsy) or at an autopsy. An autopsy report is generated after a patient's death to determine the cause of death. A pathology report focuses on microscopic (histology and cytology) findings as well as gross (overall) description of the tissues or organs. This report is related to disease findings and not laboratory findings, which are conducted on body fluids.

Radiology Report

A radiology report, completed by the radiologist, documents results of diagnostic procedures, such as x-rays, CT (computerized tomography) scans, MRI (magnetic resonance imaging) scans, nuclear medicine procedures (bone and thyroid scans), and other fluoroscopic examinations.

Discharge Summary

The discharge summary is completed on every hospitalized patient and summarizes the hospitalization. It explains why the patient was admitted, a summary of the patient's history, and a review of what occurred during the hospitalization. A discharge diagnosis is included in this report. The patient's condition upon leaving the hospital is noted.

Additional Reports

Other reports may be required concerning a patient, such as an emergency room report, psychiatric note, and special procedures, like a cardiac catheterization, or autopsy reports.

If information is not properly organized in the patient's medical record, errors can occur. It is very important that the medical assistant organize the patient's medical record according to facility policy. (See Procedure 12-2)

Filing

Choosing the type of file system for medical forms and reports, including the file folder coding system used in the office, is an important decision since all files must be maintained within that system. Some large offices hire an office consultant to set up a filing system. While the office staff are generally consulted when setting up a new file system, the decision is made by the physician and the office manager. There are three categories of files or records in a medical office: active, inactive, and closed.

- Active records relate to patients who have been seen in the past few years and are currently being treated. Each medical practice may have its own

Organize a Patient's Medical Record

OBJECTIVE: To update the patient's medical record verifying the right record and placing the information in the correct place in the record.

Equipment and Supplies
patient medical record; assorted documents for filing in record

Method

1. Verify that you have the right records for the patient record you have been given.

2. File documents given to you in the correct areas of the file, according to your facility policy for consistency. For example, file laboratory reports with other laboratory reports.

3. Return medical record to correct place in alphabetical order with other files.

---

policy regarding what constitutes an "active" file, but it is usually from one to five years.

- Inactive records relate to patients who have not been seen within the time period determined by office policy. These files are still maintained within the office but they are generally kept in a separate storage file cabinet. These patients have not received a formal notification that the physician has terminated caring for them. They may return when a medical problem develops.

- Closed records are those of patients who have actively terminated their contact with the physician. This occurs when they move away, ask to have their records sent to another physician, or death occurs. These files can be placed in storage boxes and are referred to as archives, since they are no longer needed but must be kept for legal reasons.

Fireproof cabinets are used to file documents, such as patient records, tax records, insurance policies, and canceled checks.

File Storage

Three types of file storage commonly used in a physician's office are vertical, lateral, and movable.

- Vertical—set up with two to four stacked pull-out drawers holding up to 100 files per drawer. This type of file storage system is heavy and space consuming.

- Lateral—set up with shelves allowing for easy access to files by pulling them off the shelves. This system often uses a color-coded method for visual recognition of files.

- Movable—set up with electrically powered or manually controlled file units that move on tracks in the floor. This type of open filing system is space saving since the file units can be moved close together when they are not needed. This system is also useful for books and journals since the floor can be reinforced when the track is installed.

File Folders

File folders are also designed to meet special needs. The top or side edge contains tabs at spaced intervals. These tabs are marked with identification labels. If files are stored with alternating tab cuts, it is easier to read the labels in the file drawer. The identification label is attached to the top tab in a vertical file cabinet or to the side edge of the file in a lateral file cabinet.

The patient's record may be placed within a separate tabbed folder that remains in the filing cabinet. The file folders may be color-coded to indicate the primary care physician. Each physician would be assigned a folder color. This helps keep files in order in large clinics. Professionalism discusses the importance of keeping files in order for any medical office, regardless of the size of the practice.

Professionalism

Your work reflects your professionalism. If patient records are strewn about the office, or if your system precludes your being able to pull the file you need quickly, it is a reflection on your skills as a medical assistant. If your filing system is sloppy, then you are probably sloppy too. Be sure to file all records accurately, neatly, and in a timely manner.

TABLE 12-1 Rules for Alphabetic Filing

Rules	Example
Names are filed: last name, first name, middle name (or middle initial). Each letter in the name is a separate unit.	Krause, Marvin K. is placed before Krause, Marvin L.
Initials come before a full name.	Brown, H. is placed before Brown, Henry.
Hyphenated names are treated as one unit. This applies to the names of individuals and businesses.	Amy Freeman-Smith is indexed under F for Freeman. It is considered Freemansmith for indexing purposes.
Titles (and initials) are disregarded for filing but placed in parentheses after the name.	Dr. Beth Ann Williams is indexed as Williams, Beth Ann, (Dr).
Married women are indexed using their legal name. The husband's name can be used for cross-referencing.	Mrs. Mary Jane Smith is indexed as Smith, Mary Jane (Mrs. John).
Seniority units, such as Jr. and Sr., are filed in a numerical order from first to last.	Jacob James Jurgens, Sr. comes before Jacob James Jurgens, Jr.
Numeric seniority terms are filed before alphabetic terms.	Jurgens, Jacob James III indexed before Jurgens, Jacob James, Jr.
Mac and Mc can be filed either alphabetically as they occur or grouped together depending on the preference of the office.	
Foreign language names are indexed as one unit.	Mary St. Claire is indexed as Stclaire, Mary. Carol van Damm is indexed as Vandamm, Carol.
If company names are identical, the address, by state, then city, street, may be used in the index. The ZIP code is not used to index files.	ABC Drugs, 123 Michigan Blvd., Chicago IL is indexed before ABC Drugs, 1450 N. Ash, Kalispell MT.
If individual's names are identical, use the birth date or mother's maiden name. Avoid using address since that can change.	Mark Richard Jones is indexed as Jones, Mark Richard (5/12/65) and Jones, Mark Richard (2/12/89).
Disregard apostrophes.	Megan O'Connor is indexed as OConnor, Megan.
Business organizations are indexed as they are written.	Lincoln Memorial Hospital is correct.
Disregard short terms, such as *a, and, the,* and *of.*	The Whitefish Drug Store is indexed as Whitefish Drug Store (The).
Numeric characters are indexed before alpha characters.	23rd Avenue Clinic would be indexed before the Nineteenth Street Medical Center. A separate file is set up for all numeric files.
Names with religious titles, such as Sister Mary Murphy, would be filed with the last name first, and then with the religious title.	Murphy, Sister Mary.
Compound words are filed as they are written.	South West Physician Service is filed before Southwest Physician Service.

Guides

Divider guides are used to separate files in the drawer or on the shelf. These guides are of heavy pressboard and should be placed every 1 1/2 to 2 inches to separate the file folders. The divider guide breaks the files into subsections using a letter (for example A, B, C, or A-B, Invoices) or by patient number. An out-guide is placed in the file when a file is removed to indicate where the file should be returned. The out-guide is usually a distinctive color, such as red, to indicate a file is missing.

Labels

The label on the file folder (such as the patient's name) has a main purpose of identifying what is in the file. However, the label can also include a color-coding stripe that can be used for other purposes, such as identifying the primary care physician. The label on the file drawer contains the topic and the range of files.

For example: Patient Histories

A-D

The label on the divider contains the range of files between that divider and the next.

For example: Aa-Ba

Rules for Filing

Three commonly used systems for filing are the alphabetic, numeric, and subject filing. Alphabetizing is a component of all the methods and will be explained in detail. Color-coding is used in all three systems to assist in locating files, refiling, and prevent misfiling.

Alphabetic System

Alphabetizing is the most common system for filing records in a physician's office (a hospital generally uses an ID numeric system for filing patient records). In this system, Abbott would be filed before Bacon since "A" appears before "B" in the alphabet. If the first letter is the same, then move to the second letter in the name. Abbott is filed before Acker. This does not pose problems when filing a last name since everyone understands the alphabet. However, there could be confusion when filing Jacob James Jergens, Jr. and Jacob James Jergens III, or determining how correspondence from 23rd Avenue Clinic should be filed.

The key to alphabetic filing is to divide the names and titles into units (first, second, and third). The unit is the portion of the name that is used for filing or indexing purposes. For example:

- Unit 1 Jergens
- Unit 2 Jacob
- Unit 3 James

The first letter of each unit is then used to determine where the file is to be placed. When filing a large number of files, use the first letter of the first unit and place all the files from A–Z in order. Then take each group of "A" files and use the second letter and consecutive letters to place them in order. If the entire first unit is the same, as in Smith, then move onto the second unit and third unit. For example, Smith, Loren comes before Smith, Michael, which comes before Smith, Michelle. Table 12-1 describes basic rules for alphabetic filing. Procedure 12-3 lists steps to follow when using the alphabetic filing system.

Numerical Systems

A numerical filing or patient identification system is used in hospitals and many of the larger clinics. A number is assigned to each patient's medical record. This is generally a six-digit number divided into three sections of two digits each (for example, 05-72-21). Veterans Administration hospitals use the social security number with nine digits.

There are several types of numerical filing, including straight numerical filing, filing by terminal digit, middle digit filing, unit numbering, and serial numbering.

STRAIGHT NUMERICAL FILING The simplest numerical method is the straight numerical filing system in which each record is filed sequentially based on its assigned number. The numbers used in this system begin at 01 and continue upward.

Example:	01	101	886
	02	102	887
	03	103	888
	04	104	889

In this type of system, the file space will become depleted rapidly as new files are added to one section. This requires constant re-shifting of files to make room for the new files.

TERMINAL DIGIT FILING Terminal digit filing, based on the last digits of the ID number, evenly distributes the files within the entire filing system, which eliminates the need for frequent re-shifting of files, providing enough space was designated when the filing system was set up. Filing using terminal digits requires dividing the files into 100 primary sections, starting with 00 and ending with 99. The three sections of numbers assigned to each file are designated as tertiary, secondary, and primary sections respectively. To file a record using this system, find the file section matching the patient's primary digits (21). Within that section, match up the secondary digits (72), and file the record according to the tertiary digits (05).

Example:	05	72	21
	tertiary	secondary	primary

Procedure 12-4 lists steps for using the terminal digit filing system.

Filing a Record Alphabetically

OBJECTIVE: File a patient record in the correct order, using the alphabetical method for filing.

Equipment and Supplies
patient record; alphabetical files

Method

1. Locate medical record files or medical record room.
2. Observe the name on the record to be filed.
3. Records are filed in alphabetic order by last name first, first name, then middle name or initial. Each letter in the name is a separate unit. Locate the set of records containing the same last name as the record to be filed.
4. Within the set of records containing the same last name as the record to be filed, locate the records with the same letter of the first name as the record to be filed.
5. Using the alphabet as a guide, place the record to be filed after the record that comes before it in the alphabet, but before the record that comes after it in the alphabet.
6. A name with only an initial first name is filed before a full name (Brown, H. is filed before Brown, Henry).

7. Hyphenated names are treated as one unit. (Mary Freeman-Smith is indexed as Freemansmith, Mary).
8. Disregard apostrophes (Megan O'Connor is indexed as Oconnor, Megan).
9. Titles and initials are disregarded for filing, but placed in parentheses after the name, for example, Dr. Beth Ann Williams is indexed as Williams, Beth Ann, (Dr.).
10. Married women are indexed using their legal name. The husband's name can be used for cross-referencing.
11. Seniority units, such as Jr. and Sr., are filed in numerical order from first to last.
12. Numeric seniority terms are filed before alphabetic terms.
13. After placing the file between the two records before and after it in the alphabet, check once more to be sure the file is properly placed.
14. If there is a marker or out-guide in place of the removed record, then take out the marker when replacing the file.
15. Document on the office record that the chart was filed (per office policy).

MIDDLE DIGIT FILING Using the same six-digit numbering system as with the terminal digit system, the middle digit filing system places the middle digits as the primary numbers. In this example, find the section marked 72, within that section find the 05 area, then file the record according to the tertiary digit, 21.

Example:	05	72	21
	secondary	primary	tertiary

UNIT NUMBERING This system assigns a number to patients the first time they are seen or admitted to a hospital. All other hospitalizations or hospital visits use the same number. This method requires that all the records be kept at the same location.

SERIAL NUMBERING With a serial numbering system, the patient receives a different medical record number for each hospital visit. The patient acquires multiple records that are stored at different locations. For example, a hospitalization, laboratory work, and a mammogram will all receive different numbers and be filed within their own systems.

The assigned numbers are kept in an accession record in which numbers in sequential order (1, 2, 3, 4, 5, 6 . . .) have a name placed next to them as each new name is entered. This record can also be maintained on the computer. Figure 12-5 illustrates a medical assistant filing in a medical records room.

Subject Matter

Filing by subject is used for general files, such as invoices, correspondence, resumes, and personnel records. This method is adequate as long as the files are relatively small. If these files become large, then another method, alphabetic or numerical, will have to be devised.

Filing a Record Numerically Using the Terminal Digit Filing System

OBJECTIVE: File a patient record in the correct order, using the terminal digit filing method for filing.

Equipment and supplies
patient record; numerical files

Method

1. Locate medical record files or medical record room.
2. Observe the numbers on the record to be filed.
3. Locate the set of files with the same tertiary numbers as the record to be filed (these will be the first 2 numbers on the record).
4. Within the set of records with the same tertiary numbers, locate the row of records with the same secondary numbers as the record to be filed (the secondary numbers are the second 2 numbers on the record).
5. Within the set of records with the same tertiary and secondary numbers as the record to be filed, place the record to be filed in numerical order by primary numbers (last 2 numbers on the record).
6. After placing the file in numerical order by primary numbers, check once more to be sure the file is properly placed.
7. If there is a marker or out-guide in place of the removed record, then take out the marker when replacing the file.
8. Document in the office record that the chart was filed (per office policy).

Color-Coding Systems

To decrease the number of misfiled charts and aid in file retrieval many medical record departments will use a color-coded system on their file folders. This system assigns a color for each number from 0–9. Color bars on the end of each file folder correspond to the medical record number. Usually only the three primary digits are color-coded. When files are in the correct placement, the color bands will all have the same pattern. In this manner, any misfiles are easily seen. Filing records is simplified since the correct color band can be located on the file shelf.

Color Bands

Two popular color-coding methods using a numerical system are the Ames Color File System and the Smead Manufacturing Company's method. Table 12-2 lists examples of the numerical color-coding systems used by these two systems.

There are also color-coded methods using an alphabetic system. One example is the Alpha-Z system by the Smead Manufacturing Company. This system is based on 13 colors using white letters on a colored background (for example, the white letter "A" is on a solid red background) for the first one-half of the alphabet, and the addition of a white stripe on the colored background for the second half of the alphabet (for example, the letter "N" is a red background with a white stripe).

The Alpha-Z system uses file labels to denote the patient's name, and a color label with the letter of the alphabet to indicate the index unit. For example, Emily Jane Smith would be labeled Smith, Emily Jane with an orange color block containing a white stripe and the letter "S." Two other color blocks

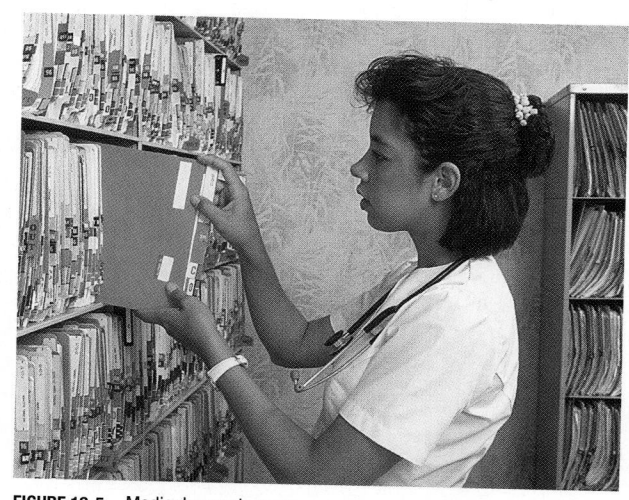

FIGURE 12-5 Medical records room.

TABLE 12-2 Numerical Color-Coding Systems

Ames Color File System	Smead Corporation System
0–red	0–yellow
1–gray	1–blue
2–blue	2–pink
3–orange	3–purple
4–purple	4–orange
5–black	5–brown
6–yellow	6–green
7–brown	7–gray
8–pink	8–red
9–green	9–black

TABLE 12-3 Alpha-Z Alphabetic Color-Coding System

Color	White Letter No Stripe	White Letter White Stripe
Red	A	N
Dark Blue	B	O
Dark Green	C	P
Light Blue	D	Q
Purple	E	R
Orange	F	S
Gray	G	T
Dark Brown	H	U
Pink	I	V
Yellow	J	W
Light Brown	K	X
Lavender	L	Y
Light Green	M	Z

would be added to the label for the secondary and tertiary letters of the index unit (in this example, "E" on a solid purple background, and "J" on a solid yellow background).

This system is ideal for the large practice with many patients having the same surnames. It can be adapted to a particular offices needs. For example, only the last name is color-coded (Joseph Evans has only one solid PURPLE color label). After the files are color-coded, they are then alphabetized within their particular "color" category.

In large practices with several physicians, each physician may have a color assigned to him or her. For example, Dr. Williams' patients might all have medical file folders with a yellow label. This color-coding system is described in Table 12-3. Figure 12-6 shows a color-coded medical record.

In some medical practices, a color-coded "year" tab is placed on folders of patients who are seen once a year. This hastens the purging of "inactive" files.

Cross-Referencing

Due to the large number of files processed in a busy office and the confusion over surnames—(for example, how are step-children's names filed for easy access?), cross-referencing of files is recommended. Cross-referencing refers to alerting the health worker that a file may be found under another name. For example, if Mrs. Henry Watts also uses her maiden name, Farideh Rahman, then a file insert into Henry Watts' file could state, "See Rahman, Farideh for Mrs. Henry Watts." Cross-referencing can be a simple, but useful tool for finding and avoiding "lost" records.

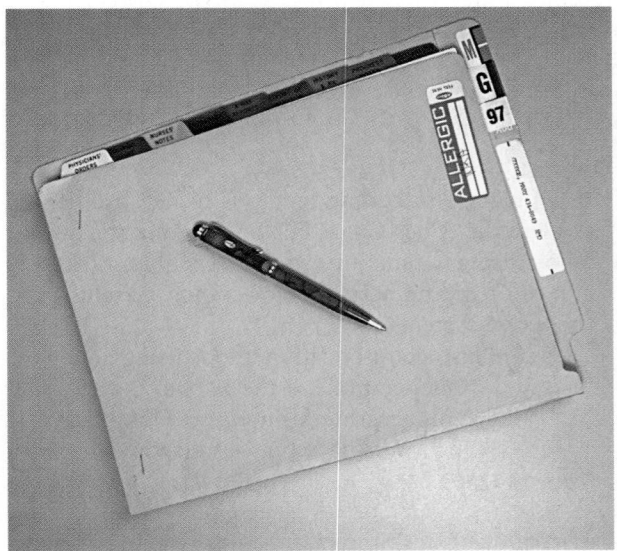

FIGURE 12-6 A color-coded record.

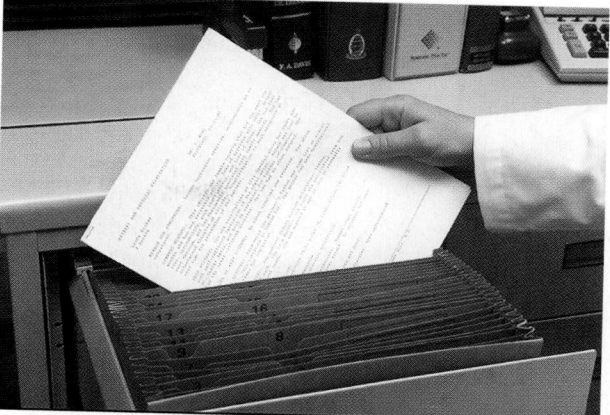

FIGURE 12-7   Tickler file using a file drawer.

Locating Missing Files

One of the most time-consuming and frustrating activities relating to medical records is locating a "missing" file. Ideally, everyone who takes a file from a cabinet should add that file name or number to a master file sheet. In addition, an out-guide should be placed in the file indicating a record was removed.

If a systematic search takes place, the file can usually be located quickly. In the case of one piece of paper that has been misfiled with other papers, it may not be located. In this case, the medical assistant will need to get another copy of the paper from the original source (for example, a laboratory or radiology report).

The best way to avoid losing a file is to file all records methodically and carefully. Guidelines 12-1 lists some ways to help you locate missing files.

Tickler Files

A tickler file is used to remind the medical assistant of an event or action that will take place at a future date. The tickler file contains patient's names and telephone numbers, dates when action or activities should occur, and actions to take. The tickler files should be reviewed on a daily basis so that actions are taken on time. For example, tickler files can be used as reminders to call patients to set appointments, to pay certain invoices, or to send fees for the physician's license renewals. Figure 12-7 is an example of a tickler file, using a file drawer. Figure 12-8 illustrates an index card tickler file.

Quality Assurance for Quality Medical Care

As discussed in Chapter 5, the primary goal of a formal quality assurance program is to improve the quality of care so that there is no difference between what should be done and what is actually being done.

Implementation of such a Quality Assurance Program (QAP) requires the development of patient-centered criteria based on acceptable standards of care. An example of this is the formalization of discharge documents from hospitals.

Incident Report

One means of documenting problem areas within the office or facility is through the incident report. In Chapter 5, an example of a typical incident report is provided. This report should be completed whenever there is an unusual occurrence, such as a fall, error in medication dispensing, needle sticks, fire, or patient complaint. The purpose is to document exactly what happened with the goal of preventing another episode.

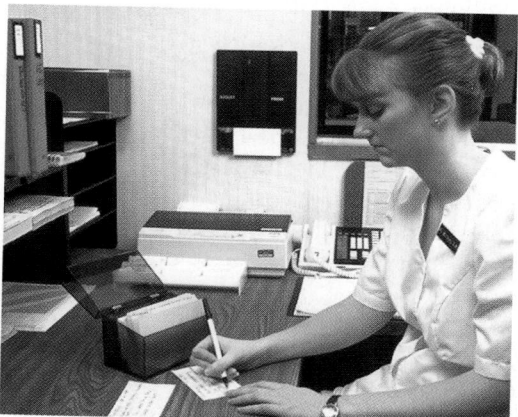

FIGURE 12-8   Index card tickler file.

Details on completing an incident report are usually included in every office's procedure manual.

Measures to Assure Quality Assurance

Quality of patient care can be assessed from within the medical profession by organized groups of physicians. It is also monitored and assessed from outside the profession through governmental or insurance provider intervention.

Joint Commission on Accreditation of Health Organizations (JCAHO)

The Joint Commission on Accreditation of Health Organizations (JCAHO), headquartered in Chicago, Illinois, is a private, nongovernmental agency that establishes guidelines for hospitals and health care agencies to follow regarding quality of care. It is supported by representatives of the American Hospital Association (AHA), American College of Surgeons, American College of Physicians, and the American Dental Association. In addition to forming guidelines for the operation of health care institutions, such as hospitals, ambulatory care facilities, and long-term care institutions, JCAHO conducts surveys and accreditation programs.

JCAHO inspectors visit a health care facility by invitation and review patient medical records, organizations of the medical staff and the general operations of the facility. Some indicators that are used during the survey and accreditation process are mortality rate, frequency of complication, nosocomial infection rate, and autopsy rate. The mortality rate refers to the number of deaths in a given population. Based on their assessment, the inspectors will issue either a full accreditation or provisional accreditation report. The Commission works with facilities to correct any deficiencies within a specified time frame.

JCAHO does not actually have authority or power to take punitive action against a physician or facility for poor treatment. However, the survey results of the JCAHO are used by other agencies, such as the Department of Health and Human Services, that do have the authority to impose a sanction or penalty.

Occupational Safety and Health Administration (OSHA)

The Occupational Safety and Health Administration (OSHA) was established by the U.S. Congress in the Occupational Safety and Health Act of 1970 "to assure so far as possible every working man and woman in the nation safe and healthful working conditions." This act covers every employer whose business affects interstate commerce.

OSHA is the federal agency that has the power to enforce regulations concerning the health and safety of employees. Every office and health care institution must be aware of OSHA recommendations and carefully monitor potential violations. For instance, the Centers for Disease Control (CDC) has issued recommendations for a set of universal precautions that all health care workers must follow when dealing with hazardous materials. The CDC has authorized OSHA to enforce these precautions.

OSHA, in cooperation with other agencies, carries out research to establish basic safety standards. OSHA inspectors carry out frequent, surprise inspections of workplaces to see that standards are maintained. OSHA safety regulations include standards for exposure to noise, asbestos, toxic chemicals, lead, pesticides and cotton dust. Violators of OSHA standards must correct the violations and pay fines if found guilty.

Since July 6, 1992, OSHA standards mandate that all health care employers must provide a means for protecting their employees from potential exposure to Hepatitis B. In fact, every health care employee must be given the choice to elect or refuse the immunization series. If refused, the employee has the right to change his or her mind and receive the immunization series at no charge. All costs associated with this immunization series must be provided by the employer.

HIPAA/Confidentiality of Records

As the demand for both access and confidentiality of medical record information grows, how does the health care provider balance the competing, often clashing, interests? The laws relating to medical recordkeeping and access have been evolving in recent years.

The privacy provisions of the federal law, the Health Insurance Portability and Accountability Act of 1996 (HIPAA), apply to health information created or maintained by health care providers who engage in certain electronic transactions, health plans, and health care clearinghouses. The Department of Health and Human Services (HHS) has issued the regulation, "Standards for Privacy of Individually Identifiable Health Information," applicable to entities covered by HIPAA. The Office for Civil Rights (OCR) is the Departmental component responsible for implementing and enforcing the privacy regulation.

The new rules require medical offices that maintain and transmit health information electronically to do the following.

- Provide reasonable and appropriate safeguards to protect the integrity and confidentiality of health care information.
- Train personnel to protect confidentiality of health care information.
- Provide policies and procedures on security and confidentiality protective measures within the medical office.

Medical information can be shared by a wide range of people, both in and out of the health care industry. Generally, access to medical records is obtained when the patient agrees to let others see them. Occasionally, patient medical information is used for health research and may be disclosed to public health agencies such as the Centers for Disease Control. Specific names are usually not given to researchers. Their use of patient information is covered by HIPAA.

Releasing Medical Records

The physician owns the medical record, but the patient has the legal right of "privileged communication" and access to his or her records. Therefore, the patient must authorize release of his or her records and state in writing that the medical records may be released. An example of a release form is seen in Figure 12-9. Since the patient has access to his or her records, the patient may also request a copy of those records. Since some records are large and require excessive duplicating time and expense, the physician may charge a fee dictated by the state to provide this service.

Health care providers have specific procedures for handling and releasing medical records because of the confidential information contained in the records and because of federal and state laws concerning HIV, mental health, and substance abuse information.

WINDY CITY CLINIC
Beth Williams, M.D.
123 Michigan Avenue
Chicago, IL 60610
(312) 123-1234

RECORDS RELEASE Date ______________

To ______________________________
Doctor

____
Address

I hereby authorize and request you to release

to ______________________________
Doctor

____
Address

all medical records in your possession concerning any examination, diagnosis, and/or treatment rendered to me during the period from __________ to __________

____
Signature of patient or closest relative

____
Relationship

______________________________ ______________________________
Signature of witness Address

FIGURE 12-9 A release form for medical records.

Persons Authorized to Release Records

Generally, only a patient can authorize the release of his or her own medical records. However, there are some exceptions to the rule and generally the following can sign a release:

- Parents of minor children
- Legal guardian
- Agent (someone you select to act on your behalf in a Health Care Power of Attorney)

Under some circumstances, a minor and not the parent must sign the release. If you have questions about who can authorize release of your patient records, check with your health care provider.

Specially Protected Medical Information

Federal law specially protects substance abuse treatment records. Some state laws specially protect HIV/AIDS information and mental health records. These laws are meant to encourage people with these problems to get the medical treatment they need. In order to obtain a copy of the records or have them sent somewhere, you may need to sign a form that specifically mentions this specially protected information.

Disclosure without Consent

Although medical records are confidential, there are times when they can be released without a patient's consent. In special cases, records are released to:

- Health care workers who have a need for the records to care for a patient.
- Qualified people or organizations that perform services, such as data processing, medical record transcription, microfilming, administrative functions, or other such related services.
- Qualified people or organizations for approved research and education functions.
- Certain government authorities, as permitted or required by law, to investigate or regulate health related issues such as child abuse, communicable diseases, and prescription drugs.
- Certain lawyers and parties in a law suit, if a patient's medical condition is an issue in the suit.

Generally, strict rules apply to those who receive medical information. For example, they are often required to have procedures to protect the patient's confidentiality and prevent release of medical information and patient identity.

Storing Medical Records

Medical records may be stored in the medical office, if there is sufficient room, or in another office or building nearby. Or, medical records storage may be outsourced to a business that specializes in managing and housing documents. Investigate the business to ensure that it is reputable and that the files will be safe and accessible. Either way, take steps to ensure that the files will be safe from fire, flood, or other damage (Legal and Ethical Issues).

Confidentiality of medical records must be maintained at all times. The medical record is the legal property of the physician. However, physicians and their staff have a responsibility to treat the medical record with care because it contains documentation of the patient's medical history. Physicians must arrange for storage facilities to keep records of inactive or closed files since they could be needed at a future date for patient care or they could be subpoenaed into court.

Medical Transcription

Medical transcription involves translating dictated or written medical information and producing a permanent record into a typed format. The information can relate to a patient's office or hospital visit, a specific hospital report such as radiology, pathology or laboratory, or a manuscript for publication.

There is an absolute need for accuracy to ensure the correct interpretation when editing the physician's dictation. The same professional standard relating to confidentiality is necessary when handling transcription, even though the transcriptionist may never see the patient.

Medical records must be professionally prepared, following appropriate formats. They should be free of errors and correctly filed. Remember medical records are always subject to possible subpoena by a court of law.

Medical Transcriptionists

Transcriptionists are medical professionals, who have excellent typing and grammar skills, knowledge of medical terminology, and a desire for accuracy. The medical transcriptionist must understand words, where and how to apply the words, as well as have proper English grammar skills. This includes an understanding of etymology, phonetics, synonyms, acronyms, antonyms, homonyms, and eponyms.

Sound-Alike Words

Caution must be used when writing words that have the same or similar sound. When taking medical dictation off a recording device, such as a dictaphone, it can be difficult to discern the term based on the physician's pronunciation. To compound the problem, many medical terms actually sound alike when spoken, but have very different meanings.

Transcriptionists must take special precautions when transcribing tapes to make sure they have heard the correct terms. In many cases, the content of the material will determine which is the correct term. For instance, mastitis, meaning an inflammation of a mammary gland, and mastoiditis, an inflammation of the mastoid bone in the middle ear, sound alike in pronunciation. However, the mammary gland in the female breast and the mastoid bone in the ear are located in different body systems and are not generally discussed in the same context.

There are other terms, such as ureter and urethra, which are organs located in close proximity to each other in the urinary system. These two terms must never be confused. When in doubt, always ask the dictating physician to clarify the term for you. You may have to look up the exact definition of the word in a medical dictionary.

Ownership of the Medical Record

The medical assistant is frequently called upon to explain the ownership of medical records and x-ray films. Patient Education explains more about dealing with patients and medical record issues. Although the

Patient Education

Many patients believe that the medical record is their property since it is a history of their medical care. The medical assistant must be able to explain that the physician owns all the equipment and files in his or her office but that patients have a right to see and have a copy of their medical records. Patients may be confused and distressed if they receive their medical record without any explanation. The physician has the responsibility of explaining the record to the patient and the medical assistant can reinforce this explanation.

patient has paid for the film, it is the property of the medical facility that performed the x-ray. Written reports prepared by the radiologist are sent to other physicians at the request of the patient but the film generally remains in the original office. The reason being, if the film remains in one location, it can always be accessed for future examination and comparison. Once it leaves the originating facility, it can be misplaced and lost.

Physicians are able to loan their films to referring physicians for further examination. The patient has to sign a release of records form for this to take place, but the film must then be returned to the original facility. Since films are a permanent record of the patient at a particular moment, they need to be preserved carefully. It is possible, in some locations, for the patient to obtain a duplicate copy of a film. The patient would have to pay for the copy to be made.

Retention and Destruction of Medical Records

From time to time in a practice, the question will arise, "How long should we keep medical records?" While we don't have definitive answers, we can provide you with the following guidelines:

- The medical record is critical in a medical liability action, and its loss may considerably harm the physician in the defense of a claim.

- To be absolutely safe, all medical records should be retained *forever*. However, in many circumstances this is impractical. It is always a good idea to keep a patient's immunization records in case they need it in the future.

- Each state varies somewhat on the legal time limits (statute of limitations) to keep records and documents. It is usually two years and begins to run at the point of discovery of damage and the connection between that damage and the treatment. In some circumstances, this

could be many years later. Special rules apply when treating a child or an incompetent patient and the time period is longer.

- Most states require all patient records be retained for two to seven years after the last treatment, or seven years after the patient reaches the age of majority (age 18 or 21 in most states), whichever comes last.

- The American Medical Association recommends keeping medical records for 10 years.

- In selected circumstances, you might consider saving the more complex records or those records with known serious patient problems for a longer period of time.

- The bottom line is there is no absolute answer and the medical assistant must be familiar with state laws.

If a physician cannot retain his or her patient records indefinitely, consideration must be given to the method of destruction. As with any office policy, a medical record destruction policy should follow a written procedure. The procedure should do the following:

- Outline the length of time records will be kept.

- Define which records will be kept on-site and which off-site.

- Designate a person to be responsible for deciding what to keep and what to purge.

- Produce a log that details which patient records have been destroyed, as well as when and how.

- Provide a method of disposal (e.g., shred, pulp, or incinerate) that destroys all information in the record. Patient confidentiality cannot be jeopardized because of an inadequate method of destruction. Many medical offices hire the services of a business that handles the destruction of medical records. That service must agree to abide by HIPAA guidelines.

SUMMARY

Handling a patient's medical record requires an efficient system, which results in few missing or misfiled records. As a medical practice grows, it may be necessary to replace an alphabetic system with a numerical or even a color-coded system. Every medical practice needs a method for alerting staff when a file has been removed from the record area. A tickler system that is used faithfully can reduce the number of omissions, such as forgetting to remind the physician to renew a medical license. Medical transcription work can be a rewarding career for a skilled typist as well.

COMPETENCY REVIEW

1. Define and spell the terms to learn for this chapter.
2. Describe where you would find Emma Holmes' file. She has not been seen by Dr. Williams for two years and there has been no communication with her. Is this an active, inactive, or closed file?
3. Set up a tickler file system for your school assignments during this semester.
4. You are missing a file for Sean Roy. Discuss what process you would use to find this file.
5. Mr. Crosby is angry and demanding that you give him his medical chart so that he can take it to another physician. How do you handle Mr. Crosby's anger and his request for his medical file?

PREPARING FOR THE CERTIFICATION EXAM

1. In filing correspondence for Janelle Louise Daniels (Mrs. Kevin Masters), 123 Valley Drive, Kalispell, MT 59999, which of the following would NOT be used as an indexing unit?
   A. Carey
   B. Daniels
   C. Jerome
   D. Masters
   E. ZIP code

2. What is the third indexing unit in the following name: Mr. Richard Allan Richards, Jr.
   A. Richards
   B. Richard
   C. Allan
   D. Jr.
   E. Mr.

3. The most commonly used filing system is based on what method?
   A. numerical
   B. color coding
   C. alphabetical
   D. unit numbering
   E. straight numbering

4. Dr. Gemma Reingold is filed as
   A. Reingold, Dr. Gemma
   B. Dr. Gemma Reingold
   C. Reingold, Gemma
   D. Reingold, Gemma (Dr.)
   E. Ms. Gemma Reingold

5. Maura Fitzpatrick has been assigned the patient ID number 239431. To search for her file, you will look under 94, then 23, then 31. What system are you using?
   A. unit numbering
   B. middle digit filing
   C. terminal digit filing
   D. straight numbering
   E. service numbering

6. Adrian Washington has been assigned a color using the Alpha-Z color-coding system. Under what color would you find his chart?
   A. lavender with white stripe
   B. light brown
   C. dark brown with white stripe
   D. yellow
   E. yellow with white stripe

7. David Jesse Montgomery III's file would be filed in what order in relation to David Jesse Montgomery, Jr.'s file?
   A. before
   B. after
   C. with David Jesse Montgomery, Jr.'s file
   D. the designations III and Jr. are ignored when filing
   E. Jr's are filed separately

8. VRT is an example of (a/an)
   A. phonetic
   B. synonym
   C. acronym
   D. antonym
   E. etymology

continued on next page

9. Transcription equipment includes all of the following EXCEPT
   A. computer
   B. typewriter
   C. transcriber
   D. word processor
   E. shredder

10. A report containing information about the tissue removed during a surgical procedure is called a/an
    A. consultation report
    B. operative note
    C. pathology report
    D. additional report
    E. history report

CRITICAL THINKING

1. How will you handle Mr. Dewey's request and unpaid balance?
2. What will you do about Mr. Dewey's missing x-ray reports?

ON THE JOB

Marissa Lopez is asked to create a patient file and records for a new patient, Jonathan Schmidt. Please walk Marissa through each step of creating a new patient file, making sure that each component of the file is complete. Use the SOAP section of this chapter as part of your solution. Show how the patient's progress will be tracked by using POMR.

INTERNET ACTIVITY

Search the Internet for the newest legislation in your home state regarding the handling of medical records. Write a summary of the article, and discuss with your class whether the legislation adds to the efficiency of dealing with medical records or creates unnecessary obstacles.

MediaLink More on managing medical records, including interactive resources, can be found on the Student CD-ROM accompanying this textbook.

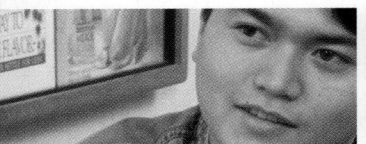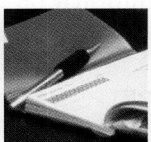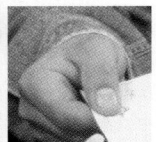

Medical Assistant Role Delineation Chart

HIGHLIGHT indicates material covered in this chapter.

ADMINISTRATIVE

Administrative Procedures

- Perform basic administrative medical assisting functions
- Schedule, coordinate and monitor appointments
- Schedule inpatient/outpatient admissions and procedures
- Understand and apply third-party guidelines
- Obtain reimbursement through accurate claims submission
- Monitor third-party reimbursement
- Understand and adhere to managed care policies and procedures
- *Negotiate managed care contracts*

Practice Finances

- Perform procedural and diagnostic coding
- Apply bookkeeping principles

- Manage accounts receivable
- *Manage accounts payable*
- *Process payroll*
- *Document and maintain accounting and banking records*
- *Develop and maintain fee schedules*
- *Manage renewals of business and professional insurance policies*
- *Manage personnel benefits and maintain records*
- *Perform marketing, financial, and strategic planning*

CLINICAL

Fundamental Principles

- Apply principles of aseptic technique and infection control
- Comply with quality assurance practices
- Screen and follow up patient test results

Diagnostic Orders

- Collect and process specimens
- Perform diagnostic tests

Patient Care

- Adhere to established patient screening procedures
- Obtain patient history and vital signs
- Prepare and maintain examination and treatment areas
- Prepare patient for examinations, procedures and treatments

- Assist with examinations, procedures and treatments
- Prepare and administer medications and immunizations
- Maintain medication and immunization records
- Recognize and respond to emergencies
- Coordinate patient care information with other health care providers
- Initiate IV and administer IV medications with appropriate training and as permitted by state law

GENERAL

Professionalism

- Display a professional manner and image
- Demonstrate initiative and responsibility
- Work as a member of the health care team
- Prioritize and perform multiple tasks
- Adapt to change
- Promote the CMA credential
- Enhance skills through continuing education
- Treat all patients with compassion and empathy
- Promote the practice through positive public relations

Communication Skills

- Recognize and respect cultural diversity
- Adapt communications to individual's ability to understand
- Use professional telephone technique

- Recognize and respond effectively to verbal, nonverbal, and written communications
- Use medical terminology appropriately
- Utilize electronic technology to receive, organize, prioritize and transmit information
- Serve as liaison

Legal Concepts

- Perform within legal and ethical boundaries
- Prepare and maintain medical records
- Document accurately
- Follow employer's established policies dealing with the health care contract
- Implement and maintain federal and state health care legislation and regulations
- Comply with established risk management and safety procedures
- Recognize professional credentialing criteria
- *Develop and maintain personnel, policy and procedure manuals*

Instruction

- Instruct individuals according to their needs
- Explain office policies and procedures
- Teach methods of health promotion and disease prevention
- Locate community resources and disseminate information
- *Develop educational materials*
- *Conduct continuing education activities*

Operational Functions

- Perform inventory of supplies and equipment
- Perform routine maintenance of administrative and clinical equipment
- Apply computer techniques to support office operations
- *Perform personnel management functions*
- *Negotiate leases and prices for equipment and supply contracts*

- *Denotes advanced skills.*

SOURCE: Reprinted by permission of the American Association of Medical Assistants from the AAMA Role Delineation Study: Occupational Analysis of the Medical Assisting Profession.

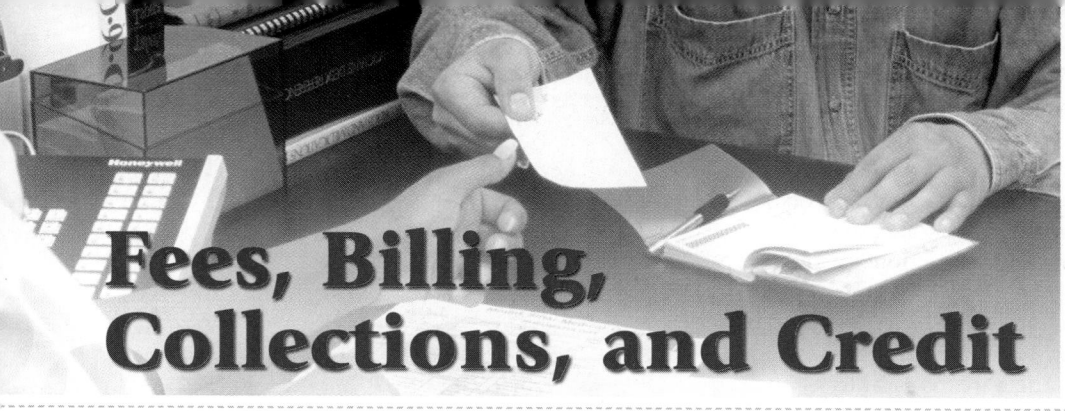

Fees, Billing, Collections, and Credit

Learning Objectives

After completing this chapter, you should be able to:

- Define and spell the terms to learn for this chapter.
- Discuss how fees are determined and be able to discuss this with patients.
- Discuss the patient information required at the time of registration and thereafter to maintain the records needed for billing.

- Discuss credit policy.
- Describe the various billing methods and preparation of billing statements.
- Discuss the collection process and the legalities involved.
- Understand the procedures for aging accounts.

OUTLINE

Professional Fees	228
Billing	229
Credit Policy	231
Collections	232
Accounting Systems	235
Bookkeeping Systems	237
Computerized Systems	243
Professional Courtesy	244

Terms to Learn

accounting	ledger card	superbill
accounts receivable	post	third-party payer
age analysis	professional courtesy (PC)	Truth in Lending Act
assignment of benefits	statute of limitations	usual, customary, and reasonable (UCR)
bookkeeping	subscriber	

Case Study

A NEW PATIENT COMES INTO your office for a new patient evaluation. This patient is a referral from another doctor, and has never been to this office before. The office policy states that any deductibles and co-payments are collected at the time of the patient visit. After submission of the bill to an insurer, the balance owed is billed to the patient, and the patient is expected to pay within 30 days.

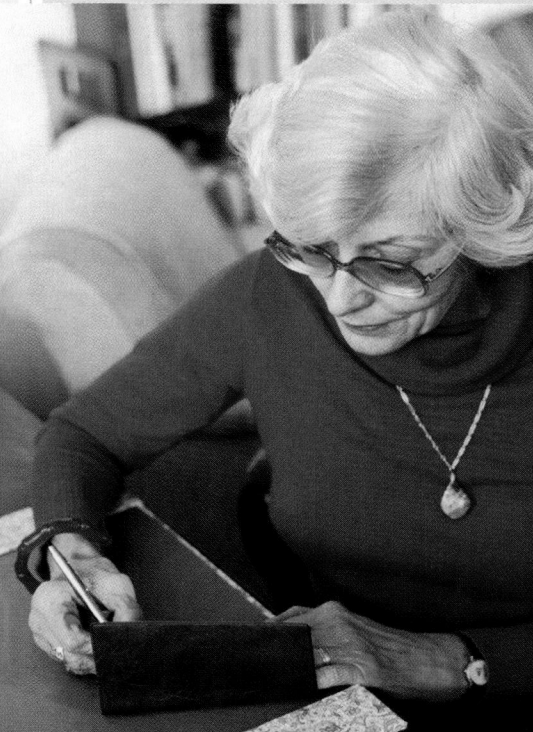

Quality service to the patient is the primary concern of any medical practice. However, revenue is also necessary to maintain a viable business. The process of setting up a fee schedule, extending credit, billing, and collection are an important part of the practice. To ensure and maintain a sound billing and collection system, the medical assistant must be aware of the importance that patients understand their financial responsibility to the doctor and to offer assistance in setting up financial arrangements.

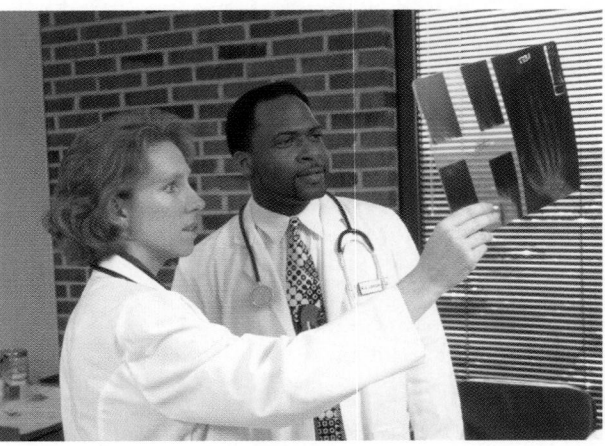

FIGURE 13-1 A physician's services frequently involve consultation with other staff members.

Professional Fees

The fee is determined by the physician or the practice's partners as a result of taking into consideration the time and services involved as well as the prevailing rate fee in the community (Figure 13-1). The economic level of the community and the average fee charged will determine the prevailing rate fee.

Fees charged for medical services are referred to as usual, customary, and reasonable.

- The usual fee is what a physician usually charges for a procedure or service.

- Customary refers to the fee charged for the same procedure by the majority of physicians with the same or similar training to perform the same procedure. This fee is also based on the socioeconomic and geographical area.

- A reasonable fee is what a physician charges for a modified procedure or service that is more difficult and requires more time and effort.

Government sponsored insurance programs maintain a record of the usual charges submitted for specific services by individual doctors. The physician will make the final determination as to what the fees for services will be. It is the medical assistant's responsibility to convey this information to the patient in a positive, responsible manner.

It is necessary to initiate a discussion of fees with patients and inform them of costs, office financial policies, and credit procedures so they can plan for medical expenses. Patients are entitled to an accurate estimate of their obligations. The medical assistant must become comfortable with these discussions. It is suggested to provide all of this information prior to the patient's first visit. This can be accomplished through the initial telephone contact and by providing a hardcopy of the materials via the U.S. Postal Service. A thorough knowledge of the physician's practice and policies will help to handle any misunderstandings, and would minimize collection problems later. Patient Education discusses more on keeping the patient informed to financial matters.

Posted information regarding payment policies and fees helps patients become aware of office procedures. It also encourages discussion of such matters. Some medical offices have a statement displayed addressing the

Patient Education

The patient must have a thorough understanding of office policy with regards to financial matters. The initial visit to the office should include information on fees, payment, and financial arrangements. This can be addressed in a patient information booklet or pamphlet given to the patient. Patients who will require surgical or other medical procedures should be made aware of fees, insurance allowances, and methods of payment. The patient must understand that he or she has the ultimate responsibility for all charges.

The informed patient will have a clear understanding of all obligations to the office and will be more likely to discuss financial arrangements. This mutual understanding helps to minimize the problems of collection for delinquent accounts.

issue of fee policy. For example, a plastic surgeon's statement may include actual fees for services. A typed fee schedule should be available for quick reference. The medical assistant, if instructed by the physician, should be able to quote fees or a range of fees from this schedule. This schedule is approved by the physician and will be updated as needed. Medical offices should post a notification that states "Payment is due on the date of service" in a prominent area for patients to view.

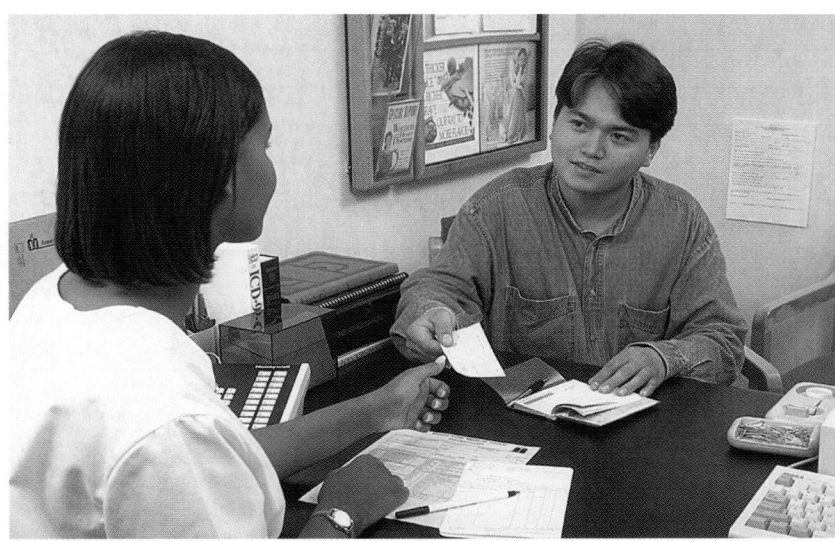

FIGURE 13-2 Payment at the time of medical service is the preferred method.

Billing

Payment of medical services can be achieved in one of three ways. First, there is payment at the time of the services, which is the preferred method (Figure 13-2). The second payment method is billing the patient for services and extending credit. The third, and usually the least desirable, is the use of outside collection assistance.

The medical assistant needs to become familiar with health insurance coverage and the differences in the various plans. As HMOs, IPAs, and PPOs become a major influence in medical practices, the levels of benefits, co-payments, and deductibles are important aspects of the fee and billing process. Patients can become easily confused about these matters, so health care providers and their staff need to be knowledgeable in these areas. See Chapter 15 for an explanation of HMOs, IPAs, and PPOs.

No matter which type of bill service is used in the medical office, each patient must sign a consent form that allows the medical office to bill the insurance carrier for services provided. This form should be placed on file and updated annually. Medicare requires specific wording on consent forms. For the most accurate wording, visit MedLearn at www.cms.gov. Each year the Center for Medicare and Medicaid Services (CMS) distributes a CD to health care providers that contains the updated fee schedule and general information on Medicare payment schedules and payment policies. The CD also provides an immediate gateway to the MedLearn Web site.

Billing Methods

The faster you bill a patient or insurance company, the faster you will receive payment. Billing methods depend on the preferences and policies of the medical office. Billing may be performed internally, generated by the physician's office, or externally, through the use of a billing service. External billing is used with large volume billing. Internal billing can include the use of the superbill, or encounter form, ledger card, and follow-up mailed statements.

Superbill/Encounter Form

The superbill (charge/encounter slip) is the document generated by the medical office and used as a charge slip, statement, and insurance reporting form (Figure 13-3). This document is a two- or three-part carbonized form that performs several functions. It provides a comprehensive list of patient services, with respective codes and fees, on which the physician indicates with a check mark the services that have been rendered. The superbill can be used to input computer information for billing, and it provides the patient with a record of the account activity (charges, payments, adjustments) for the day of service and, thus, can be used as a receipt. It also provides a record that can be used for insurance purposes. The third copy can be kept in the patient's file.

Ledger card

Statements may be handwritten, typewritten, or photocopies of the ledger card. The ledger card is used to record the charges, adjustments, and payments for the patient. The statement must be good quality and large enough to allow itemization of charges. Photocopied statements must be clear and legible and can be sent in a window envelope. Envelopes should be imprinted with ADDRESS CORRECTION REQUESTED under the return address.

Accurate information is absolutely necessary when billing patients. Good records are essential to follow-up with collections. The patient registration form is a

FIGURE 13-3 A superbill has multiple uses.

TEXAS CARDIOLOGY 877 555-1212

Patient Number	Ticket Number	Service Date	Prior Balance	Pat
Patient Name		Gender		Ins
Address		Phone		Other
SSN	Referring Dr.			Total
Primary Insurance Co.	Policy/Group ID			Paymt
Secondary Insurance Co.	Policy/Group ID			Bal Due

Location

X	Code	Service
		New Patient
	99203	Limited/Simple (30m)
	99204	Comprehensive (45m)
	99205	Complex (60m)
		New Patient Consult (Need Referring MD)
	99243	Brief (40m)
	99244	Full Consult (60m)
	99245	Very Complex (80m)
		Established Patient
	99211	Nurse Visit
	99212	Very Brief FU (10m)
	99213	Limited/Simple FU (15m)
	99214	Comprehensive FU (25m)
	99215	Complex FU (40m)
		New Cons. 2nd Opin.
	99274	Moderate 2nd Opinion
	99275	Complex 2nd Opinion
		Home Health
	99375	Home Health 30 days
		Drugs:
	J3420	B-12 Injection
	J1940	Lasix
	90724	Flu (Dx V-04.8)
	G0008	MC Flu Admin Fee
		Misc Rx ___
	90782	IM Injections
	90784	IV Injections
	A4615	O2 Cannula

Cardiologist

X	Code	Service
		Office Procedures
	93000	EKG w/ Interp
	93015	Stress Tread w/ Interp
	93040	Rhythm strip w/ Interp
	93307	2D Echo Compl.
	93320	Doppler Compl.
	93325	Color Flow Compl.
	93308	2D Echo F/U
	93321	Doppler F/U
	ES	Stress Echo
	BUB	Echo/Bubble/Doppler
		Event Monitor
	93268	Loop- Non MC
	G0005	Loop - Hookup - MC
	G0007	Loop - Interp - MC
	93012	Chest Plate Tech - Non MC
	93014	Chest Pl - Interp Non MC
	G0016	Chest Pl - Interp MC
		Holter Monitor
	93224	Holter w/ Interp Global
		Other
	92960	Cardioversion
	93734	Pacer Eval - Single
	93735	Pacer Eval - Sngl w/ Prg
	93731	Pacer Eval - Dual
	93732	Pacer Eval - Dual w/ Prg
	99499	Review outside records
	99080	Special Reports

X	Code	Service
		Diagnostic w/o Interp (Technical only)
	93005	EKG
	93017	Stress Tread
	93225	Holter Hookup
	93226	Holter Scan
	93307-TC	2D Echo
	93320-TC	Doppler Compl.
	93325-TC	Color Flow
	93308-TC	2D Echo F/U
	93321-TC	Doppler F/U
	93880-TC	Carotid Doppler
	Phys	**Interpretation**-Supervision, Interpretation & Report Only
	93010	EKG Interp & Reortt only
	TR	Regular Stress Test-S, I & R
	NU	Nuclear Stress Test–S, I & R
	ES-26	Stress Echocardiogram–S, I & R
	307	Echocardiogram 2-D
	320-26	Doppler Echocardiogram
	325-26	Color Flow
	308	Echocardiogram 2-D F/U
	321-26	Doppler F/U
	227	Holter Monitor - I & R only
	71250-26	UltraFast CT
	XXXXX	**LAB ORDERED** (see attached sheet)
	36415	VeniPuncture (non MC)
	99000	Specimen Collection (Lab)

Next Appointment: Return in: ___ (Wks) (Mo) (Yr)

BI:

Hospital Admission:
- ☐ Admit Cath
- ☐ Admit to _____ unit at:
- ☐ BAP ☐ WMC ☐ CMC ☐ SHMC
- ☐ Other: _____

Before next appointment:
- ☐ Ekg ☐ Echo ☐ Doppler ☐ CXR ☐ Event Monitor
- ☐ TM ☐ Stress Echo ☐ CFD ☐ Holter ☐ Lab

Notes:

Cardiac Diagnoses

good way to establish an information base. The following information is needed to maintain a current billing file for each patient and should be included on the registration form:

Full name of patient (If the patient is a minor, then the full name and address of the parent or guardian is also needed)

Date of birth

Address (residence and mailing address, do NOT accept a post office box only)

Telephone number (home, work, and cell phone)

Occupation and employer (employer's address and telephone number)

Nearest relative (address and telephone number)

Insurance information (company name, address, and telephone number)

Designated insurance identification number and group number

Driver's license number

If the patient and the subscriber, or the person who holds the insurance policy, are the same, this information is taken only once. If the patient is covered under a policy held by another family member (the subscriber), then the complete information is taken from the subscriber. Patient billing information should be updated every six months to one year by having patients fill out new forms.

Once the account has been set up, the medical assistant must be made aware of any changes in information. Patients should be reminded at each visit of the need to inform the office of any changes in information with particular attention to changes of address, telephone number, employer, and insurance information. A notice can be posted at the reception desk as a reminder to patients. The receptionist should also ask if the patient has any changes in information at the time the patient checks in.

Manual Billing

Manual billing was used by physician offices prior to the use of computerized billing. The bookkeeping system was all manual and all billing was generated by the office. Most medical offices have converted to computerized billing because it is more cost effective and efficient. Lifespan Considerations addresses employees that may not be computer-prepared.

Computerized Billing

Computer software is available for internal billing purposes; however, many offices with regular, monthly,

Lifespan Considerations

Since in recent years the medical office has become computerized, many older employees may not be computer-prepared. The office should provide training for these individuals so they can be a productive part of the team.

large-volume billing utilize outside computerized billing services. Many different computer programs exist and can be custom designed for the needs of the office (Figure 13-4). Database programs will include patient information, procedure and diagnosis codes, and insurance companies. Options are available to print statements, ledgers, and receipts. Professionalism has more on privacy of patient information stored on the computer.

The Billing Period: Frequency of Billing

Consistency with billing procedures is very important. The medical assistant must have a thorough understanding of office policy with regards to the timing of billing. When a billing date for an account has been established, it is extremely important not to vary the timing of the mailing statements.

There are two types of billing: once-a-month billing and cycle billing. Once-a-month billing requires that statements leave the office in time to reach the patient no later than the last day of the month. Cycle billing requires that certain portions of the accounts receivable are billed at given times during the month. For example, patients whose names begin with A-F would be billed on the first of the month, G-L on the seventh, and so on. The advantages of cycle billing over once-a-month billing are: the avoidance of once-a-month work overload, and stabilization of cash flow. The medical assistant can handle routine duties each day with the inclusion of statements, rather than intensive billing responsibilities once a month. By spacing the billing periods, more time can be given to each statement.

Patients must be made aware of the timing of billing statements. If a change is made, patients should be notified. This can be done by enclosing a notice of billing policy changes in each statement, two months prior to the change.

Billing Third-Party Payers and Minors

Third-party payers include a party or person other than the patient, such as an insurance company, who assumes responsibility for paying the patient's bill. Patient registration should include information regarding insurance. Patients should be asked to provide all insurance identification cards and copies should be made and kept in the patient's file.

A signed assignment of benefits form, can be used by the office to ensure that insurance payments are made directly to the physician. Legal and Ethical Issues has more on privacy policies and patients' rights.

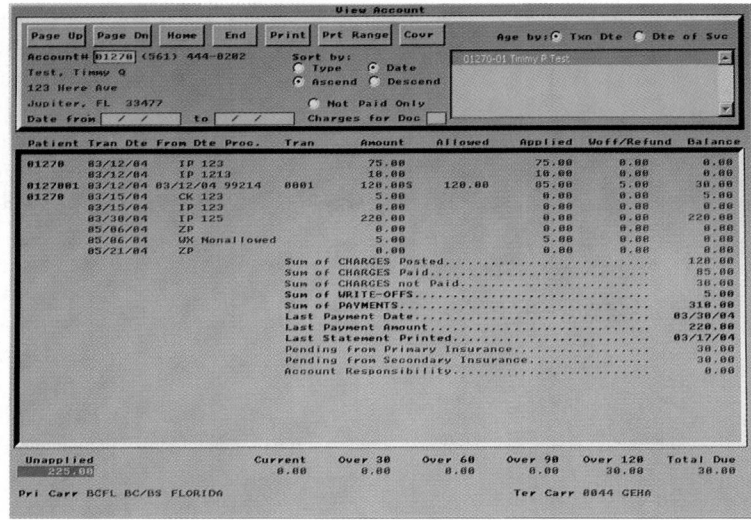

FIGURE 13-4 Computer programs can be customized to meet the medical office billing needs.

Bills for minors are addressed to parents or legal guardians (Figure 13-5). Minors are not responsible for bills unless they are declared emancipated. The parent or the subscriber to the primary insurance policy who brings the child for treatment is responsible for payment. Financial agreements between divorced or separated parents is the personal business of the parents. However, if documentation exists in the minor's file as to financial responsibility, then that party should be billed.

Credit Policy

Payment at the time of service is the ideal method of collection. The medical assistants at the front desk need to overcome any inhibitions regarding discussion of fees and payments. Patients can be informed when they call to schedule an appointment of office policies regarding payment. This is the first step in the collections process. Patients not prepared to pay at the time of service should receive a billing statement

Professionalism

Personal information about patients that is stored in the computer or on disks is just as private as information that is stored in paper files, and should be treated as such. Never allow the computer screen to be turned so that anyone but the operator can see it. Never leave the computer, even for a short time, without logging out and removing all patient information from the screen.

when they leave the office with a request to send payment immediately.

The medical assistant must find out the policies the physician wants administered and consistently and fairly maintain them. A credit policy is an important part of any accounts receivable system.

Often payment is collected upon completion of the service. When payment is deferred, credit arrangements must be made. This is best done during the patient's initial visit. All necessary information should be gathered from the patient with regard to demographics, insurance, employment, and signatures.

The medical assistant must have an understanding of the federal laws affecting credit. One of the most important is Regulation Z of the Truth in Lending Act (formerly the Consumer Protection Act of 1968) that was

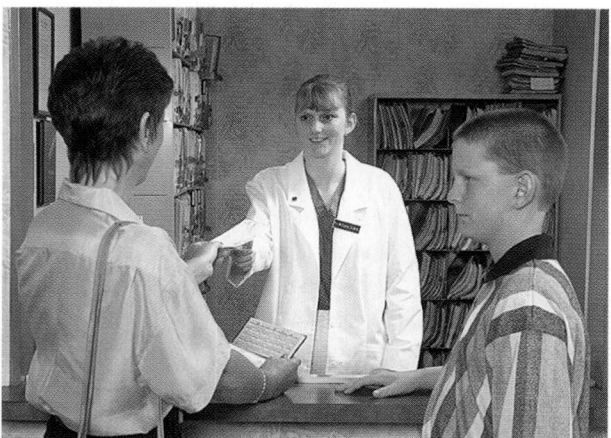

FIGURE 13-5 A parent or legal guardian is responsible for a minor's medical bills.

enacted to protect the consumer. This is an agreement between doctor and patient to accept payment in more than four installments. Under this act the physician must provide disclosure of information regarding finance charges. When there are to be no finance charges, the agreement form should be completed stating this fact. The original form is given to the patient and a copy is retained by the doctor. The disclosure must be very specific and the patient must sign it in the medical assistant's presence.

Credit bureaus operate as sources of credit data on individuals. Many of them specialize in medical and dental collections. They may supply data verifying a patient's employment, residence, and payment history. The medical office needs to be sure that it is working with a reputable credit bureau.

Collections

Every medical office should have a collection policy in place, as it is not advantageous to the office to have a haphazard method for collecting overdue accounts. The medical assistant must understand the collection policy of the medical practice and must administer it consistently and fairly according to the physician's directives. Most practices have a collection process in place that allows for timely and effective collections. Guidelines 13-1 are useful in creating and maintaining positive collection procedures.

Collection Process

Accounts that are extremely overdue become very difficult and costly to collect. Patients need to be educated on billing and collection procedures so that there is a clear understanding of the financial expectations. The patient information booklet given to new patients should have a section outlining office policy regarding billing and col-

---

13-1 GUIDELINES

Collections

- Seek immediate payment.
- Use charge slips or superbills.
- Secure accurate patient information and update as needed.
- Inform patient at the time of the appointment of possible fees and responsibility.
- Outline all fees and finance charges for the patient.
- Confirm third party responsibility.
- Bill consistently following office policy.
- Institute collection procedures as needed with personal interview, telephone calls, and letters.
- Follow up on all commitments by the patient.

lection. This information may be also distributed in a formal financial policy document. Patients need to be encouraged to openly discuss problems or questions they might have with respect to their bills.

The reasons a bill is outstanding will vary. Some reasons are:

- The patient does not feel that the bill is important.
- The patient is unable to pay (for varying reasons).
- The patient has a misunderstanding about the fee.

The medical assistant must determine, in a timely manner, the reason that payments are overdue in order to address it, and continue with the collection process. When all normal collection efforts are exhausted and the account is slated for collection, the medical office can consider a "written off" policy for a designated predetermined amount that may be forgiven and becomes lost revenue. This is only considered when the cost of the collection efforts is greater than the designated predetermined amount. For example if the patient's bill is $80.00 and the cost of collection efforts exceeds $80.00, there would be an office policy and procedure in the office manual stating the specific threshold amount for collection services.

Delinquent Accounts

Failure to collect delinquent accounts affects the medical practice in many ways. Patients who owe money may stay away from the office out of embarrassment due to their financial situation. Failure to collect delinquent accounts may imply guilt on the part of the physician as to the quality of care that the patient received. Ultimately, failure to collect delinquent accounts burdens the entire practice due to lost revenue.

Aging Accounts Receivable

It is extremely important to age all accounts receivable. Age analysis refers to the process of determining how long an account has been past due, and then instituting the necessary collection procedures. Computerized systems will allow the medical assistant to print out an aging report with a 30-day, 60-day, and 90-day and over analysis. This can be used to determine the next collection step. Manual systems may use a coding system to age accounts with various colors or flags to indicate the different ages. These may be attached directly to the patient's ledger card.

Collection Techniques

The medical office may employ several methods of collection. Reminder notices, telephone calls, collection letters, and finally a collection agency may be used. The physician decides office policy regarding collection of overdue payments; the medical assistant has responsibility to carry out the policy consistently and fairly.

A personal interview can be a very effective collection method. The patient who is seen in the office for an appointment and has an outstanding account is readily available for discussion with the office staff. This is the time to tactfully bring attention to the overdue account and to make arrangements with the patient for payment.

Reminder notices can be placed on bills when mailed to patients asking for their prompt attention to a past due bill. Other reminder notices may ask a patient to contact the office if there is a question about the past due bill. When no payment or contact is made, then a reminder letter is sent. It should not be a form letter but rather an individual letter that lets the patient know that his or her account is being reviewed and there is concern as to the unpaid debt. Tactful, professional telephone calls may also become part of the collection process and sometimes can be more effective than the letter. The last option may be the use of a collection agency when all other attempts at collection have failed.

Regulations

There are some general rules to follow when attempting to collect overdue accounts and there are laws that govern issues regarding collection such as the Fair Debt Collection Practices Act. Office staff involved with billing and collections need to be familiar with their particular state laws when applying collection techniques. Guidelines 13-2 provide basic rules to assist in the task of making collections.

| 13-2 | GUIDELINES |

Making Collections

- Never threaten an action that you do not intend to take. For example, do not tell the patient that his or her account will be handed over to a collection agency if full payment is not received by this afternoon.
- Do not make a collection telephone call before 8 A.M. or after 9 P.M., and do not call on Sundays and holidays.
- Do not make a collection call to the patient's workplace.
- Carefully identify the person accepting the telephone call. Do not discuss a delinquent account with anyone except the debtor.
- Never raise your voice, use profane language, or show anger in any way.
- Do not misrepresent yourself, by implying you are someone other than who you are.
- Do not charge interest unless the debtor has agreed to make 4 (or more) installment payments at a particular rate of interest.
- Do not harass or intimidate the debtor.

As previously stated, violation of these rules could be an offense under the Fair Debt Collection Practices Act, which is a federal law that protects debtors from harassment.

It is important not to make threatening statements that will not be pursued. Collection telephone calls must be between the hours of 8 A.M. and 9 P.M. Avoid calling debtors at their place of employment. Never use a postcard or put an overdue notice on the outside of an envelope.

Telephone Collections

A telephone call at the right time and in the right manner can be more effective than a letter. The medical assistant must be sure to make the call tactful, brief, and to the point. Make sure that all conversation is with the debtor. A firm commitment to make payment should be obtained before ending the conversation. If there is no result by the date mutually agreed upon, then the next step in the collection process must be instituted. When calling and finding the debtor is not available, only a message should be left stating that the individual needs to contact the office.

Collection Letters

The personalized letter has many advantages over the form letter. Patients who receive the personalized letter will feel that their account has been reviewed individually rather than just another form letter that has been sent to every patient with an overdue balance. The letter may be inserted with the statement. The letter should inquire why the bill has not been paid. There should be an offer to assist the patient with making payment arrangements. The letter must convey the message that action will be taken to resolve the payment obligation. Figure 13-6 provides an example of a reminder letter.

Special Problems

Even with the best billing and collection system, problems will arise making collection a challenge for the medical assistant. A "skip" is a collection problem that requires immediate action because this individual has a balance due and has moved without leaving a forwarding address. The greater the amount of time it takes to locate the "skip," the less likely you will receive payment. Skips can be traced by checking the registration form to confirm addresses, calling telephone numbers, and calling references without divulging the nature of the call. "Address Correction Requested" on the returned statement envelope may help to get the patient's statement delivered. The post office may charge a fee for "Address Correction Requested," but it is a sound investment nonetheless.

Bankruptcy

A patient who files for bankruptcy is protected by the court. When notice is received of a patient's bankruptcy, all collection attempts must cease and the medical office must file a claim for payment with the courts.

Claims against Estates

When a patient dies, a bill should be sent to the estate of the deceased. Contacting next of kin will provide

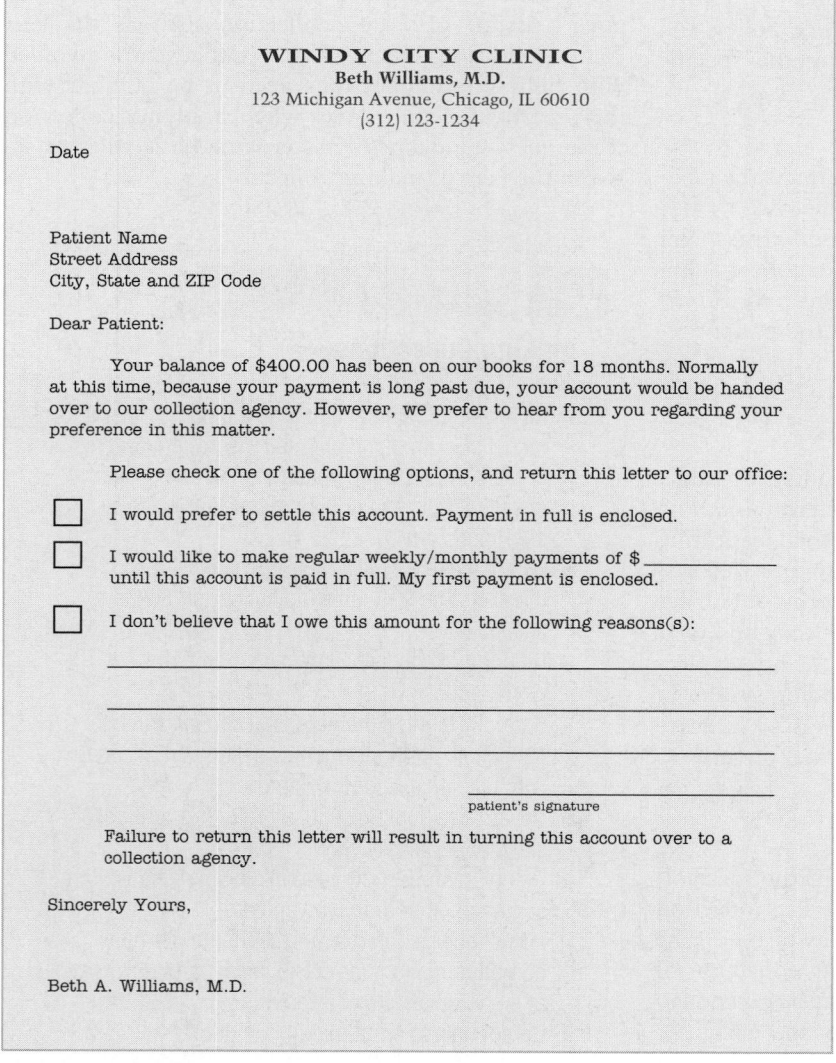

FIGURE 13-6 A reminder letter.

information regarding who is the administrator of the estate. It is important to follow up with the collection of bills to prevent any impression of physician's fault for medical care of the deceased patient.

Statute of Limitations

Statute of limitations refers to the amount of time a legal collection suit may be brought against a debtor. This will vary state to state and should be verified with state agencies. If you have aging accounts that are more than three years old, you should investigate the statute of limitations in your state before spending time, effort, and money to collect the debt.

Using a Collection Agency

Professional collection agencies are available for use when all other collection attempts fail. Be sure to review the account with the physician before turning it over for collection. The collection agency should be chosen carefully. Reputable agencies will have references that can be checked and will readily discuss their collection methods. Further checks can be done with the Better Business Bureau and national credit agencies. If possible, interview the collection agency prior to choosing one. The agency should be professional and willing to discuss collection procedures with you.

Collection agencies charge for their services either by a flat fee per account or a percentage of the amount collected. In either case, the physician's office needs to be aware of the costs involved when using this method to collect past due accounts. Be certain not to include the patient's diagnosis when turning over an account for collection. This is a violation of the patient's privacy and the HIPAA guidelines.

Once the patient is told his or her account is going to a collection agency, it must, by law, be turned over to collection. After the account has been turned over, no further collection attempts can be made by the physician's office. The collection agency will need copies of patient information, such as itemized statements showing the dates and amounts of all transactions. Again do not include the patient diagnosis. If the patient should contact the office after the account has been turned over for collection, the patient should be referred to the collection agency.

Accounting Systems

Accounting is the system of reporting the financial results of a business. The basis of accounting is the ability to make an analysis, statement, or summary about financial matters. Many physicians hire an accountant or accounting service to prepare tax returns and prepare financial statements that are used to obtain bank financing. If the physician is in a partnership with other physicians, the accountant's financial statements will assist in dividing the earnings among the partners. Providing accurate financial records to the accountant is one of the medical assistant's responsibilities.

Bookkeeping is the process of managing the accounts for a business. Bookkeeping is a continual process and should be done on a daily basis. The medical assistant or office manager may assume this duty, or the medical practice could hire a bookkeeper. All receipts and charges should be entered immediately into a daily journal, day sheet, or record. Receipts, in duplicate, must be written for all money received. One copy is given to the patient and one copy stays in the office file.

Bookkeeping is a precise skill requiring great attention to detail. Most offices use computer software for bookkeeping. However, the manual method is still used in some smaller offices. Guidelines 13-3 for manual bookkeeping provided here or those followed in your office offer sound, basic rules for the beginning or practiced bookkeeper. Preparing for Externship has more on bookkeeping and computer skills in a medical office.

13-3 GUIDELINES

Manual Bookkeeping

- Use a black pen and clear penmanship. Do not use pencil.
- Keep the columns straight with decimal points lined up.
- Check all arithmetic carefully for errors, such as misplaced decimal points or errors in adding and subtracting.
- Do not erase, write over, or use opaque correction fluid. Make all corrections by drawing a straight line through the incorrect figure and writing the correct figure above it.
- Try to work in a quiet place each day without interruptions. Bookkeeping should not be done at the front desk while answering the telephone and greeting patients.
- Pay close attention to detail.
- Form all numbers carefully to avoid errors in calculations. Use care to avoid transposing numbers (for example: 79 instead of 97).
- Always find errors as soon as they appear. Do not carry the error forward in the account books.
- Double check every entry.
- Do not discuss patient financial records with other staff members. They are confidential.

Preparing for
Externship

Before going into the externship, *every medical assistant student should be able to stroke at least 35 words per minute. This should be the minimum, and more is better. Accuracy is of paramount importance. In addition, a basic mathematics or bookkeeping course is extremely helpful, if only for learning the basic language. A course in basic computer operation is also necessary.*

Patient Accounts

The medical office is unique as a business because its services are not always paid for at the time of delivery, as would be the case in a business such as retailing. Patient accounts require careful bookkeeping. The bookkeeper or medical assistant must be sure that when insurance payments are received, they are correctly posted, or recorded, ensuring that patient's statements are accurate, and that the physician receives payments for services rendered. Most medical offices are run on a "cash" basis, which means that the charge for a medical service is entered in the financial records as income only when the payment is received. Many businesses, such as retailers and merchants, use the accrual basis of accounting for income, which enters income when the service is rendered, even if a payment has not been received. For an example of the components of a manual patient billing system, see Figure 13-7.

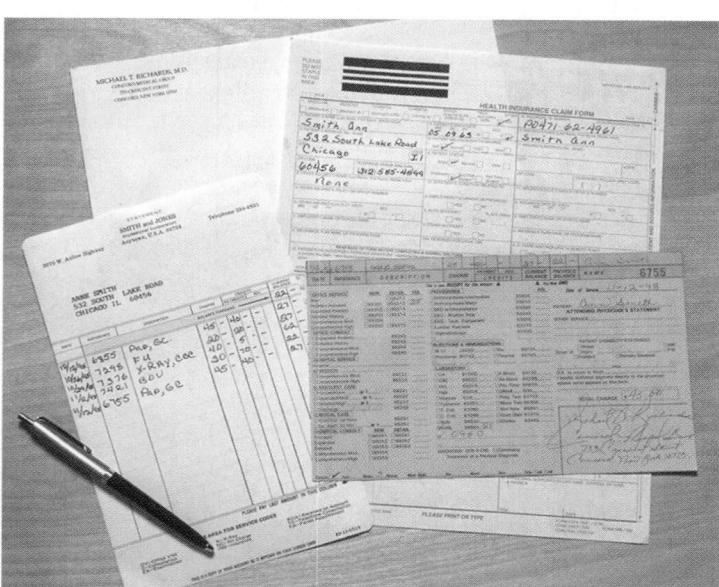

FIGURE 13-7 Components of the manual billing system.

The physician needs to be paid for the procedures done in the office. The medical assistant may need to ensure that patient accounts are in balance with financial obligations (See Procedure 13-1).

Accounts Receivable

Money owed to the physician is called accounts receivable. The accounts receivable ledger is a journal containing a record of all patients' accounts. Terms that relate to accounts receivable are:

- Credit—indicates that a payment has been received on an account or money paid. To credit an account means to record a payment to the account. A patient has a credit balance when a payment exceeds a charge.
- Debit—indicates that a charge has been entered into the account or money owed. To debit an account means to subtract from that account. In some methods of bookkeeping, debits are entered in red. If the balance of the account is negative (a debit balance), this can be indicated by placing the total in red ink or in brackets. A physician's practice usually operates with a debit balance since the total charges to patients exceed the amount paid by all the patients due to the lag time in payment from insurers and others.
- Adjustment—indicates entering a change into the account record such as a discount, write-off, or an amount not allowed by an insurance company (disallowance). A discount is entered as a credit since this amount will be subtracted from the total amount owed.
- Balance—indicates the difference between the debit (money owed) and the credit (money paid).

Accounts Receivable Insurance

Accounts receivable insurance may be purchased to protect against accounts receivable loss. The accounts receivable balance is reported each month and ledgers are kept in a secure place within the office.

Accounts Payable

Accounts payable are the amounts the physician owes to others for equipment and services that have not yet been paid. Examples of accounts payable expenditures in a medical office are:

- Office supplies, such as paper goods, day sheets, appointment cards, scheduling books.
- Medical supplies and equipment.
- Equipment repair and maintenance including housekeeping.
- Utilities such as telephone and electric.
- Taxes.
- Payroll.
- Rent.

PROCEDURE

Perform Accounts Receivable

OBJECTIVE: Demonstrate skills to ensure that patient accounts are in balance and financial obligations are met in a timely manner.

Equipment and Supplies
data; computer or ledger; telephone

Method
1. Review the accounts receivable account aging.
2. Determine if third party (insurance) payments have been received and posted to the patient accounts being reviewed.
3. Contact insurance carriers to resolve any outstanding payments, according to the facility policies.

4. Update patient account with appropriate notes.

Charting Example

Contacted Marty Shapiro at United Healthcare. He stated that check for $169 for services rendered to patient was sent on December 12, 2005. Have placed notice in tickler file to call again next week.

Records relating to accounts payable include the purchase orders, packing slips that come with the delivered goods, and the invoice requesting payment. The medical assistant, or bookkeeper, who is handling accounts payable payments must carefully document the payment made on the check stub and place the check number and date paid onto the retained invoice copy.

Bookkeeping Systems

Most medical practices today use computerized bookkeeping rather than manual. Manual bookkeeping, however, is still used in many offices where you may

work. Manual bookkeeping means that an item is entered by hand and is calculated using a hand calculator. Computerized bookkeeping is most often utilized by medical practices for efficiency and accuracy. Many software programs are available for this purpose. Medical practices use two basic types of bookkeeping systems: single-entry and double-entry. The following are examples of manual bookkeeping.

Single-Entry Bookkeeping

In a single-entry system, the bookkeeper or medical assistant records all financial transactions into the bookkeeping system just once. He or she makes a single-entry. This is a simple system to learn, inexpensive, and requires only three key records:

- Journal, or day sheet, which is also called the daily journal, or log.
- The cash payment journal. (See Figure 13-8 for an illustration of one type of cash payment record—the checkbook and stubs.)
- The accounts receivable ledger contains a record of the money owed to the physician.

Some offices will also have a journal for payroll records and petty cash (Figure 13-9). Petty cash vouchers are used to identify petty cash expenses (Figure 13-10).

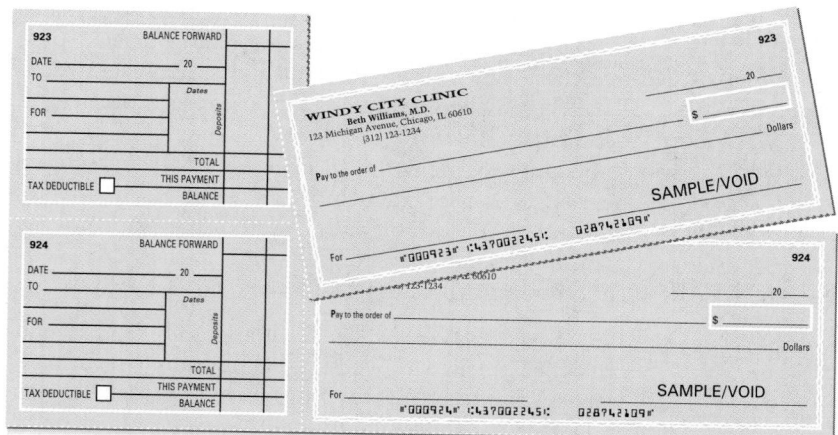

FIGURE 13-8 Cashbook and stubs are cash payment records.

Number	Date	Description	Amount	Office Expenses	Car	Misc.	Balance
	6-1	Fund established					75.00
1	6-2	Postage due	1.42	1.42			73.58
2	6-8	Taxi — (2)	8.00		8.00		65.58
3	6-10	Delivery charge	3.98			3.98	61.60
4	6-25	Supplies	11.62	11.62			49.98
		Total	25.02	13.04	8.00	3.98	
	7-1	Balance 49.98					
	ck #	790 25.02					
		75.00					

FIGURE 13-9 Petty cash record.

Double-Entry Bookkeeping

In double-entry bookkeeping, a financial transaction is recorded in two different places. This system is inexpensive but requires a trained bookkeeper.

The "double-entry" forces a balance since all accounting procedures require two entries to keep the accounting records in balance. For example, when a patient pays an outstanding bill, cash is recorded as an asset, and the receivable, which was the money owed or an asset, is eliminated.

Accounting is based on the premise that the assets of the business, less the liabilities of the business, equal the net worth of that business. This is expressed by the standard accounting formula: Assets = Liabilities + Net Worth. The double-entry system assures that the accounts are in balance.

Assets include everything owned by the medical practice such as cash, bank accounts, money owed to the physician, equipment, and real estate. Liabilities are money the medical practice owes to its creditors such as money owed for medical supplies to a vendor (supplier).

The Pegboard System (Write-It-Once System)

The Pegboard system is an old system that is rarely used. Computer software has replaced this style of bookkeeping in most physician offices, but a few offices may still utilize this system.

Amount $ 8.00   No. 2

RECEIVED OF PETTY CASH

June 8 20 08

For Dr. Williams — taxi

Charge to Medical Conference

Approved by B.F.F.

Received by Mary King

FIGURE 13-10 A petty cash voucher.

The pegboard system is used to document patient bills and payments. This system is also called the write-it-once method because a system of interrelated forms are placed onto the pegboard and used with the same master day sheet. It is an efficient system because the same data is entered on all the forms at one time. The pegboard system is inexpensive as long as all employees are trained in its use. However, be aware that the forms manufactured by one company are usually not compatible with forms from another company.

The actual pegboard is a firm-backed board that contains pegs along the left-hand side. These pegs hold the perforated edges of a day sheet (same as a daily journal) firmly onto the pegboard. Other forms can be held firmly by the pegs so when posting is done, the form, such as a superbill, will not slip.

Required Pegboard System Forms

There are four components of the pegboard system. These are

- Day sheets
- Ledger cards
- Superbill (charge/encounter slips)
- Receipt forms

These forms have a carbon ribbon attached or are on special paper which will permit entering charges, payments, and adjustments onto the master day sheet, the charge slip (superbill), and the patient's ledger card at the same time.

DAY SHEETS The day sheet component of the pegboard system is used to list or post each day's financial transactions: charges, payments, adjustments, and credits. The day sheet, one for each day of the month, must be balanced at the end of each day. The balance from the previous day is carried over to the present day's day sheet as part of the balancing process. In a large or busy practice, there may be more than one day sheet generated per day. The day sheet contains five basic sections that are described in Table 13-1.

See Figure 13-11 for an example of the accounting pegboard system. Remember that the pegboard system, using the double entry system based on the accounting equation, requires that each side of the equation must be balanced.

LEDGER CARDS Ledger cards are rarely used in modern office practice; however, it is important for the medical assistant to be aware of this form of record keeping.

Ledger cards are maintained for each patient or for a family as a whole. These provide a record of all

TABLE 13-1 Day Sheet Sections

Section	Description
Section 1	The individual transaction, such as patient charges, are posted in this column. The ledger card, charge slip, and receipt forms are used when posting in this row/column. Included in this column are: ■ Patient name ■ Description of transaction ■ Charges and credits ■ Previous and current balances
Section 2	This is the deposit portion of the day sheet. Some forms actually include a detachable slip that can be used as a deposit slip into a bank account. A payment made by the patient would also be listed under the appropriate right-hand column (cash, check, insurance).
Section 3	This is an optional column and depends on the needs of the practice. For example, it can be used to break down the type of service that was provided (office visit, office surgery, hospital visit).
Section 4	This is the totals column/row. Each of the columns feedings into the bottom section is totaled at the end of the day.
Section 5	This section is critical in checking that the accounts balance. It also keeps track of the cumulative accounts receivable figure owed by all the patients. This column is useful in determining how much money is still owed to the physician by looking at just one number.

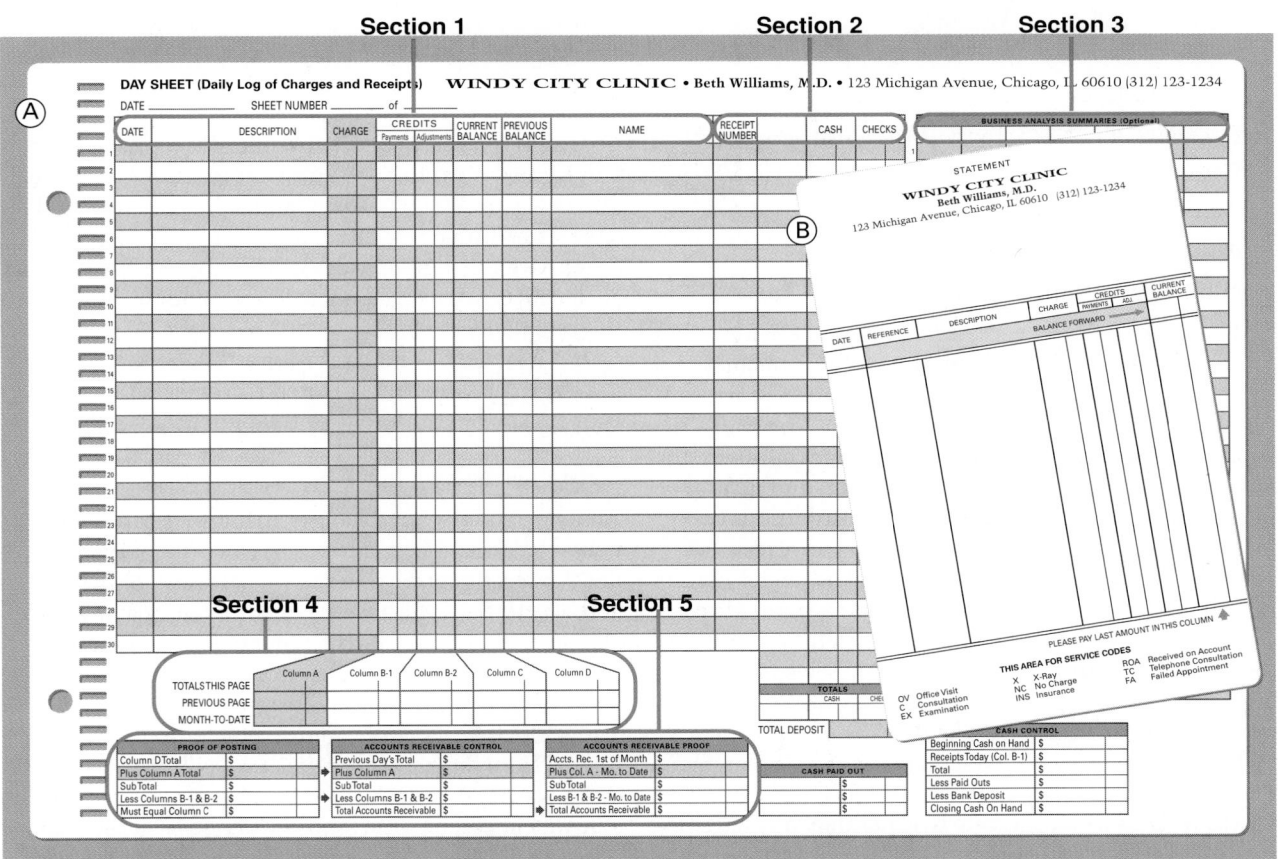

FIGURE 13-11 An accounting pegboard system showing: (A) a day sheet; and (B) a ledger card.

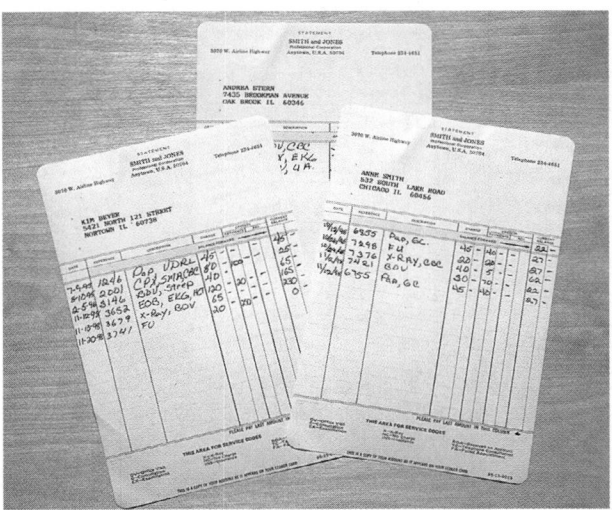

FIGURE 13-12 Examples of ledger cards.

services and charges pertaining to the patient and his or her family and can also be used as statements (Figure 13-12). The ledger card will contain all the charges for the entire family being seen by the physician. The correct charge for each individual family member must be placed next to the appropriate name so that insurance billings can be made correctly. The front of the ledger card will contain:

Name of patient

Mailing address

Description of the activity (office visit, post-op visit, prenatal visit)

Amount of the charge or payment

Adjustment(s), if any apply

Total balance due by that patient or family

The back of the ledger card includes space for information regarding the collection process. This includes the name, address, and telephone number of the employer of the person responsible for the bill, the spouse's name, address, and telephone number, the name and address of the nearest relative, and insurance information. There is also a space for additional comments such as the name of a secondary insurer.

When using the pegboard system, the ledger card is placed under the superbill (charge slip) and directly over the day sheet making sure to line up the entry line on the ledger card with the next available space on the day sheet. It is important not to miss any lines when entering information onto the day sheet.

Ledger cards can be copied and used as a statement that is sent to the patient. In offices using a computerized billing system, the bill is generated by the computer. Ledger cards are kept in a separate file container that is sized to fit them. This container is usually kept in an accessible spot close to the receptionist or person responsible for handling charges and billing.

RECEIPT FORMS A receipt form is used when a patient payment is made but no service is provided on that day. For example, a patient may come into the office or mail in a check to pay a bill. In some offices, this amount is entered onto the day sheet and ledger card, at the same time, the receipt form is completed for the patient. If the patient pays the bill with cash, a receipt is given. If the payment is made by check, the patient may use the canceled check as a receipt or may request a written receipt.

Using the Pegboard System

Every financial transaction, except the use of petty cash, is recorded on the day sheet. Each patient will have a ledger card on which individual financial activity is recorded. When the pegboard system is used, the patient's name, receipt number (the next chronological number on the day sheet), and previous balance are entered on the day sheet with a superbill attached when the patient arrives in the office. The superbill is then removed and attached to the patient's chart. After the patient is seen by the physician, the superbill is put back on the same line of the day sheet where it was originally written after placing the charge amounts next to the service rendered. Procedure 13-2 explains the pegboard system.

If the patient makes a payment in person, then issue a receipt by placing a receipt form on the pegboard in place of the superbill. Place the patient's ledger card onto the day sheet. Enter the previous balance owed on the day sheet, and calculate the new balance after this payment. On the ledger card, post the date, patient's name, a description of the transaction, such as ROA (received on account), and the amount of the payment.

If a payment is made through the mail, a receipt is not sent. The amount credited to the account will appear on the next bill sent to the patient.

Adjustments

Adjustments are any changes made that affect the patient's balance. They can occur when the physician reduces a fee, or agrees to write-off a portion of the charge and accept the insurance payment as full payment. For example, if the physician has charged $1,500 for a surgical procedure and agrees to accept the insurance payment of $1,200, then an adjustment is made for $300. The $300 appears in the adjustment column, and is subtracted from the previous balance to indicate that $1,200 is now currently owed. If the $300 was not added to the adjustment column, the totals in section 4 on the balance sheet would not balance. An adjustment or correction also has to be made to correct an error in posting.

Pegboard System

OBJECTIVE: Process patient accounts using the write-it-once system without error in posting or mathematics.

Equipment and Supplies

pegboard; superbills (charge slips); new day sheet; ledger cards for each patient scheduled during the day; calculator

Method

1. Place a new day sheet and a strip of superbills (charge slips) onto the pegboard making sure they are fastened securely into the pegs.

2. Complete all the information required at the top of the day sheet (date and page number)

3. Carry balances forward from the previous day sheet and enter it into section 4. These include "Previous Page" columns A-D, "Previous Day's Total," and "Accounts Rec. 1st of the Month," which are entered into the Accounts Receivable Control and Accounts Receivable Proof boxes. Step 3 is necessary before the day sheet is ready to use.

4. Remove the superbill from the pegboard and clip it to the front of the patient's chart. The physician will enter the procedure performed that day on the appropriate line of the superbill, fill in the diagnosis, and sign the form after he or she sees the patient. The insurance code number is included on the superbill for ease of processing. The superbill is then given to the receptionist by the medical assistant or the patient so that arrangements can be made for payment.

5. To record charges: place the ledger card under the next superbill and turn back the top two pages of the superbill. Turn back these pages to correctly line up the space for the amount to be posted on the charge slip, and through to the ledger card and day sheet. Write the amount charged, pressing firmly and evenly to press through to the forms and day sheet.

6. To record payments: When the superbill is received at the front desk, the medical assistant or receptionist will enter the correct charge next to every procedure or service and place this total on the front of the superbill. The superbill is then again placed back on the pegboard, using care to line it up on top of the correct patient's name. The ledger card is then placed under the last page of the charge slip aligning the first blank line of the ledger card with the carbonized entry strip on the superbill. On some types of superbills, you will turn back the first two pages of the superbill and enter the total charge and payment into the correct columns. Complete recording this transaction by filling in all the information that the office requires in the far right-hand columns (for example, method of payment such as cash or check).

7. To post adjustments: When an adjustment is made (for example a discount given to another health professional), the medical assistant/receptionist will enter the correct discounted amount into the computer system or subtract it from the balance due from the insurance company. If the adjustment is for non-sufficient funds, add the check amount and service fee charged by the bank to the patient balance. Always follow the facility's policy on adjustments.

8. To post collection agency payments: If the patient pays a collection agency and the collection agency forwards the money, credit that payment to the patient account and write "collection agency payment of $(amount received)" next to it.

9. If a credit balance then exists and the physician or office manager approves, issue a refund check to the patient.

Charting Example

Refunded $49 to patient for overpayment.

TABLE 13-2 Correcting Posting Errors

Date	Description	Debit	Credit Payments	Adjustments	Balance
06/19/XX	OV	25.00			25.00
06/19/XX	Error in pstg	(25.00)			0

Balancing the Day Sheets

To make sure that the accounts and entries are correct, the day sheet(s) need to be balanced at the end of the day. Use a calculator to balance day sheets and always double-check each total. When balancing the day sheet, use a calculator with paper tapes, if possible. This will allow a review of the tape for calculation errors if the figures do not balance.

When errors in posting are corrected, the corrections should be made in the same column as the original posting (Table 13-2).

The steps for balancing the day sheets are presented in Table 13-3.

Accounts Receivable Control

It is important to keep a running record of all money owed to the physician (accounts receivable). To make sure this number is accurate, an "Accounts Receivable Control" column and an "Accounts Receivable Proof" column are maintained at the bottom of the day sheet.

On the first day of the month, the day sheet being used will have a zero placed in the box marked "Previous Page." If the day sheet page is for the second of the month through the end of the month, a "Previous Page" number is brought forward from the accounts receivable total on the previous page (day before).

The columns A and B totals are brought straight across from the Proof of Posting boxes into the correct spaces in the Accounts Receivable Control section. These two figures are added together for a subtotal and then the sum of columns B1 and B2 are subtracted from this amount. This number is the new total accounts receivable figure.

The Accounts Receivable Proof is calculated in the same manner with the last box matching the last box on

TABLE 13-3 Balancing the Day Sheets

1. Total columns A, B1, B2, C, and D and place the total for each column in the boxes marked "Totals This Page." These column totals then need to be added to numbers brought forward and entered into the "Previous Page" column. This will provide the "Month to Date" total. The "Month to Date" totals are important since they indicate all the credits, charges, and transactions that have occurred from the first day of the month to the present day.

2. The Proof of Posting box is used to make sure that all entries and the totals columns are correct. The numbers used to calculate this figure are taken from the "Totals This Page" column box.
   a. Enter the amount from today's column D total, which is the sum of the previous balances into the appropriate box.
   b. Place the total for column A, which represents all the charges for this day, in the appropriate box ("Plus Column A Total") and create a subtotal by adding column D and column A totals.
   c. Add columns B1 and B2, which are both credit columns (payments and adjustments), then enter this amount in the box "Less Columns B1 and B2." This amount will then be subtracted (minus) from the subtotal of column D and column A.
   d. If the calculations have been correct, this new subtotal obtained after subtracting columns B1 and B2 should be equal to column C, which is the current balance.

   Note that when doing a proof of posting, column D is added to column A minus the sum of columns B1 and B2 and this must equal column C. Therefore, a proof of posting formula is:

   $$D + A - (B1 + B2) = C$$

   This means the previous balance (D) plus the charge (A) minus the sum of the payments and adjustments (B1 and B2) is equal to the current balance (C).

the Accounts Receivable Control for proof of posting. See Figure 13-13 for an illustration of accounts receivable control.

An accounts receivable ratio provides a measurement of how fast the outstanding accounts are being paid. The Accounts Receivable Ratio equals the Current Accounts Receivable Balance divided by the Average Gross Monthly Charges.

For example, if the current accounts receivable balance is $20,000 and the annual gross charges are $120,000, then the average monthly charges are $10,000 ($120,000 ÷ 12). The accounts receivable ratio would equal $20,000 ÷ $10,000 = 2 months.

Since a desirable accounts receivable ratio, or the amount of time it takes to have the uncollected debts paid, is two months or less, this example is at the high end of the limit. The medical assistant will have to work hard to get collections under two months.

Locating Errors

The key to error control is to prevent them in the first place. If there is a difference in the balances of the day sheet, there are several steps that can be taken to locate the error.

1. If the columns on the day sheet do not balance (using the proof of posting box at bottom of the day sheet), check all calculations. Ideally you will have saved the calculator tape. Find the difference in the balances and search for that identical amount on the ledger cards and superbill.

2. If an error is divisible by nine, it may be a transposition error. For example, if the difference in the balance is $63, you may find that you wrote $329 instead of $392.

3. Check all the columns, in particular the Previous Balance column to make sure you did not post the amount incorrectly.

4. Check the alignment of all digits to make sure a zero was not misaligned, for example in writing 200 instead of 20. One bookkeeping method for avoiding this type of error is to use a dash in the cents column instead of two zeros. Thus $45.00 would be written as $45.−.

Computerized Systems

Most offices perform the accounting function using a computer program. The computer system and program selected will depend on the needs of the office. Practice management software offers many services and can be modified to fit the needs of a particular office or specialty. When shopping for practice management software, offices often hire a consultant to evaluate the practice requirements. Specialized software is advertised in professional journals and is demonstrated at

ACCOUNTS RECEIVABLE CONTROL				
Month of __March__ , 20 − −			Accounts receivable at end of preceding month: $22,500	
	Services Rendered	Received from Patients	Adjustments Increase/ (Decrease)	Accounts Receivable Balance
1	$ 800	$ 1000		$22,300
2	$ 700	$ 400		$22,600
3	$ 900	$ 1100	($100)	$22,300
4	$1000	$ 700		$22,600

FIGURE 13-13 Accounts Receivable Control.

professional meetings for physicians and medical office personnel. Prior to making a final decision concerning office software, ask physicians' offices or practices that have similar needs for their suggestions. Another concern in choosing new software is cost. New software may require the office hardware to be upgraded. A consultant will be able to advise the office concerning these needs. The new software should contain Current Procedural Terminology (CPT) and International Classification of Diseases (ICD). The software must have these capabilities; however, this data changes yearly and the system must be able to accommodate these updates.

When using a computerized system always back up data and information on a separate disk, such as a CD-ROM that is then stored separately. Some systems also keep the information on the hard drive. Some offices keep one hard copy of printed material to be kept on file in the event the computer system goes down or there is a power failure.

HIPAA mandated the use of the computer to submit bills to insurance companies electronically. Several comprehensive software systems are available for the computer that combines many office functions into one program. These software packages will make patient appointments, keep all patient records (including lab results and x-ray reports), maintain all insurance and billing information, and perform all bookkeeping functions including insurance payments, patient payments, and accounts due. In addition, there is a function within these programs that will electronically submit the bill to an insurance clearinghouse for dissemination to the payment centers.

Most comprehensive software programs are quite expensive, so before deciding which one to buy, careful attention should be given to the needs of the office, as well as which methods the office has chosen to comply with HIPAA regulations.

To access the information in these programs, every employee must have his or her own unique, login name and password. To be in compliance with HIPAA regulations, upon leaving employment, the employee's login name and password must be rendered unusable. Only those employees with a "need" to access the information may have login names and passwords. In addition, the person responsible for providing employees with access must keep records of who accesses the information, what information was accessed, and when (date and time) information is accessed. These logs must be kept for a designated period of time, usually at least two years.

A paper backup copy of the computer files is not necessary, but a disk backup file or an off-premises electronic backup file is necessary. The process by which the backup files can or should be accessed is written into the office's policy manual, along with the

reasons and circumstances for granting access. One designated person has total access for the system and is responsible for the software, the passwords, and the backup files. This person is also documented in the office policy and procedure manual.

Professional Courtesy

Professional courtesy (PC) is typically offered by physicians to other physicians, staff, and family members, and clergy in addition to indigent patients. Professional courtesy may be rendered only at the discretion of the physician, must fall within federal guidelines, and insurance requirements, and must be recorded in the patient's record.

SUMMARY

The professional health care facility will have in place office policy regarding fee setting, billing, and collection. The medical assistant has the responsibility to carry out such policy with a professional, courteous attitude. Informed patients will have a better understanding of office expectations. This helps to lessen the

problems encountered with accounts receivable. When an account does become a collection dilemma, a series of steps can be instituted to quickly and efficiently address any problems. The goal of such policy is to protect the financial well-being and goodwill of the medical practice.

Chapter Review

COMPETENCY REVIEW

1. Define and spell the terms to learn for this chapter.
2. With a fellow student, role-play a telephone conversation you would have with Samuel Jones, a patient who is unemployed, to collect an overdue bill of 60 days for $225.
3. Write a sample collection letter from Dr. Beth Williams to Samuel Jones identified in the previous question.
4. What statements can you make to a patient to encourage payment at the time of service?
5. Discuss the ethical considerations involved when making collections.

PREPARING FOR THE CERTIFICATION EXAM

1. A patient's detailed record of financial transactions at a medical office is called a/an
   A. ledger
   B. accounts payable record
   C. register
   D. reconciliation
   E. medical record

2. Once an account has been referred for collection, the medical office should
   A. discuss payment with the patient
   B. not attempt to collect payment
   C. call the patient's employer
   D. cancel the balance
   E. send a reminder letter

3. Which form serves as the documentation of services, a billing statement, and an insurance processing form?
   A. receipt
   B. ledger
   C. account
   D. superbill
   E. credit memo

4. A "skip" has/is
   A. forgotten to pay
   B. lost his or her job
   C. moved with no forwarding address
   D. not a collection problem
   E. skipped a monthly payment

continued on next page

5. If the computer system goes down, what method would NOT be used to store electronic data?
   A. separate disk
   B. CD-ROM
   C. print a hard copy
   D. hard drive
   E. file cabinet

6. Regulation Z of the Truth in Lending Act requires physicians to outline costs, including finance charges when payment arrangements are made in
   A. two or more installments
   B. four or more installments
   C. eight or more installments
   D. three or more installments
   E. five or more installments

7. The accounts receivable record tells you
   A. how much money is owed to the practice
   B. the effectiveness of the billing system
   C. total collections divided by gross changes
   D. total collections divided by net charges
   E. how fast overdue accounts are being paid

8. Claims against estates should be
   A. canceled
   B. sent to collection
   C. discounted
   D. sent to the administrator of the estate
   E. addressed to the next of kin

9. Good bookkeeping habits include
   A. using a blue pen
   B. using a pencil to easily make changes
   C. using opaque correction fluid
   D. checking the entry once
   E. use of clear penmanship

10. The pegboard system is the same as the
    A. single-entry bookkeeping system
    B. write-it-one system
    C. computerized system
    D. write-it-now system
    E. computerized program

CRITICAL THINKING

1. What and how should you advise the patient of your credit policies to ensure the patient will understand the practice policies?

ON THE JOB

Services were rendered to Jeffrey Boylan on October 1, 2005. It is now 45 days since Mr. Boylan's received care, and he has not yet made a payment on his outstanding balance of $150.00. At this point, the office's policy requires that a reminder letter be sent. Compose a collection letter to Mr. Boylan, in accordance with HIPAA and office guidelines. Address: Mr. Jeffrey Boylan, 14 Meadow Road, Anytown, State 12345

INTERNET ACTIVITY

Your office is considering between manual and computerized accounting systems. Search the Internet for the various accounting systems. Develop an excel spreadsheet and list the manual and computerized systems found online with all necessary equipment, components, warranties, and prices.

MediaLink More on fees, billing, collections, and credit in a medical office, including interactive resources, can be found in the Student CD-ROM accompanying this textbook.

Medical Assistant Role Delineation Chart

HIGHLIGHT indicates material covered in this chapter.

ADMINISTRATIVE

Administrative Procedures

- Perform basic administrative medical assisting functions
- Schedule, coordinate and monitor appointments
- Schedule inpatient/outpatient admissions and procedures
- Understand and apply third-party guidelines
- Obtain reimbursement through accurate claims submission
- Monitor third-party reimbursement
- Understand and adhere to managed care policies and procedures
- *Negotiate managed care contracts*

Practice Finances

- Perform procedural and diagnostic coding
- Apply bookkeeping principles

- Manage accounts receivable
- *Manage accounts payable*
- *Process payroll*
- *Document and maintain accounting and banking records*
- *Develop and maintain fee schedules*
- *Manage renewals of business and professional insurance policies*
- *Manage personnel benefits and maintain records*
- *Perform marketing, financial, and strategic planning*

CLINICAL

Fundamental Principles

- Apply principles of aseptic technique and infection control
- Comply with quality assurance practices
- Screen and follow up patient test results

Diagnostic Orders

- Collect and process specimens
- Perform diagnostic tests

Patient Care

- Adhere to established patient screening procedures
- Obtain patient history and vital signs
- Prepare and maintain examination and treatment areas
- Prepare patient for examinations, procedures and treatments

- Assist with examinations, procedures and treatments
- Prepare and administer medications and immunizations
- Maintain medication and immunization records
- Recognize and respond to emergencies
- Coordinate patient care information with other health care providers
- Initiate IV and administer IV medications with appropriate training and as permitted by state law

GENERAL

Professionalism

- Display a professional manner and image
- Demonstrate initiative and responsibility
- Work as a member of the health care team
- Prioritize and perform multiple tasks
- Adapt to change
- Promote the CMA credential
- Enhance skills through continuing education
- Treat all patients with compassion and empathy
- Promote the practice through positive public relations

Communication Skills

- Recognize and respect cultural diversity
- Adapt communications to individual's ability to understand
- Use professional telephone technique

- Recognize and respond effectively to verbal, nonverbal, and written communications
- Use medical terminology appropriately
- Utilize electronic technology to receive, organize, prioritize and transmit information
- Serve as liaison

Legal Concepts

- Perform within legal and ethical boundaries
- Prepare and maintain medical records
- Document accurately
- Follow employer's established policies dealing with the health care contract
- Implement and maintain federal and state health care legislation and regulations
- Comply with established risk management and safety procedures
- Recognize professional credentialing criteria
- *Develop and maintain personnel, policy and procedure manuals*

Instruction

- Instruct individuals according to their needs
- Explain office policies and procedures
- Teach methods of health promotion and disease prevention
- Locate community resources and disseminate information
- *Develop educational materials*
- *Conduct continuing education activities*

Operational Functions

- Perform inventory of supplies and equipment
- Perform routine maintenance of administrative and clinical equipment
- Apply computer techniques to support office operations
- *Perform personnel management functions*
- *Negotiate leases and prices for equipment and supply contracts*

- *Denotes advanced skills.*

SOURCE: Reprinted by permission of the American Association of Medical Assistants from the AAMA Role Delineation Study: Occupational Analysis of the Medical Assisting Profession.

BETH WILLIAMS, MD
123 MICHIGAN AVENUE
CHICAGO, IL 60610

STATEMEN
FROM
THRU
CUST #

For *office furniture*
"000923" :437002245: 028742109"

BALANCE FORWARD   727 | 18

arch 10   20 *05*

WINDY CITY CLINIC
Beth Williams, M.D.
123 Michigan Avenue, Chicago, IL 60610
(312) 123-1234

Pay to the order of *Jamie Young*
Fifty cents only

COUNT - - - - - - - - - - - -
BALANCE $2,646.6
CREDITS $8,000.0
AID $.0
BITS $7,871.3
ARGES $5.0
ANCE $2,770.3
/CREDITS
EBITS

neman's   35 | 00
ealth Supply
              142 | 32
ndages

chapter 14

Financial Management

Learning Objectives

After completing this chapter, you should be able to:

- Define and spell the terms to learn for this chapter.
- State the correct procedure for writing a check and check stub.
- Describe the write-it-once check writing system.
- State the correct method for endorsing a check based on the guidelines issued by the federal government.
- Differentiate between the ABA number and the MICR on a check.

- State the risks associated with accepting a third-party check, cash, or check from an out-of-state bank.
- List the criteria for a negotiable instrument.
- State and describe three types of endorsements.
- List six recurring monthly expenses.
- Describe the five steps to follow when making a deposit.
- List and discuss nine steps for reconciling a bank statement.

OUTLINE

Function of Banking	248
Checks	249
Paying Bills	254
Deposits	256
Accepting Cash	257
Cash Disbursement	258
Bank Hold on Accounts	258
Bank Statement	258
Saving Documentation	259
Petty Cash	260
Payroll	260

Terms to Learn

accounts payable

accounts receivable

American Banker's Association (ABA) number

audit

canceled checks

cash disbursement

credits

debits

deposits

embezzlement

gross annual wage

Magnetic Ink Character Recognition (MICR)

negotiable instrument

payee

payer

reconciliation

signee

stop-payment order

tax withholding

third-party checks

warrant

Case Study

DR. EVERETT'S OFFICE HAS A PETTY CASH DRAWER in which Dr. Everett keeps fifty dollars to pay postage, due mail, and other incidentals. The office policy is to replace any cash taken out of the drawer with a receipt for the money taken. In this way, when the money is to be restocked, there is an account of where the fifty dollars was spent. It is the end of the month and time to get the cash for the petty cash drawer. When you count the money left and add the receipts, you find the total in the drawer is only forty dollars. Only you and Sarah, the clinic manager, have access to the drawer. You ask her about the ten missing dollars, and she says that she "borrowed" ten dollars a week ago and intends to repay the money on payday, which is a week away.

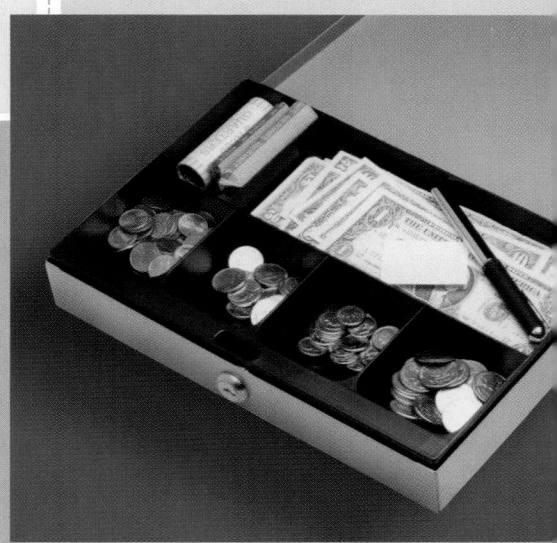

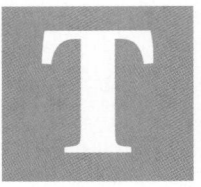

The medical assistant's responsibilities for maintaining control of the medical office's banking and accounting procedures are two-fold. First, absolute accuracy is necessary when working with bank deposits, reconciliation of funds, and all related bookkeeping activities. The second responsibility relates to the trust the physician has placed on the employee for handling cash, checks, and accounts. The medical assistant acts as the agent for the physician.

Function of Banking

The basic banking functions are depositing funds, writing checks, transferring funds between bank accounts, withdrawing funds, reconciling statements, and using banking services. Most of the funds that come into a medical office are from the collection of accounts receivable.

Money may need to be withdrawn from a checking or savings account to pay business-related expenses. Every time funds (money) are moved from one account to another or used as cash, it must be handled in a systematic manner and carefully documented. Monthly statements for both checking and savings accounts must be reconciled or balanced to determine what money or funds are available for use.

Bank records are subject to government examination since the federal government regulates banking practices. In addition, the accountant for the medical practice will need accurate records for preparation of federal tax returns. Since the medical assistant will not be present when the accountant reviews the books, all information must be clear and accurate.

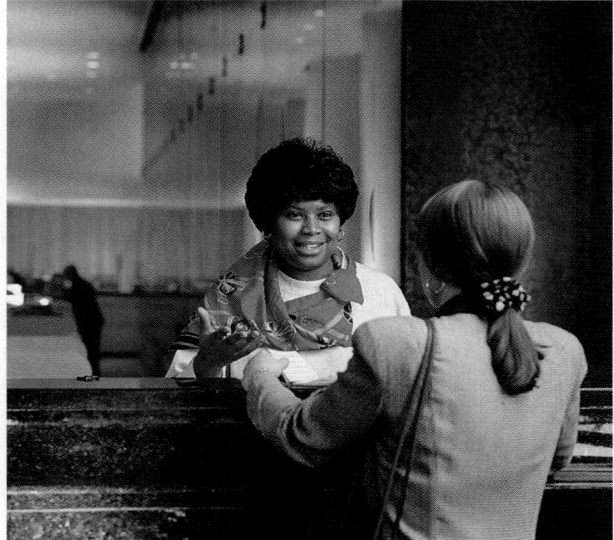

FIGURE 14-1   Bank teller assisting with customer service.

Types of Bank Accounts

Banks maintain both checking and savings accounts for their customers (Figure 14-1). A checking account allows the owner of the account to withdraw money from the account by writing checks, which are used as payment for outstanding debts (bills). Cash can also be withdrawn from a checking account. Checking accounts are not usually interest-bearing accounts. Some accounts earn interest only if there is a minimum balance in the account. Generally, the bank charges a fee, or service charge, (for example, $5.00 per month) to maintain the account.

A saving's account is an interest-bearing account in which funds not needed for daily expenses can be placed. Interest is earned monthly or quarterly. This means the bank will calculate a certain percentage (such as 3%) based on the average balance during a month and pay that amount to the account. Cash can be withdrawn from a savings account or transferred into a checking account. There is usually a limit to the number of monthly withdrawals without paying a fee.

A money market account is used more as an investment tool that usually pays a higher level of interest.

Online Banking

Most banks provide a service to their customers called "online banking." Online banking provides the customer access to his or her bank account 24-hours a day, seven days a week. By using the computer to access the World Wide Web, customers can enter the Web address for their bank's home page. This address can be obtained from the bank. Once on the bank's home page, the customer chooses "online banking." A sign-in or log-in page will appear that asks for a username and password. The username and password are usually set by the customer and are unique to each customer. Some banks also require the account number be entered.

Online banking lets customers reconcile their account, pay bills, see which checks have been processed, and check the total amount in their account. One advantage of online banking is that customers can see the bank's record of their account, and compare the bank's record to their own. Customers may see which checks have been processed and which deposits have been fully credited to their account. Another advantage of online banking is the ability to download data from the bank Web site directly to the customer's money management software program.

Online banking is a paperless system, so it is important that, when using online banking, records be kept in the office. If a bill is paid, it must be noted in the accounts payable records to ensure that the office's records always match the bank's records, and any money taken out of the account to pay a bill is posted in the office records.

Checks

A check is a written order to a bank to pay or transfer money. A check, which is payable on demand, is considered a negotiable instrument. A negotiable instrument is one that actualizes or permits the transfer of money to another person. In order to have a negotiable instrument, it must be:

- Written and signed by the maker (payer) of the check

- State a sum of money to be paid

- Payable on demand or at a fixed date in the future

- Payable to the holder (payee) of the check

Checks are supplied, for a slight charge, by the bank where the money is held or a company specializing in printing checks. These are referred to as blank checks since they contain only basic information, including the account number and name and address of the account owner.

Large medical offices that require a large supply of checks can request a business office checkbook that has several checks per page in a large bound checkbook. Medical offices can also request a duplicate or write-in-once check system. A carbon copy of the check is made when written to ensure accountability for each check.

There is standard information included on all checks regardless of the bank that issues them. This preprinted information includes:

- Name and address of the payer (person signing the check to release the money)

- Telephone number of payer (in some cases)

- Preprinted sequential number on each check

- Space to enter the full date

- American Bank Association (ABA) number

- "Pay to the order of" space in which to enter the name of the payee (the person or company to receive the money)

- Space to enter the amount of the check in writing

- Small box or space to enter the amount of the check in numbers

- Space for the signature of payer

- Preprinted name and address of bank

- Magnetic ink character recognition (MICR) figures used for bank processing of the check

The blank spaces must be completed before a bank will honor and cash the check.

Advantages of Checks

Checks are recommended for a variety of reasons, including safety of funds, convenience, ease of maintaining a record or documentation of money transfer,

reliability of records for tax purposes, summary of deposits from receipts, protection while money is in the bank account (banks carry insurance to cover loss), and stop-payment orders that can be issued by the payer to protect any lost or stolen checks.

Types of Checks

The various types of checks include cashier's checks, certified checks, bank drafts, limited checks, money orders, traveler's checks, voucher checks, and warrants. Box 14-1 lists definitions of the different types of checks. Preparing for Externship discusses the importance of knowing the different types of checks.

Warrant

A warrant is not actually a negotiable check. It is a statement issued to indicate that a debt should be paid. For example, an insurance adjuster may issue a warrant indicating that a fire insurance claim should be paid. This warrant then becomes authorization to the insurance company to issue a check as payment.

ABA Number

The American Banker's Association (ABA) number is always located in the upper right-hand corner of a printed check. It is printed as a fraction on a business check or as a straight series of numbers (1–109/210) on a personal check. The ABA originated this number to identify the area where the bank on which the check is written is located and to identify the individual bank.

Magnetic Ink Character Recognition (MICR)

Magnetic Ink Character Recognition (MICR) is a system of combining characters and numbers located at the bottom left side of checks and deposit slips. The MICR is read by high-speed machinery, increasing the speed and accuracy of processing bank statements and check sorting. It also facilitates the bookkeeping process within the bank. Printed on each check, the MICR is a form of identification for the bank and the account. The first series of numbers identifies the bank and its location. The second series of numbers identifies the individual account. During bank processing,

Prepare a Check

OBJECTIVE: Correctly prepare a check.

Equipment and Supplies
blank checks with stub or record; pen

Method

1. Move all the checks in the pad to the left so that the smallest numbered check will lay across the check register.
2. Fill in the check stub or check record before writing the check.
3. Use ink or a typewriter to complete check and stub.
4. Write the name of the payee on the "Pay to the order of" line.
5. Write out the full amount of the check on the "Pay" line.
6. Write the full date and check number in the designated boxes.
7. Write the amount of the check, using numbers in the designated area.
8. Fill in all blank spaces and leave no room for anyone to add anything. Always begin writing or figures at the extreme left of the space.
9. Date the check on the day it is written. Never postdate a check. Postdating a check means writing a future date on a check.
10. Use care when spelling the name of the payee. Do not use abbreviations or titles, such as MD. Leave no space either before or after the payee's name. If space remains after the name, draw a straight line from the name to the end of the space.
11. Make sure the dollar amount written on the second line agrees with numerical dollar amount entered in the space on the first line.
12. Use care when writing a check for less than one dollar. Write out the amount with the word "only" indicating to the reader that the amount should be noted as less than one dollar. Do not cross out the word dollars. It is not advisable to write checks for less than one dollar. In addition to the time spent bookkeeping such a small amount, many banks place a service charge for each check written. This can be costly.
13. Finally, subtract the amount of this check from the "Balance Brought Forward" line. Write this amount as the new balance forward.

additional numbers are printed across the bottom of the check to indicate the amount of the check.

Check Writing

The check writing process needs to be handled carefully to avoid errors. Methods for writing checks will vary from office to office depending upon the preferences of the physician and the accountant. Your office may use a traditional checkbook with individual checks on each page, a business office checkbook, a write-it-once system, or a computer generated check processing system. When writing a check, all the spaces must be filled in. At the top right corner is a space for the date. This is the date the check is written. The person or business to which the check is written is placed on the line following "Pay to the order of." At the end of that line is a block to put the amount of the check in numbers (for example, $100.00). The next line is the amount of the check written in words (for example, "One hundred and no/100 dollars"). A space to note what the check is for appears on the bottom left corner of the check. You might note, for example, that this check was for "office supplies." The line on the bottom right is for the writer of the check to sign. This line must be signed by the owner of the bank account, or his or her authorized agent. In some offices, the office manager is designated to sign checks for the physician.

Write-it-once System

The write-it-once system is based on the use of a check with a carbon strip on the back that allows a record to be kept of the date, check number, payee, and net amount of the check. A pegboard system (see Chapter 13), check register sheet, and checks with a carbonized writing strip on the back are used for this method. The check register sheet is placed over the pegs of a pegboard. Checks with the carbonized strip on the back edge are then placed on top of the check register, lining up the first line of the check register with the writing line of the first check. Any information that is written

BOX 14-1
Types of Checks

- **Cashier's checks** are written using the bank's own check or form and are issued by the bank. A cashier's check guarantees the money is available since the bank checks the payer's account before issuing the check. The purchaser can also pay cash to have a cashier's check issued. The funds to pay the check are debited against the payer's account when the check is issued by the bank. Cashier's checks can be requested of a bank by savings account holders who do not have a checking account. There is usually a charge for this service.

- **Certified checks** are similar to a cashier's check since the bank guarantees the money is available. A certified check is actually written on the payer's own check form. The teller will verify this check by placing an official stamp directly on the check. The bank actually withdraws the money from the payer's account when it certifies the check.

- **Bank drafts** are checks that are drawn up by a bank against funds (money) that are deposited to its account in another bank.

- **Limited checks** are issued on special check forms that contain a preprinted maximum dollar amount for which the check can be written. There may also be a time limit during which the check is valid or must be cashed. Limited checks are used for payroll checks and insurance payments.

- **Money orders** are purchased for the cash value typed on the check. Money orders can be purchased from banks, the United States Postal Service, and other authorized agents. International money orders can be purchased to be cashed in foreign countries.

A money order is purchased with cash, and there is a charge for this service. Money orders are frequently used by individuals who do not have bank accounts since it is recommended that cash not be sent through the mail. Money orders are considered safe to accept as payment since they are redeemable at the value typed on the check.

- **Traveler's checks** are familiar to most people who travel. These checks are preprinted in certain dollar amounts ($10, $20, $50, $100, $500 and $1,000) and are prepaid. Considered a safe means for carrying money when traveling, traveler's checks are also convenient since most places will accept a traveler's check and only the payer can cash it. There is a space for two signatures of the payer: one at the time of purchase and another when the check is cashed. The payee is able to check the two signatures, thus protecting the payer in the event the check is stolen or lost. People purchasing traveler's checks are advised to always sign the checks at the time of purchase before leaving the bank.

- **Voucher checks** contain three detachable sections for transaction information. This type of check is frequently used for payroll checks since additional information can be supplied to the payee. The upper portion of the check contains the actual check; the lower portion provides details about the transaction, such as any payroll deductions, account to which the check is to be credited, or reason for issuing the check; the third portion is a carbon that remains with the payer as a record of the transaction. This copy can then be filed with any additional information that is available, such as invoices or receipts.

on the check (for example, payee, dollar amounts) will then appear on the check register sheet as a permanent record.

The user must press hard when writing on this type of check so that the impression will go through to the check register underneath. The check register has space for 25 checks to be recorded on one page. Procedure 14-1 describes the check writing process using a write-it-once system.

Checks must be handwritten in ink or typewritten so they cannot be altered. Pencil is not used for check writing. The signature cannot be typewritten. Correctly written checks require legible handwriting. No blank space should be left before the name of the payee, the written dollar amount, and the numbered dollar amount. This is to prevent another person from altering any of these items. See Figure 14-2 for a sample of correctly written checks.

In some cases, the net amount of the check is imprinted by machine. All the other information is entered by hand. Checks have to be handwritten when using the write-it-once method. Checks with stubs will have to be detached from the stub for typing. However, the stub must be completed immediately.

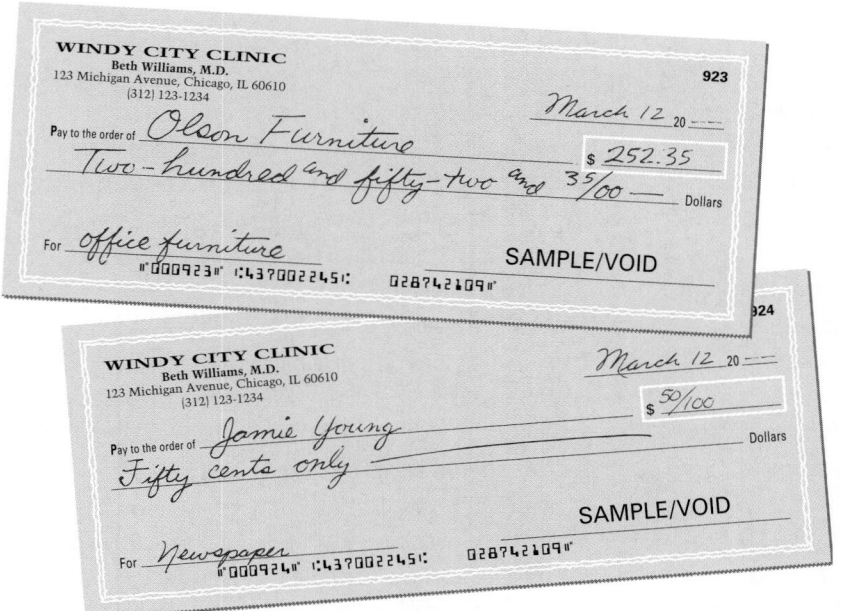

FIGURE 14-2 Correctly written checks.

Checks can be prepared ahead of time by the medical assistant and given to the physician to sign. Attach all materials, such as invoices and statements, to the check for the physician to sign. Writing a check payable to cash ("cash" checks) is not advised. These checks are easily cashed since they have no payee designated and have been signed by the payer. Banks will usually require that the person cashing this type of check endorse the check while in front of the teller. Review the guidelines for check writing to assure checks are written properly.

Errors in Writing Checks

Errors in writing checks can be handled in several ways. Do not erase on checks. They are printed on sensitive paper and erasures may not process correctly. In addition, banks are suspicious of all alterations on checks.

If there is a major error, such as writing out a different dollar amount than appears in the boxed space for the numerical amount or the payee name is written in the space meant for the handwritten dollar amount, the check is not valid. In this case, draw a line through the check and write VOID in ink in large letters on the face of the check. Keep the VOID check so that it is not considered missing when the reconciliation of the bank statement is done. If the check has already been signed, many people will tear off and discard just the signature and keep the remainder of the check for a record.

Not all errors will result in voiding the check. If the error is minor, such as writing the number "4" instead of "5," you may change the "4" to a "5" if it is still readable; the signee, the person signing the check, must then initial this change.

Accepting Checks

An office policy should be in place to guide staff about accepting checks from patients (Patient Education). It is acceptable for patients to pay for services with a personal check. Most of the accounts receivable, the outstanding bills, in a medical office are paid by checks written against the bank accounts of patients. Lifespan Considerations discusses an elderly patient's need, at times, to designate an agent to sign his or her checks.

There are some checks that most medical offices consider risky and avoid cashing. These include third-party checks, checks drawn on an out-of-town bank, overpayment of account checks, and "paid in full" checks.

Third-party checks refer to a check written by a party unknown to you. You are considered the third party in this process. The patient (the second party), the payee, has received a check from another person to pay his or her medical bill. The person who wrote the check is considered the first party. You are at risk in accepting this check since you do not know the payer who has signed the check and, thus, may have trouble collecting the money for which the check is issued.

Patient Education

The role of the medical assistant in educating the patient is twofold: to instruct the patient on the banking practices of the office and to safeguard the patient and the physician from loss of money through carelessness.

The patient may be given an informational pamphlet prepared specifically for your office with guidelines and options for payment of services. Patients should be instructed not to send cash through the mail.

In many cases, these checks will be for an amount greater than the amount of the bill and you would have to issue a refund in cash. This would require maintaining extra cash in the office, additional staff work, and may result in financial loss if the check turns out to be invalid. Therefore many offices do not accept these checks. Government checks (for example, tax refunds) and payroll checks are examples of third-party checks that are considered to be reliable.

Checks drawn on out-of-town banks are generally not accepted for payment unless identification is sought from the payee. It is difficult to collect payment if a check is not good, and it may not be easy to reach an out-of-town bank, concerning the validity of a check, prior to accepting it.

Occasionally, a patient writes a check for an overpayment of an account. This can happen accidentally if a patient has not maintained adequate records or if the patient's insurance company has also made a payment to the patient's account in the medical office. In this case, a refund needs to be made to the patient. This can be handled by issuing a refund check for the amount of overpayment or returning the incorrect check to the patient if it has not been deposited.

Checks written with the statement added "paid in full" are to be avoided. Patients sometimes write this on their check when they believe they no longer owe any money to the physician. If you deposit the check you acknowledge that this is correct. Therefore, if the patient still owes money on the bill and you deposit the check, you may have difficulty collecting any further payments.

Completing the Check Stub

A check stub can be used as a permanent record of the date, amount, payee of the check, and purpose of the check. The check stub has room to place the new balance, which is obtained by subtracting the current check from the previous balance. See Figure 14-3 for an illustration of a correctly completed check stub.

Endorsement of Checks

In order to transfer money from one person to another, the check must be endorsed. According to federal banking regulations, an endorsement is placed on the back of the check within the top one and one-half inches on the left side of the check as it is turned over. This upper left-hand corner is referred to as the "trailing edge" of a check. If the endorsement is not placed within this designated area or extends beyond the one and one-half inch mark, it can be refused by a bank. An endorsement can either be a payee's written signature or rubber-stamped. To prevent theft, checks should be endorsed "for deposit only" as soon as they arrive in the mail.

Lifespan Considerations

Sometimes an elderly person *who is physically unable to write a check, or who cannot see to write a check, will designate an agent to write and sign checks for him or her. Most often it is a family member. This is an arrangement the person has made with the bank and is a perfectly legitimate and legal way to handle finances. When money is owed to the doctor's office, it is usually the agent who will write the check for the patient, but it will be credited to the patient's account.*

It is common procedure in a medical office to endorse checks at the time they are received. This is often done with an endorsement stamp that contains the doctor's name, account number, and the name of the bank.

Endorsements are regulated by the Uniform Negotiable Instrument Act. A check that has been transferred to more than one person (third-party payer) would have more than one endorsement on the back. Types of endorsements are discussed in Table 14-1.

Mailing Checks

Care should be used when mailing checks so that the check is not visible through the envelope. Special nontransparent envelopes can be purchased. Other methods are to place the check in a piece of folded paper or to actually fold the check in half.

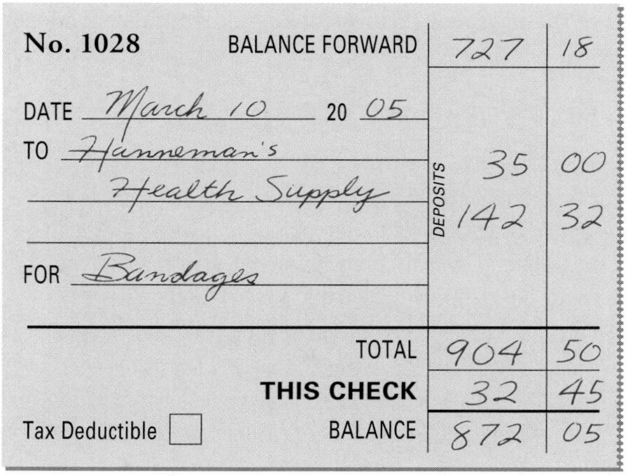
No. 1028 BALANCE FORWARD 727 18
DATE March 10 20 05
TO Hanneman's Health Supply
DEPOSITS 35 00
142 32
FOR Bandages
TOTAL 904 50
THIS CHECK 32 45
Tax Deductible ☐ BALANCE 872 05

FIGURE 14-3 Correctly completed check stub.

TABLE 14-1 Endorsements

Endorsement	Description	Example
Blank	Signature of the payee. Check can be cashed by anyone. This is not used in the business office.	Beth Williams
Full	Indicates person's name, company, account number, bank name, and payee's name.	Pay to the order of First Town Bank Beth Williams, M.D. 123-123456
Restrictive	Specifies to whom money should be paid, and the money's purpose, such as "For Deposit Only." You can rubber-stamp the physician's signature. It is considered the safest endorsement.	Pay to the order of First Town Bank For Deposit Only Beth Williams, M.D. 123-123456

Returned Checks

A check may be returned by the bank for a variety of reasons. When this occurs, a returned item notice is also included with the check detailing the reason for the return. Checks are returned, for example, when the payee name, date, or signature of payer is missing. If a check is returned with the payee's name or date missing, it is acceptable for the medical assistant to fill in the date and physician's name. If the payer's signature is missing, then the check will have to be returned to the payer. It is always wise to place a telephone call to a patient with the reasons for returning his or her check. All checks should be reviewed for either a written or stamped endorsement before depositing.

More serious reasons for the return of checks include not sufficient funds (NSF) in the payer's account or a stop-payment order issued by the payer. In the case of NSF, the payer's account does not have enough money to cover the amount of the check. You will need to contact the writer of the check and ask how he or she wishes to make the payment (Professionalism). If funds have been added to the account, the patient (payer) may ask that the check be resubmitted. To resubmit a check, call the payer's bank to determine if there are sufficient funds, write the word resubmit on both the face and the back of the check, make out another deposit slip, and resubmit. Many banks charge the account if the deposited check is NSF. Offices will then charge the patient, in addition to the amount of the NSF check, the fee charged to them by the bank and a handling charge. See Procedure 14-2 on posting non-sufficient funds checks.

Some medical offices have a policy that if a check is returned for NSF, they will not resubmit the check. They request the payment be made immediately, with either cash, a cashier's check, or money order. The returned check should be held until payment has been made. If the patient has not taken care of the bill after notification and a sufficient time have elapsed, then advise the patient in writing that the bill will be turned over to a collection agency. Some offices also charge for returned checks.

If a stop-payment order has been issued by the payer, then the bank will not allow the funds to be disbursed. The bank will indicate that you should contact the payer with the terms "refer to maker" on the item notice. This procedure is used when a check has been lost or stolen.

Professionalism

For many patients, money owed is a "touchy" and uncomfortable subject. Remember to always address this topic in a calm, nonjudgmental way. If a patient requests to make payment arrangements, comply only if the office has a policy about payment arrangements. Always follow the office policy, and never veer from the policy. In this way, your honesty in dealing with money issues will never be questioned.

Paying Bills

All bills should be paid by check for documentation and control purposes. The only exception to this policy would be very small payments, such as daily newspaper delivery and public transportation costs. In these instances, the payments could be made from petty cash. However, it is advisable that all payments, even the daily newspaper, be paid from accounts established with appropriate vendors.

PROCEDURE

Post Non-sufficient Funds Checks

OBJECTIVE: Demonstrate the process for posting non-sufficient funds (NSF) checks.

Equipment and Supplies
data; computer or ledger card; pen

Method
1. Record amount of NSF check and service fee in adjustment column on day sheet and ledger card.
2. Accurately record the NSF check to show that the amount is added to the balance, instead of subtracted from it.

3. Note the reason for the adjustment to patient account.

Charting Example
$68 plus $20 NSF check fee = $88 added to patient balance

An office policy must be established regarding how often checks are written, for example weekly, biweekly, semimonthly, or monthly. This bill-paying schedule must match a schedule of when funds are available for payment of the office expenses. For instance, your office policy may be to send all invoices to patients at the end of the month for payments that are due on the first of the next month. In this case, you would not want to write checks against your account to pay office expenses during the last week of the month since the payments from patients will not have arrived to cover your check writing.

The office banking policy should indicate who is responsible for writing and signing all checks. A smart policy is to separate the responsibilities; one person (the medical assistant) should write the checks and another person should be authorized to sign them (office manager or physician). In some medical offices, two authorized signatures are required in order to transfer funds from one account to another or to write checks over a certain dollar amount, such as $1,000.

It is not recommended to pay bills on the day they arrive since they are generally not due for 30 days. During that 30-day period, the money that is used to pay bills can remain in an interest-bearing account. The incentive to paying bills as they arrive occurs when a supplier (vendor) offers a discount if payment is included with the order or paid within ten days. Since this discount could be as much as 10 to 20 percent, it is wise to take advantage of it. Examples of recurring monthly expenses may include:

- Insurance premium(s)
- Rent or mortgage
- Waste removal
- Utilities, including telephone charges

- Housekeeping and maintenance expenses
- Laundry
- Equipment rental, such as a copy machine
- Taxes
- Maintenance contracts for equipment
- Medical and office supplies
- Postage

A schedule for paying these expenses should be kept on a master calendar or in a tickler (reminder) file. If all checks for expenses are written on a particular day of the month, a planned transfer of funds can be made from a savings account to a checking account to cover these checks.

Some offices use a tickler file to remind the bookkeeper when each bill is due. The office will have some recurrent bills that are the same amount and paid at the same time each month. One example of a recurrent bill is the office rent. The rent for the office is typically the same amount each month and is due on the same day of each month. For some offices, there may be an annual, bimonthly, or quarterly lease arrangement. In this case, the lease money may be paid up to one year in advance. The bills for the electricity, the water, the telephone, and the gas will vary in amount from month to month, but will still be due on the same day each month. These bills should be paid early enough in the month that the actual payment for the service reaches the company to which it is owed before the actual "due" date listed on the bill. It is a good idea to file these bills for payment days earlier than the actual due date so the checks or payment for them will be sent several days in advance to give the post office time to deliver the payment by the due date.

Hiring an Accountant or Bookkeeping Firm

Larger medical practices may hire an accountant or bookkeeping firm to process all checks. This is an accurate means of handling banking procedures. However, these services can be too costly for smaller medical offices. In some firms, a computerized check-writing service system is used.

Deposits

Deposits, which refer to money (cash and checks) placed into a bank account, can be made to either checking or savings accounts. Offices will vary somewhat on specific methods of handling deposits, but the following procedures are usually followed:

- Prepare and make deposits daily.
- Maintain all records of daily receipts (for checks and cash) together in a safe location.

- Compare the total on the deposit slip against the total on the day sheet.
- Keep a duplicate copy of all deposits on file in the office. Photocopy a deposit slip before submitting it to the bank. Some offices copy checks for later reference.
- Keep bank receipts of all deposits on file in the office.
- Immediately note all deposits in the checkbook.

All deposits should be made to the bank as soon as possible. Until cash and checks can be deposited, they should be stored in a secure location that is not accessible to patients.

Always compare the total credited to the accounts receivable with the total on the deposit slip. Occasionally, a check is omitted from the accounts receivable record. Numbers may be transposed when completing the deposit slip or the accounts receivable total. Using the pegboard or write-it-once system, results in a du-

---

14-3   PROCEDURE

Prepare a Deposit Slip

OBJECTIVE: Complete a bank deposit slip.

Equipment and Supplies
pen; deposit slip; checks and currency to be deposited; endorsing stamp; calculator

Method

1. Using the endorsing stamp, endorse all checks to be deposited. This means stamp the back of each check to be deposited with the endorsing stamp.
2. Complete the information on the front of the deposit slip:
   - Account name
   - Account number
   - Date of the deposit
3. If there is cash to be deposited, enter the amount of the cash in the upper right box of the deposit slip beside the "CASH" indicator. In the "CURRENCY box," list the total amount of all cash paper money to be deposited. In the "COIN" box, list the total of all the coin money to be deposited.
4. List each check to be deposited on a different line. If there are more checks than will fit on the

front, list each additional check on the reverse side of the deposit slip.
5. Beside the numbers, list who wrote the check. In the box beside the numbered box, list the amount of the check.
6. List each check in a different numbered box.
7. When all the checks to be deposited are entered on the reverse side of the deposit slip, use a calculator to add all the checks, and enter the total of the checks in the space at the bottom of the deposit slip that reads "TOTAL." This amount is also placed on the front of the deposit slip in the space that reads "TOTAL FROM REVERSE SIDE."
8. Use the calculator to add the total amount of the cash and the checks being deposited. List this amount in the space labeled TOTAL and in the space labeled NET DEPOSIT on the front of the deposit slip.
9. Place the deposit slip and the cash and checks listed on the slip in an envelope for deposit to the bank.

plicate deposit slip. Maintain an accurate balance of all accounts on a daily basis.

Completing the Deposit Slip

A deposit slip is completed every time a deposit is made into a bank account. The slip indicates the total dollar amounts of cash and checks being deposited. Entries on the slip should be printed in black ink. Currency (coins and bills) is totaled separately from checks. Each check must be entered on a different line. If there are more checks than lines provided, the excessive checks can be entered on the back of the deposit slip. The currency and coin totals and check totals are added together. Then this amount, the total for the deposit, is entered on the bottom line of the deposit slip. Procedure 14-3 lists steps for preparing deposit slips. See Figure 14-4 for an example of a deposit slip.

Check all deposits on the deposit slip against the day sheet totals. If the two figures do not match, check for the error in several ways:

- Recheck addition.
- Check each item on the deposit slip.
- Check for transposed numbers.
- If the error is still not found, subtract the difference between the deposit slip and the day sheet, then search for an item with that number.
- Check for errors of omission.

The correct order for listing money on a bank deposit is as follows: currency, coins, checks, and money orders.

Deposit to Savings Accounts

All cash and checks can also be deposited into a savings account. When the amount in a checking account becomes greater than the amount needed to cover the checks written on the account, deposits can be made into a savings account, which will have a greater interest return on the money than a checking account. When transferring funds from a checking account to a savings account, it is advisable to do so by check. This provides a record of the transaction.

A savings account is set up using a statement or a passbook, which are for maintaining a record of deposits, withdrawals, interest earned, and account balance. The passbook should be kept in a safe place

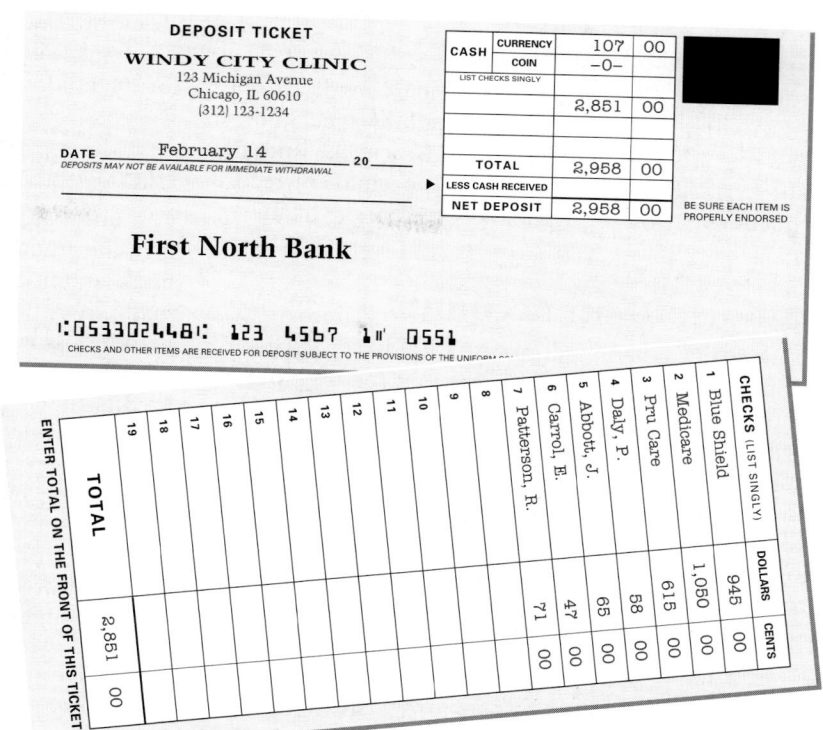

FIGURE 14-4 An example of the front and back side of a deposit slip.

designated for banking materials in the office. Statment savings accounts are sent monthly or quarterly.

Making the Deposit

Deposits can be made to both the checking and savings accounts in person, by mail, or by night depository. If a deposit is made in person, there will be an immediate receipt of deposit. A deposit by mail will result with a receipt by mail. However, cash should not be sent in the mail.

The night depository method can be set up for a business by obtaining a night depository key and depository bags with security locks. The deposit slip, cash, and checks are placed in the bag and then dropped off at the end of the day when the bank may be closed.

It is preferable that only one person be responsible for the deposits and another person be responsible for the receivable records. This separation of responsibilities is a critical method of fiscal or financial control.

Accepting Cash

Cash can be accepted as a form of payment, but this is not encouraged. Receipts must be given for all cash payments. Having large amounts of cash in an office poses a security risk and also holds the potential for the embezzlement of funds. Embezzlement is the taking of funds and involves a breach of trust. Large cash amounts may necessitate making bank deposits more than once a day.

Cash Disbursement

Cash disbursement refers to payments made to your creditors. The term "cash" is misleading since, in most cases, the disbursement is made by check, and not cash. Payment by check provides a permanent record as documentation for taxes and proof of payment.

Bank Hold on Accounts

Occasionally, a bank will place a "hold" on a checking account. A statement may appear that reads "Hold for Uncollected Funds (HCF)" when a deposit needs to "clear" so that the bank can make sure the funds (money) are present before allowing anyone to write a check on that account. This is called a "hold." The bank will not actually credit the account in which the money was deposited until the check has been processed and the funds paid to the payer's bank. These funds cannot be used by the depositor until the check or funds have cleared and the hold is removed. The bank will notify the depositor of the length of time for the hold.

Bank Statement

The purpose of a statement from the bank is to confirm the amount of funds that are in each account. The bank statement can uncover errors that have been made in either the office bookkeeping system or the bank bookkeeping system.

A monthly bank statement includes all debits and credits that have been processed. Debits are charges against an account; credits are additions to an account. The statement will include canceled checks—checks that have been processed and paid out to the medical practice's creditors by the bank. Many banks no longer return canceled checks, which indicates a further need to maintain excellent record keeping on the check stub when the check is written. Figure 14-5 is an example of a typical bank statement.

STATEMENT OF ACCOUNT

FIRST NORTH
BANK OF CHIGAGO
123 East Pearson, Chicago, IL 60611
(312) 321-1000

144808

WINDY CITY CLINIC
BETH WILLIAMS, MD
123 MICHIGAN AVENUE
CHICAGO, IL 60610

PAGE 1 OF 1
STATEMENT PERIOD
FROM 08/01/05
THRU 08/31/05
CUST # 300-30-3000

- - - - - - - - - - - - - - - ADVANTAGE CHECKING ACCOUNT - - - - - - - - - - - - - -

ACCOUNT NBR DD	12345	BEGINNING BALANCE	$2,646.63
AVG COLL BAL	$4,732.52	DEPOSITS/CREDITS	$8,000.00
MINIMUM BAL	$2,502.88	INTEREST PAID	$.00
TAX ID NUMBER	300-30-3000	CHECKS/DEBITS	$7,871.32 -
		SERVICE CHARGES	$5.00 -
		ENDING BALANCE	$2,770.31
		# DEPOSITS/CREDITS	1
		#CHECKS/DEBITS	11

DATE	DESCRIPTION		AMOUNT	BALANCE
08/01	BEGINNING BALANCE			$2,646.63
08/01	CK#	872	24.95-	2,621.68
08/06	CK#	879	3.00-	2,618.68
08/08	CK#	883	75.00-	2,543.68
08/14	CK#	885	15.80-	2,527.88
08/15	CK#	886	25.00-	2,502.88
08/19	DEPOSIT		8,000.00	10,502.88
08/26	CK#	887	32.00-	10,470.88
08/26	CK#	888	2,500.00-	7,970.88
08/28	CK#	890	70.00-	7,900.88
08/28	CK#	889	125.57-	7,775.31
08/28	CK#	884	5,000.00-	2,775.31
08/31	MONTHLY MAINTENANCE FEE		5.00-	2,770.31
08/31	ENDING BALANCE			$2,770.31

CHECK REGISTER

CHECK#	DATE	AMOUNT	CHECK#	DATE	AMOUNT
872	08/01	24.95	886	08/15	25.00
879*	08/06	3.00	887	08/26	32.00
883*	08/08	75.00	888	08/26	2,500.00
884	08/28	5,000.00	889	08/28	125.57
885	08/14	15.80	890	08/28	70.00

* INDICATES NON-CONSECUTIVE CHECK NUMBER(S)

FIGURE 14-5 A typical bank statement.

Reconciliation of Bank Statements

Reconciliation of bank statements refers to the comparison of the figures on the bank statements with the records maintained in the medical office and the adjustment of banking records so that both are in agreement. The purpose of the reconciliation of bank statements is to match the account activity and totals against the medical office records. Bank statements include the following information:

- Account number
- Average collected balance
- Minimum balance
- Tax ID number (usually the Social Security number of the physician)
- Beginning balance
- Deposit history
- Interest/credits
- Checks and debits
- Service charges
- Ending balance

Bank statements should be reconciled as soon as they are received, and errors that are found should be corrected immediately. Office policy

PROCEDURE

Reconciling a Bank Statement

OBJECTIVE: Reconcile a bank statement for a checking account.

Equipment and Supplies

current and previous bank statements; cancelled checks (if returned by the bank); checkbook stubs

Method

1. Compare the beginning balance of the current statement with the ending balance of the previous statement. These should be the same.
2. Write the current ending balance in the appropriate space on the reverse side of the bank statement.
3. Compare deposits noted on the statement against your records or receipts by making a check mark next to each correct number.
4. List separately all outstanding deposits. These are deposits made toward the end of the month that have not been included in the current statement. Add these together and place the total on the reverse side of the statement in the space provided.
5. Add the ending balance to the total of deposits not already included and write this amount on the TOTAL line.
6. Compare the value of the checks listed on the statement with the value listed in the checkbook or check stubs and place a check mark next to each correct number.
7. Note all numbers missing from the sequential list of check numbers; these are checks that have not yet cleared your bank (outstanding checks). List all outstanding checks. Add the total for outstanding checks and place that figure on the line indicated on the back of the statement.
8. Subtract the total figure for checks outstanding from the previous total on the back of the statement to determine the current balance. This amount should agree with the amount in your check book or stub balance.

Example:

1. Bank balance shown on this statement: $ _____

   ADD (+)
2. Deposits not credited in this statement, (if any) $ _____
3. TOTAL $ _____

   SUBTRACT (−)
4. Checks outstanding $ _____
5. BALANCE $ _____

Summary of RULES:

#1 Note ending statement balance.

#2 Add all deposits not yet credited.

#3 Determine subtotal of step #1 and #2.

#4 Subtract total outstanding checks.

#5 Determine balance or final total.

---

may indicate an exact date when reconciliation should take place. For better fiscal control, the person reconciling the bank statement should be someone other than the person who prepares the checks and makes the deposits. This can prevent the embezzlement of funds.

If it is an interest-bearing account, the interest earned will be on the average collected balance. It is the average amount of money in that account during the period covered by the statement. Any interest credited to the account or any service fees charged to the account, as shown on the bank statement, should be recorded in the checking account records before beginning the reconciliation.

The processed checks will be listed by number. Any checks that are listed in non-consecutive order may be indicated with an asterisk (*).

The reverse side of the bank statement includes information on how to handle errors or questions about the statement, and a form to assist in reconciling the bank statement. Procedure 14-4 lists step-by-step instructions for reconciling a bank statement.

Saving Documentation

Documents relating to banking procedures should be saved in an organized manner. In addition to banking documents, such as copies of deposit slips and check stubs, your records must include the following for verification of business expenses:

- Receipts
- Vouchers for expenses and salaries

- Invoices
- Statements from suppliers
- Proof of payments

These supporting documents should be saved in a file with check numbers of payments written on the document. After the bank statement has been reconciled each month, it should be stored with the canceled checks as further documentation of business activity. Remember that business expenses are subject to auditing by the Internal Revenue Service (IRS). Good record-keeping is essential when providing documentation to the IRS. For more on the medical assistant's responsibilities when performing banking procedures, see Legal and Ethical Issues.

Petty Cash

Petty cash is available for small purchases, reimbursements, postage due or other miscellaneous expenses within the medical office. For example, petty cash is used for postage due on certified mail received in the office, or postage due on underpaid letters received. Petty cash must be tracked and recorded in a daily financial log. To replenish petty cash, a check is written for the predetermined amount. There is usually a designated amount of cash placed in a drawer or box at the beginning of each month for this purpose. This amount will vary from office to office, depending on the needs of the office, but is usually $50 to $100. At the end of a designated period (a week, or a month), all the receipts for money taken out of the petty cash drawer will be totaled and added to the money remaining in the drawer. This total should match the amount placed in the drawer at the beginning. The cash used during the

period will then be replaced to make the total cash available in the drawer equal to the beginning amount. Petty cash is usually handled by one responsible office person and a designee in his or her absence and is kept in a secret place under lock and key.

Payroll

Payroll responsibilities include calculating payroll checks for all the staff. Some medical offices contract an independent payroll service. This may or may not include the physician, depending on how the payment system is set up. Payroll checks are generally issued weekly, biweekly, or monthly. These result in the following pay periods for a year:

Weekly—52 pay periods a year

Biweekly—26 pay periods a year

Monthly—12 pay periods a year

The physician determines the type of pay period the office will use. All employees will then be paid at the same time. Figure 14-6 is an example of an employee payroll record.

The employee's payroll check is determined by first calculating the gross annual wage before taxes and any withholdings that are taken out. Use the formula:

(Hourly wage × Number of hours worked per week) × 52 Weeks in a year = Gross pay (or Hourly wage × 2080 Full-time hours in a year = Annual pay)

The annual gross wage for an employee earning $9.00 per hour working a 40-hour week would be:

$$\$9.00 \times 40 \times 52 = \$18,720$$

annual gross wage

To determine the amount the employee earns per day, use the following formula:

(Annual gross pay ÷ 52) ÷ 5 = Day's pay

For the example above: ($18,720 ÷ 52) = $360

$$\$360 \div 5 = \$72$$

Therefore, if this employee missed a day of work, $72 would be deducted to arrive at the adjusted gross pay ($360 − $72 = $288). Occasionally, an employee will be requested to work overtime or to work more hours than normal for that pay period (a 40-hour week at 8 hours a day for 5 days per week). To calculate the overtime pay of time and a half (1 hour pay plus ½ hour pay) for an employee who worked one day of overtime at the hourly wage of $9.00, simply divide $9.00 in half ($4.50) and add that amount to the regular $9.00 hourly wage ($9.00 + $4.50 = $13.50). The payment for one hour of overtime for this employee would be $13.50 instead of the regular $9.00 payment.

Money is withheld from the employee's paycheck, depending on the taxes that must be paid by the employee and employer. This is referred to as tax withholding. For example, if the withholding tax is four percent, then this amount is calculated based on the employee's gross pay. The taxes are then subtracted from the gross or an adjusted gross pay. The amount after subtracting the withholdings is what appears on the employee's paycheck.

Government regulations require that records must be maintained for each employee relating to the following payroll items:

- Amount of gross pay
- Social Security number of the employee
- Number of exemptions of each employee (taken from W-4 form completed by the employee at the time of hire)
- Deductions for Social Security, federal, state, and city taxes
- State disability insurance and unemployment tax, where applicable

NAME __Joyce Walker__   SOCIAL SECURITY NO. __123-12-1234__
ADDRESS __22 W. Elm Avenue, Apt 3C__   DATE OF EMPLOYMENT __6-30-05__
__Goram City, MI 55555__   TELEPHONE __(010)123-4567__
EXEMPTIONS __1__   HOURLY RATE __$10.00__

HOURS REG.	HOURS O.T.	GROSS SALARY	FWT	SWT	FICA			NET SALARY	DATE	CHECK NO.
80		800 –	72–	14–	61 60			652 40	7/14	276
80		800 –	72–	14–	61 60			652 40	7/28	414
72		720 –	64 80	12 60	55 45			587 15	8/11	565
80	4	860 –	77 40	15 05	66 20			701 35	8/25	697
QUARTERLY TOTAL										
YEAR TO DATE										

FIGURE 14-6 An example of an employee payroll record.

Methods for Calculating Payroll Checks

There are several systems for calculating and issuing payroll checks. They include manual, pegboard, and computer.

Manual

Meticulous recordkeeping is necessary when performing any payroll function. Procedure 14-5 lists steps for manually generating a payroll in a medical office. Separate records are needed for documentation of the gross income, tax withholdings, and each of the checks issued for all employees. This can mean that the records for payroll are kept in more than one record book or logbook. For example, the check stub will indicate the name, date, and amount of the payroll check, while a logbook is needed to track the gross income and withholdings, which are totaled monthly, quarterly, and annually.

Pegboard

The advantage of using a pegboard (write-it-once) method is that all or most of the payroll record is in one record.

Computer

There are several software packages available that are used to calculate payroll and tax withholdings and print payroll checks. Such software programs can save time for office staff over the traditional manual method. In addition, the amounts calculated for withholding can be performed more accurately with the computer than with the manual method. In some offices, an outside payroll service is hired to process all payroll checks, withholding payments, and keep records.

Income Tax Withholding

Federal, state, and city taxes are withheld from the paycheck of the employee. These tax payments are made directly to the government. Employers have an obligation by law to withhold a portion of their employee's earnings for tax purposes, and report and forward this amount to the government. To determine the amount of money to be withheld from each paycheck, each employee must complete a W-4 form when he or she is hired (Figure 14-7). The W-4 form must include:

- Employee's name and current address
- Social Security number
- Marital status
- The number of exemptions the employee claims that should be used when calculating withheld tax money

Tables used to determine the amount of withholding are provided in the Federal Employer's Tax Guide.

Generating Payroll in a Medical Office

OBJECTIVE: Manually generate payroll.

Equipment and Supplies
pen; calculator; checkbook; employee time card; employee payroll record; payroll register; tax tables

Method
1. Gather the above equipment.
2. Using the employee time card, calculate the total number of regular hours worked and then the total number of overtime hours worked. Enter the totals obtained on the payroll register.
3. In the employee payroll record, obtain the employee's pay rate. Calculate the pay rate times the total number of regular hours worked. Next, calculate the overtime pay rate times the total number of overtime hours. Enter the totals for each on the payroll register. Add the regular hours earned and overtime hours earned and place this amount on the payroll register under the heading total gross.
4. Gather the employee payroll record and tax tables. Determine how much to withhold for federal income tax. This depends on the marital status of the employee as well as the amount of exemptions. Next, calculate the total FICA tax to be withheld for Medicare and Social Security. Enter the amounts on the payroll register.
5. Determine how much to withhold for local and state taxes. This depends on the marital status of the employee and the amount of exemptions. Enter the amounts on the payroll register.
6. Compute employer's contributions to the unemployment fund of the state of residence and FUTA. Next, document these calculations on the employer's account.
7. Determine if there are any other deductions (i.e. stock purchase plans, insurance, flexible spending account, or 401K).
8. To calculate the net earnings subtract the total amount of deductions from the gross earnings.
9. Complete the check stub and check with the required information.

See Figure 14-8 for a sample federal tax-withholding table. Tables are available for married persons, single persons, and unmarried heads of households and cover weekly, biweekly, monthly, semimonthly, and daily periods.

Social Security, Medicare, and Income Tax Withholding

The federal government mandates, or requires, the following taxes be paid: Social Security (Federal Insurance Contribution Act or FICA), Medicare, and federal income tax. These taxes are based on a percentage of the employee's total gross income (see calculation on page 260 for determining gross income). The number of exemptions claimed on the W-4 form and the marital status of the employee are taken into account when calculating the tax. The employer has an obligation to match the employee's payment for Social Security and Medicare. This means that if the employee has $100 withheld for Social Security and Medicare, the employer must match the $100 and make a total payment to the government for that employee of $200. The employer does not have to match the federal, state, and local taxes.

Deposit Requirements

The federal tax money withheld and the FICA payment are placed into a federal deposit account in a Federal Reserve Bank or into an authorized banking institution, either at the end of each period or at the end of the month. The Internal Revenue Service (IRS) has a severe penalty for failure to deposit this money.

Employers must file a quarterly report (Form 941 Employer's Quarterly Federal Tax Return) before the last day of the first month after the end of the quarter. These dates are April 30, July 31, October 31, and January 31.

Federal Unemployment Tax

Every employer must contribute to the unemployment tax act as mandated under the Federal Unemployment Tax Act (FUTA). If the employer is making payments into a state unemployment fund, this can generally be applied as credit against the FUTA tax amount.

Form W-4 (20XX)

Purpose. Complete Form W-4 so that your employer can withhold the correct federal income tax from your pay. Because your tax situation may change, you may want to refigure your withholding each year.

Exemption from withholding. If you are exempt, complete only lines 1, 2, 3, 4, and 7 and sign the form to validate it. Your exemption for 20XX expires February 16, 20XX. See Pub. 505, Tax Withholding and Estimated Tax.

Note. You cannot claim exemption from withholding if (a) your income exceeds $800 and includes more than $250 of unearned income (for example, interest and dividends) and (b) another person can claim you as a dependent on their tax return.

Basic instructions. If you are not exempt, complete the **Personal Allowances Worksheet** below. The worksheets on page 2 adjust your withholding allowances based on itemized deductions, certain credits, adjustments to income, or two-earner/two-job situations. Complete all worksheets that apply. However, you may claim fewer (or zero) allowances.

Head of household. Generally, you may claim head of household filing status on your tax return only if you are unmarried and pay more than 50% of the costs of keeping up a home for yourself and your dependent(s) or other qualifying individuals. See line E below.

Tax credits. You can take projected tax credits into account in figuring your allowable number of withholding allowances. Credits for child or dependent care expenses and the child tax credit may be claimed using the **Personal Allowances Worksheet** below. See Pub. 919, How Do I Adjust My Tax Withholding? for information on converting your other credits into withholding allowances.

Nonwage income. If you have a large amount of nonwage income, such as interest or dividends, consider making estimated tax payments using Form 1040-ES, Estimated Tax for Individuals. Otherwise, you may owe additional tax.

Two earners/two jobs. If you have a working spouse or more than one job, figure the total number of allowances you are entitled to claim on all jobs using worksheets from only one Form W-4. Your withholding usually will be most accurate when all allowances are claimed on the Form W-4 for the highest paying job and zero allowances are claimed on the others.

Nonresident alien. If you are a nonresident alien, see the Instructions for Form 8233 before completing this Form W-4.

Check your withholding. After your Form W-4 takes effect, use Pub. 919 to see how the dollar amount you are having withheld compares to your projected total tax for 20XX. See Pub. 919, especially if your earnings exceed $125,000 (Single) or $175,000 (Married).

Recent name change? If your name on line 1 differs from that shown on your social security card, call 1-800-772-1213 to initiate a name change and obtain a social security card showing your correct name.

Personal Allowances Worksheet (Keep for your records.)

A Enter "1" for **yourself** if no one else can claim you as a dependent . . . . A ____

B Enter "1" if: {
- You are single and have only one job; or
- You are married, have only one job, and your spouse does not work; or
- Your wages from a second job or your spouse's wages (or the total of both) are $1,000 or less. } . . B ____

C Enter "1" for your **spouse**. But, you may choose to enter "-0-" if you are married and have either a working spouse or more than one job. (Entering "-0-" may help you avoid having too little tax withheld.) . . . . C ____

D Enter number of **dependents** (other than your spouse or yourself) you will claim on your tax return . . . . . . D ____

E Enter "1" if you will file as **head of household** on your tax return (see conditions under **Head of household** above) . E ____

F Enter "1" if you have at least $1,500 of **child or dependent care expenses** for which you plan to claim a credit . . F ____
(**Note.** Do **not** include child support payments. See **Pub. 503,** Child and Dependent Care Expenses, for details.)

G **Child Tax Credit** (including additional child tax credit):
- If your total income will be less than $54,000 ($79,000 if married), enter "2" for each eligible child.
- If your total income will be between $54,000 and $84,000 ($79,000 and $119,000 if married), enter "1" for each eligible child plus "1" **additional** if you have four or more eligible children. . . . . G ____

H Add lines A through G and enter total here. (**Note.** This may be different from the number of exemptions you claim on your tax return.) ▶ H ____

For accuracy, complete all worksheets that apply. {
- If you plan to **itemize or claim adjustments to income** and want to reduce your withholding, see the **Deductions and Adjustments Worksheet** on page 2.
- If you have **more than one job** or are **married and you and your spouse both work** and the combined earnings from all jobs exceed $35,000 ($25,000 if married) see the **Two-Earner/Two-Job Worksheet** on page 2 to avoid having too little tax withheld.
- If **neither** of the above situations applies, **stop here** and enter the number from line H on line 5 of Form W-4 below.

Cut here and give Form W-4 to your employer. Keep the top part for your records.

Form **W-4**

Department of the Treasury
Internal Revenue Service

Employee's Withholding Allowance Certificate

▶ Whether you are entitled to claim a certain number of allowances or exemption from withholding is subject to review by the IRS. Your employer may be required to send a copy of this form to the IRS.

OMB No. 1545-0010

20XX

1 Type or print your first name and middle initial	Last name		2 Your social security number

Home address (number and street or rural route)		3 ☐ Single ☐ Married ☐ Married, but withhold at higher Single rate.
City or town, state, and ZIP code		**Note.** If married, but legally separated, or spouse is a nonresident alien, check the "Single" box.

4 If your last name differs from that shown on your social security card, check here. You must call 1-800-772-1213 for a new card. ▶ ☐

5 Total number of allowances you are claiming (from line **H** above **or** from the applicable worksheet on page 2) | 5 ____

6 Additional amount, if any, you want withheld from each paycheck . . . . | 6 $ ____

7 I claim exemption from withholding for 20XX, and I certify that I meet **both** of the following conditions for exemption.
- Last year I had a right to a refund of **all** federal income tax withheld because I had **no** tax liability **and**
- This year I expect a refund of **all** federal income tax withheld because I expect to have **no** tax liability.
If you meet both conditions, write "Exempt" here . . . . ▶ | 7 ____

Under penalties of perjury, I declare that I have examined this certificate and to the best of my knowledge and belief, it is true, correct, and complete.

Employee's signature
(Form is not valid unless you sign it.) ▶

Date ▶

8 Employer's name and address (Employer: Complete lines 8 and 10 only if sending to the IRS.)	9 Office code (optional)	10 Employer identification number (EIN)

For Privacy Act and Paperwork Reduction Act Notice, see page 2.

Cat. No. 10220Q

Form **W-4** (20XX)

FIGURE 14-7 An example of a W-4 required by the IRS.

2004 Tax Table

See the instructions for line 43 that begin on page 33 to see if you must use the Tax Table below to figure your tax.

Example. Mr. and Mrs. Brown are filing a joint return. Their taxable income on Form 1040, line 42, is $25,300. First, they find the $25,300–25,350 taxable income line. Next, they find the column for married filing jointly and read down the column. The amount shown where the taxable income line and filing status column meet is $3,084. This is the tax amount they should enter on Form 1040, line 43.

Sample Table

At least	But less than	Single	Married filing jointly *	Married filing separately	Head of a household
			Your tax is—		
25,200	25,250	3,426	3,069	3,426	3,274
25,250	25,300	3,434	3,076	3,434	3,281
25,300	25,350	3,441	3,084	3,441	3,289
25,350	25,400	3,449	3,091	3,449	3,296

If line 42 (taxable income) is— At least	But less than	And you are— Single	Married filing jointly *	Married filing separately	Head of a household
			Your tax is—		
0	5	0	0	0	0
5	15	1	1	1	1
15	25	2	2	2	2
25	50	4	4	4	4
50	75	6	6	6	6
75	100	9	9	9	9
100	125	11	11	11	11
125	150	14	14	14	14
150	175	16	16	16	16
175	200	19	19	19	19
200	225	21	21	21	21
225	250	24	24	24	24
250	275	26	26	26	26
275	300	29	29	29	29
300	325	31	31	31	31
325	350	34	34	34	34
350	375	36	36	36	36
375	400	39	39	39	39
400	425	41	41	41	41
425	450	44	44	44	44
450	475	46	46	46	46
475	500	49	49	49	49
500	525	51	51	51	51
525	550	54	54	54	54
550	575	56	56	56	56
575	600	59	59	59	59
600	625	61	61	61	61
625	650	64	64	64	64
650	675	66	66	66	66
675	700	69	69	69	69
700	725	71	71	71	71
725	750	74	74	74	74
750	775	76	76	76	76
775	800	79	79	79	79
800	825	81	81	81	81
825	850	84	84	84	84
850	875	86	86	86	86
875	900	89	89	89	89
900	925	91	91	91	91
925	950	94	94	94	94
950	975	96	96	96	96
975	1,000	99	99	99	99

1,000

At least	But less than	Single	Married filing jointly *	Married filing separately	Head of a household
1,000	1,025	101	101	101	101
1,025	1,050	104	104	104	104
1,050	1,075	106	106	106	106
1,075	1,100	109	109	109	109
1,100	1,125	111	111	111	111
1,125	1,150	114	114	114	114
1,150	1,175	116	116	116	116
1,175	1,200	119	119	119	119
1,200	1,225	121	121	121	121
1,225	1,250	124	124	124	124
1,250	1,275	126	126	126	126
1,275	1,300	129	129	129	129

If line 42 (taxable income) is— At least	But less than	And you are— Single	Married filing jointly *	Married filing separately	Head of a household
			Your tax is—		
1,300	1,325	131	131	131	131
1,325	1,350	134	134	134	134
1,350	1,375	136	136	136	136
1,375	1,400	139	139	139	139
1,400	1,425	141	141	141	141
1,425	1,450	144	144	144	144
1,450	1,475	146	146	146	146
1,475	1,500	149	149	149	149
1,500	1,525	151	151	151	151
1,525	1,550	154	154	154	154
1,550	1,575	156	156	156	156
1,575	1,600	159	159	159	159
1,600	1,625	161	161	161	161
1,625	1,650	164	164	164	164
1,650	1,675	166	166	166	166
1,675	1,700	169	169	169	169
1,700	1,725	171	171	171	171
1,725	1,750	174	174	174	174
1,750	1,775	176	176	176	176
1,775	1,800	179	179	179	179
1,800	1,825	181	181	181	181
1,825	1,850	184	184	184	184
1,850	1,875	186	186	186	186
1,875	1,900	189	189	189	189
1,900	1,925	191	191	191	191
1,925	1,950	194	194	194	194
1,950	1,975	196	196	196	196
1,975	2,000	199	199	199	199

2,000

At least	But less than	Single	Married filing jointly *	Married filing separately	Head of a household
2,000	2,025	201	201	201	201
2,025	2,050	204	204	204	204
2,050	2,075	206	206	206	206
2,075	2,100	209	209	209	209
2,100	2,125	211	211	211	211
2,125	2,150	214	214	214	214
2,150	2,175	216	216	216	216
2,175	2,200	219	219	219	219
2,200	2,225	221	221	221	221
2,225	2,250	224	224	224	224
2,250	2,275	226	226	226	226
2,275	2,300	229	229	229	229
2,300	2,325	231	231	231	231
2,325	2,350	234	234	234	234
2,350	2,375	236	236	236	236
2,375	2,400	239	239	239	239
2,400	2,425	241	241	241	241
2,425	2,450	244	244	244	244
2,450	2,475	246	246	246	246
2,475	2,500	249	249	249	249
2,500	2,525	251	251	251	251
2,525	2,550	254	254	254	254
2,550	2,575	256	256	256	256
2,575	2,600	259	259	259	259
2,600	2,625	261	261	261	261
2,625	2,650	264	264	264	264
2,650	2,675	266	266	266	266
2,675	2,700	269	269	269	269

If line 42 (taxable income) is— At least	But less than	And you are— Single	Married filing jointly *	Married filing separately	Head of a household
			Your tax is—		
2,700	2,725	271	271	271	271
2,725	2,750	274	274	274	274
2,750	2,775	276	276	276	276
2,775	2,800	279	279	279	279
2,800	2,825	281	281	281	281
2,825	2,850	284	284	284	284
2,850	2,875	286	286	286	286
2,875	2,900	289	289	289	289
2,900	2,925	291	291	291	291
2,925	2,950	294	294	294	294
2,950	2,975	296	296	296	296
2,975	3,000	299	299	299	299

3,000

At least	But less than	Single	Married filing jointly *	Married filing separately	Head of a household
3,000	3,050	303	303	303	303
3,050	3,100	308	308	308	308
3,100	3,150	313	313	313	313
3,150	3,200	318	318	318	318
3,200	3,250	323	323	323	323
3,250	3,300	328	328	328	328
3,300	3,350	333	333	333	333
3,350	3,400	338	338	338	338
3,400	3,450	343	343	343	343
3,450	3,500	348	348	348	348
3,500	3,550	353	353	353	353
3,550	3,600	358	358	358	358
3,600	3,650	363	363	363	363
3,650	3,700	368	368	368	368
3,700	3,750	373	373	373	373
3,750	3,800	378	378	378	378
3,800	3,850	383	383	383	383
3,850	3,900	388	388	388	388
3,900	3,950	393	393	393	393
3,950	4,000	398	398	398	398

4,000

At least	But less than	Single	Married filing jointly *	Married filing separately	Head of a household
4,000	4,050	403	403	403	403
4,050	4,100	408	408	408	408
4,100	4,150	413	413	413	413
4,150	4,200	418	418	418	418
4,200	4,250	423	423	423	423
4,250	4,300	428	428	428	428
4,300	4,350	433	433	433	433
4,350	4,400	438	438	438	438
4,400	4,450	443	443	443	443
4,450	4,500	448	448	448	448
4,500	4,550	453	453	453	453
4,550	4,600	458	458	458	458
4,600	4,650	463	463	463	463
4,650	4,700	468	468	468	468
4,700	4,750	473	473	473	473
4,750	4,800	478	478	478	478
4,800	4,850	483	483	483	483
4,850	4,900	488	488	488	488
4,900	4,950	493	493	493	493
4,950	5,000	498	498	498	498

(Continued on page 61)

* This column must also be used by a qualifying widow(er).

FIGURE 14-8 An example of a federal tax witholding table.

FUTA is the sole responsibility of the employer. It is based on the employee's gross income, but must not be deducted from the employee's wage.

FUTA deposits are calculated quarterly and the amount due must be paid by the last day of the first month after the quarter ends. Therefore, for the first quarter of the year ending on March 31st, the payment must be made by April 30th. An annual FUTA report must be filed to the federal government using Form 940 each year.

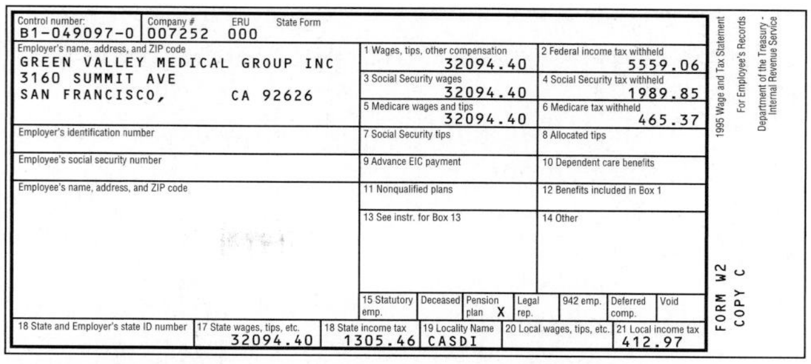
Control number: B1-049097-0 | Company # 007252 | ERU 000 | State Form
Employer's name, address, and ZIP code
GREEN VALLEY MEDICAL GROUP INC
3160 SUMMIT AVE
SAN FRANCISCO, CA 92626
1 Wages, tips, other compensation 32094.40
2 Federal income tax withheld 5559.06
3 Social Security wages 32094.40
4 Social Security tax withheld 1989.85
5 Medicare wages and tips 32094.40
6 Medicare tax withheld 465.37
Employer's identification number
7 Social Security tips
8 Allocated tips
Employee's social security number
9 Advance EIC payment
10 Dependent care benefits
Employee's name, address, and ZIP code
11 Nonqualified plans
12 Benefits included in Box 1
13 See instr. for Box 13
14 Other
15 Statutory emp. | Deceased | Pension plan X | Legal rep. | 942 emp. | Deferred comp. | Void
18 State and Employer's state ID number | 17 State wages, tips, etc. 32094.40 | 18 State income tax 1305.46 | 19 Locality Name CASDI | 20 Local wages, tips, etc. | 21 Local income tax 412.97
1995 Wage and Tax Statement
For Employee's Records
Department of the Treasury - Internal Revenue Service
FORM W2
COPY C

FIGURE 14-9 An example of a W-2 form required by the IRS.

State Unemployment Tax

All states have unemployment compensation laws. Most states require only the employer to make payments toward this fund. However, a few states require both the employer and employee to make a payment. In this case, the employer would withhold a certain calculated amount from the employee's paycheck.

In some states, the employer does not have to make a payment to unemployment compensation if there are very few employees (four or less). Each state's regulation concerning tax requirements should be checked carefully before preparing the payroll.

State Disability Insurance

Some states require a certain amount of money be withheld from the employee's check to cover a disability insurance plan. This insurance coverage assists employees in the event they become injured or disabled and unable to work. Money may also be withheld, as requested by the employee, for health, life, and disability insurances, and pension plan contributions.

Annual Tax Returns

W-2 forms must be completed at the end of each year and given to each employee. The amount of wages that were taxable under Social Security and Medicare must be listed separately on the W-2 form. The employer must provide three copies of the W-2 form to each employee from whom these taxes were withheld (one each for federal and state filing and one for the employee's file). According to the law, this form must be received by the employee by January 31. The W-2 form (Figure 14-9) lists the total gross income, total federal, state, and local taxes that were withheld, taxable fringe benefits, such as tips, and the employee's total net income for the year.

The preparation of reports to the federal government and the W-2 forms for the employees can be time-consuming and requires some training. Many offices that do not have a bookkeeper or medical assistant assigned to this duty, use the services of an accountant. The records and reports the accountant will use need to be prepared ahead of time. The pegboard system, if used, can provide summaries of the income, expenses, and payroll for the office. If a manual system is used, the totals for all the tax payment periods should be calculated for the accountant. The accountant will then audit or reexamine all the financial statements for accuracy.

SUMMARY

Banking is one of the critical office procedures, since it requires careful handling of money and records. A thorough understanding of banking procedures and terminology is vital to running on efficient medical office. Great trust is placed upon the medical assistant by the physician to handle his or her banking needs with accuracy.

Chapter Review

COMPETENCY REVIEW

1. Define and spell the terms to learn for the chapter.
2. Using your own bank statement, reconcile it to your checkbook records.
3. Create and complete a check and check stub in the amount of 65 cents drafted to Bill Jay.
4. Call a local bank and request information regarding the various options for checking and savings accounts.
5. Create a bank deposit slip for $23.10 in cash and checks for $54.00, $21.25, $110.00, $29.00, and $9.25.

1. A check that will become void if written over a certain amount is a
   A. certified check
   B. limited check
   C. cashier's check
   D. warrant
   E. deposit

2. The person who signs the check is the
   A. maker
   B. payee
   C. payer
   D. teller
   E. depositor

3. The code number found in the upper and sometimes lower right-hand corner of a printed check is the
   A. MICR
   B. withdrawal number
   C. registration number
   D. ABA number
   E. Social Security number

4. Future-dated checks are referred to as
   A. postdated
   B. old
   C. traveler's
   D. voucher
   E. predated

5. Which of the following is petty cash NOT available for?
   A. small purchase
   B. payroll
   C. postage due
   D. reimbursements
   E. other miscellaneous expenses

6. Which of the following is a FALSE statement about check stubs?
   A. stubs should have the purpose of check
   B. stubs should have the name of payee
   C. stubs should have the name of payer
   D. stubs should be filled out after removing from checkbook
   E. stubs should be retained

7. Third-party checks that are safe to accept are those that are
   A. from patients
   B. from insurance companies
   C. from vendors
   D. never to be accepted
   E. from out-of-town patients

8. Reconcile the bank statement and checkbook balance for the following: bank statement $1,200, checkbook balance $1,350, bank fees $20, outstanding checks $140 and $200. What is the correct checkbook balance?
   A. $1,200
   B. $1,310
   C. $1,330
   D. $1,350
   E. $1,430

9. What information is NOT listed on an employee's W-4 form?
   A. marital status
   B. number of exemptions
   C. salary
   D. employee's Social Security number
   E. current address

10. By law, the employer must match employee contributions on what tax?
   A. disability insurance
   B. workmans' compensation
   C. Social Security
   D. state
   E. self-employment tax

CRITICAL THINKING

1. What effect will Sara's decision to "borrow" money from petty cash have on the funds?

2. What could Sara have done differently if she wished to borrow money from petty cash?

ON THE JOB

Your office has decided that all payroll should be handled through direct deposit into the employee bank accounts. Call your bank, ask them how that procedure would be handled for a medical office. There are forms to complete and information on other bank account numbers and ABA numbers that you will need to collect and complete, according to the bank's procedures.

INTERNET ACTIVITY

Call your bank and get its online address. Then go to the Internet and access the bank's home page. If you do not have a bank account, call several local banks and go to their home pages. List the steps in setting up an online banking account.

MediaLink More on financial management, including interactive resources, can be found on the Student CD-ROM accompanying this textbook.

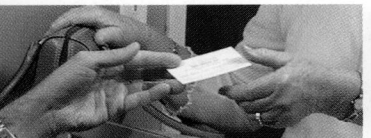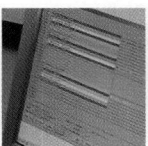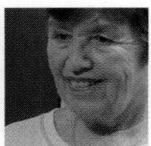

Medical Assistant Role Delineation Chart

HIGHLIGHT indicates material covered in this chapter.

ADMINISTRATIVE

Administrative Procedures

- Perform basic administrative medical assisting functions
- Schedule, coordinate and monitor appointments
- Schedule inpatient/outpatient admissions and procedures
- Understand and apply third-party guidelines
- Obtain reimbursement through accurate claims submission
- Monitor third-party reimbursement
- Understand and adhere to managed care policies and procedures
- *Negotiate managed care contracts*

Practice Finances

- Perform procedural and diagnostic coding
- Apply bookkeeping principles
- Manage accounts receivable
- *Manage accounts payable*
- *Process payroll*
- *Document and maintain accounting and banking records*
- *Develop and maintain fee schedules*
- *Manage renewals of business and professional insurance policies*
- *Manage personnel benefits and maintain records*
- *Perform marketing, financial, and strategic planning*

CLINICAL

Fundamental Principles

- Apply principles of aseptic technique and infection control
- Comply with quality assurance practices
- Screen and follow up patient test results

Diagnostic Orders

- Collect and process specimens
- Perform diagnostic tests

Patient Care

- Adhere to established patient screening procedures
- Obtain patient history and vital signs
- Prepare and maintain examination and treatment areas
- Prepare patient for examinations, procedures and treatments
- Assist with examinations, procedures and treatments
- Prepare and administer medications and immunizations
- Maintain medication and immunization records
- Recognize and respond to emergencies
- Coordinate patient care information with other health care providers
- Initiate IV and administer IV medications with appropriate training and as permitted by state law

GENERAL

Professionalism

- Display a professional manner and image
- Demonstrate initiative and responsibility
- Work as a member of the health care team
- Prioritize and perform multiple tasks
- Adapt to change
- Promote the CMA credential
- Enhance skills through continuing education
- Treat all patients with compassion and empathy
- Promote the practice through positive public relations

Communication Skills

- Recognize and respect cultural diversity
- Adapt communications to individual's ability to understand
- Use professional telephone technique
- Recognize and respond effectively to verbal, nonverbal, and written communications
- Use medical terminology appropriately
- Utilize electronic technology to receive, organize, prioritize and transmit information
- Serve as liaison

Legal Concepts

- Perform within legal and ethical boundaries
- Prepare and maintain medical records
- Document accurately
- Follow employer's established policies dealing with the health care contract
- Implement and maintain federal and state health care legislation and regulations
- Comply with established risk management and safety procedures
- Recognize professional credentialing criteria
- *Develop and maintain personnel, policy and procedure manuals*

Instruction

- Instruct individuals according to their needs
- Explain office policies and procedures
- Teach methods of health promotion and disease prevention
- Locate community resources and disseminate information
- *Develop educational materials*
- *Conduct continuing education activities*

Operational Functions

- Perform inventory of supplies and equipment
- Perform routine maintenance of administrative and clinical equipment
- Apply computer techniques to support office operations
- *Perform personnel management functions*
- *Negotiate leases and prices for equipment and supply contracts*

- *Denotes advanced skills.*

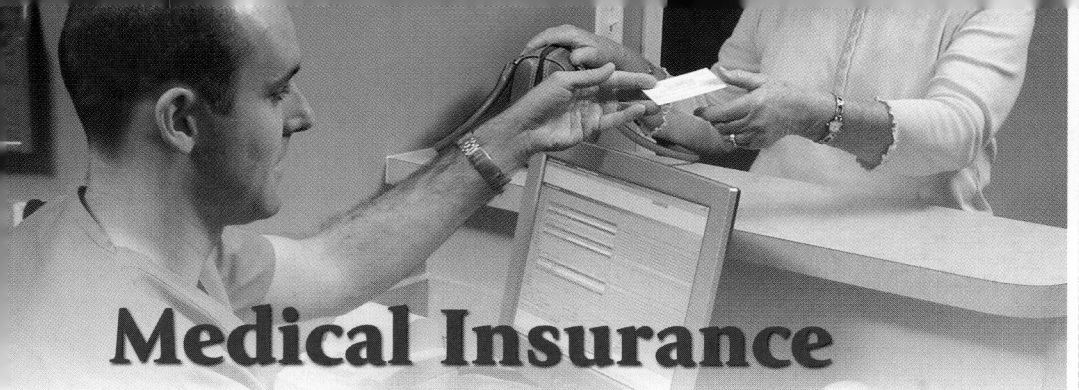

Medical Insurance

15

Learning Objectives

After completing this chapter, you should be able to:

- Define and spell the terms to learn for this chapter.

- Describe group, individual, and government-sponsored (public) health benefits and explain the differences between them.

- Explain the differences between health maintenance organizations (HMOs), preferred provider organizations (PPOs), and traditional insurance programs.

Terms to Learn

benefit period

claim

closed-panel HMO

crossover claim

deductible

exclusive provider organization (EPO)

fee schedule

health maintenance organization (HMO)

integrated delivery system (IDS)

medical foundation

open-panel HMO

point-of-service plan (POS)

preauthorization

preferred provider organization (PPO)

premium

prepaid plan

primary care physician (PCP)

referral

self-referral

subscriber

OUTLINE

Purpose of Health Insurance   270

Health Insurance and
  Availability of Health
  Insurance   270

Managed Care Organizations
  (MCOs)   270

Commercial Plans   273

Government Programs   274

Types of Health Insurance
  Benefits   276

Payment of Benefits   276

Verification of Insurance
  Benefits   279

Fee Schedules   280

Health Care Cost
  Containment   280

The Federal Register   281

Case Study

MIRIAM JONES IS THE CMA WORKING at the front desk today at Dr. Johnson's office. She is responsible for checking in patients and verifying their insurance. Jessie is a patient who arrives for an appointment. She is 16 years old and the oldest of three children in a single parent family. Jessie's mother cannot afford the insurance plan at her job. However, Jessie is able to receive medical care because she and her siblings qualify for government medical coverage.

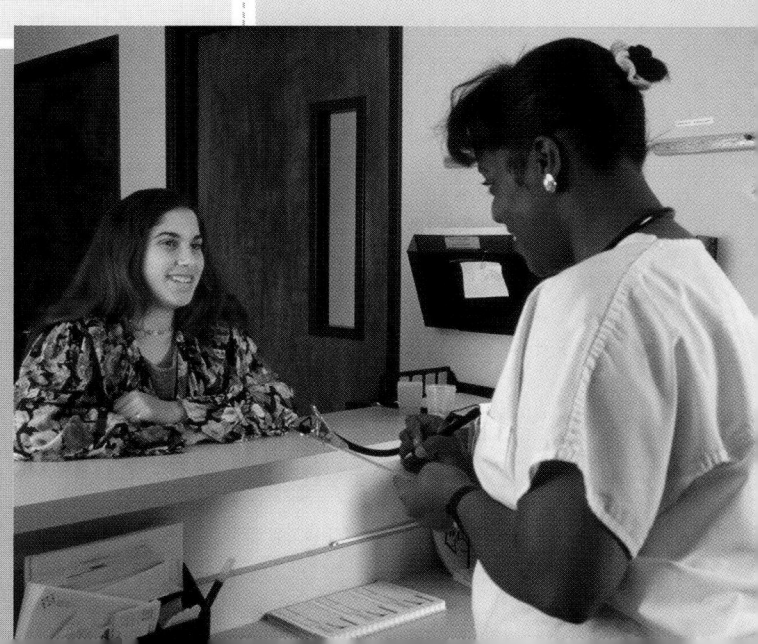

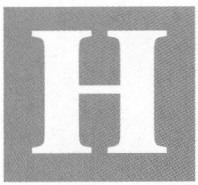

ealth insurance was originally designed to help patients with catastrophic medical expenses that occurred as a result of an unexpected illness or injury. Health benefits have existed as a contract between the subscriber (insured) and the carrier (insurance company or third party payer). The first medical or health insurance plans were not intended to cover all costs associated with health care. Over the years, insurance plans for medical and health care have expanded. As the cost of medical care has escalated, new and different types of health care plans and many regulations have also come into being. In today's medical practices, as much as 85 percent of a physician's income is paid by some form of medical insurance.

The successful medical assistant understands the importance of insurance to both the patient and the practice. He or she keeps current with regulations governing the health insurance industry and how these regulations affect the practice's reimbursements as well as the patients who are insured under the various policies available. This means the medical assistant must be able to process a written and documented request for reimbursement, or claim, for an eligible expense in a correct and timely manner.

Purpose of Health Insurance

Generally, insurance is something that provides protection against or compensation for specific types of risk, loss, or ruin. It is a contract in which an insurance company or agency agrees to pay a sum of money to the insured in the event of some contingency such as death, accident, or illness, in return for the payment of a premium by the insured. Medical insurance was not designed to cover all costs associated with health care, but to assist the patient with expenses incurred for medical treatment.

Health Insurance and Availability of Health Insurance

Health insurance includes all forms of insurance against financial loss resulting from illness or injury. These losses may include the expenses of hospitalization, surgery, and other medical services. Commercial insurance companies sell various types of medical policies. Both commercial and nonprofit programs offer essentially the same types of coverage, which are divided into four categories: regular medical expenses, hospitalization, surgery, and major medical expenses.

Hospitalization insurance includes expenses such as the cost of the hospital room and meals, use of the operating room, x-ray and laboratory fees for tests done while the insured patient is in the hospital as well as some medications and supplies. Hospitalization benefits, under insurance plans, are usually limited to a total monetary amount or a maximum number of days.

Insurance covering surgical procedures may change according to the city or state where the surgery is performed. These limits are based on "reasonable and customary" charges for various types of surgery within the region. A general statement regarding the insurers co-payment and deduction may be required by the patient as designated by the insurance carrier.

Relatively new types of insurance are the fixed payment plans. These are offered by organizations that operate their own health care facilities or that have made arrangements with a hospital or health care provider within a city or region. The fixed-payment plan offers subscribers, or members, complete medical care in return for a fixed monthly fee or semi-monthly fee. This fee is called a premium. When the premium is paid, certain benefits become available for reimbursement. Some contracts specify a maximum lifetime benefit. For example, health maintenance organizations (HMOs) base their operations on fixed prepayment plans.

Health care insurance today is available in these three common options, each having subset options discussed below:

- Managed Care—fixed, prepaid-fee plans with contracted health care providers obtained either independently or as a group.

- Group-sponsored or individual policies— purchased through commercial insurance companies.

- Government-sponsored programs—financed and regulated by federal or state governments for specific groups of people. Some examples of government-sponsored insurance include Medicare, Medicaid, workers' compensation, and military plans such as TRICARE and CHAMPVA.

Any of these plans will help with the cost of health care, but they do not cover all expenses. For any of the insurance options, the insured pays a monthly fee, or premium, for specific coverage. Often, the insured also has a deductible, or a sum of money that must be paid before the insurance plan pays benefits for services rendered. Patient Education has more on handling covered and non-covered insurance services.

Managed Care Organizations (MCOs)

Managed care organizations offer options that are available through private insurance carriers and through some government programs. This type of plan is referred

Most patients have difficulty understanding the details of health insurance. Practicing medical assistants often encounter patients who are convinced that, because they have paid premiums to the insurance company, they should pay nothing further to the provider of service. Tact and patience are essential in educating patients about covered and non-covered services.

to as a prepaid plan in that a group of physicians will have a contractual agreement to provide services to subscribers on a negotiated fee-for-service basis. A fee schedule lists the amount to be paid by the insurance company for each procedure or service subject to the managed care contract.

In some managed care situations, the patient is assigned a primary care provider (PCP), who is responsible for the overall management of the patient's health. This PCP acts as a gatekeeper, determining the medical necessity of services by specialist providers. At the same time, the managed care organization stresses the concept of wellness, often paying higher benefits for routine health maintenance (physical examinations, routine immunizations, etc.). In this manner, the managed care organization tries to decrease the number of visits a patient needs to make per calendar year for health care services of an acute nature.

The History of Managed Care Systems

America's first privately owned, prepaid medical group was founded in 1929 in Southern California. The Ross-Loos Medical Group was composed of several medical group locations and provided services to Los Angeles Department of Water and Power employees. In the 1970s, Ross-Loos merged with a health plan group in Philadelphia to become CIGNA Healthplans of California. The federal Health Maintenance Organization Act of 1973 allowed this to occur. The act:

- Provided funds (loans and grants) to assist in the development of new federally qualified HMOs.

- Required most employers with more than 25 employees to offer HMO benefits as an alternative to traditional health insurance plans.

- Established federal standards for HMOs.

In 1985, the Preferred Provider Health Care Act impacted the preferred provider organizations (PPOs). This act allowed subscribers to utilize providers outside the defined network. A 1988 amendment to the HMO Act of 1973 made similar changes to the HMO system.

Advantages and Disadvantages of Managed Care

How has managed care impacted the cost of health care? Costs have been contained by who, what, and where. This means the manage care organization has a limited number of physicians and facilities from which the patient receives services. The manage care organization also chooses the types of services the patient can or will receive. Box 15-1 lists advantages and disadvantages of managed care.

Health Maintenance Organizations (HMOs)

A health maintenance organization (HMO) is type of managed care plan in which a range of health care services by a limited group of providers (such as

---

BOX 15-1

Advantages and Disadvantages of Managed Care

Advantages
- Smaller out-of-pocket expenses for the patient.
- Patient pays a nominal co-payment.
- Some plans do not have a deductible.
- Contains health care cost.
- Payment for authorized services.
- Fee schedules are established.
- Preventive medical treatment is usually covered.

Disadvantages
- Increased amount of paperwork.
- Preauthorization requirements.
- Lower reimbursement rates.
- Limited physician choices.
- Coverage is not guaranteed to be renewed.
- Specialized care is limited at times.
- Referrals are limited at times.
- Limited flexibility.
- Non-approved or non-authorized treatments are not covered.

physicians and hospitals) are made available to plan members for a predetermined fee (the capitation rate). The HMO concept was started to control the cost explosion in health care as a result of over utilization of services. Before HMOs became so widespread, insurance companies reimbursed providers for all their charges without questioning whether the services were necessary. There was little incentive for providers to control costs. HMOs operate on a budget that is the total of their member patients' fees. For this reason, HMOs attempt to control the length of hospital stays or unnecessary surgery for their members. Two important components of an HMO are:

- All medical services are provided based upon a predetermined (per capita) fee and not on a fee-for-service basis. If the actual cost of services exceeds this predetermined (or capitation) amount, then the provider must absorb the excess in costs. This provides the incentive for the provider to control costs.

- A member patient must use the physicians and hospitals that are identified by the HMO. The HMO will pay for any covered services that are provided by designated providers, hospitals, durable medical equipment, and pharmacies. Therefore pre-approval must be granted through the primary care physician (PCP) when and if a patient has to seek consultation or medical services out of the network. The exception to this is in the case of recognized emergency services.

HMOs place an emphasis on maintaining health. Regular physical examinations and patient education are encouraged. The advantage of HMOs is the control of health costs by encouraging providers to limit unnecessary tests and procedures. Premiums therefore, are lower. The disadvantage is that providers may decide not to provide services patients need in order to cut costs.

A member patient who joins an HMO may either choose a personal physician from a list of provider physicians or be assigned a primary care physician (PCP) who is generally an internist, family practitioner, gynecologist, or pediatrician. The PCP must provide all primary care services since the HMO will not pay for the costs of a non-member provider, except in the case of an emergency. HMOs are required to tell members, in the documents regarding their coverage, of the patient's right to ask for an investigation of any problems concerning care or coverage under the HMO.

HMO Models

There are two categories of HMO models: Closed-panel HMO and open-panel HMO. In the closed-panel HMO, the clinic is owned by the HMO and the physicians are employees of the HMO. There are two types of closed-panel models: the group model HMO and staff model HMO. In the group model, the HMO may contract with physicians who are part of an independent group practice. The HMO reimburses the physician group for providing care to subscribers. The group is responsible for reimbursing the treating physician. In the staff model, the physicians are employees of the HMO. All premiums are paid to the HMO.

In the open-panel HMO, the health care providers are not employees of the HMO and do not belong to a medical group owned or managed by the HMO. There are three models under this category: direct contract model, individual practice association (IPA) model, and the network model. Individual physicians in the community provide contracted health care services to subscribers in the direct contract model. The individual practice association (IPA) model is similar to the direct contract model in that the physicians are not employees of the HMO. The difference is that the IPA can negotiate contracts and manage the capitation payment from the HMO. With the network model HMO, contracted services are provided by more than one physician group practices.

Preferred Provider Organizations (PPOs)

The "preferred provider option" means that the patient must use a medical provider (physician or hospital) who is under contract with the insurer for an agreed-on-fee. A preferred provider organization (PPO) is similar to an HMO but differs in two main areas:

- The PPO is a fee-for-service program and not based on a prepayment or capitation program such as with the HMO. Thus the physicians and hospitals, designated as a PPO, are reimbursed for each medical service they provide.

- The PPO members or enrollees are not restricted to certain designated physicians or hospitals. The PPO member may receive care from a non-PPO provider, however they will generally have to pay more when they do this.

PPOs manage cost containment in the following ways:

- They negotiate fees with providers that are less than the current market fees.

- There are financial incentives for PPO members to use a PPO provider.

- The quality and type of services offered by PPO providers are carefully monitored to maintain cost containment.

Point-of-Service Plan (POS)

To allow for more flexibility, some HMOs and PPOs have created a point-of-service plan (POS). Within this plan, patients may choose to use the panel of providers within the HMO network or to utilize the services of non-HMO providers. If the enrollee chooses to use a provider within the network, the enrollee is only responsible for the regular co-payment and no deductible amount applies. The same benefits apply if the patient is referred by a physician to a specialist outside the network (with authorization from the HMO). If an enrollee chooses to see an out-of-network provider without authorization, the enrollee may be responsible for greater out-of-pocket expenses. This is known as self-referral. The enrollee may be subject to larger deductible and coinsurance charges.

Exclusive Provider Organizations (EPOs)

Exclusive Provider Organizations (EPOs) are a combination of concepts developed by HMOs and PPOs. The EPO, a managed care system, allows the patient to only select from a defined panel of providers. This system reimburses these providers on a modified fee-for-service method, not on the basis of capitation, as in an HMO. The EPO differs from a PPO since no insurance reimbursement is made if there is a non-emergency service provided by a non-EPO provider.

Integrated Delivery System (IDS)

An organization of provider sites (e.g. ambulatory centers, clinics, or hospitals) with a contracted relationship that offer services to subscribers is known as an integrated delivery system (IDS). One such organization is a physician-hospital organization (PHO). PHOs are composed of hospital(s) and physician groups, or clinics. The PHO obtains managed care plan contracts. In this organization, the physicians are able to maintain their own practices while providing care to contracted plan members. A nonprofit IDS is a medical foundation. This type of organization contracts and acquires assets of physician practices. The foundation manages the business and clinical aspects of the practice. Other examples of IDS organizations are: management service organization (MSO), group practice without walls (GPWW), and integrated provider organization (IPO).

Commercial Plans

Group-sponsored or individual policies can be purchased through commercial insurance companies. Commercial health insurance carriers are usually for-profit organizations. These companies may offer traditional fee-for-service insurance as well as a managed care option to their subscribers. Generally, the insured pays a premium and receives coverage for specific services. Figure 15-1 shows a member insurance card, listing the name of the insured, the effective date of the coverage, and other information of importance to the health care provider.

Always ask to see your patient's insurance card. Make a copy of both sides of the card and then return

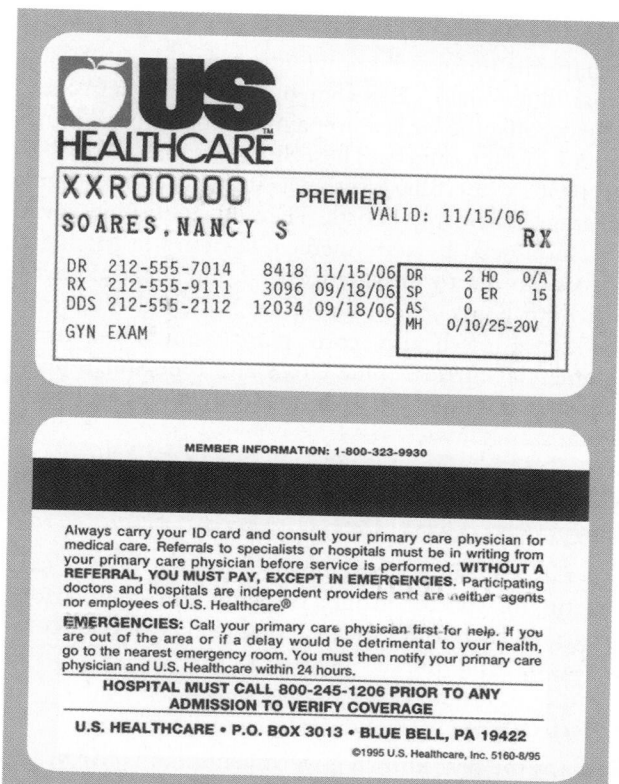

FIGURE 15-1 An insurance card front and back.

it immediately to the patient. You may also wish to write information regarding the insurance plan number on the patient's chart in addition to placing a copy of the card in the chart. Verify the patient's name with a form of photo identification. Compare the name on the insurance card with the name on the photo ID.

Become familiar with the insurance representatives who serve your area. The representatives are knowledgeable, conduct office seminars, and can answer many questions over the telephone. Professionalism has more on sources for insurance information.

Professionalism

A professional medical assistant will make every effort to stay current with health insurance procedures. There are many sources available from which you can obtain the most up-to-date information. There are also seminars and other professional development events that may address changes in insurance plans. Another source is a representative from the actual health care plan. Establish a relationship with someone at each major insurance company so that you can get accurate information.

Blue Cross/Blue Shield

Perhaps the most well known insurance plans are Blue Cross/Blue Shield plans that operate in all states and have become the largest prepayment medical insurance system in the country. These Blue plans date back to the 1930s when Blue Cross was introduced to provide coverage for hospital costs. Then in 1939, Blue Shield was sponsored by state medical societies in Michigan and California to provide medical and surgical coverage. Both plans cover all services now and offer various types of health care plans similar to other commercial carriers. Blue Cross and Blue Shield plans exist in every state and operate locally under each individual state's laws.

Government Programs

Federal and state governments provide health care benefits for specific groups of people through various programs such as Medicare, Medicaid, workers' compensation, and military plans.

Medicare

Perhaps the best known government plan is Medicare. Medicare is health insurance for the elderly that is provided by the United States government. The Medicare

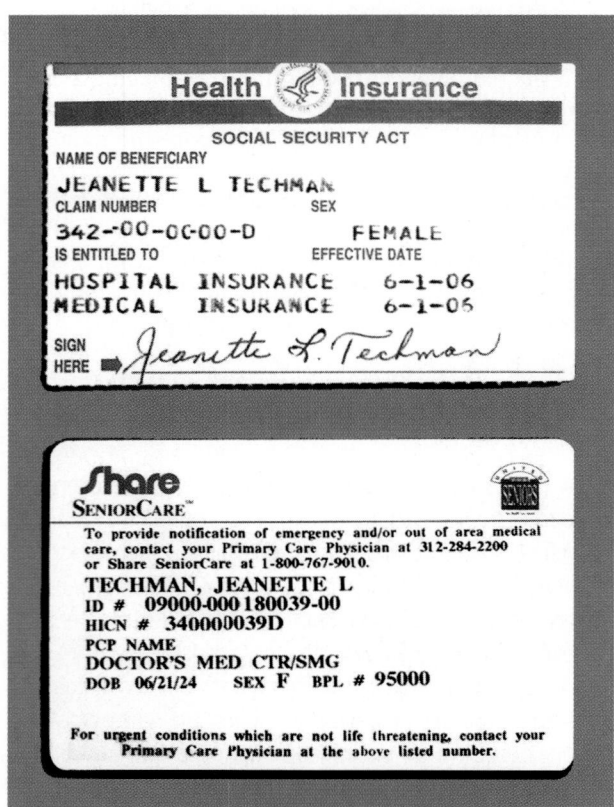

FIGURE 15-2 Medicare and supplemental private insurance cards.

system is operated by the Social Security Administration and paid for largely through Social Security funds. It is designed for persons 65 years old and older and for the severely disabled. Medicare covers approximately 32 million elderly citizens as well as two million permanently disabled persons. Eligible patients are issued a Medicare card (Figure 15-2).

Medicare is actually a two-part health care benefit system: Part A for hospital insurance and Part B for medical insurance.

Part A, which covers hospital expenses, provides coverage automatically when an insured becomes eligible for Social Security benefits. The patient must apply to receive Medicare benefits from the Social Security Administration.

Part B covers medical expenses for doctors, medical services, outpatient hospital care, durable medical equipment, and some medical services not covered by Part A. In order to qualify for Part B Medicare coverage, the insured must pay a monthly premium. This coverage is not automatic, nor does the coverage pay for all services. The patient pays a yearly deductible. After this deductible is met, Medicare will pay for 80 percent of the approved amount of covered services and the insured is liable for the 20 percent co-insurance. The 80 percent reimbursement rate of Medicare is based on their Resource-Based Relative Value Scale (RBRVS), which was developed using values for every medical and surgical procedure based on the work, practice, and malpractice expenses while accounting for regional differences. Some supplies may also be covered if found to be medically necessary for the patient.

Medicare covers all expenses for the first 60 days of hospitalization, except for an initial amount, or deductible, that is paid by the patient. Medicare will also pay for a portion of hospital costs for an additional 30 days. Medicare does not cover extended nursing-home care, or the costs of lengthy or chronic illnesses. Prescription drugs are covered under a separate medical policy.

Medicare supplements are policies that pay benefits on the co-payments and deductibles required and not paid by Medicare. Co-pay or co-payment is an amount of money the patient must pay before the insurance plan will pay. This amount can be as little as $10. Some policies require special forms to be filed before benefits can be paid to the insured. It is important for the medical assistant to check coverage with the individual carrier of the supplement policy, as the coverage provided varies widely from carrier to carrier.

Medicare deductibles, covered services, and co-payments change, so it is important to understand which services are covered under Medicare and which are not. Medical assistants should maintain their knowledge of Medicare coverages and be knowledgeable regarding the benefit period, or period of time that payments for Medicare hospital benefits are available. Lifespan Considerations has more on keeping up-to-date on Medicare guidelines.

Medicaid

While not directly a federal program, Medicaid also qualifies as government insurance. Some of the cost of the Medicaid program, designed for the medically indigent, or persons without funds, comes from state funds, with some federal money to offset costs. Federal funds may assist by supplying 50 percent to 80 percent of the cost of the state's Medicaid program. Since Medicaid is administered by individual states, the rules for eligibility and for payment vary from state to state. In most instances, however, the patient must qualify for benefits on a monthly basis. Some services require preauthorization (prior approval from the Medicaid administrator) or the cost of services will not be paid. When dealing with Medicaid patients, the medical assistant should verify coverage at each and every visit and become familiar with the policies and procedures covering Medicaid in his or her individual state.

Eligibility for Medicare does not automatically confer Medicaid eligibility. In some cases in which a person is eligible for both Medicare and Medicaid, a crossover claim is filed.

Military

Military medical benefits are also part of United States government programs. TRICARE is the U.S. Department of Defense's worldwide health care program for active duty and retired uniformed services members and their families. Box 15-2 shows TRICARE plans' coverage.

A spouse, widow, widower, children of veterans with total or permanent service-connected disabilities, and surviving spouse or dependents of veterans who have died as a result of service-connected disabilities are covered under a program called CHAMPVA (Civilian Health and Medical Program of the Veterans Administration).

Providers of service must be approved in order for the patient to receive benefits for services. Special forms are required for claim filing. Certain services require approval from the government agency responsible for administering these programs before payment can be made.

Workers' Compensation

Another type of government mandated insurance is called workers' compensation. This particular insurance is for injuries directly related to work. Payment of premiums is the employer's responsibility; the employee pays nothing. In workers' compensation cases, the provider of services must complete a report called a Surgeon's Report and must submit further reports at pre-determined intervals. In addition, if the patient re-

Lifespan
Considerations

Patients enrolled in Medicare may not be abreast of the changes that occur with their coverage. Some do not understand the difference between Medicare Part A and Part B. With changes in prescription drug coverage, your patients may be even more confused about what is covered and what is not. As a professional medical assistant, it is your responsibility to stay aware of changes that occur and explain the changes to the patients. Use the Internet and refer to the Federal Register to develop a good working knowledge of Medicare guidelines.

ceives regular care in the same practice that treats the work injury, any information connected to the injury or illness being treated under workers' compensation must be kept separate from all other patient information. Billing is to be done separately and the patient will not be billed for services. Billing statements are sent to the employer or insurer, instead. Because of the special type of documentation required for workers' compensation claims, some providers of service will not see workers' compensation patients. In some states, the patient must see physicians who specialize in these types of cases.

Disability Insurance

Disability insurance is a particular type of insurance that usually begins paying the patient (not the doctor or the hospital) after the insured has been disabled

---

BOX 15-2
Tricare

- TRICARE Prime—a managed care option similar to a civilian health maintenance organization.
- TRICARE Extra—a preferred provider option in which beneficiaries choose a doctor, hospital, or other medical provider within the TRICARE provider network.
- TRICARE Standard—a fee-for-service option.
- TRICARE For Life—an option available to Medicare-eligible beneficiaries age 65 and over.

Information is courtesy of http://www.tricareonline.com.

(unable to work) for a specific period of time. A waiting period of weeks or months before benefits are paid is not uncommon with these policies. The benefit period is the amount of time the insured will receive a monthly check after the policy begins to pay. This can be from six months to life. The payment is paid directly to the insured. This type of insurance coverage is not used for the purpose of paying medical bills. It is to be used for the income that patient has lost due to his or her disability. Most disability insurance also requires special forms to be completed by the attending physician before benefits can be paid to the insured. Before the medical assistant has the physician sign the disability insurance form, he or she needs to proofread it very carefully. After the physician has signed the disability insurance form, the medical assistant will make a copy of it and place it in the patient's medical record.

Types of Health Insurance Benefits

Many patients (and medical assistants) find the proliferation of health care policies confusing. It is important to understand what type of insurance coverage the patient has and what types of services this insurance covers. Remember, insurance is a contract between the insured (the patient or the patient's family) and the insurance company. Questions about specific coverage should be directed to the insurance carrier, as policies vary widely, even with the same carrier. Many health care providers file insurance forms for patients as a courtesy, but this service is usually not required by the insurance companies.

Legal and Ethical Issues has more about information released for insurance reimbursement.

The most basic insurance policies cover doctor office visits, hospitalization, emergency room, surgery, and wellness examinations. For coverage to be effective, the services must be performed on an inpatient basis, except surgeries may be performed as an outpatient. There may also be an annual deductible, which is the portion the patient must pay before the insurance company will pay any benefits. This type of coverage is usually the least expensive. Additionally, a fixed percentage of covered charges beyond the deductible, called coinsurance, may be required. To reduce unnecessary patient visits to the physician, insurance companies frequently require a small fee be paid at each visit, called a co-payment.

Major medical insurance covers expenses related to catastrophic illnesses or injuries. It also covers prolonged illnesses. Major medical is usually a supplemental policy to basic insurance policies. Adding this type of policy increases the premium rate the insured will pay.

Surgical insurance is just what its name implies—an insurance policy covering surgical services. These policies are not as common today as they once were; most surgical services are now covered under basic medical coverage.

Long-term care is an insurance policy designed to cover nursing home care costs. Other insurance policies have very limited coverage if any for long term care.

Dental insurance covers the dental examination, cleaning, polishing, fillings, and certain extractions. Most insurance carriers require a deductible. Depending on the insurance carrier, most procedures are covered from 50 percent to 100 percent.

Vision insurance covers the cost of an eye examination, contact lens or prescription frames and lenses. Some vision insurance policy also covers laser corrective eye surgery. The percent covered by the insurance carrier depends on the insured's policy.

International health and medical insurance covers the insured while outside of the United States in countries where the policy applies.

Student health insurance is important when the parent's insurance policy may no longer cover a child or children that are attending school. Basic insurance, major medical, or both are available. This type of coverage is usually at a reasonable rate that is affordable for the student.

Payment of Benefits

When a covered service has been rendered, the insurance carrier is obligated to pay its portion of the cost. How is this portion calculated? Many insurance carriers use the UCR (usual, customary, reasonable) method (also see Chapter 13). The URC method allows the carrier to establish a payment base for allowed or covered services. In this model, payment is set by determining:

- The usual fee a provider charges the majority of patients for a particular service.
- The geographic location of the practice and the provider's specialty.
- Any complications or unusual services or procedures.

Indemnity schedules, another means of determining the amount of payment made by an insurance carrier, are based on a maximum amount for a specific service. Payment to the provider of service is based on the lower of either the provider's submitted charge or the fee schedule. This method of payment is very common in managed care situations.

To communicate effectively and efficiently with providers of medical care, insurance companies have adopted several methods of standardizing information received. Many insurance companies, working together and separately, developed a means of calculating pricing factors in reimbursement. The results of these efforts are called Relative Value Studies (RVS). In each instance, the system takes into account the time, skill, and overhead expense of the provider as required for each service. These factors are then turned into unit counts applied to a specific service, allowing for the most efficient and effective method of calculating payment.

Since 1992, Medicare has established payment on a resource-based Relative Value Scale, which incorporates the RVS, but also allows for increases in charges tied to economic changes and other factors.

Each insurance carrier has a certain deadline for submitting insurance claims. Claims must be submitted in a timely manner in order to be processed, and if the deadline for filing has passed, no money can be recovered from the insurance carrier. It is extremely important to become familiar with these filing deadlines that vary from carrier to carrier. It is also important that the appropriate form be used for filing charges. Most carriers accept the CMS-1500 (see Chapter 16); some require forms specific to that carrier. Some carriers require supporting documentation (such as reports) that must be submitted in a timely manner.

If a patient has more than one insurance carrier, it is crucial that the primary carrier be determined for proper billing to occur. The claim must be submitted first to the primary carrier for processing, the claim must be processed, and a statement of remittance completed before the information can be sent to any secondary carrier.

Coverage for some expenses such as cosmetic surgery is excluded from policies, and are called exclusions. Payments for some medications are excluded if they are not on an approved list, called a formulary.

As with all aspects of insurance processing, accuracy and attention to detail are the primary concerns. The successful medical assistant keeps abreast of rules, regulations, and changes about insurance claims processing to prompt insurance reimbursement for the practice that is as high as is allowed for services rendered. The medical assistant will need to bill the third party payer for the patient and collect the fees owed to the physician from them. See Procedure 15-1 for performing billing and collection procedures.

Preauthorization and Precertfication

It may be necessary to seek preauthorization from the health insurance provider for certain services. Remember that part of the patient registration process is gathering all pertinent information including the insurance plan requirements. The medical assistant will need to obtain the required prior approval known as precertification or preauthorization.

Preauthorization is obtaining the permission from the insurance plan before performing a procedure or providing certain services to subscribers. It is important to find out if preauthorization is necessary prior to the patient's scheduled appointment. Involve the patient in this process; he or she may not be aware that preauthorization is necessary for the particular plan. Failure to have this permission may delay treatment. The insurance carrier may not pay all or part of the procedure or service if preauthorization is not granted beforehand. Precertification or preauthorization is usually obtained a minimum of 24 hours before a patient arrives for an office visit, hospitalization, certain procedures and treatments, and referrals to a specialist. To aquire prior authorization, the medical assistant will contact the insurance carrier, provide all of the patient information and procedure. The medical assistant should have the following information before contacting the insurance carrier:

- Patient's medical record with insurance information.
- Percertification form.
- Specific procedure or service requested, number of treatments, and period of time necessary for the treatments.
- Specific documentation by the physician in the patient's medical record supporting the requested procedure or service.
- Name, address, telephone number, and fax number of the provider who will perform the procedure or service that has been requested.

The insurance carrier will provide precertification or preauthorization information (usually a number) that will be necessary to include on the insurance

Perform Billing and Collection Procedures

OBJECTIVE: Demonstrate the ability to record payments received from a patient, to record patient information using a patient ledger card and day sheet, and to generate an insurance bill using a charge slip. Demonstrate the ability to then record a payment and provide receipt to the patient.

Equipment and Supplies
day sheet; ledger card; co-payment check; receipt book

Method
1. Pull the appropriate ledger card and place it directly on the day sheet.
2. Temporarily remove the strip of charge slips from the pegboard.
3. Enter the patient's previous balance on the day sheet. The ledger card does not extend to this column.
4. Post the date, patient's name, descriptions, and co-payment amount.
5. Calculate the new balance by subtracting the payment from the previous balance.
6. Generate an insurance bill for the remaining balance.
7. Create a receipt for the patient.

Charting Example
$20 co-pay paid by pt. at time of office visit. Allied insurance billed for balance of $79 on March 12.

---

claim. The medical assistant should make a copy of the completed precertification form and place it in the patient's medical record.

In case an insurance plan rejects the request, it may be necessary for the physician to write a letter to the carrier. With the consent of the patient, the physician should state the patient's diagnosis and professional rationale for prescribing a particular treatment. It may be helpful to recommend that the subscriber send a letter of appeal as well. A copy of the letter to the carrier must also be kept in the patient's medical record. If possible, obtain a copy of the letter of appeal from the patient to also place in the patient's medical record. The third party payers, usually insurance companies, expect medical assistants to follow their guidelines for precertification and preauthorization. See Procedure 15-2 for how to apply third party payer guidelines.

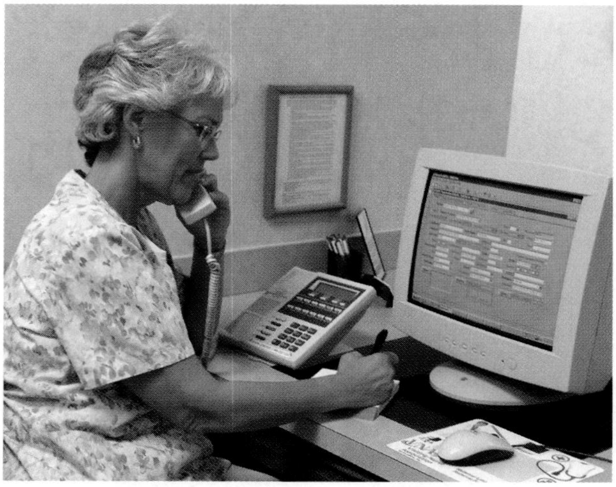

Referrals and Authorization

A patient often needs more specialized care than the family physician can provide. The patient will be referred to another physician or facility.

A referral is used to send a patient for treatment to another facility or physician. There are three types of referrals: regular, urgent, and STAT. Regular referrals are requested when the primary care physician has determined the need for a specialist to continue quality care. Regular referrals can take up to a week to obtain the authorization from the insurance plan. An urgent referral is granted for a non-life threatening need for quality of care and may take up to 48 hours to aquire prior authorization. A STAT referral is approved for life threatening quality of care. Whether the referral is regular, urgent, or STAT, it will require prior authorization direct from the insurance carrier. Prior authorization may be obtained by telephone, fax, e-mail, or in writing on specific insurance carrier forms (Figure 15-3). A medical assistant will need to always have the referral

FIGURE 15-3 A medical assistant may obtain a referral over the telephone.

PROCEDURE

Apply Third Party Guidelines

OBJECTIVE: To apply knowledge of third party guidelines to obtain prior approval for a procedure.

Equipment and Supplies

physician's report recommending procedure; telephone; notepad; pen

Method

1. Gather information about the patient
2. Locate insurance carrier's number.
3. Call carrier and introduce yourself, indicating your office.
4. Instruct carrier that physician recommends procedure, but that third party carrier requires preauthorization for the procedure.

5. Give carrier necessary information, as requested.
6. Document in patient chart preauthorization number for procedure.

Charting Example

Michelle Kimenhour preauthorized hysterectomy for pt. on September 26. Preauthorization number GAQ3498.

---

authorization prior to patient treatment and must maintain all information for insurance billing and utilization review purposes.

When a physician requests that a patient be referred to a specialist, it is important that this is documented in the patient's medical record. The appropriate paperwork must be sent to the referring physician. Referral recommendations should be in writing. When submitting the request to the health insurance plan, be sure to follow the appropriate procedures for that plan. The medical assistant should have the following information before contacting the insurance carrier:

- Patient's medical record with insurance information.
- Referral form.
- Specific procedure or service requested, number of treatments, and period of time necessary for the treatments.
- Specific documentation by the physician in the patient's medical record supporting the reason for the referral.
- Name, address, telephone number, and fax number of the provider who will be providing the procedure or service.
- Appointment date, time, and location.
- Diagnosis and procedure codes.

If certain forms are required, make sure that you have the current form and that it is filled out properly. Some requests are rejected due to incorrect or incomplete paperwork. The medical assistant should make a copy of the completed referral form and place it in the patient's medical record.

Verification of Insurance Benefits

A medical assistant will always need to confirm or verify the patient's eligibility for insurance benefits prior to the office visit for services. Verification may take time but, by performing the following guidelines, will be more effective for the insurance process.

Guidelines for insurance verification:

- Initial contact with the patient—obtain all insurance information (i.e. insurer name, guarantor name, insurance identification number, patient's address, telephone number, and birth date).
- Insurance company name, address, telephone number, fax number, co-payment fees, deductibles, and preauthorizations.
- Provide patient with written information regarding medical office policies and procedures for dealing with his or her insurance carrier.
- Discuss insurance benefits with the patient prior to services rendered.

As a medical assistant, you will need to apply managed care policies and procedures in the office as presented in Procedure 15-3. Preparing for Externship has more on working with insurance.

Apply Managed Care Policies and Procedures

OBJECTIVE: Demonstrate knowledge of managed care policies.

Equipment and Supplies
insurance card; patient record

Method
1. Greet patient and request insurance card.
2. Check card to see if coverage is current.
3. Correctly enter card information into data base.
4. Photocopy card.
5. Return card to patient.

Fee Schedules

Health care insurance providers determine fees based on several components. Determining factors include time, location of practice, type of practice, value of services, and the allowable charge. Allowable charge is the highest amount that third party payers will make for services rendered.

Health Care Cost Containment

The cost of medicine has risen steadily throughout the years. As new advances are discovered to treat and cure disease, heal injuries, and prolong life, the costs are passed on to the consumer or patient. Traditionally, medical care has been rendered on a fee-for-service

Preparing for
Externship

Part of your training as an extern will involve working with the insurance process. You may have to verify coverage, obtain preauthorizations, and request permission for referrals. Understanding the policies and procedures regarding the different plans is an on-going process. Ask questions about unfamiliar plans. Make sure you have the most current information available. Both the physician and the patient rely on those who are responsible for handling insurance in the office. The physician wants to be correctly reimbursed, and the patient does not want any unexpected costs.

basis, which was a separate charge or fee set up by individual physicians for every service. Insurance carriers initially set up their policies on this basis, as well. However, as medical care costs rose, the insurers, carriers, patients, and medical community began to offer cost-saving alternatives to higher medical costs and the escalating costs of medical premiums.

The first cost containment measure, the Peer Review Organization (PRO), was initiated when Congress amended the Social Security Act of 1972 and established the Professional Standards Review Organization (PSRO). This was a voluntary group of physicians who monitored the necessity of hospital admissions and reviewed the treatment costs and medical records of hospitals. Unfortunately, the cost of operating this system was greater than the savings that the program could generate each year. In order to establish stricter controls over Medicare reimbursement for inpatient costs, Congress created control peer review organizations (PROs). These PROs were intended to determine whether proposed services were reasonable and medically necessary and whether or not the services provided on an inpatient basis could be provided more efficiently on an outpatient basis.

As part of the cost containment process, a patient classification system was developed, which provides a means of relating the type of patients a hospital treats to the costs incurred by the hospital. Yale University developed the design of diagnosis-related groups (DRGs) in the late 1960s. The initial idea was to provide a means of monitoring the quality of care and the utilization of services in a hospital setting. Payment rates based on DRGs have now been established as the basis for a hospital's Medicare reimbursements. While DRGs have an effect on hospital reimbursements, they are not used to calculate payments made to outpatient providers. Physicians now have contracts with managed care companies and insurance companies.

The Federal Register

The *Federal Register* is a daily legal publication of the National Archives and Records Administration (NARA). The medical assistant would use this register for seeking information on Federal rules, regulations, notices, executive orders, proclamations, and Presidential documents. The *Federal Register* may be accessed through the World Wide Web, microfiche, or as a daily newspaper.

SUMMARY

Most patients coming into the medical office have some form of health care insurance. These include commercial insurers, and government plans such as Medicare, Medicaid, workers' compensation, and military insurance (TRICARE AND CHAMPVA). Many patients are members of health care plans, such as health maintenance organizations (HMOs), and preferred provider organizations (PPOs). The medical assistant should have a working knowledge of each type of insurance in order to be able to quickly and accurately process insurance forms.

Chapter Review

COMPETENCY REVIEW

1. Define and spell the terms to learn for this chapter.
2. List the three insurance options currently available.
3. What are the two important components of an HMO?
4. How does a PPO differ from an HMO?
5. What is the purpose of the peer review organization (PRO)?

PREPARING FOR THE CERTIFICATION EXAM

1. What is the term for a written and documented request for reimbursement?
   A. premium
   B. co-payment
   C. claim
   D. referral
   E. fee schedule

2. Which BEST describes health maintenance organizations?
   A. They are prepaid plans.
   B. Patients are only allowed to see physicians within the network.
   C. All HMOs are government-sponsored.
   D. Patients pay no premiums to HMOs.
   E. There is only one type of managed care plan.

3. Which government insurance provides coverage for citizens over 65 years old and the severely disabled?
   A. Medicaid
   B. TRICARE
   C. Workers' compensation
   D. Medicare
   E. Disability

4. Preauthorization is necessary in the following situations EXCEPT:
   A. referral to a specialist
   B. new treatment prescribed by the PCP
   C. making a PCP appointment for a regular physical
   D. hospital admission
   E. a medical procedure by a specialist

continued on next page

5. What is the term for an amount specified by an insurance plan that the patient must pay before the plan pays for medical services?
   A. rider
   B. deductible
   C. premium
   D. reimbursement
   E. co-payment

6. Medicare Part A covers:
   A. doctor visits
   B. hospital costs
   C. prescription drugs
   D. visits to specialists
   E. extended nursing-home care

7. Which is NOT considered a primary care physician?
   A. Chiropractor
   B. Internist
   C. Family practitioner
   D. Gynecologist
   E. Pediatrician

8. Which type of benefit begins paying the patient after the insured has been disabled and unable to work for a specific period of time?
   A. Medicaid
   B. TRICARE
   C. Medicare
   D. Workers' compensation
   E. Disability insurance

9. Which factor is NOT considered when using the UCR method to determine reimbursement rates for physicians' services?
   A. any complications or unusual services or procedures
   B. the geographic location of the practice and the provider's specialty
   C. the usual fee a provider charges the majority of patients for a particular service
   D. the subscriber's deductible amount
   E. the type of practice and its address

10. Which are NOT types of referrals?
    A. STAT and regular
    B. urgent and STAT
    C. regular and urgent
    D. regular, urgent, and life-threatening
    E. regular, urgent, and STAT

CRITICAL THINKING

1. Jessie and her siblings are eligible for what type of insurance coverage?
2. What group or groups of people qualify for this type of coverage?
3. Two years later, Jessie gets pregnant. She is not employed and her significant other does not have medical benefits. Jessie and her unborn child are able to qualify for what type of services?

INTERNET ACTIVITY

Most health insurance providers have Web sites to provide information to their members and the public. Because changes occur so quickly, important information regarding health plans is posted to keep those who are interested up to date. Conduct a search to find the Web sites for Medicare, Medicaid, a commercial insurance company, and TRICARE. List the Web site addresses and list the different plans offered by each.

ON THE JOB

Lisa Medina, CMA, processes insurance claims for a large internal medicine practice. You have recently been hired as Lisa's assistant and she has asked you to verify insurance coverage for the patients who have appointments to see Dr. Williams in the next two days. Lisa "advises" you to be careful when having to obtain preauthorizations. She hands you a list of "approved" services and tells you to use this information when calling the insurance companies.

1. Name some of the options that are possible for handling this situation.
2. For what types of services might you have to obtain preauthorizations?
3. Would Lisa's "advice" be considered fraud? Explain your response.
4. What is the proper procedure for obtaining preauthorizations?

MediaLink  More on medical insurance, including interactive resources, can be found in the Student CD-ROM accompanying this textbook.

Medical Assistant Role Delineation Chart

HIGHLIGHT indicates material covered in this chapter.

ADMINISTRATIVE

Administrative Procedures

- Perform basic administrative medical assisting functions
- Schedule, coordinate and monitor appointments
- Schedule inpatient/outpatient admissions and procedures
- Understand and apply third-party guidelines
- Obtain reimbursement through accurate claims submission
- Monitor third-party reimbursement
- Understand and adhere to managed care policies and procedures
- *Negotiate managed care contracts*

Practice Finances

- Perform procedural and diagnostic coding
- Apply bookkeeping principles

- Manage accounts receivable
- *Manage accounts payable*
- *Process payroll*
- *Document and maintain accounting and banking records*
- *Develop and maintain fee schedules*
- *Manage renewals of business and professional insurance policies*
- *Manage personnel benefits and maintain records*
- *Perform marketing, financial, and strategic planning*

CLINICAL

Fundamental Principles

- Apply principles of aseptic technique and infection control
- Comply with quality assurance practices
- Screen and follow up patient test results

Diagnostic Orders

- Collect and process specimens
- Perform diagnostic tests

Patient Care

- Adhere to established patient screening procedures
- Obtain patient history and vital signs
- Prepare and maintain examination and treatment areas
- Prepare patient for examinations, procedures and treatments

- Assist with examinations, procedures and treatments
- Prepare and administer medications and immunizations
- Maintain medication and immunization records
- Recognize and respond to emergencies
- Coordinate patient care information with other health care providers
- Initiate IV and administer IV medications with appropriate training and as permitted by state law

GENERAL

Professionalism

- Display a professional manner and image
- Demonstrate initiative and responsibility
- Work as a member of the health care team
- Prioritize and perform multiple tasks
- Adapt to change
- Promote the CMA credential
- Enhance skills through continuing education
- Treat all patients with compassion and empathy
- Promote the practice through positive public relations

Communication Skills

- Recognize and respect cultural diversity
- Adapt communications to individual's ability to understand
- Use professional telephone technique

- Recognize and respond effectively to verbal, nonverbal, and written communications
- Use medical terminology appropriately
- Utilize electronic technology to receive, organize, prioritize and transmit information
- Serve as liaison

Legal Concepts

- Perform within legal and ethical boundaries
- Prepare and maintain medical records
- Document accurately
- Follow employer's established policies dealing with the health care contract
- Implement and maintain federal and state health care legislation and regulations
- Comply with established risk management and safety procedures
- Recognize professional credentialing criteria
- *Develop and maintain personnel, policy and procedure manuals*

Instruction

- Instruct individuals according to their needs
- Explain office policies and procedures
- Teach methods of health promotion and disease prevention
- Locate community resources and disseminate information
- *Develop educational materials*
- *Conduct continuing education activities*

Operational Functions

- Perform inventory of supplies and equipment
- Perform routine maintenance of administrative and clinical equipment
- Apply computer techniques to support office operations
- *Perform personnel management functions*
- *Negotiate leases and prices for equipment and supply contracts*

- *Denotes advanced skills.*

SOURCE: Reprinted by permission of the American Association of Medical Assistants from the AAMA Role Delineation Study: Occupational Analysis of the Medical Assisting Profession.

Medical Insurance Claims

Learning Objectives

After completing this chapter, you should be able to:

- Define and spell the terms to learn for this chapter.

- Define and discuss various health insurance forms.

- Explain the differences among the discussed insurance policies.

- List the information required on a medical claim form and explain why each piece of information is needed.

- Discuss legal issues affecting medical claims submission.

- Discuss tracking insurance claims.

- Discuss insurance claims processing.

- List the reasons for insurance claims being rejected.

- Explain why insurance claim security is so important.

OUTLINE

Types of Health Insurance Claim Forms	286
Type of Claims	288
The Claim Form	290
Claims Processing	290
Claim Security	295
Tracking Claim Forms	295

Terms to Learn

assignment of benefits
benefit period
breach of confidentiality

nonparticipating provider
participating providers

preauthorization
superbill

Case Study

LEWIS JORDAN, RMA, WORKS AS DR. MILLER'S insurance clerk. His duties include verifying insurance and processing claims. Mary Free is a new patient and has an appointment to see Dr. Miller next week. She has Blue Cross/Blue Shield insurance. Mark Flannery is also a patient. He was in to see Dr. Miller last month and the claim for his care was rejected. The codes, quantities, and modifiers were all correct on the CMS-1500.

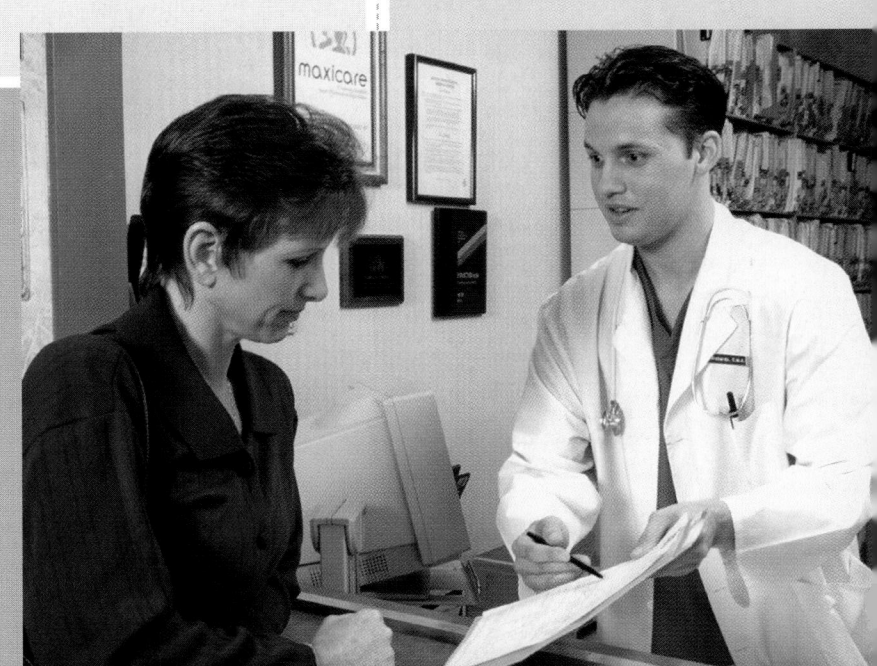

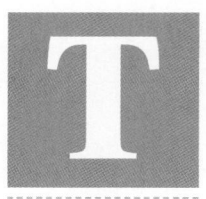

The health insurance claim form provides communication between the insurance company and physician for the patient. There are three main points to this communication process that are critical in order to receive proper reimbursement from the insurance carrier. First, the correct health insurance claim form must be used. Second, the information provided in the health insurance claim form must be accurate. One little mistake can cause the claim to be rejected. The medical assistant must always proofread the claim form before submitting it. Third, the health insurance claim form is mailed or e-mailed to the correct insurance carrier.

Types of Health Insurance Claim Forms

The CMS-1500 is the most common health insurance claim form. This form is used to file claims for physicians' services. It may be sent to the insurance carrier by standard mail or electronically. Another type of health insurance claim form is the CMS-1450 or the UB-92 (Figure 16-1). This type of form is used for services related to hospitalization. Since this type of health insurance claim form is used in a hospital setting, most medical assistants are less likely to encounter it. Most commercial insurance carriers utilize the CMS-1500 form.

Blue Cross/Blue Shield

Many Blue Cross/Blue Shield plans provide their own type of health insurance claim form. These forms are provided at the Web sites of various Blue Cross/Blue Shield plans. Depending on the type of service, the CMS-1500 or the CMS-1540 may also be used.

Managed Care

When the medical assistant is submitting a claim, he or she must find out which health insurance claim form to use. Most managed care organizations use the CMS-1500 and the CMS-1540. Using the incorrect form may cause the claim to be rejected. This will then delay payment to the physician for services rendered. Preparing for Externship has more about being familiar with the CMS-1500 form.

Medicare

Medicare deductibles, covered services, and co-payments change, so it is important to understand which services are covered under Medicare and which are not. Wise medical assistants maintain their knowledge of Medicare coverage and the benefit period, or period of time for which payments of Medicare hospital benefits are available.

The medical assistant working in a medical office needs to be familiar with the CMS-1500 claim form. This claim is used when a patient has Medicare (Figure 16-2). If the CMS-1500 claim form is not used, it will be rejected. Remember when claims are rejected, it delays payment to the physician. This claim form can be sent by standard mail or electronically.

Medicaid

Since Medicaid is administered by individual states, the rules for eligibility and for payment vary from state to state. In most instances, however, the patient must qualify for benefits on a monthly basis. Some services require preauthorization (prior approval from the Medicaid administrator) or the cost of services will not be paid. When dealing with Medicaid patients, the medical assistant should verify coverage at each and every visit and become familiar with the policies and procedures covering Medicaid in his or her individual state.

Eligibility for Medicare does not automatically confer Medicaid eligibility. In cases where a person is eligible for both Medicare and Medicaid (Medi/Medi), a crossover claim is filed.

After the patient has checked out of the office, the medical assistant will complete a CMS-1500 form. This form can be sent by standard mail or electronically depending upon the medical office.

Military

Military medical benefits are also part of government programs. There are three types of health insurance claim forms used to submit services to Tricare.

DD Form 2642 is completed and sent by the patient or a family member. This form is completed when the patient or family member is requesting payment for medical services.

CMS-1500 is completed and sent by the physician's office. Payment will be sent to the physician's office.

Preparing for Externship

It may be helpful to practice manually filling out CMS-1500 forms. Get familiar with each section and find out what information is needed to complete the forms. If you have the opportunity, use the different software packages available to submit claims. Most have tutorial software on which you can train.

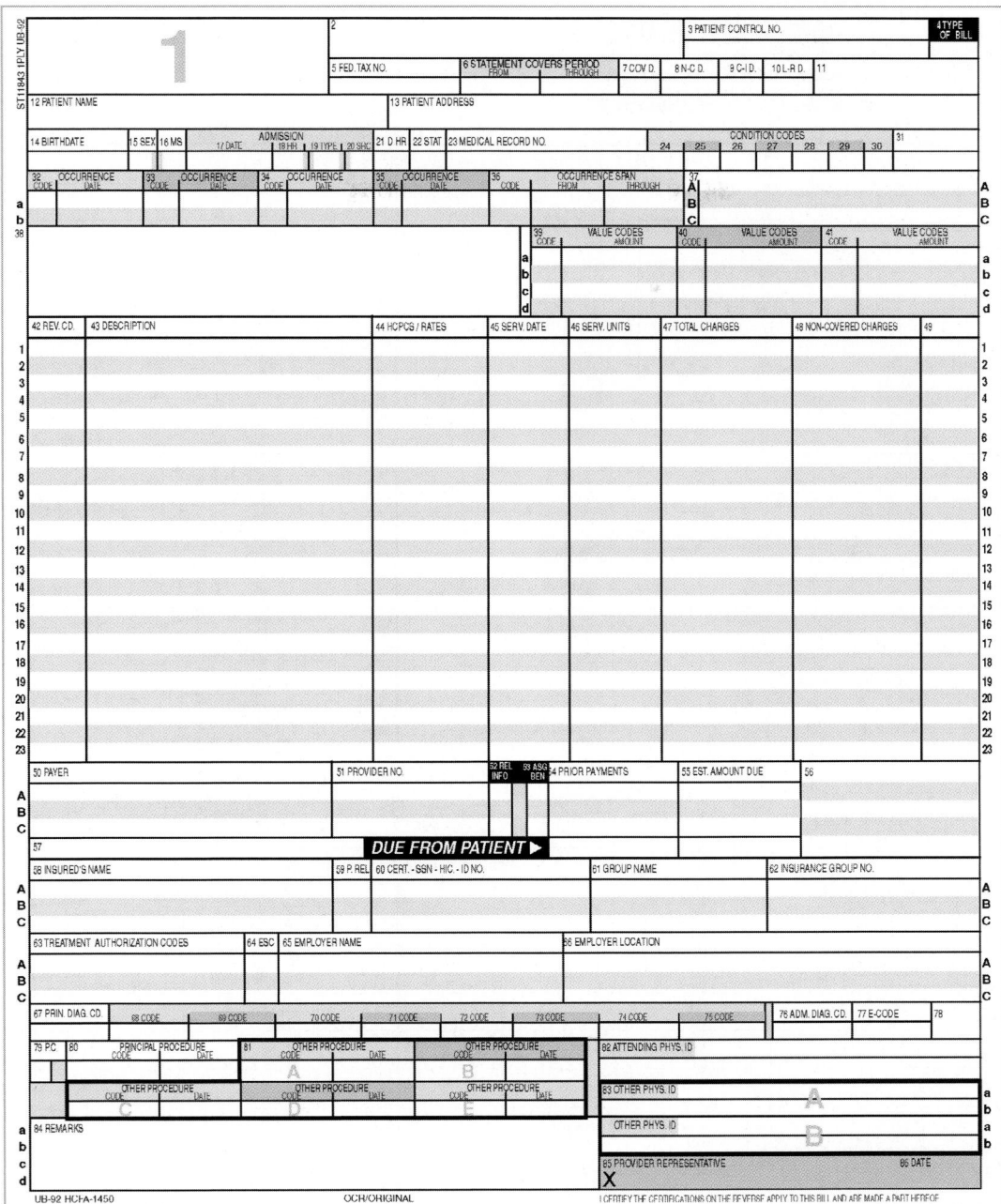

FIGURE 16-1 A CMS-1450/UB-92 health insurance claim form.

UB-92 is completed and sent by the hospital. Payment will be sent to the hospital.

Workers' Compensation

Workers' compensation is an insurance set up specifically for injuries that are related directly to work. Payment of premiums is the employer's responsibility; the employee pays nothing. Because of the particular type of documentation required for workers' compensation claims, some providers of service will not see workers' compensation patients. In some states, the patient must see physicians who specialize in these types of cases.

The most frequently used claim form is the CMS-1500, but some states or insurance carriers have a specifically designed form that must be completed. Before the medical assistant completes a claim form, he or she must investigate which claim form to use. This can be accomplished by calling the insurance carrier or checking the insurance carrier's Web site.

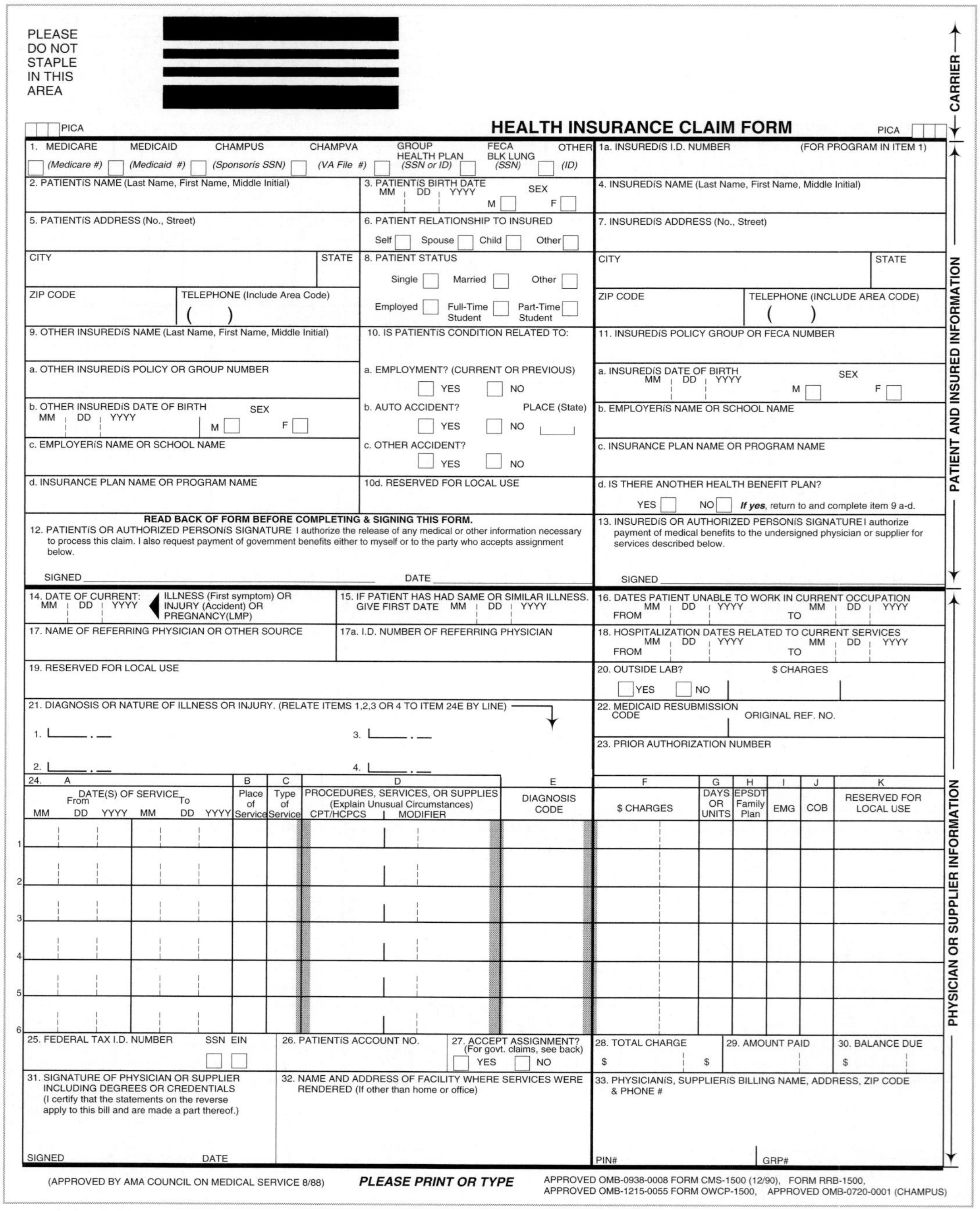

PLEASE DO NOT STAPLE IN THIS AREA

CARRIER

PICA HEALTH INSURANCE CLAIM FORM PICA

1. MEDICARE (Medicare #) MEDICAID (Medicaid #) CHAMPUS (Sponsoris SSN) CHAMPVA (VA File #) GROUP HEALTH PLAN (SSN or ID) FECA BLK LUNG (SSN) OTHER (ID)

1a. INSUREDíS I.D. NUMBER (FOR PROGRAM IN ITEM 1)

2. PATIENTíS NAME (Last Name, First Name, Middle Initial)

3. PATIENTíS BIRTH DATE MM DD YYYY SEX M F

4. INSUREDíS NAME (Last Name, First Name, Middle Initial)

5. PATIENTíS ADDRESS (No., Street)

6. PATIENT RELATIONSHIP TO INSURED Self Spouse Child Other

7. INSUREDíS ADDRESS (No., Street)

CITY STATE

8. PATIENT STATUS Single Married Other Employed Full-Time Student Part-Time Student

CITY STATE

ZIP CODE TELEPHONE (Include Area Code) ( )

ZIP CODE TELEPHONE (INCLUDE AREA CODE) ( )

9. OTHER INSUREDíS NAME (Last Name, First Name, Middle Initial)

10. IS PATIENTíS CONDITION RELATED TO:

11. INSUREDíS POLICY GROUP OR FECA NUMBER

a. OTHER INSUREDíS POLICY OR GROUP NUMBER

a. EMPLOYMENT? (CURRENT OR PREVIOUS) YES NO

a. INSUREDíS DATE OF BIRTH MM DD YYYY SEX M F

b. OTHER INSUREDíS DATE OF BIRTH MM DD YYYY SEX M F

b. AUTO ACCIDENT? YES NO PLACE (State)

b. EMPLOYERíS NAME OR SCHOOL NAME

c. EMPLOYERíS NAME OR SCHOOL NAME

c. OTHER ACCIDENT? YES NO

c. INSURANCE PLAN NAME OR PROGRAM NAME

d. INSURANCE PLAN NAME OR PROGRAM NAME

10d. RESERVED FOR LOCAL USE

d. IS THERE ANOTHER HEALTH BENEFIT PLAN? YES NO *If yes,* return to and complete item 9 a-d.

READ BACK OF FORM BEFORE COMPLETING & SIGNING THIS FORM.

12. PATIENTíS OR AUTHORIZED PERSONíS SIGNATURE I authorize the release of any medical or other information necessary to process this claim. I also request payment of government benefits either to myself or to the party who accepts assignment below.

SIGNED ______ DATE ______

13. INSUREDíS OR AUTHORIZED PERSONíS SIGNATURE I authorize payment of medical benefits to the undersigned physician or supplier for services described below.

SIGNED ______

PATIENT AND INSURED INFORMATION

14. DATE OF CURRENT: MM DD YYYY ILLNESS (First symptom) OR INJURY (Accident) OR PREGNANCY(LMP)

15. IF PATIENT HAS HAD SAME OR SIMILAR ILLNESS. GIVE FIRST DATE MM DD YYYY

16. DATES PATIENT UNABLE TO WORK IN CURRENT OCCUPATION FROM MM DD YYYY TO MM DD YYYY

17. NAME OF REFERRING PHYSICIAN OR OTHER SOURCE

17a. I.D. NUMBER OF REFERRING PHYSICIAN

18. HOSPITALIZATION DATES RELATED TO CURRENT SERVICES FROM MM DD YYYY TO MM DD YYYY

19. RESERVED FOR LOCAL USE

20. OUTSIDE LAB? YES NO $ CHARGES

21. DIAGNOSIS OR NATURE OF ILLNESS OR INJURY. (RELATE ITEMS 1,2,3 OR 4 TO ITEM 24E BY LINE)

1. ___ . ___ 3. ___ . ___

2. ___ . ___ 4. ___ . ___

22. MEDICAID RESUBMISSION CODE ORIGINAL REF. NO.

23. PRIOR AUTHORIZATION NUMBER

24. A DATE(S) OF SERVICE From MM DD YYYY To MM DD YYYY	B Place of Service	C Type of Service	D PROCEDURES, SERVICES, OR SUPPLIES (Explain Unusual Circumstances) CPT/HCPCS MODIFIER	E DIAGNOSIS CODE	F $ CHARGES	G DAYS OR UNITS	H EPSDT Family Plan	I EMG	J COB	K RESERVED FOR LOCAL USE
1										
2										
3										
4										
5										
6										

25. FEDERAL TAX I.D. NUMBER SSN EIN

26. PATIENTíS ACCOUNT NO.

27. ACCEPT ASSIGNMENT? (For govt. claims, see back) YES NO

28. TOTAL CHARGE $

29. AMOUNT PAID $

30. BALANCE DUE $

31. SIGNATURE OF PHYSICIAN OR SUPPLIER INCLUDING DEGREES OR CREDENTIALS (I certify that the statements on the reverse apply to this bill and are made a part thereof.)

SIGNED DATE

32. NAME AND ADDRESS OF FACILITY WHERE SERVICES WERE RENDERED (If other than home or office)

33. PHYSICIANíS, SUPPLIERíS BILLING NAME, ADDRESS, ZIP CODE & PHONE #

PIN# GRP#

PHYSICIAN OR SUPPLIER INFORMATION

(APPROVED BY AMA COUNCIL ON MEDICAL SERVICE 8/88) ***PLEASE PRINT OR TYPE*** APPROVED OMB-0938-0008 FORM CMS-1500 (12/90), FORM RRB-1500, APPROVED OMB-1215-0055 FORM OWCP-1500, APPROVED OMB-0720-0001 (CHAMPUS)

FIGURE 16-2 A blank CMS-1500 form.

Type of Claims

There are two methods for a medical assistant to submit claims to an insurance carrier or third-party payer. The traditional way to submit claims is by completing information on a paper claim form and mailing it to the insurance carrier. The more current and faster way to submit claims is done by using a computer to complete an electronic claim form and sending the claim electronically. The same information is provided when submitting a claim by paper or electronically.

Paper

There are only a small amount of providers who are able to submit paper claims. Paper claims are completed by the medical assistant manually. When this type of claim form is submitted, it often has errors. This means there is a greater chance for the insurance carrier to reject the claim form. The types of errors include omissions, as well as typographical, and mathematical. When a claim form has one or more errors, the claim form must be resubmitted correctly for payment. This increases the turnaround time for the medical office to receive payment and means a delayed cash flow. The patient can also be concerned when the insurance carrier has taken long to make a payment because of delays in processing a claim.

Advantages and Disadvantages of Paper Claims

The cost involved with using paper claims is minimal. The equipment and supplies needed to complete the claim forms include the claim forms and coding books. As long as the office has sufficient amount of forms, they can be accessed at any time.

The disadvantages, however, are in the cost to complete a paper claim process that includes storage space, postage, mailing, resubmission, follow-up, and copies of claim forms that are submitted and resubmitted. When the medical assistant completes a claim form manually, it must be on an original claim form. It must be legible, completed in dark ink, and printed in capital letters. This can be very time consuming. Never use punctuation, decimals, dollar signs, or correction aids. Do not tape, staple, or clip items to the claim form. Always place the necessary documentation required with the completed claim form in an envelope to be mailed and make sure the insurance address is correct.

Electronic Media Claim (EMC)

All medical offices were mandated to be in compliance with electronic filing by October 2003. Electronic claims are a way to send claims and communicate from computer to computer rather than on paper. Electronic Media Claims have fewer errors because there are fewer omissions and they are legible.

Advantages of Electronic Claims

The electronic process speeds claims processing on both the provider's end and at the insurance carrier's end. Many plans make direct electronic deposits of payments for insurance claims into the provider's bank account. Processing claims electronically decreases payment turnaround time. It also shortens the payment cycle, thereby increasing cash flow into the medical office. Sending claim forms electronically instead of by mail saves postage and labor cost for the medical office. Errors may still occur on electronic claims, so it is very important for the medical assistant to proofread all claims before submitting them.

Electronic claims submission requires the same information as on the CMS-1500 form, but instead of sending the claim form by mail, all information is sent directly to the insurance carrier's computer server. This type of submission is referred to as a paperless claim. To send a claim electronically, the medical assistant must do the following:

- Collect all information needed about the patient, including diagnostic and procedure codes as though you were completing a manual CMS-1500 form. The claim form on the screen may not be identical to a hard copy of the CMS form.

- Connect your computer to the insurance company's computer server, using instructions provided by the insurance company. Type in your identification number and password and follow the instructions and prompts on the screen.

- Fill out the claim form as you would the CMS-1500. When the insurance carrier recognizes the physician's identification number, it will automatically assign a processing number to the claim. Keep track of this number for future reference; it is your confirmation that the claim has been received. The best place to document this information is in the insurance claims log.

Software programs are available that allow claim processing without the need to re-enter some of the data more than once. It is important to be familiar with the procedures and software used to prevent delay of payment.

Disadvantages of Electronic Claims

One of the disadvantages of submitting claims electronically is the initial start-up expense. Initially, the medical office would require an Internet service provider, computer, software, printer, and backup or storage devices. Glitches may occur with the computer that delays processing time, transmission, and payments.

Transmitting Claims Electronically

Claims can be transmitted electronically in three ways. The first method is sending the transmission directly to the payer. To communicate electronically between the payer and the medical office, an electronic data exchange (EDI) information system must be utilized.

The second method is transmitting claims through a clearinghouse. The clearinghouse does not modify any of the data. It is responsible for putting the data in a format appropriate for EDI use. Clearinghouses

Most patients have difficulty understanding the details of health insurance. Practicing medical assistants often encounter patients who are convinced that, because they have paid premiums to the insurance company, they should pay nothing further to the provider of service. Tact and patience are essential in educating patients about covered and non-covered services.

eliminate the need for medical offices to have specific software that may be required by different carriers. The clearinghouse also checks each claim form for accuracy, and returns it to the medical office for correction, thereby reducing the incidence of claim rejection.

The last method is direct data entry (DDE) which is an online service provided by some carriers. The data from the claim is keyed in a specific format and then transmitted directly to the carrier.

Status of Insurance Claims

The status of insurance claims is a concern of every medical office. Lost, incomplete, or rejected claims cause delays in reimbursement to the practice. Over time, this is costly to any medical office. Errors or omission on a health care insurance claim form can cause a claim to be rejected. If this occurs, the medical assistant must investigate the reason and resubmit the claim.

Clean Claims

A health insurance claim form that has been completed correctly without any errors or omissions is called a clean claim. Clean claims are also submitted on time to the insurance carrier. The first time this claim is submitted to the insurance carrier, it is processed and payment is sent to the provider.

Dirty Claims

When a health insurance claim form is incorrect by having missing data or errors, this is considered to be a dirty claim. This will cause the claim to be rejected and when claims are rejected, payment is delayed. Delayed payments become costly to a medical office because the form must be resubmitted taking the time of a medical assistant to complete the insurance form again.

Invalid Claims

A health insurance claim form that has been completed but has some type of incorrect information is considered an invalid claim.

Denied Claims

Denied claims can occur when procedures or services are not covered by the patient's insurance policy or when the patient has not met his or her deductible. Ineligible procedures or services can also cause a claim to be denied. Patient Education discusses reviewing insurance details with patients who are not familiar with their coverage.

The Claim Form

Each time a patient is seen for services, the medial assistant must verify the insurance information in the patient's medical record. For a new patient or a patient with a new insurance card or cards, the medical assistant needs to copy the front and back of the patient's insurance card(s). After making a copy of each insurance card, the medical assistant will file it in the patient's medical record. Then, the medical assistant will verify that the patient has signed the assignment of benefits form. This form allows physicians to be paid directly from the insurance carrier. After the patient has been seen by the physician, the medical assistant can complete the CMS-1500 form. The CMS-1500 has 33 blocks of information to complete. Blocks 1 to 13 represent information about the patient's demographics and insurance carrier. Blocks 14 to 33 represent information about the patient's diagnosis, procedure(s) performed, the amount of each procedure, and the total charge. It also represents information about the physician. Procedure 16-1 reviews each step for correctly completing the CMS-1500 form.

Claims Processing

Claims are processed at insurance companies by a claims administrator. The claim form is a critical item in claims processing. While there are several forms used for claims processing, the most commonly used form was designed by the Health Care Financing Administration and is called a CMS-1500. For a claim to be processed, this form must be filled out completely and correctly. The following information is required for all claims:

- The name of the insured's insurance company
- The name of the insured
- The insured's identification number
- The address of the insured
- The telephone number of the insured

Data about the patient is also required. In general, the upper portion of the form describes the patient and the lower half of the form (separated by a heavy line) refers to the provider of services, the services provided to the patient, and the medical necessity of those services.

As with all patient information, all rules of confidentiality apply. Professionalism warns about consequences for failure of confidentiality. Therefore, the patient must sign a release of information for a claim form to be completed. To make this process simpler, many offices have a standard release form for this purpose. Once the form has been signed and is on file in the patient's record, a notation of "SIGNATURE ON FILE" may be written or typed in box 12 of the CMS-1500 form. Box 13 deals with payment of benefits. If this box

Professionalism

The professional medical assistant has access to all patient records. The records contain confidential information that only a few designated people should have access to. It is against the law to reveal any information concerning a patient or even talk about a patient's condition to the patient anywhere but in a professional setting. Be aware that neighbors, friends, may ask you about patients who have had appointments with the doctor. By law, you cannot reveal this information. HIPAA is very specific concerning confidentiality. You can be fined up to $250,000 per incident or be jailed up to 10 years for violation of HIPAA laws.

is signed, payment will frequently be made directly to the provider of services. If the box is not signed, or for a contract that cannot be assigned, payment is made to the insured. Many insurance carriers, including Medicare, allow for lifetime assignment of benefits

---

16-1 PROCEDURE

Completing the CMS-1500 Form

OBJECTIVE: Correctly complete a CMS-1500 form.

Equipment and Supplies
patient's medical record; patient's insurance information; patient's ledger card; superbill; CMS-1500 form; black ink pen; computer with a printer; or typewriter

Method
1. Box 1 refers to government medical plans. Place an "X" in the appropriate box to indicate type of coverage if applicable.
   a. Enter the identification number listed on the insurance card.
2. Enter the patient's name in the order requested on the form.
3. Enter the patient's 8-digit birth date. Place an "X" in the appropriate box that indicates patient's gender.

4. Enter the insured's name in the order requested on the form. Enter the word "SAME" if the patient and insured are the same.
5. Enter the patient's complete address and telephone number.
6. Place an "X" in the box that indicates the patient's relationship to the insured.
7. Enter the insured's complete address and telephone number.
8. Place an "X" in the box that indicates the patient's marital status. Place an "X" in the appropriate box to indicate if the patient is employed or a full-time or part-time student.

(continued)

Completing the CMS-1500 Form (continued)

9. Enter the other insured's name in the order requested on the form.
   a. Enter the other insured's policy or group number.
   b. Enter the other insured's 8-digit birth date. Place an "X" in the box that indicates the other insured's gender.
   c. Enter the other insured's employer's name or school name.
   d. Enter the other insured's insurance plan name or program name.
10. Place an "X" in either the YES or NO boxes to indicate if the patient's condition is related to:
    a. employment,
    b. auto accident, or
    c. other accident.
    d. Reserved for local use. Leave blank.
11. Enter the insured's policy group or FECA number.
    a. Enter the insured's 8-digit birth date. Place an "X" in the box that indicates the insured's gender.
    b. Enter the insured's employer's name or school name.
    c. Enter the insured's insurance plan name or program name.
    d. Place an "X" in either the YES or NO box to indicate if there is another health benefit plan. If YES, 9a to 9d must be completed.
12. In order to release and use the patient's medical information to process the claim, have the patient or authorized person sign and date in the appropriate area, or if applicable, note SIGNATURE ON FILE.
13. In order to authorize payment for the claim dispersed to the provider, have the insured or authorized person sign in the appropriate area, or if applicable, note SIGNATURE ON FILE.
14. Enter the 8-digit date of current illness, injury, or pregnancy.
15. Enter dates if patient has had same or similar condition.
16. Enter 8-digit from and to dates the patient is unable to work in his or her current occupation.
17. Enter the name of the referring physician or other source.
    a. Enter the I.D. number of the referring physician.
18. Enter the 8-digit from and to hospitalization dates related to the current services.

19. Reserved for local use. Leave blank.
20. Place an "X" in either the YES or NO box to indicate if an outside laboratory was used. Enter the amount of the charges.
21. Enter the correct ICD-9-CM code related to the diagnosis or nature of the illness or injury. Each ICD-9-CM code must be entered in priority order. Each form can only contain four ICD-9-CM codes.
22. Enter the Medicaid resubmission code and original reference number.
23. Enter the prior authorization number.
24. Enter information into columns A through K.
    A. Enter the 8-digit from and to dates the patient had services.
    B. Enter the 2-digit code for place of service.
    C. Leave blank.
    D. Enter the correct CPT/HCPCS code and modifier for procedures, services, or supplies.
    E. Enter the correct diagnosis code (1, 2, 3, or 4) that corresponds with the correct service that was rendered.
    F. Enter the charges for the service rendered.
    G. Enter the number days or units of service.
    H. Leave blank.
    I. Leave blank.
    J. Leave blank
    K. Leave blank.
25. Enter the federal tax I.D. number or Social Security Number.
26. Enter the patient's account number.
27. Place an "X" in either the YES or NO box to indicate if assignment will be accepted.
28. Enter total charges.
29. Enter amount paid.
30. Enter balance due.
31. Enter signature of physician or supplier including degrees or credentials.
32. Enter the complete name and address of the facility where the services were rendered.
33. Enter the physician's, supplier's billing name, address, zip code, and telephone number.
34. Proofread the CMS-1500 form for accuracy.
35. Make a copy of the CMS-1500 form to keep in the patient's medical record—for paper claim submissions only.
36. Enter required data into the insurance claims log.
37. Send the completed CMS-1500 form (Figure 16-3) and required documentation to the insurance carrier.

HEALTH INSURANCE CLAIM FORM

PLEASE DO NOT STAPLE IN THIS AREA

PICA [ ][ ]   HEALTH INSURANCE CLAIM FORM   PICA [ ][ ]

1. MEDICARE	MEDICAID	CHAMPUS	CHAMPVA	GROUP HEALTH PLAN	FECA BLK LUNG	OTHER	1a. INSURED'S I.D. NUMBER (FOR PROGRAM IN ITEM 1)
[X] (Medicare #)	(Medicaid #)	(Sponsor's SSN)	(VA File #)	(SSN or ID)	(SSN)	(ID)	

2. PATIENT'S NAME (Last Name, First Name, Middle Initial)
Jones, Jill

3. PATIENT'S BIRTH DATE   MM 12 DD 04 YYYY 1932   SEX M [ ] F [ ]

4. INSURED'S NAME (Last Name, First Name, Middle Initial)

5. PATIENT'S ADDRESS (No., Street)
555 High Street

6. PATIENT RELATIONSHIP TO INSURED
Self [X] Spouse [ ] Child [ ] Other [ ]

7. INSURED'S ADDRESS (No., Street)

CITY Anycity   STATE CA

8. PATIENT STATUS
Single [X] Married [ ] Other [ ]
Employed [ ] Full-Time Student [X] Part-Time Student [ ]

CITY   STATE CA

ZIP CODE 12345   TELEPHONE (Include Area Code) (805) 555-1234

ZIP CODE 12345   TELEPHONE (INCLUDE AREA CODE) (805) 555-1234

9. OTHER INSURED'S NAME (Last Name, First Name, Middle Initial)

10. IS PATIENT'S CONDITION RELATED TO:

11. INSURED'S POLICY GROUP OR FECA NUMBER

a. OTHER INSURED'S POLICY OR GROUP NUMBER

a. EMPLOYMENT? (CURRENT OR PREVIOUS)
YES [ ] NO [X]

a. INSURED'S DATE OF BIRTH   MM DD YYYY   SEX M [ ] F [ ]

b. OTHER INSURED'S DATE OF BIRTH   MM DD YYYY   SEX M [ ] F [X]

b. AUTO ACCIDENT?   PLACE (State)
YES [ ] NO [X]

b. EMPLOYER'S NAME OR SCHOOL NAME

c. EMPLOYER'S NAME OR SCHOOL NAME

c. OTHER ACCIDENT?
YES [ ] NO [X]

c. INSURANCE PLAN NAME OR PROGRAM NAME

d. INSURANCE PLAN NAME OR PROGRAM NAME

10d. RESERVED FOR LOCAL USE

d. IS THERE ANOTHER HEALTH BENEFIT PLAN?
YES [ ] NO [ ]   If yes, return to and complete item 9 a-d.

READ BACK OF FORM BEFORE COMPLETING & SIGNING THIS FORM.
12. PATIENT'S OR AUTHORIZED PERSON'S SIGNATURE I authorize the release of any medical or other information necessary to process this claim. I also request payment of government benefits either to myself or to the party who accepts assignment below.

SIGNED Signature on file   DATE 01/01/2005

13. INSURED'S OR AUTHORIZED PERSON'S SIGNATURE I authorize payment of medical benefits to the undersigned physician or supplier for services described below.

SIGNED

14. DATE OF CURRENT: MM DD YYYY   ILLNESS (First symptom) OR INJURY (Accident) OR PREGNANCY(LMP)

15. IF PATIENT HAS HAD SAME OR SIMILAR ILLNESS. GIVE FIRST DATE MM DD YYYY

16. DATES PATIENT UNABLE TO WORK IN CURRENT OCCUPATION FROM MM DD YYYY TO MM DD YYYY

17. NAME OF REFERRING PHYSICIAN OR OTHER SOURCE

17a. I.D. NUMBER OF REFERRING PHYSICIAN

18. HOSPITALIZATION DATES RELATED TO CURRENT SERVICES FROM MM DD YYYY TO MM DD YYYY

19. RESERVED FOR LOCAL USE

20. OUTSIDE LAB? $ CHARGES
YES [ ] NO [ ]

21. DIAGNOSIS OR NATURE OF ILLNESS OR INJURY. (RELATE ITEMS 1,2,3 OR 4 TO ITEM 24E BY LINE)
1. V58 . 1   3. 105 . 2
2. 787 . XX   4. ___ . ___

22. MEDICAID RESUBMISSION CODE   ORIGINAL REF. NO.

23. PRIOR AUTHORIZATION NUMBER

24. A. DATE(S) OF SERVICE From MM DD YYYY To MM DD YYYY	B. Place of Service	C. Type of Service	D. PROCEDURES, SERVICES, OR SUPPLIES (Explain Unusual Circumstances) CPT/HCPCS | MODIFIER	E. DIAGNOSIS CODE	F. $ CHARGES	G. DAYS OR UNITS	H. EPSDT Family Plan	I. EMG	J. COB	K. RESERVED FOR LOCAL USE
1 MM DD YYYY MM DD YYYY	11		J2469	1	XXXX XX	10				
2 MM DD YYYY MM DD YYYY	11		J9XXX	X	XXXX XX	X				
3 MM DD YYYY MM DD YYYY	11		GXXXX 59	1	XXXX XX	1				
4										
5										
6										

25. FEDERAL TAX I.D. NUMBER   SSN [ ] EIN [X]
123-45-6789

26. PATIENT'S ACCOUNT NO.
987654321

27. ACCEPT ASSIGNMENT? (For govt. claims, see back)
YES [X] NO [ ]

28. TOTAL CHARGE $

29. AMOUNT PAID $

30. BALANCE DUE $

31. SIGNATURE OF PHYSICIAN OR SUPPLIER INCLUDING DEGREES OR CREDENTIALS (I certify that the statements on the reverse apply to this bill and are made a part thereof.)

SIGNED On file   DATE

32. NAME AND ADDRESS OF FACILITY WHERE SERVICES WERE RENDERED (If other than home or office)

33. PHYSICIAN'S, SUPPLIER'S BILLING NAME, ADDRESS, ZIP CODE & PHONE #
Martin Smith, MD
51 Provider Dr.
Anycity, CA 12345
PIN#   GRP#

(APPROVED BY AMA COUNCIL ON MEDICAL SERVICE 8/88)   **PLEASE PRINT OR TYPE**   APPROVED OMB-0938-0008 FORM CMS-1500 (12-90), FORM RRB-1500, APPROVED OMB-1215-0055 FORM OWCP-1500, APPROVED OMB-0720-0001 (CHAMPUS)

FIGURE 16-3 A completed CMS-1500 form.

Assignment of Lifetime Medicare Benefits

Name of Beneficiary ____________________

Medicare Number ____________________

I, the undersigned, request that all authorized Medicare benefits be paid to me or on my behalf to ____________________ (Name of Physician or Supplier) for all services rendered to me by the aforementioned provider. I hereby authorize any holder of my medical records to release to the Health Care Financing Administration and its agents any information necessary to determine and secure the payment of all benefits.*

Signed ____________________ (Signature of Beneficiary) Date __________

* If you are a patient in a hospital or skilled nursing home, this authorization is in effect for the period of your confinement. Otherwise, this authorization is in effect until you choose to revoke it.

FIGURE 16-4 A Health Care Insurance Claim Form—Assignment of Lifetime Medicare.

(Figure 16-4). With a signature on one form, the notation "SIGNATURE ON FILE" can also be made in box 13. This saves the medical assistant the time required for a patient to sign an insurance claim form for each office visit. The forms, however, must be kept in the patient record and must be available at all times.

One confusing element in insurance processing is the concept of "participating" and "nonparticipating" providers. Most insurance companies will make special incentives available to those who choose to become participating providers, who can be the physician or medical facility that will accept the insurance company's allowed amount for services rendered to be payment in full (less patient co-payments). To become a participating provider, the physician completes a form and is assigned a number that is unique to the physician or practice.

With most insurance plans, payment is made directly to participating providers, while payment is made to the patient for claims of a nonparticipating provider. The nonparticipating provider bills the patient and the patient is expected to pay the charges.

There are advantages to both ways of handling insurance claims. Often, insurance companies reimburse at a lower rate than the physician bills. In this case, the physician must "write off" or agree to forfeit the amount the insurance company does not authorize. It is an expense to any practice when administrative staff (medical assistant or insurance claims processing clerk, for example) is on the payroll and need to spend time submitting and tracking insurance claims. However, payment is made directly to the physician's practice, often within a few days (especially with electronic claim submission), ensuring that large charges do not accumulate on the physician's accounts receivable. Each practice must weigh the advantages and disadvantages carefully before making a decision to become either a participating or nonparticipating practice.

Many medical offices now use a single sheet to speed the process of reimbursement. This form is called a superbill and lists the patient's name, diagnoses and treatments with additional space to fill in claim information. Some insurance carriers will accept a superbill in lieu of a claim form, although this depends on the specific carrier. Originally, superbills were created to allow patients to file their own claims; however, as insurance rules and regulations have become more complex and coding and documentation requirements more stringent, most medical practices file insurance claims for their patients as a courtesy. Lifespan Considerations has more about completing insurance claim forms.

It is important for the medical assistant to verify if a patient has primary and secondary medical insurance coverage. A patient who has health insurance coverage with more than one medical insurance plan will have one primary insurance coverage and the other insurance as secondary coverage. If the patient has coverage with his or her employer as well as his or her spouse's employer, then the patient's employer's medical insurance plan

Lifespan Considerations

***Some insurance plans** require that the subscriber fill out the claim forms. To someone, especially an older patient, who has never worked with filing claims, this can be very confusing. Because the physician cannot receive payment for services until claims are filed, it can be helpful to assist the patient in filling out the appropriate forms. Some offices do this for a small fee, while others do it at no charge. Remember to have the patient sign an authorization to release medical information before submitting any claim.*

would be primary, while the spouse's employer's medical insurance plan would be secondary. This is to prevent a person from profiting on his or her medical insurance. It also prevents double payment on services provided.

The "birthday rule" is used by insurance claims administrators to determine which parent's benefit plans will pay for the medical bills of a dependent child when the child is covered by the plans of both parents. The plan of the parent whose birthday falls earliest in the year (not the oldest parent) will be the primary plan. When parents have the same birthday, the primary medical insurance will be the one with the earliest date of inception. This rule only applies to parents who are legally married.

If the parents are divorced, the court will determine which parent's medical insurance will be primarily responsible. Just because a parent has legal custody does not mean that his or her medical insurance will be primary.

Claim Security

Confidentiality is an important issue in regards to the sensitive information that is found in a patient's medical record. Care must be taken when processing insurance claims that appropriate information is only released to the appropriate person. Security involves protection of patient information. Security is the responsibility of all who have access to patients' records. Care must be taken in the work area not to leave records unattended. When discussing patient information with insurance carriers over the telephone, it is best to be in an area where you cannot be easily overheard. It is considered to be a breach of confidentiality, or failure to keep something confidential, when patient information is released to others without authorization from the patient (Legal and Ethical Issues).

Before releasing any information regarding a patient to anyone, you must obtain a signed "Authorization for Release of Medical Information" statement. Authorization can be given by having the patient sign block 12, Patient's or Authorized Person's Signature, on the CMS-1500. A practice can also create its own release form. It is good routine to have the patient renew this authorization annually.

Another element of claim security is making sure electronic data containing health information about a patient is secure when stored on a computer network. A firewall is used to prevent unauthorized access from another computer system to the data stored on the computer network.

Tracking Claim Forms

When a medical assistant is submitting paper claims, he or she must have a tracking system in place to follow up on claims that have been submitted. An insurance

claims log is used for this purpose. An insurance claims log can be documented manually or it may be kept on a computerized spreadsheet. It gives the medical assistant the status of a claim quickly. After the medical assistant completes a claim form, he or she then enters data into the insurance claims log. The data entered at this time includes the patient's name, date of service, insurance carrier, date the claim was submitted, and amount of the claim submitted. When the medical assistant follows up on the claim, the date must be documented on the insurance claims log. Once the medical assistant receives payment on the claim, this date must also be documented on the insurance claims log. The difference between the submitted and paid amounts is also documented on the insurance claims log. After the claim is paid in full, the medical assistant can highlight that section of the insurance claims log to indicate that the claim is completely processed.

Claim Form Rejection

Occasionally, if a claim is not correct in some way, the insurance company will reject the claim. Some of the most common reasons for claim rejection include:

- Incorrect or missing patient registration information (name, address, insurance number)
- Incorrect or missing name of a referring physician
- Incorrect or missing diagnosis code
- Overlapping, incorrect, or duplicate dates of service
- Incorrect place of service
- Invalid, incorrect, or missing procedure code
- Incorrect or missing number of days or units
- Incorrect or missing modifier

If a claim is rejected for any reason, it must be corrected and resubmitted to the insurance carrier. There are usually time limits for refiling rejected claims, so the medical assistant must be very aware of these deadlines and resubmit the claims before the time has expired. Expired claims will not be processed by the insurance carrier and will ultimately cost the practice money.

As a precaution, the medical assistant must review every claim for accuracy prior to submitting it. While no one process or procedure can guarantee that a claim will never be rejected or reviewed, a careful, studious approach to the claims process can ensure greater accuracy.

Preventing Claim Form Rejection

To prevent a claim from being rejected, the medical assistant must have all the books and equipment readily available. When he or she is filing insurance claim forms, the medical assistant must carefully review each claim before it is submitted. Limiting distractions that occur in the medical office can also help the medical assistant ensure the claim form is correct and complete. Having time to focus on claims processing is not always possible, but if the office team works together, it can be accommodated. Having a certain time period each day set aside for working on claims and not doing other tasks, can help the medical assistant complete the forms correctly and, most of the time, faster. Lastly, have another medical office staff member review each insurance claim form before it is submitted. A second set of eyes may notice errors or omissions not detected by the person processing the forms.

SUMMARY

The health insurance claim form provides communication between the insurance company and physician for the patient. When the medical assistant is submitting a claim, he or she must find out which health insurance claim form to use. The most commonly used form is the CMS-1500 claim form. Claims are submitted in paper form or electronically. The medical assistant must be familiar with how to complete the CMS-1500 form.

Chapter Review

COMPETENCY REVIEW

1. Define and spell the terms to learn for this chapter.
2. Explain the "birthday rule."
3. What is the name of the standardized form used to submit insurance claims? What information must be included on this form?
4. List the reasons a claim may be rejected.
5. Use the health insurance claim forms shown in Figures 16-4 and 16-5 to complete the forms for: Jane Doe, address 123 Main Street, Anytown, ST 60000, U.S.A., telephone 444-555-1234, S/S # 123-45-6789, DOB (date of birth) 1/15/1973. She is single and self-insured. Jane Doe's insurance number is the same as her social security number. Jane saw Dr. Brent Smith for the first time on May 27, 2005 and he diagnosed her with primary hypertension. Jane paid $40.00 for the office visit. Jane's account number is 00321. Dr. Smith is located at 555 Frances Street, Anytown, ST 60000, U.S.A., telephone 444-555-1111, Federal Tax ID # 000000000.

PREPARING FOR THE CERTIFICATION EXAM

1. What information is not required for completing a CMS-1500?
   A. the number of people in the household
   B. the name of the insured
   C. the name of the insured's insurance company
   D. the insured's identification number
   E. the telephone number of the insured

2. Once a patient has signed a release of information statement, what may be written in box 12 of the CMS-1500?
   A. BENEFITS ASSIGNED
   B. CONFIDENTIAL
   C. SIGNATURE ON FILE
   D. PERMISSION GRANTED
   E. the patient must sign each time

continued on next page

3. Which form allows a medical office to use a single sheet that lists the patient's name, diagnoses, treatments, and claim information?
   A. charge sheet
   B. CMS-1500
   C. superclaim
   D. reimbursement form
   E. superbill

4. Which is NOT a reason a claim may be rejected?
   A. overlapping dates of service
   B. missing name of a referring physician
   C. incorrect place of service
   D. incorrect patient telephone number
   E. correct diagnosis is given

5. The CMS-1500 claim form
   A. is accepted by every insurance company.
   B. must be filled out by the patient
   C. must be filled out by the provider
   D. is accepted as a standard submission (claim) form by most carriers
   E. is never used

6. Which is filed when a patient is eligible for both Medicare and Medicaid?
   A. CMS-1500
   B. HCFA-1500
   C. superbill
   D. crossover claim
   E. DD form 2642

7. Which insurance is mandated by the federal government to cover those who have received injuries directly related to work?
   A. Blue Cross/Blue Shield
   B. disability insurance
   C. workers' compensation
   D. Medicaid
   E. CHAMPUS

8. Which is a reason a claim might be rejected?
   A. appropriate diagnosis code
   B. missing procedure code
   C. correct place of service
   D. correct date of service
   E. correct social security number

9. When a health insurance claim form has missing data or errors, this is considered to be a?
   A. clean claim
   B. invalid claim
   C. dirty claim
   D. denied claim
   E. rejected claim

10. Electronic claim submission
    A. is difficult and costly
    B. cannot be completed by a medical assistant
    C. is referred to as a paperless claim
    D. increases the time it takes to pay a claim
    E. frequently have errors

CRITICAL THINKING

1. What steps should Lewis take to verify Mary Free's insurance?
2. List some reasons the claim for Mark's care could have been rejected.

ON THE JOB

Drake Scott, CMA, is responsible for processing insurance claims for a large medical clinic. You have just hired Anne Obermark, CMA to work with Drake in processing insurance claims. You determined that Anne will be responsible for tracking claims.

1. Why is it important for Anne to track insurance claims processed through the clinic?
2. What kind of information should the insurance claim log contain?
3. When Anne checks the insurance claim log, she finds five claims that have not been paid in the past three months. What should Anne do?

INTERNET ACTIVITY

There are many software packages available to help complete and submit insurance claims. Conduct a search to find 5 such packages. List the unique features, similar features, and cost.

 MediaLink More on medical insurance claims, including interactive resources, can be found on the Student CD-ROM accompanying this textbook.

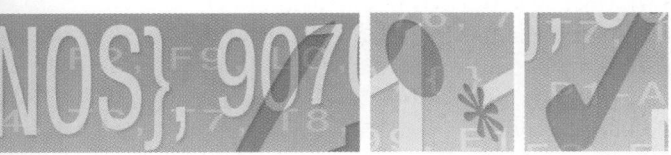

Medical Assistant Role Delineation Chart

HIGHLIGHT indicates material covered in this chapter.

ADMINISTRATIVE

Administrative Procedures
- Perform basic administrative medical assisting functions
- Schedule, coordinate and monitor appointments
- Schedule inpatient/outpatient admissions and procedures
- Understand and apply third-party guidelines
- Obtain reimbursement through accurate claims submission
- Monitor third-party reimbursement
- Understand and adhere to managed care policies and procedures
- *Negotiate managed care contracts*

Practice Finances
- Perform procedural and diagnostic coding
- Apply bookkeeping principles

- Manage accounts receivable
- *Manage accounts payable*
- *Process payroll*
- *Document and maintain accounting and banking records*
- *Develop and maintain fee schedules*
- *Manage renewals of business and professional insurance policies*
- *Manage personnel benefits and maintain records*
- *Perform marketing, financial, and strategic planning*

CLINICAL

Fundamental Principles
- Apply principles of aseptic technique and infection control
- Comply with quality assurance practices
- Screen and follow up patient test results

Diagnostic Orders
- Collect and process specimens
- Perform diagnostic tests

Patient Care
- Adhere to established patient screening procedures
- Obtain patient history and vital signs
- Prepare and maintain examination and treatment areas
- Prepare patient for examinations, procedures and treatments

- Assist with examinations, procedures and treatments
- Prepare and administer medications and immunizations
- Maintain medication and immunization records
- Recognize and respond to emergencies
- Coordinate patient care information with other health care providers
- Initiate IV and administer IV medications with appropriate training and as permitted by state law

GENERAL

Professionalism
- Display a professional manner and image
- Demonstrate initiative and responsibility
- Work as a member of the health care team
- Prioritize and perform multiple tasks
- Adapt to change
- Promote the CMA credential
- Enhance skills through continuing education
- Treat all patients with compassion and empathy
- Promote the practice through positive public relations

Communication Skills
- Recognize and respect cultural diversity
- Adapt communications to individual's ability to understand
- Use professional telephone technique

- Recognize and respond effectively to verbal, nonverbal, and written communications
- Use medical terminology appropriately
- Utilize electronic technology to receive, organize, prioritize and transmit information
- Serve as liaison

Legal Concepts
- Perform within legal and ethical boundaries
- Prepare and maintain medical records
- Document accurately
- Follow employer's established policies dealing with the health care contract
- Implement and maintain federal and state health care legislation and regulations
- Comply with established risk management and safety procedures
- Recognize professional credentialing criteria
- *Develop and maintain personnel, policy and procedure manuals*

Instruction
- Instruct individuals according to their needs
- Explain office policies and procedures
- Teach methods of health promotion and disease prevention
- Locate community resources and disseminate information
- *Develop educational materials*
- *Conduct continuing education activities*

Operational Functions
- Perform inventory of supplies and equipment
- Perform routine maintenance of administrative and clinical equipment
- Apply computer techniques to support office operations
- *Perform personnel management functions*
- *Negotiate leases and prices for equipment and supply contracts*

- *Denotes advanced skills.*

SOURCE: Reprinted by permission of the American Association of Medical Assistants from the AAMA Role Delineation Study: Occupational Analysis of the Medical Assisting Profession.

Medical Coding

Learning Objectives

After completing this chapter, you should be able to:

- Define and spell the terms to learn for this chapter.
- Describe the purpose of diagnosis coding.
- Correctly apply the principles of ICD-9-CM coding.

- Describe the purpose of CPT coding.
- Correctly apply the principles of CPT coding.
- Discuss basic coding rules for CPT.

OUTLINE

Insurance Coding	300
Understanding the ICD-9-CM	300
Procedure Coding	303
Getting to Know the CPT	305
Insurance Fraud	308
Compliance Plan	311

Terms to Learn

Current Procedural Terminology (CPT)

Evaluation and Management (E/M)

International Classification of Diseases, Ninth Revision Clinical Modification (ICD-9-CM)

International Classification of Diseases, Tenth Revision (ICD-10)

modifier

principal diagnosis

procedural coding

symbol

World Health Organization (WHO)

Case Study

CASEY ALLEN, A 5-MONTH OLD MALE, WAS seen by Dr. Adams for chronic otitis media. This was the child's third bout in the last 10 months. Dr. Adams recommended bilateral myringotomies and tube placement. The physician also ordered an audiogram. The insurance company denied the claim, stating the procedure code was wrong for the diagnosis.

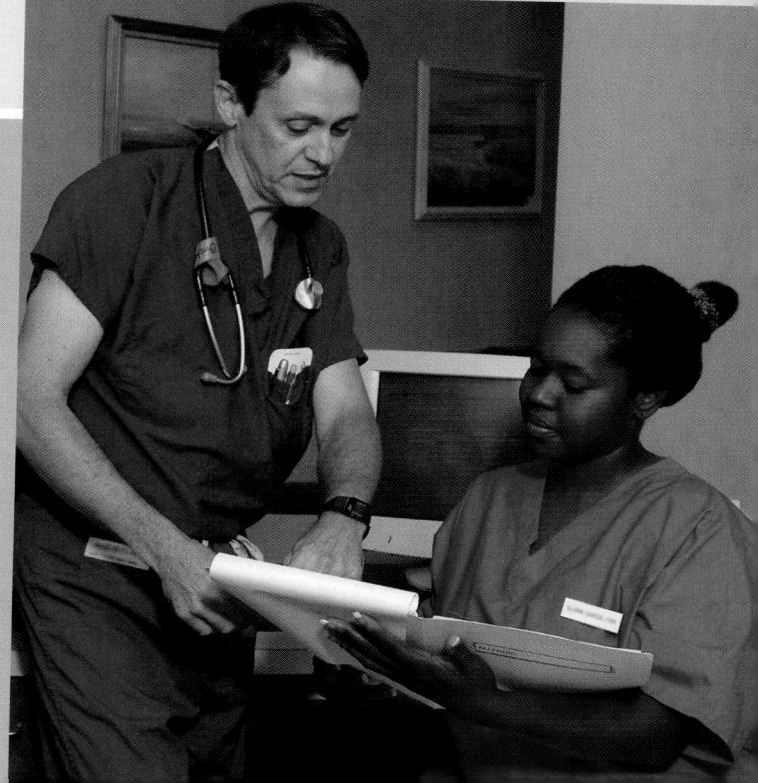

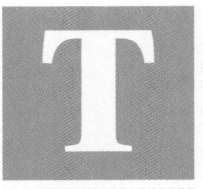

The process of insurance billing includes the accurate identification of the diagnostic, procedure, and service codes on the medical insurance claim form. The diagnostic code is located in the International Classification of Disease, Ninth Revision Clinical Modifications (ICD-9-CM) listing. The procedure and service codes are located in the Current Procedural Terminology (CPT) listing. Each individual code specifically represents a numeric or alphanumeric identification for insurance carriers and aids in obtaining the maximum reimbursement. The medical assistant will need to identify the appropriate codes, which reflect the correct diagnosis and the procedure or service performed, in order to maintain sound billing practices.

Insurance Coding

Proper coding of insurance claims is the basis of the practice income. Incorrect coding will cause delays or denials in reimbursement. Anytime the medical assistant does not observe clear and concise documentation in the patient's medical record to support the ICD-9-CM or CPT code, he or she must consult the physician for further clarification. To be proficient in coding, the medical assistant must also have a good understanding of medical terminology, diseases, procedures, as well as anatomy and physiology. Having a medical dictionary is a handy resource for any medical assistant who is coding. Another helpful resource is the Internet. Having access to the Internet allows the medical assistant to research a disease or procedure he or she does not understand. The Health Insurance Portability and Accountability Act of 1996 (HIPAA) requires correct coding of services and may sanction providers who do not comply with the rules. It is important for the medical assistant to understand how to code and bill with accuracy. In addition, HIPAA requires the use of the

CMS-1500 form for Medicare billing, and for most providers, for all medical billing, as well as electronic submission of all bills. In many ambulatory care settings, the process of insurance coding begins with identifying and recording the appropriate diagnosis, procedure, or service codes on the superbill (Figure 17-1). The superbill is a document generated by the medical office and used as a charge slip, statement, and insurance reporting form. It is important for the codes on the superbill to be updated each year when the medical office receives the newest published coding books.

This document provides a comprehensive list of patient procedures, services, and diagnoses with respective codes and fees on which the physician indicates the services rendered. The superbill is used as a reference base for traditional paper insurance forms and electronic claims (Figure 17-2). Lifespan Considerations emphasizes the importance of understanding the superbill to advise patients, especially the elderly.

History of Coding

In 1937, the *International List of Causes of Death* was introduced. Then in 1948, the World Health Organization (WHO) published the *International Classification of Diseases*. This provided a revised list of the first classification system. In the United States, the Department of Health and Human Services published the ICD-9-CM (International Classification of Diseases, Ninth Clinical Modification) in 1979. By 1988, the Medicare Catastrophic Coverage Act was passed. This law made it a requirement for physicians to use diagnosis codes to receive Medicare reimbursement. Coding has gradually grown from a new office task to a career that requires extensive training and knowledge of both the medical and insurance professions. Coding is so important to proper fee reimbursement that an office may offer a bonus payment to its insurance coders if their insurance processing results in increased and accurate collections for the physician's practice. For information about becoming a certified medical coding specialist, contact the American Health Information Management Association (AHIMA) and the American Academy of Professional Coders (AAPC).

Lifespan
Considerations

Elderly patients and caregivers of patients may not understand the diagnosis as stated on the superbill. The medical assistant can help the patient or patient's parent with any questions he or she may have concerning the superbill.

Understanding the ICD-9-CM

Upon the physician evaluation, each patient will be diagnosed in medical terms. These medical terms are converted into numeric and alphanumeric diagnosis codes. The diagnosis codes are systematically classified in the International Classification of Disease, published by a specialized agency for health of the United Nations known as the World Health Organization (WHO).

WINDY CITY CLINIC
Beth Williams, M.D.
123 Michigan Avenue, Chicago, IL 60610
(312) 123-1234

UROLOGIC GYNECOLOGY
GENERAL GYNECOLOGY
OBSTETRICS

ID.# 20-1342846

No. 4815

PATIENT INFORMATION

PATIENT'S LAST NAME		FIRST	INITIAL	BIRTHDATE	SEX ☐ MALE ☐ FEMALE	TODAY'S DATE / /
ADDRESS	CITY	STATE	ZIP	RELATION TO SUBSCRIBER		REFERRING PHYSICIAN
SUBSCRIBER or POLICY HOLDER				INSURANCE		
ADDRESS	CITY	STATE	ZIP	INSURANCE ID.#	COVERAGE CODE	GROUP

OTHER HEALTH COVERAGE?
☐ NO
☐ YES   IDENTIFY

DISABILITY RELATED TO:
☐ ACCIDENT   ☐ PREGNANCY
☐ INDEPENDENT   ☐ OTHER

DATE SYMPTOMS APPEARED, INCEPTION OF PREGNANCY, OR
ACCIDENT OCCURED: / /

ASSIGNMENT and RELEASE: *I hereby assign my insurance benefits to be paid directly to the undersigned physician. I am financially responsible for noncovered services. I also authorize the physician to release any information required to process this claim.*

SIGNATURE OF PATIENT (or Parent, if Minor) _____   DATE / /

	PROCEDURES	CPT-Mod	AMOUNT		PROCEDURES	CPT-Mod	AMOUNT		PROCEDURES	CPT-Mod	AMOUNT
	A. OFFICE VISITS			31	Post-Partum	59430		60	PG Test, Urine	86006	
1	New GYN, Limited	90010			**F. GYN PROCEDURES**			61	Antigen Test	86006	
2	New GYN, Intermediate	90015		32	Irrigation of Vagina	57150*		62	Cytopathology Smear	88155	
3	New GYN, Extensive	90017		33	Insert Pessary	57160*		63	Specimen Handling	99000	
4	New GYN, Comprehensive	90020		34	Pessary Supplies	99070			**I. MISCELLANEOUS**		
5	Return GYN, Minimal	90030		35	Colposcopy	57452		64	Surgical Tray	99070	
6	Return GYN, Brief	90040		36	Biopsy, Cervix	57500		65	Therapeutic Injection	90782	
7	Return GYN, Limited	90050		37	Biopsy, Vagina	57100		66	Injection, Kenalog	J1870	
8	Return GYN, Intermediate	90060		38	Biopsy, Vulva	56600		67	Injection, Xylocaine	J3480	
9	Return GYN, Extended	90070		39	Biopsy, Endometrium	58100		68	Injection, Estrogen	J2655	
10	Return GYN, Comprehensive	90080		40	Biopsy, Skin			69	Injection, Progesterone	J2675	
11	Return GYN, Post-Operative	99024			0.5 cm.	11420		70	Injection, Vitamin B12	P4320	
	B. CONSULTATION				0.6 to 1.0 cm.	11421		71	Special Reports	99080	
12	GYN Consultation, Limited	90600			1.1 to 2.0 cm.	11423					
13	GYN Consultation, Intermed.	90605		41	Cryotherapy, Cervix	57511					
14	GYN Consultation, Compreh.	90620		42	Destruct. Condyloma	56501					
15	GYN Consultation, Complex	90630		43	Diaphragm Fitting	57170					
16	Second Opinion Surgery	90653		44	Diaphragm Supplies	99070					
	C. TELEPHONE CONSULTATION			45	IUD Insertion	58300					
17	Telephone Consult., Simple	99013		46	IUD Supplies	99070					
18	Telephone Consult., Intermed.	99014		47	IUD Removal	58301					
19	Telephone Consult., Compreh.	99015			**G. UROLOGIC PROCEDURES**						
	D. SPECIAL SERVICES			48	Urethral Dilation	53660					
20	ER Service after Office Hrs.	99064		49	Urethral Dilation, Repeat	53661					
21	ER Service during Office Hrs.	99065		50	Bladder Instillation	51700					
22	Night Call before 10 pm	99050		51	Periurethral Injection	53665					
23	Night Call after 10 pm	99052		52	Simple Catheterization	53670					
24	Sunday or Holiday Service	99054		53	Manual Electric Stimulation	97118					
25	Office Non-Schedule	99058			**H. LAB**						
	E. OB CARE			54	Urine Analysis	81000					
26	Prenatal Dx, Consultation	90620		55	Urine Culture	87068					
27	Initial OB, NOrmal	59400		56	Hematocrit	85015					
28	Initial OB, High Risk	59400.22		57	Hemogram	85021					
29	Return OB, Normal	59420		58	Commercial-Lat.	87087			TODAY'S TOTAL FEE	$	
30	Return OB, High Risk	59420.22		59	Wet Mount	87210					

	DIAGNOSIS	CODE		DIAGNOSIS	CODE		DIAGNOSIS	CODE		DIAGNOSIS	CODE
	Abortion:			Breasts	216.5		Galactorrhea	676.6		Pregnancy Postpartum	V24.2
	Threatened	640.0		Vulva	221.2		Hemorrhoids	455.0		Rectocele	618.0
	Incomplete	637.1		Breast Disorder (Mass)	611.72		Hypertension	401		Retention of Urine	788.2
	Habitual	646.3		Bronchitis	491		Incontinence of Urine	788.3		Stress Incontinence	625.6
	Abnormal Urination	788.6		Carcinoma In Situ:			Interstitial Cystitis	595.1		Urethral Stricture	598
	Abnormal PAP Smear	795.0		Cervix	233.1		Irritable Colon	564.1		Urethral Syndrome	597.81
	Adenomyosis	617.0		Uterus	233.2		Irregular Menstrual Cycle	626.4		Uterine Leiomyoma	218
	Adnexal MAss	625.8		Female Genital Organs	233.3		Malignant Neoplasm:			Uterine Prolapse:	
	Amenorrhera	626.0		Cervical Dysplasia	622.1		Cervix	180.9		Incomplete	618.2
	Anemia	285.9		Cervicitis	616.0		Uterus	182.0		Complete	618.3
	Arthritis	716.9		Contraceptive Management	V25.0		Ovary	183.0		Vaginal Discharge-Non Specific	623.5
	Artificial Menopause	627.4		Cystocele	618.0		Vagina	184.0		Vaginal Enterocele	618.6
	Asthma-Hayfever	493.0		Cystourethritis	595.0		Vulva	184.4		Vaginal Prolapse	618.0
	Atrophic Vaginitis	627.3		Diabetes Melliuts	250.0		Menopausal Syndrome	627.2		Vaginal Vault Prolapse Post	
	Bartholin Abscess	616.3		Thyroid Disorder	246.9		Menometrorrhagia	626.2		Hysterectomy	618.5
	Benign Neoplasm:			Dysmenorrhea	625.3		Oligomenorrhea	626.1		Vulvovaginitis:	
	Cervix	219.0		Dyspareunia	625.0		Obesity	278.0		Non Specific	616.1
	Uterus	219.1		Dysuria	788.1		Ovarian Cyst	620.2		Candida	112.1
	Ovary	220		Ectopic Pregnancy	617.0		Pelvic Inflammatory Disease	614.9		Trichomonas	131.01
	Vagina	221.1		Endometriosis	617.9		Pelvic Peritoneal Adhesions	614.6			
	Vulva	221.2		Enuresis-Unstable Bladder	788.3		Polycystic Ovaries	256.4			
	Benign Neoplasm of Skin:			Frequency of Urination	788.4		Postmenopausal Bleeding	627.1			
	Buttocks	216.5		Functional Disorder:			Post-Op Wound Infection	998.5			
	Abdomen	216.5		Bladder Instability	596.5		Pregnancy Prenatal	V22			

| **MISCELLANEOUS DIAGNOSIS** | DOCTOR'S SIGNATURE |
| | DATE / / |

SERVICES PERFORMED AT: ☐ Office ☐ Emergency Room
☐ **WINDY CITY CLINIC**
123 Michigan Avenue, Chicago, IL 60610
(312) 123-1234
☐ Hospital Calls at $_____ per Visit

ADMITTED _____ / /
DISCHARGED _____ / /

RETURN VISIT INFORMATION
15 • 30 • 45 • 60
_____ DAYS _____ WEEKS _____ MONTHS ☐ WILL CALL
Procedure:

ACCEPT ASSIGNMENT
☐ YES
☐ NO

INSTRUCTIONS TO PATIENT FOR FILING INSURANCE CLAIMS

1. Complete patient information portion of this form.
2. Sign and date.
3. Mail this form directly to your insurance company with your own insurance company's form.
4. Patients with health care insurance please remember:
   A. Professional services are charged to the patient, and not to the insurance company.
   B. Insured patients are expected to take care of their fees as services are rendered.
   C. This office cannot accept responsibility for collecting your insurance claim or for negotiating a settlement on a disputed claim.
   D. You are responsible for payment of your account.

TODAY'S FEE	$
OLD BALANCE	$
ADJUSTMENTS	$
TOTAL DUE	$
AMOUNT RECEIVED TODAY	$
☐ CASH ☐ CHECK ☐ C.C.	
NEW BALANCE	$

FIGURE 17-1   An example of a superbill.

WHO accumulates all of the diagnoses reported on claim forms and places the diagnostic codes into a computerized database. This database tracks statistical information, such as morbidity data.

Every year ICD-9-CM codes are updated. The newly published codes are available to the public on or before October 1st. Every medical office should use the newest published copy of the ICD-9-CM (Figure 17-3)

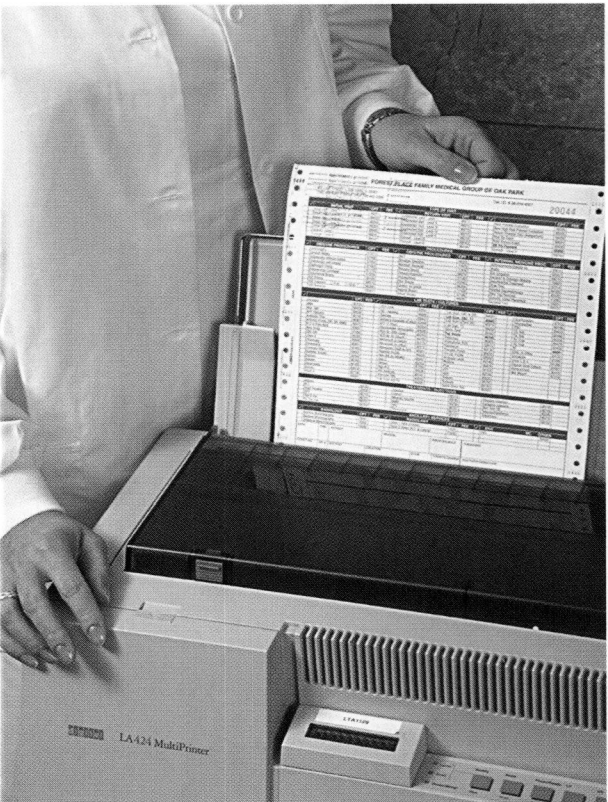

FIGURE 17-2 A computer generated superbill.

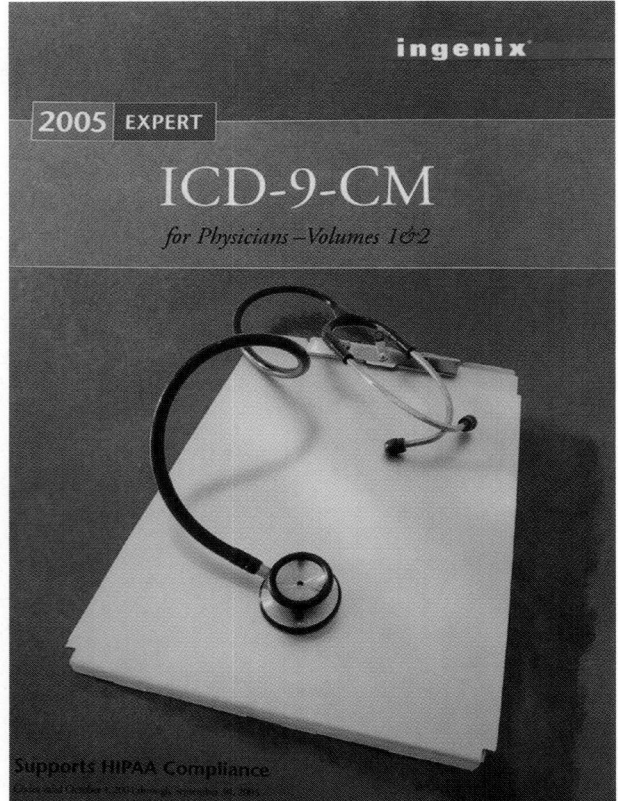

FIGURE 17-3 ICD-9 Code Book.

to perform coding. If the newest published copy of the ICD-9-CM is not used, this could cause the claim to be rejected because of incorrect coding.

Formats and Conventions of ICD-9-CM

ICD-9-CM (International Classification of Diseases, Ninth Clinical Modification) provides numeric and alphanumeric codes for patient diagnoses. In order for an insurance payment to be processed appropriately, the diagnosis code must appear on a claim form and must support the medical necessity of the procedure code (service rendered).

The ICD-9-CM coding manual contains three volumes of information. Volume III deals with inpatient diagnosis and treatment and is used to code inpatient hospital-billed procedures. It is not used in most ambulatory care settings. Therefore, we will concentrate on Volumes I, the Tabular List, and Volume II, the Alphabetic Index.

Volume I (the Tabular List) contains 17 chapters of disease and injury codes and supplementary classifications for V and E codes. It also contains five appendices. In the Tabular List, codes are arranged in numerical order.

Volume II or the Alphabetic Index, lists the disease and injuries that are in the Tabular List in alphabetical order. In addition, Volume II contains an index of poisoning and adverse effects of chemicals and drugs and an index of injuries caused by external efforts, such as accidents.

Steps in ICD Coding

To understand how to code diagnoses, it is important that the medical assistant understand the organization of the ICD-9-CM. Diagnoses are given a three-digit main code, with fourth and fifth digits when required for certain conditions that define the code to the highest level of specificity. To code properly, it is necessary to begin with Volume II, the Alphabetic Index. Diagnoses and conditions are located alphabetically by condition, not body system. Therefore, when trying to find a code for a closed fracture of the right arm, the coder would begin by looking for the key word "fracture." This term is listed in bold type. The coder would next locate the word "arm." A code number of 818.0 is given. Next, the coder would turn to the numeric index (Volume I, Tabular List) and find the code number 818.0. After reading the description, the code 818.0 is determined to be the correct one. However, the diagnosis may need greater specification that requires an additional fifth digit to designate the specific bone of the arm that contains the fracture. Special notes and symbols used in ICD-9-CM coding, such as not otherwise specified (NOS), are listed as reference material in the code books and should be used only when a higher level of specificity is not available.

When coding for claim reimbursement, the medical assistant must also understand the significance of a principal diagnosis. The principal diagnosis is the reason the patient sought care on a particular date. Principal diagnosis is used when performing coding in the hospital setting and when a final diagnosis was unable to be determined without further patient follow-up. The primary diagnosis represents the patient's major health problem for that particular claim. This is important when you file a claim for a patient who has more than one diagnosis, for example cancer and a urinary tract infection (UTI). If the UTI is unrelated to the cancer, and the cancer will not affect the treatment or recovery from the UTI, then the code used for that claim would be UTI. Any other diagnoses treated at that time (up to four) must also be listed. For example, if a diabetic patient is seen for an ear infection, the ear infection is the primary diagnosis, while diabetes is a secondary diagnosis.

Special Codes

The ICD-9-CM coding system also allows for visits (V codes) not directly related to illness or injury or to add supportive information to patient family or personal history. The codes are used to describe a person who may not have a current illness, but uses the health care system for some specific purpose, such as well-baby care, birth control advice, pregnancy test, or immunizations. The codes are also used as supportive information when some circumstance or problem is present that may influence the patient's health, but is not in itself a current illness or problem, such as an allergy to penicillin.

The ICD-9-CM manual also uses tables for certain diseases and conditions. A diagnosis of hypertension, for example, must be coded from the hypertension table. A neoplasm, whether benign or malignant, must be coded from the neoplasm table, and the morphology (behavior) of the neoplasm is coded from a morphology table (M code). Additionally, adverse reactions or poisoning are listed in a section listing various drugs and other agents. Again, the medical assistant should become familiar with the organization of the ICD-9-CM manual in order to code diagnoses properly and correctly. Procedure 17-1 provides steps on how to assign the correct ICD-9-CM codes.

E codes (Figure 17-4) are used to describe external causes of injury and poisoning or adverse effect. These codes may not be used as primary or principal diagnoses (they do not stand alone). E codes are used as additional information regarding a particular diagnosis and to further define the cause of a poisoning or adverse effects, such as therapeutic use, attempted suicide, or accidental. For example, a drug overdose can be either accidental or taken as a suicide attempt. The use of E codes (E930–E949) is mandatory when coding the use of drugs.

Abbreviations, Symbols, and Other Conventions

Instructional notes are included in the listings to guide the user on how to accurately code. Following are some examples:

NEC—Not elsewhere classifiable

NOS—Not otherwise specified

[]—Brackets enclose synonyms, alternative terminology, or explanatory phrases

()—Parentheses enclose supplementary words, called nonessential modifiers, that may be present in the narrative description of a disease without affecting the code assignment

}—The brace encloses a series of terms, each of which is modified by the statement appearing to the right of the brace

● bullet—Indicates a new code

▲—Indicates a revision in the Tabular List and a code change in the Alphabetic index

►◄—Indicates revised text

Boldface type—Used for all codes and titles in the Tabular List

Italicized type—Used for all exclusion notes and to identify codes that should not be used for describing the primary diagnosis

ICD-10

The diagnosis codes in the International Classification of Diseases, Tenth Revision (ICD-10) contain increased specificity and include recently discovered or diagnosed diseases. The ICD-10 has more codes as well as organizational and content modifications and new features.

Procedure Coding

Required elements for reimbursement from insurance carriers are based on a coding system that converts uniform descriptions of medical, surgical, and diagnostic services into numbers. This system, developed by the American Medical Association (AMA) in 1966, allows providers to communicate the procedures and services provided to the patient with increased accuracy. Reimbursement is based on codes submitted for services rendered. The process of transferring a narrative description of procedures into numbers is referred to as procedure coding.

SUPPLEMENTARY CLASSIFICATION OF EXTERNAL CAUSES OF INJURY AND POISONING (E800-E999)

This section is provided to permit the classification of environmental events, circumstances, and conditions as the cause of injury, poisoning, and other adverse effects. Where a code from this section is applicable, it is intended that it shall be used in addition to a code from one of the main chapters of ICD-9-CM, indicating the nature of the condition. Certain other conditions which may be stated to be due to external causes are classified in Chapters 1 to 16 of ICD-9-CM. For these, the "E" code classification should be used as an additional code for more detailed analysis.

Machinery accidents [other than those connected with transport] are classifiable to category E919, in which the fourth-digit allows a broad classification of the type of machinery involved. If a more detailed classification of type of machinery is required, it is suggested that the "Classification of Industrial Accidents according to Agency," prepared by the International Labor Office, be used in addition. This is reproduced in Appendix D for optional use.

Categories for "late effects" of accidents and other external causes are to be found at E929, E959, E969, E977, E989, and E999.

DEFINITIONS AND EXAMPLES RELATED TO TRANSPORT ACCIDENTS

(a) A **transport accident** (E800-E848) is any accident involving a device designed primarily for, or being used at the time primarily for, conveying persons or goods from one place to another.

> INCLUDES   accidents involving:
> aircraft and spacecraft (E840-E845)
> watercraft (E830-E838)
> motor vehicle (E810-E825)
> railway (E800-E807)
> other road vehicles (E826-E829)

In classifying accidents which involve more than one kind of transport, the above order of precedence of transport accidents should be used.

Accidents involving agricultural and construction machines, such as tractors, cranes, and bulldozers, are regarded as transport accidents only when these vehicles are under their own power on a highway [otherwise the vehicles are regarded as machinery]. Vehicles which can travel on land or water, such as hovercraft and other amphibious vehicles, are regarded as watercraft when on the water, as motor vehicles when on the highway, and as off-road motor vehicles when on land, but off the highway.

> EXCLUDES   accidents:
> in sports which involve the use of transport but where the transport vehicle itself was not involved in the accident
> involving vehicles which are part of industrial equipment used entirely on industrial premises
> occurring during transportation but unrelated to the hazards associated with the means of transportation [e.g., injuries received in a fight on board ship; transport vehicle involved in a cataclysm such as an earthquake]
> to persons engaged in the maintenance or repair of transport equipment or vehicle not in motion, unless injured by another vehicle in motion

(b) A **railway accident** is a transport accident involving a railway train or other railway vehicle operated on rails, whether in motion or not.

> EXCLUDES   accidents:
> in repair shops
> in roundhouse or on turntable
> on railway premises but not involving a train or other railway vehicle

(c) A **railway train** or **railway vehicle** is any device with or without cars coupled to it, designed for traffic on a railway.

> INCLUDES   interurban:
> electric car   } (operated chiefly on its
> streetcar   } own right-of-way, not open to other traffic)
> railway train, any power [diesel] [electric] [steam]
> funicular
> monorail or two-rail
> subterranean or elevated
> other vehicle designed to run on a railway track

> EXCLUDES   *interurban electric cars [streetcars] specified to be operating on a right-of-way that forms part of the public street or highway [definition (n)]*

(d) A **railway** or **railroad** is a right-of-way designed for traffic on rails, which is used by carriages or wagons transporting passengers or freight, and by other rolling stock, and which is not open to other public vehicular traffic.

(e) A **motor vehicle accident** is a transport accident involving a motor vehicle. It is defined as a motor vehicle traffic accident or as a motor vehicle nontraffic accident according to whether the accident occurs on a public highway or elsewhere.

> EXCLUDES   *injury or damage due to cataclysm*
> *injury or damage while a motor vehicle, not under its own power, is being loaded on, or unloaded from, another conveyance*

(f) A **motor vehicle traffic accident** is any motor vehicle accident occurring on a public highway [i.e., originating, terminating, or involving a vehicle partially on the highway]. A motor vehicle accident is assumed to have occurred on the highway unless another place is specified, except in the case of accidents involving only off-road motor vehicles which are classified as nontraffic accidents unless the contrary is stated.

(g) A **motor vehicle nontraffic accident** is any motor vehicle accident which occurs entirely in any place other than a public highway.

(h) A **public highway** [**trafficway**] or **street** is the entire width between property lines [or other boundary lines] of every way or place, of which any part is open to the use of the public for purposes of vehicular traffic as a matter of right or custom. A **roadway** is that part of the public highway designed, improved, and ordinarily used, for vehicular travel.

> INCLUDES   approaches (public) to:
> docks
> public building
> station

> EXCLUDES   *driveway (private)*
> *parking lot*
> *ramp*
> *roads in:*
> *airfield*
> *farm*
> *industrial premises*
> *mine*
> *private grounds*
> *quarry*

✓4th Fourth-digit Required   ►◄ Revised Text   ● New Code   ▲ Revised Code Title

---

FIGURE 17-4   An E-code section of the ICD-9-CM. Printed with permission from Ingenix, Inc. Copyright © 2004.

ICD-9-CM Coding

OBJECTIVE: Accurately assign an ICD-9-CM code.

Equipment and Supplies

patient's medical record; patient's insurance card; computer with printer or typewriter; medical billing software; current ICD-9-CM coding book; medical reference material; superbill with the doctor's diagnosis

Method

1. Locate the condition or diagnosis on the superbill or in the patient's medical record.
2. In Volume II (Alphabetic Index) of the ICD-9-CM book, locate the condition or diagnosis. (A condition may be expressed as: a noun, an adjective, or an eponym)
3. Examine the diagnostic statement to determine if the main term specifically describes that disease. If it does not, then look at the modifiers listed under that main term to find a more specific code. Also read any notes or cross references that may apply.
4. Then, locate the code in Volume I (Tabular Index).
5. Match the code description in the Tabular Index with the diagnosis in the patient's medical record.
6. Any of the codes from 0021.0 through V 82.9 in ICD-9-CM can be used to describe the main reason for the patient's office visit.
7. First list the ICD-9-CM code for the condition, problem, or diagnosis that is the main reason for the visit. Then, list coexisting conditions under additional codes.

8. Use codes at their highest level—5th digit codes first, then 4th digit, 3rd digit, and so on.
9. Do not code questionable or probable diagnoses, or the rule-out (R/O) diagnosis. One of the signs or symptoms of the R/O diagnosis will have to be identified by the physician as the reason for the office visit. For example, in R/O cystic fibrosis, the symptom of dyspnea would be coded until a definitive diagnosis of cystic fibrosis is made.
10. V codes describe factors that influence the health status of the patient, such as pregnancy test or vaccination, and are not used to code current illnesses. V codes are located in Volume II.
11. E codes are used for identifying external environmental events or conditions as the cause of injury, some adverse effect, or poisoning. For example, a drug overdose, either accidental or taken as a suicide attempt. The use of E codes (E 930-E 949) is mandatory when coding the use of drugs.
12. M codes, in Appendix A of Volume I, relate to the morphology of neoplasms. Morphology codes are not used as the primary diagnosis code; they are listed after the ICD-9-CM code. Each M code begins with the letter "M." The M codes cannot be used on claims for patient billing.
13. List all diagnosis codes (up to four) on the insurance claim form.

Healthcare Common Procedure Coding System (HCPCS) Sections

To report services and procedures for Medicaid and Medicare patient, the Healthcare Common Procedure Coding System (HCPCS) is used. There are two coding levels (Level I and Level II) available in HCPCS. Level I provides the same codes from the Current Procedural Terminology (CPT) manual, which provides procedure and service codes. Level II has codes that are not available in the CPT. This part has twenty-two sections that contain five-digit alphanumeric codes (Figure 17-5). These codes are for items that Medicare covers, such as

materials, supplies, and injections. Each Level II code begins with a letter with four numbers behind it. E1280 is an example of a Level II HCPCS code. HCPCS also has modifiers. Each modifier consists of two letters. These can also be used in addition to the modifiers from the CPT manual.

Getting to Know the CPT

In order to maximize reimbursements for a particular practice, the medical assistant must be familiar with CPT codes and how they are used. Codes are reviewed

Durable Medical Equipment

E1231 — E1520

[Y] **E1231** Wheelchair, pediatric size, tilt-in-space, rigid, adjustable, with seating system
MED: 100-3, 280.1

[Y] **E1232** Wheelchair, pediatric size, tilt-in-space, folding, adjustable, with seating system
MED: 100-3, 280.1

[Y] **E1233** Wheelchair, pediatric size, tilt-in-space, rigid, adjustable, without seating system
MED: 100-3, 280.1

[Y] **E1234** Wheelchair, pediatric size, tilt-in-space, folding, adjustable, without seating system
MED: 100-3, 280.1

[Y] **E1235** Wheelchair, pediatric size, rigid, adjustable, with seating system
MED: 100-3, 280.1

[Y] **E1236** Wheelchair, pediatric size, folding, adjustable, with seating system
MED: 100-3, 280.1

[Y] **E1237** Wheelchair, pediatric size, rigid, adjustable, without seating system
MED: 100-3, 280.1

[Y] **E1238** Wheelchair, pediatric size, folding, adjustable, without seating system
MED: 100-3, 280.1

● **E1239** Power wheelchair, pediatric size, not otherwise specified

WHEELCHAIR — LIGHTWEIGHT

[A] **E1240** Lightweight wheelchair; detachable arms, desk or full-length, swing-away, detachable, elevating legrest
MED: 100-3, 280.1

[A] **E1250** Lightweight wheelchair; fixed full-length arms, swing-away, detachable footrests
MED: 100-3, 280.1
See code(s): K0003

[A] **E1260** Lightweight wheelchair; detachable arms, desk or full-length, swing-away, detachable, footrests
MED: 100-3, 280.1
See code(s): K0003

[A] **E1270** Lightweight wheelchair; fixed full-length arms, swing-away, detachable elevating legrests
MED: 100-3, 280.1

WHEELCHAIR — HEAVY-DUTY

[A] **E1280** Heavy-duty wheelchair; detachable arms, desk or full-length, elevating legrests
MED: 100-3, 280.1

[A] **E1285** Heavy-duty wheelchair; fixed full-length arms, swing-away, detachable footrests
MED: 100-3, 280.1
See code(s): K0006

[A] **E1290** Heavy-duty wheelchair; detachable arms, desk or full-length, swing-away, detachable footrests
MED: 100-3, 280.1
See code(s): K0006

[A] **E1295** Heavy-duty wheelchair; fixed full-length arms, elevating legrests
MED: 100-3, 280.1

[Y] **E1296** Special wheelchair seat height from floor
MED: 100-3, 280.3

[Y] **E1297** Special wheelchair seat depth, by upholstery
MED: 100-3, 280.3

[Y] **E1298** Special wheelchair seat depth and/or width, by construction
MED: 100-3, 280.3

WHIRLPOOL — EQUIPMENT

[E] **E1300** Whirlpool, portable (overtub type)
MED: 100-3, 280.1

[Y] **E1310** Whirlpool, nonportable (built-in type)
MED: 100-3, 280.1

REPAIRS AND REPLACEMENT SUPPLIES

[Y] [☑] **E1340** Repair or nonroutine service for durable medical equipment requiring the skill of a technician, labor component, per 15 minutes
Medicare jurisdiction: local carrier if repair of implanted DME.
MED: 100-2, 15, 110.2

ADDITIONAL OXYGEN RELATED EQUIPMENT

[Y] **E1353** Regulator
MED: 100-3, 240.2

[Y] **E1355** Stand/rack
MED: 100-3, 240.2

[Y] **E1372** Immersion external heater for nebulizer
MED: 100-3, 240.2

[Y] **E1390** Oxygen concentrator, single delivery port, capable of delivering 85 percent or greater oxygen concentration at the prescribed flow rate
MED: 100-3, 240.2

[Y] [☑] **E1391** Oxygen concentrator, dual delivery port, capable of delivering 85 percent or greater oxygen concentration at the prescribed flow rate, each
MED: 100-3, 240.2

[N] **E1399** Durable medical equipment, miscellaneous
Determine if an alternative HCPCS Level II or a CPT code better describes the service being reported. This code should be used only if a more specific code is unavailable. Medicare jurisdiction: local carrier if repair or implanted DME.

[Y] **E1405** Oxygen and water vapor enriching system with heated delivery
MED: 100-3, 240.2; 100-4, 20, 20; 100-4, 20, 20.4

[Y] **E1406** Oxygen and water vapor enriching system without heated delivery
MED: 100-3, 240.2; 100-4, 20, 20; 100-4, 20, 20.4

ARTIFICIAL KIDNEY MACHINES AND ACCESSORIES

For glucose monitors, see A4253–A4256. For supplies for ESRD, see procedure codes A4651–A4929.

[A] **E1500** Centrifuge, for dialysis

[A] **E1510** Kidney, dialysate delivery system kidney machine, pump recirculating, air removal system, flowrate meter, power off, heater and temp control with alarm, IV poles, pressure gauge, concentrate container

[A] **E1520** Heparin infusion pump for hemodialysis

▨ Special Coverage Instructions	Noncovered by Medicare	Carrier Discretion	☑ Quantity Alert	● New Code	○ Reinstated Code	▲ Revised Code

FIGURE 17-5   HCPCS Level II sections. Printed with permission from Ingenix, Inc. Copyright © 2004.

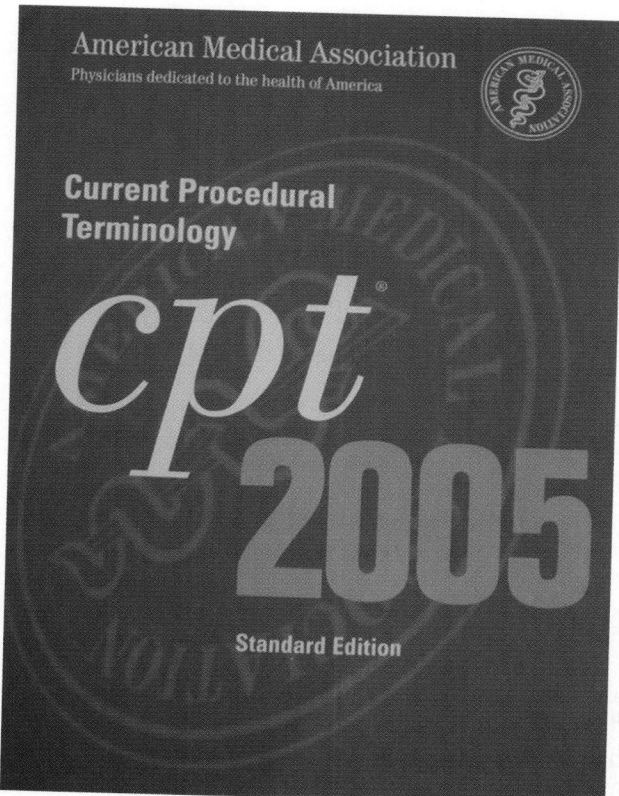

FIGURE 17-6 CPT coding book.

and updated on a yearly basis. Coding from the most current edition of the CPT manual is essential (Figure 17-6). The CPT manual is available for purchase from the AMA.

The CPT manual is organized numerically or alphanumerically in sections according to classified types of service (Table 17-1). The most commonly used codes for Evaluation and Management (E/M) services (office visits, consultations, the physician's component for emergency services and inpatient hospital care, etc.) are located in the front of the book. Codes for anesthesia, surgery, radiology, pathology and laboratory, and miscellaneous medical services

follow. Several appendices follow, including a complete list of all modifiers used in CPT with descriptions, as well as a quick reference summary of codes that have been added, deleted, or revised. Patient Education discusses the need for the medical assistant to understand the codes to inform patients of the codes' meanings.

Understanding Evaluation and Management

For a beginning coder, the most complex section of the CPT coding system is the Evaluation and Management Services. E/M, as it is referred to, is based on the following criteria: history of the patient, complexity of the examination, and the degree of difficulty in medical decision-making. Of these three factors, the medical decision-making factor can be the most complex.

Levels of Evaluation and Management

The four levels of decision-making are: straightforward, low complex, moderate complex, and high complex. The E/M codes are service oriented and were designed to link the procedure or diagnosis with the amount of time it takes the physician to diagnosis and treat the patient. For coding purposes, all patients are either an established patient or a new patient. It is important to understand the difference between a new and established patient, a consultation and a referral, and to be sure the proper place of service (office, hospital, skilled nursing facility, emergency department) is coded. Take a few moments to look through the CPT manual to become familiar with its structure and how codes are presented. Commonly accepted descriptions of services or procedures are presented after the code number. There are two types of codes listed. One type stands alone; the other is indented. Only the codes that stand alone have full descriptions. Indented codes include only that portion of the stand-alone code before the semicolon. This is an extremely important concept to remember.

Patient Education

Procedure and diagnosis coding is required for billing purposes and physician orders of extended services. The diagnosis code reflects detailed information about the illness or injury converted to numeric form. The procedure code reflects detailed information about the service provided utilizing levels of care. Patients may have questions concerning "all those numbers" and their meaning. The medical assistant can explain the codes used and that they are used for billing purposes.

Procedures and services are listed by name of service or procedure, anatomic site, condition or disease, synonym, eponym, or abbreviation. In order to code services correctly, locate the desired procedure in the index at the back of the CPT manual. Often a single code is given, although ranges of possible codes (joined with a hyphen) are presented and should be utilized, if necessary.

Modifiers

There are times when it is necessary to report a service not contained in the CPT manual. These procedures may be reported using the "unlisted procedure" code for that particular section, or by use of a modifier—a two-digit code preceded by a hyphen that clarifies the procedure. This is used in circumstances when the procedure code does not accurately describe the procedure. The two-digit modifier provides additional information about services provided to a patient. For example, the most common modifier is "50," which indicates the procedure was bilateral and done at the same time, such as bilateral myringtomies and tube insertion. The two-digit code for this procedure would be listed followed by a hyphen and the number 50. When using multiple modifiers always list the modifier -99 first. This indicates to the person checking the claim that multiple modifiers are being used (Figure 17-7).

Medical Coding

The medicine section of the CPT manual is organized according to body system, not disease. This section of the manual also includes codes for noninvasive procedures and treatment procedures. Included in this section are many diagnostic tests, such as an EKG, and many procedures (noninvasive) performed in a physician's office. If the procedure is invasive, meaning that it enters the skin (other than by injection) or a body cavity, it is found in the surgical section of the manual. Procedure 17-2 reviews examples for assigning CPT codes.

Symbols

Symbols are used in the CPT manual to distinguish changes or give instructions to be used when coding. These symbols add additional information or instructions for proper coding of certain procedures. It is imperative that the coder be familiar with the symbols and their meaning in order to accurately code procedures.

Insurance Fraud

Unfortunately, insurance fraud occurs on a regular basis. The Centers for Medicare and Medicaid Services Web site (http://www.cms.hhs.gov/providers/fraud/) has information to help you better understand insurance fraud. Even though this information comes strictly from the Centers for Medicare and Medicaid Services Web site, it can also apply to other insurance carriers.

Medicare Definition of Fraud

As a medical assistant, it is important to understand insurance fraud. Insurance fraud is often committed within the Medicare system. "Fraud" is an intentional representation that an individual knows to be false or does not believe to be true and makes, knowing that the representation could result in some unauthorized benefit to him or herself or some other person.

The most frequent kind of fraud arises from false statements or misrepresentations that claim to provide proof to entitlement or payment under the Medicare program. The violator may be a physician or other practitioner, a hospital or other institutional provider, a clinical laboratory or other supplier, an employee of any provider, a billing service, a beneficiary, a Medicare carrier employee, or any person in a position to file a claim for Medicare benefits. Under the broad definition of fraud are other violations, including the offering or acceptance of kickbacks and the routine waiver of co-payments.

Fraud schemes range from those perpetrated by individuals acting alone to broad-based activities by institutions or groups of individuals, sometimes employing sophisticated telemarketing and other promotional techniques to lure consumers into serving

TABLE 17-1	CPT Manual: Examples of Sections and Codes

CPT Section	Code
Evaluation and Management	99200–99499
Anesthesia	00100–01999
Surgery	10000–69999
Radiology	70000–79999
Pathology and Laboratory	80000–89999
Medical Services	90700–99999

Symbols

▲ Revised Code
● New Code
▶◀ New or Revised Text
⊃ Reference to *CPT Assistant, CPT Changes Book*
✛ Add-on Code
⊘ Exemptions to Modifier 51
⊙ Conscious Sedation

Modifiers (See Appendix A for Definitions)

21 Prolonged Evaluation and Management Services
22 Unusual Procedural Services
23 Unusual Anesthesia
24 Unrelated Evaluation and Management Service by the Same Physician During a Postoperative Period
25 Significant, Separately Identifiable Evaluation and Management Service by the Same Physician on the Same Day of the Procedure or Other Service
26 Professional Component
32 Mandated Services
47 Anesthesia by Surgeon
50 Bilateral Procedure
51 Multiple Procedures
52 Reduced Services
53 Discontinued Procedure
54 Surgical Care Only
55 Postoperative Management Only
56 Preoperative Management Only
57 Decision for Surgery
58 Staged or Related Procedure or Service by the Same Physician During the Postoperative Period
59 Distinct Procedural Service
62 Two Surgeons
63 Procedure Performed on Infants
66 Surgical Team
76 Repeat Procedure by Same Physician
77 Repeat Procedure by Another Physician
78 Return to the Operating Room for a Related Procedure During the Postoperative Period
79 Unrelated Procedure or Service by the Same Physician During the Postoperative Period
80 Assistant Surgeon
81 Minimum Assistant Surgeon
82 Assistant Surgeon (when qualified resident surgeon not available)
90 Reference (Outside) Laboratory
91 Repeat Clinical Diagnostic Laboratory Test
99 Multiple Modifiers

Physical Status Modifiers

P1-A normal healthy patient
P2-A patient with mild systemic disease
P3-A patient with severe systemic disease
P4-A patient with severe systemic disease that is a constant threat to life
P5-A moribund patient who is not expected to survive without the operation
P6-A declared brain-dead patient whose organs are being removed for donor purposes

Modifiers Approved for Hospital Outpatient Use Level I (CPT)

25 Significant, Separately Identifiable Evaluation and Management Service by the Same Physician on the Same Day of the Procedure or Other Service
27 Multiple Outpatient Hospital E/M Encounters on the Same Date
50 Bilateral Procedure
52 Reduced Services
58 Staged or Related Procedure or Service by the Same Physician During the Postoperative Period
59 Distinct Procedural Service
73 Discontinued Out-Patient Procedure Prior to Anesthesia Administration
74 Discontinued Out-Patient Procedure After Anesthesia Administration
76 Repeat Procedure by Same Physician
77 Repeat Procedure by Another Physician
78 Return to the Operating Room for a Related Procedure During the Postoperative Period
79 Unrelated Procedure or Service by the Same Physician During the Postoperative Period
91 Repeat Clinical Diagnostic Laboratory Test

Level II (HCPCS/National)

LT Left side (used to identify procedures performed on the left side of the body)
RT Right side (used to identify procedures performed on the right side of the body)
E1 Upper left, eyelid
E2 Lower left, eyelid
E3 Upper right, eyelid
E4 Lower right, eyelid
FA Left hand, thumb
F1 Left hand, second digit
F2 Left hand, third digit
F3 Left hand, fourth digit
F4 Left hand, fifth digit
F5 Right hand, thumb
F6 Right hand, second digit
F7 Right hand, third digit
F8 Right hand, fourth digit
F9 Right hand, fifth digit
LC Left circumflex, coronary artery (Hospitals use with codes 92980-92984, 92995, 92996)
LD Left anterior descending coronary artery (Hospitals use with codes 92980-92984, 92995, 92996)
RC Right coronary artery (Hospitals use with codes 92980-92984, 92995, 92996)
QM Ambulance service provided under arrangement by a provider of services
QN Ambulance service furnished directly by a provider of services
TA Left foot, great toe
T1 Left foot, second digit
T2 Left foot, third digit
T3 Left foot, fourth digit
T4 Left foot, fifth digit
T5 Right foot, great toe
T6 Right foot, second digit
T7 Right foot, third digit
T8 Right foot, fourth digit
T9 Right foot, fifth digit

FIGURE 17-7 Modifier page from the CPT. Printed with permission by the American Medical Association. Copyright © 2004.

Assigning a CPT Code

OBJECTIVE: Accurately assign a CPT code.

Equipment and Supplies

patient's medical record; computer; medical billing software; current CPT coding book; superbill with procedure marked

Method

1. Locate the completed procedure on the superbill.
2. If the only procedure done was a physician visit, locate CPT codes 99200–99499 in the front of the CPT coding book.
3. Determine by the patient's medical record whether this office visit was a first time visit or a follow-up visit.
4. Also determine by the patient's medical record whether this visit was done by the patient's attending physician, or whether it was done by a consulting physician.
5. Note where the visit took place (nursing home, hospital, emergency room, office, etc.).
6. After locating the place of service set of codes in the CPT book, locate the level of the visit within the place of service set of codes. It may be necessary to study the patient's personal, family, and social history, the physical examination, and determine which and how many tests were done in order to determine the correct level of service. This is one of the most important codes you can list because improper level of service billing can result in nonpayment of the bill, and can also result in very large monetary fines.
7. If there was a surgical procedure, these will be in the code section between 10000 and 69999 of the CPT book. For these codes, locate the surgical procedure and read the operative report. For some situations, the anesthetic for the surgery is included in the surgery code. In other cases, the anesthesia must be billed as a separate code. In addition, some surgical procedure groups are billed under one code, while others are billed as separate procedures. It will usually be necessary to read the operative report to determine which situation applies.
8. Some equipment used in surgery is billable under the 10000 to 69999 codes, while other equipment is billed separately.
9. Any radiological procedure is billed under the codes 70000 to 79999, including x-rays, diagnostic ultrasound, angiography, and computerized tomography.
10. Locate the procedure done in the section 70000 to 79999.
11. In the appropriate section, locate the part of the body to which the procedure was done.
12. Last, locate the correct procedure, being careful to note if the test was bilateral, unilateral, or if there were two different views done.
13. If a laboratory test was run, or if a specimen was sent to the laboratory for pathology inspection, the code will be under 80000 to 89999.
14. If the test was a laboratory test, it will be in the first part of this section. It is necessary to know what test was done, and whether the test is a "panel," which contains many tests within one ordered block, or if the test is organ-specific or disease-specific.
15. In addition, if the test was actually done by an outside laboratory, then the test itself cannot be billed. However, the cost of the venipuncture to obtain the specimen and the cost of transporting the specimen to the laboratory, if it was transported by the physician's staff, may be billed.
16. In some cases, some medicines can be billed to insurance. Some general rules apply to most billable medicines.
17. Usually billed medicines must be injected, not administered orally.
18. Many specialized procedures, such as ophthalmology services and pulmonary tests and services, can be billed under the CPT codes.
19. Always compare the final CPT codes with the ICD codes before finalizing the bill. There must be a logical "match." For example, if the patient was seen in the physician's office for removal of a foreign body in the ear, the visit can be billed, but the blood sugar done at the same time cannot be billed under a diagnosis of foreign body in the ear.

as the unwitting tools in the schemes. Seldom do perpetrators target only one insurer or either the public or private sector exclusively. Rather, most are defrauding several private and public sector victims, such as Medicare, simultaneously. According to a 1993 survey by the Health Insurance Association of America for private insurers' health care fraud investigations, overall health care fraud activity broke down as follows:

- 43%—Fraudulent diagnosis
- 34%—Billing for services not rendered
- 21%—Waiver of patient deductibles and co-payments
- 2%—Other

In Medicare, the most common forms of fraud include:

- Billing insurance companies for services not furnished
- Misrepresenting the diagnosis to justify payment
- Soliciting, offering, or receiving a kickback
- Billing for separate services that are usually bundled in a single procedure code
- Falsifying certificates of medical necessity, plans of treatment, and medical records to justify payment
- Billing for a service not furnished as billed; i.e., "upcoding"

Fraud Tips

The Centers for Medicare and Medicaid Services Web site also offers consumers and patients information to help them identify fraud. The medical assistant can also watch for the following items, whether the provider is telling the patient, or you are asked to relay this information to the patient:

- The test is free; he only needs your Medicare number for his records.
- Medicare wants you to have the item or service.
- They know how to get Medicare to pay for it.
- The more tests they provide, the cheaper they are.
- The equipment or service is free; it won't cost you anything.

Consumers should also be suspicious of medical offices or employers who do the following:

- Routinely waive co-payments without checking on ability to pay
- Advertise "free" consultations to Medicare beneficiaries

Professionalism

The medical record must reflect all services and care for which the insurance company is billed. If a provider is found to have billed for services not received, or if a provider is found to have billed for a more complicated or expensive service than was actually received, the penalty will be denial of the claim, or worse, monetary sanctions and even prison. If the medical assistant believes that such a bill is being submitted, he or she should discuss the situation with the physician in order to be assured that the care being delivered is, in fact, the service being billed.

- Claim they represent Medicare
- Use pressure or scare tactics to sell high priced medical services or diagnostic tests
- Bill Medicare for services the patient does not recall receiving
- Use telemarketing and door-to-door selling as marketing tools

Professionalism discusses the importance of reflecting correct billing practices in the medical record. Box 17-1 lists information on how to report suspected fraud.

Compliance Plan

Each medical office should have a compliance plan. A medical office without a compliance plan may be at risk for liability issues. It also demonstrates to the physician, fraud investigators, or insurance carriers that the medical office is attempting to locate and correct errors. Having a compliance plan gives the staff members of the medical office a process of locating, correcting, and preventing practices that are illegal. Health and Human Services Office of Inspector General provides compliance guidance for fraud prevention and detection. The following are basic components for an effective compliance plan:

- Conducting periodic audits of billing and coding practices
- Developing written standards and procedures for compliance
- Training and educating staff members on procedures

BOX 17-1
How to Report Suspected Fraud

Before you get in touch with your state Medicaid agency, contact or call the National Fraud Hotline and be ready to provide as much information as possible, including:

- The name of the Medicaid client
- The client's Medicaid card number
- The name of the doctor, hospital, or other health care provider
- The date of service
- The amount of money that Medicaid approved and may have paid
- A description of the acts that you suspect involve fraud or abuse

Who to Contact

Contact Your State Agency Directly—Medicaid is a joint Federal and State-funded program. Although the Federal Government requires that certain persons be eligible for Medicaid benefits and sets standards for quality of care, the States carry out most of the day-to-day business of Medicaid. If you suspect that fraud is being committed against Medicaid, first get in touch with the Program Integrity contact at your State Medicaid Agency. A list of *State Medicaid Contacts* has the names of the Program Integrity contact that you should use to report suspected fraud, whether it involves a person, a company, or an agency.

Call the OIG National Fraud Hotline—A second way to report suspected fraud in Medicaid is to call the Office of Inspector General's (OIG) *National Fraud Hotline* **1-800-HHS-TIPS (1-800-447-8477)**. This hotline handles calls about both Medicaid and Medicare, but it is not as direct as calling your state contact.

- Investigating violations and disclosing incidents to appropriate government agencies
- Discussing in staff meetings how to avoid erroneous or fraudulent conduct

As a medical assistant, it is important to research and understand practice standards so that the medical office is in compliance with various regulations.

Legal and Ethical Issues

Federal regulations on coding are specific and require full compliance. Coding of procedures and diagnoses must be supported by the documentation in the patient record. Providers as well as medical staff may be sanctioned with fines or prison terms if improper coding is discovered to increase reimbursement.

Coding Compliance

Reasonability of accurate documentation, completion of health insurance claim forms, and regulation compliance falls ultimately on the physician. It is the medical assistant's responsibility to make certain these responsibilities are followed (Legal and Ethical Issues).

Code Linkage

When the medical assistant is completing the health insurance claim form, it is critical for the diagnosis to be related to the procedure. An example of code linkage would be a diagnosis of diabetes mellitus and a glucose tolerance test. However, a diagnosis of hypertension and a procedure to remove five skin tags cannot be linked in a health insurance claim form because there is no connection between the patient's diagnosis and the procedure the physician performed. Coding inaccuracies such as this can result in minor to severe penalties.

SUMMARY

Most patients coming into the medical office have some form of health care insurance. The medical assistant should have a general overview of the coding process, using the procedure coding process (CPT codes) and diagnostic coding (ICD-9-CM) in order to be able to assist the medical coder if necessary.

Chapter Review

COMPETENCY REVIEW

1. Define and spell the terms to learn for this chapter.
2. Describe what steps you would take to determine if a patient has insurance coverage.
3. What code book is used to code a diagnosis?
4. What code book is used to code an office visit and procedure?
5. Explain the difference between a primary and secondary diagnosis, using the example of stroke and hypertension.

PREPARING FOR THE CERTIFICATION EXAM

1. Which describes transforming verbal descriptions into numerical designations?
   A. grouping
   B. coding
   C. classifying
   D. modifying
   E. rider

2. In ICD-9-CM coding conventions, E codes
   A. stand alone
   B. are required for all diagnoses
   C. give external causes or factors for illness or injury
   D. should never be used with V codes
   E. are the same as CPT codes

3. CPT stands for
   A. current physician's terminology
   B. current procedure terminology
   C. current procedural terminology
   D. current procedural term
   E. current procedural timetable

4. In CPT coding conventions, modifiers are used to
   A. explain unusual circumstances
   B. list a patient's treatment options
   C. frustrate a medical assistant
   D. communicate with the insurance company via electronic billing
   E. make the coding statement grammatically correct

5. The CMS-1500 claim form
   A. is accepted by most insurance companies in the United States
   B. must be filled out by the patient
   C. must be filled out by the provider
   D. is accepted as a standard submission (claim) form by most carriers
   E. is never used

continued on next page

6. In CPT coding conventions,
   A. both inpatient and outpatient visits use the same code
   B. inpatient visit codes are different from outpatient visit codes
   C. a complicated system is used to determine whether services were rendered on an inpatient or outpatient basis
   D. a call to the insurance company is required to determine which code to use
   E. all codes are the same as ICD-9-CM

7. ICD-9-CM codes
   A. may require a fifth digit for detail
   B. never require a fifth digit for detail
   C. always require a V code to support the diagnosis
   D. may be coded directly from Volume II
   E. should always be initialed by the physician

8. Which of the following is NOT true of diagnoses coding?
   A. the medical assistant needs to understand the ICD-9-CM
   B. diagnosis are given in three, four, or five digits
   C. always code to the highest level of specificity
   D. to code properly, start with Volume II
   E. Volume II is the numeric index

9. Which of the following is NOT true of CPT coding?
   A. the CPT coding book is updated yearly
   B. the CPT coding book is organized numerically
   C. CPT codes can be obtained from outdated CPT coding books
   D. the CPT coding book is organized alphanumerically
   E. E/M codes are located in the front of the CPT coding book

10. Electronic claim submission
   A. is difficult and costly
   B. is mandated by HIPAA for most medical providers
   C. is only done on rare occasions in most medical practices
   D. increases the time it takes for an insurance carrier to pay a claim
   E. does not require diagnosis codes

CRITICAL THINKING

1. What would the CPT code be for an audiogram?
2. How can a medical assistant made sure a diagnosis code is correct on the CMS-1500 before submitting it to the insurance carrier?
3. What is the diagnosis code for chronic otitis media?

ON THE JOB

Lisa Medina, certified medical coding specialist, processes insurance claims for a large internal medicine practice. You have recently been hired as Lisa's assistant and she has asked you to verify the accuracy of a group of claim forms. As you review the forms, you notice that one of the doctors regularly checks the superbill used in the office at one evaluation/management code level higher than the actual level of service provided.

1. Name some of the options that are possible for handling this situation.
2. Tell which option you would select.
3. Give three reasons for your selection of this particular option.
4. Whose advice might you seek before acting on your choice?

INTERNET ACTIVITY

There are many places to purchase ICD-9-CM and CPT coding books. Search the Internet to find the cost of the ICD-9-CM and CPT coding books and coding software. What month are the new editions of the ICD-9-CM and CPT coding books available?

MediaLink  More on medical coding, including interactive resources, can be found on the Student CD-ROM accompanying this textbook.

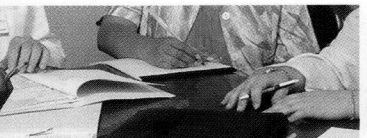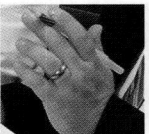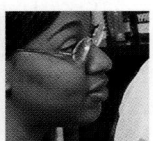

Medical Assistant Role Delineation Chart

HIGHLIGHT indicates material covered in this chapter.

ADMINISTRATIVE

Administrative Procedures

- Perform basic administrative medical assisting functions
- Schedule, coordinate and monitor appointments
- Schedule inpatient/outpatient admissions and procedures
- Understand and apply third-party guidelines
- Obtain reimbursement through accurate claims submission
- Monitor third-party reimbursement
- Understand and adhere to managed care policies and procedures
- *Negotiate managed care contracts*

Practice Finances

- Perform procedural and diagnostic coding
- Apply bookkeeping principles

- Manage accounts receivable
- *Manage accounts payable*
- *Process payroll*
- *Document and maintain accounting and banking records*
- *Develop and maintain fee schedules*
- *Manage renewals of business and professional insurance policies*
- *Manage personnel benefits and maintain records*
- *Perform marketing, financial, and strategic planning*

CLINICAL

Fundamental Principles

- Apply principles of aseptic technique and infection control
- Comply with quality assurance practices
- Screen and follow up patient test results

Diagnostic Orders

- Collect and process specimens
- Perform diagnostic tests

Patient Care

- Adhere to established patient screening procedures
- Obtain patient history and vital signs
- Prepare and maintain examination and treatment areas
- Prepare patient for examinations, procedures and treatments

- Assist with examinations, procedures and treatments
- Prepare and administer medications and immunizations
- Maintain medication and immunization records
- Recognize and respond to emergencies
- Coordinate patient care information with other health care providers
- Initiate IV and administer IV medications with appropriate training and as permitted by state law

GENERAL

Professionalism

- Display a professional manner and image
- Demonstrate initiative and responsibility
- Work as a member of the health care team
- Prioritize and perform multiple tasks
- Adapt to change
- Promote the CMA credential
- Enhance skills through continuing education
- Treat all patients with compassion and empathy
- Promote the practice through positive public relations

Communication Skills

- Recognize and respect cultural diversity
- Adapt communications to individual's ability to understand
- Use professional telephone technique

- Recognize and respond effectively to verbal, nonverbal, and written communications
- Use medical terminology appropriately
- Utilize electronic technology to receive, organize, prioritize and transmit information
- Serve as liaison

Legal Concepts

- Perform within legal and ethical boundaries
- Prepare and maintain medical records
- Document accurately
- Follow employer's established policies dealing with the health care contract
- Implement and maintain federal and state health care legislation and regulations
- Comply with established risk management and safety procedures
- Recognize professional credentialing criteria
- *Develop and maintain personnel, policy and procedure manuals*

Instruction

- Instruct individuals according to their needs
- Explain office policies and procedures
- Teach methods of health promotion and disease prevention
- Locate community resources and disseminate information
- *Develop educational materials*
- *Conduct continuing education activities*

Operational Functions

- Perform inventory of supplies and equipment
- Perform routine maintenance of administrative and clinical equipment
- Apply computer techniques to support office operations
- *Perform personnel management functions*
- *Negotiate leases and prices for equipment and supply contracts*

■ *Denotes advanced skills.*

SOURCE: Reprinted by permission of the American Association of Medical Assistants from the AAMA Role Delineation Study: Occupational Analysis of the Medical Assisting Profession.

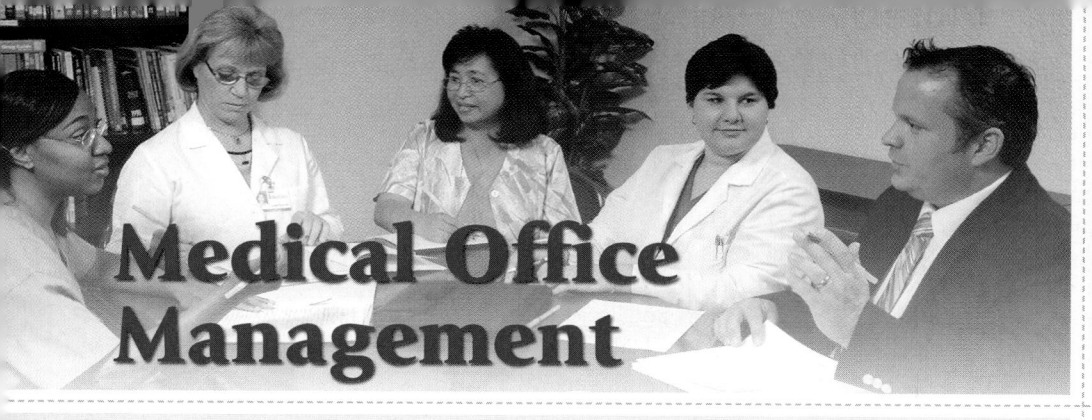

chapter 18

Medical Office Management

Learning Objectives

After reading this chapter, you should be able to:

- Define and spell the terms to learn for this chapter.
- Define the systems approach to management.
- List and discuss the personnel management duties as they relate to the medical office.
- Discuss the elements of monthly planning including holding staff meetings.
- Describe time management principles and how a TO DO list would enhance office organization.

- Differentiate between the employee policy manual and the office procedures manual.
- Describe ten responsibilities in assisting the physician to set up a medical meeting.
- Discuss how to perform basic library research to assist the physician in a medical paper development.
- List five items that belong in a patient information booklet.

Terms to Learn

colleague	grievance	seniority
discriminatory	probationary	solvent

Case Study

MARSHA BROWN IS AN OFFICE MANAGER at the Main Street Clinic. The clinic's business has been growing steadily, and the office is in need of a new medical assistant. Marsha decided to put an advertisement in the local newspaper and received many resumes in response to the ad. She took a couple of days to sort through the resumes, removing all that did not have appropriate backgrounds for the position. On Monday, she called several individuals who had the best resumes and set up interviews for the week.

Her first interview went very well, but it was difficult to read the application form that was completed. The second applicant was wearing a tongue ring during the interview, and at times, it was very difficult to understand her speech. The third applicant had the least experience, but looked very professional, wrote neatly, and spoke well. The next week, Marsha called the third applicant and offered her the position.

OUTLINE

Systems Approach to Office Management	318
The Office Manager	319
Leadership Styles	322
Creating a Team Atmosphere	323
Hiring Procedures: Selecting the Right Staff Members	324
Orientation and Training	326
Using Performance Evaluation Effectively	328
Time Management	330
Personnel Policy Manual	331
Office Procedures Manual	332
Medical Meetings and Speaking Engagements	332
Patient Information Booklet	333
Medical Practice Marketing and Customer Service	333

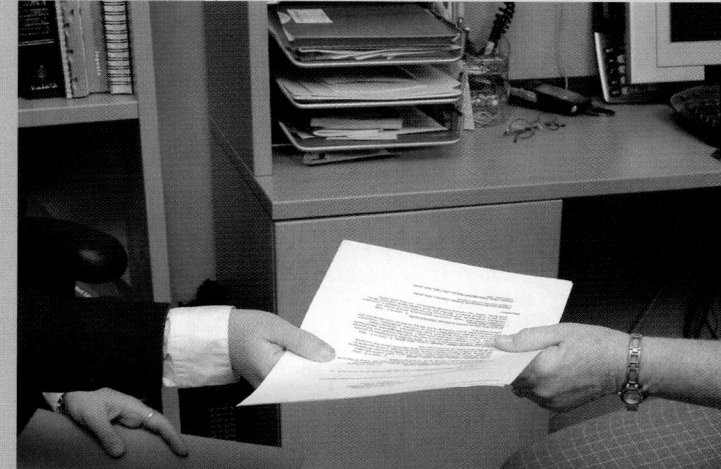

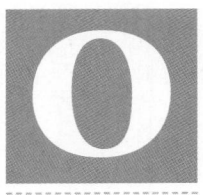Office management requires special administrative and people skills. Office management cannot be discussed without discussing time management. Careful planning of activities, delegation of tasks, and effective use of all personnel involve careful attention to how time is managed. Several documents are important for a smooth running medical office. These include the personnel policy manual, a procedures manual, and patient information booklets.

Systems Approach to Office Management

Current management philosophy recommends a systematic approach when managing a medical office. Under this approach, the functions of an office are categorized into systems that must function simultaneously and be integrated into a whole system, the medical office. For example, the administrative component of a medical office can be divided into the following systems:

- Personnel management
- Financial management (including banking, billing, collections, and insurance)
- Scheduling
- Facility and equipment management (including computers)
- Communications (written and oral including patient education)
- Legal concepts

The clinical component of managing an office can be considered a system by itself. Brief descriptions of the various systems that form the medical practice follow.

Personnel Management Responsibilities

Personnel management duties include recruitment and selection, probation, performance and salary review, discipline, and maintenance of employee records.

The recruitment and selection process is used when a medical practice needs to replace a staff member who has left or when more staff is needed for an expanding practice. All new employees are entitled to an orientation to their new position and duties. Large offices and clinics often have formal orientation training sessions that employees attend before beginning their day-to-day assignments.

Personnel management usually requires an annual salary review of each employee at which time, if the employee's performance has been acceptable, a merit raise in salary is granted. However, there will be times when it is necessary to discipline an employee during these reviews. These topics will be discussed in greater detail further in the chapter.

Employee Records

There are records that are required by law to be maintained for every employee. These include the following payroll records.

- Social Security number of the employee
- Number of exemptions claimed by the employee (W-4 form)
- Gross salary amount (salary before taxes are removed)
- Deductions for Social Security taxes, federal, state, and city withholding taxes, state disability tax, and state unemployment tax, if applicable.

Payroll is discussed further in Chapter 14.

Financial Management

Financial management includes banking, billing, collections, and insurance collections. This critical area is responsible for generating the income necessary to keep the practice solvent or capable of paying its bills and salaries. Fees, billings, collections, and credit are discussed in Chapter 13. Financial management, including employee record keeping, is discussed in Chapter 14.

Scheduling

The scheduling process involves using a systematic method for patient appointments. This is discussed in Chapter 8. Scheduling also includes managing staff work hours and vacation periods.

Facility and Equipment Management

Facility and equipment management includes facility layout and planning, inventory, maintaining safety and OSHA standards, and equipment replacement. This is discussed in Chapter 5. Computer use in the medical office is presented in Chapter 11.

Clinical Office Management

Apart from the administrative aspects of medical office management, there is also the clinical aspect. Managing the clinical aspect of a medical office requires a wide variety of duties, including the training of any new clinical personnel, keeping track of medical supplies and purchasing supplies when the stock is low, and making sure that the physician's requests are met and that proper procedures are followed. It is often within the clinical office duties that the office manager will have to handle safety issues and OSHA regulations. Because of the many duties required in managing the clinical aspect of the office, it is not uncommon to find that an office has a separate supervisor who will take on those duties to reduce the workload of the general office manager.

Communication

Written communication skills are presented in Chapter 4, oral communication, including verbal and nonverbal, in Chapter 10, and patient education in Chapter 50.

Legal Concepts

Physicians have their own personal attorney to assist with handling legal documents and issues. However, medical assistants must have an understanding of legal terminology. Legal and ethical issues are discussed fully in Chapter 3.

The Office Manager

The office manager acts as a coordinator for the business activities conducted in the office. Each office varies somewhat; however, the general duties include:

- Acting as liaison between staff and physician/ employer.
- Conducting performance and salary reviews.
- Delegating responsibilities to staff.
- Developing and training staff.
- Improving office efficiency.
- Maintaining office procedure manual.
- Planning and conducting staff meetings.
- Preparing patient education materials.
- Providing guidelines for patient education.
- Recruiting, hiring, and firing.
- Supervising cash, banking, and payroll operations.
- Supervising employees on a day-to-day basis.

- Supervising the purchase and storage of equipment and supplies.
- Training new personnel.

Along with knowledge of the clinical skills needed to run an efficient medical office, an office manager needs effective administrative and people skills. Medical assistants who have demonstrated these skills may seek to be promoted into this position. Other qualities or skills observed in good managers are:

- Ability to enforce policy, when necessary
- Ability to organize
- Ability to resolve conflicts
- Creativity
- Diplomacy
- Excellent judgment
- Flexibility
- Leadership/take charge initiative
- Objectivity
- Sense of fairness
- Willingness to continue to learn

The office manager's time is generally spent on administrative and employee issues. The employees, on the other hand, spend most of their time working with patients. A good office manager does not strive to become "the boss" but, rather, to establish and implement a team approach to management by including all staff in the decision-making process. Ultimately, the manager must make the final decision in conjunction with the physician/employer, but compliance with decisions is much greater when employees have had the opportunity to participate. Table 18-1 describes responsibilities

TABLE 18-1 Manager's Responsibilities to Employee and Physician/Employer

Employee	Physician/Employer
Interview	Increase efficiency of office.
Hire/terminate	Meet with physician to discuss problems/plans.
Orientate/train	Manage calendar for physician.
Arrange work schedules	Assist with meetings.
Arrange vacation coverage	Update physician on insurance changes related to Medicare fee schedules.
Conduct performance evaluations	Order CPT and ICD code books and current pharmacology books annually.
Consult with physician regarding salary increases	Renew insurance policies and pay premiums.

Professionalism

> **The office manager has an important** position in the office and should always set the standard of professionalism. He or she is usually the role model for the office staff. Office managers must dress appropriately and take firm charge of the medical office, while always treating their staff, patients, and physician and employer with the utmost courtesy and respect.

the office manager has to the employees and to the physician. Professionalism discusses more on being an office manager.

Many office managers are promoted based on seniority—a status gained by being the individual who has worked for the physician the longest. This is not always a wise practice since not everyone is a skilled manager. When no internal candidate is available with the necessary skills or interest for the office manager position, then the physician/employer will have to seek an outside candidate. This is usually handled by placing an advertisement in the medical help wanted sections of the local newspaper. In some cases, the physicians' colleagues (fellow members of the profession) will recommend a qualified candidate for the position.

Monthly Planning

The office manager may wish to develop a system in which the entire month is laid out on a calendar. All physicians' conferences, staff meetings, vacations, accountant meetings, and other vendor visits should be noted. One of the office manager's tasks will be to approve and decline vacation requests from staff members. It is important to list staff vacations on a

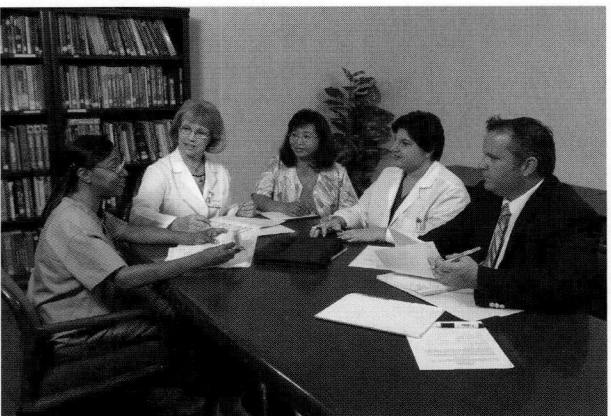

FIGURE 18-1 Regular staff meetings will help the efficiency of the medical office staff.

calendar because it helps to prevent overlapping of vacations, which can leave an office short-staffed. This calendar should be placed in an accessible location. It may be helpful to purchase an erasable-style wall calendar so that corrections and changes can be made easily.

The manager will create and update the physician's own calendar. It is not necessary to include staff vacations on the physician's calendar. However, the office manager's own vacation schedule and days off should be included in the physician's calendar.

Many physicians carry a personal pocket or electronic calendar in which they enter all patient hospital visits and meetings. It is wise to compare the office calendar with the physician's calendar on a periodic basis so that the office's master calendar can be updated.

Staff Meetings

Lack of communication between the staff and management is a common complaint in a medical office. Staff members wish to have direct communication with the physician, but this is often not possible in a large practice. The office manager can help to resolve this problem by requesting the physician(s) to attend all or part of the regularly scheduled staff meetings, if this is not already being done. Many of the best ideas for office improvement are a result of suggestions made at staff meetings (Figure 18-1).

Staff meetings should be held on a regular basis. If it is necessary to hold weekly meetings because of the nature of the practice, then the physician(s) should be invited monthly to accommodate his or her busy schedule.

Meetings may need to be scheduled during a time period in which the staff's hours overlap, either due to shift changes or staggered hours. For instance, if the practice is open from 9:00 A.M. to 9:00 P.M. on Thursdays, the meetings could be scheduled for 4:30 P.M. or 5:00 P.M. when all staff would be present. Generally, staff members are compensated when they arrive before or remain after working hours to attend staff meetings.

The office manager usually conducts staff meetings and facilitates team interaction. The office manager determines the time and date for the meeting, and also prepares the agenda, frequently with input from the physician and other staff. The key to a good meeting is a concise agenda that identifies items for discussion, such as staff responsibilities, and limits the time allotted. Focusing staff meetings and discussions in this way limits the amount of time wasted. Generally, minutes are recorded for future reference and distributed for review prior to the next meeting. See Box 18-1 for an example of an office staff meeting agenda. Procedure 18-1 shows how to prepare and hold a staff meeting.

Motivating Employees

Motivating employees is vital to maintaining a positive working environment and an efficiently run medical office. Respect, ownership of personal space or environment, a sense of affiliation with the practice, fair compensation, acknowledgement, recognition, emotional rewards, honesty, visibility at the top, empathy, trust, safety, and equal treatment of all staff are a few items that employees expect from management.

Respect from their management is a basic need of all employees. As their manager, greet them with a pleasant manner and always acknowledge their hard work. Listen to them when they need to talk and take their suggestions into consideration. Satisfied employees are one of the best resources that the office manager has in running an efficient medical office.

In the medical office, it is often that many people share one space. If possible, provide some personal space for each employee. This would preferably be a desk, but it may just be a small table or a locker located somewhere in the office. Allow employees to place pictures in the area in which they work most often. This makes the employee feel settled, and in turn, tends to produce a greater level of productivity.

Creating a sense of affiliation to the medical office is often achieveable by making simple considerations. Sharing in the highlights of staff member's lives, such as throwing a small birthday celebration or recognizing a special event (marriage or birth of a child),

BOX 18-1
Staff Meeting Agenda

Windy City Clinic
Staff Meeting Agenda
Date: December 19, 20XX
Time: 4:30–5:30 P.M.
Place: Staff Conference Room

Time	Agenda	Person Responsible
4:30	Introduction of new staff	M. King/ Office Manager
	Review of last meeting's minutes	
4:35	Discussion of new policies	
4:45	Problems with insurance	L. Turner/Insurance Coding Clerk
4:55	OSHA protocol for needlesticks	K. Wall/Lab Tech
5:05	Vacation schedules	M. King
5:10	New office location	Dr. Williams
5:20	New business meeting adjourned	Mary King

18-1 PROCEDURE

Staff Meeting Procedures

OBJECTIVE: Explain and present the necessary steps to preparing and running a staff meeting.

Equipment and Supplies
agenda items received from staff; meeting agenda; means of keeping time (watch, clock, stopwatch, etc.); room for the meeting; any audio/visual equipment that may be needed

Method
1. One week before the meeting, request agenda items from the staff.
2. Before the meeting, create a meeting agenda with all topics that need to be discussed. On the agenda include the date, time, and place of the meeting. List who will be running (facilitating) the meeting. This is most often the office manager. Assign a length of time to each topic and who will be responsible for that topic.
3. On the day of the meeting, start the meeting on time.
4. Begin by briefly covering the last meeting.
5. Try to keep each topic to its allowed amount of time.
6. Allow for time at the end of the meeting to have open discussion of any new business.
7. Adjourn the meeting. Try to stay on schedule as much as possible.
8. After the meeting, the minutes of the meeting should be typed and distributed to all involved.

help employees feel part of the office community or "family." Bringing the staff together outside of the office with special events, such as a company picnic, can also increase the sense of affiliation.

Generally, employees will want to feel that they are being compensated sufficiently for the amount of work they produce. If an employee feels that he or she is doing the quality and quantity of work that is required and that it is not reflected in his or her pay, the employee will most likely seek a position elsewhere. As an office manager, one of your responsibilities will be to make sure that your staff is being appropriately compensated.

There are other awards beyond pay. Employees need encouragement and recognition. Present them with items that praise their work, such as awards for meeting or exceeding set goals.

Communication is key to managing an efficient office and maintaining a cohesive work atmosphere. Employees like honest, straight talk from their employers. It is important to realize that in an office, secrets breed distrust. It is always best for employees to receive news from their manager rather than through rumors. Keep your staff informed of the good and the bad issues affecting the practice.

It is essential as the manager to be available to the employees. Being visible to your employees creates a positive rapport and any problems that may arise can often be dealt with swiftly and efficiently. Do not hide in the manager's office, staying busy with business affairs.

An office manager can often gain a great deal of loyalty from his or her employees through empathy. Though the office manager is a figure of authority to the employee, honest communication and a sincere regard for the employee's well being goes a long way in creating a comfortable and productive work place.

Leadership Styles

The ability to make appropriate calls of judgment, the willingness to learn new ideas, staying calm during stressful situations, and good listening skills are all attributes of good leaders. As an office manager, you will be the team leader of the medical office. Think back to good managers that you have had in the past. What attributes made them good managers? Was it their knowledge, or was it that they were easy to approach? If you think back, you may find traits in former managers that you can incorporate to create your version of an office manager.

The four standard types of leaders are authoritarian, democratic, permissive, and bureaucratic. Each type of leader has different distinctions and motivators. Knowledge of different management styles may help you fine-tune your own management style and give you ideas on how to benefit your employees.

Authoritarian leaders tend to be very direct. They will make most of their decisions on their own without the input of others. They will probably not be team players so much as solid leaders. Authoritarian leaders tend to want respect and obedience from their staff members and may even use fear to achieve staff obedience. The need for power and absolute authority often drives this type of leader. Authoritarian leaders work best in times of great stress and crisis situations.

A democratic leader will concentrate more on the relations between staff members and emphasize teamwork within the office. He or she tends to be motivated from within to provide a comfortable work environment for all. With a leader of this style, you will often find very open communication. Democratic leaders are more receptive to new ideas from staff members, which helps create an atmosphere of cooperation among the staff, instituting greater participation in the decision-making process. This style of leadership often leads to a contented staff.

Permissive leaders are very open with the staff. They are not strict with rules and policies. Like the democratic leader, the permissive leader is self-motivated. In many situations, he or she will let the staff make their own decisions and will not interfere with staff processes. However, medical offices need to keep an ordered environment and at times, permissive leadership can lead to disorganization and even hazardous conditions.

Bureaucratic leaders are very strong at enforcing rules. Their motivation comes from external means. They prefer to rely on established management methods for office matters. Bureaucratic leaders tend to be rigid and set in their ways. There is a level of insecurity in bureaucratic leaders because they do not trust themselves in making decisions that will affect the office. The staff often will find the bureaucratic leader to be very distant and formal.

Each type of leadership style has its benefits and its downfalls. The best leaders will use a combination of styles, depending upon the situations that they must face.

For any manager to do a proper job, he or she must establish a level of power to enact and enforce the rules necessary to run an efficient medical office. There are several different types of authoritative power that a manager may establish. One type uses the power of rewards. This type of power incorporates rewards or some type of enticement in exchange for better job performance and teamwork. When managers use rewards to exact better productivity from their employees, they are exercising a form of power over their employees. The degree to which this works will depend on the level of reward that the employee receives.

There are other types of power used by individuals in authoritative positions. Legitimate power is given to people based upon their title. The president of a company will hold legitimate power, the power of the title of president. Expert power is given to those who have a great deal of knowledge. This is earned through experience and education. Referent power is given out of high regard and respect. It comes with a person's likeability and even his or her success in the field. Informative power is a type of power that most individuals have experienced at some point in their lives. It is the power wielded by those with information that others want or need. Connective power—the idea that if you know the right people you can get what you need—is one reason to network at local organizations. As a student, it is never too early to start making connections.

With all power comes the ability to abuse or overuse it. The effects of overuse of power will depend on the type of power wielded by the individual. With reward power, one downfall is that the employees can become reliant upon rewards. Once this happens, the power becomes coercive, which is a negative power because it uses fear to motivate employees. The employee may be afraid of punishment or the manager may withhold certain rewards to gain cooperation. Also there is the possibility of jealousy among the employees; they may have the perception that someone is getting more attention or rewards than someone else. With coercive power, a misuse can lead to distrust and fear of the manager and of other employees. Misused legitimate power leads to fear of the person with the title or even the title itself. In the misuse of informative power, you will often see avoidance, a sense of unfairness, and a bit of hostility. Expert, referent, and connective powers all tend to lead to the same effects when misused. There is a perceived level of manipulation and intrusion among those affected.

Creating a Team Atmosphere

For a medical office to run at its most efficient level, the staff must work as a team. This can be difficult to manage on the part of the office manager. The office manager is in charge of strengthening and enhancing the team atmosphere. The following are some factors that must come together to create a successful office team:

- Size—the smaller a team, the better it will work together.
- Team personalities—it is inadvisable to put together a team made of the same personalities.

- Responsible team members—all members of the team must be accountable for their actions.
- Unified team approach—team members must come together to face the project with the same purpose and goals.

Every team must have its leader. It is important that the office manager realize that he or she is the team leader. Managers should treat all members of a team equally. Showing favoritism to one or two employees can easily break down the team atmosphere that has been created.

Managers also need to show that they are an integral part of the team. It will make employees more confident and content in their jobs to know that their manager is willing to help out with employee duties when assistance is needed.

In some medical offices, it may also be necessary to have several levels of leaders in the office team. There may be a leader of the front desk part of the team and a leader of the clinical part of the team. All leaders within the team must be highly organized and have a good deal of energy to help to keep the team unified and productive.

Team Size

The size of a group can greatly affect the dynamics of how it will work. Small groups often will be very intimate. Close bonds may form, but because of the small group dynamics, they also tend to be very unstable. However, as groups grow larger, they tend to become more stable, but at a loss of group intimacy. This information is important to know when assembling a team. You will find that the smaller a group, the more relaxed the atmosphere will be, whereas a larger group will have a more rigid structure. Similar to group size and structure, the smaller the office, the easier going it may be. Larger multi-physician offices tend to be much more formal and systematic.

Team Personality and Skills

Creating a team atmosphere will begin as early as the hiring process. Staff who feel they have no say in the people being hired tend to have a harder time adjusting to the presence of a new staff member. One way to minimize staff frictions would be to allow some staff members to help in the hiring process. It is important that the staff understand what you, as the office manager, are looking for in potential employees. They may be able to provide same insight into the personality of the job candidate, which would be helpful in maintaining a cohesive team atmosphere. Ultimately, the office manager and physician will have the final say in the hiring of the candidate, but this process lets the staff know that their opinion also matters.

It takes the right mix of people to create a strong team. It is never a good idea to fill an office with

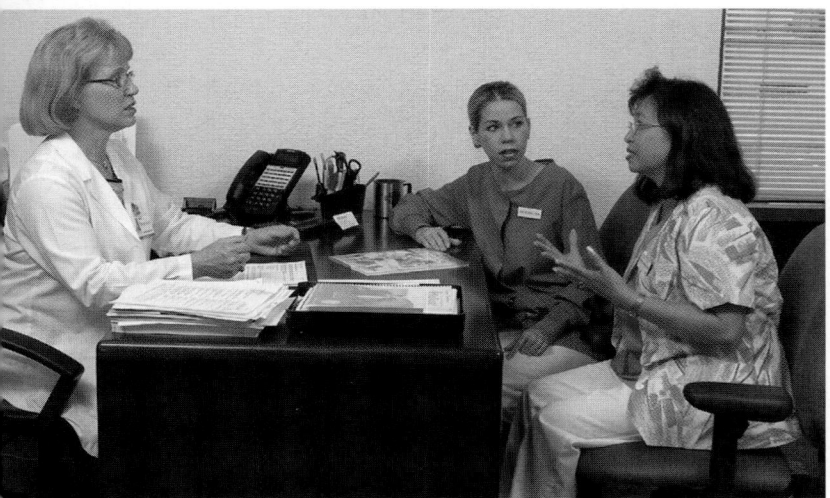

FIGURE 18-2 A medical office requires teamwork.

people who are of similar personality types and leadership styles. Often, similar weaknesses will manifest in the day-to-day business of the office, which defeats the goal of efficiency and teamwork. A manager should look for staff members who complement each other's talents and traits. For example, one member of the staff who is really good with computers but is weak in filing will be complemented by a staff member who is weak in computers but an excellent filer. Creating this mix will give you the foundation for a strong team (Figure 18-2).

You will find that within any given team, the different team members will take on various roles. These roles can be of a task-oriented nature, or they may be more nurturing. Some of the task-oriented roles include the information seeker, the information giver, the coordinator, the energizer, the evaluator/critic, and the recorder. These roles all focus on the goal that the team is working towards. The nurturing roles may include the encourager, the harmonizer, the compromiser, and the follower. A team member may take on one or many roles within the team.

Team Accountability

As a team, members must hold each other accountable for their actions. If something goes wrong, the team must come together to locate and fix the problem. This means that the team should not attack or try to blame a problem on any one member, but that they must find where, as a team, they lost track and how they can prevent a similar problem from reccuring.

Team Purpose and Goals

The team must find a way to work together. Ensuring that you have the correct personalities and talents matched up is a good start. Encourage team members to concentrate on a single goal. Successful teams work with the same purpose in mind and approach a problem or task using similar means. That way there is little conflict among the team as they work out problems that may get in the way of achieving their goal.

Any team will have some weaknesses. It is important for the office manager to monitor the progress of the team. You may find in a medical office that has employees who are strictly clinical and employees who are strictly clerical, that instead of working as one whole team, the tendency for these groups to divide themselves into two separate teams. The employees may feel comfortable with this, but this type of division usually puts strains on running the practice. As the office manager, you will need to prevent this from happening. When possible, it is a good idea to have staff members who are strictly front office employees switch places occasionally with those who are only accustomed to back office duties. This will help them to reexperience the duties and responsibilities of the office as a whole. When other options aren't working toward the goal of a cohesive team, the manager may wish to use team-building exercises. There are many companies that specialize in helping office managers pull their team together.

Hiring Procedures: Selecting the Right Staff Members

There will be times when the office manager will need to hire new staff. It may be that someone has left the office or that a new position has been created. Recruitment can begin in-house, which means that the job vacancy is posted within the medical office before the position is advertised elsewhere. An existing employee may apply for the vacant positions. If there are no interested or qualified internal candidates, several methods may be used to seek applicants.

Advertising the Position

There are many ways of advertising for open positions. These include placement of newspaper and trade journal ads, professional organizations, the Internet, formal training programs, and employment agencies, which charge a fee to be paid by the employer to the agency if an agency's candidate is hired. Local training programs in colleges are also excellent resources.

In most cases, the newspaper will often be the best way to reach your local population. However, Internet resources are becoming increasingly popular. There are many online providers that offer options for job advertisements. Remember to describe the position accurately. This will prevent the office from receiving too many resumes that do not pertain to the advertised position. If you are too general in your description, you may receive an excess of applicants. However, being too specific can cause the opposite problem: you may receive very few individuals applying for the position.

Once you have advertised and received resumes, then you will begin the task of sorting through the applicants' resumes. Each office manager has his or her own way of doing this, but some of the most commonly used sorting methods include first removing any resumes that have obvious errors, such as poor grammar and spelling errors. Next, many office managers will remove all resumes that do not show the appropriate background for the position that has been advertised. Once those resumes have been weeded out, office managers are usually left with the candidates that they believe show the most promise for the position. At this point, the interview process begins.

The Interview

Before each interview, it is good practice to have all applicants fill out a job application form (Figure 18-3). You may choose to send this to the applicant by mail and have them bring it with them to the interview. However, there are benefits to having the applicant fill out the form at the time of the interview. You will be able to see how the applicant handles filling out forms under a time constraint. You will also get a visual of the applicant's handwriting. It is important to see whether or not they have legible handwriting since most of these potential employee's will be writing directly into charts and must have legible handwriting. The last thing that you will learn from this process is how adept they are at completing a requested task. Do they take shortcuts, or do they complete every line? This can be an indication of how they handle on-the-spot tasks that may need to be resolved quickly and efficiently.

While interviewing, it is important to remember what you can and cannot ask an applicant. When interviewing, remember to assess important aspects of the applicant. How is he or she dressed? Does he or she reflect a professional appearance? Is the resume neatly prepared? This will give you insight into the type of employee

the applicant will make and whether he or she will fit into your current team. You will need to keep in mind the fair-employment practice (FEP) laws that affect hiring. Title VII of the Civil Rights Act of 1964, later amended as the Equal Employment Opportunity Act of 1972 (and further amended in 1990), prohibits asking applicants questions about their race, color, sex, religion, and national origin both during the interview and on the application. For example, asking a female applicant questions such as, "Did you have difficulty finding a baby-sitter today?" or "Do you plan to have children?" is considered discriminatory or prejudicial treatment and is therefore against the law.

Learning important information about applicants is key to making sure that they would be a good fit for your practice. You may want to ask them about past office experience, and want to know what types of physicians the applicant has worked with before.

EMPLOYMENT APPLICATION FORM

Directions: Answer all questions using black ink (print).

PERSONAL NAME

(LAST)	(FIRST)	(MI)
ADDRESS-STREET	CITY	STATE ZIP

PHONE NUMBER: SOCIAL SECURITY NUMBER:

POSITION DESIRED:

EXPECTED SALARY OR HOURLY WAGE:

EDUCATION

NAME OF SCHOOL	ADDRESS	DATE(S)	DEGREE/CERTIFICATE
HIGH SCHOOL			
VOCATIONAL/TECHNICAL			
COLLEGE			
OTHER			

WORK EXPERIENCE – Give present position (or last position held first).

JOB TITLE:	EMPLOYER	ADDRESS	DATES
DUTIES PERFORMED:			
JOB TITLE:	EMPLOYER	ADDRESS	DATES
DUTIES PERFORMED:			
JOB TITLE:	EMPLOYER	ADDRESS	DATES
DUTIES PERFORMED:			

REFERENCES – List three persons (other than relatives) who have known you for at least 2 years

NAME/TITLE	ADDRESS	TELEPHONE NUMBER

APPLICANT'S SIGNATURE _____

Date

FIGURE 18-3   A standard employment application form may be used.

Another good idea is to test applicants' ability to think on their feet. It has been an increasing practice to give applicants off-the-cuff questions to see how they respond. You are not looking for a correct answer, but only wish to see how they reason through the question. Do they give up and guess, or do they try to make a logical guess by thinking through the possibilities? Many managers will also give applicants situational questions. You may wish to ask how they would handle a patient that is upset about a test result.

As discussed in team building, it is sometimes a good idea to allow certain staff members to ask questions of the applicant. Again, staff members can give input whether or not the applicant will fit with the other staff.

It is important to find the right employee for the position. Always remember to look beyond experience and knowledge to the personality that will come with the applicant's experience. Sometimes it is better to hire someone with a little less experience to maintain a positive team atmosphere.

References

The next step in the selection process is to check references of the applicants. This is done by conducting a brief telephone interview with the person(s) referenced by the applicant. After interviewing all the applicants that interest you and checking their references, it will be time to decide whom to hire. You may choose to have your top applicants come back for second interviews. During this time, you may wish to have the physician in or other staff members interview the applicant.

Hiring

Once you have verified the references of your applicants, you can begin the process of selecting your top choices for the position. It may be that you call your top choice and offer them the position, but find that they decline your offer. You would then need to offer the position to your next choice.

After an applicant has accepted the position, all other applicants should be notified, either by telephone or in writing, that the position is filled. The new employee should receive a written confirmation of the job offer along with the salary. The office manager will usually sign this letter.

The first three months (90 days) is usually a probationary or trial period for all new employees. This time frame allows the supervisor to observe the new employee at work and to determine if the new employee is suited to the position for which he or she was hired. During this probationary period an employee can be terminated without cause. After 90 days, the employer must show just cause, or reason, to dismiss an employee. Absenteeism, poor performance, or violations of OSHA and safety standards are examples of just cause.

Orientation and Training

If you were to take a poll of new employees and ask what was most frustrating about their first days on the job, they would reply "lack of orientation." An effective manager will have an organized, efficient method of orientation and training for all new hires. The time and effort will pay off in the long run.

What issues should be covered in orientation? The following list shows the minimum subjects that should be covered for all new hires.

- Work hours and schedule
- Office layout (include the locations of the restrooms and breakrooms)
- Dress code
- Lunch break
- Job description
- All employment records—including I-9's (Figure 18-4), emergency contact information, insurance enrollment, etc.
- OSHA Bloodborne Pathogens Standards and Universal Precautions—including request for a waiver form for Hepatitis B vaccine
- Fire safety—locations of fire extinguishers (Figure 18-5), exit procedures, stairwell locations (Figure 18-6)
- Confidentiality—signature on confidentiality statement
- Policy and Procedure Manual—employee should read and sign a statement that the document has been read and understood
- Physician's work preferences—explain the way the physician prefers to work; if a team approach is used, examples should be provided to help the medical assistant understand his or her role

Smaller offices with fewer employees may conduct orientation sessions on-the-job as the new employee begins working. This is not ideal but often necessary. Orientation materials and a schedule can be developed to assist in this training process.

While some of these issues should have been covered during the interview process, many new employees need to be reminded. The pressure of the interview often causes applicants to forget important issues. Reiterating these issues during orientation can prevent confusion and errors. A confident employee is an efficient employee. Legal and Ethical Issues discusses the importance of confidentiality in the workplace.

U.S. Department of Justice
Immigration and Naturalization Service

OMB No. 1115-0136

Employment Eligibility Verification

Please read instructions carefully before completing this form. The instructions must be available during completion of this form. ANTI-DISCRIMINATION NOTICE: It is illegal to discriminate against work eligible individuals. Employers CANNOT specify which document(s) they will accept from an employee. The refusal to hire an individual because of a future expiration date may also constitute illegal discrimination.

Section 1. Employee Information and Verification. To be completed and signed by employee at the time employment begins.

Print Name: Last	First	Middle Initial	Maiden Name
Address (Street Name and Number)		Apt. #	Date of Birth (month/day/year)
City	State	Zip Code	Social Security #

I am aware that federal law provides for imprisonment and/or fines for false statements or use of false documents in connection with the completion of this form.

I attest, under penalty of perjury, that I am (check one of the following):

☐ A citizen or national of the United States
☐ A Lawful Permanent Resident (Alien # A_____)
☐ An alien authorized to work until ___/___/___
(Alien # or Admission #) _____

Employee's Signature	Date (month/day/year)

Preparer and/or Translator Certification. (To be completed and signed if Section 1 is prepared by a person other than the employee.) I attest, under penalty of perjury, that I have assisted in the completion of this form and that to the best of my knowledge the information is true and correct.

Preparer's/Translator's Signature	Print Name
Address (Street Name and Number, City, State, Zip Code)	Date (month/day/year)

Section 2. Employer Review and Verification. To be completed and signed by employer. Examine one document from List A OR examine one document from List B and one from List C, as listed on the reverse of this form, and record the title, number and expiration date, if any, of the document(s)

List A	OR	List B	AND	List C
Document title:_____		_____		_____
Issuing authority: _____		_____		_____
Document #: _____		_____		_____
Expiration Date (if any): ___/___/___		___/___/___		___/___/___
Document #: _____				
Expiration Date (if any): ___/___/___				

CERTIFICATION - I attest, under penalty of perjury, that I have examined the document(s) presented by the above-named employee, that the above-listed document(s) appear to be genuine and to relate to the employee named, that the employee began employment on (month/day/year) ___/___/___ and that to the best of my knowledge the employee is eligible to work in the United States. (State employment agencies may omit the date the employee began employment.)

Signature of Employer or Authorized Representative	Print Name	Title
Business or Organization Name	Address (Street Name and Number, City, State, Zip Code)	Date (month/day/year)

Section 3. Updating and Reverification. To be completed and signed by employer.

A. New Name (if applicable)	B. Date of rehire (month/day/year) (if applicable)

C. If employee's previous grant of work authorization has expired, provide the information below for the document that establishes current employment eligibility.

Document Title:_____ Document #: _____ Expiration Date (if any): ___/___/___

I attest, under penalty of perjury, that to the best of my knowledge, this employee is eligible to work in the United States, and if the employee presented document(s), the document(s) I have examined appear to be genuine and to relate to the individual.

Signature of Employer or Authorized Representative	Date (month/day/year)

Form I-9 (Rev. 11-21-91)N Page 2

FIGURE 18-4 A standard I-9 form.

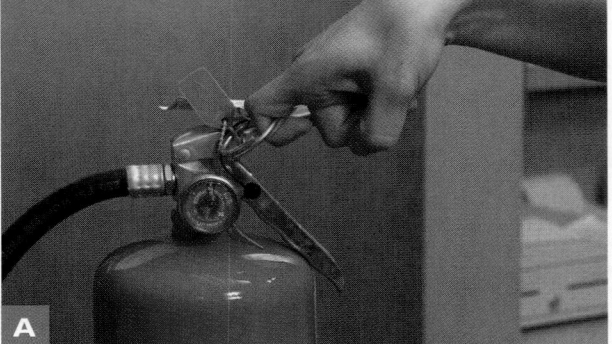

(A) Pull the pin on the upper handle of the fire extinguisher.

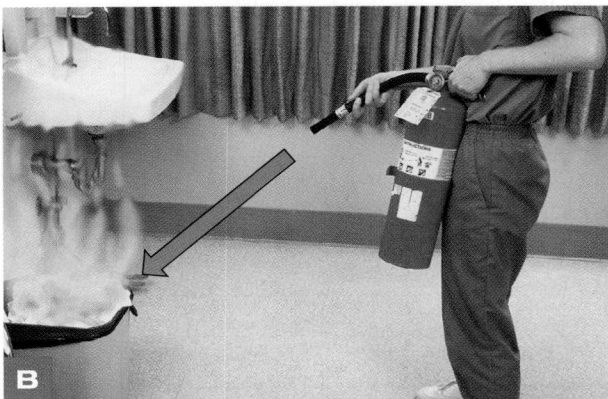

(B) Aim low toward the base of the fire.

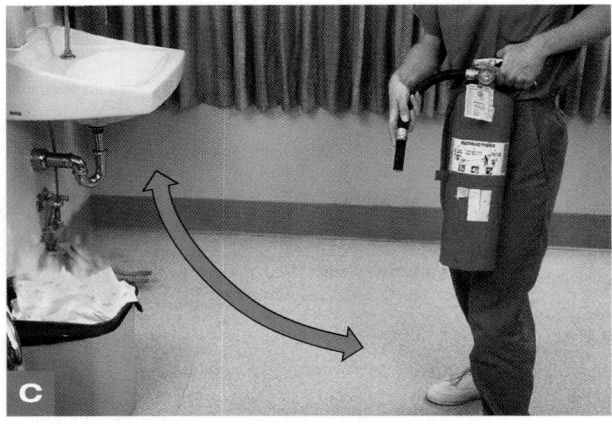

(C) Sweep the area from side to side.

FIGURE 18-5 It is important for new employees to know the location of all fire extinguishers.

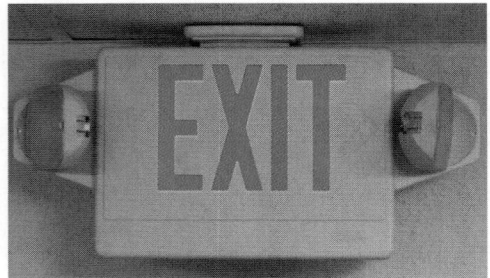

FIGURE 18-6 New employees should be shown all exits in case of an emergency.

Using Performance Evaluation Effectively

All employees need feedback on how well they are performing in their assigned positions. In addition, management needs opportunities to introduce new goals for their staff. The employee, in return, can have the chance to voice concerns and suggestions for increasing the morale and productivity of the staff. Regular evaluations offer the chance for a productive give-and-take beyond the day-to-day interactions.

When it comes to any evaluation, preparation is the key. As the office manager, you do not want to go into an evaluation unprepared. This will only set you up for problems. The appraisal should be given in a nonjudgmental manner. The manager should not take the stance of "the boss" versus the employee, but rather be open to understanding any problems the employee may be experiencing. Discussion of the job description and required duties should allow the employee to voice any frustration. At the same time, the manager should reinforce what is expected of the staff member. Teamwork should be emphasized.

The manager needs to sit down and look at the employee's performance as a whole. Reexamine the employee's job description and identify the most important aspects of the position. You will then want to rate the employee on those points. Look at whether the employee's performance was outstanding, good, average, poor, or unacceptable. Once you have evaluated these particulars, you can examine the whole of the employee's performance. How does he or she get along with the other members of the office team?

In this general evaluation of the employee, it is also important to give him or her goals to meet before the next evaluation. Mention areas in which the employee may want to improve work performance. If possible, you will always want to end the evaluation meeting on a good note. It is ideal that the employee leave the meeting with the feeling that something valuable was gained from the review.

In situations where employees are not performing up to the standard set for them, the performance evaluation may satisfy the legal requirements for documentation for rightful termination. If you are giving an employee a poor evaluation, it is a good idea to warn the employee at the start of the meeting. This will prevent the employee from being surprised when you begin to explain the problems with his or her performance.

Most employees look at an evaluation as the chance to ask for a raise in pay. When writing a personnel manual, there should be a delineation of the types of reviews and the time intervals at which they will be given. Following is a list of different types of reviews.

- Orientation or training—Every few days ask the employee how the training is going. Make sure he or she has the materials, equipment and supplies needed to perform the job. Ask the employee if he or she has any questions regarding policy and if supervision is being provided.
- Routine performance review—Reviews are normally performed at 90-day, six-month and yearly intervals. Approximately one hour should be devoted to this meeting. These reviews should not come as a surprise to the employee. They should be stated in the policy manual. Many offices offer the staff member the opportunity to do a self-evaluation prior to the meeting. This allows the employee the chance to think about his or her performance thus far. Figure 18-7 is an example of a form that may be used in a routine evaluation.
- Poor performance reviews—These are held when there have been obvious deficiencies in the performance of the employee. They offer the opportunity to help the employee improve. Conversely, they document the poor performance and set the stage for dismissal.

Should salary reviews be tied to the performance evaluation? There are several schools of thought regarding this issue. Whatever the policy of the office, fair and equal standards should be set.

What should the manager hope to accomplish with the meeting? It is important to target specific areas of performance. Following are some questions to ask in order to achieve effective management goals.

- How can improvement be achieved?
- How can you as the manager help the improvement?
- How can you remain fair and even in your opinion?
- How will you handle the possibility of a negative response from the employee?

Box 18-2 is a list of possible topics to cover during the review. Finally, as in all aspects of medical office management, document all that is said during the evaluation. Be mindful to document only objective facts and statements made and leave personal opinions aside.

Discipline and Probation

Occasionally it is necessary to discipline an employee. Due to the sensitive nature of medical work, there are certain situations that can result in immediate discharge. These include intoxication, drug use, breach of confidentiality, and sleeping on the job. The employee must be sent home on suspension while the incident is investigated. If the facts prove to be true, then the employee is dismissed.

BOX 18-2
Topics of Review for Front Office Personnel

Telephone technique

Balance of cash box daily

Accurate filing

Appointment scheduling

General

Treats patients with respect

Prioritizing of tasks

Makes efficient use of time

Works neatly

Follows directions

Cheerful and interested in the patient's comfort

Is punctual and has achieved good attendance

Uses good grammar

Appropriate appearance and hygiene

Works as a team member

Additional Topics for Medical Assistant's Review

Charts accurately

Anticipates the needs of the doctor

Is knowledgeable about procedures

PERFORMANCE EVALUATION AND DEVELOPMENT PLAN
(OFFICE AND CLERICAL)

NAME:_____ DATE OF EVALUATION:_____

DATE OF HIRE:_____ DEPARTMENT:_____

JOB TITLE:_____ SUPERVISOR:_____

DATE APPOINTED THIS JOB:_____ MANAGER:_____

LAST REVIEW DATE:_____ LAST REVIEW RATING:_____

NEXT REVIEW DATE:_____ CURRENT REVIEW RATING:_____

PURPOSE

The purpose of this evaluation is to:
1. SET GOALS WITHIN SCOPE OF PRESENT JOB.
2. COMMUNICATE OPENLY ABOUT PERFORMANCE.
3. EVALUATE PAST PERFORMANCE.
4. DISCUSS FUTURE DEVELOPMENT PLANS FOR GROWTH.

INSTRUCTIONS

1. Supervisor to review form prior to completion. If specific iter they should be left blank.
2. Supervisor and employee to review job description prior to
3. In "COMMENTS" section supervisor may indicate which fac more heavily weighted in this particular evaluation.
4. Comments should be specific and job-related. All appropri should be commented on to some degree.

I. POSITION OBJECTIVES AND MAJOR RESPONSIBILITIES: Summ

II. ACCOMPLISHMENTS AND/OR IMPROVEMENTS: What specific a has employee made since last review with respect to set goals?

PLEASE CONSIDER THE EMPLOYEE'S DEMONSTRATED PERFORMANCE A CLOSELY DESCRIBES THAT PERFORMANCE.

4 - Performance consistently far exceeds expectations and requirements.
3 - Performance consistently exceeds normal expectations and job require
2 - Performance consistently meets expectations and job requirements.
1 - Performance usually meets expectations and minimum job requireme
0 - Performance does not meet job requirements.

– CONTINUED, NEXT PAGE –

ORDER # 72-119 • PERSONNEL RECORDS SYSTEM • © 1987 BIBBERO SYSTEMS, INC. • PETALUMA, CA • TO REORDER CALL TOLL FREE: (800)

7. DEPENDABILITY: Consider attendance, punctuality, idle time and reliance which can be placed on employee to persevere and carry through to completion all assigned tasks.

○ 0   ○ 1   ○ 2   ○ 3   ○ 4

8. COMPLIANCE WITH COMPANY POLICIES: Does the employee comply with rules and regulations which apply to safety, fair employment practices and general administrative procedure?

○ 0   ○ 1   ○ 2   ○ 3   ○ 4

9. SPECIFIC PERFORMANCE

	0	1	2	3	4	COMMENTS
A. Ability to handle scheduling:						
B. Willingness to work OT when necessary:						
C. Handling of calls and follow-up:						
D. Maintenance of equipment:						
E. Ability to handle patient complaints:						
F. Tact in dealing with patients:						
G. Speed (in specific technical procedures):						
H. Secretarial accuracy:						
I. Professional terminology:						
J. Assisting procedures:						
K. Laboratory techniques:						
L. X-ray techniques:						
M. Physical therapy:						
N. Collections:						
O. Medical Insurace:						
P. Bookkeeping:						

10. PERSONAL

	0	1	2	3	4	COMMENTS
A. Grooming:						
B. Professional conduct:						
C. Energy, enthusiasm:						
D. Ability to handle stress:						

ADDITIONAL COMMENTS:_____

– CONTINUED, NEXT PAGE –

ORDER # 72-119 • PERSONNEL RECORDS SYSTEM • © 1987 BIBBERO SYSTEMS, INC. • PETALUMA, CA • TO REORDER CALL TOLL FREE: (800) BIBBERO (800 242-23'6) OR FAX (800) 242-9330

FIGURE 18-7 There are standard employee performance evaluation forms that may be used.

For frequent tardiness or absenteeism, an employee may be placed on probation and told that if the situation occurs again, the employee will be discharged. In some facilities, both verbal and written warnings are issued before corrective action is taken. Investigating every employee incident prevents someone being falsely fired. For instance, diabetic employees may appear to be on drugs when they are, in fact, having a diabetic reaction.

Any employee incident must be carefully documented with the time, date, and an objective statement about what happened and then placed into the employee's file. Document the incident immediately after it has occurred. It is always better to have a witness present when dismissing an employee.

Time Management

One of the greatest attributes of an effective office manager is the ability to successfully manage time. If the manager is organized, the office is usually organized. Time management requires the ability to prioritize the important tasks and to complete them on schedule. This is quite different from doing every task as it comes along. The office manager generally has little control over the tasks presented. The control is in how the tasks are handled and delegated.

One of the main responsibilities of the office manager/medical assistant is to manage all the peripheral office functions so that the physician is free to concentrate on practicing medicine. It is possible for the physician to gain an hour each day to devote to administrative and patient related tasks that only he or she can do, because tasks, such as opening the daily mail, searching for a drug sample to give to a patient, and dealing with pharmaceutical and other sales representatives, are handled by the office manager.

Before establishing a time management system, it is important to define the office goals with the physician. Physicians' goals vary from complex to simple and from long-term to short-term. These goals may include collecting all payments at the time of delivery of services, re-organizing or computerizing billing, limiting the practice, adding a partner or new service, writing a textbook, or plans for early retirement.

One of the dangers of strictly adhering to time management and goal-setting practices is that by totally concentrating on organizing the office, the patient may be forgotten in the process. The main concern should be to always take care of a patient who is waiting at the reception desk before straightening up the work area.

After the goals have been established, priorities can be set. The office manager/medical assistant can establish a priority list of the goals. A priority list is a composite of all the tasks that need to be accomplished to actualize each goal. These can be placed on a TO DO list as they come to the office manager's attention. Each item is assigned a priority designation of 1, 2, or 3, depending on how critical the item is to complete the task. For example, ordering supplies that are running out is a number 1, while rearranging a linen cupboard or a file drawer might be a number 3. Number 1 priority items must be done first and number 3 last. It is often tempting to do the easier tasks first since they take less time and show an immediate accomplishment. Good use of time management would determine that the inventory order should be placed immediately and the number 3 priority items be delegated to someone else or completed later, if necessary. It is a good idea to date a TO DO list and to cross off or check items as they are accomplished. Box 18-3 shows an example of one type of TO DO list.

Make every attempt to complete each task, such as handling paper, only once. As mail is opened, it needs to be quickly sorted according to importance, handled, and processed. Mail should be handled immediately, if possible.

BOX 18-3
Medical Office TO DO List

Priority	TO DO _____ Date: _____
2	Order paper supplies
1	Arrange Dr. Williams' air transportation to medical convention next week
2	Prepare performance appraisal for J. Jones
3	Reorganize storeroom
1	Type convention speech
1	Place ad for new medical assistant
3	Ask Janet to remove old magazines from reception room
1	Call for PAP test report for Ms. Kohut
2	Block out schedule book for next quarter
1	Prepare agenda for Thursday's staff meeting

When leaving a telephone message, it is advisable to record detailed voice mail messages, whenever possible, since it can actually save time. Leaving a detailed message during the first call can prevent having to make another telephone call. An exception would be when calling a patient. The patient's confidentiality should be protected. See Chapter 6 for more information regarding voice messaging.

Never trust anything to memory in the medical office. Always write down all instructions from the physician, information from the patient, another employee, or supplier. It is better to maintain one small record book and keep all notations in that book rather than have several pieces of paper with information that can be misplaced. Many medical assistants carry a small notepad and pen in their pocket at all times.

Some offices require that the in-basket of the day's mail and incoming laboratory reports be emptied before the end of the day. This is a good time management technique to develop.

Personnel Policy Manual

The personnel policy manual, also known as the employee handbook, contains information for the employee about the employer-employee relationship, the work environment, and the expectations of the particular medical facility. This manual contains general information about office policies relating to dress and behavior codes, punctuality, office safety, and the role of the employee in an emergency, such as a fire. OSHA guidelines and Standard Precautions are included. It usually describes the circumstances or grounds for dismissal, such as sleeping, drinking, or swearing on the job.

Employees may be given specific information about the following issues or benefits.

- Compensation and reimbursement for work-related activities, such as attending conventions and courses (CEU/degree), and parking fees
- Emergency leave
- Grievance (complaint) process
- Health benefits
- Holidays
- Jury duty
- Overtime policy
- Pension plan
- Performance review and evaluation
- Probationary period
- Sick leave
- Termination of employment
- Vacation
- Work hours, including flex time

An office manager will find that an updated policy manual can be a useful tool when providing employee counseling. A well-designed policy manual remains flexible enough in its design to allow for revisions, if and when policies change. Small office policy manuals consist of several pages that are copied on-site. In large practices, the manual may be bound and copied at a printing service.

The employee handbook is often the first piece of office literature that the employee is asked to read. Employees should be asked to sign a statement indicating they have read and understood the information contained in it.

Office Procedures Manual

All offices should have a procedures manual describing how to carry out tasks within a particular medical practice. The office procedures manual varies in content from the personnel policy manual. Detailed descriptions of the standard operating procedure (SOP) and how to perform both administrative and clinical tasks are included in this manual.

Policy refers to a plan of action, such as "It is office policy that all employees receive hepatitis B (HBV) vaccination." The procedure will describe the steps to be performed to carry out the policy. For example, "a

series of three injections of HBV will be administered over a seven-month period of time, free of charge, to the employee." The terms policy and procedure are used interchangeably in many office.

The primary functions of a procedures manual are: (1) list the tasks to be performed within the office; (2) standardize the procedure for each task; and (3) describe job responsibilities and titles. The procedures manual, when properly updated, is an excellent reference tool for the new employee since it provides guidelines for performing specific tasks. Temporary or substitute employees also find it valuable.

Ideally, the procedure manual is contained in a loose-leaf binder that allows the addition of new pages for ease of updating. Each policy is numbered and dated. As the policy is updated, the number remains the same but the date changes to indicate the revision. The manual should be clearly labeled and available for employees to read.

New policies and procedures are usually distributed or posted for employees in addition to being added to the policy and procedures manuals. In some offices, staff are asked to initial the corner of the policy indicating they have read it.

Table 18-2 contains a list of information that should be included in a procedure's manual. Completing and updating a procedures manual is often a job function of the medical assistant or the office manager. While one person may have responsibility for development of the manual, good manuals are the result of the input from a variety of personnel. The physician should always provide the final review of all policies and procedures.

Medical Meetings and Speaking Engagements

The medical assistant may be asked to assist the physician in the travel arrangements for medical meetings or in the preparation of medical speaking engagements. Travel arrangements may include making hotel, flight, and car reservations, and sometimes typing a travel itinerary for the trip. Preparation for medical speaking engagements may require the medical assistant to do research for a physician's speech or to create certain documents such as handouts and computer presentations.

When making the travel arrangements, the physician may wish to use a local travel agent or one of the many Internet sites available for booking flights and hotels. It is important to find out what the physician's preferences are before making any plans. The physician may prefer a non-smoking hotel room and only business class flight tickets. Make sure the reservations are what he or she wants.

TABLE 18-2 Contents of an Office Procedure Manual

Content	Description
Job Description	Every position including office manager, medical assistant, nurses, technician, housekeeping personnel, and custodian.
Routine Office Tasks	Clinical tasks such as venipuncture, taking vital signs, EKGs, assisting with physical examinations, assisting with PAP test and other laboratory tests.
Special Procedures	Surgical tray set-up for individual physicians, assisting with special exams such as proctological exams, using specialized equipment such as ultrasound.
Emergency Procedures	Protocol for handling telephone and office emergencies, description of equipment used for emergency care such as mouth shield for CPR, proper sequence for alerting physician and 911 emergencies.
Quality Assurance	Procedures for maintaining quality control over all laboratory testing and procedures.
OSHA Compliance	Compliance regarding needles, other sharps, specimens, personal protective equipment, regulated waste control, HBV vaccine, laundry disposal, and contaminated equipment.

When putting together the travel itinerary, obtain all of the flight, hotel, car rental, and meeting or engagement information. Flight information includes travel dates, airline name, flight number, and departure and arrival times. The hotel information includes the hotel name, address, telephone number, reservation dates and confirmation number. Also assemble car rental reservations and any information pertinent to the meeting that the physician is attending. Keep a copy of the itinerary at the office and give a copy to the physician.

When helping a physician to prepare for a speaking engagement, you can help in a variety of capacities. It may include doing research. Be sure to provide all source material with any research that you reference and cite. The physician may ask you to create handouts for his or her presentation. The physician may also ask you to create a computer presentation. There are different software programs that will assist you in creating a presentation.

Patient Information Booklet

Many medical practices use a professional advertising service to develop informational brochures as a marketing tool. However, a patient information booklet or a variety of patient teaching materials can be developed in-house. These materials should provide patient information regarding office hours, payment guidelines, appointment and cancellation policy, the telephone answering service, information about the physician(s), directions to the facility, and parking information. A good patient information booklet can reduce the number of questions by telephone from patients, enhance the office's image, and reduce the number of patients who fail to follow instructions.

Instruction booklets for patients with special needs or to teach methods of disease prevention can be developed using a format and design described in Procedure 18-2. The patient information booklet should be handed to each new patient at the time of registration or mailed prior to the first appointment. Patient information materials never replace the need for personal instructions to the patient. They augment or reinforce patient teaching. Patient Education includes more about patient information booklets.

Medical Practice Marketing and Customer Service

Marketing is a subject that most office managers do not think much about when running a medical office. Marketing a medical practice involves various activities to promote the services of a physician or group of physicians to a population of patients. Marketing can promote a new office and improve the image of an established office to compete with the new offices and

Developing a Patient Information Booklet

OBJECTIVE: Develop a booklet to inform patients about services provided by your medical office.

Equipment and Supplies
computer; design software (if including images); high quality paper; printer (or an independent printing service)

Method

1. Make the booklet as appealing as possible. Allow white space around all the edges. Use large print for the elderly reader's benefit. The booklet should be small enough that it will fit easily into a pocket or purse.
2. Write the booklet with the reader in mind. Avoid the use of technical medical terms. Never use medical abbreviations in patient literature.
3. Avoid long paragraphs of explanation. Keep the sentences short and concise.
4. Provide a listing of the regular office hours.
5. List any special services offered by the practice or clinic such as patient education classes or blood pressure testing programs.
6. Explain the procedure for having a prescription refilled.
7. Explain the procedure for processing medical insurance forms.
8. Include a general statement about payment of fees, especially if payment is expected at the time of delivery of services. Specific fees are not discussed in patient brochures.
9. Provide information about the physician and the staff. For example, "Dr. Williams is in general practice specializing in family practice. Our pediatrician is Dr. Conway. Our physicians are on staff at two hospitals: Northwestern Memorial Hospital and Children's Memorial Hospital." The name and telephone number of the office manager, the personnel responsible for insurance processing and the patient educator should be included.
10. State what procedure to follow in case of an emergency. For example, instruct the patients to call 911 if the emergency is life threatening. Also provide a 24-hour emergency telephone number. Request the patient to keep this number near his or her telephone.
11. Include a telephone number at the end of the brochure in the event there are additional questions.
12. End the brochure by thanking the patient for taking the time to read the literature.

---

to retain patients. There are many ways that marketing can impact a medical office. Customer service can be a valuable marketing tool.

The Target Market

In marketing a medical office or facility, one of the first things to look at is the target market of the physician(s). What kinds of services are being offered? This can affect the physician's office location. A new geriatric medical practice has a better chance of doing well if it is located near retirement communities rather than with young families. The services of the office should match the area in which it is located.

After assessing the target market and the needs of the target group, types of services the practice could offer can be determined. Services may include new procedures that could benefit patients' needs.

Once you have determined your services, then a plan must be developed and put into place. The first step will be to look for any problems or opportunities that may come about in the execution of the plan. The plan should describe what steps need to be implemented, who is responsible, and a time frame. A plan must be thought through and in place before you begin to follow and execute it. Many ventures have failed due to poor planning. When the plan has been executed, it is a good idea to go back and review if the plan met expectations or not. Make note of any particular problems that may have arisen and positives that may have been learned in the process.

Patients need an introduction to all the caregivers they come into contact with in the office. Employees should always identify themselves to patients. Many patients need further education about the functions that individual employees are able to perform.

Patient information booklets are one of the best ways to educate the patient about the functions of the staff and medical office. While verbal instructions are still necessary, the booklets can enhance learning. Medical assistants need to involve the entire staff in the production of patient literature.

Marketing the Practice

There are many ways to promote a medical practice. Some marketing plans may require budgets for expenses to implement the plan. However, some marketing tools available to physicians and medical practices are free or at low-cost

Free Marketing and Public Relations

One of the best ways of promoting a practice is by word of mouth, which is completely free. Many patients choose their physician based upon friends and family recommending their own physician. Word of mouth is built upon a base of good customer service, which will be discussed later in the chapter.

Another method of promoting a practice is through public relation activities such as local charities and events. Involvement in the community will spread the office's name and show that you are a participating member of the community. Goodwill in the community can translate into growing the practice.

Web Sites

Building a practice Web site is a relatively new marketing tool for medical professionals. This can be done using simple Web site building software or hiring a Web site firm. It is important to plan what should be included on the Web site. The main objective of the site needs to be determined. What is the site's function? Is it only providing information regarding the practice? Would the patient to be able to access different forms and procedure instructions? Will patients be able to request appointments online? Remember to keep the site easy to use. Graphics and colors need to be simple and pleasing to the eye.

You will then have to choose a Web server to support your site. There are many options that will need to be researched. Some are free, but they will add advertisements to your site. Others will require a fee.

Customer Service

One of your most potent marketing tools will depend entirely upon your customer service. Just as word of mouth can bring you many customers, it can also drive them away if poor services are provided.

The patient, like a customer, will respond positively or negatively to his or her experience at the medical office. What impression does the patient have? Is the staff helpful? Is the staff attentive and considerate of the patient's time and condition? It is important that all patients are treated with respect and concern. Box 18-4 includes phrases that will leave the patient with a poor view of a medical office's customer service abilities.

BOX 18-4

Phrases that Decrease Customer Service Level

"I don't know."

"It's not my fault."

"What do you want?"

"I can't."

"It's not my job."

"You're wrong."

"It's not my problem."

SUMMARY

A smooth running office requires attention to many factors, including staff training, good time management skill, up-to-date policy and procedure manuals, and careful attention to detail. A medical office requires the same management skills that any business organization uses. Maintaining good customer service is key to keeping a contented patient base while enhancing the possibility of growing the practice.

COMPETENCY REVIEW

1. Define and spell the terms to learn for this chapter.
2. Prepare an office procedure for any one of the following tasks: appointment scheduling, patient reception process, taking vital signs, OSHA guidelines.
3. Prepare a monthly calendar for the month of December showing staff vacations and office coverage.
4. Develop a patient information booklet for your own physician's practice.
5. Prepare an employee policy for taking vacation days.

PREPARING FOR THE CERTIFICATION EXAM

1. Which of the following is a purpose of the procedure manual?
   A. standardization of procedures
   B. listing of job descriptions
   C. listing of tasks to perform within the office
   D. marketing tool
   E. listing of hospitals and clinics

2. An employee policy describing the grievance process should be contained in the
   A. general policy manual
   B. personnel policy manual
   C. employee handbook
   D. patient information booklet
   E. physician/employer file

3. What law affects the hiring of a new employee?
   A. OSHA
   B. EEOA
   C. Title VII of the Civil Rights Act
   D. EEOC
   E. AMA

4. A systems approach to office management is
   A. using outside consultants for all financial and business operations
   B. performing individual office functions in isolation
   C. integrating functions
   D. not advisable in the office setting
   E. is the only way to manage

5. Arranging staff vacation coverage is usually the responsibility of the
   A. physician
   B. individual who is going on vacation
   C. office manager
   D. medical assistant
   E. nurse

6. The purpose of a performance evaluation is to
   A. positively encourage the continued improvement of the employee's performance
   B. negotiate a salary increase
   C. find any fault(s) in an employee's performance
   D. provide a document to compare one employee's performance with another employee's performance
   E. improve office moral

7. Employee records must be kept for all of the following EXCEPT
   A. Social Security Number
   B. net salary
   C. gross salary
   D. number of claimed exemptions (W-4 form)
   E. deductions

8. Patient instruction booklets should be used
   A. in place of individual instructions
   B. to avoid contact with difficult patients
   C. to prevent lawsuits
   D. to standardize instructions
   E. only with hearing-impaired patients

9. A new employee's probationary period is usually
   A. 30 days
   B. 2 months
   C. 3 months
   D. 6 months
   E. 1 year

10. Seniority refers to the person in the organization who
    A. is the oldest
    B. is in the highest position of power
    C. has been recognized the most for achievement
    D. has been with the company the longest
    E. will be the first to leave the office

CRITICAL THINKING

1. Where else could Marsha have advertised the job opening?
2. How could she have sorted the resumes further?
3. Why was it important for Marsha to know about the applicant's handwriting?
4. Was it appropriate for the second interviewee to wear a tongue ring? Why or why not?
5. Do you think that Marsha made the right choice from the three applicants?

ON THE JOB

Sarah Egan is the office manager in Dr. Williams' practice. Nell Jacobs, who has worked as a medical assistant in the office for one year, has frequently been absent or tardy on Mondays. Sarah suspects that Nell has a drinking problem. However, Nell has never arrived at the office intoxicated—until today. Sarah has just observed Nell stumbling in the parking lot when getting out of her car. Her speech is slurred and her breath has a fruity odor that Sarah thinks could be alcohol. Nell doesn't appear to understand anything that Sarah is saying to her.

1. Given the situation, as the office manager, what should Sarah do immediately regarding Nell?
2. If Sarah decides to send Nell home, should she call Nell's husband to come and get her, or, perhaps, insist that Nell go home in a cab?
3. Does Sarah have an obligation to tell Dr. Williams about her suspicions regarding Nell?
4. Should this incident become part of Nell's employment record?
5. Is this incident grounds for firing an employee?
6. Because Nell is a medical assistant and works with patients, is it within Sarah's rights to demand a blood and urine screening for alcohol and drugs?
7. Should the police be notified of the incident?
8. If Nell is indeed intoxicated or under the influence of drugs, is Sarah obligated to refer Nell to counseling at an alcohol and drug rehabilitation facility?

INTERNET ACTIVITY

Research the different methods that the Internet provides for advertising job opportunities available at your medical office.

MediaLink More on medical office management, including interactive resources, can be found on the Student CD-ROM accompanying this textbook.

Unit Three

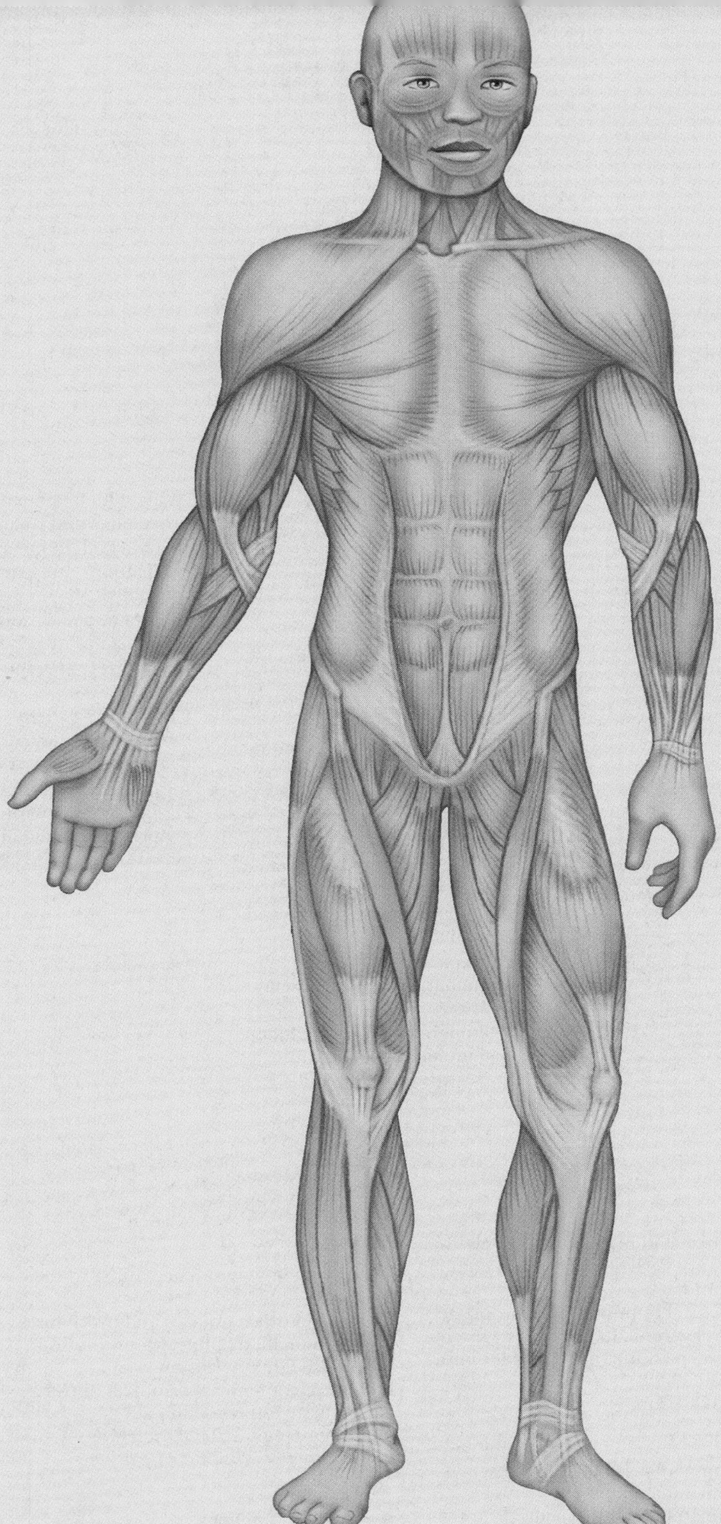

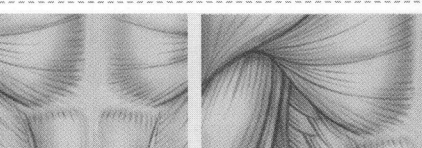

Anatomy and Physiology

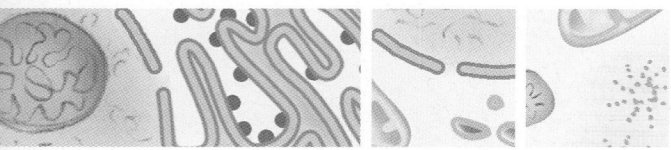

Medical Assistant Role Delineation Chart

HIGHLIGHT indicates material covered in this chapter.

ADMINISTRATIVE

Administrative Procedures

- Perform basic administrative medical assisting functions
- Schedule, coordinate and monitor appointments
- Schedule inpatient/outpatient admissions and procedures
- Understand and apply third-party guidelines
- Obtain reimbursement through accurate claims submission
- Monitor third-party reimbursement
- Understand and adhere to managed care policies and procedures
- *Negotiate managed care contracts*

Practice Finances

- Perform procedural and diagnostic coding
- Apply bookkeeping principles

- Manage accounts receivable
- *Manage accounts payable*
- *Process payroll*
- *Document and maintain accounting and banking records*
- *Develop and maintain fee schedules*
- *Manage renewals of business and professional insurance policies*
- *Manage personnel benefits and maintain records*
- *Perform marketing, financial, and strategic planning*

CLINICAL

Fundamental Principles

- Apply principles of aseptic technique and infection control
- Comply with quality assurance practices
- Screen and follow up patient test results

Diagnostic Orders

- Collect and process specimens
- Perform diagnostic tests

Patient Care

- Adhere to established patient screening procedures
- Obtain patient history and vital signs
- Prepare and maintain examination and treatment areas
- Prepare patient for examinations, procedures and treatments

- Assist with examinations, procedures and treatments
- Prepare and administer medications and immunizations
- Maintain medication and immunization records
- Recognize and respond to emergencies
- Coordinate patient care information with other health care providers
- Initiate IV and administer IV medications with appropriate training and as permitted by state law

GENERAL

Professionalism

- Display a professional manner and image
- Demonstrate initiative and responsibility
- Work as a member of the health care team
- Prioritize and perform multiple tasks
- Adapt to change
- Promote the CMA credential
- Enhance skills through continuing education
- Treat all patients with compassion and empathy
- Promote the practice through positive public relations

Communication Skills

- Recognize and respect cultural diversity
- Adapt communications to individual's ability to understand
- Use professional telephone technique

- Recognize and respond effectively to verbal, nonverbal, and written communications
- Use medical terminology appropriately
- Utilize electronic technology to receive, organize, prioritize and transmit information
- Serve as liaison

Legal Concepts

- Perform within legal and ethical boundaries
- Prepare and maintain medical records
- Document accurately
- Follow employer's established policies dealing with the health care contract
- Implement and maintain federal and state health care legislation and regulations
- Comply with established risk management and safety procedures
- Recognize professional credentialing criteria
- *Develop and maintain personnel, policy and procedure manuals*

Instruction

- Instruct individuals according to their needs
- Explain office policies and procedures
- Teach methods of health promotion and disease prevention
- Locate community resources and disseminate information
- *Develop educational materials*
- *Conduct continuing education activities*

Operational Functions

- Perform inventory of supplies and equipment
- Perform routine maintenance of administrative and clinical equipment
- Apply computer techniques to support office operations
- *Perform personnel management functions*
- *Negotiate leases and prices for equipment and supply contracts*

- *Denotes advanced skills.*

chapter 19

Body Structure and Function

Learning Objectives

After completing this chapter, you should be able to:

- Define and spell the terms to learn for this chapter.
- List the systems of the body and identify the organs located in each system.
- Discuss the structural unit of the cell and briefly explain the function of each of its components.
- Explain anatomical locations and positions and define the terms used

- to describe direction, planes, and cavities of the body.
- Briefly explain the differences between passive and active transport.
- Discuss genetics, genetic engineering, genetic fingerprinting, and the role genetics plays in disease.
- Identify common genetic and congenital disorders.

OUTLINE

The Human Body: Levels of Organization   342

Anatomical Locations and Positions   350

Chemistry   354

Genetics and Heredity   355

Terms to Learn

active transport
anatomical position
anatomy
atom
cavities
cell
cell membrane
cilia
cytokinesis
cytoplasm
diaphragm

DNA (deoxyribonucleic acid)
electrolyte
genetics
homeostasis
lysosomes
meiosis
mitochondrion
mitosis
molecule
nucleus

organelles
organs
passive transport
pathophysiology
physiology
ribosome
RNA (ribonucleic acid)
selective permeability
system
tissue

Case Study

DR. NANCY MENENDEZ SAW MICKEY SCHULTZ IN THE CLINIC for abdominal pain. The pain was centered in the epigastric region, and Dr. Menendez needed to determine if the pain was cardiac or gastrointestinal in origin. She ordered a variety of tests to ensure that there were no chemical changes, musculoskeletal origins, or blockages in the soft tissue causing the pain. Eventually, the pain was determined to be caused by a peptic ulcer in the stomach.

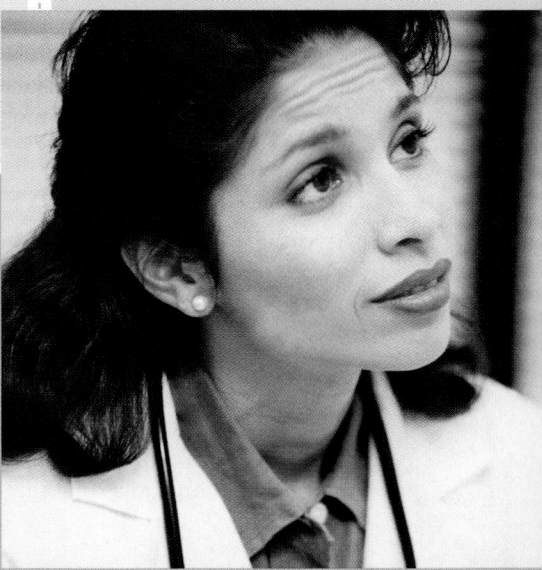

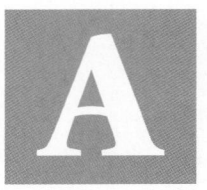natomy can be defined as the study of the structure of an organism. The word *anatomy* is derived from a Greek word meaning "to cut up" (to dissect). Physiology can be defined as the study of the function of the organism. Aging or a malfunction of a part of the body can lead to diseases or disorders. The study of these diseases or disorders is called pathophysiology.

The human body consists of a series of increasingly complex and larger systems. The basis of the structure of the body is the atom, which makes up molecules. Molecules form organelles, which form cells. A group of cells forms tissues, which create organs. Then organ systems combine to form the completion of the organism (the body). By adjusting for constant changes, all of these systems work together to maintain balance or equilibrium. This is known as homeostasis. Homeostasis is one of the fundamental characteristics of living things. It refers to the maintenance of the internal environment within tolerable limits. All sorts of factors affect the suitability of our body fluids to sustain life; these include properties such as temperature, salinity, acidity, and the concentrations of nutrients and wastes. Because these properties affect the chemical reactions that keep us alive, we have built-in physiological mechanisms to maintain them at desirable levels.

When a change occurs in the body, the body can respond in either of two general ways. In negative feedback, the body responds in such a way as to reverse the direction of change. Because this tends to keep things constant, it allows us to maintain homeostasis. On the other hand, positive feedback is also possible. This means that if a change occurs in some variable, the response is to change that variable even more in the same direction. This has a destabilizing effect, so it does not result in homeostasis. Positive feedback is used in certain situations where rapid change is desirable. The nervous system and the endocrine system have the main responsibility for maintaining homeostasis.

The body responds to changes from stimuli, either internal or external. Usually the change is accomplished by a negative feedback mechanism. This means the body's response reverses the stimulus to assist in maintaining homeostasis. For example, if your body temperature rises on a hot day, sweating occurs. This helps to decrease the body's temperature. But, with continued, excessive sweating, dehydration could result. To prevent dehydration, thirst occurs. As the thirst is quenched (through fluid intake), the body's temperature again rises. Thus, sweating and thirst assist in maintaining homeostasis.

In positive feedback, the response to the stimulus does not cause the reversal of the stimulus, but instead actually causes it to continue. One example is childbirth. As oxytocin is secreted, the uterus contracts. As the uterus contracts and the cervix begins to stretch, more oxytocin is secreted. The cycle continues. When delivery of baby and placenta is completed, the sequence is interrupted.

The Human Body: Levels of Organization

The human body is organized in different levels (see Figure 19-1). These include atoms (the smallest unit), molecules, cells, tissues, organs, systems, and finally the body. As you study the body, you will find that organ systems often depend on each other, or at least assist each other, in completing the required functions for a healthy life.

Atoms

The first level of organization of the human body consists of atoms. The atom is the smallest chemical unit of matter. Chemical elements are made up of atoms, and the number of protons, neutrons, and electrons that are contained within creates each element. An element cannot be separated into substances that differ from itself by use of ordinary chemical means. A compound is composed of two or more parts that combine in definite proportions by weight.

Atoms are composed of three types of particles: protons, neutrons, and electrons. Protons and neutrons are responsible for most of the atomic mass. The mass of an electron is very small. Both the protons and neutrons reside in the nucleus. Protons have a positive (+) charge, neutrons have no charge—they are neutral. Electrons reside in orbitals around the nucleus. They have a negative charge (−). The number of protons determines the atomic number. The number of protons in an element is constant, but neutron number may vary, so mass number may also vary.

Molecules

A molecule is the smallest part of a substance called a compound that can still be considered that substance. For example, a molecule of water is the smallest bit of water that is still water. A molecule of a substance cannot be seen by the naked eye—a drop of water is made up of many, many molecules of water. Molecules are composed of atoms joined together chemically. Molecules do not have an electrical charge.

Scientists believe that molecules are always moving. They can be solids, liquids, or gases, and those that move the most are the farthest apart when they are gases. Molecules are closest together and move the most slowly when they are solids. Molecules whose movement is between those of gases and those of solids are liquids. A formula tells what elements make up a molecule. For example, a molecule of water is made up of two hydrogen atoms and one oxygen atom. The formula for a molecule

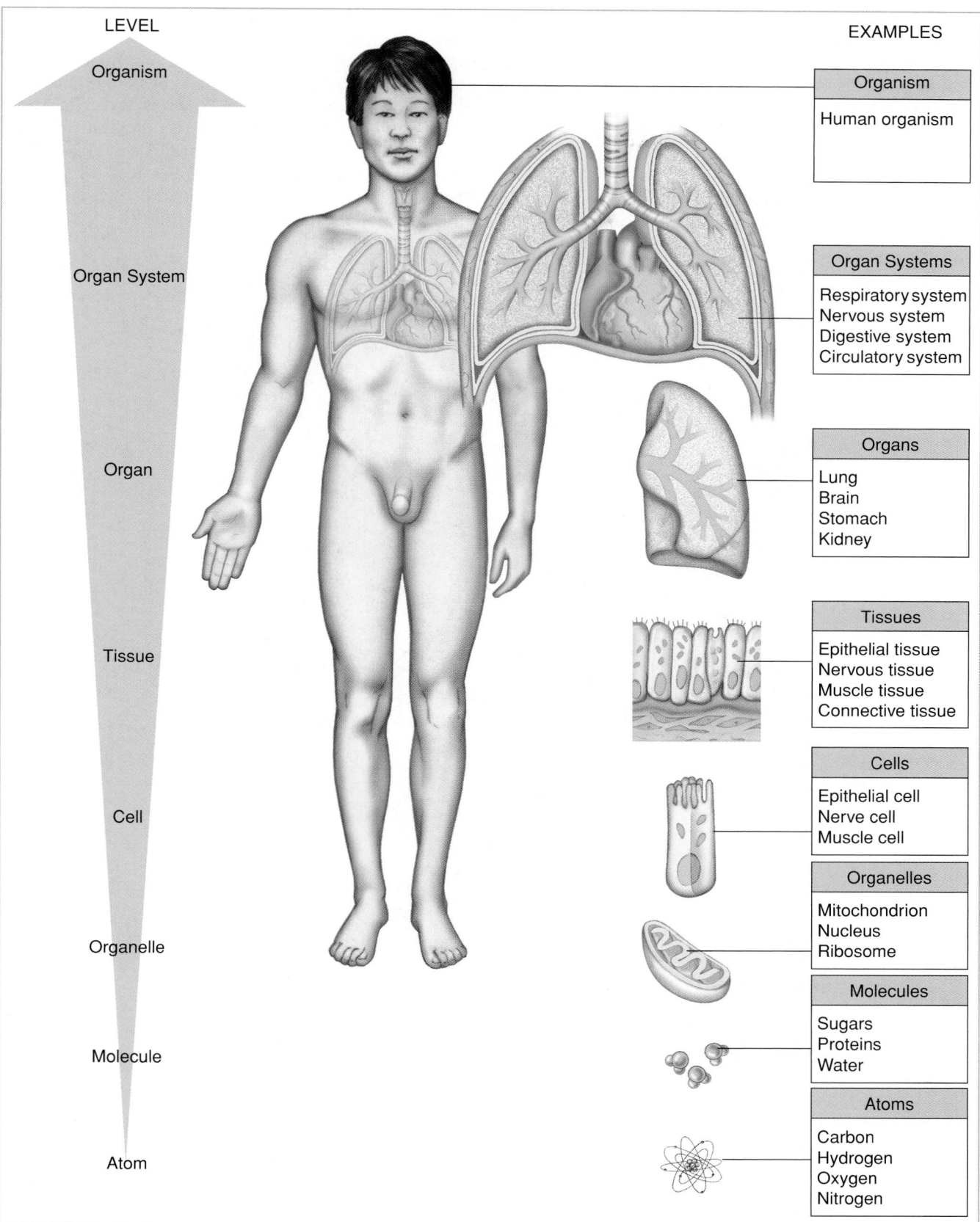

LEVEL

Organism

Organ System

Organ

Tissue

Cell

Organelle

Molecule

Atom

EXAMPLES

Organism

Human organism

Organ Systems

Respiratory system
Nervous system
Digestive system
Circulatory system

Organs

Lung
Brain
Stomach
Kidney

Tissues

Epithelial tissue
Nervous tissue
Muscle tissue
Connective tissue

Cells

Epithelial cell
Nerve cell
Muscle cell

Organelles

Mitochondrion
Nucleus
Ribosome

Molecules

Sugars
Proteins
Water

Atoms

Carbon
Hydrogen
Oxygen
Nitrogen

FIGURE 19-1 Organization of the human body.

of water is H_2O. Finally, molecules come in different sizes and molecular weights. Because of this, their atoms can be arranged in different ways. Molecules in substances can be split up in chemical reactions to form other molecules. They can also recombine into larger molecules or be broken down into smaller molecules.

Cells

The cell is one of the most basic units of life, and cells are often described as the basic building blocks of the human body (see Figure 19-2). There are millions of different types of cells. Some cells are organisms unto themselves, such as microscopic amoebas and bacteria cells. Other cells only function as part of a larger organism, such as the cells that make up your body. The cell is the smallest unit of life in our bodies. The body has brain cells, skin cells, liver cells, stomach cells, and the list goes on. All of these cells have unique functions and features, and all have some recognizable similarities.

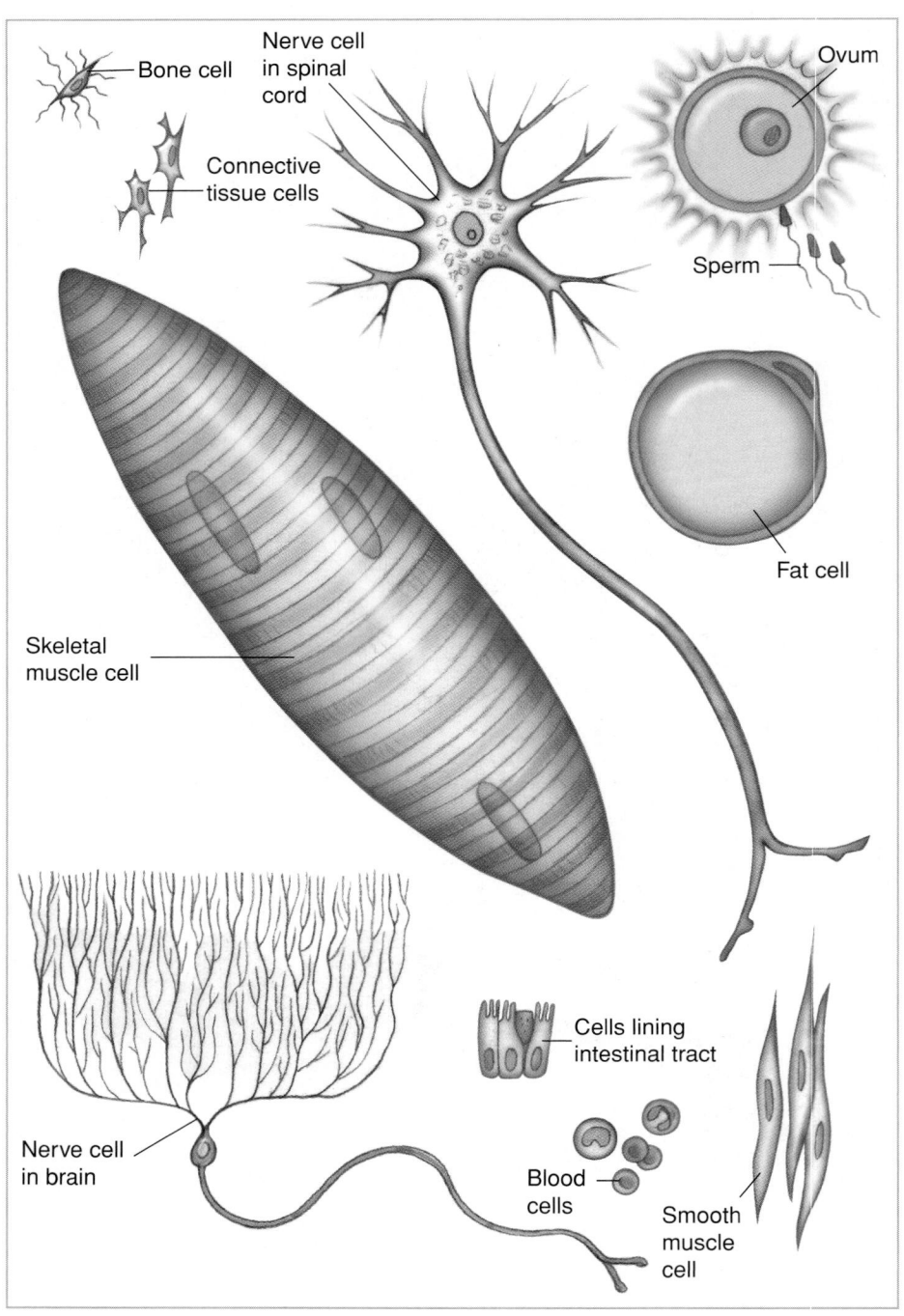

FIGURE 19-2   Cells are often described as the basic building blocks of the human body. There are millions of different cells.

All cells have a "skin," called the cell membrane, that protects them from the outside environment. The cell membrane regulates the movement of water, nutrients, and wastes into and out of the cell. Inside of the cell membrane are the working parts of the cell. At the center of the cell is the cell nucleus. The cell nucleus contains the cell's DNA (deoxyribonucleic acid), the genetic code that coordinates protein synthesis. In addition to the nucleus, there are many organelles inside of the cell—small structures that help carry out the day-to-day operations of the cell. One important cellular organelle is the ribosome. Ribosomes participate in protein synthesis. The transcription phase of protein synthesis takes places in the cell nucleus. After this step is complete, the RNA (ribonucleic acid) leaves the nucleus and travels to the cell's ribosomes, where translation occurs. Another important cellular organelle is the mitochondrion. Mitochondria (many mitochondrion) are often referred to as the power plants of the cell because many of the reactions that produce energy take place in mitochondria. Also important in the life of a cell are the lysosomes. Lysosomes are organelles that contain enzymes that aid in the digestion of nutrient molecules and other materials. Figure 19-3 shows the major parts of the cell and the structures located within each individual cell.

Cell Membrane

The cell membrane is a lipid bilayer that allows for selective permeability, meaning it allows certain substances to enter the cell and prevents others from entering. It is responsible for controlling transport in and out of the cell and for helping to maintain the cell's shape.

Cytoplasm

Cytoplasm is basically the substance that fills the cell. It is a jelly-like material that is 80 percent water and usually clear in color. It is more like a viscous (thick) gel than a watery substance, but it liquefies when shaken or stirred. Cytoplasm, which can also be referred to as cytosol, means "cell substance." This name is very fitting because cytoplasm is the substance of life that serves as a molecular soup in which all of the cell's organelles are suspended and held together by a fatty membrane. The cytoplasm is found inside the cell membrane, surrounding the nuclear envelope and the cytoplasmic organelles. Cytoplasm is also the home of the cytoskeleton, a network of cytoplasmic filaments that are responsible for the movement of the cell and give the cell its shape. The cytoplasm contains dissolved nutrients and helps dissolve waste products. The cytoplasm helps materials move around the cell by moving and churning through

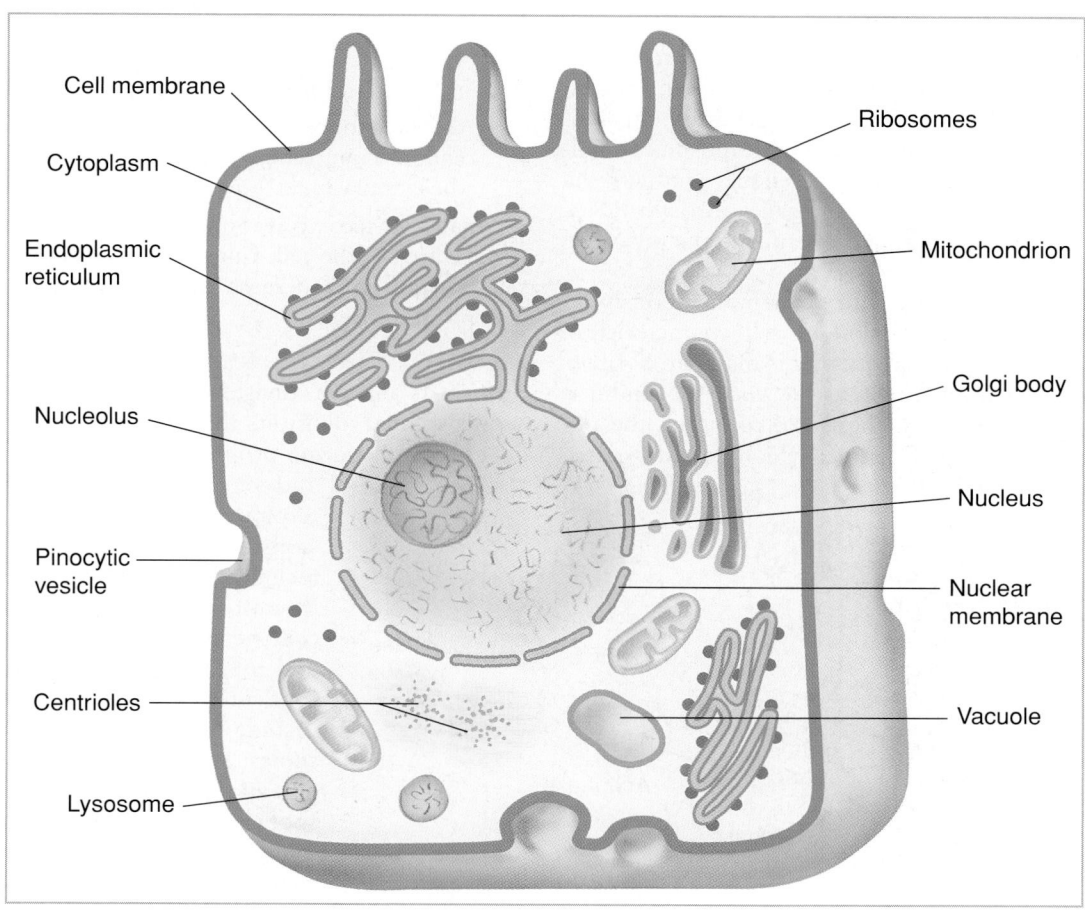

FIGURE 19-3 Major parts of the cell and the structures located inside the cell.

a process called *cytoplasmic streaming*. The nucleus often flows with the cytoplasm changing the shape as it moves. The cytoplasm contains many salts and is an excellent conductor of electricity, which therefore creates a medium for the vesicles, or mechanics of the cell. The function of the cytoplasm and the organelles within it are critical to the cell's survival.

Nucleus

The nucleus, which is known as the control center of the cell, is a remarkable organelle because it forms the package for our genes and their controlling factors. Its functions include the storage of genes on chromosomes, organization of genes into chromosomes to allow cell division, transport of genetic products via nuclear pores, production of messages through RNA, production of ribosomes, and organizing the uncoiling of DNA to replicate key genes.

The nucleus is necessary for growth, metabolism reproduction, and transmission of cell characteristics. Within the nucleus is a sphere that is made up of fibers and granules. This is known as the *nucleolus* and it is necessary for protein synthesis. Surrounding the nucleus is the nuclear membrane, which contains chromosomes. These thread-like structures are made up of DNA that can be described as a double helix. This means that it is formed from two long chains of nucleic acid that twist around each other. Nucleic acid, present in chromosomes of cells, is the chemical basis of heredity. The DNA provides the cell's genetic makeup, or "blueprint." DNA is absolutely necessary for cell reproduction. RNA is a single chain of chemical bases. RNA molecules direct the formation of proteins. The two types of RNA are mRNA and tRNA. Each of these is important for protein synthesis.

The portions of the cell that provide for work and storage include the following:

- Endoplasmic reticulum—This is a network of tubules through the nucleus and cytoplasm.
- Mitochondria—Mitochondria supply most of the ATP (energy) so they are referred to as the "power house" of the cell.
- Golgi apparatus—The Golgi apparatus is a series of flat, membranous sacs. It secretes substances such as mucus.
- Lysosomes—Lysosomes contain digestive enzymes. They phagocytize bacteria. (*Phag/o* means "to ingest or engulf" or "to eat.")
- Centrioles—The function of centrioles is to organize the spindle fibers during cell division. Centrioles are necessary for mitosis.
- Ribosomes—Ribosomes are the site of protein synthesis. Some are located on the surface of the rough endoplasmic reticulum. Some float freely within the cytoplasm.

Small hair-like projections, called cilia, increase the surface area of the cell. Cilia propel substances along a cell's surface and increase the cell's ability to absorb water and nutrients.

Mitosis and Cell Division

Mitosis is nuclear division plus cytokinesis, or the actual cellular division, that produces two identical daughter cells during prophase, metaphase, anaphase, and telophase (see Figure 19-4). Interphase is often included in discussions of mitosis, but interphase is technically not part of the process of mitosis. During interphase, the cell is engaged in metabolic activity and preparing for mitosis (the next four phases that lead up to and include nuclear division). Chromosomes are not clearly distinguishable in the nucleus, although a dark spot called the nucleolus may be visible. The cell may contain a pair of centrioles, which are organizational

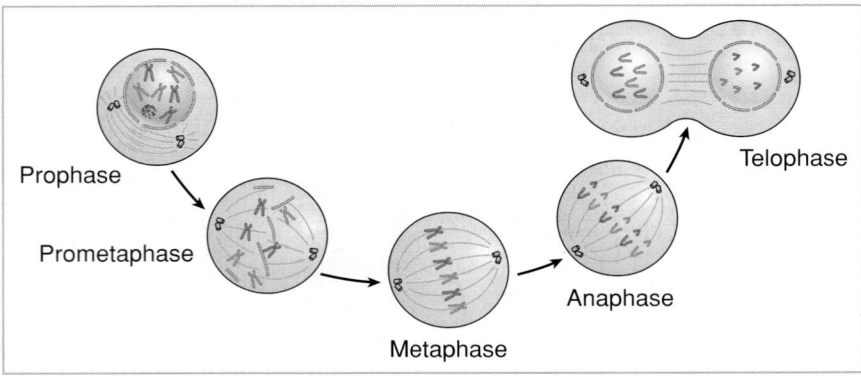

Prophase
Prometaphase
Metaphase
Anaphase
Telophase

FIGURE 19-4 Stages of mitosis.

sites for microtubules. Chromatin in the nucleus begins to condense and becomes visible in the light microscope as chromosomes. The nucleolus disappears. Centrioles begin moving to opposite ends of the cell and fibers extend from the centromeres. Some fibers cross the cell to form the mitotic spindle. During the prophase, the nuclear membrane disperses. Proteins attach to the centromeres, creating the kinetochores. Microtubules attach at the kinetochores and the chromosomes begin moving.

During the metaphase, spindle fibers align the chromosomes along the middle of the cell nucleus. This line is referred to as the metaphase plate. This organization helps to ensure that in the next phase, when the chromosomes are separated, each new nucleus will receive one copy of each chromosome.

Anaphase occurs when the paired chromosomes separate at the kinetochores and move to opposite sides of the cell. Motion results from a combination of kinetochore movement along the spindle. This is followed by the telophase. During this process, the chromatids arrive at opposite poles of the cell, and new membranes form around the daughter nuclei. The chromosomes then disperse and are no longer visible under the light microscope. The spindle fibers also disperse, and cytokinesis, or the partitioning of the cell, may also begin during this stage.

Meiosis

Meiosis is a two-part cell division process in organisms that sexually reproduce which results in gametes with one-half the number of chromosomes of the parent cell. Meiosis I encompasses four stages: prophase I, metaphase I, anaphase I, and telophase I. The largest differences between mitosis and meiosis occur in prophase I. Prophase I is usually longer in duration when compared to prophase in mitosis and it is usually much more complex. It can take days for prophase I to complete. It is estimated that prophase I accounts for some 85 to 95 percent of the total time for meiosis. Metaphase I is of much shorter duration and complexity when compared to prophase I. Anaphase I is also very similar to anaphase in mitosis. Likewise, telophase I is similar to telophase in mitosis. Meiosis II is the second part of the meiotic process. Much of the process is similar to mitosis and meiosis I. In prophase II, if needed, the nuclear membrane and nuclei break up while the spindle "network" appears and the chromosomes begin migrating to the metaphase II plate (at the cell's equator). During metaphase II, the chromosomes line up at the metaphase II plate at the cell's center. The kinetochores of the sister chromatids point toward opposite poles. In anaphase II, the sister chromatids separate and move toward the opposite cell poles. And in telophase II, distinct nuclei form at the opposite poles and cytokinesis occurs. Finally, at the end of meiosis II, there are four daughter cells each with one-half the number of chromosomes of the original parent cell.

Tissues

A grouping of cells creates a tissue. Each tissue performs a specialized function, depending on the types of cells that create it. There are four types of tissues in the body: epithelial, connective, muscle, and nerve (see Figure 19-5).

Epithelial Tissue

Epithelial tissue is a flat arrangement of cells that forms the skin, lines and covers the organs, lines the walls of cavities, and forms tubes, ducts, and some glands. Epithelial cells have four functions: protection, absorption, secretion, and excretion.

Connective Tissue

Connective tissue is the most abundant tissue in the body. All parts of the body have connective tissue either assisting in the construction of or holding different organs in place. Bones are dense connective tissue. Tendons (the structures that hold muscle to bone) and muscle sheaths are other examples of connective tissue. Blood is also a type of connective tissue. Blood is the only liquid tissue in the body.

Muscle Tissue

Muscle is used for movement. The primary function of muscle tissue is to contract or shorten. The three types of muscle tissue are skeletal, smooth, and cardiac. Skeletal muscle tissue is part of the skeleton and assists with voluntary movement of the body. The tissue is striated, meaning that it appears to have stripes.

Smooth muscle tissue is found in the viscera (internal organs). It is nonstriated and is involuntary muscle. It is not controlled through active participation of movement. An example of this is peristalsis (wave-like contractions) such as occurs during the movement of food through the intestinal tract.

Cardiac muscle tissue is found only in the heart. The cardiac muscle is called the *myocardium* and has the function of pumping blood.

Nerve Tissue

Nerve tissue is the functional part of the nervous system. Neurons, or nerve cells, have the properties of excitability, which means they are active, and conductivity, which means that they transmit impulses.

Body Organs and Systems

The human body is made up of organs, which are groups of tissues that serve a common purpose or function. When a group of organs works together to perform a specific function, it is called a system (see Figure 19-6).

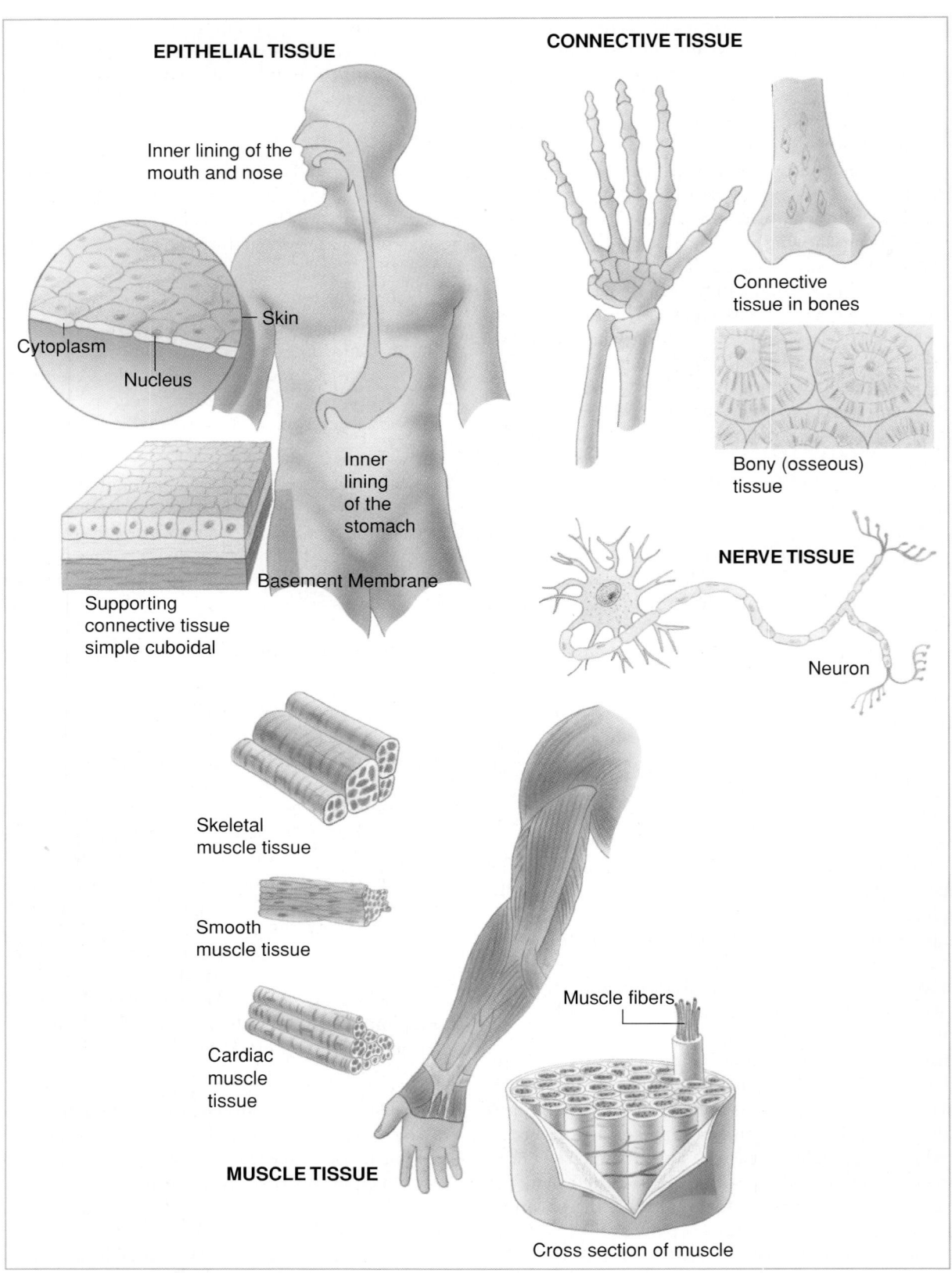

EPITHELIAL TISSUE

Inner lining of the mouth and nose

Cytoplasm

Nucleus

Skin

Inner lining of the stomach

Basement Membrane

Supporting connective tissue simple cuboidal

CONNECTIVE TISSUE

Connective tissue in bones

Bony (osseous) tissue

NERVE TISSUE

Neuron

Skeletal muscle tissue

Smooth muscle tissue

Cardiac muscle tissue

Muscle fibers

MUSCLE TISSUE

Cross section of muscle

FIGURE 19-5 Types of tissue in the human body.

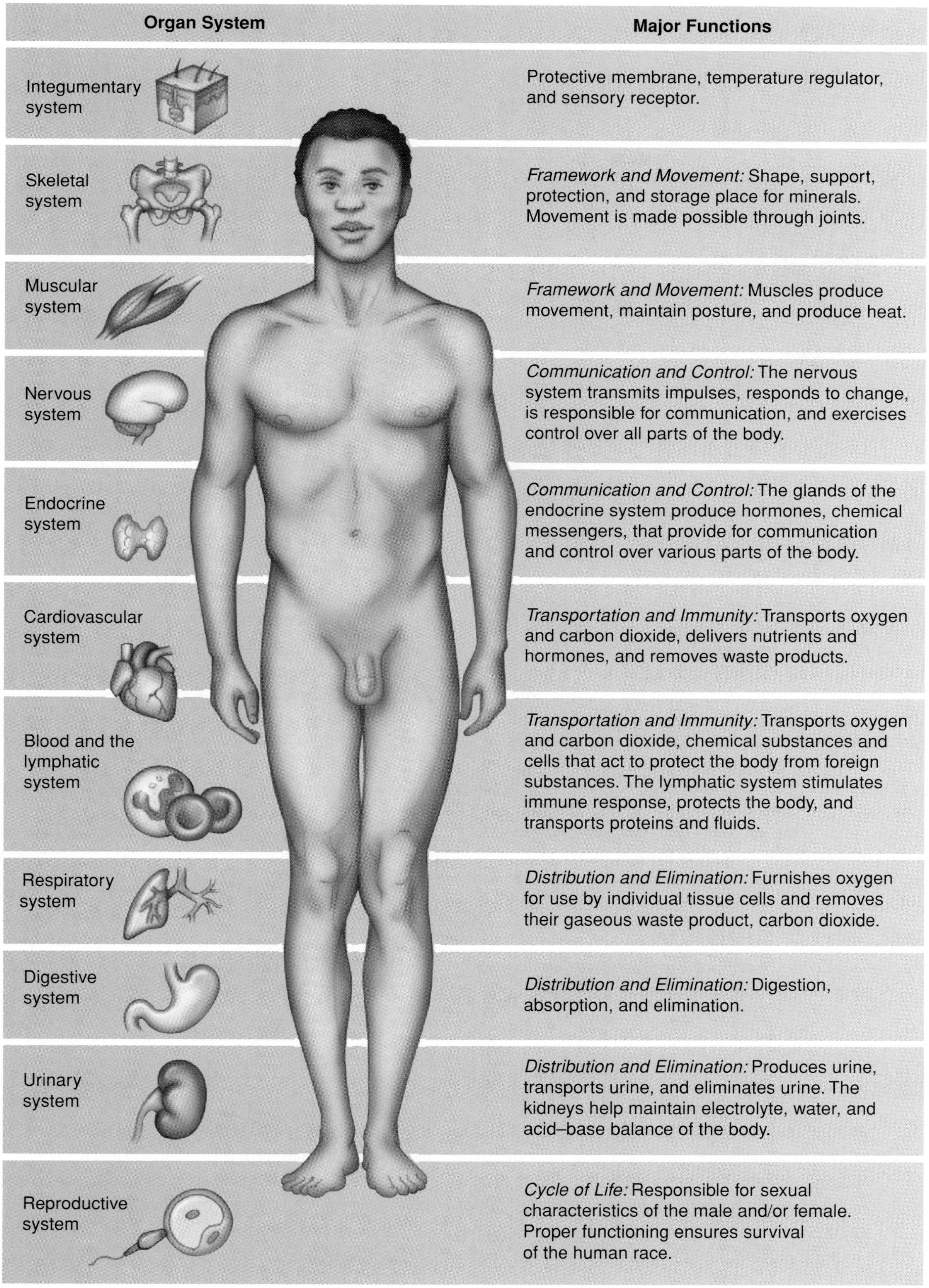

Organ System	Major Functions
Integumentary system	Protective membrane, temperature regulator, and sensory receptor.
Skeletal system	*Framework and Movement:* Shape, support, protection, and storage place for minerals. Movement is made possible through joints.
Muscular system	*Framework and Movement:* Muscles produce movement, maintain posture, and produce heat.
Nervous system	*Communication and Control:* The nervous system transmits impulses, responds to change, is responsible for communication, and exercises control over all parts of the body.
Endocrine system	*Communication and Control:* The glands of the endocrine system produce hormones, chemical messengers, that provide for communication and control over various parts of the body.
Cardiovascular system	*Transportation and Immunity:* Transports oxygen and carbon dioxide, delivers nutrients and hormones, and removes waste products.
Blood and the lymphatic system	*Transportation and Immunity:* Transports oxygen and carbon dioxide, chemical substances and cells that act to protect the body from foreign substances. The lymphatic system stimulates immune response, protects the body, and transports proteins and fluids.
Respiratory system	*Distribution and Elimination:* Furnishes oxygen for use by individual tissue cells and removes their gaseous waste product, carbon dioxide.
Digestive system	*Distribution and Elimination:* Digestion, absorption, and elimination.
Urinary system	*Distribution and Elimination:* Produces urine, transports urine, and eliminates urine. The kidneys help maintain electrolyte, water, and acid–base balance of the body.
Reproductive system	*Cycle of Life:* Responsible for sexual characteristics of the male and/or female. Proper functioning ensures survival of the human race.

FIGURE 19-6   Organ systems of the human body with major functions.

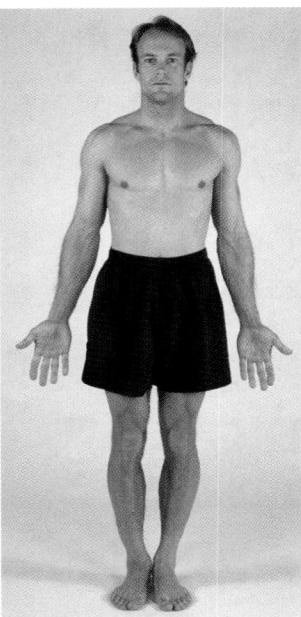

FIGURE 19-7 Anatomical position.

Anatomical Locations and Positions

In discussing the anatomy and physiology of the body, specific terms are used to determine relationships of the parts of the body. For example, in the anatomical position (see Figure 19-7), the body is assumed to be standing, with the feet together, the arms to the side, and the head, eyes, and palms of the hands facing forward. To ensure consistency of description, it is important to keep the anatomical position constantly in mind. This last point is an important one, because in the normal relaxed position of the body, the thumb points anteriorly. In anatomical parlance, the thumb is a lateral structure, not an anterior one. (Note, however, as discussed in Patient Education, that your patients may not understand this terminology.)

Directions of the Body

Directional terms describe the positions of structures relative to other structures or locations in the body.

The directional anatomical terms are shown in Figure 19-8 and include the following:

- Superior or cranial: toward the head end of the body; upper (example: the hand is part of the superior extremity)
- Inferior or caudal: away from the head; lower (example: the foot is part of the inferior extremity)
- Anterior or ventral: front (example: the kneecap is located on the anterior side of the leg)
- Posterior or dorsal: back (example: the shoulder blades are located on the posterior side of the body)
- Medial: toward the midline of the body (example: the middle toe is located at the medial side of the foot)
- Lateral: away from the midline of the body (example: the little toe is located at the lateral side of the foot)
- Proximal: toward or nearest the trunk or the point of origin of a part (example: the proximal end of the femur joins with the pelvic bone)
- Distal: away from or farthest from the trunk or the point or origin of a part (example: the hand is located at the distal end of the forearm)

Planes of the Body

Medical professionals often refer to sections of the body in terms of anatomical planes (flat surfaces). These planes are imaginary lines—vertical or horizontal—drawn through an upright body. The following terms are used to describe a specific body part (see Figure 19-9):

- Coronal plane (frontal plane): A vertical plane running from side to side; divides the body or any of its parts into anterior and posterior portions.
- Sagittal plane (median plane): A vertical plane running from front to back; divides the body or any of its parts into right and left sides.
- Axial plane (transverse plane): A horizontal plane; divides the body or any of its parts into upper and lower parts.

Patient Education

As a medical assistant, you will become accustomed to using medical language. Remember that the patient may not understand medical terminology and will thus require explanations. You may be asked to explain prescription instructions or procedure preparations to patients. Always use terms that the patient understands, yet without making the patient feel you are talking down to him or her. Ask the patient for confirmation of his or her understanding of the information. An informed patient will be more compliant. Document patient education on the chart.

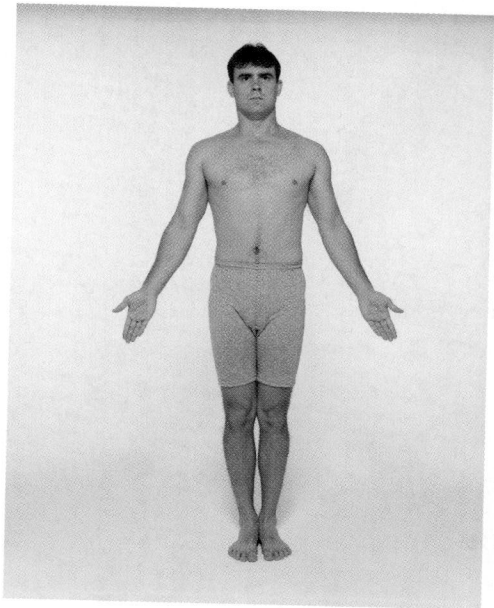

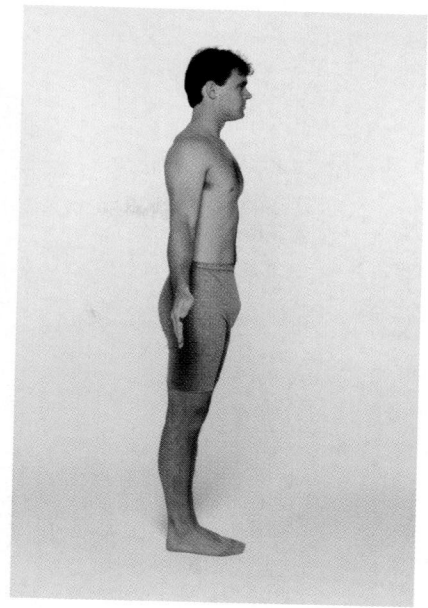

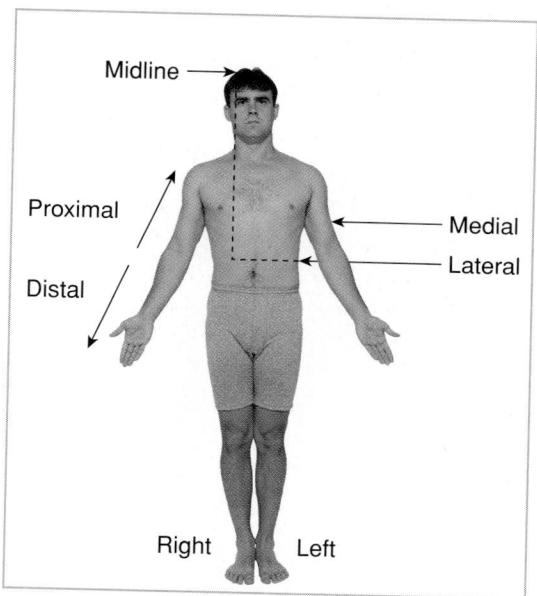

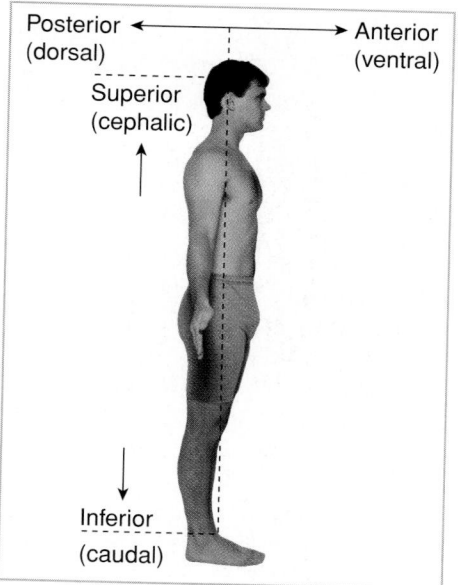

FIGURE 19-8 Directional anatomical terms.

Body Cavities and Abdominal Regions

The cavities, or spaces, of the body contain the internal organs, or viscera (see Figure 19-10). The two main cavities are called the *ventral* and *dorsal cavities*. The ventral is the larger cavity and is subdivided into two parts (thoracic and abdominopelvic cavities) by the diaphragm, a dome-shaped respiratory muscle. The thoracic cavity consists of the upper ventral, or chest, cavity and contains the heart, lungs, trachea, esophagus, large blood vessels, and nerves. The thoracic cavity is bound laterally by the ribs (covered by costal pleura) and the diaphragm caudally (covered by diaphragmatic pleura).

The abdominopelvic cavity is the lower part of the ventral cavity. It can be further divided into two portions: the abdominal portion and the pelvic portion. The abdominal cavity contains most of the gastrointestinal tract as well as the kidneys and adrenal glands. The abdominal cavity is bound cranially by the diaphragm, laterally by the body wall, and caudally by the pelvic cavity. The pelvic cavity contains most of the urogenital system as well as the rectum. The pelvic cavity is bounded cranially by the abdominal cavity, dorsally by the sacrum, and laterally by the pelvis. The dorsal cavity is the smaller of the two main cavities. As its name implies, it contains organs lying more posterior in the body. The dorsal cavity,

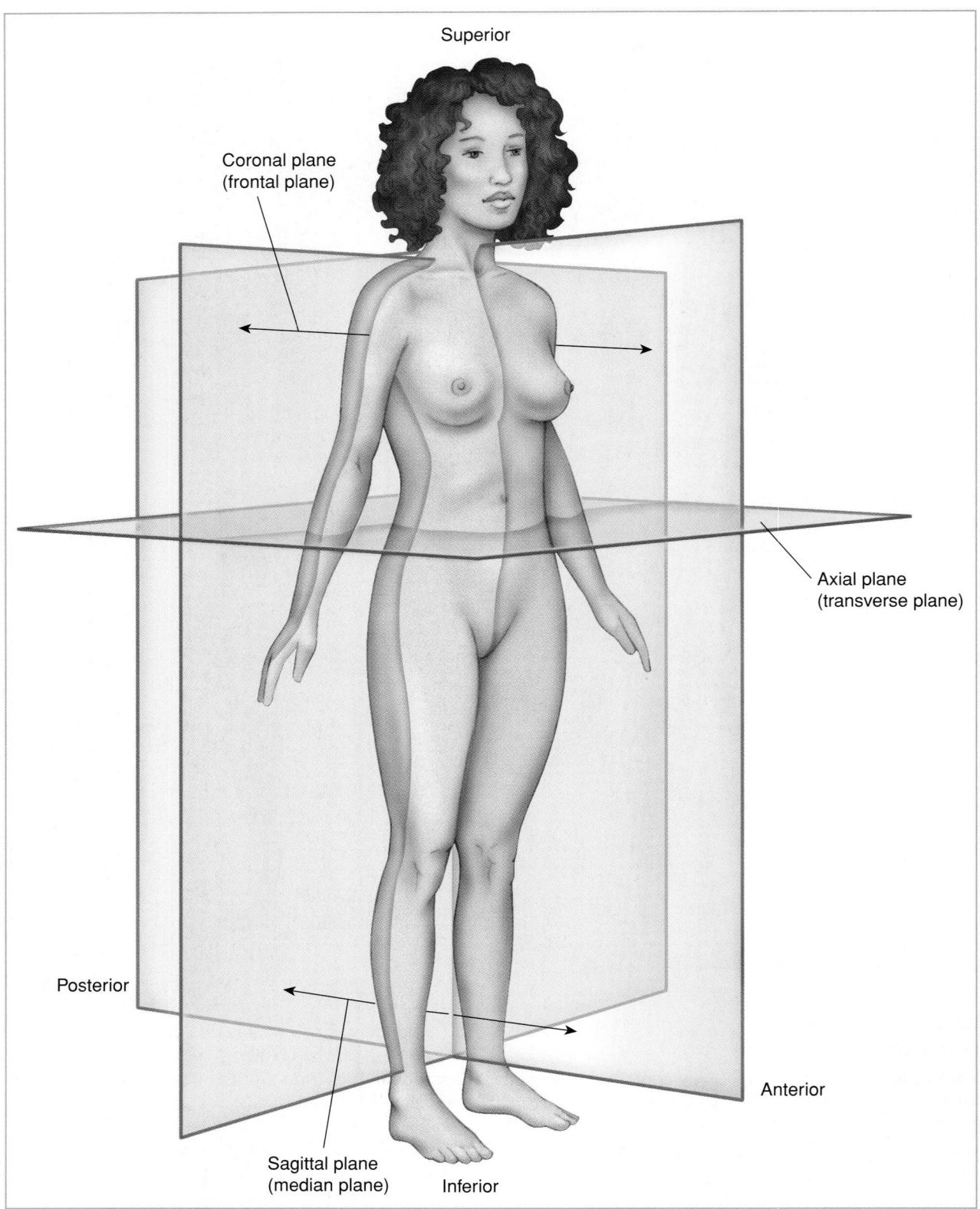

Superior

Coronal plane
(frontal plane)

Axial plane
(transverse plane)

Posterior

Anterior

Sagittal plane
(median plane)

Inferior

FIGURE 19-9 Anatomical planes.

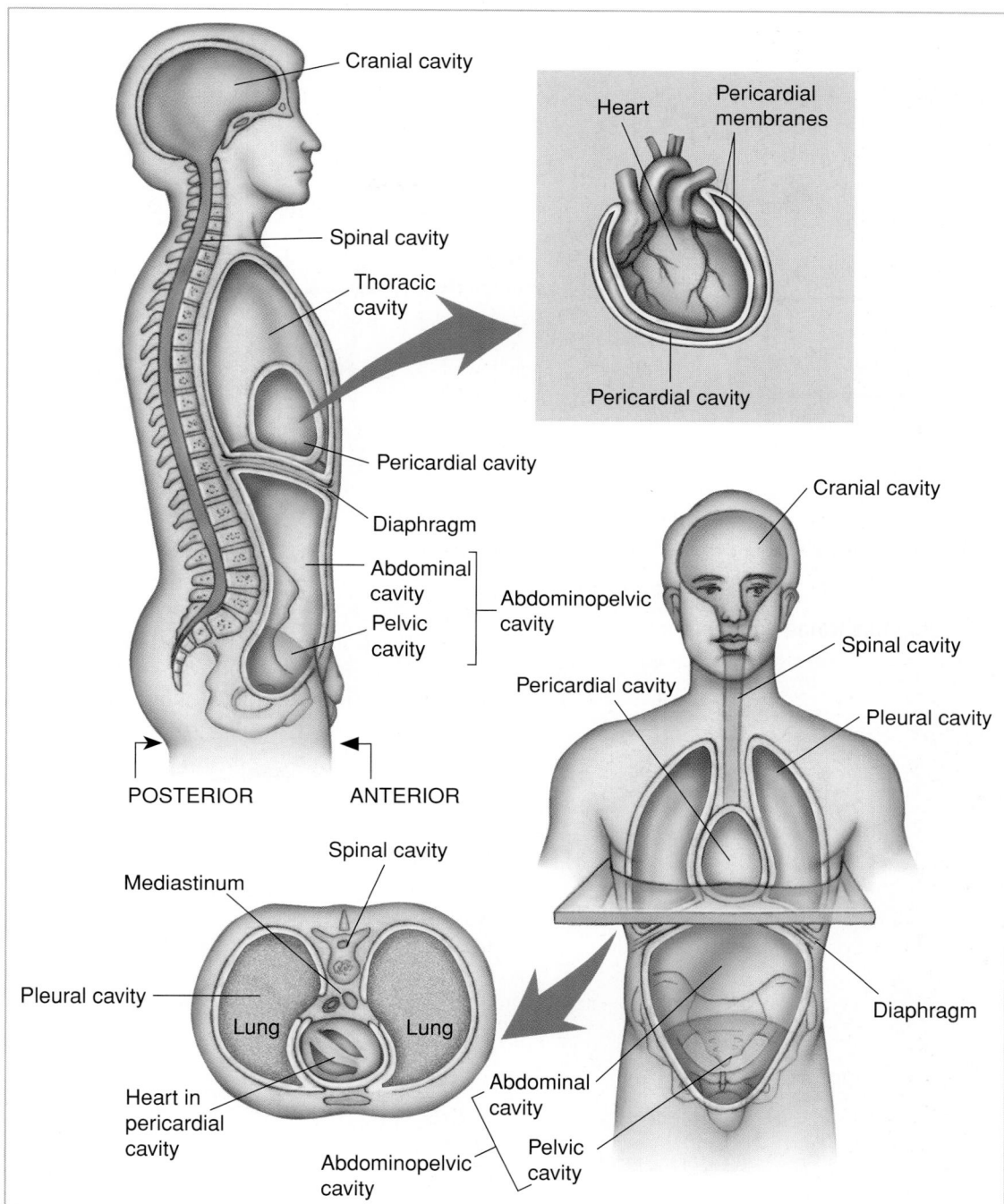

FIGURE 19-10 Body cavities.

again, can be divided into two portions. The upper portion, or the cranial cavity, houses the brain, and the lower portion, or vertebral canal houses the spinal cord.

Abdominal Regions and Quadrants

The abdominopelvic cavity, which can be seen in Figure 19-11, is frequently divided into nine regions, including:

- Right and left hypochondriac
- Right and left lumbar
- Right and left iliac
- Epigastric
- Umbilical
- Hypogastric

The abdomen is also divided into four quadrants. These are:

- Right upper quadrant (RUQ)
- Left upper quadrant (LUQ)
- Right lower quadrant (RLQ)
- Left lower quadrant (LLQ)

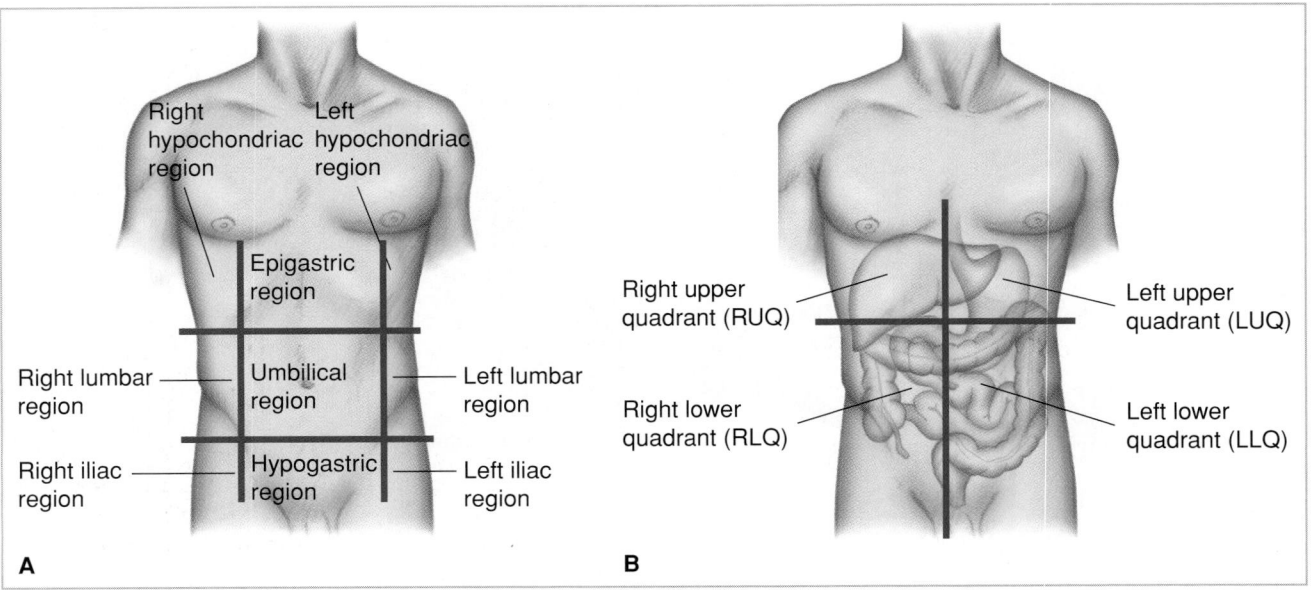

FIGURE 19-11 (A) The nine regions of the abdominopelvic cavity. (B) The four quadrants of the abdomen.

TABLE 19-1	**Frequently Noted Landmarks**
Landmark/Term	**Refers to**
Antecubital	Bend of the elbow
Axillary	Armpit
Buccal	Cheek
Cervical	Neck
Deltoid	Shoulder
Femoral	Thigh
Gluteal	Buttocks
Hepatic	Liver
Lumbar	Lower back
Occipital	Back of the head
Patellar	Kneecap
Popliteal	Behind the knee
Pulmonary	Lungs
Renal	Kidney
Sural	Calf of the leg
Thoracic	Chest
Volar (palmer)	Palm of the hand

Landmarks

The body has many landmarks. Table 19-1 provides a listing of the most frequently noted landmarks. Landmark terms should be used when charting information or when relaying information to other health care personnel.

Chemistry

Cells must receive nourishment and also eliminate wastes. For this to occur, materials must be transported to and from the cell, or even within the cell. There are two mechanisms in which this occurs. The first, which does not require energy from the cell, is through passive

Cultural Considerations

An interpreter might be needed for patients who speak a language other than English, or who perhaps have English as a second language. Dictionaries can assist the staff with commonly used words and may be purchased from local bookstores. Anything that can be done to make the patient more at ease in your office setting will be beneficial.

transport Passive transport may involve any number of processes, including the following:

- Diffusion: This is movement of dissolved particles from an area of greater concentration to an area of lesser concentration. This action requires no cell energy.

- Osmosis: This is a type of diffusion in which water is pulled through a semipermeable membrane. Molecules are again transported from an area of greater concentration to an area of lesser concentration. This also requires no cell energy.

- Filtration: In filtration, dissolved particles are diffused through membranes but only mechanical pressure is required. Whether or not filtration occurs depends on the size of the cell's pores. Only liquids are allowed through the barrier.

The second method by which cells may become nourished and their wastes eliminated is through **active transport**. Active transport requires energy to carry material from areas of lesser concentration to an area of greater concentration. In this method, the cell is able to obtain what it requires from the tissue fluid. These mechanisms include:

- Phagocytosis: In this method, the cell engulfs a solid particle, such as bacteria.

- Pinocytosis: In this method, the cell "drinks" the fluid required.

Electrolytes

Electrolyte is a "medical/scientific" term for salts, specifically ions. The term *electrolyte* means that this ion is electrically charged and moves to either a negative (cathode) or positive (anode) electrode. Ions that move to the cathode are positively charged and are called *cations*. Ions that move to the anode and are negatively charged are called *anions*. Body fluids, such as blood, plasma, and interstitial fluid (the fluid between cells), are like seawater and have a high concentration of sodium chloride. The electrolytes in sodium chloride include sodium ion (Na^+), the cation, and chloride ion (Cl), the anion. The major electrolytes in the human body include sodium (Na^+), potassium (K^+), chloride (Cl), calcium (Ca), magnesium (Mg), bicarbonate (HCO_3), phosphate (PO_4), and sulfate (SO_4).

Electrolytes are important because they are what your cells (especially nerve, heart, muscle) use to maintain voltages across their cell membranes and to carry electrical impulses (nerve impulses, muscle contractions) across themselves and to other cells. Your kidneys work to keep the electrolyte concentrations in your blood constant despite changes in your body. For example, when you exercise heavily, you lose electrolytes in your sweat, particularly sodium and potassium. These electrolytes must be replaced to keep the electrolyte concentrations of your body fluids constant. Therefore, many sports drinks have sodium chloride or potassium chloride added to them. They also have sugar and flavorings to provide your body with extra energy and to make the drink taste better.

Genetics and Heredity

Genetics is the study of the makeup of animals or plants. DNA carries all the information needed for protein synthesis and replication of cells. In living organisms DNA is organized in chromosomes and is located in the nucleus of each cell.

Genetic Engineering

Genetic engineering is defined as making or changing an organism's DNA. There are many forms of genetic engineering, some occurring naturally whereas others are human-made. Genetic engineering in the current state is a relatively new science, the effects of which are not yet known. This causes controversy as to whether or not genetic engineering is safe or ethical.

Genetic engineering has been going on for years in the form of natural selection and artificial breeding. Natural selection, or "survival of the fittest" as it is sometimes known, occurs when the environment chooses the traits that are best suited to the current environment and allows animals with those traits to reproductively mature and reproduce. This changing of the genes within a species is nature's way of ensuring survival. Artificial breeding is human intervention in the process of natural selection. Humans choose traits for an animal that they think are beneficial and then breed those traits into the animal's offspring. An example of this is domestic dogs, all of which are descended from the wolf family through artificial breeding.

Genetic Fingerprinting

The chemical structure of everyone's DNA is the same. The only difference between people (or any animal) is the order of the base pairs. There are so many millions of base pairs in each person's DNA that although—it is possible to have the exact same DNA sequences—it is very unlikely. This means that every person has a different sequence from which he or she can be identified. DNA fingerprinting is carried out by obtaining a small amount of the person's DNA, usually from hair, sexual fluid, blood, or saliva, but any part of a human can be used. This piece of DNA is put through various tests to extract and isolate part of the strand of DNA. This is done by using chemicals such as enzymes and by using electricity to separate the different parts of DNA. This process results in a profile of the person that matches one person and one person only; the only exception to this is for identical twins. The sample is analyzed by a picture showing the DNA patterns in the form of an x-ray photo. If the two patterns from the two DNA samples match, they are very likely to have come from the same person. In the case of proving parentage, DNA from the child is matched to that of the people requesting the test. The tests show the relationship of the people to the particular child by matching both the maternal (mother's) and paternal (father's) DNA fingerprints to the child's. If the DNA fingerprint shows significant similarities, then the people having the test are the parents.

Genetics, Heredity, and Disease

Heredity is the genetic transmission from parent to child. The genes for certain traits are passed down in families from parents to children, and hereditary traits are determined by specific genes.

Individuals carry two genes for each trait, one from the mother's egg and one from the father's sperm. When an individual reproduces, the two genes split up (segregate) and end up in separate gametes.

Genetic Disorders

Genetic disorders are medical conditions caused by mutations in a gene or a set of genes. Mutations are changes in the DNA sequence of a gene. They can happen at any time, from when we are a single cell to when we are 90—or even older! Some people say that there are disorder genes. It is not a gene or genes, however, that cause the illness, but a mutation that causes the normal genes to operate improperly. It is better to say that mutated genes cause genetic disorders. A genetic disorder that is present at birth is frequently referred to as a *congenital disorder*. They may also be called *birth defects*. Listed here are some of the more common congenital disorders:

- Albinism is a congenital, but nonpathological disorder. A recessive gene mutation causes hereditary lack of pigment in the skin, hair, and eyes.

The patient may complain of photophobia and is prone to sunburn because protective melanin is not present.

- Attention deficit hyperactivity disorder (ADHD) is a disease that can affect both children and adults. It is characterized by the person having difficulty organizing and completing a task. The cause may be due to genetic factors, and it is 10 times more prevalent in boys than in girls. There is no known cure, but treatment often includes medications or counseling. Abstinence from certain foods or food additives may be recommended if these are determined to be a part of the cause of hyperactivity. However, symptoms may subside or even disappear with time.

- Cleft palate is a congenital defect in the roof of the mouth that occurs when the palatine bones of the skull do not close properly. The cleft causes a passageway between the mouth and nasal cavities. It may also be associated with a cleft upper lip, and it affects females more often than males. Initially, the infant has special needs for feeding. Surgical repairs are usually performed within the first year of life and are generally successful in repairing the defect.

- Color deficiency is a disorder that was previously called color blindness. It often entails difficulty in distinguishing between reds and greens. It is an inherited, sex-linked disorder, usually passed from mother to son. In total color deficiency, the person is unable to perceive any color at all due to a defect in or absence of cones in the retina.

- Cystic fibrosis (CF) is a chronic and progressive disease usually diagnosed in childhood that causes mucus to become thick, dry, and sticky. The mucus builds up and clogs passages in many of the body's organs, but primarily the lungs and the pancreas. In the lungs, the mucus can lead to serious breathing problems and lung disease. In the pancreas, the mucus can lead to malnutrition and problems with growth and development. People with CF have an average life expectancy of about 32 years, although new treatments offer hope for longer and healthier lives.

- Down syndrome (trisomy 21) is a disorder caused by the person having an extra chromosome, usually number 21 (hence, the name). A few of the major features seen include marked sloping of the forehead, a short broad hand with a single palmer crease (known as a simian crease), and a flat nose. A mother who gives birth after the age of 40 has a higher risk at delivering an infant with Down syndrome. Amniocentesis is generally used as a tool for diagnosing this disorder.

- Fragile X syndrome, also known as Martin-Bell syndrome, Marker X syndrome, and FRAXA syndrome, is the most common form of inherited mental retardation. Individuals with this condition have developmental delays, variable levels of mental retardation, and behavioral and emotional difficulties. They may also have characteristic physical traits. Generally, males are affected with moderate mental retardation and females with mild mental retardation. Fragile X is caused by a mutation in the FMR-1 gene, located on the X chromosome. The role of this gene is unclear, but it is probably important in early development.

- Hemochromatosis is an inherited disorder of excessive body accumulation of iron. It is common among the white population, affecting approximately 1 in 400 individuals of European ancestry. Hemochromatosis patients are believed to absorb excessive amounts of iron from the diet. Since the human body has limited ways of eliminating the absorbed iron, the iron accumulates over time in the liver, bone marrow, pancreas, skin, and testicles. This accumulation of iron in these organs causes them to function poorly. Patients with early hemochromatosis have no symptoms and are unaware of their condition. The disease may be discovered when elevated iron blood levels are noted as a result of routine blood testing. In males, symptoms may not appear until 40 to 50 years of age. Iron deposits in the skin cause darkening of the skin. Because females lose iron through menstrual blood loss, they develop organ damage from iron accumulation 15 to 20 years later than men on average.

- Hemophilia is a hereditary, sex-linked disorder in which the blood coagulation time is greatly increased. It is due to a recessive gene mutation in the X chromosome. Females carry the recessive gene and transmit the disorder to their male offspring.

- Klinefelter's syndrome is a congenital endocrine disorder. Primary testicular failure occurs that usually is not evident until puberty. The testes are small and firm and gynecomastia may be present. The boy has abnormally long legs. This disorder also can lead to subnormal intelligence.

- Muscular dystrophy is a genetic disease characterized by a gradual atrophy and weakening of the muscle. It is more frequent in males. The most common type is Duchenne's Muscular dystrophy, which accounts for 50% of all cases. The onset is at an early age, and the patient is usually confined to a wheelchair by the age of 12. Death often occurs within 10 to 15 years of onset of symptoms. Unfortunately, there is no successful

Professionalism

A large part of the medical assistant's job is taking messages for the physician. This means that the medical assistant may speak to a patient, gather data for the physician, and then transcribe the information. When doing this, it is essential to first confirm the spelling of the patient's name and the birth date. Many offices use the birth date as a double check to ensure that the correct medical record is accessed. The patient's chief complaint or question is listed first, along with pertinent information about his or her complaint, the medications being taken, and any questions. Be sure that all of the writing is legible and that the message is timed, dated, and signed. Many offices have specific protocols regarding taking messages, the form on which the message is written, and the method of delivering the messages to the physician. These messages are part of the medical record, and should never be scratched out or scribbled on, and should always look professional. Never write messages on scraps of paper. Use the appropriate forms provided by your work facility.

treatment, although physical therapy and exercise are recommended to prevent more atrophy of muscles.

- PKU (phenylketonuria) is due to a recessive gene mutation. A defective enzyme causes the body to be unable to oxidize an amino acid, known as phenylalanine, to tyrosine. If the condition is not treated early, mental retardation occurs due to brain damage. Many states require testing at birth to detect PKU.

- Sickle cell anemia is a hereditary, chronic form of anemia that is due to a recessive gene mutation. It affects millions of people throughout the world and it is particularly common among people whose ancestors came from sub-Saharan Africa; Spanish-speaking regions (South America, Cuba, Central America); Saudi Arabia; India; and Mediterranean countries, such as Turkey, Greece, and Italy. In the United States, sickle cell disease occurs in about 1 in every 500 African-American births and 1 in every 1,000 to 1,400 Hispanic-American births. Erythrocytes, which are usually round, "sickle out," meaning that they take on a half-moon shape. The abnormally shaped cells block blood vessels and can cause a sickle cell "crisis" during times of stress or illness. Sickle cell crisis is characterized by joint pain, thrombosis, and fever.

- Spina bifida is a congenital neural tube defect. The posterior vertebral arch has a developmental anomaly. In some cases, the spinal cord and its membranes may protrude. Most often the abnormality occurs in the lumbar region.
- Talipes (clubfoot) is a congenital deformity of the foot. Treatment may include casting of the foot or special orthopedic shoes to assist with walking.
- Tay-Sachs disease (TSD) is an inherited disorder that tends to affect people of central and northern European Jewish (Ashkenazi) or French-Canadian ancestry. The faulty gene targets the nervous system. Symptoms first appear at around 6 months of age in a previously healthy baby. Over a short period of time, the baby stops moving and smiling, becomes paralyzed, and eventually dies. Most children with TSD die before their fifth birthday. There is no cure.
- Turner's syndrome is a congenital disorder caused by failure of the ovaries to respond to the stimulation of pituitary hormones. Intelligence may be impaired, amenorrhea may be present, and the patient is usually short in stature.

SUMMARY

In this chapter, you have learned of the organizational components of the body. A group of cells with similar functions forms tissues, and tissues with similar functions form organs. These organs then form systems that make up the human body. As each of these systems performs its function, the body can remain in homeostasis. Although disease processes may occur, the body is remarkable in its ability to fight off infections, or in some cases, as in cellular development, even regenerate.

Chapter Review

COMPETENCY REVIEW

1. Define and spell the terms to learn for this chapter.
2. What does the term anatomy mean?
3. What is the substance within the cell called?
4. What are the three types of muscle tissue?
5. What are the four functions of epithelial tissue?
6. What are the two properties of nerve tissue?
7. Which part of the cell is known as the control center?
8. Name the three distinct cavities of the ventral cavity.
9. What is the plane that vertically divides the body into right and left sides?
10. Where is cardiac muscle located?

PREPARING FOR THE CERTIFICATION EXAM

1. What is the basic structural unit of the body?
   A. tissue
   B. organ system
   C. cell
   D. molecule
   E. electrolyte

2. Which plane divides the body into superior and inferior parts?
   A. frontal
   B. midsagittal
   C. sagittal
   D. transverse

3. The cavity containing the heart and lungs is the
   A. abdominopelvic cavity
   B. dorsal cavity
   C. buccal cavity
   D. thoracic cavity

4. Which type of tissue is the most widespread and abundant tissue in the body?
   A. muscle tissue
   B. connective tissue
   C. nervous tissue
   D. epithelial tissue

continued on next page

5. Which plane divides the body into anterior and posterior parts?
   A. sagittal
   B. coronal
   C. transverse
   D. midsagittal

6. Which term means nearer the point of attachment?
   A. proximal
   B. distal
   C. ventral
   D. dorsal
   E. lateral

7. Which of the following would NOT describe smooth muscle?
   A. found in the heart
   B. involuntary
   C. nonstriated
   D. found in visceral organs

8. Which cell organelle phagocytizes bacteria?
   A. endoplasmic reticulum
   B. lysosomes
   C. mitochondria
   D. ribosomes

9. The cell membrane allows diffusion of dissolved particles through membranes while requiring mechanical pressure. This is known as
   A. filtration
   B. facilitated diffusion
   C. osmosis
   D. phagocytosis

10. Homeostasis means
   A. blood stoppage
   B. spreading
   C. maintaining inner balance
   D. study of the function of an organism

CRITICAL THINKING

1. Where is the epigastric region?

2. If Dr. Menendez ordered a test that required the patient to be supine, how would you position the patient?

3. Visualize the imaginary lines dividing the abdomen into quadrants. In which quadrant would Mr. Schultz's pain be localized?

ON THE JOB

Ben is a medical assistant who is taking a medical history on Tyler Jackson. Tyler has a lot of bruises on his left calf on the outside as a result of falling down the stairs. He also has a fracture on his right arm closer to the wrist as a result of the same fall.

1. How would Ben chart these injuries on the medical record using correct directional terms?

INTERNET ACTIVITY

Use the Internet to look up different anatomical direction descriptions (such as lateral wrist).

MediaLink  More on body structure and function, including interactive resources, can be found on the Student CD-ROM accompanying this textbook.

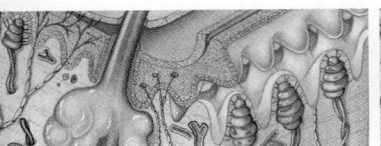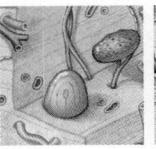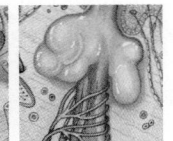

Medical Assistant Role Delineation Chart

HIGHLIGHT indicates material covered in this chapter.

ADMINISTRATIVE

Administrative Procedures

- Perform basic administrative medical assisting functions
- Schedule, coordinate and monitor appointments
- Schedule inpatient/outpatient admissions and procedures
- Understand and apply third-party guidelines
- Obtain reimbursement through accurate claims submission
- Monitor third-party reimbursement
- Understand and adhere to managed care policies and procedures
- *Negotiate managed care contracts*

Practice Finances

- Perform procedural and diagnostic coding
- Apply bookkeeping principles

- Manage accounts receivable
- *Manage accounts payable*
- *Process payroll*
- *Document and maintain accounting and banking records*
- *Develop and maintain fee schedules*
- *Manage renewals of business and professional insurance policies*
- *Manage personnel benefits and maintain records*
- *Perform marketing, financial, and strategic planning*

CLINICAL

Fundamental Principles

- Apply principles of aseptic technique and infection control
- Comply with quality assurance practices
- Screen and follow up patient test results

Diagnostic Orders

- Collect and process specimens
- Perform diagnostic tests

Patient Care

- Adhere to established patient screening procedures
- Obtain patient history and vital signs
- Prepare and maintain examination and treatment areas
- Prepare patient for examinations, procedures and treatments

- Assist with examinations, procedures and treatments
- Prepare and administer medications and immunizations
- Maintain medication and immunization records
- Recognize and respond to emergencies
- Coordinate patient care information with other health care providers
- Initiate IV and administer IV medications with appropriate training and as permitted by state law

GENERAL

Professionalism

- Display a professional manner and image
- Demonstrate initiative and responsibility
- Work as a member of the health care team
- Prioritize and perform multiple tasks
- Adapt to change
- Promote the CMA credential
- Enhance skills through continuing education
- Treat all patients with compassion and empathy
- Promote the practice through positive public relations

Communication Skills

- Recognize and respect cultural diversity
- Adapt communications to individual's ability to understand
- Use professional telephone technique

- Recognize and respond effectively to verbal, nonverbal, and written communications
- Use medical terminology appropriately
- Utilize electronic technology to receive, organize, prioritize and transmit information
- Serve as liaison

Legal Concepts

- Perform within legal and ethical boundaries
- Prepare and maintain medical records
- Document accurately
- Follow employer's established policies dealing with the health care contract
- Implement and maintain federal and state health care legislation and regulations
- Comply with established risk management and safety procedures
- Recognize professional credentialing criteria
- *Develop and maintain personnel, policy and procedure manuals*

Instruction

- Instruct individuals according to their needs
- Explain office policies and procedures
- Teach methods of health promotion and disease prevention
- Locate community resources and disseminate information
- *Develop educational materials*
- *Conduct continuing education activities*

Operational Functions

- Perform inventory of supplies and equipment
- Perform routine maintenance of administrative and clinical equipment
- Apply computer techniques to support office operations
- *Perform personnel management functions*
- *Negotiate leases and prices for equipment and supply contracts*

- *Denotes advanced skills.*

SOURCE: Reprinted by permission of the American Association of Medical Assistants from the AAMA Role Delineation Study: Occupational Analysis of the Medical Assisting Profession.

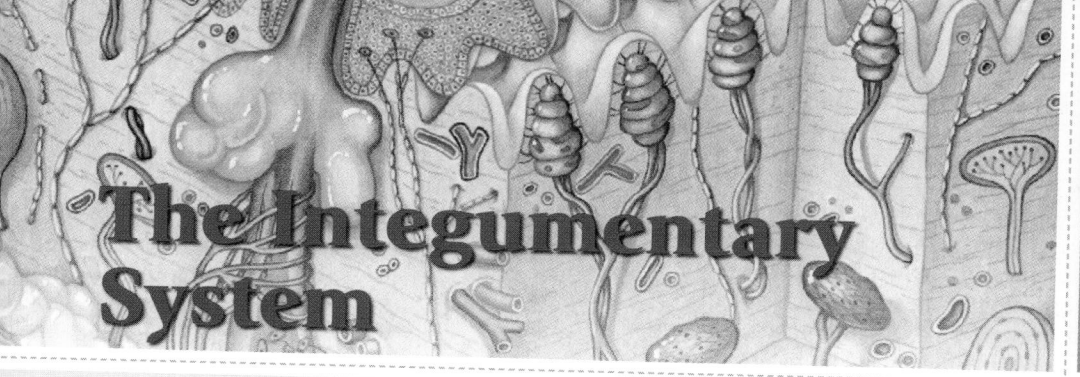

The Integumentary System

Learning Objectives

After completing this chapter, you should be able to:

- Define and spell the terms to learn for this chapter.
- Describe the integumentary system and identify its accessory structures.
- List the functions of the skin.
- Explain skin differences of the child and the older adult.
- Identify and explain common disorders associated with the integumentary system.

OUTLINE

Overview of the Integumentary System	362
Functions of the Integumentary System	362
Layers of the Skin	362
Accessory Structures of the Skin	363
Common Disorders Associated with the Integumentary System	364

Terms to Learn

acne vulgaris
alopecia
cellulitis
contact dermatitis
decubitus ulcer
dermis
eczema
epidermis

folliculitis
herpes simplex
herpes zoster
impetigo
malignant melanoma
pediculosis
psoriasis

rosacea
scabies
sebaceous glands
squamous cell carcinoma
sudoriferous glands
sweat glands
wart

Case Study

CELINE JACKSON IS A 42-YEAR-OLD FEMALE seen by Dr. Black for moderate itching of her fist, with small vesicles on her forearms and redness and swelling on bilateral hands and arms. When questioned, she states that she was working in her backyard, which opens into a wooded area. Although she was not specifically looking, she knows that there is poison ivy growing in the wooded area. There is no redness or itching anywhere else, and she has no history of other allergies and does not take any medications.

Dr. Black diagnoses her with contact dermatitis poison ivy and treats her with antiallergy medicines and corticosteroid therapy. Temovate cream to be applied to the irritated areas twice a day and a Medrol dose pack (low-dose oral steroids) to take as directed.

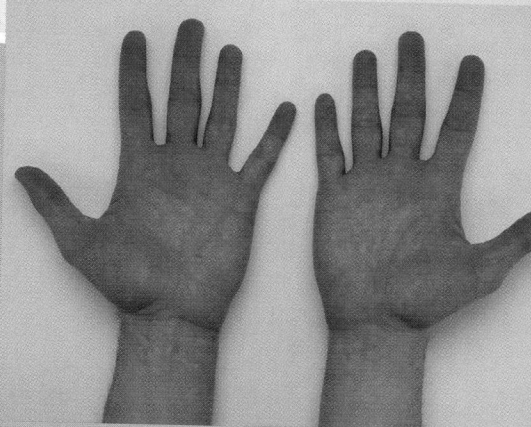

Overview of the Integumentary System

The integumentary system consists of the skin, which is the largest organ in the body. The skin contains 12 to 15 percent of the body's weight, and has a surface area of 1 to 2 meters. Skin is continuous with, but structurally distinct from, mucous membranes that line the mouth, anus, urethra, and vagina. Two distinct layers occur in the skin: the dermis and epidermis. The basic cell type of the epidermis is the keratinocyte, which contains keratin, a fibrous protein. Basal cells are the innermost layer of the epidermis. Melanocytes produce the pigment melanin, and are also located in the inner layer of the epidermis. The dermis, which consists of connective tissue, is located under the epidermis, and contains nerve endings, sensory receptors, capillaries, and elastic fibers. The skin is innervated from the nervous system, and is well supplied by blood vessels from the circulatory system. The accessory structures in the integumentary system include the hair, nails, sebaceous (oil) glands, and sweat glands.

Functions of the Integumentary System

The integumentary system has multiple roles in homeostasis, including protection, temperature regulation, sensory reception, and secretion. All body systems work in an interconnected manner in order to maintain the internal conditions essential to the function of the body.

Protection

The skin serves as a protective membrane, providing a barrier over the internal compartments of the body that serves to hold potential harmful agents (such as bacteria, viruses, pollution) outside of the body. The thicker coverings of the skin protect the more delicate structures below from harm. By producing melanin (pigment) the external skin coverings protect the underlying structures from ultraviolet light's harmful rays while producing vitamin D, which works in conjunction with calcium for multiple body processes. The skin also protects the body from excess fluid and electrolyte loss while providing a reservoir for emergency supplies of nutrients and fluids.

Regulation

The skin also serves as a temperature regulator. When the body is too warm, the skin notifies the rest of the body, so sweating begins for cooling and the vascular system dilates and sends blood to the surface to cool the interior. When the body is too cool, the skin notifies the body so that the circulatory system constricts the blood vessels for heat conservation, and the muscles begin shivering to produce extra warmth.

Sensory Reception

Millions of sensory receptors (nerves) are located in the skin for the sensations of pain, touch, heat, cold, and pressure. The nerve endings in the skin are specialized to react to specific sensory stimulation (temperature, pressure, etc.) and send that information to the cerebral cortex of the brain. When the message reaches the brain, the necessary response is triggered. For example, if the hand touches a hot plate, the message goes to the brain that the hand is on the hot plate, then the brain sends the message back to the hand to move off the plate.

Secretion

The skin contains millions of sweat glands, which secrete perspiration or sweat, and sebaceous glands, which secrete oil for lubrication. Perspiration is mostly water with a small amount of salt and other chemical compounds. If the secretions are allowed to accumulate, especially among body hair in the axillary region, then bacteria grow, creating body odor. Sebaceous glands produce sebum, which acts to protect the body from dehydration and the possible absorption of harmful substances.

Layers of the Skin

The skin is composed of two layers: the epidermis and the dermis (see Figure 20-1).

The Epidermis

The epidermis is divided into four layers or strata: the stratum corneum, stratums lucidum, stratum granulosum, and stratum germinativum.

Stratum Corneum

The stratum corneum is the outermost layer of skin consisting of dead cells filled with a protein called keratin. It forms a protective covering for the body, and the thickness of the layer depends on the part of the body. Because of the ongoing pressure on their surfaces, the soles of the feet and the palms of the hands have thicker layers than do the eyelids or forehead.

Stratum Lucidum

The stratum lucidum is a translucent layer lying directly beneath the stratum corneum. In thinner skin, it is often absent. Cells in this layer are either dead or dying.

Stratum Granulosum

The stratum granulosum consists of several layers of living cells that are becoming part of the stratum lucidum and stratum corneum. These cells are actively becoming keratinized or hardened, after they lose their nuclei.

Stratum Germinativum

The stratum germinativum is made of several layers of living cells, still capable of mitosis, or cell division. This layer, occasionally referred to as the mucosum, is most responsible for the regeneration of the epidermis. If damage, such as a severe burn, occurs to this layer, the skin is unable to regenerate itself, and skin grafting must be done. This layer also contains the melanocytes, the cells that produce melanin, the pigment that gives the skin its color.

The Dermis

The dermis is also known as the "true skin." It is composed of connective tissue containing nerves and nerve endings, blood vessels, sebaceous and sweat glands, hair follicles, and lymph vessels. The dermis is divided into two layers, the papillary, or upper, layer and the reticular, or lower, layer. The papillary layer is arranged in parallel layers of microscopic papillae. These papillae are what form the ridges that are fingerprints. The reticular layer is composed of white fibrous tissues, which support blood vessels. Underneath, the dermis is attached to the subcutaneous tissue, which supports, nourishes, insulates, and cushions the skin.

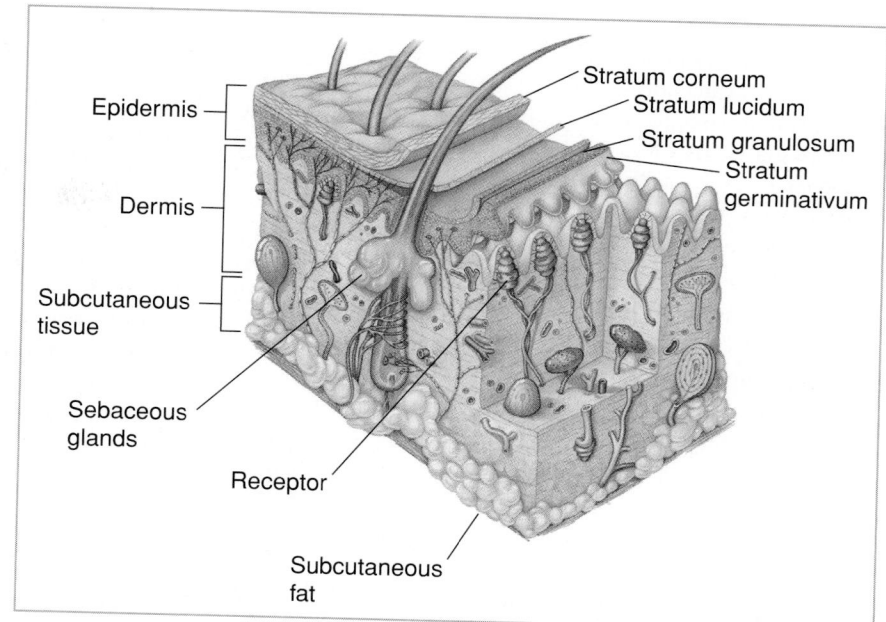

FIGURE 20-1 The integument: the epidermis, dermis, subcutaneous tissue, and its appendages.

Accessory Structures of the Skin

The accessory structures of the skin include the hair follicles, nails, sebaceous glands, and sweat glands. Hair follicles are tube-like depressions located in the dermis of the skin (see Figure 20-1). The shaft is the visible portion of the hair. The root is embedded within the follicle. At the base of each follicle is the hair papilla, which is a loop of capillaries enclosed in the connective tissue. The pilomotor muscle is attached to the side of each follicle. Contraction of the pilomotor muscle causes "goose pimples" or the sensation of the hair "standing on end." This is both a result of an emotional reaction and the skin's attempt at self-warming. The entire body has a very thin layer of hair, except for the palms of the hands and the soles of the feet. Hair is thicker on the scalp than on other portions of the body. The hair around the eyes, ears, and nose serves to filter out foreign particles and prevent their entrance into the sensory organs. Hair color is a result of genetics, and is determined by the amount of pigmentation within the hair shaft. Gray hair has little or no pigmentation. Hair grows about one-half inch a month, and cutting the hair does not affect its growth rate.

Nails

Fingers and toenails are horny cell structures of the epidermis and are composed of hard keratin. The nail consists of the body, the root, and the matrix, or nail bed (see Figure 20-2). The lunula is the crescent-shaped white area at the base of the nail. Average nail growth is about 1 mm per week. A lost fingernail may take 3½ to 5½ months to regrow, while a lost toenail may take as long as 6 to 8 months to regrow. Nail growth is affected by disease and hormonal insufficiencies.

Sebaceous Glands

The sebaceous glands are located in the dermis. They secrete an oily substance called sebum that is made of fat (lipids) and the debris of dead fat-producing cells. Sebum acts to protect and waterproof hair and skin. Sebaceous glands can usually be found in hair-covered areas where they are contained in hair follicles, but can also be found in the hairless areas of the lips, eyelids, penis, labia

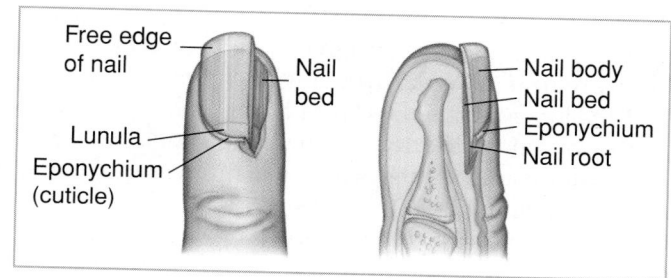

FIGURE 20-2 The fingernail, an appendage of the integument.

minora, and nipples. Sebaceous glands that are found in hair follicles deposit sebum on the hairs and bring it to the skin surface along the hair shaft. At the hairless areas, sebum rises to the surface through ducts. The sebaceous glands of a fetus *in utero* secrete a substance called *vernix caseosa*, a "waxy" or "cheesy" white substance found coating the skin of the newborn baby.

Typically, sebaceous glands can be involved in skin problems such as acne, which is studied and treated by dermatologists. A blocked sebaceous gland can result in a sebaceous cyst.

Sudoriferous (Sweat) Glands

Sudoriferous, or sweat glands, occur in nearly all regions of the skin, but are most numerous in the palms and soles. Each gland consists of a tiny tube that originates as a ball-shaped coil in the dermis or subcutaneous layer of the skin. The coiled portion of the gland is closed at its deep end and is lined with sweat-producing cells. Some sweat glands, the "apocrine glands," respond to emotional stress. Apocrine secretions typically have odors, and the glands are considered to be scent glands. They begin to function at puberty and are responsible for some skin regions becoming moist when a person is emotionally upset, frightened, or experiencing pain. They are also active when a person is sexually stimulated. In adults, the apocrine glands are most numerous in the armpits, groin, and the regions around the nipples. They are usually associated with hair follicles. Other sweat glands, the "eccrine glands," are not connected to hair follicles. They function throughout life by responding to elevated body temperature due to environmental heat or physical exercise. These glands are common on the forehead, neck, and back, where they produce profuse sweating on hot days and when a person is physically active. They also are responsible for the moisture that may appear on the palms and soles when a person is emotionally stressed.

Common Disorders Associated with the Integumentary System

Skin is vulnerable to many disorders because it is the most exposed of all the body systems.

Skin Cancer

Skin cancer is the most common of all human cancers, and some form of skin cancer is diagnosed in more than 1 million people in the United States each year. It is the type of cancer that occurs when normal cells undergo a transformation during which they grow and multiply without normal controls. As the cells multiply, they form a mass called a tumor. Tumors of the skin are often referred to as lesions, and tumors are cancerous only if they are malignant. This means that they encroach on and invade neighboring tissues, especially lymph nodes, because of their uncontrolled growth.

Skin cancers are of three major types: basal cell, squamous cell, and melanoma. The vast majority of skin cancers are basal cell carcinomas or squamous cell carcinomas. While malignant, these are unlikely to spread to other parts of the body. They may be locally disfiguring if not treated early. A small but significant number of skin cancers are malignant melanomas. Malignant melanoma is a highly aggressive cancer that tends to spread to other parts of the body. These cancers may be fatal if not treated early. Like many cancers, skin cancers start as precancerous lesions. These precancerous lesions are changes in skin that are not cancer, but could become cancer over time. Health care professionals often refer to these changes as dysplasia. One example of this is a dysplastic neve, or an abnormal mole. These can develop into melanoma over time. Moles are simply growths on the skin. They are very common. Very few moles become cancerous. Dysplastic nevi are not cancer, but they can become cancer. People with dysplastic nevi often have a lot of them, perhaps as many as 100 or more. They are usually irregular in shape, with notched or fading borders, and may be flat or raised, and the surface may be smooth or rough ("pebbly").

Signs and Symptoms

Nonmelanoma skin cancer may appear as a change in the skin, such as a growth, an irritation or sore that does not heal, or a change in a wart or mole. Basal cell carcinoma usually affects the head, neck, back, chest, or shoulders. The nose is the most common site. Signs of basal cell carcinoma can vary and may include skin changes such as a:

- Firm, pearly bump with tiny blood vessels in a spiderlike appearance (telangiectasias)
- Red, tender, flat spot that bleeds easily
- Small, fleshy bump with a smooth, pearly appearance, often with a depressed center
- Smooth, shiny bump that may look like a mole or cyst
- Scar-like patch of skin, especially on the face, that is firm to the touch
- Bump that itches, bleeds, crusts over, and then repeats the cycle and has not healed in 3 weeks
- Change in the size, shape, or color of a wart or mole

Treatment

The goals of treatment for nonmelanoma skin cancer are to remove the entire skin cancer and a margin of skin tissue around the cancer to reduce the chance of recurrence, to preserve nearby skin tissue that is free of cancer, and to minimize scarring after surgery. Treatment for nonmelanoma skin cancer depends on the size

THE CHILD

- In children, skin conditions can be acute or chronic, local or systemic, and some can be congenital. Age-related skin conditions, include milia (the white pimples occurring in newborns) and acne.
- Skin infections in children present as systemic infections with symptoms such as fever and malaise. Because the sebaceous glands do not produce sebum until the child is about 8 to 10 years old, a child's skin is drier and chaps more easily. For that reason, it is important to teach children good hygiene habits at an early age.

THE OLDER ADULT

- As a person ages, the papilla grow less dense and the skin becomes looser. There is less collagen and fewer elastic fibers in the upper dermis, and the skin loses its elastic tone, causing wrinkles to occur more easily. The occurrence of premalignant and malignant skin lesions may also increase with aging, especially on the nose, eyelids, and cheeks. Eighty percent of skin cancers found in older adults are basal cell carcinomas.
- By age 50, approximately half of adults have some gray hair. The scalp hair continues to thin in men and women as aging progresses, and the hair becomes dry and brittle. The nails may flatten and become more discolored, dry, and brittle.

and location of the cancer, whether it is basal cell or squamous cell, and the age and overall health of the patient. Because skin cancer usually grows slowly, it often can be detected and successfully treated early in its development. The most common treatment is surgery to destroy or remove the entire skin growth, including a margin of cancer-free tissue around the growth. Most surgical treatments are very effective, with cure rates higher than 90 percent.

Squamous Cell Carcinoma

Squamous cell carcinoma is a malignant tumor that affects the middle layer of the skin. Any change in an existing wart, mole, or other skin lesion, or the development of a new growth that ulcerates and does not heal well, could indicate skin cancer. This type of cancer has a high cure rate if it is treated early, but neglect can allow the cancer to spread, causing great disability or even death. It is important to note that more than 90 percent of skin cancers occur on areas of the skin that are regularly exposed to sunlight or other ultraviolet radiation. This is considered the primary cause of all squamous cell carcinomas. Other risks include genetic predisposition (skin cancers are more common in those who have light-colored skin, blue or green eyes, and blond or red hair), chemical pollution, and overexposure to x-rays or other forms of radiation. Exposure to arsenic, which may be present in some herbicides, presents another risk for development of skin cancers.

Squamous cell cancer is more aggressive than basal cell cancer, but still may be relatively slow growing. It is more likely than basal cell cancer to spread (metastasize) to other locations, including internal organs. Squamous cell cancer is usually painless initially, but may become painful with the development of ulcers that do not heal. This cancer may begin in normal skin; in the skin of a burn, injury, or scar; or at a site of

Patient Education

Skin care is a very important part of hygiene. Patients should be taught that they should moisturize their skin on a daily basis, or more often as necessary. Sunscreen is one of the easiest ways to avoid skin cancer, and teaching patients about using adequate sun protection may be one duty of the medical assistant. Write down the correct sun protection factor prescribed by the physician so that the patient can easily locate the appropriate lotion in the store. Patients should be taught to avoid sunburn as much as possible. Some medications can increase the risk of sunburn, and education for patients who take these medications is extremely important.

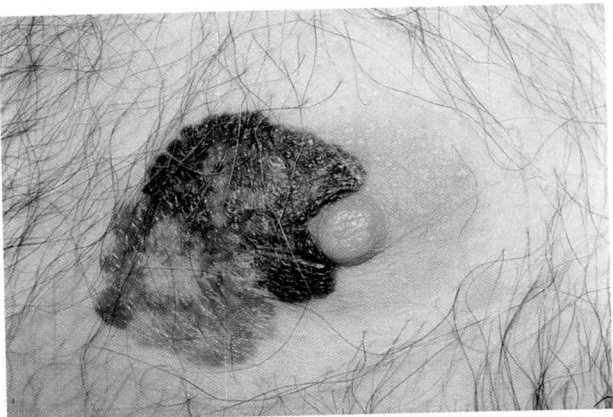

FIGURE 20-3 Melanoma.

chronic inflammation (which may occur with many skin disorders). It most often originates from sun-damaged skin areas, such as actinic keratosis. It usually begins after age 50.

Symptoms include any skin lesion, growth, or bump that is small, firm, reddened, nodular, coned, or flat in shape. Also, if the surface is scaly or crusted and the lesion or growth is located on the face, ears, neck, hands, or arms, there is a good possibility it is a squamous cell carcinoma. Occasionally the growth may occur on the lip, mouth, tongue, or genitals.

The treatment varies with the tumor's size, depth, location, and how much it has spread or metastasized. Surgical removal of the tumor, which may include removal of the skin around the tumor (wide excision), is often recommended. Microscopic shaving (Mohs' surgery) may remove small tumors. Skin grafting may be needed if wide areas of skin are removed. The tumor may also be reduced in size by radiation treatments. Chemotherapy can be used if surgery and radiation fail, but it is usually minimally effective.

Melanoma

Malignant melanoma is a type of cancer arising from the melanocyte cells of the skin (see Figure 20-3). Melanocytes are cells in the skin that produce a pigment called *melanin*. Malignant melanoma develops when the melanocytes no longer respond to the normal control mechanisms of cellular growth. They may then invade nearby structures or spread to other organs in the body (metastasis), where again they invade and compromise the function of that organ. The primary tumor begins in the skin, often from the melanocytes of a preexisting mole. Once it becomes invasive, it may progress beyond the site of origin to the regional lymph nodes or travel to other organ systems in the body and become systemic in nature. Cancer, as it invades in its place of origin, may also work its way into blood vessels. If this occurs, it provides yet another route for the cancer to spread to other organs of the body. When the cancer spreads elsewhere in the body, it has become systemic in extent and the tumor appearing elsewhere is known as a *metastasis*.

Untreated malignant melanoma follows a classic progression. It begins and grows locally, penetrating vertically. It may be carried via the lymph to the regional nodes, known as regional metastasis. It may go from the lymph to the bloodstream or penetrate blood vessels, allowing it a direct route to go elsewhere in the body. When systemic disease or distant metastases occur, melanoma commonly involves the lung, brain, liver, or occasionally bone. The malignancy causes death when its uncontrolled growth compromises vital organ function.

The predisposing causes to the development of malignant melanoma are environmental and genetic. A small percentage of melanomas arise within burn scar tissue. As of 2003, researchers did not fully understand the relationship between deep burns and an increased risk of skin cancer. Malignant melanomas are usually diagnosed by using the ABCDE rule (see Table 20-1), which is an excellent way of identifying changes of significance in a mole. This includes checking the mole for the following: asymmetry, border irregularity, color variegation, diameter greater than 6 mm (0.24 in.), and elevation above surrounding tissue.

Another summary of important changes in a mole is the Glasgow seven-point scale. The symptoms and signs, which are listed below, can occur anywhere on the skin, including the palms of the hands, soles of the feet, and also the nail beds. In this scheme, change is

TABLE 20-1	The ABCDEs of Melanoma Changes in a Mole
A—Asymmetry	The mole does not have two halves that match each other.
B—Border	The border is ragged, notched, or blurred together.
C—Color	Color is uneven; shades of black, brown, or tan are present; there may be areas of white, red, or blue present.
D—Diameter	There may be a change in size, and the mole is typically greater than 6 mm in diameter.
E—Elevation	The mole sits above the surrounding tissue.

emphasized along with size. Bleeding and sensory changes are relatively late symptoms.

- Change in size
- Change in shape
- Change in color
- Inflammation
- Crusting and bleeding
- Sensory change
- Diameter greater than 7 mm (0.28 in.)

The key to successful treatment of melanoma is early diagnosis. Patients identified with localized, thin, small lesions nearly always survive. For those with advanced lesions, the outcome is poor in spite of progress in systemic therapy.

Acne Vulgaris

Acne vulgaris (acne) is a common skin condition that occurs when oil and dead skin cells clog the skin's pores (see Figure 20-4). These clogs cause blemishes in the skin that are often red and swollen, and it most often affects teens, with more than 85 percent of them developing at least a mild form of this condition. Severe acne can mean hundreds of pimples or sores that can cover the face, neck, chest, and back. While mild acne is merely annoying, severe acne can lead to emotional and physical scars. Most people outgrow acne by the time they are in their 40s and 50s.

Acne develops most often on the face, neck, chest, shoulders, or back and can range from mild to severe. It can last for a few months, many years, or come and go your entire life. In a mild case of acne, only whiteheads and blackheads may be present. At times, these may develop into an infection in the skin pore (pimple). Severe acne can produce hundreds of pimples that cover large areas of skin. Cystic lesions are pimples that are large and deep. These lesions are often painful and can leave scars on your skin. Acne can also lead to low self-esteem and sometimes depression. These conditions need treatment along with the acne.

Treatment for acne depends greatly on whether the person has a mild, moderate, or severe form. Sometimes the health care provider will combine treatments to get the best results and to avoid developing drug resistant bacteria. Treatment could include lotions or gels applied to blemishes or sometimes entire areas of skin, such as the chest or back (topical medications) and oral antibiotics.

Alopecia

Alopecia (see Figure 20-5) is baldness or loss of hair. The most common form is male-pattern baldness (also known as androgenic alopecia), but both women and men can experience hair loss. Alopecia areata is another type of hair loss, involving patches of baldness

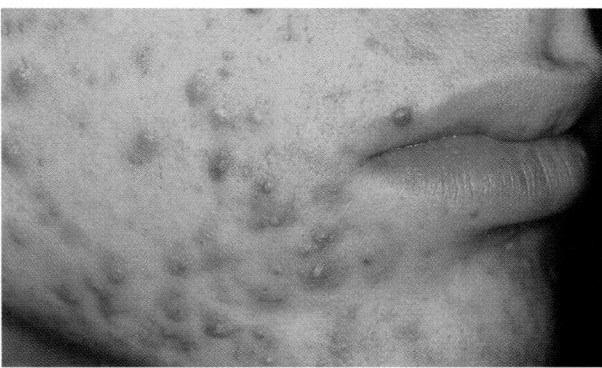

FIGURE 20-4 Acne vulgaris.

that may come and go. It affects about 1 in 100 people, mostly teenagers and young adults. In some cases, hair loss is a side effect of having cancer treatment drugs, but in many cases the hair grows back. Male-pattern baldness is hereditary, which means it runs in families. It usually starts to happen around the late 20s and 30s although this can vary. By the age of 60, most men have some degree of hair loss. It is called male-pattern baldness because it tends to follow a set pattern. The first stage is usually a receding hairline, followed by thinning of the hair on the crown and temples. When these two areas meet in the middle, there is a horseshoe shape of hair around the back and sides of the head. Eventually the person may be completely bald. Women's hair gradually thins with age but they only tend to lose hair from the top of the head. This usually becomes more noticeable after menopause. It is called androgenetic alopecia, or female-pattern hair loss, and also tends to run in families.

Alopecia areata causes patches of baldness that are about the size of a large coin. They usually appear on the scalp but can occur anywhere on the body, including the beard, eyebrows, and eyelashes. There are usually no other symptoms.

If the hair loss is caused by an infection, or other condition such as anemia, it can be treated to prevent

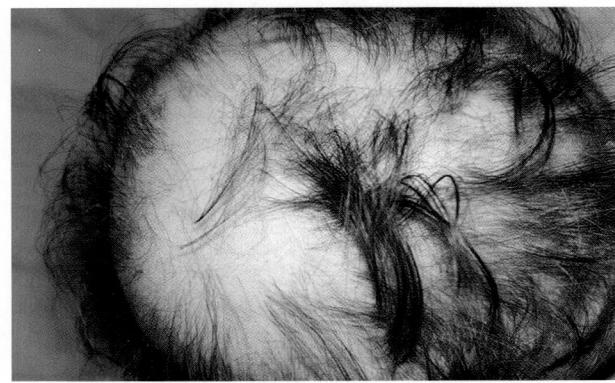

FIGURE 20-5 Alopecia.

further hair loss. In some cases, including after cancer treatment, hair may start to grow again. Drugs are available to treat male-pattern and female-pattern baldness but they do not work for everyone and the effects are not long lasting. There are also lotions that can be rubbed on the scalp, although these do not work for everyone nor do they have long-lasting effects. Shampoos and formulas are available for improving circulation to the scalp, and some people try herbal treatments. Unfortunately, hair loss can lead to problems with confidence and self-esteem.

Cellulitis

Cellulitis is an acute spreading bacterial infection below the surface of the skin characterized by redness (erythema), warmth, swelling, and pain. It can also cause fever, chills, and enlarged lymph nodes (see Figure 20-6). Cellulitis commonly appears in areas where there is a break in the skin from an abrasion, a cut, or a skin ulcer. It can also be due to local trauma, such as an animal bite. Only rarely is cellulitis due to the bacteremic spread of infection, that is, bacteria arriving from a distant source via the bloodstream.

Risk factors for cellulitis include diabetes and impairment of the immune system (from, for example, HIV/AIDS or immunosuppressant drugs). Cellulitis is not contagious because it is an infection of the skin's deeper layers, the dermis and subcutaneous tissue, and the skin's top layer (the epidermis) provides a cover over the infection.

The main bacterium that causes cellulitis is staph (*Staphylococcus aureus*), and strep (Group A Streptococcus) is the next most common cause. It can be caused by many other types of bacteria. In children under six, H. flu (*Haemophilus influenzae*) can cause cellulitis, especially on the face, arms, and upper torso. Cellulitis from a dog or cat bite or scratch may be caused by the *Pasteurella multocida* bacteria. Cellulitis after an injury from a saltwater fish or shellfish can be due to *Erysipelothrix rhusiopathiae*. These same bacteria can also cause cellulitis after a skin injury on the farm, especially while working with pigs or poultry.

Antibiotics such as derivatives of penicillin that are most effective against the staph germ are used to treat cellulitis. If other bacteria, as determined by culture tests, turn out to be the cause, or if patients are allergic to penicillin, other appropriate antibiotics are substituted.

Contact Dermatitis

Contact dermatitis is an allergic reaction of the skin caused by irritating substances coming in contact with it. Most frequently, the obvious response is red, irritated skin, but vesicles (small blisters) and rash may also result. Oftentimes, the skin itches, and pain may also be present. Serious allergic reactions may result in urticaria, or hives.

Causes of contact dermatitis often include exposures to poison ivy, poison oak, nickel (especially on jewelry or jean snaps), lotions, detergents, or other chemicals. Most of these allergic reactions are treated with antihistamines (antiallergy medicines) and topical corticosteroid creams to reduce the inflammation. Widespread or excessively uncomfortable reactions may also be treated with systemic corticosteroids (oral medications) that help to further decrease the inflammation caused by the allergic reaction.

Decubitus Ulcer

Decubitus ulcers, also called pressure sores or bedsores, refer to an area of skin and tissue that breaks down. These typically happen when constant pressure is maintained on a specific area of the skin, such as on the coccyx in a patient lying in bed for too long a period of time without being repositioned. The constant pressure on the area decreases the blood supply, caus-

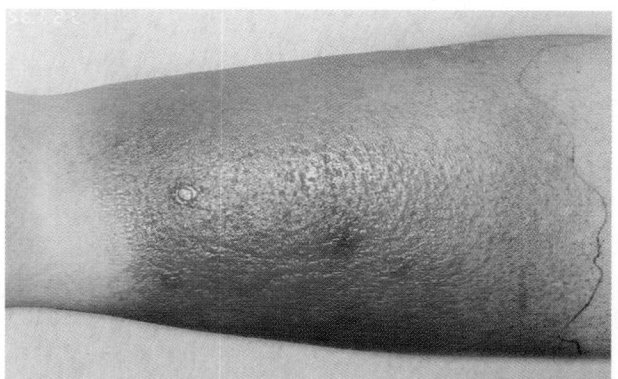

FIGURE 20-6 Cellulitis.

ing death to the affected tissue. The most common location for a decubitus ulcer to occur is over bony prominences, such as the coccyx, hips, heels, ankles, shoulders, back, and the back of the head.

According to the National Pressure Ulcer Advisory Panel, the four stages of decubitus ulcers include:

- Stage I: A reddened area on the skin that does not blanch (turn white) when pressed. This is an early stage, and if the pressure is kept off of the area, healing may occur.
- Stage II: The skin has a blister or an open sore. The area around the site may be red and irritated.
- Stage III: The skin breakdown looks like a crater with damage to the tissue below the skin.
- Stage IV: The wound becomes so deep that there is damage to the tissues beneath the initial ulcer, including damage to bone and muscle.

Treatment of decubitus ulcers starts with relieving the pressure. Special pillows, cushions, and sheepskin are frequently used to ensure that there is no pressure on the area. Regular repositioning must be routine. Decubitus ulcers are typically debrided, that is, cleaned of all the toxins and then medicated and covered with special gauze dressings to help in healing. Protecting the wound from any further injury is essential in order to protect the patient from infections and other serious complications and systemic sepsis.

Eczema

Eczema, called atopic dermatitis, is a chronic skin condition caused by an allergic-type reaction on the skin. It is characterized by scaling, itching, and rashes. Typically, there is a family history of allergies and eczema, and the patient may also suffer from other allergic conditions. Eczema is most common in infants, and about half of the cases disappear by age 3. Adults may also suffer from chronic episodes of eczema.

Treatment of eczema often depends on the stage, or appearance, of the lesions that have formed on the skin. These lesions range from dry and scaly, to "weeping." Weeping lesions are treated with mild soaps and dressings, whereas severe cases and dry scaly lesions may be treated with mild, anti-itch lotions or low-potency topical corticosteroids. Chronically thickened areas may be treated with ointments or creams that contain tar compounds, medium- to high-potency corticosteroids, and lubricating ingredients. Very severe cases may require systemic corticosteroids and topical immunomodulators (TIMs).

Folliculitis

Folliculitis is an inflammation or infection of hair follicles. While folliculitis can occur anywhere there is body hair, it most often appears in areas that become irritated by shaving, the rubbing of clothes, or where

follicles and pores are blocked by oils and dirt. Common sites of folliculitis include the face, the scalp, under the arms, and on the legs.

The appearance of folliculitis may vary from person to person, but generally the symptoms include a reddened rash; raised, red, often pus-filled lesions around hair follicles (pimples); pimples that eventually crust over and occur in areas of a high concentration of hair follicles such as the face (especially in the area of men's beards and moustaches), under the arms, on the scalp, and in the groin; and itching at the site of the rash and pimples.

Diagnosis of folliculitis is generally made by examining the appearance of the skin. On occasion, a skin biopsy will be done, not to diagnosis the folliculitis but to rule out other types of skin lesions. A culture of the lesion may show which bacteria or fungus has caused the infection.

Treatment for folliculitis generally involves taking steps to minimize damage to hair follicles by avoiding clothing that will rub against the skin, damaging hair follicles, shaving with an electric razor as opposed to a blade razor, and keeping the skin clean using soap and water and skin cleansers. When folliculitis is present, treatment usually includes the application of antibiotic ointments.

Herpes Simplex

Herpes simplex is an infection that primarily affects the mouth or genital area. There are two different strains of herpes simplex viruses:

- Herpes simplex virus type 1 (HSV-1) is usually associated with infections of the lips, mouth, and face. It is the most common herpes simplex virus and is usually acquired in childhood. HSV-1 often causes lesions inside the mouth such as cold sores (fever blisters) and is transmitted by contact with infected saliva. By adulthood, up to 90 percent of individuals will have antibodies to HSV-1.

- Herpes simplex virus type 2 (HSV-2) is sexually transmitted. Symptoms include genital ulcers or sores. In addition to oral and genital lesions, the virus can also lead to complications such as meningoencephalitis (infection of the lining of the brain and the brain itself) or cause an infection of the eye, in particular the conjunctiva and cornea. However, some people have HSV-2 but do not display symptoms. Up to 30 percent of U.S. adults have antibodies against HSV-2. Cross-infection of type 1 and 2 viruses may occur from oral–genital contact.

A finger infection, called herpetic whitlow, is another form of herpes infection. It usually affects health care providers who are exposed to oral secretions during procedures. Sometimes, young children contract the disease.

A herpes virus can infect the fetus and cause congenital abnormalities. It may also be transmitted to a newborn during vaginal delivery in mothers infected with herpes viruses, particularly if the mother has active infection at the time. It can also be transmitted even in the absence of symptoms or visible lesions. Symptoms of herpes simplex include:

- Mouth sores
- Genital lesions—may be preceded by burning or tingling sensation
- Blisters or ulcers—most frequent on the mouth, lips, and gums or genitalia
- Fever blisters
- Fever—may be present especially during the first episode
- Enlargement of lymph nodes in the neck or groin

Some cases of herpes simplex are relatively mild and may not require treatment. In severe or prolonged cases, however, or in individuals who are immunosuppressed or who have frequent recurrences, antiviral medications such as acyclovir may be used. In individuals with more than six recurrences of genital herpes per year, chronic antiviral medications may be offered to reduce recurrences.

Herpes Zoster

Herpes zoster, which is also known as *shingles*, is a viral infection that causes a painful rash. It is caused by the varicella-zoster virus, the same virus that causes chickenpox. After you've had chickenpox, the virus lies dormant in your nerves. Years later, the virus may reactivate as shingles. Although painful, typically this condition isn't a serious one. Sometimes, however, the rash can lead to a debilitating complication called postherpetic neuralgia. This condition causes the skin to remain painful and sensitive to touch for months or even years after the rash clears up. Early treatment can help shorten a shingles infection and reduce the risk of complications.

The signs and symptoms of herpes zoster may include pain, burning, tingling, itching, numbness or extreme sensitivity in a certain part of the body, a red rash with fluid-filled blisters that begins a few days after the pain, fever, headache, chills, and an upset stomach. Typically, the rash occurs on only one side of the body. It often appears as a band of blisters that wraps from the middle of your back around one side of your chest to your breastbone, following the path of the nerve where the virus had been dormant.

Although the herpes zoster rash may resemble chickenpox, the virus typically causes more pain and less itching the second time around. And while an episode of herpes zoster usually heals on its own within a few weeks, prompt treatment can ease pain, speed healing, and reduce the risk of complications. Complications are more likely for people who have weak immune systems and people older than age 65.

Doctors typically prescribe oral antiviral medications, preferably beginning within 48 to 72 hours of the first sign of the rash. Sometimes, antiviral medications are combined with corticosteroids to reduce swelling and pain. If the pain is severe—particularly if the patient develops postherpetic neuralgia—the health care provider may prescribe oral analgesics or a skin patch that contains a pain-relieving medication.

Impetigo

Impetigo is a skin infection caused by bacteria. It is most common in children and is contagious. Impetigo forms round, crusted (see Figure 20-7), oozing spots that grow larger day by day. It may affect the skin anywhere on the body but commonly occurs in the area around the nose and mouth. Impetigo is characterized by blisters that may burst, ooze fluid, and develop a honey-colored crust. Impetigo may itch, and it can be spread by scratching. The infection usually spreads along the edges of an affected area, but may also spread to other areas of the body. While the bacteria causing impetigo may have been caught from someone else with impetigo or boils, impetigo usually begins out of the blue without any apparent source of infection.

Antibiotics taken by mouth usually clear up impetigo in 4 or 5 days.

Pediculosis

Pediculosis is an infestation of the hairy parts of the body or clothing with the eggs, larvae or adults of lice (see Figure 20-8). The crawling stages of this insect feed on human blood, which can result in severe itching. Head lice are usually located on the scalp, crab lice in the pubic area, and body lice along seams of clothing. Body lice travel to the skin to feed and return back to the clothing. Anyone may become louse infested under suitable conditions of exposure. Pediculosis is easily transmitted from person to person during direct contact. Head lice infestations are frequently found in school settings or institutions. Crab lice infestations can be found among sexually active individuals. Body lice infestation can be found in people living in crowded, unsanitary conditions where clothing is infrequently changed or laundered.

For both head lice and body lice, transmission can occur during direct contact with an infested individual. Sharing of clothing and combs or brushes may also result in transmission of these insects. Although other means are possible, crab lice are most often transmitted through sexual contact. Usually, the first indication of an infestation is itching or scratching in the area of the body where the lice feed. Scratching at the back of the head or around the ears should lead to an examination for head louse eggs (nits) on the hair. Itching around the genital area should lead to an examination for crab lice or their eggs. (See Legal and Ethical Issues for a discussion of a patient's right to privacy during an examination.) Scratching can be sufficiently intense to result in secondary bacterial infection in these areas.

Medicated shampoos or cream rinses containing pyrethrins are preferred for treating people with head lice. Lindane-based shampoos are also available but not recommended for infants, young children, and pregnant or lactating women. Products containing pyrethrins are available over the counter, but those containing lindane are available only through a physician's prescription. Retreatment after 7 to 10 days is recommended to ensure that no eggs have survived. Nit combs are available to help remove nits from hair. Dose and duration of shampoo treatment should be followed carefully according to label instructions.

Psoriasis

Psoriasis is characterized by frequent episodes of redness, itching, and thick, dry scales on the skin. It is a common condition that affects approximately 3 millions Americans, beginning most commonly between the ages of 1 and 35. It is believed to be genetic, but

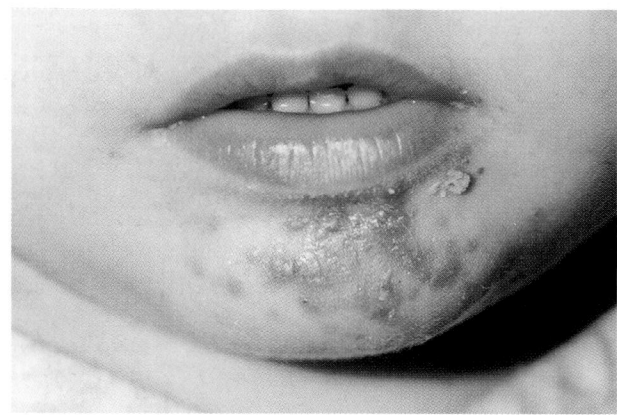

FIGURE 20-7 Impetigo.

also has characteristics related to autoimmune disorders. Typically, the movement of new skins from the lower layers of the skin to the top takes about a month. In psoriasis, however, the cells move in a few days, causing a buildup of dead skin cells and the formation of thick scales. The condition is most commonly seen on the trunk, elbows, knees, scalp, skin folds, and fingernails, but can appear on any area of the skin.

The onset of psoriasis can be gradual or abrupt. Typically, it appears for a time, then goes away for a while. Medications, viral or bacterial infections, excessive alcohol consumption, obesity, lack of sunlight, sunburn, stress, general poor health, cold climate, and frequent skin friction are associated causes of flares. Psoriasis is not contagious.

The treatment of psoriasis depends on the extent and severity of the disorder. Lesions can be serious and extensive enough to require hospitalization. When the case is severe and widespread, large quantities of fluid can be lost, causing dehydration and severe secondary infections that can be serious. Treatment involves analgesics, sedation, intravenous fluids, retinoids (such as Retin-A) and antibiotics. Mild cases are treated at

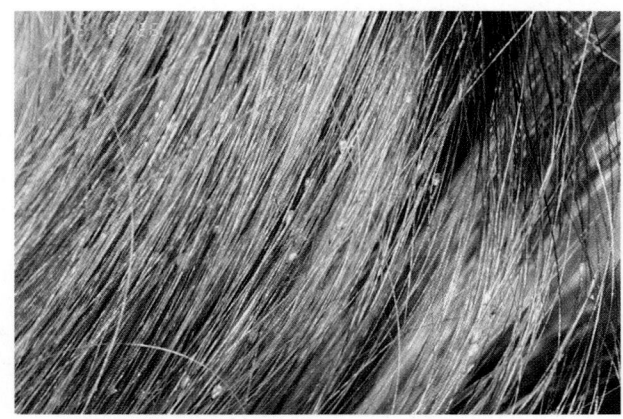

FIGURE 20-8 Pediculosis capitis.

home with topical medications such as prescription or nonprescription dandruff shampoos, cortisone or other corticosteroids, and antifungal medications.

Rosacea

Rosacea is a chronic and potentially life-disruptive disorder primarily of the facial skin, often characterized by flare-ups and remissions. It typically begins after age 30 as a redness on the cheeks, nose, chin, or fore-

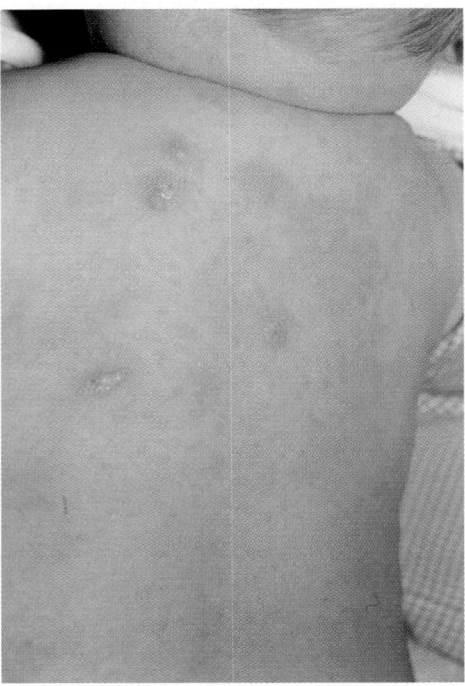

FIGURE 20-9 Scabies.

head that may come and go. In some cases, rosacea may also occur on the neck, chest, scalp, or ears. Symptoms of rosacea can include redness on the cheeks, nose, chin, or forehead, small visible blood vessels on the face, bumps or pimples on the face, and watery or irritated eyes. Over time, the redness becomes ruddier and more persistent. Left untreated, bumps and pimples often develop, and in severe cases the nose may grow swollen and bumpy from excess tissue. This condition affects an estimated 14 million Americans— and most of them don't know they have it.

Although rosacea can affect all segments of the population, individuals with fair skin who tend to flush or blush easily are believed to be at greatest risk. The disease is more frequently diagnosed in women, but more severe symptoms tend to be seen in men— perhaps because they often delay seeking medical help until the disorder reaches advanced stages.

Although there is no cure for rosacea and the cause is unknown, medical therapy is available to control or reverse its signs and symptoms. Individuals who suspect they may have rosacea are urged to see a dermatologist or other knowledgeable physician for diagnosis and appropriate treatment.

Scabies

Scabies is a contagious disorder of the skin (see Figure 20-9) caused by very small, wingless insects or mites called the human itch mite or scabies itch mite *Sarcoptes scabiei* var. *hominis* (Hering). The female insect burrows into the skin where she lays one to three eggs daily. A very small, hard-to-see, zigzag blister usually marks the trail of the insect as she lays her eggs. Other more obvious symptoms are an intense itching (especially at night) and a red rash that can occur at the area that has been scratched. The most common locations for scabies are on the sides of fingers, between the fingers, on the backs of the hands, on the wrists, heels, elbows, armpits, and inner thighs, and around the waist (belt line). If untreated, the female will continue to lay eggs for about 5 weeks. The eggs hatch and the new mites begin the cycle all over again. The mites themselves are too small to be seen without magnification. One of the biggest problems with scabies always has been misdiagnosis. Scabies is spread by personal contact, such as by shaking hands or sleeping together or by close contact with infected articles such as clothing, bedding, or towels. It is usually found where people are crowded together or have frequent contact, and is most common among schoolchildren, families, roommates, and sexual partners. Scabies can be spread by the insect itself or by the egg. Prompt action is required to rid a person of the insects and eggs. Sulfur has been used (6 to 10 percent in lotion or cream) since Roman times as a scabicide; however, some patients may be allergic to sulfur.

Warts

Warts are a type of infection caused by viruses in the human papillomavirus (HPV) family. There are at least 60 types of HPV viruses. Warts can grow on all parts of the body, including the skin, the inside of the mouth, the genitals, and the rectal area. Warts located on the skin can be passed from one person to another when that person touches the warts. It is also possible to get warts from using towels or other objects that were used by a person who has warts. Often warts disappear on their own, although it may take many months, or even years, for the warts to go away; sometimes they never disappear.

Burns

Burns occur when heat, chemicals, or electricity destroys a portion of the skin. Burns are classified as either partial thickness or full thickness. Partial-thickness burns, previously known as first- and second-degree burns, destroy only a portion of the skin. These burns can be painful, may blister, and have a chance of recovery, depending on the amount of skin burned and the depth of the burn. Examples of partial-thickness burns include sunburn, scalds, and chemical burns. Full-thickness burns, previously called third-degree burns, destroy the entirety of the skin in a specified location. These burns are usually not initially painful, because the nerve endings in the skin have also been destroyed. Full-thickness burns are typically caused by direct exposure to fire. Recovery from full-thickness burns is possible,

Professionalism

While in a professional environment, courtesy and manners are very essential to the medical assistant's practice. Unless instructed to do otherwise, always call adult patients (especially the elderly) by Mr., Mrs., or Ms. Using the phrases "please" and "thank you" also helps to establish you as a courteous, caring professional. Never address any patient by the endearments of "honey" or "sweetie." Although some individuals may find this cute, many others will find the phraseology demeaning. Convey an attitude of being caring, professional, and sincere. Speak in full sentences, using complete words and avoiding slang, and your patients will know that you truly are a professional.

but the chances tend to decrease significantly if the burn covers a large area. The usual cause of death from burns is by infections that set in as the skin can no longer perform its protective function.

The extent of the body surface areas affected and the severity of a burn are often the most important factors in predicting the risk of death resulting from burn injuries. Several factors are used to determine the severity of this injury, including the patient's age, size and depth of the burn, and the location of the burn.

SUMMARY

The skin provides many protective functions for the body, including preventing infection and preserving the internal environment. Skin also helps to promote optimum temperature levels. Disorders of the skin can be uncomfortable, but most can be treated without too much discomfort.

Chapter Review

COMPETENCY REVIEW

1. Define and spell the terms to learn for this chapter.
2. What is the primary organ of the integumentary system?
3. Name the four accessory structures of the integumentary system.
4. Name the four functions of the skin.
5. Name the two layers of the skin.
6. What is the protein substance in the dead cells of the epidermis that serves as a protective mechanism?
7. Name the four layers of the epidermis.

8. What is the name of the cresecent-shaped area of the nail?
9. What is the name of the cell that gives color to the skin?
10. What are the ABCDEs of skin cancer?

1. The black pigment that gives skin its color is
   A. basal layer
   B. keratin
   C. melanin
   D. cyano
   E. chloro

2. The dermis layer of the skin contains
   A. keratin
   B. melanin
   C. stratified squamous epithelium
   D. blood vessels
   E. basal layer

3. The medical term for a dangerous form of skin cancer caused by an overgrowth of melanin-producing cells is
   A. Kaposi's sarcoma
   B. malignant melanoma
   C. basal cell carcinoma
   D. squamous cell carcinoma
   E. lupus erythematosus

4. Urticaria is the medical term for
   A. ringworm
   B. hives
   C. verruca
   D. furuncle
   E. scabies

5. A chronic inflammatory condition consisting of crusty, silvery papules forming patches with pink, circular borders is called
   A. eczema
   B. psoriasis
   C. cellulitis
   D. scleroderma
   E. neoplasm

6. Which is not a function of the skin?
   A. protection
   B. sensation
   C. regulation
   D. germination
   E. secretion

7. What type of decubitus is a red place over a bony prominence that does not blanch?
   A. stage I
   B. stage II
   C. stage III
   D. stage IV
   E. This is not a decubitus.

8. What kind of burn destroys all the layers of skin?
   A. chemical
   B. second degree
   C. partial thickness
   D. full thickness
   E. electrical

9. What is the name of a common skin condition that occurs when oil and dead skin cells clog the skin pores?
   A. acne vulgaris
   B. contact dermatitis
   C. eczema
   D. psoriasis
   E. pediculosis

10. What is another medical term for shingles?
    A. impetigo
    B. pediculosis
    C. herpes zoster
    D. herpes simplex
    E. psoriasis

CRITICAL THINKING

1. If the patient had been aware of poison ivy in her environment, what are three precautions that she could have followed to either decrease or prevent her exposure to the poison ivy?

2. Why was the patient given topical steroids for her poison ivy rash?

INTERNET ACTIVITY

Several organizations have been established to help in the prevention and treatment of diseases affecting the integumentary system. Perform an Internet search to learn more about these organizations and what each provides to people afflicted with specific skin disorders.

 MediaLink More on the integumentary system, including interactive resources, can be found on the Student CD-ROM accompanying this textbook.

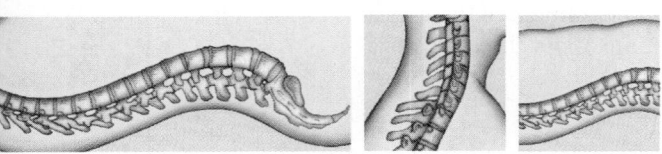

Medical Assistant Role Delineation Chart

HIGHLIGHT indicates material covered in this chapter.

ADMINISTRATIVE

Administrative Procedures

- Perform basic administrative medical assisting functions
- Schedule, coordinate and monitor appointments
- Schedule inpatient/outpatient admissions and procedures
- Understand and apply third-party guidelines
- Obtain reimbursement through accurate claims submission
- Monitor third-party reimbursement
- Understand and adhere to managed care policies and procedures
- *Negotiate managed care contracts*

Practice Finances

- Perform procedural and diagnostic coding
- Apply bookkeeping principles

- Manage accounts receivable
- *Manage accounts payable*
- *Process payroll*
- *Document and maintain accounting and banking records*
- *Develop and maintain fee schedules*
- *Manage renewals of business and professional insurance policies*
- *Manage personnel benefits and maintain records*
- *Perform marketing, financial, and strategic planning*

CLINICAL

Fundamental Principles

- Apply principles of aseptic technique and infection control
- Comply with quality assurance practices
- Screen and follow up patient test results

Diagnostic Orders

- Collect and process specimens
- Perform diagnostic tests

Patient Care

- Adhere to established patient screening procedures
- Obtain patient history and vital signs
- Prepare and maintain examination and treatment areas
- Prepare patient for examinations, procedures and treatments

- Assist with examinations, procedures and treatments
- Prepare and administer medications and immunizations
- Maintain medication and immunization records
- Recognize and respond to emergencies
- Coordinate patient care information with other health care providers
- Initiate IV and administer IV medications with appropriate training and as permitted by state law

GENERAL

Professionalism

- Display a professional manner and image
- Demonstrate initiative and responsibility
- Work as a member of the health care team
- Prioritize and perform multiple tasks
- Adapt to change
- Promote the CMA credential
- Enhance skills through continuing education
- Treat all patients with compassion and empathy
- Promote the practice through positive public relations

Communication Skills

- Recognize and respect cultural diversity
- Adapt communications to individual's ability to understand
- Use professional telephone technique

- Recognize and respond effectively to verbal, nonverbal, and written communications
- Use medical terminology appropriately
- Utilize electronic technology to receive, organize, prioritize and transmit information
- Serve as liaison

Legal Concepts

- Perform within legal and ethical boundaries
- Prepare and maintain medical records
- Document accurately
- Follow employer's established policies dealing with the health care contract
- Implement and maintain federal and state health care legislation and regulations
- Comply with established risk management and safety procedures
- Recognize professional credentialing criteria
- *Develop and maintain personnel, policy and procedure manuals*

Instruction

- Instruct individuals according to their needs
- Explain office policies and procedures
- Teach methods of health promotion and disease prevention
- Locate community resources and disseminate information
- *Develop educational materials*
- *Conduct continuing education activities*

Operational Functions

- Perform inventory of supplies and equipment
- Perform routine maintenance of administrative and clinical equipment
- Apply computer techniques to support office operations
- *Perform personnel management functions*
- *Negotiate leases and prices for equipment and supply contracts*

- *Denotes advanced skills.*

SOURCE: Reprinted by permission of the American Association of Medical Assistants from the AAMA Role Delineation Study: Occupational Analysis of the Medical Assisting Profession.

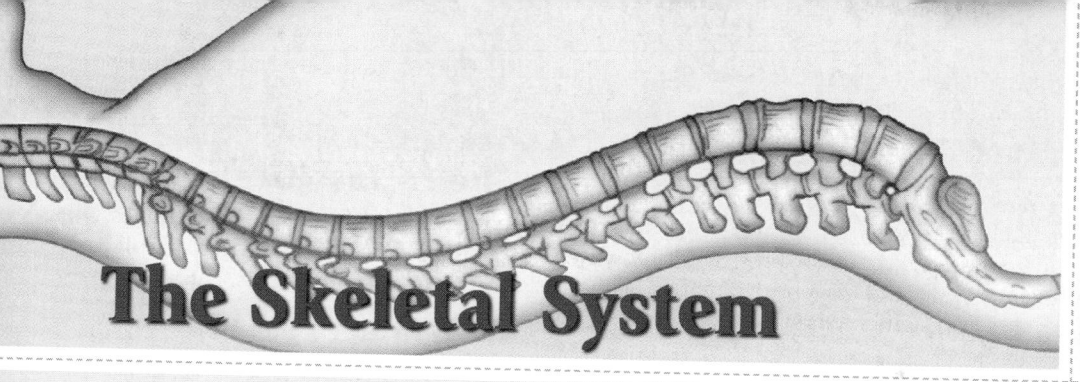

The Skeletal System

Learning Objectives

After completing this chapter, you should be able to:

- Define and spell the terms to learn for this chapter.
- Describe the skeletal system of the body.
- Explain various types of body movement.
- Discuss the vertebral column and explain its function.
- Identify abnormal curvatures of the spine.
- Discuss the male and female pelvis and explain the differences between them.
- List and explain common disorders of the skeletal system.
- Identify various types of fractures.

OUTLINE

Bones and Their Classification	378
Joints and Movement	380
The Axial Skeleton	381
The Appendicular Skeleton	383
Common Disorders Associated with the Skeletal System	383

Terms to Learn

abduction
adduction
amphiarthrotic joint
appendicular skeleton
arthritis
articulation
axial skeleton
bursitis
cancellous (spongy) bone
circumduction
compact bone

diaphysis
diarthrotic joint
dislocation
dorsiflexion
endosteum
epiphysis
eversion
extension
flexion
gout
inversion

medullary canal
osteoarthritis
osteoporosis
periosteum
pronation
protraction
retraction
rheumatoid arthritis
rotation
supination
synarthrotic joint

Case Study

JOSEPHINE IS A 62-YEAR-OLD FEMALE seen by Dr. Penningworth for a chief complaint of constant back pain, the development of a humpback, and loss of height. She is postmenopausal, has been a two-pack-a-day smoker for 45 years and drinks three beers a day. She also has a history of asthma and has regularly taken steroids in the past. She has broken her hip once and her wrist once. Dr. Penningworth diagnosed Josephine as having osteoporosis and kyphosis. He prescribed increased calcium, vitamin D, and Fosamax. He also prescribed physical therapy to develop a home exercise program focusing on weight-bearing exercises.

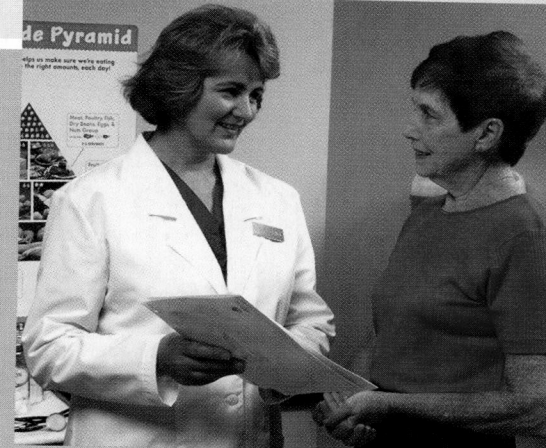

The skeletal system makes up the framework of the body. The skeletal system has 206 bones. The rest of the skeletal system is composed of cartilage and ligaments. There are two different divisions of the skeletal system: the axial skeleton, consisting of 80 bones from the axis of the body, including the skull and vertebral system, and the appendicular skeleton, which consists of the remaining 126 bones, including the extremities (see Figure 21-1).

Bones and Their Classification

The primary organs of the skeletal system are the bones, which consist of 50 percent water and 50 percent solid matter. The solid matter, or osseous tissue, is made of calcified, rigid tissue. Bones are classified according

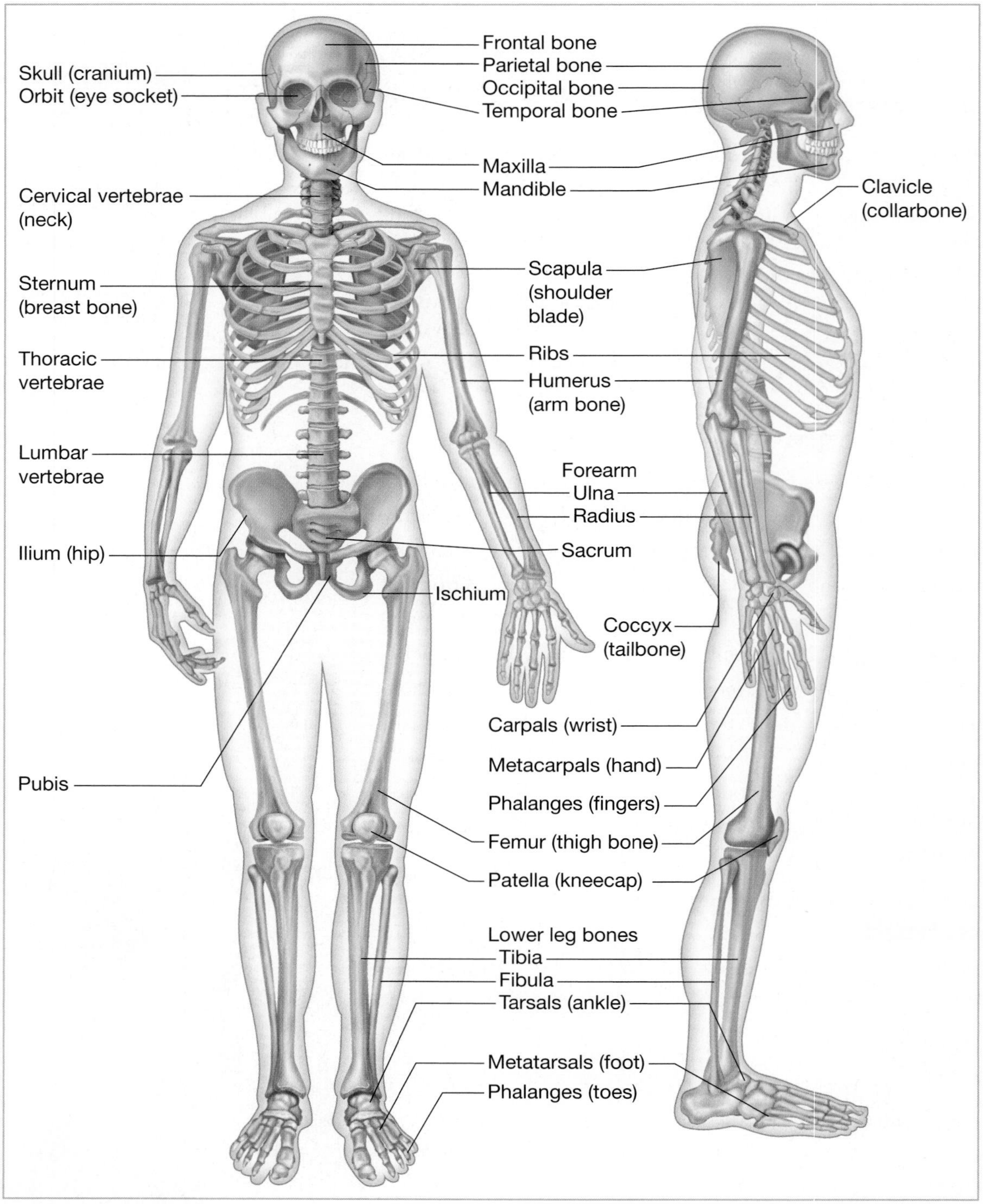

Frontal bone
Parietal bone
Skull (cranium)
Occipital bone
Orbit (eye socket)
Temporal bone

Maxilla
Mandible

Clavicle
(collarbone)

Cervical vertebrae
(neck)

Scapula
(shoulder
blade)

Sternum
(breast bone)

Thoracic
vertebrae

Ribs
Humerus
(arm bone)

Lumbar
vertebrae

Forearm
Ulna
Radius

Ilium (hip)

Sacrum

Ischium

Coccyx
(tailbone)

Pubis

Carpals (wrist)

Metacarpals (hand)

Phalanges (fingers)

Femur (thigh bone)

Patella (kneecap)

Lower leg bones
Tibia
Fibula
Tarsals (ankle)

Metatarsals (foot)
Phalanges (toes)

FIGURE 21-1 The human skeleton.

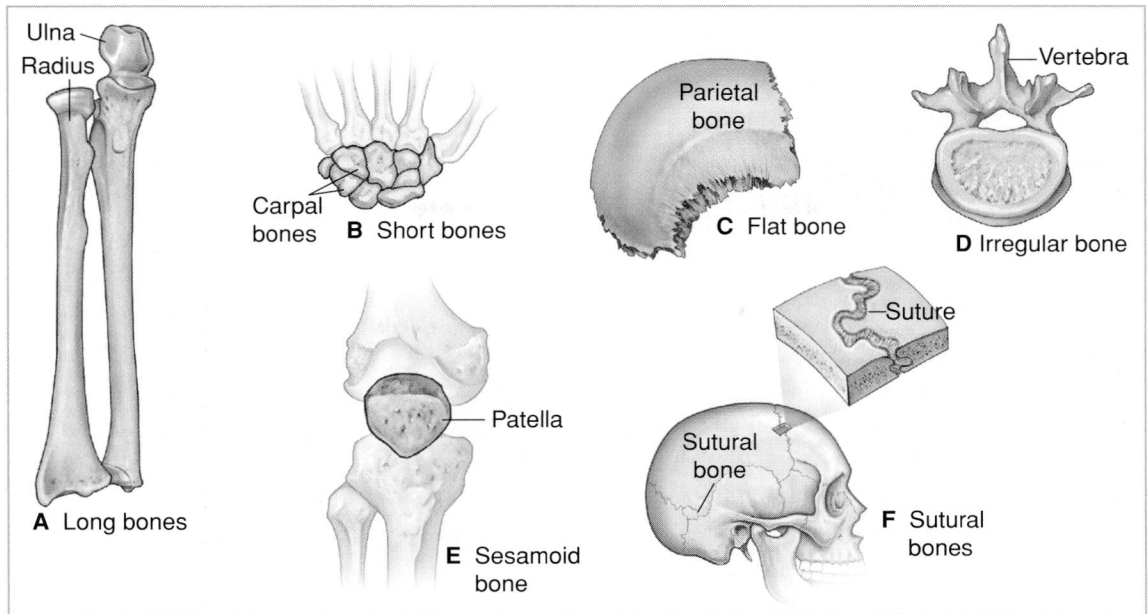

FIGURE 21-2 Classification of bones by shape.

to shape (see Figure 21-2). The six common shapes of bones are long, short, flat, irregular, sesamoid, and sutural (wormian) bones.

Functions of Bones

The bones of the skeleton have six main functions:

- Providing shape, support, and the framework of the body
- Providing protection for the body's internal organs

- Serving as a storage place for mineral salts, calcium, and phosphorus
- Playing an important role in the formation of blood cells as hemopoiesis takes place in the bone marrow
- Providing an area for the attachment of skeletal muscle
- Helping to make movement possible through articulation

Lifespan
Considerations

THE CHILD

- *Bones develop from cartilage. Babies are born with a large amount of cartilage and more bones than adults. These bones eventually fuse together to form the normal number of adult bones. Bone tissue begins to develop at the center of the cartilage, and blood vessels carry nutrients to the developing bone. As more bone tissue is formed, the bones grow longer. Eventually, the center of the bone is fully formed.*
- *A baby's bones are soft, but they gradually become harder as more minerals are deposited. This hardening process is called* ossification.
- *As a child grows, new bone tissue is made between the head of the bone and its shaft in special areas called* growth plates *or* growth zones. *This is how children grow taller.*

THE OLDER ADULT

- *Women build bone until about age 35 and then begin to lose about 1 percent of their bone mass annually. Men start losing bone mass approximately 10 to 20 years later. During the aging process, most of the skeletal system changes are a result of changes in connective tissue. Most bone loss is due to the loss of bone mineral content, especially calcium salts later in life. The calcium salts are deposited in the bone matrix and the cartilage becomes hard and brittle.*
- *As individuals age, they begin to have less joint movement, thus an increase in joint diseases, such as arthritis, begins to occur.*
- *Because of impaired functioning of the osteoblasts, which are the cells present in the bones, in the older adult, bone healing is slower than in children.*

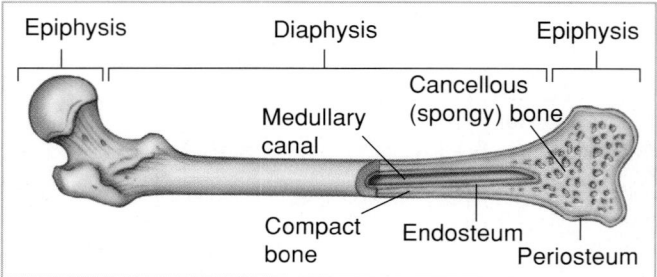

FIGURE 21-3 The features found in a long bone.

Structure of a Long Bone

Long bones, such as the tibia, femur, humerus, or radius, have most of the features found in all bones (see Figure 21-3). These features include the following:

- Epiphysis—the ends of a developing bone

- Diaphysis—the shaft of the long bone

- Periosteum—membrane that forms the covering of bones, except at their articular surfaces

- Compact bone—the dense, hard layer of bone tissue

- Medullary canal—the narrow space or cavity throughout the length of the diaphysis. The medullary canal contains yellow bone marrow, which is made of fat cells

- Endosteum—the tough, connective tissue membrane lining the medullary canal and containing the bone marrow

- Cancellous or spongy bone—the reticular tissue that makes up most of the volume of bone. The spongy bone contains red bone marrow, which manufactures most of the red blood cells found in the body and is found in the long bone.

TABLE 21-1	**Bone Markings**
Tuberosity	Large rounded projection that may be roughened
Crest	Narrow, usually prominent, ridge of bone
Trochanter	Very large, blunt, irregularly shaped process (bony projection)
Line	Narrow ridge of bone that is less prominent than a crest
Tubercle	Small rounded process
Epicondyle	Raised area on or above a condyle
Spine	Sharp, slender, often pointed process

See Lifestyle Considerations for information about the skeletal systems of children and older adults.

Bone Markings

The markings of bones are used to indicate the position of different structural features of the bones. These features mark the attachment of tendons and ligaments to muscles, joining of bones, and as passageways for blood vessels and nerves (see Table 21-1).

Joints and Movement

A joint, which is also called an articulation, is located at the place where two bones connect (see Figure 21-4). The positioning of the bones at the joint determines the type of movement that the joint performs. Because of this, joints are always classified according to the type of movement they provide. A joint that produces no movement is called a synarthrotic joint. While the bones may actually touch, there is no joint cavity. An example of a synarthrosis is the bones in the cranium. Amphiarthrotic joints permit very slight movement. An example of this joint is the vertebrae. Diarthrotic joints allow for free movement in a variety of directions. Examples of this type of joint are the elbow, wrist, hip, and knee.

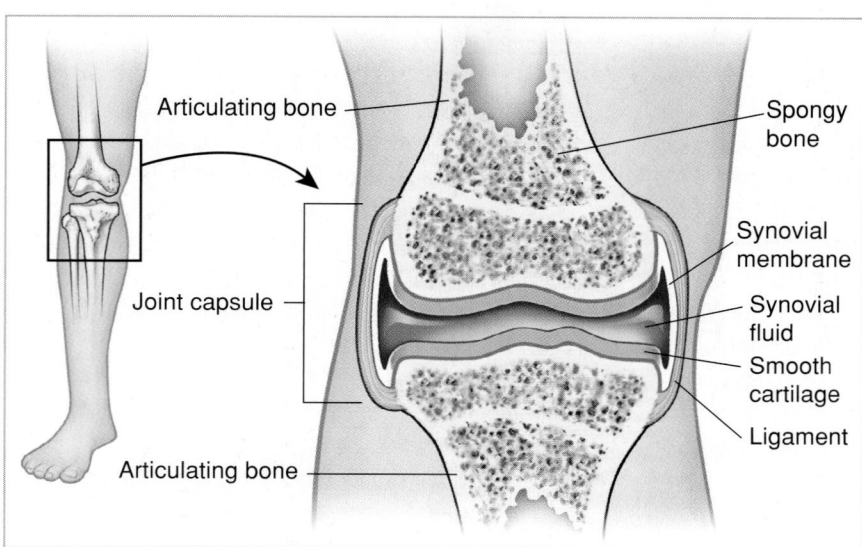

FIGURE 21-4 Typical joint.

Professionalism

The diarthrotic joint allows for several types of body movement. These movements, which can be seen in Figure 21-5, include the following:

- Abduction—movement of a body part *away* from the midline
- Adduction—movement of a body part *toward* the midline
- Circumduction—the process of moving a body part in a circular motion
- Dorsiflexion—the process of bending a body part backward
- Eversion—the process of turning outward
- Extension—the process of straightening a flexed limb
- Flexion—the process of bending (or curving) the spine
- Inversion—the process of turning inward
- Pronation—the process of lying prone or face down; the process of turning the hand so that the palm points downward
- Protraction—the process of moving a body part forward
- Retraction—the process of moving a body part backward
- Rotation—the process of moving a body part around a central axis

- Supination—the process of lying supine or face upward; also the process of turning the palm or foot upward

The Axial Skeleton

The axial skeleton is the central portion of the skeleton (see Figure 21-6). It consists of the skull, the sternum, the ribs, the vertebrae, the sacrum, and the coccyx. Twenty-two bones form the skull, 8 of which are located in the cranium and 14 that form the face (see Figure 21-7).

The vertebral column, which houses the spinal cord, consists of a series of vertebrae that are connected in

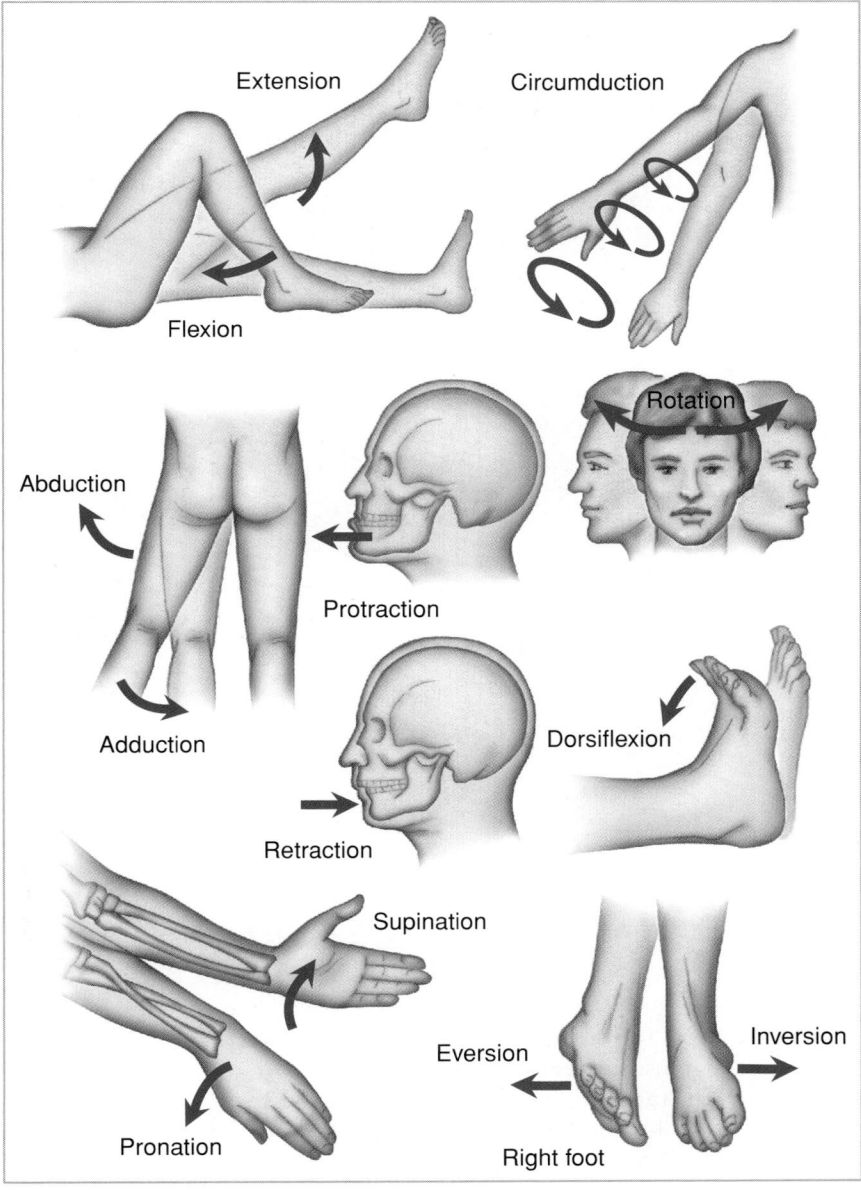

FIGURE 21-5   Types of body movements.

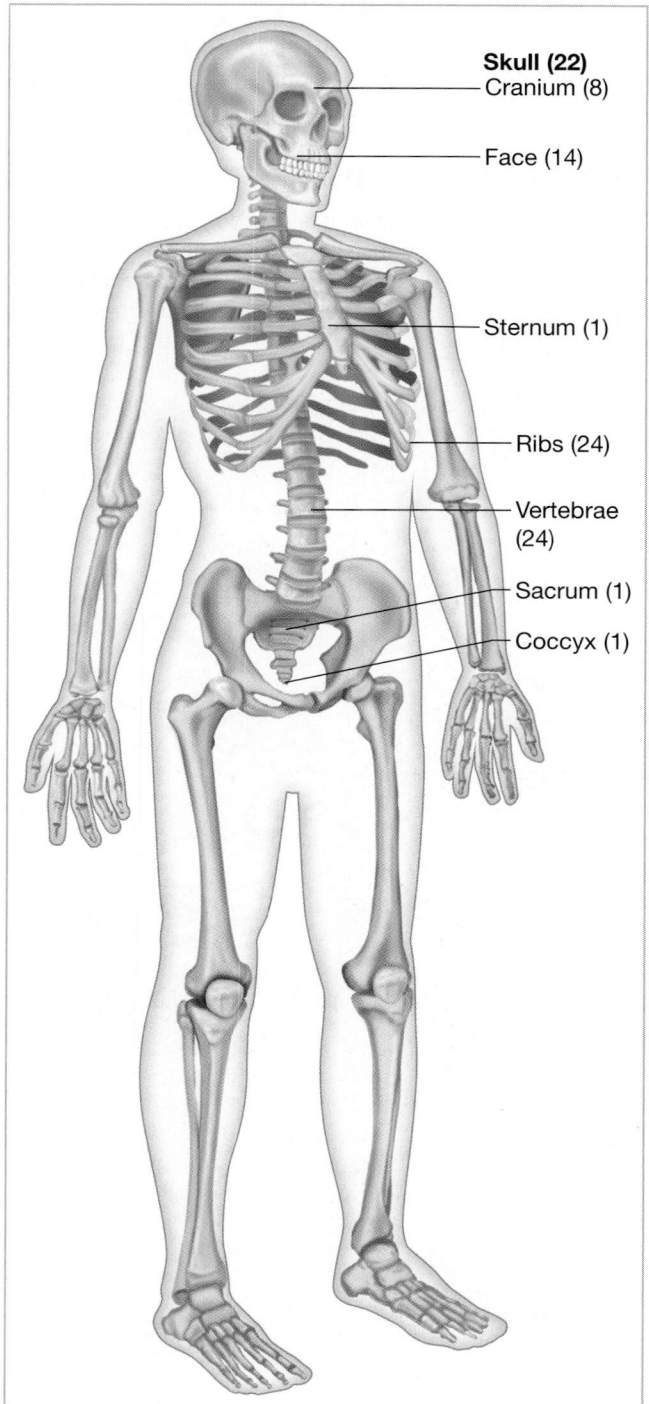

FIGURE 21-6 The axial skeleton.

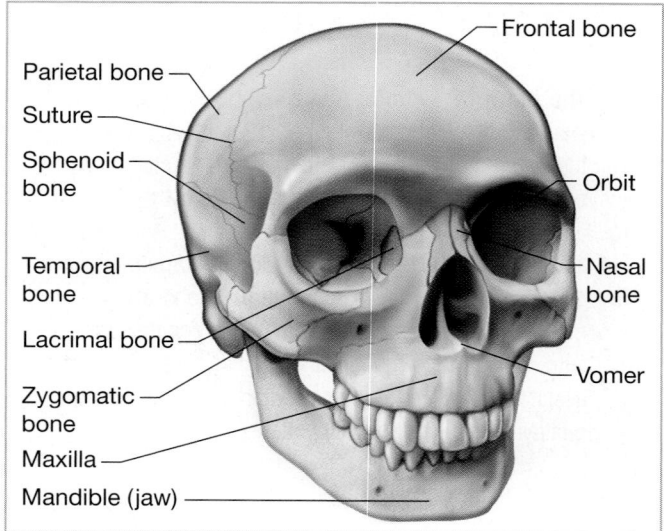

FIGURE 21-7 The cranial and facial bones.

The bones of the rib cage, which are also part of the axial skeleton and which can be seen in Figure 21-9, serve as protection for the vital organs, such as the heart and lungs. There are a total of 12 pairs of ribs.

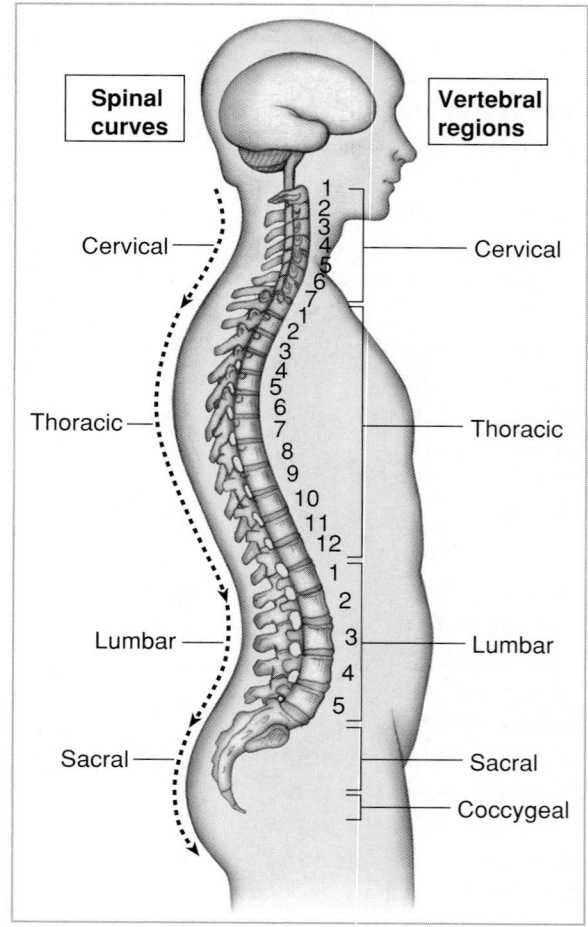

FIGURE 21-8 Vertebral regions showing the four spinal curves.

such a way as to form four spinal curves (see Figure 21-8). These curves are referred to as cervical, thoracic, lumbar, and sacral. The vertebrae are divided into five regions: the cervical, consisting of the first 7 vertebrae; the thoracic, which include the next 12 vertebrae; the 5 lumbar vertebrae; the sacral, and the coccyx, or tailbone.

On the posterior, or back side, the ribs articulate with the thoracic vertebrae. Anteriorly, or in front, 10 pair of ribs articulate with the sternum, which consists of the manubrium, body, and xiphoid process. Two pairs of ribs are called the floating ribs because they are attached only to the spinal vertebrae. There are three pairs of false ribs. They are called false because their cartilages do not reach the sternum directly. Instead, the cartilages of the three false ribs, which are located above the floating ribs, join the cartilages attached to the seven pairs of true ribs above. The true ribs attach both to the sternum and to the spinal vertebrae, while the false and the floating ribs have no cartilaginous attachments to the sternum at all. The three pair of false ribs are joined together on the anterior side of the body with the costal cartilage.

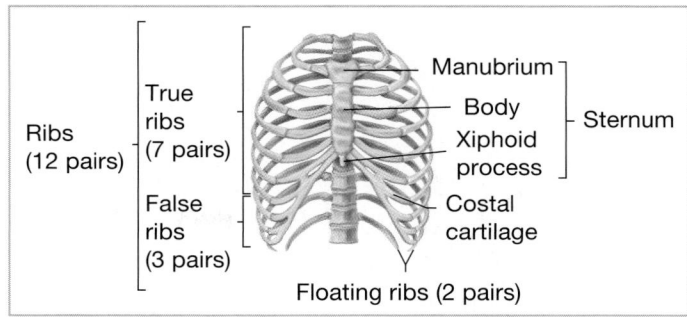

FIGURE 21-9 The rib cage.

The Appendicular Skeleton

The appendicular skeleton, which is responsible for body movement, consists of the upper and lower extremities, the pectoral girdle, and the pelvic girdle. The upper extremities include the pectoral girdle, consisting of the clavicles and the scapula. The bones of the upper extremities include the humerus, radius, ulna, carpals, metacarpals, and phalanges. The bones of the lower extremities include the femur, patella, tibia, fibula, tarsals, metatarsals, and phalanges (see Figure 21-10).

The pelvis, which is also part of the appendicular skeleton, forms the lower portion of the trunk of the body. It is easy to visualize the pelvis as a basin, with the posterior being formed by the sacrum and coccyx, and the hipbones forming the sides and front. The hipbones that help to form the bony pelvis are the ileum, the pubis, and the ischium (Figure 21-10C). In childhood, these bones are separate, but they fuse in adulthood.

The male pelvis (see Figure 21-11A) is shaped like a funnel, with the inferior outlet being significantly more narrow than seen in the female. It is stronger and heav-ier, and is more suited for lifting and running than is the female pelvis, which is shaped more like a basin than is the male pelvis. It may be oval to round and is wider than the male pelvis. The female pelvis, which can be seen in Figure 21-11B, is constructed to accommodate a fetus during pregnancy and then facilitate its downward passage through the pelvic cavity during the birth process. The female pelvis is lighter and broader than the male pelvis.

Common Disorders Associated with the Skeletal System

Various pathological conditions are associated with the skeletal system (see Table 21-2). (See Patient Education for information about teaching patients how to maintain bone health and prevent bone loss.)

Abnormal Curvature of the Spine

There are three common abnormal curvatures of the spine: scoliosis, lordosis, and kyphosis (see Figure 21-12). Scoliosis is an abnormal lateral curvature of the spine. This condition usually appears during adolescence, during periods of rapid growth. Treatment modalities may include the application of a brace or cast, traction, electrical stimulation, or surgery.

Patient Education

Medical assistants teach patients how to maintain bone health and prevent bone loss. Education can include information about dietary supplementation, exercise, lifestyle modification, and hormone replacement. When adults have healthy bones, they stand a smaller chance of developing bone fractures. Exercise and healthy nutrition can also help children to develop healthy bones and healthy habits to help prevent bone disease later in life. Any patient, regardless of his or her current state of bone health, can benefit from education and simple lifestyle changes.

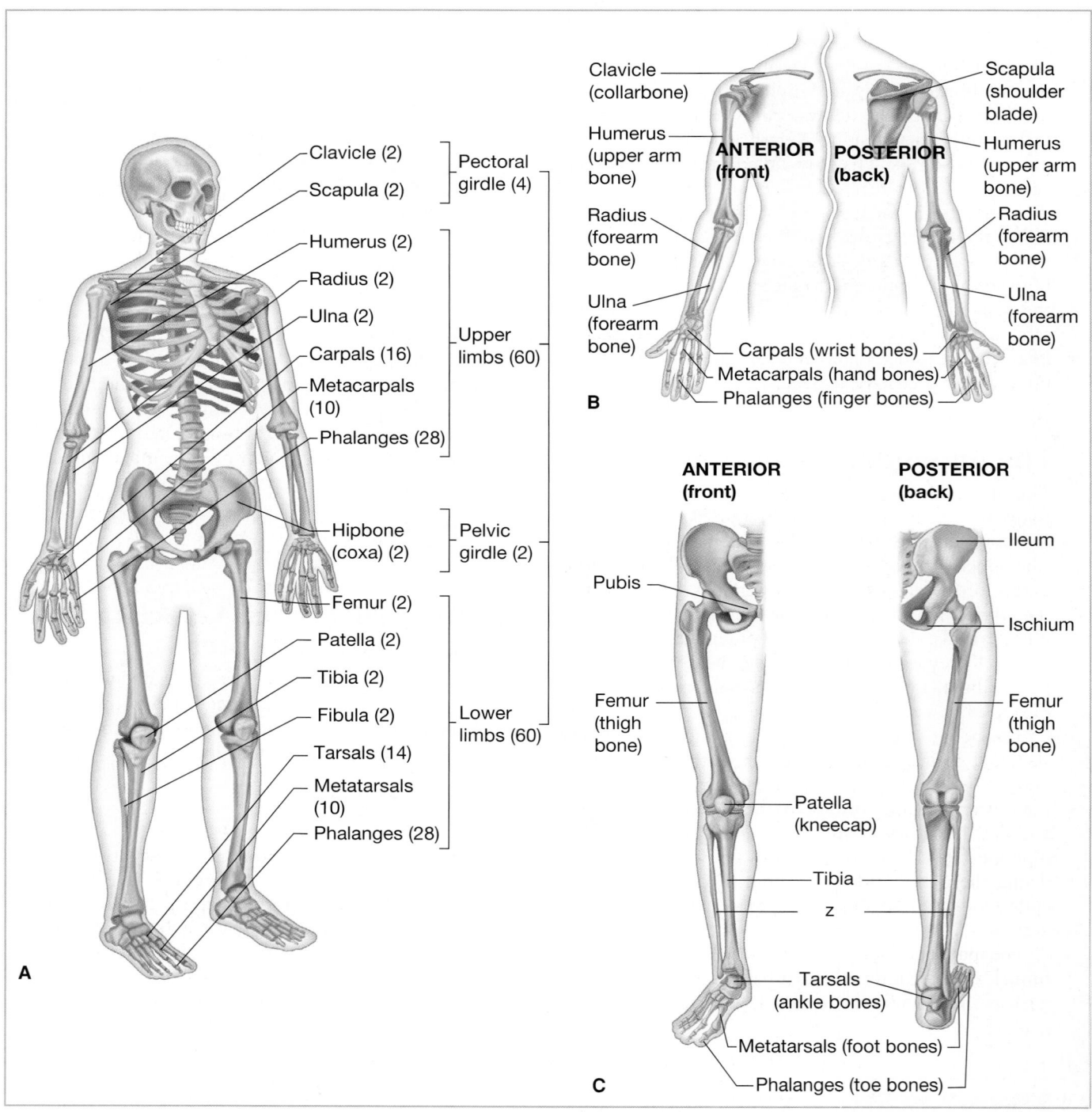

Clavicle (2)
Scapula (2)
} Pectoral girdle (4)

Humerus (2)
Radius (2)
Ulna (2)
Carpals (16)
Metacarpals (10)
Phalanges (28)
} Upper limbs (60)

Hipbone (coxa) (2)
} Pelvic girdle (2)

Femur (2)
Patella (2)
Tibia (2)
Fibula (2)
Tarsals (14)
Metatarsals (10)
Phalanges (28)
} Lower limbs (60)

A

Clavicle (collarbone)
Humerus (upper arm bone)
Radius (forearm bone)
Ulna (forearm bone)

ANTERIOR (front) POSTERIOR (back)

Scapula (shoulder blade)
Humerus (upper arm bone)
Radius (forearm bone)
Ulna (forearm bone)

Carpals (wrist bones)
Metacarpals (hand bones)
Phalanges (finger bones)

B

ANTERIOR (front) POSTERIOR (back)

Pubis
Femur (thigh bone)
Patella (kneecap)
Tibia
z
Tarsals (ankle bones)
Metatarsals (foot bones)
Phalanges (toe bones)

Ileum
Ischium
Femur (thigh bone)

C

FIGURE 21-10 (A) The appendicular skeleton. (B) Bones of the upper extremities. (C) Bones of the lower extremities.

Lordosis, also known as "swayback," is a condition in which the abdomen and buttocks protrude due to an exaggerated lumbar curvature. Lordosis is most commonly treated with physical therapy activities. Finally, kyphosis, sometimes referred to as "humpback," is a result of the normal thoracic curvature becoming exaggerated due to a congenital defect, disease process (such as tuberculosis, syphilis, or malignancy), compression fracture, faulty posture, osteoarthritis, rheumatoid arthritis, rickets, osteoporosis, or other conditions.

Arthritis

Arthritis is the inflammation of one or more joint. Various disease processes cause arthritis, including joint injury, autoimmune disorders, and wear and tear

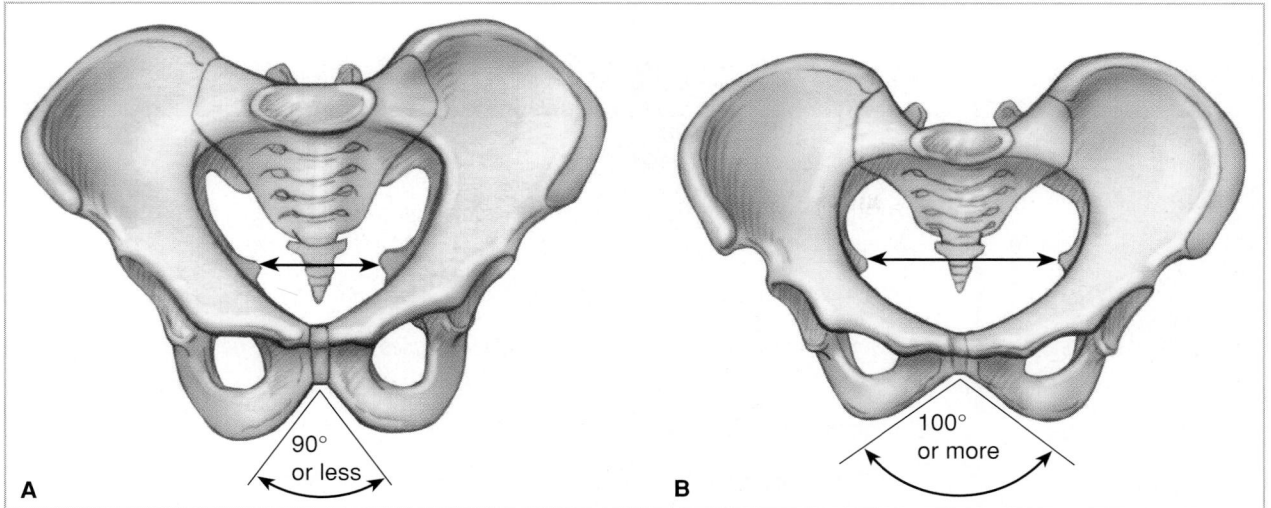

FIGURE 21-11 (A) The male pelvis; (B) the female pelvis.

on the joints. It is a condition that can occur in any individual of any age, although it most commonly occurs in older adults. Symptoms of arthritis include joint pain and swelling, morning stiffness, warmth and redness around a joint, and decreased ability to move the joint.

The treatment for arthritis varies, depending on the cause, the severity of the disease, the joints affected, and the age, occupation, and daily activities of the patient. Treatment is aimed at pain reduction and preventing further disability. Simple modifications in daily activities, including adequate rest and appropriate forms of exercise, may help to reduce the symptoms. Low-impact aerobic exercise (such as swimming) may relieve joint strain. Other times, more extensive therapies, including the application of heat or cold, joint protection, medications, and surgery, may be used. Medications to reduce joint pain and swelling include acetaminophen, aspirin, nonsteroidal anti-inflammatory drugs (NSAIDs), corticosteroids, and other immunosuppressive drugs. There are also "antibiologic" drugs, still fairly new, which can help reduce inflammation. These medications are administered by injection or intravenously.

Osteoarthritis

Osteoarthritis is the most common type of arthritis resulting from years of wear and tear on joints (see Figure 21-13). It most frequently occurs in the elderly in the hips, knees, and finger

joints. Obesity, a history of trauma, and various genetic and metabolic diseases increase the risk of osteoarthritis.

Rheumatoid Arthritis

Rheumatoid arthritis is an autoimmune disorder in which the joints may actually become deformed due to the inflammation (see Figure 21-14). This formation can be typically seen in the hands; however, rheumatoid arthritis may affect other parts of the body.

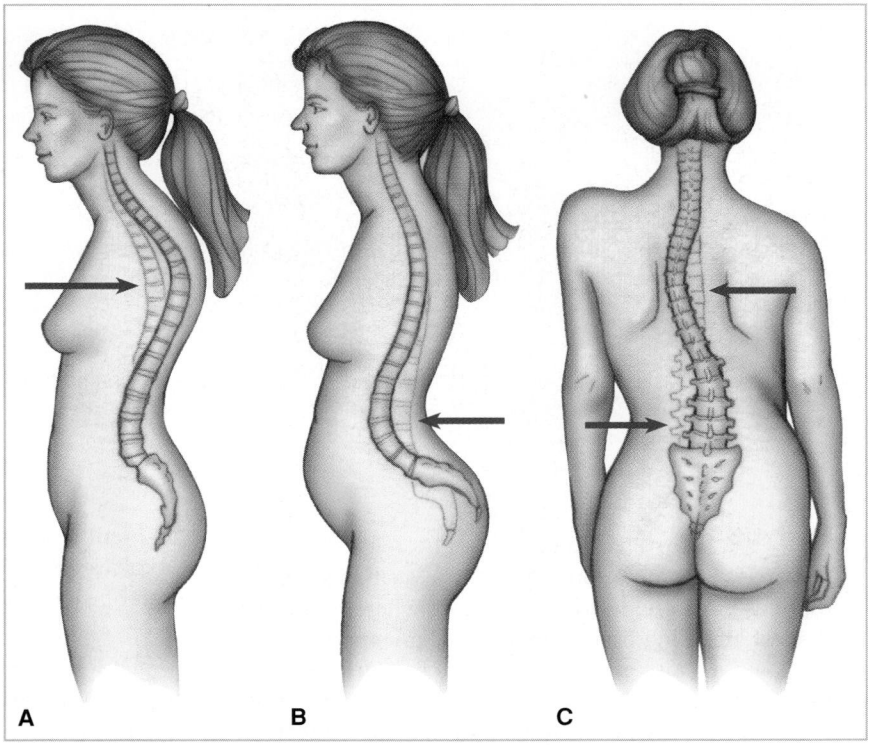

FIGURE 21-12 Abnormal curvatures of the spine: (A) kyphosis; (B) lordosis; (C) scoliosis.

TABLE 21-2 Disorders of the Skeletal System

Disorder	Description
Arthritis	Inflammation of the bone joints
Bunion	Enlargement of the joint at the base of the great toe caused by inflammation of the bursa of the great toe
Bursitis	Inflammation of the bursa, the connective tissue surrounding a joint
Carpal tunnel syndrome	Pain caused by compression of the nerve as it passes between the bones and tendons of the wrist
Gout	Inflammation of the joints caused by excessive uric acid
Kyphosis	Abnormal increase in the outward curvature of the thoracic spine; also known as hunchback or humpback
Lordosis	Abnormal increase in the forward curvature of the lumbar spine; also known as swayback
Osteoarthritis	Noninflammatory type of arthritis resulting in degeneration of the bones and joints, especially those bearing weight
Osteomalacia	Softening of the bones caused by a deficiency of phosphorus or calcium; it is thought that in children the cause is insufficient sunlight and vitamin D
Osteomyelitis	Inflammation of the bone and bone marrow due to infection; can be difficult to treat
Osteoporosis	Decrease in bone mass that results in a thinning and weakening of the bone with resulting fractures; the bones become more porous, especially in the spine and pelvis
Paget's disease	A fairly common metabolic disease of the bone from unknown causes; it usually attacks middle-aged and elderly people and is characterized by bone destruction and deformity
Rheumatoid arthritis	Chronic form of arthritis with inflammation of the joints, swelling, stiffness, pain, and changes in the cartilage that can result in crippling deformities
Rickets	Deficiency in calcium and vitamin D in early childhood that results in bone deformities, especially bowed legs
Ruptured intervertebral disk	Herniation or outpouching of a disk between two vertebrae; also called a slipped or herniated disk
Scoliosis	Abnormal lateral curvature of the spine
Spinal stenosis	Narrowing of the spinal canal causing pressure on the cord and nerves

Bursitis

Bursitis is inflammation of the bursa, a small sac of fluid that cushions and lubricates an area where joint-related tissues, including bones, tendons, ligaments, muscles, or skin, rub against one another. It occurs most frequently in the elbow, knee, shoulder, and hip, and is generally the result of overuse and trauma to joints. The most common signs and symptoms include joint pain, swelling, and tenderness surrounding the joint. Treatment usually involves rest, pain medication, steroid injections, aspiration of excess fluid from the bursa, and antibiotics.

Carpal Tunnel Syndrome

The carpal tunnel is a narrow passageway about the diameter of the thumb located on the palm side of the wrist. The tunnel protects the main nerve to the hand

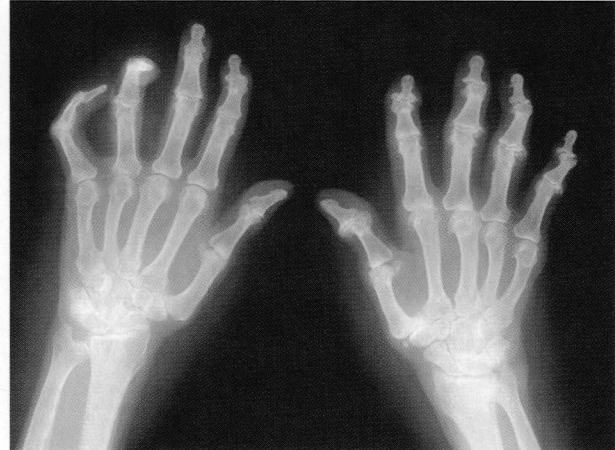

FIGURE 21-13   X-ray showing typical joint changes associated with osteoarthritis.

and the nine tendons that bend the fingers. When pressure is placed on this nerve (the median nerve), pain is produced along with numbness and hand weakness.

Injury or trauma to the areas, including repetitive movement of the wrists, can cause swelling of the tissues that surround the nerve, causing the known symptoms of carpal tunnel syndrome. Repetitive movements might be caused by sports such as racquetball or tennis, or activities such as sewing, keyboarding, driving, assembly-line work, painting, writing, the use of hand tools or vibrating tools, or other similar activities.

The most common age of occurrence of carpal tunnel syndrome is between ages 30 and 60. It occurs more commonly in women than men. Certain conditions increase the risk of carpal tunnel syndrome, including obesity, diabetes, and rheumatoid arthritis. Proper treatment can alleviate the symptoms of pain and numbness, and can restore the normal use of the wrists. Treatment can include the application of wrist splints at night for several weeks. Hot and cold compresses may also be used. Another important treatment is the evaluation of the working environment. Individuals should ensure that their wrists are held relatively straight during keyboarding and other activities. If the wrists are hyperextended (bent backwards), the chance for carpal tunnel syndrome increases. Many other specialized tools are available that can be used to decrease wrist stress.

Medications used in the treatment of carpal tunnel syndrome include the use of NSAIDs such as ibuprofen or naproxen. Injections of corticosteroids can also help decrease the symptoms. If these measures do not provide significant relief, then a surgical procedure that decreases the pressure on the median nerve is about 85 percent effective in relieving carpal tunnel symptoms. The healing process from the surgery may take several months, so the results are not immediately seen.

Fractures

Fractures or bone breaks, are classified based on their external appearance, the site of the fracture, and the nature of the crack or break in the bone. The different types of fractures, some of which are illustrated in Figure 21-15, include:

- Closed: Also known as a simple fracture, this type of fracture does not involve a break in the skin. It is completely internal.
- Open (compound): These are more dangerous fractures because of the projection of the fracture through the skin. Because the integrity of the skin and other tissues is damaged in this type of fracture, there is a greater risk of infection or hemorrhage than with a closed fracture.

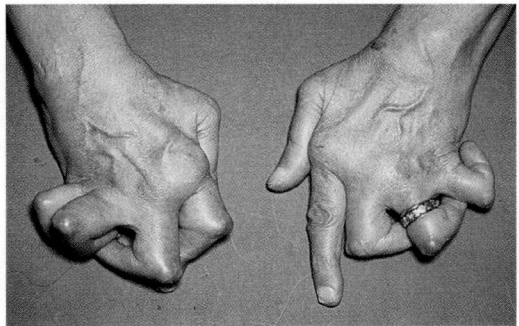

FIGURE 21-14   Typical hand deformities associated with rheumatoid arthritis.

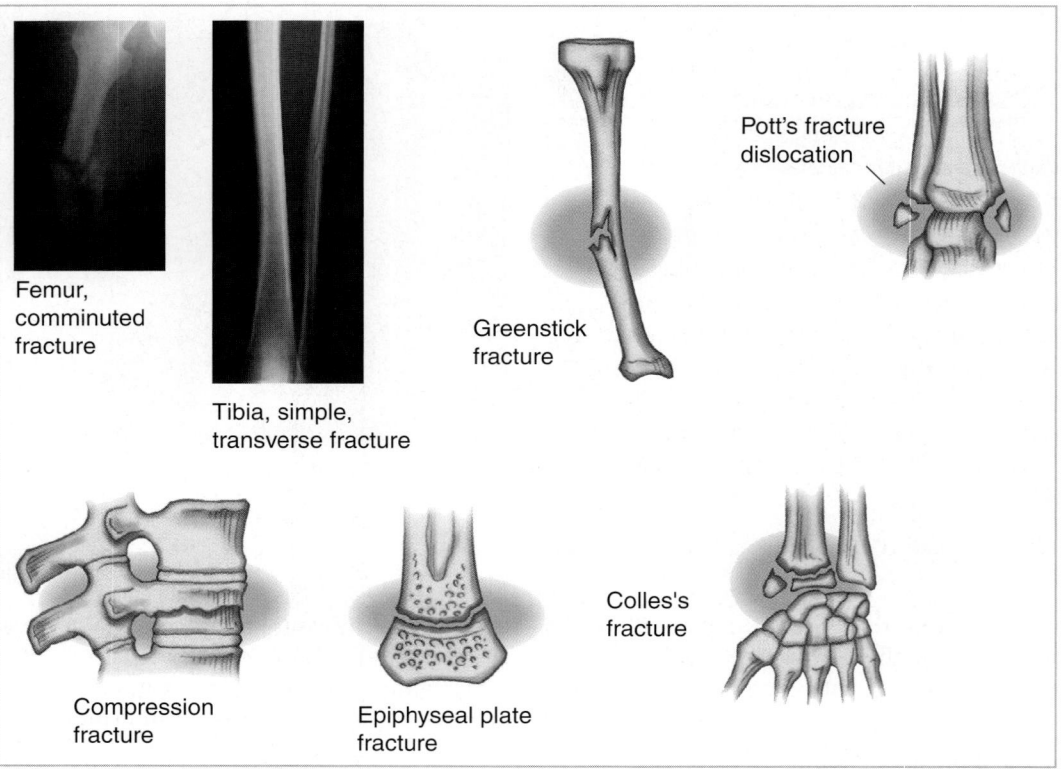

FIGURE 21-15 Various types of fractures.

- Comminuted: In this type of fracture, part of the bone is shattered into a multitude of bony fragments.

- Transverse: These fractures break the shaft of the bone across its longitudinal access.

- Greenstick: This type of fracture usually occurs in young children, whose bones are still relatively

soft. In a greenstick fracture, only one side of the shaft is broken; the other side is bent, similar to breaking a green stick.

- Spiral: Spiral fractures are spread along the length of a bone, and are produced by twisting stresses.

- Colles's: Colles's fracture is frequently the result of reaching forward to stop or cushion a fall. This fracture is exemplified by a break in the distal portion of the radius. Colles's fractures are most frequently seen in children and the elderly.

- Pott's: These are fractures that occur in the ankle and affect both bones of the lower leg (the tibia and fibula).

- Compression: Compression fractures occur in the vertebrae after severe stress, such as when someone falls and "sits down" with a significant amount of force.

- Epiphyseal: These fractures are commonly seen in children in areas where the matrix is undergoing calcification and the chondrocytes are dying.

Dislocations

As discussed earlier, joints are areas where two or more bones come together. If a sudden impact injures a joint, the bones that meet at that joint may become dislocated, or not connected. That means the bones are no longer in their normal position. Usually the joint capsule and ligaments tear when a joint becomes dislocated, and often the nerves are injured.

Dislocations usually occur following a blow, fall, or other trauma. The dislocated joint may be visibly out of place, discolored, or misshapen, limited in movement, swollen or bruised, and intensely painful, especially if the person tries to use the joint or bear weight on it.

Gout

Gout is a disease caused by the formation of crystals in the joints, leading to inflammation. It is most commonly seen in men over the age of 40, and the most frequent joint affected is the great toe. Medications are available to treat gout, and a diet rich in colorful fruits and vegetables helps to decrease the symptoms of gout.

Osteoporosis

Osteoporosis is characterized by the progression of loss of bone density and the thinning of bone tissue. This condition is seen most commonly in older adults, especially postmenopausal women and in individuals who do not consume enough calcium. If there is not enough calcium in the diet, then the body appropriates calcium from the bones to continue the many chemical reactions requiring calcium. Vitamin D is required for the processing of calcium.

Osteoporosis affects more than 25 million Americans, mostly women ages 50 to 70 years old. Individuals with osteoporosis are subject to increased fracture potential, especially in the hips, vertebrae, and wrists.

Individuals are at a higher risk of this disease if they have a family history of osteoporosis. Others who may also be at risk include people who tend not to do weight-bearing exercises as part of their lifestyle, Cau-

Cultural Considerations

Although Caucasian women have a higher risk of osteoporosis, the disease also affects other races. It is important to teach all women, and men, the risk factors for osteoporosis and the prevention of osteoporosis. Any individual who is slender is at a greater risk for osteoporosis, but larger individuals may also be at risk. It is also important to double check the patient's past medical history. Any individual who has taken steroids over a long period of time is at risk, and the physician should be alerted.

casian females who have never been pregnant and are experiencing early menopause, individuals who have a history of frequent corticosteroid use, and those people who smoke, drink alcohol, have a diet high in salt, caffeine, or fat, or have an insufficient intake of calcium or vitamin D (Cultural Considerations). The risk in these populations can be decreased by increasing calcium and vitamin D intake, decreasing risk-increasing behaviors, and engaging in daily weight-bearing exercise.

Diagnosis of osteoporosis is done by bone density testing. Treatments include calcium and vitamin D supplementation, medications to help preserve calcium, hormone replacement, and exercise.

SUMMARY

The skeletal system makes up the framework of the human body. Consisting of 206 bones and cartilage and ligaments this system is responsible for providing shape and support, protecting internal organs, and serving as a storage place for mineral salts, calcium, and phosphorus. The skeletal system also plays an important role in the formation of blood cells and in providing an area for the attachment of skeletal muscles.

Chapter Review

COMPETENCY REVIEW

1. Define and spell the terms to learn for this chapter.
2. Name the two main divisions of the skeletal system.
3. Name the five classifications of bone and give an example of each.
4. Discuss the six main functions of the skeletal system.

5. Name the three classifications of joints.
6. What is abduction?
7. What is adduction?
8. What is extension?
9. What is the medical term for lying face down?
10. What is arthritis?

PREPARING FOR THE CERTIFICATION EXAM

1. Which of the following bones is NOT one of the lower extremity bones?
   A. femur
   B. patella
   C. tibia
   D. ulna
   E. tarsal

2. A wrist fracture is
   A. comminuted
   B. compound
   C. transverse
   D. greenstick
   E. Colles's

3. Backward bending movement at a joint is called
   A. circumduction
   B. inversion
   C. dorsiflexion
   D. supination
   E. plantar flexion

4. Which of the following bones is NOT one of the bones of the upper extremities?
   A. fibula
   B. clavicle
   C. scapula
   D. humerus
   E. radius

5. Which of the following bones is NOT one of the cranial bones?
   A. temporal
   B. vomer
   C. occipital
   D. parietal
   E. sphenoid

6. The cheekbones are the
   A. mandibular bones
   B. maxillary bones
   C. palatine bones
   D. zygomatic bones
   E. lacrimal bones

7. How many bones are in the lumbar vertebrae?
   A. 1
   B. 3
   C. 5
   D. 7
   E. 12

8. The end of a long bone is called the
   A. epiphysis
   B. diaphysis
   C. periosteum
   D. mediastinum
   E. cartilage

9. What is the name of the membrane that forms the covering of bones, except at their articular surfaces?
   A. epiphysis
   B. diaphysis
   C. periosteum
   D. mediastinum
   E. cartilage

10. Which of the following is NOT a division of the spine?
    A. lumbar
    B. thoracic
    C. parietal
    D. cervical
    E. sacral

CRITICAL THINKING

1. If Josephine has broken her wrist, what is the most likely type of fracture she sustained?

2. Why did the physician order physical therapy?

3. What other lifestyle changes could Josephine make to slow the development of her osteoporosis?

INTERNET ACTIVITY

Do an internet search to look up the National Osteoporosis Association. Research the association to see what information they provide for both patients and health care providers. Utilize this information to learn how to teach a patient about osteoporosis.

MediaLink More on the skeletal system, including interactive resources, can be found on the Student CD-ROM accompanying this textbook.

throughout the body. Muscles made from these types of cells include those found in the walls of blood vessels, the urinary bladder, and the digestive system.

Skeletal muscles allow movement by being attached to bones in the body. Skeletal muscles control voluntary movements, which can be consciously controlled. Skeletal muscles are made up of cylindrical fibers that are found in the locomotive system. The nucleus of each cell tends to be toward the edge of each cell and the cells are striated.

Cardiac muscles are roughly quadrangular in shape and have a single central nucleus. The cells form a network of branching fibers. The muscles are cross striated and are involuntary. The muscles are found in the heart. Muscle tissues are supplied with nerve fibers that carry messages to and from the central nervous system (brain and spinal cord).

Finally, it is important to note that muscles are composed of about 75 percent water, 20 percent protein, and about 5 percent carbohydrates, lipids, inorganic salts, and nonprotein nitrogenous compounds. The composition does vary in the different muscles.

Energy Production for Muscle

Muscles use energy in the form of ATP (adenosine triphosphate), which is a type of chemical energy needed for sustained or repeated muscular contractions. To make the ATP, thus creating an atmosphere in which the muscle cells can make this energy, the muscle must do the following:

- Break down the creatine phosphate, which is a protein that stores extra phosphate groups. This is a very fast way for the muscles to produce energy.
- Carry out anaerobic respiration by which glucose is broken down to lactic acid, thus forming the ATP.
- Carry out aerobic respiration, by which glucose, glycogen, fats, and amino acids are broken down in the presence of oxygen, thus leading to the production of ATP.

Oxygen Debt and Muscle Fatigue

When skeletal muscles are used for more than a minute or two, a condition called oxygen debt may occur. Simply put, this means that if your body is working hard, and you are breathing in a lot of oxygen, your body may not be able to absorb enough to cope with the level of activity. If this happens, your body is mainly utilizing the anaerobic energy system and, as a result, lactic acid builds up as an undesirable waste product. This system can only be sustained for about 60 seconds, depending on the individual, before severe fatigue sets in, making it very difficult to recover. The amount of oxygen "owed" to the body in order to recover is called the oxygen debt.

Muscle fatigue, which is often accompanied by muscle cramps, occurs when a muscle has lost its ability to contract. Like oxygen debt, it usually develops as a result of an accumulation of lactic acid. It may also occur if the blood supply to a muscle is stopped or interrupted, or if a motor neuron loses its ability to release acetylcholine into the muscle fibers.

Structure of Skeletal Muscles

Skeletal muscle is also known as striated muscle or voluntary muscle (see Figure 22-3). Skeletal muscle is controlled by the conscious part of the brain, and each of these muscles attaches to bones. There are 600 different skeletal muscles that are responsible for the movement of the body through contractility, extensibility, and elasticity. When viewed under a microscope, skeletal muscle has a cross-striped appearance, which is the reason why skeletal muscle is also known as striated muscle. Various sizes, shapes, and fiber arrangements create a variety of muscles that can each perform a specific function for its use in the body.

Several coverings made up of connective tissue are associated with skeletal muscle. The fascia is the structure covering the entire skeletal muscle and separating the muscles from one another. Muscles, which are surrounded by a thin covering called the epimysium, are attached to bones by structures called tendons. The aponeurosis is a wide, thin, sheet-like tendon, made up of fibrous connective tissue, that typically attaches muscles to other muscles. The perimysium, also made up of connective tissue,

Professionalism

Because there are going to be unhappy patients, and physicians, in any medical practice, it is important to realize that most of the time, individuals who complain about service are not attacking the person responding to their call, but are instead venting their frustration, because they do not understand something. As a professional, it is important for you to understand that listening and learning go hand-in-hand. If a person is upset or concerned about his or her health, instead of getting angry, take the time to "listen," and try to focus on how you can best meet that person's needs.

is responsible for dividing a muscle into sections called fascicles. The endomysium is the covering made up of connective tissue that surrounds the individual muscle cell.

Attachments to Skeletal Muscles

The actions of the skeletal muscles depend greatly on what the skeletal muscles are attached to. The origins and insertions are the locations at which skeletal muscles attach. The origin is the attachment to the bone that is more fixed, or still, while the insertion is the attachment point on the bone that moves.

Muscles and nerves function together as a motor unit. Skeletal muscles require innervation to contract. To complete such a task, these muscles must move as a single unit. The three types of skeletal muscle units include:

- Antagonist—a muscle that counteracts, or opposes, the action of another muscle

- Prime mover—a muscle that is the primary actor in a given movement. This is the muscle that produces the movement in muscle contraction

- Synergist—a muscle that acts with another muscle to produce movement

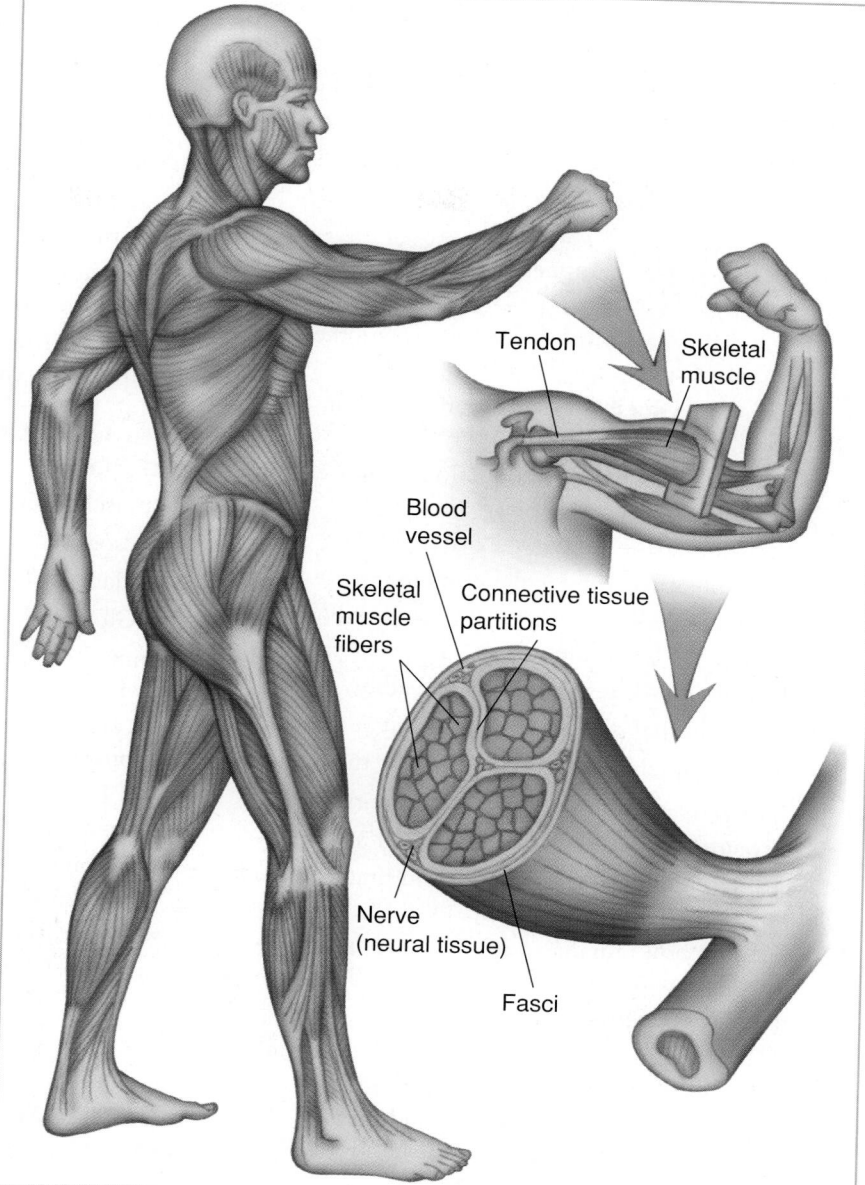

FIGURE 22-3   A skeletal muscle consists of a group of fibers held together by connective tissue. It is enclosed in a fibrous sheath (fascia).

Labels in figure: Tendon · Skeletal muscle · Blood vessel · Skeletal muscle fibers · Connective tissue partitions · Nerve (neural tissue) · Fasci

Major Skeletal Muscles

When describing the major skeletal muscles, it is important to remember that these muscles are often identified according to their location, size, action, shape, or number of attachments of the muscle. They are usually listed in the following groups:

- Muscles of the head
- Muscles of the arm, wrist, hand, and fingers
- Respiratory muscles
- Abdominal muscles
- Muscles of the pectoral girdle
- Muscles of the leg, ankle, and foot.

Muscles of the Head

The muscles of the head include those that move the head, provide facial expressions, and move the jaw. They include the following muscles:

- Sternocleidomastoid—pulls the head from side to side and head to chest
- Splenulus capitis—rotates the head and allows it to bend to the side

The muscles that provide for facial expression include the following:

- Frontalis—raises the eyebrows
- Orbicularis oris—allows the lips to pucker
- Orbicularis oculi—allows the eyes to close

- Zygomaticus—pulls the corners of the mouth up
- Platysma—pulls the corners of the mouth down

The muscles of the jaw allow for chewing, or mastication. They include the following:

- Masseter and temporalis—close the jaw

Muscles of the Arm, Wrist, Hand, and Fingers

Muscles that move the upper extremity include those in the arm and forearm:

- Pectoralis major—pulls the arm across the chest and also rotates and adducts the arms
- Latissimus dorsi—provides for extension, adduction, and rotation of the arm inwardly
- Deltoid—provides for abduction and extension of the arm at the shoulder
- Subscapularis—rotates the arm medially
- Infraspinatus—rotates the arm laterally
- Biceps brachii—flexes the arm at the elbow and rotates the hand laterally
- Brachialis—flexes the arm at the elbow
- Brachioradialis—flexes the forearm at the elbow
- Triceps brachii—extends the arm at the elbow
- Supinator—rotates the forearm laterally
- Pronator teres—rotates the forearm medially

Muscles that move the wrist, hand, and fingers include the following:

- Flexor carpi radialis and flexor carpi ulnaris—flex and abduct the wrist
- Palmaris longus—flexes the wrist
- Flexor digitorum profundus—flexes the distal joints of the fingers, but not the thumb
- Extensor carpi radialis longae and brevis—extend the wrist and abduct the hand
- Extensor carpi ulnaris—extends the wrist
- Extensor digitorum—extends the fingers, but not the thumb

Respiratory Muscles

The muscles of respiration include the following:

- Diaphragm—separates the thoracic cavity from the abdominal cavity and its contraction causes the process of inspiration
- External and internal intercostals—contraction of these muscles expands and lowers the ribs during breathing

Abdominal Muscles

The muscles of the abdominal wall include the following:

- External and internal obliques—compress the abdominal wall
- Transverse abdominis—also compresses the abdominal wall
- Rectus abdominis—flexes the vertebral column and compresses the abdominal wall

Muscles of the Pectoral Girdle

The muscles that move the pectoral girdle, or shoulder, include the following:

- Trapezius—raises the arms and pulls the shoulders downward
- Pectoralis minor—pulls the scapula downward and raises the ribs

Muscles of the Leg, Ankle, and Foot

The muscles that move the leg include the following:

- Psoas major—flexes the thigh
- Iliacus—also flexes the thigh
- Gluteus maximus—extends the thigh

The muscles that move the ankle and foot include the following:

- Gastrocnemius—flexes the foot and aids in pushing the body forward
- Tibialis anterior—causes dorsiflexion and inversion of the foot
- Peroneus—everts the foot and helps bring about plantar flexion
- Flexor and extensor digitorum longus—flexes and extends the toes and assists in other movements of the feet

---

Common Disorders Associated with the Muscular System

Muscular disorders are characterized by abnormalities of muscle fibers. In addition, many neurological disorders, such as lesions of the central or peripheral nervous system and abnormalities of neuromuscular transmission, can also produce symptoms that are primarily muscular. Other systemic disorders, including those that are frequently seen in conditions of the cardiovascular, respiratory, and endocrine systems, frequently mimic muscular disorders but do not directly affect muscular function. These systemic disorders account for more than half of muscular complaints.

Difficulty in walking, unsteadiness with occasional falls, and joint stiffness with leg pains, especially at night, may also be due to conditions affecting the skeletal system, such as degenerative joint disease and rheumatoid arthritis. Significant degenerative joint disease can limit mobility by producing structural spinal

Medical assistants teach patients how to maintain good posture and a healthy attitude toward exercise. Education can include information about dietary supplementation, exercise, and lifestyle modification. When adults maintain a healthy attitude toward exercise, they stand less chance of developing disorders that will negatively affect them and their muscular system in later life.

Exercise and healthy nutrition can also help children to develop healthy habits to prevent muscle weakness and other disorders later in life. Expectant parents can also prevent pain and hardships by testing their unborn infants for possible congenital and neuromuscular diseases prior to birth.

changes and joint symptoms in the limbs and occasionally by damaging the spinal cord, nerve roots, and peripheral nerves.

Atrophy

Atrophy occurs with the disuse of muscles over a long period of time. Oftentimes, atrophy is caused by bed rest and immobility, which cause a loss of muscle mass and strength. If the atrophy is caused by a specific treatment (such as a cast or traction), some atrophy can be minimized by the practice of isometric exercises of the immobilized limb. Isometric exercise uses active muscle contractions performed against stable resistance—for example, tightening the muscles of the thighs or the buttocks. Active exercise of uninjured limbs helps prevent atrophy.

Lipoatrophy, which is a type of atrophy that can occur at a site of insulin or corticosteroid injections, is the atrophy of fat tissue. It is also known as lipodystrophy.

Fibromyalgia

Fibromyalgia is a widespread musculoskeletal pain and fatigue disorder affecting an estimated 3 million individuals in the United States, generally women more than men. Symptoms include mild to severe muscle pain and fatigue, sleep disorders, irritable bowel syndrome, depression, and chronic headaches. There is no obvious known cause of fibromyalgia, but there is evidence pointing to a genetic predisposition that creates a neuromuscular/neuroendocrine abnormality that disturbs the usual sensory perception, especially to pain signals.

The American College of Rheumatology (ACR) has identified specific criteria for fibromyalgia. The ACR states that a patient must show pain at 11 of 18 trigger points to be considered for a diagnosis of fibromyalgia. The patient must also have a history of widespread pain lasting at least 3 months.

Treatment is geared toward improving the quality of sleep and reducing pain. Sleep is important for many body functions, including tissue repair and antibody production, so the disruption of sleep will directly affect the quality of life in a patient with fibromyalgia. Frequently, the medications prescribed for fibromyalgia include muscle relaxants, antidepressants, antianxiety medications, and anti-inflammatories. Other treatments frequently employed include chiropracty, acupuncture, acupressure, relaxation techniques, and massage.

Muscle Cramps and Pain

Muscle cramps or pain in the absence of electrolyte or pH disturbance commonly indicates a peripheral nerve disorder and less commonly an abnormality in muscle fibers. Intense pain that is most prominent in proximal muscles in the morning may indicate polymyalgia rheumatica. Pain in localized muscle regions may indicate fibromyalgia. Pain largely restricted to muscle groups and periarticular tissue may indicate diffuse arthritic disease with limited muscle function.

Muscular Dystrophy

Muscular dystrophy (MD) is one of a group of genetic diseases characterized by progressive weakness and degeneration of the skeletal or voluntary muscles that

Cultural Considerations

Some cultures, such as those seen in the Far East, include exercise and holistic health as a way of life. Hence, many of the citizens of those countries may experience fewer problems affecting the muscular system. It is important for the medical assistant to be sensitive to the beliefs of patients from different cultures and to gain an understanding of how culture may play a role in their daily lives.

control movement. The muscles of the heart and some other involuntary muscles are also affected in some forms of muscular dystrophy, and a few forms involve other organs as well. The major forms of muscular dystrophy include:

- Duchenne's muscular dystrophy
- Becker's muscular dystrophy
- Limb-girdle muscular dystrophy
- Facioscapulohumeral muscular dystrophy
- Congenital muscular dystrophy
- Oculopharyngeal muscular dystrophy
- Distal muscular dystrophy
- Emery-Dreifuss muscular dystrophy
- Myotonic dystrophy

Muscular dystrophy can affect people of all ages. Although some forms first become apparent in infancy or childhood, others may not appear until middle age or later. Duchenne's muscular dystrophy is the most common kind of muscular dystrophy affecting children. Myotonic dystrophy is the most common of these diseases in adults.

There is no specific treatment for any of the forms of muscular dystrophy. Physical therapy to prevent contractures (a condition in which shortened muscles around joints cause abnormal and sometimes painful positioning of the joints), orthoses (orthopedic appliances used for support), and corrective orthopedic surgery may be needed to improve the quality of life in some cases. The cardiac problems that occur with Emery-Dreifuss muscular dystrophy and myotonic dystrophy may require a pacemaker. The myotonia (delayed relaxation of a muscle after a strong contraction) occurring in myotonic dystrophy may be treated with medications such as phenytoin or quinine.

The prognosis (outlook) with muscular dystrophy varies according to the type of muscular dystrophy and the progression of the disorder. Some cases may be mild and very slowly progressive with normal life span, while other cases may have more marked progression of muscle weakness, functional disability, and loss of ambulation. Life expectancy depends on the degree of progression and late respiratory deficit. In Duchenne's muscular dystrophy, death usually occurs in the late teens to early 20s.

Myasthenia Gravis

Myasthenia gravis (MG) is a chronic neuromuscular disease characterized by varying degrees of weakness of the skeletal or voluntary muscles of the body. The muscle weakness increases during periods of activity and improves after periods of rest. MG most commonly occurs in young adult women and older men but can occur at any age. Although MG may affect any voluntary muscle, certain muscles, including those that control eye movements, eyelids, chewing, swallowing, coughing, and facial expressions, are more often affected. Weakness may also occur in the muscles that control breathing and arm and leg movements. The muscles involved in MG vary from one individual to the next.

Today, MG is well controlled. Therapies include medications such as anticholinesterase agents, prednisone, cyclosporine, and azathioprine; thymectomy, which is the surgical removal of the thymus gland; plasmapheresis, a procedure in which abnormal antibodies are removed from blood plasma; and high-dose intravenous immunoglobulin, which modifies the immune system. A physician will determine which treatment option is best for each patient depending on the severity of the weakness, which muscles are affected, and the patient's age and other associated medical problems.

With treatment, most MG patients will have excellent improvement of their muscle weakness. In some patients, MG may go into remission and muscle weakness may disappear completely. In a few cases, MG may cause severe weakness resulting in acute respiratory failure; however, most patients can expect to lead normal or nearly normal lives.

Sprains and Strains

A sprain is an injury to a ligament—a stretching or a tearing—whereas a strain is an injury to either a muscle or a tendon. Depending on the severity of the injury, a strain may be a simple overstretching of the muscle or tendon, or it can result in a partial or complete tear.

Sprains

Typically, sprains occur when people fall and land on an outstretched arm, slide into base, land on the side of their foot, or twist a knee with the foot planted firmly on the ground. This results in an overstretching or tearing of the ligament supporting that joint.

Although sprains can occur in both the upper and lower parts of the body, the most common site is the ankle. Ankle sprains are the most common injury in the United States and often occur during sports or recreational activities.

The usual signs and symptoms include pain, swelling, bruising, and loss of the ability to move and use the joint (called functional ability). However, these signs and symptoms can vary in intensity, depending on the severity of the sprain. Sometimes people feel a pop or tear when the injury happens. In general, a grade I or mild sprain causes overstretching or slight tearing of the ligaments with no joint instability. A person with a mild sprain usually experiences minimal pain, swelling, and little or no loss of functional ability. Bruising is absent or slight, and the person is usually able to put weight on the affected joint. A grade II or moderate sprain causes partial tearing of the ligament and is characterized by bruising, moderate pain, and swelling. A person with a moderate sprain usually has some difficulty putting weight on the affected joint and experiences some loss of function. An x-ray or MRI may be needed.

People who sustain a grade III or severe sprain completely tear or rupture a ligament. Pain, swelling, and bruising are usually severe, and the patient is unable to put weight on the joint. An x-ray is usually taken to rule out a broken bone.

When diagnosing any sprain, the doctor will ask the patient to explain how the injury happened. The doctor will examine the affected joint and check its stability and its ability to move and bear weight.

Strains

A strain is caused by twisting or pulling a muscle or tendon. Strains can be acute or chronic. An acute strain is caused by trauma or an injury such as a blow to the body; it can also be caused by improperly lifting heavy objects or overstressing the muscles. Chronic strains are usually the result of overuse—prolonged, repetitive movement of the muscles and tendons.

Two common sites for a strain are the back and the hamstring muscle (located in the back of the thigh). Contact sports such as soccer, football, hockey, boxing, and wrestling put people at risk for strains. Gymnastics, tennis, rowing, golf, and other sports that require extensive gripping can increase the risk of hand and forearm strains. Elbow strains sometimes occur in people who participate in racquet sports, throwing, and contact sports.

Typically, people with a strain experience pain, muscle spasm, and muscle weakness. They can also have localized swelling, cramping, or inflammation and, with a minor or moderate strain, usually some loss of muscle function.

Tendonitis

A tendon is the end part of a muscle that attaches the muscle to the bone. The normally very elastic and soft muscle tapers off at the end to form the much more dense and stiff tendon. While this density makes the tendons stronger, the lack of elasticity of the tendon and the constant pulling on its attachment to the bone with movement make it much more susceptible to a low level of tearing at a microscopic level. This tearing will produce the inflammation and irritation known as tendonitis. Often spelled *tendinitis,* either spelling is correct for this condition. Tendonitis is usually seen after excessive repetitive movement with which the tendon gradually becomes tighter until the fibers start to tear. For example, a person who plays tennis may overuse the muscles of the elbow through hitting the ball repetitively and cause tendonitis, or inflammation, to the area.

The most common tendon areas that become inflamed are the elbow, wrist, biceps, shoulder (including rotator cuff attachments), leg, knee (patellar), ankle, hip, and Achilles. Of course, tendonitis varies with each person, because it strikes the areas used most. The symptoms can also vary from an achy pain and stiffness in the local area of the tendon, to a burning that surrounds the whole joint around the inflamed tendon. With this condition, the pain is usually worse during and after activity, and the tendon and joint area can become stiffer the following day.

With proper care for the area, the pain in the tendon should lessen over 3 weeks, but it should be noted that the healing of the area continues and does not peak until at least 6 weeks following the initial injury. This is due to scar tissue formation, which initially acts like the glue to bond the tissue back together. Scar tissue will continue to form past 6 weeks in some cases and as long as a year in severe cases. After 6 months this condition is considered chronic and much more difficult to treat. The initial approach to treating tendonitis is to support and protect the tendons by bracing any areas of the tendon that are being pulled on during use. It is important to loosen up the tendon, reduce the pain, and minimize any inflammation.

Tetanus

Tetanus is an often fatal infectious disease caused by the bacteria *Clostridium tetani,* which usually enters the body through a puncture, cut, or open wound. It is characterized by profoundly painful spasms of muscles, including "locking" of the jaw so that the mouth cannot open (*lockjaw*). *Clostridium tetani* releases a toxin that affects the motor nerves (the nerves that stimulate the muscles).

Prevention of tetanus is aided by immediately cleaning and covering any open wound and by vaccination. All children should be immunized against tetanus by receiving a full series of 5 DPT vaccinations ("baby

Preparing for
Externship

One hallmark of a professional is the ability to seek the cause of problems and solve problems for patients without ever fixing blame on any specific individual. Frustrated patients are not interested in who is responsible for something that has gone wrong, but are instead concerned about having their problem resolved. Because humans work in the medical field, mistakes will happen. Be sure to focus on defining the problem and a remedy to the problem rather than trying to place the blame.

shots"), which generally are started at 2 months of age and completed at about 5 years of age. Tetanus and diphtheria toxoid (Td) is now recommended at 11 to 12 years of age if at least 5 years have elapsed since the last dose of tetanus and diphtheria toxoid-containing vaccine.

Follow-up booster vaccination is recommended every 10 years thereafter (i.e., 21 years old, 31 years old, etc.). Although a 10-year period of protection exists after the basic childhood series is completed (at age 11 to 12), should a potentially contaminated wound occur during the second half of this block of time (i.e., at ages 5 to 12), an "early" booster may be given and the 10-year "clock" is then reset. It is important to remember that unvaccinated people who get a puncture wound or cut should get tetanus immunoglobulin and a series of tetanus shots immediately. People who have been immunized but are unsure of when their last tetanus shot was should get a booster.

SUMMARY

The muscular system is composed of specialized cells called muscle fibers. These fibers, when brought together, form muscle, which makes up about 42 percent of a person's total body weight. In order for our muscles to perform properly, which is to create movement, maintain posture and stability, and aid in heat production, they must be supplied with proper nutrition and oxygen.

Chapter Review

COMPETENCY REVIEW

1. Define and spell the terms to learn for this chapter.
2. Name the three types of muscle tissue.
3. What are the two points of attachment for muscles.
4. What are the other names for skeletal muscle?
5. What are the three parts of muscle?
6. What are other names for smooth muscle?
7. Give examples of internal organs with smooth muscle.
8. What is the name of heart muscle?
9. What is a special property of cardiac muscle?
10. What are the three primary functions of muscle?

PREPARING FOR THE CERTIFICATION EXAM

1. Aponeuroses are
   A. flattened tendons attaching muscles
   B. striated muscles
   C. smooth muscles
   D. bones of the lower extremities
   E. bones of the upper extremities

2. Which of the following is NOT a type of muscle tissue?
   A. clavicle
   B. smooth
   C. visceral
   D. striated
   E. cardiac

3. The muscle that separates the thoracic and abdominal cavities is the
   A. psoas major
   B. psoas minor
   C. diaphragm
   D. epiglottis
   E. biceps

4. The predominant function of the muscular system is
   A. heat production
   B. contractibility
   C. elasticity
   D. posture
   E. stability

continued on next page

5. The term used to describe the muscle's maintenance of posture through contraction is
   A. tonicity
   B. movement
   C. elasticity
   D. contractibility
   E. movability

6. A condition that occurs due to the disuse of muscles over a long period of time is called
   A. fibromyalgia
   B. myasthenia gravis
   C. atrophy
   D. muscular dystrophy
   E. tendonitis

7. How many types of muscle tissues are there?
   A. two
   B. three
   C. four
   D. five
   E. six

8. The structure covering the entire skeletal muscle and separating them from one another is called the
   A. perimysium
   B. endomysium
   C. fascicle
   D. fascia
   E. epimysium

9. What form of muscular dystrophy usually leads to death between the late teens and the early 20s?
   A. Duchenne's muscular dystrophy
   B. Becker's muscular dystrophy
   C. limb-girdle muscular dystrophy
   D. facioscapulohumeral muscular dystrophy
   E. congenital muscular dystrophy

10. What is the name of the chronic neuromuscular disease characterized by varying degrees of weakness of the skeletal or voluntary muscles of the body?
   A. fibromyalgia
   B. myasthenia gravis
   C. muscular dystrophy
   D. atrophy
   E. melanoma

CRITICAL THINKING

1. What were the symptoms that clued the doctor in to a diagnosis of Duchenne's muscular dystrophy?

2. Why will Robert benefit from physical therapy?

INTERNET ACTIVITY

Do an Internet search to learn about resources for families who have members with muscular dystrophy.

MediaLink More on the muscular system, including interactive resources, can be found on the Student CD-ROM accompanying this textbook.

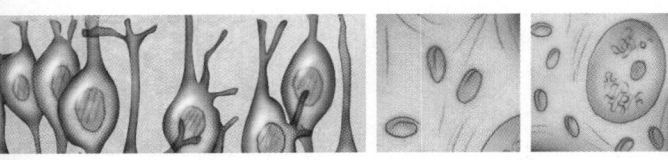

Medical Assistant Role Delineation Chart

HIGHLIGHT indicates material covered in this chapter.

ADMINISTRATIVE

Administrative Procedures
- Perform basic administrative medical assisting functions
- Schedule, coordinate and monitor appointments
- Schedule inpatient/outpatient admissions and procedures
- Understand and apply third-party guidelines
- Obtain reimbursement through accurate claims submission
- Monitor third-party reimbursement
- Understand and adhere to managed care policies and procedures
- *Negotiate managed care contracts*

Practice Finances
- Perform procedural and diagnostic coding
- Apply bookkeeping principles

- Manage accounts receivable
- *Manage accounts payable*
- *Process payroll*
- *Document and maintain accounting and banking records*
- *Develop and maintain fee schedules*
- *Manage renewals of business and professional insurance policies*
- *Manage personnel benefits and maintain records*
- *Perform marketing, financial, and strategic planning*

CLINICAL

Fundamental Principles
- Apply principles of aseptic technique and infection control
- Comply with quality assurance practices
- Screen and follow up patient test results

Diagnostic Orders
- Collect and process specimens
- Perform diagnostic tests

Patient Care
- Adhere to established patient screening procedures
- Obtain patient history and vital signs
- Prepare and maintain examination and treatment areas
- Prepare patient for examinations, procedures and treatments

- Assist with examinations, procedures and treatments
- Prepare and administer medications and immunizations
- Maintain medication and immunization records
- Recognize and respond to emergencies
- Coordinate patient care information with other health care providers
- Initiate IV and administer IV medications with appropriate training and as permitted by state law

GENERAL

Professionalism
- Display a professional manner and image
- Demonstrate initiative and responsibility
- Work as a member of the health care team
- Prioritize and perform multiple tasks
- Adapt to change
- Promote the CMA credential
- Enhance skills through continuing education
- Treat all patients with compassion and empathy
- Promote the practice through positive public relations

Communication Skills
- Recognize and respect cultural diversity
- Adapt communications to individual's ability to understand
- Use professional telephone technique

- Recognize and respond effectively to verbal, nonverbal, and written communications
- Use medical terminology appropriately
- Utilize electronic technology to receive, organize, prioritize and transmit information
- Serve as liaison

Legal Concepts
- Perform within legal and ethical boundaries
- Prepare and maintain medical records
- Document accurately
- Follow employer's established policies dealing with the health care contract
- Implement and maintain federal and state health care legislation and regulations
- Comply with established risk management and safety procedures
- Recognize professional credentialing criteria
- *Develop and maintain personnel, policy and procedure manuals*

Instruction
- Instruct individuals according to their needs
- Explain office policies and procedures
- Teach methods of health promotion and disease prevention
- Locate community resources and disseminate information
- *Develop educational materials*
- *Conduct continuing education activities*

Operational Functions
- Perform inventory of supplies and equipment
- Perform routine maintenance of administrative and clinical equipment
- Apply computer techniques to support office operations
- *Perform personnel management functions*
- *Negotiate leases and prices for equipment and supply contracts*

- *Denotes advanced skills.*

SOURCE: Reprinted by permission of the American Association of Medical Assistants from the AAMA Role Delineation Study: Occupational Analysis of the Medical Assisting Profession.

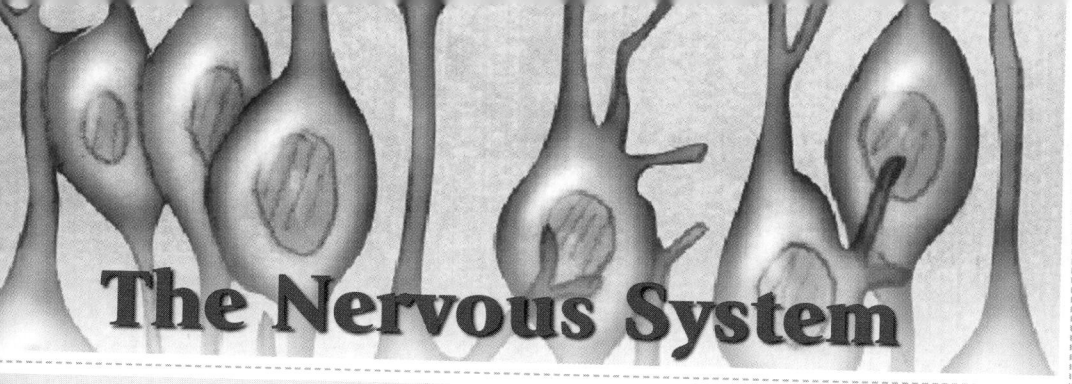

The Nervous System

Learning Objectives

After completing this chapter, you should be able to:

- Define and spell the terms to learn in this chapter.
- Identify and discuss the structures that make up the nervous system.
- Explain how nerve impulses are transmitted.
- State the functions of the central nervous system, the peripheral nervous system, and the autonomic nervous system, and distinguish the differences between each.
- Identify and explain common disorders associated with the nervous system.

OUTLINE

Functions of the Nervous System	407
Neurons	407
Nerve Fibers, Nerves, and Tracts	407
Nerve Impulses and Synapses	408
Central Nervous System	408
Peripheral Nervous System	411
Autonomic Nervous System	414
Common Disorders Associated with the Nervous System	415

Terms to Learn

Alzheimer's disease

amyotrophic lateral sclerosis (ALS)

Bell's palsy

cerebrospinal fluid

encephalitis

epilepsy

headache

meningitis

multiple sclerosis (MS)

neuralgia

paraplegia

Parkinson's disease

quadriplegia

sciatica

seizure

spina bifida

stroke

Case Study

EMILY MONTERO IS A 73-YEAR-OLD FEMALE who presents at Dr. Esso's office complaining of a new onset of left-sided weakness and drooping of the side of her face. This started about 2 hours ago with a headache, and she is experiencing progressively worsening symptoms. Her blood pressure is 172/108, and her pulse is rapid and thready. She denies pain other than her headache.

Dr. Esso immediately has his medical assistant call 911 and arrange for transport to the emergency room. Mrs. Montero receives a CT scan that shows a thrombus in her brain with no other acute abnormalities seen. She is given thrombolytics (clotbusters) and is admitted to the ICU. Eventually, she is put on a rehabilitation service, and returns to Dr. Esso's office 12 weeks later with a slight limp and no other difficulties.

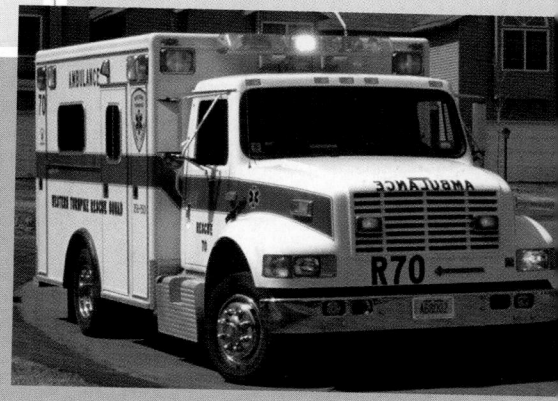

 he nervous system is the body's information gatherer, storage center, and control system (see Figure 23-1). Its overall function is to collect information about external conditions in relation to the body's external state, to analyze this information, and to initiate appropriate responses to satisfy certain needs.

The most powerful of these needs is survival. The nerves do not form one single system, but several systems that are interrelated. Some of these are physically separate, others are different in function only. The brain and spinal cord make up the central nervous system. The peripheral nervous system is responsible for the body functions that are not under conscious control, such as the heartbeat or the digestive system. The

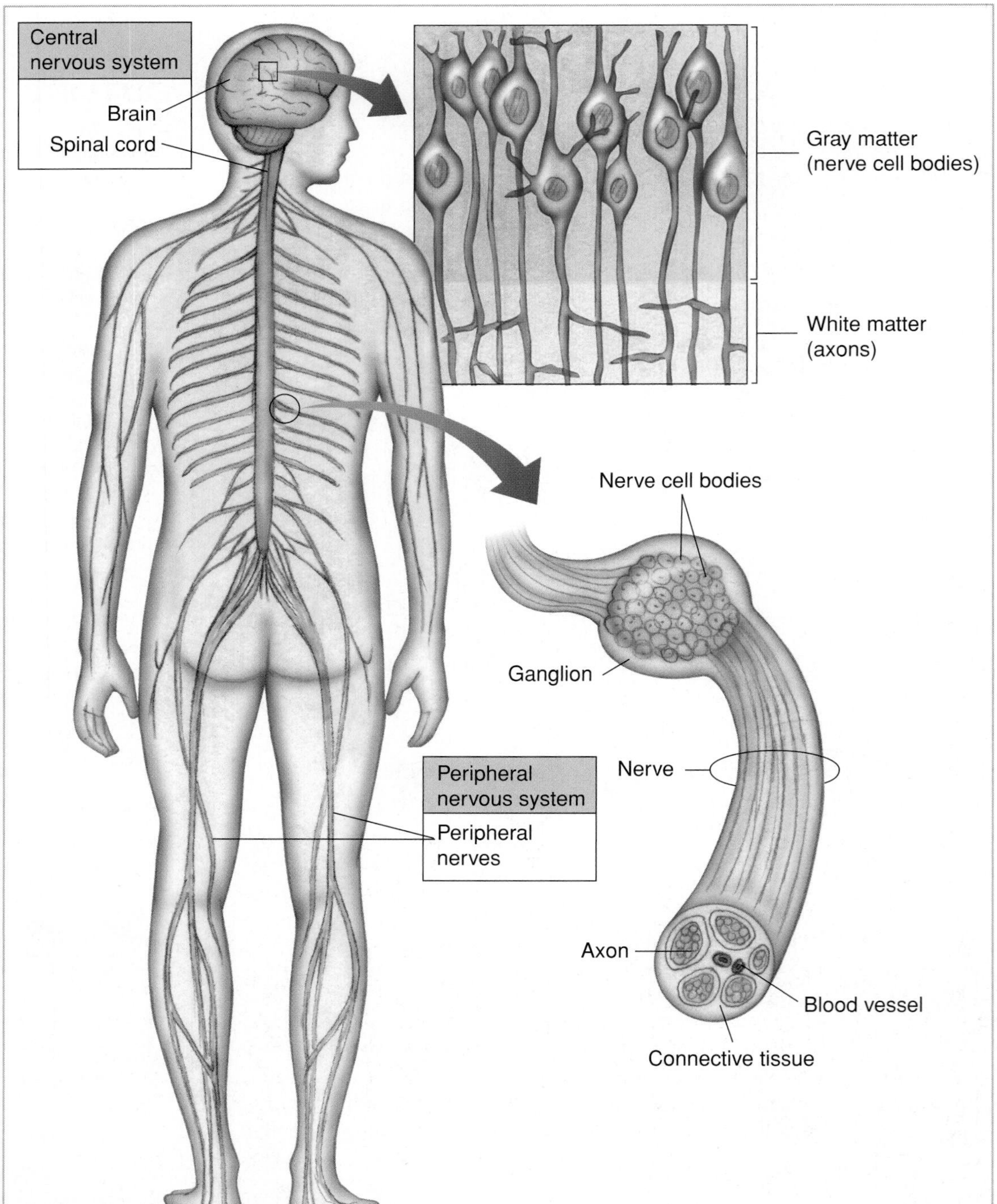

Central nervous system

Brain

Spinal cord

Gray matter (nerve cell bodies)

White matter (axons)

Nerve cell bodies

Ganglion

Nerve

Peripheral nervous system

Peripheral nerves

Axon

Blood vessel

Connective tissue

FIGURE 23-1 The nervous system.

smooth operation of the peripheral nervous system is achieved by dividing it into sympathetic and parasympathetic systems. These systems have opposing actions and check on each other to provide a balance. The nervous system uses electrical impulses, which travel along the length of the cells. The cell processes information from the sensory nerves and initiates an action within milliseconds. These impulses travel at up to 250 miles per hour, while other systems such as the endocrine system may take many hours to respond with hormones.

Functions of the Nervous System

The nervous system is responsible for three separate functions: (1) It detects and interprets sensory information. (2) It then takes that information and makes decisions about how it is being received. (3) Finally, it carries out a motor function based on the decisions made.

Neurons

All nervous system tissues are made of up neurons, or nerve cells, and their supporting tissues, called neuroglia. The neuron (see Figure 23-2) is the structural and functional unit of the nervous system. These cells are specialized conductors of impulses that enable the body to interact with its internal and external environments. There are three types of neurons: motor neurons, sensory neurons and interneurons. (For development of the nervous system in children and changes with aging, see Lifespan Considerations).

The motor neurons cause the muscles to contract and the glands to secrete their products and organs to perform their functions. They also inhibit the actions of glands and organs, controlling most of the body's functions. Motor neurons are called *efferent*, meaning that they transmit messages away from the cell body to the muscles and organs. Motor nerves have a nucleated cell body with processes extending away from the cell body. The processes, or "nerve fibers," are called the axon and dendrites. Neurons typically have several dendrites and one axon. The dendrites carry impulses to the cell body, and the axon carries impulses away from it. Most axons are covered with a fatty insulating substance called the myelin sheath. Axons with an intact myelin sheath transmit faster than those without. The axons and dendrites, along with the membrane of the cell body, provide the main receptive surfaces of the neuron to which processes from other neurons communicate.

Sensory neurons differ from motor neurons in that they do not have dendrites. They process and transmit sensory information to the cell body with sheathed, axon-resembling peripheral processes. They

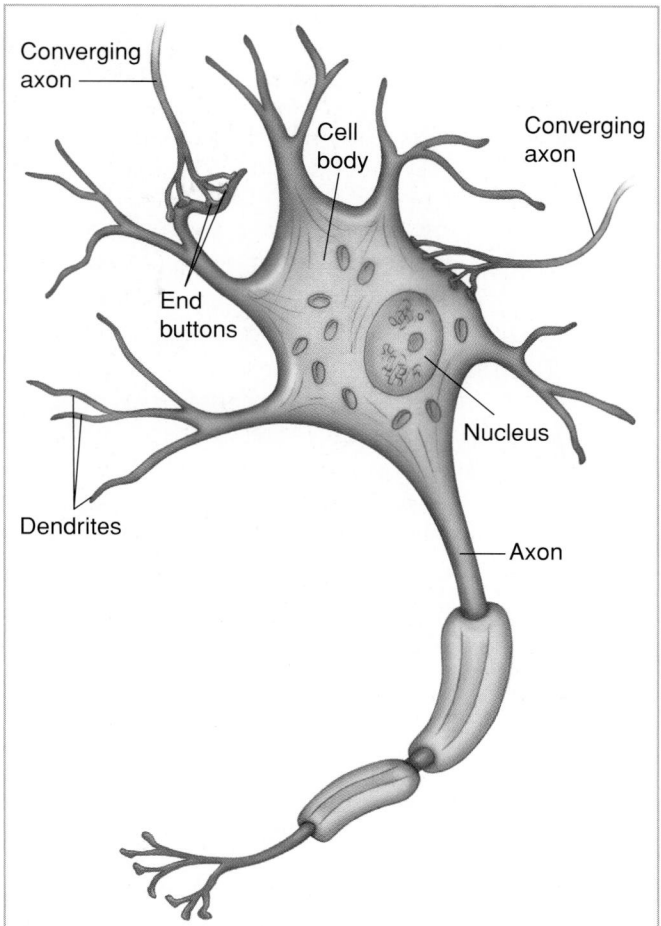

FIGURE 23-2 A neuron (nerve cell) with two converging axons.

are attached to sensor receptors and transmit impulses to the central nervous system. As a result, the central nervous system will stimulate motor neurons in response, causing movement. Sensory neurons are often called *afferent* neurons, since they carry impulses to the cell body and the central nervous system.

Interneurons are also known as associative neurons and are housed entirely within the central nervous system. They mediate impulses between the motor and sensory neurons.

Nerve Fibers, Nerves, and Tracts

A nerve fiber is a single elongated process, usually an axon or peripheral process. Each nerve fiber is wrapped in a protective membrane called a *sheath*. Schwann cells create the myelin sheath. Not all nerve cells have myelin sheaths. Damage to nerve cells without a myelin sheath is permanent, because regeneration of the nerve cell can only happen when Schwann cells are present. Cells without the Schwann cells and the myelin sheath are called unmyelinated cells. Unmyelinated cells have a very thin sheath that provides minimal protection.

THE CHILD

- The development of the child's nervous system begins at about 6 weeks. By the time the child is born, the baby's brain waves can be measured. As the child grows, regular neurological testing can provide the physician with important information that indicates various neurological disorders. Testing of the child's nervous system includes testing the newborn's reflexes, as well as testing the child as he or she grows. This includes testing of the mental status, motor functions and balance, and the sensory system.

THE OLDER ADULT

- In individuals who do not have neurological disease, intellectual performance tends to be maintained until at least age 80. However, tasks may take longer to perform because of some slowing in central processing. Verbal skills are well maintained until age 70, after which, some healthy elderly persons gradually develop a reduction in vocabulary, a tendency to make semantic errors, and abnormal pronunciation. Other age-related changes are subtle but can be detected as difficulty learning, especially languages, and forgetfulness in noncritical areas. However, this mild forgetfulness is unlike dementia in that it does not impair recall of important memories or affect function.
- With normal aging, the number of nerve cells in the brain decreases. From age 20 or 30 to age 90, brain weight declines by about 10 percent, and the area of the cerebral ventricles relative to the entire brain may increase three to four times.

Typically, the nerves in the peripheral nervous system are myelinated, and those in the central nervous system are not.

A nerve is a bundle of nerve fibers, located outside the brain and spinal cord, connecting various parts of the body. Afferent, or sensory, nerves carry messages to the central nervous system, and efferent, or motor, nerves carry messages from the central nervous system. There are also mixed nerves, which can be both afferent and efferent (sensory and motor).

Groups of nerve fibers within the central nervous system are referred to as *tracts*. To be a tract, all of the nerves included must have the same origin, function, and termination. The spinal cord contains afferent (sensory) tracts ascending to the brain and efferent (motor) tracts descending from the brain. The brain contains numerous tracts, including the *corpus callosum*, which is the largest, and which joins the right and left hemispheres of the brain.

a nerve fiber is based on the "all or none" principle, meaning, that either there is a response or there isn't. The receptor must receive sufficient stimulation to send the impulse, or the impulse is not transmitted to the brain. Each receptor has its own threshold at which it will react to a stimulus, and each will only respond when its threshold is reached. Impulses travel from the receptors down the dendrites to the cell body, and then down the axon of the nerve to the synapse. The end of the axon is knob shaped, and there are specialized cells at that knob which secrete neurotransmitters (nerve system chemicals) that travel across the synapse to the dendrites of the next nerve, where the entire process repeats itself until the synapse ends at a motor plate attached to a muscle, creating movement. The space at the end of the synapse is called the *synaptic cleft*. The neurotransmitters reach the synaptic cleft, where they cause another chemical–electrical change, causing the next nerve cell to react.

Nerve Impulses and Synapses

A receptor is the point where a stimulation of the nerve occurs. There are many types of sensory receptors, starting from the very simple nerves that receive pain to very complex receptors, including those in the retina of the eye, which collect all the input necessary for sight. Receptors are typically function specific (pain, heat, cold, sharp), and they react by initiating a chemical change, or impulse. The transmission of an impulse by

Central Nervous System

The central nervous system (CNS) (Figure 23-3) encompasses the brain and spinal cord (see Figure 23-1). The CNS receives impulses from the entire body, processes the information, and responds with the appropriate action. Activity may be conscious or unconscious, depending on the source of the sensory stimulus. Both the brain and the spinal cord are divided into gray matter and white matter. Gray matter is the unsheathed cell bodies and true dendrites. The white matter consists of the myelinated nerve fibers. In the spinal cord, the arrangement of the gray and white matter is in an H-shaped fashion, with the gray matter forming the core of the spinal cord, surrounded by the white matter. In the brain, the reverse arrangement is true; the white matter forms the core of the brain with the gray matter surrounding the cortex (surface layer).

Brain

Millions of nerve cells and fibers make up the brain. It is the largest mass of nervous tissue in the body, weighing about 1,380 grams in males, and 1,250 grams in females. When fully developed, the brain fills the cranial cavity and is enclosed by three membranes, or meninges. The meninges, from the inside moving outward, are the pia mater, the arachnoid, and the dura mater. The major divisions of the brain are the cerebrum, the diencephalon, the brainstem, which consists of the midbrain and the hindbrain. The hindbrain includes the cerebellum, the pons, the medulla oblongata, and the reticular formation (see Figure 23-4).

Cerebrum

The cerebrum, which develops from the front portion of the forebrain, is the largest part of the mature brain. It consists of two large masses, called *cerebral hemispheres,* that are almost

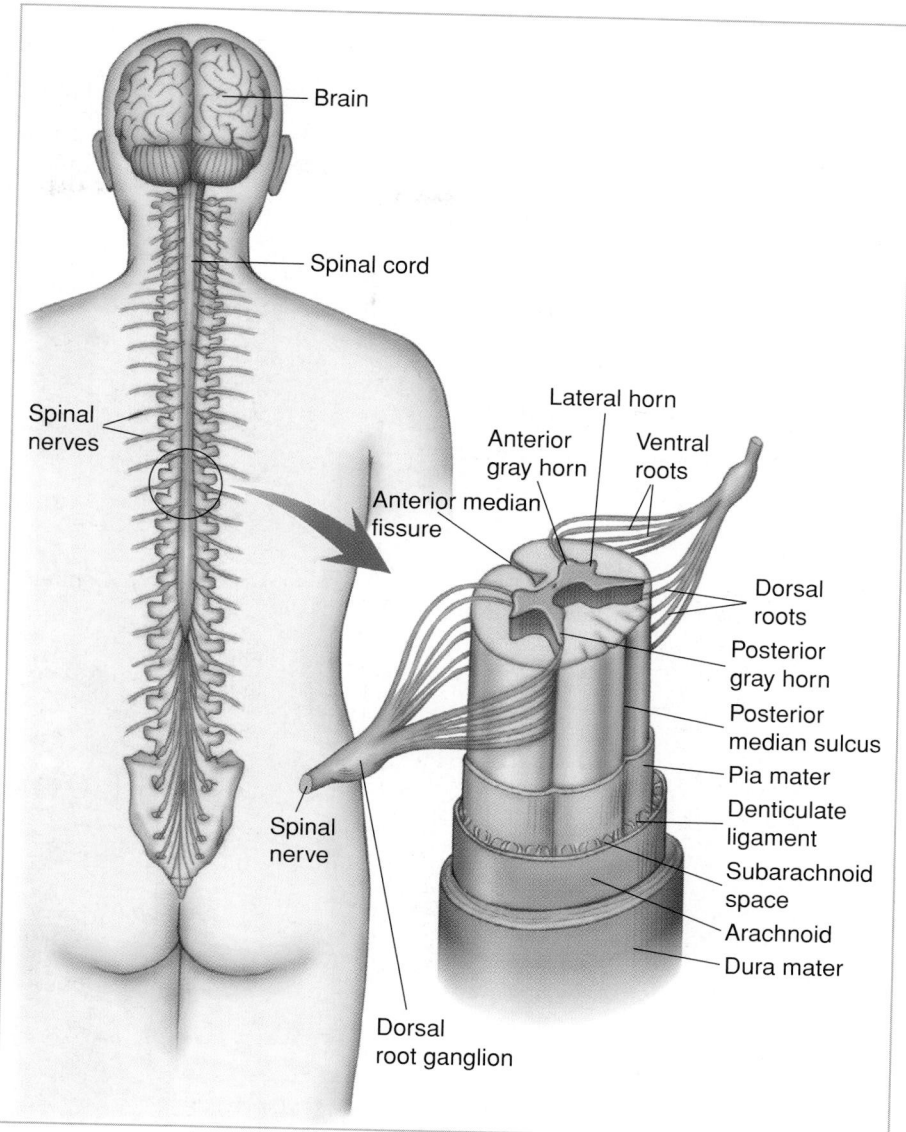

FIGURE 23-3 The central nervous system.

mirror images of each other. They are connected by a deep bridge of nerve fibers called the *corpus callosum* and are separated by a layer called the *falx cerebri.* The surface of the cerebrum is marked by numerous ridges or *convolutions,* called *gyri,* that are separated by grooves. A shallow groove is called a *sulcus,* and a very deep one is a *fissure.* A *longitudinal* fissure separates the right and left hemispheres of the cerebrum, and a *transverse* fissure separates the cerebrum from the cerebellum. Various sulci divide each hemisphere into *lobes* (sometimes called *poles*). The four lobes are named for the skull bones under which they rest: the frontal lobe, the parietal lobe, the temporal lobe, the occipital lobe, and the insula. The cerebrum is concerned with the higher brain functions of interpreting sensory impulses and initiating muscle movement. It stores information and uses it to process reasoning. It also functions in determining intelligence and personality.

LOBES OF THE CEREBRUM As previously stated, there are four lobes located in the cerebrum. The frontal lobe is located in front of the central sulcus and is concerned with reasoning, planning, parts of speech and movement, emotions, and problem solving. The parietal lobe is located behind the central sulcus and is concerned with perception of stimuli related to touch, pressure, temperature, and pain. The temporal lobe is located below the lateral fissure and it is concerned with perception and recognition of auditory stimuli (hearing) and memory. The occipital lobe, which is located at the back of the brain, behind the parietal lobe and temporal lobe, is concerned with many aspects of vision.

CORTEX AND VENTRICLES The outermost layer that surrounds the cerebrum is called the cerebral cortex. Composed of gray matter and containing neuron cell bodies and dendrites, the cortex contains nearly

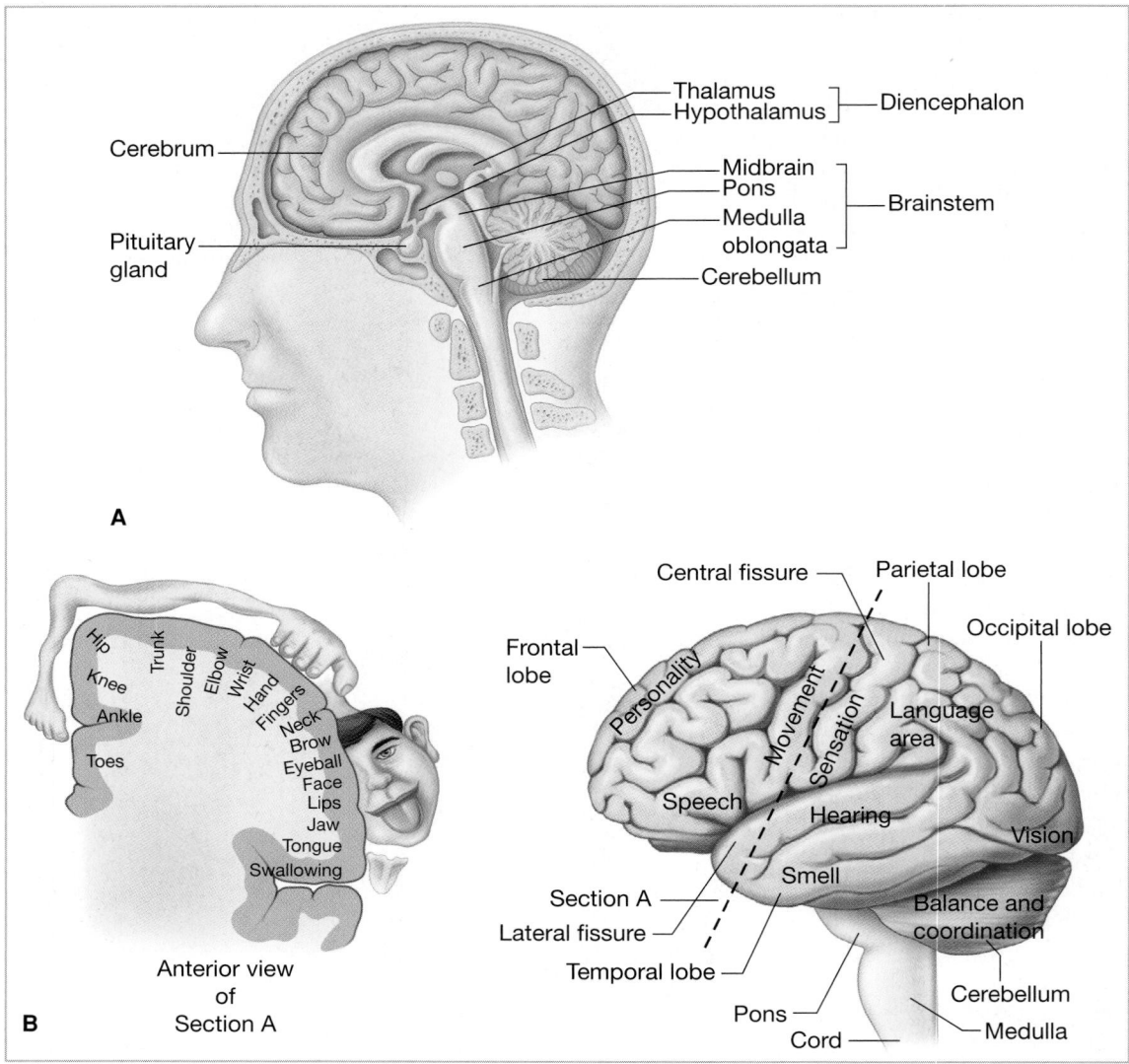

FIGURE 23-4   (A) Sagittal section of the brain. (B) Lateral view of the brain.

75 percent of all neurons in the entire nervous system. Just below the cerebral cortex is white matter. In addition to interpreting sensory information and initiating body movements, the cerebral cortex is also responsible for storing memories and creating emotions.

Within the cerebral hemispheres and brainstem are a series of cavities called *ventricles*. These spaces are contiguous with the central canal of the spinal cord and, like the spinal cord, they are filled with cerebrospinal fluid. The largest of the ventricles are the first and second (lateral) ventricles, which extend into the cerebral hemispheres and occupy portions of the frontal, temporal, and occipital lobes. The third ventricle is in a narrow space in the midline of the brain and connects with the lateral ventricles through openings in the front of it, which are called interventricular foramina. The fourth ventricle is located in the brainstem, just in front of the cerebellum. It is connected to the third ventricle by a narrow canal, the *cerebral aqueduct* (aqueduct of Sylvius), which passes lengthwise through the brainstem. This ventricle is contiguous with the central canal of the spinal cord and has openings in its roof that lead into the meninges (membranes that cover the brain and spinal cord).

Diencephalon

The diencephalon contains the thalamus and hypothalamus. The thalamus, which is the largest of the two divisions of the diencephalon, acts as a telephone line of sorts, allowing information to get through to the cerebral cortex. It also relays motor impulses from the cerebellum and the basal ganglia to the motor areas of the cortex. Some impulses related to emotional behavior are also passed through the thalamus to the cerebral cortex.

The hypothalamus is important for regulating hormones, hunger, thirst, and arousal. Located inferior to the thalamus, it functions as a regulator of autonomic nervous activity associated with behavior and emotional expression. The hypothalamus also produces neurosecretions to control water balance, glucose and fat metabolism, the regulation of body temperature, and other metabolic activities. It also produces hormones for the posterior pituitary gland and manages secretions from the anterior and posterior pituitary glands. The pituitary gland is attached to the inferior side of the hypothalamus by the infundibulum.

Brainstem

The brainstem consists of the midbrain and the hindbrain. Just as the name suggests, the brainstem resembles the stem of a branch. The midbrain is the upper part of the branch that is connected to the forebrain. This region of the brain sends and receives information. Data from our senses, such as the eyes and ears, are sent to this area and then directed to the forebrain.

The hindbrain makes up the lower portion of the brainstem and consists of four units. The medulla oblongata controls involuntary functions such as digestion and breathing. The second unit of the hindbrain, the pons, also assists in controlling these functions. The third unit, the cerebellum, is responsible for the coordination of movement. The fourth unit is the reticular form action, which is responsible for sleep.

MEDULLA OBLONGATA The medulla oblongata connects the brain and the spinal cord. This area is also known as the brainstem and all afferent and efferent nerve tracts from the spinal cord either pass through or terminate in the medulla oblongata. The medulla's functions are the control of breathing, swallowing, coughing, sneezing, and vomiting. Centers in the medulla are responsible for regulating arterial blood pressure and contributing to the control of the circulation of blood.

PONS The pons is a broad band of white matter anterior to the cerebellum and between the midbrain and medulla oblongata. The pons has fiber tracks that link the cerebellum and medulla to higher cortical areas.

CEREBELLUM The cerebellum, which is located in the back of the skull below the cerebrum and behind the pons and medulla oblongata, is the largest part of the hindbrain. The surface of the cerebellum has a large cortex of gray cell bodies with nerve fibers and white matter on its interior. The cerebellum functions in balance and coordination of voluntary movement.

RETICULAR FORMATION The reticular formation is a diffuse network of small groups of cells bodies and their processes located in and around the brainstem. The reticular formation is responsible for sleep, wakefulness, and some reflex activities of the spinal nerves.

Spinal Cord

The spinal cord extends from the medulla oblongata down past the vertebrae and the tailbone, terminating at the cauda equine (which means "horse's tail"), infe-rior to the spine. The spinal cord has an H-shaped central portion of gray matter surrounded by white matter. The white matter consists of nerve tracts and fibers that send sensory input to the brain and conduct motor impulses from the brain back to the body. Other fibers connect nerve cells from one area of the cord to other areas of the cord. The function of the spinal cord is to conduct sensory impulses from the body to the brain and send motor impulses from the brain to the body. The spinal cord also serves as a reflex center for nerve impulses that do not need to pass through the brain.

Cerebrospinal Fluid

Although it is colorless in appearance, cerebrospinal fluid is often considered to be the "blood" of the nervous system. Produced by the choroid plexus, which is located in the ventricles of the brain, the cerebrospinal fluid moves from the ventricles into the connecting canal, and then through the spinal canal and the subarachnoid space that surround the brain. Cerebrospinal fluid has several functions, including serving as a cushion to protect the brain and spinal cord floating in the fluid, and nourishing the brain and spinal cord with oxygen and glucose. It also contains several neurotransmitters, including monoamines, acetylcholine, and neuropeptides.

Peripheral Nervous System

The peripheral nervous system (PNS), which also includes the somatic nervous system, is one of the two major divisions of the nervous system. The other is the central nervous system which is made up of the brain and spinal cord. The nerves in the peripheral nervous system connect the central nervous system to sensory organs (such as the eye and ear), other organs of the body, muscles, blood vessels, and glands.

The somatic nervous system is the part of the PNS that is associated with the voluntary control of body movements through the action of skeletal muscles. It consists of afferent fibers, which receive information from external sources, and efferent fibers, which are responsible for muscle contraction. It is the part of the peripheral nervous system that is made up of 12 cranial nerves from the brain, 31 pairs of spinal nerves from the spinal cord, and all of their branches.

The 12 cranial nerves and the spinal nerves and roots are called the autonomic nerves. The autonomic nerves are concerned with automatic functions of the body. Specifically, autonomic nerves are involved with the regulation of the heart muscle, the tiny muscles lining the walls of blood vessels, and glands.

Cranial Nerves

The cranial nerves are composed of 12 pairs of nerves that emanate from the nervous tissue of the brain (see Figure 23-5). To reach their targets, they must

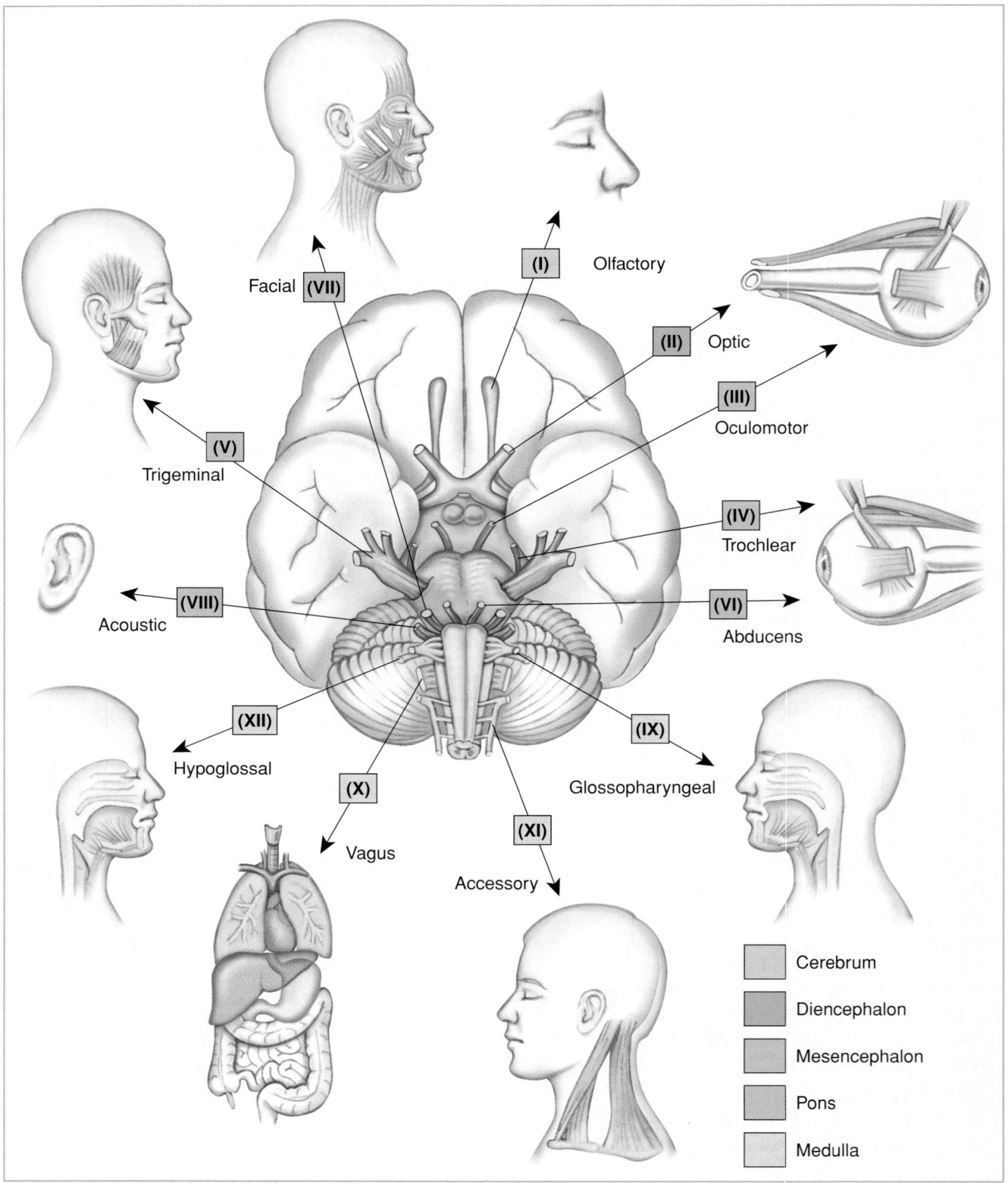

Facial **(VII)**

(I) Olfactory

(II) Optic

(III) Oculomotor

(V) Trigeminal

(IV) Trochlear

(VIII) Acoustic

(VI) Abducens

(XII) Hypoglossal

(IX) Glossopharyngeal

(X) Vagus

(XI) Accessory

Cerebrum

Diencephalon

Mesencephalon

Pons

Medulla

FIGURE 23-5 The relationship of the 12 cranial nerves to specific regions of the brain.

TABLE 23-1 **The 12 Pairs of Cranial Nerves**

Brain Region	Cranial Nerve Number	Cranial Nerve Name	General Function
Telencephalon	I	Olfactory	Olfaction (smell)
Diencephalon	II	Optic	Vision
Midbrain	III	Oculomotor	Eye movement (most of our eye movements are commanded through this nerve)
	IV	Trochlear	Eye movement (only one eyeball muscle, the trochlear muscle, is controlled through this nerve)
	V	Trigeminal	Sensation of face and mouth Mastication (chewing) commands
Pons	VI	Abducens	Eye movement (only one eyeball muscle, the lateral rectus muscle, is controlled through this nerve)
	VII	Facial	Facial muscle contraction Some taste sensation Some glandular innervation
	VIII	Acoustic or vestibulocochlear	Senses from our ears: hearing and balance
	IX	Glossopharyngeal	Some taste Some swallowing muscles
Medulla (and spinal cord for CN XI)	X	Vagus	Involuntary functions, it has a role in heart rate and breathing rate Some taste Some swallowing muscles and laryngeal muscles
	XI	Spinal accessory	Some laryngeal muscles Some muscles of the back and neck
	XII	Hypoglossal	Movement of tongue

ultimately exit and enter the cranium through openings in the skull. Hence, their name is derived from their association with the cranium. The function (see Table 23-1) of the cranial nerves is for the most part similar to the spinal nerves, the nerves that are associated with the spinal cord. The motor components of the cranial nerves are derived from cells that are located in the brain. These cells send their axons out of the cranium where they will ultimately control muscle, such as eye movements; glandular tissue, as in the salivary glands; or specialized muscle, like that found in the heart or stomach. The sensory compo-

nents of cranial nerves originate from collections of cells that are located outside the brain. These collections of nerve cell bodies are called *sensory ganglia*. They are essentially the same functionally and anatomically as the dorsal root ganglia that are associated with the spinal cord. In general, sensory ganglia of the cranial nerves send out a branch that divides into two branches: a branch that enters the brain and one that is connected to a sensory organ. Examples of sensory organs are pressure or pain sensors in the skin and more specialized ones such as taste receptors of the tongue. Electrical impulses are transmitted from the sensory organ through the ganglia and into the brain via the sensory branch that enters the brain. In summary, the motor components of cranial nerves transmit nerve impulses from the brain to target tissue outside of the brain, while components transmit nerve impulses from sensory organs to the brain.

Spinal Nerves

Thirty-one pairs of spinal nerves originate from the spinal cord. They are all mixed nerves, and they provide a two-way communication system between the spinal cord and parts of the arms, legs, neck, and trunk of the body. Although spinal nerves do not have individual names, they are grouped according to the level from which they stem, and each nerve is numbered in sequence. Hence, there are 8 pairs of *cervical nerves* (numbered C1–C8), 12 pairs of *thoracic nerves* (T1–T12), 5 pairs of *lumbar nerves* (L1–L5), 5 pairs of *sacral nerves* (S1–S5), and 1 pair of *coccygeal nerves*. The nerves coming from the upper part of the spinal cord pass outward nearly horizontally, while those from the lower regions descend at sharp angles. This is derived from the consequence of growth. In early life, the spinal cord extends the entire length of the vertebral column, but with age, the column grows faster than the cord. As a result, the adult spinal cord ends at the level between the first and second lumbar vertebrae, so the lumbar, sacral, and coccygeal nerves descend to their exits beyond the end of the cord.

Autonomic Nervous System

The autonomic nervous system (ANS) is a regulatory structure that helps people adapt to changes in their environment. It adjusts or modifies some functions in response to stress. It also helps to regulate the size of blood vessels and blood pressure, the heart's electrical activity and ability to contract, and the flow of air in the lungs. The ANS also regulates the movement and work of the stomach, intestine and salivary glands, the secretion of insulin, and the urinary and sexual functions. The ANS acts through a balance of its two components, the sympathetic nervous system and the parasympathetic nervous system.

Sympathetic and Parasympathetic Nervous Systems

As we have already stated, the autonomic nervous system is divided into two subsystems, the sympathetic and the parasympathetic, which work in tandem, either in a synergistic or an antagonistic way. The sympathetic system is responsible for providing the responses and energy needed to cope with stressful situations such as fear or extremes of physical activity. In response to such stress, the sympathetic system raises blood pressure, heart rate, and the blood supply to the skeletal muscles at the expense of the gastrointestinal tract, kidneys, and skin; dilates both the pupils and the bronchioles, providing improved vision and oxygenation; and generates needed energy by stimulating glycogenolysis in the liver and lipolysis in adipose tissue. In general, it serves to stimulate organs and to mobilize energy.

Between stressful situations, the body needs to rest, recover, and gain new energy. These tasks are under the control of the parasympathetic system, which lowers the heart rate and blood pressure, diverts blood back to the skin and the gastrointestinal tract, contracts the pupils and bronchioles, stimulates salivary gland secretion, and accelerates peristalsis. The parasympathetic system influences organs toward restoration and the saving of energy. Table 23-2 provides a summary of some of

TABLE 23-2 Summary of the Effects of the Sympathetic and Parasympathetic Nervous Systems

Sympathetic	Structure	Parasympathetic
Rate increased	Heart	Rate decreased
Force increased	Heart	Force decreased
Bronchial muscle relaxed	Lungs	Bronchial muscle contracted
Pupil dilation	Eye	Pupil constriction
Motility reduced	Intestine	Digestion increased
Sphincter closed	Bladder	Sphincter relaxed
Decreased urine secretion	Kidneys	Increased urine secretion

the effects of both the sympathetic and the parasympathetic nervous system.

Common Disorders Associated with the Nervous System

The nervous system involves a complex interaction between special elements designed to originate or to carry unique electrochemical charges to and from the various organs within the body. Like its endocrine counterpart, the nervous system initiates and regulates body functions and ensures its owner of an awareness of his or her surrounding environment.

Alzheimer's Disease

Alzheimer's disease is a progressive, degenerative disease of the brain characterized by loss of memory and other cognitive functions. Alzheimer's affects an individual's ability to carry out daily activity. It affects the parts of the brain that control thought, memory, and language. Alzheimer's is not a normal part of aging, although it does affect over 4 million people. The symptoms start slowly, with the first signs typically being mild forgetfulness, especially about more recent events. Such difficulties may not be serious and the patient and family may write them off as the normal consequences of growing older. However, as the disease progresses, the symptoms are more easily noticed by family members and the individual. They lose the ability to think clearly and may begin to forget how to do basic tasks such as brushing their teeth or combing their hair. They may begin to have problems being able to speak clearly, understand, read, or write. As the disease progresses, they may being to wander and change their behavior, becoming aggressive, agitated, or depressed, or have more difficulty swallowing. As the disease destroys the nervous system, they will eventually be unable to speak, walk, sit or swallow and will require complete and total care.

At this time, there is no definitive known cause of Alzheimer's, or the other related dementias. Family history plays a role, as does age and activity. There are medications that are used for patients in early Alzheimer's (those who can function, but are impaired). These medications can slow the progression of the disease, but stopping the medications will restart the previous speed at which the disease was progressing.

Amyotrophic Lateral Sclerosis

Amyotrophic lateral sclerosis (ALS) is a disease of unknown cause, that breaks down tissues in the nervous system, and affects the nerves responsible for movement. It is also known as motor neuron disease and Lou Gehrig's disease, after the baseball player whose career

it ended. It is a disease of the motor neurons, that is, those nerve cells reaching from the brain to the spinal cord (upper motor neurons) and the spinal cord to the peripheral nerves (lower motor neurons) that control muscle movement. In ALS, for unknown reasons, these neurons die, leading to a progressive loss of the ability to move virtually any of the muscles in the body. ALS affects "voluntary" muscles, those controlled by conscious thought, such as the arm, leg, and trunk muscles. ALS, in and of itself, does not affect sensation, thought processes, the heart muscle, or the "smooth" muscle of the digestive system, bladder, and other internal organs. Most people with ALS retain function of their eye muscles as well. However, various forms of ALS may be associated with a loss of intellectual function (dementia) or sensory symptoms.

Bell's Palsy

Bell's palsy is a weakness or paralysis of the muscles that control expression on one side of your face. The disorder results from damage to a facial nerve, one of which runs beneath each ear to the muscles on the same side of your face. The condition may result in a droopy appearance of your face, which can be a blow to your self-esteem. Most often, Bell's palsy isn't serious. The disorder clears up on its own within weeks or months for most people. In some cases, doctors prescribe a corticosteroid medication within the first few days, hoping to increase the likelihood of a good recovery. Bell's palsy, also called facial palsy, is named for Dr. Charles Bell, of Edinburgh, Scotland, who first described the condition in 1882. About 40,000 people in the United States experience Bell's palsy each year. The problem can occur at any age.

Encephalitis

Encephalitis is an inflammation in the brain. The most common causes of encephalitis are viral infections. Symptoms include fever, headache, vomiting, photophobia (sensitivity to light), stiff neck and back, confusion, drowsiness, clumsiness, and irritability. If there is a loss of consciousness, poor responsiveness, seizures, muscle weakness, or impaired judgment, emergency care is required, because these symptoms indicate a life-threatening turn in the disease. There are approximately 1,500 cases per year in the United States, with the most frequently affected individuals being the elderly and infants. Treatment for encephalitis includes antiviral medications, antibiotics, anticonvulsants for seizures, steroids to decrease inflammation, and sedatives for irritability and agitation. Fever may be treated with over-the-counter medications. Typically, individuals with encephalitis or meningitis are hospitalized.

Epilepsy and Seizure Disorders

Epilepsy is a common neurological disorder that results when something interferes with electrical impulses in the brain. In this disorder, the nervous system produces intense, abnormal bursts of electrical activity in the brain, which can lead to seizures. Seizures temporarily interfere with muscle control, movement, speech, vision, or awareness. Having seizures can be terrifying, especially if they are severe. Fortunately, treatment is available to reduce the abnormal electrical impulses in your brain and control seizures. Epilepsy is not a form of mental retardation or mental illness and is not contagious. The cause of epilepsy is not always clear. Less than one-half of people with epilepsy have an identifiable, primary cause. Epilepsy is sometimes the result of another condition, such as head injury, brain tumor, brain infection, or stroke.

Seizure disorders can affect about one-half of a percent of the population. Seizures can also accompany epilepsy, which can affect people of all ages. Some individuals only have one seizure, while others may have repeated episodes. The most common test used to diagnose seizures is an electroencephalogram (EEG). Brain scans (CT scans) are also used to rule out anomalies in brain structure. For most individuals with epilepsy, the seizures are controlled by medications. These medications are typically taken for life, and the control of the seizures will be compromised if they stop taking the medications. More severe cases might require surgical intervention.

Headaches

Recurring headache may be the most common reason for seeking medical care. Headaches account for about 10 million visits to physicians' offices each year—not counting visits to nonphysicians, chiropractors, hypnotists, or other health care providers who offer headache relief. But as common as the condition is, it is still in many respects a mystery. Researchers are not exactly sure what causes headaches or which people are more susceptible, though they believe a biological predisposition may be responsible and that overuse of pain-relievers and caffeine can make them worse. Likewise, doctors cannot always tell what kind of headache an individual has and therefore what kind of medicine would be best. Headaches are described in various ways, including the use of such terms as tension headache, muscle contraction headache, stress headache, daily chronic headache, migraine headache, and cluster headache. Specialists also deal with post-traumatic headache and disease-related headache.

Types of Headaches

In 1988, the International Headache Society (IHS) developed the criteria most often used to differentiate the verious type of headaches from one another. They are based on clinical features of the headache, including the number of attacks per month, length of time per attack, pain characteristics, and accompanying symptoms. The types of headaches include migraine, tension, cluster, and post-traumatic.

MIGRAINE HEADACHES In the United States, it is estimated that 17.6 percent of women and 5.7 percent of men have one or more migraine headaches a year, with half of all the 8.7 million women who suffer from mild to moderate migraines saying they have more than one migraine each month. It is thought that hormones cause the higher frequency of migraines in women. The characteristic that usually distinguishes migraine from other types of headache is pain experienced on one side of the head behind the eye.

TENSION HEADACHES Muscle contraction headache, stress headache, ordinary headache, psychomyogenic headache, and idiopathic headache are some of the many other names for tension headache. A mild to moderate squeezing or pressing pain that is steady and nonthrobbing on both sides of the head, back of the neck, and possibly the facial area characterizes a typical attack. It can last from an hour to several hours or more and may occur once or twice a week. They can either be an episodic tension headache or a chronic tension headache. The problem is considered episodic if 10 such headaches have occurred any time previously. Sensitivity to light or sound may also be part of this kind of headache. To be labeled chronic the headache must occur more than 15 times a month. It is important to note that a tension headache can occur at any age. It is often hereditary. Sore and contracted neck, shoulder, and/or back muscles usually accompany it. As with both migraine and tension headache, people suffering from daily chronic headache often overuse painkillers like aspirin or prescription drugs. The overuse of medication, and of caffeine, is believed to be a major causative factor in daily chronic headache.

CLUSTER HEADACHES Unlike migraine, which primarily affects women, cluster headache mainly affects men. Although the exact U.S. incidence is not known, an estimated 500,000 to 2 million Americans experience cluster headaches. These excruciatingly painful headaches occur in bursts every year or two, seemingly more often in the spring and autumn than any other time. The cluster period usually lasts between 2 and 3 months. The penetrating and mostly nonthrobbing pain is often felt behind the eyes or in the temples. Attacks can last from 45 minutes to 2 hours and tend to occur at night. Individuals who smoke cigarettes or drink alcohol excessively are more likely to suffer cluster headaches. Many cluster headache sufferers also have peptic ulcers. Women who have cluster headaches may also have a history of migraine.

POST-TRAUMATIC HEADACHES As many as half of all people who suffer a head or neck injury will develop one or more headache patterns after the primary injury has healed. Symptoms are the same as those of migraine or tension headache. Certain areas of the head may also be sensitive to touch. The condition seems to be unrelated to the amount or severity of damage caused by the primary injury. Symptoms usually develop 24 to 48 hours after the trauma, but can develop later.

Meningitis

Meningitis is an infection of the meninges that surround and protect the brain and spinal cord. Symptoms, which may occur without warning, include high fever, severe and persistent headache, neck stiffness, and nausea and vomiting. Changes in behavior, sleepiness, and difficulty waking indicate an emergency situation requiring immediate medical involvement. Typically, meningitis is caused by a bacterial or viral infection, and lasts about 10 days. Meningitis can be fatal, so medical intervention is mandatory.

Multiple Sclerosis

Multiple Sclerosis (MS) is a chronic, potentially debilitating disease that affects the brain and spinal cord, and there is no known cure. MS is an autoimmune disease, in which the body actually attacks itself. In MS, the body directs the antibodies and white cells to attack the myelin sheath surrounding the nerves in the brain and spinal

Cultural Considerations

There are many cultural stereotypes about neurological diseases. Some individuals may consider these diseases as a "curse" or a weakness" and may not volunteer a lot of information about such disorders. Respect their beliefs, and focus on supporting your patients and their families. Be very careful about asking questions, and make sure that questions are focused on the disease and may not be construed as being judgmental.

cord. This causes inflammation and injury to the sheath and the nerves, and later on, scarring may result. Because of these effects, the transmission of nerve impulses is impeded, resulting in difficulty with movement, vision, or sensation. Symptoms, which may vary with each attack, include weakness, paralysis, or tremor of one or more extremities; muscle spasticity; numbness, decreased, or abnormal sensation in any area; and urinary hesitancy, urgency, or frequency. Fever can also worsen attacks, as can hot baths, sun exposure and stress.

Neuralgia

Neuralgia is an intense burning or stabbing pain caused by irritation of or damage to a nerve. The pain is usually brief but may be severe. It often feels as if it is shooting along the course of the affected nerve. The causes of neuralgia are varied. Chemical irritation, inflammation, trauma (including surgery), compression by nearby structures such as tumors, and infections may all lead to neuralgia. In many cases, however, the cause is unknown or unidentifiable.

Treatment of neuralgia is aimed at reversing or controlling the cause of the nerve problem (if identified) as well as providing pain relief. Therefore, the treatment varies depending on the cause, location, and severity of the pain and other factors. Even if the cause of the neuralgia is never identified, the condition may improve spontaneously or disappear with time. The cause, if known, should be treated. This may include surgical removal of tumors, or surgical separation of the nerve from blood vessels or other structures that compress it.

Preparing for
Externship

In preparing for externship, the medical assistant should focus on learning how to respond to individuals who don't appear "normal." Different patient presentations are seen in neurological practices, especially patients who may have a history of strokes, epilepsy, dementia, or brain trauma. It is especially important to realize that just because an individual is unable to speak clearly or make sense, inside, his or her brain may work perfectly, and it is only the outward expression that is compromised. Never speak poorly of an individual who has a different presentation, especially in his or her presence or that of the family. There is no way for the medical assistant to know exactly what is going on inside the patient's mind.

Mild over-the-counter analgesics such as aspirin, acetaminophen, or ibuprofen may be helpful for mild pain. Narcotic analgesics such as codeine may be needed for a short time to control severe pain. These traditional painkillers, however, often have disappointing results. Other treatments may include nerve blocks, local injections of anesthetic agents, or surgical procedures to decrease sensitivity of the nerve. Some procedures involve the ablation (surgical destruction) of the affected nerve using different methods, such as local radio-frequency, heat, balloon compression, and injection of chemicals.

Paraplegia and Quadriplegia

A lesion of the spinal cord can result in paralysis of certain areas of the body, along with the corresponding loss of sensation. Paraplegia refers to paralysis from approximately the waist down, and quadriplegia refers to paralysis from approximately the shoulders down. Most spinal cord injuries result in loss of sensation and function below the level of injury, including loss of controlled function of the bladder and bowel. Due to the decreased movement and inability to walk, paraplegia may cause numerous medical complications, many of which can be prevented with good nursing care. Complications include pressure sores (decubitus), thrombosis, and pneumonia. Physiotherapy, apart from in assisting in movement, may aid in preventing these complications.

Parkinson's Disease

Parkinson's disease is a progressive disorder, with no known cure, caused by degeneration of the nerve cells in the parts of the brain that control movement. Because of the degeneration, there is a shortage of the neurotransmitter dopamine, causing the movement impairments that characterize the disease.

Parkinson's typically presents as a tremor of a limb, especially when the body is at rest. The tremor usually begins on one side, is localized to one limb, and is usually seen in the hand. Other common symptoms include (slow movement) (bradykinesia) or an inability to move (akinesia) rigid limbs, a shuffling gait, and a stooped posture. Other frequent signs of Parkinson's include reduced facial expression (the "mask") and a soft voice. The disease may also cause depression, personality change, dementia, sleep disturbances, speech impairment, and sexual difficulties. Parkinson's tends to worsen over time.

Sciatica

Sciatica, or pain along the large sciatic nerve that runs from the lower back down the back of each leg, is a relatively common form of low back pain and leg pain. This pain along the sciatic nerve can be caused when a root that helps form the sciatic nerve is pinched or irritated. It is usually caused by pressure on the sciatic nerve from a herniated disk (also referred to as a ruptured disk, pinched nerve, slipped disk, etc.). The problem is often diagnosed as a *radiculopathy,* meaning that a disk has protruded from its normal position in the vertebral column and is putting pressure on the radicular nerve (nerve root) in the lower back, which forms part of the sciatic nerve. Sciatica occurs most frequently in people between 30 and 50 years of age. Often a particular event or injury does not cause sciatica; instead, it may develop as a result of general wear and tear on the structures of the lower spine. The vast majority of people who experience sciatica get better with time (usually a few weeks or months) and find pain relief with nonsurgical treatments.

Spina Bifida

Spina bifida is the most frequently occurring, permanently disabling, and devastating of all birth defects. It affects approximately 1 out of every 1,000 newborns in the United States. More children have spina bifida than have muscular dystrophy, multiple sclerosis, and cystic fibrosis combined. It results from the failure of the spine to close properly during the first month of pregnancy. In severe cases, the spinal cord protrudes through the back and may be covered by skin or a thin membrane. Surgery to close a newborn's back is generally performed within 24 hours after birth to minimize the risk of infection and to preserve existing function in the spinal cord. Because of the paralysis resulting from the damage to the spinal cord, people born with spina bifida may need surgeries and other extensive medical care. The condition can also cause bowel and bladder complications. A large percentage of children born with spina bifida also have hydrocephalus, the accumulation of fluid in the brain. Hydrocephalus is controlled by a surgical procedure called *shunting* that relieves the fluid buildup in the brain by redirecting it into the abdominal area. Most children born with spina bifida live well into adulthood as a result of today's sophisticated medical techniques.

Stroke

A stroke known in medicine as a cerebrovascular accident (CVA), is the third leading cause of death in the United States. Death occurs to brain tissue when the blood supply to a part of the brain is decreased, either by a clot or by hemorrhage. Brain cells can die when their oxygen supply is interrupted for more than a few minutes, so speed in diagnosis and treatment is extremely important. One common cause of stroke is atherosclerosis, or narrowing of the arteries by fatty plaques. At other times, the flow of blood over the plaque causes the release of clotting factors, which leads to a blood clot that can block the flow of blood to a specific part of the brain, causing a stroke.

SUMMARY

The nervous system is a very complex communication system that affects all functions in the body. The structure and function of the nervous system, while initially seeming complex, provides for an efficient system of stimulus recognition and motor reaction for the entire body. The brain and the central nervous system collect, interpret, and coordinates all sensory input and responses performed by the peripheral nervous system. The destruction of the myelin sheath is detrimental to the functioning of the entire system. Neurological disorders must be recognized and reported to the appropriate professionals in a very timely manner to prevent long-lasting disability.

- -

Chapter Review

COMPETENCY REVIEW

1. Define and spell the terms to learn for this chapter.
2. What are the two divisions of the nervous system?
3. What are the structural and functional units of the nervous system?
4. What is an axon?
5. What is a neuron?

6. What are the parts of the central nervous system?
7. What are the functions of the hypothalamus?
8. What are the functions of the medulla oblongata?
9. What are three functions of the spinal cord?
10. What are three functions of the central nervous system?

PREPARING FOR THE CERTIFICATION EXAM

1. The first cranial nerve (olfactory) is concerned with
   A. sense of taste
   B. sense of smell
   C. sense of hearing and equilibrium
   D. chief sensory nerve of face and head
   E. sense of sight

2. The cerebrum is the largest part of the mature brain. Which of the following is NOT a part of the cerebrum?
   A. frontal lobe
   B. parietal lobe
   C. cerebellar hemisphere
   D. temporal lobe
   E. occipital lobe

3. The junction between two nerve endings that permits the transmission of a nerve impulse to continue is the
   A. gap
   B. synapse
   C. connectors
   D. receptors
   E. sensors

4. The cranial nerve that supplies most of the organs in the abdominal cavity and the thoracic cavity is the
   A. acoustic
   B. glossopharyngeal
   C. vagus
   D. spinal accessory
   E. hypoglossal

5. Afferent neurons
   A. carry impulses away from the brain and spinal cord
   B. carry impulses to the brain and spinal cord
   C. carry sensory impulses
   D. exist only in the central nervous system
   E. are stimulated only as part of the sympathetic nervous system

6. What chemicals are found in the synapse of the nerves?
   A. endorphins
   B. efferent transmitters
   C. afferent transmitters
   D. neurotransmitters
   E. adrenalin

7. The 12 cranial nerves are located within what part of the nervous system?
   A. central nervous system
   B. peripheral nervous system
   C. autonomic nervous system
   D. voluntary nervous system
   E. sympathetic nervous system

8. The membrane surrounding the brain and spinal cord is called the
   A. vertebrae
   B. cranium
   C. cranial nerves
   D. meninges
   E. pons

9. Which portion of the brain controls respiration, heart rate, and blood pressure?
   A. thalamus
   B. hypothalamus
   C. medulla oblongata
   D. brainstem
   E. cerebrum

10. The portion of the brain controlling motor function is the
    A. frontal lobe
    B. parietal lobe
    C. occipital lobe
    D. temporal lobe
    E. cerebellum

CRITICAL THINKING

1. Why did Dr. Esso send Mrs. Montero to the hospital via the 911 emergency number?

2. Why did Mrs. Montero receive clot-busting drugs?

3. What cardiovascular symptoms were present that led Dr. Esso to think that his patient may have suffered a stroke?

INTERNET ACTIVITY

Do an Internet search to learn about Alzheimer's support groups.

 MediaLink More in the nervous system, including interactive resources, can be found on the Student CD-ROM accompanying this textbook.

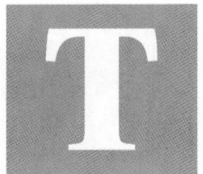his chapter discusses the special senses, which include the structures and organs that make it possible for us to see, hear, smell, taste, and feel different sensations.

The Eye and the Sense of Vision

The eye is a fluid-filled and spherical-shaped organ, composed of special anatomical structures that work together in order to facilitate sight. Light passes through the cornea, pupil, lens, and the vitreous body to stimulate sensory receptors on the retina. Vision is made possible by the coordinated actions of the nerves that control the movement of the eyeball, the amount of light admitted by the pupil, the focusing of the light on the retina by the lens, and the transmission of the resulting impulses to the brain.

Anatomy of the Eye

The eye may be broken down into three separate compartments. The first section includes the cavity, which houses the eyeball. Each eyeball has both a front, or anterior, cavity that is filled with a watery fluid called the aqueous humor, and a posterior, or back, section, which is located behind the lens and is filled with a very thick fluid called the vitreous humor (see Figure 24-1).

The eye is also composed of a wall that has three separate layers. The outer layer houses two structures that play a key role in allowing light to enter the eye. These include the sclera, or "white" part of the eye,

and the cornea, frequently referred to as the "window" of the eye, because it allows the light to enter.

The middle layer of the eye is composed of those structures that are primarily concerned with supplying rich blood to the eye. These include the choroids, which line the sclera and absorb extra light entering the eye; the ciliary body, the structure responsible for holding and moving the lens; and the iris, which contains the pupil, or "hole" in the iris, and which is responsible for controlling the amount of light entering the eye. The pigment or eye color is also located in the middle layer.

The third, or inner, layer of the eye is the retina. This structure is concerned with allowing a person to see visual images through the use of rods and cones that act as visual receptors. The lens focuses and sharpens the light onto the retina. The function of the lens is to sharpen the focus of the light on the retina. This process is called *accommodation*. This is a reflexive function of the body and is combined with the changes in the size of the pupil, the curvature of the lens, and the convergence of the optic axis to maintain the image in the same area on both retinae. The eye also accommodates for distance and depth perception.

The second section of the eye is concerned with those structures that help to protect the eye and provide for visual acuity. These structures include the eyelids, the conjunctiva, the lacrimal apparatus, and the extrinsic eye muscles.

The eyelids close over the eyeball, protecting the eye from intense light, foreign matter, and impacts. They also keep the eye moist by preventing the tears from evaporating. The margins (or the edges) of the superior and inferior palpebrae (the moving parts of the eyelids) have eyelashes that protect the eye from foreign matter. The opening between the eyelids is called the palpebral fissure, which allows light to reach the inner eye. The canthus is the place where the superior and inferior palpebrae meet, also known as the corner of the eye.

The tissue located on the underside of the eyelid and the anterior, or front, portion of the eyeball is a mucous membrane called the conjunctiva. This membrane acts as a protective covering for the exposed surface of the eyeball.

The lacrimal apparatus includes all of the structures that produce, store, and remove the tears that cleanse and lubricate the eye. They include the lacrimal gland located above the outer corner of the eye, which secretes tears through lacrimal

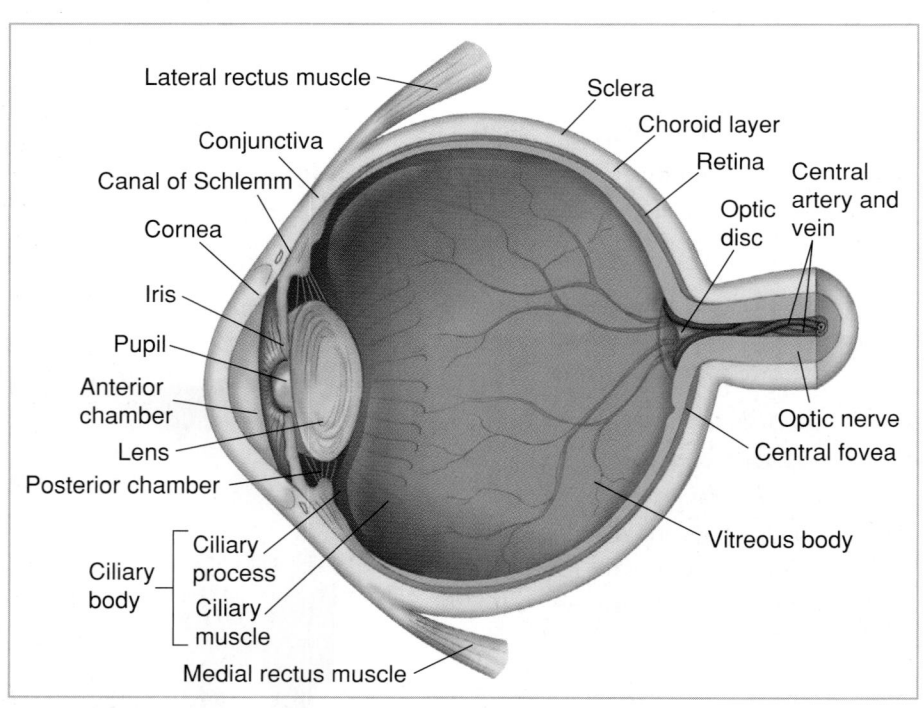

FIGURE 24-1 The eyeball and its anatomical structures.

Labels: Lateral rectus muscle, Conjunctiva, Canal of Schlemm, Cornea, Iris, Pupil, Anterior chamber, Lens, Posterior chamber, Ciliary body, Ciliary process, Ciliary muscle, Medial rectus muscle, Sclera, Choroid layer, Retina, Optic disc, Central artery and vein, Optic nerve, Central fovea, Vitreous body

As with all of the body systems, the process of aging also affects our senses of sight, hearing, smell, taste, and touch. As such, specific developmental changes begin from the time of early embryonic development and continue throughout one's life.

- Special sense organs are formed early in embryonic development. Maternal infections during the first 5 or 6 weeks of pregnancy may cause visual abnormalities, such as strabismus, as well as sensorineural deafness and other congenital ear problems, in the developing child.

- The developing infant has poor visual acuity, is often farsighted, and lacks color vision and depth perception at birth. The eye continues to grow and mature until the eighth or ninth year of life.

- The newborn infant can hear sounds, but initial responses are reflexive. By the toddler stage, the child is listening critically and beginning to imitate sounds as language development begins.

- Taste and smell are most acute at birth and decrease in sensitivity after the age of 40 as the number of olfactory and gustatory receptors decreases.

- Problems of aging associated with vision include presbyopia; glaucoma, which is the main cause of blindness in the United States; cataracts; and arteriosclerosis of the eye's blood vessels.

- Sensorineural deafness, or presbycusis, is a normal consequence of aging.

---

ducts found on the surface of the conjunctiva of the upper lid, and the lacrimal canaliculi, which are located at the inner corner of each eye and are responsible for collecting tears and then draining them into the lacrimal sac. The lacrimal sac empties into the nasolacrimal duct, which empties the tears into the nasal cavity (see Figure 24-2).

The six short extrinsic eye muscles connect the eyeball to the orbital cavity, providing it with support and rotary movement. Four of these muscles are straight, called rectus muscles, and two are oblique, or slanted, muscles.

The third section of the eye is primarily concerned with the path that is taken in order for an image to be seen by the person. Visual receptors are activated, thus allowing information to be sent by way of the optic nerve. Parts of this nerve are located at the base of the brain, the area of the brain responsible for vision. Vision occurs when the image is focused on the optic disc, which transfers the image to the optic chiasm and then to the optic nerve to the brain for interpretation of the image's impulses.

Common Disorders Associated with the Eye

Several different types of disorders can affect the eye. These conditions range from an inability to focus correctly on an object to irregularities found in the actual structures that make up the eye. These conditions include refractive errors, age-related disorders, and infections.

Refractive Errors

The most common disorders of the eye are refractive errors, which are caused as a result of the eye no longer being able to focus effectively on an object.

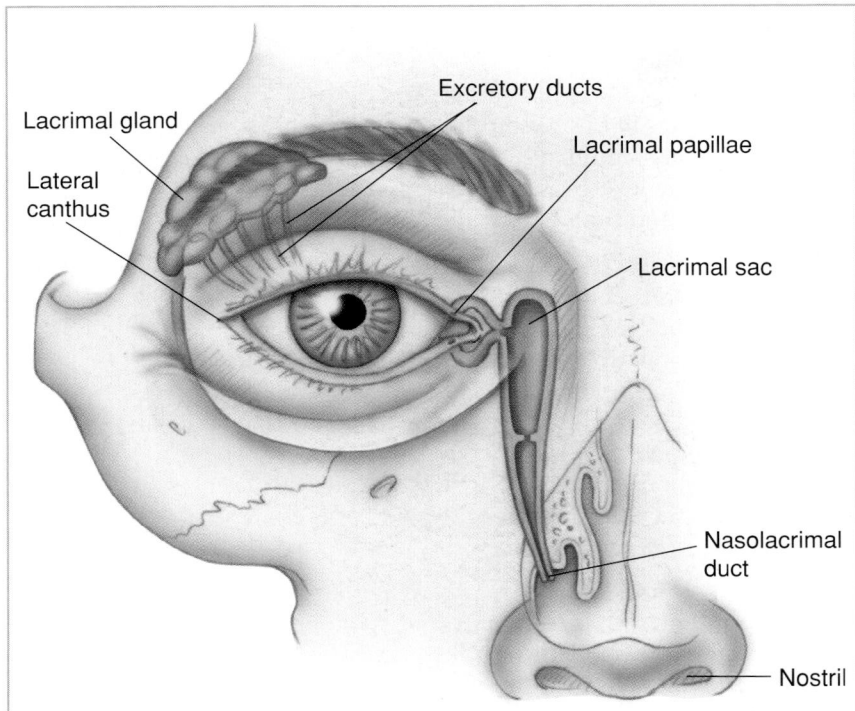

FIGURE 24-2 The lacrimal apparatus and its anatomical structure.

The majority of refractive errors can be corrected by adding a corrective lens (glasses or contact lenses) to help refocus the light correctly on the retina. Other options for correction of refractive errors include radial keratotomy (RK) and the Lasik procedure (laser surgery that reshapes the cornea of the eye and corrects imperfections in the cornea). The three most common refractive errors include myopia, or near-sightedness, which occurs when the lens focuses the light in front of the retina; hyperopia, or farsightedness, caused by the lens focusing behind the retina; and presbyopia, a disorder that causes the loss of lens elasticity as a result of aging. Treatments for these refractive errors generally include contact lenses and eyeglasses.

Another common disorder of the eyes is strabismus, or crossed eyes. In this condition, the eyes are not able to focus on the same image. Treatment usually includes eyeglasses, eye exercises, wearing a patch over the stronger eye, and surgery to realign the eyes.

Astigmatism and Amblyopia

Astigmatism is a condition caused by irregularities of the cornea, thus leading to blurred images during near or distant vision. Treatment generally includes corrective lenses or surgery to reshape the cornea. Amblyopia, or "lazy eye," is a disorder seen in children that is caused by the eye muscles being weaker in one eye. The primary treatment is to wear a patch over the stronger eye to strengthen the muscles of the weaker eye.

Cataracts

A cataract is a clouding over the lens that prevents light from entering. Over time, and without proper treatment, images begin to look fuzzy. The cataract may cloud the lens so severely that vision becomes impossible. Although we do not know for sure what causes cataracts to occur, physicians believe there may be a correlation between their incidence and smoking, diabetes, and excessive exposure to sunlight. For early or immature cataracts, the use of eyeglasses, magnifying lenses, or stronger lighting is frequently used to aid vision. However, if these measures do not improve vision, surgery is the recommended treatment. Cataract removal is one of the most common surgeries performed in the United States. It is also one of the safest and most effective, with a complete cure rate of 90 percent in most cases.

Conjunctivitis

Conjunctivitis, commonly referred to as "pink eye," is an inflammation of the conjunctiva, the tissue that lines the inside of the eyelid. It is frequently caused by a virus, bacteria, irritating substances, such as shampoos, dirt, or smoke, or sexually transmitted infections (STIs). It is one of the most common and treatable eye infections seen in both children and adults. Conjunctivitis is highly contagious and can be easily spread from person to person. Early recognition of the symptoms is extremely important. Some of the most commonly seen symptoms include redness in the sclera of the eye, an increase in the amount of tears being produced, the presence of a thick yellow discharge that crusts over the eyelashes, itchy eyes, burning in the eyes, blurred vision, and an increased sensitivity to light.

Early recognition of the symptoms and early treatment, including administration of antihistamines or antibiotics by an ophthalmologist or family physician, are important. Cure is almost always 100 percent.

Glaucoma

Glaucoma is a condition caused by an increase in the amount of pressure being built up in the eye, which leads to an excessive amount of aqueous humor. If left untreated, the pressure can lead to damage of the optic nerve, resulting in blindness.

There are two basic types of glaucoma. In open-angle glaucoma, pressure builds up very slowly, causing a slow drainage of aqueous humor from the anterior segment of the eye. However, in acute-angle closure glaucoma, which is considered much more serious, the space between the iris and the cornea decreases, causing a greater degree of pressure to build.

Glaucoma affects people of all ages and all races. There are no symptoms of glaucoma, so it must be diagnosed by pressure testing in a doctor's office. About 80,000 people are totally blind, another 250,000 are blind in one eye, and over 1.2 million people have some degree of visual loss as a result of glaucoma.

Disorders Affecting the Retina

Several disorders affect the retina, but two of the most severe include retinal detachment and macular degeneration. While considered fairly rare and primarily affecting people as they age, a detached retina occurs when the retina separates from the underlying choroid layer. When such a separation occurs, vision becomes damaged. However, if the detachment is detected early, the separation can be repaired and the vision spared. In cases where the retina has already separated and become detached, vision can frequently be restored by surgery and laser therapy.

Macular degeneration, which is caused by a deterioration of the central portion of the retina, is an incurable disease of the eye that affects more than 10 million Americans, and is considered one of the leading causes of blindness in Americans over the age of 55.

There are two types of macular degeneration: dry and wet. Of these, 85 to 90 percent are the dry (atrophic) type. In the dry type of macular degeneration, small yellow deposits (*drusen*) form under the macula. This phenomena leads to a thinning and drying out of the macula. The amount of loss of central vision is directly related to the location and the amount of retinal thinning caused by the drusen. This form of macular degeneration has a slower progression than does the wet type. Sometimes, however, dry macular degeneration will turn into wet degeneration. There is no known treatment or cure for dry macular degeneration.

In the 10 percent of the cases of wet macular degeneration, abnormal new blood vessels, called subretinal neovascularizations, grow underneath the retina and the macula. These new blood vessels may then bleed and leak fluid, causing the macula to bulge or lift up, distorting or destroying the central vision. Vision loss may be rapid and severe. If performed early, laser surgery may halt the progression of wet macular degeneration, thus preventing a total loss of vision. There is no guarantee, however, that this will preserve vision, but it is the best treatment.

Corneal Abrasion

The cornea, which is located at the front of the eye, may become the site of lesions or abrasions. These can be a direct result of an injury, an infection, or sometimes both. A corneal abrasion is a very painful condition. The patient will be very sensitive to light and will have difficulty opening the affected eye. The usual treatment is visual rest and mild analgesic. If the abrasion becomes infected, treatment generally consists of antibiotics in the form of drops or ointment and the use of an eye patch.

Hordeolums

Also known as a "sty," hordeolums are considered very common and frequently contagious. Structurally, they appear as a pus-filled swelling located near the roots of the eyelash. They are often caused by a bacterial infection and are generally predisposed by blocked or in-

fected eyelid glands or inflammation of the eyelids. Contaminated fingers that touch the eye area may also cause the infection. Painful hordeolums can also occur internally within the eyelids, usually in association with a blocked gland that provides lubrication for the eyelid. Hordeolums may resolve on their own; however, a warm, wet compress applied to the area may help relieve the pain. Antibiotics may be taken orally or antibiotic ointments applied topically to aid in the healing.

Legal and Ethical Issues

Be clear on the rules for driving in your state in order to help patients who have visual difficulties. If the patient cannot see clearly, then the physician should instruct him or her regarding local laws and the dangers of driving. Help the patient by having a list of community resources available that provide transportation when necessary. As vision decreases, the patient will need to rely on community resources for activities of daily living. Be sure those resources are readily available so that the patient can take immediate steps to access them. It is unsafe for patients with limited visual abilities to operate any motorized vehicle.

Professionalism

The professional medical assistant will occasionally have days on which the physician is seeing patients later than their appointments. This can create discomfort for both the patients and the medical assistant. Explain to patients that the physician is running behind, and give them the option to reschedule their appointment. If they choose to wait, be sure to move them to an exam room as quickly as possible, and plan ahead as much as possible to help the physician be as efficient as possible. Explaining to patients that the physician is providing the same care to other patients that he or she will provide to them will help to alleviate their frustrations with the delays. Always remember that if patients verbalize their frustrations about the delay, their attack is never personal; instead, they are just venting their frustration.

The Ear and the Sense of Hearing

The ear is the site of hearing and equilibrium. There are specialized anatomical structures that receive the vibration of sound and are also sensitive to gravity and the movements of the head. These structures are connected to the eighth cranial nerve by special nerve fibers.

Anatomy of the Ear

The ear consists of three separate sections: the external ear, the part visible to the outside; the middle ear, the part responsible for transmitting sounds to the inner ear; and the inner ear, which houses the receptors responsible for providing hearing and equilibrium, or balance (see Figure 24-3).

The External Ear

The external ear is the visible portion of the ear. The appendage on the side of the head consists of the pinna (auricle), the auditory canal (the auditory meatus), and the tympanic membrane (eardrum). The auricle collects sounds waves and then directs them through the auditory canal to the tympanic membrane. The auditory canal is about 2.5 cm long and is S shaped. The tympanic membrane separates the external ear from the middle ear.

The Middle Ear

The function of the middle ear is to transmit sound vibrations, provide equalization of air pressure on both sides of the tympanic membrane, and protect the ossicles from potentially damaging loud sounds. It is a tiny cavity of the temporal bone of the skill, located inside the tympanic membrane. This structure contains three small bones, or ossicles, that are necessary for hearing. The three bones are the malleus (hammer), the incus (anvil), and the stapes (stirrup). The names are indicative of their shapes. These bones react to the vibrations of the sound waves and mechanically transmit the vibrations from the tympanic membrane to the bones in the order presented. The oval window is a small opening on the cochlea, which marks the beginning of the inner ear. During transmission, the tympanic vibrations may be amplified as much as 22 times their original force.

The Inner Ear

The inner ear consists of a membranous labyrinth (maze) located within a bony labyrinth. The bony labyrinth has three divisions: the cochlea, the vestibule, and the three semicircular canals. The perilymph separates the membranous labyrinth from the bony labyrinth. The cochlear duct is one membranous division, located inside the cochlea, and the semicircular ducts are other divisions, located inside the semicircular canals. The final divisions of the membranous labyrinth are the utricle and the saccule, small sac-like structures located in the vestibule. Tiny hair cells that sense movement are located inside the inner ear, functioning as the receptors for hearing and equilibrium (balance).

The Cochlea

The cochlea is a spiral-shaped bony structure that resembles a snail's shell (see Figure 24-4). The spiral cavity of the bony cochlea contains three tube-like channels that run the entire length of the spiral. The three channels are the scala vestibule, the scala tympani, and the cochlear duct. The organ of Corti contains the hair cell sensory receptors used for the sense of hearing. The organ of Corti is located in the cochlear duct on the floor, also known as the basilar membrane. The perilymph (a pale fluid) fills the scala tympani and the scala vestibule, helping to transmit wound waves. Endolymph fills the cochlear duct and protects the hair cells, while assisting with the sense of hearing.

Common Disorders Associated with the Middle Ear

Many of the disorders affecting our hearing are inflammatory and often occur in the middle ear where sounds are transmitted and in the inner ear, at the point where balance

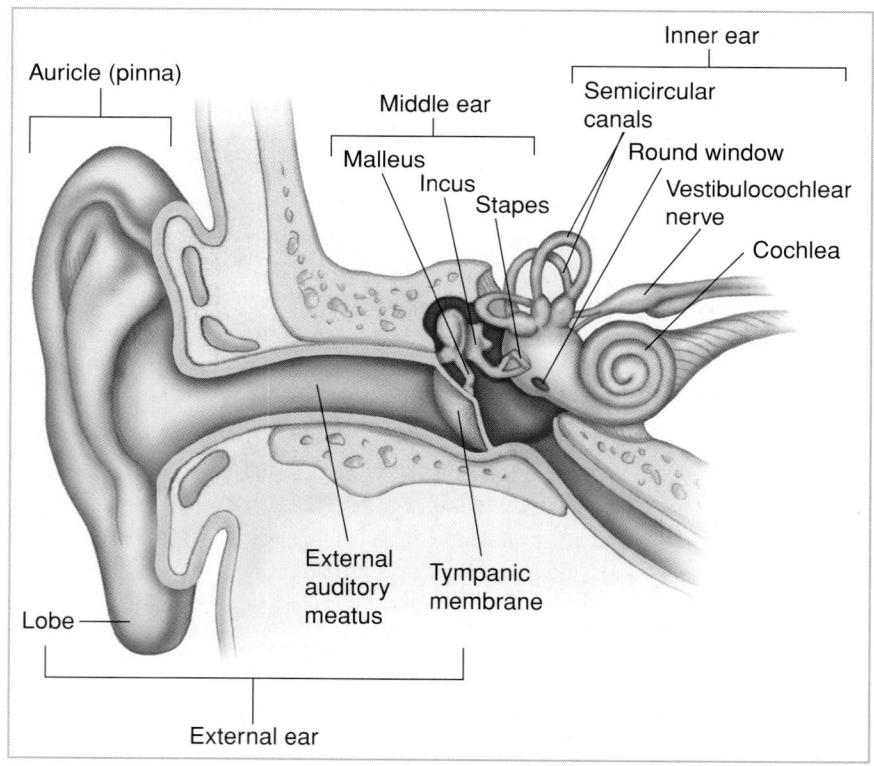

FIGURE 24-3 The ear and its anatomical structures.

and equilibrium take place. The most common inflammatory disorder affecting the middle ear is otitis media, and the most frequently encountered condition affecting the inner ear is Ménière's disease.

Otitis Media

Otitis is an inflammation of the ear. Otitis externa is an inflammation of the outer ear (swimmer's ear). Otitis media is inflammation of the middle ear. This inflammation can be caused by viral or bacterial infections, some related to sore throats, colds, or breathing problems.

Children suffer from otitis media more frequently than do adults. This is due to the size of the eustachian tube leading from the ear to the pharynx. If there is any swelling in the tissues that surround this tube, it can close, decreasing the ability of the ear to drain. If the naturally occurring fluids remain in ear, they can become a source of infection. The eustachian tube in children is also straighter than that of an adult, so a child drinking a bottle while lying down stands a greater chance of the fluids flowing backwards up the tube and into the middle ear.

The main goal of treating otitis media is to rid the middle ear of infection before more serious complications set in. Treatment usually involves eliminating the causes of the infection, killing any invading bacteria, boosting the immune system, and reducing swelling in the eustachian tubes. This is frequently accomplished through the introduction of oral antibiotics and decongestants, such as pseudoephedrine. In cases where the otitis media is more acute and there is thick effusion and poor eustachian tube function, daily or every other day tubal insufflation may be in order. Persistent serous fluid may be removed by needle aspiration, but thick mucoid or organized blood must be removed by myringotomy if it has not cleared after 2 or 3 weeks of intensive therapy.

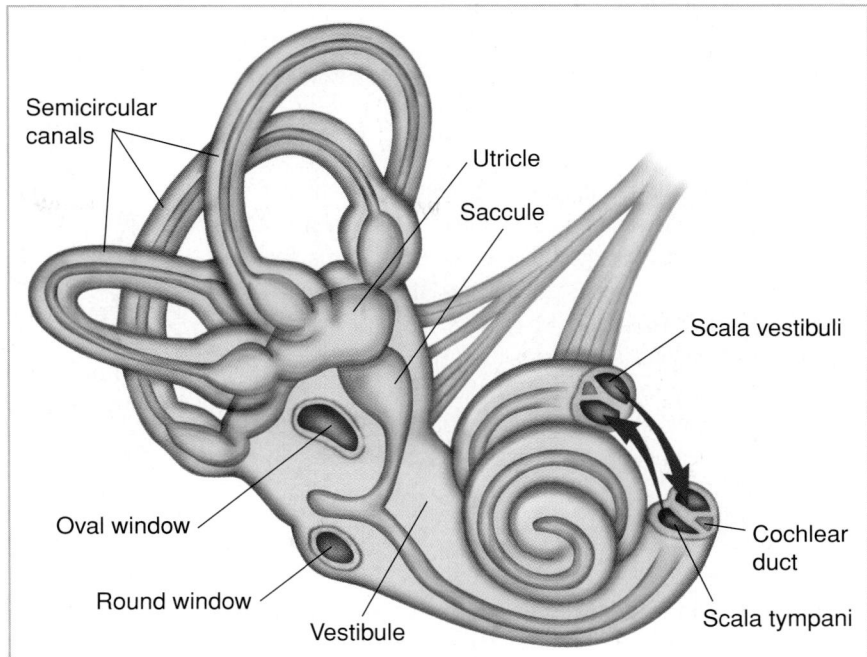

FIGURE 24-4 The cochlea.

Otosclerosis

Otosclerosis, which is frequently hereditary, is a condition that occurs when the tissue surrounding the bone of the stapes grows abnormally around it. When this happens, the overgrowth of the tissue prevents the stapes from transmitting sound vibrations to the inner ear. The result is profound hearing loss involving one or both ears.

Common Disorders Associated with the Inner Ear

The inner ear, as we have previously discussed, is most responsible for helping us to maintain our equilibrium and balance. Because of that, many of the disorders inherent to the inner ear are often accompanied by severe dizziness, ringing in the ears, and a loss of balance.

Ménière's Disease

Ménière's disease is a condition of the inner ear that causes a host of symptoms including vertigo (severe

---

Patient **Education**

The parents of small children should be instructed to never allow their children to lie down while drinking a bottle. When a child drinks while supine the chances of getting middle ear infections increase. Instead, the child should be at a 30-degree angle at least while drinking a bottle and left in that position for a few minutes after drinking.

dizziness), tinnitus (ringing in the ears), fluctuating hearing loss, and a possible sensation of pressure or pain in the affected ear. The disease is named after the French physician Prosper Ménière, who first described the syndrome in 1861.

Symptoms of Ménière's disease, which often occur suddenly and can arise daily or infrequently, are associated with a change in fluid volume within the labyrinth portion of the inner ear. Many experts on Ménière's disease think that a rupture of the membranous labyrinth allows the endolymph and the perilymph to mix. This mixing may be the cause of the symptoms. There are other possible causes, including bacterial or viral infections, environmental factors, and noise pollution.

Although there is no known cure for Ménière's disease, symptoms of the disease can be controlled by reducing the body's retention of fluids, eating a low-salt diet, with no caffeine or alcohol, and possibly using diuretic drugs. Other medication changes that may be beneficial include those that control allergies and improve the blood circulation in the inner ear. Eliminating tobacco use and reducing stress levels are additional ways to reduce the severity of these symptoms.

Presbycusis

Presbycusis is a type of hearing loss involving the gradual deterioration of the sensory receptors located in the cochlea. Seen most frequently in older adults—and affecting approximately 25 percent of people by the time they reach the age of 60 to 70—it affects more men than women. It generally occurs in both ears, causing the patient to have problems hearing high-pitched tones as well as the normal verbal sounds heard during conversation and talking. Factors that lead to presbycusis include long exposures to loud noises, infection, injury, and, in some cases, side effects caused by cer-

tain medications. Treatment is generally to assist hearing loss by the use of a hearing aid.

Tinnitus

Tinnitus is a symptom associated with many forms of hearing loss. It can also be a symptom of other health problems. According to estimates by the American Tinnitus Association, at least 12 million Americans have tinnitus. Of these, at least 1 million experience it so severely that it interferes with their daily activities. People with severe cases of tinnitus may find it difficult to hear, work, or even sleep.

Tinnitus is frequently caused by hearing loss, loud noises, medicines, and other health problems, such as allergies, tumors, and problems arising from the cardiovascular system. If a physician suspects tinnitus, he or she may refer the patient to an otolaryngologist for diagnosis or an audiologist who will test the patient's hearing. Although there is no cure for tinnitus, scientists and doctors have discovered several treatments that may provide some relief. The most common of these include the use of hearing aids, maskers, or small electronic devices that are worn by the patient to help mask the sounds, and medications, such as antiarrhythmics and antidepressants.

Impacted Cerumen

Cerumen is a complex mixture of lipids, including waxy compounds produced by the sebaceous glands of the external auditory meatus as a mean of protecting the epithelial lining of the tract. Impacted cerumen, or wax, in the ear is a frequent occurrence in which the wax becomes so hard that it obstructs the auditory canal. It generally affects older adults and is frequently exacerbated by their use of cotton-tipped swabs to clean their ears. Treatment includes "softening" the wax, so that it may be removed by an ear syringe. If left untreated, impacted cerumen can lead to hearing loss or tinnitus.

Audiology and Hearing Loss

Audiology is the study of hearing disorders. Sustained noise over 85 decibels can cause permanent hearing loss, and the risk doubles with each 5-decibel increase.

The two most common types of hearing loss are conductive hearing loss, which may develop when sound waves have no way of being conducted through the ear and are often temporary, and sensorineural hearing loss, which occurs when neural structures of the ear become damaged, eventually leading to permanent deafness.

The Senses of Taste and Smell

Our sense of smell is dependent on olfactory cells, which are located high in the roof of the nasal cavity. This means that they respond to changes in chemical concentrations. Once a smell receptor is activated, it then sends information to the olfactory nerves, located in different areas of the brain (see Figure 24-5).

The sense of taste and the sense of smell work close together to create a combined effect that is interpreted by the brain. Therefore, when you smell something, some of the tiny molecules move from the nose down into the mouth region, thus stimulating the taste buds. In actuality, part of what we refer to as smell is really taste.

Taste buds, which are tiny bumps located on the tongue, are microscopic, so they cannot be seen by the naked eye (see Figure 24-6). Some can be found on the roof of the mouth, while others are located in the walls of the throat. Each of these buds is made up of cells that function as taste receptors. There are four types of taste cells, with each one of them functioning as an individual group of chemicals that ultimately provides us with different tastes. They include the sweet taste cells, located on the tip of the tongue; the sour taste cells, located on the sides of the tongue; the salty taste cells, located on the tip and sides of the tongue; and the bitter taste cells, located at the back of the tongue.

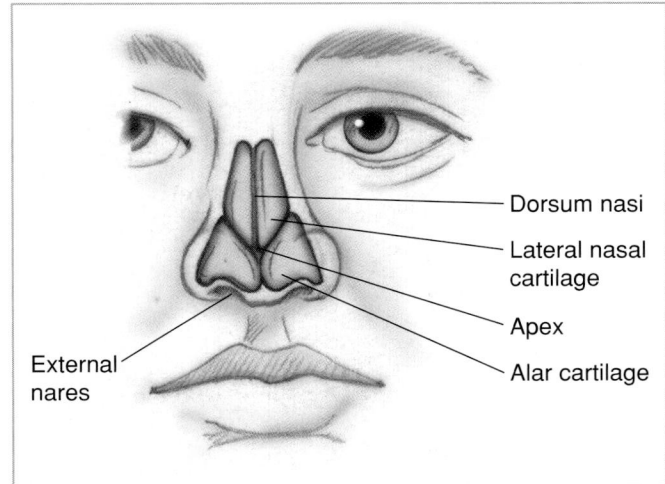

FIGURE 24-5   Nasal cartilages and external structures.

endings that are very sensitive to pain. However, the tongue is not as good at sensing hot or cold. That's why it seems so easy to burn the mouth when something is eaten that is really hot.

The Sense of Touch

Touch is our oldest, most primitive and pervasive sense. It is the first sense we experience in the womb and the last one we lose before death. And while the other four senses (sight, hearing, smell, and taste) are located in specific parts of the body, the sense of touch is found all over. This is because touch originates in the bottom layer of the skin, called the dermis. The dermis is filled with many tiny nerve endings called receptors that provide information about the things with which the body comes in contact (see Figure 24-7). They do this by carrying touch information to the spinal cord, which, in turn, sends messages to the brain where the feeling is registered.

Some areas of the body are more sensitive than others because they have more nerve endings. A good example of this is the pain that is felt when you accidentally bite down on your tongue. The pain occurs because the sides of the tongue have a lot of nerve

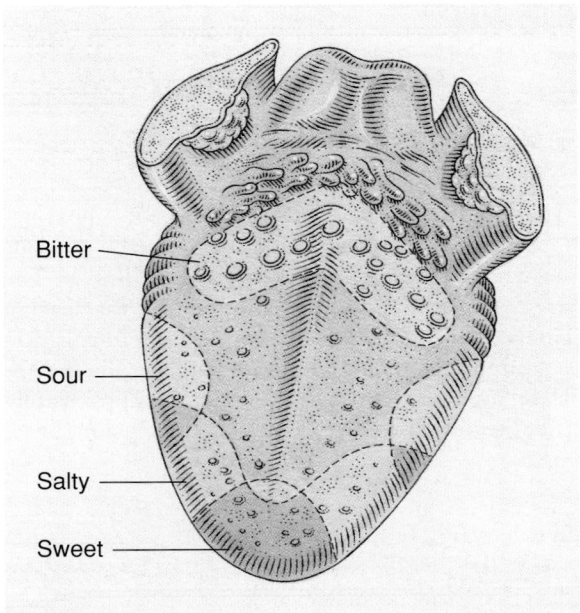

FIGURE 24-6   Tongue and taste buds.

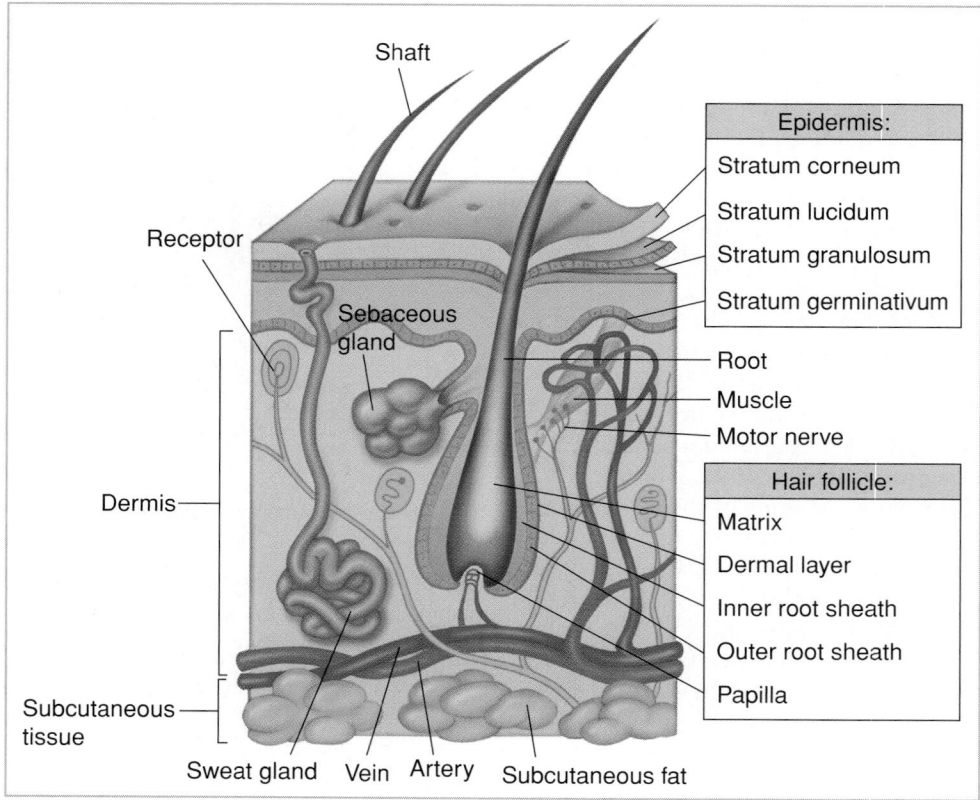

FIGURE 24-7 Layers of the skin showing receptors.

SUMMARY

The special senses, which include vision, hearing, smell, and taste, are special extensions of the nervous system, while the sense of touch is found all over. The eyes are responsible for vision and the ears for hearing and balance, and both systems require the integration of specialized cells that collaborate and provide the appropriate input so that the brain can appropriately interpret the data it receives. The senses of vision, hear-

ing, taste, and smell are all activated through the brain and the nervous system. The sense of touch originates in the dermis, where nerve endings process and transfer information to the spinal cord, which sends messages to the brain where the feeling is registered. During the aging process, all of these systems can decline significantly, greatly affecting the activities and quality of life.

Chapter Review

COMPETENCY REVIEW

1. Define and spell the terms to learn for this chapter.
2. What structures are contained in the middle layer of the eye?
3. What are the external structures of the ear?
4. What are the functions of the muscles of the eye?
5. What is the inner layer of the eye called?
6. What are the functions of the ear?
7. What are the three ossicles of the ear?
8. What is the bony labyrinth?
9. What is the most common "waxy" fluid found in the ear?
10. How many different types of taste cells are located on the tongue?

PREPARING FOR THE CERTIFICATION EXAM

1. What is the name of the substance that fills the anterior cavity that houses the eyeball?
   A. vitreous humor
   B. nasolacrimal fluids
   C. aqueous humor
   D. lacrimal glands
   E. lacrimal fluids

2. The structure of the eye that lines the sclera and absorbs extra light entering the eye is called the
   A. pupil
   B. aqueous humor
   C. retina
   D. ciliary body
   E. choroid

3. Refractive errors are defects in visual acuity. The eye has lost its ability to effectively focus light on the surface of the retina. Which of the following is NOT a refractive error?
   A. hyperopia (farsightedness)
   B. astigmatism
   C. presbyopia
   D. myopia (nearsightedness)
   E. glaucoma

4. A condition of the eye with excessive intraocular pressure that can damage the retina and the optic nerve, often causing blindness, is
   A. glaucoma
   B. cataracts
   C. retinal detachment
   D. astigmatism
   E. corneal ulcers

5. A highly contagious condition of the eye, often caused by a bacterial infection and generally predisposed by blocked or infected eyelid glands, is called
   A. corneal abrasion
   B. astigmatism
   C. hordeolum
   D. conjunctivitis
   E. macular degeneration

6. The mucous membranes that line the inner surfaces of the eyelids are called the
   A. retina
   B. sclera
   C. lens
   D. conjunctiva
   E. iris

7. A condition that is frequently hereditary, and occurs as a result of bone tissue growing abnormally around the stapes is called
   A. otitis externa
   B. otitis media
   C. otosclerosis
   D. Ménière's disease
   E. swimmer's ear

8. Symptoms of Ménière's disease include all of the following EXCEPT
   A. nausea and vomiting
   B. vertigo
   C. pain and pressure in the affected ear
   D. tinnitus
   E. eustachian tube dysfunction

9. All of the following are ossicles of the ear are EXCEPT
   A. cochlea
   B. malleus
   C. incus
   D. stapes
   E. anvil

10. Which taste cell is located on the tip of the tongue?
    A. bitter
    B. sour
    C. sweet
    D. salty
    E. bittersweet

CRITICAL THINKING

1. Why do young children get otitis media more frequently than adults?
2. Why do you think this patient refuses to eat when her ears hurt?
3. Why would acetaminophen (Tylenol) be prescribed for this patient?

INTERNET ACTIVITY

Do an Internet search on Lasik surgery to learn more about the procedure.

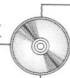 **MediaLink** More on the special senses, including interactive resources, can be found on the Student CD-ROM accompanying this textbook.

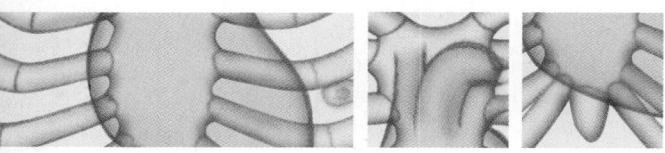

Medical Assistant Role Delineation Chart

HIGHLIGHT indicates material covered in this chapter.

ADMINISTRATIVE

Administrative Procedures

- Perform basic administrative medical assisting functions
- Schedule, coordinate and monitor appointments
- Schedule inpatient/outpatient admissions and procedures
- Understand and apply third-party guidelines
- Obtain reimbursement through accurate claims submission
- Monitor third-party reimbursement
- Understand and adhere to managed care policies and procedures
- *Negotiate managed care contracts*

Practice Finances

- Perform procedural and diagnostic coding
- Apply bookkeeping principles

- Manage accounts receivable
- *Manage accounts payable*
- *Process payroll*
- *Document and maintain accounting and banking records*
- *Develop and maintain fee schedules*
- *Manage renewals of business and professional insurance policies*
- *Manage personnel benefits and maintain records*
- *Perform marketing, financial, and strategic planning*

CLINICAL

Fundamental Principles

- Apply principles of aseptic technique and infection control
- Comply with quality assurance practices
- Screen and follow up patient test results

Diagnostic Orders

- Collect and process specimens
- Perform diagnostic tests

Patient Care

- Adhere to established patient screening procedures
- Obtain patient history and vital signs
- Prepare and maintain examination and treatment areas
- Prepare patient for examinations, procedures and treatments

- Assist with examinations, procedures and treatments
- Prepare and administer medications and immunizations
- Maintain medication and immunization records
- Recognize and respond to emergencies
- Coordinate patient care information with other health care providers
- Initiate IV and administer IV medications with appropriate training and as permitted by state law

GENERAL

Professionalism

- Display a professional manner and image
- Demonstrate initiative and responsibility
- Work as a member of the health care team
- Prioritize and perform multiple tasks
- Adapt to change
- Promote the CMA credential
- Enhance skills through continuing education
- Treat all patients with compassion and empathy
- Promote the practice through positive public relations

Communication Skills

- Recognize and respect cultural diversity
- Adapt communications to individual's ability to understand
- Use professional telephone technique

- Recognize and respond effectively to verbal, nonverbal, and written communications
- Use medical terminology appropriately
- Utilize electronic technology to receive, organize, prioritize and transmit information
- Serve as liaison

Legal Concepts

- Perform within legal and ethical boundaries
- Prepare and maintain medical records
- Document accurately
- Follow employer's established policies dealing with the health care contract
- Implement and maintain federal and state health care legislation and regulations
- Comply with established risk management and safety procedures
- Recognize professional credentialing criteria
- *Develop and maintain personnel, policy and procedure manuals*

Instruction

- Instruct individuals according to their needs
- Explain office policies and procedures
- Teach methods of health promotion and disease prevention
- Locate community resources and disseminate information
- *Develop educational materials*
- *Conduct continuing education activities*

Operational Functions

- Perform inventory of supplies and equipment
- Perform routine maintenance of administrative and clinical equipment
- Apply computer techniques to support office operations
- *Perform personnel management functions*
- *Negotiate leases and prices for equipment and supply contracts*

- *Denotes advanced skills.*

SOURCE: Reprinted by permission of the American Association of Medical Assistants from the AAMA Role Delineation Study: Occupational Analysis of the Medical Assisting Profession.

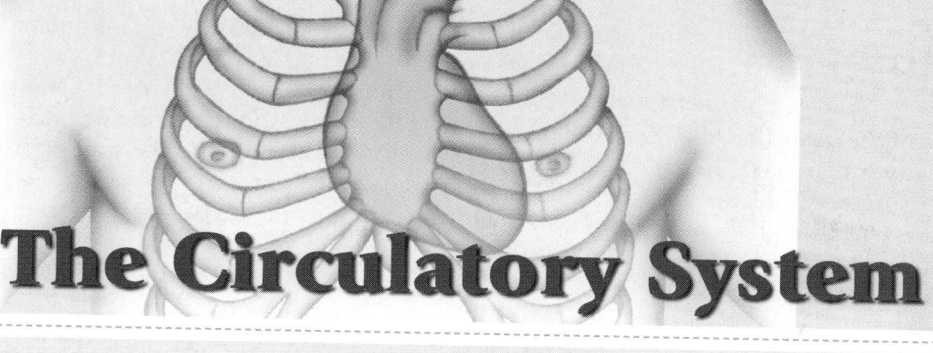

The Circulatory System

Learning Objectives

After completing this chapter, you should be able to:

- Define and spell the terms to learn for this chapter.
- Identify the organs that make up the circulatory system.
- Identify the structures that make up the heart and briefly explain the function of each.
- Explain the conduction system of the heart.
- Explain the functions of the arteries, veins, and capillaries.
- List and describe the components of blood.

- State the difference between Rh-positive blood and Rh-negative blood.
- Discuss the importance of blood typing and cite which blood types are compatible.
- Identify the organs of the lymphatic system and cite the location and function of each.
- Define lymph and explain how it is circulated throughout the body.
- Identify and explain common disorders associated with the circulatory system.

OUTLINE

Overview of the Circulatory System — 436

The Heart — 436

Blood Vessels — 439

Blood Pressure — 440

Pulmonary and Systemic Circulation — 442

Blood — 442

Hemostasis and Bleeding Control — 446

Blood Types — 446

The Lymphatic System — 448

Common Disorders Associated with the Circulatory System — 450

Terms to Learn

anemia	coronary heart disease	myocardial infarction
aneurysm	diastolic blood pressure	myocardium
angioplasty	dyspnea	pericardium
arrhythmia	endocardium	platelets
arteriosclerosis	erythrocytes	Purkinje fibers
atherosclerosis	heart murmur	RhoGAM
atria	hemostasis	sinoatrial node
atrioventricular node	hypertension	systolic blood pressure
bicuspid valve	hypotension	tachycardia
bradycardia	leukemia	thrombophlebitis
bundle of His	leukocytes	tricuspid valve
congestive heart failure	lymph	ventricles

Case Study

JOE FRANCISCO IS A 79-YEAR-OLD who comes to Dr. Schaffer's office complaining of chest pain. Joe has a history of multiple cardiac issues including hypertension and hyperlipidemia. Mr. Francisco is 85 pounds overweight. Dr. Schaffer asks his medical assistant to give Joe one sublingual nitroglycerin and to do an electrocardiogram. His vital signs are blood pressure 150/95; pulse 88; respirations 18. Oxygen is started at 2 liters per minute.

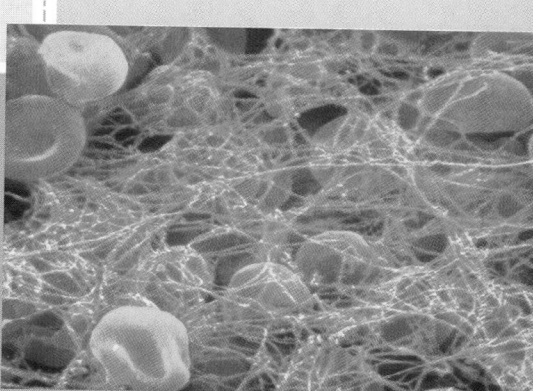

Overview of the Circulatory System

The circulatory system consists of the heart, the blood vessels, the blood, and the structures that make up the lymphatic system. The heart is responsible for the movement of blood through the arterial and vascular system throughout the entire body, providing oxygenation and the removal of waste for the entire body, while the lymphatic system, which is a subsystem of the circulatory system, acts as the body's transportation system. The lymphatic system is also responsible for defending the body against disease-causing agents, called pathogens.

The Heart

The heart is a four-chambered muscular pump lying just left of the midline of the chest (mediastinum), beneath the sternum (see Figure 25-1), and consisting of three linings: the outer lining, called the pericardium; the middle layer, or heart muscle, called the myocardium; and the innermost lining, called the endocardium (see Figure 25-2). Most of the heart is made of cardiac muscle, which is the only muscle with automaticity, meaning

that the contractions are controlled by the autonomic nervous system.

The human heart is about the size of a fist and weighs approximately 9 ounces. It is cone shaped, with the apex at the most inferior point and the wider portion of the cone shape at the top.

Four chambers make up the heart, with the right side working to move blood from the body to the lungs, and the left side of the heart pumping the blood back to the body (see Figure 25-3).

The left and right sides of the heart are separated by a wall called the septum. The two upper chambers are called the atria (singular is *atrium*) and are receiving chambers. The lower two chambers pump blood out of the heart and are called the ventricles.

Blood Flow through the Heart

The right atrium is the first chamber that blood comes into as it enters the heart. This is the smallest chamber with the thinnest wall, and it is responsible for receiving all of the blood from the body via the superior vena cava and the inferior vena cava. The valve (or entryway) from the right atrium to the right ventricle is called the tricuspid valve.

After going through the tricuspid valve, the blood enters the right ventricle. This chamber is more muscular

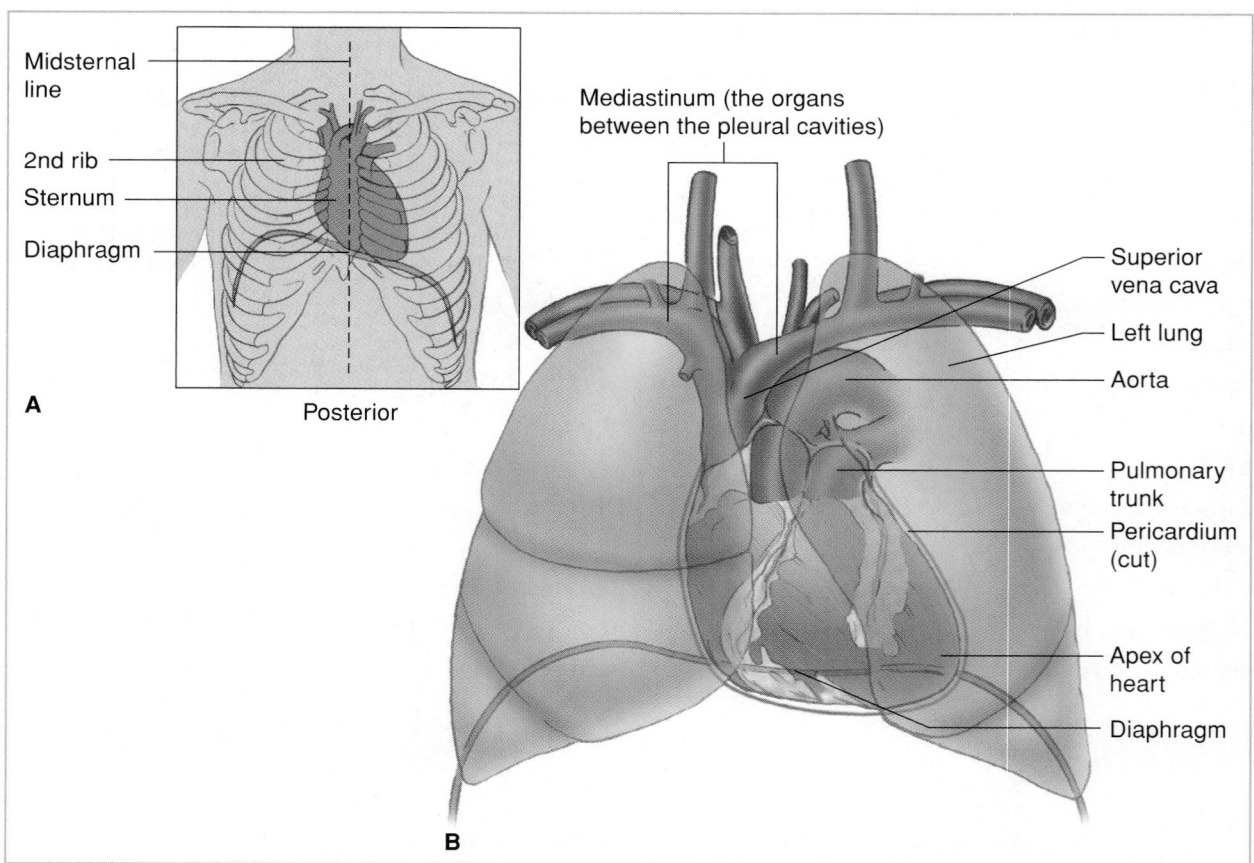

FIGURE 25-1 Location of the heart in the chest cavity.

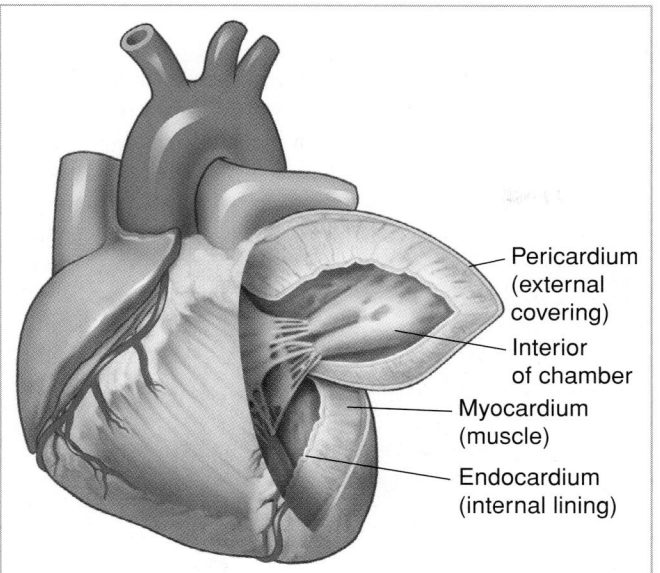

FIGURE 25-2 Linings of the heart.

Labels for Figure 25-2:
Pericardium (external covering)
Interior of chamber
Myocardium (muscle)
Endocardium (internal lining)

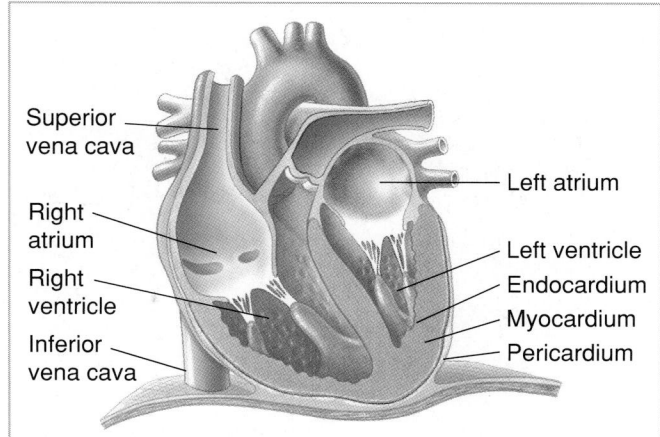

FIGURE 25-3 The heart: interior view of the heart chambers.

Labels for Figure 25-3:
Superior vena cava
Right atrium
Right ventricle
Inferior vena cava
Left atrium
Left ventricle
Endocardium
Myocardium
Pericardium

than the right atrium. Blood leaves the right ventricle through the pulmonary valve to go to the lungs, via the pulmonary artery, where the carbon dioxide and waste material from the blood are exchanged for oxygen.

On its return from the lungs, blood enters the left atrium via the pulmonary vein. This atrium is more heavily muscled than is the right atrium. The blood leaves the left atrium through the mitral, or bicuspid valve.

The final stop within the heart for the blood is the powerhouse chamber, the left ventricle. The walls of this chamber are highly muscular, so they can pump blood out from the heart to the farthest reaches of the body. When the blood leaves the left ventricle through the aortic valve, it enters the aorta, to begin its journey to the body. The aorta is the largest artery in the body. Figure 25-4 shows the flow of blood through the heart.

It is important to note that during the time the blood is making its way through the heart, the valves are functioning as "doorways" for the blood to move through the chamber, thus never allowing the blood to flow backward (see Figure 25-5). A damaged or diseased valve can allow blood to escape and moves backward through the valves and is known as a heart murmur.

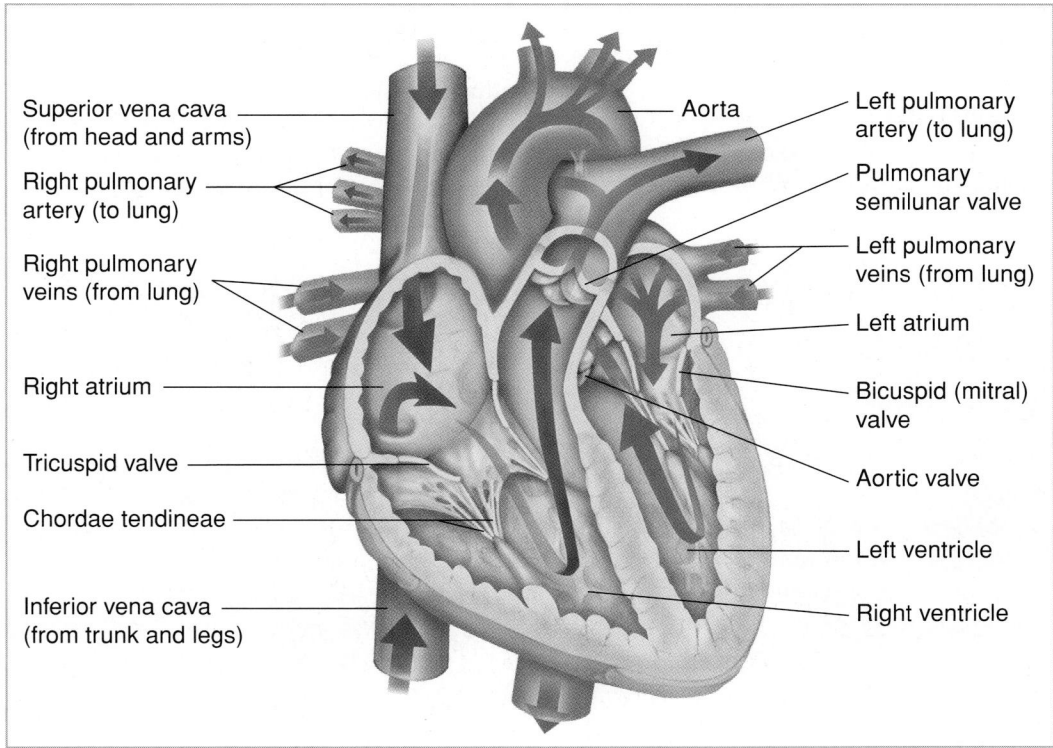

FIGURE 25-4 The flow of blood through the heart.

Labels for Figure 25-4:
Superior vena cava (from head and arms)
Right pulmonary artery (to lung)
Right pulmonary veins (from lung)
Right atrium
Tricuspid valve
Chordae tendineae
Inferior vena cava (from trunk and legs)
Aorta
Left pulmonary artery (to lung)
Pulmonary semilunar valve
Left pulmonary veins (from lung)
Left atrium
Bicuspid (mitral) valve
Aortic valve
Left ventricle
Right ventricle

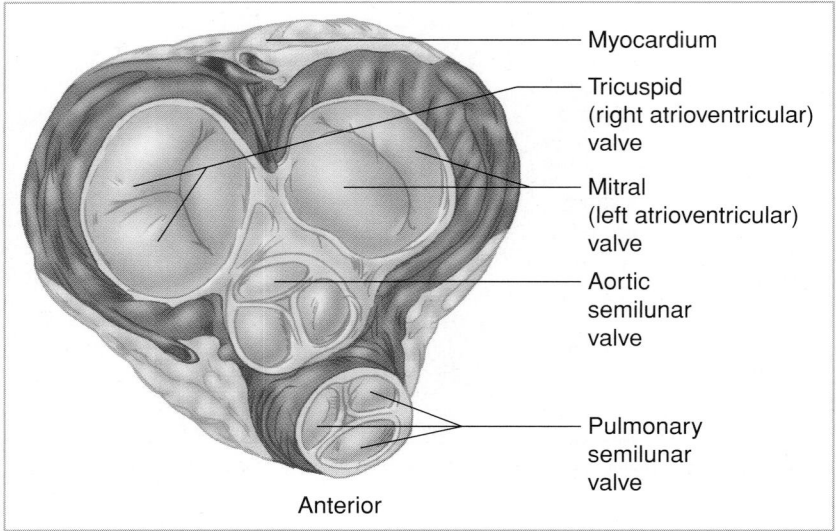

Myocardium

Tricuspid
(right atrioventricular)
valve

Mitral
(left atrioventricular)
valve

Aortic
semilunar
valve

Pulmonary
semilunar
valve

Anterior

FIGURE 25-5 The valves of the heart.

Physiology of the Heart

The heart is a strong muscle, moving blood out from the left ventricle to the entire body with very little obvious effort. The opening of the valves allows the chambers to pump the blood out and receive the next flow of blood into the chamber between contractions. The mechanical, or pump, action of the heart is the cardiac muscle contraction. When the chamber is full, the valves close, prohibiting backflow of blood into the previous chamber. The sounds heard when listening to the heart, auscultation, are made by the valves as they snap shut.

Vascular System of the Heart

The dense muscularity of the heart requires its own vascular system. The coronary arteries, which can be seen in Figure 25-6, supply the heart with blood, and the coronary veins drain the blood into the coronary sinus and then back into the right atrium for oxygenation. When these vessels are occluded (blocked), the heart muscle can be starved for oxygen, causing chest pain, and if the lack of oxygen occurs over a long period of time, then heart muscle damage or death will occur.

Conduction System of the Heart

Cardiac muscle has the property of automaticity. This means that the heart is able to determine its rate and rhythm by way of the autonomic nervous system. Three areas have specialized neuromuscular tissues that initiate the heartbeat. They are the sinoatrial node (SA node), the atrioventricular node (AV node), and the atrioventricular bundle, also known as the bundle of His. Figure 25-7 shows the conduction system of the heart.

The sinoatrial node is also called the "pacemaker." It is located in the upper wall of the right atrium, just blow the opening of the superior vena cava. The SA node is responsible for initiating the heartbeat. The electrical impulses discharged by the SA node are distributed to the right and left atria, causing contractions of the atria. Heart rates initiated by the SA node are typically 60 to 80 beats per minute in a healthy adult at rest.

The atrioventricular node is located beneath the endocardium of the right atrium. It is a "gatekeeper," responsible for transmitting impulses from the SA

Lifespan
Considerations

THE CHILD
- The development of the circulatory system begins with the development of the fetal heart during the first 2 months of gestation, and the newborn's circulation begins to function just after birth.
- Children have a smaller circulatory system, and their vital signs are typically different than those of adults. Their blood pressure will typically be higher than that of an adult, as will their pulse and respiratory rates.

THE OLDER ADULT
- Cardiac and other circulatory changes once attributed to aging may be minimized with appropriate lifestyle modifications.
- Reduced blood flow, elevated blood lipids, and defective endothelial repair that can be seen in aging may accelerate the course of circulatory disease.

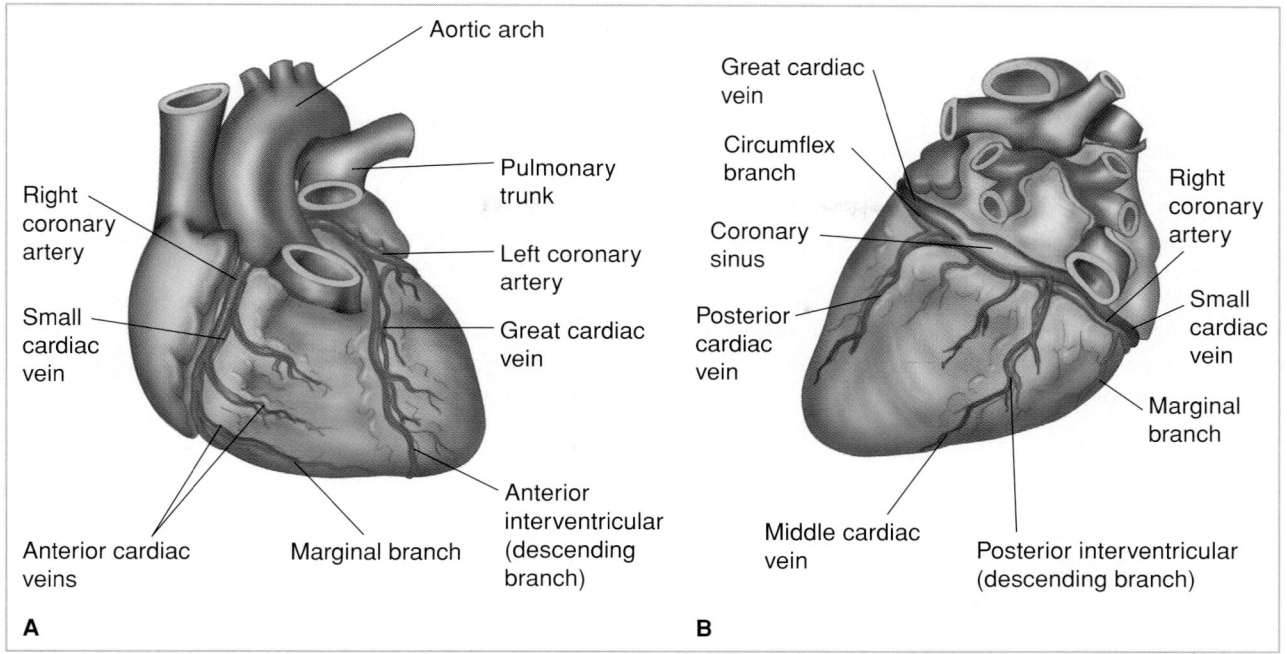

FIGURE 25-6 Coronary circulation. (A) Coronary vessels portraying the complexity and extent of the coronary circulation; (B) coronary vessels that supply the anterior surface of the heart.

node to the inferior portions of the heart. The Purkinje fibers are specialized conductive fibers located within the walls of the ventricles. They are responsible for relaying cardiac impulses to the cells of the ventricles, which allow the ventricles to contract.

The final part of the electrical system of the heart is the AV bundle or the bundle of His. The AV bundle extends from the AV node into the intraventricular septum (the wall separating the right and left ventricles), where it branches off, sending a branch to each ventricle. The Purkinje system includes the bundle of His and the peripheral fibers. These fibers end in the ventricular muscles where they cause the strong ventricular muscle contractions.

The Cardiac Cycle

The cardiac cycle includes all of the events that occur during one complete heartbeat. On the average, the heart beats about 70 times per minute, although adult heart rates can vary from 60 to 110 beats per minutes.

The cardiac cycle has three phases. Phase 1, called *atrial systole,* takes about 0.15 second. During this phase, both atria are contracted, while the ventricles are relaxed. Phase 2 is called *ventricular systole.* It takes about 0.30 second to complete. During this phase, both ventricles are contracted, while the atria are relaxed. The third phase of the cycle is called *atrial and ventricular diastole*. It is the longest phase, taking about 0.40 second to complete. During this phase, both atria and ventricles are relaxed and the pressure in the heart chambers is low. Blood returning to the heart from the superior and inferior venae cavae and the pulmonary veins fills the right and left atria and flows passively into the ventricles.

Heart Sounds

A heartbeat produces the familiar "LUB-DUP" sounds as the chambers contract and the valves close. The first heart sound, "lub," is heard when the ventricles contract and the AV valves close. This sound lasts longest and has a lower pitch. The second heart sound, "dup," is heard when the relaxation of the ventricles allows the semilunar valves to close.

In some cases, the valves may become ineffective, causing a clicking or swishing sound after the "lub." This is called a heart murmur. These "leaky" valves do not close completely and allow blood to pass back into the atria or into the ventricles.

Blood Vessels

Blood vessels, which include arteries, arterioles, veins, venules, and capillaries, are responsible for forming a closed pathway that carries blood from the heart to all the cells of the body, and then back again.

The Arteries

The arteries are the vessels that carry the blood away from the heart. There are arteries that carry oxygenated and deoxygenated blood, making it important to remember that arteries always move away from the heart (see Figure 25-8). The arteries are elastic tubes that expand when there is pressure (during the contraction of the heart) and then relax between beats. Because of this expansion and recoil, arteries are an easy place to record the rate of the heart, by palpating the pulse. Some of the most common sites for palpating an artery to obtain an accurate pulse rate include the following locations (see Figure 25-9):

- Radial—found in the lateral wrist, just proximal to the thumb
- Brachial—located in the antecubital space of the elbow, commonly used for taking blood pressures.

It can also be found between the biceps and triceps muscle in pediatric and thinner adult patients

- Carotid—located in the lateral neck; this site is most commonly used in emergency situations
- Temporal—located in the temple area
- Femoral—found in the groin
- Popliteal—located behind the knee on the posteromedial aspect
- Dorsalis pedis—found on the upper surface of the foot
- Anterior tibial—located in the ankle medial to the Achilles tendon.

Veins

The vessels that transport blood from peripheral tissues to the heart are the veins (see Figure 25-10). Veins have thin walls that contain valves that force blood to flow toward the heart and prevent blood from pooling in the lower extremities. Veins have elastic walls, similar to the arteries, but the pressure in the veins is significantly lower than in the arteries. Veins are more superficial than arteries, and are used as phlebotomy sites for obtaining blood specimens, and as sites to administer intravenous (IV) medications.

Capillaries

Capillaries are microscopic blood vessels that have single-celled walls located in the tissues (see Figure 25-11). Oxygenated blood travels through the arterioles to capillaries and on to the tissue cells, where the oxygen is deposited and waste material is picked up. The capillaries transport carbon dioxide and waste material in the blood to the small venules and on to the veins returning to the heart.

Blood Pressure

Blood pressure is defined as the measurement of the force applied to the walls of the arteries. The pressure is determined by the force and amount of blood pumped and by the size and flexibility of the arteries.

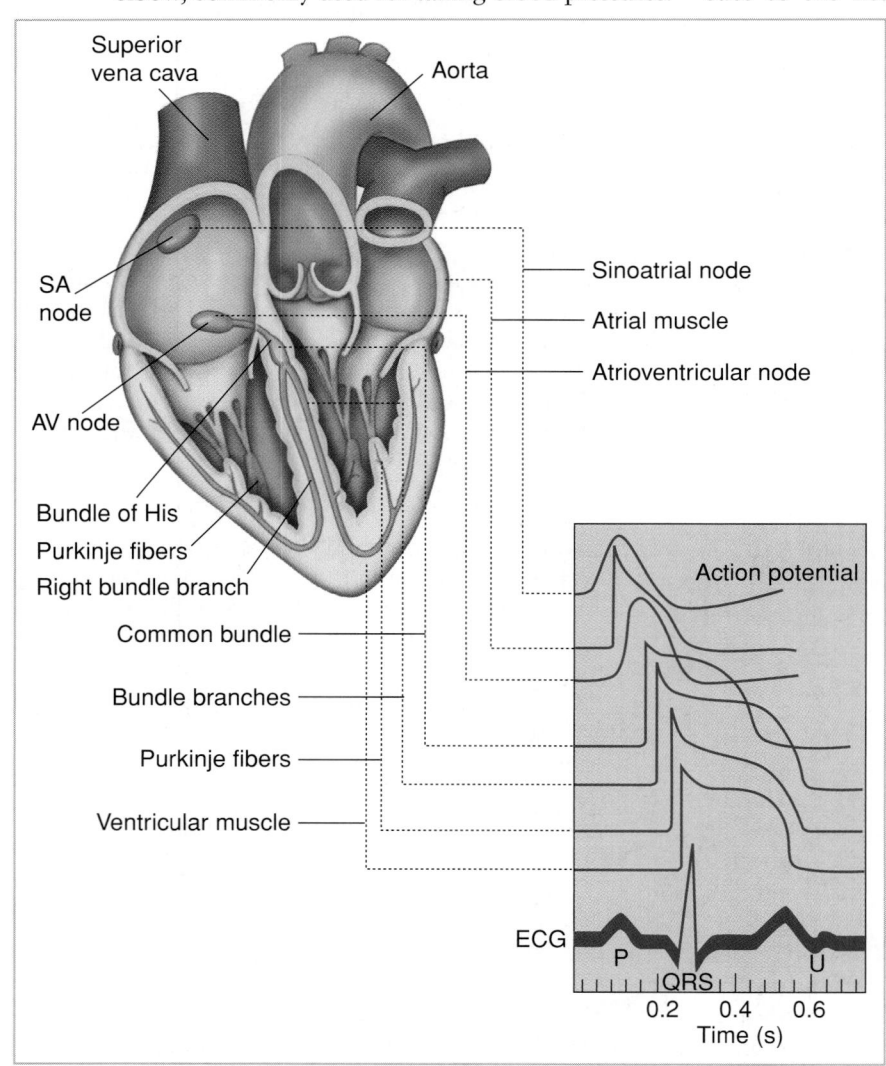

FIGURE 25-7 The conduction system of the heart. Action potentials for the SA and AV nodes, other parts of the conduction system, and the atrial and ventricular muscles are shown along with the correlation to recorded electrical activity (electrocardiogram ECG [EKG]).

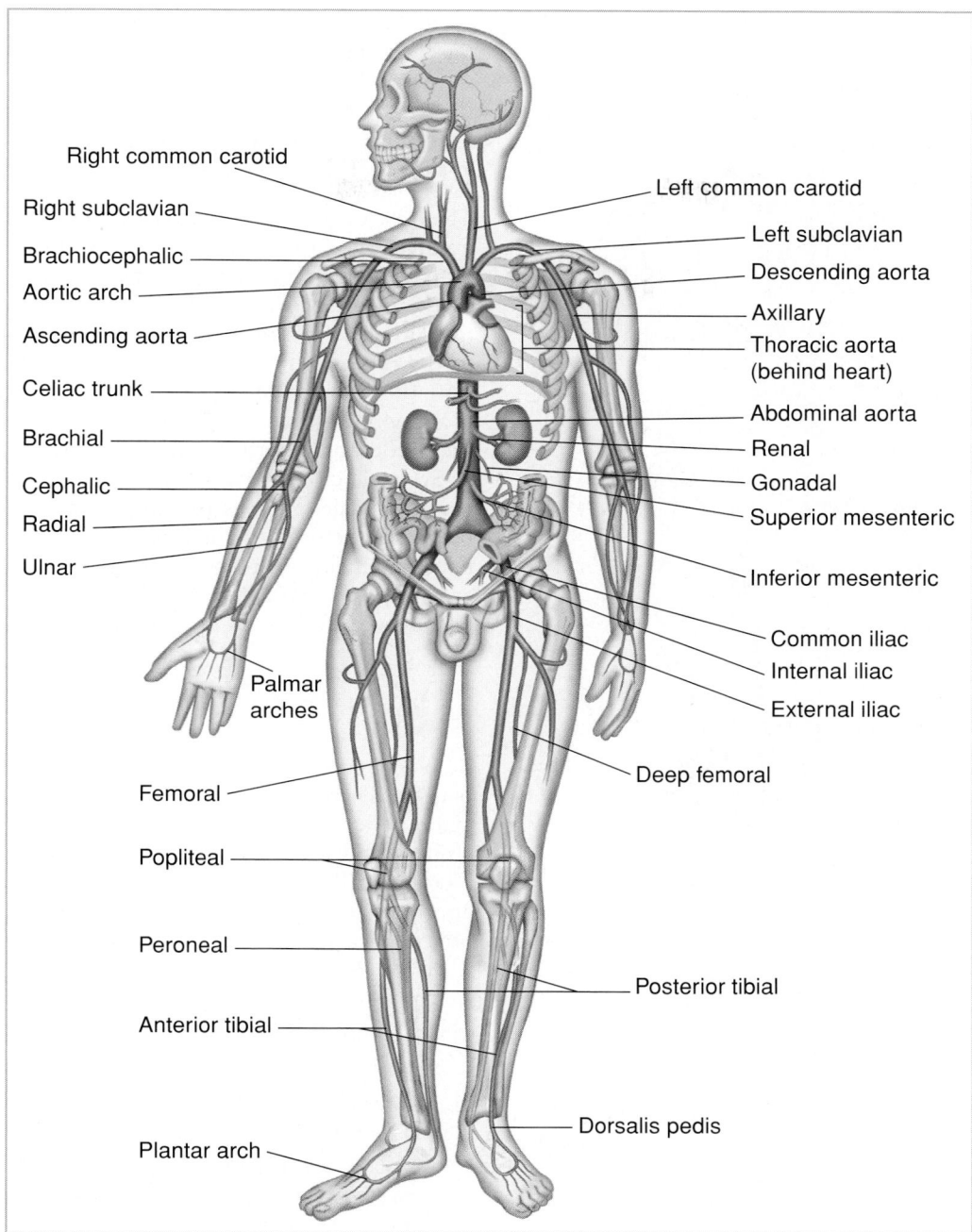

FIGURE 25-8 An overview of the arterial system.

Blood pressure is continually changing depending on activity, temperature, diet, emotional state, posture, physical condition, and medication use.

Blood pressure is usually measured in the brachial artery with a sphygmomanometer, an instrument that records changes in terms of millimeters of mercury. A blood pressure cuff connected to the sphygmomanometer is wrapped around the patient's arm, and a stethoscope is placed over the brachial artery. The blood pressure cuff is inflated until no blood flows through it; thus, no sounds can be heard through the stethoscope. The cuff pressure is then gradually lowered. *Korotkoff sounds* are the sounds heard during the measurement of blood pressure, and up to five phases or sounds may be heard. The first phase heard is when the systolic pressure is recorded. As the pressure in the cuff is lowered still more, the Korotkoff sounds change tone and loudness. When the cuff

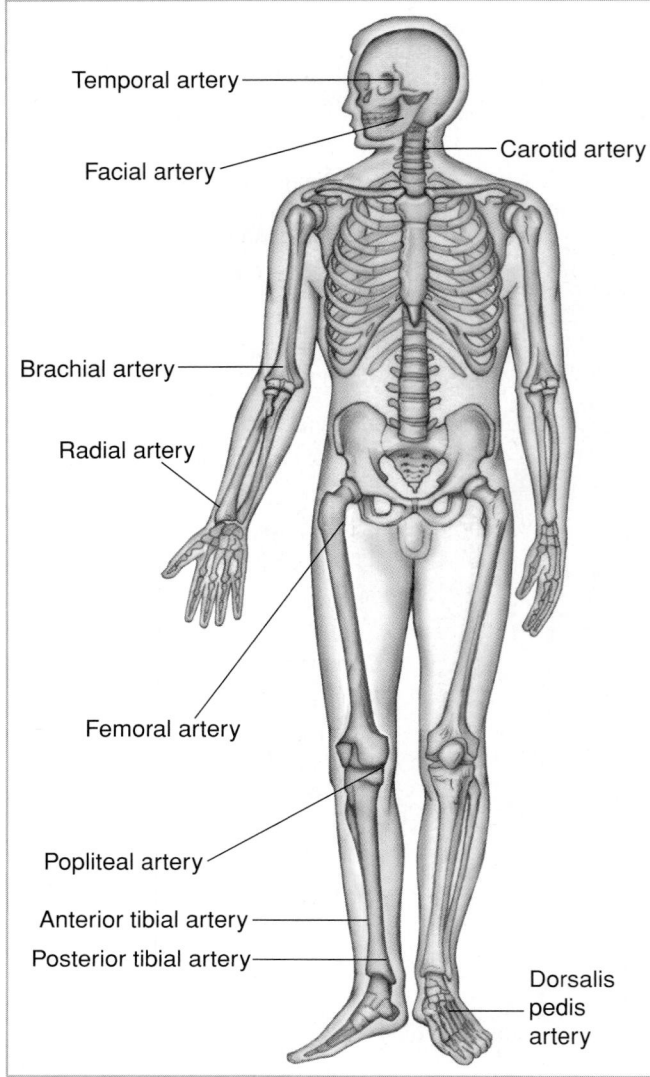

FIGURE 25-9 The primary pulse points of the body.

Temporal artery

Facial artery

Carotid artery

Brachial artery

Radial artery

Femoral artery

Popliteal artery

Anterior tibial artery

Posterior tibial artery

Dorsalis pedis artery

pressure no longer constricts the brachial artery, no sound is heard. The cuff pressure at which the Korotkoff sounds disappear is the diastolic pressure.

The average resting blood pressure for a young adult is 120/80. The higher number is the systolic blood pressure, that is, the pressure recorded in an artery when the left ventricle contracts. The lower number is the diastolic blood pressure, the pressure recorded in an artery when the left ventricle relaxes. The recorded measurement is written one above the other, with the systolic number on top and the diastolic number on the bottom. For example, a blood pressure measurement of 120/80 mmHg (millimeters of mercury) is expressed verbally as "120 over 80."

Pulse Pressure

The pulse pressure is the difference between the systolic and diastolic blood pressure. Normal pulse pressure is 30 to 50 points. The pulse pressure is an indication of the tone of the arterial walls.

Pulmonary and Systemic Circulation

The flow of the blood through the circulatory system involves the blood making its way through the pulmonary system and through the systemic circulation of the body (see Figure 25-12). Pulmonary circulation involves the route the blood takes from the heart to the lungs and back to the heart again. The function of pulmonary circulation is to oxygenate the blood while allowing for the carbon dioxide to leave the blood and enter the lungs to be exhaled.

Systemic circulation involves the route blood takes from the time it leaves the heart, travels through the body, and returns to the heart. The function of systemic circulation is to deliver oxygen and other nutrients to body cells, while carbon dioxide and waste products from the cells are picked up.

Blood

Blood is a type of connective tissue made up of cells and plasma. There are three types of blood cells; erythrocytes, which are the red blood cells, leukocytes are the white blood cells; and platelets. The fluid part of the blood is called *plasma*. While the average adult has approximately 5 liters of blood, a person's blood volume may vary depending on his or her size, the amount

Professionalism

The professional medical assistant takes pride in his or her appearance. Long hair should be tied back so there is no chance of contaminating hair with any specimens or other fluids. Jewelry should be restrained and kept at a minimum. Rings and bracelets especially should be kept at a minimum because of the issues of frequent hand washings and wearing latex gloves. Long sleeves should not hang off the arms where they could get wet with frequent hand washing or possibly touch specimens. If the clinic uniform is scrubs, the scrubs should be pressed and worn with pride. In a situation where the environment is cool, it is generally acceptable to wear a plain t-shirt underneath the scrub top for extra warmth. White lab coats should be bleached so as to remove stains.

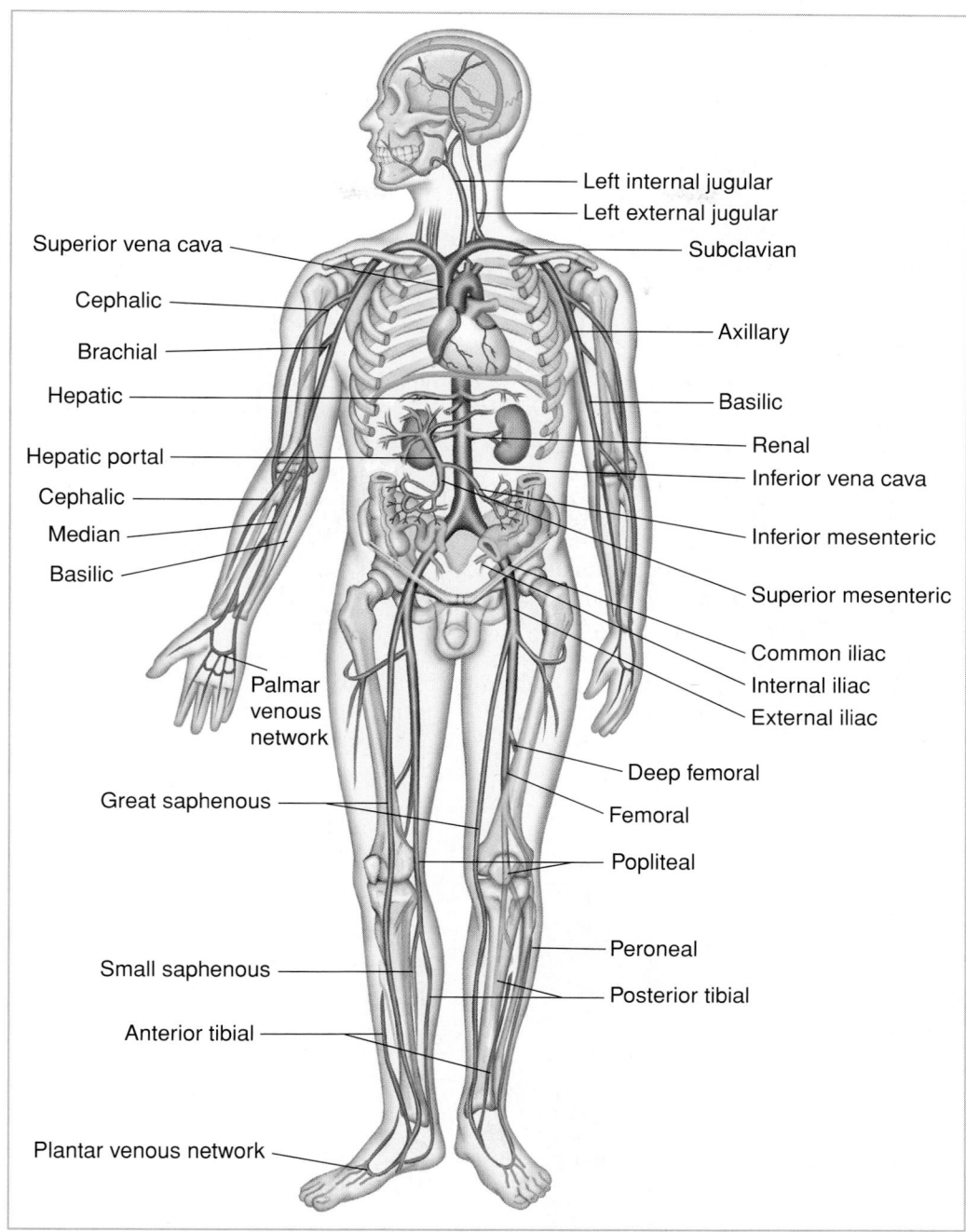

FIGURE 25-10 An overview of the venous circulation.

of adipose tissue, and hydration. The formation of blood cells (hematopoiesis) in adults primarily occurs in the bone marrow.

Composition of Blood

When a fresh blood sample is spun in a centrifuge tube, the blood separates into three layers. The lower layer in the tube is composed of red blood cells, the middle *buffy coat* layer contains the white blood cells and platelets, and the top layer is plasma. The percentage of blood attributed to red blood cells is called the *hematocrit*. Plasma contains a variety of inorganic and organic molecules dissolved or suspended in water. Plasma accounts for about 55 percent of the total volume of whole blood. Figure 25-13 shows the formed elements of blood, including erythrocytes, leukocytes (neutrophils, eosinophils, basophils, lymphocytes, and monocytes), and thrombocytes (platelets).

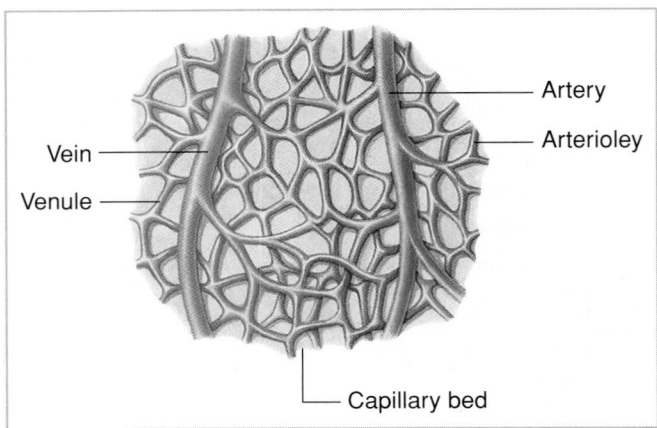

FIGURE 25-11 The capillaries.

Red Blood Cells

Red blood cells (RBCs), or erythrocytes, are produced in the red bone marrow. They are biconcave-shaped cells that are small enough to pass through capillaries. Mature red blood cells do not contain nuclei in order to make room for a red pigment called *hemoglobin*. The function of hemoglobin is to carry oxygen. A RBC count refers to the number of red blood cells in 1 cubic millimeter of blood. This count is normally between 4 million and 6.5 million red blood cells. A low RBC in-dicates a decreased ability of the red blood cell to carry oxygen, a condition referred to as anemia.

White Blood Cells

White blood cells, called leukocytes, differ from red blood cells in that they are usually larger, have a nucleus, lack hemoglobin, and are translucent unless stained. They are also not as numerous as red blood cells; there are normally only 5,000 to 11,000 per cubic millimeter of blood. White blood cells fight infection and in this way are important contributors to homeostasis.

Leukocytes are divided into two categories: *Granulocytes* have granules in their cytoplasm, are visible after staining, and include neutrophils, eosinophils, and basophils. Monocytes and lymphocytes are *agranulocytes*, which do not contain granules.

A differential white blood cell count allows the number of each of the five types of leukocytes to be measured. An increase or decrease in percentages may be indicative of infection or disease.

Blood Platelets

Platelets are fragments of cells (thrombocytes) that are found in the bloodstream. Thrombocytes control bleeding by forming a clot (coagulation) at the point of injury. A normal platelet count is between 130,000 and 360,000 platelets per cubic millimeter of blood.

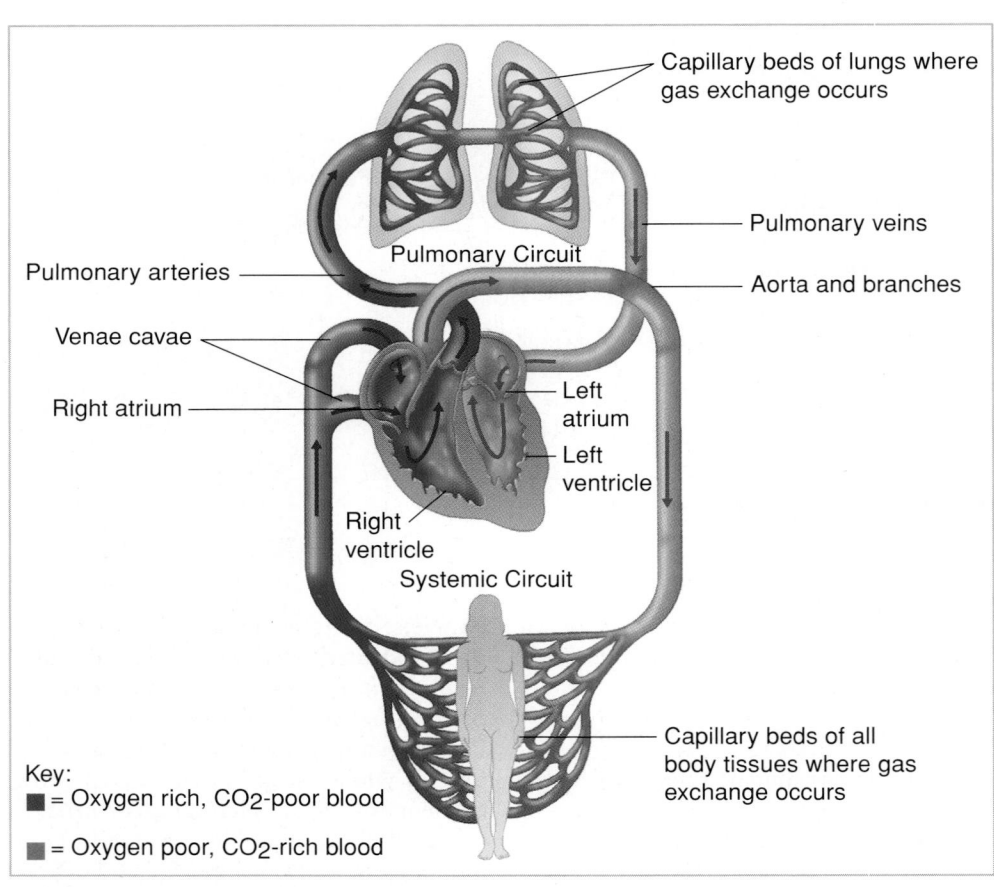

FIGURE 25-12 Systemic and pulmonary circulation.

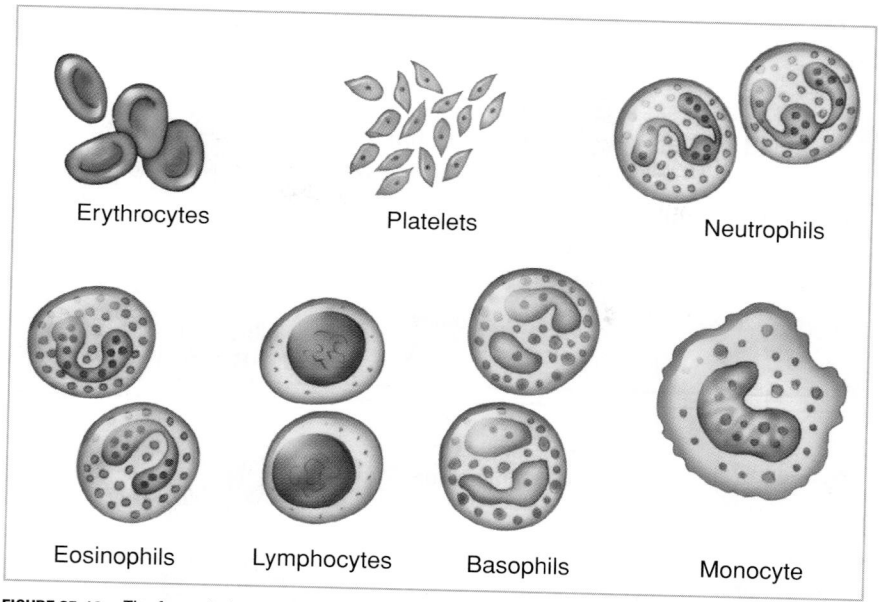

FIGURE 25-13 The formed elements of blood: erythrocytes, leukocytes (neutrophils, eosinophils, basophils, lymphocytes, and monocytes), and thrombocytes (platelets).

Blood Plasma

Plasma is the liquid portion of the blood consisting of 90 percent water. The other 10 percent is a mixture of proteins, nutrients, gases, electrolytes, fats, hormones, enzymes, and waste products. Albumin is the most abundant protein found in plasma and it functions to help maintain the fluid volume in the blood to control blood pressure. Fibrinogen, used in clot formation, and globulins, some of which are antibodies and some are molecule transporters, are the other proteins found in plasma.

Functions of Blood

Blood has three major functions: transportation, defense, and regulation.

Transportation

Blood moves from the heart to all the organs, where gas and nutrient exchange with the tissues takes place across thin capillary walls. Hemoglobin transports oxygen to the cells and picks up carbon dioxide. The blood then transports oxygen from the lungs and nutrients from the digestive tract and delivers these to the tissues. The waste material is removed from the blood and excreted by the kidneys. Various organs and tissues also secrete hormones into the blood, and the blood transports these to other organs and tissues, where they serve as signals that influence cellular metabolism.

Defense

Leukocytes defend the body against invasions by pathogens, microscopic infectious agents, such as bacteria and viruses. This is accomplished in several ways. Neutrophils and monocytes are capable of engulfing and destroying pathogens (*phagocytosis*). Lymphocytes are able to produce and secrete antibodies into the blood. Antibodies incapacitate the pathogens, making

them vulnerable to destruction. Another method of defense has to do with blood clotting. When an injury occurs, platelets form a clot, thus preventing blood loss. Coagulation involves platelets and the plasma protein fibrinogen forming a barrier to seal the wound. Without the clotting of blood, we could bleed to death even from a tiny cut.

Regulation

Blood helps to regulate body temperature by picking up heat, mostly from active muscles and then distributing it throughout the body. If the blood is too warm, the heat dissipates from dilated blood vessels in the skin, and the

Legal and Ethical Issues

When providing care and treatment to a patient with a disorder of the circulatory system, it is important for the medical assistant to be mindful of the patient's privacy. Patient privacy is a serious issue and, as such, the government has enacted HIPAA regulations that provide for patient rights and protection. In the office, when you are talking to a patient either directly or on the telephone, you must ensure that other patients cannot hear your conversation. Charts should always be turned so that no one walking by can see any personal information on them. Never leave schedules or charts in a place where nonemployees might be able to see them.

fetus generally does not suffer from these antibodies due to the length of time it takes for the mother's body to generate them, if a second Rh-positive fetus is conceived, the fetus's blood will be attacked by the antibodies almost immediately. The main reason that this occurs is because the blood cells of the baby and mother do not mix until birth. Thus, the first child is not usually affected. When this occurs, it can lead to a serious condition called erythroblastosis fetalis in which the baby is born severely anemic. The condition can be prevented by administering the drug RhoGAM to the Rh-negative mother, which will inhibit the production of antibodies against the Rh antigen.

The Lymphatic System

The lymphatic system is a subsystem of both the circulatory system and the immune system. Its primary responsibility is to defend the body from foreign invasion by disease-causing agents such as viruses, bacteria, or fungi. It consists macroscopically of the bone marrow, spleen, thymus gland, lymph nodes, tonsils, appendix, and a few other organs.

The lymphatic system, which is seen in Figure 25-15, contains a network of vessels that assists in circulating body fluids. These vessels transport excess fluids away from interstitial spaces in body tissue and return it to the bloodstream. Lymphatic vessels prevent the backflow of the lymph fluid. They have specialized organs called lymph nodes that filter out destroyed microorganisms.

The function of the lymphatic system is seen most easily at the microscopic level. Blood cells are produced in the marrow of human bone. When mature, white blood cells actively seek out possible pathogens or unknown substances, they attack directly or provide for the removal of this substance. If a white blood cell is alerted to the presence of unwanted bacteria in the blood, it will find this bacteria and surround it. After a type of white blood cell, called a T cell, has the bacteria trapped, it releases a deadly toxin that destroys the bacteria by breaking its outer membrane.

Tissue Fluid, Lymph, and Lymph Nodes

Lymph is a clear fluid that travels through the body's arteries and circulates through the tissues in order to cleanse them and keep them firm. It then drains away through the lymphatic system. Lymph nodes are the filters along the lymphatic system. Their job is to filter out and trap bacteria, viruses, cancer cells, and other unwanted substances, and to make sure they are safely eliminated from the body. Also traveling through the arteries is fresh blood, which brings oxygen and other nutrients to all parts of the body (see Figure 25-16).

After lymph enters the lymphatic vessels, which contain valves that prevent its backflow, the lymph is pushed through the vessels by the movement of skeletal muscles. If lymph is not pushed through a lymphatic vessel, a leakage can occur, causing the surrounding tissue to swell and eventually leading to a condition called *edema.*

Cultural Considerations

When working with patients of different cultures, try to obtain information about cultural habits, especially those related to diet. Oftentimes, teaching for dietary adaptations is focused on a "traditional American" diet—one that not all patients follow. Ask the patient what types of foods they eat and how those foods are prepared. Then it is easier to assist the patient in making dietary modifications to create a more healthful diet without deviating from their own cultural norms. Other modifications include exercise, and it is important to help patients find activities that are appropriate for their cultural expectations.

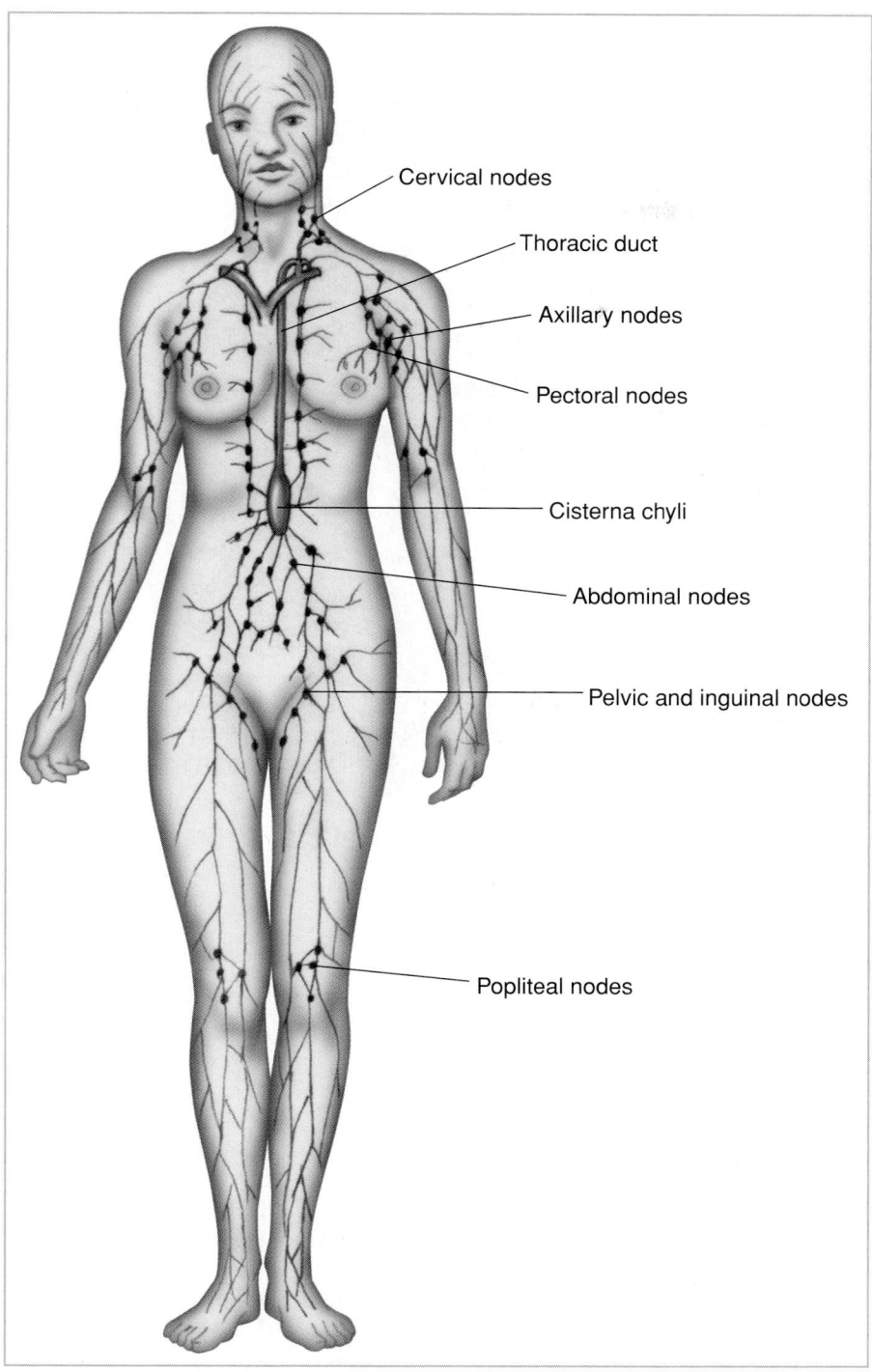

FIGURE 25-15 The lymphatic system.

Labels in figure:
Cervical nodes
Thoracic duct
Axillary nodes
Pectoral nodes
Cisterna chyli
Abdominal nodes
Pelvic and inguinal nodes
Popliteal nodes

Thymus and Spleen

The thymus, which lies just above the heart, and the spleen, located in the upper left portion of the abdominal cavity and considered the largest lymphatic organ, are both part of the lymphatic system. While the thymus carries out many of the same functions as the lymph nodes, it is also responsible for the production of lymphocytes and the hormone called thymosin, which stimulates the production of mature lymphocytes.

The spleen also plays an important part in a person's immune system and helps the body fight infection. Like the lymph nodes, the spleen contains antibody-producing lymphocytes. These antibodies weaken or kill bacteria, viruses, and other organisms that cause infection. Also, if the blood passing through the spleen carries damaged cells, white blood cells called macrophages in the spleen will destroy them and clear them from the bloodstream.

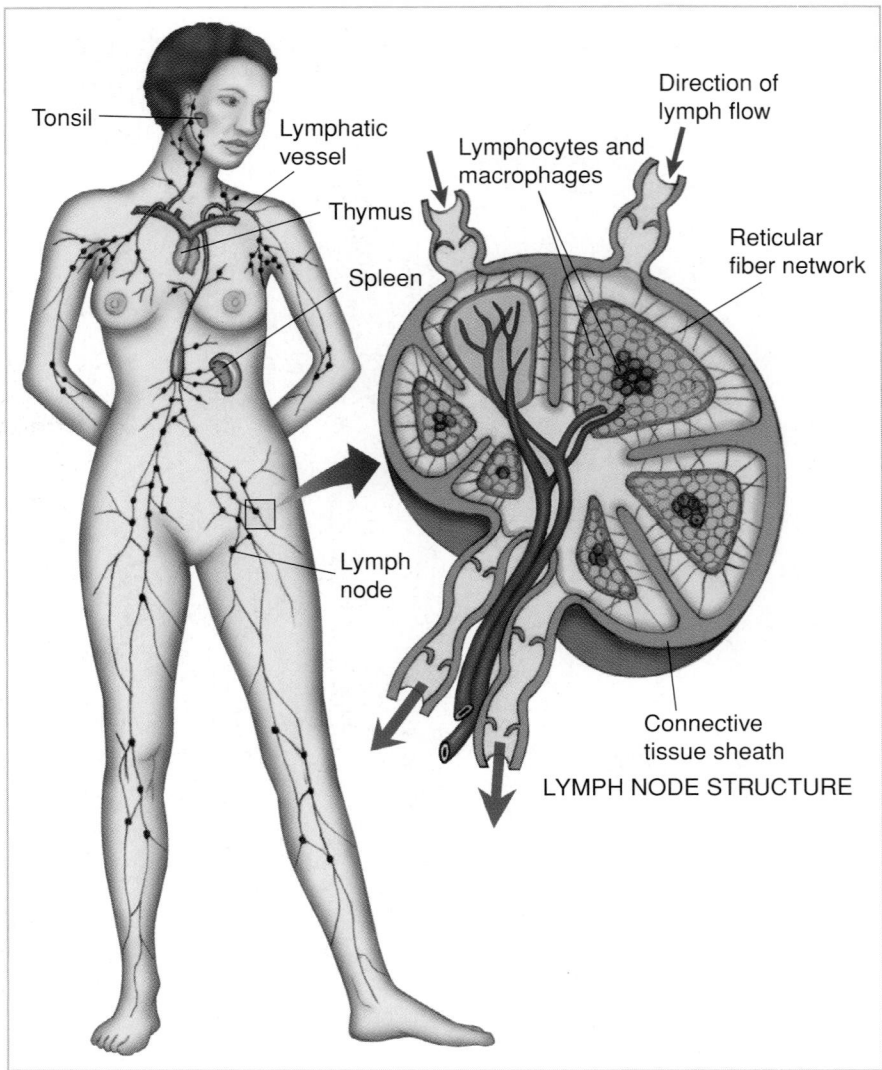

FIGURE 25-16 The tonsils, lymph nodes, thymus, spleen, and lymphatic vessels with an expanded view of a lymph node.

Common Disorders Associated with the Circulatory System

Disorders of the circulatory system are very common in the United States. Many are the result of a combination of lifestyle (lack of exercise, stress, obesity) and genetics.

Coronary Heart Disease

Coronary heart disease (CHD), also known as *coronary artery disease (CAD)*, is considered one of the most common forms of heart disease. This heart disease is due to a narrowing of the coronary arteries that supply blood to the heart. CHD is a more progressive disease that, if left untreated, can lead to a higher risk of myocardial infarction, or heart attack, and possibly sudden death.

Considered one of the leading causes of death in the United States for both men and women, according to the American Heart Association, at least two people per minute in the United States suffer from a CHD-related event, and someone dies about once a minute from cardiac events. During middle age, men have about a 40 to 49 percent risk of a cardiac event, and women have a 32 percent risk. After menopause, the risk increases for women to the same risk level as men.

CHD affects people of all races. It can be caused by lifestyle factors, including obesity, unhealthy diet choices, lack of exercise, and stress, as well as by genetic factors. High levels of lipoproteins or LDL cholesterol are associated with increased deposits on the interior of the arteries, leading to increased CHD. Total cholesterol should be below 200 mg/dL, and the HDL cholesterol (good cholesterol) should be above 35 mg/dL. Steps people can take to increase the HDL cholesterol and decrease total cholesterol include daily aerobic exercise, a dietary increase of vegetables and grain products, weight loss, and smoking cessation.

Atherosclerosis

Atherosclerosis, or narrowing of the vessel lumen of the arteries, results from a buildup of fatty material and plaque within the vessel (see Figure 25-17). It is the leading cause of CHD. As the coronary arteries become narrower and constricted, the flow of blood within the coronary arteries can slow or stop. Blood clots can form as a result of restricted blood flow. The arteries of the heart can narrow to the point that it becomes totally blocked. Plaque that breaks loose forms an embolus that can move and occlude a narrow vessel, causing death to the area supplied by that vessel.

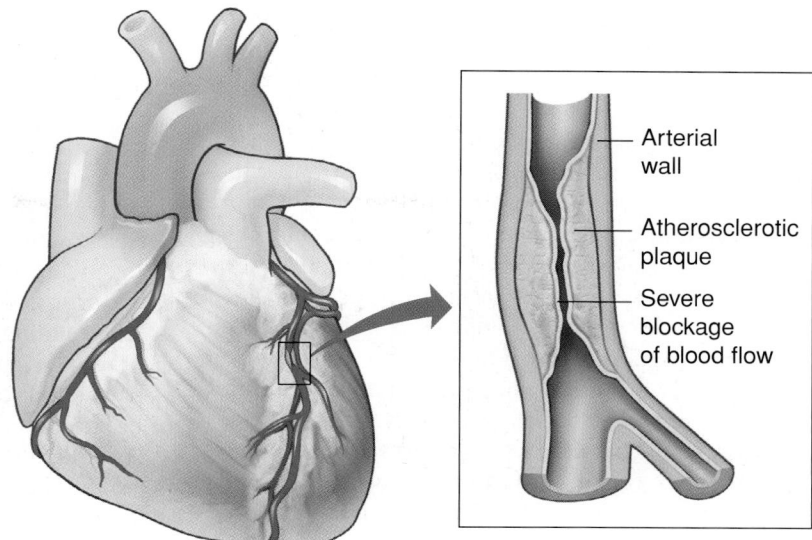

FIGURE 25-17 An atherosclerotic artery.

Small blockages may not always affect the heart's performance. When the heart needs more oxygen-rich blood than the vessels can supply, chest pain or other warning symptoms may occur. This commonly occurs during exercise or other activity. The pain that results is called angina. If the blockage is large, the anginal pain can occur with little or no activity. This pain is known as unstable angina. Sometimes, with unstable angina, the flow of blood to the heart is so limited that the person is restricted in his or her daily activities due to the chest pain. Typically, anginal pain decreases with rest and oxygen, but unrelieved angina is a common symptom of impending myocardial infarction.

Arteriosclerosis

Often referred to as "hardening of the arteries," arteriosclerosis is a term used to describe the thickening and loss of elasticity of the arteries. It is a condition that occurs over a period of many years during which the arteries of the circulatory system develop areas that become hard and brittle due to deposits of calcium on the walls. It can involve the arteries of the brain, kidneys, and upper and lower extremities.

A number of factors are causative for arteriosclerosis, including hypertension, diabetes mellitus, smoking, and obesity. Since this disease occurs within the body where it cannot be seen, it is not always recognized early or easily. There are, however, a series of signs and symptoms that should warn the individual and his or her physician. These include high blood pressure, recurrent kidney infections, and impaired circulation, particularly to the fingers and toes, due to peripheral vascular disease. Once recognized, arteriosclerosis can be treated through relieving symptoms and causes. And although several drugs for treating arteriosclerosis are on the market, it is most important to prevent its occurrence by treating the causative factors.

Heart Attack (Myocardial Infarction)

A heart attack or myocardial infarction (MI) occurs when the blood supply to a part of the myocardium is severely reduced or stopped (see Figure 25-18). The blockage is usually due to atherosclerosis, preventing blood flow in the coronary arteries. The accumulated plaque can even tear loose or rupture and trigger a blood clot that blocks the artery. This event is called a coronary thrombosis or coronary occlusion. If the blood supply is cut off, then the muscle tissues fed by that artery suffer irreversible injury and die. Depending on the extent of the injury, disability or death can result.

The most common symptom of an MI is chest pain. Angina is often described as a crushing or squeezing pain, with a feeling of fullness, heaviness, or aching in the center of the chest that may radiate down the arm or into the neck or back. Men experience chest pain as

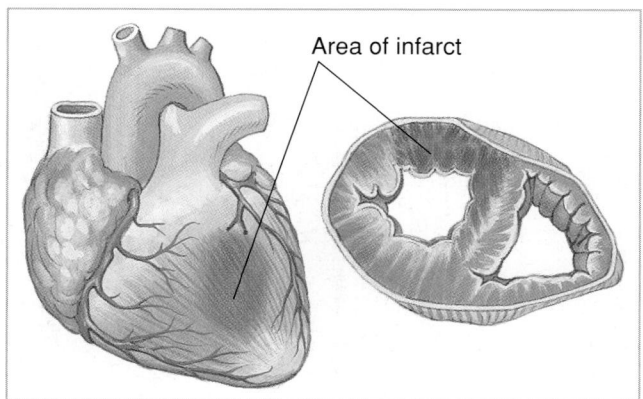

FIGURE 25-18 Cross-section of myocardial infarction.

a symptom of a MI more frequently than do women. However, women do experience the other symptoms of a MI—shortness of breath, diaphoresis, pain or discomfort in the arms, back or jaw, dizziness, fainting, nausea, and a sense of impending doom. Each person experiences their own set of symptoms with an MI—anytime any of these symptoms are present for more than 2 minutes, immediate emergency treatment must be started. Waiting to treat the symptoms increases the chances of serious disability or death.

Treatment for an MI, when sought quickly, can benefit most patients. Cardiopulmonary resuscitation (CPR) and defibrillation within the first few minutes increase the survival rate. Thrombolytics ("clot-busters") can stop some heart attacks in progress. Angioplasty, surgical vessel repair, is frequently used to reopen blocked coronary arteries, and stents are used to hold the arteries open. If more conservative measures fail, or if the heart attack is too severe, open heart surgery will be attempted to bypass the blocked artery using a vein from the leg or arm, called a coronary artery bypass graft (CABG).

The most important key for heart attack survival is immediate intervention. Patients need to be educated on the necessity of seeking medical assistance immediately when they have any symptoms of a heart attack. Delay because "it's just indigestion" only decreases the patient's chance of survival.

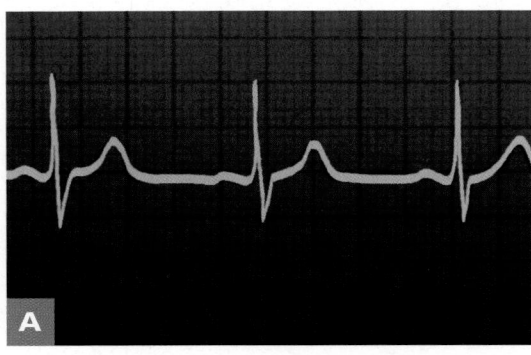

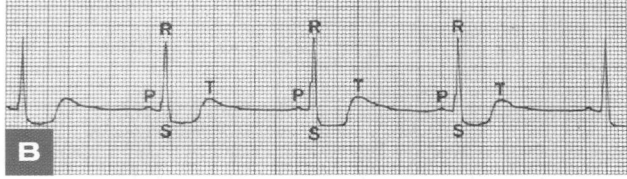

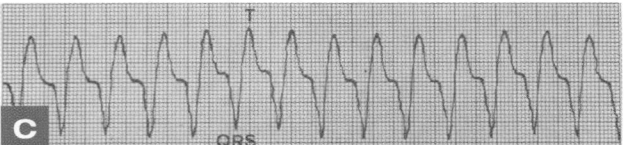

FIGURE 25-19 (A) Example of normal heart rhythm. (B) Example of sinus bradycardia. (C) Example of ventricular tachycardia.

Congestive Heart Failure

Congestive heart failure (CHF), or heart failure, is a condition in which the heart cannot pump enough blood to the body's other organs. This can result from any number of other conditions, including coronary artery disease, past heart attack, hypertension, heart valve disease due to past rheumatic fever or other causes, primary diseases of the heart muscle itself, heart defects present at birth, and any infection of the heart valves or heart muscle, such as endocarditis and myocarditis.

The "failing" heart keeps working but not as efficiently as it should. People with heart failure cannot exert themselves because they become extremely short of breath and tired.

As blood flowing out of the heart slows, blood returning to the heart through the veins backs up, causing congestion in the tissues. Often swelling, or edema, results. Most often there is edema in the legs and ankles, but it can also occur in other parts of the body, too. Sometimes fluid collects in the lungs and interferes with breathing, causing shortness of breath, which becomes more pronounced when a person is lying down. Heart failure also affects the kidneys' ability to dispose of sodium and water. The retained water increases the edema.

Congestive heart failure usually requires a treatment program consisting of rest, proper diet, modified daily activities, and medications such as angiotensin-converting enzyme (ACE) inhibitors, beta blockers, digitalis, diuretics, and vasodilators.

When a specific cause of CHF is discovered, it should be treated or, if possible, corrected. For example, some cases of congestive heart failure can be treated by treating high blood pressure. If the heart failure is caused by an abnormal heart valve, the valve can be surgically replaced.

Arrhythmia

An arrhythmia is an irregular heartbeat caused by a disturbance of normal electrical activity of the heart. There are two types of arrhythmias: tachycardias, or fast rhythms, and bradycardias, or slow heart rates. Tachycardia is an abnormally fast heartbeat of more than 100 beats per minute. The rhythm may be regular or irregular, but, if it is too fast, it may not allow the ventricles of the heart to fill properly, causing a lack of oxygen to the brain and body. Some tachycardias have such high rates that they can be fatal if not treated immediately. Bradycardia is an abnormally slow heart rate, less than 60 beats per minute, which may be regular or irregular. Figure 25-19 shows examples of normal heart rhythm and two examples of arrhythmias, sinus bradycardia and ventricular tachycardia.

While the causes of an arrhythmia may vary, both tachycardias and bradycardias produce similar symptoms, including dizziness, palpitations, shortness of breath, fatigue, weakness, angina, and fainting.

Arrhythmias can be life threatening, especially when they significantly impact the pumping function of the heart. If the oxygen supply to the brain and major organs is interrupted for more than a few minutes, death can occur. Most arrhythmias are caused by heart diseases, including CHD, heart valve disease, heart failure, or infections such as endocarditis.

Carditis (Endocarditis, Myocarditis, Pericarditis)

Carditis is an inflammation of the heart. It is more accurately referred to as endocarditis, myocarditis, or pericarditis, depending on the layer of the heart that is affected.

Endocarditis refers to an inflammation of the lining of the heart, including the heart valves. It is most commonly caused by a bacterial infection and frequently affects patients with existing abnormal conditions of their heart valves. Persons who suffer from this life-threatening condition may experience weakness, fever, diaphoresis or excessive sweating, dyspnea or difficulty breathing, and the formation of embolisms that lodge in other organs. Treatment generally consists of antibiotics given intravenously followed by the administration of oral antibiotics over a 6-week period.

When inflammation of the muscular layer of the heart occurs, the condition is referred to as *myocarditis*. Considered relatively uncommon, myocarditis is a very serious condition that, if left untreated, can also lead to death. The most common cause of myocarditis is a viral infection; however, exposure to bacteria and certain drugs, chemicals, and allergens may also lead to its development. Symptoms generally include palpitations or chest pains that closely resemble a heart attack, fever, dyspnea, general fatigue and malaise, and fainting. The person may also experience a decreased urine output. The best treatment for myocarditis includes reduction of the inflammation, bed rest, and a low-sodium diet.

When the inflammation affects the pericardium, that is, the membrane that surrounds the heart, the condition is known as *pericarditis*. It is most commonly seen as a complication of a viral or bacterial infection. Symptoms of this deadly condition frequently include sharp, stabbing chest pain, fatigue, fever, and dyspnea, especially while lying down. Treatment frequently includes analgesics, diuretics to help reduce the amount of fluid around the heart, and antibiotics to decrease the inflammation. Chronic cases of pericarditis may necessitate pericardiocentesis to remove fluid around the heart.

Thrombophlebitis

Thrombo means "clot"; *phlebitis* is the inflammation of a vein. Thrombophlebitis occurs when a blood clot causes inflammation in one or more veins, typically, those in the lower extremities (see Figure 25-20). On rare occasions, thrombophlebitis can also affect the veins in

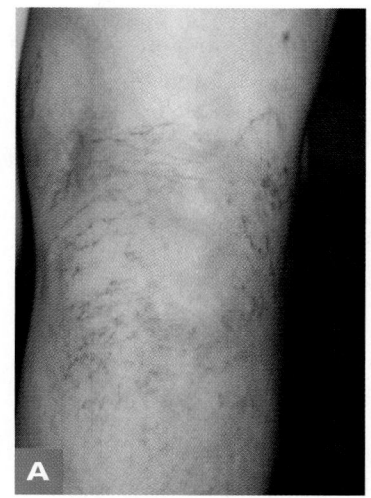

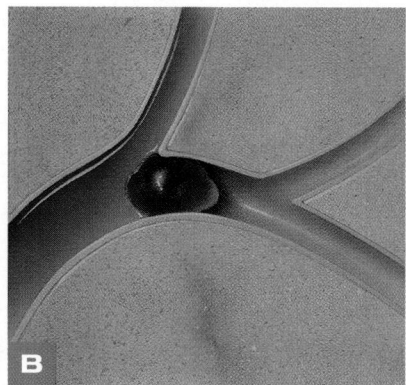

FIGURE 25-20 Example of thrombophlebitis: (A) superficial thrombophlebitis of the leg; (B) cross-section of vein where thrombophlebitis is present.

the upper extremities. The affected vein may be near the surface of the skin (superficial thrombophlebitis) or deep within a muscle (deep venous thrombosis). A clot in a deep vein increases the risk of serious health problems, including the possibility that a dislodged clot will travel to the lungs and block an artery (pulmonary embolism).

Thrombophlebitis is often caused by prolonged inactivity, such as sitting during a long period of travel in an airplane or automobile, by trauma, or from lengthy bed rest following surgery. Such inactivity decreases blood flow through the veins and may cause a clot to form. Paralysis and the use of oral contraceptives or hormone replacement therapy may also lead to thrombophlebitis. A history of varicose veins or an inherited tendency for blood clots can also place someone at higher risk for thrombophlebitis.

If thrombophlebitis occurs in a superficial vein, the physician generally recommends self-care steps that include the application of heat to the pain area, elevation of the affected limb, and the use of nonsteroidal anti-inflammatory drugs, such as aspirin. The condition usually subsides within a week or two. In more severe cases, as in deep venous thrombosis, an injection of a blood-thinning (anticoagulant) medication often prevents the clot from growing. Additional treatments may include the application of support stockings, in order to constrict the superficial veins and increase blood flow in the deep veins, and varicose vein ligation or stripping, in which the doctor surgically removes the varicose veins that causes pain or recurrent thrombophlebitis. In the most severe cases, a thrombectomy or bypass surgery may be required in order to remove an acute clot blocking a pelvic vein or an abdominal vein.

The most common signs and symptoms of thrombophlebitis include redness, swelling, warmth, tenderness, and a dull ache or pain in the affected area. When a superficial vein is affected, a red, hard and tender cord may also be present just under the surface of the skin. When a deep vein is affected, the leg may become swollen, tender, and painful, particularly when the person stands or walks.

Varicose Veins

Varicose veins are gnarled, enlarged veins. They are usually dilated and twisted, usually involving the superficial veins in the leg. These visible and bulging veins are often linked with symptoms such as tired, heavy, or aching limbs. This may be due to prolonged periods of standing, pregnancy or aging. In severe cases, varicose veins can rupture, or form open sores, called varicose ulcers, on the skin.

Varicose veins occur when the valves in the veins malfunction. As one gets older, the veins tend to lose elasticity, causing them to stretch. Blood pools in the veins, causing the veins to become engorged with deoxygenated blood.

Treatment for varicose veins falls into two categories: relief of the symptoms and ligation, or removal of the affected veins. Symptom relief includes such measures as moderate exercise, avoiding long periods of standing, elevating the legs, and wearing support stockings, which compress the veins and hold them in

Preparing for
Externship

In preparing for an externship, medical assistants should examine their wardrobes, particularly their uniforms. Expensive clothing is not necessary; however, the medical assistant should appear in professional attire, that is, uniforms or street clothes that are pressed, mended, and appear to be cared for. In any clinical environment, closed-toe shoes and socks are mandatory. Open-toed shoes or bare legs are never acceptable.

place. Cosmetic treatments may be used to decrease the size and visibility of the affected veins.

Anemia

Anemia is a condition in which there are abnormally low numbers of healthy red blood cells circulating in the body. More specifically, it is the result of low amounts of hemoglobin or abnormal hemoglobin in the red blood cells. Hemoglobin is the iron-containing pigment of the red blood cells that carries oxygen from the lungs to the tissues. Often considered the most common dysfunction of the red blood cells, it affects about 3.5 million Americans.

The three general causes of anemia are (1) decreased healthy red cell production by the bone marrow, (2) increased erythrocyte destruction, or hemolysis, and (3) blood loss from heavy menstrual periods or internal bleeding. A diet lacking in certain vitamins and minerals can also slow down the production of hemoglobin.

Some of the more common symptoms of anemia include fatigue, weakness, fainting, breathlessness, heart palpitations and tachycardia, dizziness, headache, ringing in the ears, difficulty sleeping, and trouble concentrating.

Types of Anemia

There are several types of anemia. Some forms of this condition may be inherited, while others are brought on by poor nutrition or toxins.

IRON DEFICIENCY ANEMIA The body needs iron for hemoglobin production. Low hemoglobin results in pale red blood cells with a reduced capacity to transport oxygen. In general, most people need just 1 milligram of iron daily. Menstruating or pregnant women may require iron supplements.

VITAMIN DEFICIENCY ANEMIAS Vitamin B_{12} is also essential for normal hemoglobin production. However, some people can't readily absorb B_{12}. The result is a vitamin B_{12} deficiency, or a condition known as *pernicious anemia.*

HEMOLYTIC ANEMIAS Anemia caused by the premature destruction of red blood cells is known as hemolytic anemia. In this type of anemia, antibodies produced by the immune system damage red blood cells. This condition is sometimes associated with disorders such as lupus or lymphoma. Toxic materials, such as lead, copper, and benzene, can also lead to the destruction of red blood cells.

SICKLE CELL ANEMIA Sickle cell anemia, which is characterized by a sickle-shaped red blood cell, is also known as hemoglobin S disease. This is a serious, life-threatening inherited form of anemia, and persons with the disease often suffer from pain in the joints and bones. Infections and heart failure can also occur. Sickle cell anemia occurs in about 0.6 percent of the population, and is highest among African Americans.

APLASTIC ANEMIA This is one of the deadliest and most rare forms of anemia, affecting only one to six people per million. The condition results from an unexplained failure of the bone marrow to produce certain types of blood cells. Instead, fat cells replace bone marrow.

Aplastic anemia is usually found in adolescents and young adults. Symptoms can include bleeding in the mucous membranes, infections with high fevers, pallor, and dyspnea. Injury to the bone marrow or chemicals, such as benzene and certain pesticides, can cause this type of anemia.

Treatments for Anemia

The treatment for anemia will depend on the type and cause. In some cases, injections of vitamin B_{12} may be necessary or specific medications that suppress the body's immune system may need to be eliminated. Blood transfusions, painkilling drugs, and antibiotics may also be required.

Leukemia

Leukemia is a malignant cancer of the bone marrow and blood and, like all cancers, it involves the uncontrolled growth of abnormal cells. In most cancers, these out-of-control cells form tumors, but in leukemia, the problem is with the white blood cells.

There are four major types of leukemia, and this cancer can be acute or chronic. Acute leukemias progress rapidly and cause a marked increase of cells that do not develop normally and never become functional. The leukemia cells crowd out the normal healthy blood cells, increasing the risk of anemia and infection. Patients with acute leukemia also lack platelets that help blood to clot, so they may bleed extensively. Chronic leukemias worsen gradually because the abnormal cells accumulate over time and affect other body tissues.

Leukemia is classified by the type of leukocyte affected. When it strikes the lymphoid cells, it is called lymphocytic leukemia. When it strikes the myeloid cells, it is called myeloid or myelogenous leukemia.

The symptoms of the disease are broad. These include excessive bruising, fatigue, weakness, dyspnea, bleeding of the mucous membranes, bone and joint pain, abdominal pain, weight loss, abdominal bleeding, and enlargement of the lymph nodes, spleen, and/or liver. Anemia and frequent infections are common.

Treatments for Leukemia

There are three major approaches to treating leukemia, depending on the severity and phase of the disease. These include chemotherapy to kill leukemia cells using strong anticancer drugs, radiation therapy to kill cancer cells by exposure to high-energy radiation, and bone marrow transplantation.

Aneurysm

An aneurysm is an abnormal widening or ballooning of a portion of an artery, related to weakness in the wall of the blood vessel. Some common locations for aneurysms include the aorta (major artery from the heart), brain (cerebral aneurysm), leg (popliteal artery aneurysm), and intestine (mesenteric artery aneurysm).

Aneurysms can be congenital or acquired. The cause of aneurysms is unknown; however, defects in some of the components of the artery wall may be responsible. High blood pressure and atherosclerotic disease may also contribute to the formation of certain types of aneurysms.

The symptoms of an aneurysm will vary depending on its location. Swelling with a throbbing mass at the site of an aneurysm is often seen if it occurs near the body's surface. Unfortunately, aneurysms within the body or brain often have no symptoms, and frequently go undetected until it is too late.

Surgical intervention may be indicated to repair the vessel and prevent rupturing. Some people may also be candidates for stent placement. This procedure involves the use of a tube placed inside the vessel with specialized catheters that are introduced through arteries at the groin.

Cerebrovascular Accident

A cerebrovascular accident (CVA), or stroke, occurs when the blood supply to part of the brain is suddenly interrupted by an occlusion of a blood vessel (ischemia or embolism) or a ruptured blood vessel (hemorrhage) in the brain. Brain cells die when they no longer receive oxygen and nutrients from the blood. The symptoms of a CVA include sudden numbness or weakness on one side of the body, sudden confusion or trouble speaking, sudden vision problems, severe dizziness, loss of balance or coordination, or sudden severe headaches.

Therapies to prevent a first or recurrent CVA are based on managing an individual's underlying risk factors, such as hypertension, atrial fibrillation, and diabetes. Permanent neurological damage may be avoided with prompt treatment of the underlying cause. Post-CVA rehabilitation helps individuals overcome speech, movement, and mobility disabilities resulting from damage to the affected side of the brain. Drug therapy includes the administration of antithrombotics and thrombolytics.

Hypertension

Hypertension (high blood pressure) is a term used to describe a blood pressure that is higher than 140/90. When the blood vessels can become rigid and constricted, the pressure within the vessels increases. When this force stays high for a period of time, the diagnosis of hypertension is made. Hypertension has few if any symptoms, thus is it called the "silent killer." If left untreated, hypertension can lead to kidney failure, stroke, heart attack, peripheral artery disease, and eye damage.

TABLE 25-2 **Disorders of the Cardiovascular System**

Disorder	Description
Anemia	A reduction in the number of circulating red blood cells per cubic millimeter of blood. It is not a disease but a symptom of disease.
Aneurysm	An abnormal dilation of a blood vessel, usually an artery, due to a congenital weakness or defect in the wall of the vessel.
Angina pectoris	Condition in which there is severe pain with a sensation of constriction around the heart. It is caused by a deficiency of oxygen to the heart muscle.
Angioma	Tumor, usually benign, consisting of blood vessels.
Angiospasm	Spasm of contraction of blood vessels.
Aortic aneurysm	Localized, abnormal dilation of the aorta, causing pressure on the trachea, esophagus, veins, or nerves. This is due to a weakness in the wall of the blood vessels.
Aortic insufficiency	A failure of the aortic valve to close completely, which results in leaking and inefficient heart action.
Aortic stenosis	Condition caused by a narrowing of the aorta.
Arrhythmia	An irregularity in the heartbeat or action.
Arterial embolism	Blood clot moving within an artery. This can occur as a result of arteriosclerosis.
Arteriosclerosis	Thickening, hardening, and loss of elasticity of the walls of arteries.
Atherosclerosis	This is the most common form of arteriosclerosis. It is caused by the formation of yellowish plaques of cholesterol building up on the inner walls of the arteries.
Bradycardia	An abnormally slow heart rate (under 60 beats per minute).
Congenital heart disease	Heart defects that are present at birth, such as patent ductus arteriosus, in which the opening between the pulmonary artery and the aorta fails to close at birth. This condition requires surgery.
Congestive heart failure	Pathological condition of the heart in which there is a reduced outflow of blood from the left side of the heart. This results in weakness, breathlessness, and edema.
Coronary artery disease	A narrowing of the coronary arteries that is sufficient enough to prevent adequate blood supply to the myocardium.
Coronary thrombosis	Blood clot in a coronary vessel of the heart causing the vessel to close completely or partially.
Embolus	Obstruction of a blood vessel by a blood clot that moves from another area.
Endocarditis	Inflammation of the membrane lining the heart. May be due to microorganisms or to an abnormal immunological response.
Fibrillation	Abnormal quivering or contractions of heart fibers. When this occurs within the fibers of the ventricle of the heart, arrest and death can occur. Emergency equipment to defibrillate, or convert the heart to a normal beat, will be necessary.

(continued)

TABLE 25-2 Disorders of the Cardiovascular System *(continued)*

Disorder	Description
Hypertensive heart disease	Heart disease as a result of persistently high blood pressure that damages the blood vessels and ultimately the heart.
Hypotension	A decrease in blood pressure. This can occur in shock, infection, anemia, cancer, or as death approaches.
Infarct	Area of tissue within an organ or part that undergoes necrosis (death) following the cessation of the blood supply.
Ischemia	A localized and temporary deficiency of blood supply due to an obstruction to the circulation.
Mitral stenosis	Narrowing of the opening (orifice) of the mitral valve, which causes an obstruction in the flow of blood from the atrium to the ventricle on the left side of the heart.
Mitral valve prolapse (MVP)	Common and serious condition in which the cusp of the mitral valve drops back (prolapses) into the left atrium during systole.
Murmur	A soft blowing or rasping sound heard upon auscultation of the heart.
Myocardial infarction	Condition caused by the partial or complete occlusion or closing of one or more of the coronary arteries. Symptoms include a squeezing pain or heavy pressure in the middle of the chest. A delay in treatment could result in death. This is also referred to as MI or heart attack.
Myocarditis	An inflammation of the myocardial lining of the heart resulting in an extremely weak and rapid beat, and irregular pulse.
Patent ducts arteriosus	Congenital presence of a connection between the pulmonary artery and the aorta that remains after birth. This condition is normal in the fetus.
Pericarditis	Inflammatory process or disease of the pericardium.
Phlebitis	Inflammation of a vein.
Reynaud's phenomenon	Intermittent attacks of pallor or cyanosis of the fingers and toes associated with the cold or emotional distress. There may also be numbness, pain, and burning during the attacks. It may be caused by decreased circulation due to smoking.
Rheumatic heart disease	Valvular heart disease as a result of having had rheumatic fever.
Tetralogy of Fallot	Combination of four symptoms (tetralogy), resulting in pulmonary stenosis, a septal defect, abnormal blood supply to the aorta, and the hypertrophy of the right ventricle. A congenital defect that is present at birth and needs immediate surgery to correct.
Thrombophlebitis	Inflammation and clotting of blood within a vein.
Thrombus	A blood clot.
Varicose veins	Swollen and distended veins, usually in the legs, resulting from pressure, such as occurs during a pregnancy.

Hypertension can be controlled by a variety of methods, including antihypertensive and diuretic medications, dietary changes, and exercise.

Prehypertension

A newer classification of hypertension is *prehypertension*. This diagnosis is used on individuals who are over 18 years old with a blood pressure that ranges from 120/80 to 139/89 mmHg. This diagnosis was deemed necessary for prevention and treatment of hypertension by the Joint National Committee of the National Institutes of Health National Heart, Lung, and Blood Institute (NHLBI) seventh report. According to the NIH/ NHLBI report, adults at the upper end of the prehypertension blood pressure range are twice as likely to progress to hypertension than those with lower blood pressures. The committee recommends lifestyle changes, including reducing dietary fat and sodium, increasing exercise, and limiting alcohol consumption.

Hypotension

Hypotension, or low blood pressure, is an abnormal condition in which a person's blood pressure is much lower than usual, generally below 90/60 mmHg. When blood pressure drops significantly, blood flow to the heart, brain, and other vital organs is inadequate.

Low blood pressure can also be a sign of a well-conditioned heart in those who get regular aerobic exercise, such as running. In these individuals, the myocardium is able to produce strong contractions to easily pump the blood through the body.

A sudden significant drop in blood pressure is a warning that the body is not receiving enough oxygen and is in danger of shutting down. Normal body functions like breathing, movement, and brain function can be impaired and damage can occur. Rapid drops in blood pressure that threaten life can occur due to loss of blood, shock, severe infections, or low body temperature due to cold exposure. Emergency treatment for these conditions raises blood pressure to a more normal level.

Other causes of hypotension include dehydration, heart failure, heart attack, changes in the heart's rhythm (arrhythmias), syncope (fainting), anaphylaxis, and drug overdose. Another common cause type of low blood pressure is orthostatic hypotension, which results from a sudden change in body position, usually moving from lying down to an upright position.

For more information on disorders, see Table 25-2.

SUMMARY

The circulatory system is concerned with the body's ability to circulate blood, oxygen, nutrients, and other substances. The structures that carry on these processes include the heart and the blood vessels. The heart is a pump used to move oxygen and nutrients to the body and waste and carbon dioxide back to the lungs for excretion from the body. Arteries carry blood away from the heart to the body; the exchange of oxygen and carbon dioxide and carbon dioxide and waste happens in the capillaries, then the veins carry the blood back to the heart and lungs. The lymphatic system acts as a defense system for the body, as well as a means of circulating blood, oxygen, and other fluids throughout the entire body.

Chapter Review

COMPETENCY REVIEW

1. Define and spell the terms to learn for this chapter.
2. Name the components of the circulatory system.
3. Name the three layers of the heart.
4. Name the upper chambers of the heart.
5. Name the lower chambers of the heart.
6. What role do the arteries play in circulation?
7. What role do the veins play in circulation?
8. Name the heart's pacemaker.
9. Define blood pressure.
10. Define pulse pressure.

PREPARING FOR THE CERTIFICATION EXAM

1. Another name for the mitral valve of the heart is the
   A. tricuspid
   B. pulmonary semilunar
   C. bicuspid
   D. aortic semilunar
   E. intraventricular septum

2. Blood enters the right atrium of the heart through the
   A. pulmonary artery
   B. superior and inferior venae cavae
   C. pulmonary veins
   D. descending aorta
   E. coronary artery

3. What are the two lower chambers of the heart called?
   A. superior and inferior venae cavae
   B. right and left pulmonary arteries
   C. right and left pulmonary veins
   D. right and left ventricles
   E. right and left atria

4. The inner layer of the heart is called the
   A. pericardium
   B. myocardium
   C. apex
   D. endocardium
   E. mediastinum

5. The largest artery in the body is the
   A. superior vena cava
   B. aorta
   C. pulmonary artery
   D. pulmonary vein
   E. jugular

6. The blood pressure that is considered hypertension is
   A. 90/60
   B. 120/40
   C. 120/80
   D. 130/85
   E. 160/90

7. Bradycardia means
   A. abnormally fast heartbeat
   B. abnormally slow heartbeat
   C. average heartbeat
   D. diseased heart
   E. throbbing pulse

8. The artery at the wrist where the pulse is taken is the
   A. radial artery
   B. temporal artery
   C. carotid artery
   D. facial artery
   E. femoral artery

9. What is another term for red blood cells?
   A. erythrocytes
   B. leukocytes
   C. platelets
   D. monocytes
   E. thrombocytes

10. What is a person with type AB blood often referred to as?
    A. universal donor
    B. universal recipient
    C. double antigen donor
    D. double antibody donor
    E. double antigen–antibody recipient

CRITICAL THINKING

1. What are signs and symptoms of angina?
2. Why was the patient given nitroglycerin?
3. If the patient does not get relief from his chest pain, what should he do next?

INTERNET ACTIVITY

Access one of the many "health heart" websites and see what type of education that they provide for their readers. What are some good points of the sites you access?

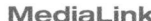 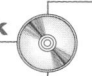 More on the Circulatory System, including interactive resources, can be found on the Student CD-Rom accompanying this textbook.

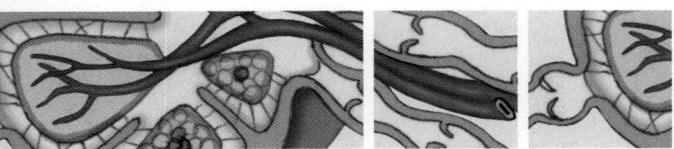

Medical Assistant Role Delineation Chart

HIGHLIGHT indicates material covered in this chapter.

ADMINISTRATIVE

Administrative Procedures

- Perform basic administrative medical assisting functions
- Schedule, coordinate and monitor appointments
- Schedule inpatient/outpatient admissions and procedures
- Understand and apply third-party guidelines
- Obtain reimbursement through accurate claims submission
- Monitor third-party reimbursement
- Understand and adhere to managed care policies and procedures
- *Negotiate managed care contracts*

Practice Finances

- Perform procedural and diagnostic coding
- Apply bookkeeping principles

- Manage accounts receivable
- *Manage accounts payable*
- *Process payroll*
- *Document and maintain accounting and banking records*
- *Develop and maintain fee schedules*
- *Manage renewals of business and professional insurance policies*
- *Manage personnel benefits and maintain records*
- *Perform marketing, financial, and strategic planning*

CLINICAL

Fundamental Principles

- Apply principles of aseptic technique and infection control
- Comply with quality assurance practices
- Screen and follow up patient test results

Diagnostic Orders

- Collect and process specimens
- Perform diagnostic tests

Patient Care

- Adhere to established patient screening procedures
- Obtain patient history and vital signs
- Prepare and maintain examination and treatment areas
- Prepare patient for examinations, procedures and treatments

- Assist with examinations, procedures and treatments
- Prepare and administer medications and immunizations
- Maintain medication and immunization records
- Recognize and respond to emergencies
- Coordinate patient care information with other health care providers
- Initiate IV and administer IV medications with appropriate training and as permitted by state law

GENERAL

Professionalism

- Display a professional manner and image
- Demonstrate initiative and responsibility
- Work as a member of the health care team
- Prioritize and perform multiple tasks
- Adapt to change
- Promote the CMA credential
- Enhance skills through continuing education
- Treat all patients with compassion and empathy
- Promote the practice through positive public relations

Communication Skills

- Recognize and respect cultural diversity
- Adapt communications to individual's ability to understand
- Use professional telephone technique

- Recognize and respond effectively to verbal, nonverbal, and written communications
- Use medical terminology appropriately
- Utilize electronic technology to receive, organize, prioritize and transmit information
- Serve as liaison

Legal Concepts

- Perform within legal and ethical boundaries
- Prepare and maintain medical records
- Document accurately
- Follow employer's established policies dealing with the health care contract
- Implement and maintain federal and state health care legislation and regulations
- Comply with established risk management and safety procedures
- Recognize professional credentialing criteria
- *Develop and maintain personnel, policy and procedure manuals*

Instruction

- Instruct individuals according to their needs
- Explain office policies and procedures
- Teach methods of health promotion and disease prevention
- Locate community resources and disseminate information
- *Develop educational materials*
- *Conduct continuing education activities*

Operational Functions

- Perform inventory of supplies and equipment
- Perform routine maintenance of administrative and clinical equipment
- Apply computer techniques to support office operations
- *Perform personnel management functions*
- *Negotiate leases and prices for equipment and supply contracts*

- *Denotes advanced skills.*

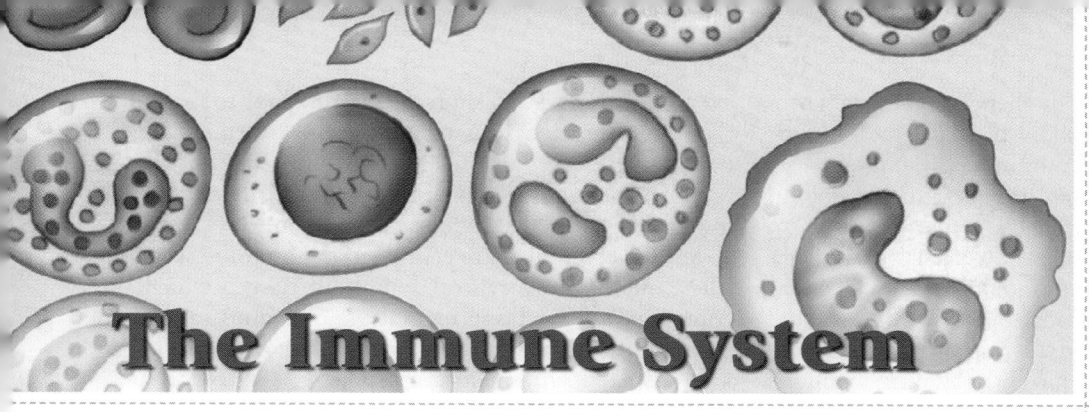

The Immune System

Learning Objectives

After completing this chapter, you should be able to:

- Explain the immune system and its response.
- Identify and discuss the anatomy of the immune system.
- Discuss the functions of the immune system.
- List and briefly discuss disorders of the immune system.

OUTLINE

Anatomy of the Immune
System   462

The Immune System
and the Body's Defense   464

Common Disorders
Associated
with the Immune
System   465

Terms to Learn

active immunity

antibodies

antigen

B lymphocytes

chemotherapy

chronic fatigue syndrome (CFS)

complement

cortex

germinal centers

immune response

immune system

infectious mononucleosis

leukocytes

lymphedema

lymphocytes

medulla

metastasis

neutrophils

oncogenes

phagocytes

radiation therapy

rheumatoid arthritis

systemic lupus erythematosus (SLC)

T lymphocytes

trabeculae

Case Study

JULIE IS A 62-YEAR-OLD FEMALE SEEN BY THE PHYSICIAN. She has been suffering from what appears to be a multitude of individual problems, including low blood pressure, cold and flu-like symptoms, extreme fatigue, and what she describes as "hot" and "cold flashes." Upon a thorough physical exam, which includes a complete blood cell count and an evaluation of her entire treatment history, Julie is diagnosed with CFS. As part of her care, Julie's doctor has informed her that she must take an active role in her treatment. This includes getting plenty of rest and monitoring her for any additional viral infections.

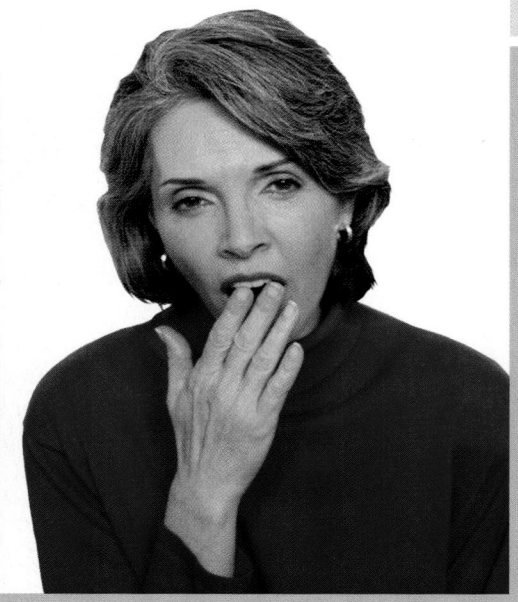

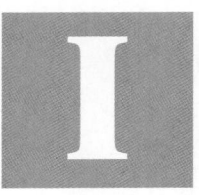

Inside the body there is an amazing protection mechanism called the immune system. The immune system consists of the tissues, organs, and physiological processes used by the body to identify abnormal cells, foreign substances, and foreign tissues, such as transplants, and defend against those substances that might be harmful to the body. It is a protective mechanism designed to defend the body against invaders. Those invaders can be bacteria, microbes, viruses, toxins, and parasites. To understand the power of the immune system, all one has to do is look at what happens to a living being once it dies. When a person dies, the immune system shuts down. In a matter of hours, the body is invaded by all sorts of bacteria, microbes, and parasites. None of these things are able to enter when the immune system is working properly; how-

ever, once this system shuts down, the door to many of the invading microorganisms is wide open. Once a person is deceased, it only takes a short time for these organisms to completely dismantle the body and carry it away, until all that is left is a skeleton.

Several structures are central to the immune system. These include the central lymphoid tissue, which is comprised of the bone marrow and thymus, and the peripheral lymphoid tissue, consisting of the lymph nodes, spleen, and mucosa-associated lymphoid tissue.

Anatomy of the Immune System

The immune system operates throughout the body. There are, however, certain sites where the cells of the immune system are organized into specific structures. These are classified as central lymphoid tissue and peripheral lymphoid tissue. All of these structures are also part of the lymphatic system (see Figure 26-1), which is a subsystem of the circulatory system. The primary responsibility of the lymphatic system is to defend the body from foreign invasion by disease-causing agents such as viruses, bacteria, or fungi. The lymphatic system consists macroscopically of the bone marrow, spleen, thymus gland, lymph nodes, tonsils, appendix, and a few other organs.

Central Lymphoid Tissue

The central lymphoid tissue consists of the bone marrow and the thymus. The bone marrow contains stem cells that create all the cells in the immune system. The bone marrow is also the origin of the red blood cells, the white blood cells, and the platelets. During a procedure called hematopoiesis, the bone marrow–derived cells either become mature cells of the immune system or precursors of cells that will mature in a place other than the bone marrow. The bone marrow produces B cells, natural killer cells, granulocyte and red blood cells, and platelets.

The thymus gland is located posterior to the sternum, in the anterior mediastinum. It enlarges during childhood, but begins to shrink again after maturity. It continues to function even though the size is small throughout life. It is arranged into an outer cortex and an internal medulla. Immature lymphoid cells enter the cortex and reproduce and mature, then move to the medulla where they reenter the circulation. The thymus manufactures infection fighting T cells and helps distinguish normal T cells from those that attack the body's own tissues.

Peripheral Lymphatic System

The peripheral lymphatic system consists of the lymph nodes, spleen, and other lymphoid tissue. (refer back to Figure 25-18 in the previous chapter). The lymphatic system is also composed of lymphatic capillaries, lymphatic vessels, and lymphatic ducts.

Lymph Nodes

Lymph nodes can take on many different sizes and shapes, but most are bean shaped and are about 1 inch in length. The node is covered thickly with a fibrous capsule and is subdivided into different compartments by inward-pointing trabeculae. As with many organs, the lymph node has two basic parts, the cortex and the medulla. The cortex is populated mainly with lymphocytes. The germinal centers are the primary resting place for B-cell lymphocytes, which are the cells responsible for production of circulating antibodies. In the event of an infecting antigen, these B lymphocytes will rapidly undergo mitosis and divide. Each unique kind of B cell produces only one type of antibody. Thus, by dividing, they can produce large quantities of a specific antibody to seek out and help destroy the antigen. The rest of the cortex contains T lymphocytes, that is, cells that circulate through the lymph nodes, bloodstream, and lymphatic ducts to seek out any infection. The medulla of the lymph nodes is primarily made up of macrophages attached to reticular fibers.

Lymph nodes have two functions. First, the phagocytic cells act as filters for particulate matter and microorganisms. The phagocytic cells are also called macrophages, and are one type of B cell. These cells destroy the invading cells.

The second function of lymph nodes has to do with the development of antigens. The antigens act as "invaders" to inhibit such substances as bacteria, viruses, or other toxic substances that may have breached the other protective mechanisms of the body, possibly causing infection or inflammation.

Spleen

Located in the upper left quadrant of the abdomen, the spleen is responsible for receiving blood from an artery off of the aorta. After passing through an intricate meshwork of tiny blood vessels, the blood continues to the liver. The blood vessels of the spleen are surrounded by nests of B lymphocytes, mainly of the memory type. As the blood slowly moves through the spleen, it is monitored by T cells for any non–self-invaders. If some suspicious cell or molecule is detected, it is presented to the B cells for a match to an appropriate memory B cell. Once a matching B cell is activated, the cell divides rapidly and begins producing antibodies directed against the invading antigen.

The spleen blood vessels are also lined with macrophages, which swallow and digest debris in the blood such as worn-out red blood cells and platelets. In a disease such as mononucleosis, the macrophages in the spleen become overactive and trap a higher number of

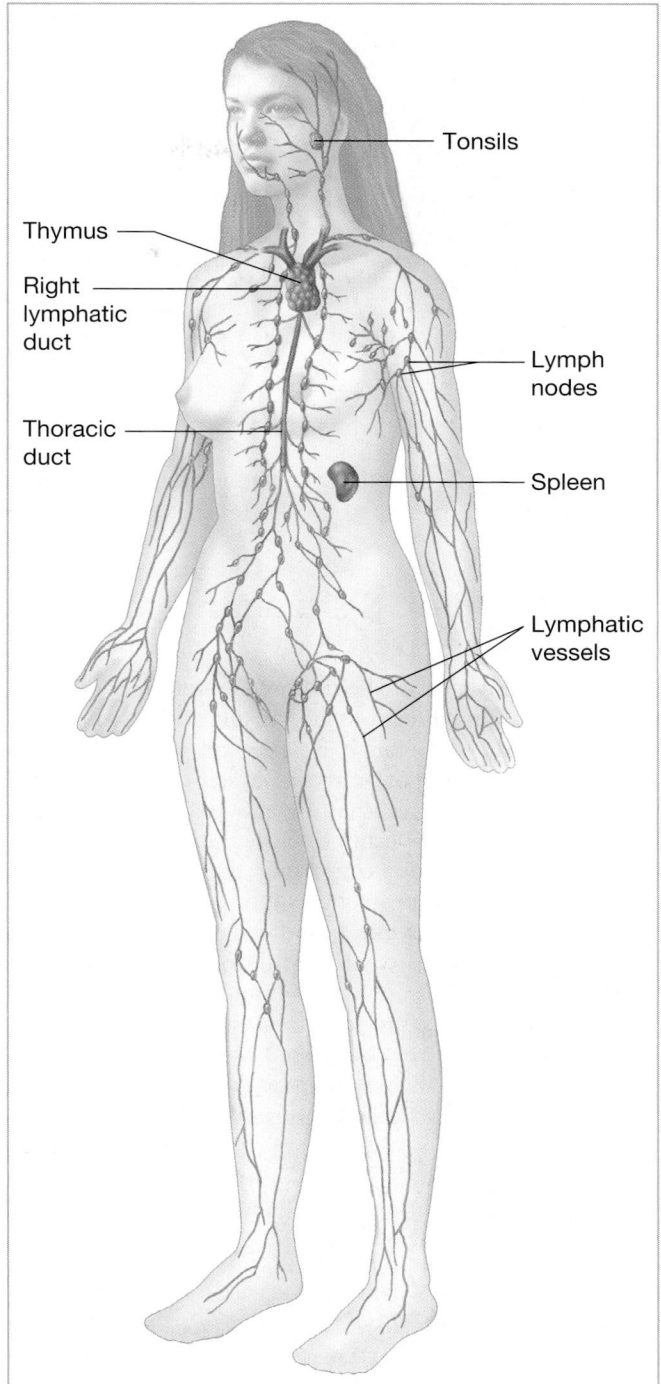

FIGURE 26-1 Components of the lymphatic system.

white blood cells. In the process, the spleen becomes swollen and may even rupture.

Tonsils

The tonsils are located in the depressions of the mucous membranes of the face and the pharynx (see Figure 26-2). There are three sets: the palatine, the pharyngeal, and the lingual. The function of the tonsils

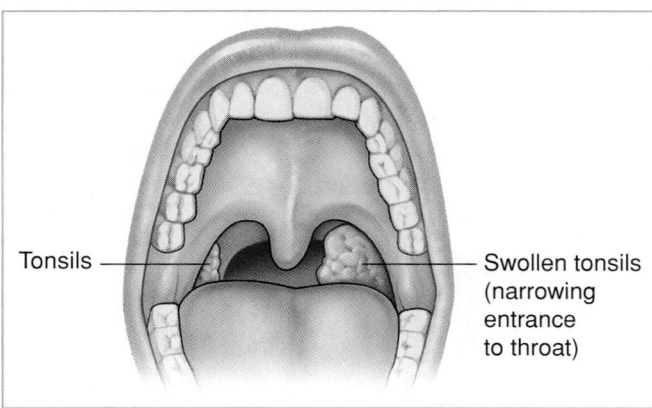

FIGURE 26-2 Tonsils—normal and enlarged.

is to filter bacteria and aid in the formation of white blood cells.

The Immune System and the Body's Defense

As previously noted, the immune system is the body's defense against infectious organisms and other pathogenic invaders. Through a series of steps called the immune response, the immune system attacks organisms and substances that invade body systems and cause disease. This occurs because the network of cells, tissues, and organs comprising the immune system works together to protect the body.

Leukocytes, or white blood cells (WBCs), combine to seek out and destroy harmful organisms. There are two types of WBCs: phagocytes and lymphocytes. The phagocytes attack the invading organism. A number of different cells are considered phagocytes; however, the most common are neutrophils, which primarily fight off bacteria. Lymphocytes allow the body to re-

Professionalism

As a medical assistant, you work under the license of the physician. You are a team member with the physician, but still subordinate to physicians and their levels of education. Always address physicians by their title and name, for example, "Dr. Morales." Even if the physician has invited you to call him or her by their first name, never do so in front of a patient. This can undermine the doctor–patient relationship. Physicians refer to each other as Doctor "so-and-so" when talking to their patients, and the staff should take their cue from the physician. They have earned the right to be called "Dr." and the medical assistant should honor that right.

member and recognize previous invading organisms. There are two kinds of lymphocytes: B lymphocytes and the T lymphocytes. Lymphocytes start out in the bone marrow and either stay there and mature into B cells, or they leave for the thymus gland, where they mature into T cells. B lymphocytes and T lymphocytes have separate responsibilities within the immune system. The B lymphocytes seek out the invading organisms and send defenses to attach onto them; the T cells destroy the organisms that the B lymphocytes identified.

How Immunity Works: Antigens versus Antibodies

When a foreign substance invades the body, it is called an antigen. When an antigen is detected, several types of cells work together to recognize and respond to it. These cells trigger the B lymphocytes to produce antibodies. This occurs through a process known as *humoral immunity*. Antibodies are specialized proteins that lock onto specific antigens. Immunoglobulins are glycoproteins that function as antibodies. The terms *antibody* and *immunoglobulin* are often used interchangeably. They are found in the blood and tissue fluids, as well as many secretions. Structurally they are globulins, which means they are synthesized and secreted by plasma cells that are derived from the B cells of the immune system. B cells are activated upon binding to their specific antigen and differentiate into plasma cells. In some cases the interaction of the B cell with a T cell is also necessary.

Once the B lymphocytes have produced antibodies, they continue to exist in a person's body. That means if the same antigen is presented to the immune system again, the antibodies are already there. That is why if a person becomes ill with a specific disease, such as chickenpox, that person typically will not get sick from it again. This is also why we use immunizations to prevent getting certain diseases. Immunizations, which are also called vaccinations, help protect a person from a specific disease. When an individual is given an immunization, that person is also receiving a vaccine that contains fragments of a disease organism or small amounts of a weakened disease organism. The vaccine causes the person's immune system to develop antibodies that can subsequently recognize and attack the organism if he or she is exposed to it. Sometimes an immunization does not completely prevent the disease, but it will significantly reduce its severity. More information on immunizations will be covered in Chapter 49.

Although antibodies can recognize an antigen and lock onto it, they are not capable of destroying it without help. That is the job of the T cells. The T cells are part of the system that destroys antigens that have been tagged by antibodies or cells that have been infected or somehow changed. T cells are also involved in assisting other cells, such as phagocytes. Antibodies can also neutralize toxins produced by different organisms. Finally, antibodies can activate a group of proteins called complement that are also part of the immune system. Complement assists in destroying bacteria, viruses, or infected cells. All of these specialized cells and parts of the immune system offer the body protection against disease. This protection is called *immunity*. There are three types of immunity: innate, active, and passive.

Innate Immunity

Everyone is born with innate, or natural, immunity. Because of that fact, many of the viruses and bacteria that affect other species are not capable of harming human beings. For example, the viruses that cause leukemia in cats or distemper in dogs do not affect humans. The way in which innate immunity works to protect humans against illnesses that affects other species also works to protect nonhumans against human diseases. For example, the HIV/AIDS virus is not capable of making cats or dogs sick. Innate immunity also includes the external barriers of the body, including the skin and mucous membranes that line the nose, throat, and gastrointestinal tract, all of which are the body's first line of defense in preventing diseases from entering it. If this outer defensive wall is broken, such as when a person cuts himself or herself, the skin attempts to heal the break quickly, and special immune cells on the skin attack invading microorganisms.

Active Immunity

The introduction of immunity by infection or with a vaccine is called active immunity. Active immunity is permanent, meaning that the individual is protected from the disease all of his or her life. Acquired active immunity occurs when the person is exposed to a live pathogen, develops the disease, and becomes immune as a result of the primary immune response. Artificially acquired active immunity can be induced by a vaccine, a substance that contains the antigen. A vaccine stimulates a primary response against the antigen without causing symptoms of the disease.

Passive Immunity

Passive immunity is "borrowed" from another source and only lasts for a short time. For example, antibodies in a mother's breast milk provide an infant with temporary immunity to diseases to which the mother has been exposed. This can help protect the infant against infection during the early years of childhood.

It is important to remember that everyone's immune system is different. Some people never seem to get infections, whereas others seem to be sick all the time. As a person gets older, he or she usually becomes immune to more germs as the immune system comes into contact with more and more of them. That's why adults and teens tend to get fewer colds than children; their bodies have learned to recognize and immediately attack many of the viruses that cause colds.

Common Disorders Associated with the Immune System

Immune system disorders occur when the immune response is inappropriate, excessive, or lacking. And lack of one or more components of the immune system can result in any number of immunodeficiency disorders. Disorders may be inherited, acquired through infection or other illness, or produced as an inadvertent side effect of certain drug treatments. (See Table 26-1).

Allergies

Allergies are disorders of the immune system. Most allergic reactions are a result of an immune system that responds to a "false alarm." When a harmless substance such as dust, mold, or pollen is encountered by a person who is allergic to that substance, the immune system may react dramatically, by producing antibodies that "attack" the allergen (substances that produce allergic reactions). The result of an allergen entering a susceptible person's body may include wheezing, itching, runny nose, watery or itchy eyes, and other symptoms.

Cultural Considerations

Because some diseases of the immune system appear to have psychological implications associated with them, many cultures also see them as disorders that can be avoided. In fact, some physicians view some of these disorders, such as chronic fatigue syndrome, as more "psychosomatic" than physical. Providing emotional support and knowledge of resources may help patients with these illnesses to rebuild a support system and a new community for themselves. The most important help the medical assistant can give these individuals is the feeling that they can be self-sufficient and that they are not alone in the world, even though the medical assistant must be certain to maintain a professional relationship with the patient.

TABLE 26-1   Disorders of the Lymphatic System

Disorder	Description
Acquired immune deficiency syndrome (AIDS)	A disease that involves a defect in the cell-mediated immunity system. A syndrome of opportunistic infections occurs in the final stages of infection with the human immunodeficiency virus (HIV). This virus attacks T4 lymphocytes and destroys them, which reduces the person's ability to fight infection.
AIDS-related complex (ARC)	A complex of symptoms that appears in the early stages of AIDS. This is a positive test for the virus but only mild symptoms of weight loss, fatigue, skin rash, and anorexia.
Elephantiasis	Inflammation, obstruction, and destruction of the lymph vessels, which results in enlarged tissues due to edema.
Epstein-Barr virus	Virus believed to be the cause of infections mononucleosis.
Hodgkin's disease	Lymphatic system disease that can result in solid tumors in any lymphoid tissue.
Lymphadenitis	Inflammation of the lymph glands. Referred to as swollen glands.
Lymphangioma	A benign mass of lymphatic vessels.
Lymphoma	Malignant tumor of the lymph nodes and tissue.
Lymphosarcoma	Malignant disease of the lymphatic tissue.
Mononucleosis	Acute infections disease with a large number of atypical lymphocytes. Caused by the Epstein-Barr virus. There may be abnormal liver function and spleen enlargement.
Multiple sclerosis	Autoimmune disorder of the central nervous system in which the myelin sheath of nerves is attacked.
Non-Hodgkin's lymphoma	Malignant, solid tumors of lymphoid tissue.
Peritonsillar abscess	Infection of the tissues between the tonsils and the pharynx. Also called quinsy sore throat.
Sarcoidosis	Inflammatory disease of the lymph system in which lesions may appear in the liver, skin, lungs, lymph nodes, spleen, eyes, and small bones of the hands and feet.
Splenomegaly	Enlargement of the spleen.
Systemic lupus erythematosus (SLE)	A chronic autoimmune disorder of connective tissue that causes injury to the skin, joints, kidneys, mucous membranes, and nervous system.
Thymoma	Malignant tumor of the thymus gland.

Allergies are rarely cured, but many medications, supplements, and treatment options are available to help relieve allergy symptoms. The best way to treat an allergic reaction is for a person to stay away from the offending allergen. If that is not possible, treatment may include the use of antihistamines or decongestants to help combat allergy symptoms. Other forms of treatment for some types of airborne allergens may include the use of air filters and dehumidifiers. There are also various ways to cope with allergic symptoms other than traditional medical treatment and medications. Those methods often include the use of acupressure and chiropractic treatments. In severe cases, treatment may only be identified through specific allergy testing and desensitization. See Chapter 35, for more information on allergies.

Cancer

Cancer is actually a group of many related diseases that all have to do with cells. Cells are the very small units that make up all living things, including the human body. Each person's body has billions of cells. Cancer cells are not normal; instead, they grow and spread very fast. Normal body cells grow and, through mitosis, divide and know to stop growing. Over time, they also die. Unlike these normal cells, cancer cells just continue to grow and divide out of control and do not die.

Cancer cells usually group or clump together to form tumors. A growing tumor becomes a lump of cancer cells that can destroy the normal cells around the tumor and damage the body's healthy tissues. Sometimes the cancer cells break away from the original tumor and travel to other areas of the body, where they keep growing and can go on to form new tumors. That occurs through a process known as metastasis.

Causes and Treatment of Cancer

While the causes of cancer are relatively unknown, there are certain risk factors that may make predisposed person to cancer. These include the presence of a suppressed immune system, radiation, tobacco, and some viruses.

Cancer may be treated with surgery, chemotherapy, radiation, or sometimes a combination of all of these treatments. The choice of treatment generally depends on the type of cancer someone has and the stage of the tumor, meaning how much and to where, if at all, the cancer has spread within the body. Surgery is the oldest form of treatment for cancer. Three out of every five people with cancer may require surgery to remove the cancer. During surgery some healthy cells or tissue may also be removed to make sure that all the cancer is removed.

Chemotherapy involves the use of anticancer drugs to treat the cancerous growth or tumor. These medicines are sometimes taken as a pill, but are usually given intravenously. Chemotherapy is usually given over a number of weeks to months. Often, a permanent IV catheter is placed under the skin into a larger blood vessel of the upper chest. This way, a person can easily get several courses of chemotherapy and other medicines through this catheter without having a new IV needle inserted. The catheter remains under the skin until the cancer treatment is completed. Radiation therapy may also be used to treat cancer. It uses high-energy waves, such as x-rays, to damage and destroy the cancer cells. This form of treatment may cause tumors to shrink and, in some cases, disappear completely. Radiation therapy is one of the most common treatments for cancer.

Cancer and the Immune System

When the immune system is at its peak, it recognizes, attacks, and destroys the cancerous cells before potentially deadly growth and multiplication of the cancer

can occur. However, when not destroyed immediately by the immune system, the new cancer cells avoid the usual controls on growth and multiplication in normal cells. The growth begins when the genes controlling cell growth and multiplication, called oncogenes, are transformed by cancer-causing agents, called carcinogens, into cancer cells.

Normal cells can undergo a malignant change to become cancer-infested cells. These small groups of abnormal cancer cells divide more rapidly than the normal surrounding cells. The fast multiplication results in invasion and destruction of normal body cells.

Cancerous cells act as uncontrollable parasites, consuming needed nutrients while contributing nothing except malnutrition. If not killed and removed, these cancerous cells can then metastasize via the bloodstream and lymphatic system to other parts of the body from their original site and potentially be fatal if they cause organs to fail.

The immune response is critical to beating or controlling cancer because cancerous tumors develop and multiply when the white immune cells fail to recognize, respond, and kill the cancerous cell invaders. If not at its peak, the immune response often fails to respond in a timely manner when overwhelmed due to the massive number of corrupted cancer cells that have multiplied rapidly when undetected and unchecked. When the immune response is in peak condition, it is better able to recognize the cancerous cells quickly and respond to kill the health invaders rapidly in most instances. A suppressed or impaired immune response exposes a body to both development and spread (metastasis) of too-often deadly cancer cells in the body.

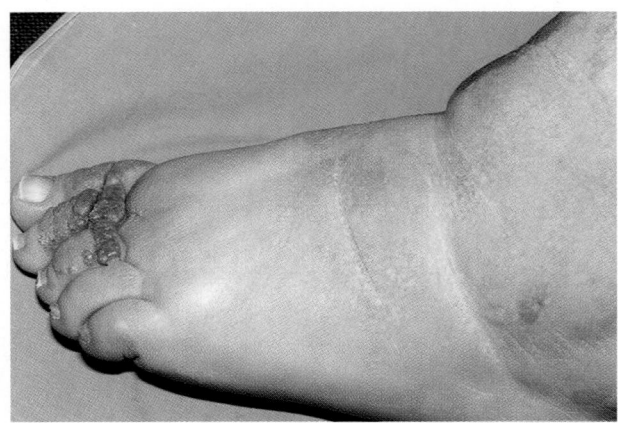

FIGURE 26-3 Chronic lymphedema.

Chronic Fatigue Syndrome

While there is no known single cause of chronic fatigue syndrome (CFS), some authorities believe it is a condition shared by many different underlying diseases rather than an entity unto itself. Others believe it is caused by a defect of the immune system. Hormonal deficits, low blood pressure, and viral infections have been studied as possible causes or contributors. There has also been some correlation between chronic single or multiple viral infections, but CFS has also been identified in the absence of any apparent viral infection. Food allergies are commonly associated with this disorder, as is candidiasis, intestinal parasites, and toxic chemical exposure.

The goal in any treatment regimen for CFS generally begins with the patient undergoing a thorough evaluation of his or her prior treatment history. And the treatment plan must also take into consideration the patient's ability to optimize sleep quality and quantity. Educating the patient with emphasis on becoming an active participant of his or her own treatment is extremely important in the treatment of CFS.

Infectious Mononucleosis

Infectious mononucleosis is a viral infection caused by the Epstein-Barr virus (EBV), which is part of the herpes family of diseases. It is characterized by an increase of white blood cells that are mononuclear, that is, containing a single nucleus. For that reason, this disease is frequently referred to as "mono." Because it often develops in young adults between the ages of 15 and 24 and is frequently spread through saliva, mono is also commonly referred to as the "kissing disease." The illness is less severe in young children and the incubation period for mono is generally between 4 and 8 weeks. Symptoms include fever, fatigue, sore throat, and swollen lymph glands. There is usually no treatment for this disorder except getting plenty of rest, gargling with saltwater or using throat lozenges to soothe a sore throat, taking aspirin or acetaminophen to reduce fever and relieve a sore throat and headache. If left untreated, mono can lead to liver inflammation or hepatitis and enlargement of the spleen; recovery from mono generally occurs within several weeks. However, for some people, it may take as long as several months before they regain their normal energy levels.

Lymphedema

Lymphedema is a condition that occurs from a damaged or dysfunctional lymphatic system (see Figure 26-3). There are two different types of lymphedema. The first, called primary lymphedema, can be hereditary. Each stage of the disease is called by a different name. It is known as Milroy's disease or syndrome when it expresses itself at birth or in the very early years. Meige lymphedema, also known as lymphedema praecox, generally begins sometime during puberty. Lymphedema tarda begins in or around middle age. Lymphedema that has not expressed itself as an active condition is referred to as latent lymphedema. Primary lymphedema can also be congenital. Secondary lymphedema is generally caused by an obstruction, or damage to, or injury to the lymph system that leads to an interruption of the normal lymphatic flow.

Causes of congenital primary lymphedema can be a developmental disorder of the lymphatics, *in utero* infection, injury, or delivery difficulties. The causes of secondary lymphedema are multiple. Infections from insect bites, serious wounds, or burns can cause lymphedema when they damage or destroy lymphatics as can any type of serious injury. Radiation for cancer treatments is also a cause. Outside the tropics the number one cause of secondary lymphedema is the removal of lymph nodes for cancer biopsies. Through improved techniques of small-needle biopsies, radiological diagnostic improvements, and site-specific node biopsies, there has been a marked decrease in secondary lymphedema.

The preferred treatment for lymphedema is decongestive therapy. The forms of therapy are complete decongestive therapy (CDT) or manual decongestive therapy (MDT). CDT is used primarily in the treatment of lymphedema and venous insufficiency edema. It is a combination of MDT, bandaging exercises, and skin care. CDT may also involve breathing exercises, compressive garments, and dietary measures. A frequent indication for CDT is lymphedema caused by irradiation or surgery due to cancer. It can relieve edema, fibrosis and the accompanying pain and discomfort. Other treatments include the use of compression pumps, surgery, and newer approaches such as the use of lasers, liposuction, and even acupuncture.

Rheumatoid Arthritis

Rheumatoid arthritis is a chronic disease that causes great suffering, reduced quality of life, major financial outlays, and loss of income due to functional impairment and the prospect of invalidity. One person out of every 100 suffers from chronic rheumatoid arthritis. It is a condition that occurs when the body's immune defenses attack tissue in the joints, leading to pain and degeneration of the articular cartilage. The disease or its treatment also increases mortality, and patients with rheumatoid arthritis often have a shorter life expectancy than their healthy peers. Drugs used to limit the symptoms have a limited effect and do not improve the long-term prognosis.

The treatment of rheumatoid arthritis is based on medical treatment and providing the patient with advice about how to facilitate daily activities. While preventive treatment of persons who may be genetically exposed to the disease is currently not an issue, persons with a family history of rheumatoid arthritis are four times more at risk of developing the disease than others. It is also important to note that treating the symptoms is only part of the regime for the rheumatoid arthritis patient. Maintenance of articular, or joint, function is equally important.

Systemic Lupus Erythematosus

Systemic lupus erythematosus or SLE is one of a group of illnesses called autoimmune diseases. One of the ways in which the immune system works is by producing antibodies that allow the cells of the immune system to destroy the invading organisms such as viruses and bacteria. Sometimes, the immune system starts to make antibodies that stick to the body's own cells. These antibodies are called *autoantibodies* and when they stick to the body's own cells they can cause an inflammatory reaction, which results in damage to the cells. This is what occurs with SLE. Patients suffering from SLE produce abnormal antibodies in their blood that target tissues within their own body rather than foreign infectious agents. SLE is called a "systemic" disorder because its effects can show in many parts of

the body, that is, it is systemwide. *Lupus* refers to a type of skin rash and *erythematosus* means "red." SLE can produce many different symptoms and can imitate many other diseases. Many patients with SLE have pain and swelling in the joints. They may also suffer from general fatigue, fever, chills, and headache.

About one-fifth of SLE patients have round (discoid) lesions that are raised and scaly. This condition is known as discoid lupus erythematosus. If left untreated, these lesions grow and can cause severe scarring.

A condition that may be present with lupus is vasculitis, or inflamed blood vessels. The inflammation may cause red marks in any area of the body. Sometimes deep red lumps appear, especially on the leg, where they may develop into ulcers. In some people, reddish-purple lesions appear on the tips of the fingers and toes.

Ninety percent of patients with SLE are women and it is more common before menopause. There is a genetic component to SLE because there is a higher risk of developing SLE if a close family member also has it.

Unfortunately, there is no cure for most autoimmune diseases and SLE is no different. Treatment is usually aimed at reducing the immune response using drugs such as steroids. It is important to note that SLE is a chronic, lifelong condition that is characterized by periods of remission and relapse. The course in any individual is difficult to predict but with immediate treatment, most patients have a normal life span.

Patient Education

Patients who take medication for a chronic or other disease must be educated that they need to be extremely compliant when taking their medications. They need to take all of the medications exactly as prescribed, every day, without exception. This requires dedication on the part of the patient. If the patient is not compliant with the regimen, the medications may not be effective in treating the disease and a relapse may occur.

SUMMARY

The immune system is the body's defense against infectious organisms and other pathogenic invaders, keeping the body healthy. There are three types of immunity: innate, active, and passive. Immune system disorders occur when the immune response is inappropriate, excessive, or lacking. Disorders may be inherited, acquired through infection or other illness, or produced as an inadvertent side effect of certain drug treatments.

Chapter Review

COMPETENCY REVIEW

1. Define and spell the terms to learn for this chapter.
2. What is the function of leukocytes?
3. What is the most common type of leukocyte?
4. What is the main function of the immune system?
5. Name the three accessory organs of the lymphatic system.
6. What is the difference between innate immunity and active immunity?
7. What does the central lymphoid tissue include?
8. What does the peripheral lymphoid tissue include?
9. What is the spleen responsible for?
10. What role do phagocytes perform?

PREPARING FOR THE CERTIFICATION EXAM

1. What structures are responsible for allowing the body to remember and recognize previous invaders?
   A. neutrophils
   B. lymphocytes
   C. phagocytes
   D. antigens
   E. antibodies

2. Accessory lymph organs include
   A. pharynx, larynx, trachea, and bronchi
   B. liver, gallbladder, and pancreas
   C. tonsils, spleen, and thymus gland
   D. lymphatic duct, thoracic duct, and lymph nodes
   E. ureters, urethra, and kidneys.

3. Humoral immunity refers to
   A. the binding of an antigen with an antibody
   B. the production of plasma lymphocytes or B cells
   C. the production of lymphocytes or T cells
   D. a severe reaction to an antigen
   E. a hypersensitivity to an allergen

4. An autoimmune viral disease characterized by an increase of white blood cells is
   A. allergies
   B. Epstein-Barr virus
   C. lymphedema
   D. rheumatoid arthritis
   E. Infectious mononucleosis

5. Which organ has a secondary purpose of the destruction of red blood cells?
   A. thymus
   B. bone marrow
   C. spleen
   D. tonsils
   E. liver

6. What condition of the immune system creates autoantibodies that stick to the body's own cells, causing an inflammatory reaction that eventually causes damage to the cells?
   A. chronic fatigue syndrome
   B. systemic lupus erythematosus
   C. cancer
   D. lymphedema
   E. infectious mononucleosis

continued on next page

7. What disorder do some authorities believe is a condition shared by many different underlying diseases, rather than an entity onto itself?
   A. cancer
   B. chronic fatigue syndrome
   C. rheumatoid arthritis
   D. SLE
   E. lymphedema

8. What disorder can produce all sorts of symptoms and can initiate many other diseases?
   A. cancer
   B. systemic lupus erythematosis
   C. CFS
   D. Infectious mononucleosis
   E. lymphedema

9. What organ manufactures infection-fighting T cells and helps distinguish normal T cells from those that attack the body's own tissues?
   A. spleen
   B. thyroid
   C. thymus
   D. pancreas
   E. large intestine

10. When expressing itself at birth or in the very early years, lymphedema is known as
   A. Milroy's disease
   B. Meige lymphedema
   C. lymphedema praecox
   D. lymphedema tarda
   E. latent lymphedema

CRITICAL THINKING

1. Why was it important to note that Julie was having many cold and flu-like symptoms?

2. Why did the physician order a complete blood cell count?

3. Why did the physician tell Julie to get plenty of rest and decide to monitor her for any other viral infections?

INTERNET ACTIVITY

Do an Internet search for chronic fatigue syndrome services in your hometown. What resources are available in your area?

 MediaLink   More on the immune system, including interactive resources, can be found on the Student CD-Rom accompanying this textbook.

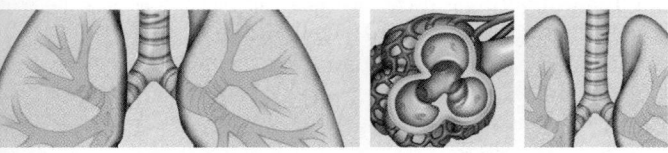

Medical Assistant Role Delineation Chart

HIGHLIGHT indicates material covered in this chapter.

ADMINISTRATIVE

Administrative Procedures

- Perform basic administrative medical assisting functions
- Schedule, coordinate and monitor appointments
- Schedule inpatient/outpatient admissions and procedures
- Understand and apply third-party guidelines
- Obtain reimbursement through accurate claims submission
- Monitor third-party reimbursement
- Understand and adhere to managed care policies and procedures
- *Negotiate managed care contracts*

Practice Finances

- Perform procedural and diagnostic coding
- Apply bookkeeping principles

- Manage accounts receivable
- *Manage accounts payable*
- *Process payroll*
- *Document and maintain accounting and banking records*
- *Develop and maintain fee schedules*
- *Manage renewals of business and professional insurance policies*
- *Manage personnel benefits and maintain records*
- *Perform marketing, financial, and strategic planning*

CLINICAL

Fundamental Principles

- Apply principles of aseptic technique and infection control
- Comply with quality assurance practices
- Screen and follow up patient test results

Diagnostic Orders

- Collect and process specimens
- Perform diagnostic tests

Patient Care

- Adhere to established patient screening procedures
- Obtain patient history and vital signs
- Prepare and maintain examination and treatment areas
- Prepare patient for examinations, procedures and treatments

- Assist with examinations, procedures and treatments
- Prepare and administer medications and immunizations
- Maintain medication and immunization records
- Recognize and respond to emergencies
- Coordinate patient care information with other health care providers
- Initiate IV and administer IV medications with appropriate training and as permitted by state law

GENERAL

Professionalism

- Display a professional manner and image
- Demonstrate initiative and responsibility
- Work as a member of the health care team
- Prioritize and perform multiple tasks
- Adapt to change
- Promote the CMA credential
- Enhance skills through continuing education
- Treat all patients with compassion and empathy
- Promote the practice through positive public relations

Communication Skills

- Recognize and respect cultural diversity
- Adapt communications to individual's ability to understand
- Use professional telephone technique

- Recognize and respond effectively to verbal, nonverbal, and written communications
- Use medical terminology appropriately
- Utilize electronic technology to receive, organize, prioritize and transmit information
- Serve as liaison

Legal Concepts

- Perform within legal and ethical boundaries
- Prepare and maintain medical records
- Document accurately
- Follow employer's established policies dealing with the health care contract
- Implement and maintain federal and state health care legislation and regulations
- Comply with established risk management and safety procedures
- Recognize professional credentialing criteria
- *Develop and maintain personnel, policy and procedure manuals*

Instruction

- Instruct individuals according to their needs
- Explain office policies and procedures
- Teach methods of health promotion and disease prevention
- Locate community resources and disseminate information
- *Develop educational materials*
- *Conduct continuing education activities*

Operational Functions

- Perform inventory of supplies and equipment
- Perform routine maintenance of administrative and clinical equipment
- Apply computer techniques to support office operations
- *Perform personnel management functions*
- *Negotiate leases and prices for equipment and supply contracts*

- *Denotes advanced skills.*

SOURCE: Reprinted by permission of the American Association of Medical Assistants from the AAMA Role Delineation Study: Occupational Analysis of the Medical Assisting Profession.

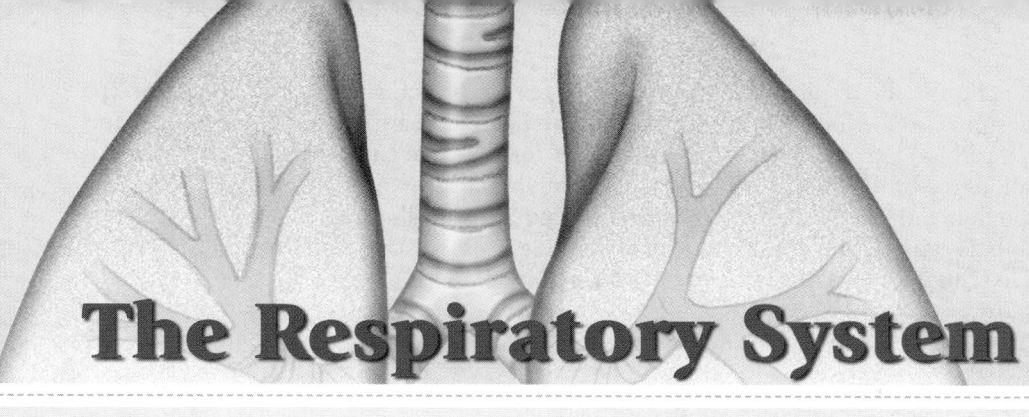

The Respiratory System

Learning Objectives

After completing this chapter, you should be able to:

- Define and spell the terms to learn for this chapter.
- Explain the purpose and function of the respiratory system.
- List and explain the structures and functions of the organs of the respiratory system.
- Explain the different respiratory volumes and capacities.
- Identify and discuss common disorders associated with the respiratory system.

OUTLINE

Organs of the Respiratory System   474

Mechanism of Breathing   478

Respiratory Volumes and Capacities   479

Common Disorders Associated with the Respiratory System   480

Terms to Learn

asthma

atmospheric pressure

bronchitis

chronic obstructive pulmonary disease (COPD)

cilia

common cold

cyanosis

cystic fibrosis (CF)

emphysema

hay fever

hemoptysis

influenza

Legionnaire's disease

lung cancer

pleurisy

pneumonia

pulmonary edema

pulmonary embolism (PE)

severe acute respiratory syndrome (SARS)

sinusitis

tuberculosis (TB)

Case Study

JOE F. IS A 65-YEAR-OLD MALE being seen in your clinic for minor shortness of breath. Upon taking his medical history, it is learned that he has a distant history of "some asthma" and has been a two-pack-a-day smoker for 40 years. He has recently been coughing up greenish-tinted sputum. He denies any exposure to tuberculosis or other infectious diseases. Sputum cultures, chest x-rays, and pulmonary function tests indicate a bacterial infection, no masses or infiltrates in the lungs, and decreased forced expiratory volumes and a low FEV_1/FEC ratio. The physician diagnoses COPD with an overlying bacterial bronchial infection. The patient is started on Levaquin, 500 mg a day, as an antibiotic; albuterol, two puffs every 4 hours or as needed; Tessalon for his cough; and guaifenesin, 600 mg twice a day. In 2 weeks, the patient reports back, stating he feels better, is breathing much better, and rarely coughs. He is beginning to cut back on his tobacco usage.

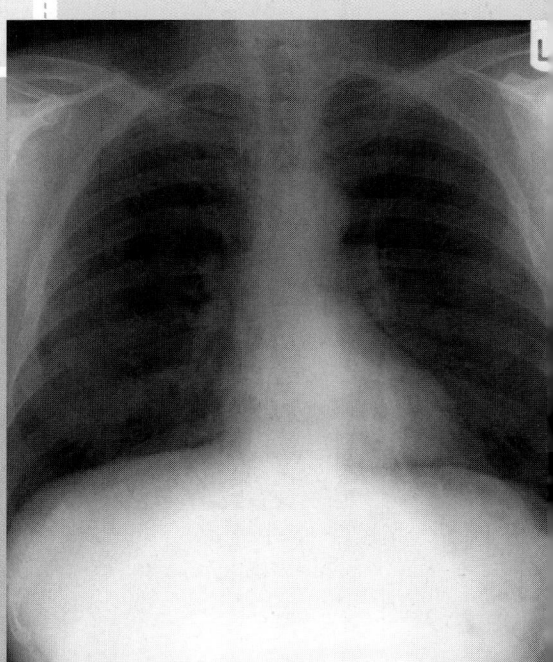

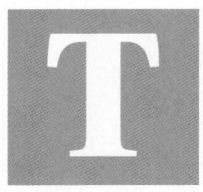he primary function of the respiratory system is to supply the blood with oxygen so the blood can deliver oxygen to all parts of the body. It does this through breathing. When we breathe, we inhale oxygen and exhale carbon dioxide. This exchange of gases is the respiratory system's means of getting oxygen to the blood.

Respiration is achieved through the mouth, nose, trachea, lungs, and diaphragm. Oxygen enters the respiratory system through the mouth and the nose. The oxygen then passes through the larynx (where speech sounds are produced) and the trachea, which is a tube that enters the chest cavity. In the chest cavity, the trachea splits into two smaller tubes called the bronchi. Each bronchus then divides again, forming the bronchial tubes. The bronchial tubes lead directly into the lungs where they divide into many smaller tubes, which connect to tiny sacs called alveoli. The average adult's lungs contain about 600 million of these spongy, air-filled sacs that are surrounded by capillaries. The alveoli are the final branchings of the respiratory tree and perform gas exchange for the lungs. The inhaled oxygen passes into the alveoli and then diffuses through the capillaries into the arterial blood. Meanwhile, the waste-rich blood from the veins releases its carbon dioxide into the alveoli. The carbon dioxide follows the same path out of the lungs when you exhale.

The diaphragm's job is to help pump the carbon dioxide out of the lungs and pull the oxygen into the lungs. The diaphragm is a sheet of muscles that lie across the bottom of the chest cavity.

Organs of the Respiratory System

The organs of the respiratory system extend from the nose to the lungs and are divided into the upper and lower respiratory tracts (see Figure 27-1). The upper respiratory tract consists of the nose and the pharynx, or throat. The lower respiratory tract includes the larynx, or voice box; the trachea, or windpipe, which splits into two main branches called bronchi;

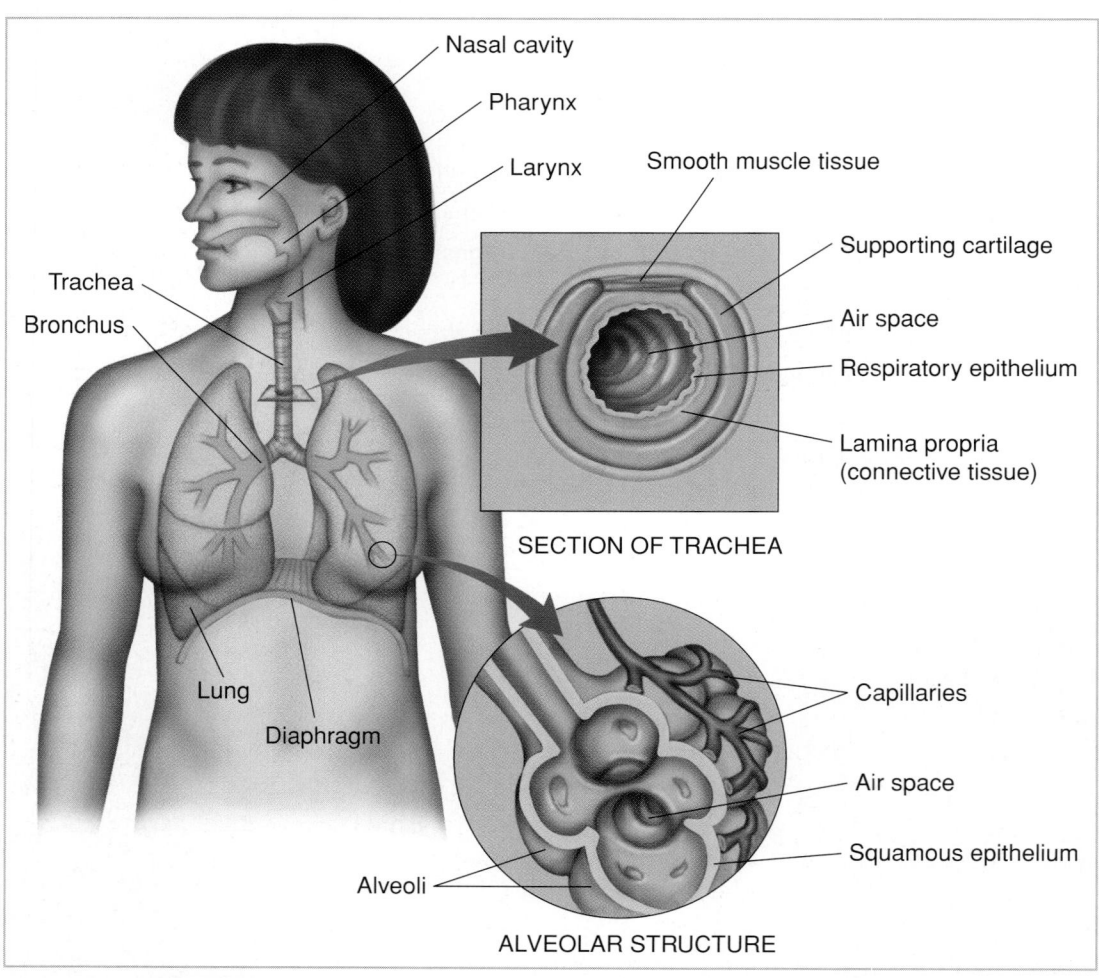

FIGURE 27-1   The respiratory system: nasal cavity, pharynx, larynx, trachea, bronchus, and lung with expanded views of the trachea and alveolar structure.

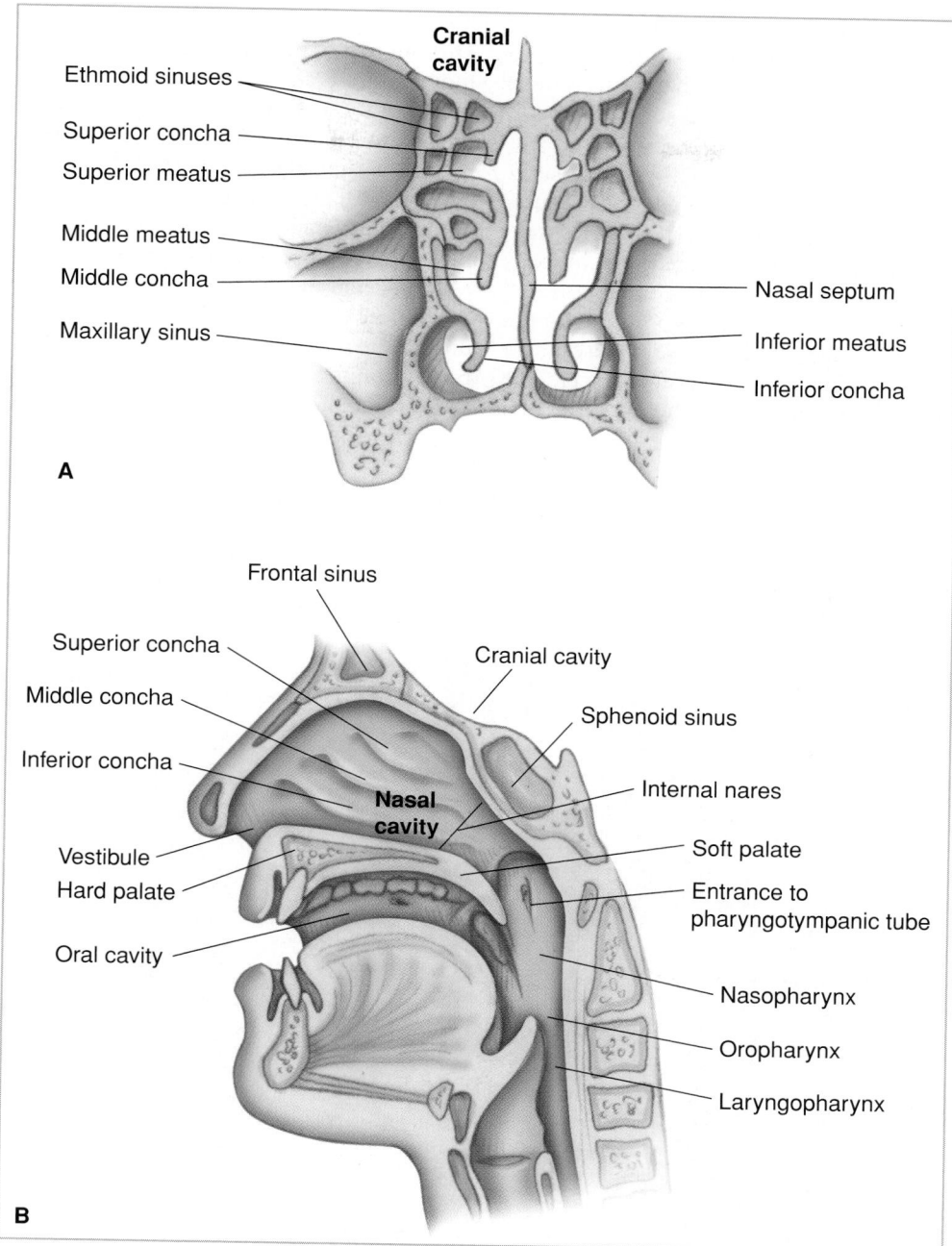

FIGURE 27-2 The nasal cavity and pharynx: (A) meatuses and positions of the entrance to the ethmoid and maxillary sinuses; (B) sagittal section of the nasal cavity and pharynx.

tiny branches of the bronchi called bronchioles; and the lungs, a pair of sac-like, spongy organs. The nose, pharynx, larynx, trachea, bronchi, and bronchioles conduct air to and from the lungs. The lungs interact with the circulatory system to deliver oxygen and remove carbon dioxide.

Nose

The nose is the organ of smell, and also part of the apparatus of respiration and voice (see Figure 27-2). In addition to being our organ of smell, it is also respon-

sible for performing several other functions, including being a passageway for air to move; warming and moistening inhaled air; using hair-like projections, called cilia, to trap and prevent dust, pollens, and other foreign matter from entering the nasal cavity; and assisting in the making of sounds that occur during speaking and singing. Considered anatomically, the nose is divided into an external portion—the visible projection portion, to which the term *nose* is popularly restricted—and an internal portion, consisting of two principal cavities, or nasal fossae, separated from each other by a vertical septum, and subdivided by spongy or turbinated bones that project from the outer wall into three passages, or meatuses, with which various sinuses in the ethmoid, sphenoid, frontal, and superior maxillary bones communicate by narrow apertures.

The external entrances of the nose are called nares. The inside structure of the nose includes the septum, which divides the nose into right and left sides. The septum is a cartilaginous wall. It is also lined with mucous membranes. Each side of the nose has three conchae (inferior, middle, and superior), which connect with the eustachian tube (to the ear) the paranasal sinuses (also known as "the sinuses") and nasolacrimal ducts. The nasolacrimal ducts drain fluid from the eyes into the

nose, explaining why your nose runs when you cry. Turbinates also are present, forming a "maze" for air to move around, allowing for warming of the air and removal of foreign particles by the mucus produced from the mucous membranes. The nose is separated from the mouth by the palatine bones of the skull.

The nasal mucosa produces about one quart per day of mucus, which is used to moisten the air moving through the nose and also to trap pollens, dust, and other foreign matter traveling through the nose.

The nose also drains the four pairs of paranasal sinuses. The maxillary sinuses are located over the medial portion on the cheekbones, while the frontal sinuses are found over the eyebrows. The ethmoidal sinuses reside

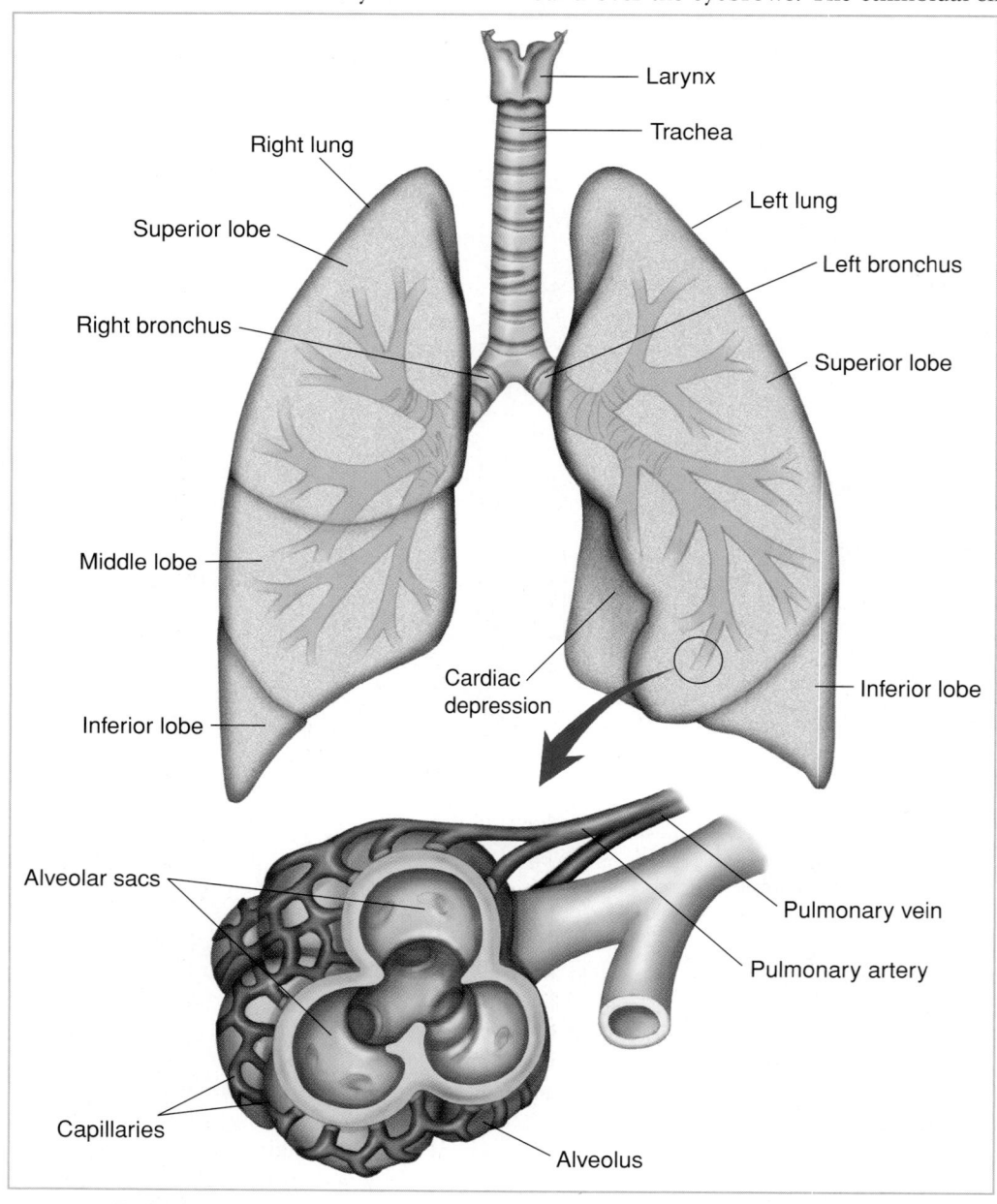

FIGURE 27-3 The larynx, trachea, bronchi, and lungs with an expanded view showing the structures of an alveolus and the pulmonary blood vessels.

in the area between and behind the eyes and the sphenoidal sinuses are located behind the ethmoidal sinuses. The sinuses decrease the weight of the skull with the creation of "air pockets" and also aid in phonation.

Pharynx

The pharynx is the musculo-membranous tube approximately 5 inches long that stretches from the base of the skull to the cervical spine and connects to the trachea and esophagus. The major functions of the pharynx include being a passageway for air and food and assisting in the production and sound of speech.

The pharynx has three parts: the nasopharynx, connects with the nose; the oropharynx, which connects with the back of the mouth; and the laryngopharynx, which is where the pharynx is located. Three paired sets of tonsils reside in the pharynx. The adenoids are located behind the nose and are often blamed for snoring, especially in children. The palatine tonsils are in the oropharynx and are often referred to as "the tonsils," and are located on either side of the throat on the anterior portion of the oropharynx. The lingual tonsils are located at the base of the tongue. The tonsils are part of the immune system and help in infection control.

Larynx

The larynx is also known as the voice box (see Figure 27-3). It is a muscular, cartilaginous structure lined with mucous membrane and connected to the inferior (lower) end of the pharynx. The larynx has several cartilaginous structures to help protect it from trauma. The thyroid cartilage is the largest of the cartilage structures, and is also known as the "Adam's apple." The epiglottic cartilage is also known as the epiglottis. Its function is to cover the trachea (windpipe) during swallowing so that food is all directed down the esophagus to the stomach rather than down the trachea and into the lungs. The cricoid cartilage is the lowest cartilage in the larynx. It is C shaped and wraps around the larynx to protect it from pressure. The "opening" in the "C" allows for large boluses of food to be swallowed down the esophagus. The inside of the larynx contains the false and true vocal folds and the entrance of the glottis—the opening between the vocal folds through which air passes.

The larynx functions in the production of vocal sounds. If the larynx is relaxed, then low sounds are produced. If it is tense, then higher pitched notes occur. The nose, mouth, pharynx, and bony sinuses impact the other aspects of speaking and singing.

Trachea

The trachea is also known as the windpipe (Figure 27-3). It is a cartilaginous tube that extends between the larynx to the main bronchi, and is about 1 inch wide and 4.5 inches long. Like the larynx, it has C-rings of cartilage that protect its structure and shape.

Lifespan
Considerations

THE CHILD
- Infants born before the age of 24 weeks gestation are frequently administered a product called surfactant, which the body produces in more mature lungs to help increase the surface tension of the fluid lining in the alveoli, making oxygen exchange more efficient. By administering this fluid to more immature lungs, there is a decrease in the occurrence of respiratory distress syndrome and lung damage in these infants.
- A newborn has a respiratory rate of 30 to 80 breaths per minute. As the infant matures, the respiratory rate drops to 20 to 40 by the first birthday. A 5-year-old has a respiratory rate of approximately 20 to 25 breaths per minute, while a 15-year-old usually demonstrates a rate of 15 to 20 breaths per minute. Healthy adults also breathe in the range of 15 to 20 breath per minute.

THE OLDER ADULT
- Older adults may increase their respiratory rates as the cumulative effects of pollution, smoking, and disease begin to wear on the integrity of the tissues. Mucous membranes produce less mucus, and the cilia decrease in their function. As a result, less foreign matter is trapped prior to entering the lungs and an increase in infections results.
- With skeletal changes of aging, oftentimes breathing in the elderly is diaphragm based rather than rib based, decreasing the tidal volume of external respiration. The lungs also lose their flexibility and become stiffer, so the volume of air that can be moved decreases. As a result, older adults are less able to move out foreign and disease-causing materials, and are more susceptible to bronchitis and pneumonia.

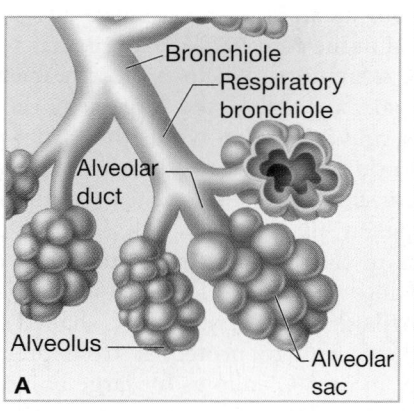
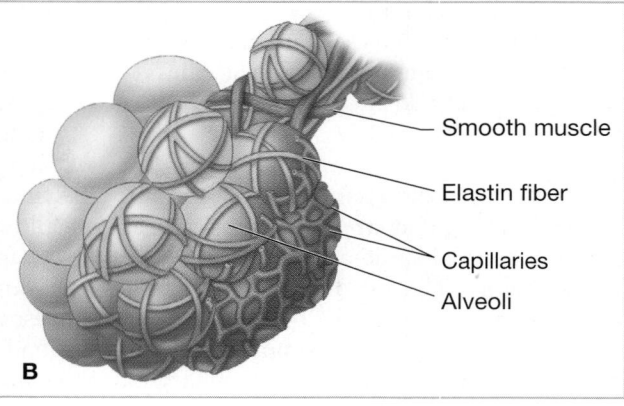

FIGURE 27-4 (A) Alveolar sac; (B) alveoli with capillaries.

The interior is lined with mucous membrane and cilia to trap foreign matter. One of the most important functions of the trachea is to transfer oxygen to the lungs and carbon dioxide from the lungs; in other words, breathing.

Bronchi

The bronchi are the two main branches of the trachea that stretch between the trachea and the lungs (Figure 27-3). These structures are responsible for providing a passageway for air between the trachea and the lungs. The right bronchus is the longer, larger branch moving down the right side of the heart. The left bronchus is shorter and more vertical, as it makes room for the heart in the chest cavity. After entering the lungs at the hilum, the lungs subdivide into the bronchial tree, which continues to branch into smaller and small branches called bronchioles. Eventually, those bronchioles terminate at the alveoli. The alveoli are small air sacs that support a network of capillaries used for oxygen and carbon dioxide transfer (see Figure 27-4). In healthy individuals, the alveoli resemble small balloons that inflate and deflate as air moves in and out. The bronchial tubes are lined with a mucous membranes and cilia to assist in removing foreign matter prior to its entry into the lungs.

Lungs

The lungs are large, conical-shaped, lobed organs in the chest (Figure 27-3). At birth the lungs are pinkish in color, but as adulthood approaches, the lungs turn a dark, slate gray color. The lungs are porous and spongy in texture and highly elastic. The right lung is made up of three lobes, called the upper, middle, and lower lobes, and weighs about 625 grams, whereas the left lung weighs 567 grams and only has two lobes: upper and lower. Each lung is between 10 and 12 inches in length, and they are separated by the mediastinum. The mediastinum contains the heart, trachea, esophagus, and blood vessels.

Pleura, thin sheets of epithelium sometimes referred to as pleural membranes, cover the outer surface of the lungs and the inside of the thoracic cavity. The gap between the pleura is called the pleural space. The pleura produce a lubricating fluid called surfactant that fills the pleural space. Surfactant helps the lungs glide smoothly in the chest cavity during inhalation and exhalation.

The lungs have three important roles: to supply oxygen, remove wastes and toxins, and defend against hostile intruders.

The lungs have three dozen distinct types of cells. Some of these cells scavenge foreign matter. Others have cilia that sweep the mucous membranes lining the smallest air passages. Some cells act on blood pressure control, while others spot infection invaders.

Mechanism of Breathing

Ventilation is the term used for movement to and from the alveoli. The two aspects of ventilation are inhalation and exhalation, which are brought about by the nervous system and the respiratory muscles. The respiratory centers are located in the brainstem, specifically, in the medulla oblongata and the pons. The respiratory muscles are the diaphragm and the internal and external intercostal muscles. The diaphragm is a dome-shaped muscle below the lungs. When it contracts, the diaphragm flattens and moves downward. The intercostal muscles are found between the ribs. The external intercostal muscles pull the ribs upward and outward, and the internal intercostal muscles pull the ribs downward and inward. Ventilation is the result of the respiratory muscles producing changes in the pressure within the alveoli and bronchial tree. Breathing involves three important pressure measurements:

- Atmospheric pressure—the pressure of the air around us. At sea level the atmospheric pressure is 760 mmHg; at higher altitudes the pressure is lower.

- Intrapleural pressure—the pressure within the potential pleural space between the parietal and visceral pleura. This space is a potential rather than a real space. Intrapleural pressure is always slightly below atmospheric pressure. This is called negative pressure because the elastic lungs are always tending to collapse and pull the visceral pleura away from the parietal pleura. The serous fluid, however, prevents separation of the pleural membranes.
- Intrapulmonic pressure—the pressure within the bronchial tree and alveoli. This pressure fluctuates below and above atmospheric pressure during each cycle of breathing.

Inhalation

Inhalation, which is also called *inspiration*, involves a precise sequence of events. The nervous system sends an impulse to the diaphragm and external intercostal muscles. The diaphragm flattens, which increases the top-to-bottom length of the thorax. Contraction elevates the ribs and increases the size of the thorax from the front to the back and from side to side. This increase in the size of the chest cavity reduces pressure within it, and what follows is an active process through which air moves into the lungs.

Expiration

Quiet *expiration* is ordinarily a passive process. During expiration the thorax returns to its resting size and shape. Elastic recoil of lung tissues aids in expiration. However, expiratory muscles used in forceful expiration are the internal intercostals and abdominal muscles. Reduction of the size of the thoracic cavity builds pressure and air leaves the lungs. Figure 27-5 shows how the actual mechanism of breathing takes place.

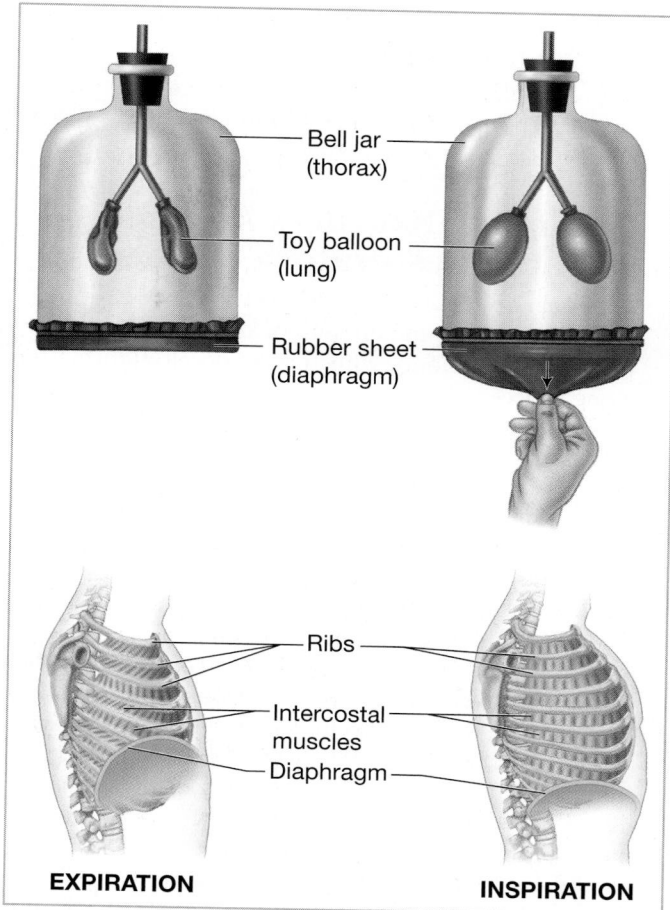

FIGURE 27-5 Mechanism of breathing.

Respiratory Volumes and Capacities

During the act of breathing, different volumes of air are moving in and out at different capacities, and these capacities can be calculated by adding specific respiratory volumes together. For example, when measuring lung volume, the following volumes would be used:

- Tidal volume (V_T) = volume of air entering or leaving the lungs during a single breath.
- Inspiratory reserve volume (IRV) = volume of air that can be inspired over and above the resting tidal volume
- Expiratory reserve volume (ERV) = volume of air that can be expired after a normal expiration

- Residual volume (RV) = volume of air remaining in the lungs after a maximal expiration, which can be estimated as 25 percent of the vital capacity

When measuring lung capacities, the following measurements would be used:

- Inspiratory capacity (IC) = maximum volume that can be inspired after a normal expiration = VT + IRV
- Vital capacity (VC) = maximum volume that can be expired after a maximal inspiration = VT + IRV + ERV
- Functional residual capacity (FRC) = volume of air left in the lungs after a normal expiration = ERV + RV
- Total lung capacity (TLC) = volume of the lungs when fully inflated = VC + RV (or $1.25 \times$ VC)

When measuring a person's respiratory volume and capacity, other measurements may be used including the following:

- Respiratory rate (f) = number of breaths per minute
- Minute ventilation (V_E) = total volume of air expired per minute = $V_T \times f$

- Dead space (V_D) = volume of inspired air that is not available for gas exchange
- Alveolar ventilation (V_A) = volume of air that reaches the alveoli per minute = $(V_T - V_D) \times f$

Common Disorders Associated with the Respiratory System

Pulmonary diseases have a wide range of presentation, from life-threatening to mildly irritating. Many are present in childhood, while others develop during the aging process.

Asthma

Asthma is a chronic, inflammatory disease. It is typically caused when allergens or other irritating substances cause swelling in the lining of the trachea and bronchial tubes, aggravating sensitive tissues. The tissues create mucus in an attempt to trap the offending intruder, which can cause coughing or a sense of struggling to breathe. This, in turn, causes more swelling, which causes more mucous production. It becomes a vicious cycle. Most individuals with asthma carry an inhaler of a beta-2 medication called albuterol or pirbuterol. This medication is a rescue medicine used during an asthma episode. Long-term, preventive medications are also used, including long-acting beta-2 medications (such as Serevent [salmeterol]), leukotrienes (Singulair), and inhaled corticosteroids (Flovent, Intal, beclomethasone). These medications do not stop an already occurring asthma episode, but must be used on a daily basis to keep medication levels in the tissues at an effective level for preventing the asthma episodes. In an asthma exacerbation, prescribers will give the patient steroids, such as prednisone, to help reduce the inflammation and allow the patient to heal faster with fewer complications.

Asthma is related to the same process that causes allergic reactions, so the two disorders are usually related. Asthma can have its onset during childhood, but adult-onset asthma is also common.

Chronic Obstructive Pulmonary Disease

Chronic obstructive pulmonary disease (COPD) is comprised primarily of two related diseases: chronic bronchitis and emphysema. In both diseases, there is chronic obstruction of the flow of air through the airways and out of the lungs, and the obstruction generally is permanent and progressive over time. Smoking is responsible for 90 percent of COPD in United States. Although not all cigarette smokers will develop COPD, it is estimated that 15 percent will. Smokers with COPD have higher death rates than nonsmokers with COPD. They also have more frequent respiratory symptoms (coughing, shortness of breath, etc.) and more deterioration in lung function than nonsmokers. Air pollution and some occupational pollutants such as cadmium and silica may increase the risk of COPD.

COPD usually is first diagnosed on the basis of a medical history that discloses many of the symptoms of COPD and a physical examination that discloses signs of COPD. Other tests to diagnose COPD include chest x-ray, computerized tomography (CT or CAT scan) of the chest, tests of lung function (pulmonary function tests), and the measurement of oxygen and carbon dioxide levels in the blood.

The goals of COPD treatment include prevention of further deterioration in lung function, alleviation of symptoms, and improvement in the performance of daily activities and quality of life. The treatment strategies include quitting smoking, taking medications to dilate airways (bronchodilators) and decrease airway inflammation, vaccinating against influenza and pneumonia, regular oxygen supplementation, and pulmonary rehabilitation.

Bronchitis

Bronchitis is a respiratory disease in which the mucous membrane in the lungs' bronchial passages becomes inflamed. As the irritated membrane swells and grows thicker, it narrows or shuts off the tiny airways in the lungs, resulting in coughing spells accompanied by thick phlegm and breathlessness. The disease comes in two forms: acute (lasting less than 6 weeks) and chronic (reoccurring frequently for more than 2 years). In addition, people with asthma also experience an inflammation of the lining of the bronchial tubes called asthmatic bronchitis.

Acute bronchitis is generally caused by lung infections. In most cases the infection is viral in origin, but sometimes it is caused by bacteria. Chronic bronchitis may be caused by repeated attacks of acute bronchitis, which weaken and irritate bronchial airways over time, and by industrial pollution. Chronic bronchitis is found in higher than normal rates among coal miners, grain handlers, metal molders, and other people who are continually exposed to dust. But the chief cause is heavy, long-term smoking, which irritates the bronchial tubes and causes them to produce excess mucus. The symptoms of chronic bronchitis are also worsened by air pollution.

Symptoms of acute bronchitis include a hacking cough; appearance of yellow, white, or green phlegm, usually appearing 24 to 48 hours after a cough; fever and chills; soreness and tightness in the chest; some pain below the breastbone during deep breathing; and some shortness of breath. Symptoms of chronic bronchitis generally include a persistent cough that produces yellow, white, or green phlegm (for at least 3 months of the year, and for more than two consecutive years) and sometimes wheezing, and breathlessness.

Conventional treatment for acute bronchitis may consist of simple measures such as getting plenty of rest, drinking lots of fluids, avoiding smoke and fumes, and possibly getting a prescription for an inhaled bronchodilator and/or cough syrup. In severe cases of chronic bronchitis, inhaled or oral steroids to reduce inflammation or supplemental oxygen may be necessary. In severe cases of chronic bronchitis with COPD, a physician may prescribe oxygen therapy, either on a continuous or as-needed basis.

Emphysema

Emphysema is a long-term, progressive disease of the lung that primarily causes shortness of breath. In people with emphysema, the lung tissues necessary to support the physical shape and function of the lung are destroyed. It is considered an obstructive lung disease because the destruction of lung tissue around smaller airways, called bronchioles, makes these airways unable to hold their shape properly when you exhale.

Tobacco smoking is by far the most dangerous reason why people develop emphysema, and it is also the most preventable cause. Other risk factors include a deficiency of an enzyme called alpha$_1$-antitrypsin, air pollution, airway reactivity, heredity, gender (male), and age.

Shortness of breath is the most common symptom of emphysema. Cough, sometimes caused by the production of mucus, and wheezing may also be symptoms of emphysema. A tolerance for exercise may also decrease over time. Emphysema usually develops slowly. There may not be any acute episodes of shortness of breath. Slow deterioration is the rule, and it may go unnoticed.

Treatment for emphysema can take many forms and different approaches to treatment are available. Generally, a doctor will prescribe these treatments in

a stepwise approach, depending on the severity of the condition. Smoking cessation is a treatment that most doctors require of people with emphysema. Quitting smoking may halt the progression of the disease and should improve the function of the lungs to some extent. Bronchodilating medications, which cause the air passages to open more fully and allow better air exchange, are usually the first medications that a physician will prescribe. Other medications that may be prescribed include steroids and antibiotics. In cases where there is shortness of breath, oxygen may also be a prescribed treatment, and in very severe cases, surgery may be required. This may involve the actual removal of a lung.

Common Cold

A common cold is an infection of the upper respiratory tract. Because any one of more than 200 viruses

Patient Education

Patients with pulmonary diseases must be educated on the need to be aware of their respiratory status and to alter their daily activities accordingly. Environmental irritants such as smoke, pollution, and allergens will irritate respiratory symptoms and should be avoided. Compliance with medication instructions is another way in which patients can avoid exacerbations of their disease. If prescribed medications do not relieve their symptoms, then the patient should contact the office for further instructions.

Patients who have pulmonary diseases are also at higher risk for developing bronchitis and pneumonia. Because they may be unable to clear their secretions, and because of inflammation blocking the bronchial tubes, an increased amount of bacteria can collect in the bases of the lungs and thrive in the dark, stagnant environment. As a result, these patients should avoid other individuals who are sick.

can cause a common cold, symptoms tend to vary greatly. The symptoms of a common cold usually appear about 1 to 3 days after exposure to a cold virus. Signs and symptoms may include a runny or stuffy nose, itchy or sore throat, cough, congestion, slight body aches or a mild headache, sneezing, watery eyes, low-grade fever of less than 102°F, and mild fatigue. Discharge from the nose may become thicker and yellow or green in color as a common cold runs its course. What makes a cold different from other viral infections is that generally a high fever does not accompany a cold. A person is also unlikely to experience significant fatigue from a common cold.

Although more than 200 viruses can cause a common cold, the rhinovirus is the most common culprit. Many cold viruses are highly contagious. Although a common cold can spread through sneezing and coughing, it often spreads by hand-to-hand contact with someone who has a cold or by using shared objects, such as utensils, towels, toys, or telephones.

There is no cure for the common cold. Antibiotics are of no use against cold viruses, and over-the-counter cold preparations will not cure a common cold or make it go away any sooner. However, over-the-counter medications can relieve some symptoms. For fever, sore throat, and headache, mild pain relievers may help. For runny nose and nasal congestion, antihistamines or decongestants may be useful. Because so many different viruses can cause a common cold, no effective vaccine has been developed. However, there are some common-sense precautions a person can follow that will help to slow the spread of cold viruses. These include washing their hands; scrubbing countertops clean, especially when someone in the household has a common cold; using tissues to sneeze and cough into and then discarding them right away; and not sharing drinking glasses or other utensils with family members who may be sick.

Cystic Fibrosis

Cystic fibrosis (CF) is a chronic and progressive disease usually diagnosed in childhood that causes mucus to become thick, dry, and sticky. The mucus builds up and clogs passages in many of the body's organs, but primarily the lungs and the pancreas. In the lungs, the mucus can lead to serious breathing problems and lung disease. In the pancreas, the mucus can lead to malnutrition and problems with growth and development. People with CF have an average life expectancy of about 32 years, although new treatments offer hope for longer and healthier lives. It is an incurable genetic disorder that occurs when a child inherits a specific defect in the cystic fibrosis transmembrane regulator (CFTR) gene from both parents. If the gene defect is inherited from only one parent, the child will not have the disease but is considered a carrier. Symptoms of cystic fibrosis are usually caused by the production of thick, sticky mucus. Symptoms vary from person to person and are not always present at birth; in some people, symptoms may be very mild and not be noticed or develop until later in childhood or early adulthood. The goal of treatment for CF is to manage symptoms and prevent complications.

Hay Fever

Hay fever, which is also called seasonal allergic rhinitis or pollinosis, is a seasonal allergy causing inflammation of the mucous membranes of the nose and eyes. About 26.1 million Americans experience hay fever symptoms each year. During the seasons when plants are pollinating, people breathe in the pollen and have an allergic reaction to it. Some of the symptoms of hay fever include repeated and prolonged sneezing; a stuffy and watery nose; redness, swelling, and itching of the eyes; itching of the nose, throat, and mouth; and itching of the ears or other ear problems. Sometimes breathing difficulties occur at night. Coughing is sometimes a symptom and is a result of postnasal dripping of clear mucus. Loss of smell is common and sometimes loss of taste occurs. In severe conditions, nose bleeding occurs.

Hay fever is best controlled by avoiding the substance that causes a reaction, and using medications that counteract the histamine that is released during the reaction. In more severe cases, corticosteroids may be also be used. The best way to control hay fever is by removing pollen from the air by means of air conditioners and filters.

Influenza

Influenza, commonly called the flu, is an illness caused by viruses that infect the respiratory tract. Compared with most other viral respiratory infections, such as the common cold, influenza (flu) infection often causes a more severe illness.

Influenza viruses continually change over time, usually by mutation. This constant changing enables the virus to evade the immune system of its host, so that people are susceptible to influenza virus infection throughout life.

Typical symptoms of influenza include fever (usually 100°F to 103°F in adults and often even higher in children), respiratory symptoms such as cough, sore throat, and runny or stuffy nose, headache, muscle aches, and extreme fatigue. Although nausea, vomiting and diarrhea can sometimes accompany influenza infection, especially in children, gastrointestinal symptoms are rarely prominent. The term "stomach flu" is a misnomer that is sometimes used to describe gastrointestinal illnesses caused by other microorganisms.

Most people who get the flu recover completely in 1 to 2 weeks, but some people develop serious and potentially life-threatening medical complications, such as pneumonia.

Legionnaire's Disease

Legionnaire's disease is a type of pneumonia or lung infection. It causes 2 percent of pneumonia cases that need hospital treatment. The disease came to be known as Legionnaire's disease, or legionellosis, in 1976. More than 40 different strains of the Legionella germ have now been discovered. Outbreaks of the disease tend to occur in healthy people staying in hotels or other buildings in which the cooling systems or showers have become contaminated by Legionella germs. They may also occur as single cases in which the source of the germs is uncertain. About three-quarters of all cases in the United States occur as isolated instances rather than as epidemics. It usually affects middle-aged or elderly people and it more commonly affects smokers or people with other respiratory problems.

The symptoms of the disease generally start 2 to 10 days after a person has been infected. They include high fever with sweating, severe headache, shortness of breath, a worsening cough, with greenish thick mucus (can be bloodstained), and muscle aches and pains. In severe cases, other systems of the body may be affected, leading to diarrhea, vomiting, mental confusion, and kidney and liver damage. The most serious effects are on the lungs. The mortality rate in previously fit and well people is about 10 percent. Many people experience fatigue, lack of energy,

and difficulty concentrating for some time after recovering from the disease. Joint pain and muscle weakness are also fairly common. These symptoms may last for some months or less commonly for a year or two.

Treatment normally includes antibiotics. In some cases, where the patient experiences difficulty breathing, intensive care with ventilation may be necessary, especially if the pneumonia is severe.

Lung Cancer

Lung cancer is the leading cause of cancer deaths in both women and men in the United States and throughout the world.

Smoking is the most significant cause of lung cancer. About 85 percent of lung cancers occur in a smoker or former smoker. The risk of developing lung cancer is related to the number of cigarettes smoked, the age at which a person started smoking, and how long a person has smoked (or had smoked before quitting). Other causes of lung cancer include passive smoking. Air pollution from motor vehicles, factories, asbestos exposure, and the presence of other lung diseases may increase the risk for lung cancer.

The most widely used therapies for lung cancer are surgery, chemotherapy, and radiation therapy.

Pleurisy

Pleurisy is an inflammation of the membrane that surrounds and protects the lungs (the pleura). The condition, which is also called *pleuritis*, is a disorder that generally stems from an existing respiratory infection, disease, or injury. In people who have otherwise good health, respiratory infections or pneumonia are the main causes of pleurisy.

A variety of conditions can give rise to pleurisy. These include infections, such as pneumonia, tuberculosis, and other bacterial or viral respiratory infections; immune disorders, including systemic lupus erythematosus, rheumatoid arthritis, and sarcoidosis; and other diseases, including pancreatitis, liver cirrhosis,

Professionalism

and heart or kidney failure. Pleurisy may also result from an injury.

The chief symptom of pleurisy is sudden, intense chest pain that is usually located over the area of inflammation. Although the pain can be constant, it is usually most severe when the lungs move during breathing, coughing, sneezing, or even talking. In some cases the pain may be felt in other areas such as the neck, shoulder, or abdomen (referred pain). Another indication of pleurisy is that holding one's breath or exerting pressure against the chest causes pain relief.

Pleurisy is also characterized by certain respiratory symptoms. In response to the pain, pleurisy patients commonly have a rapid, shallow breathing pattern. If severe breathing difficulties persist, patients may experience a blue-colored complexion (cyanosis).

The pain of pleurisy is usually treated with analgesic and anti-inflammatory drugs, such as acetaminophen. People with pleurisy may also receive relief from lying on the painful side. Sometimes, a painful cough will be controlled with codeine-based cough syrups. However, as the pain eases, a person with pleurisy should try to breathe deeply and cough to clear any congestion, otherwise pneumonia may occur.

Pneumonia

Pneumonia is an inflammation of the lung or lungs, caused by bacteria, viruses, fungi, or chemical irritants. The most common bacterial cause of pneumonia in the United States is *Streptococcus pneumoniae* (pneumococcus). Oftentimes, pneumonia follows influenza in the elderly and debilitated. Symptoms include a productive cough with greenish mucus or pus-like sputum, fever, chills, fatigue, chest pain, and muscle aches. Diagnostic indicators include chest auscultation with a stethoscope, sputum cultures, and chest x-rays. Treatment of pneumonia includes drinking fluids, rest, antibiotics, and nonprescription drugs for pain relief. Supportive care includes oxygen therapy and respiratory treatments to thin out and remove secretions as necessary.

Pulmonary Edema

Pulmonary edema is a condition in which fluid accumulates in the lungs, usually because the heart's left ventricle does not pump adequately. Pulmonary edema can be a chronic condition, or it can develop suddenly and quickly become life threatening.

Most cases of pulmonary edema are caused by failure of the heart's main chamber, the left ventricle. It can be brought on by an acute heart attack, severe ischemia, volume overload of the heart's left ventricle, and mitral stenosis. Non-heart-related pulmonary edema is caused by lung problems such as pneumonia, an excess of intravenous fluids, some types of kidney disease, bad burns, liver disease, nutritional problems, and Hodgkin's disease.

Early symptoms of pulmonary edema include shortness of breath upon exertion, sudden respiratory distress after sleep, difficulty breathing, except when sitting upright, and coughing. In cases of severe pulmonary edema, the symptoms may worsen and will frequently include labored and rapid breathing; frothy, bloody fluid containing pus coughed from the lungs (sputum); a fast pulse and possibly serious disturbances in the heart's rhythm; cold, clammy, sweaty, and bluish skin; and a drop in blood pressure resulting in a thready pulse.

Pulmonary edema requires immediate emergency treatment. Treatment includes placing the patient in a sitting position and, in some cases, oxygen, assisted or mechanical ventilation, and drug therapy. The goal of treatment is to reduce the amount of fluid in the lungs, to improve gas exchange and heart function, and, where possible, to correct the underlying disease.

Pulmonary Embolism

A pulmonary embolism (PE) is a blood clot in the lung. It usually comes from smaller vessels in the leg, pelvis, arms, or heart. The clot travels through the vessels of the lung continuing to reach smaller vessels until it becomes wedged in a vessel that is too small to allow it to continue farther. The clot gets wedged and prevents any further blood from traveling to that section of the lung. When no blood reaches a section of the lung, that portion of the lung suffers an infarct, meaning it dies because no blood or oxygen is reaching it. This is referred to as a pulmonary (or lung) infarct.

Several factors can make someone more susceptible to developing a blood clot that can eventually break loose and travel to the lung. These factors may include immobilization due to illness or injury, or prolonged sitting, such as on an airplane or a long car trip, which allows the blood to sit in the legs and increases the risk of clot formation. Other factors are recent surgery, trauma or injury (especially to the legs), obesity, heart disease, burns, and a previous history of blood clot in the legs.

There are specific symptoms that may indicate that a PE has occurred. These include chest pain that is very sharp and stabbing in nature, has a sudden onset, and is worse when taking a deep breath; shortness of breath; anxiety or apprehension; dry cough; sweating; and passing out.

For someone who is critically ill and may have severe shortness of breath, low blood pressure, and low oxygen concentrations, the treatment may be much more aggressive, and often includes medications to elevate the blood pressure and increase the oxygen in the blood. Additional treatment might also include the use of "clot-buster" medications to help dissolve the emboli, and blood pressure elevators to raise the blood pressure. In cases where the PE is not as severe, oxygen therapy and the administration of blood-thinning medications are generally all that are needed.

Severe Acute Respiratory Syndrome

Severe acute respiratory syndrome (SARS) is a newly identified respiratory illness that first infected people in parts of Asia, North America, and Europe in early 2003. SARS is caused by a previously unknown type of coronavirus, a family of viruses that often cause mild to moderate upper respiratory illness, such as the common cold. This new virus is known as SARS-CoV. It is possible that outbreaks of SARS may be seasonal, appearing during winter months. Experts believe SARS may have first developed in animals, since the virus has been found in civets—a cat-like wild animal that is eaten as a delicacy in China.

The World Health Organization (WHO) reported that 8,096 people became sick with SARS, 774 of whom died, in the first outbreak. In 2004, China reported five confirmed and four possible cases of SARS by April 30. By May 18, 2004, WHO reported that the outbreak had been contained.

Like most respiratory illnesses, SARS is spread mainly through contact with infected saliva or droplets from coughing. You cannot get SARS from brief, casual exposure to an infected person, such as passing someone on the street. Close proximity, that is, less than 3 feet, or contact is probably necessary to become infected. Close contact includes living with or caring for a person who has SARS or having direct contact with saliva or respiratory droplets from an infected person. Treatment of SARS usually consists of antibiotics, antiviral medications, and steroids.

Sinusitis

Sinusitis is an infection or inflammation of the mucous membranes that line the inside of the nose and sinuses. Sinuses are hollow spaces, or cavities, located around your eyes, cheeks, and nose. When a mucous membrane becomes inflamed, it swells, blocking the drainage of fluid from the sinuses into the nose and throat, which causes pressure and pain in the sinuses. Bacteria and fungus are more likely to grow in sinuses that are unable to drain properly.

Sinuses can become blocked during a viral infection such as a cold, and sinus inflammation and infection can develop as a result. One key distinction between a cold and sinusitis is that cold symptoms, including a stuffy nose, begin to improve within 5 to 7 days. Sinusitis symptoms last longer and get worse after 7 days. There are two types of sinusitis: acute (sudden) and chronic (long term). With chronic sinusitis, a person is never really free from symptoms and always has a low level of sinusitis symptoms.

Pain and pressure in the face along with a stuffy or runny nose are the main symptoms of sinusitis. You also may have a yellow or greenish discharge from your nose. Leaning forward or moving your head often increases facial pain and pressure. The location of pain and tenderness may depend on which sinus is affected. Pain over the cheeks and upper teeth is often caused by maxillary sinus inflammation. Pain in the forehead, above the eyebrow, may be caused by frontal sinus inflammation. Pain behind the eyes, on top of the head, or in both temples may be caused by sphenoid sinus inflammation. And pain around or behind the eyes is caused by ethmoid sinus inflammation.

Sinusitis is generally treated with medications and home treatment measures, such as applying moist heat to the face. The goals of treatment for sinusitis are to improve drainage of mucus and reduce swelling in the sinuses, relieve pain and pressure, clear up any infection, prevent the formation of scar tissue, and avoid permanent damage to the tissues lining the nose and sinuses. Medications may also be used to treat sinusitis, especially when it is caused by a bacterial infection. There are varying lengths of treatment with medications—as short as 3 days or lasting as long as several weeks or more. The medications most often used to treat the condition include a combination of antibiotics, decongestants, analgesics, corticosteroids, and mucolytics.

Tuberculosis

Tuberculosis (TB) is a contagious disease caused by the bacillus *Mycobacterium tuberculosis*. The bacteria are spread from person to person by inhaling droplets infected with the bacteria. This often happens when an individual with this bacteria coughs, sneezes, or laughs, spreading those bacteria for others to breathe.

TB bacteria can grow anywhere in the body, but are most commonly found in the lungs. They produce granulomas (granular tumors) in the infected tissues. Symptoms for lung infections include coughing, hemoptysis (coughing up blood), white/gray frothy sputum, and night sweats. Other symptoms can include fatigue, chills, weakness, and anorexia.

Diagnosis is done by chest x-ray and sputum culture. The PPD skin test is done to see if an individual has ever been exposed to the bacteria, but is not indicative of whether the person actually has the disease.

Treatment of this disease is long term, usually taking 9 to 12 months to eradicate the bacteria. The first period requires that individuals take respiratory precautions to prevent the spread of the bacteria. Antibiotics are used to begin eradication of the bacteria, usually rifampin, isoniazid, and ethambutol HCl. After the patient shows negative sputum cultures, they will still need to continue antibiotic treatment for another 6 to 9 months to prevent multi-drug-resistant TB that is more difficult to treat.

Individuals who are immunocompromised, such as the homeless, those with AIDS, infants, the elderly, and individuals on chemotherapy, are the most at risk for developing TB.

SUMMARY

The respiratory system is made of a system of tubes lined with mucous membranes and cilia, which serve a protective function. The function of the system is external, internal, and cellular respiration. Multiple disease processes can result from infection and inflammation within the system.

Chapter Review

COMPETENCY REVIEW

1. Define and spell the terms to learn for this chapter.
2. List the organs of the respiratory system.
3. What is the primary function of the respiratory system?
4. What does atmospheric pressure represent?
5. What are the five functions of the nose?
6. What are the three functions of the pharynx?
7. What is the function of the epiglottis?
8. Describe the bronchi. What are the differences between the left and right bronchus?
9. What are the alveoli?
10. What does tidal volume represent?

PREPARING FOR THE CERTIFICATION EXAM

1. What organ is responsible for being a passageway for air and food and also assists in the production and sound of speech?
   A. pharynx
   B. nares
   C. trachea
   D. bronchi
   E. epiglottis

2. The sac that encases the lungs is called the
   A. thorax
   B. pleura
   C. bronchiole
   D. pneumoderma
   E. pneumocardium

3. Another name for the windpipe is the
   A. bronchial tube
   B. trachea
   C. larynx
   D. pharynx
   E. epiglottis

4. The function of the epiglottis is to
   A. aid in swallowing
   B. aid in speaking
   C. prevent swallowing
   D. prevent aspiration
   E. aid in aspiration

continued on next page

5. A genetic condition characterized by the production of thick sticky mucus is called
   A. asthma
   B. pneumonia
   C. cystic fibrosis
   D. COPD
   E. tuberculosis

6. The volume of air remaining in the lungs after a maximal expiration is called the
   A. tidal volume
   B. inspiratory reserve volume
   C. expiratory reserve volume
   D. residual volume
   E. vital capacity

7. What term is used to describe the number of breaths per minute?
   A. ventilation rate
   B. respiratory rate
   C. alveolar ventilation rate
   D. minute ventilation
   E. respiratory ventilation

8. Bronchitis is
   A. inflammation of the bronchial tubes
   B. constriction of the bronchial tubes
   C. destruction of the bronchial tubes
   D. seen only in the elderly
   E. seen only in infants

9. What disease is smoking most responsible for causing in the United States?
   A. asthma
   B. COPD
   C. cystic fibrosis
   D. pneumonia
   E. tuberculosis

10. Tuberculosis is spread by
    A. touching the infected person
    B. breathing an allergen
    C. breathing infected droplets
    D. the casual handshake
    E. smoking

CRITICAL THINKING

1. What could Joe have done early on to reduce his chances of getting COPD?
2. Why did the physician prescribe an antibiotic for Joe?
3. Why did the physician prescribe two puffs of albuterol every 4 hours?

INTERNET ACTIVITY

Do an Internet search for COPD services in your hometown and see what resources are available in your area.

MediaLink More on the respiratory system, including interactive resources, can be found on the Student CD-ROM accompanying this textbook.

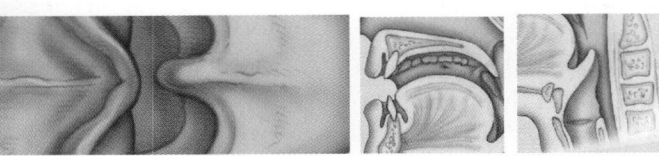

Medical Assistant Role Delineation Chart

HIGHLIGHT indicates material covered in this chapter.

ADMINISTRATIVE

Administrative Procedures

- Perform basic administrative medical assisting functions
- Schedule, coordinate and monitor appointments
- Schedule inpatient/outpatient admissions and procedures
- Understand and apply third-party guidelines
- Obtain reimbursement through accurate claims submission
- Monitor third-party reimbursement
- Understand and adhere to managed care policies and procedures
- *Negotiate managed care contracts*

Practice Finances

- Perform procedural and diagnostic coding
- Apply bookkeeping principles

- Manage accounts receivable
- *Manage accounts payable*
- *Process payroll*
- *Document and maintain accounting and banking records*
- *Develop and maintain fee schedules*
- *Manage renewals of business and professional insurance policies*
- *Manage personnel benefits and maintain records*
- *Perform marketing, financial, and strategic planning*

CLINICAL

Fundamental Principles

- Apply principles of aseptic technique and infection control
- Comply with quality assurance practices
- Screen and follow up patient test results

Diagnostic Orders

- Collect and process specimens
- Perform diagnostic tests

Patient Care

- Adhere to established patient screening procedures
- Obtain patient history and vital signs
- Prepare and maintain examination and treatment areas
- Prepare patient for examinations, procedures and treatments

- Assist with examinations, procedures and treatments
- Prepare and administer medications and immunizations
- Maintain medication and immunization records
- Recognize and respond to emergencies
- Coordinate patient care information with other health care providers
- Initiate IV and administer IV medications with appropriate training and as permitted by state law

GENERAL

Professionalism

- Display a professional manner and image
- Demonstrate initiative and responsibility
- Work as a member of the health care team
- Prioritize and perform multiple tasks
- Adapt to change
- Promote the CMA credential
- Enhance skills through continuing education
- Treat all patients with compassion and empathy
- Promote the practice through positive public relations

Communication Skills

- Recognize and respect cultural diversity
- Adapt communications to individual's ability to understand
- Use professional telephone technique

- Recognize and respond effectively to verbal, nonverbal, and written communications
- Use medical terminology appropriately
- Utilize electronic technology to receive, organize, prioritize and transmit information
- Serve as liaison

Legal Concepts

- Perform within legal and ethical boundaries
- Prepare and maintain medical records
- Document accurately
- Follow employer's established policies dealing with the health care contract
- Implement and maintain federal and state health care legislation and regulations
- Comply with established risk management and safety procedures
- Recognize professional credentialing criteria
- *Develop and maintain personnel, policy and procedure manuals*

Instruction

- Instruct individuals according to their needs
- Explain office policies and procedures
- Teach methods of health promotion and disease prevention
- Locate community resources and disseminate information
- *Develop educational materials*
- *Conduct continuing education activities*

Operational Functions

- Perform inventory of supplies and equipment
- Perform routine maintenance of administrative and clinical equipment
- Apply computer techniques to support office operations
- *Perform personnel management functions*
- *Negotiate leases and prices for equipment and supply contracts*

- *Denotes advanced skills.*

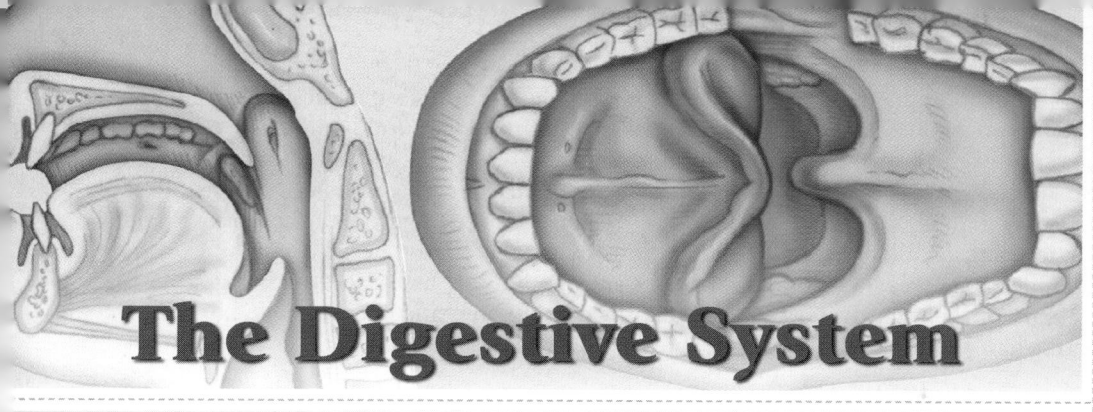

The Digestive System

Learning Objectives

After completing this chapter, you should be able to:

- Define and spell the terms to learn for this chapter.
- Describe the purpose and function of the digestive system.
- Identify the primary organs of the digestive system and briefly explain the function of each.
- Name the two sets of teeth with which a person is born.

- Discuss the three main portions of a tooth.
- Identify the accessory organs of the digestive system and state the function of each.
- Briefly explain common disorders associated with the digestive system.

OUTLINE

Organs of the Digestive System   491

Common Disorders Associated with the Digestive System   495

Terms to Learn

appendicitis
cirrhosis
colitis
colorectal cancer
constipation
Crohn's disease
diarrhea
diverticulitis

diverticulosis
gastroesophageal reflux disease (GERD)
hemorrhoid
hernia
hiatal hernia
inguinal hernia

irritable bowel syndrome (IBS)
oral cancer
pancreatic cancer
peptic ulcer disease (PUD)
pyloric stenosis
stomach ulcers

Case Study

NATE SYLVANS IS A 38-YEAR-OLD MALE seen by Dr. Sammons. He is complaining of "a lot of heartburn" and frequent "belching." He admits to being under a lot of pressure at work lately, and has a frequent dull aching pain in his stomach and back. Pain is localized in the midepigastrium. Mr. Sylvans is diagnosed with an acute gastric ulcer after receiving an upper GI series, gastric analysis and histology with culture, indicating no presence of *H. pylori* bacteria.

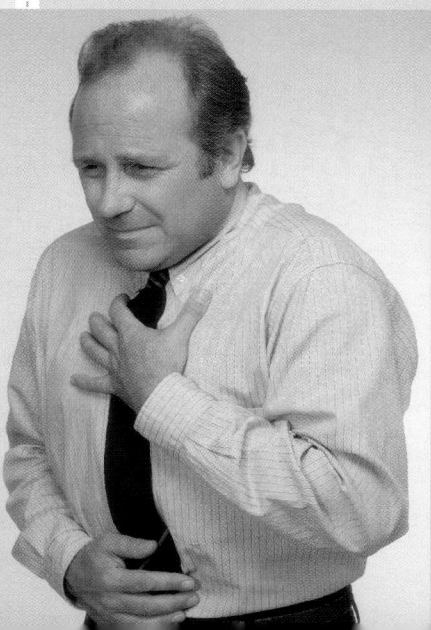

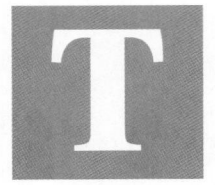he digestive system contains those organs that are responsible for getting food into and out of the body and for making use of it. These organs include the salivary glands, the mouth, esophagus, stomach, small intestine, liver, gallbladder, pancreas, colon, rectum, and anus. The main part of the digestive system is the digestive tract. This is like a long tube, some 30 feet long in adults, through the middle of the body. It starts at the mouth, where food and drink enter the body, and finishes at the anus, where leftover food and wastes leave the body. The three main functions of the digestive system include digestion, absorption, and elimination (by means of urine or feces). Each of the various organs commonly associated with digestion is described in this chapter, and the organs of digestion are shown in Figure 28-1.

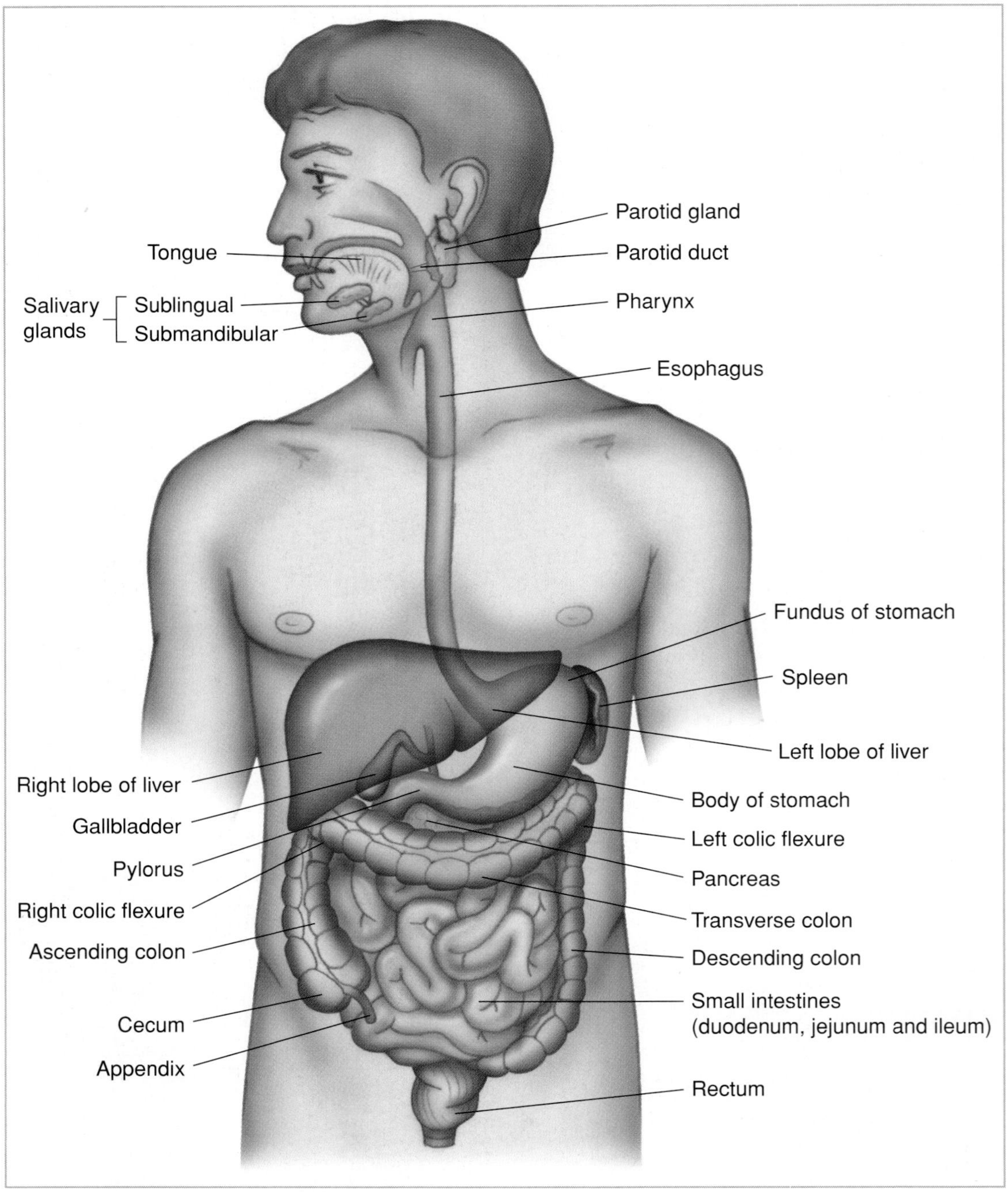

Tongue

Salivary glands
— Sublingual
— Submandibular

Parotid gland

Parotid duct

Pharynx

Esophagus

Fundus of stomach

Spleen

Left lobe of liver

Right lobe of liver

Gallbladder

Pylorus

Right colic flexure

Ascending colon

Cecum

Appendix

Body of stomach

Left colic flexure

Pancreas

Transverse colon

Descending colon

Small intestines
(duodenum, jejunum and ileum)

Rectum

FIGURE 28-1 The digestive system.

Organs of the Digestive System

The digestive system is a series of hollow organs joined in a long, twisting tube from the mouth to the anus. Inside this tube is a lining called the mucosa. In the mouth, stomach, and small intestine, the mucosa contains tiny glands that produce juices to help digest food.

Mouth

The mouth is the cavity formed by the palate (roof), the lips and cheeks on the sides, and the tongue on the floor (see Figure 28-2). The oral cavity (the mouth) contains the teeth and the salivary glands. The cheeks form the lateral walls and are continuous with the lips. The vestibule includes the space between the cheeks and the teeth. The gingivae (gums) surround the neck of the teeth, helping to hold the teeth in place. The hard and soft palates form a roof for the oral cavity, and the tongue is connected to the floor of the mouth by the lingual frenulum. The tongue is made of skeletal muscle and is covered with mucous membrane. The tongue can be divided into the rear portion called the root, the central body, and the pointed tip. Papillae (elevations) and taste buds are located on the surface of the tongue. There are four types of taste buds—sweet, salt, sour, and bitter. Three pairs of salivary glands secrete saliva into the oral cavity. They are called the parotid, sublingual, and submandibular glands. The posterior margins of the soft palate support the muscular pharyngeal arches, which function in swallowing and phonation, and the uvula—the dangling tissue hanging down from the center of the pharyngeal arches. The line formed by the pharyngeal arches and the uvula separates the oral cavity from the pharynx. Digestion begins in the mouth with the process of mastication (chewing) and the secretion of saliva, which moistens the food and starts the chemical breakdown of food. The combination of the chewing action and the saliva helps to form the food into a bolus (ball) for swallowing.

Teeth

Humans have two sets of teeth: 28 deciduous teeth (the baby teeth) and 32 permanent teeth (see Figure 28-3). The 28 deciduous teeth include 8 incisors, 4 canines (cuspids), and 8 molars. The permanent teeth include 8 incisors, 4 canines, 8 premolars, and 12 molars. The incisors are so named because of their sharp, cutting edge used for biting food. The incisors are the four front teeth of the dental arch. The upper incisors are larger and stronger than the lower ones.

The canine teeth are also known as the cuspids. These teeth have their roots stuck deeply into the bones of the jaw. The upper canines are also known as the "eye teeth" and are larger than the lower canines. The lower canines are also known as the "stomach teeth."

The premolar teeth are situated lateral to, and behind, the canine teeth. They are also known as the bicuspid teeth and are smaller and shorter than the canine teeth. There are four premolars in each arch. The molar teeth are the largest teeth in the permanent set and are adapted to grinding and pounding food. An adult has 12 molars, six in each arch, placed posterior to the premolars.

The deciduous teeth are smaller than the permanent teeth, but generally resemble the permanent teeth on a smaller scale.

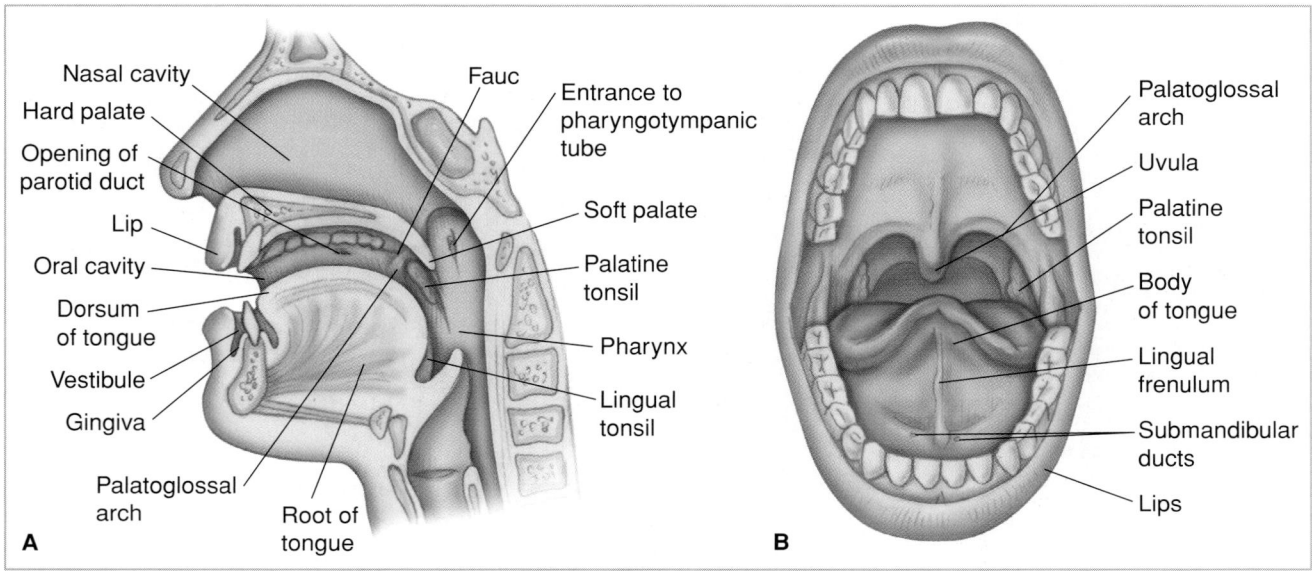

FIGURE 28-2   The oral cavity: (A) sagittal section; (B) anterior view as seen through the open mouth.

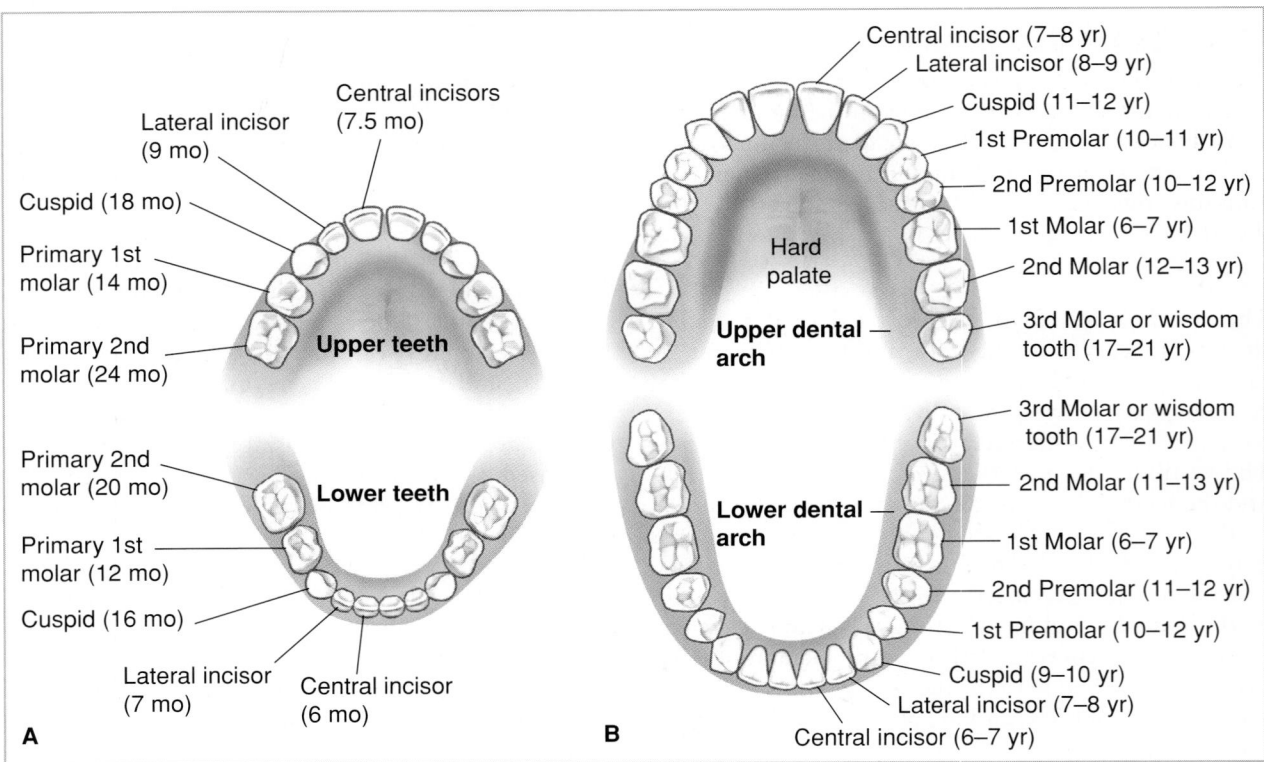

FIGURE 28-3 Deciduous and permanent teeth: (A) deciduous teeth, with the age at eruption given in months; (B) permanent teeth, with the age at eruption given in years.

Each tooth consists of three main portions: the crown (the part above the gum); the root (embedded in the gums); and the neck, the part between the root and the crown (see Figure 28-4). The root of each tooth sits in a bony socket called the alveolus. Collagen fibers of the periodontal ligament extend from the dentin of the root to the bone of the alveolus, creating a strong

articulation known as a gomphosis (that binds the teeth to the bony sockets in the maxillary bone and mandible). A layer of cementum covers the dentin of the root, providing protection and firmly anchoring the periodontal ligament. The solid portion of the tooth consists of the dentin, which forms the bulk of the tooth, and the enamel, which covers the exposed

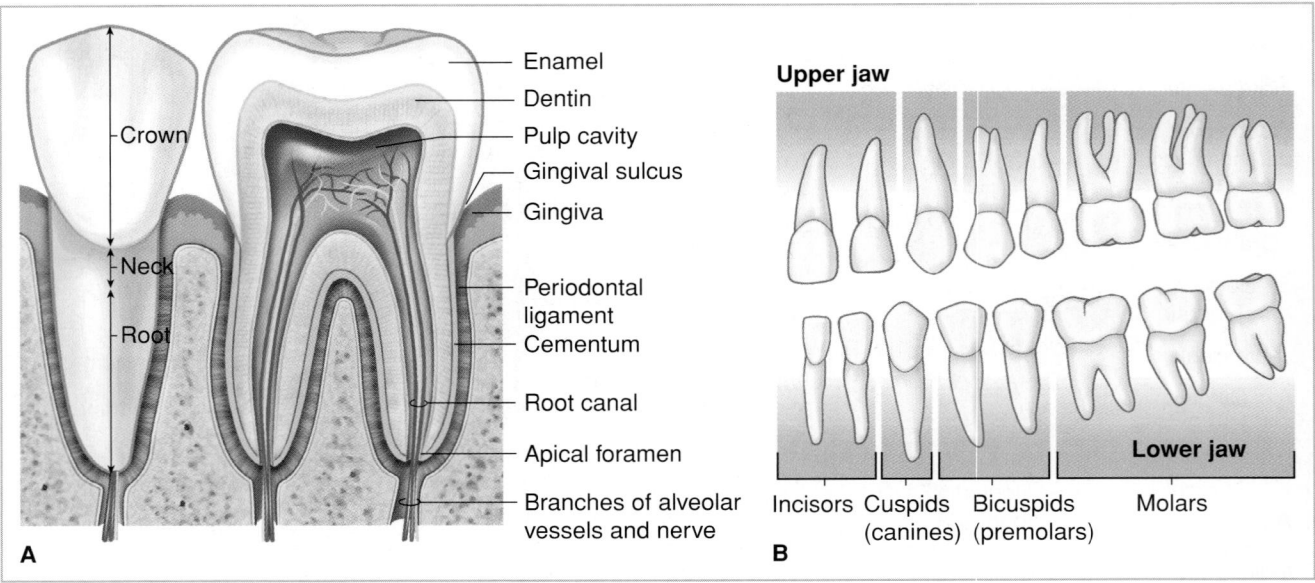

FIGURE 28-4 Teeth: (A) a diagrammatic section through a typical adult tooth; (B) the adult teeth.

part of the crown. The enamel is the hardest and most compact part of the tooth. The cementum is a think layer of bone, deposited on the surface of the root. The neck of the tooth is the part between the crown and the root. The gingiva is the soft tissue of the gum that surrounds the neck. A shallow groove called the gingival sulcus surrounds the neck of each tooth.

Teeth erupt from the gums when there is sufficient calcification for the tooth to be able to tolerate the stress that it will be subjected to later on. Deciduous teeth erupt from the gums starting at about 7 months and finishing at about age 2½. The permanent teeth erupt at about the following ages:

First molars	6th to 7th year
Two central incisors	7th to 8th year
Two lateral incisors	8th to 9th year
First premolars	10th to 11th year
Second premolars	10th to 12th year
Canines	11th to 12th year
Second molars	12th to 13th year
Third molars	17th to 21st year

Pharynx

The pharynx lies posterior to the mouth and is the beginning of the tube leading to the stomach. The pharynx is used by both the respiratory system and the digestive system. Both the larynx and the esophagus begin in the pharynx. Anything that is swallowed passes through the pharynx into the esophagus reflexively. Muscular constructions move the ball of food into the esophagus while closing the trachea to prevent food from entering the trachea.

Esophagus

The esophagus is a collapsible tube, about 10 inches long, that starts at the pharynx and ends at the stomach. Food is carried down the esophagus by a series of muscular contractions called peristalsis. These wave-like contractions will move the bolus of food along through the entire digestive system.

Stomach

The stomach is a large sac-like organ that holds food for the beginning of the digestive process (see Figure 28-5). The stomach holds about 1 to 1.5 liters of food and fluid at a time. The stomach secretes hydrochloric acid and gastric juices to convert food into a semiliquid state to be passed into the small intestine for further digestion.

Small Intestine

The small intestine is 21 feet long, and about 1 inch in diameter (see Figure 28-6). The opening of the small

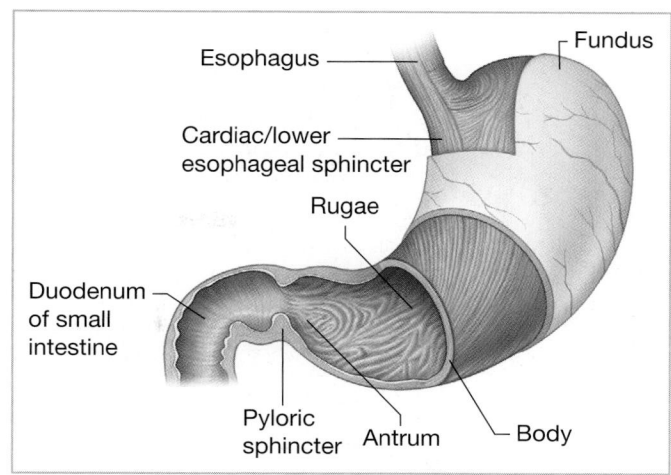

FIGURE 28-5 Stomach.

intestine, the pyloric sphincter, is at the base of the stomach. The first 12 inches of the small intestine is the duodenum, the second 8 feet is called the jejunum, and the ileum consists of the last 12 feet of intestine. Semi-liquid food (now called *chime*) is received from the stomach through the pylorus and mixed with bile from the liver and gallbladder along with pancreatic juice from the pancreas. Digestion and absorption of nutrients occur in the small intestine. Nutrients are absorbed into tiny capillaries and lymph vessels located in the walls of the small intestine and transmitted to the body cells via the circulatory system.

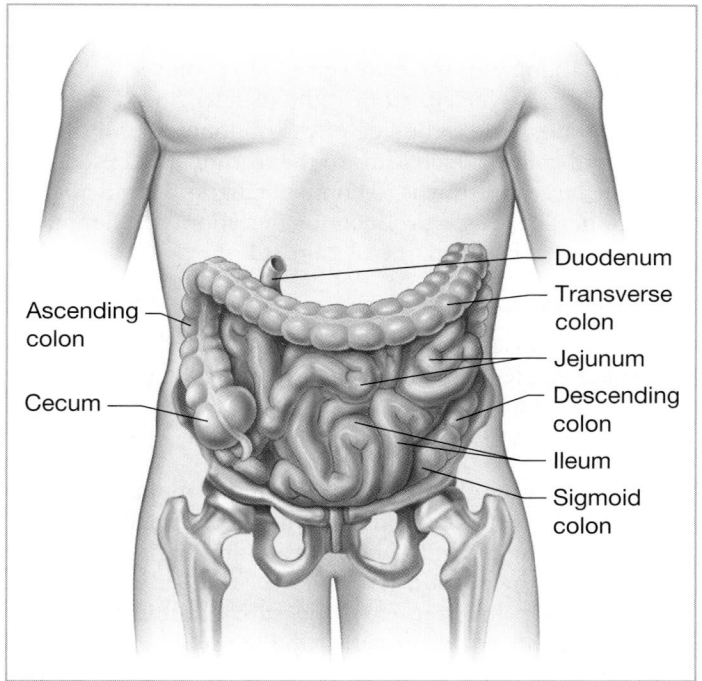

FIGURE 28-6 Small intestine.

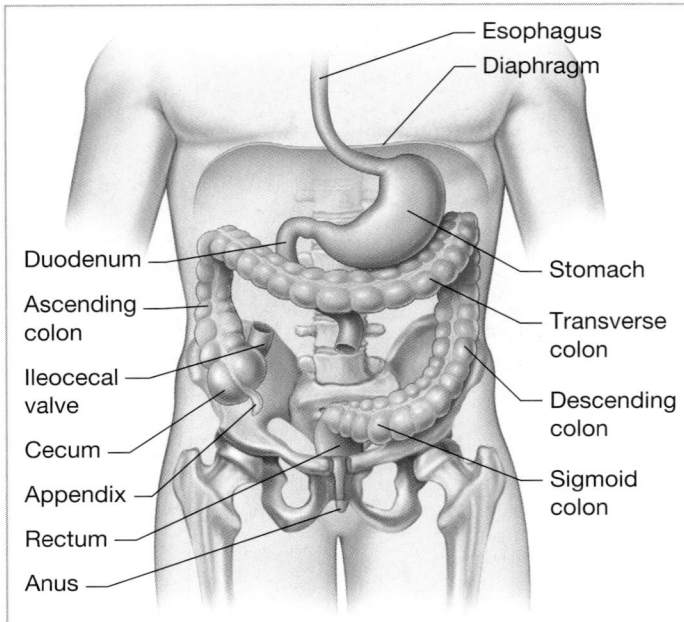

FIGURE 28-7 Large intestine (colon).

Large Intestine

The small intestine terminates at the ileocecal orifice at the large intestine. The large intestine starts at this terminus, and continues through the cecum (a small pouch about 3 inches long), the colon, the rectum, and the anal canal (see Figure 28-7). The large intestine is 5 feet long and about 2.5 inches in diameter. The appendix is a small appendage attached to the cecum that has no known function in humans. The colon makes up the bulk of the large intestine and is divided into several parts: the ascending colon (on the right side of the abdomen), the transverse colon (moves across the body transversely from right to left), the descending colon (on the right side of the abdomen), and the sigmoid colon, which leads to the rectum. The function of the large intestine is to complete digestion and absorption. The waste products of digestion are eliminated from the body via the rectum and the anus.

Accessory Organs

The accessory organs of digestion include the salivary glands, the gallbladder, the liver, and the pancreas (see Figure 28-8).

Salivary Glands

The salivary glands are located in the mouth, and produce saliva in response to the sight, smell, taste, or mental images of food. There are three pairs of salivary glands: the parotid (located on either side of the face slightly below the ear), the submandibular (located on the floor of the mouth), and the sublingual (located below the tongue). All of the salivary glands secrete saliva through openings into the mouth. Saliva con-

tains amylase—an enzyme that helps to start the break down of carbohydrates.

Gallbladder

The gallbladder is a membranous sac where bile is stored and concentrated. Any bile stored in the gallbladder is 10 times more concentrated than bile not stored in the gallbladder. Because of the function of concentrating bile, gallstones can occur, as can inflammation of the gallbladder. This condition is called cholelithiasis.

Liver

The liver is located on the upper right quadrant of the abdomen. It is the largest glandular organ and weight about 3.5 pounds. The liver plays an essential role in the metabolism of carbohydrates, fats, and proteins. The liver changes glucose to glycogen, and stores that glycogen as a product of carbohydrate metabolism.

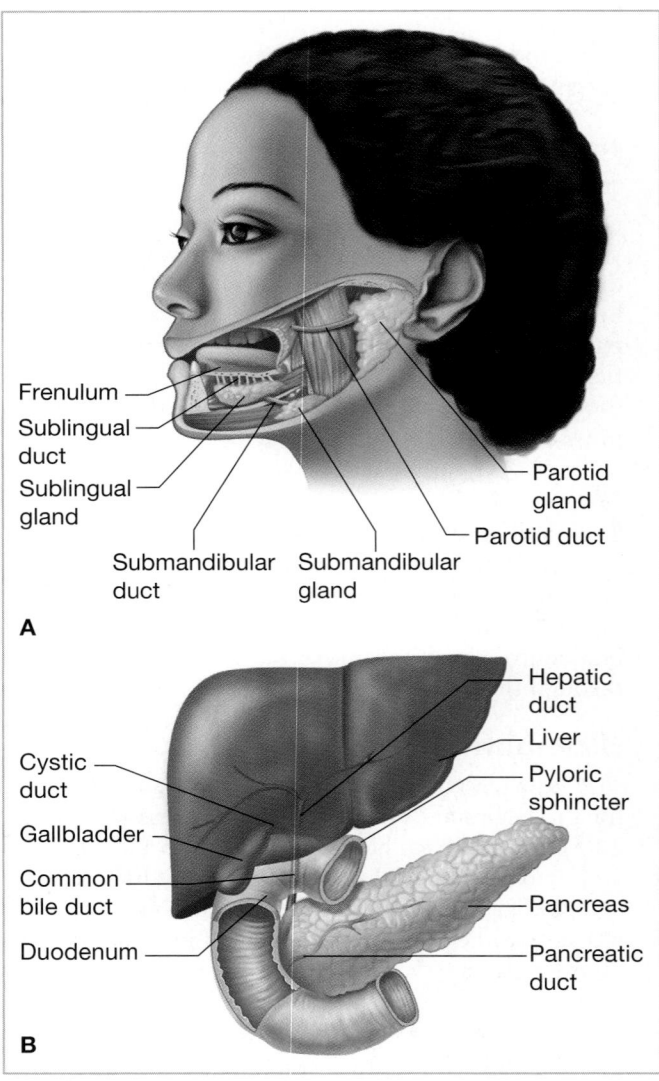

FIGURE 28-8 (A) Salivary glands; (B) gallbladder, liver, and pancreas.

The liver produces bile, which emulsifies fats for fat metabolism before releasing the products into the bloodstream. For protein metabolism, the liver acts as a storage place for the components of proteins, so the body can break down or build up proteins as it requires.

The liver manufactures four important substances for the function of the body:

- Bile—emulsifies fats
- Fibrinogen and prothrombin—essential for blood clotting
- Heparin—prevents the clotting of blood
- Blood proteins—albumin, gamma globulin

The liver also stores iron and the vitamins B_{12}, A, D, E, and K. The liver produces body heat and detoxifies the body from substances such as drugs and alcohol.

Pancreas

The pancreas is a long, elongated gland situated behind the stomach that secretes pancreatic juice into the small intestine. The pancreas is 6 to 9 inches long and contains cells that produce digestive enzymes. Other cells in the pancreas secrete the hormones insulin and glucagon, which lower and raise glucose levels in the blood.

Common Disorders Associated with the Digestive System

Digestive disorders range from the occasional upset stomach, heartburn, and nausea to the more serious and life-threatening colorectal cancer. These disorders encompass the gastrointestinal tract as well as the liver, gallbladder, and pancreas. Most digestive disorders and diseases are complex, with subtle symptoms, and the causes of many remain unknown (see Table 28-1). Some may be genetic or develop from multiple factors such as stress, fatigue, diet, or smoking. Alcohol abuse also poses a risk for digestive disorders. Diagnosis of a digestive disorder requires a thorough and accurate medical history and physical examination. Some may need to undergo more extensive diagnostic evaluations including laboratory tests, endoscopic procedures, and imaging techniques.

Appendicitis

The appendix is a small, tube-like structure attached to the first part of the large intestine, also called the colon. The appendix is located in the lower right portion of the abdomen. It has no known function, and removal of this structure appears to cause no change in digestive function. Appendicitis is an inflammation of the appendix.

Lifespan
Considerations

THE CHILD

- A child's digestive system continues to develop throughout the first year of life. Many environmental factors can stress a child's digestive system. Aside from the dietary factors, children are exposed to heavy metals, pollutants, solvents, and carcinogens found in food, water, air, medicine, and plastics that can injure the digestive system.

- Digestive disorders affecting infants and children range from simple problems that most children experience from time to time, such as vomiting or diarrhea, to more serious (and possibly life-threatening) birth defects such as tracheoesophageal fistula, or illnesses such as appendicitis.

- Digestive and liver disorders can have significant effects on the health of a child. A healthy digestive system processes the foods and liquids that we eat, replenishing vitamins, minerals, proteins, carbohydrates, and fats that are vital for the body to function properly. Occasional vomiting or diarrhea may lead to dehydration; however, long-term problems with the digestive system and/or liver can deplete these important nutrients, causing malnutrition that affects a child's physical and mental growth and development.

THE OLDER ADULT

- The digestive system becomes less motile with aging, as muscle contractions become weaker. Glandular secretions decrease, causing a drier mouth and a lower volume of gastric juices. Nutrient absorption decreases due to the atrophy of the mucosal lining. Because of age and continued use, the gums recede and the tooth surfaces wear down. There may be a loss of taste, and food preferences may change.

- Gastric motor activity slows, causing delayed gastric emptying and decrease in hunger contractions. Although there are no significant changes in the small intestine, the muscle layer and the blood flow through the large intestine begin to decline. Constipation can be a frequent problem, especially because of a decrease in dietary and fluid intake.

TABLE 28-1 Disorders and Pathology of the Digestive System

Disorder/Pathology	Description
Anorexia	Loss of appetite that can accompany other conditions such as a gastrointestinal (GI) upset.
Ascites	Collection or accumulation of fluid in the peritoneal cavity.
Bulimia	Eating disorder that is characterized by recurrent binge eating and then purging of the food with laxatives and vomiting.
Cholecystitis	Inflammation of the gallbladder.
Cholelithiasis	Formation or presence of stones or calculi in the gallbladder or common bile duct.
Cirrhosis	Chronic disease of the liver.
Cleft lip	Congenital condition in which the upper lip fails to come together. This is often seen along with cleft palate and is corrected with surgery.
Cleft plate	Congenital condition in which the roof of the mouth has a split or fissure. It is corrected with surgery.
Constipation	Experiencing difficulty in defecation or infrequent defecation.
Crohn's disease	Form of chronic inflammatory bowel disease affecting the ileum or colon. Also called regional ileitis.
Diarrhea	Passing of frequent, watery bowel movements. Usually accompanies gastrointestinal (GI) disorders.
Diverticulitis	Inflammation of a diverticulum or sac in the intestinal tract, especially in the colon.
Dyspepsia	Indigestion.
Emesis	Vomiting usually with some force.
Enteritis	Inflammation of only the small intestine.
Esophageal stricture	Narrowing of the esophagus, which makes the flow of foods and fluids difficult.
Fissure	Crack-like split in the rectum or anal canal or roof of mouth.
Fistula	Abnormal tube-like passage from one body cavity to another.
Gastritis	Inflammation of the stomach, which can result in pain, tenderness, nausea, and vomiting.
Gastroenteritis	Inflammation of the stomach and small intestine.
Halitosis	Bad or offensive breath, which is often a sign of disease.
Hepatitis	Inflammation of the liver.
Ileitis	Inflammation of the ileum of the small intestine.
Inflammatory bowel syndrome	Ulceration of the mucous membranes of the colon of unknown origin. Also known as ulcerative colitis.

(continued)

TABLE 28-1 **Disorders and Pathology of the Digestive System** (*continued*)

Disorder/Pathology	Description
Inguinal hernia	Hernia or outpouching of intestines into the inguinal region of the body. May require surgical correction.
Intussusception	Result of the intestine slipping or telescoping into another section of intestine just below it. More common in children.
Irritable bowel syndrome	Disturbance in the functions of the intestine from unknown causes. Symptoms generally include abdominal discomfort and an alteration in bowel activity.
Malabsorption syndrome	Inadequate absorption of nutrients from the intestinal tract. May be caused by a variety of diseases and disorders, such as infections and pancreatic deficiency.
Peptic ulcer	Ulcer occurring in the lower portion of the esophagus, stomach, and duodenum thought to be caused by the acid of gastric juices. Some peptic ulcers are now successfully treated with antibiotics.
Pilonidal cyst	Cyst in the sacrococcygeal region due to tissue being trapped below the skin.
Polyphagia	To eat excessively.
Polyps	Small tumors that contain a pedicle or foot-like attachment in the mucous membranes of the large intestine (colon).
Reflux esophagitis	Acid from the stomach backs up into the esophagus causing inflammation and pain. Also called GERD (gastroesophageal reflux disease).
Regurgitation	Return of fluids and solids from the stomach into the mouth. Similar to emesis but without the force.
Ulcerative colitis	Ulceration of the mucous membranes of the colon of unknown source. Also known as inflammatory bowel disease.
Volvulus	Condition in which the bowel twists upon itself and causes an obstruction. Painful and requires immediate surgery.

Once it starts, there is no effective medical therapy, so appendicitis is considered a medical emergency. When treated promptly, most patients recover without difficulty. If treatment is delayed, however, the appendix can burst, causing infection and even death. Anyone can get appendicitis, but it occurs most often between the ages of 10 and 30. The cause of appendicitis relates to blockage of the inside of the appendix, known as the lumen. This blockage leads to increased pressure, impaired blood flow, and inflammation.

Appendicitis is the most common acute surgical emergency of the abdomen. The appendix is almost always removed, even if it is found to be normal. With complete removal, any later episodes of pain will not be attributed to appendicitis. If the diagnosis is uncertain, people may be watched and sometimes treated with antibiotics. This approach is taken when the doctor suspects that the patient's symptoms may have a nonsurgical or treatable cause. If the cause of the pain is infectious, symptoms resolve with intravenous antibiotics and intravenous fluids.

Cirrhosis

Cirrhosis is a potentially life-threatening condition that occurs when scarring damages the liver. This scarring (also called *fibrosis*) replaces healthy tissue and prevents the liver from working normally. Cirrhosis usually develops after years of liver inflammation.

Cirrhosis can have many causes. Some people have cirrhosis without an obvious cause (cryptogenic cirrhosis). In the United States, the major causes of cirrhosis are drinking excessive amounts of alcohol over many years or having certain forms of viral hepatitis (mainly hepatitis B or C). Cirrhosis may be caused by a condition in which too much fat is stored in the liver, or when the ducts that carry bile out of the liver become inflamed and blocked. The latter may be related to a problem with the immune system. Another type of cirrhosis can be caused as a result of the immune system attacking the liver, a condition known as autoimmune hepatitis. Sometimes cirrhosis can be caused by an inherited disease, such as cystic fibrosis.

In many cases, symptoms develop only after the disease progresses. They may include fluid buildup in the legs (edema) and abdomen (ascites), fatigue, yellowing of the skin (jaundice), itching, nosebleeds, redness of the palms, bleeding from enlarged veins in the digestive tract, easy bruising, weight loss and muscle loss, abdominal pain, frequent infections, and confusion.

Treatment focuses on avoiding substances that can further damage the liver, especially alcohol and nonsteroidal anti-inflammatory drugs; making dietary changes; and using medications, surgery, and other treatment to prevent and treat complications. A liver transplant may be considered when liver damage is severe.

Colitis

Colitis is an inflammation of the large intestine that may be caused by many different disease processes, including acute and chronic infections, primary inflammatory disorders (ulcerative colitis, Crohn's colitis, lymphocytic and collagenous colitis), lack of blood flow (ischemic colitis), and history of radiation to the large bowel. Symptoms can include abdominal pain, diarrhea, dehydration, abdominal bloating, increased intestinal gas, and bloody stools. The disorder may be identified by flexible sigmoidoscopy or colonoscopy. In both of these tests, a flexible tube is inserted in the rectum, and specific areas of the colon are evaluated. Biopsies taken during these tests may show changes related to inflammation. Other studies that can iden-

tify colitis include barium enema, abdominal CT scan, abdominal MRI, and abdominal x-ray. Treatment is directed at the underlying cause of disease, whether it is infection, inflammation, lack of blood flow, or another cause.

Colorectal Cancer

Colon cancer is cancer of the large intestine (colon), the lower part of the digestive system. Rectal cancer is cancer of the last 8 to 10 inches of the colon. Together, they are often referred to as colorectal cancers, and they make up the second-leading cause of cancer-related deaths in the United States. Only lung cancer claims more lives.

Most cases of colon cancer begin as small, noncancerous (benign) clumps of cells called adenomatous polyps. Over time some of these polyps become cancerous. The polyps may be small and produce few, if any, symptoms; therefore, regular screening tests are important to help prevent colon cancer. If signs and symptoms of cancer do appear, they may include a change in bowel habits, blood in the stool, persistent cramping, gas, or abdominal pain.

Screening tests, along with a few simple changes in your diet and lifestyle, can dramatically reduce a person's overall risk of developing colon cancer. The type of treatment the physician recommends will depend largely on the stage of the cancer. The three primary treatment options are surgery, chemotherapy, and radiation. Surgery is the main treatment for colorectal cancer. How much of the colon is removed and whether other therapies, such as radiation or chemotherapy, are an option will be determined depending on how far the cancer has penetrated into the wall of the bowel and whether it has spread to the lymph nodes or other parts of the body.

Constipation

Constipation occurs when stools are difficult to pass. Constipation is said to be present if a person has two or fewer bowel movements each week or has two or more of the following problems at least 25% of the time: straining, a feeling of not completely emptying the bowels, and hard or pellet-like stools. Lack of fiber and dehydration are common causes of constipation. Other causes may include irritable bowel syndrome, travel or other changes in one's daily routine, lack of exercise, immobility caused by illness or aging, medication use, overuse of laxatives, and pregnancy. Constipation may occur with cramping and pain in the rectum caused by the strain of trying to pass hard, dry stools. There may also be some bloating and nausea. Sometimes there may be small amounts of bright red blood on the stool or on the toilet tissue, caused by bleeding hemorrhoids or a slight tearing of the anus (anal fissure) as the stool

Preparing for
Externship

Communicating with patients can be challenging, especially with those individuals who may have difficulties hearing or understanding. Communicating can be extra difficult for individuals who are not native to the area in which they live. Be sure to speak slowly and very clearly, and encourage patients and families to repeat your instructions to be sure that they understand.

is pushed through the anus. This should stop when the constipation is controlled.

Constipation can usually be treated effectively at home, often through exercise, good nutritional habits, and a change of lifestyle that provides for a scheduled time each day for bowel movements. Laxatives may also be used.

Crohn's Disease

Crohn's disease is a chronic inflammatory disease of the intestines. It primarily causes ulcerations, or breaks in the lining of the small and large intestines, but can affect the digestive system anywhere from the mouth to the anus. Crohn's disease is related closely to another chronic inflammatory condition that involves only the colon called ulcerative colitis. Together, Crohn's disease and ulcerative colitis are frequently referred to as inflammatory bowel disease (IBD). They affect approximately 500,000 to 2 million people in the United States. Crohn's disease also tends to be more common in relatives of patients with Crohn's disease or ulcerative colitis.

The cause of Crohn's disease is unknown. Some scientists suspect that infection by certain bacteria, such as strains of mycobacterium, may be the cause of Crohn's disease. Crohn's disease is not contagious. Although diet may affect the symptoms in patients with Crohn's disease, it is unlikely that diet is responsible for the disease.

Common symptoms of Crohn's disease include abdominal pain, diarrhea, and weight loss. Less common symptoms include poor appetite, fever, night sweats, rectal pain, and rectal bleeding. Patients with mild or no symptoms may not need treatment. Patients whose disease is in remission (where symptoms are absent) also may not need treatment. There is no medication that can cure Crohn's disease. Patients with Crohn's disease typically will experience periods of relapse (worsening of inflammation) followed by periods of remission (reduced inflammation) lasting months to years.

Because there is no cure for Crohn's disease, the goals of treatment are to induce remissions, maintain remissions, minimize side effects of treatment, and improve the quality of life. Treatment of Crohn's disease and ulcerative colitis with medications is similar though not always identical. These medications may include anti-inflammatory agents such as 5-ASA compounds, corticosteroids, topical antibiotics, or immunomodulators.

Diarrhea

Diarrhea is an increase in the frequency of bowel movements or a decrease in the form of stool (greater looseness of stool). Although changes in frequency of bowel movements and looseness of stools can vary in-

Professionalism

Ensuring that patients and their families understand instructions and explanations can present difficulties. Never address any patient with nicknames such as "sweetie" or "honey." Many individuals consider these terms derisive and unprofessional. Instead, address all adults as Mr. or Ms. or Mrs. unless otherwise instructed. If you are working in an office where English is the primary language and your first language is not English, or if you have a heavy regional accent not native to your office, practice speaking very clearly so that those who have hearing difficulties can still understand your instructions. Supplement verbal instructions with clearly written instructions to help increase understanding. Be sure all explanations are not in medical terminology, but do not oversimplify so that the patients feel "talked down to."

dependently of each other, changes usually occur in both.

Diarrhea generally is divided into two types, acute and chronic. Acute diarrhea lasts a few days or up to a week. Chronic diarrhea can be defined in several ways but almost always lasts more than 3 weeks. It is important to distinguish between acute and chronic diarrhea because they usually have different causes, require different diagnostic tests, and require different treatment.

The most common cause of acute diarrhea is infection—viral, bacterial, and parasitic. Bacteria can also cause acute food poisoning. A third important cause of acute diarrhea is medications.

Diarrhea is usually treated through the use of absorbents and antimotility medications. Absorbents are compounds that absorb water. When they are taken orally, they bind water in the small intestine and colon and make diarrheal stools less watery. They also may bind toxic chemicals produced by bacteria that cause the small intestine to secrete fluid; however, the importance of toxin binding in reducing diarrhea is unclear. Antimotility medications are drugs that relax the muscles of the small intestine or the colon. Relaxation results in slower flow of intestinal contents. Slower flow allows more time for water to be absorbed from the intestine and colon and reduces the water content of stool. Cramps, due to spasm of the intestinal muscles, also are relieved by the muscular relaxation.

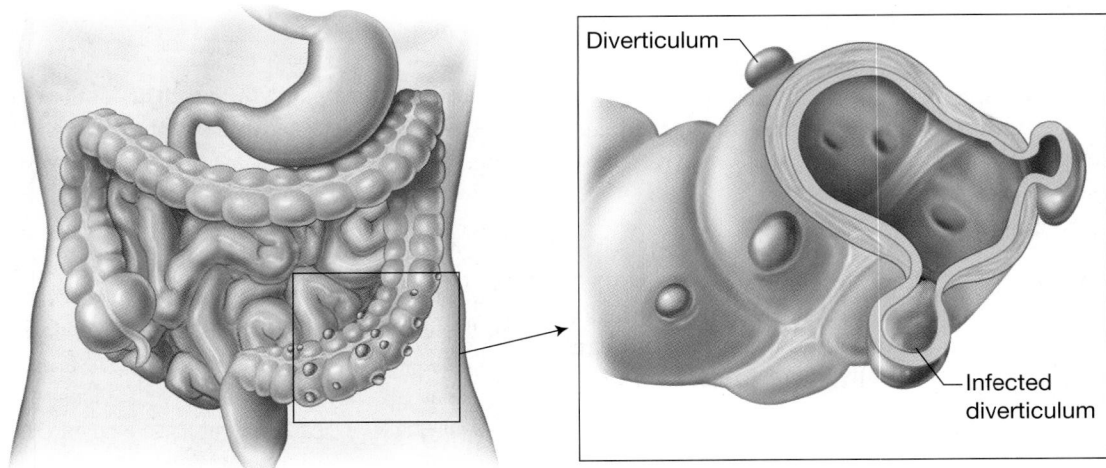

FIGURE 28-9   Colon with diverticulosis. An infected diverticulum is called diverticulitis.

Diverticulitis

Diverticulitis is an inflammation of a small pouch or sac of the walls called a diverticulum that may occur in the wall of the colon (see Figure 28-9). The exact cause of diverticulitis is not known, but generally begins when stool lodges in the diverticula. Infection can lead to complications, including swelling or rupture. Symptoms include pain, fever, chills, cramping, bloating, constipation, or diarrhea. The treatment will depend on the severity of the condition.

Diverticulosis

Diverticulosis is the condition of having diverticula, or small outpouchings, from the large intestine, the colon (see Figure 28-9). It can occur anywhere in the colon

but it is most typical in the sigmoid colon, the S-shaped segment of the colon located in the left lower part of the abdomen. The incidence of diverticulosis increases with age. This is because age causes a weakening of the walls of the colon and this weakening permits the formation of diverticula. By age 80, most people have diverticulosis.

A key factor promoting the formation of diverticulosis is elevated pressure within the colon. The pressure within the colon is raised when a person is constipated and has to push down to pass small, hard bits of stool.

Most patients with diverticulosis have few or no symptoms although some have mild symptoms including abdominal cramping and bloating. This condition does, however, set the stage for inflammation and infection of the outpouching, a condition called diverticulitis.

The best way to avoid developing diverticulosis is to eat a healthy diet with plenty of fiber. A diet high in fiber keeps the bowels moving, keeps the pressure within the colon within normal limits, and slows or stops the formation of diverticula.

Gastroesophageal Reflux Disease

Gastroesophageal reflux disease (GERD) occurs when the muscle at the superior portion of the stomach (the cardiac sphincter) does not close tightly, or relaxes inappropriately, allowing for a "backwash" of gastric fluids and stomach contents back up the esophagus and into the throat. Individuals with GERD may have symptoms, but there are also quite a few incidences where the patient is symptom free. Symptoms may include heartburn, sore throat, hoarse voice, bad taste in the patient's mouth, belching, and regurgitation of food. If not treated, the patient may begin to suffer from reflux esophagitis, a potentially serious disease resulting from damage to the tissues of the esophagus

Legal and Ethical Issues

Some digestive disorders, such as stomach ulcers, IBS, and GERD, may be associated with a person's lifestyle. Your role, as a member of the health care profession, is to provide care and assist with the treatment of your patients, and it is never acceptable, nor appropriate, to judge or make reference to how a person chooses to live his or her life. You are, however, when required, expected to provide patients with information and education regarding how they can best manage their conditions and, at the same time, live a long and productive life.

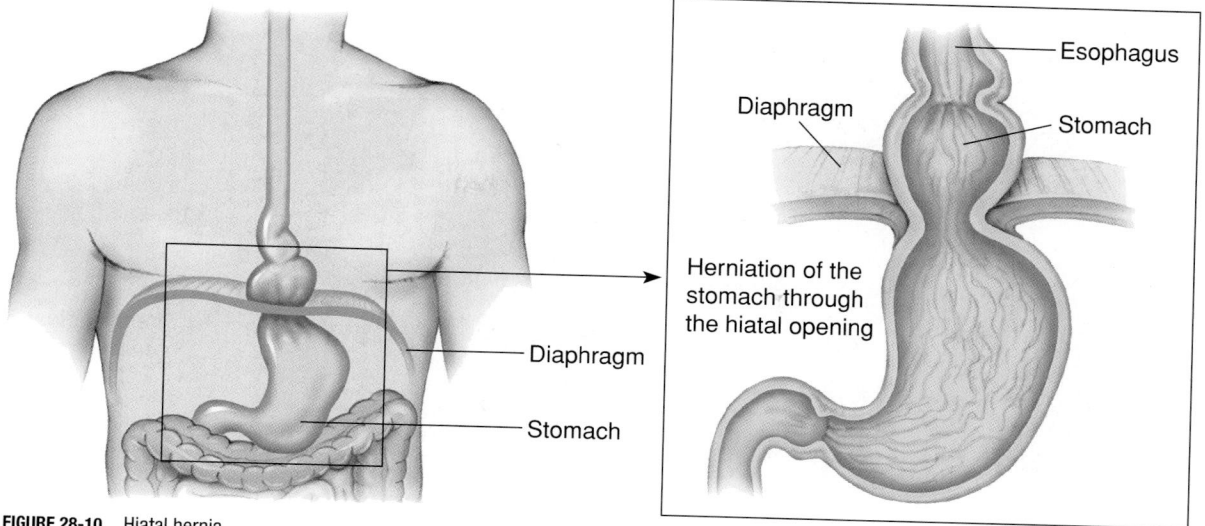

FIGURE 28-10 Hiatal hernia.

by the acidic fluids from the stomach. Barrett's esophagitis, a precancerous condition can also be a result of GERD, and must be treated. Other possible results of long-term, untreated GERD include perforation of the esophagus, esophageal cancer, esophageal stricture (abnormal narrowing of the esophagus), and esophageal ulcers.

Treatment of GERD relies on medications that block the production of hydrochloric acid (the chief digestive acid) and that protect the mucosa of the esophagus. Other simple treatments taught to patients include not lying down until at least 3 hours after eating, weight loss, sleeping on a bed that has the head raised 6 inches, and sleeping on the left side. If medications and basic treatments do not work, surgery called a fundoplication, which tightens the cardiac sphincter and its surrounding tissues, can be performed. Strictures are treated with dilation, or expansion, of the narrowed area.

Hemorrhoids

A hemorrhoid is a dilated, or enlarged, vein in the walls of the anus and sometimes around the rectum, usually caused by untreated constipation but occasionally associated with chronic diarrhea. Symptoms start with bleeding after defecation. If untreated, hemorrhoids can worsen, protruding from the anus. In their worst stage, they must be returned to the anal cavity manually. Fissures can develop, and these may cause intense discomfort. Treatment is by changing the diet to prevent constipation and avoid further irritation, the use of topical medication, and sometimes surgery or sclerotherapy.

Hernia

A hernia is an abnormal protrusion of an organ, or part of an organ through the wall of the body cavity where

it is located. The most common types of abdominal hernias are hiatal hernias and inguinal hernias.

Hiatal Hernia

Hiatal hernia is a condition in which the upper portion of the stomach protrudes into the chest cavity through an opening of the diaphragm called the esophageal hiatus (see Figure 28-10). This opening usually is large enough to accommodate the esophagus alone. With weakening and enlargement, however, the opening (or herniation) can allow upward passage or even entrapment of the upper stomach above the diaphragm. Hiatal hernia is a common condition. By age 60, up to 60 percent of people have it to some degree.

Suspected causes or contributing factors of hiatal hernia include obesity, poor seated posture (such as slouching), frequent coughing, straining with constipation, frequent bending over or heavy lifting, heredity, smoking, and congenital defects.

Some of the symptoms that may be present include chest pain or pressure, heartburn, difficulty swallowing, coughing, belching, and hiccups. Hiatal hernia also causes symptoms of discomfort when it is associated with gastroesophageal reflux disease. GERD is characterized by the upwelling of stomach acids and digestive enzymes into the esophagus through a weakened sphincter that is supposed to act as a one-way valve between the esophagus and stomach. Hiatal hernia is thought to contribute to the weakening of this sphincter muscle.

Inguinal Hernia

An inguinal hernia occurs when tissue or part of the intestine pushes through a weak spot in the abdominal wall in the groin area, causing a bulge in the groin or scrotum (see Figure 28-11).

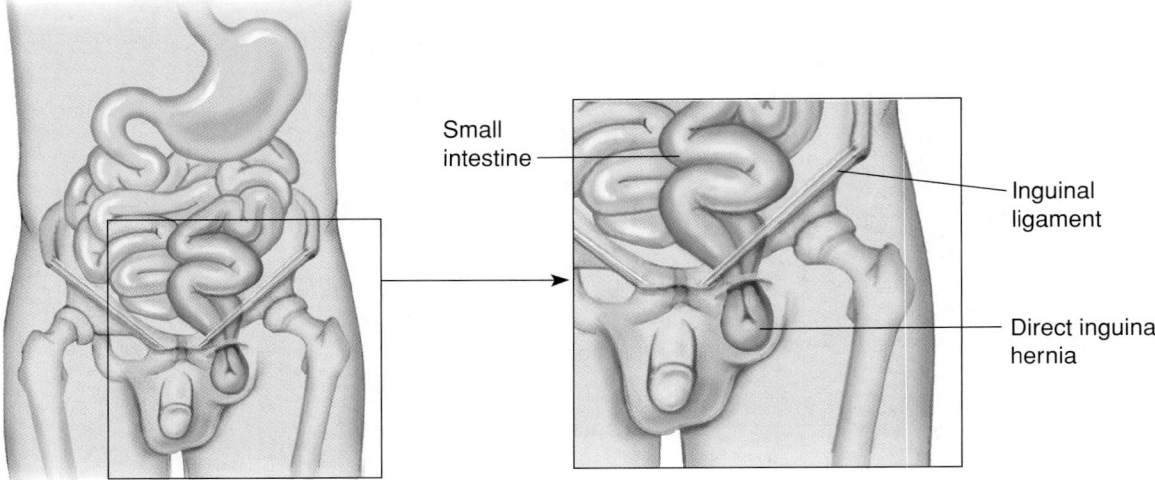

FIGURE 28-11 Inguinal hernia.

The bulge may appear gradually over a period of several weeks or months, or it may form suddenly after you have been lifting heavy weights, coughing, bending, straining, or laughing. Many hernias flatten when you lie down. Pain and discomfort may also be present and is usually worse when a person bends or lifts an object. While men may have pain or discomfort in the scrotum, many hernias do not cause any pain. Nausea and vomiting may also be present if part of the intestine bulges outside the abdomen and becomes trapped (incarcerated) in the hernia.

Other symptoms of a hernia may include heaviness, swelling, and a tugging or burning sensation in the area of the hernia, scrotum, or inner thigh. Males may have a swollen scrotum, and females may have a bulge in the large fold of skin (labia) surrounding the vagina. Discomfort and aching are relieved only when the person lies down. This is often the case as the hernia grows larger.

Surgery is the only treatment and cure for inguinal hernia. Hernia repair is one of the most common surgeries done in the United States. About 750,000 people have hernia repairs each year. However, if an inguinal hernia does not cause any symptoms, it may not need treatment.

Irritable Bowel Syndrome

Irritable bowel syndrome (IBS) is a common intestinal condition characterized by abdominal pain and cramps, changes in bowel movements (diarrhea, constipation, or both), gassiness, bloating, and nausea. Other symptoms—which vary from person to person—include cramps, a powerful and uncontrollable urge to defecate (urgency), passage of a sticky fluid (mucus) during bowel movements, or the feeling after finishing a bowel movement that the bowels are still not com-

pletely empty. There is no cure for IBS. Much about the condition remains unknown or poorly understood; however, dietary changes, drugs, and psychological treatment are often able to eliminate or substantially reduce its symptoms. The symptoms of IBS tend to rise and fall in intensity rather than growing steadily worse over time.

Researchers remain unsure about the cause or causes of IBS. It is called a functional disorder because it is thought to result from changes in the activity of the major part of the large intestine (the colon). Stress is an important factor in IBS because of the close nervous system connections between the brain and the intestines. Although researchers do not yet understand all of the links between changes in the nervous system and IBS, they point out the similarities between mild digestive upsets and IBS. Just as healthy people can feel nauseated or have an upset stomach when under stress, people with IBS react the same way, but to a greater degree. Finally, IBS symptoms sometimes intensify during menstruation, which suggests that female reproductive hormones are another trigger.

Dietary changes, sometimes supplemented by drugs or psychotherapy, are considered keys to the successful treatment of IBS.

Oral Cancer

Oral cancer starts in the cells of the mouth (oral cavity). Almost all cases of oral cancer start in the flat squamous cells that line the mouth. Squamous cell carcinoma can start on the lips, inside the lips and cheeks (buccal mucosa), the gums (gingiva), the front two-thirds of the tongue, the tissue under the tongue (the floor of the mouth), the tissue behind the wisdom teeth, and the bony roof of the mouth (hard palate).

There is no single cause of oral cancer, but several factors appear to increase the risk of developing it. These include age, particularly after 50; gender—more men develop oral cancer; smoking, particularly if combined with heavy alcohol consumption; chewing tobacco or using snuff; heavy alcohol consumption, particularly if combined with smoking; excessive sun exposure to the lips; some medical problems in the mouth tissues; and chewing betel nut.

The signs and symptoms of oral cancer can be seen and felt quite early. Pain is very rare in early oral cancer, but any sore, irritation, or swelling in the mouth or lump on the neck that lasts longer than 2 weeks should be checked by a doctor or dentist. Velvety red or white patches in the mouth may also indicate a precancerous condition. Sores or wart-like patches on the lip, a persistent sore throat, sores under dentures, a lump in the lip, tongue, or neck, and trouble chewing, swallowing, or speaking are all symptoms.

Treatment of oral cancer will depend on the extent of the condition. Surgery to remove part or all of the tumor and some surrounding tissue may be required. Radiation and chemotherapy, that is, the use of drugs or medications that interfere with the cancer cell's ability to grow and spread, may also be used in the treatment of oral cancer.

Pancreatic Cancer

The most common type of pancreatic cancer arises from the exocrine glands and is called adenocarcinoma of the pancreas. The endocrine glands of the pancreas can give rise to a completely different type of cancer, referred to as pancreatic neuroendocrine carcinoma or islet cell tumor, which is considered very rare. In 2004, approximately 31,800 people in the United States were diagnosed with pancreatic cancer, and approximately 31,200 people died of this disease. These numbers reflect the challenge in treating pancreatic cancer and the relative lack of curative options.

The symptoms of pancreatic cancer are generally vague and can easily be attributed to other less serious and more common conditions. This lack of specific symptoms explains the high number of people who have a more advanced stage of the disease when pancreatic cancer is eventually discovered. The main symptoms include pain in the abdomen, the back, or both; weight loss, often associated with loss of appetite; bloating; diarrhea or fatty bowel movements that float in water; and jaundice or yellowing of the skin.

Complete surgical removal of the cancer is the only known cure for pancreatic cancer. Only 15 to 20 percent of people with pancreatic cancer have disease that

Cultural Considerations

Culture seems to play a major role in how people eat and view disorders of their digestive system. Hindus, for example, believe in fasting and in eating a specific way. While Americans may believe such a lifestyle could lead to digestive problems, the Hindu religion believes their dietary experiences are part of what makes them at one with God. Other cultures, such as those in the Far East, believe that alternative medicine therapies, such as acupuncture, homeopathy, meditation, and biofeedback, are frequently more useful than western medicine in treating disorders of the digestive system. While there may appear to be many cultural stereotypes regarding specific diseases of the digestive system, as a member of the health care team, it is important to remember to always respect a person's beliefs and focus on supporting and treating the patient. When asking questions or assisting in a treatment, make sure that the questions are not disrespectful and your care is directed at the "total" patient, and not just the disease.

Patient Education

When teaching patients about a bland diet, it is important to take their cultural preferences into consideration. Be sure patients understand which foods in their diet are appropriate and which should be temporarily avoided. This may require asking patients or their families for more information regarding their dietary preferences. It is also important to be sure that all patients understand the need to avoid alcohol and tobacco until their conditions have healed.

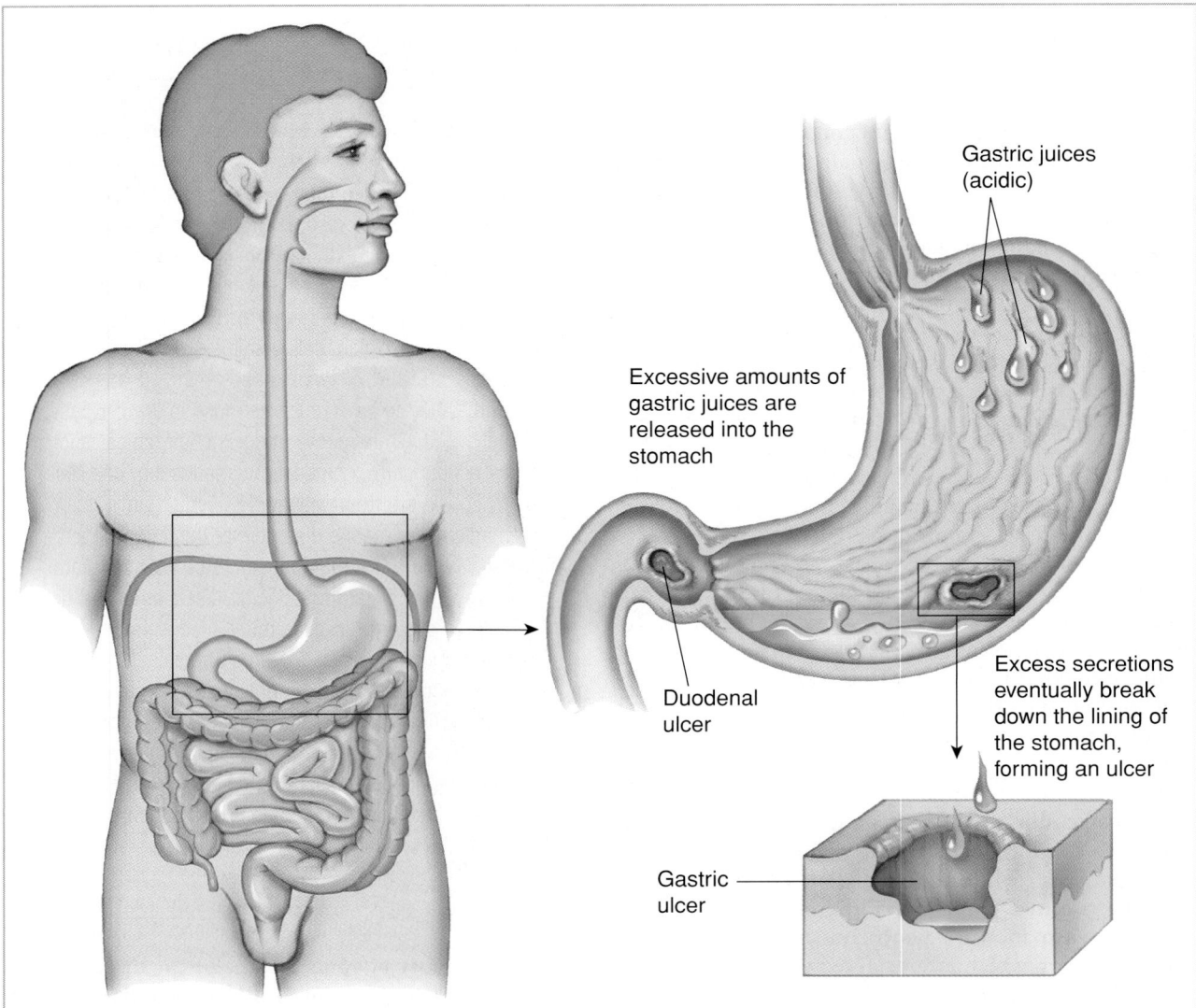

FIGURE 28-12 Peptic ulcer disease (PUD).

can be surgically removed at the time of diagnosis. Depending on how advanced the cancer is, chemotherapy and radiation therapy may also be included in the treatment of pancreatic cancer.

Peptic Ulcer Disease

Peptic ulcer disease (PUD) occurs when there is a disruption in the lining of the esophagus, stomach, or duodenum (see Figure 28-12). The most frequent location for PUD is in the duodenum (the upper part of the small intestine). Peptic ulcers (ones that occur in the stomach) are also common.

Peptic ulcers are most likely caused by an imbalance between acid and pepsin (a stomach acid) secretion and the defenses of the mucosal lining. Inflammation results, causing some of the discomfort. This inflammation may be caused or aggravated by aspirin or nonsteroidal anti-inflammatories (NSAIDs) such as ibuprofen. Because of the resulting erosion of the stomach mucosa, a bacteria

called *Helicobacter pylori* can cause infection, further aggravating the situation.

The most common symptoms of PUD are abdominal pain, nausea, vomiting, and weight loss. Esophageal ulcers often include heartburn and chest pain. Other symptoms that may occur include black, tar-like or maroon stools (indicating old blood), fresh blood in the stool, and a burning or gnawing pain in the stomach or the back.

Prevention of ulcers includes avoiding alcohol and tobacco, and limiting the use of NSAIDs and aspirin. Spicy foods do not cause ulcers, but can aggravate the condition.

Treatment of PUD depends on the cause. Any medications that may be causing or aggravating the condition need to be changed. Tobacco use and alcohol should be avoided because they delay healing. Medications that speed healing will be prescribed to protect the stomach from the stomach acid by either decreasing or stopping the secretion of stomach acids. Severe cases might require surgery.

Pyloric Stenosis

Pyloric stenosis is a condition in which a baby's pylorus gradually swells and thickens, which interferes with food entering the intestine. The pylorus is the connection between the stomach and the first part of the small intestine (duodenum). It can occur any time between birth and 5 months of age. However, it most commonly develops about 3 weeks after birth.

Vomiting all or most of feedings on a repeated basis is the main symptom of pyloric stenosis. The vomiting usually starts gradually and gets worse over time. As the pylorus becomes tighter, the vomiting becomes more frequent and more forceful. As the vomiting continues, the baby will lose weight, develop symptoms of not getting enough fluids (dehydration), be sleepier than normal, and be very fussy when awake.

Pyloric stenosis is always treated with surgery (pyloromyotomy). Once the baby has the surgery, the disorder usually will not develop again.

Stomach Ulcers

The stomach produces acid to break down food during the digestive process. The stomach and upper part of the small intestine (duodenum) are protected from the acid by a lining of sticky fluid (mucus). If this lining is damaged, the sensitive tissue underneath is exposed to acid. Irritation of the wall tissue in the stomach and duodenum may cause a stomach ulcer to form. Bacteria may also cause *stomach ulcers.*

Stomach or gastric ulcers are more common in people over the age of 50. Mild symptoms may be mistaken for indigestion or heartburn. Symptoms of a stomach ulcer that may occur include any or all of the following:

- Pain, or a burning sensation (similar to indigestion) in the upper abdomen and sometimes the lower chest. The pain from a duodenal ulcer can be worse when the stomach is empty and is relieved by eating, but then recurs a few hours afterward
- Pain that is often made worse by eating
- Difficulty swallowing or regurgitation (bringing up swallowed food into the mouth)
- Bloating, retching, and feeling sick, particularly after eating
- Vomiting and nausea
- Loss of appetite and weight loss

Severe ulcers may be very painful and bleed. Bleeding can indicate a serious problem—the ulcer may have burrowed through the stomach or duodenal wall, or it may be blocking the path of food trying to leave the stomach. Sometimes the stomach acid or the ulcer itself breaks a blood vessel in the lining of the stomach or duodenum.

If long-term treatment with aspirin or another (NSAID) is the cause, ulcer-healing drugs and additional drugs to protect the lining of the stomach and duodenum are advised. Antibiotics may be given to treat *H. pyloric* infections. Occasionally surgery is recommended if the ulcer does not respond to medication. This may include one of the following options:

- Vagotomy: cutting the vagus nerve that links the stomach to the brain. This reduces acid production
- Antrectomy: removal of the lower part of the stomach that produces the hormone that causes the stomach to produce digestive juices
- Pyloroplasty: enlarging the opening into the duodenum and small intestine to allow the contents of the stomach to move more freely

SUMMARY

The digestive system consists of a single tube starting at the mouth and ending at the rectum. Its function is to process food and other nutritional sources for energy for the body. The primary digestive system consists of the mouth, the pharynx, the esophagus, the stomach, the small intestine, the large intestine, and the rectum. The accessory organs of digestion include the salivary glands, pancreas, liver, and gallbladder.

Chapter Review

COMPETENCY REVIEW

1. Define and spell the terms to learn for this chapter.
2. Name the primary organs associated with digestion.
3. What are the four accessory organs of digestion?

4. What are the three main functions of the digestive system?
5. What is the first portion of the intestine called?
6. The large intestine can be divided into four distinct sections. Name them.
7. What is the function of the gallbladder?
8. What sac-like organ holds food for the beginning of the digestive process?
9. How many deciduous teeth is a person born with?
10. What essential role does the liver play?

PREPARING FOR THE CERTIFICATION EXAM

1. The medical term for gallstones is:
   A. cholecystectomy
   B. cholecystotomy
   C. choledochal
   D. cholelithiasis
   E. choledochectomy

2. The muscle at the superior portion of the stomach is the
   A. pyloric sphincter
   B. esophageal sphincter
   C. cardiac sphincter
   D. gallbladder
   E. fundus

3. Which substance is not produced by the liver?
   A. heparin
   B. bile
   C. hydrochloric acid
   D. fibrogen and prothrombin
   E. blood proteins

4. Which is not a component of the small intestine?
   A. jejunum
   B. ileum
   C. duodenum
   D. cecum
   E. pyloric sphincter

5. What is the function of the gallbladder?
   A. production of bile
   B. storage of bile
   C. production of pepsin
   D. production of insulin
   E. storage of insulin

6. How many permanent teeth does the body produce?
   A. 20
   B. 24
   C. 28
   D. 32
   E. 36

7. A potentially life-threatening condition that occurs when scarring damages the liver is
   A. pancreatitis
   B. cirrhosis
   C. cholecystitis
   D. colitis
   E. stomatitis

8. An inflammation of the large intestine that may be caused by many different disease processes is
   A. pancreatitis
   B. cirrhosis
   C. cholecystitis
   D. colitis
   E. stomatitis

9. Symptoms of Crohn's disease include all of the following EXCEPT
   A. abdominal pain
   B. diarrhea
   C. weight loss
   D. night sweats
   E. constipation

10. GERD occurs when the muscle of what organ does not close tightly?
    A. stomach
    B. liver
    C. gallbladder
    D. pancreas
    E. large intestine

CRITICAL THINKING

1. Why did the physician order a gastric analysis and histology with culture?

2. What type of diet will the physician prescribe for Mr. Sylvans? Why?

3. What steps can Mr. Sylvans take to lower his risk of any future episodes of pain and discomfort from his condition?

INTERNET ACTIVITY

Do an Internet search on peptic ulcer disease.

MediaLink  More on the digestive system, including interactive resources, can be found on the Student CD-ROM accompanying this textbook.

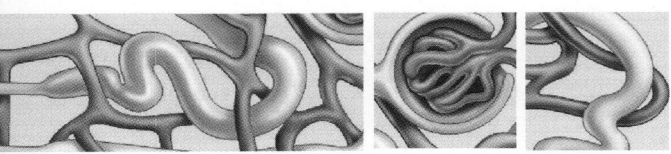

Medical Assistant Role Delineation Chart

HIGHLIGHT indicates material covered in this chapter.

ADMINISTRATIVE

Administrative Procedures

- Perform basic administrative medical assisting functions
- Schedule, coordinate and monitor appointments
- Schedule inpatient/outpatient admissions and procedures
- Understand and apply third-party guidelines
- Obtain reimbursement through accurate claims submission
- Monitor third-party reimbursement
- Understand and adhere to managed care policies and procedures
- *Negotiate managed care contracts*

Practice Finances

- Perform procedural and diagnostic coding
- Apply bookkeeping principles

- Manage accounts receivable
- *Manage accounts payable*
- *Process payroll*
- *Document and maintain accounting and banking records*
- *Develop and maintain fee schedules*
- *Manage renewals of business and professional insurance policies*
- *Manage personnel benefits and maintain records*
- *Perform marketing, financial, and strategic planning*

CLINICAL

Fundamental Principles

- Apply principles of aseptic technique and infection control
- Comply with quality assurance practices
- Screen and follow up patient test results

Diagnostic Orders

- Collect and process specimens
- Perform diagnostic tests

Patient Care

- Adhere to established patient screening procedures
- Obtain patient history and vital signs
- Prepare and maintain examination and treatment areas
- Prepare patient for examinations, procedures and treatments

- Assist with examinations, procedures and treatments
- Prepare and administer medications and immunizations
- Maintain medication and immunization records
- Recognize and respond to emergencies
- Coordinate patient care information with other health care providers
- Initiate IV and administer IV medications with appropriate training and as permitted by state law

GENERAL

Professionalism

- Display a professional manner and image
- Demonstrate initiative and responsibility
- Work as a member of the health care team
- Prioritize and perform multiple tasks
- Adapt to change
- Promote the CMA credential
- Enhance skills through continuing education
- Treat all patients with compassion and empathy
- Promote the practice through positive public relations

Communication Skills

- Recognize and respect cultural diversity
- Adapt communications to individual's ability to understand
- Use professional telephone technique

- Recognize and respond effectively to verbal, nonverbal, and written communications
- Use medical terminology appropriately
- Utilize electronic technology to receive, organize, prioritize and transmit information
- Serve as liaison

Legal Concepts

- Perform within legal and ethical boundaries
- Prepare and maintain medical records
- Document accurately
- Follow employer's established policies dealing with the health care contract
- Implement and maintain federal and state health care legislation and regulations
- Comply with established risk management and safety procedures
- Recognize professional credentialing criteria
- *Develop and maintain personnel, policy and procedure manuals*

Instruction

- Instruct individuals according to their needs
- Explain office policies and procedures
- Teach methods of health promotion and disease prevention
- Locate community resources and disseminate information
- *Develop educational materials*
- *Conduct continuing education activities*

Operational Functions

- Perform inventory of supplies and equipment
- Perform routine maintenance of administrative and clinical equipment
- Apply computer techniques to support office operations
- *Perform personnel management functions*
- *Negotiate leases and prices for equipment and supply contracts*

- *Denotes advanced skills.*

SOURCE: Reprinted by permission of the American Association of Medical Assistants from the AAMA Role Delineation Study: Occupational Analysis of the Medical Assisting Profession.

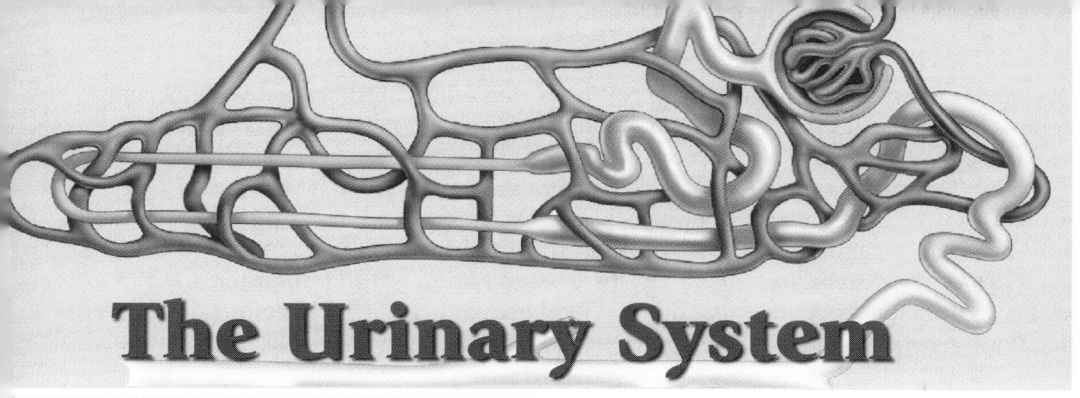

The Urinary System

Learning Objectives

After completing this chapter, you should be able to:

- Define and spell the terms to learn for this chapter.

- Describe the purpose and function of the urinary system.

- Identify the individual organs of the urinary system and briefly explain the function of each.

- List and discuss the three processes involved in the formation of urine.

- Explain the normal constituents of urine.

- List and briefly explain common disorders associated with the urinary system.

OUTLINE

Organs of the Urinary
System   511

Urine   512

Common Disorders
Associated with the
Urinary System   513

Terms to Learn

acute renal failure

ascites

chronic renal failure

cortex

cystitis

dialysis

glomerulonephritis

hilum

incontinence

interstitial cystitis (IC)

kidney stones

kidneys

lithotripsy

medulla

nephrons

polycystic kidney disease (PKD)

pyelonephritis

renal calculi

renal pelvis

ureters

urethra

urinary bladder

urinary meatus

Case Study

MARTIN TEVIA ARRIVED AT THE EMERGENCY ROOM with severe right-sided flank pain and visible blood in his urine. He states that he has no previous history of kidney problems and no pelvic pain or difficulty urinating. He is sweating, nauseated and continues to complain of extreme pain. Mr. Tevia was diagnosed with a kidney stone (renal calculi) located in the right renal ureter. He receives IV fluids and pain medication. He eventually passes the stone and is discharged to home with instructions to follow up with a urologist in 1 week.

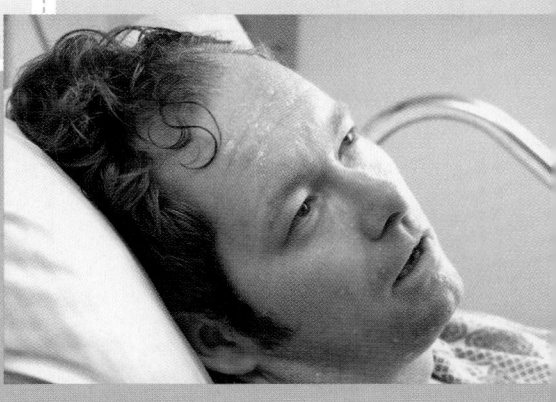

The urinary system consists of organs that produce and excrete urine from the body (see Figure 29-1). Urine is a transparent yellow fluid containing unwanted wastes, mostly excess water, salts, and nitrogen compounds. The primary organs of the system are the kidneys, which continuously filter substances from the blood and produce urine. Urine flows from the kidneys through two long, thin tubes called ureters. With the aid of gravity and wave-like contractions, the ureters transport the urine to the bladder, a muscular vessel. The normal adult bladder can store up to about 0.5 liter (1 pint) of urine, which it excretes through the tube-like urethra.

In addition to producing and excreting urine from the body, the urinary system is also responsible for regulating blood volume and blood pressure by adjusting the volume of water lost in the urine and releasing the

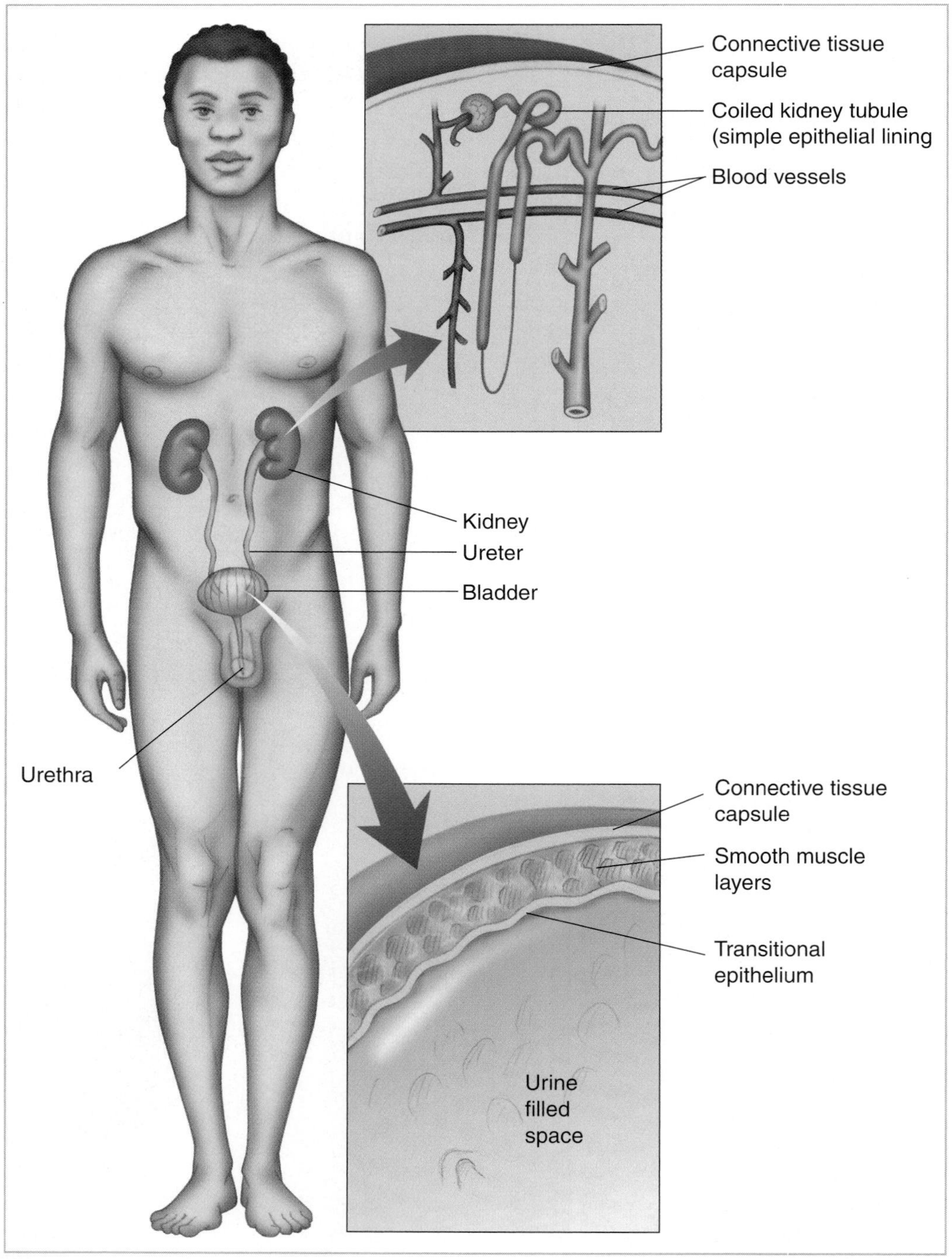

Connective tissue capsule

Coiled kidney tubule (simple epithelial lining

Blood vessels

Kidney

Ureter

Bladder

Urethra

Connective tissue capsule

Smooth muscle layers

Transitional epithelium

Urine filled space

FIGURE 29-1   The urinary system: kidneys, ureters, bladder, and urethra with expanded view of a nephron and the urine-filled space within a bladder.

hormones erythropoietin and rennin. It is also responsible for regulating blood concentrations of sodium, potassium, chloride, and other ions by controlling the quantities lost in the urine. By doing this, the urinary system is able to conserve valuable nutrients by selectively preventing losses while eliminating waste products.

Organs of the Urinary System

The components of the urinary system include the kidneys, which are the primary organs of the system; the ureters, which transport urine from the kidney to the urinary bladder; the urinary bladder, which is a temporary storage reservoir for urine; and the urethra, which is the final passageway for the flow of urine. The flow of urine through the urethra is controlled by an involuntary internal urethral sphincter and voluntary external urethral sphincter.

Kidneys

The kidneys are paired, bean-shaped organs located at the back of the abdominal cavity, retroperitoneal between the 12th thoracic and 3rd lumbar vertebrae (see Figure 29-2). They lie on either side of the spinal column in the flank area, against the muscles of the back. Each kidney has three capsules surrounding it: the true capsule, the perirenal fat, and the renal fascia. The true capsule is a smooth, fibrous connective membrane that loosely adheres to the surface of the kidney. Surrounding that is the adipose capsule (the perirenal fat) that embeds the kidney in fatty tissue, providing a layer of protection. The renal fascia is a sheath of fibrous tissue that anchors the kidney to the surrounding structures and ensures that the normal position is maintained.

External Structure of the Kidney

The concave border of each kidney has a notch called the hilum. The hilum is the entrance for the renal artery and vein, nerves, and the lymphatic vessels. The hilum also houses the opening for the ureters, where it connects with the renal pelvis, which is a sac-like collecting area for urine.

Internal Structure of the Kidney

Two distinct parts of the kidney are visible on a cross section, the cortex (the outer layer) and the medulla (the middle portion). The arteries, veins, convoluted tubules, and glomerular capsules are found in the cortex, and the renal pyramids are found in the medulla.

Nephrons

Microscopic examination of the kidney reveals about 1 million nephrons, which is the functional unit of the kidney (see Figure 29-3). Each nephron contains a renal corpuscle and a tubule. The nephron removes the waste products of metabolism from the blood plasma. The waste products are urea, uric acid, and creatinine, along with sodium, chloride, and potassium ions and ketone bodies. Nephrons help the body to maintain fluid balance by helping regulate the amount of fluid and electrolytes reabsorbed into the blood and how much is excreted. Approximately 1,000 to 1,200 mL of blood passes through the kidney per minute; at that rate, about 1.5 million millileters of blood passes through the kidneys each day. The renal corpuscle consists of the glomerulus and the Bowman's capsule. The Bowman's capsule has a tubule extending from it called the proximal convoluted tubule, which becomes the loop of Henle and then the distal convoluted tubule, which opens into a collecting tubule.

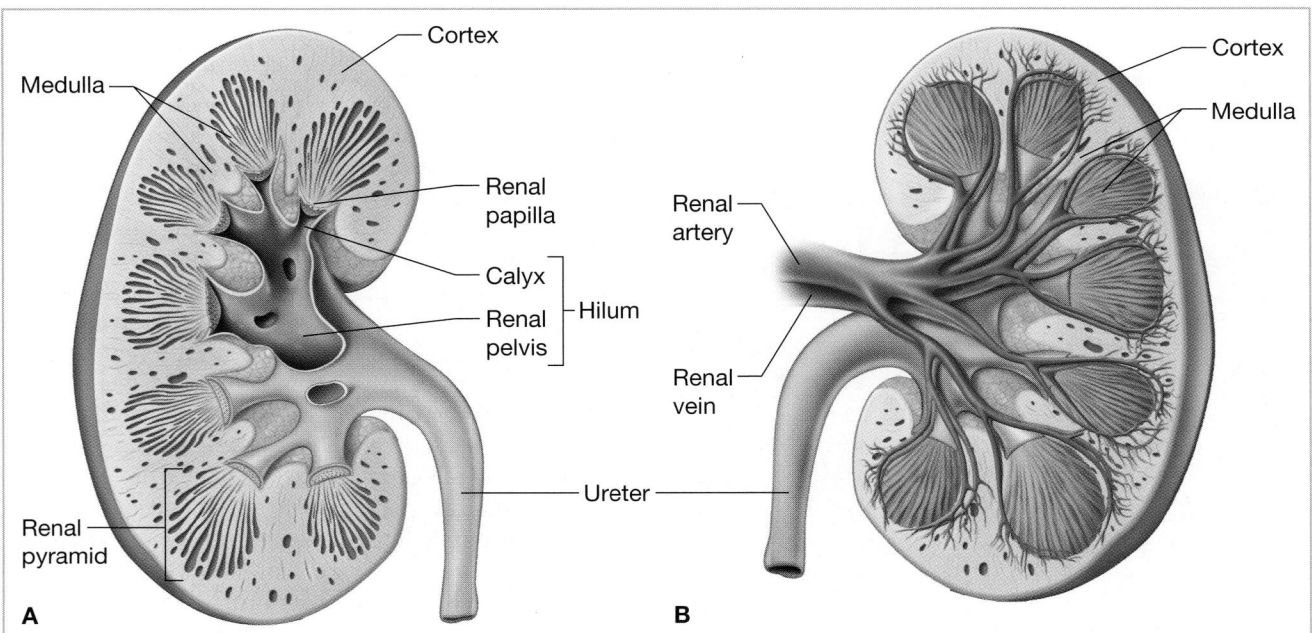

FIGURE 29-2 (A) Sectioned kidney; (B) renal artery and vein.

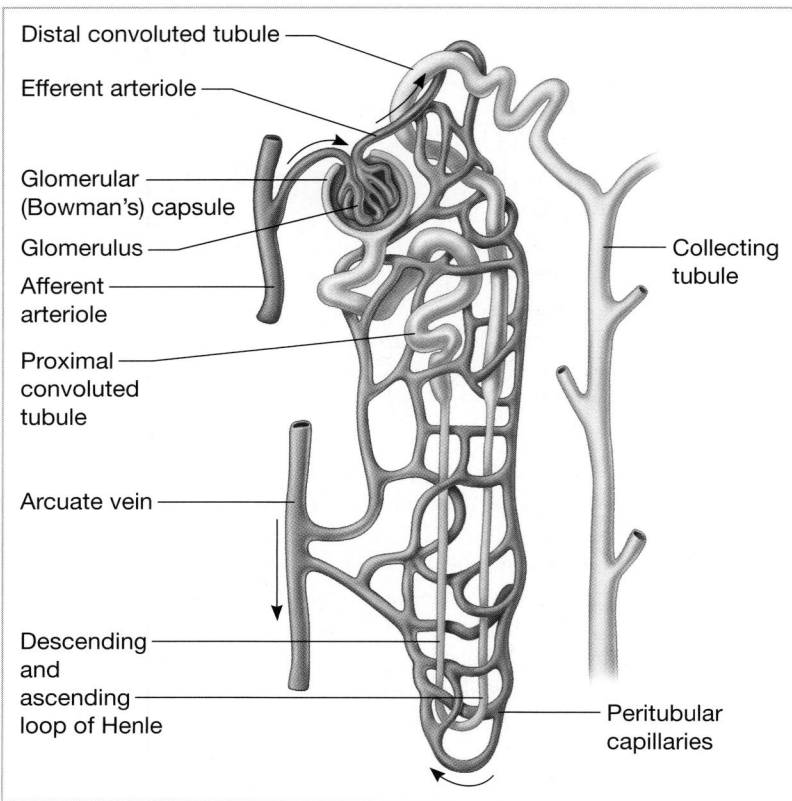

Distal convoluted tubule

Efferent arteriole

Glomerular (Bowman's) capsule

Glomerulus

Afferent arteriole

Proximal convoluted tubule

Arcuate vein

Descending and ascending loop of Henle

Collecting tubule

Peritubular capillaries

FIGURE 29-3 The structure of a nephron.

Ureters

The ureters are tubes that carry the newly formed urine from each kidney down to the bladder. There is one ureter from each kidney to the bladder. Each ureter is 28 to 34 cm long and has a diameter of 1 mm to 1 cm. There are three layers to the ureter wall: an inner coat of mucous membrane, a middle coat of smooth muscle, and an outer layer of fibrous tissue.

Legal and Ethical Issues

Patient privacy is always of utmost concern *in any part of the medical field. Never leave a telephone message stating the results of any test, or even stating the type of test a patient had. All messages should simply request that the patient call you back during office hours. Never leave any more information, even on a cell phone. By following this procedure, you will avoid violating HIPAA regulations.*

Urinary Bladder

The urinary bladder is the muscular sac that serves as a reservoir for urine. It is located in the pelvic cavity. The wall of the bladder consists of four layers: an inner layer of epithelium, a muscular coat of smooth muscle, an outer layer made of longitudinal muscle, and a fibrous layer. When the bladder is empty, the wall of the bladder feels firm because the walls of the bladder are thick. As the bladder becomes more full, it stretches so it can hold the urine present, and the walls become thinner.

Urethra

The urethra is the musculomembranous tube extending from the bladder to the urinary meatus, the external opening of the urinary system. The male urethra is approximately 20 cm long and has three sections, the prostatic, membranous, and penile sections. In males, the urethra transports both urine and semen. In females, the urethra is approximately 3 cm long, and its external opening is situated between the clitoris and the opening of the vagina. In females, the urethra transports only urine.

Urine

The formation of urine has three processes: filtration, reabsorption, and tubular secretion (see Figure 29-4). During filtration, or glomerular excretion, blood pressure forces all the small molecules in the blood into the lumen of the nephron through the pores both in the walls of the glomerular capillaries and in the wall of the Bowman's capsule. The filtrate has the same concentration of dissolved substances as the blood minus the formed elements and the plasma proteins that are too large to fit through the pores of the capillaries and the Bowman's capsule. As the filtrate passes through the tubules of the nephron, water and many dissolved materials are reabsorbed by the blood. In fact, during the filtrate's passage through the tubules up to 99 percent of the water is reabsorbed. In addition, the tubules also remove substances from the blood. This process, called tubular secretion, supplements the initial glomerular filtration. Water and some selected substances are reabsorbed from the filtrate by the capillaries surrounding the nephrons. Other substances, such as hydrogen ions and uric acid, will be transported into the filtrate, now known as urine.

Urine consists of 95 percent water and 5 percent solid substances. The average normal adult feels a need to void, or urinate, when the bladder contains 300 to 350 mL of urine. Typically, about 1,000 to 1,500 mL of urine is voided daily, depending on fluid intake. Normal urine is clear (not cloudy), straw colored, and has a faintly aromatic odor, with a specific gravity of 1.003 to 1.030 and a slightly acidic pH of about 6. Specific gravity measures the kidney's ability to concentrate or dilute urine in relation to plasma. Because urine is a solution of minerals, salts, and compounds dissolved in water, the specific gravity is greater than 1.000. The more concentrated the urine, the higher the urine specific gravity. An adult's kidneys have a remarkable ability to concentrate or dilute urine. In infants, the range for specific gravity is less because immature kidneys are not able to concentrate urine as effectively as mature kidneys.

Common Disorders Associated with the Urinary System

Compromised kidneys, and even healthy kidneys, can suffer from a variety of conditions that can affect an individual's lifestyle and activities of daily living (see Table 29-1)

Cystitis

Cystitis is an inflammation of the bladder, usually occurring as a result of ascending urinary tract infections. Cystitis occurs when bacteria, causing irritation and inflammation, infect the lower urinary tract. Most cases of urinary tract infection are caused by *Escherichia coli* (*E. coli*), a bacterium found in the lower gastrointestinal system.

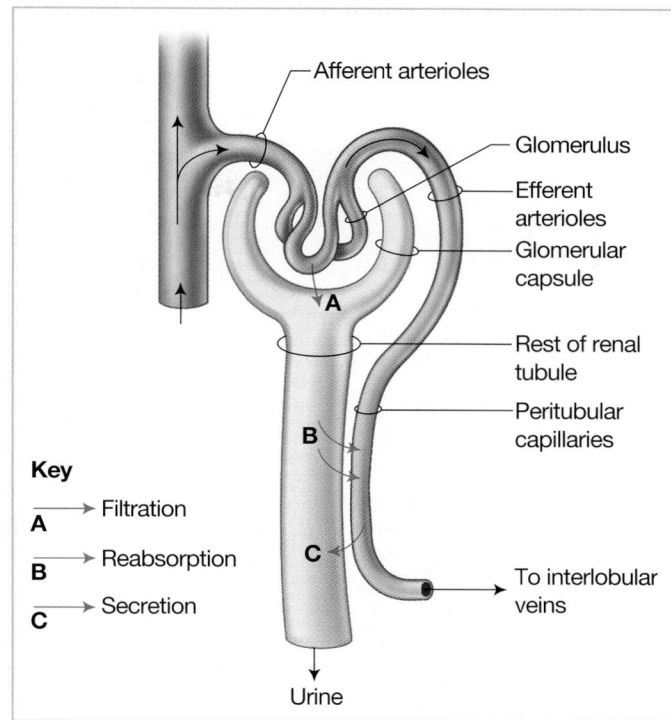

FIGURE 29-4 Schematic view of the three stages of urine production: (A) filtration; (B) reabsorption; (C) secretion.

Urinary tract infections are common, especially in sexually active women ages 20 to 50, but they can happen in anyone. Women are more frequently affected, secondary to the anatomy of the perineum, improper personal hygiene, and the short length of the urethra.

Lifespan
Considerations

THE CHILD
- At about 10 weeks gestation, the kidneys begin forming urine. By 3 months gestation, the fetus actually begins to secrete small quantities of urine. Quantities continue to increase during the rest of fetal development. However, a newborn's kidneys are not able to concentrate urine. Because of this, newborns and even older infants are more prone to fluid volume excess or dehydration. Extreme changes in temperature and fluid intake must be avoided until their kidneys are better able to adjust for fluid needs. Because of the lack of fat pads in the flank, the kidneys of small children are more susceptible to trauma.
- Small children, especially those wearing diapers, are susceptible to urinary tract infections. It is especially important that the diaper area be cleaned regularly and appropriately to prevent urinary tract infections.

THE OLDER ADULT
- As people age, the kidneys begin to lose mass as the blood vessels degenerate. The kidneys lose their ability to filter as well, and their ability to conserve water and sodium decreases. This means that dehydration can happen more quickly. In addition, the tubules' ability to balance the pH of the body decreases, as well as the ability to balance electrolytes. As a result, acid–base imbalances can happen much more easily. There is also a loss of muscle tone in the ureters, bladder, and urethra. Bladder capacity is reduced by as much as 50 percent, causing more frequent trips to the bathroom. In some adults, urge incontinence (the inability to voluntarily retain urine) is a big concern.

TABLE 29-1 Disorders of the Urinary System

Disorder	Description
Anuria	No urine formed by the kidneys and a complete lack of urine excretion.
Bladder neck obstruction	Blockage of the bladder outlet.
Dysuria	Painful or difficult urination.
Enuresis	Involuntary discharge of urine after the age by which bladder control should have been established. This usually occurs by the age of 5. Also called bed-wetting at night.
Glomerulonephritis	Inflammation of the kidney (primarily of the glomerulus). Since the glomerular membrane is inflamed, it becomes more permeable and this results in protein (proteinuria) and blood (hematuria) in the urine.
Hematuria	A condition of blood in the urine. This is a symptom of a disease process.
Hypospadius	A congenital opening of the male urethra on the underside of the penis.
Interstitial cystitis	Disease of an unknown cause in which there is inflammation and irritation of the bladder. It is most commonly seen in middle-aged women.
Nocturia	Excessive urination during the night. This may or may not be abnormal.
Pyelitis	Inflammation of the renal pelvis.
Pyelonephritis	Inflammation of the renal pelvis and the kidney. This is one of the most common types of kidney disease. It may be the result of a lower urinary tract infection that moved up to the kidney via the ureters. There may be large quantities of white blood cells and bacteria in the urine. Hematuria may also be present. This condition can occur whenever there is an untreated or persistent case of cystitis.
Pyuria	Presence of pus in the urine.
Renal colic	Pain caused by a kidney stone. This type of pain can be excruciating and generally requires medical treatment.

Sexual activity can introduce bacteria into the urethra. Bacteria in the bladder are often removed through urination, but occasionally, the bacteria reproduce more quickly than they are washed away, causing an infection. In men, cystitis is usually secondary to another infection, such as epididymitis, prostatitis, gonorrhea, syphilis, or kidney stones.

Frequently, the most common symptoms of cystitis are urgency and frequency. Urgency is a need to void immediately. Frequency is the need to void frequently. Another common symptom of cystitis is painful urination. Occasionally, the patient may suffer from chills and fever. If the cystitis is chronic, then dysuria (burning urination) may be the only symptom. Urinary tract infections are treated with antibiotics and antispasmodics.

Interstitial cystitis (IC) is a painful inflammation of the bladder wall. Ninety percent of the 450,000 people who suffer from this condition are women. The cause is unknown. The symptoms can be mild to severe, but IC does not respond to typical antibiotic therapy.

Glomerulonephritis

Glomerulonephritis is a type of kidney disease that hampers the kidneys' ability to remove waste and excess fluids. Also called glomerular disease, glomerulonephritis can be acute, referring to a sudden attack of inflammation, or chronic, which comes on gradually. Glomerular disease can be part of a systemic disease, such as lupus or diabetes, or it can be a disease by itself, called primary glomerulonephritis. Glomerulonephritis can lead to kidney failure.

Proper hygiene is one component of prevention of urinary tract infections. Women should always wipe from front to back with white, unscented toilet paper after using the toilet to decrease the incidence of transmission of bacteria to the ureters. Also, after sexual intercourse, women should urinate as soon as possible. Bubble baths have also been implicated as an irritant to the urinary system.

The proper intake of fluids is the best mechanism of keeping the urinary system healthy. Individuals should drink at least 64 ounces of water every 24 hours to keep the kidneys working properly and to eliminate toxins. This helps not only prevent urinary tract infections, but also decreases the incidence of kidney stones since the stones are not able to grow as large if the kidneys are properly flushed.

There are many causes of glomerulonephritis. They include those related to infections, immune diseases, inflammation of the blood vessels (vasculitis) and conditions that scar the glomeruli. Chronic glomerulonephritis sometimes develops after a bout of acute glomerulonephritis. Infrequently, chronic glomerulonephritis runs in families. In many cases, the specific cause is unknown.

Signs and symptoms of glomerulonephritis may depend on whether the patient has the acute or chronic form, and the cause. The first indication that something is wrong may come from symptoms or from the results of a routine urinalysis. Signs and symptoms may include cola-colored or diluted iced-tea-colored urine from red blood cells in the urine (hematuria), foam in the toilet water from protein in the urine (proteinuria), high blood pressure (hypertension), fluid retention (edema) with swelling evident in the face, hands, feet, and abdomen, fatigue from anemia or kidney failure, and less frequent urination than usual.

Some cases of acute glomerulonephritis, especially those that follow a strep infection, often improve on their own and require no specific treatment. Other treatments may include the use of diuretics, angiotensin-converting enzyme (ACE) inhibitors, calcium channel blockers, and beta blockers.

Incontinence

More common in women who have had children, incontinence is the involuntary and unpredictable flow of urine. Stress incontinence is the most common, and happens when sneezing, laughing, or other causes of intra-abdominal pressure cause the involuntary release of urine. Urge incontinence occurs when the bladder contracts without warning. Leakage will occur if the patient is not able to respond to that need immediately. Overflow incontinence happens when a blockage prohibits normal emptying. The bladder simply overflows. Incontinence is diagnosed by a urologist, and treatment may include medications, surgery, and pelvic floor exercises.

Kidney Stones

Kidney stones, or renal calculi, are caused by deposits of mineral salts in the kidney (see Figure 29-5). The stones are usually benign when still in the kidney, but can pass into the ureter, slowing down or blocking urine flow. Because the stones have a rough surface, they irritate and scratch the ureters, causing bleeding. The kidney becomes irritated due to the bleeding and

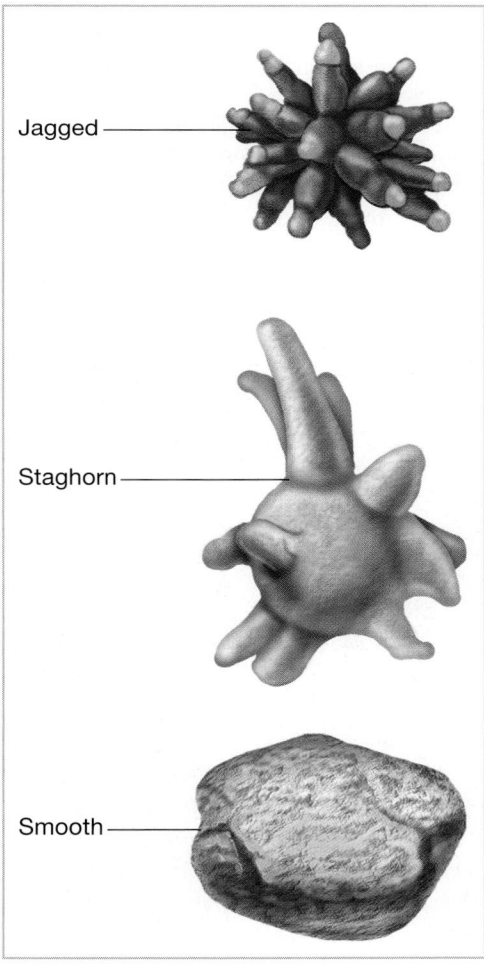

Jagged

Staghorn

Smooth

FIGURE 29-5 Types of kidney stones found in an adult.

the decreased urine flow, causing pain and spasms. Kidney stones are painful, and a person suffering from one presents with flank pain along with possible nausea and vomiting. On urinalysis, hematuria is usually present.

Kidney stones afflict about 10 percent of the people in the United States, and men are more often afflicted than women. A person with a family history of kidney stones is more likely to have stones that someone with no family history. Urinary tract infections, kidney disorders, and metabolic disorders, such as hyperparathyroidism are linked to kidney stones.

Most kidney stones are made of calcium oxalate. Calcium from food is absorbed in excess, and then excreted

into the urine. There, it combines with oxalates, and creates the stones. Individuals with this type of stone are advised to control their intake of foods containing calcium and oxalate. Foods containing oxalate include beets, chocolate, tea, coffee, cola, nuts, rhubarb, strawberries, tea, wheat bran, and spinach. To prevent stone formation, individuals should drink enough fluid to produce at least 2 quarts of urine each day.

Many kidney stones are able to pass out of the body without physician intervention. Stones that cause lasting symptoms or other complications may require treatment, including lithotripsy. There are two types of lithotripsy, extracorporeal shock wave lithotripsy and percutaneous ultrasonic lithotripsy. Both procedures involve passing shock waves through the body that will cause the stone to break down. Other procedures require surgical intervention to either retrieve or disintegrate the stone. Stones that do not pass can either cause infection, or, if they completely block the ureter, hydronephrosis, which can eventually cause kidney damage.

Polycystic Kidney Disease

Polycystic kidney disease (PKD) is a disorder in which clusters of cysts develop primarily within the kidneys. Cysts are noncancerous (benign) round sacs of waterlike fluid. The disease is not limited to the kidneys, although the kidneys usually are the most severely affected organs. The disease can cause cysts to develop in your liver, pancreas, membranes that surround your brain and central nervous system, and seminal vesicles. PKD affects more than 12 million people worldwide. The disease varies greatly in its severity, and some complications are preventable. Regular checkups can lead to treatments to reduce damage to your kidneys from complications, such as high blood pressure. The greatest risk for people with polycystic kidney disease is developing high blood pressure. Kidney failure also is common with PKD.

Signs and symptoms of polycystic kidney disease may include high blood pressure, back or side pain related to enlarged kidneys, abdominal pain, an increase in the size of the abdomen, blood in the urine, kidney stones, kidney failure, kidney infections, and headache.

Treating polycystic kidney disease involves dealing with and treating the signs, symptoms, and complications of high blood pressure, pain, bladder and kidney infections, blood in the urine, and kidney failure.

Pyelonephritis

Pyelonephritis is an infection of the kidney and renal pelvis. It may have a sudden onset, or be a chronic condition. Bacteria entering the kidneys from the bladder, usually *E. coli*, causes pyelonephritis. This may be a result of the same mechanisms as seen in cystitis. Sometimes, pyelonephritis is caused by an indwelling urinary

Professionalism

catheter and cystoscopy (visualization of the urinary bladder and urethra with a special instrument). Other causes include prostate enlargement and kidney stones. Symptoms of pyelonephritis include back, side, and groin pain; urgency and frequency; pain and burning during urination; fever; nausea and vomiting; and blood and pus in the urine.

Antibiotics are used to treat pyelonephritis. If pyelonephritis is left untreated, scarring may result and could cause permanent kidney damage.

Renal Failure

The two types of renal failure are acute and chronic. Acute renal failure occurs when something causes a change in the filtering function of the kidneys, altering the ability of the kidneys to maintain normal body function. A blockage, toxins, or a sudden loss of blood flow to the kidneys can cause acute renal failure. People who have other kidney diseases are at a greater risk for acute renal failure.

There are no immediate signs of acute kidney failure, but, over time, urine output is decreased, resulting in increased fluid buildup in the tissues. Common symptoms include irregular heart rate, ascites (fluid in the abdomen), and swelling in the extremities.

In chronic renal failure, there is a gradual and progressive loss of kidney function. Renal failure may be mild or severe. Typically, it takes a period of years for the renal failure to progress. Symptoms may be mild or nonexistent until at least 10 percent of the kidney function is lost. Diabetes and hypertension are the two most common causes of chronic renal failure in the United States. About 2 out of every 1,000 people in the United States have chronic renal failure.

The goal of treatment for chronic renal failure is to identify and treat the reversible causes if the kidney fails. Then, treatment focuses on preventing fluid volume excesses while the kidneys have a chance to heal and resume their normal function. If normal function cannot be regained, then dialysis may be necessary (see Figure 29-6). Dialysis uses a filter other than the kidneys to remove toxins and maintain water balance. The two types of dialysis are hemodialysis and peritoneal dialysis. Hemodialysis uses a machine that cleans the blood outside of the body. A specialized catheter, called a shunt, is inserted in the patient's arm or leg. The shunt is accessed with special tubing that carries

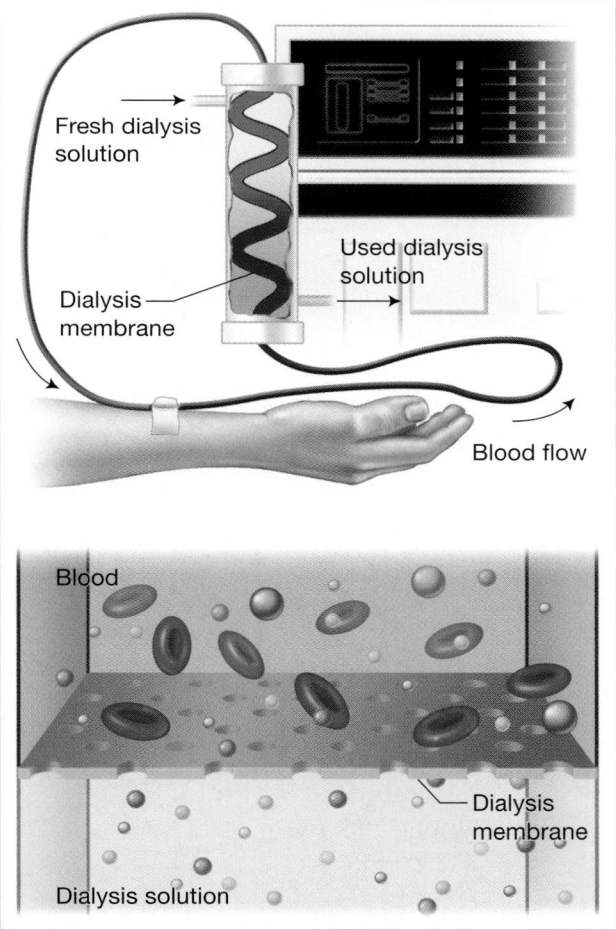

FIGURE 29-6 Dialysis machine showing diffusion of concentrations, which are the same, between the patient's blood and dialysis solution.

the blood to the machines that filter and clean the blood and then return the blood back to the body. Patients receiving hemodialysis must go to a special center three times a week for 2 to 3 hours at a time.

The other type of dialysis is called peritoneal dialysis. Peritoneal dialysis is done through the tissues of the abdomen, where a dialysis fluid is instilled in the stomach, left for a period of time while the membranes in the abdomen filter toxins, and then the fluid is re-moved. These patients can be dialyzed at home or in any environment.

Some patients may receive a kidney transplant, in which a donor kidney is inserted into the patient's body, with the blood vessels and ureters attached to the patient's already existing structures. Kidney transplant recipients must take antirejection drugs for their lifetime following the transplant. Kidney transplants are the second most common transplant in the United States.

SUMMARY

The urinary tract can present many challenges both for the patient and for the medical assistant. One of the most common reasons patients come into the medical office is to seek help for a urinary tract infection. Oftentimes called the excretory system, the function of the urinary system is to help clean wastes from the bloodstream and then carry those wastes outside the body via the kidneys and bladder, through the urethra.

Chapter Review

COMPETENCY REVIEW

1. Define and spell the terms to learn for this chapter.
2. List the organs of the urinary system.
3. What are the vital functions of the urinary system?
4. Define renal pelvis.
5. In what portion of the kidney is the medulla located?
6. What is the vital function of the nephrons?
7. What are the three processes of urine formation?
8. What is the major organ of the urinary system?
9. Define ureter.
10. How much urine is formed daily?

PREPARING FOR THE CERTIFICATION EXAM

1. The part of the urinary tract that collects urine in the bladder is the
   A. ureter
   B. bladder
   C. urethra
   D. jejunum
   E. renal pelvis

2. The condition in which an individual experiences an involuntary and unpredictable flow of urine is called
   A. constipation
   B. incontinence
   C. dysuria
   D. urethral pressure
   E. anuria

3. A urinary tract disease that causes inflammation of the bladder is
   A. pyelonephritis
   B. glomerulonephritis
   C. polycystic kidney disease
   D. cystitis
   E. renal calculus

4. The anatomical structure that is the functional unit of the kidney is the
   A. nephrons
   B. ureter
   C. bladder
   D. urethra
   E. renal pelvis

continued on next page

5. The anatomical structure of the urinary system that is responsible for carrying urine from the bladder to the outside of the body is the
   A. nephrons
   B. ureter
   C. bladder
   D. urethra
   E. renal pelvis

6. The function of a diuretic is to
   A. treat kidney infections
   B. treat cystitis
   C. remove fluid from the body
   D. add fluid to the body
   E. eliminate kidney stones

7. Chronic renal failure is treated by
   A. lithotripsy
   B. cystoscopy
   C. dialysis
   D. radiology
   E. diuretics

8. Kidney stones are caused by deposits of
   A. mineral salts
   B. proteins
   C. phosphorus
   D. sodium
   E. potassium

9. A procedure that uses a telescopic lens to visualize the urethra and the urinary bladder is called
   A. laparoscopy
   B. cystoscopy
   C. endoscopy
   D. arthroscopy
   E. telescopy

10. A disease that causes a gradual and progressive loss of kidney function is called
   A. acute renal failure
   B. chronic renal failure
   C. polycystic nephritis
   D. cystitis
   E. glomerulonephritis

CRITICAL THINKING

1. During the urinalysis, what substance was found in Mr. Tevia's specimen?

2. If Mr. Tevia had not been able to pass his kidney stone, what would have been a possible treatment for him?

3. What type of dietary instructions should Mr. Tevia receive?

INTERNET ACTIVITY

Use the Internet to learn about types of incontinence and their treatment.

 MediaLink More on the urinary system, including interactive resources, can be found on the Student CD-ROM accompanying this textbook.

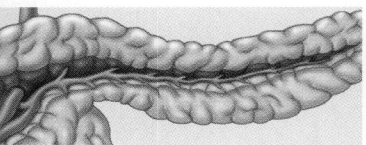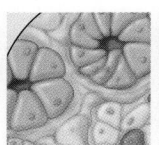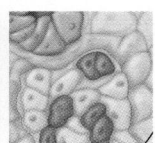

Medical Assistant Role Delineation Chart

HIGHLIGHT indicates material covered in this chapter.

ADMINISTRATIVE

Administrative Procedures

- Perform basic administrative medical assisting functions
- Schedule, coordinate and monitor appointments
- Schedule inpatient/outpatient admissions and procedures
- Understand and apply third-party guidelines
- Obtain reimbursement through accurate claims submission
- Monitor third-party reimbursement
- Understand and adhere to managed care policies and procedures
- *Negotiate managed care contracts*

Practice Finances

- Perform procedural and diagnostic coding
- Apply bookkeeping principles

- Manage accounts receivable
- *Manage accounts payable*
- *Process payroll*
- *Document and maintain accounting and banking records*
- *Develop and maintain fee schedules*
- *Manage renewals of business and professional insurance policies*
- *Manage personnel benefits and maintain records*
- *Perform marketing, financial, and strategic planning*

CLINICAL

Fundamental Principles

- Apply principles of aseptic technique and infection control
- Comply with quality assurance practices
- Screen and follow up patient test results

Diagnostic Orders

- Collect and process specimens
- Perform diagnostic tests

Patient Care

- Adhere to established patient screening procedures
- Obtain patient history and vital signs
- Prepare and maintain examination and treatment areas
- Prepare patient for examinations, procedures and treatments

- Assist with examinations, procedures and treatments
- Prepare and administer medications and immunizations
- Maintain medication and immunization records
- Recognize and respond to emergencies
- Coordinate patient care information with other health care providers
- Initiate IV and administer IV medications with appropriate training and as permitted by state law

GENERAL

Professionalism

- Display a professional manner and image
- Demonstrate initiative and responsibility
- Work as a member of the health care team
- Prioritize and perform multiple tasks
- Adapt to change
- Promote the CMA credential
- Enhance skills through continuing education
- Treat all patients with compassion and empathy
- Promote the practice through positive public relations

Communication Skills

- Recognize and respect cultural diversity
- Adapt communications to individual's ability to understand
- Use professional telephone technique

- Recognize and respond effectively to verbal, nonverbal, and written communications
- Use medical terminology appropriately
- Utilize electronic technology to receive, organize, prioritize and transmit information
- Serve as liaison

Legal Concepts

- Perform within legal and ethical boundaries
- Prepare and maintain medical records
- Document accurately
- Follow employer's established policies dealing with the health care contract
- Implement and maintain federal and state health care legislation and regulations
- Comply with established risk management and safety procedures
- Recognize professional credentialing criteria
- *Develop and maintain personnel, policy and procedure manuals*

Instruction

- Instruct individuals according to their needs
- Explain office policies and procedures
- Teach methods of health promotion and disease prevention
- Locate community resources and disseminate information
- *Develop educational materials*
- *Conduct continuing education activities*

Operational Functions

- Perform inventory of supplies and equipment
- Perform routine maintenance of administrative and clinical equipment
- Apply computer techniques to support office operations
- *Perform personnel management functions*
- *Negotiate leases and prices for equipment and supply contracts*

- *Denotes advanced skills.*

SOURCE: Reprinted by permission of the American Association of Medical Assistants from the AAMA Role Delineation Study: Occupational Analysis of the Medical Assisting Profession.

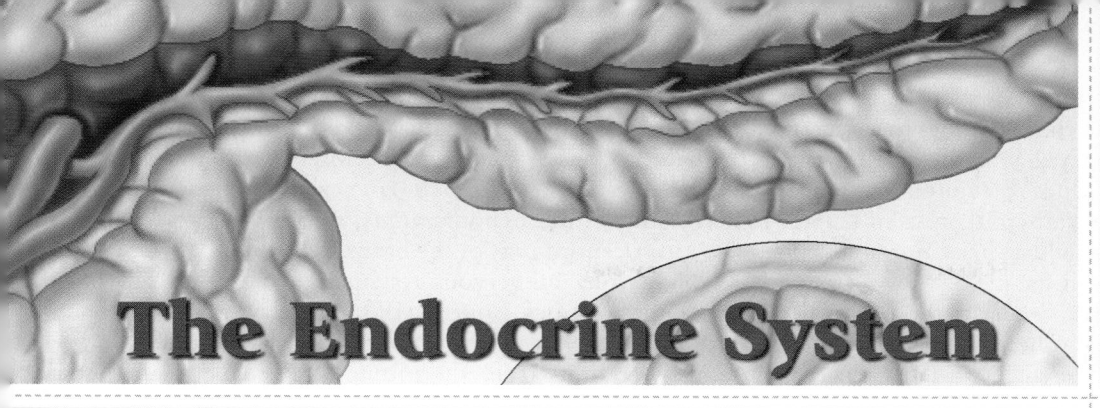

chapter 30

The Endocrine System

Learning Objectives

After completing this chapter, you should be able to:

- Define and spell the terms to learn for this chapter.
- Describe the primary glands of the endocrine system.
- Explain the vital function of the endocrine system.
- State the primary functions of the endocrine glands.
- Identify and state the functions of the various hormones secreted by the endocrine glands.
- Identify and explain common disorders associated with the endocrine system.

OUTLINE

Pituitary Gland	523
Pineal Gland	524
Thyroid Gland	524
Parathyroid Glands	524
Pancreas (Islets of Langerhans)	525
Adrenal Glands	525
Ovaries	527
Testes	527
Placenta	527
Gastrointestinal Mucosa	527
Thymus Gland	527
Common Disorders Associated with the Endocrine System	527

Terms to Learn

acromegaly
Addison's disease
cardiomegaly
Cushing's disease
diabetes mellitus
dwarfism
exophthalmos

gestational diabetes
gigantism
goiter
Graves' disease
Hashimoto's thyroiditis
hyperthyroidism
hypothyroidism

insulin-dependent diabetes mellitus (IDDM)
lipolysis
myxedema
non–insulin-dependent diabetes mellitus (NIDDM)

Case Study

12-YEAR-OLD FORREST DISER PRESENTED to the pediatrician's office with a 2-month history of weight loss, fatigue, polyuria, and polydipsia. Family history is significant for several relatives with type 1 diabetes mellitus. In the office, the patient was found to have hyperglycemia with a fasting blood sample, and glucosuria on a urine dipstick test. He was admitted to the hospital, where type 1 diabetes mellitus was diagnosed. After 3 days, he was discharged from the hospital on an insulin protocol of twice a day insulin injections and glucose monitoring. The patient and his family were educated on diet, exercise, symptoms of hypoglycemic coma, and the long-term complications of diabetes mellitus. He was placed on a 2,000-calorie diabetic diet with three meals and two snacks a day.

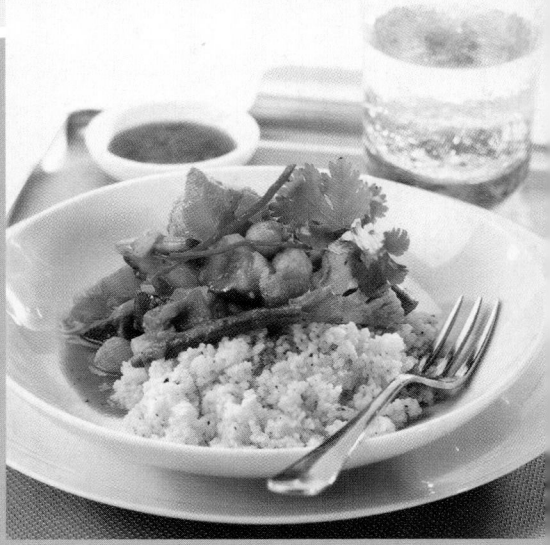

he endocrine system is made up of glands and the hormones they secrete. The primary glands of the endocrine system include the pituitary, pineal, thyroid, parathyroid, islets of Langerhans, adrenals, ovaries in the female, and testes in the male.

The vital function of this system is the production and regulation of hormones. A hormone is the chemical substance that regulates different body function. Hormones are the chemical messengers that regular growth, development, mood, tissue function, metabolism, and sexual function in both males and females.

Many disorders are associated with a hypersecretion or hyposecretion of hormones of the endocrine system. Controlling the secretion of specific hormones can help treat many of those hormonal conditions or disorders.

The nervous system works closely with the endocrine system in the maintenance of homeostasis. For example, the hypothalamus, which is located in the lower central part of the brain, is the link between the endocrine and nervous systems. The nerve cells in the hypothalamus control the pituitary gland by producing chemicals that suppress or stimulate hormone secretions from the pituitary. The hypothalamus synthesizes and secretes releasing hormones such as thyrotropin-releasing hormone (TRH) and gonadotropin-releasing hormone (GTRH), and releasing factors such as corticotropin-releasing hormone (CRF), growth hormone-releasing factor (GHRF),

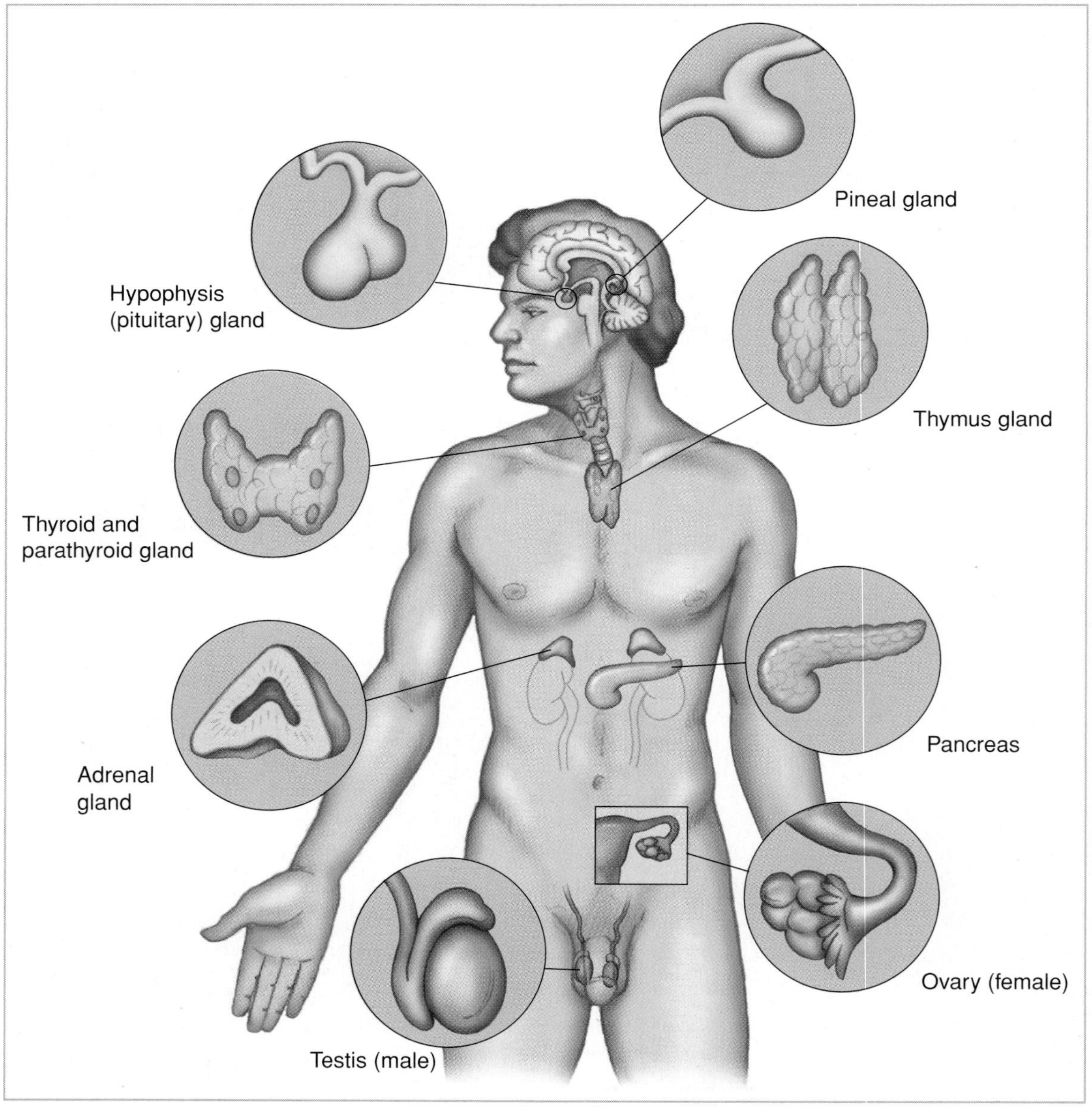

Hypophysis (pituitary) gland

Pineal gland

Thymus gland

Thyroid and parathyroid gland

Adrenal gland

Pancreas

Testis (male)

Ovary (female)

FIGURE 30-1   The primary glands of the endocrine system.

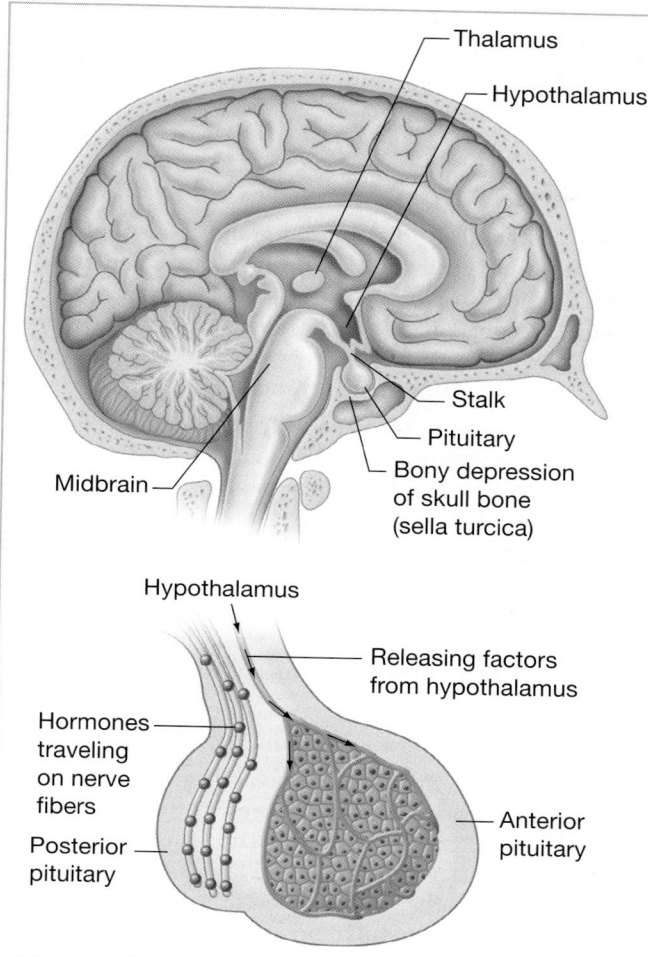

FIGURE 30-2 The pituitary gland and its relation to the brain.

prolactin-releasing factor (PRF), and melanocyte-stimulating releasing factor (MRF). The secretion of the hormones norepinephrine and epinephrine is also controlled by the hypothalamus, which exerts direct nervous control over the anterior pituitary and the adrenal medulla. Figure 30-1 illustrates the primary glands of the endocrine system.

Pituitary Gland

The pituitary gland (see Figure 30-2), is located near the base of the brain in a small depression of the sphenoid bone called the sella turcica. It is attached to the hypothalamus by the infundibulum stalk. The pituitary, which consists of both an anterior lobe and a posterior lobe, is called the master gland of the body, because it regulates all of the other endocrine glands.

Anterior Lobe

The adenohypophysis or anterior lobe (see Figure 30-3) secretes several hormones that are essential for the growth and development of bones, muscles, other or-gans, sex glands, the thyroid gland, and the adrenal cortex. The hormones produced in the anterior lobe of the pituitary gland include the following:

- Growth hormone (also called somatotrophic hormone)—essential for the growth and development of bones, muscles, and other organs. Growth hormone enhances protein synthesis, decreases glucose use, and promotes the destruction of fats (lipolysis). Hyposecretion of this hormone results in dwarfism; conversely, hypersecretion leads to gigantism during early life, and acromegaly in adults.

- Adrenocorticotropin I—essential for the growth and development of the middle and inner parts of the adrenal cortex. The glucocorticoids cortisol and corticosteroid are secreted by the adrenal cortex.

- Thyroid-stimulating hormone—controls the growth and development of the thyroid gland. It also stimulates the production of thyroxine and triiodothyronine, influencing the body's metabolic processes and metabolism.

- Follicle-stimulating hormone—a gonadotropic hormone that is responsible for stimulating the growth of ovarian follicles in females and the production of sperm in males.

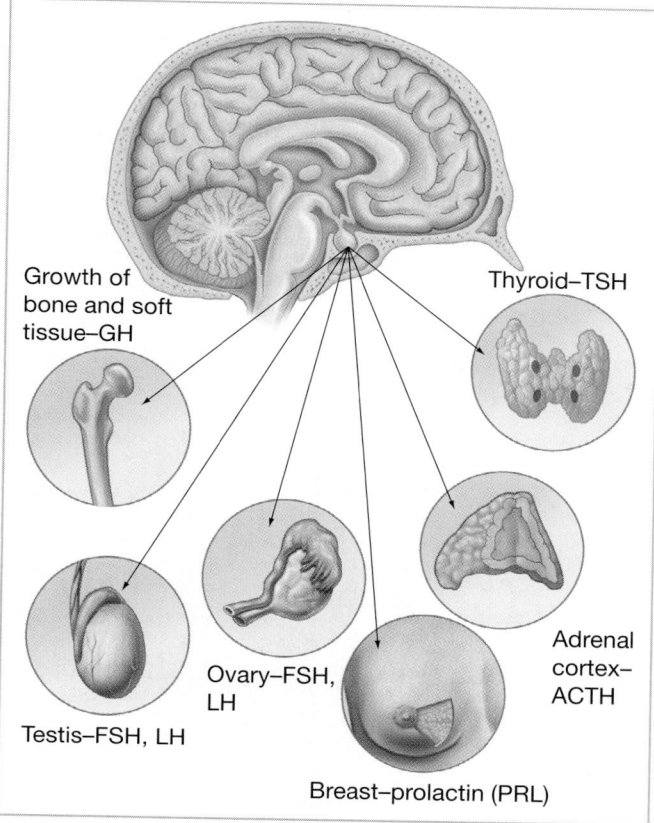

FIGURE 30-3 The anterior pituitary gland and its target organs.

- Luteinizing hormone—gonadotropic hormone that is responsible for the maturation process in the ovarian follicles and for stimulating the development of the corpus luteum in the female. In the male, LH is responsible for the production of testosterone.
- Prolactin (also known as lactogenic hormone)—a gonadotropic hormone that stimulates the mammary glands to produce milk after childbirth.
- Melanocyte-stimulating hormone—controls skin pigmentation. The deposit of melanin helps protect skin after exposure to sunlight.

Posterior Lobe

The posterior lobe of the pituitary gland is also known as the neurohypophysis. It secretes two hormones:

- Antidiuretic hormone (ADH)—also known as vasopressin, it is responsible for stimulating the reabsorption of water by the kidneys, so that less fluid is eliminated. In doing this, the blood pressure can be elevated. If this hormone is undersecreted, a condition known as diabetes insipidus will result.
- Oxytocin—responsible for stimulating the uterus for contraction during labor and childbirth and for stimulating the mammary glands to release milk after delivery.

Pineal Gland

The pineal gland is located at the posterior end of the corpus callosum in the brain. It secretes melatonin and serotonin. Melatonin is released at night and helps with sleep and the release of gonadotropin. Serotonin is a neurotransmitter, vasoconstrictor, and smooth muscle stimulant. Depression is commonly associated with the hormone serotonin.

Thyroid Gland

Located in the neck, the thyroid gland is responsible for metabolism (see Figure 30-4). It is located anterior to the trachea, just below the thyroid cartilage. The thyroid is approximately 5 cm long and 3 cm wide, and weighs about 30 grams. The thyroid gland is responsible for secreting three hormones:

- Thyroxine (T_4)—essential for the maintenance and regulation of the basal metabolic rate (BMR). Thyroxine influences growth and development, both physical and mental, as well as the metabolism of fats, proteins, carbohydrates, water, vitamins, and minerals. In thyroid dysfunction, it can be replaced with medications. Disorders resulting from hyposecretion of thyroxine include cretinism, myxedema, and Hashimoto's disease.
- Triiodothyronine (T_3)—influences the BMR.
- Calcitonin—influences bone and calcium metabolism. During infancy, if there is not enough calcitonin, cretinism may occur, causing mental retardation. Myxedema and Hashimoto's disease are also results of hyposecretion of calcitonin, along with its companion hormones, T_3 and T_4.

Hypersecretion of T_3 and T_4 is called *hyperthyroidism* (thyrotoxicosis). Other disorders resulting from hypersecretion of T_3 and T_4 include Graves' disease, exophthalmic goiter, toxic goiter, and Basedow's disease.

Parathyroid Glands

The four parathyroid glands are located around the dorsal and lower aspect of the thyroid gland (see Figure 30-5). Each parathyroid gland is about 6 mm in diameter and weighs about 0.033 grams. The parathyroids secrete parathormone (PTH). PTH is responsible for the maintenance of normal serum calcium levels, along with that of phosphorus. Hyposecretion of PTH may result in hypoparathyroidism, causing tetany (twitching of muscles or nerves). Hypersecretion of PTH may result in hyperparathyroidism, which can result in osteoporosis, kidney stones, and hypercalcemia.

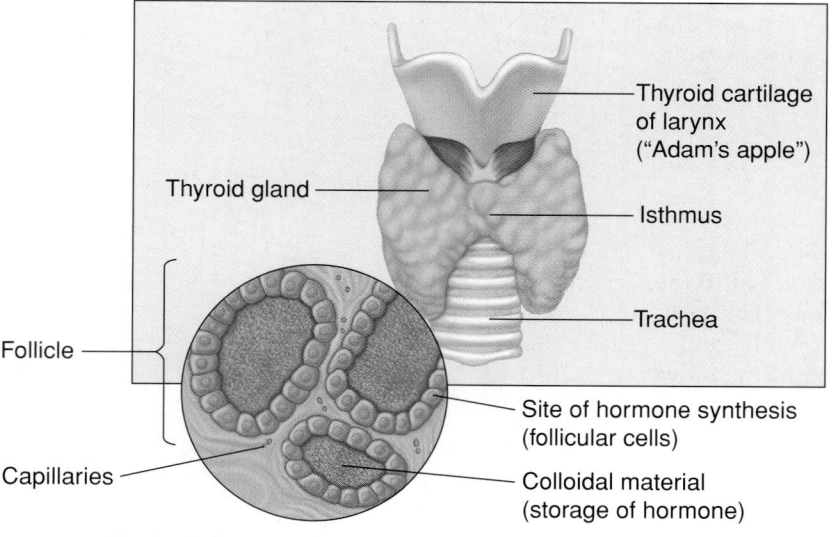

Thyroid cartilage of larynx ("Adam's apple")

Thyroid gland

Isthmus

Trachea

Follicle

Site of hormone synthesis (follicular cells)

Capillaries

Colloidal material (storage of hormone)

FIGURE 30-4   The thyroid gland.

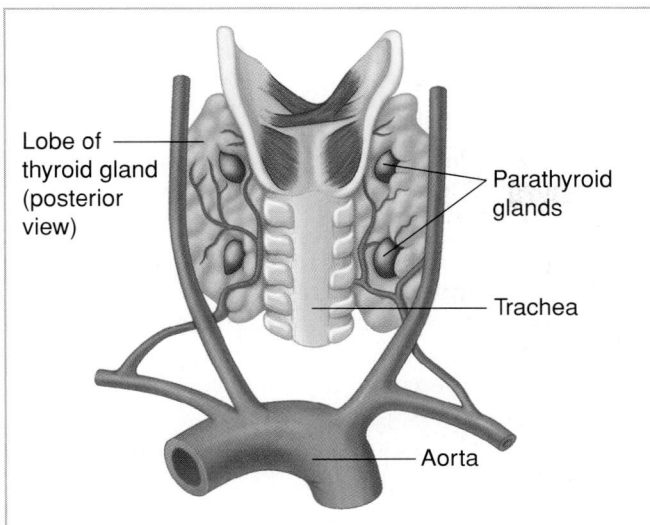

FIGURE 30-5 Parathyroid glands.

Pancreas (Islets of Langerhans)

The islets of Langerhans are small clusters of cells located within the pancreas (see Figure 30-6). Three types of cells make up the islets of Langerhans: the alpha, beta, and delta cells. The alpha cells secrete the hormone glucagon, which helps break down glycogen to glucose, increasing blood sugar. The beta cells secrete the hormone insulin, which lowers blood sugar. Normal fasting blood sugar is 70 to 110 mg/dL. In individuals who do not produce enough insulin, a synthetic insulin can be injected subcutaneously to help control the blood sugar. Hyposecretion of insulin results in diabetes mellitus. Hypersecretion results in hyperinsulinemia. The delta cells secrete somatostatin, which suppresses the release of glucagon and insulin.

Adrenal Glands

The adrenal glands are located on top of each kidney (see Figure 30-7). Each gland is triangle shaped and consists of an outer portion (cortex) and an inner portion (medulla).

Adrenal Cortex

The adrenal cortex secretes the groups of hormones called glucocorticoids (cortisol and corticosterone), mineralocorticoids (aldosterone), and androgens. These hormones are essential to life, and are described here:

- Cortisol—the principal steroid secreted by the cortex. It is responsible for regulating carbohydrate, protein, and fat metabolism. It also stimulates the output of glucose from the liver, increasing the blood sugar level. Cortisol also promotes the transport of amino acids into extracellular tissue for energy stores, and it influences the effectiveness of the catecholamines such as dopamine, epinephrine, and norepinephrine. The final critical function of cortisol is as an anti-inflammatory. Hyposecretion of cortisol may result in Addison's disease. Hypersecretion of cortisol may result in Cushing's disease.

- Corticosterone—essential for the normal use of carbohydrates, the absorption of glucose, and gluconeogenesis.

- Aldosterone—the principal mineralocorticoid secreted by the adrenal cortex. Aldosterone is essential in regulating electrolyte and water balance by promoting sodium and chloride retention and potassium excretion. A reduced plasma volume may result from hyposecretion of aldosterone. Hypersecretion of the hormone may result in primary aldosteronism.

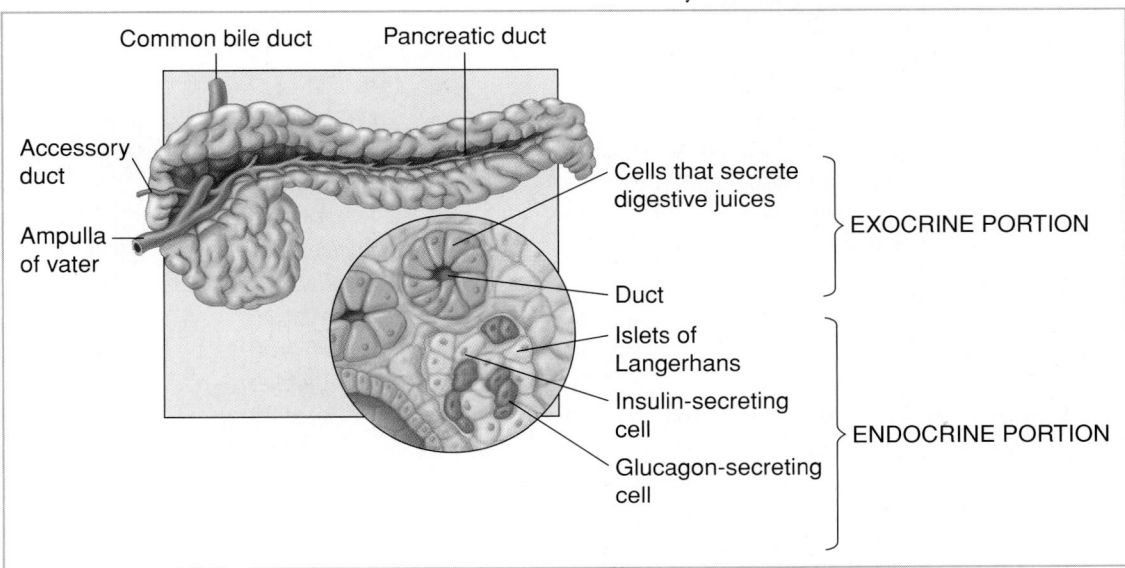

FIGURE 30-6 The pancreas—an endocrine and exocrine gland.

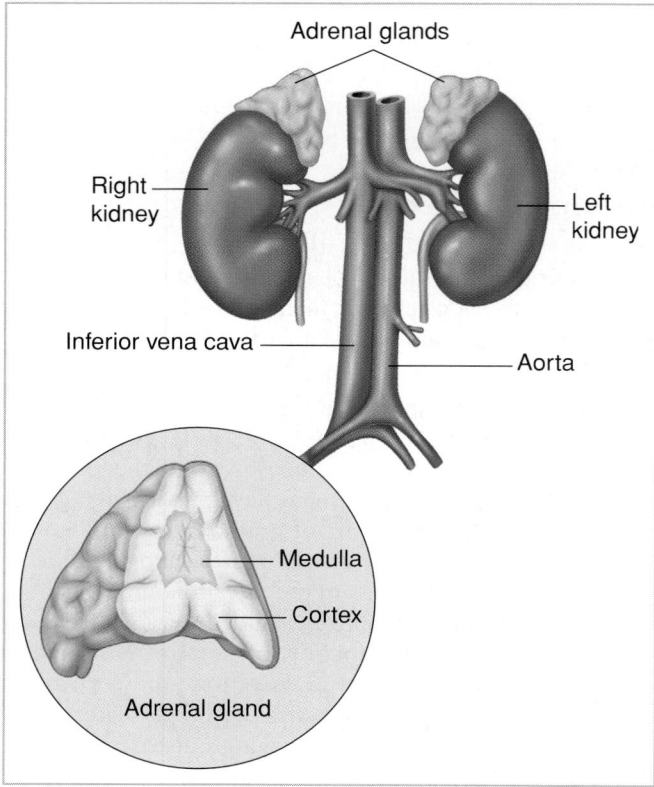

FIGURE 30-7 The adrenal glands.

- Androgens—Androgens are hormones that promote the development of male characteristics. The two main hormones are testosterone and an-

drosterone. These hormones cause the development of secondary sex characteristics.

Adrenal Medulla

The adrenal medulla synthesizes, secretes, and stores catecholamine. The primary catecholamines are dopamine, epinephrine, and norepinephrine:

- Dopamine—responsible for causing vasoconstriction, so that the blood pressure is increased. As a result, cardiac output is increased, and urine production is also stimulated. Synthetic dopamine can be administered in the treatment of shock.

- Epinephrine—also known as adrenaline, this catecholamine is responsible for the "fight or flight" syndrome, as regulated by the sympathetic nervous system. In times of stress, epinephrine causes peripheral vasoconstriction, dilation of the pupils, decreased salivation, decreased GI motility, and increased heart rate. It also elevates the blood pressure and dilates the bronchial tubes. It helps the body to get ready to flee in times of emergency. Epinephrine can be synthetically produced and administered in emergency situations, such as cardiac arrest or allergic reaction.

- Norepinephrine—also acts on the sympathetic nervous system by causing vasoconstriction, elevating systolic and diastolic blood pressure, and increasing the heart rate and cardiac output, while also increasing glycogenolysis.

Lifespan Considerations

THE CHILD

- Most of the structures and glands of the endocrine system develop during the first 3 months of pregnancy. During pregnancy, the hormones that cross the placental barrier protect the fetus. Because of maternal hormones, both male and female newborns may have swelling of the breasts and genitalia.

- Excessive production of growth hormone (GH) can cause gigantism. Insufficient production can cause dwarfism. The anterior lobe of the pituitary produces growth hormone.

- Diabetes mellitus is the most common endocrine system disorder of childhood. The rate of diabetes is highest among 5- to 7-year-olds and 11- to 13-year-olds. Individuals with childhood-onset diabetes mellitus typically lack the ability to secrete insulin.

Management of diabetes in children is somewhat challenging, because diet, exercise, and medication must be continually adjusted to meet the changing needs of the growing child.

THE OLDER ADULT

- The number of tissue receptors decreases with age, diminishing the body's response to hormones. Also, when the elderly develop diabetes, they typically have the ability to produce insulin, but not in sufficient quantities to manage blood sugar adequately.

- Other risk factors associated with the older adult and the development of diabetes, include age-related insulin resistance, heredity, decreased physical activity, multiple diseases, polypharmacy, obesity, and life stressors.

- Other changes in older adults include a decrease in estrogen production in females as a result of menopause, resulting in increased risk of heart disease and increased occurrence of osteoporosis.

Ovaries

The ovaries produce estrogens and progesterone (see Figure 30-8). Estrogen is the female sex hormone secreted by the graafian follicles of the ovaries. Progesterone is secreted by the corpus luteum and is a steroid hormone. These hormones are needed for promoting the growth, development, and maintenance of secondary female sex organs and characteristics. Other functions of these hormones include uterine pregnancy preparation and mammary gland preparation, and they also play a vital role in a woman's emotional well-being and sexual drive.

Testes

The testes are located in the male scrotum and produce the male hormone testosterone, which is essential for the normal growth and development of the male accessory sex organ (see Figure 30-9). Testosterone is necessary for the reproductive act of copulation.

Placenta

Only present during pregnancy, the placenta produces chorionic gonadotropin hormone, estrogen, and progesterone. Besides acting as an endocrine gland, the placenta is the spongy structure that joins the mother and the child and provides the blood supply between the two.

Gastrointestinal Mucosa

The mucosa of the pyloric area of the stomach secretes the hormone gastrin. Gastrin stimulates gastric acid secretion in the stomach, gallbladder, pancreas, and small intestine.

Secretin is secreted by the mucosa of the duodenum and jejunum. Secretin stimulates pancreatic juice, bile, and intestinal secretions. Pancreozymin-cholecystokinin, which stimulates the pancreas, is also secreted by duodenal mucosa, as is enterogastrone, a hormone that regulates gastric secretions.

Thymus Gland

The thymus gland is actually composed of lymphoid tissue and is located in the mediastinal cavity, in front of and above the heart (see Figure 30-10). The thymus is part of the lymphatic system, but also functions as an endocrine gland by releasing thymosin and thymopoietin. Thymosin promotes the maturation of T lymphocytes. Thymopoietin influences the production of lymphocyte precursors and aids in their process of becoming T lymphocytes.

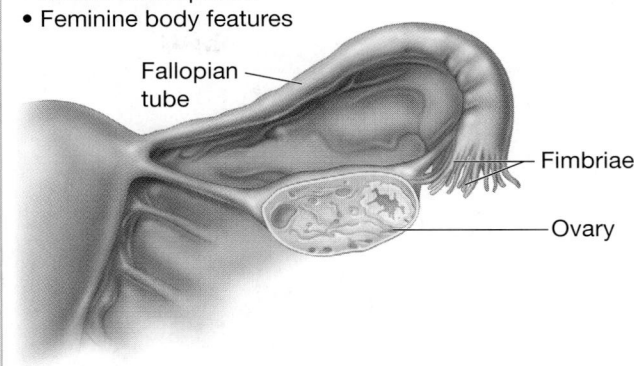

Female Secondary Sex Characteristics
- Sexual desire
- Body hair growth
- Breast development
- Feminine body features

Fallopian tube

Fimbriae

Ovary

FIGURE 30-8 Structure and functions of the ovary.

Common Disorders Associated with the Endocrine System

A variety of diseases are related to disorders of the endocrine system (see Table 30-1). Most are treated medically; however, there are a few surgical options.

Acromegaly

Acromegaly is a hormonal disorder that results when the pituitary gland produces excess growth hormone (GH). It most commonly affects middle-aged adults and can result in serious illness and premature death. The most serious health consequences of acromegaly are diabetes mellitus, hypertension, and increased risk of cardiovascular disease.

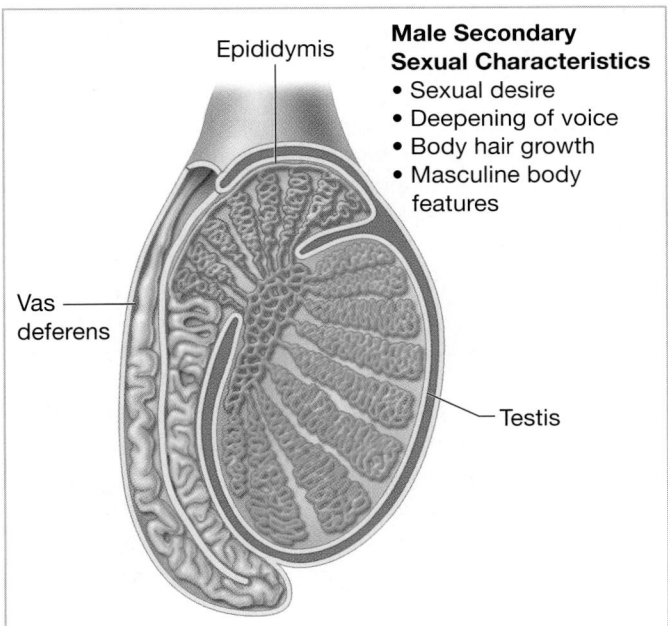

Epididymis

Male Secondary Sexual Characteristics
- Sexual desire
- Deepening of voice
- Body hair growth
- Masculine body features

Vas deferens

Testis

FIGURE 30-9 Structure and function of male testes.

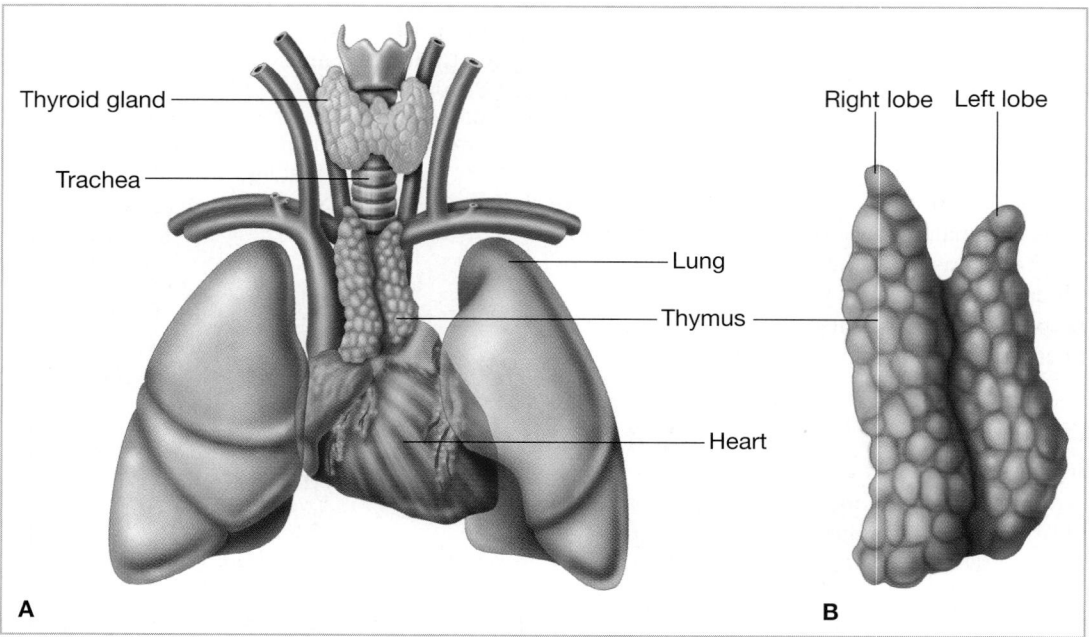

FIGURE 30-10 The thymus gland: (A) appearance and position; (B) with anatomical structures.

Common symptoms of acromegaly are the abnormal growth of the hands and feet. Soft tissue swelling of the hands and feet is often an early feature, with patients noticing a change in ring or shoe size. Gradually, bony changes alter the patient's facial features: the brow and lower jaw protrude, the nasal bone enlarges, and spacing of the teeth increases. Overgrowth of bone and cartilage often leads to arthritis. When tissue thickens, it may trap nerves, causing carpal tunnel syndrome, characterized by numbness and weakness of the hands. Other symptoms of acromegaly include thick, coarse, oily skin; skin tags; enlarged lips, nose, and tongue; deepening of the voice due to enlarged sinuses and vocal cords; snoring due to upper airway obstruction; excessive sweating and skin odor; fatigue and weakness; headaches; impaired vision; abnormalities of the menstrual cycle and sometimes breast discharge in women; and impotence in men. There may be enlargement of body organs, including the liver, spleen, kidneys, and heart.

Preparing for Externship

Part of preparing for externship is examining your own values, how you work with others, and how you view others. As a professional, all patients must be treated with equal respect, regardless of how they might treat you. Learning to do this is part of the process of developing as a professional.

The goals of treatment for acromegaly are to reduce GH production to normal levels, to relieve the pressure that the growing pituitary tumor exerts on the surrounding brain areas, to preserve normal pituitary function, and to reverse or ameliorate the symptoms of acromegaly. Currently, treatment options include surgical removal of the tumor, drug therapy, and radiation therapy of the pituitary.

Addison's Disease

Addison's disease occurs when the cortex of the adrenal gland is damaged, decreasing the production of adrenocortical hormones. This is usually an autoimmune disease, where the body attacks itself. Other causes of Addison's disease include infection of the adrenal glands, cancer, or hemorrhage into the glands.

Addison's disease can occur at any age, including infancy, and is equally prevalent in both men and women. It is rare, occurring in 1 in 100,000 Americans. Signs and symptoms of Addison's disease include weight loss, anorexia, weakness and lethargy, increased pigmentation of the skin and mucous membranes, hypoglycemia, joint and muscle aches, persistent fever, nausea, vomiting, diarrhea, and abdominal discomfort.

Most of the signs and symptoms occur over several months; however, they may occasionally appear quite suddenly. Addison's disease is diagnosed by blood and urine tests that measure the amount of corticosteroid hormones present. With a diagnosis of Addison's disease, the level of corticosteroids is very low.

Treatment consists of replacement of adrenocortical hormones and supplemental sodium. The patient and family are taught the importance of lifelong treatment

TABLE 30-1   Disorders of the Endocrine System

Disorder	Description
Acidosis	Excessive acidity of bodily fluids due to the accumulation of acids, as in diabetic acidosis.
Acromogaly	Chronic disease of middle-aged persons that results in an elongation and enlargement of the bones of the head and extremities. There can also be mood changes.
Addison's disease	A disease resulting from a deficiency in adrenocortical hormones. There may be an increased pigmentation of the skin, generalized weakness, and weight loss.
Adenoma	A neoplasm or tumor of a gland.
Cretinism	Congenital condition due to a lack of thyroid, which may result in arrested physical and mental development.
Cushing's syndrome	Set of symptoms that result from hypersecretion of the adrenal cortex. This may be the result of a tumor of the adrenal glands. The syndrome may present symptoms of weakness, edema, excess hair growth, skin discoloration, and osteoporosis.
Diabetes insipidus (DI)	Disorder caused by the inadequate secretion of the antidiuretic hormone ADH by the posterior lobe of the pituitary gland. There may be polyuria and polydipsia.
Diabetes mellitus (DM)	Chronic disorder of carbohydrate metabolism which results in hyperglycemia and glycosuria. Type 1 diabetes mellitus (IDDM) involves insulin dependency, which requires that the patient take daily injections of insulin. Type 2 (NIDDM) patients may not be insulin dependent.
Diabetic retinopathy	Secondary complication of diabetes mellitus (DM) that affects the blood vessels of the retina, resulting in visual changes and even blindness.
Dwarfism	Condition of being abnormally small. It may be the result of a hereditary condition or an endocrine dysfunction.
Gigantism	Excessive development of long bones of the body due to overproduction of the growth hormone by the pituitary gland.
Goiter	Enlargement of the thyroid gland.
Graves' disease	Disease that results from an overactivity of the thyroid gland and can result in a crisis situation. Also called hyperthyroidism.
Hashimoto's disease	A chronic form of thyroiditis.
Hirsutism	Condition of having an excessive amount of hair on the body. This term is used to describe females who have the adult male pattern of hair growth. Can be the result of a hormonal imbalance.
Hypercalcemia	Condition of having an excessive amount of calcium in the blood.
Hyperglycemia	Having an excessive amount of glucose (sugar) in the blood.
Hyperkalemia	Condition of having an excessive amount of potassium in the blood.
Hyperthyroidism	Condition that results from overactivity of the thyroid gland. Also called Graves' disease.
Hypothyroidism	Result of a deficiency in secretion by the thyroid gland. This results in a lowered basal metabolism rate with obesity, dry skin, slow pulse, low blood pressure, sluggishness, and goiter. Treatment is replacement with synthetic thyroid hormone.

(continued)

TABLE 30-1   Disorders of the Endocrine System *(continued)*

Disorder	Description
Ketoacidosis	Acidosis due to an excess of ketone bodies (waste products) that can result in death for the diabetic patient if not reversed.
Myasthenia gravis	Condition in which there is great muscular weakness and progressive fatigue. There may be difficulty in chewing and swallowing and drooping eyelids. If a thymoma is causing the problem, it can be treated with removal of the thymus gland.
Myxedema	Condition resulting from a hypofunction of the thyroid gland. Symptoms can include anemia, slow speech, enlarged tongue and facial features, edematous skin, drowsiness, and mental apathy.
Thyrotoxicosis	Condition that results from overproduction of the thyroid gland. Symptoms include a rapid heart action, tremors, enlarged thyroid gland, exophthalmos, and weight loss.
von Rechlinghausen's disease	Excessive production of parathyroid hormone that results in degeneration of the bones.

and intramuscular hydrocortisone injections. The patient needs to always carry medical identification.

Cushing's Disease

Cushing's disease is a rare disorder than develops when there is too much cortisol (see Figure 30-11). ACTH releases cortisol as a result of stimulation of the pituitary. Symptoms of Cushing's syndrome include weight gain, skin changes, and fatigue. Results of the disease include diabetes, high blood pressure, depression, and osteoporosis. Cushing's disease can cause death if it is not treated. Treatments include surgery and radiation.

Legal and Ethical Issues

Each state has its own laws regarding individuals with diabetes driving school buses and other forms of public transportation. It is important to understand the regulations in your state. In some states, if there is evidence that the diabetes is controlled, then the individual may be allowed to drive one of these means of transportation. These individuals do typically need regular monitoring with the appropriate documentation sent to the authorities. The medical assistant is often integral in maintaining these records.

Diabetes Mellitus

Patients with diabetes mellitus have an inability to produce enough insulin to properly control their blood sugar levels. Insulin is a hormone that converts sugar and starches into the energy that the body needs.

Diabetes is a silent disease, especially adult-onset diabetes, which may not be detected until it has become advanced. According to the American Diabetes Association, approximately 11.1 million people have been diagnosed with diabetes, but an estimated 5.9 million individuals are undiagnosed.

Classic symptoms of diabetes are polyuria (frequent urination), polydipsia (excessive thirst), and polyphagia (excessive hunger). Other symptoms include weakness, weight loss, lethargy, anorexia, irritability, dry skin, vaginal yeast infections in women, recurrent infections, and abdominal cramps.

There are three types of diabetes. Juvenile diabetes is also known as type 1 diabetes. This is typically diagnosed in children who cannot produce sufficient quantities if any, of insulin. These individuals are typically dependent on insulin injections for the duration of their life. Type 1 diabetes is also known as insulin-dependent diabetes mellitus (IDDM).

Type 2 diabetes is also known as non–insulin-dependent diabetes mellitus (NIDDM) or adult-onset diabetes. Typically, type 2 diabetes is diagnosed later in life and is the most common form of the disease. It results from insulin resistance combined with a relative insulin deficiency. There is a very strong correlation between obesity and type 2 diabetes. People who are

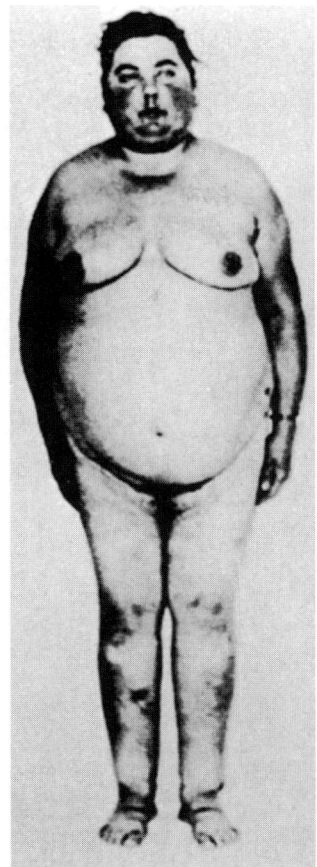
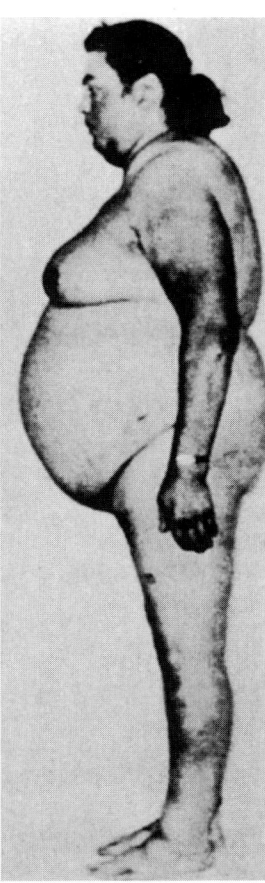

FIGURE 30-11 Cushing's syndrome patient showing round, red face; stocky neck; and marked obesity of the trunk with protruding abdomen. Note bruises on trunk and legs and also stretch marks. Note fat pads above the collar bone and on the back of the neck, which produces the "buffalo hump."

overweight may make sufficient insulin for their ideal body weight, but their body cannot make enough insulin to compensate for extra weight.

Type 2 diabetes is treated with diet and exercise, along with the administration of oral hypoglycemic medications to help control the blood sugar levels. It may also be possible to prevent type 2 diabetes with modest lifestyle changes, including healthy diet choices, exercise, and weight management.

Gestational diabetes is pregnancy-related diabetes. Typically, this type of diabetes disappears after the pregnancy is completed, but occasionally precipitates ongoing type 2 diabetes. During pregnancy, this pa-

tient may have to monitor her diet and blood sugar, and she may need to give herself insulin injections on a daily basis.

Dwarfism

Dwarfism refers to a group of conditions characterized by shorter than normal skeletal growth. This shortness can be manifested in the arms and legs or trunk. More than 300 conditions can cause abnormal skeletal growth and dwarfism. Achondroplasia is the most common type of short-limb dwarfism, occurring in 1 in 25,000 children with both sexes at equal risk. This type of skeletal dysplasia (abnormal skeletal growth) is usually diagnosed at birth.

The majority of children born with the disorder have average-sized parents. The child may experience a delay in developing motor skills, such as controlling the movements of the head, but intellectual development is normal in children with achondroplasia. The average final height for a person with this condition is 130 cm for men and 125 cm for women. Short-statured people lead normal, fulfilled lives. Achieving higher levels of

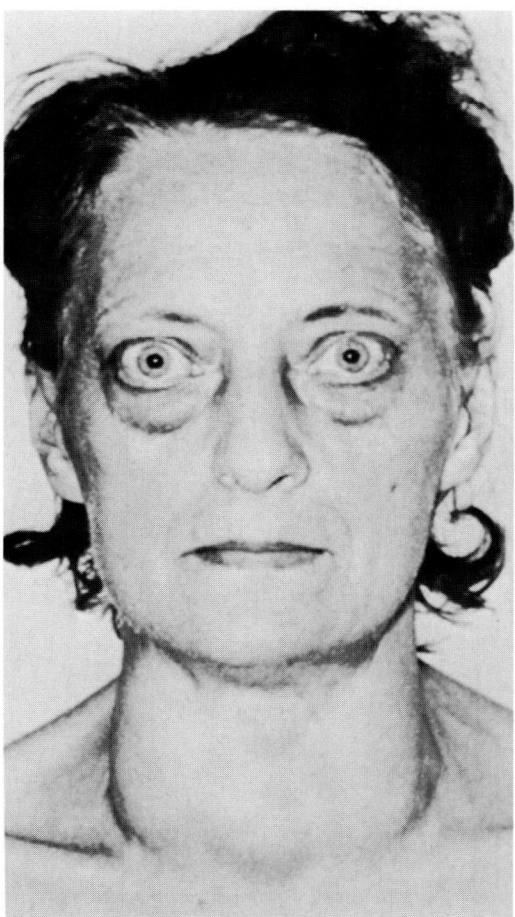

FIGURE 30-12   A patient with exophthalmos.

growth plates, which causes overgrowth of the long bones and very tall stature. The vertical growth in height that marks this condition is also accompanied by growth in muscles and organs, which makes the child extremely large for his or her age. The disorder can also delay puberty.

The cause of excess growth hormone secretion is most often a pituitary gland tumor. Gigantism may also be caused by an underlying medical condition such as multiple endocrine neoplasia. Pituitary tumors are never malignant (cancerous). If excessive secretion of growth hormone occurs after normal bone growth has stopped, the condition is known as acromegaly. Treatments for gigantism include radiation therapy and surgical removal of the tumor.

Hyperthyroidism

In hyperthyroidism, the thyroid hormone levels are elevated. The symptoms of elevated thyroid levels include nervousness, heart palpitations, tremors, sweating, increased activity in the intestinal tract, changes in menstruation, and weight loss. Sometimes, there is a feeling of anxiousness or restlessness, along with changes in the fingernails and hair. Palpitations may be presented, along with possible enlargement of the heart. A condition known as exophthalmos may also affect the eyes. In this disease, the eyeball may protrude beyond its normal protective orbit when the tissues behind swell (see Figure 30-12).

education and career and personal ambitions is not limited by stature.

The physical characteristics of a person born with achondroplasia include a trunk of normal length; disproportionately short arms and legs; bowed legs; reduced joint mobility in the elbow, while other joints seem overly flexible, or "double jointed," because of loose ligaments; shortened hands and feet; large head; flat midface and crowded teeth, because of a small upper jaw; prominent forehead; and flattened bridge of the nose.

There is no cure for achondroplasia. Treatment focuses on the prevention, management, and treatment of medical complications as well as social and family support. Surgery may be advised to relieve pressure on the nervous system, generally at the base of the skull and lower back, or to open obstructed airways by removing the adenoids. Dental and orthodontic work may be necessary to correct malocclusion and ensure dental health.

Gigantism

Gigantism is an excessive secretion of growth hormone during childhood before the closure of the bone

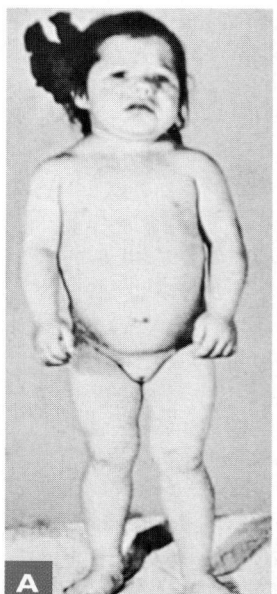
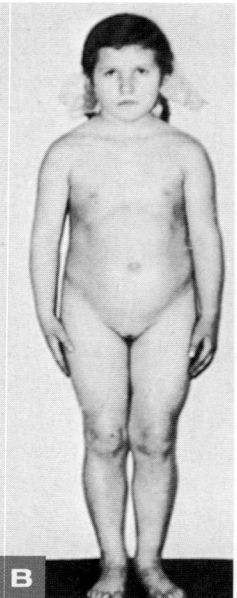

FIGURE 30-13   (A) A 6-year old child with congenital hypothyroidism, cretinism, exhibiting marked mental and physical retardation. (B) The same patient after 3 years of thyroxine therapy, which resulted in a spurt of growth and regression of pathological manifestations. Mental retardation is delayed.

Graves' disease is the most common cause of hyperthyroidism. It is an autoimmune disorder when the antibodies produced by the immune system stimulate the thyroid to produce too much thyroxine. Other forms of hyperthyroidism may be caused by thyroiditis (inflammation of the thyroid gland) or benign or malignant tumors.

Hyperthyroidism can lead to a rapid heart rate, atrial fibrillation, and congestive heart failure. Other complications include osteoporosis (weak, brittle bones), bulging red or swollen eyes, sensitivity to light or blurring and double vision.

Hyperthyroidism is treated with antithyroid medications, radioactive iodine to destroy the thyroid, or surgery (thyroidectomy). If the thyroid is removed or destroyed, then lifelong thyroid replacement therapy must be initiated.

Hypothyroidism

In hypothyroidism, the thyroid does not produce adequate amounts of the thyroid hormones. Because hypothyroidism develops slowly, only about half of the 7 million cases in the United States are diagnosed early. Figure 30-13 shows an example of a child born with hypothyroidism.

Symptoms initially tend to be subtle, including fatigue, decreased concentration, intolerance to cold environments, constipation, loss of appetite, muscle cramping, stiffness, and weight gain. Other symptoms may include hair loss, dry skin, and nail changes. Untreated hypothyroidism can lead to other conditions because the constant stimulation to release more thyroid hormones can cause the thyroid gland to enlarge. This condition is called a goiter (see Figure 30-14). The most common cause of a goiter is Hashimoto's thyroiditis, an autoimmune inflammation of the thyroid. If hypothyroidism goes untreated, there is an associated risk of heart disease, due to the high levels of low-density lipoproteins (LDL—bad cholesterol) that can occur. Cardiomegaly (an enlarged heart) can also occur.

Other complications of hypothyroidism include depression, decreased sexual desire, and slowed mental functioning. Myxedema is a rare, life-threatening condition that is a result of long-term, untreated hypothyroidism (see Figure 30-15). The symptoms of myxedema include intense cold intolerance and drowsiness followed by profound lethargy and unconsciousness. A myxedema coma can be triggered

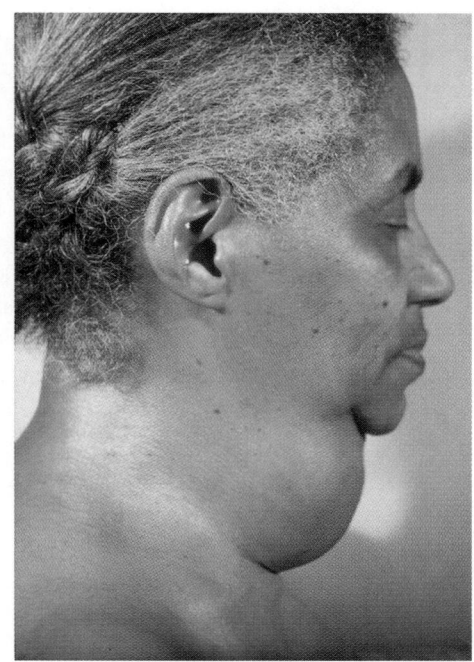

FIGURE 30-14 Goiter.

by sedatives, infection, or other stress. Emergency treatment should be initiated immediately if these symptoms are observed.

Typical treatment for hypothyroidism involves the daily use of a synthetic thyroid hormone called levothyroxine (Synthroid, Levothroid). This oral hormone reduces the symptoms of hypothyroidism, especially in the areas of fatigue, weight loss, and decrease of cholesterol levels. This medication must be taken on a routine basis; it should be monitored regularly with blood work and the dosage adjusted as necessary. Thyroid supplementation is a lifelong therapy.

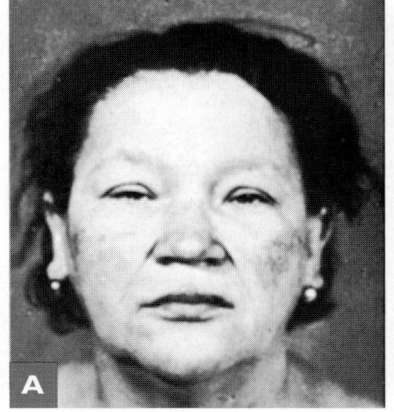 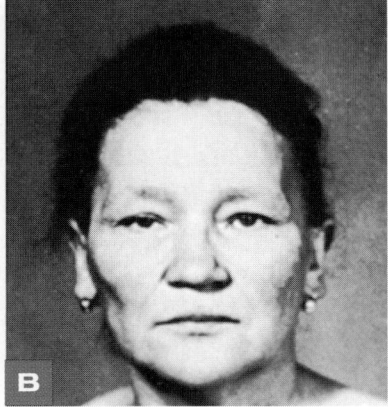

FIGURE 30-15 (A) A 62-year-old patient with myxedema exhibiting marked edema of the face and a somnolent look. The hair is stiff and without luster. (B) The same patient after 3 months of treatment with thyroxine.

SUMMARY

The endocrine system releases the hormones that keep the body in its proper balance, helping to maintain homeostasis. These hormones regulate growth, development, mood, tissue function, metabolism, and sexual function. This is achieved by a close working relationship with the nervous system.

Chapter Review

COMPETENCY REVIEW

1. Define and spell the terms to learn for this chapter.
2. What is the vital function of the endocrine system?
3. Why is the pituitary gland known as the master gland of the body?
4. What hormones are secreted by the thyroid gland?
5. What is the function of insulin?
6. What are the four functions of cortisol?
7. Name three functions of the hormone epinephrine.
8. Name the catecholamines synthesized, secreted, and stored by the adrenal medulla.
9. What hormones do the ovaries secrete?
10. Name two hormones secreted by the thymus.

PREPARING FOR THE CERTIFICATION EXAM

1. Which of the following organs/structures is/are NOT found in the endocrine system?
   A. pineal
   B. ovaries
   C. thymus
   D. testes
   E. spleen

2. Graves' disease is a result of the dysfunction of what structure?
   A. pituitary
   B. thymus
   C. ovary
   D. thyroid
   E. adrenal gland

continued on next page

3. The endocrine gland that is responsible for stimulating growth with the growth hormone (GH) is the
   A. parathyroid
   B. pancreas
   C. pituitary posterior lobe
   D. pituitary anterior lobe
   E. adrenal cortex

4. The result of inadequate secretion of the antidiuretic hormone from the pituitary gland is
   A. diabetes insipidus
   B. diabetes mellitus
   C. tetany
   D. exophthalmos
   E. Addison's disease

5. A chronic form of thyroiditis is
   A. myasthenia gravis
   B. myxedema
   C. Graves' disease
   D. Hashimoto's disease
   E. ketoacidosis

6. One of the leading causes of type 2 diabetes is
   A. excessive secretion of insulin
   B. obesity
   C. pancreatectomy
   D. high-protein diets
   E. inadequate control of type 1 diabetes

7. Individuals with hypothyroidism should expect to take medications to treat the disorder for
   A. 1–2 weeks
   B. 10 days
   C. 1 year
   D. 5 years
   E. the remainder of their lives

8. The function of aldosterone is
   A. development of male secondary sex characteristics
   B. development of female secondary sex characteristics
   C. water and electrolyte balance
   D. to suppress the release of glucagon and insulin
   E. to regulate the release of gonadotropin

9. The islets of Langerhans are found in the
   A. parathyroid glands
   B. anterior pituitary
   C. gastric mucosa
   D. pancreas
   E. posterior pituitary

10. Excessive secretion of growth hormone (GH) will result in
    A. exophthalmos
    B. dwarfism
    C. Simmonds' disease
    D. Cushing's syndrome
    E. gigantism

CRITICAL THINKING

1. List the symptoms that were indicative of the final diagnosis.
2. What is the difference between type 1 diabetes and type 2 diabetes?
3. Can this patient stop taking his insulin? Why?
4. This patient wants to play baseball with his friends. What adjustments will he need to make to be able to participate?

INTERNET ACTIVITY

Do an Internet search to learn about support groups for individuals with diabetes. What kind of support is available for people with this disorder?

MediaLink More on the endocrine system, including interactive resources, can be found on the Student CD-ROM accompanying this textbook.

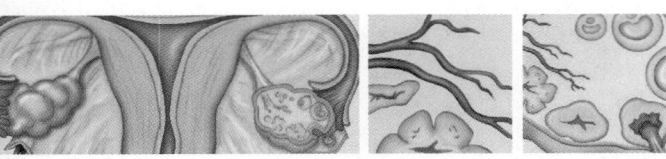

Medical Assistant Role Delineation Chart

HIGHLIGHT indicates material covered in this chapter.

ADMINISTRATIVE

Administrative Procedures

- Perform basic administrative medical assisting functions
- Schedule, coordinate and monitor appointments
- Schedule inpatient/outpatient admissions and procedures
- Understand and apply third-party guidelines
- Obtain reimbursement through accurate claims submission
- Monitor third-party reimbursement
- Understand and adhere to managed care policies and procedures
- *Negotiate managed care contracts*

Practice Finances

- Perform procedural and diagnostic coding
- Apply bookkeeping principles

- Manage accounts receivable
- *Manage accounts payable*
- *Process payroll*
- *Document and maintain accounting and banking records*
- *Develop and maintain fee schedules*
- *Manage renewals of business and professional insurance policies*
- *Manage personnel benefits and maintain records*
- *Perform marketing, financial, and strategic planning*

CLINICAL

Fundamental Principles

- Apply principles of aseptic technique and infection control
- Comply with quality assurance practices
- Screen and follow up patient test results

Diagnostic Orders

- Collect and process specimens
- Perform diagnostic tests

Patient Care

- Adhere to established patient screening procedures
- Obtain patient history and vital signs
- Prepare and maintain examination and treatment areas
- Prepare patient for examinations, procedures and treatments

- Assist with examinations, procedures and treatments
- Prepare and administer medications and immunizations
- Maintain medication and immunization records
- Recognize and respond to emergencies
- Coordinate patient care information with other health care providers
- Initiate IV and administer IV medications with appropriate training and as permitted by state law

GENERAL

Professionalism

- Display a professional manner and image
- Demonstrate initiative and responsibility
- Work as a member of the health care team
- Prioritize and perform multiple tasks
- Adapt to change
- Promote the CMA credential
- Enhance skills through continuing education
- Treat all patients with compassion and empathy
- Promote the practice through positive public relations

Communication Skills

- Recognize and respect cultural diversity
- Adapt communications to individual's ability to understand
- Use professional telephone technique

- Recognize and respond effectively to verbal, nonverbal, and written communications
- Use medical terminology appropriately
- Utilize electronic technology to receive, organize, prioritize and transmit information
- Serve as liaison

Legal Concepts

- Perform within legal and ethical boundaries
- Prepare and maintain medical records
- Document accurately
- Follow employer's established policies dealing with the health care contract
- Implement and maintain federal and state health care legislation and regulations
- Comply with established risk management and safety procedures
- Recognize professional credentialing criteria
- *Develop and maintain personnel, policy and procedure manuals*

Instruction

- Instruct individuals according to their needs
- Explain office policies and procedures
- Teach methods of health promotion and disease prevention
- Locate community resources and disseminate information
- *Develop educational materials*
- *Conduct continuing education activities*

Operational Functions

- Perform inventory of supplies and equipment
- Perform routine maintenance of administrative and clinical equipment
- Apply computer techniques to support office operations
- *Perform personnel management functions*
- *Negotiate leases and prices for equipment and supply contracts*

- *Denotes advanced skills.*

SOURCE: Reprinted by permission of the American Association of Medical Assistants from the AAMA Role Delineation Study: Occupational Analysis of the Medical Assisting Profession.

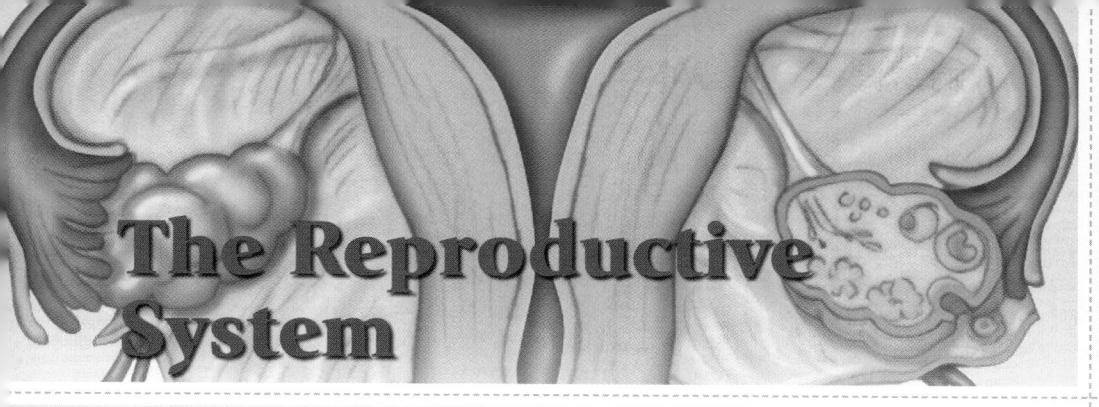

chapter 31

The Reproductive System

Learning Objectives

After completing this chapter, you should be able to:

- Define and spell the terms to learn for this chapter.
- Explain the purpose and function of the female reproductive system.
- Identify the structures of the female reproductive system and briefly explain the function of each.
- Explain the menstrual cycle.
- Explain the purpose and function of the male reproductive system.
- Identify the male external organs of reproduction and explain the function of each.
- Identify and state the function of the testes, epididymis, ductus deferens, seminal vesicles, prostate gland, bulbourethral glands, and the urethra.
- List common disorders associated with the female and male reproductive systems.

OUTLINE

Female Reproductive System	538
The Menstrual Cycle	542
Male Reproductive System	542
Common Disorders Associated with the Female Reproductive System	544
Common Disorders Associated with the Male Reproductive System	554

Terms to Learn

benign prostatic hyperplasia (BPH)

breast cancer

cervical cancer

cervicitis

circumcision

dysmenorrhea

endometriosis

epididymitis

episiotomy

erectile dysfunction (ED)

fibrocystic breast disease

hydrocele

hysterectomy

myomectomy

ovarian cancer

ovarian cysts

ovulation

pelvic inflammatory disease (PID)

perineum

premenstrual syndrome (PMS)

prostate cancer

sexually transmitted infection (STI)

urethritis

uterine cancer

uterine fibroids

vaginitis

Case Study

MARK SANSONE IS AN 85-YEAR-OLD MAN seen in the clinic with complaints of difficulty with urination. He needs to urinate often, especially at night; has difficulty starting his stream; has urgency; and has experienced a decrease in the size and force of his stream. The physician does a full physical on Mr. Sansone, including a PSA test, urinalysis, and digital rectal exam. He is diagnosed with benign prostatic hyperplasia and given a prescription. Mr. Sansone is to follow up with the physician in 6 months.

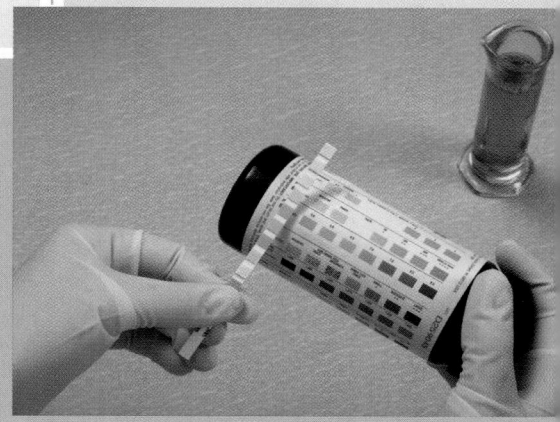

Female Reproductive System

The female reproductive system consists of the ovaries, which are the primary sex organs, and the accessory sex organs, which include the fallopian (uterine) tubes, the uterus, the vagina, the vulva, and the breasts (see Figure 31-1). The vital function of the female reproductive system is to perpetuate the species through sexual (germ cell) reproduction.

Uterus

The uterus is a hollow, pear-shaped, muscular organ located in the anterior portion of the pelvic cavity, between the sacrum and the symphysis pubis, above the bladder and in front of the rectum. There are three identifiable areas: the upper portion, called the body, the central portion, which is called the isthmus, and the neck, which is called the cervix. The fundus is the bulging surface of the body extending from the internal os (mouth) of the cervix upward above the fallopian tube. A number of ligaments support the uterus and hold it in place: two broad ligaments, two round ligaments, and two uterosacral ligaments. There are also ligaments that attach the uterus to the bladder. The normal position of the uterus is tilted, with the cervix pointing toward the sacrum and the fundus toward the suprapubic region. Generally, the normal uterus is about 8 cm long and 2.5 cm thick (see Figure 31-2).

The uterine wall has three layers: the perimetrium (the outer wall), the myometrium (the muscular middle layer), and the endometrium (the mucous membrane lining the inner surface). The endometrium is composed of columnar epithelium and connective tissue and is supplied with arterial blood. The endometrium undergoes marked changes in response to hormonal stimulation during the menstrual cycle.

The uterus has three primary functions. It is the site for cyclic discharge of blood fluid as evidenced by the changes in the endometrium in response to hormonal changes. It is also the site of nourishment and protection of the fetus during pregnancy. Finally, during labor, the myometrium contracts rhythmically to expel the fetus from the uterus.

As a result of weakness of any of the supporting ligaments, the uterus may become malpositioned. This may be caused by trauma, a disease process in the uterus, or as a result of multiple pregnancies. The more common abnormal positions of the uterus include anteflexion, which is the bending forward of the uterus at its body and neck; retroflexion, which is the bending backward of the uterus at any angle with the cervix unchanged from its normal position; anteversion, which is the process of turning the fundus toward the pubis, with the cervix tilted up toward the sacrum; and retroversion, which is the process of turning the uterus backward, with the cervix pointing forward toward the symphysis pubis.

Fallopian Tubes

The fallopian tubes, also called the uterine tubes or the oviducts, extend laterally from either side of the uterus near each ovary. Their function is to serve as ducts to move the ovum from the ovary to the uterus and to move sperm from the uterus toward the ovary. Each tube is about 11.5 cm long and 6 mm wide and is composed of three layers. The serous layer is the

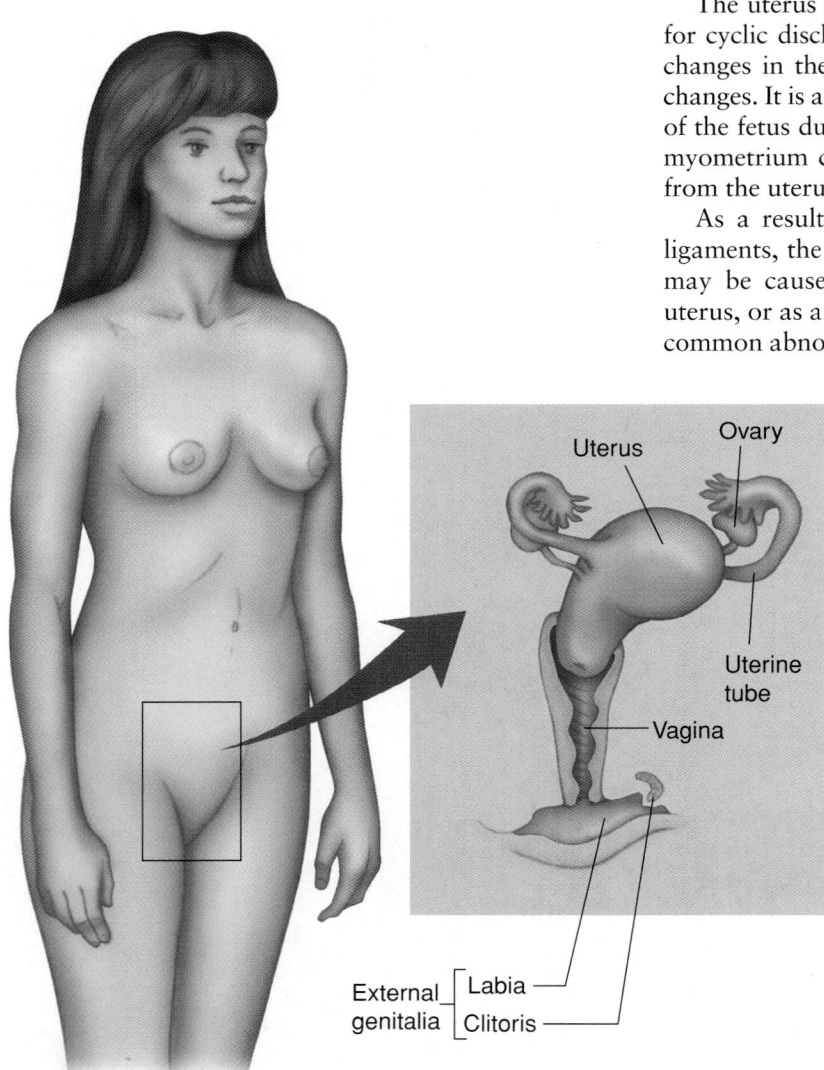

FIGURE 31-1 The female reproductive system.

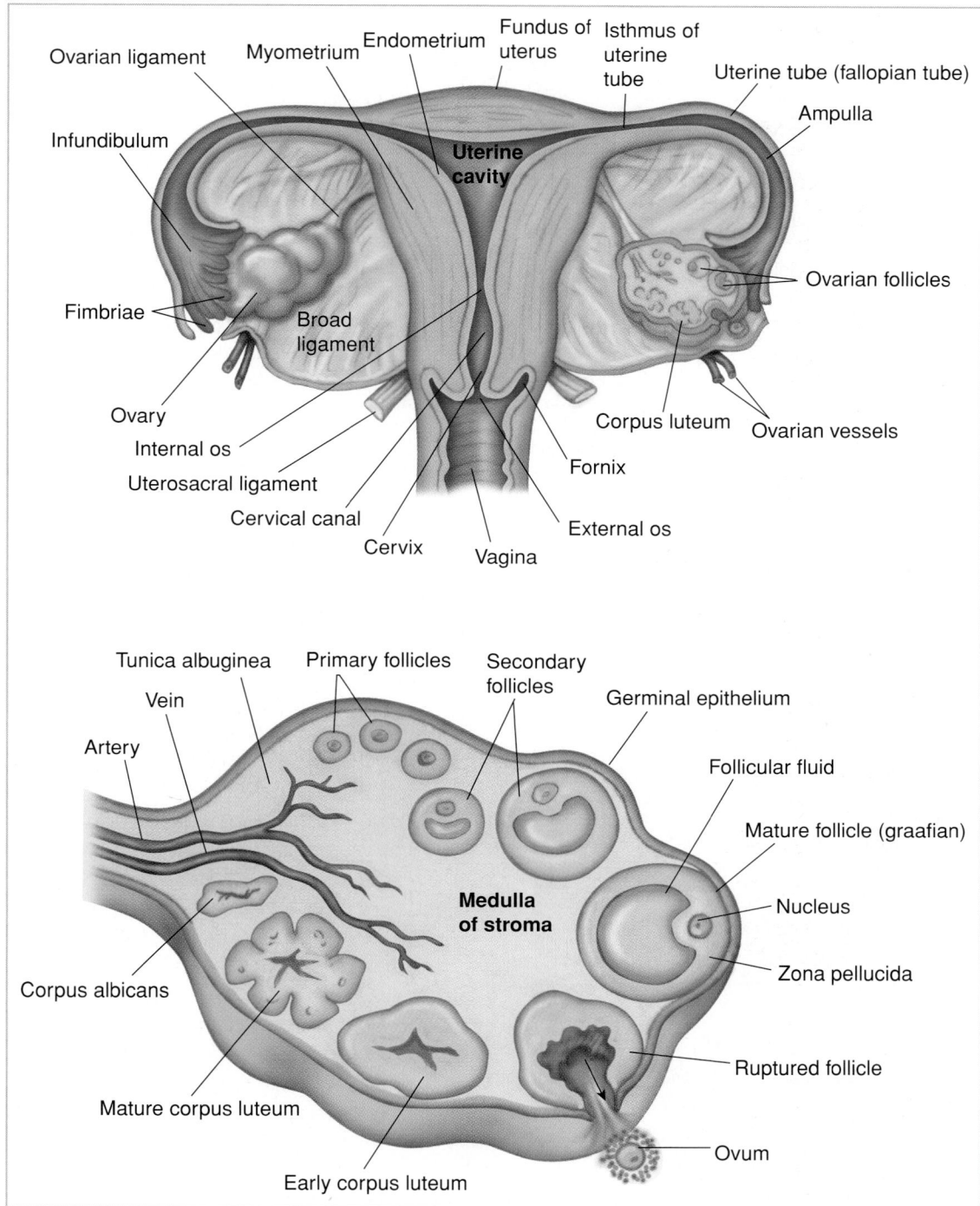

FIGURE 31-2   The uterus, ovaries, and associated structures, with expanded view of a mammalian ovary showing stages of graafian follicle and ovum development.

outermost layer made of connective tissue. The middle layer is the muscular layer, made of circular and longitudinal smooth muscle. The mucosa is the inner layer, consisting of simple columnar epithelium.

The isthmus is the constricted portion of the tube nearest the uterus. The tube extends laterally from the isthmus to the ampulla, where it widens. The tube continues to widen until it gains a funnel-shaped opening at the infundibulum called the ostium. Each ostium is surrounded by fimbriae, finger-like processes that help propel the ovum toward the tube after discharge from the uterus.

Ovaries

The two ovaries, located on either side of the uterus, are almond-shaped organs attached to the uterus by

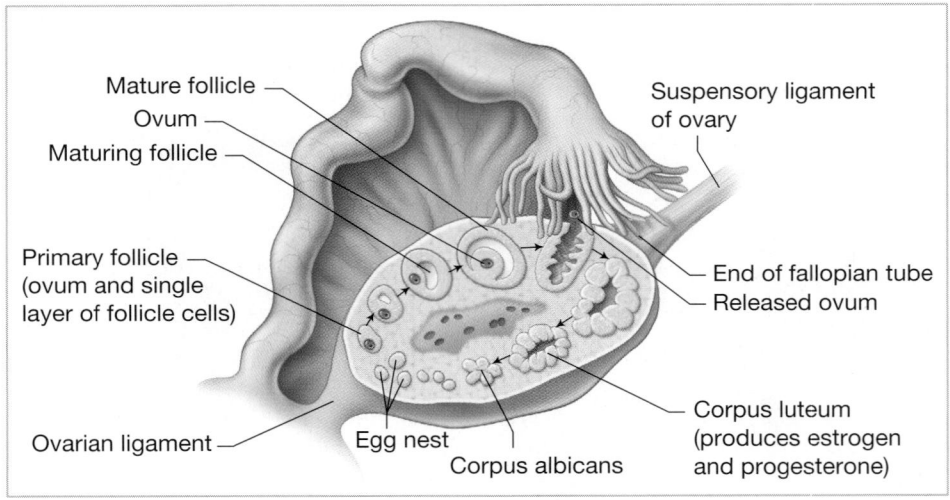

FIGURE 31-3 The ovary.

the ovarian ligament (see Figure 31-3). They lie close to the fimbriae of the fallopian tubes. The anterior border of each ovary is connected to the posterior layer of the broad ligament by the mesovarium. On the sides, they are attached by the suspensory liga- ments. Each ovary is about 4 cm long, 2 cm wide, and 1.5 cm thick.

There are two distinct microscopic divisions of the ovary: the cortex (the outer layer) and the medulla (in- ner layer). The cortex contains small secretory sacs

Lifespan
Considerations

THE CHILD
- *Every child develops according to his or her own biological clock. Puberty is triggered when the pituitary gland signals the body to release hormones. Hormones in turn stimulate the growth and development of the reproductive organs. Estrogen and testosterone spur the development of the child's secondary sex characteristics, such as breast development in girls and the growth of facial hair in boys. Fluctuating levels of hormones may also bring on adolescent mood swings.*

THE OLDER ADULT
- *The most dramatic age-related changes in the reproductive system occur with women at menopause when their estrogen production ceases and they lose their capacity to reproduce. The menopause in which the cycle of ovulation ceases occurs between the ages of 45 and 52 years.*
- *The lower estrogen levels also cause atrophic changes in the uterus and vagina. The uterine lin- ing thins and the elasticity decreases. Vaginal se- cretions are reduced. Common symptoms include hot flashes, palpitations, irritability, headaches, depression, fatigue, weight gain, insomnia, night sweats, forgetfulness, and inability to concentrate. The vaginal walls become thinner and less elastic and there is a decrease in lubrication.*
- *In the years following menopause, the circulating follicle-stimulating hormone (FSH) and luteinizing hormones (LH) are greatly increased. Over subse- quent years, FSH and LH levels fall slowly before leveling off about 30 years after menopause. These hormonal changes cause a relaxation of lig- aments and a loss of muscular tone that alter the contour of the breast. Women also face an in- creased risk for osteoporosis, heart attack, stroke, and possibly Alzheimer's disease.*
- *In men, the decline in reproductive ability is more gradual. The testes secrete testosterone and pro- duce spermatozoa. With aging, the rate of sperm production slows although there are few changes in sperm number so this does not affect fertility. However, there may be an increase in chromoso- mal abnormalities. By the age of 85 there is a 35 percent decrease in the level of testosterone and a reduction in the size of the testes. The amount of fluid ejaculated remains the same. Declining levels of testosterone may be partly responsible for losses in muscle strength.*

called follicles, which hold the ova in differing stages of development. The different stages are the primary, growing, and graafian. The ovarian medulla contains connective tissue, nerves, blood and lymphatic vessels, and some smooth muscles at the hilus.

The functions of the ovaries are to produce ova (eggs, or reproductive cells) and to produce hormones. The activity of the ovaries is controlled by the anterior lobe of the pituitary, which produces the gonadotropic hormones, FSH (follicle-stimulating hormone) and luteinizing hormone (LH). FSH is instrumental in the development of the follicle nurturing the ovum. Luteinizing hormone stimulates the development of the corpus luteum, a small mass of cells that develops after the release of the ovum. Each month, a graafian follicle ruptures on the ovarian cortex, and an ovum releases into the pelvic cavity and into the fallopian tube. This process is known as ovulation. In the average normal woman, more than 400 ova may be produced during the reproductive years.

The hormones estrogen and progesterone are also produced by the ovaries. These two hormones play key roles in the reproductive system. Estrogen is the female sex hormone secreted by the follicles. Progesterone is a steroid hormone secreted by the corpus luteum. Both hormones are responsible for promoting growth, development, and maintenance of the female secondary sex characteristics and organs. They prepare the uterus for pregnancy, promote development of the mammary glands, and play a major role in a woman's emotional well-being and sexual drive.

Vagina

The vagina is a musculomembranous tube extending from the vestibule to the uterus. Typically, the vagina is 10 to 15 cm in length and is situated between the bladder and the rectum. It is lined by mucous membrane and squamous epithelium. There is a fold of membrane called the hymen that partially covers the external opening of the vagina.

The vagina has three basic functions. It is the organ of female copulation, the passageway for discharge of menstruation, and the passageway for the birth of the fetus.

Vulva

The vulva consists of the five organs that comprise the external female genitalia. These include the following structures:

- Mons pubis: The pad of fatty, triangular-shaped fatty tissue that is covered with hair after puberty. It is the rounded area over the symphysis pubis.
- Labia majora: The two folds of adipose tissue that are lip-like structures lying on either side of the vaginal opening.

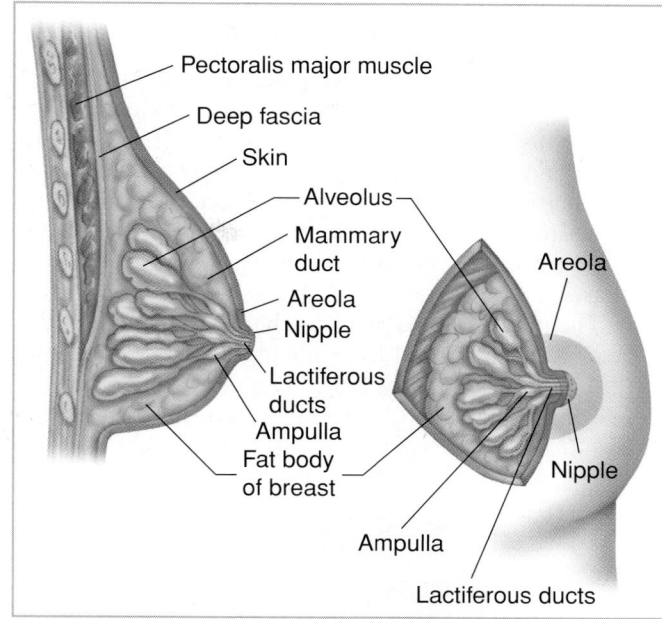

FIGURE 31-4 The breast.

- Labia minora: The two thin folds of skin within the labia majora enclosing the vestibule.
- Vestibule: The cleft between the labia minora, approximately 4 to 5 cm long and about 2 cm wide. There are four structures in the vestibule: the urethra (the external opening of the urinary system), the vagina, and the two excretory glands of the Bartholin's glands.
- Clitoris: Small organ of sensitive erectile tissue that is analogous to the penis of the male.

Between the vulva and the anus is an external region known as the perineum, which is composed of muscle covered with skin. Sometimes during labor, this area is incised by the physician in a process called episiotomy, which is performed in order to prevent tearing of the perineum during delivery.

Breast

The breasts, or mammary glands, are compound alveolar structures consisting of 15 to 12 glandular tissue lobes separated by septa of connecting tissue (see Figure 31-4). The areola is the dark, pigmented area found in the skin of each breast, and the nipple is the elevated area in the center of the areola. During pregnancy, the areola changes from pinkish in color to a darker brown or reddish color. The areola is supplied with a row of small sebaceous glands that secrete an oil that keeps it resilient. The lactiferous glands consist of 20 to 24 glands in the areola of the nipple and during lactation will provide milk to a suckling infant. Prolactin is the hormone produced by the anterior lobe of the pituitary that stimulates the mammary glands to produce milk after childbirth. The other hormones that play a role in milk production include insulin and glucocorticoids.

The Menstrual Cycle

The onset of the menstrual cycle, called the menarche, occurs at the age of puberty, and the cessation is called menopause. Typically, the menstrual cycle lasts about 28 days, with a cycle of a repetitive series of changes to the uterine tissue, breasts, and vagina. There are four phases to the menstrual cycle: menstruation, proliferation, luteal (or secretory), and the premenstrual (or ischemic) phases.

The menstruation phase is characterized by the discharge of blood fluid from the uterus by a shedding of the endometrium. This phase averages 4 to 5 days. The first day of the blood discharge is considered the first day of the cycle. The proliferation phase is characterized by the thickening and vascularization of the endometrium, along with the maturing of the ovarian follicle. This phase begins on about the fifth day of the cycle and lasts until the eruption of the graafian follicle, about day 14.

The luteal or secretory phase is characterized by the continued thickening of the endometrium, while the glands in the endometrium become tortuous, and by the appearance of coiled arteries in the tissue. The endometrium becomes edematous (swollen and fluid filled). During this phase, the body is preparing for a possible pregnancy by getting the endometrium ready to support the early developmental phase of an embryo. The corpus luteum in the ovary is developing and secreting progesterone at this time. The progesterone level is at its highest during this phase, and the estrogen level begins to decrease.

During the premenstrual, or ischemic, phase, the coiled arteries become constricted, the endometrium becomes anemic and begins to shrink, and the corpus luteum decreases in functional activity. This phase lasts about 2 days and ends with the onset of menstruation.

Male Reproductive System

The male reproductive system consists of the testes; various ducts; the urethra; accessory glands, which include the bulbourethral, prostate, and the seminal vesicles; and the supporting structures and accessory sex organs, the scrotum and the penis (see Figure 31-5). The vital function of the male reproductive system is to provide the sperm cells necessary to fertilize the ovum, thereby perpetuating the species.

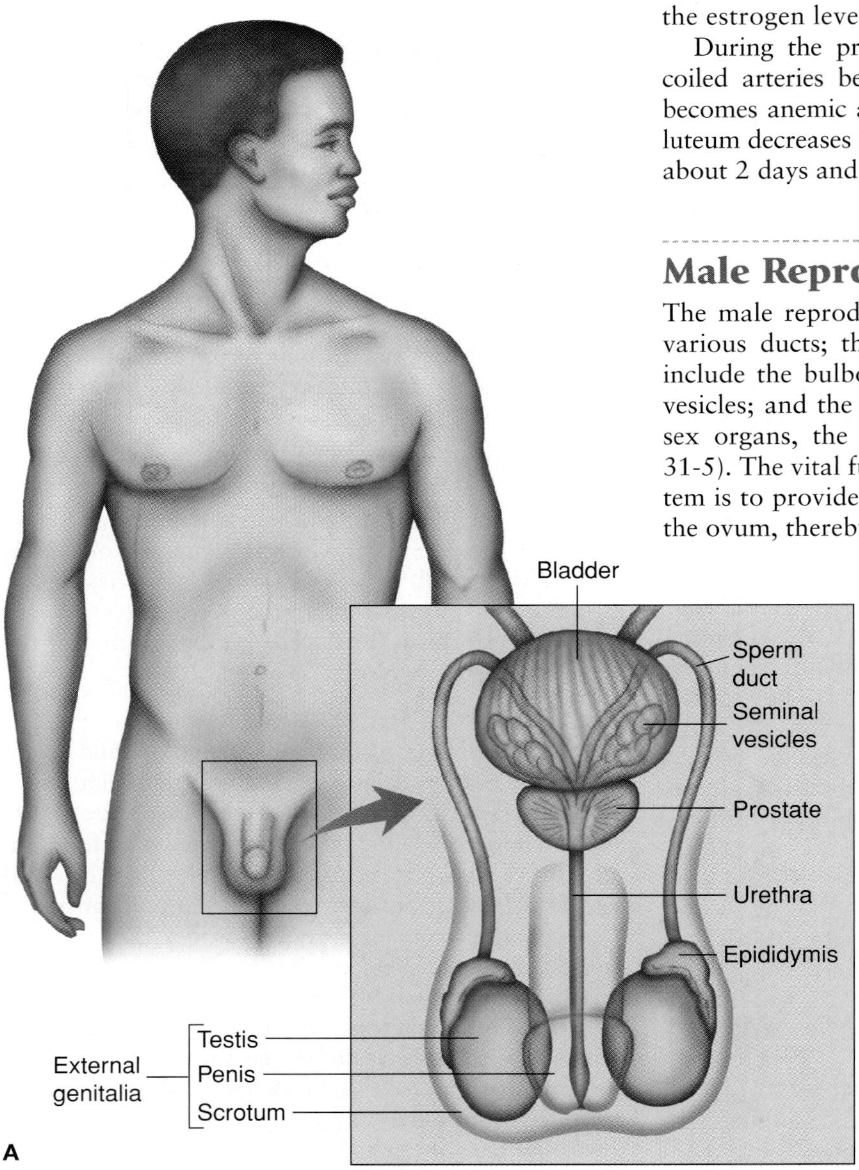

FIGURE 31-5 (A) The male reproductive system: sperm duct, seminal vesicles, prostate, urethra, epididymis, and external genitalia.

External Organs

In the male, the scrotum and the penis are the external organs of reproduction. The scrotum is a pouch-like structure, located behind the penis. It is suspended from the perineal region and is divided into two sacs by a septum, one containing each of the two testes along with the epididymis, the connecting tube to the rest of the reproductive system. The tissues of the scrotum have fibers of smooth muscle that contract in the absence of sufficient heat, giving the scrotum a wrinkled appearance. This contractile action brings the testes closer to the perineum, helping them to absorb sufficient body heat to maintain the viability of the spermatozoa.

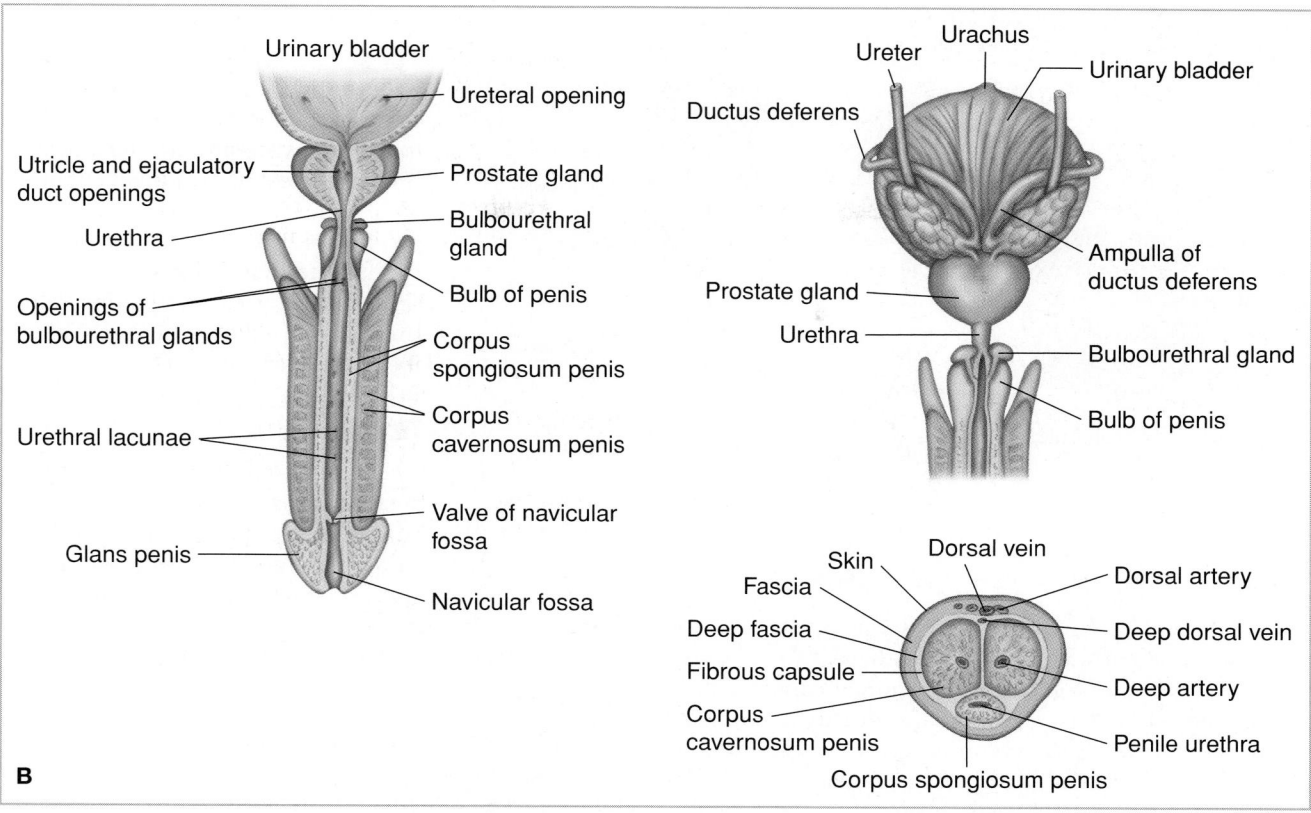

FIGURE 31-5 (B) The structures of the bladder, prostate gland, and penis.

The penis is the male external sex organ and is composed of erectile tissue and covered with skin. The size and shape of the penis varies with an average erect penis being about 15 to 20 cm in length. There are three longitudinal columns of erectile tissues capable of significant enlargement when engorged with blood, such as during sexual stimulation. Two of these columns are called the *corpora cavernosa penis*. The third column is called the *corpus spongiosum*. The corpus spongiosum extends at its distal end into the glans penis, the cone-shaped head at the end of the penis, and the site of the urethral orifice. The penis is covered with a loose fold of skin called the foreskin or prepuce. The foreskin contains glands that secrete a lubricating fluid called smegma. During a procedure called a circumcision, the foreskin is removed. This is often performed for medical, cultural, or religious reasons.

The erectile state in the penis occurs when sexual stimulation causes large quantities of blood from dilated arteries supplying the penis to fill the cavernous spaces in the erectile tissue. When the arteries constrict, the pressure on the veins in the area is reduced, allowing more blood to leave the penis than can enter it, allowing it to return to its previous size. The functions of the penis are to serve as the male organ for intercourse or copulation, and as the site of the orifice for the elimination of urine and semen from the body.

Internal Organs

The two oval-shaped organs located in the scrotum are called the testes. Each testes is about 4 cm long and 2.5 cm wide. The interior of each is divided into about 250 wedge-shaped lobes by fibrous tissues. The seminiferous tubules are located within each lobe of the testes. This is the site of the development of the spermatozoa, the male reproductive cells (see Figure 31-6). Other cells within the testes produce the male sex hormone, testosterone. Testosterone is responsible for the development of the normal secondary sex characteristics during puberty. Testosterone also places a vital role in the erection process and is necessary for the reproductive act. Additionally, it also affects the growth of hair on the face, muscular development, and vocal timbre. The seminiferous tubules form a network in the testes and they connect with the efferent ductus to leave the testes and enter the epididymis.

Each testes is connected to the epididymis, a coiled tube lying in the posterior aspect of the testes. Each epididymis is between 13 and 20 feet in length, but is coiled into a space that is less than 5 cm in length, and ends at the ductus deferens. The function of the epididymis is the maturation of sperm and is the first part of the duct system through which the sperm pass in their travels to the urethra.

The ductus deferens (vas deferens) is a slim, muscular tube that is about 45 cm in length and is continuous

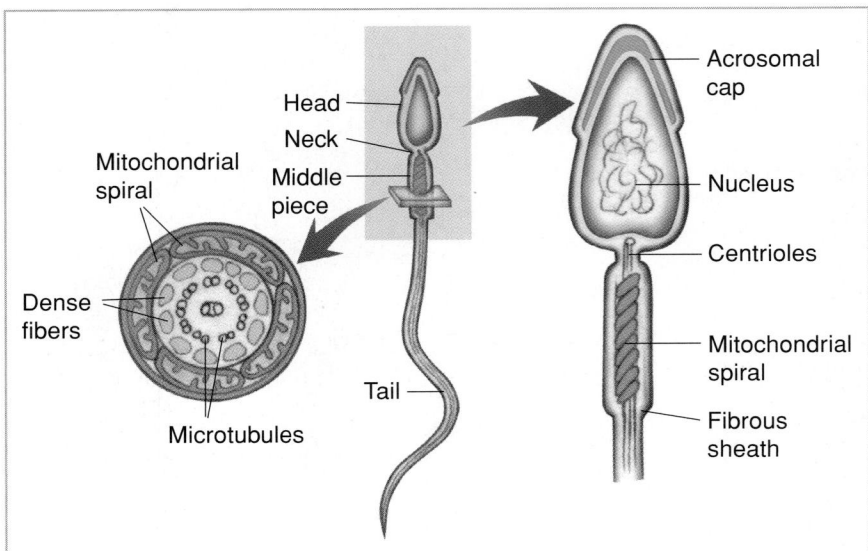

FIGURE 31-6   The basic structure of a spermatozoon (sperm).

Prostate Gland

The prostate gland is about 4 cm wide and weighs about 20 grams. It wraps around the urethra, similar to a donut wrapping around a straw. It is composed of glandular, connective, and muscular tissue and lies behind the urinary bladder. It surrounds the first 2.5 cm of the urethra and secretes an alkaline fluid that aids in maintaining the viability of the spermatozoa.

Bulbourethral Glands (Cowper's Glands)

The bulbourethral glands are two small, pea-sized glands located inferior to the prostate and on either side of the urethra. A 2.5-cm duct connects them with the wall of the urethra, where they can secrete a mucous secretion into the seminal fluid before ejaculation.

Urethra

The male urethra is approximately 20 cm long, and is divided into three sections: the prostatic, the membranous, and the penile. The urethra extends from the bladder to the urethral orifice at the end of the penis. The functions of the urethra in the male are the expulsion of urine and semen from the body.

with the epididymis. It is the excretory duct of the testes and extends from the point adjacent to the testes and enters the abdomen at the inguinal canal. A duct from the seminal vesicle joins the ductus deferens at the inguinal canal. Between the testes and the internal inguinal ring (part of the abdomen), the ductus deferens is contained within a structure known as the spermatic cord. The spermatic cord also contains arteries, veins, lymphatic vessels, and nerves.

The two seminal vesicles are connected by a narrow duct to the ductus deferens, which then forms the ejaculatory duct, a short tube that penetrates the base of the prostate gland and opens into the prostate portion of the urethra. The seminal vesicles produce an alkaline fluid that becomes part of the seminal fluid or semen.

Common Disorders Associated with the Female Reproductive System

Disorders that may affect the proper functioning of the reproductive system range from abnormal hormone secretion and breast diseases, to sexually transmitted infections, the presence of cancerous tissue in a region, and all inflammations, infections, and disorders in between. Many of those problems frequently affect fertility and the actual process of being able to reproduce. (see Table 31-1 lists common disorders and pathology of the female reproductive system).

Breast Cancer

Breast cancer is cancer arising in breast tissue (see Figure 31-7). Although it is primarily a disease of women, about 1 percent of breast cancers occur in men. It is the most common type of cancer in women and is the second leading cause of death by cancer in women, following only lung cancer.

The breasts are made of fat, glands, and connective (fibrous) tissue. They have several lobes, which are divided into lobules and end in the milk glands. Tiny ducts run from the many tiny glands, connect together, and end in

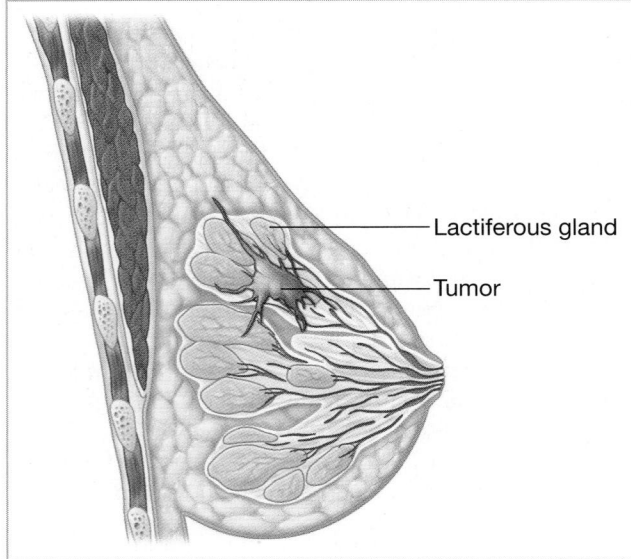

FIGURE 31-7   Breast cancer. Tumor is growing within a milk gland.

TABLE 31-1 Disorders of the Female Reproductive System

Disorder	Description
Abruptio placenta	An emergency condition in which the placenta tears away from the uterine wall before the 20th week of pregnancy. This requires immediate delivery of the baby.
Amenorrhea	An absence of menstruation, which can be the result of many factors, including pregnancy, menopause, and dieting.
Breech presentation	Position of the fetus within the uterus in which the buttocks or feet are presented first for delivery rather than the head.
Carcinoma *in situ*	Malignant tumor that has not extended beyond the original site.
Cervical cancer	A malignant growth in the cervix of the uterus. This is an especially difficult type of cancer to treat, and causes 5 percent of the cancer deaths in women. Pap tests have helped to detect early cervical cancer.
Cervical polyps	Fibrous or mucous tumor or growth found in the cervix of the uterus. These are removed surgically if there is a danger that they will become malignant.
Cervicitis	Inflammation of the cervix of the uterus.
Choriocarcinoma	A rare type of cancer of the uterus that may occur following a normal pregnancy or abortion.
Condyloma	A wart-like growth on the external genitalia.
Cystocele	Hernia or outpouching of the bladder that protrudes into the vagina. This may cause urinary frequency and urgency.
Dysmenorrhea	Painful cramping that is associated with menstruation.
Eclampsia	Convulsive seizures and coma occurring between the 20th week of pregnancy and the first week of postpartum.
Ectopic	A fetus that becomes abnormally implanted outside the uterine cavity. This is a condition requiring immediate surgery.
Endometrial cancer	Cancer of the endometrial lining of the uterus.
Fibroid tumor	Benign tumor or growth that contains fiber-like tissue. Uterine fibroid tumors are the most common tumors in women.
Mastitis	Inflammation of the breast, which is common during lactation but can occur at any age.
Menorrhagia	Excessive bleeding during the menstrual period. Can be either in the total number of days or the amount of blood or both.
Ovarian carcinoma	Cancer of the ovary.
Ovarian cyst	Sac that develops within the ovary.
Pelvic inflammatory disease (PID)	Any inflammation of the female reproductive organs, generally bacterial in nature.
Placenta previa	When the placenta has become attached to the lower portion of the uterus and, in turn, blocks the birth canal.

(continued)

TABLE 31-1 Disorders of the Female Reproductive System (*continued*)

Disorder	Description
Preeclampsia	Toxemia of pregnancy that if untreated can result in true eclampsia. Symptoms include hypertension, headaches, albumin in the urine, and edema.
Premature birth	Delivery in which the infant (neonate) is born before the 37th week of gestation (pregnancy).
Premenstrual syndrome (PMS)	Symptoms that develop just prior to the onset of a menstrual period, which can include irritability, headache, tender breasts, and anxiety.
Prolapsed uterus	A fallen uterus that can cause the cervix to protrude through the vaginal opening. It is generally caused by weakened muscles from vaginal delivery or as a result of pelvic tumors pressing down.
Rh factor	A condition that can develop in a baby when the mother's blood type is Rh negative and the father's is Rh positive. The baby's red blood cells can be destroyed as a result of this condition. Treatment is early diagnosis and blood transfusion.
Salpingitis	Inflammation of the fallopian tube or tubes.
Spontaneous abortion	Loss of a fetus without any artificial aid. Also called a miscarriage.
Stillbirth	Birth in which the fetus dies before or at the time of delivery.
Toxic shock syndrome	Rare and sometimes fatal staphylococcus infection that generally occurs in menstruating women.
Tubal pregnancy	Implantation of a fetus within the fallopian tube instead of the uterus. This requires immediate surgery.
Vaginitis	Inflammation of the vagina, generally caused by a microorganism.

the nipple. These ducts are where 80 percent of breast cancers occur. Cancer may also develop in the lobules. Another type of breast cancer is inflammatory breast cancer. The most serious cancers are metastatic cancers, meaning that the cancer has spread from the place where it started into other tissues. The most common place for breast cancer to metastasize is into the lymph nodes under the arm or above the collarbone on the same side as the cancer. Other common sites of breast cancer metastasis are the brain, the bones, and the liver.

Family history has long been known to be a risk factor for breast cancer. The risk is highest if the affected relative developed breast cancer at a young age or if she is a close relative such as a mother, sister, daughter, or aunt. Hormonal influences also play a role in the development of breast cancer. Women who start their periods at an early age or experience a late menopause have a higher risk of developing breast cancer. Conversely, being older at your first menstrual period and early menopause tend to protect one from breast cancer.

Early breast cancer has no symptoms, and it is not painful. Most breast cancer is discovered before symptoms are present, either by finding an abnormality on a mammography or feeling a breast lump. A lump located under the arm or above the collarbone that does not go away may be an indication of the presence of breast cancer. Other possible symptoms are breast discharge, nipple inversion, or changes in the skin overlying the breast.

Most breast lumps are not cancerous; however, all breast lumps should be evaluated by a physician. Breast discharge is a common problem and is rarely a symptom of cancer. Discharge is of most concern if it is from only one breast or if it is bloody. In any case, all breast discharge should also be evaluated. Nipple inversion is a common variant of normal nipples, but nipple inversion that is a new development can be of concern. And any changes in the skin of the breast that include redness, changes in texture, and puckering should also be evaluated.

In this disease, patient preference plays a major role in decisions regarding treatment, and treatment depends on several factors, including the type of breast cancer, the hormone receptor status of the tumor, the stage of the tumor, the size of the breast, and the person's general health, age, and menstrual status (has or has not been through menopause). Radiation therapy is used to kill tumor cells if there are any left after surgery. Chemotherapy may also be used to kill the cancer cells or stop them from growing. Hormonal therapy may also be given.

Surgery is the mainstay and, in many cases, the best form of therapy for breast cancer. The choice as to which type of surgery is based on a number of factors, including the size and location of the tumor, the type of tumor, and the person's overall health and personal wishes. Breast-sparing surgery, such as a lumpectomy, is often possible. Other more radical treatment may include a simple mastectomy, a modified radical mastectomy, and, in the most severe cases, a radical mastectomy, which is complete removal of the breast.

Cervical Cancer

Cervical cancer is the rapid, uncontrolled growth of severely abnormal cells on the cervix. There are two main types of cervical cancer: squamous cell (epidermoid) cervical cancer and adenocarcinoma cervical cancer. Fortunately, when detected at an early stage, cervical cancer is highly curable. Pap test screening, when done regularly, is the single most important tool for preventing cervical cancer because it can detect abnormal cervical cell changes before they become cancerous, when treatment is most effective.

Several factors may play a role in causing cervical cancer. These include smoking or a history of smoking, having an impaired immune system, such as from having human immunodeficiency virus (HIV) or human papillomavirus (HPV), and using birth control pills for more than 5 years.

Because abnormal cervical cell changes rarely cause symptoms, it is important to have regular Pap test screening. As cervical cell changes progress to cervical cancer, symptoms may develop. These often include abnormal vaginal bleeding or a significant unexplained change in your menstrual cycle pain during sexual intercourse, and abnormal vaginal discharge containing mucus that may be tinged with blood. Symptoms that may occur when cervical cancer has progressed may include anemia because of abnormal vaginal bleeding, ongoing pelvic, leg, or back pain, urinary problems because of blockage of a kidney or ureter, leakage of urine or fecal content into the vagina because an abnormal opening (fistula) has developed between the vagina and the bladder or rectum, and weight loss.

Cervical cancer detected in its early stages can be cured with treatment and close follow-up. The treatment may include surgery to remove the cancer, radiation therapy to treat other organs affected by the cancer, or chemotherapy to treat cancer that has spread or metastasized. The treatment may be a single

therapy or a combination of any of these. The choice of treatment and the long-term outcome depend on the type and stage of cancer. A person's age, overall health, quality of life, and desire to be able to have children are almost always considered.

Cervicitis

Cervicitis is an inflammation of the cervix. Most cases are caused by infection with sexually transmitted infections, including gonorrhea and chlamydia. Most often, there are no signs and symptoms, and the patient may first learn of the condition as a result of a Pap test or a biopsy for another condition. If symptoms are present, they may include vaginal discharge that is grayish or yellow, possibly with an odor; frequent, painful urination; pain during intercourse; and vaginal bleeding after intercourse, between menstrual periods, or after menopause.

Successful treatment of cervicitis involves addressing the cause of the inflammation. In most cases, antibiotics are used to clear an underlying bacterial infection. If the cause is viral, such as genital herpes, the treatment is an antiviral medication. However, antiviral medication does not cure herpes, which is a chronic condition. The person's sexual partner may also be treated to prevent reinfection.

Dysmenorrhea

Dysmenorrhea is the presence of painful cramps during menstruation. More than half of all girls and women suffer from some form of dysmenorrhea, which is often associated with a dull or throbbing pain that usually centers in the lower midabdomen, radiating toward the lower back or thighs. Menstruating women of any age can experience cramps, and while the pain may be only mild for some women, others may experience severe discomfort that can significantly interfere with everyday activities for several days each month.

In addition to cramping, some women may experience nausea and vomiting, diarrhea, irritability, sweating, or dizziness. Cramps usually last for 2 or 3 days at the beginning of each menstrual period, and many women often notice their painful periods disappear after they have their first child. This is probably due to the stretching of the opening of the uterus or because the birth improves the uterine blood supply and muscle activity.

Dysmenorrhea is controlled by treating the underlying disorder. This may include the use of nonsteroidal anti-inflammatory drugs (NSAIDs), which prevent or decrease the formation of prostaglandins. For more severe pain, prescription-strength ibuprofen (Motrin) is available. These drugs are usually begun at the first sign of the period and taken for a day or two. There are many different types of NSAIDs, and women may find that one works better for them than the others.

New studies of a drug patch containing glyceryl trinitrate to treat dysmenorrhea suggest that it also may help ease pain. Other treatments may include simply changing the position of the body, changes in dietary intake of fibers, fats, calcium, and carbohydrates, and using visualization and guided imagery to help relieve and ease the cramps. Aromatherapy and massage may ease pain for some women. Others find that imagining a white light hovering over the painful area can actually lessen the pain for brief periods. Acupuncture and Chinese herbs are other popular alternative treatments for cramps.

Endometriosis

Endometriosis occurs when the endometrium, which is the tissue that lines the inside of the uterus, travels outside the uterus. In a women with endometriosis, the tissue is found in the pelvis or abdominal cavity. This tissue reacts to the changing levels of estrogen, but cannot be sloughed off with the tissues inside the uterus. This tissue still causes bleeding and forms scars and adhesions. Typically, this is what causes daily or monthly cyclic pain.

Symptoms of endometriosis include blood in the urine, difficulty urinating, dyspareunia (painful intercourse), heavy menstrual bleeding, irregular periods, nausea and vomiting, pelvic pain after intercourse or exercise, and dysmenorrhea. The symptoms of endometriosis tend to decrease after menopause, when the involved tissues shrink.

Although the cause of endometriosis is unknown, several theories have been proposed. One theory is that delayed childbearing increases the risk for endometriosis. Another is that during menstruation, some of the endometrial tissue backs up through the fallopian tubes into the abdomen. Genetics may also play a role.

Early diagnosis and treatment may limit cell growth and help prevent adhesions, while pregnancy, oral contraceptives, and other hormones seem to delay its onset. Treatment with medication focuses on treating the discomfort. Surgery is generally reserved for women with severe endometriosis. Conservative surgery will attempt to remove or destroy all of the endometriotic tissue existing outside the uterus, remove adhesions, and restore the pelvic anatomy. More extensive surgery will be done for women with severe symptoms or disease and no desire to bear children. Typically, a total hysterectomy (removal of the uterus, ovaries and fallopian tubes along with any adhesions) will be performed. Hormonal replacement will be lifelong after the removal of the ovaries.

Fibrocystic Breast Disease

Fibrocystic breast disease involves common, benign changes in the tissues of the breast (see Figure 31-8). The condition is so commonly found in normal breasts, it is believed to be a normal variant. Other related terms that refer to this disorder include mammary dysplasia, benign breast disease, and diffuse cystic mastopathy. The cause is not completely understood; however, the changes are believed to be associated with ovarian hormones since the condition usually subsides with menopause and may vary in consistency during the menstrual cycle.

The incidence of fibrocystic breast disease is estimated to be more than 60 percent of all women. It is common in women between the ages of 30 and 50, and rare in postmenopausal women. The risk factors may include family history and diet. Symptoms may range from mild to severe, and frequently include a dense, irregular and bumpy "cobblestone" consistency in the breast tissue, breast discomfort that is persistent or that occurs intermittently, and a feeling of fullness in the breasts. There may also be premenstrual tenderness and swelling and nipple sensation changes, such as itching.

Treatment of this disorder often involves self-care, dietary restrictions to eliminate caffeine, performing a breast self-exam monthly, and wearing a well-fitted bra to provide good breast support. Oral contraceptives may also be prescribed because they often decrease the symptoms.

Ovarian Cancer

Ovarian cancer starts in the cells of the ovary or ovaries. There are three main types of ovarian cancer, depending on the type of cell where the cancer starts: epithelial cell cancer, which starts in the outer covering of the ovary and is the most common type of ovarian cancer; germ cell tumors that start in the egg cells within the ovary and generally occur in younger women, even in children; and stromal tumors, which start in the cells that form the structural framework of the ovary. Ovarian cancer can develop for a long time without causing any signs or symptoms. When symptoms do start, they are often vague and easily mistaken for more common illnesses. Most women with ovarian cancer have advanced disease at the time of their diagnosis.

Symptoms of early-stage ovarian cancer frequently include mild abdominal discomfort or pain, abdominal swelling, change in bowel habits, feeling full after a light meal, indigestion, gas, an upset stomach, a feeling that the bowel has not completely emptied, nausea and vomiting, constant tiredness, pain in lower back or leg, abnormal menstrual or vaginal bleeding, more frequent urination, and pain during intercourse. Symptoms of advanced ovarian cancer may cause a buildup of fluid in the abdomen, shortness of breath and a dry persistent cough, nausea and vomiting, abdominal tumors, and weight loss.

Treatment is based on the type, grade, and stage of the cancer, and it may include surgery to remove the tumor and some surrounding tissue, radiation therapy, and chemotherapy. Complementary therapies, such as medi-

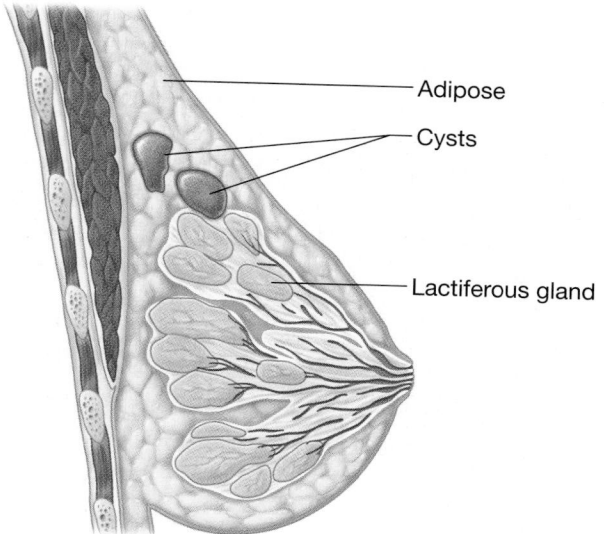

FIGURE 31-8 Fibrocystic breast disease.

tation and supportive therapies, are also encouraged as part of the treatment for ovarian cancer. Alternative therapies, such as traditional Chinese medicines or special diets, are sometimes used; however, their effectiveness in the treatment of cancer is not completely known.

Ovarian Cysts

Ovarian cysts are sacs filled with fluid or a semisolid material that develops on or within the ovary. Typically, ovarian cysts are not disease related and disappear on their own. During the days preceding ovulation, a follicle grows. At the time of expected ovulation, the follicle fails to rupture and release an egg. Instead of being reabsorbed, the fluid within the follicle persists and forms a cyst. Functional cysts usually disappear within 60 days without treatment and are relatively common. They occur most often during childbearing years, that is, puberty to menopause, but may occur at any time. No known risk factors have been identified. Functional ovarian cysts should not to be confused with other disease conditions involving ovarian cysts, specifically benign cysts of different types that must be treated to resolve, true ovarian

Patient Education

When caring for a patient dealing with a disorder or a condition of the reproductive system, the medical assistant has a responsibility to be knowledgeable about the structures affected by these disorders and, just as important, to be knowledgeable about the emotional and psychosocial aspects associated with many of these disorders. As a member of the health care team, your role is to provide the patient with basic information that will assist him or her in understanding how to live with the situation. Oftentimes, this involves teaching the patient about lifestyle changes, nutrition, and how to deal with change and new challenges that directly affect their lifestyles.

Professionalism

tumors, including ovarian cancer, or hormonal conditions such as polycystic ovarian disease.

Oftentimes, there are no symptoms; however, if symptoms are present, they generally include constant, dull aching pelvic pain, pain with intercourse or pelvic pain during movement, pelvic pain shortly after beginning or ending a menstrual period, and abdominal bloating or distention.

Functional ovarian cysts generally disappear within 60 days without any treatment. Oral contraceptive pills may be prescribed to help establish normal cycles and decrease the development of functional ovarian cysts. Ovarian cysts that do not appear to be functional may require surgical removal by laparoscopy or exploratory laparotomy. Surgical removal is often necessary if a cyst is larger than 6 cm or that persists for longer than 6 weeks. Other medical treatment may be recommended if other disorders are found to be the cause of ovarian cysts, such as polycystic ovary disease.

Pelvic Inflammatory Disease

The most common and serious complication of sexually transmitted infections (STIs) among women is pelvic inflammatory disease (PID). This condition is an infection of the upper genital area and occurs when disease-carrying organisms migrate upward from the urethra and cervix into the upper genital area. PID can affect the uterus, ovaries, and fallopian tubes. If untreated this disease can cause scarring, which can lead to infertility, tubal pregnancy, chronic pelvic pain, and other serious consequences.

Many different organisms can cause PID, but most cases are associated with gonorrhea and genital chlamydial infections, two common STIs. After a period of time, the infection spreads to other cells and organs, causing more infection and scarring.

The major symptoms of PID are lower abdominal pain and abnormal vaginal discharge. Other symptoms such as fever, pain in the right upper quadrant, painful intercourse, and irregular menstrual bleeding may also be present. PID may be very painful, or may have few if any symptoms even though it can seriously damage the reproductive organs.

Premenstrual Syndrome

Premenstrual syndrome (PMS) is a condition affecting women that may cause annoying symptoms including constipation, diarrhea, nausea, anorexia, appetite cravings, headache, backache, muscular aches, edema, insomnia, clumsiness, malaise, irritability, indecisiveness, mental confusion, and depression. There is no specific known cause, but it is believed that there is a relationship to the amount of prostaglandin and estrogen produced (see Figure 31-9). It is estimated that 85 percent of women who menstruate are affected by PMS. However, only 5 to 10 percent of menstruating women are severely impaired by PMS. There is no known reason why some women are affected, while others are not.

Some recommendations may help to decrease the severity of PMS symptoms. These include eating a healthy diet high in vegetables and fruits and low in starches, sugars, sodium, fat, caffeine, and alcohol; performing regular aerobic exercise; including enough vitamins and minerals, especially B vitamins, calcium, and magnesium in the diet; and using relaxation therapy and stress management techniques. Some herbal treatments have also been reported as helpful, including chasteberry and black cohosh. Medications may be used to help decrease and control the symptoms of PMS as well.

Sexually Transmitted Infections

Sexually transmitted infection (STI) is a term used to describe more than 20 different infections that are transmitted through exchange of semen, blood, and other body fluids; or by direct contact with the affected body areas of people with STIs. Sexually transmitted infections are also called venereal diseases. The Centers for Disease Control and Prevention (CDC) has reported

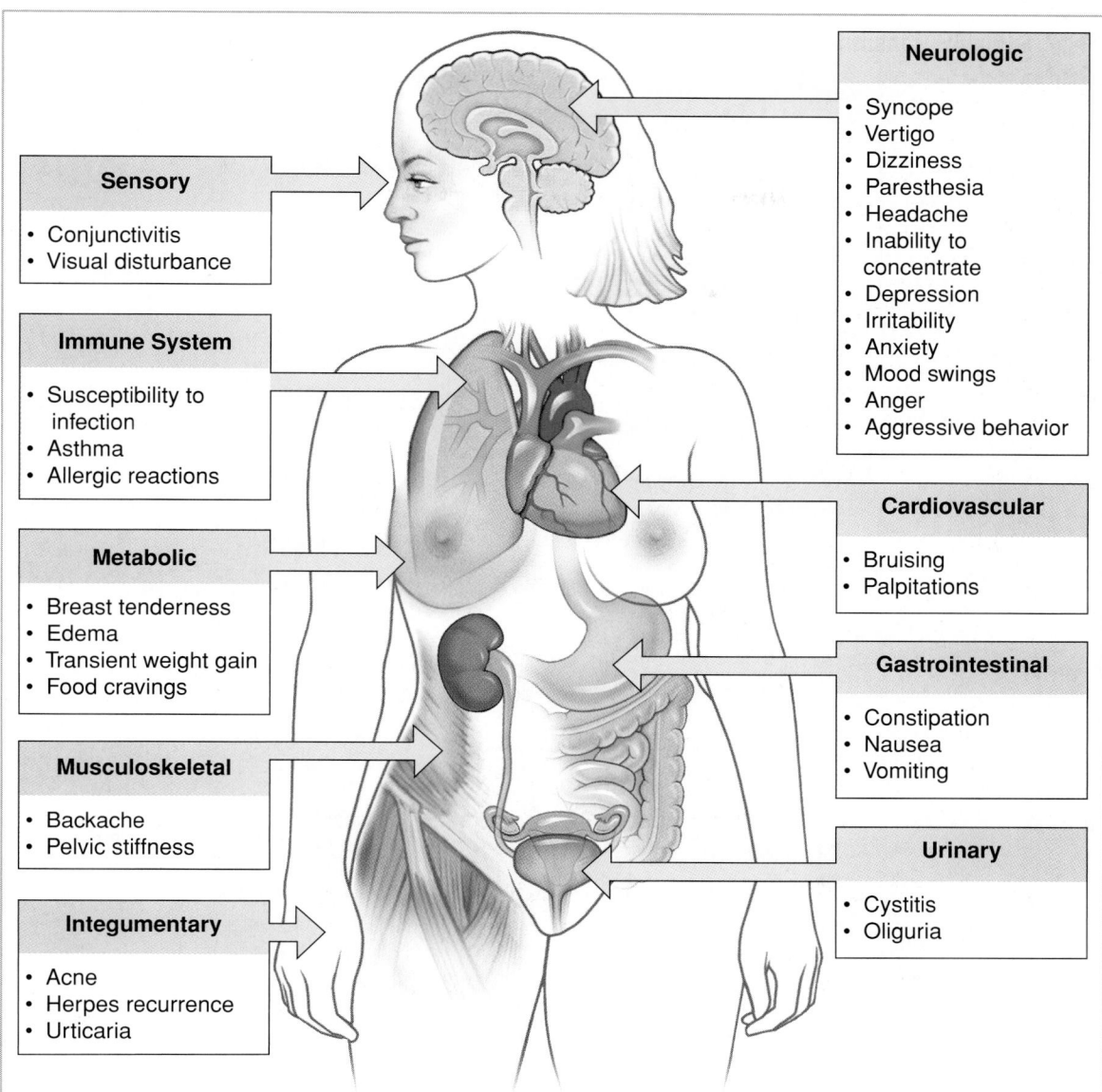

Sensory

- Conjunctivitis
- Visual disturbance

Immune System

- Susceptibility to infection
- Asthma
- Allergic reactions

Metabolic

- Breast tenderness
- Edema
- Transient weight gain
- Food cravings

Musculoskeletal

- Backache
- Pelvic stiffness

Integumentary

- Acne
- Herpes recurrence
- Urticaria

Neurologic

- Syncope
- Vertigo
- Dizziness
- Paresthesia
- Headache
- Inability to concentrate
- Depression
- Irritability
- Anxiety
- Mood swings
- Anger
- Aggressive behavior

Cardiovascular

- Bruising
- Palpitations

Gastrointestinal

- Constipation
- Nausea
- Vomiting

Urinary

- Cystitis
- Oliguria

FIGURE 31-9 Multisystem effects of premenstrual syndrome.

that 85 percent of the most prevalent infectious diseases in the United States are sexually transmitted. The rate of STIs in this country is 50 to 100 times higher than that of any other industrialized nation. One in four sexually active Americans will be affected by an STI at some time in his or her life. They can have very painful long-term consequences as well as immediate health problems. They can cause birth defects, blindness, bone deformities, brain damage, cancer, heart disease, infertility and other abnormalities of the reproductive system, mental retardation, and death. Some of the most common and potentially serious STIs in the United States include chlamydia, human papillomavirus (HPV), genital herpes, gonorrhea, syphilis, and HIV infection.

The symptoms of STIs vary somewhat according to the disease agent, the sex of the patient, and the body systems affected. Some are easy to identify, while others

produce infections that may either go unnoticed for some time or are easy to confuse with other diseases. Syphilis in particular can be confused with disorders ranging from infectious mononucleosis to allergic reactions to prescription medications. In addition, the incubation period of STIs varies. Some produce symptoms close enough to the time of sexual contact, often less than 48 hours. Others may have an even longer incubation period, so that the patient may not recognize the early symptoms as those of a sexually transmitted infection. Some symptoms of STIs that affect the genitals and reproductive organs include bleeding not associated with menstruating, abnormal vaginal discharge, vaginal burning, itching, pain in the pelvic area while having sex, discharge from the tip of the penis, swelling of the lymph nodes near the groin area, and in males and females, painful or burning sensations when urinating.

TABLE 31-2 Sexually Transmitted Infections

Disease	Description
Acquired immune deficiency syndrome (AIDS)	The final stage of infection from the human immunodeficiency virus (HIV). At present there is no cure.
Candidiasis	A yeast-like infection of the skin and mucous membranes that can result in white plaques on the tongue and vagina.
Chancroid	Highly infectious nonsyphilitic ulcer.
Chlamydial infection	Parasitic microorganism causing genital infections in males and females. Can lead to pelvic inflammatory disease (PID) in females and eventual infertility.
Genital herpes	Growths and elevations of warts on the genitalia of both males and females that can lead to cancer of the cervix in females. These painful vesicles on the skin and mucosa erupt periodically and can be transmitted through the placenta or at birth.
Genital warts	Growths and elevations of warts on the genitalia of both males and females that can lead to cancer of the cervix in females. There is currently no cure.
Gonorrhea	Sexually transmitted inflammation of the mucous membranes of either sex. Can be passed on to an infant during the birth process.
Hepatitis	Infectious, inflammatory disease of the liver. Hepatitis B and C types are spread by contact with blood and bodily fluids of an infected person.
Syphilis	Infectious, chronic, venereal disease that can involve any organ. May exist for years without symptoms.
Trichomoniasis	Genitourinary infection that is usually without symptoms (asymptomatic) in both males and females. In women the disease can produce itching and/or burning, a foul-smelling discharge, and results in vaginitis.

Both men and women may also develop skin rashes, sores, bumps, or blisters near the mouth or genitals. Other symptoms of STIs are systemic, which means that they affect the body as a whole. These symptoms may include fever, chills, and similar flu-like symptoms, skin rashes over large parts of the body, arthritis-like pains or aching in the joints, and throat swelling and redness that lasts for 3 weeks or longer.

Although self-care can relieve some of the pain and symptoms of STIs, other symptoms often require immediate medical attention, such as antibiotics, which are used to treat gonorrhea, chlamydia, syphilis, and other STIs caused by bacteria. What is most important to note is that the risk of becoming infected with an STI can be reduced or eliminated by changing certain personal behaviors. Abstaining from sexual relations or maintaining a mutually monogamous relationship with a partner are considered legitimate options. Avoiding sexual contact with partners who are known to be infected with an STI, whose health status is unknown, who abuse drugs, or who are involved in prostitution are also considered ways in which the risk of becoming infected with an STI can be decreased or eradicated completely. (See Table 31-2 for more information about sexually transmitted infections.)

Uterine Cancer

Uterine cancer (endometrial cancer) starts in the cells of the lining of the uterus. In most cases, it develops in the glandular tissue of the endometrium and is called adenocarcinoma. If the cancer is found and treated early, treatment is usually very successful. There is no single cause of uterine cancer; however, some factors appear to increase the risk of developing it. These include age, particularly in women over 50, obesity, childlessness, reaching menopause later than average, prolonged use of medications with the hormone estrogen, and the taking of the drug tamoxifen.

Many of the signs and symptoms of uterine cancer may be associated with other disorders of the female reproductive system. These frequently include bleeding between menstrual periods, heavy bleeding or spotting during periods or after menopause, bleeding after intercourse, and a foul discharge. Other symptoms may include a yellow watery discharge, cramping pain, pressure in the abdomen or pelvis, back, or legs, and discomfort over the pubic area.

Treatment of uterine cancer will depend on the type, grade, and stage of the cancer. These treatments may include any one, or a combination of, surgery, radiation therapy, or chemotherapy.

Uterine Fibroids

Uterine fibroids are benign growths or tumors made up of muscle cells and other tissues that grow within the wall of the uterus (see Figure 31-10). Fibroids can grow as a single growth or as a cluster of tumors. They can be seed sized or the size of a grapefruit. They are common in women of childbearing age, and African-American women are more likely to get them than women of other racial groups. African-American women also tend to get fibroids at an earlier age than do women of other races. There also appears to be a higher risk for fibroids with women who are overweight or obese. Women who have given birth appear to be at a lower risk for fibroids. There is no known cause of uterine fibroids and they can be frustrating to endure because there are few treatment options.

The symptoms that may occur with uterine fibroids include heavy bleeding or painful periods; bleeding between periods, feeling of fullness in the pelvic area, frequent urination, pain during sex, lower back pain, and reproductive problems, including infertility or early onset of labor. Although the cause of fibroids is unknown, it may be a combination of hormones, genetics and environmental factors. Fibroids usually shrink or disappear after menopause, but not always.

Patients who have mild symptoms may only require over-the-counter medications for pain relief and relief of inflammation. Those who require more relief may require *gonadotropin releasing hormone agonists* (GnRHa). These drugs will decrease the size of the fibroids. Side effects can include hot flashes, depression, insomnia, decreased libido, and joint pain. *Antihormonal* agents may stop or slow the growth of fibroids. These drugs only offer temporary relief from the symptoms of the fibroids, because the symptoms will restart as soon the therapy is discontinued.

Two types of surgery are used to treat fibroids. A myomectomy removes the fibroids without taking the healthy tissue of the uterus. This may be done either by laparotomy or as an open surgery. A hysterectomy removes the entire uterus.

Vaginitis

Vaginitis is an inflammation of the vagina that can result in discharge, itching, or pain. The cause is usually

a change in the normal balance of vaginal bacteria or an infection. Vaginitis can also result from reduced estrogen levels after menopause. The most common types of vaginitis are bacterial vaginitis, yeast infections, trichomoniasis, and atrophic vaginitis. The signs and symptoms of vaginitis may include any change in color, odor, or amount of discharge from the vagina, vaginal itching or irritation, pain during intercourse, painful urination, and light vaginal bleeding.

Treatment depends on the type of vaginitis, present. For bacterial vaginitis, vaginal gels or creams may be prescribed. Yeast infections are usually treated with

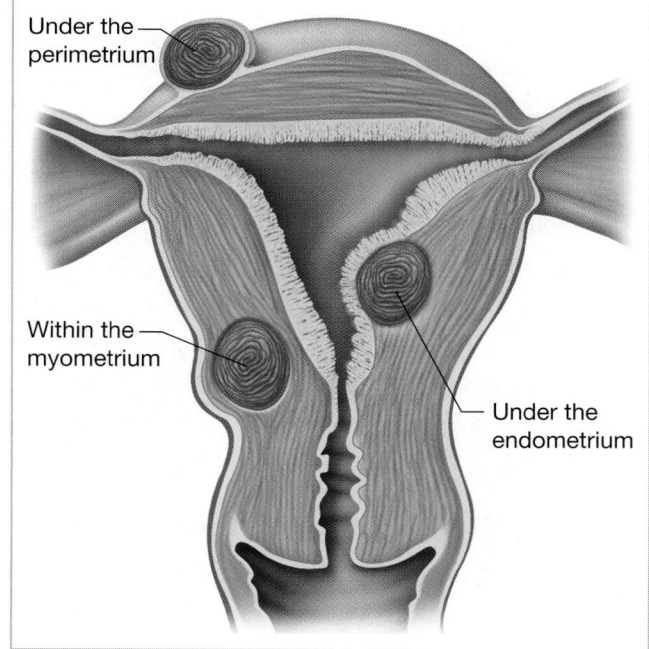

FIGURE 31-10 Types of uterine fibroid tumors.

antifungal creams or suppositories. Trichomoniasis is frequently treated with Flagyl (metronidazole). And atrophic vaginitis is generally treated with estrogen.

Common Disorders Associated with the Male Reproductive System

The male reproductive system is essential to reproduction. It is also related to the male excretion, or urinary, system, and many of the disorders affect both systems. Conditions range from inflammatory, such as epididymitis, and infectious diseases, such as those classified as STIs, to other, more life-threatening diseases and disorders such as prostate cancer and testicular cancer. (See Table 31-3 for more information about disorders of the male reproductive system.)

Benign Prostatic Hyperplasia

Benign prostatic hyperplasia (BPH), also known as benign prostatic hypertrophy, is an enlargement of the

TABLE 31-3 Disorders of the Male Reproductive System

Disorder	Description
Anorchism	A congenital absence of one or both testes.
Aspermia	The lack of, or failure to, eject sperm.
Azoospermia	Absence of sperm in the semen.
Balanitis	Infammation of the skin covering the glans penis.
Benign prostatic hypertrophy	Enlargement of the prostate gland commonly seen in males over age 50.
Carcinoma of the testes	Cancer of one or both testes.
Cryptorchidism	Failure of the testes to descend into the scrotal sac before birth. Generally, the testes will descend permanently before the boy is 1 year old. A surgical procedure called an orchidopecy may be required to bring the testes down into the scrotum permanently and secure them permanently. Failure of the testes to descend could result in sterility in the male.
Epididymitis	Inflammation of the epididymis that causes pain and swelling in the inguinal area.
Epispadias	Congenital opening of the male urethra on the dorsal surface of the penis.
Hydrocele	Accumulation of fluid within the testes.
Hypospadias	Congenital opening of the male urethra on the underside of the penis.
Impotence	Inability to copulate due to inability to maintain an erection or to achieve orgasm.
Perineum	In the male, the external region between the scrotum and the anus.
Phimosis	Narrowing of the foreskin over the glans penis that results in difficulty with hygiene. The condition can lead to infection or difficulty with urination. The condition is treated with circumcision, the surgical removal of the foreskin.
Prostate cancer	A slow-growing cancer that affects a large number of males after age 50. The PSA (prostate-specific antigen) test is used to assist in early detection of this disease.
Prostatic hyperplasia	Abnormal cell growth within the prostate.
Prostatitis	An inflamed condition of the prostate gland that may be the result of infection.
Varicocele	Enlargement of the veins of the spermatic cord that commonly occurs on the left side of adolescent males. This seldom needs treatment.

prostate gland that may occur in men who are 50 years of age and older (see Figure 31-11). By age 60, four out of five men may have an enlarged prostate. As the prostate enlarges, it compresses the urethra, thereby restricting the normal flow of urine. The restriction generally causes a number of symptoms, including a condition known as prostatism. Prostatism is any collection of the prostate gland that interferes with the flow of urine from the bladder.

Symptoms usually include a weak or hard-to-start urine stream; a feeling that the bladder is not empty; a need to urinate often, especially at night; a feeling of urgency (the sudden need to urinate right away); abdominal straining; interruption of the stream; acute urinary retention; and recurrent urinary infections.

Treatment for BPH may include drug therapy, nonsurgical procedures, and surgery. Medications either work by reducing the size of the prostate (finasteride) or by relaxing the smooth muscle of the prostate and the bladder neck to improve urine flow and reduce bladder outlet obstruction.

Epididymitis

Epididymitis is an inflammation or infection of the epididymis, which is the long coiled tube attached to the upper part of each testicle, and where mature sperm are stored before ejaculation. It is the most common cause of pain in the scrotum. The acute form is usually associated with the most severe pain and swelling. If symptoms last for more than 6 weeks after treatment begins, the condition is considered chronic.

Epididymitis can occur any time after the onset of puberty, but is most common between the ages of 18 and 40. Factors that increase the risk of developing epididymitis include infection of the bladder, kidney, prostate, or urinary tract, the presence of other recent illness, a narrowing of the urethra, and use of a urethral catheter.

Although epididymitis can be caused by the same organisms that cause some STIs or occur after prostate surgery, the condition is generally due to pus-generating bacteria associated with infections in other parts of the body. It can also be caused by injury or infection of the scrotum or by irritation from urine that has accumulated in the vas deferens. It is characterized by sudden redness and swelling of the scrotum. The affected testicle is hard and sore, and the other testicle may feel tender. The patient has chills and fever and usually has acute urethritis, or inflammation of the urethra. Enlarged lymph nodes in the groin may also cause scrotal pain that intensifies throughout the day and may become so severe that walking normally becomes impossible.

Because this disorder that affects both testicles can make a man sterile, antibiotic therapy must be initiated as soon as symptoms appear. To prevent reinfection, medication must be taken exactly as prescribed, even if

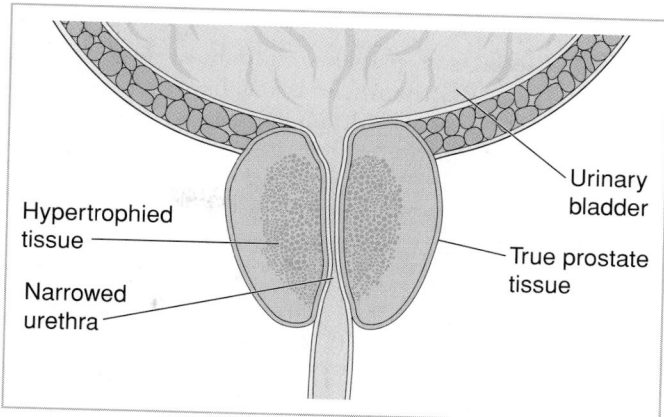

FIGURE 31-11 Benign prostatic hyperplasia.

the patient's symptoms disappear or he begins to feel better. Over-the-counter anti-inflammatories can relieve pain but should not be used without the approval of a family physician or urologist. Bed rest is also recommended until symptoms subside, and patients are advised to wear athletic supporters when they resume normal activities. If pain is severe, a local anesthetic such as lidocaine (Xylocaine) may be injected directly into the spermatic cord.

Erectile Dysfunction

Erectile dysfunction (ED) is the inability to achieve or maintain an erection sufficient for sexual intercourse. It occurs when not enough blood is supplied to the penis, when the smooth muscle in the penis fails to relax, or when the penis does not retain the blood that flows into it. According to studies at the National Institutes of Health, 5 percent of men have some degree of erectile dysfunction at age 40, and approximately 15 to 25 percent at age 65 and older. Although the likelihood of erectile dysfunction increases with age, it is not an inevitable part of aging. About 80 percent of erectile dysfunction has a physical cause that can be addressed.

Risk factors for ED include hypertension, hyperlipidemia, endocrine disorders, low testosterone, thyroid disease, diabetes, coronary artery disease, peripheral vascular disease, anemia, medications, smoking, alcohol abuse, surgical procedures, neurological conditions, and psychiatric illness.

ED can affect relationships and men should discuss the issue with their partners as well as seek medical advice. A medical evaluation is done when a man expresses his concern about his condition with his physician. Underlying causative factors should be treated.

Treatment may include medication therapy, medication changes, or other treatments that include devices (the vacuum constriction device), urethral and penile injection therapies, and surgical therapies, including a penile prosthesis.

Hydrocele

A hydrocele is a painless buildup of watery fluid around one or both testicles that causes the scrotum or groin area to swell. Although this swelling may be unsightly and uncomfortable, it is not painful and generally is not dangerous. A hydrocele can be present at birth (congenital) or can develop after birth (acquired). With a congenital hydrocele, the normal process of testicle migration and closure of the space around the testicles is interrupted. The space may not close, or the closure may be delayed. A hydrocele occurs when fluid from the abdominal cavity fills this space.

The symptom of a congenital hydrocele is a swollen scrotum or groin area. The scrotum may have a bluish tinge. The swelling is painless, may be soft or firm, and cannot be reduced by changing its position or gently pushing it up. It may also be small in the morning and gradually increase in size throughout the day, and may be translucent. If pain is present, it may indicate the presence of an inguinal hernia, injury to the testicles, or some other problem.

For a congenital hydrocele that remains the same size or gets smaller, aggressive treatment is not recommended. It generally will go away by age 1 or 2. The focus should be on watching the hydrocele for any changes. However, surgery generally is necessary if a hydrocele varies in size, does not go away by the age of 1 or 2, comes and goes, or feels firm.

Prostate Cancer

Prostate cancer is a malignant tumor that grows in the prostate gland. It is the most common cancer found in American men. By age 50, one in four American men have some cancerous cells in the prostate gland. By age 80, the ratio increases to one in two. The average age of diagnosis is 70. Prostate cancer is the second leading cause of cancer death in men, exceeded only by lung cancer. However, only 1 in 32 men with a diagnosis of cancer actually dies from prostate cancer.

Prostate cancer can grow slowly for many years, but it occasionally will grow quickly and spread (metastasize) to other parts of the body. Men may or may not have symptoms of prostate cancer. For those who do, the more common symptoms are dull pain in the lower pelvic area; general pain in the lower back, hips, and upper thighs; blood in the urine or semen; dribbling when urinating; erectile dysfunction; frequent urination, especially at night; painful urination and/or ejaculation; smaller stream of urine or urgent need to urinate; and loss of appetite and weight. If the cancer has spread to other parts of the body, there may be persistent bone pain, occasional nerve loss, or a loss of bladder function.

Some risk factors that are associated with prostate cancer these include advanced age, eating a diet that is high in animal fats, being of the African and Northern European ethnic group, the presence of a family history of cancer, and a history of vasectomy, smoking, or cadmium exposure.

Depending on the type and stage of the prostate cancer, treatment options may include any one or all of the following: chemotherapy, cryosurgery to freeze cancer cells, external radiation to the prostate and pelvis, hormone therapy, radioactive implants in the prostate, surgery to remove part of all of the prostate and the surrounding tissue, surgical removal of the testes to block testosterone production, and watchful waiting and monitoring only. Hormone and chemotherapy are used for men with advanced cancer. The focus of hormone therapy is to reduce the body's production of testosterone, which should slow the growth of the cancer.

SUMMARY

The reproductive system functions both for reproduction and maintaining the secondary sex characteristics for both males and females. The female reproductive system is cyclic, with an approximate 28-day cycle as the body prepares itself for reproduction. The male reproductive system produces sperm on a regular basis and is not reliant on any cycle for reproduction.

Chapter Review

COMPETENCY REVIEW

1. Define and spell the terms to learn for this chapter.
2. What is another term for the fallopian tube?
3. What are the three identifiable areas of the uterus?
4. What is the function of the ovaries?
5. What are the three functions of the vagina?

6. What are the two principal hormones in the female reproductive system?
7. What is the vital function of the male reproductive system?
8. What are the two functions of the penis?
9. What are the two functions of the male urethra?
10. What is the function of the seminal vesicles?

PREPARING FOR THE CERTIFICATION EXAM

1. A condition that is caused when the endometrium travels outside the uterus is called
   A. pelvic inflammatory disease
   B. endometriosis
   C. sexually transmitted infection (STIs)
   D. myometriosis
   E. salmonella infection

2. The most common complication of an STI is
   A. pelvic inflammatory disease
   B. endometriosis
   C. myometriosis
   D. ovarian dysfunction
   E. fallopian tube dysfunction

3. The male reproductive system does NOT include the
   A. ureters
   B. urethra
   C. vas deferens
   D. prostate
   E. testes

4. The upper portion of the uterus is called the
   A. fundus
   B. corpus
   C. ovum
   D. cervix
   E. vulva

5. The more common abnormal positions of the uterus include all of the following EXCEPT
   A. anteversion
   B. retroversion
   C. anteflexion
   D. retroflexion
   E. introversion

6. Surgical removal of the fallopian tube and ovary is called
   A. panhysterosalpingo-oophorectomy
   B. oophorectomy
   C. salpingo-oophorectomy
   D. panhysterectomy
   E. laparoscopy

7. The male sperm, in the form of semen, are nourished by a fluid in the
   A. seminal vesicles
   B. epididymis
   C. prostate gland
   D. urethra
   E. vas deferens

8. The vas deferens in the male reproductive system is also known as the
   A. vasectomy
   B. ductus deferens
   C. spermatic cord
   D. scrotum
   E. phimosis

9. The testes produce
   A. progesterone
   B. estrogen
   C. testosterone
   D. oxytocin
   E. prolactin

10. The hormone that stimulates the production of milk in a mother postdelivery is
    A. progesterone
    B. estrogen
    C. testosterone
    D. oxytocin
    E. Prolactin

CRITICAL THINKING

1. Why did the physician include a PSA and digital rectal exam for Mr. Sansone.

2. If Mr. Sansone has BPH, does he have prostate cancer?

3. Why was Mr. Sansone having difficulty starting his stream of urine and having urgency to urinate?

INTERNET ACTIVITY

Do an Internet search of the National Breast Cancer Foundation and other breast cancer awareness organizations. Research the following regarding breast cancer: cancer myths, early detection, and up-and-coming research.

MediaLink  More on the repoductive system, including interactive resources, can be found on the Student CD-ROM accompanying this textbook.

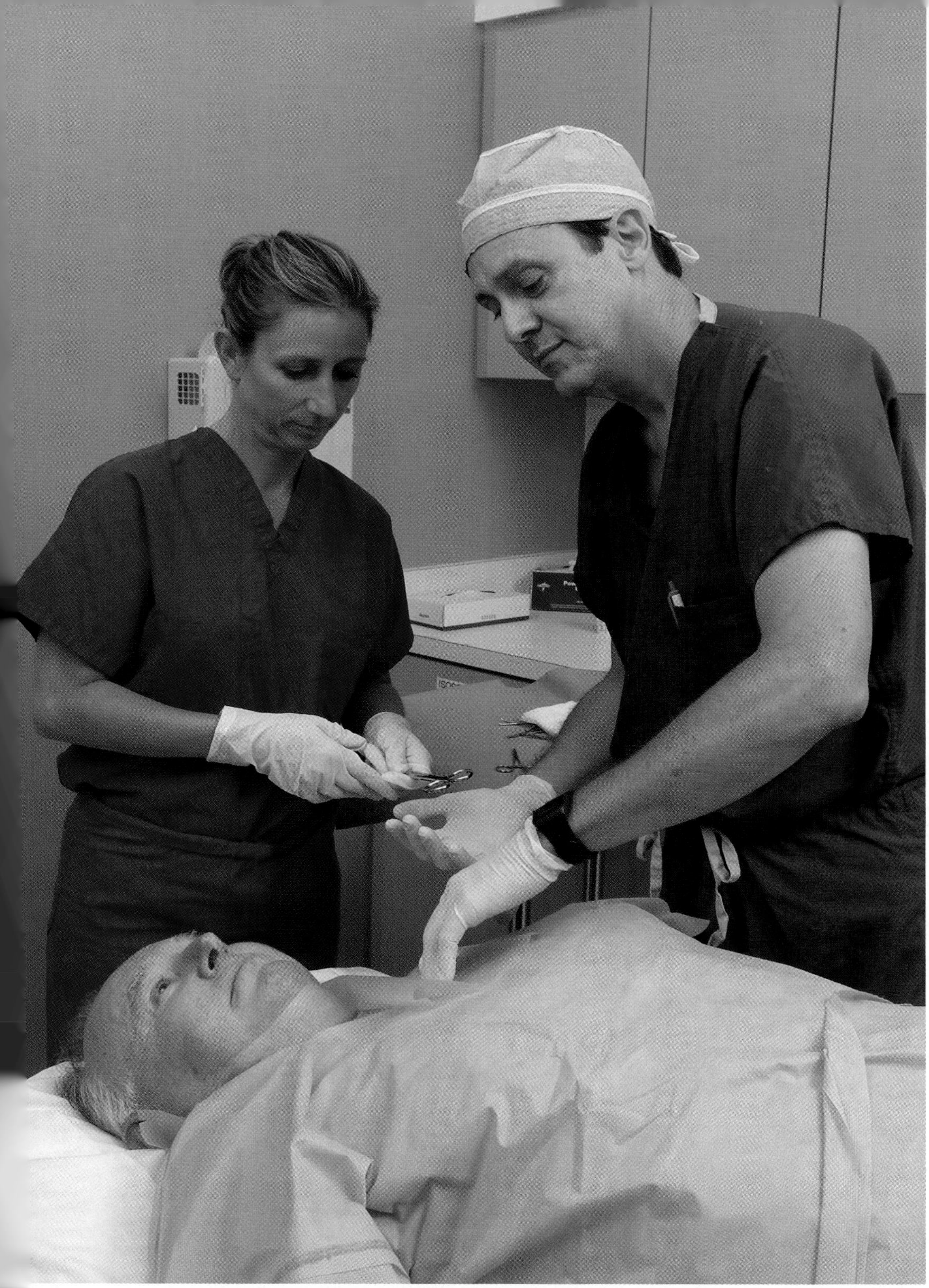

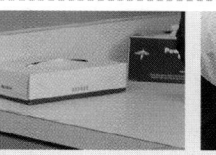
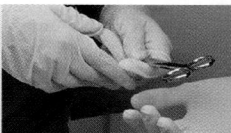

Unit Four

Clinical Medical Assisting

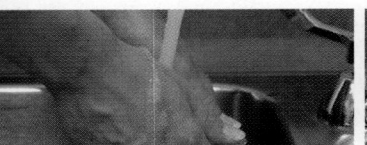 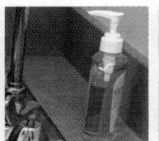 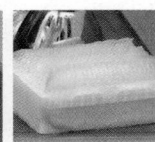

Medical Assistant Role Delineation Chart

HIGHLIGHT indicates material covered in this chapter.

ADMINISTRATIVE

Administrative Procedures

- Perform basic administrative medical assisting functions
- Schedule, coordinate and monitor appointments
- Schedule inpatient/outpatient admissions and procedures
- Understand and apply third-party guidelines
- Obtain reimbursement through accurate claims submission
- Monitor third-party reimbursement
- Understand and adhere to managed care policies and procedures
- *Negotiate managed care contracts*

Practice Finances

- Perform procedural and diagnostic coding
- Apply bookkeeping principles

- Manage accounts receivable
- *Manage accounts payable*
- *Process payroll*
- *Document and maintain accounting and banking records*
- *Develop and maintain fee schedules*
- *Manage renewals of business and professional insurance policies*
- *Manage personnel benefits and maintain records*
- *Perform marketing, financial, and strategic planning*

CLINICAL

Fundamental Principles

- Apply principles of aseptic technique and infection control
- Comply with quality assurance practices
- Screen and follow up patient test results

Diagnostic Orders

- Collect and process specimens
- Perform diagnostic tests

Patient Care

- Adhere to established patient screening procedures
- Obtain patient history and vital signs
- Prepare and maintain examination and treatment areas
- Prepare patient for examinations, procedures and treatments

- Assist with examinations, procedures and treatments
- Prepare and administer medications and immunizations
- Maintain medication and immunization records
- Recognize and respond to emergencies
- Coordinate patient care information with other health care providers
- Initiate IV and administer IV medications with appropriate training and as permitted by state law

GENERAL

Professionalism

- Display a professional manner and image
- Demonstrate initiative and responsibility
- Work as a member of the health care team
- Prioritize and perform multiple tasks
- Adapt to change
- Promote the CMA credential
- Enhance skills through continuing education
- Treat all patients with compassion and empathy
- Promote the practice through positive public relations

Communication Skills

- Recognize and respect cultural diversity
- Adapt communications to individual's ability to understand
- Use professional telephone technique

- Recognize and respond effectively to verbal, nonverbal, and written communications
- Use medical terminology appropriately
- Utilize electronic technology to receive, organize, prioritize and transmit information
- Serve as liaison

Legal Concepts

- Perform within legal and ethical boundaries
- Prepare and maintain medical records
- Document accurately
- Follow employer's established policies dealing with the health care contract
- Implement and maintain federal and state health care legislation and regulations
- Comply with established risk management and safety procedures
- Recognize professional credentialing criteria
- *Develop and maintain personnel, policy and procedure manuals*

Instruction

- Instruct individuals according to their needs
- Explain office policies and procedures
- Teach methods of health promotion and disease prevention
- Locate community resources and disseminate information
- *Develop educational materials*
- *Conduct continuing education activities*

Operational Functions

- Perform inventory of supplies and equipment
- Perform routine maintenance of administrative and clinical equipment
- Apply computer techniques to support office operations
- *Perform personnel management functions*
- *Negotiate leases and prices for equipment and supply contracts*

- *Denotes advanced skills.*

SOURCE: Reprinted by permission of the American Association of Medical Assistants from the AAMA Role Delineation Study: Occupational Analysis of the Medical Assisting Profession.

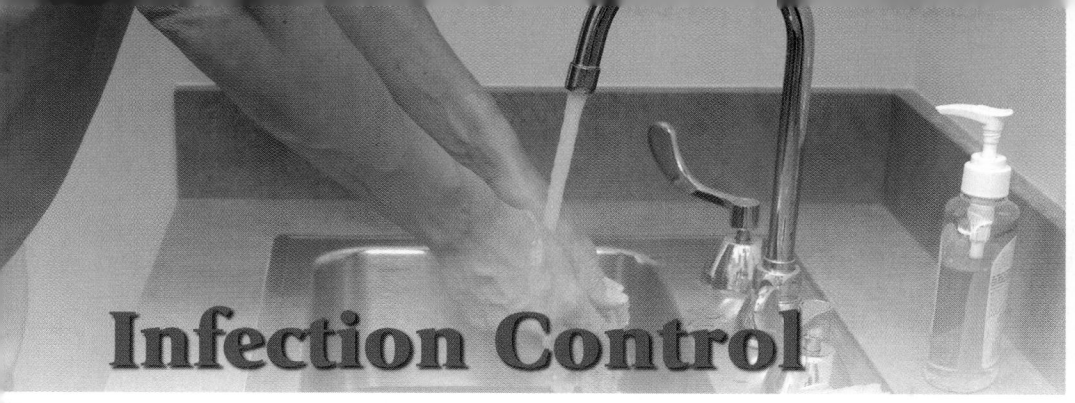

Infection Control

Learning Objectives

After completing this chapter, you should be able to:

- Define and spell the terms to learn for this chapter.
- Describe the conditions required for the infection process to occur.
- Discuss the steps to follow concerning Standard Precautions.
- Define medical asepsis.
- Explain the correct procedure for hand washing.

- Define surgical asepsis.
- Explain the difference between sanitization, disinfection, and sterilization.
- Describe the means of transmission for HIV.
- Discuss the modes of transmission for the different types of hepatitis.

OUTLINE

History of Asepsis	562
Microorganisms	562
The Infection Control System	564
Universal Precautions	565
Hepatitis and AIDS	582
Bioterrorism	585

Terms to Learn

aerobic	incubation	portal of entry
anaerobic	medical asepsis	portal of exit
antibodies	nosocomial infection	reservoir
aseptic	opportunistic infections	sanitization
bactericidal	pathogens	sterilization
bloodborne pathogens	permeable	surgical asepsis
immunity	phagocytosis	susceptible host

Case Study

A PATIENT COMES TO YOUR OFFICE stating that he has had some unusual symptoms recently, and after surfing the Internet, he found that the symptoms strongly suggest HIV. He admits to having an unprotected sexual relationship recently, as well as being an IV drug user.

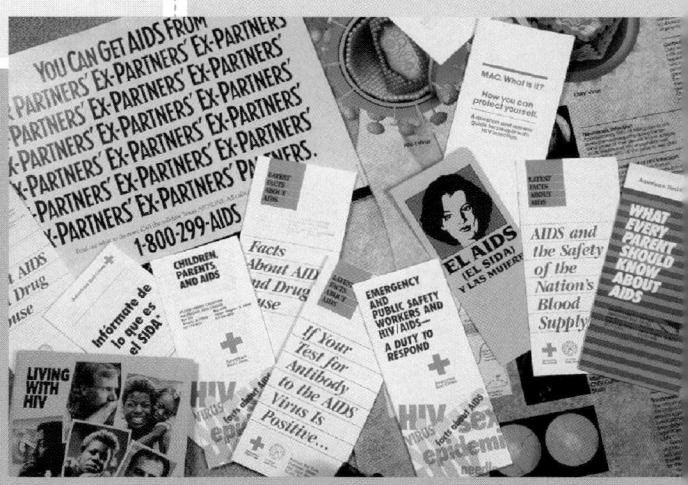

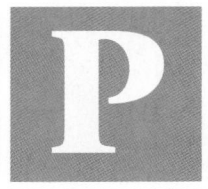**P**athogenic, or disease-producing organisms, are everywhere. The healthy individual has some resistance to pathogens. However, pathogens are especially important to control in the medical office setting because patients who may already be suffering from a disease are more susceptible to new infections. The medical assistant must be aware of how easily pathogens can be spread from one person to another or from an inanimate object to a person because lack of knowledge can cause infections to occur.

History of Asepsis

Methods for controlling the spread of infection were used before early man understood the infection process. Religions, such as the Jewish faith, emphasize the careful preparation and cleanliness associated with foods. About 500 years ago, microorganisms known as germs were suspected to be the cause of some diseases. But it was not until 100 years ago that Semmelweiss, Lister, and Pasteur (discussed in Chapter 2) contributed solid research to our understanding of germ theory.

Louis Pasteur discovered that many diseases are caused by bacteria and that bacteria can be killed by excess heat. The use of heat to kill germs in milk is called *pasteurization* in his honor. Joseph Lister discovered that germs could be killed using carbolic acid. He was the first to insist on cleaning surgical wounds by spraying the surrounding tissue with carbolic acid. This introduced the principles of aseptic, or germ-free, technique in surgery. Lister introduced the concept of clean techniques in hospitals, which greatly reduced the death rate from amputations from 45 to 15 percent. Semmelweiss taught his medical students to wash their hands before delivering babies. Prior to this time, physicians would go from an autopsy directly to delivery of an infant—without washing their hands. This simple precaution of hand washing had an immediate effect on reducing the death rate from puerperal sepsis (childbed fever) in new mothers.

Today, we have a better understanding of germs and bacteria thanks to high-powered microscopes. Sophisticated equipment is used to disinfect and sterilize equipment and materials. However, sterilization is meaningless if good aseptic technique is not practiced. With the advent of communicable diseases such as hepatitis, acquired immunodeficiency syndrome (AIDS), and tuberculosis (TB) the need to adhere to aseptic technique has become critical.

Microorganisms

Microorganisms are small, living organisms that can only be seen with the aid of a microscope. Microorganisms that are normally found on the skin, in the urinary and gastrointestinal tract, and in the respiratory tract are known as normal flora for these areas. They do not cause diseases as long as they are not transferred to another part of the body.

Microorganisms, also called microbes, include bacteria, fungi, protozoa, and viruses. The sizes of microorganisms can be expressed in micrometers. A micrometer is one-millionth of a meter or one-thousandth of a millimeter. Refer to Figure 32-1 for an illustration of

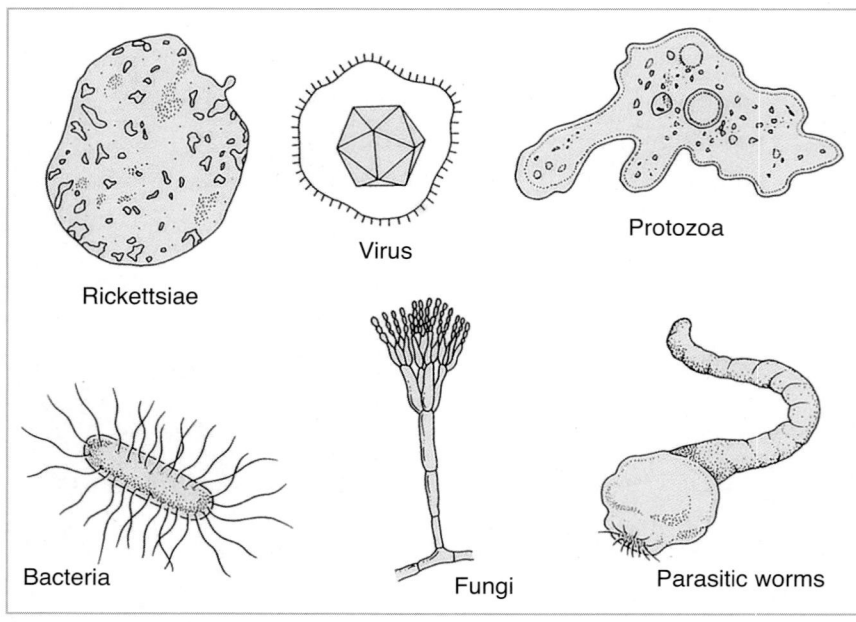

FIGURE 32-1 Pathogens.

pathogens. The study of each type of microorganism represents a separate science:

- Bacteriology—the study of bacteria
- Mycology—the study of fungi
- Protozoology—the study of protozoa
- Virology—the study of viruses

How Microorganisms Grow

Microorganisms occur everywhere in nature and have several requirements to grow: food, moisture, darkness, and a suitable temperature. In addition, some bacteria are aerobic (require oxygen to live) or anaerobic (not requiring oxygen to live). Refer to Table 32-1 for the conditions necessary for the growth of bacteria.

Some microorganisms, such as certain types of fungi and bacteria, are necessary for normal body function. For example, normal flora within the digestive system breaks down food and converts unused food into waste products. In some cases the normal flora will invade areas of the body where they do not belong and, thus, they become pathogens, which are disease-producing microorganisms. For example, *Escherichia coli* (*E. coli*), a normal bacteria within the colon, aids in food digestion. When *E. coli* moves into the bladder or bloodstream, through improper hygiene habits, such as improper (or lack of) hand washing, it can cause urinary and blood infections. Those microorganisms which are capable of producing disease (pathogens) grow best at body temperature (98.6°F), destroy and use human tissue as food, and give off waste toxins that are absorbed and poison the body.

Transmission

Scientists have determined that certain germs can multiply every 12 minutes. If not controlled, germs may spread infection and diseases rapidly from one person to another. The principles of asepsis are applied in the hospital setting to prevent the spread of nosocomial infections. These are infections acquired while in a medical facility. The bacteria were not in the body at the time the patient came into the facility, but were introduced into the body due to poor aseptic technique. The same emphasis on halting the spread of infection takes place in the medical office setting.

The presence of a pathogenic organism, or microorganism, is not enough to cause an infection to occur. Several factors must be in place for infection to occur. These are often referred to as the chain of infection:

1. The pathogen present in the reservoir host is the beginning of the chain of infection. This host not only is infected with the pathogen, but is also the source of transfer of that pathogen. The host (unknowingly) provides nourishment and sustenance for the microorganism, thus allowing it to grow.

TABLE 32-1 Conditions Required for Bacterial Growth

Condition	Explanation
Moisture	Bacteria grow best in moist areas: skin, mucous membranes, wet dressings, wounds, dirty instruments.
Temperature	Thrive at body temperature (98.6°F). Low temperatures (32°F and below) retard, but do not kill, bacterial growth. A temperature of 107°F and above will kill most bacteria.
Oxygen	Aerobic bacteria require an oxygen supply to live. Anaerobic bacteria can survive without oxygen.
Light	Darkness favors the growth of bacteria. Bacteria will die if exposed to direct sunlight or light.

2. For the pathogen to be spread, there must be a portal of exit from the reservoir host. The means of exit includes the respiratory, intestinal, urinary, and reproductive tracts of the body. An open wound is also an excellent portal of exit.

3. Next, there must be a means of transmission for the pathogen from one person to another. This can be through direct contact, either with the infected person or with the discharge or excreta of the infected person. The transmission can also be by indirect contact, such as air droplets from a cough or sneeze, or even by touching a contaminated object. Other methods of indirect contact can be through contaminated food, or even through insects.

4. A portal of entry into a new host is required. This is the means by which the pathogens enter the body. These include the respiratory, urinary, and reproductive tracts, skin and mucous membranes, or blood, for example.

5. A susceptible host must now be available and capable of being infected by the pathogen. For a host to be susceptible, it must be unable to fight off infection. Some things that cause susceptibility include poor health, poor hygiene, or poor nutrition. Stress may also be a factor.

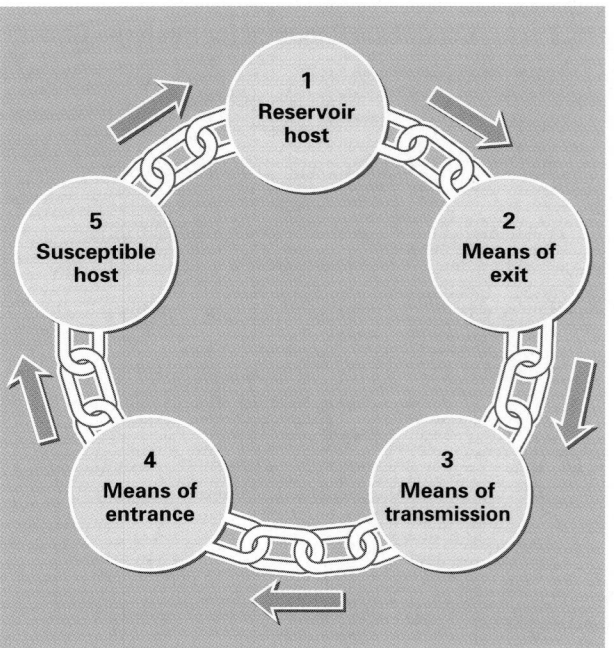

FIGURE 32-2 Chain of infection.

When another reservoir host is found, the chain begins again. Figure 32-2 illustrates the chain of infection.

Fortunately, if the chain is broken, infection does not occur. For instance, the chain may be broken at the reservoir by means of the use of medical asepsis, good

TABLE 32-2	**Stages of the Infection Process**
Stage	**Description**
Invasion	Pathogen enters the body through the portal of entry: respiratory, digestive, reproductive, urinary tracts, and skin.
Multiplication	Reproduction of pathogens.
Incubation period	May vary from several days to months or years during which time the disease is developing but no symptoms appear.
Prodromal period	First mild signs and symptoms appear; a highly contagious period.
Acute period	Signs and symptoms are evident and most severes.
Recovery period	Signs and symptoms begin to subside.

employee health, or use of Standard Precautions. In fact, attaining medical asepsis through proper hand hygiene is the most important method for the reduction of spread of infections.

Microorganisms normally found on the skin may enter the body through a portal of entry and then become pathogens. Portals of entry can occur when the skin is cut, as in a surgical incision; when an injury causes a skin break; or during any invasive procedure, such as the insertion of a needle in venipuncture. The stages of the infection process are described in Table 32-2. These stages include invasion by the pathogen, multiplication (reproduction) of the pathogens, an incubation period, a prodromal period, an acute period, and finally the recovery period.

Once the infection process has begun, it can be broken at any point, thus preventing the spread of the bacteria to another person. For example, after coughing, effective hand hygiene could prevent the spread of the microorganisms to another person or to an inanimate object that could become a means of transmission.

The Infection Control System

The body has several natural defense mechanisms to prevent the spread of infection. These include:

- Dietary intake of sufficient nutrients to promote health
- Age of the person—the young and aged are more susceptible to diseases of the immune system due to immaturity of the immune system in the young and decrease in effectiveness of the system in the aged
- Adequate amount of rest

Mechanisms that promote the spread of infection include:

- Presence of other disease processes in the body—diseases such as diabetes and pneumonia can weaken the system.
- Genetic inheritance of a disease, such as cystic fibrosis, can leave the body in a more susceptible state for infections.

The spread of infection can be prevented in two ways: by preventing the spread of the causative microorganisms and by destroying the microorganisms themselves.

Prevention

The human body has several natural barriers to infection. These include the skin, mucous membranes, gastrointestinal tract, and lymphoid and blood system. The largest natural barrier to infection is the intact skin. The acid pH of the skin inhibits bacterial action. Mucous membranes lining the body's orifices and its respiratory, digestive, reproductive, and urinary tracts also assist in repelling microorganisms. The gastrointestinal tract, containing hydrochloric acid (HCl), causes a bactericidal action that destroys disease-producing bacteria.

Lymphatic System and Blood System

The lymphatic system and blood produce antibodies that protect the body from disease. The composition of the lymph varies in different parts of the body. Leukocytes (white blood cells) actively fight pathogenic microorganisms with the process of phagocytosis. The process of phagocytosis is shown in Figure 32-3. During the process of inflammation, phagocytes engulf, digest, and destroy pathogens. Lymphocytes produce antibodies during the antigen–antibody reaction.

Antigen–Antibody Reaction

Lymphocytes produce antibodies during the antigen–antibody reaction. Antibodies, which are protein substances produced by lymphocytes in the spleen, lymph nodes and tissue, and the bone marrow, react in response to antigens (foreign substances). Antibodies have the ability to neutralize antigens or make them more susceptible to phagocytosis. The antigen–antibody reaction then occurs in response to an invasion of antigens. The body has a natural protective mechanism called immunity. Immunity, a resistance to disease, is said to have occurred when enough antibodies have been produced to provide protection for weeks, months, or years.

Immunity can either be genetic or acquired. Genetic immunity does not involve antibodies. Species immunity, which is passed on genetically, protects humans from certain animal diseases such as chicken cholera. It also protects animals from certain human diseases such as measles and influenza. Acquired immunity, on the other hand, does involve the development of antibodies. This type of immunity may be acquired through active or passive means. Passive immunity develops when antibodies are artificially introduced into the body, and provides only temporary immunity. There are two types of active immunity: natural (person is born with this immunity) and artificial (from an immunization or having had the disease such as with measles). Active immunity provides long-term immunity because the body produces its own antibodies.

Active and passive immunity can be produced by both natural and acquired methods. Natural active immunity results from having recovered from a disease, such as measles, or being exposed to disease and becoming a carrier, such as in tuberculosis.

Artificial active immunity is the result of receiving vaccinations with inactivated (dead) or attenuated (weakened) organisms. For example, inactivated vaccines include influenza, whooping cough, typhoid, and the polio vaccine (Salk). Examples of attenuated vaccines are measles, polio (Sabin), smallpox, German

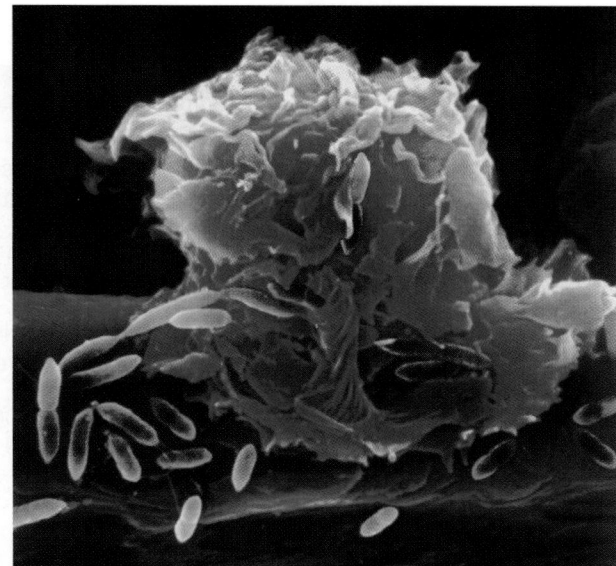

FIGURE 32-3 Phagocytosis.

measles (rubella), and mumps. Natural passive immunity is produced when a mother's antibodies cross the placental barrier and protect the fetus in the womb. Artificial passive immunity is produced by injecting a commercially prepared product to produce antibodies. Gamma globulin, used to prevent viral hepatitis, is an example. The various types of acquired immunity are described in Table 32-3.

Inflammatory Process

The body may react to the invasion of a foreign substance, such as bacteria or virus, with an acute inflammatory process. This process produces dilation of blood vessels due to an increased blood flow, production of watery fluids and materials (exudates), and the invasion of monocytes and neutrophils into the injured tissues to produce phagocytosis. This action of phagocytosis is necessary for repair of tissues. The signs and symptoms of the inflammatory process may be local or systemic.

The four cardinal signs of inflammation are redness, heat, swelling, and pain. These signs are localized at the site of injury and may also be accompanied by stiffness at the site. Systemic symptoms may vary according to the part of the body which is affected. See Table 32-4 for a description of this process.

Universal Precautions

The Centers for Disease Control and Prevention (CDC) in 1994 issued new isolation guidelines that emphasize two tiers of approach to infection control. The first and most important tier, or level, contains precautions designed to care for all patients in a health

TABLE 32-5 Standard Precautions—Equipment and Situations

Precaution	Description
Gloves	Must be worn when in contact with blood; all body fluids, secretions, and excretions (except sweat) regardless of whether or not they contain visible blood; mucous membranes; nonintact skin; and contaminated articles.
Gown	Must be worn during procedures (or situations) in which there may be exposure to blood, body fluids, mucous membranes, or draining wounds. Wash hands after removing gown.
Mask/protective eyewear	Must be worn during procedures that are likely to generate droplets of blood or body fluids (splashes or sprays), for instance, when a patient is coughing excessively.
Hand hygiene	Hands must be washed both before and after gloves are removed. Hands must be washed immediately if contaminated with blood or body fluids, between patient contact, and when indicated to prevent transfer of microorganisms between other patients and the environment.
Transportation	Precautions must be taken when transporting a patient to minimize the risk of transmitting microorganisms to other patients or environmental surfaces or equipment.
Multiple-use equipment	Common multiple-use equipment, such as blood pressure cuffs or stethoscopes, must be cleaned and disinfected after use or when they become soiled with bodily fluids or blood. Single-use items are discarded.
Needles and sharp instruments	Must be discarded into a puncture-proof container. Needles should not be recapped.

currents. Airborne Precautions include isolation of the patient in a private room if hospitalized, with a mask and protective gown used by all health care workers. Hands must be washed before gloving and after gloves are removed. The transport of the patient should be as limited as possible with the patient wearing a mask during transport. All reusable patient care equipment should be cleaned and disinfected before use on another patient. Disposable items should be used if available.

- Droplet Precautions are used for patients known or suspected to be infected with microorganisms transmitted by droplets generated by a patient during coughing, sneezing, talking, or performance of procedures that induce coughing. Examples of these illnesses include invasive *Haemophilus influenzae* Type b disease (meningitis, pneumonia), invasive *Neisseria meningitis* disease (meningitis, pneumonia, and sepsis), diphtheria, pertussis, streptococcal pneumonia, scarlet fever, mumps, and rubella. Precautions include isolation of the patient in a private room if hospitalized. Hands must be washed before and after gloves are worn. Gloves and gowns must be worn if coming into contact with body fluids or blood of the patient. A

mask should be worn if the medical assistant is within 3 feet of the patient and transport of the patient should be limited. All reusable equipment should be cleaned and disinfected.

- Contact Precautions are used for patients known to be infected with a microorganism that is not easily treated with antibiotics and which can be transmitted easily between the patient and health care worker or from patient to patient. Examples of these illnesses include enteric (intestinal) infections, gastrointestinal, respiratory, skin, or wound infections, diphtheria, herpes simplex virus, impetigo, hepatitis A, scabies, pediculosis, and herpes zoster. Precautions include isolation of the patient in a private room if hospitalized. Gloves and gowns must be worn if coming into contact with the patient. A mask and eyewear should be worn if there is potential for exposure to infectious body materials and fluids. When possible, use disposable equipment. If not available, clean and disinfect equipment before use for another patient.

Be aware that some communicable diseases may be transmitted by more than one method. For example, influenza can be transmitted by direct or indirect contact, and chickenpox can be transmitted by direct, indirect contact, or droplets.

The CDC's Standard Precautions are similar to Universal Precautions since both are directed at blood and body fluids that contain blood. However, the CDC's Standard Precautions are broader since they include precautions for any moist body substance. Standard Precautions are used in hospitals, whereas Universal Precautions are used in the medical office.

OSHA

The CDC precautions are required and enforced by the Occupational Safety and Health Administration (OSHA). On December 2, 1991, OSHA issued its final standard on occupational bloodborne pathogens, which resulted from a concern that health care workers face a significant health risk from occupational exposure to bloodborne pathogens, or disease-producing organisms transmitted via the blood.

This OSHA directive is aimed at minimizing exposure of health care workers to hepatitis B virus (HBV) and human immunodeficiency virus (HIV). The OSHA federal standard is now a law which states that Universal Precautions against transmission of bloodborne pathogens cannot just be recommended. They are law and must be observed by employers of health care personnel. All health care agencies were required to comply with this law by July 6, 1992.

The OSHA guidelines apply to facilities in which the employees could be "reasonably anticipated" to come into contact with potentially infectious materials: body fluids, saliva, and tissues. An exposure control program must be implemented in each facility. This includes:

- Exposure determination—job classifications and probability of exposure

- Method of compliance—documentation of safety measures that would decrease the risk of exposure

- Postexposure evaluation—specifies procedures in the event of exposure

For protection, engineering controls are the responsibility of the employer. These would include such items as availability of sharps containers, sinks and running water, and biohazard containers. Work practice controls are the responsibility of the employee. These include your use of such items as sharps containers and PPE. (See Procedure 32-1 for disposing of infectious waste.)

Disposal of Infectious Wastes and Substances

OBJECTIVE: Student will perform procedure without errors.

Equipment and Supplies

infectious waste container with lid marked appropriately with Universal Biohazard symbol and label; red disposal plastic liners.

Method

1. Check to ensure that infectious waste container is lined with red disposal plastic bag.
2. Discard any infectious waste into the infectious waste container.
3. Make sure that all liquid waste is already contained in a closable device before putting it into the infectious waste container.
4. Do not put contaminated glass into the infectious container. Instead, all glass should be placed into a puncture-proof or very highly puncture-resistant container for disposal; small glass items can be deposited into a sharps container for disposal.
5. When the infectious waste container becomes full, the red trash bag should be closed, either tied with a securing knot, twist-tied, or otherwise secured to protect the trash handling personnel and others in the environment from exposure to their contents.
6. Make sure that the contents of the red bags are completely contained inside the the closed bag.
7. Make sure red bags are not overstuffed so that they cannot be closed, ruptured when handled or lifted, opened, or anything leaking from them.
8. Do not mix non-infectious trash in the same large bin, container, or dumpster with infectious waste or trash.
9. Make sure there are no sharps put into infectious bag, or if they are, that they are contained in a designated sharps container.
10. Make sure there is no glass of any kind placed into the infectious bag.
11. Closed red bags should be transported from the point of waste generation to a dirty utility room/area and stored in a designated holding area away from access by other than authorized staff until transported from the facility; never store trash in hallways, entrances, corridors or other areas accessible to and used by public.

Physical and Chemical Barriers

Effective physical and chemical barriers are used to maintain infection control. The development of a nosocomial infection, or hospital/medical facility–acquired infection, is prevented when careful medical and surgical asepsis is maintained.

Medical Asepsis

Medical asepsis refers to the destruction of organisms after they leave the body. Techniques such as hand hygiene, using disposable equipment, and wearing gloves can help reduce the number and transfer of pathogens. Aseptic technique is a means of reducing the transfer of pathogens in the medical office.

Ordinary hygiene habits of everyday life are a form of medical asepsis. These include hand washing when handling food or after using the bathroom and covering one's mouth during a cough or sneeze. One of the most effective means of reducing pathogenic transmission is through hand hygiene. This is considered the first stage of infection control since the hands are a primary method for infection to transfer from the host to the receiver. To keep the skin free of harmful organisms, there must be frequent hand washing using a disinfectant soap, friction, and warm running water. Jewelry, such as rings, allows germs to hide and grow. See Figure 32-5 for an illustration of jewelry that is likely to catch pathogens. Jewelry should be removed (as in Figure 32-5C) prior to hand washing or applying gloves.

Situations involving medical asepsis would include but are not limited to taking oral, aural, and rectal temperatures; obtaining throat or vaginal cultures or smears; obtaining urine, stool, or sputum specimens; administering medications; and cleaning treatment rooms.

Aseptic techniques that can cause a break in the chain of infection include:

- Washing hands before and after any contact with patients or equipment

- Handling all specimens and materials as though they contain pathogens
- Using gloves to protect yourself when handling contaminated articles or materials, such as specimens
- Not wearing jewelry that can attract and harbor bacteria
- Using disposable equipment whenever possible. Dispose of all equipment properly after use
- Cleaning all nondisposable equipment as soon as possible after patient use, using approved disinfectant
- Using only clean or sterile supplies for each patient
- Using a protective covering over your clothes if there is any danger of contaminated materials or supplies coming into contact with your uniform
- Discarding items that fall on the floor if they cannot be cleaned. Any item dropped on the floor must be resterilized or disinfected prior to use. All floors are considered contaminated. If in doubt, throw it out!
- Placing all wet or damp dressings and bandages in a waterproof bag to protect the persons handling the garbage

Medical asepsis also relates to other aspects of the facility, not just to the equipment and instruments. Having proper ventilation in all areas of the office will also assist in decreasing the transfer of microorganisms. All examination rooms should be cleaned with an approved disinfectant after each patient contact. Checking and emptying trash cans, replacing sharps containers in a timely manner, and observing for any insect infestation are also means of maintaining medical asepsis.

Some offices have one seating area for "well patients" and another for "sick patients." For example, a patient who is returning for a follow-up visit is seated in one area, while a patient with symptoms of the flu is

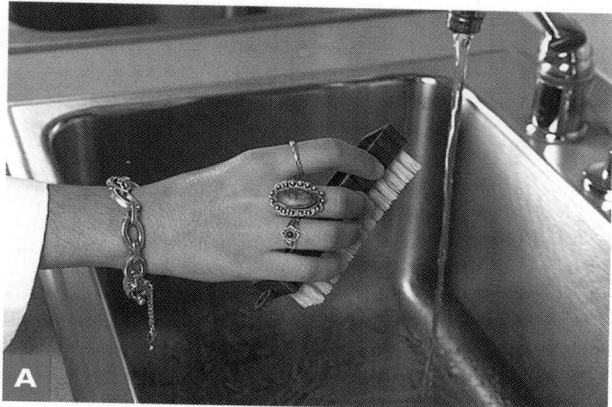
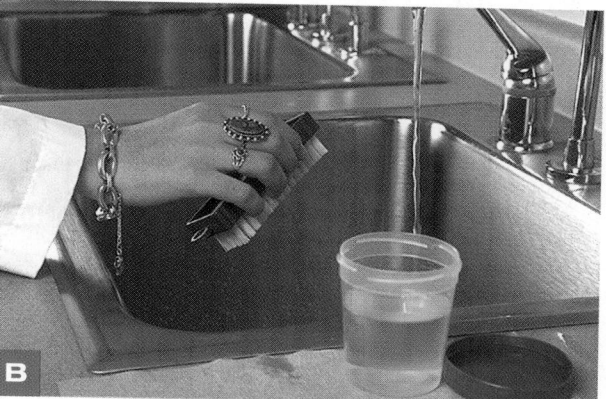
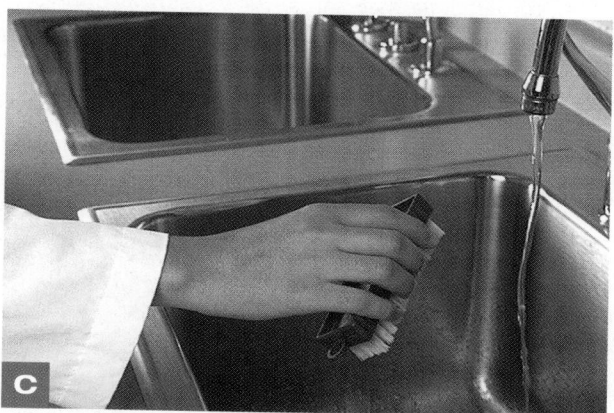

FIGURE 32-5 Jewelry provides places for pathogens to hide and grow.

Professionalism

Wearing excessive jewelry, long fingernails, or long hair can cause contamination. Allow your patients and coworkers to view you as someone who maintains good technique at all times.

Maintaining confidentiality is absolutely necessary at all times for the medical professional. Allow your patients and coworkers to view you as someone who can be trusted.

seated in another area. This helps to decrease the chance of cross-contamination.

HAND HYGIENE Frequent and diligent hand washing provides the first defense against the spread of disease and should be done often. Refer to Figure 32-6 for a demonstration of proper hand washing technique and to Procedure 32-2 for proper hand washing procedure.

Alcohol-Based Hand Rubs The CDC has presented some new guidelines concerning the use of alcohol-based

Hand Washing

OBJECTIVE: Perform hand washing procedure without error.

Equipment and Supplies

soap in liquid soap dispenser; nail brush or orange cuticle stick; hot running water; paper towels; waste container

Method

1. Remove jewelry (includes rings with the exception of wedding band, watch, bracelets).
   Rationale: Jewelry has crevices and grooves that can harbor bacteria and dirt.
2. Stand at sink without allowing clothing to touch sink. Turn water on using paper towel (Figure 32-6A). Adjust running water to moderately warm temperature.
   Rationale: Hot water may burn skin and cold water will not allow soap lather to form. Improper water temperature can cause chapping and cracking of skin, which allows pathogens to enter.
3. Discard paper towel.
   Rationale: Avoid direct contact with contaminated sinks and faucets. Paper towel becomes contaminated after touching the faucet(s).
4. Wet hands under running water and place liquid soap (size of a nickel or 1 teaspoon) into palm of hand (Figures 32-6B and C). If using bar soap, keep the bar in hands and use enough soap to form a lather. Work soap into a lather by moving it over palms, sides, and backs—the entire surface—of both hands for 2 minutes. Use a circular motion and friction. Interlace fingers and move soapy water between them (Figure 32-6C).

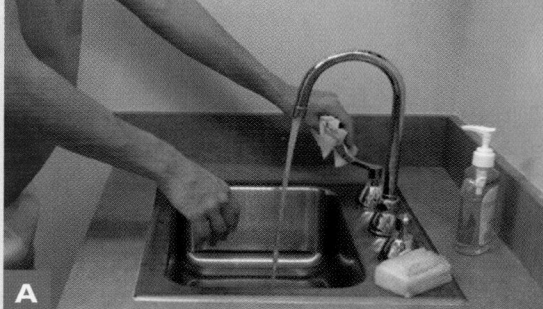
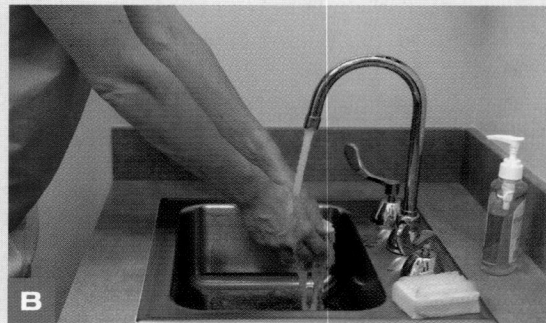
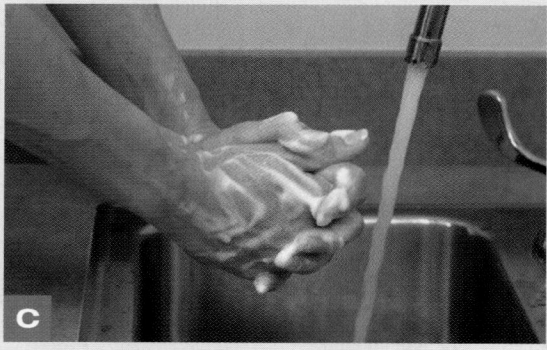
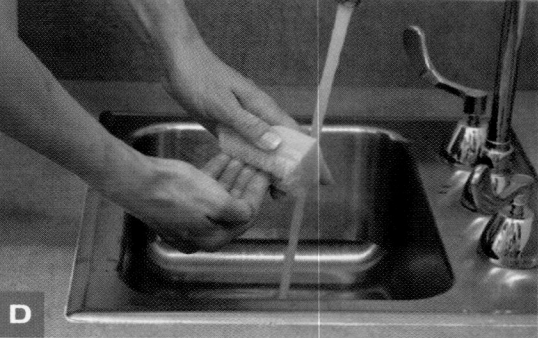

FIGURE 32-6 Hand hygiene. (A) Turn water on using paper towel. (B) Wet hand and arms downward. (C) Add soap and interlace fingers and thumbs. (D) Use hand brush to clean fingernails.

Rationale: Friction assists in removing organisms and dirt. If the soap bar falls into the sink or onto the floor during the procedure, the medical assistant must start over again. Only use bar soap if liquid soap is unavailable. Soap bars allow the growth of bacteria to occur and must be thoroughly rinsed after each use.

5. Keep hands pointed downward with hands and forearms below elbow level during the entire hand washing procedure.
Rationale: Water will run off hands and not back up onto arms for further contamination.

6. Use hand brush and/or orange cuticle stick to clean under fingernails (Figure 32-6D). Thoroughly scrub wedding band if present.
Rationale: Running water and soap may not be sufficient to remove dirt particles under nails.

7. Rinse hands under running water with fingers pointed down using care not to touch the sink or faucets (Figure 32-6E).
Rationale: The sink is not sterile (only clean), so contaminants may be present. Running water will wash away dirt and organisms.

8. Reapply soap and wash wrists and forearms for 1 more minute using circular motions (Figure 32-6F).

9. Rinse hands under running water.

10. Dry hands thoroughly with paper towel (Figure 32-6G). Discard paper towel.

11. Using a dry paper towel, turn faucet off (Figure 32-6H).
Rationale: The paper towel, will protect clean hands from coming into contact with contaminated faucet handles.

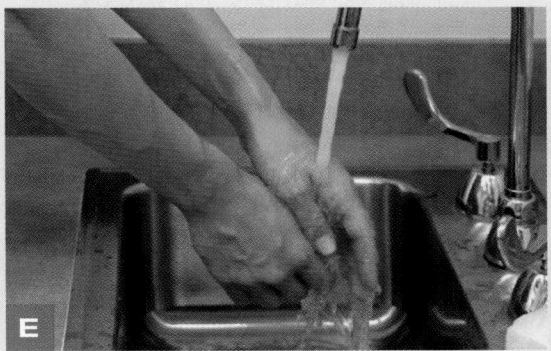
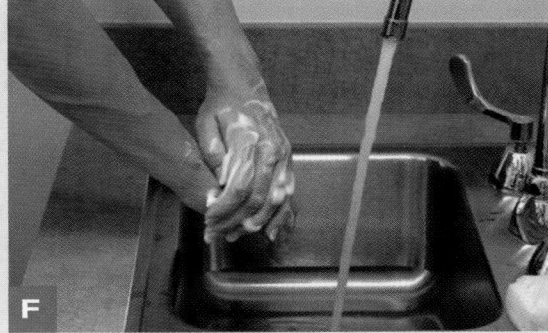
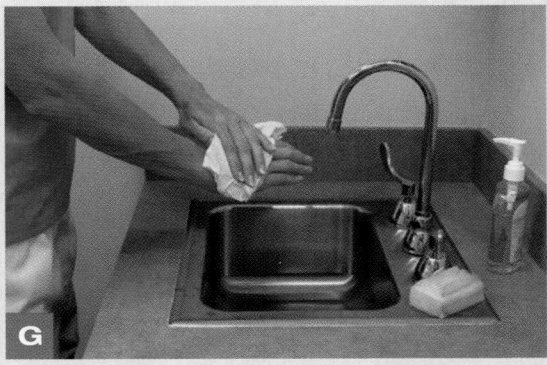
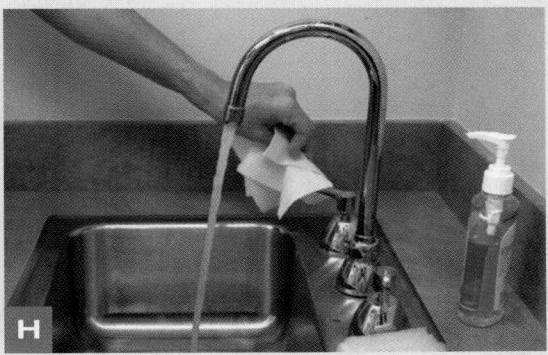

FIGURE 32-6 (*continued*) (E) Rinse hands keeping them lower than elbows. (F) Reapply soap and wash wrists and forearms. (G) Rinse and then dry hands with paper towel. (H) Turn the water off using a dry paper towel.

hand rubs. These rubs have the advantage of not requiring rinsing, and many contain emollients that prevent drying of the skin. A disadvantage, however, is that they are more expensive than hand soaps and may cause stinging if there is an abrasion on the skin.

The guidelines suggest that the alcohol-based hand rubs can be used at the times usually required for hand washing. However, the hands should be washed with soap and water if they are visibly soiled with dirt or body fluids and before eating and after using the restroom.

As with regular hand washing, jewelry should be removed prior to using the hand rubs. Approximately 2 to 3 mL of the gel should be placed in the palm of the hand, and thoroughly spread over the surface of both hands up to one-half inch above the wrist. Continue to rub the hands together until dry, approximately 15 to 30 seconds.

PROTECTIVE CLOTHING AND EQUIPMENT Protective clothing, such as gowns, gloves, and masks, are worn for two reasons:

1. To protect the patient from any microorganisms that might be present on the health care worker's street clothing
2. To protect the health care worker from carrying microorganisms away from the patient

In addition, protective devices, such as gloves and masks, assist in protecting the health care worker from contamination with bloodborne pathogens. Nonsterile gowning technique is used for procedures, such as drawing blood, specimen collection, infant handling, and when in contact with a patient who is in isolation. Figure 32-7 illustrates nonsterile gown technique. You will not need each piece of PPE for every procedure. PPE should be chosen in consideration of the possibility of contamination.

If wearing more than one piece of PPE, maintain medical asepsis when removing it. Remove your gloves first. Do not reach around to untie the gown or mask with your contaminated gloves. This would transfer contaminants to your uniform. After removing gloves, next remove the gown, and lastly remove the mask. (When wearing the mask, it should fit snugly over the nose, mouth, and chin.) Wash your hands after completion of any procedure, including removal of PPE.

Figure 32-8 shows proper technique for putting on an isolation gown and Figure 32-9 illustrates how to remove an isolation gown. The proper step-by-step technique for removing gloves is shown in Figure 32-10.

Surgical Asepsis

Surgical asepsis refers to the techniques practiced to maintain a sterile environment. It is the destruction of organisms before they enter the body.

Three important steps methods are used to reach sterility, which is the absence of microorganisms. These methods for preventing the spread of disease in the medical office are sanitization, disinfection, and sterilization. Sanitization inhibits or inactivates pathogens by means of scrubbing and washing items. Disinfection destroys most or all pathogens on

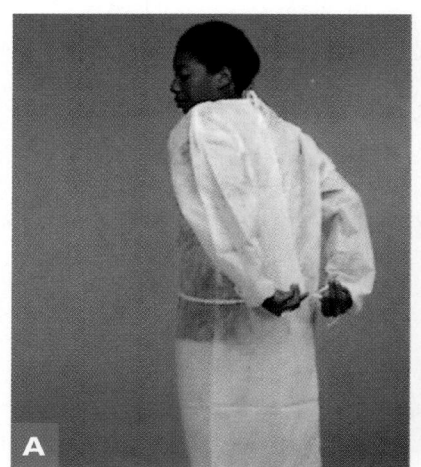
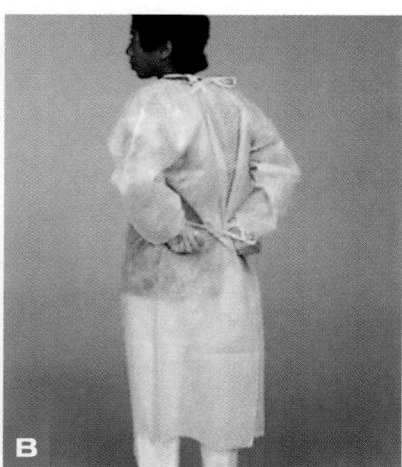
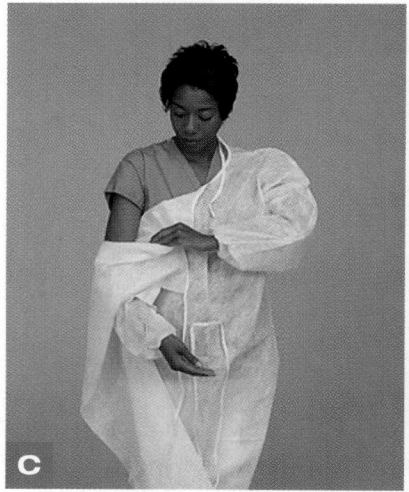
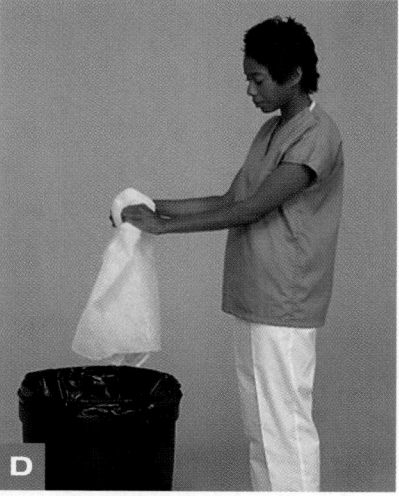

FIGURE 32-7 Technique for donning and removing a nonsterile gown. (A) Tie the neck piece of the gown and overlap the flaps. (B) Tie the gown securely at the waist. If gloves are to be worn, put them on now. (C) To take off a gown, remove and dispose of gloves properly if you are wearing them. Untie neck and waist. Grasp shoulders. Turn gown inside out as you remove it. (D) Fold up the gown and discard. Do not reuse a gown. Wash your hands.

inanimate objects with the use of chemicals such as iodine, chlorine, alcohol, and phenol. Sterilization is the destruction of all living organisms and spores with the use of pressurized steam, extreme temperatures, or radiation.

SANITIZATION Sanitization inhibits or inactivates pathogens by means of careful scrubbing of equipment and instruments using a brush and detergent with a neutral pH, such as a soapless soap, and then rinsing in hot water and air drying. Although sanitization cleans items, microorganisms and bacteria are not destroyed. This process can be used for supplies and equipment that do not come into direct contact with the patient or that touch only the skin surface. If contaminated material cannot be sanitized immediately, then it should be soaked in detergent and water according to the manufacturer's instructions.

Another means of sanitizing equipment is with the use of ultrasound. In this case the instruments and equipment are placed into a bath tank and sound waves vibrate to break up the contamination. The articles are then rinsed thoroughly. Always follow the instructions of your facility procedure manual regarding the proper procedure for sanitizing instruments. See Procedure 32-3 for one method of sanitizing instruments.

DISINFECTION Disinfection involves a soaking and wiping process. Disinfection destroys or inhibits the activity of disease-causing organisms. Disinfecting agents include chemical germicides, flowing steam, and boiling water. Chemical germicides are used to disinfect heat-perishable objects in the medical office, including some rubber and plastic items, and to clean floors and office furniture. Two common disinfectants are zephiran chloride and chlorophenol.

Disinfectants can eliminate many organisms, but are not effective against spores (the dormant stage of some bacteria), spore-forming bacteria, and some viruses. Disinfectants, alcohol, and Betadine are used when preparing a patient's skin for surgical procedures or injections since antiseptics prevent the growth of some microorganisms. Some disinfectants, however, while effective on objects, may be too strong to use on patients (for example, formaldehyde).

Contaminated instruments and equipment are completely immersed in a germicidal solution according to the manufacturer's instructions from 1 to 10 hours. They are then rinsed in water. (Instruments are rinsed in distilled water to prevent rust and corrosion.) Instruments must be dried after disinfection and rinsing.

Objects that come into contact with mucous membranes, such as vaginal speculums, laryngoscopes, or thermometers, should be disinfected or even sterilized,

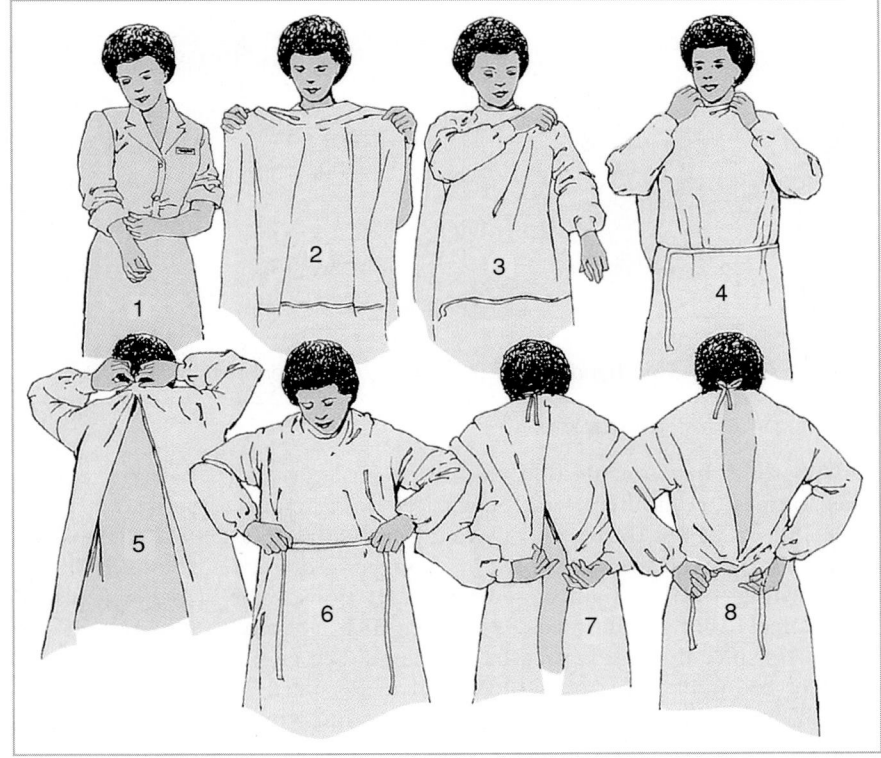

FIGURE 32-8 Putting on an isolation gown.

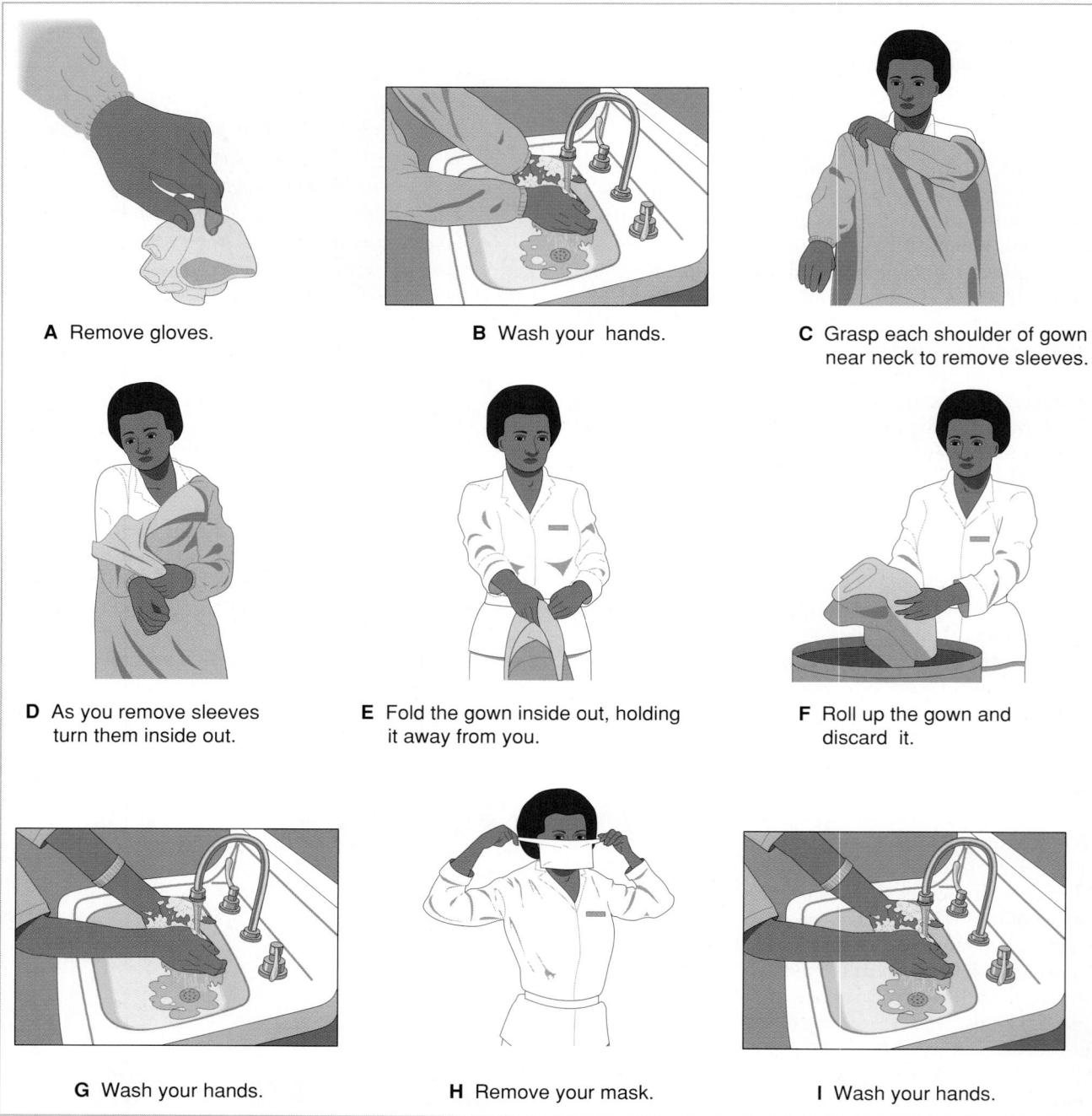

A Remove gloves.

B Wash your hands.

C Grasp each shoulder of gown near neck to remove sleeves.

D As you remove sleeves turn them inside out.

E Fold the gown inside out, holding it away from you.

F Roll up the gown and discard it.

G Wash your hands.

H Remove your mask.

I Wash your hands.

FIGURE 32-9 Removing an isolation gown.

if possible. Instruments that cannot be soaked, such as scopes, computers, and electrical instruments, should be wiped thoroughly with a germicidal solution. Germicidal solutions must be changed frequently according to the manufacturer's instructions. The chemical disinfection process is referred to as a "cold" process since no heat is used or generated. See Figure 32-11 for an example of a cold chemical sterilizer.

Chemical disinfectants used for soaking and wiping include soap, alcohol, phenol, acid, alkalines (such as bleach), and formaldehyde. Some of these are described in Table 32-6.

A means of disinfection that is used in operating rooms is ultraviolet rays. Equipment that cannot be soaked is placed under the ultraviolet lamps for a specified period of time. This will kill microorganisms.

Although not effective for viruses (such as hepatitis) or for destroying spores, boiling water can be used as a means of disinfection. Moist heat of up to 212°F will kill most pathogens. Sterilization cannot occur at

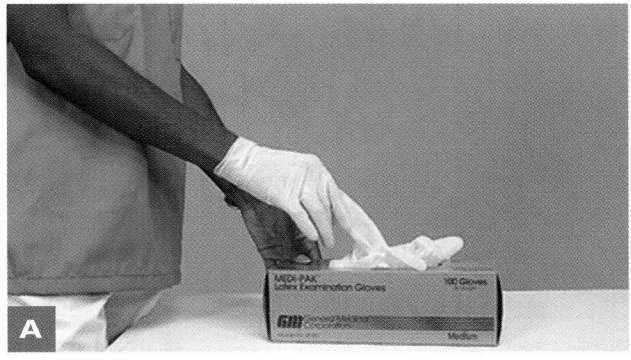

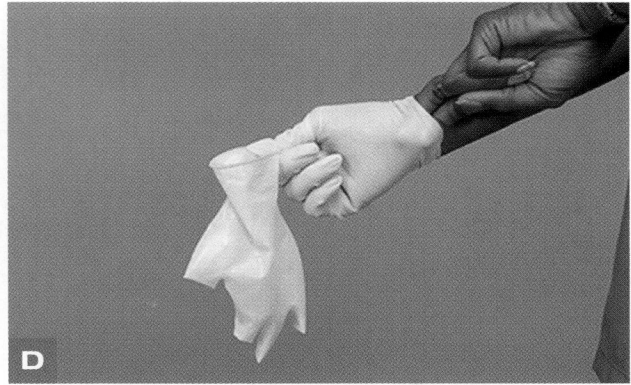

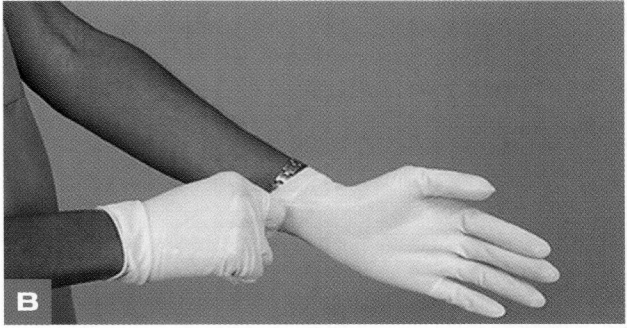

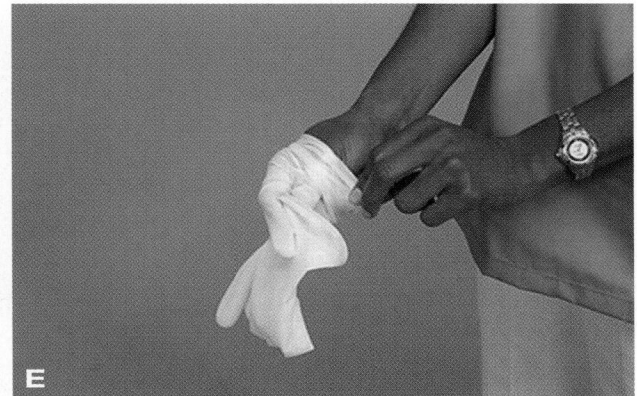

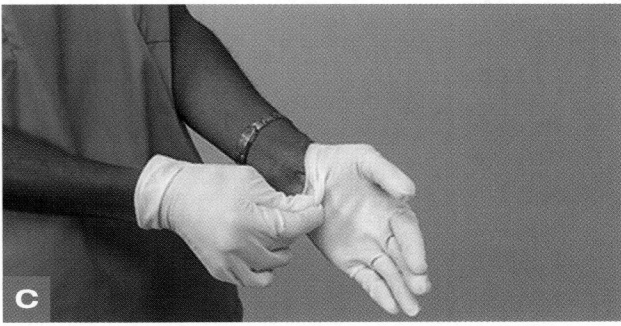

FIGURE 32-10 Removing gloves. (A) Use a clean pair of gloves for each patient contact. (B) Grasp the glove just below the cuff. (C) Pull the glove over your hand while turning the glove inside out. (D) Place the ungloved index finger and middle finger inside cuff of the glove, turning the cuff downward. (E) Pull the cuff and glove inside out as your remove your hand from the glove.

this temperature. Stainless steel, glassware, and instruments can be boiled without damage. The articles are submerged in a container filled with cold water. (Distilled water should be used when boiling instruments or stainless steel to prevent sediment or deposits from forming.) The water must completely cover the articles to be disinfected. The water is then brought to the boiling point and continues to boil for 20 to 30 minutes for disinfection. When the boiling time has elapsed, the disinfected materials are allowed to cool. To maintain disinfection, they must be touched only with sterile forceps.

STERILIZATION Sterilization kills all microorganisms, both pathogenic and nonpathogenic. The use of heat (steam or dry), chemicals, high-velocity electron

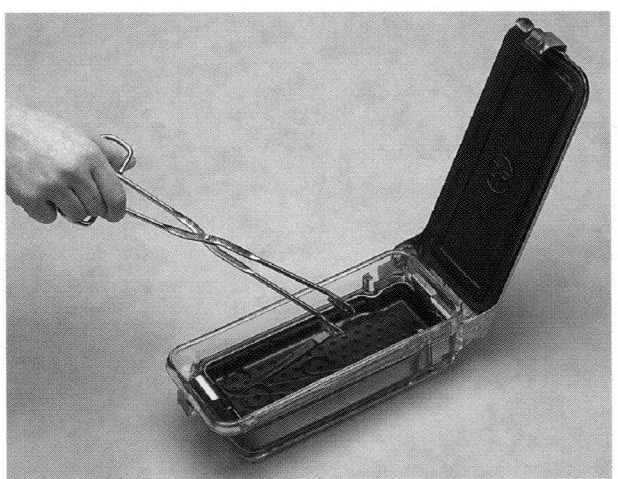

FIGURE 32-11 Cold chemical sterilizer.

Sanitizing Instruments

OBJECTIVE: Learn to clean and sanitize instruments with no visible contamination remaining.

Equipment and Supplies

disposable gloves; rubber (utility) gloves; plastic brush; towel; sink; running water; container to hold all the instruments; low-sudsing (low-pH) detergent or germicidal agent

Note: Instruments should be rinsed under warm running water immediately after surgery to remove gross blood, body fluids, and tissue. If it is not possible to clean them immediately, instruments should be submerged in water containing a low-pH detergent.

Method

1. Apply both disposable and rubber gloves.
   Rationale: Instruments have sharp edges that can cut through disposable gloves. Instruments are contaminated with blood and other waste materials.
2. Place a low-sudsing (low-pH) detergent or germicidal agent in a large container with water. Rinse all instruments.
   Rationale: This will clean off gross blood and waste products. A low-pH detergent prevents staining on stainless steel surfaces.
3. Rinse instruments in clear water in either sink or container. Delicate and sharp instru-

ments should be separated from general instruments.
4. Scrub each instrument individually with brush and detergent under running water. Open instruments to thoroughly scrub all serrated edges and hinge areas.
   Rationale: Blood and other debris collect in hinges and cracks and on serrated edges.
5. Rinse instruments thoroughly under hot water.
   Rationale: Any detergent left on an instrument will prevent the disinfection process.
6. If instruments cannot be cleaned immediately after use, then soak them in a solution of water and a blood solvent. When ready to wash instruments begin with step 1.
   Rationale: Soaking instruments prevents blood and other organic material from hardening. Hardened blood is difficult to remove.
7. After thoroughly rinsing cleaned instruments, roll them in a towel to dry them.
   Rationale: Drying instruments prevents rust.
8. Check condition of all instruments for defects or remaining soil.
9. Wrap instrument(s) for sterilization.

---

bombardment, or ultraviolet light radiation are used for this process. Heat sterilization, produced by an autoclave under steam pressure, is able to kill spores, bacteria, and other microorganisms. Dry heat is used for dense ointments such as petroleum jelly.

All supplies including dressings, needles, and instruments that come into contact with internal body tissue or an open wound must be sterile. Once a sterile article is touched by hands or another unsterile object, it is considered contaminated. Sterile gloves must be used when touching sterilized items. The procedure for applying gloves (whether sterile or nonsterile) is sometimes referred to as *donning*.

AUTOCLAVE   The methods used for sterilization include the autoclave and chemical (cold) sterilization. The autoclave process is an effective means of

sterilization in the medical office. Types of autoclaving include steam under pressure, dry heat (320°F for 1 hour), dry gas, or radiation.

Autoclaving destroys organisms by causing them to explode. This method of sterilization requires 15 pounds of pressure and a temperature of 250°F to 270°F depending on the manufacturer's recommendations. Distilled water must be used in the steam autoclave. The autoclave consists of an outer chamber (jacket), that creates a buildup of steam that is forced into an inner chamber, into which the materials to be sterilized are placed. Figure 32-12 shows an example of an autoclave. Depending on the model type, there may be three gauges on the autoclave: (1) a jacket pressure gauge to indicate pressure in the outer chamber, (2) a chamber pressure gauge to indicate the steam pressure in the inner chamber, and (3) a temperature gauge to

TABLE 32-6 **Disinfection Methods**

Method	Description and Use
Alcohol (70% isopropyl)	Used for skin surfaces, equipment such as stethoscopes and thermometers, and table surfaces Causes damage to rubber products, lens, and plastic Flammable
Chlorine (sodium hypochlorite or bleach)	Use in dilution of 1:10 (1 part bleach to 10 parts water) Used to eliminate a broad spectrum of microorganisms Has a corrosive effect on instruments, rubber, and plastic products Can cause skin irritation Inexpensive
Formaldehyde	Used to disinfect and sterilize Dangerous product that is regulated by OSHA—must have clearly marked labels
Hydrogen peroxide	Effective disinfectant for use only on nonhuman surfaces and products May damage rubber, plastics, and metals
Glutaraldehyde	Effective against viruses, bacteria, fungi and some spores Regulated by OSHA—must have clearly marked labels and be used in well-ventilated area Must wear gloves and masks when using

indicate the temperature in the inner chamber in which items are placed. Some models have only one gauge.

The microorganisms are killed in autoclaving by the condensation of steam on each of the items, not by the heat produced. Heat is actually transferred to the items by way of the steam condensation. Steam sterilization is not effective if air pockets are present within the surgical packs. A pump within the autoclave will first remove air from the chamber. The pressure level and temperature levels within the autoclave chamber can be built up only after the air is removed. Therefore, the gauges indicating pressure and temperature must be monitored by the medical assistant. Table 32-7 describes autoclave sterilization time requirements. Always read and follow the manufacturer's instructions for use and maintenance prior to using any piece of electrical equipment.

The autoclave should be thoroughly cleaned (sanitized) and free of any materials or lint before using. If detergent or other cleaner is used for cleaning, the autoclave should be completely rinsed before placing objects into it. The air exhaust valve must be cleaned and free of lint after each use.

The wrapping in which the instruments and materials to be sterilized, such as dressings, are placed must be permeable, or allow steam to pass through, and be strong enough to hold together during the

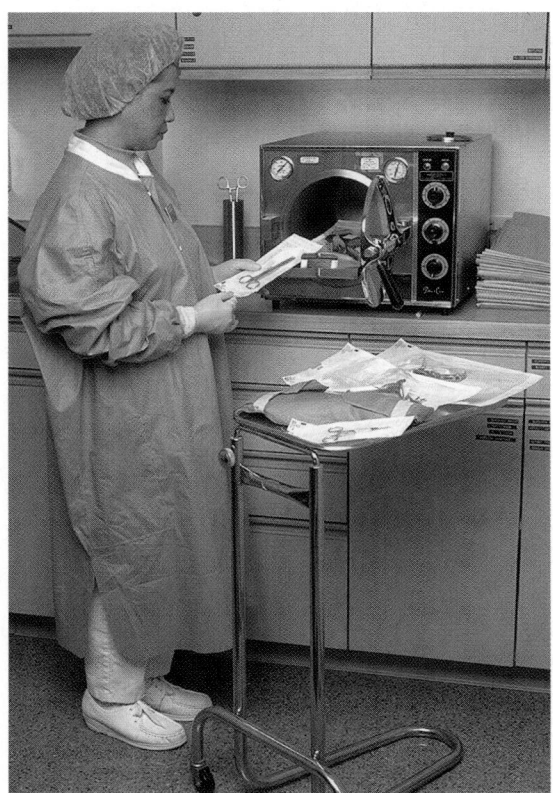

FIGURE 32-12 An autoclave.

TABLE 32-7 Sterilization Time Requirements

Time	Article
15 minutes	Glassware Metal instruments—open tray or individual wrapping with hinges open Syringes (unassembled) Needles
20 minutes	Instruments—partial metal in double-thickness wrapper or covered tray Rubber products: gloves, tubing, catheters wrapped or unwrapped Solutions in a flask (50–100 mL)
30 minutes	Dressings—small packs in paper or muslin Solutions in a flask (500–1,000 mL) Syringes—unassembled, individually wrapped in gauze Syringes—unassembled, individually wrapped in glass tubes Needles—individually packaged in paper or glass tubes Sutures—wrapped in paper or muslin Instrument and treatment trays—wrapped in paper or muslin Gauze—loosely packed
60 minutes	Petroleum jelly—in dry heat

steam process. Wrapping materials include heavy paper, muslin, plastic, and stainless steel containers. The wrapping generally consists of two layers of permeable materials. All items must be completely covered with the wrapping material and fastened with tape that states the date of sterilization and identifies the item. Instruments with hinges should be open, the tubing free of any kinks, and syringes unassembled before wrapping. Refer to Procedure 32-4 and Figure 32-13 for wrapping of instruments for the autoclave.

Refer to Figure 32-14 for a display of autoclave indicator tapes. The lines on the tape change color during the autoclaving process and indicate that exposure to the correct temperature has occurred.

Sterilization pouches or bags are often used for individual instruments. Careful inspection must be made to make sure the bag has not ruptured or been punctured during the autoclave process. Small, lightweight instruments are suitable for pouches. The pouches have sterilization indicators both inside and outside the bag.

Instruments that will be used immediately can be placed in perforated trays and autoclaved unwrapped. The lid for the tray is placed next to the open tray of instruments. The lid is immediately placed over the instruments after sterilization. A towel is usually placed under the instruments to absorb moisture during autoclaving.

Items should be wrapped in individual packs that can be handled for storage and use by their outer wrapping without contaminating the inner items. When the autoclaved package is opened, the contents are removed without contaminating them.

Containers and jars of supplies should be placed on their sides for full sterilization to occur. Solutions should be autoclaved separately since they may boil over during autoclaving. The lid of plastic containers and bags will become sealed upon sterilization.

The autoclave chamber must not be overloaded or the steam will not be able to penetrate the wrapping and sterilize the instruments and materials. Items should be placed on their edges to permit the proper penetration with moisture and heat.

The time or pressure required for autoclaving, according to the manufacturer's recommendations, must never be shortened. If proper timing and pressure are not observed when autoclaving, the items will not be sterilized.

At intervals an independent company should check the operation of the autoclave. Your office can continue to autoclave items as usual, but one item is chosen to be sent to an outside lab where it is checked for sterility. These checks are necessary to determine that the autoclave is working properly. For instance, if the steam levels or temperatures being used are inadequate, autoclaved items might not be completely sterilized.

Drying Autoclaved Goods   After the autoclave process is complete, the drying process is almost as important as the correct temperature and pressure in autoclaving. Wetness on items ("wet packs") can cause a break in sterility since moisture will allow bacteria to grow and be transmitted into the inside of the package. Wet packs can be avoided by allowing for a drying period at the end of autoclaving. To do this, open the door of the autoclave ¾ inch (but no more) just before the drying cycle on the autoclave. Run the dry cycle according to the manufacturer's directions.

Sterilization Indicators   Indicators are used to signify sterilization. Indicators come in a variety of types

PROCEDURE

Wrapping Instruments for Autoclaving

OBJECTIVE: Wrap and label instruments properly.

Equipment and Supplies

wrapping material; instrument(s) for autoclaving; sterilization indicator strips; autoclave tape

Method

1. Wash your hands.
2. Place a square of wrapping material on the table so that is appears as a "diamond" shape when you look at it. Be sure the wrapping material is large enough to cover the entire article being wrapped.
3. Place the item in the center of the wrapping material. If hinged items are included, be sure the instrument is in the open position. If sharp instruments are being autoclaved, place the tip in a piece of gauze to prevent puncture through the material.
4. Place the indicator strip in the center of the packet.
5. Fold the bottom point of the wrapping material up and over the instruments. Fold a small portion of the point back over so that it can be used to pick up the paper when it is unwrapped (Figure 32-13A).
6. Fold the right side of the wrapping paper over until it covers the instrument(s). Fold a small portion of the point back over as in the previous step.
7. Fold the left side of the wrapping paper over until it covers the instrument(s). Fold a small portion of the point back over as in the previous step (Figure 32-13B).
8. Now fold the bottom of the package up. Continue folding until you have reached the top point (Figure 32-13C).
9. Be sure the pack is folded "snugly."
10. Secure by using a piece of autoclave tape (Figure 32-13D).
11. Label the package with the name of the item(s) inside, your initials, and the date.
12. If bags are used for the autoclaving procedure, place the item and an indicator strip, inside the bag. (If the item has a sharp point, wrap the point in a piece of gauze.)
13. Seal the bag. Label the bag with the name of the item(s) inside, your initial, and the date.

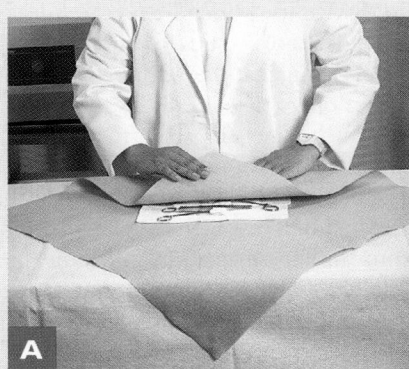

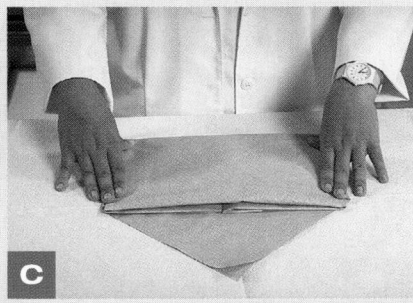

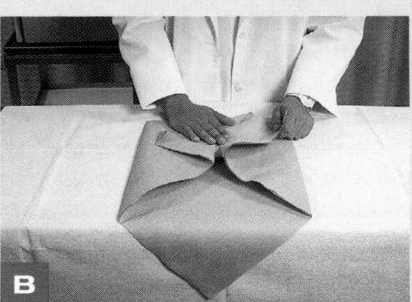

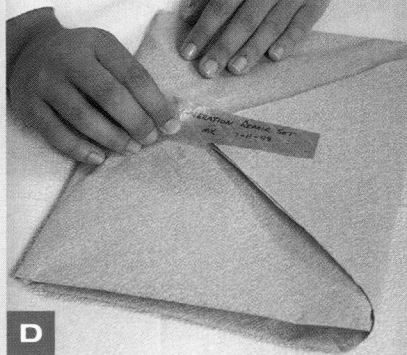

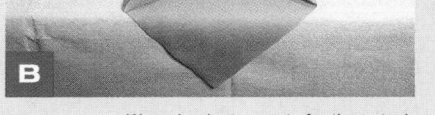

FIGURE 32-13   Wrapping instruments for the autoclave.

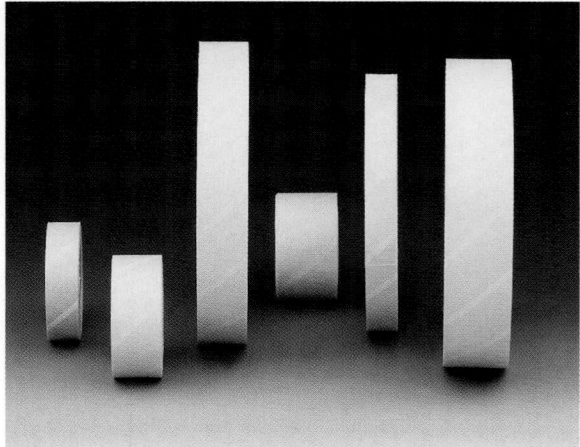

FIGURE 32-14 Autoclave indicator tapes.

including strips and tape. OK strips are placed inside the wrapper or in the chamber. Note that the change of color or dots appearing in an indicator indicate that the inner contents have been exposed to the conditions for sterility: correct temperature, correct time, and exposure to moisture. Figure 32-15 shows sterility check strips.

Shelf-Life Autoclaved packages are stored with the date visible and the item with the oldest date in front of the stack so that it is used first. Instruments are considered sterile for 21 to 30 days (21 days in plastic bags and 30 days in muslin), with a shelf life of approximately 1 month. Shelf life is dependent on the type of wrapper used. The individual manufacturer's guidelines should be followed concerning when to reclean and resterilize the item. Autoclaved items cannot be reautoclaved in the same packages without washing, rinsing, drying and rewrapping each item.

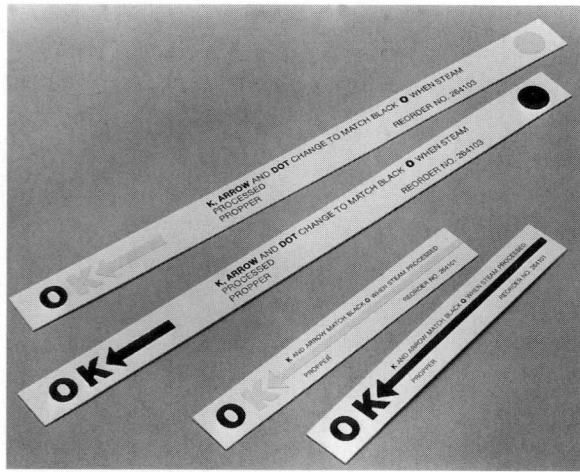

FIGURE 32-15 Sterility check strips.

Hepatitis and AIDS

Two diseases that require special attention during a discussion of infection control are hepatitis and AIDS because both of these diseases affect several million people. Hepatitis is a viral disease of the liver resulting in inflammation and infection. Forms of hepatitis are A, B, C, D, and E.

Hepatitis A (Acute Infective Hepatitis)

Hepatitis A (HAV) is transmitted by fecal waste contamination of food and the water supply. This occurs when food and water become contaminated with the fecal waste products of animals or humans. The incubation period, or period of time during which the disease develops after exposure to symptoms, is from 14 to 50 days with a very slow onset of symptoms. Symptoms include fever, loss of appetite, jaundice, nausea, vomiting, malaise, dark urine, and whitish stools. A vaccination is available that prevents infection by HAV.

Hepatitis B (Serum Hepatitis)

Hepatitis B, also called HBV, is transmitted through body fluids, including blood, semen, saliva, and breast milk, that are contaminated with the virus. This potentially fatal disease can be passed from one drug user to another when sharing a contaminated needle. Hepatitis B is on the increase due to its appearance in persons with HIV and AIDS. The incubation period for this liver infection is 60 to 90 days with a rapid onset of symptoms. HBV symptoms include fever, chills, diarrhea with clay-colored stools, nausea and vomiting, orange-brown urine, headache, anorexia, enlarged liver, and jaundice.

The diagnosis of HBV is made through a liver biopsy to identify the virus. Treatment for all forms of hepatitis is a high-protein diet and rest. Treatment for HBV may last for several weeks with the possibility of relapse.

Two types of vaccine are available for HBV: one made from human serum and the other a synthetic product. HBV vaccine is administered in three doses; the second dose 1 month after the first and the third dose 5 months later.

Pediatricians and health officials are now recommending that infants and adolescents be vaccinated for hepatitis B due to the rising incidence of this disease. The schedule for infants is for the first dose to be given at time of birth.

Any personnel with a high risk of contact with blood/body fluids should be encouraged to receive the vaccination against hepatitis B. However, it is not required. If the employee decides not to receive the vaccination, a disclaimer must be signed and placed in the employee file. The disclaimer allows for the possibility that the employee might decide at a later date to receive the vaccine.

Some people should not receive the vaccine. These include someone who is sensitive to yeast or any of the other components found in the vaccine. If a woman is pregnant, or plans to attempt to become pregnant within the next 6 months, she should not receive the vaccine. Others, such as breast-feeding mothers or people with heart diseases, should also be cautious about receiving the vaccine. Occasionally side effects occur; they usually include swelling, pain or redness at the injection site, and flu-like symptoms.

Hepatitis C

Hepatitis C, also referred to as non-A and non-B hepatitis, is the most common form of new hepatitis cases every year. The symptoms and treatment are similar to those of hepatitis B. A patient may be a carrier of hepatitis C and not be aware of it. Treatments are available, yet liver damage, liver failure, and cancer can occur.

Hepatitis D

Hepatitis D, also called delta hepatitis, is the most recently identified form of hepatitis. The symptoms of this form of hepatitis can be more severe than those of other forms of hepatitis. Hepatitis D is spread through the use of intravenous drugs and intimate contact. There is a rapid growth of this form of hepatitis due to the increased number of HIV and AIDS cases in which it is seen.

Hepatitis E

Hepatitis E is the result of exposure to food contaminated with human feces. It is a major infectious disease in developing countries due to poor sanitary conditions.

HIV and AIDS

Human immunodeficiency virus (HIV) is the virus that causes acquired immunodeficiency syndrome (AIDS) (Figure 32-16). AIDS was first identified in the United States in 1981. Since it was first identified, it is thought that more than 1 million people are living with HIV in the United States and that more than half a million have died after developing AIDS. At the present time, AIDS is considered the fifth leading cause of death in the United States in persons between the ages of 25 and 44. More than 47 million people worldwide have been infected with HIV since the start of the epidemic.

This infectious virus causes the immune system, which is the body's shield against infection, to break down and eventually become ineffective by invading the body's macrophages and T cells, which fight disease. When the T cells are invaded, they render the macrophages useless for fighting off pathogenic invasions.

The various means by which the AIDS virus can enter the body are listed here:

- Vaginal, anal, or oral intercourse with a person who has the virus

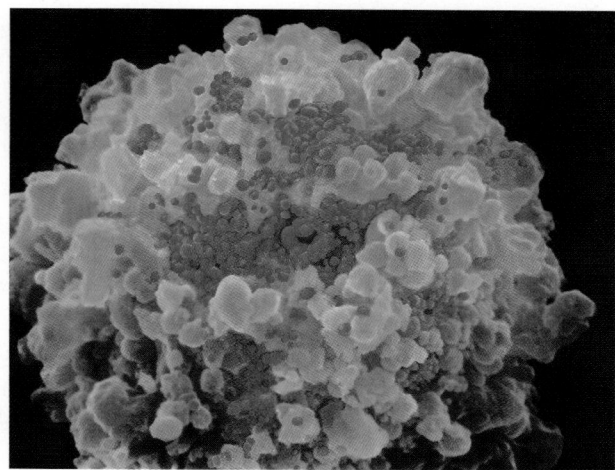

FIGURE 32-16 The AIDS virus.

- Sharing needles or syringes with a person who has the virus
- Receiving transfusions of blood or blood products donated by someone who has the virus
- Receiving organ transplants from a donor who has the virus
- Contaminating open wounds or sores with blood, semen, or vaginal secretions infected with the virus
- Having artificial insemination with the sperm of a man who has the virus
- Being born to a mother who is infected with the virus
- Being an infant who is breast-fed by a woman who is infected with the virus

HIV cannot survive on inanimate objects. The virus can, however, survive well in body fluids such as blood, semen, and vaginal secretions. The virus can stay in cells for months and even years. During this time the cells will replicate, or reproduce, themselves. The body's defensive T cells are eventually destroyed by the new viral cells.

Some HIV victims will develop AIDS-related complex (ARC), which has less serious symptoms than AIDS. ARC symptoms include loss of appetite and weight loss, diarrhea, skin rash, fatigue, night sweating, swollen lymph glands, and poor resistance to infection.

Not all HIV patients develop AIDS or any other HIV-related condition. Estimates, according to the CDC, range from 50 to 90 percent of patients developing full-blown AIDS. It may take 8 to 10 years for symptoms of HIV infection to develop and 12 years or more for symptoms of AIDS to develop. The stages of HIV infection are as follows:

- After becoming infected with HIV, it may take a person 6 weeks to 3 years to develop antibodies (which means they will not test positive for HIV).

Before developing these antibodies, some people with HIV have symptoms that are usually brief but not severe. These might include slight fever, headaches, fatigue, and swollen glands for a few weeks.

- After antibodies develop, the person will test positive for HIV. another period with no symptoms may occur. This "incubation period" can last several years. Even though there are no symptoms, the immune system becomes increasingly damaged during this time.

- Next, a person with HIV may experience a long period of swelling of the lymph glands in the throat, armpits, and groin. This condition is called *persistent generalized lymphadenopathy* and may last a number of years.

- When HIV has seriously damaged the immune system, ARC may occur. These symptoms can include a white coating of the mouth and throat (thrush), similar infections of the skin and mucous membranes of the anus and genital area, and severe viral infections such as herpes.

- The final stage of an HIV infection (AIDS) includes a variety of viral, fungal, bacterial, and parasitic infections, nervous disorders, and cancers.

When these infections are present in the healthy body they can be overcome by the immune system. However, in the AIDS patient, the immune system is no longer effective and, hence, the infections become life threatening. The immune system can be suppressed for many reasons, such as stress, poor nutrition, or an infection such as HIV. During this time, the patient is more susceptible to infections. These are known as opportunistic infections. This means the infection, having the advantage of the suppressed immune system, is taking the opportunity to make the patient sick. Opportunistic diseases for AIDS patients include:

- *Pneumocystis carinii* pneumonia (PCP)

- Kaposi's sarcoma, a type of skin cancer

- Toxoplasmosis, an infestation of parasites that infect the brain and central nervous system

Tuberculosis (TB) is seen with increasing frequency among persons infected with HIV. HIV infection is one of the strongest known risk factors for the progression of TB from infection to disease. However, of the diseases associated with HIV infection, TB is one of the few that is transmissible, treatable, and preventable.

AIDS is diagnosed based on several factors: functioning ability of the immune system based on tests such as T-cell counts, the presence of one or more opportunistic infections, and the presence of HIV antibodies. The HIV or AIDS antibody test, known as ELISA (enzyme-linked immunosorbent assay), is used as a screening test. With a positive ELISA, a patient is said to be HIV positive or HIV antibody positive. The Western blot test is used to confirm results of the ELISA.

HIV does not survive well outside the human body, and it is not transmitted through air, food, water, pets, or bugs. The virus has been found in tears, saliva, urine, and breast milk. HIV is destroyed by a 1:10 household bleach solution or an application of heat treatment at 132°F (56°C) for 10 minutes. Standard Precautions, which include the use of aseptic technique, gloving, and careful handling of needles and syringes to avoid puncture wounds, can prevent health care workers from contracting the virus.

People at the highest risk for HIV infection include men and women who engage in unprotected sex, intravenous drug users who share needles, sexual partners of those who engage in high-risk activity, infants born to HIV-positive mothers, and people who received blood transfusions or clotting factors between 1977 and 1985 (prior to current screening processes for blood).

The symptoms of AIDS are:

- T-cell count less than 200 (normal range for T cells is 500 cells per cubic millimeter of blood)

- Unexplained weight loss of 10 to 15 pounds in less than 2 months that is not associated with diet or exercise

- Long-lasting occurrences of diarrhea

- Unexplained fever, chills, and drenching night sweats for more than 2 weeks

- Unexplained extreme fatigue

- Swelling or hardening of lymph glands located in the throat, groin, or armpit

- Periods of continued, deep, dry coughing that are not due to other illnesses or smoking

- Increased shortness of breath

TABLE 32-8   Caring for Someone with AIDS

To protect themselves from infection, caregivers should be reminded to do the following:

- Handle all needles with care. Never replace caps back on needles or remove needles from syringes. Dispose of all needles in puncture-proof containers out of the reach of children.
- Wear latex or rubber gloves when in contact with blood, blood-tinged body fluids, urine, feces, or vomit.
- Wash hands after removing gloves.
- Any cut, open sore, or breaks on exposed skin of either the patient or caregiver should be covered with a bandage.
- Flush all liquid waste containing blood down the toilet using care to avoid splashing during pouring. Nonflushable items such as paper towels, sanitary pads and tampons, wound dressings, or items soiled with blood, semen, or vaginal fluid should be enclosed in a plastic bag and tightly sealed. Check with your local health department or physician to determine trash disposal regulations for your area.
- Use a disinfection solution of one part bleach to 10 parts water to disinfect such items as floors, showers, tubs, and sinks. Discard solution in the toilet after using.

To protect the person with AIDS from infection:

- If the caregiver has a cold or flu, and there is no one else available to care for the AIDS patient, a surgical-type mask should be worn.
- Wash your hands before touching the AIDS patient.
- Anyone with boils, fever blisters (herpes simplex), or shingles (zoster) should avoid close contact with the patient.
- Gloves should be worn if the caregiver has a rash or sores on his or her hands.
- Persons living with or caring for an AIDS patient should have received all the recommended childhood immunizations and booster shots, including the hepatitis vaccine.
- The AIDS patient should not be in the same room with a person who has, or is recovering from, chickenpox.

The caregiver should:

- Call the local AIDS service organization for support.
- Seek the help of clergy, counselors, and other health care professionals to help cope with feelings of frustration and stress.
- Not be afraid to touch the person with AIDS.
- Encourage the patient to become involved in his or her own care. Assist them in being active as long as possible.
- Not be afraid to discuss the disease with the patient.

When patients come in for HIV or AIDS testing, they should receive counseling from the physician before and after the test. The counseling should include information on methods for safer sex.

For more information on HIV or AIDS, write to the CDC National AIDS Clearinghouse, P.O. Box 6003, Rockville, MD 20849-6003 or call 1-800-458-5231. The Spanish hotline is 1-800-344-7432. The deaf access hotline is 1-900-AIDS-TTY.

- Appearance of discolored or purplish growths on the skin or inside the mouth
- Unexplained bleeding from growths on the skin, mucous membranes, or from any opening on the body
- Severe numbness or pain in the hands and feet, loss of motor control and reflex, paralysis, or loss of muscular strength
- Altered state of consciousness, personality change, or mental deterioration

There is currently no cure for AIDS. However, several treatment regimens are used that can help delay the progression of the disease and improve the quality of life for those living with the symptoms. These include the main form of treatment, antiviral therapy, which suppresses the replication of the HIV virus in individuals. Supportive measures to improve the quality of life for the AIDS patient include delivery of home meals, nutritional supplements, and hospice care.

The medical assistant may be asked to provide information to a caregiver regarding caring for an AIDS patient. Such recommendations are presented in Table 32-8.

Bioterrorism

In recent years the threat of bioterrorism has become more prevalent in our nation. The spread of toxic microorganisms could occur very quickly and become widespread.

One threat is from anthrax. This acute, infectious disease can be passed from animal to man by contact with animal hair or waste. This disease can attack the lungs, causing symptoms from respiratory distress to coma. Penicillin, tetracyclines, and erythromycin are antibiotics of choice for treatment. Isolation Precautions must be maintained, including incineration of contaminated materials.

Another threat is from smallpox (sometimes referred to as variola). This is an acute, contagious disease that can be quickly spread from person to person. Until the mid-1900s, smallpox vaccinations were recommended for the general public. Eventually it seemed that smallpox had been eradicated, as no new cases had been reported, yet the danger of an outbreak could still occur. Some of the symptoms include macules, papules, vesicles, pustules, and crusts. Vaccinations are available and have been given to military personnel and to medical personnel who might come into contact with the virus. At present widespread vaccination has not again been recommended.

SUMMARY

Good aseptic technique is everybody's business. The medical assistant is often the first barrier against infection in the office. The meticulous attention given to sterilization of all reusable materials and equipment is often the full responsibility of the medical assistant. This is a serious responsibility. All who handle waste products must be trained in safety measures such as Standard Precautions. Always document waste removal.

When practicing aseptic technique, know the right way to do something and then never deviate from that method. Never take shortcuts with asepsis.

Chapter Review

COMPETENCY REVIEW

1. Define and spell the terms to learn for this chapter.
2. How does the age of the person affect susceptibility to infections?
3. List three natural barriers to infection.
4. List the four cardinal signs of infection.
5. List three examples of body fluids included in Standard Precautions.
6. A sterilized package has reached its expiration date. What should you do?
7. What solution of household bleach has been found to be effective in destroying HIV?
8. What test would be ordered after the ELISA test shows a patient is HIV positive?
9. List examples of PPE.

PREPARING FOR THE CERTIFICATION EXAM

1. A commonly used disinfectant is:
   A. formaldehyde
   B. Lysol
   C. 70% alcohol
   D. soap
   E. phenol

2. Most sterilization indicators operate on what principle?
   A. Color change will revert back when item is contaminated.
   B. Original color reappears after 6 weeks.
   C. Color change indicates the package has been properly sealed.
   D. Color change indicates sterilization is complete.
   E. Color change occurs at the beginning of the process.

3. Dry heat sterilization is used for:
   A. plastic items
   B. dressings
   C. gloves
   D. surgical instruments
   E. ointments and powders

4. Steam under pressure, dry heat, and chemical-gas mixtures are used in:
   A. disinfection
   B. sterilization
   C. sanitization
   D. cleaning
   E. fumigation

continued on next page

5. Before removing sterilized items from the auto-clave, they should be allowed to:
   A. change color
   B. cool
   C. dry
   D. depressurize
   E. all of the above

6. Sterile materials which are wrapped in paper or cloth can be stored for:
   A. 1 year
   B. only 10 days
   C. 6 months
   D. 21 to 30 days
   E. 2 years

7. Instruments that are being disinfected in boiling water should remain immersed for NOT less than
   A. 90 minutes
   B. 60 minutes
   C. 20 to 30 minutes
   D. 45 minutes
   E. 15 minutes

8. After the autoclave temperature reaches 250°F, the timer for sterilizing wrapped surgical instruments should be set for:
   A. 10 minutes   D. 50 minutes
   B. 15 minutes   E. 60 minutes
   C. 30 minutes

9. Which of the following is NOT a cause of incomplete sterilization when using the autoclave?
   A. trapping pockets of air in the autoclave
   B. setting the timer before the correct temperature has been reached
   C. opening the door completely during the drying cycle
   D. placing instruments overlapping one another
   E. placing only one instrument in each packet

10. What conditions are necessary for bacterial growth to occur?
    A. moisture
    B. body temperature
    C. oxygen
    D. light
    E. all of the above

CRITICAL THINKING

1. How do you treat and react to this patient in comparison to the way you would treat some other patient who complained of a wound infection?

2. Is any extra protection needed when you draw blood from this patient?

3. Whom in your office would need to know about the patient's signs and symptoms, and his concerns about his condition?

ON THE JOB

Emma Brown, 70 years old, is caring for her 78-year-old husband, George Brown. Mr. Brown, a diabetic, has been hospitalized with a recurring infection that may lead to amputation of his right leg. Mr. Brown's physical condition may not be able to withstand another massive leg infection. He has been placed on antibiotics and his leg is now healing. Mrs. Brown will require instructions on irrigating the leg wound and changing her husband's dressing. When the leg wound was cultured, *E. coli* was present. Mrs. Brown mentioned to the medical assistant that she is concerned about her own health since she has a colostomy.

What is your response?

1. What patient education is required for Mrs. Brown regarding the procedure to be used in caring for her husband?

2. Is it possible that the *E. coli* was transmitted from Ms. Brown's colostomy site to her husband's leg wound? Explain.

INTERNET ACTIVITY

Research Kaposi's sarcoma on the Internet.

 MediaLink More on the infection control, including interactive resources, can be found on the Student CD-ROM accompanying this textbook.

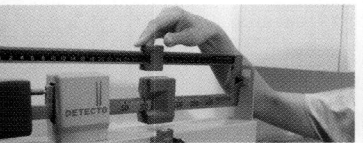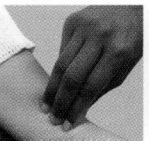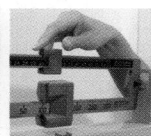

Medical Assistant Role Delineation Chart

HIGHLIGHT indicates material covered in this chapter.

ADMINISTRATIVE

Administrative Procedures

- Perform basic administrative medical assisting functions
- Schedule, coordinate and monitor appointments
- Schedule inpatient/outpatient admissions and procedures
- Understand and apply third-party guidelines
- Obtain reimbursement through accurate claims submission
- Monitor third-party reimbursement
- Understand and adhere to managed care policies and procedures
- *Negotiate managed care contracts*

Practice Finances

- Perform procedural and diagnostic coding
- Apply bookkeeping principles

- Manage accounts receivable
- *Manage accounts payable*
- *Process payroll*
- *Document and maintain accounting and banking records*
- *Develop and maintain fee schedules*
- *Manage renewals of business and professional insurance policies*
- *Manage personnel benefits and maintain records*
- *Perform marketing, financial, and strategic planning*

CLINICAL

Fundamental Principles

- Apply principles of aseptic technique and infection control
- Comply with quality assurance practices
- Screen and follow up patient test results

Diagnostic Orders

- Collect and process specimens
- Perform diagnostic tests

Patient Care

- Adhere to established patient screening procedures
- Obtain patient history and vital signs
- Prepare and maintain examination and treatment areas
- Prepare patient for examinations, procedures and treatments

- Assist with examinations, procedures and treatments
- Prepare and administer medications and immunizations
- Maintain medication and immunization records
- Recognize and respond to emergencies
- Coordinate patient care information with other health care providers
- Initiate IV and administer IV medications with appropriate training and as permitted by state law

GENERAL

Professionalism

- Display a professional manner and image
- Demonstrate initiative and responsibility
- Work as a member of the health care team
- Prioritize and perform multiple tasks
- Adapt to change
- Promote the CMA credential
- Enhance skills through continuing education
- Treat all patients with compassion and empathy
- Promote the practice through positive public relations

Communication Skills

- Recognize and respect cultural diversity
- Adapt communications to individual's ability to understand
- Use professional telephone technique

- Recognize and respond effectively to verbal, nonverbal, and written communications
- Use medical terminology appropriately
- Utilize electronic technology to receive, organize, prioritize and transmit information
- Serve as liaison

Legal Concepts

- Perform within legal and ethical boundaries
- Prepare and maintain medical records
- Document accurately
- Follow employer's established policies dealing with the health care contract
- Implement and maintain federal and state health care legislation and regulations
- Comply with established risk management and safety procedures
- Recognize professional credentialing criteria
- *Develop and maintain personnel, policy and procedure manuals*

Instruction

- Instruct individuals according to their needs
- Explain office policies and procedures
- Teach methods of health promotion and disease prevention
- Locate community resources and disseminate information
- *Develop educational materials*
- *Conduct continuing education activities*

Operational Functions

- Perform inventory of supplies and equipment
- Perform routine maintenance of administrative and clinical equipment
- Apply computer techniques to support office operations
- *Perform personnel management functions*
- *Negotiate leases and prices for equipment and supply contracts*

- *Denotes advanced skills.*

SOURCE: Reprinted by permission of the American Association of Medical Assistants from the AAMA Role Delineation Study: Occupational Analysis of the Medical Assisting Profession.

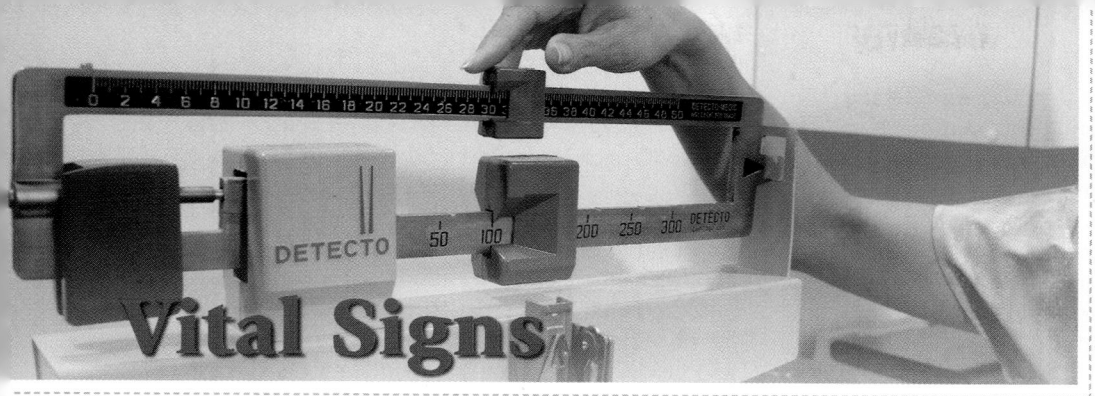

Vital Signs

Learning Objectives

After completing this chapter, the student will be able to:

- Define and spell the terms to learn for this chapter.
- List and describe the components of a medical history.
- State the normal values of temperature, pulse, respiratory rates, and blood pressure.
- List 10 conditions that cause the body temperature to increase or decrease.
- State three situations in which measuring an oral, rectal, and axillary temperature should be avoided.
- List and describe the seven pulse sites.

- Describe the respiratory rate range for the various age groups.
- Discuss the five phases of the Korotkoff sounds.
- Explain the four physiological factors that affect blood pressure.
- Convert temperature readings from degrees Fahrenheit (F) to degrees Centigrade (C) (and vice versa).
- Convert weight in pounds to kilograms (and vice versa).
- Convert height from inches to centimeters (and vice versa).

OUTLINE

Interviewing the Patient	590
Patient History	591
Correct Documentation	593
Measuring Weight and Height	593
Vital Signs	595
Temperature	596
Pulse	606
Respiration	612
Blood Pressure	616
Pain	623
Body Fat Measurement	626

Terms to Learn

acute pain	differential diagnosis	phantom pain
afebrile	eupnea	prognosis
anthropometry	febrile	pulse deficit
apical	intractable pain	pulse pressure
apnea	medical diagnosis	pyrexia
asymptomatic	metabolism	radiating pain
bounding pulse	objective symptom	referred pain
chronic pain	oximetry	subjective symptoms
clinical diagnosis	oxygen saturation	thready pulse
cyanosis	palpatory method	vital signs
diagnosis		

Case Study

MR. WADE, AGE 60, IS A NEW PATIENT with an appointment to see Dr. Welch for an annual physical. Mary Fox, CMA, will be preparing him for his physical and taking his vital signs. Although he is dapper in appearance and cheerful in his demeanor, Mr. Wade becomes apprehensive when Mary mentions having his vital signs taken. She explains that she will weigh him and measure his height before she takes his vital signs. Mr. Wade admits that he detests having his blood pressure taken. She takes TPR, and Ht. Wt. He mentions again that he "hates the squeezing feeling you get when the thing is pumped up." When she begins to take his blood pressure he stands up and is extremely agitated and very embarrassed.

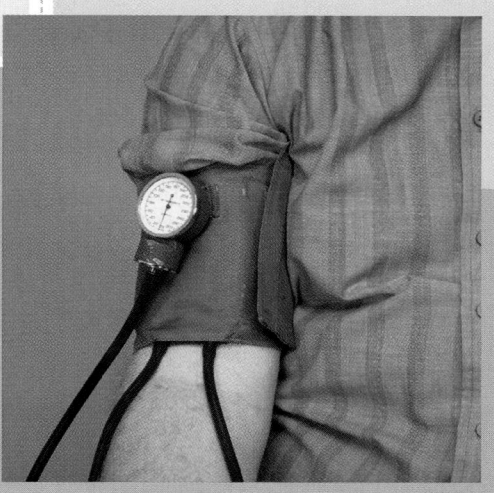

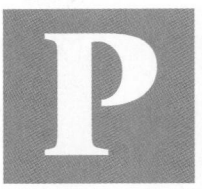**P**atient care depends on effective communication. The patient's medical history is a formal, enduring legal document that makes information available to provide quality health care. Various members of the health care team record information and submit tests results that become a permanent part of the medical history. Confidentiality of patient information must be safeguarded at all levels. Accuracy in testing, clear documentation, and timely charting are necessary to ensure quality care for the patient. Client records are maintained for a number of reasons including planning patient care, auditing health agencies for quality assurance information, gathering research data, educating future health care providers, obtaining reimbursement for services, providing legal documentation of care, and analyzing health care to assist in planning for future health care needs.

A patient comes to a physician either for an annual physical to establish a baseline of results that can be used in the event of later illnesses, for early detection of disease, and for disease prevention. In addition, a physician visit may be scheduled to diagnose a set of symptoms and seek treatment. Each time a patient is seen by the physician, makes a call to the office, has laboratory work done, has a prescription ordered, or receives patient education, the information is recorded in the medical record or chart. At any time a health care provider involved in the patient's care can pick up the chart and read what has been done in the past to treat the patient or what is to be done in the future, thereby ensuring continuity of care.

Although diagnosis (determination of the cause and nature of a disease) and treatment of the problem are the main goals, a final or medical diagnosis is arrived at after all tests, procedures, and examinations are complete. A clinical diagnosis or working diagnosis is a preliminary presumptive diagnosis made by the physician based on the health history and physical examination. A differential diagnosis is the determination of which one of several diseases is the cause of a problem. Once the medical diagnosis is made (and sometimes this is not possible), the prognosis is made. Prognosis is the prediction of the course of the disease and the recovery rate. During the course of the disease or condition, the physician will monitor the patient's progress and adjust treatment as needed.

Interaction with the patient begins with making the appointment. From this point on the medical assistant has the chance to establish a positive, empathetic relationship with the patient by acting in a professional, warm manner. Before a patient has a physical examination or is seen by the physician, a medical history must be obtained. The initial patient interview is conducted by the medical assistant and the information gathered be-

comes part of the permanent medical history. Health history forms vary from brief to comprehensive depending on the physician specialty and choice of the facility.

After initial data have been gathered, the patient's vital signs, height, and weight are assessed. Then the physician examines the patient and records the information obtained. In this chapter the components of a medical history, interviewing patients, and rules for charting, measuring vital signs, and recording height and weight will be discussed. Chapter 34 includes a more detailed discussion of assisting with physical examinations along with more detail about types of medical records.

Interviewing the Patient

A patient's medical history provides information about current and past illnesses and treatments that the physician utilizes to provide care. Information gathered during the initial interview forms the basis of this vital document.

Privacy

The patient is entitled to privacy during the interviewing process. The federal government's Health Insurance Portability and Accountability Act (HIPAA) mandates that facilities make every effort to preserve confidentiality of patient information. The Patient's Bill of Rights reminds health care workers that patients have the right to respectful, considerate care. The interview should be done in an area that ensures privacy and freedom from interruption. Patients may feel more comfortable sharing details about their health and private life if they have a sense of confidentiality and privacy.

Effective Communication

The goal of the patient interview is to obtain information about the patient's condition while establishing rapport and a positive relationship. Review Chapter 4, for discussion of communication techniques, styles, barriers, and questioning skills before continuing with this chapter. Follow these steps in interviewing a patient:

- Review the patient's chart before meeting the patient and plan the interview.
- Greet the patient by name (Mrs. Jones) and give your name.
- Maintain a professional demeanor.
- Ask permission to interview the patient to help him or her feel more in control.
- Use "icebreaker" comments to help put the patient at ease (weather, sports, etc.).
- Provide privacy during the interview.

- Be aware of verbal and nonverbal cues.
- Avoid making judgmental responses.
- Avoid providing medical assurances.
- Treat sensitive topics with respect, keeping in mind cultural and personal biases.
- Summarize important points.
- Document according to facility policy.

Patient History

Before the physician can adequately assess the patient's condition, a past medical history is obtained from the patient. This history assists the physician in assessing the patient's general health status and helps determine a diagnosis of the patient's present problem or condition. Although each office or facility has preferences regarding the specific format of the health history form, the following information is standard:

- Intake or registration form—demographic information, name, address, sex, age, DOB, education, occupation, SS number, insurance information, racial or ethnic background, marital status, number of children and nearest relative
- Medical history—chief complaint, present illness, past medical history, family history, social or personal history, review of systems or systems assessment, result of general physical
- Test results—requested by physician and performed in the office or elsewhere (blood, urine, x-rays, scans, etc.)
- Records from other physicians or facilities—received with patient's written permission
- Diagnosis and detailed treatment plan—determined by the physician
- Operative reports—on all procedures and surgeries including treatment and follow-up care information
- Informed consent forms—signed by patient indicating understanding of and granting permission for specific treatments including possible outcomes
- Hospital discharge summary—if patient was hospitalized, includes pertinent information about hospital stay including reason for admission, procedures, treatments, medications, care plans, and outcomes
- Correspondence—written information stamped with date received in office

WINDY CITY CLINIC
Beth Williams, M.D.
123 Michigan Avenue
Chicago, IL 60610
(312) 123-1234

Name ______ Date:
Social Security No. ______ Date of Birth ______
Occupation ______
Date of Last Physical ______
☐ Single ☐ Married ☐ Divorced ☐ Widowed
Weight Today ______ 1 Year Ago ______
Military Services ☐ Yes ☐ No; When and Where ______

Please answer the following questions. Where boxes are provided to check, place a check mark in the box in front of the disease or condition which you have had. *THIS FORM MUST BE COMPLETED AND RETURNED TO THE CLINIC AT LEAST 1 WEEK PRIOR TO YOUR APPOINTMENT.*

FAMILY HISTORY:

Relative	If Living, Give Present Age.	If Deceased, At What Age?	Cause of Death
Father			
Mother			
Siblings ☐M☐F			
☐M☐F			
☐M☐F			
☐M☐F			
☐M☐F			
☐M☐F			

HAS ANY RELATIVE EVER HAD? (Check boxes that apply)

	Relationship		Relationship
☐ Asthma		☐ Hay fever	
☐ Cancer		☐ Ulcers	
☐ Tumor		☐ Kidney disease	
☐ Leukemia		☐ Kidney stones	
☐ Bleeding problems		☐ Gall stones	
☐ Anemia		☐ Lung disease	
☐ Diabetes		☐ Mental disorders	
☐ Gout		☐ Suicide	
☐ Rheumatism or arthritis		☐ Typhoid disease	
☐ High blood pressure		☐ Migraine	
☐ Heart disease		☐ Tuberculosis	
☐ Strokes		☐ Asthma	
☐ Epilepsy		☐ Allergies	
☐ Emphysema		☐ Other	

HAVE YOU HAD A FAMILY HISTORY OF? (Check boxes that apply)
☐ Heart disease ☐ Cancer ☐ Stroke ☐ Allergies

FIGURE 33-1 Patient's medical history.

Many medical offices give new patients the history form to complete when the patient arrives for the first visit with the physician (Figure 33-1). If the patient is expected to complete a history form, then the medical assistant is responsible for making sure that the patient understands the terminology and how to answer the questions.

Some medical offices send the health history form to the patient's residence with a request that the form be completed and submitted when the patient comes for the first visit. This allows patients the opportunity to check their own records for important dates and the names and dosages of medications they are taking. When the form is sent to the patient ahead of time, many offices request patients come to the office a half hour before the actual examination by the physician. This permits the medical assistant to verify that the form is complete, get information required for billing and insurance, or to help patients who require assistance completing the form.

Some physicians prefer to take all of the components of the medical history directly from the patient. On some medical history forms, there are specific questions geared to the physician's specialty. A cardiologist, for example, may require a more extensive history relating to the cardiovascular system. Whether the patient completes the form at home or in the office, it is important to mark any sections the patient is to skip. Particular care should be taken to assist patients who may be embarrassed that they are unable to complete the form themselves due to frailty, disability, or because they are unable to read. The medical assistant must stress the importance of filling out the form completely.

The patient history should include the following six areas:

1. Chief complaint
2. Present illness
3. Past medical history
4. Family medical history
5. Social history or personal history
6. Assessment of body systems (review of symptoms) performed by physician in the office

Chief Complaint

The chief complaint (CC)is also referred to as the presenting problem. The chief complaint is the reason for the office visit. It usually consists of one or two signs or symptoms. Symptoms are either subjective or objective. Subjective symptoms are felt by the patient but not apparent to an observer, such as vertigo or pain, and cannot be measured. Objective symptoms are felt by the patient and are apparent to observers, such as a rash or fever, and they can be measured. The chief complaint is usually stated in the patient's own words such as "I'm having trouble sleeping" or "I'm out of breath after climbing only two or three stairs." It is important to ask the following questions to obtain more complete information:

- *What?* What is the patient experiencing? What makes it worse or relieves it?
- *When?* When did it start (onset)? How long does it last (duration)?
- *Where?* Where is the symptom located? How intense is it?

Because only the physician is able to diagnose patient's problems, the medical assistant does not use diagnostic terms when recording the chief complaint. The patient's own words are used to describe the problem.

- *Correct documentation:*
  10/23/XX Pt. c/o "dying of thirst all the time" and unusual weight loss during past month.
- *Incorrect documentation:*
  10/23/XX Pt. experiencing excessive thirst and unusual weight loss indicative of diabetes.

Present Illness

The present illness (PI) provides a more complete, expansive description of the chief complaint. The PI component of the health history must contain a detailed description of the symptom(s), including the onset, duration, and intensity of each. Each symptom should be documented as to its relationship to the chief complaint. For example, a patient who came to the office with a chief complaint of "dull aching pain in left side of belly" may add that it happens every time she eats popcorn or nuts and has occurred monthly for the past 6 months. This information amplifies the CC.

Past Medical History

This part of the medical history includes all diseases and medical problems the patient has experienced in the past. Past illnesses or injuries can affect present health. Dates of major illnesses, hospitalizations, and surgeries and current medications are noted whenever possible. Patients often forget to tell the physician how much aspirin or other over-the-counter (OTC) drugs they take. Remind patients that aspirin is considered a drug even though it may be purchased over the counter. Aspirin can duplicate other medication the physician may prescribe or interfere with the treatment of conditions such as gastric ulcers. Today herbal supplements are used by many, and the patient should be queried about what vitamins and supplements they are taking. Interactions between herbal supplements and other medications are possible. A complete past medical history will include information about the following items:

- Childhood diseases
- Major illnesses
- Injuries
- Hospitalization
- Surgeries
- Allergies
- Immunizations
- Current and past medications (prescription and OTC)
- Last examination

Family Medical History

The family history is a record of the health problems of the patient's blood relatives. Blood relatives include the patient's mother, father, sisters, brothers, grandparents, aunts, and uncles related by birth. Information on blood relatives should include their current health, major health problems, and cause of death. Family medical histories focus on diseases that may be inherited such as diabetes mellitus (DM), seizures, heart disease, hypertension (elevated blood pressure), and some types of cancer.

Social History or Personal History

Personal histories include lifestyle patterns that could affect the health status of the patient, for example smoking, drinking, and using recreational drugs. The patient's occupation, marital status, and sexual preferences are also noted along with the patient's type of diet choices, frequency of exercise, sleep habits, and other health habits. Information about the patient's previous occupation(s) (if the patient has had several occupations) and lifelong hobbies, or interests, often provide helpful information. Box 33-1 provides a list of questions that are included on the patient history form or might be asked to gain a good personal history from a patient.

Assessment of Body Systems (Review of Systems)

The physician conducts this assessment immediately prior to or during the physical examination. This review of systems (ROS) consists of a systematic review of all body systems, beginning with the head and neck area and working downward to the feet through all the body systems. This will be discussed in depth in Chapter 34.

Correct Documentation

A patient's chart is a vital document and an integral part of their health care. Chapter 34 will discuss different methods for documentation. Regardless of the method used, the following guidelines must be followed when recording information in a patient's medical record.

- Date and time every entry (while timing may not be required in the medical office, it is in hospital and ambulatory care settings).
- Write legibly.
- Use permanent dark ink.
- Use medical terminology and accepted abbreviations.
- Use correct spelling.
- Sign every entry.
- Accurately document information (stick to facts not opinion).
- Document in proper sequence in which events occurred.
- Document appropriate information concerning health and care given.

BOX 33-1
Personal History Questions

1. What was the last grade you attended in school?
2. What is your occupation?
3. How long have you done that type of work?
4. Have you been exposed to any toxic or harmful substances such as dust, chemicals, cleaning fluids/fumes, smoke, radiation, pesticides, or paint at work? At home?
5. What do you usually eat for breakfast?
6. Have you gained or lost 10 or more pounds during the past year? Is there a reason?
7. Do you follow a low-fat diet? Low salt?
8. What do you do for exercise? How often?
9. How much alcohol do you drink a day? A month? Preferred drink?
10. Do you smoke cigarettes? If yes, how many packs a day? Filtered?
11. Do you smoke a pipe, cigars, or chew tobacco? If yes, how much?
12. How many cups of coffee do you drink a day? Tea? Soft drinks with caffeine?
13. Have you ever used heroin, cocaine, or LSD? OTC drugs? Laxatives? How often?
14. Do you have unusual stress at home or work?
15. What are your hobbies?

- Be concise.
- Correct errors only by drawing a single line through the incorrect entry and initialing it. Then record corrected entry.

Refer to Box 33-2 for the six C's of charting which provides a summary of the charting guidelines.

Measuring Weight and Height

Weight and height are two important measurements even though they are not considered vital signs in the true sense of the term. These measurements are called anthropometric measurements since they relate to anthropometry, the science of size, proportion, weight, and height.

Weight and height can provide indications of a person's general health. Infants who fail to gain weight or "fail to thrive" need close supervision of weight gains and losses. The diagnosis of hormonal imbalances in children resulting in abnormal growth patterns can be picked up through routine comparisons of the child's height and weight against national growth charts. See Chapter 37 for measuring height, weight, chest, and head circumference in infants and small children.

Diabetic patients, pregnant women, cardiac patients, patients with fluid retention, and patients suffering from eating disorders such as bulimia and obesity need to have frequent weight monitoring.

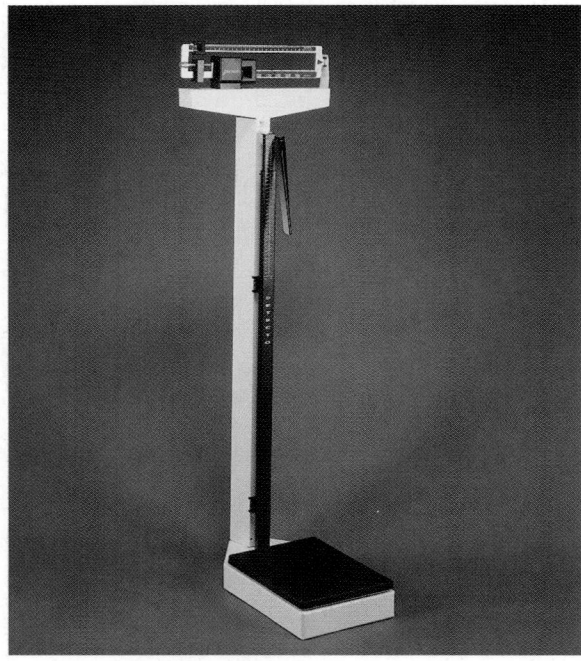

FIGURE 33-2 Upright scale.

Weight

Patients prefer privacy when having their body measurements taken. They can remain fully clothed for this procedure. Indicate on the medical record if measurements were taken with clothes on or off. Patients are weighed and measured with shoes off.

Scales may be calibrated in either kilograms (metric weight) or pounds (Figure 33-2). In some cases, a scale will have a ruled panel that can be flipped up to reveal both pounds and kilograms. However, the medical assistant must know how to do conversions from pounds into kilograms and vice versa. Table 33-1 contains conversion charts to be used when converting a weight from kilograms to pounds or from pounds to kilograms. Procedure 33-1 lists the steps for obtaining the weight and height of a patient. Patients who cannot stand may be weighed on a chair or bed scale (Figure 33-3).

Height

Patient's height is measured without shoes with the heel, buttocks, and back of head touching the measuring stick or bar. The L-shaped arm is raised and lowered until it rests on the top of the head, not on the top of the hair (Figure 33-4). The height is then taken and may be recorded in inches and feet or centimeters. To convert inches and feet to centimeters multiply by 2.5. To convert from centimeters to inches, divide by 2.5. Older patients and women should be measured yearly to observe for signs of osteoporosis.

TABLE 33-1
Conversion Chart for Pounds and Kilograms

TO CONVERT KILOGRAMS TO POUNDS (kg to lb)

1 kilogram (kg) = 2.2 pounds (lbs)

Multiply the number of kilograms by 2.2 lbs.
Example: If a patient weighs 64 kilograms, multiply 64 by 2.2.

$64 \times 2.2 = 140.8$ or 141 pounds

TO CONVERT POUNDS TO KILOGRAMS (lb to kg)

1 pound = 0.45 kilograms

Multiply the number of pounds by 0.45.
Example: If a patient weighs 130 pounds, multiply 130 by 0.45.

$130 \times 0.45 = 58.5$ or 59 kilograms

PROCEDURE

Measuring Adult Weight and Height

OBJECTIVE: Obtain height and weight measurements and perform math conversions.

Equipment and Supplies

balance scale with bar to measure height; paper towel; pen; patient record

Method

1. Perform hand hygiene.
2. Identify the patient.
3. Explain procedure to the patient.
4. For patients who wish to remove shoes, place a paper towel on the scale. Heavy objects such as keys should be removed and female patients should set their purses aside.
5. Set all the weights to zero. Balance the scale by adjusting the small knob at one end until the balance bar pointer floats in the center of the frame. (A coin can be used to make this adjustment.)
6. Assist the patient onto the scale.
7. Ask the patient to stand still.
8. First move the large weight into the groove closest to the weight you estimate for the patient. If the balance bar pointer touches the bottom of the bar then move the large weight back one notch. Move the small weight by tapping it gently until it reaches a point in which the pointer floats in the center of the frame.
9. Leave the weights in place.

Continue with Height

10. Ask the patient to place his or her back to the scale, stand erect, and look straight ahead.

11. Raise the height bar in a collapsed position making sure the tip is over the patient's head.
12. Open the bar into the horizontal position and bring it down gently to touch the top of the patient's head. Leave this setting in place.
13. Assist the patient in stepping off the scale.
14. Read the weight scale by adding the number at the large weight to the number behind the small weight to the nearest ¼ pound. For example, 150 pounds at the large weight and 23½ at the small weight 173½ pounds.
15. Record this measurement on the patient's record.
16. Read the height as marked behind the movable level of the ruled bar. Record this measurement to the nearest ¼ inch on the patient's record. (Convert inches to feet by dividing by 12. Chart height in feet and inches.)
17. Return the weights to zero and the height bar to the normal position.
18. Discard paper towel.
19. Perform hand hygiene.

Charting Example

2/14/XX	wt. 140¼ lbs with shoes; ht. 5′7″ = (67 inches)
	M. King, CMA

Vital Signs

A healthy human body regulates itself. Vital signs are indicators of the body's ability to maintain homeostasis. Temperature (T), pulse (P), respiration (R), and blood pressure (BP) measurements are considered vital signs since they measure some of the body's vital functions and provide necessary information about the patient's physical well-being. Pain is considered by many to be the fifth vital sign with assessment taking place at the same time as the other vital signs are evaluated. Vital signs are routinely measured by medical assistants before physical examinations. Care must be taken to be accurate and efficient so the reading or results reflect a true picture of the patient's condition.

Along with the physiology behind body temperature, pulse rate, respirations, blood pressure, and measurement of weight and height, this chapter discusses the normal or average readings for all vital signs at varying ages. Different methods and types of equipment for measuring temperature, pulse rate, respirations, and blood pressure are discussed along with guidelines and ways for choosing the best methods and equipment.

When temperature, pulse, and respirations are measured at the same time, it is referred to as *TPR*. During some office visits only one of the vital signs

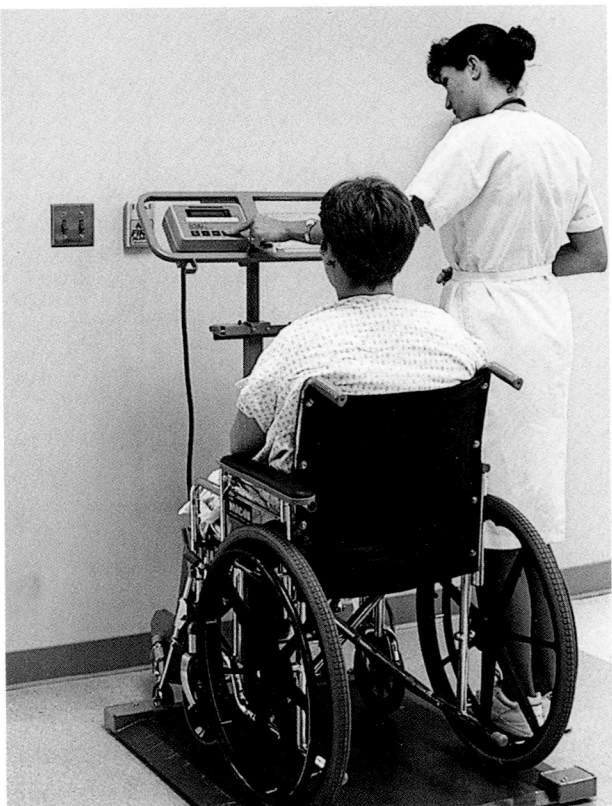

FIGURE 33-3 Chair scale.

of heat lost from the body. The physical and chemical process that produces heat is known as metabolism. The hypothalamus, a portion of the brain that controls autonomic nervous system functions, is able to adjust the body temperature as the need for more or less heat production occurs during the day. For example, when a jogger is running on a hot day, the body's cooling mechanism reacts to this by creating perspiration, which evaporates and removes some of the excess heat the jogger experiences. Heat is also lost from the body through radiation, the transfer of heat from one object to another; by convection, the dispersion of heat by air currents; and by conduction, transfer of heat from a hotter molecule or body to a cooler molecule or substance (a patient with high fever is placed in cool water).

Temperature: Normal Values and Terms

The average body temperature of a healthy person is 98.6°F or 37°C, and may vary by 1°F (0.6°C) either up or down during the day. There is normally only a 1°F to 2°F variance throughout the day. While a slight variance in body temperature (diurnal rhythm) is not a cause for alarm, it is important to remember that greater body temperature variations from normal are

may be measured, for example, blood pressure in a patient with hypertension. Factors influencing readings and procedures with step-by-step instructions for accurately and efficiently measuring vital signs are thoroughly presented.

Note: All health care professionals are required to use Standard Precautions to maintain infection control while measuring vital signs. The details of Standard Precautions will not be repeated for each procedure. The medical assistant is expected to know and continually apply the techniques recommended by the Centers for Disease Control and Prevention as discussed in Chapter 32.

Temperature

An understanding of the way the body maintains a balance between the amount of heat produced and the amount of heat lost is important for the medical assistant. Other factors that inform and assist the medical assistant to measure temperature accurately include knowledge of normal readings, factors that influence readings, how to select and use the proper thermometer, and how to clean and care for equipment.

Physiology of Body Temperature

Body temperature is regulated through balancing the amount of heat produced in the body with the amount

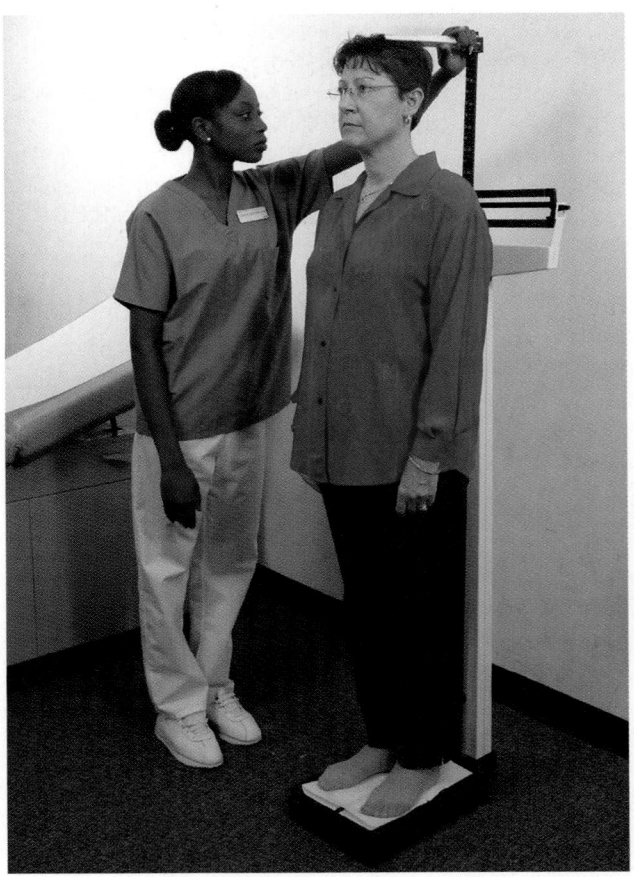

FIGURE 33-4 Height bar attached to the scale used for measuring adult and child height.

TABLE 33-2 Factors Affecting Body Temperature

Cause	Description
Time of day	Body temperature is lower in the morning on wakening when metabolism is still slow. The lowest body temperature is between 2 A.M. and 6 A.M. The highest body temperature usually occurs in the evening between 5 P.M. and 8 P.M. Daily variation in oral temperature can range from 97.6°F to 99.6°F (36.4°C to 37.3°C).
Age	Infants and children normally have a higher body temperature than adults due to immature heat regulation. Children often spike a fever late in the day. Older adults usually have lower than normal body temperature.
Gender	Women may experience a slight increase in body temperature at time of ovulation.
Physical exercise	Body temperature will rise with exercise due to increased muscle contraction.
Emotions	Emotions such as crying and anger can cause an increase in body temperature.
Pregnancy	An increase in metabolism during pregnancy may cause the body temperature to rise.
Environmental changes	Hot weather can cause serious consequences in older adults whose bodies are unable to regulate body temperature due to a decreased metabolism. Exposure to cold may lower body temperature.
Infection	An elevated temperature may be one of the first signs of an infection. A fever is body's way of fighting or killing off infectious organisms.
Drugs	Drugs may increase muscular activity or metabolism, which in turn increases temperature. Antipyretic (fever-reducing) drugs such as aspirin lower the above-normal temperature.
Food	The process of eating may also raise the body temperature. Fasting decreases metabolism, which will lower body temperature.

often the first sign of illness or disease. Body temperature is lowest on rising in the morning and rises in late afternoon. Table 33-2 describes some causes of variations in body temperature.

Always be alert for all causes of changes in body temperature. For example, an infant's elevated temperature during an examination may be due to the infant's crying and not due to an illness. Always ask whether the patient has taken aspirin or Tylenol, which lower the temperature. Older adults who normally have body temperatures below normal may be ill even when their temperature is within a normal range for adults.

Fever

Fever or pyrexia is a body temperature above 100.4°F (38°C). At this point it can be stated that the body is producing greater heat than it is losing and is febrile. Absence of a fever is afebrile. When the body temperature exceeds 105.8°F (41°C), a serious condition known as hyperpyrexia or hyperthermia develops. Temperatures at this level may result in seizures in infants and small children. Body temperature above 109.4°F (43°C) is usually fatal.

It can be a result of hyperthermia. (Refer to Lifespan Considerations.) There are four common types of fevers:

- Intermittent fever—body temperature alternates between fever and normal or subnormal
- Remittent fever—wide range of temperature fluctuations over a 24-hour period
- Relapsing fever—short febrile periods of a few days with a few days of normal temperature readings
- Constant fever—body temperature fluctuates small amount but is always above normal

Clinical signs of fever include increased heart rate, increased respiratory rate, shivering, chills, and sweating. Hyperthermia symptoms include cessation of sweating, loss of coordination, drowsiness, convulsions, and death. Each year children left in overheated cars die from hyperthermia.

Hypothermia

The reverse of a fever is a subnormal temperature or hypothermia. This occurs when the temperature falls below 97°F (36°C). At this point, the body is losing more heat than it is producing. This occurs in cases of exposure and near-drowning in cold water. In general, a temperature below 93.2°F (34°C) is fatal. Clinical signs of hypothermia are decreased pulse and respirations; pale, waxy, cool skin; lack of muscle coordination; and drowsiness progressing to coma and death.

Sites for Measuring Body Temperature

Body temperature can be taken in a variety of ways including oral (mouth), aural (ear) or tympanic, axillary (under the arm), and rectal (rectum).

Normal Values

The normal temperature based on statistical averages for each of the sites where temperature can be measured is:

Oral	98.6°F (37°C)
Rectal	99.6°F (37.6°C)
Axillary	97.6°F (36.4°C)
Ear (aural)	98.6°F (37°C)

As these figures indicate, the temperature obtained through the rectal method registers 1°F (or 0.6°C) higher than the oral temperature. Axillary temperatures register 1°F (0.6°C) lower than oral temperatures. The medical assistant must document if the temperature was taken rectally by the abbreviation "R" or axillary by the abbreviation "AX." In addition, body temperature can be measured on the surface of the body on the forehead, which is useful when assessing the temperature of children and infants.

Oral

The oral method of temperature measurement is most commonly used. There is a potential for error with this method, however, because the patient may not form a tight closure over the thermometer. This allows air to enter the mouth and give a false temperature reading. In documenting this measurement, no designation needs to be used to indicate that it was taken by the oral route. The thermometer is inserted under the tongue on either side of the frenulum linguae. This is the longitudinal fold of mucous membrane. For an accurate measurement, the patient must be advised not to talk during the procedure. Oral temperature should only be measured if 30 minutes have passed since the patient has taken fluids or smoked.

Aural (Eardrum)/Tympanic

One of the newest technologies for accurate temperature measurement involves the aural site. This method uses the tympanic membrane area at the end of the external auditory canal for an instantaneous temperature measurement. The tympanic thermometer provides a closed cavity within the easily accessible ear. The aural method is now considered to be an accurate means of temperature measurement due to the eardrum's proximity to a blood supply and to the hypothalamus. This method also poses the fewest problems with Standard Precautions.

Axillary (Under the Arm)

The axillary method has proven to be the least accurate of the temperature measurement sites. It is the recommended site for small children unable to understand how to hold an oral thermometer in their mouth if a tympanic membrane thermometer is not available. The axillary site is recommended for patients who have had oral surgery, any situation in which the patient may bite the oral thermometer, and mouth-breathing patients. The axillary temperature reading is affected by perspiration. The underarm area should be dry for an accurate reading.

Rectal

The rectal route is considered more reliable than the oral method. The mucous membrane lining of the rectum does not come into contact with air, which could interfere with accuracy, as do the oral and axillary

TABLE 33-3 Selecting a Method for Measuring Body Temperature

Method	Advisable	Inadvisable
Oral	Most adults and children who are able to follow instructions	Patients who have had oral surgery, mouth sores, dyspnea; uncooperative patients; patients on oxygen; infants and small children; patient's with facial paralysis or nasal obstruction
Rectal	Infants and small children; patients who have had oral surgery; mouth-breathing patients; unconscious patients	Active children; fragile newborns
Axillary	Small children	Patients who cannot form an airtight seal around the thermometer
Tympanic (aural)	Small children	Patient with in-the-ear hearing aids or ear infections

routes. The rectal route is advised for unconscious patients, infants, small children, and mouth-breathing patients. The rectal method should be avoided when there is a danger of rectal wall perforation.

Use the guidelines given in Table 33-3 to determine which method to use when measuring a patient's body temperature.

Fahrenheit/Celsius Conversions

The Fahrenheit (F) scale of temperature measurement is widely used throughout the United States. However, some physicians use the Celsius (or centigrade) (C) scale. Figure 33-5 shows examples of Fahrenheit and Celsius in non-mercury thermometers. To convert degrees Fahrenheit to Celsius, subtract 32, and then multiply by 5/9. To convert degrees Celsius to Fahrenheit, multiply by 9/5, and then add 32. See Figure 33-6 for a Fahrenheit/Celsius conversion chart and Table 33-4 for temperature scale conversion formulas and examples.

Non-mercury — Calibrations — Stem

Bulb

94 6 8 100 2 4 6 8 110

6 8 100

Normal body temperature is 98.6 degress Fahrenheit and is written 98.6°F.

Non-mercury — Stem

Bulb

35 36 38 39 40 41 42 43

36 38

Normal body temperature is 37 degrees centigrade (Celsius) and is written 37°C.

FIGURE 33-5 Fahrenheit and centigrade thermometers.

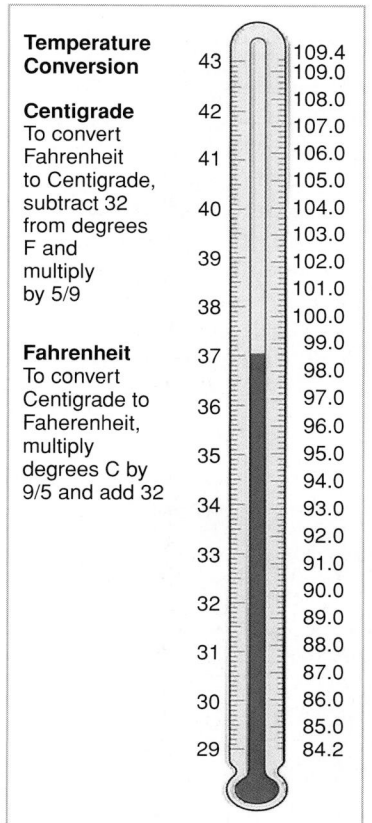

Temperature Conversion

Centigrade
To convert Fahrenheit to Centigrade, subtract 32 from degrees F and multiply by 5/9

Fahrenheit
To convert Centigrade to Faherenheit, multiply degrees C by 9/5 and add 32

43	109.4 / 109.0
42	108.0 / 107.0
41	106.0 / 105.0
40	104.0 / 103.0
39	102.0 / 101.0
38	100.0
37	99.0 / 98.0
36	97.0 / 96.0
35	95.0 / 94.0
34	93.0 / 92.0
33	91.0 / 90.0
32	89.0
31	88.0 / 87.0
30	86.0 / 85.0
29	84.2

FIGURE 33-6 Fahrenheit/centigrade conversion.

TABLE 33-4 **Temperature Scale Conversion Formulas**

Scale	Conversion Formula	Example
Centigrade	(F − 32) × 5/9 = C	101°F − 32 = 69 × 5/9 = 38°C
Fahrenheit	(C × 9/5) + 32 = F	38.3°C × 9/5 = 69 + 32 = 101°F

Types of Thermometers

Four types of thermometers are available for measuring body temperature: non-mercury glass thermometers, electronic thermometers, tympanic membrane thermometers, and disposable thermometers. Figure 33-7 shows an example of a digital electronic thermometer.

Note: Mercury thermometers are no longer widely used in the health care environment due to the potential danger of mercury and the frequency of breakage. Mercury is toxic and can be harmful to humans and animals. Several cities have banned the sale of mercury thermometers and some areas have thermometer exchange programs, in which an individual brings in a mercury thermometer and is given a non-mercury one in exchange. This book will use non-mercury thermometers in its discussion of assessing body temperatures.

Non-Mercury Glass Thermometers

Non-mercury glass thermometers are available in two shapes to measure temperature using the oral, rectal, and axillary methods. Mercury has been replaced by safer chemicals and glass has been replaced by plastic in many cases. The oral thermometer has a long, slender tip that fits easily under the tongue. A thermometer with a stubby or pear-shaped tip is available that can be used for taking oral, axillary, and rectal temperatures. Some thermometers may have a blue dot that indicates the thermometer is for oral use or a red dot indicating rectal use. (Refer to Patient Education.)

The shaft or stem of the thermometer is calibrated in tenths (0.2, 0.4, 0.6, and so on) of degrees, with each short line representing two-tenths (0.2) of a degree. A whole degree is marked with a long line. The even-numbered degrees are printed on the thermometer. The average normal body temperature (97.6–99.6) is indicated by an arrow on the thermometer.

When reading the thermometer, it should be held between the thumb and index finger, at eye level, by the stem end (Figure 33-8). While looking at the edge of the thermometer, keep the lines at the top of the edge and the numbers at the bottom. The stem is then gently rotated until the silver column can be seen in the middle of the lines and numbers. The point where the silver line stops is read for the body temperature at each two-tenths of a degree. When the silver line appears between two markings, the temperature is read at the next higher two-tenths of a degree.

The temperature reading is then recorded. The temperature must be carefully charted with absolute accuracy. Always record tenths of degrees of temperature in even numbers when using a non-mercury glass thermometer.

THERMOMETER SHEATHS Plastic disposable slip-on sheaths are available to use with both oral and rectal glass thermometers (Figure 33-9). The sheath

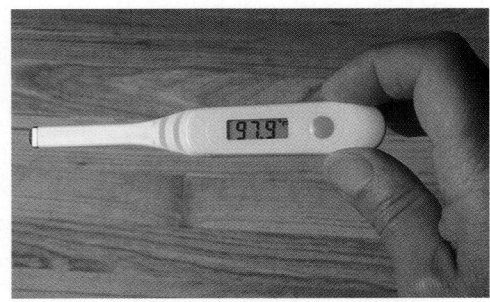

FIGURE 33-7 Example of a digital electronic oral thermometer.

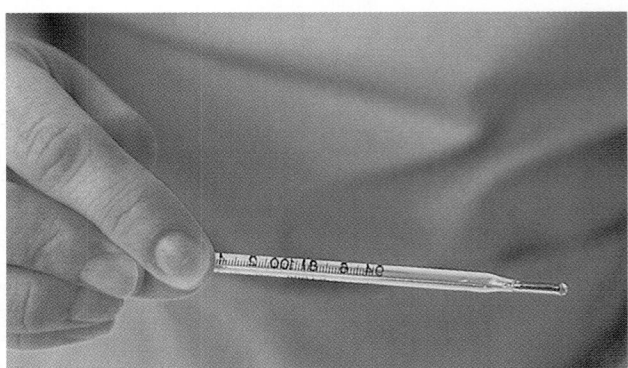

FIGURE 33-8 Reading a clinical thermometer.

The medical assistant acts as the resource person for instructing the patient on the correct use of equipment, such as the thermometer, to ensure accuracy in reporting temperatures to the physician.

Teaching methods include verbal instructions, demonstration and return demonstration, educational pamphlets, and drawings, when necessary, depending on what you are teaching and the patient's educational and motivational level.

Patients must be cautioned that an abnormal vital sign, such as an elevated temperature, should not be ignored with a "wait and see" attitude since a prolonged high fever can result in brain damage and even death.

Patient education will vary. For example, patients suffering from cardiovascular disease should be taught to take their own pulse and to detect abnormalities in pulse rate, rhythm, and volume. Hypertensive patients should be taught the symptoms and causes of high blood pressure and how to monitor their own blood pressure. In addition, patient education is needed to alert the patient to risk prevention, dietary control, and the role of exercise, lifestyle choices, and compliance with drug therapy.

comes in a small paper envelope and slips over the tip of the thermometer. The sheath provides a sanitary protective covering and is discarded after use. When using a rectal thermometer, a lubricant is always used over the sheath for ease of insertion into the rectum.

The sheath is removed from the thermometer by pulling on the tear tab, which inverts the plastic thus protecting the medical assistant's hands from coming into contact with contamination. Remove and properly dispose of the sheath in a hazardous waste container. After the temperature is read, clean and disinfect the thermometer since mucous membranes may still come into contact with it.

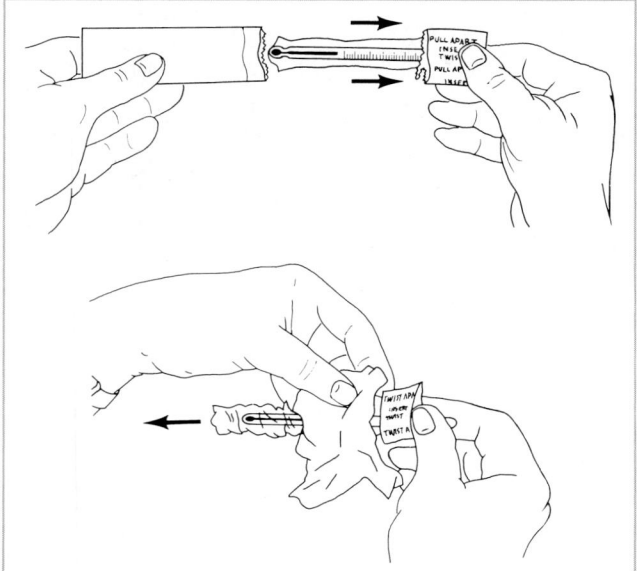

FIGURE 33-9   Using a thermometer sheath.

Figure 33-10 illustrates the steps followed in taking an oral temperature. See Procedure 33-2 for instructions on measuring an oral temperature using a non-mercury thermometer. Figure 33-11 provides an example of how to chart temperature readings.

A rectal thermometer has a small, round bulb that is inserted gently into the rectum. This thermometer may be marked "for rectal use" on its stem and have a red dot indicating the rectal route should be used. It is not safe to use an oral thermometer to take a rectal temperature because the long slender tip may injure tender rectal mucous membranes or may break off in the rectum. Procedure 33-3 provides the steps for measuring rectal temperature using a non-mercury thermometer.

CLEANING AND STORING NON-MERCURY GLASS THERMOMETERS   The non-mercury glass thermometer must be cleaned and soaked in a disinfectant after each use. The thermometer is then stored in a proper container. Procedure 33-4 lists the steps for cleaning and storing glass thermometers.

Electronic or Digital Thermometers

The electronic thermometer is very popular. It is considered accurate, easy to read, sanitary, fast, and requires no cleaning or disinfection. Electronic thermometers are battery operated with digital windows for easy viewing and reading (Figure 33-12). They can accurately register body temperature within a few seconds.

The electronic thermometer consists of a metal probe that is color coded: blue for oral and red for rectal. The probe is attached to the battery unit by a flexible cord. A nonflexible plastic disposable cover fits over the probe to provide each patient with a sanitary

text continues on page 605

PROCEDURE

Measuring Oral Temperatures Using a Glass Non-Mercury Thermometer

OBJECTIVE: Accurately perform all steps of the procedure and provide an accurate temperature reading.

Equipment and Supplies

oral glass non-mercury thermometer; disposable plastic thermometer sheath; watch with second hand; biohazardous waste container; patient's record; paper and pen/pencil

Method

1. Perform hand hygiene.
2. Apply gloves.
3. Identify patient.
   Note: To avoid error, call patient by name and check against the name on the patient's record.
4. Ask if patient has recently taken a hot or cold drink or smoked within last 30 minutes.
   Rationale: Hot and cold liquids will affect temperature in the mouth.
5. Take thermometer out of container. Do not touch bulb end with fingers. If thermometer is stored in a disinfectant, then rinse thoroughly under cool water.
6. Inspect thermometer for any chipped areas or other defects (Figure 33-10A). Discard if damaged.
7. Read the thermometer. If it is not at 95°F, then shake down to that point by firmly holding the end of the glass shaft between the thumb and index finger. Firmly snap the wrist to shake (Figure 33-10B).
8. Place plastic sheath on thermometer. Make sure that sheath is tightly in place on the thermometer.
9. Place bulb end of thermometer encased in plastic sheath sublingually (under the tongue) in patient's mouth (Figure 33-10C).
   Rationale: The space on either side of the frenulum linguae is close to numerous small

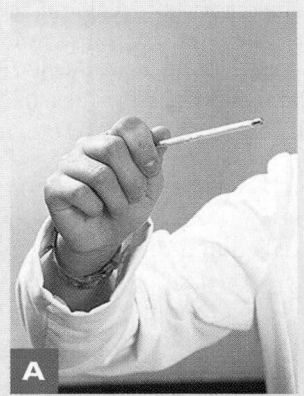 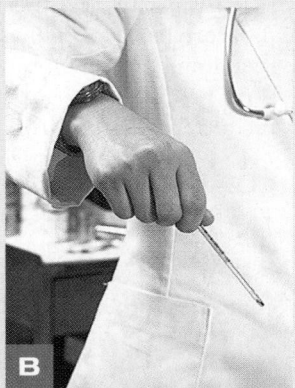 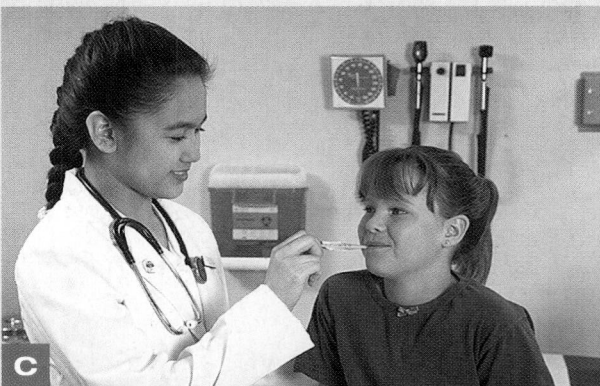

FIGURE 33-10   Taking an oral temperature. (A) Inspect the thermometer. (B) Shake down the thermometer. (C) Place the thermometer under the tongue after inserting it into thermometer sheath.

blood vessels, which will provide an accurate indication of body temperature.

10. Ask the patient to close his or her mouth over the thermometer and hold it in place without biting down. It helps to tell the patient to suck the thermometer rather than to clamp it between the teeth.

11. Leave the thermometer in place for at least 3 minutes.
Rationale: It takes at least 3 minutes for an accurate oral reading to take place. The medical assistant can use this time to take the pulse and respiratory rate.

12. Remove and read the thermometer (Figure 33-10D). If the thermometer reads less than 97°F, shake down the thermometer and reinsert for an additional few minutes.

13. Reread the thermometer and write the reading on a piece of paper.

14. Holding tightly by the stem end of the glass shaft pull the plastic sheath off thermometer and discard the sheath in a biohazardous waste container.
Rationale: The plastic sheath has come into contact with the patient's mucous membranes.

15. Follow the procedure for temporary storage of soiled thermometers.

16. Remove gloves and place in biohazardous waste container.

17. Wash hands.

18. Record temperature in patient's record.

19. Follow procedure for cleaning and disinfecting soiled thermometers (Figure 33-10E).

Charting Example

10/23/XX	4:00 P.M. 99°F

M. King, CMA

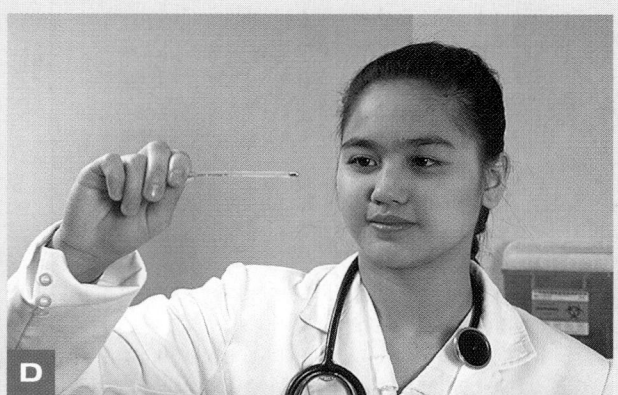
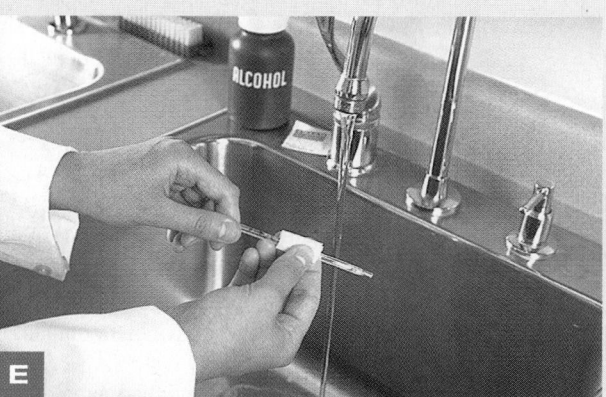

FIGURE 33-10 (*continued*) (D) Medical assistant reads the thermometer. (E) Thermometer is washed with soap and water.

Measuring Rectal Temperatures Using a Glass Non-Mercury Thermometer

OBJECTIVE: Accurately perform all steps of the procedure and provide an accurate temperature reading.

Equipment and Supplies

rectal non-mercury glass thermometer; disposable thermometer sheath; disposable gloves; patient's record; paper and pen/pencil; tissue; watch with second hand; water-soluble lubricant; biohazardous waste container

Method

1. Perform hand hygiene.
2. Apply gloves.
3. Identify patient.
   Note: To avoid error, call the patient by name and check against the name on the patient's record.
4. Explain procedure. If the patient is a child, explain the procedure to both the parent and child.
5. Place small amount of lubricant on a tissue.
   Rationale: Tissue will serve to keep the work area clean and also as a temporary receptacle for the prepared thermometer.
6. Remove the rectal thermometer from its container by holding the stem end only.
7. Inspect thermometer for any cracks or defects. Discard if damaged.
8. Read the thermometer. If it is not at 95°F, then shake down to that point by firmly holding the end of the glass shaft between the thumb and index finger. Firmly snap the wrist to shake down.
9. Place plastic sheath on thermometer, making sure that it is tightly in place.
10. Apply lubricant to thermometer by rolling bulb end in lubricant on tissue. Leave thermometer on the tissue.
    Rationale: Lubricant allows the thermometer to be inserted easily with reduced chance for injury to mucous membranes. Tissue provides a clean surface for temporary storage of prepared thermometer.
11. Instruct patient to remove appropriate clothing so that rectal area can be accessed. Provide privacy for patient.
12. Assist patient onto examining table and cover with sheet/drape.
    Rationale: Protect patient's modesty.
13. Instruct patient to lie on left side with top leg bent (Sim's position).
14. With one hand raise the upper buttock to expose the anus or anal opening. If unable to see the anal opening, ask the patient to bear down slightly. This will expose the opening.
15. With other hand, gently insert lubricated thermometer 1½ inches into anal canal. Do not force the thermometer into the anal canal. Rotating the thermometer may make insertion easier.
16. Hold the thermometer in place for 3 minutes.
17. Withdraw thermometer.
18. Dispose of the plastic sheath in biohazardous waste container.
19. Read thermometer.
20. Reread thermometer and write the reading on a piece of paper.
21. Place thermometer back on tissue or in a temporary storage container. Never place soiled thermometer on unprotected surface.
22. Wipe anus from front to back to remove any excess lubricant.
23. Assist patient from the examination table. Instruct the patient to dress, and assist the patient if necessary.
24. Follow the procedure for temporary storage of soiled thermometers.
25. Remove gloves and place in biohazardous waste container.
26. Perform hand hygiene.
27. Record temperature in patient's record using (R) to indicate a rectal reading.
28. Follow procedure for cleaning and disinfecting soiled thermometers.

Charting Example

2/14/XX	4:00 P.M. Temp. 99.6°R
	M. King, CMA

PROCEDURE

Cleaning and Storing Glass Non-Mercury Thermometers

OBJECTIVE: Correctly clean, inspect, disinfect, and store non-mercury thermometers, observing aseptic and safety precautions as prescribed by Standard Precautions.

Equipment and Supplies

70% isopropyl alcohol or other disinfectant for thermometer use; container with soiled thermometer(s); cotton balls; soap; utility or disposable gloves; water; biohazardous waste container

Method

1. Perform hand hygiene.
2. Apply gloves according to office policy.
   Rationale: Universal Precautions are used to provide protection from contaminated mucous membrane products on soiled thermometer.
3. Take soiled thermometer(s) to sink.
4. Liberally apply soap and water to cotton balls. Holding thermometer by stem, wipe from stem end to bulb by applying friction and rotating the glass stem.
   Rationale: Friction will assist in dislodging contamination from calibrated markings.
5. Discard cotton balls into container.
6. Hold stem of thermometer while rinsing under cool running water.
7. Inspect thermometer for cleanliness. Note condition of thermometer and discard if damaged. If soil remains, repeat steps 4 through 6.

8. Holding the stem tightly between thumb and index finger shake down to at least 95°F by a quick snapping motion of the wrist.
   Rationale: A wet thermometer may slip out of the hand while shaking down. Thermometer needs to be prepared for next use.
9. Place thermometer in a container filled with disinfectant.
   Rationale: Thermometer must be completely covered with disinfectant and allowed to remain in solution for at least 20 minutes to be considered disinfected.
   Note: Disinfection in liquid cannot take place without thorough soap and water cleaning first.
10. When all thermometers have been cleaned and placed in disinfectant, then clean the soiled thermometer container using soap, water, and disinfectant.
11. Using correct procedure, remove and discard gloves into waste container.
12. Wash hands.
13. Set timer for 20 minutes.
    Rationale: Timer should not be touched until hands have been washed to avoid contamination of timer.
14. After 20 minutes have elapsed, wash hands, rinse thermometers under cool water, and place in sterile storage container.

---

thermometer (Figure 33-13). This plastic-covered probe is inserted under the patient's tongue or rectally like a non-mercury thermometer.

The medical assistant will hold the thermometer in place since the reading is performed quickly. The unit

Date	TPR	Initials
9/9/98	100⁶ Ⓡ – 72 – 20	BF

FIGURE 33-11 Charting temperature.

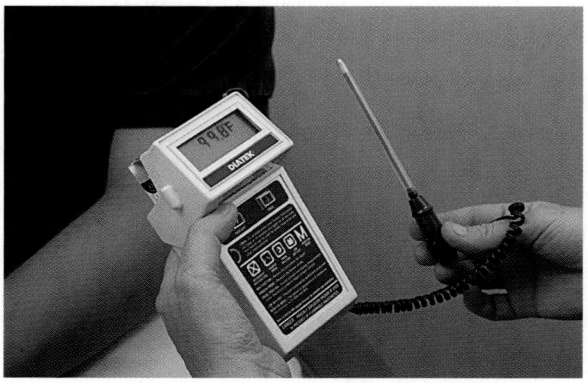

FIGURE 33-12 Electronic thermometers have a large window, making them easy to read.

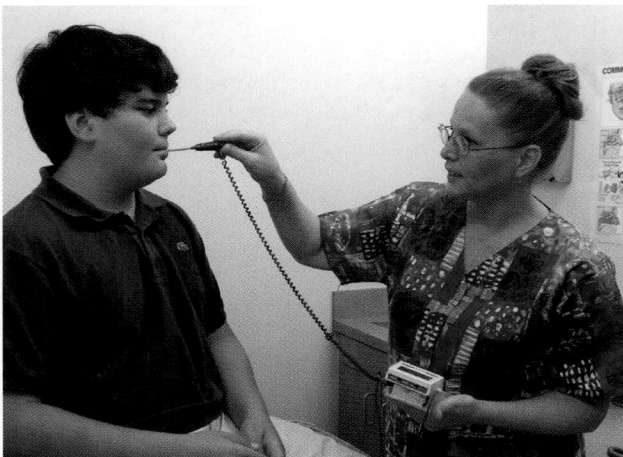

FIGURE 33-13 The disposable cover, also referred to as a sheath, provides sanitary protection for patient.

will emit a signal when the temperature has registered. The plastic probe shield is then popped into a biohazardous waste container and the probe is replaced into the battery-powered storage unit. Procedure 33-5 provides the steps for measuring an oral temperature with a digital or electronic thermometer.

The electronic thermometer can be used for oral, rectal, and axillary body temperature readings. The blue oral probe is generally used for taking oral and axillary temperatures. Rectal temperatures, taken using the red probe, require lubrication on the tip of the probe. The rectal probe is inserted ½ inch into the adult rectum and ¼ inch into the child's. The probe may have to be angled slightly to ensure contact with the rectal mucosa.

These units are time saving but expensive. They are used in medical offices, hospitals, and clinics but rarely by patients in their homes due to cost. The battery-operated unit must be readjusted at intervals to maintain accuracy. The unit should always be returned to the charging stand after each use to maintain the battery.

Tympanic Thermometers

The tympanic membrane thermometer is used for an aural temperature. The tympanic membrane or aural thermometer is so named because it is able to detect heat waves within the ear canal and near the eardrum. The thermometer calculates the body temperature from the energy generated by these heat waves. Figure 33-15 shows an example of a tympanic membrane thermometer, and Procedure 33-6 lists the steps required to obtain a temperature reading using a tympanic thermometer.

Axillary Temperature

The axillary area, under the arm is easily accessible and offers no possibility of rectal perforation or broken oral thermometers. It is used in assessing body temperature in newborns, infants, children, and adults with jaw impairments or surgery and those who are irrational. The process for measuring axillary temperature is given in Procedure 33-7. Figure 33-16 shows an example of a non-mercury thermometer.

Disposable Thermometers

There are several types of disposable thermometers. A chemical disposable thermometer uses liquid dots or heat-sensitive bars or patches applied to the forehead. They change color to indicate body temperature. Some are single use and others may be reused several times. Figure 33-17 shows an example of a disposable thermometer with chemical dots. The reading is taken by noting the highest reading among the dots that have changed color. Figure 33-18 shows temperature-sensitive tape being used to measure temperature. It is held in place for about 15 seconds and is read by the color change on the strip. Both of these methods are excellent when dealing with small children or large numbers of patients who need to be evaluated.

Pulse

Pulse rate is a measurement of the number of times the heart beats per minute (bpm). It is the wave of blood created each time the left ventricle of the heart contracts. Between contractions the heart rests. Each pulse beat represents one cardiac cycle or one heartbeat. In a healthy person the heart normally beats around 70 times per minute. An increased oxygen requirement will cause an increase in heart rate and result in a faster pulse rate. For instance, a jogger starts out at a slow pace and as the pace increases muscles will need more oxygen to produce energy, thus the heart rate (pulse) will increase as will the rate of breathing (respiratory rate). A pulse rate above 100 bpm is tachycardia; a rate below 60 bpm is referred to as bradycardia.

Factors Influencing Pulse Rates

The pulse rate is influenced by several factors including exercise, age, gender, size, physical conditions, disease states, medications, and feelings such as depression, fear, anxiety, and anger. Table 33-5 describes factors that influence pulse rate, and Table 33-6 lists average pulse rates for different age groups.

Characteristics of Pulse

Four characteristics need to be noted and recorded when observing pulse rate: rate, volume, rhythm, and compliance of the arterial wall.

1. Rate describes the number of pulse beats per minute.

text continues on page 610

Measuring Oral Temperature Using an Electronic or Digital Thermometer

OBJECTIVE: Accurately perform all steps of the procedure and provide an accurate temperature reading.

Equipment and Supplies
electronic or digital thermometer (rechargeable); probe cover; waste container; pen; patient's chart

Method
1. Perform hand hygiene.
2. Assemble equipment.
3. Identify patient and explain procedure.
4. Remove thermometer unit from base and attach probe (blue for oral).
5. Remove thermometer probe from holder.
6. Insert thermometer probe into disposable tip box to secure tip (Figure 33-14A).
7. Insert into patient's mouth on either side of frenulum linguae and instruct patient to close mouth.
8. When temperature signal is seen or heard, remove thermometer from patient's mouth and read the result in the LED window.
9. Dispose of thermometer tip into waste container. (Figure 33-14B)
10. Return thermometer probe to storage place (Figure 33-14C).
11. Replace unit on the rechargeable base.
12. Perform hand hygiene.
13. Document results.

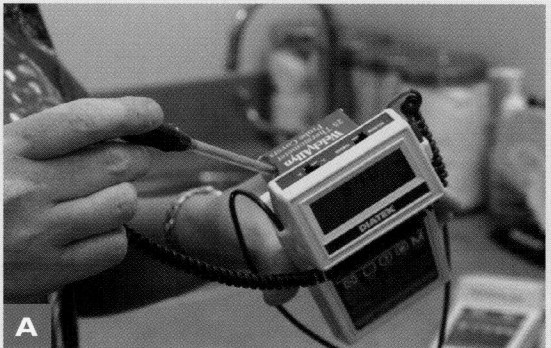

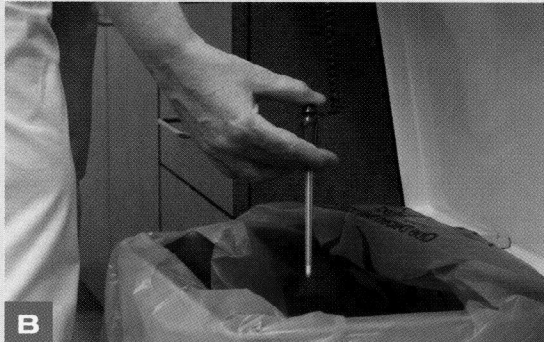

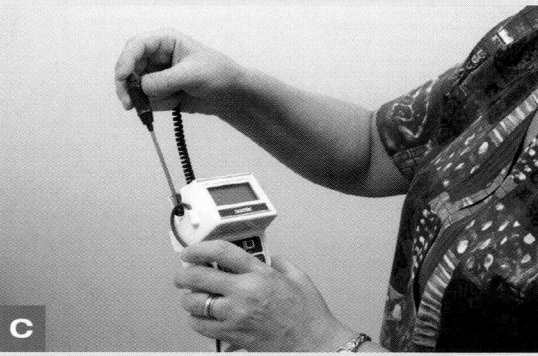

FIGURE 33-14 Using the electronic thermometer. (A) Insert probe into probe cover. (B) After measuring the temperature, press to eject the probe cover. (C) Replace the probe into the holder.

PROCEDURE

Measuring Temperature Using an Aural (Tympanic Membrane) Thermometer

OBJECTIVE: Accurately perform all steps of the procedure and provide an accurate temperature reading.

Equipment and Supplies
tympanic membrane thermometer; disposable protective probe cover; paper and pen/pencil; patient record; biohazardous waste container

Method
1. Perform hand hygiene.
2. Identify patient.
   Note: To avoid error, call patient by name and check against the name on the patient's record.
3. Explain procedure to patient.
4. Remove thermometer from its base. The display will read "ready."
5. Attach disposable probe cover to the earpiece.
   Rationale: The probe cover will assist in keeping the probe free of contamination.
6. With one hand gently pull upward on the patient's outer ear if an adult or pull back and downward if an infant or child.
   Rationale: This pulling mechanism will straighten the ear canal for ease of insertion.
7. Gently insert the plastic-covered tip of the probe into ear canal.
   Rationale: The ear canal opening is then sealed so that air will not enter and affect the temperature reading.

8. Press the scan button, which activates the thermometer.
   Rationale: An infrared beam is activated that measures the heat waves in 1 to 2 seconds.
9. Observe the temperature reading in the display window.
10. Gently withdraw the thermometer.
11. Eject the used probe cover into a biohazardous waste container by pressing the eject button.
    Rationale: The medical assistant's hands should not come in contact with the contaminated probe cover.
12. Record temperature using the designation (T) indicating a tympanic temperature.
    Note: Tympanic thermometers can be set to correlate with either an oral or rectal reading. Generally, the oral mode in which 98.6°F is considered normal is used.
13. Return the tympanic thermometer to its base.

Charting Example

10/23/XX	4:00 P.M.	Temp. 99.2°F

M. King, CMA

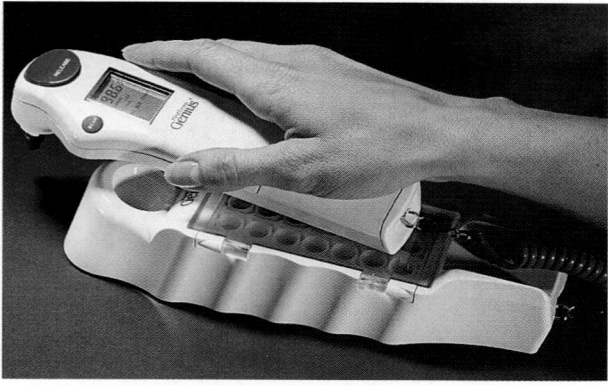

FIGURE 33-15 Tympanic thermometer.

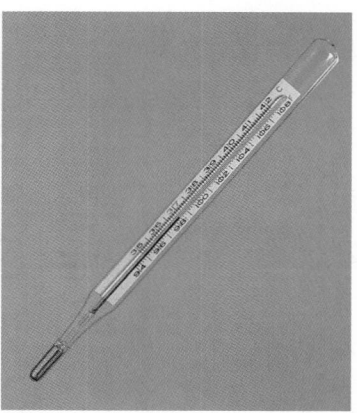

FIGURE 33-16 Mercury-free glass thermometer.

PROCEDURE

Measuring Axillary Temperature

OBJECTIVE: Accurately perform all steps of the procedure and provide an accurate temperature reading.

Equipment and Supplies

oral non-mercury glass thermometer; paper and pen/pencil; patient's record; tissue; watch with second hand; biohazardous waste container

Method

1. Perform hand hygiene.
2. Identify patient.
   Note: To avoid error, call patient by name and check against the name on the patient's record.
3. Explain procedure. If patient is a child then explain procedure to both the parent and child.
4. Take thermometer out of container. Do not touch bulb end with fingers. If thermometer is stored in a disinfectant, then rinse thoroughly under cool water.
5. Inspect thermometer for any chipped areas or other defects. Discard if damaged.
6. Read the thermometer. If it is not at 95°F, then shake down to that point by firmly holding the end of the glass shaft between the thumb and index finger. Firmly snap the wrist to shake down.
7. Ask patient to expose axilla. If patient is an infant or child, ask parent to take child's arm out of clothing to expose axilla.
8. Using tissue pat axilla dry of perspiration.
   Rationale: Perspiration will interfere with thermometer coming into tight contact with skin.
9. Place bulb end of thermometer into the axillary space. Make sure the bulb comes into contact with the patient's skin.

Rationale: Temperature cannot register unless patient's skin touches thermometer.
10. Ask patient to remain still and hold the arm tightly next to the body while the temperature registers. Caution patient not to apply so much pressure that the thermometer breaks.
11. Leave thermometer in place for 6 to 9 minutes. Children need to be carefully monitored during this time. Do not leave any patient unattended.
12. Medical assistant can take pulse and respirations while patient is holding thermometer under axilla.
13. Remove thermometer after designated number of minutes has elapsed, read it, and wipe dry with tissue.
    Note: If thermometer reads less than 96°F, shake down and reinsert for an additional few minutes.
14. Reread thermometer and write the reading on a piece of paper.
15. Follow the procedure for temporary storage of soiled thermometers.
16. Wash hands.
17. Record temperature in patient's record.
18. Follow procedure for cleaning and disinfecting soiled thermometers.

Charting Example

2/14/XX	4:00 P.M.	Temp. 97.0° AX
		M. King, CMA

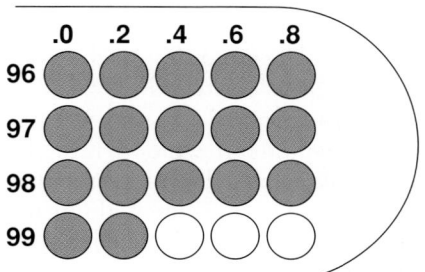

FIGURE 33-17 Disposable thermometer with chemical dots.

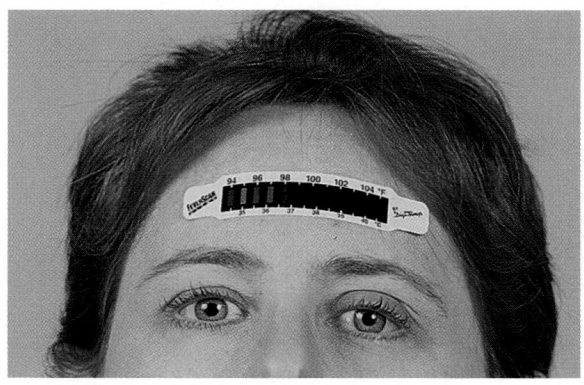

FIGURE 33-18 Temperature-sensitive skin tape.

TABLE 33-5 Factors that Influence Pulse Rate

Exercise	Activity increases body's requirements. Rate may increase 20–30 bpm.
Age	As age increases, pulse rate decreases. Infants and children have a faster pulse rate than adults.
Gender	Female pulse rate is around 10 bpm higher than a male of the same age.
Size	Pulse rate is proportionate to the size of the body. Heat loss is greater in a small body, resulting in the heart pumping faster to compensate. Larger males will have slower pulse rates than smaller males. During sleep and rest the pulse rate may drop to 50–60 bpm.
Physical condition	Athletes and people in good physical condition have lower pulse rates. The lower rate is due to a more efficient circulatory system. Pulse rate of 60 or below can be normal for athletes.
Disease conditions	Increased pulse rate in thyroid disease, fever, and shock due to increased metabolism.
Medications	Many medications can either raise or lower the pulse rate. Medications such as digoxin are given to regulate the heartbeat. Caffeine and nicotine can increase the heart rate in certain people. Recreational drugs such as cocaine and speed increase the pulse rate.
Depression	May lower the pulse rate.
Fear, anxiety, anger	May raise the pulse rate.

2. Volume or force refers to the strength of the pulse. This is noted as a full or bounding pulse indicating an increase in blood volume; a strong or normal amount of force or blood volume; or a weak or thready (barely perceptible) force or blood volume. Volume is influenced by the forcefulness of the heartbeat, the condition of the arterial walls, and dehydration. A variance in intensity of the pulse may indicate heart disease.

TABLE 33-6 Average Pulse Rates by Age

Less than 1 year	120–160 bpm
2–6 years	80–120 bpm
6–10 years	80–100 bpm
11–16 years	70–90 bpm
Adult	60–80 bpm
Older adult	50–65 bpm

3. Rhythm refers to the regularity, or equal spacing, of all the beats of the pulse. Normally, the intervals between each heartbeat are of the same duration. A pulse with an irregular rhythm is known as a dysrhythmia or arrhythmia. The irregular rhythm may be random irregular beats or a predictable pattern of irregular beats. It is not considered abnormal if the heart occasionally skips a beat. This is referred to as an intermittent pulse. Exercise or drinking a caffeine-rich beverage may cause this to occur. When arrhythmia occurs on a consistent basis, it may indicate heart disease and should be brought to the attention of the physician. If an irregular pulse is detected, the apical pulse should be assessed. In addition, the physician may want to order an ECG to further assess the arrhythmia.

4. Compliance of the arteries refers to their ability to expand and relax. The condition of the arterial wall should be felt as elastic and soft. With age arteries lose their elasticity and greater force is required to pump the blood into the arteries. A pulse taken in a blood vessel that feels hard and rope-like is considered abnormal and may indicate heart disease such as arteriosclerosis.

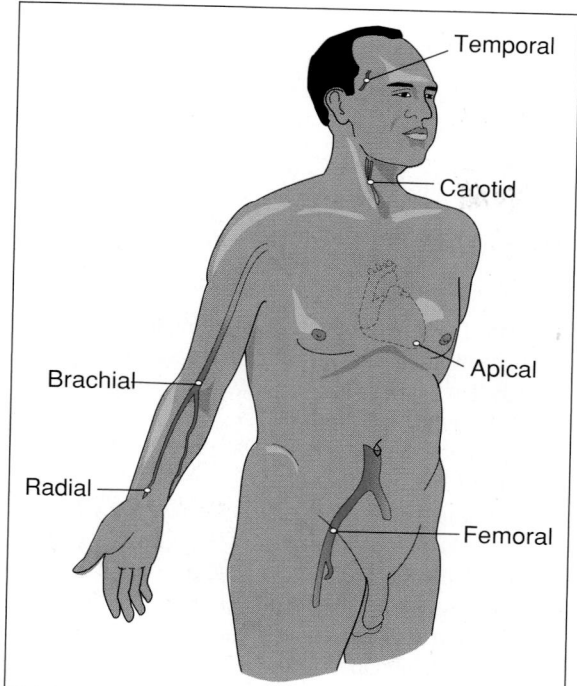

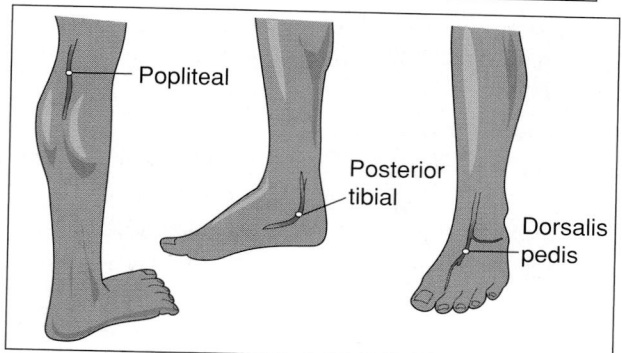

FIGURE 33-19   Nine sites for measuring pulse.

TABLE 33-7   Location of Common Pulse Sites

Site	Location
Radial	Thumb side of wrist about 1 inch below base of thumb (most frequently used site)
Brachial	Inner (antecubital fossa/space) aspect of the elbow (pulse heard when taking BP)
Carotid	At side of neck between larynx and sternocleidomastoid muscle (pulse used in CPR; pressing both carotids at the same time can cause a reflex drop in BP and pulse)
Temporal	At side of head just above the ear
Femoral	In groin where femoral artery passes to leg
Popliteal	Behind the knee; pulse is located deeply behind the knee and can be felt when knee is slightly bent
Posterior tibial	On medial surface of ankle near ankle bone
Dorsalis pedis	On top of foot slightly lateral to midline; helps assess adequate circulation to foot
Apical	At apex of heart left of sternum 4th or 5th intercostal space below the nipple

Pulse Sites

There are nine areas in the body where the pulse can be easily measured. These pulse sites are radial, brachial, carotid, temporal, femoral, popliteal, posterior tibial, dorsalis pedis, and apical (Figure 33-19). Table 33-7 describes the nine common pulse sites.

Procedure 33-8 provides the steps for accurately measuring a radial pulse. Figure 33-20 shows a medical assistant measuring a patient's radial pulse as described in the procedure, and Figure 33-21 illustrates the location of pulse sites on an actual patient.

Apical Heart Rate

The apical heart rate is the heart rate counted at the apex of the heart. It can only be heard with a stethoscope placed over the apex. This is considered to be a very accurate heart rate. The apical rate is taken in infants and young children. The physician may also re-

quest an apical rate be taken when a patient is on heart medications.

An apical-radial pulse rate may be taken to determine if there is a difference between the pulse rates taken at the two sites. An apical-radial pulse must be taken for a full minute. Normally the pulse rates should be the same. The radial pulse is never greater than the apical pulse. The difference between the two readings is called the pulse deficit. Refer to Procedure 33-9 for taking an apical-radial pulse. This measurement requires two people: one to take the radial pulse and one to take the apical pulse. When only one person is doing the procedure, the apical pulse is taken first and then the radial pulse rate. When taking an apical-radial pulse, have only one

PROCEDURE

Measuring Radial Pulse Rate

OBJECTIVE: Accurately perform all steps of the procedure and provide an accurate radial pulse reading.

Equipment and Supplies
paper and pen/pencil; patient's record; watch with second hand

Method
1. Perform hand hygiene.
2. Identify patient.
   Note: To avoid error, call patient by name and check against the name on the patient's record.
3. Explain procedure.
4. Ask the patient about any recent physical activity or smoking.
   Rationale: Exertion can increase pulse rate. Wait 10 minutes after physical exertion of patient to take pulse.
5. Ask patient to sit down and place arm in a comfortable, supported position. The hand should be at chest level with the palm down.
6. Place finger tips on radial artery on thumb side of wrist.

Note: Do not use thumb when taking pulse because the pulse in your thumb may be felt in addition to patient's pulse in wrist.
7. Check quality of pulse.
8. Start counting pulse beats when second hand on watch is at 3, 6, 9, or 12.
   Rationale: One minute is easier to observe at these points.
9. Count the pulse for 1 full minute. The number will always be an even number.
10. Write the pulse beats per minute immediately on a piece of paper.
11. Perform hand hygiene.
12. Record the pulse beats per minute in patient's record, describing any abnormalities in pulse rate.

Charting Example

2/14/XX	4:00 P.M.	Pulse 72	Regular and strong
			M. King, CMA

---

person responsible for using the watch. This person will raise one finger or nod the head when counting begins and lower the finger or nod again when a minute has passed. Coordination of timing is good when using this method.

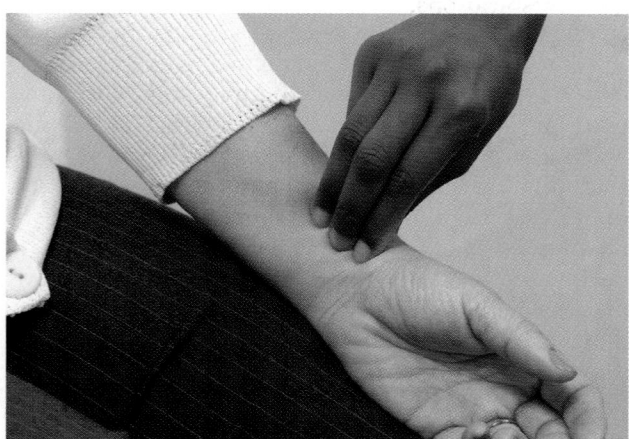

FIGURE 33-20 Measuring a patient's radial pulse.

Respiration

Respiration, or the act of breathing, is the exchange of oxygen and carbon dioxide (CO_2) between the atmosphere and the body cells. It consists of one expiration or exhalation and one inspiration or inhalation. This is called the respiratory cycle.

Physiology of Respiration

During the process of inspiration, oxygen, which is necessary for body cells and life, is taken into the lungs. The diaphragm moves downward, intercostal muscles move outward, and the lungs expand in order to take oxygen into the lungs. During expiration air containing carbon dioxide is expelled from the lungs as a waste product. The diaphragm moves upward and the lungs deflate.

The respiratory process is both external and internal. The external respiratory process is an exchange of oxygen and carbon dioxide between the alveoli, the minute air sacs of the lungs, and the blood. The

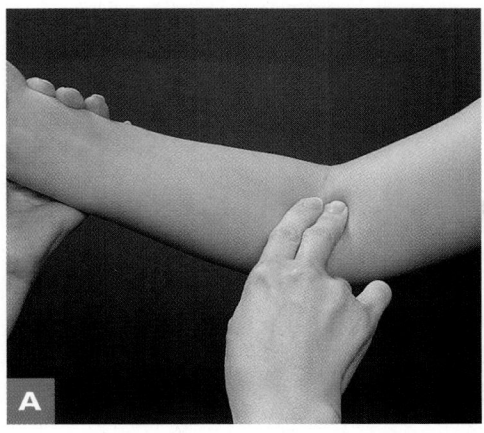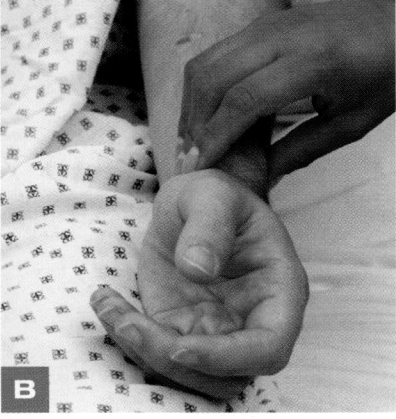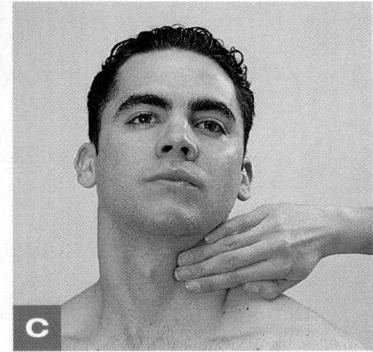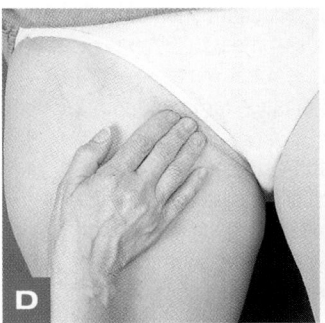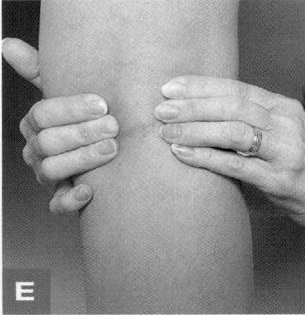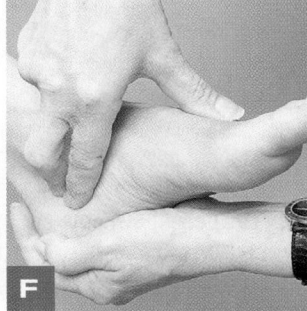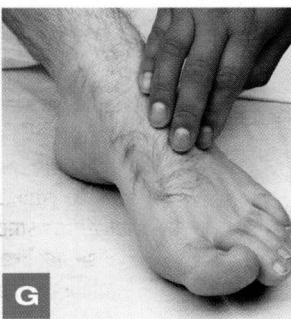

FIGURE 33-21 Measuring pulses. (A) Brachial, (B) radial, (C) carotid, (D) femoral, (E) popliteal, (F) posterior tibial, and (G) pedal (dorsalis pedis).

internal respiratory process takes place when blood in the capillaries comes into contact with the alveoli where it picks up oxygen and carries it to cells throughout the body. Carbon dioxide is thrown off as a waste product and then carried back to the lungs, where it is exhaled. The process then begins all over again with inhalation.

The medulla oblongata located in the base of the brain contains the respiratory, cardiac, and vasomotor centers. When the medulla oblongata receives a message indicating there is a buildup of carbon dioxide, this message is translated by the brain into a need for increased respiration to occur. Breathing is actually controlled by the involuntary nervous system. However, breathing is also under some control of the voluntary nervous system.

Characteristics of Respiration

When counting a patient's respiration rate, watch or feel the rise and fall of the chest. Each rise and fall is one respiration. Do not take respiration measurements immediately after the patient has experienced exertion, such as climbing stairs, unless so ordered.

Because patients have some control over their respiration, it is advisable to take a respiratory count without the patient's awareness. It is recommended that respirations be counted while appearing to count the pulse. This will result in a more accurate indication of the true respiratory rate.

The pulse and respiratory rate are usually taken at the same time. However, it is never permissible to take the respiratory rate and multiply it by four to estimate a pulse rate. Likewise the respiratory rate cannot be determined by dividing the pulse rate by four. Refer to Procedure 33-10 for measuring patient's respirations.

When counting respirations several characteristics should be noted: rate, rhythm, depth, and quality or characteristics of breathing.

Respiratory Rate

Rate refers to the number of respirations per minute and can be described as normal, rapid, or slow. The adult normal range of respirations is 14 to 20 cycles per minute. A respiratory rate of below 12 (bradypnea) or above 40 (tachypnea) in an adult should be considered a serious symptom. Rapid respirations are usually shallow in depth. Apnea means lacking of breathing and eupnea means normal breathing.

Children have a much more rapid rate of breathing than adults with an average of 30 to 50 cycles per

Measuring Apical-Radial Pulse (Two-Person)

OBJECTIVE: Accurately perform all steps of the procedure and provide an accurate apical-radial pulse reading.

Equipment and Supplies

stethoscope; alcohol wipe/cotton balls with isopropyl alcohol 70%; paper and pen/pencil; patient's record; watch with second hand

Method

1. Perform hand hygiene.
2. Prepare stethoscope using alcohol wipe or cotton balls with alcohol on earpieces and diaphragm of scope.
   Rationale: To prevent carrying organisms into ear canal of medical assistant or between patients.
3. Identify patient.
   Note: To avoid error, call patient by name and check against the name on the patient's record.
4. Explain procedure. If patient is a child, explain procedure to both the parent and child.
5. Uncover left side of patient's chest. Provide privacy with a drape, if necessary.
6. First person places earpieces of stethoscope in ears with opening in tips forward.
7. Locate apex of patient's heart by palpating to left fifth intercostal space (between fifth and sixth ribs) at the midclavicular line. This is found just below the nipple.
8. Warm chestpiece by holding in the palm of hand before placing onto patient's chest.
   Rationale: This is a comfort measure for the patient. A cold stethoscope can be startling to the patient and may cause a faster heart beat.

9. Second person locates radial pulse in the thumb side of wrist 1 inch below base of thumb.
10. First person places the chestpiece of stethoscope at apex of heart. When the heartbeat is heard, a nod is made to the second person and counting begins. Ideally, the count should begin when the second hand is at the 3, 6, 9, or 12.
11. Count for 1 full minute.
    Note: Both systole and diastole (or lubb/dubb) count as one beat.
12. Remove stethoscope and earpieces.
13. Record the rate and quality of heartbeats. Include both apical and radial rates using the designation "AP." Calculate the pulse deficit by subtracting the radial pulse rate from the apical pulse rate.
    Note: A pulse deficit may indicate that the heart contractions are not strong enough to produce a palpable radial pulse.
14. Assist the patient with replacement of clothing, if necessary. Assist patient from the examining table.
15. Wipe earpieces and chestpiece of stethoscope with alcohol wipes or cotton balls and alcohol.
    Rationale: Prevent cross-contamination.
16. Perform hand hygiene.

Charting Example

2/14/XX	4:00 P.M.	82/78 AP Pulse deficit 4. Quality of beat strong.

M. King, CMA

TABLE 33-8	**Respiratory Rate Ranges of Various Age Groups**
Newborn	30–50
1 year old	20–40
2–10 years	20–30
11–18 years	18–24
Adult	14–20

minute. Table 33-8 lists respiratory rates for various age groups.

The respiratory rate is usually at a 1:4 proportion of the pulse rate. Many factors affect the respiratory rate. Some of these include an elevated temperature, age, pain, and medical conditions such as asthma. An elevated temperature in both adults and children can result in an elevated respiratory rate. Extreme pain may also cause respirations to increase. The respiratory rate is also affected by both emotional and physical conditions. Table 33-9 lists situations that may cause an alteration in the respiratory rate.

PROCEDURE

Measuring Respirations

OBJECTIVE: Accurately perform all steps of the procedure and provide an accurate respiration measurement.

Equipment and Supplies
watch with sweep second hand

Method
1. Perform hand hygiene.
2. Identify patient.
3. Assist patient into a comfortable position.
4. Place your hand on the patient's wrist in position to take the pulse.
5. Count each breathing cycle by observing and/or feeling the rise and fall of the chest or upper abdomen.
6. Count for 1 full minute using a watch with a sweep second hand. If the rate is atypical, or unusual, in any way, take it for another minute.
7. Record respiratory rate in patient's record noting date, time, any abnormality in rate, rhythm, and depth, and your signature.

Charting Example

2/14/XX	4:00 P.M.	Resp. 20 and regular
		M. King, CMA

Rhythm

Rhythm is the breathing pattern that occurs at either regular or irregular intervals. In regular rhythm, inspirations and expirations should be the same in rate and depth. In an irregular breathing pattern, the amount of air inhaled and exhaled and the rate of respirations per minute will vary.

If the breathing rhythm appears irregular after 1 minute of observation, then respirations should be observed for several more minutes for comparison purposes. Patients with emphysema, an abnormal pulmonary condition, may experience no difficulty with inhalation but may struggle to fully exhale. Asthma may also cause an irregularity in breathing rhythm.

Depth

The depth of respiration refers to the volume of air being inhaled and exhaled. It is described as either shallow or deep. Shallow respirations with a rapid rate occur in some disease conditions such as high fever, shock, and severe pain. Hyperventilation refers to deep rapid respirations while hypoventilation refers to shallow respirations.

When a patient is unable to take in enough oxygen during inhalation, the skin and nail beds may appear bluish in color. This is called cyanosis and is due to the increase of carbon dioxide (CO_2) in the blood. In this situation, both the depth of respiration and cyanosis must be noted in the patient's record. Chronic obstructive pulmonary disease (COPD) is one of the

TABLE 33-9 Situations Causing Changes in Respiratory Rate

Increased Rate	Decreased Rate
Allergic reactions	Certain drugs (for example, morphine)
Certain drugs (for example, epinephrine)	Decrease of CO_2 in blood
Disease (for example, asthma, heart disease)	Disease (stroke, coma)
Exercise	
Excitement/anger	
Fever	
Hemorrhage	
High altitudes	
Nervousness	
Obstruction of air passage	
Pain	
Shock	

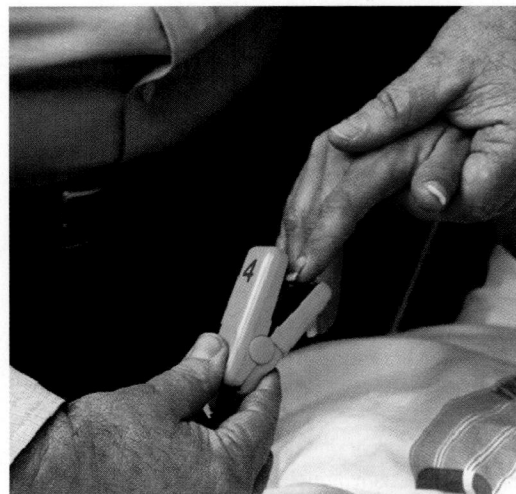

FIGURE 33-22 Pulse oximeter: The sensor probe is applied securely, flush with skin, making sure that both sensor probes are aligned directly opposite each other.

leading causes of disability and affects approximately 17 million Americans. Cigarette smoking, air pollution, and occupational exposure to dust and fumes are some of the leading causes of this disease. COPD is the result of chronic bronchitis, asthma, emphysema, and heart disease.

Respiratory Quality

Respiratory quality or character refers to breathing patterns that differ from normal effortless breathing. Labored breathing refers to respirations that require greater effort from the patient.

Breath Sounds

Normal respirations have no noticeable sound. Breath sounds occur in some disease conditions. Terms for describing breath sounds include the following:

1. Stridor, a shrill, harsh sound is heard more clearly during inspiration. This sound may be heard in children with croup and patients with laryngeal obstruction.

2. Stertorous sounds are noisy breathing sounds such as those heard in snoring.

3. Crackles or rales consist of crackling sounds resembling crushing tissue paper. They are caused by fluid accumulation in the airways and are heard with some types of pneumonia.

4. Rhonchi, which are also called gurgles, are rattling, whistling sounds made in the throat. This sound may be heard in a patient with a tracheostomy who requires suctioning of mucus.

5. Wheezes are high-pitched, whistling sounds made when airways become obstructed or severely narrowed, as in asthma or COPD.

6. Cheyne-Stokes breathing is irregular breathing that may be slow and shallow at first, then becomes faster and deeper, and then may stop for a few seconds and begin the pattern again. This type of respiration maybe seen in certain patients with cerebral, cardiac, or pulmonary diseases.

7. Bubbling breathing sounds like gurgling sounds, as if air is passing through moist secretions in the respiratory tract.

Oxygen Saturation

Oximetry is the process of measuring the oxygen saturation of arterial blood. An oximeter is a photoelectric device that measures oxygen saturation by recording the amount of light transmitted or reflected by deoxygenated (venous) blood versus oxygenated hemoglobin in arterial blood. A pulse oximeter is a noninvasive method of indicating the arterial oxygen saturation of a patient's functional hemoglobin (oxygen-carrying molecules in blood). Refer to Figure 33-22 for an example of a pulse oximeter being applied to patient's finger to measure the oxygen saturation level (SaO_2). It is important to align the sensor probes directly opposite each other. Procedure 33-11 lists the steps for measuring oxygen saturation. Normal values for SaO_2 are 95% to 100% while a level below 70% is life threatening.

Blood Pressure

The measurement of blood pressure (BP) is an important vital sign to aid in diagnosis and treatment and is therefore taken routinely. Many medical conditions can be indicated by either a rise or fall in blood pressure. The condition of high blood pressure known as hypertension is often asymptomatic (without any symptoms). An abnormal blood pressure reading can be the first indication of this condition. It is also known as essential hypertension, while secondary hypertension is due to an underlying cause such as renal disease, pregnancy, or an endocrine disorder. Symptoms of hypertension are headache, blurred vision, chest pain, or no symptoms at all, which is why it is known as the silent killer. Hypotension is low blood pressure and may be due to emotional shock, trauma, and central nervous system disorders. Symptoms of hypotension are dizziness and syncope (fainting). (Refer to Legal and Ethical Issues.)

Physiology of Blood Pressure

Blood pressure is actually caused by the action of the blood moving against the walls of the arteries. Blood is pushed out of the heart and into the aorta and pul-

Measuring Oxygen Saturation Using a Pulse Oximeter

OBJECTIVE: Correctly measure arterial blood oxygen saturation.

Equipment and Supplies

pulse oximeter; alcohol wipe; towel; nail polish remover as needed; patient's chart

Method

1. Perform hand hygiene and explain procedure to patient.
2. Observe infection control procedures as needed.
3. Select appropriate size sensor (pediatric, small or large).
4. Clean site with alcohol.
5. If patient is female and is wearing nail polish it may be necessary to remove it because polish interferes with accuracy of measurements.
6. Apply sensor and connect to pulse oximeter, making sure it is correctly aligned.
7. Turn on machine according to manufacturer's directions. (A beep will indicate each arterial pulsation.) Patient movement may be interpreted as arterial pulsations.
8. Take reading and document.

Charting Example

11/29/XX | (S_{AO_2}) Blood oxygen saturation 89%.

M. King, CMA

---

monary arteries as the ventricles contract. This, in turn, exerts continuous pressure on the walls of the arteries. Refer to Figure 33-23 to review the blood flow of the heart.

Blood Pressure Readings

Blood pressure levels are taken at two different points called *readings*. The two blood pressure readings are systolic pressure, or the highest pressure that occurs as the heart is contracting, and diastolic pressure, which is the lowest pressure level that occurs when the heart is relaxed (the ventricle is at rest). The pulse beat is felt at the systolic pressure level and is absent at the diastolic pressure level.

Pulse pressure is the difference between the systolic and diastolic readings. This is found by subtracting the diastolic reading from the systolic reading. A pulse pressure that is greater than 50 mmHg or less than 30 mmHg is considered to be abnormal. For instance, if the blood pressure is 130/82, the pulse pressure would be 48, which is still within the range considered normal. Extremes of pulse pressure can result in stroke or shock.

Korotkoff Sounds

Korotkoff sounds are the sounds actually heard as the arterial wall distends during the compression of the blood pressure cuff. The sounds were first classified into five different phases by Russian neurologist Nicolai Korotkoff.

When the blood pressure cuff is first inflated, no sound can be heard because the brachial artery is compressed. As air is slowly removed from the cuff during deflation, the Korotkoff sounds become audible. The deflation of air should be at the rate of 2 to 3 mmHg

Legal and Ethical Issues

The medical assistant has an ethical responsibility to use careful, proper technique when performing procedures to measure vital signs since an incorrect reading could lead to misdiagnosis and result in serious consequences for the patient. Proper technique includes allowing enough time for the temperature to register, using a watch with a second hand when taking pulse and respiration, and never guessing the time when measuring pulse and respirations, to name just a few. Incorrect documentation of vital signs can lead to serious complications for the patient and legal consequences for the physician and the medical assistant.

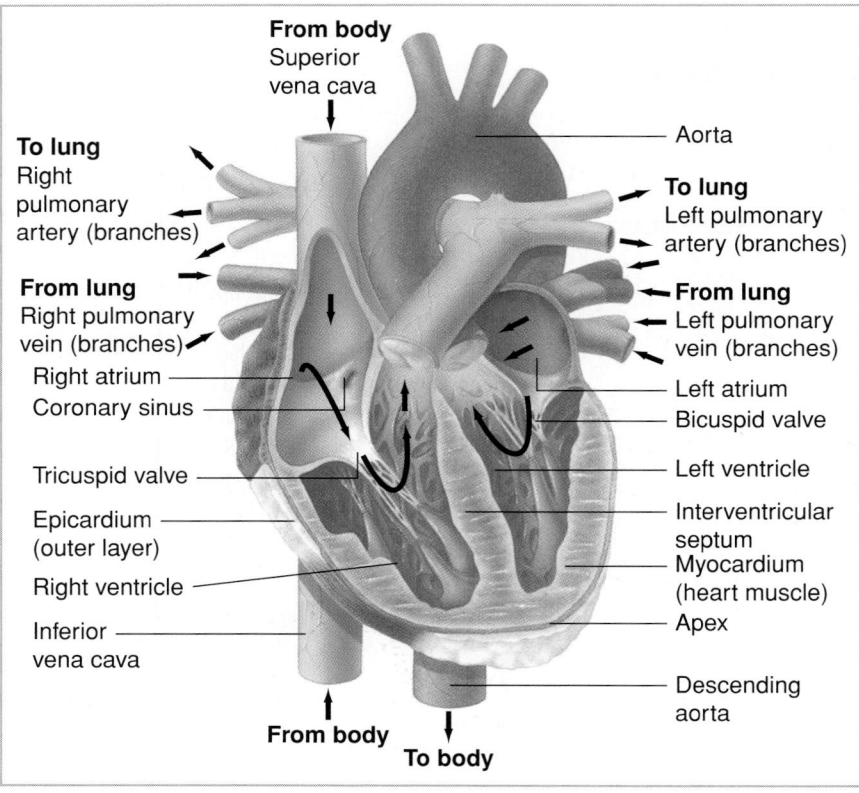

FIGURE 33-23 Circulation of blood through the heart.

the last sound is heard. Some facilities and physicians measure the diastolic pressure at the fourth Korotkoff phase where the sound changes from a clear tapping or thumping sound to a more muffled softer sound. When the fourth sound is used as the diastolic pressure three readings are often made: systolic, first diastolic (fourth Korotkoff sound), and second diastolic (last sound). Korotkoff sounds are described in Table 33-10.

Readings of blood pressure are in millimeters (mm) of mercury (Hg) The abbreviations *mm* and *Hg* are not necessary when recording the blood pressure readings. The actual blood pressure is recorded using just the systolic or highest pressure reading, over the diastolic or lowest reading. For example, 120/80 would be considered a normal blood pressure reading for an adult. Generally, a range of normal is used for blood pressure readings since slight variations can occur among normal healthy adults. A deviation, either a rise or fall, from the patient's baseline measurement of 20 to 30 mmHg can be significant for that patient.

per heartbeat. The medical assistant should practice taking blood pressure readings slowly in order to be able to identify each phase. The systolic pressure is the first distinct clear tapping sound that is heard, and the diastolic pressure is the pressure at which

Blood pressure readings should routinely be started at age 5 as part of the school physical or earlier if medically

TABLE 33-10 **Five Phases of Korotkoff Sounds**

Phase I	This is the first faint sound heard as the cuff is deflated. Record this reading as the systolic pressure reading. The cuff must be inflated to a high enough level to hear this first sound during relaxation.
Phase II	The second phase occurs as the cuff continues to be deflated and blood flows through the artery. This sound has a swishing quality. The cuff has to be slowly deflated in order to hear this soft sound. An **ausculatory gap** is said to have occurred if there is a total loss of sound at this stage which then reoccurs later. An ausculatory gap can occur in certain cases of heart disease and hypertension. An auscultatory gap should be reported to the physician.
Phase III	During this phase the sound will become less muffled and develop a crisp tapping sound as the blood flow moves easily through the artery. If the BP cuff was not inflated enough to hear the Phase I sound, then the Phase III sound may be heard and incorrectly stated as the systolic reading.
Phase IV	The sound will now begin to fade and become muffled. The American Heart Association, which believes Phase IV is the best indicator of the diastolic pressure, recommends the reading at this phase be recorded as the diastolic pressure for a child.
Phase V	Sound will disappear at this phase. Some physician's want both phase IV and phase V recorded for the diastolic pressure reading (for example, 120/78/74 rather than 120/74).

TABLE 33-11 New Blood Pressure Guidelines

New Classification (2003)		Previous Classification
140/90 or above	Hypertension	High blood pressure > 140/90
120/80 to 139/89	Prehypertension	Borderline 130–139/85–89
119/79 or below	Normal	Normal 129/84 or below
		Optimal 120/80 or below

necessary. Patients should have a complete physical to see why their blood pressure is elevated. Patients with a sustained high blood pressure measurement may require further diagnostic evaluation for the presence of other disease conditions, as well as medication to lower the blood pressure. Controlling blood pressure can lower the incidence of stroke and heart attack.

If a patient's blood pressure deviates from the normal range, he or she should be tested again. Many patients experience "white coat syndrome." They are so apprehensive about visiting the physician and having blood pressure taken that the results are extremely elevated. Often these same individuals, when tested at home, are within the normal range. Being empathetic and sensitive to their problems may help you obtain a better reading. Ideally, blood pressure is taken while the patient is sitting with both feet flat on the floor since crossed knees may result in elevated readings. If the patient's condition warrants, blood pressure may be measured lying down but should be charted accordingly.

New Guidelines for Blood Pressure

In 2003 new guidelines for blood pressure were established in the Seventh Report of the Joint National Committee (JCN7) on the Prevention, Detection, Evaluation and Treatment of High Blood Pressure published by the National Institute of Health, U.S. Department of Health and Human Services. The normal blood pressure range for an adult should be below 119/79. Refer to Table 33-11 for the complete list of new values recommended by the JCN7.

Average normal blood pressure readings are listed in Table 33-12. While an average blood pressure is listed for a newborn, blood pressure readings are not generally taken on infants. Monitors are used on the very young.

Factors Affecting Blood Pressure

Physiological factors affecting blood pressure include volume or amount of blood in the arteries, peripheral resistance of the vessels, condition of the heart muscle, and the elasticity of vessels. These four factors are discussed in Table 33-13.

Many other factors may affect blood pressure. Two of these are gender and age. Women generally have a lower blood pressure than men. Blood pressure is lowest at birth and tends to increase as people age. The time of day can also cause blood pressure variations. For example, blood pressure is usually at its lowest point early in the morning just before awakening.

Activities such as standing, sitting, or lying down can affect blood pressure. When blood pressure is measured while the patient is in an erect position, it is referred to as an orthostatic blood pressure reading. Orthostatic hypotension refers to the lowered blood pressure that occurs when a patient moves from a lying down to an erect position. Sudden movement or a sudden change in position, with a resulting fall in blood pressure is referred to as postural hypotension.

The pressure reading in the right arm is usually 3 to 4 mmHg higher than in the left arm. Numerous situations that cause changes in blood pressure readings are listed in Table 33-14. Terms relating to abnormal blood pressure readings are described in Table 33-15.

Blood pressure is a routinely taken vital sign. It is especially important for patients with the following characteristics or conditions:

1. Patients on antihypertensive drugs
2. Patients with a history of heart disease, kidney disease, stroke or hypertension

TABLE 33-12 Average Normal Blood Pressure Readings

Newborn	75/55
6–9 years of age	90/55
10–15 years of age	100/65
16 years to adulthood	118/76
Adult	120/80

TABLE 33-13	**Physiological Factors Affecting Blood Pressure**
Volume of blood	Increase of blood volume increases the BP. Decrease of blood volume decreases BP. *Example:* Hemorrhage causes volume and BP to drop.
Peripheral resistance	Relates to the size of the lumen, the cavity or space, within blood vessels and amount of blood flowing through it. *Example:* The smaller the size of the lumen, the greater the resistance to blood flow. Fatty cholesterol deposits result in high BP due to narrowing of the lumen.
Condition of heart muscle	Strength of heart muscle affects volume of blood flow. The pumping action of the heart and how efficiently it does the job affect the BP. *Example:* A weak heart muscle can cause an increase or decrease in BP.
Elasticity of vessels	The ability of blood vessels to expand and contract decreases with age. *Example:* Nonelastic blood vessels, as in arteriosclerosis, cause an elevated BP.

TABLE 33-14 **Causes of Blood Pressure Variations**

Elevated/ Increased BP	Lowered/ Decreased BP
Anger	Anemia
Certain drug therapies, nicotine, caffeine	Approaching death
Endocrine disorders (hyperthyroidism)	Cancer
Exercise	Certain drug therapies (antihypertensives, narcotics, analgesics, diuretics)
Fear, excitement	Decreased arterial blood volume (hemorrhage)
Heart and liver disease	Decreased arterial BP
Increased arterial BP	Dehydration
Late pregnancy	Massive heart attack
Lying down position with legs elevated	Middle pregnancy
Obesity	Pain
Renal disease	Shock
Right arm	Starvation
Rigidity of blood vessels	Sudden postural changes
Smoking	Thyroid and adrenal disorders
Stress, anxiety	Time of day (during sleep and early morning)
Vasoconstriction or narrowing of peripheral blood vessels	Weak heart

3. Patients receiving a complete physical examination, including children

4. Pregnant women

5. Preoperative and postoperative patients

6. Patients who are bleeding or in shock

7. Patients with symptoms of a neurological disorder

8. Patients experiencing allergic reactions

Blood pressure readings, as with all vital signs, should be interpreted using the patient's baseline measurement. This means that a previously taken blood pressure reading, when the patient was not ill, is used as that patient's "normal" measurement. All subsequent readings are then compared to that patient's "normal" baseline reading.

Equipment for Measuring Blood Pressure

Two pieces of equipment are necessary for measuring blood pressure: a sphygmomanometer and a stethoscope. The sphygmomanometer is the instrument used for measuring the pressure the blood exerts against the

TABLE 33-15 Terms Related to Abnormal Blood Pressure Readings

Hypertension	A condition in which the patient's blood pressure is consistently above the norm for his or her age group. Also called high blood pressure. Below 120/80 is the baseline.
Benign	Slow-onset elevated blood pressure without symptoms.
Essential	This is a primary hypertension of unknown cause. It may be genetically determined.
Secondary	Elevated blood pressure associated with other conditions such as renal disease, pregnancy, arteriosclerosis, and obesity.
Malignant	Rapidly developing elevated blood pressure that may become fatal if not treated immediately.
Renal	Elevated blood pressure as a result of kidney disease.
Hypotension	Condition of abnormally low blood pressure that may be caused by shock, hemorrhage, and central nervous system (CNS) disorders.
Orthostatic	A temporary fall in blood pressure that occurs when a patient rapidly moves from a lying to a standing position. Dizziness and blurred vision can also be present.
Postural	A temporary fall in blood pressure from standing motionless for extended periods of time.

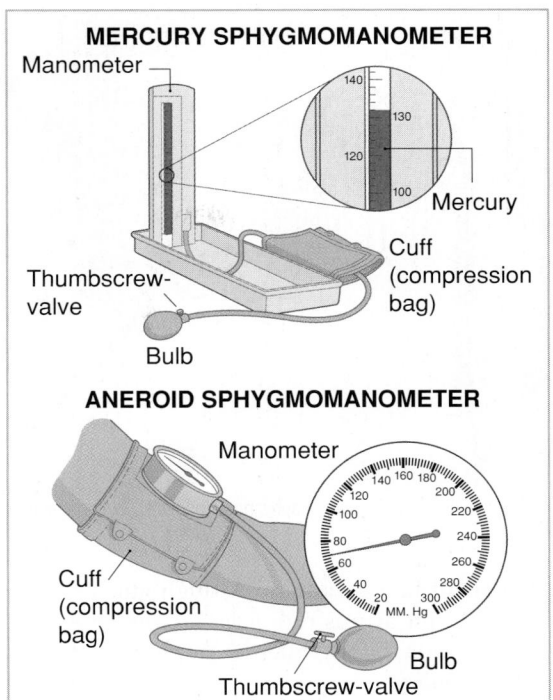

FIGURE 33-24 Sphygmomanometers are used to measure blood pressure and may be either mercury or aneroid.

walls of the artery (Figure 33-24). The stethoscope is a diagnostic instrument that amplifies sound. It is used to detect sounds produced by blood pressure as well as the heart and other internal organs such as the stomach.

Sphygmomanometers

The components of a sphygmomanometer are manometer, inflatable rubber bladder, cuff, and bulb. The manometer is a scale that registers the actual pressure reading. The core of the blood pressure cuff is the rubber bladder, which, when inflated, distends to temporarily constrict blood circulation in the arm. A soft material cuff covers the bladder and is placed next to the skin of the patient. The pressure bulb has a thumbscrew attached to a control valve that allows for inflation and deflation of the cuff.

The size of the blood pressure cuff is important. Three sizes are available: pediatric, large arm adult, and thigh (Figure 33-25). Blood pressure cuffs are not generally used on infants. The pediatric cuff can also

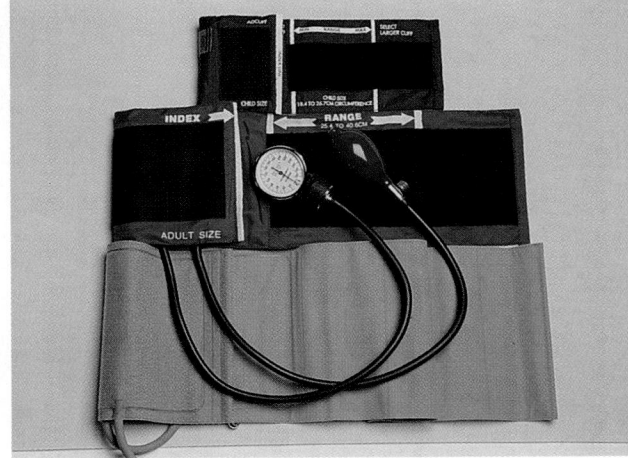

FIGURE 33-25 Three standard sizes of cuffs: a small cuff for a child or frail adult; a normal adult size; and a large size for measuring blood pressure on the leg or on the arm of an obese adult.

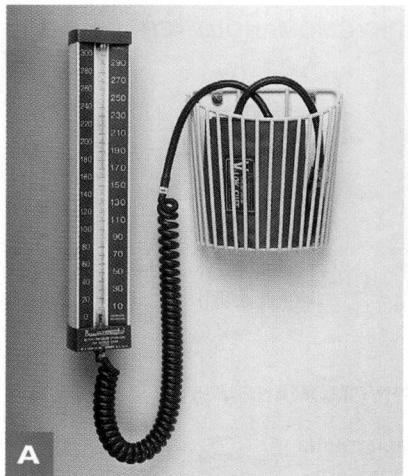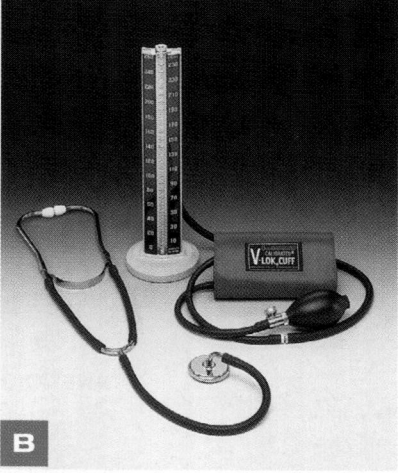

FIGURE 33-26 (A) Wall-mounted mercury sphygmomanometer. (B) Portable mercury sphygmomanometer.

be used on small-limbed adults. A thigh cuff is available when an adult arm is too large for the large arm cuff. When using a thigh cuff, the popliteal artery is palpated for a pulse.

The two types of sphygmomanometers are mercury and aneroid. A discussion follows with illustrations of portable and wall-mounted versions of each type.

MERCURY SPHYGMOMANOMETER The mercury sphygmomanometers are widely used and are found on the walls in many physicians offices (Figure 33-26). It contains a column of mercury that rises as the pressure bulb is pressed and the rubber bladder inflated. A calibrated scale runs down both sides of the mercury column. The reading is taken at eye level at the top of the mercury line next to a calibrated scale. This type of instrument must be placed vertically on the wall or on

a flat, level surface so that the mercury will rise in a vertical position. Periodic recalibration is necessary for accuracy.

ANEROID SPHYGMOMANOME-TER The aneroid sphygmomanometer has a round dial that contains a scale calibrated in millimeters (mm) and a needle to register the reading (Figure 33-27). The needle must be at zero before starting the procedure. The aneroid sphygmomanometer should be recalibrated for accuracy every year by using a mercury manometer as the model. This instrument is easily portable. Some facilities and many individuals use electronic blood pressure devices. The home units are relatively inexpensive and are easy to use.

Stethoscopes

The stethoscope is used to detect sounds produced by blood pressure. This instrument consists of a chestpiece containing a diaphragm and/or bell, flexible tubing, binaurals, a spring mechanism, and earpieces. The key components of the stethoscope are described in Table 33-16 and shown in Figure 33-28. Stethoscopes are also used to measure apical pulse and listen to chest sounds.

Measuring Blood Pressure

After greeting the patient, attempt to relax him or her by explaining in a calm, quiet manner that the procedure is not painful and what it will entail. Most patients have had BP measured previously. Ask the patient if he or she knows what the previous reading was or if there is have a history of hypertension. This will guide you when you have to inflate the cuff (30 mm over systolic pressure). If this is this first time taking a reading on a new patient, you should take a BP reading on each arm. After inflating the cuff to the level recommended by your physician (180 in some offices) and the pulse beat is audible, deflate the cuff and begin inflating again 20 to 30 mm higher than previously. Do not comment on the BP reading to the patient unless the physician has instructed you to. Remember it is the physician's duty to explain the results. Figure 33-29 for an illustration of measuring a patient's blood pressure.

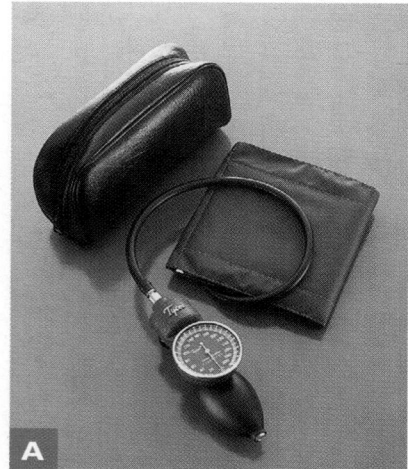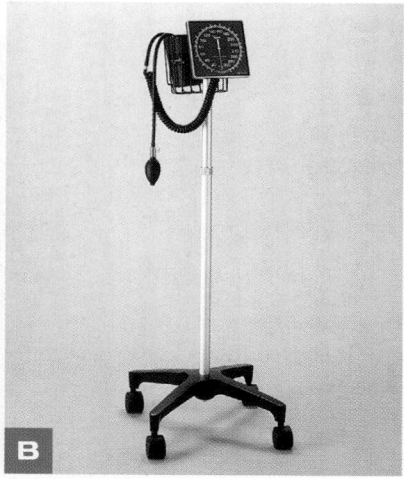

FIGURE 33-27 (A) Portable aneroid sphygmomanometer. (B) Portable aneroid sphygmomanometer on wheels.

TABLE 33-16 Components of the Stethoscope

Chestpiece	Portion of the instrument that is placed over the site where the sound is to be heard. May consist of a diaphragm or a bell or both.
Diaphragm	A disc-like sound sensor which picks up both low and high-pitched sound frequencies. More useful for high sounds such as bowel and lung sounds.
Bell	A hollow, curved bell or cup shaped sound sensor which may have one, two, or three "heads" which are useful in picking up sounds of the cardiovascular system.
Flexible tubing	Rubber or plastic tubing to carry the sound from the patient to the binaurals. The usual length of tubing is 12 to 14 inches. You may prefer using longer tubing up to 22 inches. However, some of the sound clarity is lost as the tubing becomes longer.
Binaurals	Rigid small metal tubes that connect the tubing to the earpieces.
Spring mechanism	Flexible external metal spring that holds the binaural steady so that the earpiece will remain in the ear.
Earpieces	Molded plastic tips which attach to the end of the binaurals and are placed in the medical assistant's ears

Estimated Systolic Pressure

The palpatory method of feeling the radial pulse while the blood pressure cuff is deflating can be used to determine systolic pressure. This method cannot be used to determine the diastolic pressure or to hear the Korotkoff sounds. However, it is useful when a student is learning to take blood pressure readings. The level of inflation necessary to hear the first sound in phase I can be determined by using the palpatory method, which is explained in Procedure 33-12. Procedure 33-13 lists the steps to correctly measure a systolic and diastolic blood pressure.

Causes of Error in Blood Pressure Measurements

Accuracy is very important is evaluation of blood pressure. Many conclusions about a patient's health are made based on a BP assessment. Being in a hurry and failing to allow sufficient time to elapse before retaking a reading are common errors. Table 33-17 describes causes of errors in taking blood pressure readings. Blood pressure measurement is not used solely to determine if hypertension exists. Abnormal blood pressure measurements are found with other conditions including kidney disease and stress.

Pain

Pain is often considered the fifth vital sign. Many patients will not mention pain unless they are specifically asked about it. Pain is a universal symptom we all have experienced. It is extremely subjective and personal and it can overpower and change one's life. No two individuals experience pain in the same way. If the patient says he or she is in pain, the caregiver must accept his or her word because this is a subjective symptom. When documenting a patient's description of pain, the caregiver must use the patient's own words. For example, if the patient complains of a "sharp, knife-like stabbing pain in the belly" that is how it should be written in the chart.

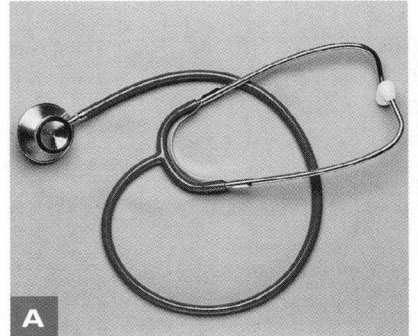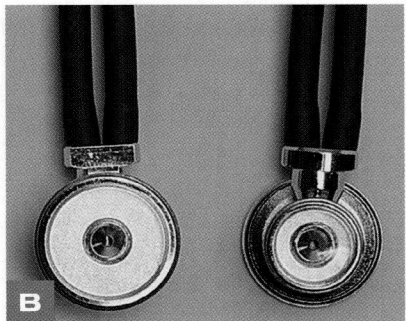

FIGURE 33-28 (A) Stethoscope with both a bell and flat-disc amplifier. (B) Close-up of a flat-disc amplifier on left and a bell amplifier on right.

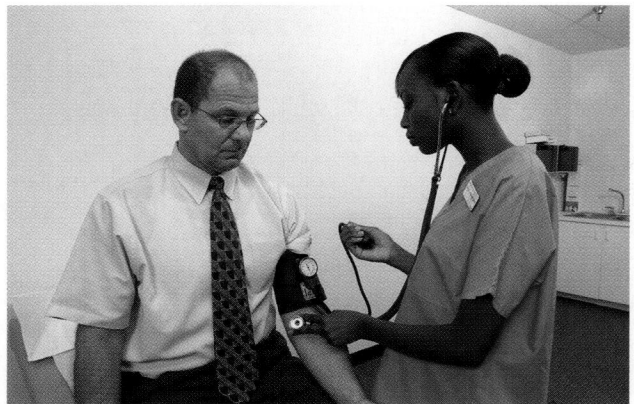

FIGURE 33-29 Measuring a patient's blood pressure.

Pain is difficult to describe. It is important for medical personnel to have a vocabulary of terms and to observe for nonverbal signs when discussing pain with a patient. Signs such as grimacing or moaning or grasping a particular body part are forms of nonverbal communication. Use of a numerical pain measurement scale with 1 being no pain and 10 being extreme pain can be useful. For children and non-English speaking patients, scales with happy and sad faces are available. The goal of assessing pain is to find a treatment or means to relieve the discomfort. Assessment of pain is also important after treatment plans have been initiated.

Types of Pain

Pain may be acute or chronic. Acute pain is expected pain associated with trauma or surgery that lasts through the recovery of that condition. Chronic pain is long-term pain that persists over 6 months and interferes with functions of life. Pain can be categorized by where it seems to becoming from, for example, deep in the organs or on the surface of the body. Pain is also described by where it is felt in the body. Radiating pain spreads out from an area. For instance, pain from a heart attack is felt in the chest and down the right arm. Referred pain is pain in an area away from the tissue causing the problem. An example of this would be gallbladder pain, which may be felt in the right shoulder. Intractable pain is overwhelming, difficult to relieve, and all consuming like the pain associated with end-stage cancer. Phantom pain is a sensation felt in a missing body part after it has been removed. Other terms such as *dull, achy, throbbing, cramping,* or *stabbing* may be used by patients to describe their pain.

Pain threshold is the amount of pain stimulation required for an individual to feel pain. It is generally fairly consistent from person to person but it can change with other circumstances. For example, a sprained ankle hurts, but if the patient is emotionally upset and depressed it may bother him more than normal.

33-12 | **PROCEDURE**

Measuring Systolic Blood Pressure Using Palpatory Method

OBJECTIVE: Obtain an accurate systolic reading.

Equipment and Supplies
sphygmomanometer; stethoscope; 70% isopropyl alcohol; alcohol sponges or cotton balls; paper and pen/pencil; patient's record
Note: American Heart Association recommends that approximate systolic BP be determined first by palpating radial pulse, then pumping up cuff until pulse in no longer felt. This is standard procedure in many cases.

Method
1. Place the blood pressure cuff in the usual position on the upper arm.
2. Locate the radial pulse on the thumb side of the wrist.
3. Inflate the blood pressure cuff until the pulse disappears and note the reading on the manometer.
4. Reinflate the cuff until the pulse once again disappears, and inflate another 30 mmHg to get above the systolic pressure.
5. Slowly deflate the cuff while keeping fingers on the pulse. The point at which the pulse is felt is the systolic pressure.
6. Remember this number if you are going to take a brachial artery blood pressure reading immediately. Write the number on paper if there will be a delay before you can take the complete blood pressure.

Charting Example
Note: This number is not usually charted since it is only used to estimate the systolic BP.

Measuring Blood Pressure

OBJECTIVE: Obtain an accurate systolic and diastolic reading.

Equipment and Supplies

sphygmomanometer; stethoscope; 70% isopropyl alcohol; alcohol sponges or cotton balls; paper and pen/pencil; patient's record

Method

1. Perform hand hygiene.
2. Assemble equipment. Thoroughly cleanse the earpieces, bell, and diaphragm pieces of the stethoscope. Use an alcohol sponge or cotton ball with 70% isopropyl alcohol. Allow alcohol to dry.
3. Identify patient verbally and explain the procedure.
4. Assist the patient into a comfortable position. BP is usually taken with patient in sitting position. However, the patient may be lying down, sitting, or standing. If taken while the patient is lying down or standing, note this in the chart. Inform the doctor since the pressure changes in different positions. The patient's arms should not be higher than heart level.
5. Place the mercury sphygmomanometer on a solid surface with the gauge within 3 feet for easy viewing. The sphygmomanometer should be able to be read by the medical assistant, but not by the patient.
6. Uncover the patient's arm by asking patient to roll back sleeve 5 inches above the elbow. If the sleeve becomes constricting when rolled back, ask patient to slip the arm out of the sleeve. Never take a blood pressure reading through clothing.
7. Have patient straighten arm with palms up. Apply the cuff of the sphygmomanometer over the brachial artery 1 to 2 inches above the antecubital space (bend in the elbow). Many cuffs are marked with arrows or circles to be placed over the artery. Hold the edge of the cuff in place as you wrap the remainder of the cuff tightly around the arm. If the cuff has a Velcro closure, press it into place at the end of the cuff.
8. Palpate with your finger tips to locate the brachial artery in the antecubital space.
9. Place earpieces in your ears and the diaphragm (or bell) of the stethoscope over the area where you feel the brachial artery pulsing. Hold the diaphragm in place with one hand on the chestpiece without placing your thumb over the diaphragm. The stethoscope tubing should hang freely and not touch any object or the patient during the reading.
10. Close the thumbscrew on the hand bulb by turning clockwise with your dominant hand. Close the thumbscrew just enough so that no air can leak out. Do not close so tightly that you will have difficulty reopening it with one hand.
11. Pump air into the cuff quickly and evenly until the level of mercury is 20 to 30 mmHg above the previously measured BP or the palpatory method. Some physicians prefer inflating the cuff to 180 mmHg as a starting point.
12. Slowly turn the thumbscrew counterclockwise with your dominant hand. Allow the pressure reading to fall only 2 to 3 mmHg at a time.
13. Listen for the point at which the first clear sound is heard (phase I of the Korotkoff sounds). Note where this occurred on the mercury column (or spring gauge scale on an aneroid manometer). This is the systolic pressure.
14. Slowly continue to allow the cuff to deflate. The sounds will change from loud to murmur and then fade away (phases I, II, III, and IV of Korotkoff sounds). Read the mercury column (or spring gauge scale) at the point where the sound is muffled or dull. This is the diastolic pressure (phase IV of Korotkoff sounds).
15. Continue to deflate the cuff and read the mercury column (or spring gauge scale on aneroid manometer) until the sound is gone. This is phase V of the Korotkoff sounds. Many physicians will want both phase IV and phase V reported for the diastolic reading.
16. Quickly open the thumbscrew all the way to release the air and deflate the cuff.
17. If you are unsure about the BP reading, wait at least a minute or two before taking a second reading. Never take more than two readings in one arm since blood stasis may have occurred, resulting in an inaccurate reading.
18. Immediately write the BP as a fraction on paper. You may inform the patient of the reading if this is the policy in your office.
19. Remove the cuff.
20. Clean the earpieces of the stethoscope with an alcohol sponge.
21. Wash hands.
22. Chart the results including the date, time, BP reading and your name.

Charting Example

2/14/XX	9:00 A.M.	B/P 134/88 left arm, sitting
		M. King, CMA

TABLE 33-17 Causes of Error in Blood Pressure Readings

Equipment	Cuff is improper size. The cuff bladder should be 20 percent wider than the diameter of the extremity where cuff is placed. Large cuffs for obese arms and small cuffs for children should be available in all offices; air leaks around the valve may cause mercury to drop suddenly; air leaks in the cuff bladder delay the inflation rate and could give a false high reading. Air leaks may also occur along the tubing if it is old or worn; mercury column is not calibrated to the zero point; velcro may be worn and does not hold.
Procedure	Patient's arm is not uncovered; medical assistant is too far away from manometer to accurately read gauge; cuff is improperly applied (too loose or too small); cuff is not centered over the brachial artery, 1 to 2 inches above bend in the elbow; end of the cuff is not secured tightly; part of stethoscope tubing or chestpiece touches the blood pressure cuff while taking the pressure reading; failure to locate brachial pulse before placing stethoscope in position; the rubber bladder in the cuff was not deflated completely before beginning the procedure; valve on bulb is not completely closed before beginning to pump air into cuff; cuff was not inflated to a level 20 to 30 mmHg above the palpated or previously measured systolic pressure or 200 mmHg; deflation occurs too rapidly to accurately determine the sounds; the arm used for the reading is not at the same level as the heart. The arm cannot be held above the level of the heart; failed to wait 1 to 2 minutes before taking second reading; failed to notice the auscultatory gap.
Patient	Patient is nervous or anxious, resulting in a false high reading; patient's arm is too large for accurate reading with available equipment.

Pain tolerance is the amount and duration of pain a person can experience before requiring intervention and relief. This also varies with the individual and cultural and psychological circumstances. (Refer to Cultural Considerations.)

Cultural Considerations

Pain is influenced by the ethnic and cultural background of the patient. Caregivers also have their own set of attitudes and beliefs related to pain. How one behaves when in pain is learned in the cultural environment. One culture may be overtly expressive when in pain, while another culture values the stoic silent suffering response to pain. As medical assistants we need to examine our own beliefs and attitudes about pain and objectively relate to the patient in distress. Understanding cultural differences and our own attitudes will aid in providing better care for the patient in pain.

Body Fat Measurement

Metabolism is the sum of all the biochemical and physiological processes that take place in the body and are needed to grow and maintain life. Basal metabolism is the rate of metabolism when the body is awake and at rest. The amount of calories one takes in should equal the number of calories of energy expended or a weight gain will result. The ideal weight is the weight at which the individual maintains optimal heath. The ideal weight values vary with age, sex, body build, and standardized charts. There are many methods for measuring the percentage of body fat. Some are expensive and time consuming, for example, underwater weighing or x-ray absorptiometry methods. Two easier and more practical methods are the skin-fold test and the calculation of body mass index (BMI) method.

Skin-Fold Fat Measurement

The skin-fold measurement of body fat involves using special skin calipers to measure the thickness of fat folds in three areas: triceps, suprailiac, and subscapular areas. Figure 33-30 illustrates the use of calipers to measure the triceps fat fold. Each of the designated areas is measured, and a reading from the instrument is taken. After all readings are complete, calculations are made and the results are recorded. For example, an acceptable result in a female in the triceps area would be 12 to 25 percent body fat or 9 to 17 mm.

Body Mass Index

Body mass (BMI) index is calculated using

- Patient's height in meters (1 m = 3.3 ft or 39.6 inches)
- Patient's weight in kilograms (1 kg = 2.2 lb)
- The following formula: BMI = weight in kilograms/height in meters squared

A nomogram may be used to calculate a BMI (see Chapter 47). Use a ruler to make an imaginary line between your height on the right and weight on the left. A BMI of 19 to 22 is most desirable. A reading over 30 is considered obese.

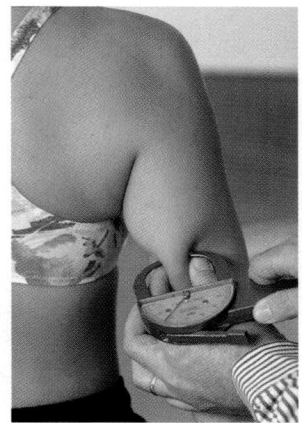

FIGURE 33-30 Measuring body fat using calipers on the triceps of a patient.

SUMMARY

Patient interviewing and correct documentation in a medical history or record are of vital importance to the health of the patient and the quality of health care provided by the physician. Privacy, empathy, and confidentiality are important goals to keep in mind when interviewing and assisting patients.

Vital signs are an important objective indication of the patient's overall physical condition. One vital sign measurement taken alone does not necessarily provide a complete picture. The medical assistant must be able to skillfully take all vital measurements and be able to assess what she or he is observing such as the rate, rhythm, and depth of respirations. Other factors such as age, gender, nervousness, and physical condition of the patient may affect vital sign readings. Measurements such as height and weight are an important part of patient examination. At times additional assessments of BMI or skin-fold fat percentage may be requested. Assessing pain, the fifth vital sign, helps provide additional information to aid in the delivery of health care.

The accuracy of obtaining and recording vital sign measurements is critical for the ultimate diagnosis and treatment of the patient. Communication skills, while important in all aspects of medical assisting work, are essential when obtaining vital measurements. A positive and sincere approach in interacting with the patient may be enough to put the patient at ease and result in obtaining more valid vital sign measurements.

Chapter Review

COMPETENCY REVIEW

1. Define and spell the terms to learn for this chapter.
2. Name five factors that affect body temperature.
3. Name four types of fever.
4. What is hypothermia?
5. What is the desirable range for blood pressure in an adult?
6. What level does a pulse oximeter measure?
7. List the six Cs of charting.

PREPARING FOR THE CERTIFICATION EXAM

1. Dinesha Reynolds has an oral temperature of 100.8°F. The medical term for this is:
   A. pyuria
   B. purulent
   C. hyperpyrexia
   D. pyrexia
   E. hypotension

2. Which of the following is NOT considered a vital sign?
   A. body temperature
   B. weight
   C. blood pressure
   D. respiration
   E. Stridor

continued on next page

3. What is considered the least accurate indicator of temperature?
   A. axilla
   B. oral
   C. eardrum
   D. rectum
   E. all are equally accurate

4. The ratio of pulse to respirations is usually:
   A. 1:5
   B. 1:4
   C. 1:3
   D. 1:2
   E. 1:6

5. During which phase of the Korotkoff sounds will the sound fade and become muffled?
   A. phase I
   B. phase II
   C. phase III
   D. phase IV
   E. phase V

6. Blood pressure that becomes low when a patient assumes an erect position is called:
   A. postural hypertension
   B. orthostatic hypertension
   C. essential hypertension
   D. orthostatic hypotension
   E. postural hypotension

7. Mr. Daniels weighs 83.92 kg. How many pounds does he weigh?
   A. 185 lb
   B. 195 lb
   C. 180 lb
   D. 200 lb
   E. 210 lb

8. The normal pulse rate (beats per minute) for adults is:
   A. 40–60
   B. 60–80
   C. 80–100
   D. 100–120
   E. 120–160

9. When taking an oral temperature, the thermometer should be left in the mouth for at least how many minutes?
   A. 3 minutes
   B. 5 minutes
   C. 10 minutes
   D. 12 minutes
   E. 15 minutes

10. When taking a rectal temperature, the thermometer should be left in the rectum for how many minutes?
   A. 3 minutes
   B. 5 minutes
   C. 10 minutes
   D. 12 minutes
   E. 15 minutes

CRITICAL THINKING

1. What should Mary say to Mr. Wade to relieve his anxiety?

2. Mary tries to measure the BP again after she has spoken to Mr. Wade and relayed the importance of the test. He begins to sweat profusely and is unable to remain still long enough for her to get an accurate reading. What should she do now?

3. What is considered the normal range for blood pressure? How does a patient's anxiety affect vital sign values?

4. Dr. Welch comes in, greets Mr. Wade, and begins to take his medical history and to get to know him. Mary hasn't told him about Mr. Wade's reaction to the blood pressure evaluation. How would you handle this situation?

5. How should Mary document the patient's chart?

ON THE JOB

Lakisha Smith is working in an OB/GYN clinic affiliated with a major teaching hospital. Her general responsibilities include registering patients, handling phone calls when the receptionist is on a break, escorting patients into the examination room, taking vital signs, running selected laboratory tests, setting up the clinic examination rooms for gynecological examinations, and providing patient education.

The morning's schedule of patients/visitors follows:

9:00 Adele Bishop   New mother checkup

9:15 Amy Campbell   First OB visit

9:30

9:45 Maria Lopez   OB patient in last month of pregnancy

10:00 Meg Rivers   Regular OB checkup

10:15 Vanessa Brown   New gynecology patient w/ovarian cyst

10:30

10:45 Tiffany Baker   Regular OB checkup

11:00 Vern Simmons   Pelvic inflammatory disease

11:15 Latonya Pike   1st visit after miscarriage

11:30 Emma Thompson Yearly check-up, gynecology patient

12:00 Lunch break

During the morning the following occurs:

When Maria Lopez arrives, she tells Lakisha that she has been bleeding since the weekend.

A pharmaceutical representative comes in at 10:00 A.M. and asks to see the doctor.

Supplies are delivered that must be signed for.

Dr. Williams is called away to perform a delivery at 11:00 A.M.

Vital signs including TPR, BP, and weight are taken for all OB patients.

Urinalysis is performed by another medical assistant assigned to the clinic laboratory.

What is your response?

1. How should Lakisha handle the pharmaceutical representative?
2. Should Maria Lopez's bleeding be considered an emergency? If so, what is Lakisha's responsibility?
3. What is the correct procedure for signing for and checking in medical supplies?
4. Since Dr. Williams was called away for a delivery, how should the patients be rescheduled? What about the patients who are already in the waiting room?

INTERNET ACTIVITY

Go to the American Heart Association website and look for dietary guidelines for hypertension.

 MediaLink More on the vital signs, including interactive resources, can be found on the Student CD-ROM accompanying this textbook.

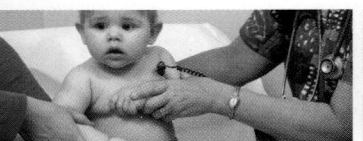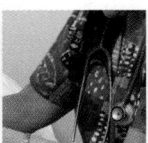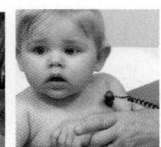

Medical Assistant Role Delineation Chart

HIGHLIGHT indicates material covered in this chapter.

ADMINISTRATIVE

Administrative Procedures

- Perform basic administrative medical assisting functions
- Schedule, coordinate and monitor appointments
- Schedule inpatient/outpatient admissions and procedures
- Understand and apply third-party guidelines
- Obtain reimbursement through accurate claims submission
- Monitor third-party reimbursement
- Understand and adhere to managed care policies and procedures
- *Negotiate managed care contracts*

Practice Finances

- Perform procedural and diagnostic coding
- Apply bookkeeping principles

- Manage accounts receivable
- *Manage accounts payable*
- *Process payroll*
- *Document and maintain accounting and banking records*
- *Develop and maintain fee schedules*
- *Manage renewals of business and professional insurance policies*
- *Manage personnel benefits and maintain records*
- *Perform marketing, financial, and strategic planning*

CLINICAL

Fundamental Principles

- Apply principles of aseptic technique and infection control
- Comply with quality assurance practices
- Screen and follow up patient test results

Diagnostic Orders

- Collect and process specimens
- Perform diagnostic tests

Patient Care

- Adhere to established patient screening procedures
- Obtain patient history and vital signs
- Prepare and maintain examination and treatment areas
- Prepare patient for examinations, procedures and treatments

- Assist with examinations, procedures and treatments
- Prepare and administer medications and immunizations
- Maintain medication and immunization records
- Recognize and respond to emergencies
- Coordinate patient care information with other health care providers
- Initiate IV and administer IV medications with appropriate training and as permitted by state law

GENERAL

Professionalism

- Display a professional manner and image
- Demonstrate initiative and responsibility
- Work as a member of the health care team
- Prioritize and perform multiple tasks
- Adapt to change
- Promote the CMA credential
- Enhance skills through continuing education
- Treat all patients with compassion and empathy
- Promote the practice through positive public relations

Communication Skills

- Recognize and respect cultural diversity
- Adapt communications to individual's ability to understand
- Use professional telephone technique

- Recognize and respond effectively to verbal, nonverbal, and written communications
- Use medical terminology appropriately
- Utilize electronic technology to receive, organize, prioritize and transmit information
- Serve as liaison

Legal Concepts

- Perform within legal and ethical boundaries
- Prepare and maintain medical records
- Document accurately
- Follow employer's established policies dealing with the health care contract
- Implement and maintain federal and state health care legislation and regulations
- Comply with established risk management and safety procedures
- Recognize professional credentialing criteria
- *Develop and maintain personnel, policy and procedure manuals*

Instruction

- Instruct individuals according to their needs
- Explain office policies and procedures
- Teach methods of health promotion and disease prevention
- Locate community resources and disseminate information
- *Develop educational materials*
- *Conduct continuing education activities*

Operational Functions

- Perform inventory of supplies and equipment
- Perform routine maintenance of administrative and clinical equipment
- Apply computer techniques to support office operations
- *Perform personnel management functions*
- *Negotiate leases and prices for equipment and supply contracts*

- *Denotes advanced skills.*

SOURCE: Reprinted by permission of the American Association of Medical Assistants from the AAMA Role Delineation Study: Occupational Analysis of the Medical Assisting Profession.

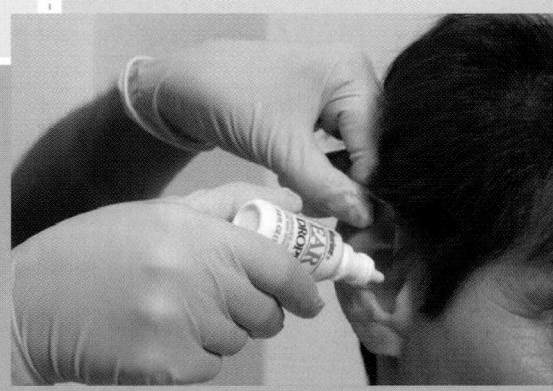

Assisting with Physical Examinations

Learning Objectives

After completing this chapter, you should be able to:

- Define and spell the terms to learn for this chapter.
- Discuss the steps to take in preparing a patient for a physical examination.
- List and describe nine patient examination positions that are used during a physical examination.
- Explain concepts of properly draping patients.
- Describe the six examination methods used by physicians.
- Recognize six pieces of equipment commonly used during a physical examination.
- List laboratory and diagnostic tests that may be ordered as part of a complete physical examination.
- Discuss the problem-oriented medical record.
- Describe the four components of the SOAP charting method.
- Explain the sequence of a routine physical examination.

OUTLINE

Preparing the Exam Room 632

Equipment and Supplies
Used for Physical
Examinations 634

Examination Methods
Used by the Physician 635

Adult Examination 639

Assisting the Physician
with a Physical Exam 640

Sequence of Examination
Procedures 645

Documentation of Patient
Medical Information 651

Terms to Learn

alopecia
amplify
auscultation
bimanual
chronological
goiter
goniometer
hirsutism
inspection
laryngeal mirror

manipulation
mensuration
objective
palpation
patellar
percussion
problem-oriented
medical record (POMR)
reflex hammer
scoliosis

SOAP
source-oriented medical
record (SOMR)
speculum
subjective
tongue depressor
tuning fork
turgor
vaginal speculum

Case Study

JERRY EVERSON, CMA, HAS BEEN ASSIGNED TO ASSIST DR. WILLIAMS with Mrs. Lewis's complete physical examination today. Her vital signs were T = 99.2, P = 62, R = 16, and BP = 148/92. There was cerumen (earwax) in the left ear, which Dr. Williams irrigated. Mrs. Lewis stated she is allergic to penicillin. Blood was drawn for a complete blood count (CBC), a urine specimen was sent to the lab, and a Pap test was done. Mrs. Lewis was also scheduled for a mammogram at the radiology facility.

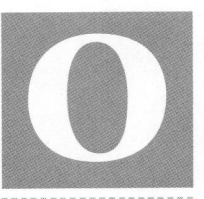One of the key responsibilities of the medical assistant is assisting the physician with a patient's physical exam. The medical assistant's role in the patient physical exam includes interviewing the patient, documenting patient information, preparing the exam room prior to the patient visit, positioning and draping the patient, assisting the physician during the examination, cleaning the room after the visit, and instrument care. Other duties include maintaining supplies, ensuring safety of patient and coworkers through adherence to infection control standards, observing confidentiality and patient privacy, and performing these functions in a professional, competent, empathetic manner. Chapter 33 covered information on patient interviewing, an overall discussion of the main components of a medical history, and guidelines for charting. This chapter will expand information on types of documentation formats and the process of patient physical examination.

Preparing the Exam Room

Preparing for the next patient begins immediately after the previous patient leaves the examining room. A medical assistant should never take a patient to an examination room that has not been cleaned. Patients do not want to watch a medical assistant clean the examination room, see items used on or by other patients, or be exposed to chemicals used to clean the examination room. Patients expect the examination room to be clean and clutter free. The medical assistant is responsible for cleaning the room between patients and preparing the room for each patient. (Refer to Lifespan Considerations.)

Immediately after the patient leaves the room, the used gown should be rolled up into a ball shape and placed in the laundry receptacle. If the used gown is disposable, it should also be rolled up into a ball shape but placed in the appropriate waste container. The used examination table paper and drape must also be removed by rolling it up into a ball shape and disposing of it in the appropriate waste container. By carefully rolling these items into a ball and keeping the contaminated items away from his or her uniform, the medical assistant prevents microorganism from being spread. After removing the used examination table paper, the medical assistant must clean the examination table, allow it to dry, and recover it with clean, new paper. The pillow cover should be disposed of following Universal Precautions and replaced with a new one. Disposable equipment used during the examination is discarded in the appropriate containers. Reusable equipment is taken (following Universal Precautions) to the appropriate area for cleaning and disinfection. All surfaces in the examination room should be disinfected with an appropriate cleaner to prepare the room for the next patient. There should be no evidence of any other patient's presence when a new patient is taken into an exam room. All biohazard containers should be closed, and, if full, the bag should be sealed and removed from the room to the appropriate holding area per Occupational Safety and Health Administration (OSHA) regulations. See Procedure 34-1, Cleaning the Examination Room.

Lifespan
Considerations

Care and consideration should be used when dealing with all patients; however, children, adolescents, and older adults may need additional assistance.

THE CHILD
Children require a little extra time and understanding. Explain in very simple, age-appropriate terms exactly what you want them to do, and plan to talk to the child during any special procedures.

THE ADOLESCENT
Adolescents may also require a little extra time. It is important for the medical assistant to take the time to ask adolescents questions and to get them involved with their medical care. Never use "baby talk" with adolescents because it offends them.

THE OLDER ADULT
Older adults tend to accept examinations as "necessary." Be sure to carefully explain the examination, in terms they understand, so that they are comfortable with what is expected. If older adults need help disrobing, be sure to protect their privacy while assisting them, and be very respectful of their need for modesty. Be sure there is a safe step when they need to climb up on the exam table. Providing a supporting hand will help to stabilize the patient when getting up and down from the table.

PROCEDURE

Cleaning the Examination Room

OBJECTIVE: Clean an examination room to instructor specifications.

Equipment and Supplies
disinfectant; paper towels; disposable gloves; examination table; pillow; disposable gown

Method
1. Perform hand hygiene.
2. Put on a clean pair of disposable gloves.
3. Roll soiled disposable gown into a ball shape and dispose of in the appropriate waste container.
4. Roll soiled examination table paper into a ball shape and dispose of in the appropriate waste container.
5. Remove soiled pillow cover and dispose of it in the appropriate waste container.
6. Remove any other soiled items or equipment from the examination room.
7. Clean examination table and cabinet surfaces with disinfectant and paper towels.
8. Dispose of soiled paper towels in the appropriate waste container.
9. Remove soiled gloves and dispose in the appropriate waste container.
10. Perform hand hygiene.
11. Put clean paper on the examination table.
12. Put a new pillow covering over the pillow.
13. Make sure the examination room is clean and clutter and odor free.

Examination Room Features

The number of examination rooms available to a physician varies depending on the medical office. If a physician has his or her own practice, there may be two to four examination rooms. A physician who belongs to a group practice may have only two examination rooms designated to him or her. Each medical office may have different types and sizes of rooms available (Figure 34-1). The standard examination room is most often used and is furnished with an examination table (with stirrups in a practice performing pelvic exams), a pillow, a footstool, a supply cupboard, a trash can, hazardous waste and sharps containers, a rolling stool, and a chair. Sometimes, a writing surface and a sink are also present. For specialist physicians, special chairs or other diagnostic equipment specific to the practice may also be present. Physicians in specialized practices such as ophthalmology will require specialized furniture and equipment.

The size of the examination room varies from medical office to medical office. Renting office space can be very expensive for a medical office, so rooms are often designed to be just big enough for the patient, the physician, the medical assistant, and the equipment discussed above. The examination room, however, should be spacious enough that the patient, the physician, and the medical assistant do not feel confined.

Examination Room Safety

Examination rooms must follow the standards required by the Americans with Disabilities Act (ADA). These standards address the width of doorways and hallways; placement of door handles, grab bars, and handrails; spatial accommodations for patients in wheelchairs; floor surfaces; and much more. For further information about the ADA Standards for Accessible Design visit www.usdoj.gov/crt/ada/stdspdf.htm.

If a medical assistant witnesses any unsafe situation, he or she should take care of the situation immediately. Examples of unsafe situations include clutter in the hallway or examination room, a spill on the floor, and an extension cord lying in the middle of a dirty utility room. A patient or staff member of the medical office could trip or slip on any of these items and be injured. All furniture in the examination room should be check routinely. Any item such as a broken drawer, a sharp

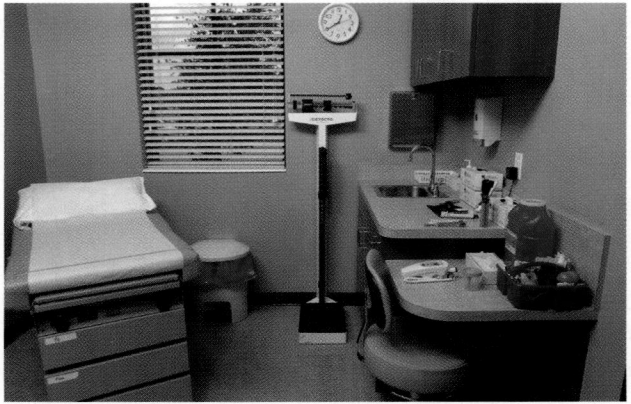

FIGURE 34-1 Examination room.

edge on the countertop, or a broken hinge on a door should be reported immediately. If it is unable to be repaired immediately, the medical assistant needs to document the situation in the maintenance log book.

Most examination rooms have electrical cords running from an outlet to a piece of medical equipment. There can also be cables running to a computer or other medical devices. It is important for the medical assistant to make sure all electrical cords and cables are secured to the floor or wall. Unsecured electrical cords or cables represent an unsafe situation for patients of medical office staff.

All instruments and equipment needed for the examination should be ready for the physician. This equipment should not be left within reach of the patient. If an examination light is present, the medical assistant is responsible for positioning the light so that it provides correct illumination for the physician, but not so that it could fall on the patient or cause a burn. Gooseneck lamps are especially prone to tipping over, so caution should be exercised.

Medical assistants should ensure their own safety by using proper body mechanics when moving or assisting patients. Proper body mechanics should be used in all aspects of patient care including front office work.

Patient Comfort

Patients often change into thin, disposable gowns while waiting for the physician, so the medical assistant needs to make sure the room is warm enough for the patient. Most medical offices keep the thermostat around 71°F to 73°F. If the thermostat is set on the reading established by the physician or office manager

Cultural Considerations

It is very important to be aware of the cultural norms of the patients seen in the office. Some cultures require that only members of the same sex be in the exam room during an examination, especially when disrobing is required. In working with individuals from other cultures, sometimes obtaining a clear history can be difficult, either due to language difficulties, or misunderstandings as to why the medical assistant is asking these questions. If the patient seems reluctant to answer questions, then notify the physician of the difficulty. The physician may be more successful in obtaining information due to cultural barriers.

and the patient is still cold, the medical assistant can give the patient a blanket, a sheet, or a disposable sheet to help keep warm. A patient may already be uncomfortable being in a thin, disposable gown and if also feeling cold, he or she can become anxious and agitated. This does not lead to a pleasant experience for the patient and is poor customer service.

When the patient enters the examination room, it should smell fresh and have been cleaned. A well-ventilated examination room can help decrease offensive odors. These offensive odors can come from sweat, urine, feces, vomit, blood, and infectious wounds. If there is an offensive odor in the examination room after the patient leaves, the medical assistant must find the item causing the offensive odor and properly dispose of it. If a chair smells from sweat it needs to be removed from the examination room and replaced with a new chair until the soiled chair is clean and ready to be used again. Items soaked in urine, feces, blood, and/or infectious waste will need to be double bagged and taken to the dirty utility room to be stored. When the medical assistant eliminates the sources of offensive odors, he or she can then concentrate on removing the offensive odor that may linger in the air. This can be accomplished by disinfecting all surfaces and using a room deodorizer and air freshener.

Patient Privacy

Patients expect privacy, especially when in the examination room. If a patient needs to wear a gown during the examination, the medical assistant must make sure one is available and explain to the patient whether it should open to the front or back. The medical assistant should also tell the patient where his or her clothes can be kept during the examination. Properly draping patients to protect their sense of modesty is vitally important to their sense of well-being during an examination. Draping techniques will be discussed fully later in this chapter. (Refer to Cultural Considerations.)

The medical assistant should never stay in the room with a patient who is disrobing unless the patient needs assistance. Once the medical assistant leaves the examination room, he or she should not reenter without knocking and receiving permission from the patient to enter. If a patient is in the middle of getting dressed and the medical assistant knocks and just walks in the examination room without permission, the patient may become very upset or embarrassed and, again, this is poor customer service.

Equipment and Supplies Used for Physical Examinations

The physician's hands are the primary tool used for the physical exam, but special instruments are also used to help with the exam and diagnosis. These include the ophthalmoscope, otoscope, reflex hammer, pinwheel, stethoscope, sphygmomanometer, tuning fork, laryngeal mirror, and tape measure. Supplies are generally considered disposable items that are replaced as they are used in the exam room. Refer to Figure 34-2 for examples of equipment and supplies necessary for a health examination.

Equipment

Here is a description of the equipment usually found in an examining room:

- Ophthalmoscope: The ophthalmoscope is used to examine the interior of the eye, especially the retina. Light is focused through a magnifying lens onto the inner surfaces of the eye to check for abnormalities. Position the patient in a sitting position and looking straight ahead during this exam. Chapter 36 of this text covers eye and ear examinations in detail.

- Otoscope: The otoscope is used to examine the ears. The light is focused through the disposable speculum to examine the outer ear, then the tympanic membrane (eardrum). A speculum is any instrument used to view a body cavity. The long, pointed speculum on the otoscope can be replaced with a short, wide disposable speculum for visualization of the lining of the nose and other internal structures of the nose.

- Reflex Hammer and Pinwheel: The reflex hammer is sometimes called a percussion hammer. It has a hard rubber, triangular head used for testing reflexes. This instrument is commonly used to check the patellar reflex of the knee and may also be used to check the reflex of the Achilles tendon (in the ankle) or the elbows. The pinwheel has sharp points and is used for testing sensory perception.

- Stethoscope: The stethoscope is used to amplify sounds in the body, such as the heart, lungs, and abdomen. It is made of two earpieces connected by rubber tubing to a chestpiece with a bell and/or diaphragm to amplify sound. Stethoscopes are discussed in more detail in Chapter 33.

- Sphygmomanometer: This is a blood pressure measuring device that may be portable or attached to the wall. Refer to Chapter 33 for further discussion of sphygmomanometers.

- Tuning fork: The tuning fork is a metal instrument that has with two prongs extending from the handle, designed to vibrate at a specific frequency. Tuning forks come in different sizes, and each size produces a different pitch level. The tuning fork is used to test the patient's hearing ability by making a humming sound that can be heard and felt when struck.

- Laryngeal mirror: The laryngeal mirror is a small mirror attached to a long handle that is used to visualize the larynx. Warming the laryngeal mirror can help prevent fogging. Warming can be done by using warmers, by running warm water over the mirror, or by briefly holding the mirror close to the exam light.

- Tape measure: A tape measure is used to measure a body part such as the chest or head in an infant and must be bendable and plastic. It should also indicate inches and centimeters.

Supplies

Supplies are the disposable items used for patient examination and treatment. Supplies include examination table paper, drapes and various dressings and bandages, tongue depressors, disposable gloves, both sterile and nonsterile, syringes and needles, and alcohol pads to name a few. A tongue depressor is a thin, flat, disposable wooden blade used to press down the tongue to observe the mouth and throat.

Ordering supplies and stocking the exam rooms are important to patient care and maintaining work flow. Delaying a procedure while you run for something that should have been there can put the patient at risk, delay schedules, and be annoying to all. An overall supply list is good office policy. Once an item is down to half a box or bottle, a new one should be placed in the exam room as a backup. An inventory system should contain the following information:

- List of supplies used in your facility
- Each supplier's name, address, telephone number, and contact person
- Amount of each supply used monthly
- How often to reorder

Refer to Table 34-1 for descriptions of additional supplies and equipment commonly present in exam rooms.

Examination Methods Used by the Physician

The hands of the physician are used during the various methods of examination. Some of these methods require pieces of equipment to be used as well. There are six commonly used methods of physical examination: inspection, palpation, percussion, auscultation, mensuration, and manipulation. As the physician enters the room, these methods of examination are already in use. As the physician is greeting the patient, he or she is evaluating speech, social response, and general behavior. Once the review of systems (ROS) begins, many of the following examination methods are employed—some at

Supplies		Purpose
Flashlight or penlight	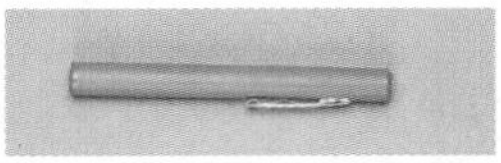	To assist viewing of the pharynx and cervix or to determine the reactions of the pupils of the eye
Laryngeal or dental mirror	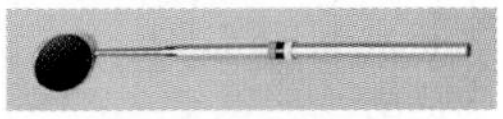	To observe the pharynx and oral cavity
Nasal speculum	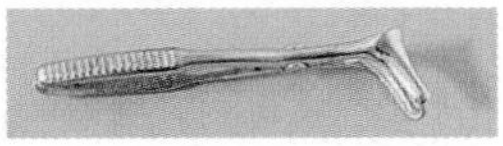	To permit visualization of the lower and middle turbinates; usually, a penlight is used for illumination
Ophthalmoscope	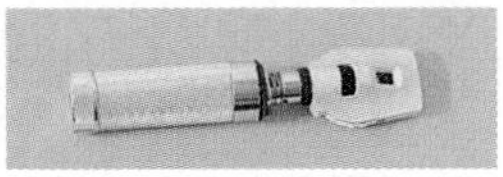	A lighted instrument to visualize the interior of the eye
Otoscope	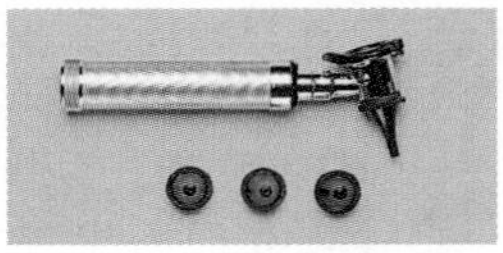	A lighted instrument to visualize the eardrum and external auditory canal (a nasal speculum may be attached to the otoscope to inspect the nasal cavities)
Percussion (reflex) hammer	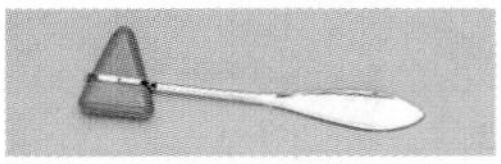	An instrument with a rubber head to test reflexes
Tuning fork	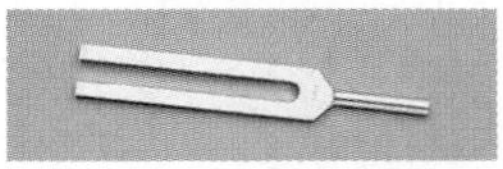	A two-pronged metal instrument used to test hearing acuity and vibratory sense
Vaginal speculum	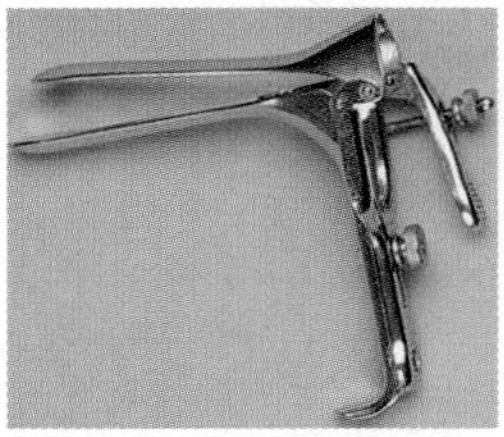	To assess the cervix and the vagina
Cotton applicators	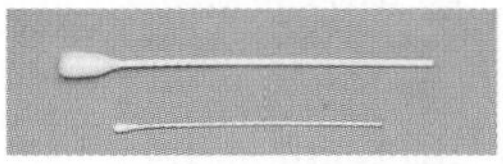	To obtain specimens
Disposable pads	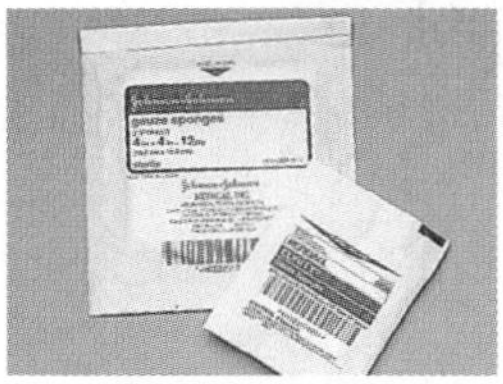	To absorb liquid
Gloves	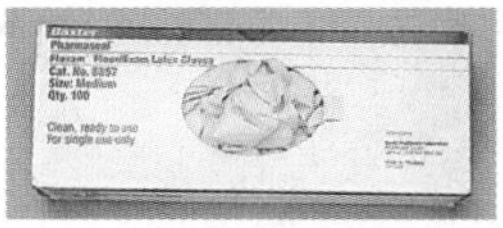	To protect the nurse
Lubricant	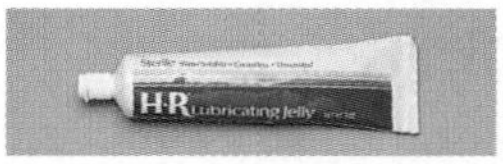	To ease insertion of instruments (e.g., vaginal speculum)
Tongue blades (depressors)	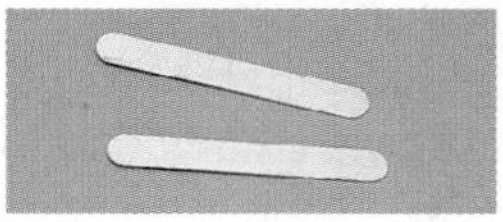	To depress the tongue during assessment of the mouth and pharynx

FIGURE 34-2 Equipment and supplies used for a health examination.

TABLE 34-1 Typical Examining Room Equipment and Supplies

Equipment/Supply	Use
Alcohol wipes	Disinfect and cleanse skin before injections and phlebotomy.
Balance scale	Take patient's weight and height.
Bandages (small)	Applied after taking blood sample and some injections.
Batteries and light bulbs	Extra batteries and light bulbs are required for lighted equipment.
Betadine (or other topical antiseptic)	Used to disinfect skin before minor surgery.
Biohazard waste container	Closed rigid container with biohazardous labeling and appropriate red waste bags.
Cotton balls (sterile and nonsterile)	Used to apply antiseptic or to clean the skin.
Cotton-tipped swabs (sterile and nonsterile)	Used to clean recessed areas, to apply medications and lubricant, and to obtain specimens from the throat and other orifices.
Drapes	Disposable paper or cloth sheet used to cover patient during examination.
Emesis basin	Kidney-shaped receptacle for body drainage, such as sputum, and for used instruments.
Fixative spray	Used to preserve slides.
Gauze dressings (4 × 4 or 3 × 4)	Applied to dress small wounds.
Gloves (nonsterile disposable)	Worn by all staff to protect against microorganisms and bloodborne pathogens.
Gloves (sterile disposable)	Worn when performing minor surgery and handling sterile materials.
Gooseneck lamp	Movable light used to focus on a body area for increased visibility.
Hydrogen peroxide (H_2O_2)	Used to clean open wounds.
Irrigation syringe	Used to wash cerumen (earwax) out of ear canal or to irrigate wounds.
Lubricant	Water-soluble gel applied to physician's glove, speculum, or rectal thermometer to reduce friction during insertion. Prevents damage to delicate mucous membranes.
Soap dispenser	Used to dispense germicidal soap for hand washing between each patient.
Sphygmomanometer	Machine used to measure blood pressure.
Tape	Used to secure dressings.
Tape measure	Measure lesions, head circumference, body measurements.
Thermometers of various types	Measure temperature.
Tissues	Wipe body secretions.
Tongue depressor	Wooden blade used to hold patient's tongue down while examining mouth and throat.
Vaginal speculum	Instrument used to expand vaginal opening to view cervix.

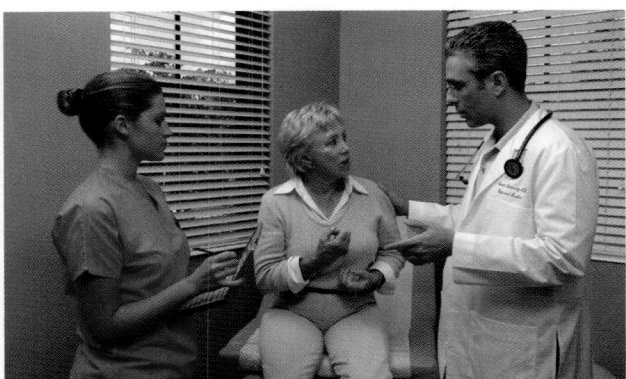

FIGURE 34-3 Inspection is one method of examination used in a health exam.

Palpation

Palpation is performed by using the hands to feel the skin and accessible underlying organs. Other areas examined by palpation include the axilla (armpits), neck, and chest. Palpation is used to determine any unusual tenderness, size, shape, and texture. Oftentimes, abnormalities and masses in the abdomen can be discovered through palpation. Refer to Figure 34-4 for examples of light palpation using one hand and bimanual, or two-handed, deep palpation.

Percussion

Percussion refers to use of the fingertips to tap the body lightly but sharply to gain information about the position and size of the underlying body parts, To do this, two fingers of one hand are placed on the patient's skin and then struck with the index and middle finger of the other hand. The physician uses his or her fingers to percuss the chest wall and abdomen by gentle thumping or tapping, which produces a standard sound or vibrations. An alteration of this sound or vibration aids in determining the presence of fluid or pus in a cavity. Figure 34-5 illustrates percussion on a patient's back.

the same time. All contribute salient information about the patient's general overall health.

Inspection

A physician inspects the patient by visually examining the exterior surface of the body. At the same time the general state of health, overall demeanor, grooming, and social interactions are observed. Some interior portions of the body, including the throat, eyes, ears, vaginal wall, cervix, and rectum may be inspected using special instruments. Notes are made of any unusual color, size, shape, position, or symmetry of the areas being inspected (Figure 34-3).

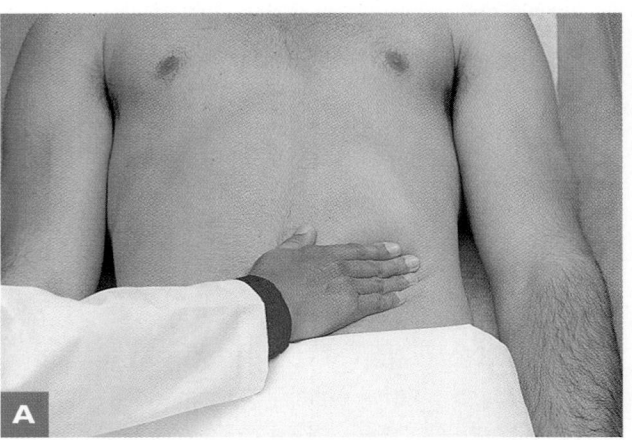

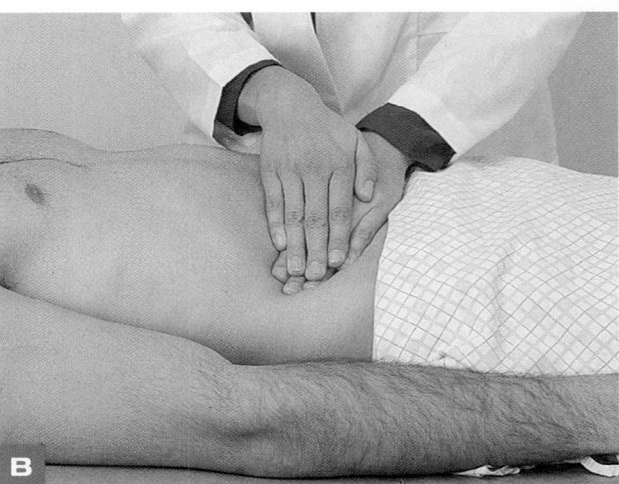

FIGURE 34-4 (A) An example of light palpation of the abdomen. (B) The physician uses two hands for deep bimanual palpation.

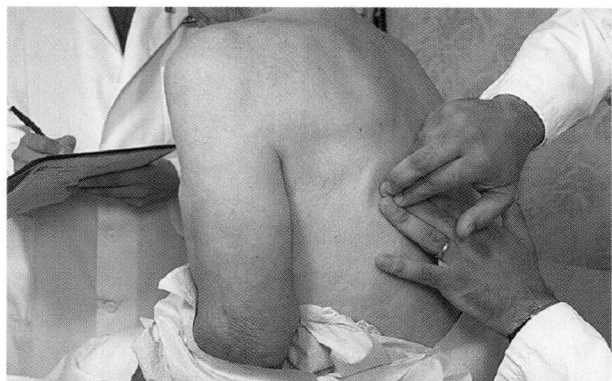

FIGURE 34-5 The physician uses percussion—tapping—to detect sound or vibration.

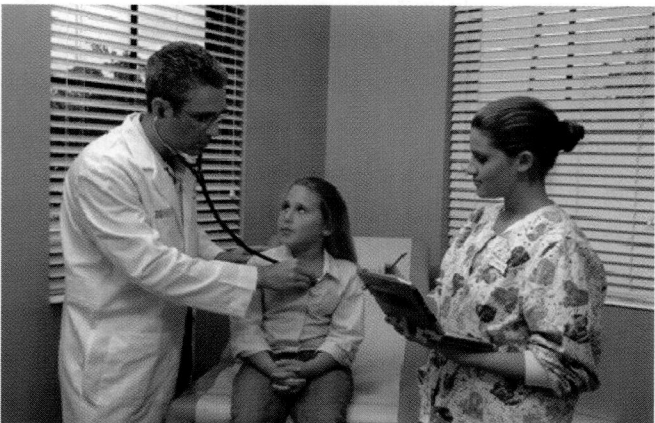

FIGURE 34-7 The physician uses auscultation to listen to a patient's heart.

The reflex hammer is used to test the reflexes of the body. As part of the neurological test, the physician gently taps the reflex hammer once against the tendon reflex at the bottom of the patellar (kneecap) bone (Figure 34-6).

Auscultation

Auscultation means to listen to sounds that are found within the body. Sounds made by the heart, lungs, stomach, and bowel are assessed for strength, presence or absence, and rhythm. These sounds must be differentiated from normal body sounds by the physician. These sounds can be heard by using the auscultation method of examination (Figure 34-7). A stethoscope is usually used to amplify (make louder) body sounds; however, auscultation can also be performed by placing the ear directly over the body surface.

Mensuration

Mensuration is the use of special tools to measure the body or specific parts. These special tools include a scale, tape measure, and calipers. To determine a patient's weight, a scale is used. A tape measure would be used to determine a patient's height, to measure an infant's head and chest circumference and the abdomen, the diameter of a limb, the length of a limb, or the length and width of a wound. A goniometer is used to measure range of motion of a joint (Figure 34-8). Calipers are used to determine the amount of body fat.

Manipulation

Manipulation is passively assessing the range of motion of a joint. When a physician is performing this examination method, he or she may palpate the joint for abnormalities and warmth. Neurologists and orthopedists may use this method to evaluate patients who want to return to work after accidents or illness or for insurance company's records.

Adult Examination

Patient visits to physician offices are scheduled for a variety of reasons, including illness, emergency, and routine checkups. Typically a physical examination is

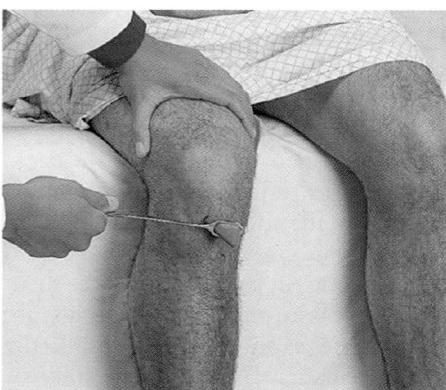

FIGURE 34-6 Testing the patellar reflex with a percussion hammer.

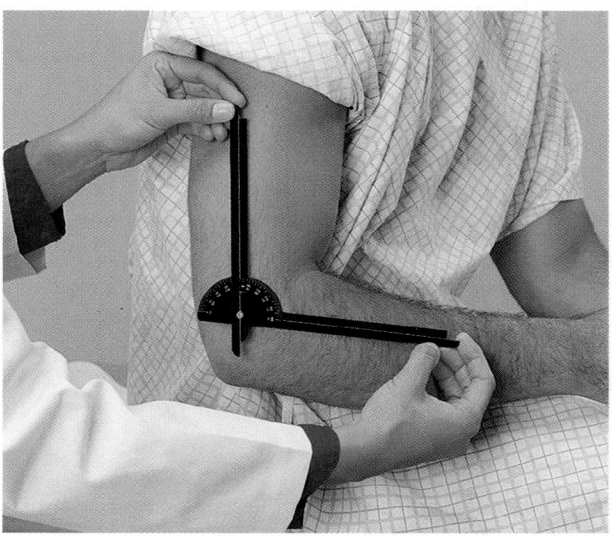

FIGURE 34-8 Mensuration—physician uses a goniometer to measure range of motion in a joint.

done as part of each visit. The length, extent, and type of exam will be determined by the reason for the visit and the specialty of the physician. The purpose of the physical examination is to assess as much of the body as possible during the visit to help diagnose new diseases and to measure the effectiveness of the current plan of care of previously diagnosed issues. The physical examination may also include laboratory and diagnostic tests, such as blood work and x-rays.

Oftentimes, patients will have a routine physical examination with no presenting, or chief, complaint. This is a time when it is especially important for the physician to have up-to-date medical records to compare the current physical exam with previous ones. The physician will be looking for weight changes, blood pressure variances, or other conditions requiring more frequent evaluations.

Other patients will be seen by the physician to diagnose a problem. The physician will analyze the information gained during the physical exam and combine it with the past medical history, laboratory findings, and other medical information to determine a diagnosis. Only the physician may actually diagnose a condition. The medical assistant's role in this process is to assist the physician in obtaining correct, current data.

Sometimes, the symptoms a patient demonstrates can be indicative of more than one diagnosis. At this time, the physician will have to make a differential diagnosis. The physician will then begin to rule out (R/O) diagnoses in an attempt to determine the most correct one. It is important to remember that when coding for insurance purposes, the R/O diagnosis may not be used. The actual diagnosis must be used.

Assisting the Physician with a Physical Exam

The physician, not the medical assistant, will actually perform the physical examination, but the medical assistant will help the physician in the following ways:

1. Position and drape the patient for examination. If the patient is elderly or has a disability, then help the patient to maintain the correct position.

2. Hand instruments, equipment, and other medical supplies to the physician.

3. Document and label specimens.

4. Offer reassurance to the patient.

5. Act as a witness to the behavior of the physician and the patient.

6. Carry out treatment plans, such as providing patient education, applying dressings, and administering medications.

7. Schedule diagnostic tests as ordered by the physician.

Table 34-2 lists the methods and equipment used to examine the areas/parts of the body during a complete physical examination.

Patient Preparation

Patient preparation consists of obtaining the patient's medical history, acquiring the chief complaint, measuring vital signs including height and weight, and assisting the patient to prepare for the visit with the physician. For specific information in obtaining vital signs, see Chapter 33. All vital signs should be entered on the chart prior to the time the physician sees the patient.

The patient's level of anxiety should be assessed. If the patient seems extremely nervous or ill at ease, then the medical assistant must attempt to allow the patient to express these feelings. Unusual nervousness should be reported to the physician.

It is important for the medical assistant to prepare the patient for any task or procedure before it is performed in the medical clinic. Each task or procedure must be communicated to the patient in a warm, caring, simple, and direct manner. Patients are usually more cooperative when approached in this manner. Elderly, frail patients and children should not be left unattended. If the medical assistant is unable to remain in the room, a family member should be asked to sit with the patient until the doctor begins the examination.

Depending on the physician's and patient's gender, a medical assistant may be requested during certain examinations. For example, if a male physician needs to perform a gynecological examination, he would request a female medical assistant to be in the examination room to serve as a witness. This method protects both the physician and patient from accusations of unethical behavior.

Patients should be requested to empty their bladder prior to undressing, and instructions for obtaining a urine sample should be given when required. Obtaining urine specimens will be fully discussed in Chapter 42 of this text. Be sure that patients know how to find their way back to the appropriate exam room from the restroom. All specimen collection containers should be appropriately labeled.

The medical assistant should provide a patient gown and drape for all examinations. Depending on the type of exam, all clothing, including underwear, should be removed, and the patient should wear the patient gown. It is especially important to be sure that the patient knows whether to leave the gown open at the front or the back. For problem-specific exams, only part of the clothing (such as all clothing above the waist) may need to be removed. In this case, patient gowns and drapes should still be provided. Depending on patient needs, the medical assistant may need to assist the patient with disrobing or climbing onto the exam table. Be especially cautious when assisting patients onto a step stool or other step to access the table, because this is a time when accidental falls may happen.

Area	Body Part	Method/Equipment
Head	Skull, hair, scalp	Inspection and palpation
Ears	Ear canals, eardrum	Inspection with otoscope and tuning fork
Eyes	Visual acuity	Vision chart, Snellen eye chart Inspection with ophthalmoscope
Nose	Nasal passages	Inspection with otoscope and nasal speculum
Mouth and throat (pharynx)	Mucous membranes, lips, gums, teeth, tongue, pharynx	Inspection with laryngeal mirror, flashlight, tongue blade Palpation and inspection
Neck	Thyroid gland, trachea, and cervical lymph nodes; carotid artery	Palpation, auscultation, and inspection
Back and spine	Muscles, spinal cord	Inspection, palpation, and percussion
Chest and lungs	Heart, lungs	Stethoscope Inspection, percussion, palpation, and auscultation
Breasts	Breast tissue, nipples	Palpation
Heart	Heart sounds, apical pulse	Auscultation with stethoscope
Abdomen	Bowel sounds Symmetry Presence of air masses, enlargement Uterus	Auscultation Inspection Percussion Palpation Palpation Stethoscope
Inguinal area	Inguinal nodes hernia	Palpation
Genitalia	*Female:* cervix and vagina *Male:* penis, scrotum, prostate gland	Inspection using vaginal speculum Palpation
Rectal	Anus Rectum	Inspection Inspection using proctoscope
Legs	Circulation Pulse sites	Inspection Palpation
Musculoskeletal system	Muscle strength Gait abnormalities	Inspection Palpation
Neurological examination	Reflexes	Percussion hammer, pinwheel

Professional etiquette demands that the medical assistant and other office personnel always knock and wait for a response before entering a patient room. This prevents surprising a patient, and ensures patient comfort at all times. Be sure to keep the doors of exam rooms closed while patients are waiting to provide for patient privacy and respect.

Draping the Patient

Drapes are sheets used to protect patient privacy and keep the patient warm. When used properly, they cover all but the part of the patient being examined. Typically, drapes are smaller than bed sheets, although they are often made of the same material or may be disposable. Protecting a patient's modesty as much as possible

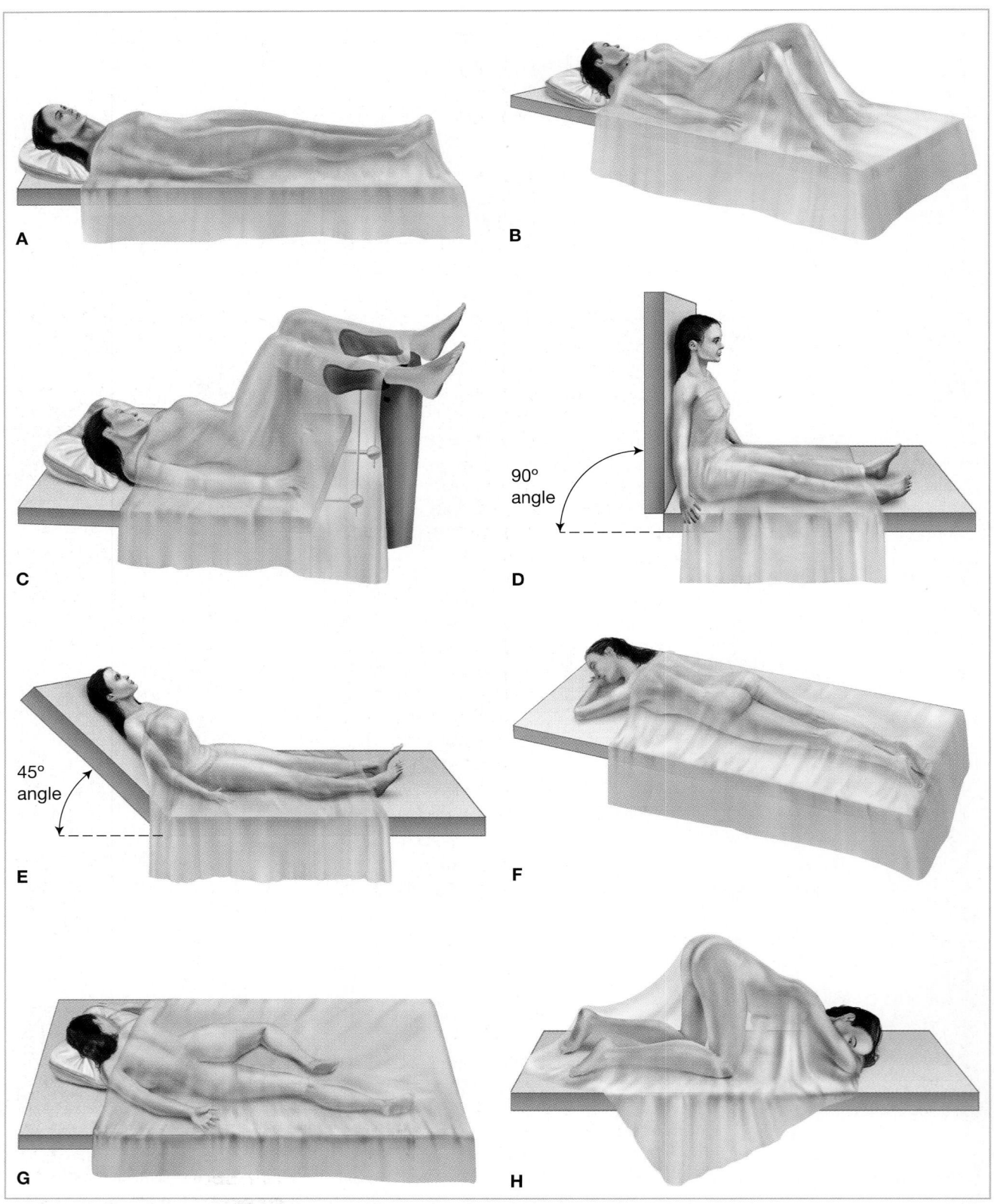

FIGURE 34-9 (A) The supine or horizontal recumbent position. (B) Dorsal recumbent position. (C) Lithotomy position. (D) Fowler's position. (E) Semi-Fowler's position. (F) Prone position. (G) Sims' or lateral position. (H) Knee-chest position.

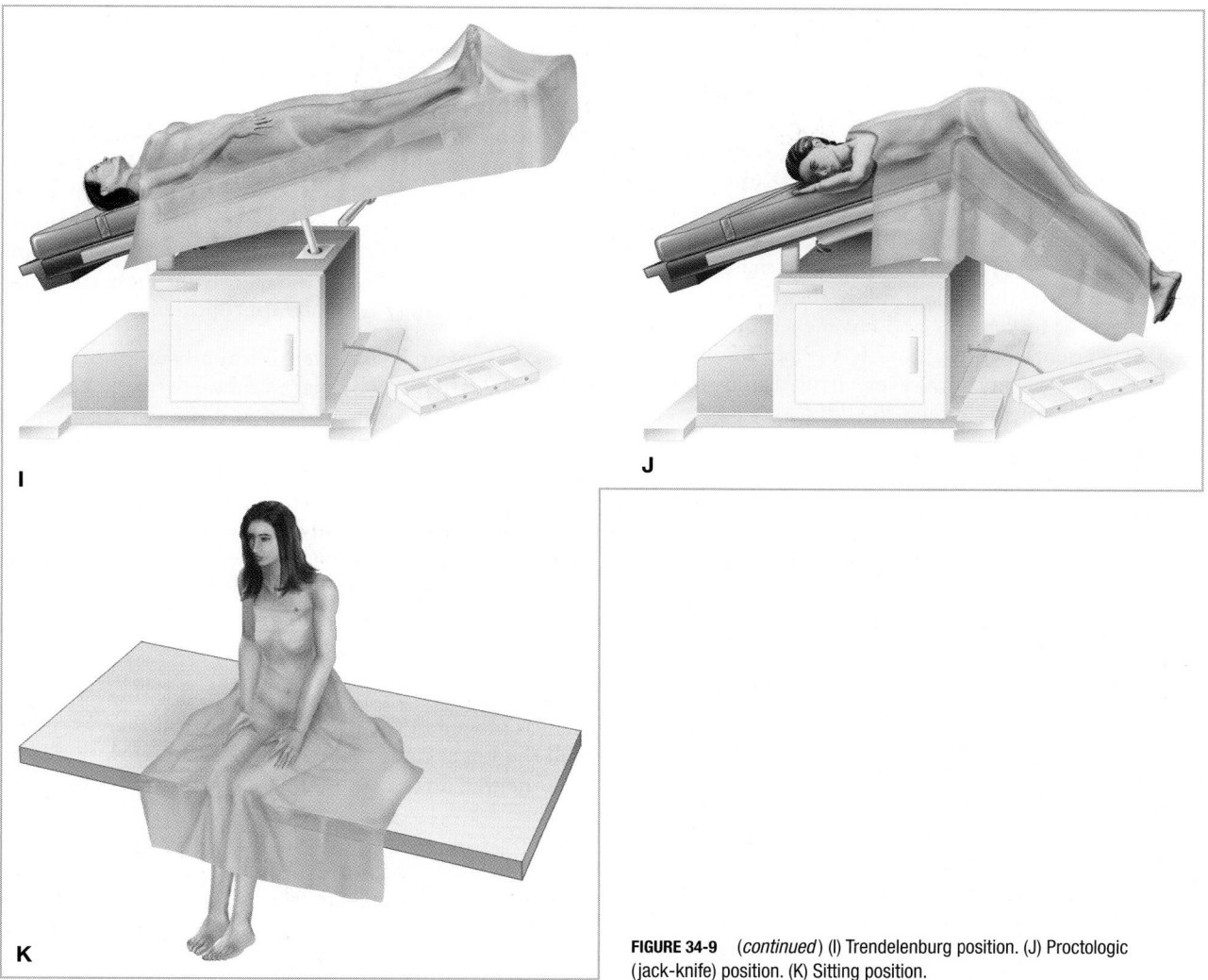

FIGURE 34-9 (*continued*) (I) Trendelenburg position. (J) Proctologic (jack-knife) position. (K) Sitting position.

is important to ensure patient comfort and compliance with uncomfortable positions and examinations. However, the drape must not obstruct the visibility of the physician or interfere with the examination.

During sterile procedures, sterile drapes may be used to protect the surgical area from contamination and to provide a sterile surface for instruments, suture materials, and dressings. They also function to protect the patient from blood or drainage during the procedure. Sterile drapes will be placed around a surgical site in such a manner to expose only the site of incision using sterile surgical technique.

Positioning the Patient

The medical assistant will help the physician with the physical examination by positioning the patient. Nine standard positions are used for a variety of medical and surgical examinations and procedures. They are supine or horizontal recumbent, dorsal recumbent, lithotomy, Fowler's, semi-Fowler's, prone, Sims', knee-chest, and Trendelenburg. Complete familiarity with each position

is necessary. As a medical assistant you will need to give patients clear directions on how to assume each position while gently guiding them and protecting their safety. If a patient must turn from back to stomach or vice versa, always be sure to stand alongside the exam table and have the patient turn toward you so you can prevent him or her from falling off the exam table. Each position will be considered in the following paragraphs.

SUPINE In the supine position, also known as the horizontal recumbent position, the patient lies flat on his or her back with hands at the sides (Figure 34-9A). Be sure that the patient's feet are supported by extending the table. This position is used to examine anything on the anterior or ventral surface of the body (head, chest, stomach, etc.) and for certain types of x-rays. The patient should be draped from the chest, down over the feet. You will expose any areas necessary during the exam as indicated by the physician. This position may not be comfortable for patients who are short of breath or who have lower back problems. Placing a pillow under their heads and under knees may be more comfortable for them.

DORSAL RECUMBENT   In this position the patient is lying flat on the back with knees bent and feet flat on the table (Figure 34-9B). This position relieves strain on the lower back and relaxes abdominal muscles. The dorsal recumbent position is used to inspect the head, neck, chest, and vaginal, rectal, or perineal areas. This position can be used for digital exams of the vagina and rectum. To drape the patient, place the drape at the patient's neck or underarms and cover the body down to the feet. Patients with leg problems may find this uncomfortable. Patients with severe arthritis may find this position more tolerable than the lithotomy position.

LITHOTOMY   The lithotomy position is similar to the dorsal recumbent position except the patient's feet are placed in stirrups attached to the side of the table (Figure 34-9C). The stirrups must be locked in place. The patient may need assistance placing her feet in the stirrup. After the feet are in place in the stirrups, the patient is instructed to slide down until buttocks are positioned at the edge of the table. The patient is draped from under the arms to the ankles. This position is used for vaginal examinations requiring the use of a vaginal speculum (instrument to hold open the walls of the vagina) and for Pap smears.

It is uncomfortable for the patient to maintain this position for any length of time, therefore the patient's feet should not be placed in stirrups until the physician is in the room and ready to begin the vaginal examination. Patients with severe arthritis or those who are severely obese or at the end of pregnancy may find this position impossible. The dorsal recumbent may be used instead with physician permission.

FOWLER'S   In this position the patient sits on the examination table with the head of the table raised to a 90-degree angle (Figure 34-9D). If the patient is able, he or she may be seated on the edge of the table with feet over the edge in an upright position. This position is useful for examinations of the head, neck, and upper body. Patients who have difficulty breathing in the supine position may find this position more comfortable. The drape should be placed over the patient's lap covering the legs.

SEMI-FOWLER'S   The semi-Fowler's position is similar to the Fowler's position but the head of the table is at a 45-degree angle (Figure 34-9E) instead of 90. This position is used for post surgical exams, patients with breathing difficulties or those suffering from general malaise. The drape should be placed over the patient's lap covering the legs. Fowler's or semi-Fowler's positions are more comfortable for patients with lower back injury or breathing difficulties.

PRONE   The prone position requires the patient to lie face down, flat on the stomach or the ventral surface of the body, with the head turned to the side and arms either alongside the body or crossed under the head (Figure 34-9F). It is the opposite of the supine position. The drape should cover the patient from upper back to over the feet. This position is used for back exams and certain types of surgery. The prone position is unsuitable for patients with breathing problems, women in late-term pregnancies, or the elderly. In these cases the Sims' position may be more appropriate.

SIMS'   The Sims' or lateral recumbent position requires the patient to be placed on the left side with the right leg sharply bent upward and the left leg slightly bent (Figure 34-9G). The patient's weight is mainly on the chest area. The right arm is flexed next to the head for support. The patient is draped from under arm to below the knees on an angle. This allows the physician to raise a small section of the drape while keeping the rest of patient covered. This position is used for rectal exams, rectal temperatures, enemas, and perineal and pelvic exams.

KNEE-CHEST   In the knee-chest position, the patient is placed in the prone position and then asked to pull the knees up to a kneeling position with thighs at a 90-degree angle to the table and buttocks in the air (Figure 34-9H). The head is turned to one side and arms may be placed under the head or on either side of the head for comfort and support. Most patients need assistance to assume this position correctly and should never be left unattended in this position at any time. It is uncomfortable and embarrassing, so the patient should not be made to assume the knee-chest position until necessary during the examination. This position is used for proctologic exams, sigmoidoscopy procedures, and rectal and vaginal exams. The drape should be placed from upper back at an angle covering the anal area. A fenestrated drape (a drape with a precut opening in the appropriate area) may be used. Many physicians have proctologic tables available for this type of exam. This specialized exam table can be elevated in the middle, which places the patient so he or she is bent at the hips with head and feet lowered. It is much easier on the patient than the knee-chest position.

TRENDELENBURG   This position is not normally used in a physician's office except in cases of shock or low blood pressure. For this position the patient is placed in the supine position and the end of the table is raised to about a 30-degree angle with the patient's legs bent at the knees over the end of the table (Figure 34-9I). This position is also used for abdominal surgeries. The patient is draped from underarms to below the knees.

PROCTOLOGIC The proctologic (jack-knife) position is used for proctologic examinations with a sigmoidoscope. It is similar to the knee-chest position, but with a greater bend at hips (Figure 34-9J). Patients will lie face down with hips at hinge of table. A special exam table may then be tipped downward.

SITTING This position is used to examine the head and chest (anterior and posterior). The patient sits upright with legs over the side of the examination table (Figure 34-9K).

Always explain to the patient why he or she is being placed in a specific position and the purpose of the drapes. Be sure that the patient is never left in an uncomfortable position any longer than is necessary, and assist the patient when a position change is required. Some of the positions can be very embarrassing to a patient. A medical assistant must be professional at all times to prevent the patient from being uncomfortable and self-conscious. A patient will be less embarrassed if the medical assistant explains why the patient needs to be in that particular position; therefore, it is essential for a medical assistant to understand why it is necessary to place a patient in a certain position for a specific procedure. Physicians expect the medical assistant to have the patient in the correct position for a procedure. The patient will also think the medical assistant does not know what he or she is doing; this can cause the patient to lose trust and faith in you as a medical assistant and possibly cause the patient to become more apprehensive than he or she is already. (Refer to Patient Education.)

Some examinations and positions may be uncomfortable to a patient. The medical assistant must always explain to the patient the events that will occur during the physical examination. This allows the patient time to prepare as well as to ask any questions. The medical assistant must also be truthful when preparing a patient for a physical examination. If a certain part of the physical examination is going to make the patient uncomfortable, the medical assistant must be honest and explain this to the patient so the patient can be prepared and more willing to cooperate during the physical examination. For example, if a female patient is having a Pap smear, the medical assistant needs to explain to the patient that when the physician inserts the vaginal speculum into the vagina she might feel some pressure in that area. How do you think the patient would feel if the medical assistant never told her that this might happen? The patient could feel angry and upset. The patient may not trust the medical assistant anymore because the medical assistant did not tell her what could be happening to her and her body. This is just one example of how a patient could be made uncomfortable when the medical assistant is not communicating effectively with the patient.

Some positions are also uncomfortable to patients because of health reasons. If a patient has low back pain, he or she may not be able to sit for a long time. If a patient with COPD is in the supine position and having difficulties breathing, the medical assistant should immediately help the patient to a semi-Fowler's position so he or she can breathe better. When a medical assistant is aware of the patient's medical history, he or she can make the patient more comfortable.

Laboratory and Diagnostic Tests

Laboratory and other diagnostic tests may be ordered as an adjunct to the physician's exam. Some of these tests, such as a urinalysis or electrocardiogram, may be conducted in the office on the day of the examination, and others, such as x-rays, may be scheduled by appointment with a separate laboratory or diagnostic facility. Table 34-3 gives examples of tests that might be ordered as part of a complete examination.

Sequence of Examination Procedures

Individual physicians will instruct their medical assistant as to the specific order of the physical examination. Typically, they will discuss the past medical history, chief complaint and the history of the current illness first, and then do a review of systems (ROS), a

TABLE 34-3 Laboratory and Diagnostic Tests

Tests	Description
Blood chemistry profile	Package (or panel) of chemistry tests that provides overview of patient's body chemistries. Less expensive than performing individual tests
SMA-12 (or Chem 12)	Panel of 12 chemistry tests
SMAC (or Chem 20)	Panel of 20 tests
Complete blood count (CBC) including a differential count	Includes red blood count (RBC), white blood count (WBC), hemoglobin (Hg), hematocrit (Hct), RBC indices, platelets, and differential. The differential count indicates abnormalities of RBCs, platelets, and types of WBCs
Electrocardiogram (ECG/EKG)	Record of electrical activity of the heart. Useful in diagnosis of heart muscle damage causing disruption of electrical activity of the heart and abnormal cardiac rhythm
Pulmonary function test (PFT)	Breathing equipment used to determine respiratory function and measure lung volume and gas exchange
Sedimentation rate (Sed rate, ESR)	Measures the rate at which erythrocytes (RBCs) settle out of blood in 1 hour. Inflammatory conditions will cause RBCs to settle faster since they are heavier and the Sed rate will be higher than normal
Visual acuity	Sharpness of vision
Vital signs	Measurements of signs of life, which include temperature, pulse, respirations, and blood pressure
Weight and height	Anthropometric measurements of the human body
X-rays	Radiology studies of body parts (for example, chest and spine)

head-to-toe exam, but this will vary among physicians. The following is a common sequence for an examination: skin→hair→nails→head→neck→eyes→ears →nose→mouth→throat→arms→heart→chest→lungs →breasts→abdomen→genitalia→rectum→legs→feet→ neurological system. Figure 34-10 is an example of a ROS sheet that will be documented by the physician as this portion of the exam is completed. Refer to Procedure 34-2 for steps required to assist with a complete physical examination. During the examination the physician will wear the appropriate personal protective equipment (PPE).

A word about medical terminology and abbreviations is appropriate before considering individual sections of the review of systems. Every medical assistant must have excellent medical terminology skills and be thoroughly familiar with correct usage and spelling of abbreviations. The proper usage, pronunciation, and spelling of medical terms are critical to your functioning professionally as a medical assistant. If you encounter words you are unsure of, look them up when time permits. Never guess at the meaning. When reading a

physician's order and you are unsure of the abbreviation used, look it up or ask. While many terms and abbreviations are fairly generic and widely used, others pertain to specific specialties and may be unfamiliar.

Review of Systems

- Skin: The physician will inspect and palpate the skin, taking special note of the condition of the skin. This is an important aspect of the physical examination because it can indicate the patient's nutritional status and level of hydration. The color, temperature, texture, and turgor of the skin are assessed. Turgor refers to the resistance of the skin when grasped between fingers. Turgor is decreased in dehydration and increased in edema.

- Hair: The color, texture, distribution, quantity, and growth pattern of the hair are assessed. Certain diseases such as hyperthyroidism can cause alopecia (hair loss). Excessive facial hair in a female is known as hirsutism and may indicate hormonal imbalance.

REVIEW OF SYSTEMS

Name _____ **Date** _____
Doctor's notes _____

MUSCULOSKELETAL
1. _____ aching muscles or joints
2. _____ swollen joints
3. _____ back or shoulder pains
4. _____ painful feet
5. _____ handicapped

SKIN
6. _____ skin problems
7. _____ itching or burning skin
8. _____ bleeds easily
9. _____ bruises easily

NEUROLOGICAL
10. _____ faintness
11. _____ numbness
12. _____ convulsions
13. _____ change in handwriting
14. _____ trembles

MOOD
15. _____ nervous with strangers
16. _____ difficulty in making decisions
17. _____ lack of concentration or memory
18. _____ lonely or depressed
19. _____ cries often
20. _____ hopeless outlook
21. _____ difficulty relaxing
22. _____ worries a lot
23. _____ frightening dreams or thoughts
24. _____ shy or sensitive
25. _____ dislikes criticism
26. _____ loses temper
27. _____ annoyed by little things
28. _____ work or family problems
29. _____ sexual difficulties
30. _____ considered suicide
31. _____ desired psychiatric help

GENERAL
32. _____ weight changes
33. _____ tends to be hot or cold
34. _____ loss of interest in eating
35. _____ always hungry
36. _____ more thirsty lately
37. _____ armpits or groin swelling
38. _____ fatigue
39. _____ sleeping difficulties
40. _____ exercises less than 3 times per week
41. _____ cigarettes——cigars/pipes——don't smoke
42. _____ two or more alcoholic drinks per day
43. _____ over 6 cups of coffee/tea per day
44. _____ uses sleeping pills, marijuana, tranquilizers
45. _____ has used hard drugs
46. _____ drives vehicle over 25,000 miles per year
47. _____ never——sometimes——always wears seat belts
48. _____ visited in the last 6 months

DIGESTIVE
49. _____ heartburn
50. _____ bloated stomach
51. _____ belching
52. _____ stomach pains
53. _____ nausea
54. _____ vomited blood
55. _____ difficulty swallowing
56. _____ constipation
57. _____ loose bowels
58. _____ black stools
59. _____ grey stools
60. _____ pain in rectum
61. _____ rectal bleeding

URINARY
62. _____ night frequency
63. _____ day frequency
64. _____ wets pants or bed
65. _____ burning on urination
66. _____ brown, black or bloody urine
67. _____ difficulty starting urine
68. _____ urgency

MALE GENITAL
69. _____ weak urine stream
70. _____ prostate trouble
71. _____ burning or discharge
72. _____ lumps on testicles
73. _____ painful testicles

FEMALE GENITAL
74. __/__/__ last menstrual period
75. _____ post-menopausal or hysterectomy
76. _____ noticed vaginal bleeding
77. _____ abnormal LMP
78. _____ heavy bleeding during periods
79. _____ bleeding between periods
80. _____ bleeding after intercourse
81. _____ recent vaginal itching/discharge
82. _____ no monthly breast exam
83. _____ lump or pain in breasts
84. _____ complications with birth control
85. __/__/__ last Pap test

OBSTETRIC HISTORY
86. _____ gravida
87. _____ para
88. _____ pre-term
89. _____ miscarriages
90. _____ still births
91. _____ has had an abortion

HEAD and NECK
92. _____ frequent headaches
93. _____ neck pains
94. _____ neck lumps or swelling

EYES
95. _____ wears glasses
96. _____ blurry vision
97. _____ eyesight worsening
98. _____ sees double
99. _____ sees halo
100. _____ eye pains or itching
101. _____ watering eyes
102. _____ eye trouble

EARS
103. _____ hearing difficulties
104. _____ earaches
105. _____ running ears
106. _____ buzzing in ears
107. _____ motion sickness

MOUTH
108. _____ dental problems
109. _____ swellings on gums or jaws
110. _____ sore tongue
111. _____ taste changes

NOSE and THROAT
112. _____ congested nose
113. _____ running nose
114. _____ sneezing spells
115. _____ headcolds
116. _____ nose bleeds
117. _____ sore throat
118. _____ enlarged tonsils
119. _____ hoarse voice

RESPIRATORY
120. _____ wheezes or gasps
121. _____ coughing spells
122. _____ coughs up phlegm
123. _____ coughed up blood
124. _____ chest colds
125. _____ excessive sweating, night sweats

CARDIOVASCULAR
126. _____ high blood pressure
127. _____ racing heart
128. _____ chest pains
129. _____ dizzy spells
130. _____ shortness of breath
131. _____ shortness of breath at night
132. _____ more pillows to breathe
133. _____ swollen feet or ankles
134. _____ leg cramps
135. _____ heart murmur

Special problems or symptoms: _____

Patient's Signature: _____

FIGURE 34-10 An example of a medical history sheet used by the physician to record the review of systems (ROS).

- Nails: Color, texture, symmetry, shape, and size are assessed for possible circulation problem, fungus, or infections. Brittle, grooved, or lined nails may indicate local or systemic conditions.

- Head: The shape, size, and symmetry of the head are assessed. The scalp is also assessed for parasites (nits and lice), lesions, flakes, and irritations. The face of a patient reveals much about his or her state of health and stress level. Bruises or other signs of trauma may be indications of abuse. Specific questions by the physician during an examination may shed light on potential abuse problems.

- Neck: The neck is assessed for range of motion, texture, color, lumps, masses, pulsations, and swelling. The physician will also assess the carotid pulse, lymph nodes, thyroid gland, and trachea. Asking a patient to swallow while palpating the thyroid gland helps detect lumps or enlargement of the thyroid gland or goiter.

- Eyes: Prior to the physician seeing the patient, the medical assistant will test the patient's distance vision by using a Snellen chart, near vision using a Jaeger reading card, and color vision using the Ishihara test book. The physician will examine visual fields, pupils reaction to light, and the internal and external structures of the eye. The internal examination is accomplished with an ophthalmoscope. The color of the sclera or white of the eye is evaluated for signs of jaundice. Eye movements are noted as well. (Refer to Preparing for Externship.)

- Ears: The physician will examine the internal and external ear for color, size, shape, and position.

Assisting with a Complete Physical Examination

OBJECTIVE: Assist with physical examination by preparing the necessary equipment, while observing proper sequencing and ensuring patient safety with limited direction.

Equipment and Supplies

Note: Equipment and supplies will vary, depending on the type and purpose of the examination and personal preferences of the physician.

alcohol swabs; drape; emesis basin; examination table with clean sheet; disposable gloves; laryngeal mirror; lubricant; nasal speculum; ophthalmoscope; otoscope; pillow (with clean cover); reflex hammer; scale with height rod; Snellen chart (vision); sphygmomanometer; stethoscope; tape measure; thermometer; tissues; tongue depressors; tuning fork; urine specimen container

Method

1. Perform hand hygiene.
2. Assemble all equipment in examining room.
3. Identify the patient and explain the procedure. Patients should always be accompanied into the examining room.
4. For comfort and efficiency during the examination, the patient should have an empty bladder. If a urine sample is needed for testing, provide the patient with a urine specimen container and instructions at this time. Otherwise, simply offer the patient the opportunity to use the bathroom now.
5. Take vital signs and measurements (temperature, pulse, respirations, blood pressure, height, and weight). Document these data in the patient's record or on a complaint slip immediately.
6. Provide the patient with a gown and drape and give instructions on undressing. Have patient wear gown with opening in front if this is appropriate. Allow patient to undress in privacy.
   Rationale: Gowns that are open in the front provide easier access to the patient's chest and abdomen.
7. Have patient sit on the side of the examination table with legs hanging over the side. Place a drape sheet over the patient's legs.
   Rationale: This position provides easy access to the patient when the physician examines the head, eyes, ears, nose, mouth, neck, throat, breasts, axilla (armpit), chest, and heart.
   Note: The physician may prefer to examine the female breasts and axilla when the patient is in a reclining position.
8. Tell the physician that the patient is ready. A female medical assistant should remain in the room if the patient is a female and the physician is a male or if the physician needs assistance.
9. Assist the physician as needed. The patient may require assistance during position changes.
10. Use gloves when handling used equipment that may contain biohazardous materials, such as the laryngeal mirror. The mirror and other contaminated equipment are placed in the emesis basin until they can be carried to the decontamination area.
11. As the physician progresses from one section of the body to the next during the ROS, reposition the drape to expose only the portion of the patient's body being examined. Label all specimen slides as soon as possible. Use gloves when handling specimens.
12. When the examination is complete, assist the patient to sit up slowly.
    Note: Some patients experience dizziness if they sit up suddenly. When removing legs from stirrups, take both legs down together to prevent strain on hips and back.
13. Assist the patient off the examination table, as necessary.
14. Ask the patient if he or she requires help dressing. If no help is needed, allow the patient to dress in privacy.
15. Instruct the patient where to go after dressing.
16. After the patient has left the examination room, discard all disposable materials into the appropriate sharps and waste containers. Ideally, sharps should be disposed of as they are used to prevent injury to the patient. Remove soiled linens and place them in the laundry container. Reusable equipment is removed to a decontamination area to be cleaned and disinfected or sterilized.
17. Resupply the examination room.
18. Clean the examination table and replace the soiled linens and gowns.
19. Complete any documentation on the patient's record or the complaint slip.

Charting Example

2/14/XX	3:00 P.M.

CPX by Dr. Williams. Pt. referred to clinic lab for CBC, UA, and mammogram. Pt. to return in 1 week to discuss results. Appointment made for 2/21/XX.

M. King, CMA

Note: The physician will document his or her findings from the CPX on the patient record.

The physician will use tuning forks and whispering to assess the patient's hearing. The ear canals are examined with an otoscope for signs of foreign bodies or excess cerumen or earwax.

- Nose: The internal and external nose will be examined for color and symmetry. The physician will also assess the patient's sense of smell. If drainage is observed, the physician will note the amount, color, and consistency. Red swollen mucosa with yellow to greenish discharge indicates infection.

- Mouth: The physician will assess the lips and inside the mouth for symmetry, moisture, color, and lesions. The tongue texture, color, size, shape, symmetry, movement, and position will be assessed. The number of teeth as well as the color and condition will be noted. Adequate oral hygiene is important to a patient's overall health. Patients should be reminded to schedule regular dental care and cleaning. Gums should be pink and healthy and not prone to bleeding.

- Throat: When the physician asks the patient to say "ah", this gives the physician an opportunity to assess the uvula, tonsils, and throat for color, size, shape, symmetry, and movement, using the tongue depressor. The physician will also check the patient's gag reflex.

- Arms: The joints and pulses of the arms as well as the strength and range of motion will be assessed by the physician.

- Heart: Using a stethoscope the physician will auscultate the sounds of the heart noting the rate, rhythm, pitch, and quality. The physician will then place the stethoscope over various areas of the patient's heart and listen. Any murmurs detected will be noted.

- Chest: The chest wall will be assessed for symmetry during inspiration and expiration. It will also be assessed for pain, tenderness, lesions, lumps, and temperature. Postural abnormalities such as scoliosis or curvature of the spine may be noted as well.

- Lungs: Using a stethoscope the physician will auscultate the patient's breath sounds noting rate, rhythm, pitch, depth, and location.

- Breasts: The physician will assess the breasts of both males and females. The breasts will be assessed for size, shape, symmetry, and texture. Any discharge, lumps, masses, pain, or tenderness will be noted.

- Abdomen: The abdomen is assessed for symmetry, texture, temperature, and movement. Using a stethoscope the physician will auscultate the

patient's bowel sounds for frequency, pitch, gurgling, and clicking sounds. The abdomen is visually divided into four quadrants: right and left upper quadrants and right and left lower quadrants. Next, the organs in each quadrant are percussed and palpated for signs of masses, position of organs, and muscle tone.

- Genitalia: The physician will assess the internal and external genitalia of a female patient. For the male patient the physician will assess the external genitalia and perform a testicular examination. These examinations will be discussed more fully in Chapter 35.

- Rectum: To assess the rectum for lesions or masses, the physician will perform a digital rectal examination. Most physicians require anyone over 40 years of age to have a digital rectal exam for early detection of colorectal cancer. A stool sample may be gathered for occult or hidden blood at the same time.

- Legs and feet: The joints and pulses of the legs and feet as well as the strength and range of motion will be assessed by the physician. Other postural problems may be noted.

- Neurological system: The physician will examine each reflex for appropriate response. The physician will also observe the patient's gait, facial expressions, sensation response, speech, and movement. Table 34-4 presents a synopsis of the review of systems. Table 34-5 presents a typical sequence of procedures to be preformed and the person responsible for completing the procedure. Procedure 34-3 lists the steps for interviewing a patient to obtain medical information and prepare for a physical examination.

TABLE 34-4 Review of Systems (ROS)

Head	Headaches, sinus pain, masses, alopecia (unusual hair loss), dizziness, injury, or trauma
Eyes	Visual acuity, blurred vision, burning, halo effect, tearing, photophobia (sensitivity to light), discharge, redness, jaundice (yellowing of skin and sclera), known eye diseases, date of last eye exam, prescription glasses, contact lenses
Ears	Tinnitus or ringing in the ears, dizziness, hearing loss, discharge, ear infections, exposure to loud noise on a regular basis
Nose	Allergies, obstruction, sense of smell, pain, discharge
Mouth	Dental work, dentures, gums, sense of taste, teeth, salivation (producing saliva), dryness of mouth, tongue, leukoplakia (white patches, possibly cancerous), gingivitis
Throat	Hoarseness, laryngitis (loss of voice), redness, speech defect, masses, pain
Neck	Tenderness, pain, swelling, difficulty swallowing, enlarged nodes
Respiratory	Dyspnea (labored breathing), cough, asthma, wheezing, allergies, hemoptysis (coughing up blood), chest pain, night sweats, orthopnea (difficulty breathing while lying down), shortness of breath (SOB)
Cardiovascular (CV)	Chest pain, hypertension, peripheral edema, cyanosis, fainting, dizziness, heart murmurs, palpitations, arrhythmias
Gastrointestinal (GI)	Nausea, vomiting, anorexia (loss of appetite), bulimia (eating disorder—binge eating followed by purging), indigestion, diarrhea, constipation, hemorrhoids, presence of blood in stool, number of bowel movements daily, hematemesis (vomiting blood)
Genitourinary (GU)	History of urinary tract infection, frequency, hesitation, oliguria (reduced urine), hematuria (blood in urine), dysuria (difficult or painful urination), renal colic (kidney pain), stones, discharge, nocturia (urination during the night)
Female reproductive	Menstrual history, obstetric history, leukorrhea (white discharge), itching, pain, discharge, date of last Pap test, breast self-exam history, sexual habits, menopause symptoms, last mammogram (breast exam)
Male reproductive	Prostate problems, testicular self-exam, discharge, sexual habits, frequency of urination, decreased stream, nocturia, impotence
Endocrine	Growth and development, goiter, excessive thirst, intolerance to temperature change, hormone therapy, diabetes symptoms, irregular menses, symptoms of thyroid disorders
Skin	Rash, urticaria (hives), texture, moles, infection, redness, jaundice, cyanosis, allergies, dry/oily, acne
Musculoskeletal (MS)	Joint pain, swelling, weakness, stiffness, numbness, muscle pain, fractures, discoloration, edema
Neurologic	Fainting, loss of consciousness, headaches, tremor, nervousness, paralysis, pain, memory loss
Psychiatric	Mental health history, emotional stability, depression, stress
General	Weight gain or loss, sleep habits, fatigue, eating habits, smoking, work environment

Documentation of Patient Medical Information

Many different formats are used for recording medical information. Each practice will have its own format specific to its needs. One format is the chronological record, which follows the patient over a period of time, with each visit consisting of a new entry by date, rather than by symptoms or diagnosis. Although this is one of the most common types of medical records, it does make some diagnoses, such as hypertension, more difficult to "catch." For such diagnoses, a problem-oriented medical record might be more appropriate.

Problem-Oriented Medical Record

The problem-oriented medical record (POMR) was developed by Dr. Lawrence Weed in 1970, and is used to identify patient problems and chart by those problems. It is important to note that everyone in the office should chart with the same system.

The functional aspect of this type of charting is the patient problem list found at the front of the chart (Figure 34-11). As new problems and diagnoses are identified, they are noted on the problem list, helping the provider to identify trends in the patient's medical history or emerging diagnoses. POMR also helps providers or physicians who do not already know a specific patient obtain a "snapshot" regarding previous visits and problems at a glance. A POMR has four parts:

- Database: Consists of the physical examination and patient history and results of baseline laboratory or diagnostic procedures.
- Problem list: List of patient problems that is kept in the front of the chart much like a table of contents would be. The problem list assigns each problem a number with the date. The problem can be further explained by information in the database. Each problem the patient has experienced is titled and numbered in the problem list. Because each patient problem is numbered, that number can be referenced throughout the medical record when needed. Throughout the rest of the history, problems are referred to numerically. If one is resolved, the date of resolution is placed next to the problem listed. If a new problem arises, it is assigned a number and listed with the date.
- Plan: Indicates a written plan for each numbered problem identified on the problem list. The plan may include other tests to be ordered, treatment plans, or plans for patient education about specific problems. The treatment plan is a

TABLE 34-5	Sequence of Physical Examination Procedures
1. Registration	Receptionist/ medical assistant
2. History	Receptionist/ medical assistant
3. Urine specimen	Medical assistant or laboratory technician
4. Blood specimen	Medical assistant or laboratory technician
5. Vital signs	Medical assistant
6. Weight and height	Medical assistant
7. Visual acuity	Medical assistant
8. Electrocardiogram	Medical assistant
9. X-ray	X-ray technician (provided x-ray room is available; otherwise x-ray completed before the patient's visit)
10. Preparation of patient	Medical assistant

very important part of the medical record because it tells what has been done for the patient. Each treatment plan should have a title and should reference the problem number with which it is associated.

- Progress notes: Made up of several sections with the first initial spelling out the word SOAP. Thus, this portion of the POMR is known as SOAP notes. Sometimes E is added to SOAP if evaluation is completed. All progress notes should be in chronological order. Each progress note will also reference the patient problem number. The progress note follows a specific format.

Soap Charting

The SOAP charting method is distinct because of the four parts of the approach. The "S" in SOAP identifies the subjective information gathered from the patient—the things that the patient believes they are seeing a physician for—usually the same as a chief complaint. The "O" stands for objective, the data gathered during the visit—such as vital signs, weight change, fevers,

Interview New Patient to Obtain Medical History Information and Prepare for Physical Examination

OBJECTIVE: Obtain pertinent patient information for medical history to assist physician to establish cause and treatment of present illness. Include chief complaint (CC), present illness (PI), past history (PH), social or personal history (SH), and family history (FH).

Note: This may be performed on a fellow student.

Equipment and Supplies
medical history form; clipboard; pen (black and red); scale; equipment for vital signs; urine container; gown; drape

Method
1. Identify patient, greet warmly, and identify yourself
2. Explain what you are going to do and what you want the patient to do and why.
3. Provide a private area to conduct the interview.
4. Ask patient to fill in the patient data portion of the form consisting of demographic information. (Be sure to use terminology the patient can understand and speak in a clear voice.) Be ready to assist or do it for the patient if he or she seems unable to complete the form.
5. Review the portion of the form completed; ask for any additional information necessary.
6. Ask for the reason for being at the physician's office that day, that is, the chief complaint (CC).
7. Record CC in patient's own words as appropriate.
8. Ask the patient other open-ended questions to gather more information about CC to record under present illness (PI). Use observation skills during interview.
9. Gather other information on PH, FH, and SH and document in patient's record.
10. Ask patient about allergies. Record in red ink as required by office policy (usually on first page of medical history).
11. Note any other observations or information you feel relevant (such as illness at home or loss of loved one).
12. Record all information using correct charting guidelines.
13. Correct any errors using one line through error and date; initial them. Record correct information.
14. Ask patient to provide urine specimen if required or ask the patient to empty bladder.
15. Explain what clothes you wish the patient to remove; where you want the opening of the exam gown; and where you want the patient to sit and wait.
16. Explain what procedures will follow (physician will be in shortly, etc.).
17. Place patient history in designated place for physician.

---

blood work, and other measurable data. The "A" is for assessment, the physician's preliminary diagnosis. The "P" indicates the section of the chart discussing the plan of care for this patient. The SOAP method of documenting in a medical record is described in Table 34-6.

A problem list for the patient in the example given in Table 34-6 might appear as:

- *Problem List*

  2/14/XX

  Problem No. 1: Diabetes

  Problem No. 2: Hypertension, essential

- *Plan*

  2/14/XX

  Problem No. 1: Diabetic exchange diet

  Regular insulin, 20 units SC q AM

  Monitor blood sugar levels during day

  Problem No. 2: Norvasc 2.5 mg. daily

  Monitor blood pressure weekly

- *Progress Note*

  2/14/XX

  Problem No. 1: Diabetes

| NAME _____ AGE _____ |
| OCCUPATION _____ SOC. SEC.# _____ |

	BLOOD PRESSURE	VISION Without Glasses	Diagnostic Tests	Results
Height ____	**Sitting** R / :L /	Far R20/ L20/ Near R / L /		
Weight ____				
Build ____		**With Glasses**		
(Sm.Med.Lg.Obese.)	**Standing** R / :L /	Far R20/ L20/ Near R / L /		
Pulse ____		Tonometry R ___ L ___		
Resp. ____	**Lying** R / :L /	Colorvision ____ (Ishihara plates missed)		
Temp. ____		Peripheral Fields R ___ L ___		

	250	500	1000	2000	4000	8000
AUDIOMETRIC TESTING R	___	___	___	___	___	___
L	___	___	___	___	___	___
Gross Hearing _____						

PULMONARY FUNCTION

Initial Problem List

_____
_____
_____
_____
_____

Employment status _____ Physician's signature _____
DATE _____

FIGURE 34-11 An example of a medical history sheet to list patient problems.

S – Patient states thirst has diminished and hunger lessened

O – Urine +2, FBS positive, gained 4 pounds in past 3 weeks, skin turgor good

A – Diet and medication effective

P – Continue medication, monitor blood sugar level daily, adjust insulin levels per instruction, return visit in 2 weeks

Problem No. 2: Hypertension

S – Patient states no complaints related to high blood pressure

O – BP 138/86, down 10 points in past 3 weeks

A – Medication effective

P – Continue with medication and patient monitor of BP weekly. Come in for check in 2 weeks

The POMR and SOAP methods can be combined in one chart, making for a very concise, clear set of information on any patient.

Source-Oriented Medical Record

The source-oriented medical record (SOMR) is a common method utilized in medical clinics. Patient

TABLE 34-6 SOAP Charting for 1/24/XX

S	Subjective symptoms provided by the patient and/or family. The actual patient's words are recorded	"I'm thirsty and eating all the time but I'm not gaining any weight. I feel tired all the time."
O	Objective findings from vital signs, physical examination, and laboratory and diagnostic tests	B/P: 158/96; T: 98°F; P: 76; R: 16 Skin turgor (resiliency) poor. Wt. 10# less than 6 weeks ago Urine 4+ sugar, FBS positive
A	Assessment, including the physician's diagnosis	Uncontrolled diabetes
P	Plan including recommended treatments, further tests, medications, consultation, surgery, physical therapy	Dx: Lab tests for diabetes Tx: Begin diabetic diet and insulin Instruct on diet and exercise follow-up

information is placed in the medical record in reverse chronological order and organized in different sections. Each office determines which sections to be used and in what order they are to appear in the medical chart. The sections commonly used include history and physical, insurance, progress notes, medications, laboratory, and consultations. The most recent information is seen first in each section of the medical record. This method makes it complicated to identify and locate past medical problems, treatments, and results. Progress notes are included with each patient encounter whether it is an office visit, telephone call, or written communication.

Electronic Medical Records

Computer software programs have been developed to simulate a paper medical record. More and more medical clinics are using electronic medical records (EMRs). Medical clinics that are considered paperless use computers and computer software to complete scheduling and billing, completing insurance and submitting insurance forms, and documenting in the medical record. Handheld computer devices are being used in many facilities to input information directly into the patient's computerized record. It is critical for the medical clinic to have policies and procedures outlining security measures, confidentiality, and data backup methods.

EMRs have several advantages:

1. Medical staff is able to access the electronic medical record anywhere in the clinic.
2. Able to share the medical record with other medical staff.
3. Lost or misfiled medical records are eliminated.
4. Medical record is continuously updated.
5. Provides reminders and alerts for the medical staff.

6. A storage room for medical records is eliminated.
7. Documentation is legible, faster, and easier.

Disadvantages of EMR:

1. Security
2. Confidentiality
3. Electric and equipment failures
4. Equipment and software start-up costs

When writing in the medical record, it is especially important that the medical assistant be very clear and concise in the information provided. The information provided must also be complete and in chronological order. This is called the "six Cs of charting": clear, concise, complete, client's words, confidentiality, and chronological order. Each line in the progress note should be filled out completely, using a black ink pen, and using correct spelling. It is especially important to write neatly and legibly. Guidelines 34-1 lists important charting guidelines.

If there is an error when writing the information, draw a single line through the error, date and initial the error, write the word *error* above the incorrect information, and then write the correct information. Never scribble out an error or try to write over the incorrect information.

The patient's chart is typically placed in a rack outside the door of the examination room. Special care should be taken to maintain the patient's privacy by making sure the chart is closed and any identifiable information is facing the door, not out to the hallway where another individual might see it. HIPAA regulations must be followed at all times. If a patient requests to read his or her chart, the most appropriate response is to politely inform the patient that you will relay the request to the physician. The physician is the most appropriate individual to discuss the medical record with the patient.

GUIDELINES   **Charting**

1. Double check to make sure that you have the correct patient chart.
2. Use dark ink, preferably black, and write legibly. Printing is preferred if one's handwriting is difficult to read.
3. The patient's name should appear on each page of the record. Many offices will have a device that stamps the patient's name and identification number onto paper.
4. Every entry must be dated and initialed by the person writing in the record. The full name of the person initialing the document should either be in the medical record or on file in the physician's office.
5. Entries should be brief but complete.
6. Use only accepted medical abbreviations known by the general staff and correctly spell all medical terms.

See Appendix B for a list of commonly used medical abbreviations.

7. Never erase, use a liquid eraser, or in any way remove information from a medical record. The accepted method of correcting medical records is described fully in Chapter 12.
8. Document all telephone calls relating to the patient in the medical record as well as other correspondence.
9. Document any action(s) taken as a result of telephone conversations.
10. Document all missed appointments.
11. Document any incidences of noncompliance.
12. Document every circumstance of patient education.
13. Do not record personal opinion, speculations, or judgments.

SUMMARY

The atmosphere provided by the medical assistant, whose responsibilities include preparation of the exam room and the medical record, creates a patient's first impression of a physician's office. The ability to anticipate the physician's needs during the exam is acquired with experience. Patient safety and comfort during the exam are a priority, because they allow the physician to efficiently complete the examination while obtaining the most accurate data. The medical assistant's role before, during, and after the examination is to ensure that the medical record, the patient, and the equipment are completely prepared and ready for the exam. Accuracy and thoroughness are imperative to providing quality medical care.

Chapter Review

COMPETENCY REVIEW

1. Define and spell the terms to learn for this chapter.
2. Prepare exam room for a physical examination.
3. Identify instruments and equipment used by the physician when completing a physical examination.
4. Prepare a patient for a physical exam.
5. Demonstrate knowledge of positions used for physical examinations.
6. Correctly document a patient office visit using both chronological and problem-oriented medical records.

PREPARING FOR THE CERTIFICATION EXAM

1. For a routine physical examination, the medical assistant will have all of the following ready, EXCEPT:
   A. reflex hammer
   B. laryngeal mirror
   C. otoscope
   D. irrigation syringe
   E. stethoscope

2. Distinguishing between two diseases by contrasting their symptoms is called:
   A. chemical diagnosis
   B. physical diagnosis
   C. differential diagnosis
   D. laboratory diagnosis
   E. radiologic diagnosis

   continued on next page

3. Which of the following is considered a blood chemistry test?
   A. ECG
   B. EKG
   C. PFT
   D. SMAK
   E. SMAC

4. The position the patient is placed in for a pelvic exam is:
   A. semi-Fowler's
   B. lithotomy
   C. knee-chest
   D. prone
   E. jack-knife

5. Which position is NOT used when a patient is having a sigmoidoscopic examination?
   A. semi-Fowler's
   B. dorsal recumbent
   C. knee-chest
   D. jack-knife
   E. proctologic

6. Listening to the sound made when the body is being struck is called:
   A. palpation
   B. auscultation
   C. inspection
   D. percussion
   E. menstruation

7. The actual method of documentation in using the problem-oriented medical record (POMR) uses _____ charting:
   A. CC
   B. PI
   C. ROS
   D. SOAP
   E. ABS

8. Four standard examination methods used when a physician conducts a physical examination are:
   A. inspection, palpation, percussion, and auscultation
   B. anthropomorphic, palpation, percussion, and auscultation
   C. inspection, percussion, auscultation, and anthropomorphic
   D. percussion, pertussis, external, and internal
   E. auscultation, pertussis, palpation, and inspection

9. The primary reason to position a patient seated on an examination table with legs hanging over the side during a complete physical examination is to:
   A. let the patient's legs relax
   B. provide for easy access to the patient for the physician
   C. protect the physician from being kicked during the examination
   D. allow for unencumbered reflex examination
   E. maximize the privacy for the undressed but draped patient

10. Which of the following is NOT considered one of the six Cs of charting?
    A. clear
    B. concise
    C. complete
    D. chronological order
    E. compromise

CRITICAL THINKING

1. How should Jerry prepare the examining room for Mrs. Lewis's complete physical examination?

2. What instruments are needed?

3. How should Mrs. Lewis be positioned?

4. If Jerry is a male medical assistant, what type of assistance should Jerry give Dr. Williams during the exam?

5. How should this visit be charted? Which part of the examination is Jerry responsible for charting? Dr. Williams?

ON THE JOB

Elizabeth Smith, CMA, just started working for Dr. Williams today. The first task he gave Elizabeth was to make sure each exam room had the correct supplies. After she completed that task, Dr. Williams had her prepare the examining room for his next patient.

1. What supplies should an examining room typically have in it?
2. What is the function of the supplies in a typical examining room?
3. How should Elizabeth prepare the examining room for Dr. Williams's next patient?

INTERNET ACTIVITY

Perform an Internet search looking for examples of the various types of electronic medical record systems available for a medical office.

MediaLink More on assisting with physical examinations, including interactive resources, can be found on the Student CD-ROM accompanying this textbook.

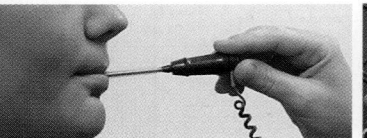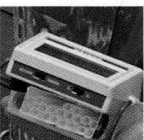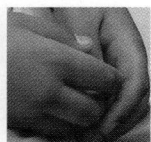

Medical Assistant Role Delineation Chart

HIGHLIGHT indicates material covered in this chapter.

ADMINISTRATIVE

Administrative Procedures

- Perform basic administrative medical assisting functions
- Schedule, coordinate and monitor appointments
- Schedule inpatient/outpatient admissions and procedures
- Understand and apply third-party guidelines
- Obtain reimbursement through accurate claims submission
- Monitor third-party reimbursement
- Understand and adhere to managed care policies and procedures
- *Negotiate managed care contracts*

Practice Finances

- Perform procedural and diagnostic coding
- Apply bookkeeping principles

- Manage accounts receivable
- *Manage accounts payable*
- *Process payroll*
- *Document and maintain accounting and banking records*
- *Develop and maintain fee schedules*
- *Manage renewals of business and professional insurance policies*
- *Manage personnel benefits and maintain records*
- *Perform marketing, financial, and strategic planning*

CLINICAL

Fundamental Principles

- Apply principles of aseptic technique and infection control
- Comply with quality assurance practices
- Screen and follow up patient test results

Diagnostic Orders

- Collect and process specimens
- Perform diagnostic tests

Patient Care

- Adhere to established patient screening procedures
- Obtain patient history and vital signs
- Prepare and maintain examination and treatment areas
- Prepare patient for examinations, procedures and treatments

- Assist with examinations, procedures and treatments
- Prepare and administer medications and immunizations
- Maintain medication and immunization records
- Recognize and respond to emergencies
- Coordinate patient care information with other health care providers
- Initiate IV and administer IV medications with appropriate training and as permitted by state law

GENERAL

Professionalism

- Display a professional manner and image
- Demonstrate initiative and responsibility
- Work as a member of the health care team
- Prioritize and perform multiple tasks
- Adapt to change
- Promote the CMA credential
- Enhance skills through continuing education
- Treat all patients with compassion and empathy
- Promote the practice through positive public relations

Communication Skills

- Recognize and respect cultural diversity
- Adapt communications to individual's ability to understand
- Use professional telephone technique

- Recognize and respond effectively to verbal, nonverbal, and written communications
- Use medical terminology appropriately
- Utilize electronic technology to receive, organize, prioritize and transmit information
- Serve as liaison

Legal Concepts

- Perform within legal and ethical boundaries
- Prepare and maintain medical records
- Document accurately
- Follow employer's established policies dealing with the health care contract
- Implement and maintain federal and state health care legislation and regulations
- Comply with established risk management and safety procedures
- Recognize professional credentialing criteria
- *Develop and maintain personnel, policy and procedure manuals*

Instruction

- Instruct individuals according to their needs
- Explain office policies and procedures
- Teach methods of health promotion and disease prevention
- Locate community resources and disseminate information
- *Develop educational materials*
- *Conduct continuing education activities*

Operational Functions

- Perform inventory of supplies and equipment
- Perform routine maintenance of administrative and clinical equipment
- Apply computer techniques to support office operations
- *Perform personnel management functions*
- *Negotiate leases and prices for equipment and supply contracts*

- *Denotes advanced skills.*

SOURCE: Reprinted by permission of the American Association of Medical Assistants from the AAMA Role Delineation Study: Occupational Analysis of the Medical Assisting Profession.

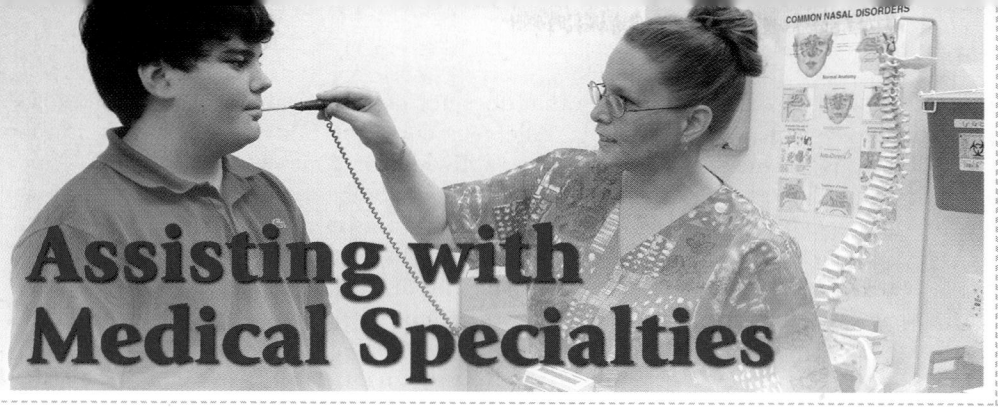

Assisting with Medical Specialties

Learning Objectives

After completing this chapter, you should be able to:

- Define and spell the terms to learn for this chapter.
- Prepare patients for examinations and diagnostic procedures.
- Assist the physician with examinations and treatments.
- Perform selected diagnostic tests.
- Instruct patients with special procedures.
- Follow up with patients' test results.
- Document special procedures accurately.

Terms to Learn

allergen
anaphylactic shock
angina
atherosclerosis
benign
carcinoma in situ
cerebral spinal fluid (CSF)
colic
desensitizing injection
diaphoresis
dysplasia

dyspnea
embolus
eosinophil
flatus
fundus
gonads
histamine
hypersensitivity
ischemia
lochia
malignant

myocardial infarction (MI)
nonsteroidal anti-inflammatory drugs (NSAIDs)
parturition
puerperium
referred
thrombus
venom
wheal

OUTLINE

Allergy	660
Dermatology	662
Cardiovascular System	663
Endocrinology	669
Gastrointestinal System	672
Lymphatic System	677
Musculoskeletal System	678
Nervous System	679
Reproductive Systems	684
Female Reproductive System	684
Male Reproductive System	695
Sexually Transmitted Diseases (STDs)	696
Urinary System	699

Case Study

BRIAN JOHNSON, A 35-YEAR-OLD construction worker, is scheduled for a physical examination as part of a pre-employment physical. He appears muscular and physically fit. Susan Clark, CMA, asks Mr. Johnson if he has any problems or symptoms as she prepares him for his physical. He states that he has no complaints. However, his physical examination indicates that he has rhinitis, reddened, irritated eyes, some wheezing, and he admits he is a heavy smoker. Mr. Johnson's blood pressure is 140/88, his ECG is normal, and his height and weight are average.

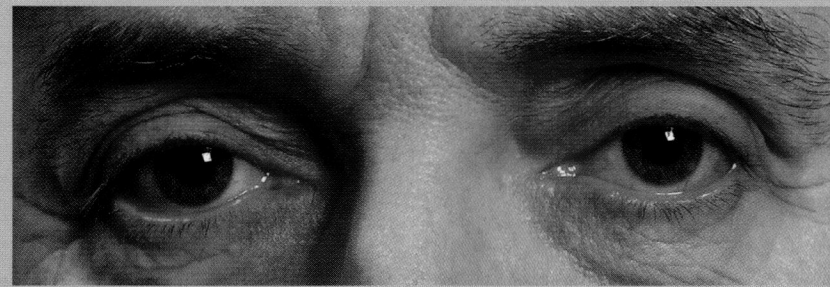

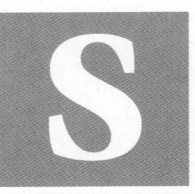

Special examinations and procedures relating to specific body systems are commonly performed in the medical office. The most commonly performed examinations include: pediatric, gynecologic, prenatal, proctoscopic, and sigmoidoscopic. Discussion of some of these examinations, along with a review of procedures and tests related to specific body systems, is presented in this chapter.

The role of the medical assistant is to assist the physician during special examinations and procedures and to instruct the patient before, during, and after many of these procedures. Though some of the procedures discussed throughout this chapter are performed in the hospital setting, the medical assistant, as one of the prime educators of the patient, must know and understand a vast amount of medical information regarding these procedures.

Working as a medical assistant will bring you into contact with a variety of conditions and diseases. Whether the conditions are acute (rapid onset) or chronic (long lasting or recurring) patients will exhibit a wide range of reactions such as fear, anger, and frustration. They deserve your empathy and support.

Allergy

An allergy is an abnormal response or hypersensitivity to a substance (allergen), such as a medication or pollen that does not normally cause a reaction in most people. Allergens enter the body through inhalation, injection, swallowing, or contact with the skin. Any substance in the environment, such as pollen, certain foods, insect venom (poison), animal dander or saliva, can cause an allergy in sensitive persons. Allergic reactions may be localized, such as a mosquito bite, or systemic, such as asthma or anaphylactic shock, both of which can be life threatening. An antigen is a substance, usually protein in nature, which induces the production of antibodies. An antibody is a protein substance produced in the body in response to a foreign invading substance (antigen). In a normal immune reaction, the foreign substance (antigen) and the specific antibody unite and are excreted from the body. The allergic interaction of an antigen and antibody causes the release of histamine, which is the substance that produces signs and symptoms of allergies. The symptoms of allergies consist of a local or systemic inflammatory reaction, which is characterized by redness, edema, and heat. Respiratory symptoms include wheezing, sneezing, coughing, and nasal congestion.

Allergic conditions include eczema, allergic rhinitis, hay fever, bronchial asthma, urticaria (hives), and food allergies. See Table 35-1 for information on common types of allergies. An increase in the blood eosinophil level may occur with allergies. An eosinophil is a granular white cell that captures invading microorganisms and antibody-anitgen reactions through phagocytosis (engulfing or eating).

TABLE 35-1	**Common Types of Allergies**
Allergy	**Description**
Allergic rhinitis	Inflammation of the nasal mucosa that results in nasal congestion, rhinorrhea (runny nose), sneezing, and itching of the nose. Seasonal allergic rhinitis, such as hay fever, occurs only during certain seasons of the year. Children suffering from this type of allergy may rub their nose in an upward movement, called the "allergic salute."
Asthma	A condition seen most frequently in childhood in which wheezing, coughing, and dyspnea are the major symptoms. Asthmatic attacks may be caused by allergens inhaled from air, food, and drugs. The patient's airway is affected by constriction of the bronchial passages. Treatment is medication and control of the causative factors.
Contact dermatitis	Inflammation and irritation of the skin due to contact with an irritating substance, such as soap, perfume, cosmetics, plastics, dyes, and plants, such as poison ivy. Treatment consists of topical and systemic medications and removal of the causative item.
Eczema	A superficial dermatitis accompanied by papules, vesicles, and crusting. The condition can be acute or chronic.
Urticaria	A skin eruption of pale reddish wheals (circular elevations of the skin) with severe itching. It is usually associated with a food allergy, stress, or drug reactions. Also called hives.

The treatment for allergies consists of medications, such as the antihistamine *Benadryl,* allergy testing, and desensitization. Desensitizing injections involve administering minute amounts of the allergen into the patient's system over an extended period of time and are used to develop a tolerance for the allergen in the patient. Desensitization is necessary if the allergic reactions significantly interfere with the patient's lifestyle or is life threatening. Figure 35-1 shows a young patient receiving an allergy injection.

Anaphylactic Shock

In some persons, a life-threatening allergic reaction called anaphylactic shock can occur. Insect stings (for example, bees and wasps) and allergies to drugs, such as penicillin, can cause severe reactions. The symptoms include acute respiratory distress, edema, hypotension, rash, tachycardia, pale cool skin, convulsions, and cyanosis. This condition can result in circulatory and respiratory changes. It requires emergency treatment consisting of medication, such as epinephrine, to relax smooth muscles in the airways and, in some cases, endotracheal intubation and mechanical ventilation. (The terms adrenalin and epinephrine are used interchangeably.) If no treatment is received, unconsciousness and death may result in a short period of time.

Anaphylaxis is an emergency situation that requires medical intervention. Patients with hypersensitivity to insect venom or foods, such as peanuts, must carry an anaphylactic shock kit containing a self-injecting dose of epinephrine. The kit should be worn by the patient at all times. In case of anaphylaxis, either the patient can self-administer or a witness may perform the intervention. Patient and family education on the use of epinephrine for anaphylaxis is extremely important. All allergy patients should be instructed to read labels of foods, herbal products, and over-the-counter medications carefully. You should remind those with severe food allergies to check with their server or host about food ingredients that could be harmful if not fatal to them.

Allergy Testing

Testing is ordered by the physician to determine a patient's sensitivities to allergens. The methods used include scratch or skin testing, intradermal tests, patch tests, and radioallergosorbenttest (RAST).

Scratch Test

The scratch method of allergy testing is usually performed on the patient's back or arms (Figure 35-2). The skin is divided into small squares, which are approximately one inch apart, and labeled with a ballpoint pen to indicate which allergen is being used. A drop of allergen is placed onto the skin at the appropriately labeled site, then the skin is scratched with a needle or lancet. A new needle or lancet is used for each allergen tested. Many scratch tests using different

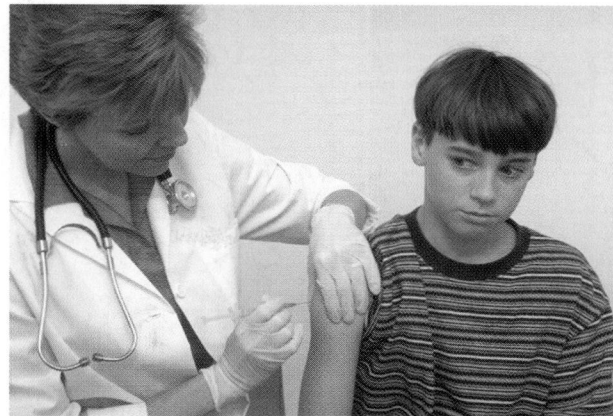

FIGURE 35-1 An allergy injection is used to desensitize an allergen.

allergens can be performed at the same time. If a wheal forms within 15 minutes after placing an allergen on the skin, an allergy is indicated (Figure 35-3). A wheal is a small, round raised area that may be accompanied by itching. The patient should be advised to remain in the physician's office for at least 30 minutes after the testing has been completed in the event there is a delayed allergic reaction to the testing.

Intradermal Test

Intradermal allergy testing is performed by injecting 0.01 to 0.02 mL of an allergen extract into the anterior surface of the forearm. Several tests (10 to 18) can be performed on each arm. A red wheal is a positive sign. An intradermal test is considered more accurate than a scratch test. See Chapter 49 for a more detailed description of intradermal injections.

Patch Test

The patch test consists of placing a small amount of the allergen onto the anterior forearm and then covering this with a plastic wrap. Several patch tests can be

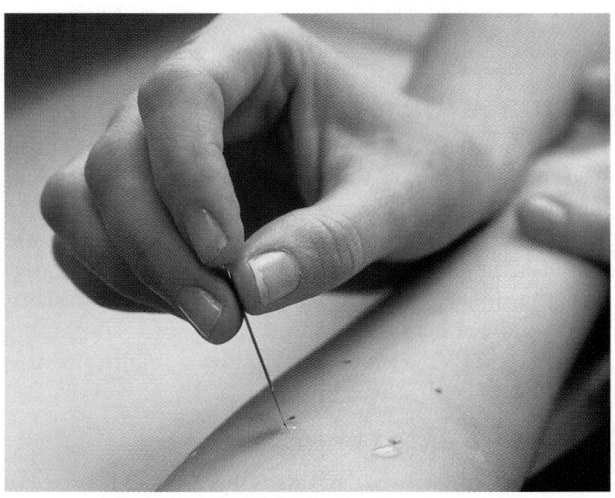

FIGURE 35-2 A scratch test of allergens is performed on a patient's arm.

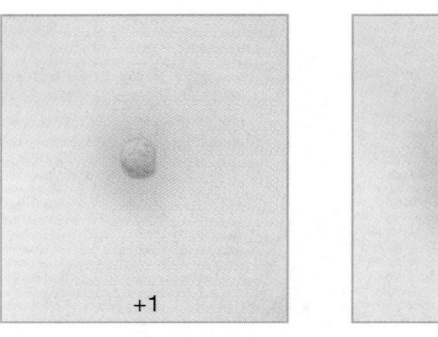
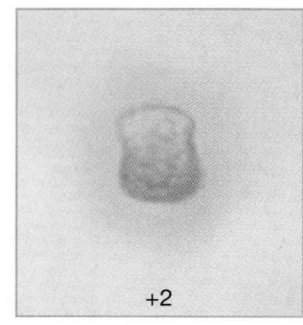
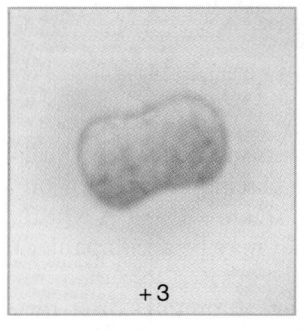
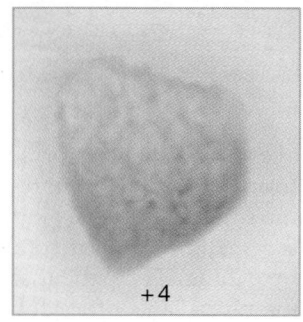

FIGURE 35-3 Wheals form in reaction to scratch testing of allergens.

performed at the same time and these are read after the patches have remained in place for 24 to 48 hours. Patch tests are used to detect the causative agents in contact dermatitis.

RAST Test

Radioallergosorbent test (RAST) measures blood levels of antibodies to particular antigens. A venipuncture is performed on the patient and the sample is sent to a laboratory where it is exposed to a variety of suspected allergens and the levels of antibodies are measured. This test is expensive but more sensitive and useful for patients who have dermatological problems or cannot stop taking allergy medication safely in order to have one of the other tests performed.

Dermatology

The skin and its accessory structures—sweat glands, oil glands, nails, and hair—are known as the integumentary system. The sense organs, which respond to changes in temperature, pain, touch, and pressure, are located in this system. The skin consists of the epidermis (thin outer membrane), the dermis (middle, fibrous layer), and subcutaneous (innermost layer containing fatty tissue) layers. Medical conditions relating to this system occur in all three layers.

Common Skin Disorders

Most skin conditions and diseases are diagnosed, in part, by observing the lesion. Skin lesions can occur whenever the normal surface of the skin is invaded or changed. A skin lesion is not always a sign of disease, such as seen with a non-cancerous nodule. There is generally some discoloration or change from the normal coloration.

Some of the more common lesions are illustrated in Figure 35-4 (dermatology skin lesions). These terms should be used when charting information relating to any skin lesions.

Bacteria, viruses, and parasites can all invade the skin if its protective barrier is broken down. Inflammatory skin disorders result in swelling, redness, and often itching over the affected site. These conditions include cellulitis, decubitus ulcers, psoriasis, acne vulgaris, and scleroderma.

- Cellulitis or erysipelas is an inflammation of the cellular or connective tissue caused by either staphylococcus or streptococcus infection of a cut or lesion. Treatment consists of antibiotics and application of warm compresses.

- Decubitus ulcers, also called bedsores, are open sores caused by pressure over bony prominences on the body due to a lack of blood flow. These can appear in bedridden patients who lie in one position too long. Treatment consists of relieving the pressure through frequent turning and exercise of the patient, thorough cleansing of the wound, and topical antibiotics. Deep ulcers may require surgical debridement (removal of dead tissue).

- Psoriasis is a chronic inflammatory condition consisting of discrete red or pink lesions covered with silver scaling. Psoriasis is non contagious and is thought to be an autoimmune disease. Treatment consists of topical ointments, and in some severe cases, ultraviolet light therapy.

- Acne vulgaris is an inflammatory disease of the sebaceous glands and hair follicles that results in papules and pustules. Treatment consists of thorough cleansing and systemic and topical antibiotics.

- Scleroderma is a chronic, progressive autoimmune disease that affects the blood vessels and connective tissue of the skin and other organs. Integumentary symptoms include hardening of the skin, pallor, edema, and fixating of skin to subcutaneous tissues. There is no known cause and no cure.

Dermatological Neoplasms

Neoplasms or tumors can be either benign (non-cancerous) or malignant (cancerous). Neoplasms are biopsied by surgically removing a small amount of tissue for testing. Benign growths may grow in size but are usually encapsulated. Malignant growths are invasive and tend to take over surrounding tissues. Invasion of area tissue takes place when malignant cells break through the basement membrane separating epithelial cells from connective tissue below. Cancer cells then may invade blood and lymphatic tissue and spread to other areas of the body. See Table 35-2 for a list of of different types of neoplasms and corresponding descriptions.

To determine a course of treatment, a physician must grade and stage the malignancy. Grading is done by a pathologist, who examines the tissue removed during biopsy. The pathologist examines the tissue to see how closely cells resemble normal cells in the tissue. The less closely cells resemble normal cells or the less differentiated cells are, the poorer the prognosis for the patient. Staging a tumor uses the results of diagnostic tests such as bone and liver scans and other information gathered from the physical examination to determine the size, depth, and degree of spread of the initial tumor. Treatment of a malignant tumor is usually surgical removal of the tumor and follow-up treatment is based on the results of all the tests performed. Benign tumors may also require surgical removal if they impair normal functioning of an organ.

When patients hear the term "tumor" they immediately think of cancer. Since a tumor can be either benign or malignant, it is advisable not to use the general term "tumor" when talking to a patient. Oncology is the branch of medicine dealing with malignant neoplasms. Cancer therapy, consisting of chemotherapy (toxic drugs), radiation, cryotherapy, and radiotherapy is used in the treatment of cancer.

Diagnostic Procedures

A variety of diagnostic tests and procedures are used when treating disorders of the integumentary system. These are described in Table 35-3. These procedures are performed by the physician with the assistance of the medical assistant. The physician may order a wound culture to determine the causative agent and best antibiotic to treat an infected wound. Procedure 35-1 provides the steps necessary to obtain a culture of a wound.

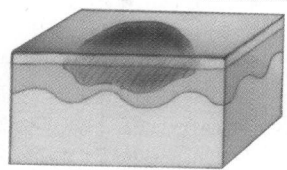

A macule is a discolored spot on the skin; freckle.

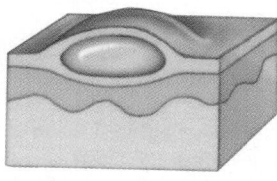

A wheal is a localized, evanescent elevation of the skin that is often accompanied by itching; urticaria.

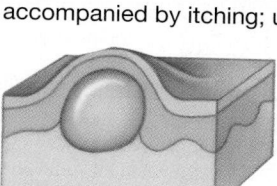

A papule is a solid, circumscribed, elevated area on the skin; pimple.

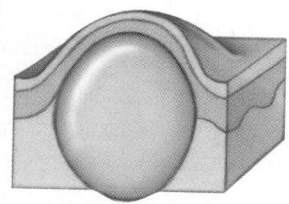

A nodule is a larger papule; acne vulgaris.

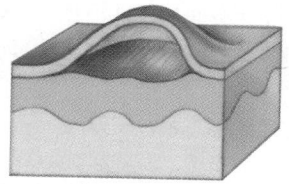

A vesicle is a small fluid filled sac; blister. A bulla is a large vesicle.

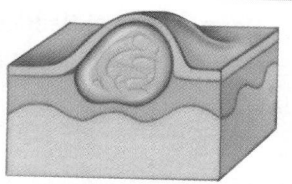

A pustule is a small, elevated, circumscribed lesion of the skin that is filled with pus; varicella (chickenpox).

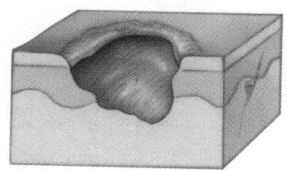

An erosion or ulcer is an eating or gnawing away of tissue; decubitus ulcer.

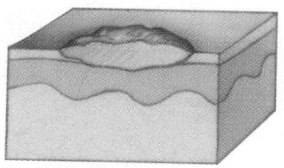

A crust is a dry, serous or seropurulent, brown, yellow, red, or green exudation that is seen in secondary lesions; eczema.

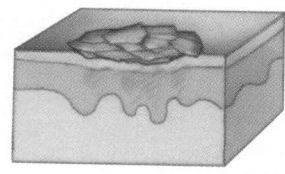

A scale is a thin, dry flake of cornified epithelial cells.

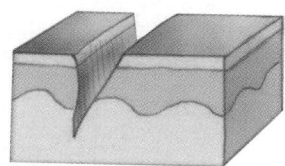

A fissure is a crack-like sore or slit that extends through the epidermis into the dermis; athlete's foot.

FIGURE 35-4 Skin signs are objective evidence of an illness or disorder. They can be seen, measured, or felt.

Cardiovascular System

A study of the cardiovascular or circulatory system is called *cardiology*. This system includes the heart and blood vessels. For a review of anatomy and physiology of the cardiovascular system, see Chapter 25.

TABLE 35-2 Dermatological Neoplasms

Benign (Non-Cancerous) Neoplasms	Description
Dermatofibroma	A fibrous tumor of the skin. It is painless, round, firm, red, and generally found on extremities.
Hemangioma	Benign tumor of dilated vessels.
Keloid	The formation of a scar after an injury or surgery that results in a raised, thickened, red area.
Keratosis	Overgrowth or thickening of cells in the epithelium located in the epidermis of the skin.
Leukoplakia	A change in the mucous membrane that results in thick, white, patches on the mucous membrane of the tongue and cheek. It is considered precancerous and is associated with smoking.
Lipoma	Fatty tumor that generally does not metastasize (spread).
Nevus	A pigmented (colored) congenital skin blemish. It is usually benign but may become cancerous. Also called a birthmark or mole.

Malignant (Cancerous) Neoplasms	Description
Basal cell carcinoma	An epithelial tumor of the basal cell layer of the epidermis. A frequent type of skin cancer that rarely metastasizes.
Karposi's sarcoma	A form of skin cancer frequently seen in acquired immune deficiency syndrome (AIDS) patients. It consists of brownish-purple papules that spread from the skin.
Malignant melanoma	A dangerous form of skin cancer caused by an overgrowth of melanin in the skin. It may metastasize.
Squamous cell carcinoma	Epidermal cancer that may go into deeper tissue but does not generally metastasize.

Cardiovascular disease is the most frequent cause of death and illness in the United States, regardless of gender. Working as a medical assistant in any specialty, you will care for patients with heart disease. It is important that you recognize the signs and symptoms of heart disease. You must also be able to explain and perform diagnostic procedures and tests associated with the circulatory system. Chapter 45 discusses performing routine tests such as ECG and Holter Monitoring.

The symptoms of cardiovascular disease and disorders are varied due to the wide range of precipitating causes such as poor circulation, defective heart valves, conduction defect, and blood clots in the heart layers or blood vessels. The most common symptoms of cardiovascular disorders are:

- Chest pain (crushing type of pain)
- Cyanosis (bluish skin color due to lack of oxygen in the tissues)
- Diaphoresis (excessive sweating)
- Dyspnea (difficult breathing)
- Edema
- Irregular heartbeat

Procedures and diagnostic tests related to the cardiovascular system are listed in Table 35-4.

TABLE 35-3 Procedures and Diagnostic Tests Relating to the Integumentary System

Procedure/Test	Description
Adipectomy	Surgical removal of fat.
Biopsy	Removal of a piece of tissue by syringe and needle, knife, punch, or brush to examine under a microscope as an aid diagnosis.
Cauterization	The destruction of tissue with a caustic chemical, electrical current, freezing, or hot iron.
Chemobrasion	Abrasion of skin using chemicals; also called chemical peel.
Cryosurgery	The use of extreme cold to freeze and destroy tissue.
Curettage	The removal of superficial skin lesions with a curette or scraper.
Debridement	The removal of foreign material or dead tissue from a wound.
Dermabrasion	Abrasion or rubbing, using wire brushes or sandpaper.
Dermatoplasty	The transplantation of skin or skin grafting. May be used to treat large birthmarks (hemangiomas) and burns.
Electrocautery	To destroy tissue with an electric current.
Exfoliative cytology	Scraping cells from tissue and then examining them under a microscope.
Frozen section	Taking a thin piece of tissue from a frozen specimen for rapid examination under a microscope. Often performed during a surgical procedure to detect cancer.
Fungal scrapings (FS)	Scrapings taken with a curette from lesions, placed on a growth medium and examined under the microscope to identify fungal growth.
Incision and drainage (I&D)	Making an incision to create an opening for the drainage of material, such as pus.
Laser therapy	Removal of skin lesions and birthmarks using a laser that emits intense heat and power at close range. The laser converts frequencies of light into one small beam.
Lipectomy	Surgical removal of fat.
Marsupialization	Creating a pouch to promote drainage by surgically opening a closed area, such as a cyst.
Needle biopsy	Using a sterile needle to remove tissue for examination under a microscope.
Plication	Taking tucks surgically in a structure to shorten it.
Rhytidectomy	Surgical removal of excess skin to eliminate wrinkles. Commonly referred to as a facelift.
Skin grafts	The transfer of skin from a normal area to cover another site. Used to treat burn victims and after some surgical procedures.
Sweat test	Test performed on sweat to see the level of chloride. There is an increase in skin chloride in some diseases such as cystic fibrosis.
Tzanck test	A microscopic examination of a small piece of tissue that has been surgically scraped from a pustule. The specimen is placed on a slide and stained; then the type of viral infection can be identified.

Taking a Wound Culture

OBJECTIVE: Obtain a sample from a wound by using a swab technique without error.

Equipment and Supplies

gloves; culture tube with sterile swab and transport media; tape for dressing; sterile water for cleansing wound; sterile 4 × 4 gauze dressing; hazardous waste container; bag for soiled dressing; prepared label for culture tube or pen for labeling tube

Method

1. Perform hand hygiene.
2. Assemble equipment.
3. Identify patient and explain procedure.
4. Apply gloves.
5. Remove dressing, noting amount and type of exudate and place in bag.
6. Observe wound for redness, crusting, swelling, and odor.
7. Using a sterile swab, place it in the wound using a wiping motion. Place the swab in the sterile culture tube. Crush the ampule of preservative that is in the culture tube and seal the tube. Label the culture tube with patient's name, identification number, and date.
8. Remove gloves, perform hand hygiene, and apply sterile gloves.
9. Clean the wound using sterile water and 4 × 4 gauze squares.
10. Apply sterile dressing over the wound.
11. Instruct patient in wound care.
12. Remove gloves and dispose of them properly in hazardous waste container.
13. Chart the procedure.

Charting Example

2/14/XX	3:30 P.M.

Small amount of exudate obtained from open wound on L. ankle using sterile swab. Tube labeled and sent to lab. Wound cleaned and dressed. Erythema surrounding wound site. No odor noted. Home care instructions given.

M. King, CMA

Coronary Artery Disease

Coronary artery disease (CAD) usually results from atherosclerosis (build up of fatty material and plaque in the arteries), particularly the coronary arteries. As the coronary arteries narrow, the blood flow to the heart muscle is lessened and angina (suffocating pain) may occur. If enough of the heart muscle is denied oxygen-rich blood supply, a myocardial infarction (MI) or heart attack may occur. Classic symptoms are pain in the left arm and jaw, sweating, and crushing or squeezing sensation. In females, the symptoms vary widely and often go undetected because it has been commonly believed that CAD is a man's disease. One in ten American women 45 to 64 have some sort of heart disease, and the number affected increases to one in four over 65 years of age.

Congestive Heart Failure

Congestive heart failure (CHF) may result from ischemia (reduced blood supply) to the heart muscle. Symptoms of CHF are shortness of breath and swollen feet and ankles (Figure 35-5). These symptoms occur because the heart muscle becomes weakened and is less able to pump blood to the rest of the body. The American Heart Association reports that every 29 seconds someone in the United States has a CHF-related event, and every minute someone dies from this event.

Risk Factors

Understanding the risk factors associated with heart disease will help you to educate your patients. Patients with multiple risk factors are not only at risk for heart attack, but also for cerebral vascular accidents (CVA) or stroke due to blood clots traveling to the brain. There is evidence that cardiac changes that were once associated with aging can be modified by changes in lifestyle and personal habits. Reducing fat intake, monitoring sodium intake, exercising regularly, refraining from smoking, moderating alcohol intake, and managing stress help to promote good cardiovascular health. Physicians monitor blood pressure and blood lipid levels of patients as part of annual physical examinations.

The National Cholesterol Education Program recommends more intensive treatment, such as drug therapy for individuals at a moderately high to high risk of having a heart attack. Research indicates that the more you lower low-density lipids (LDL or bad

TABLE 35-4 Procedures and Diagnostic Tests Relating to the Cardiovascular System

Procedure/Test	Description
Aneurysmectomy	The surgical removal of the sac of an aneurysm, which is an abnormal dilation of a blood vessel.
Angiography	X-rays taken after the injection of opaque material into a blood vessel. They can be performed on the aorta as an aortic angiogram, on the heart as an angiocardiogram, and on the brain as a cerebral angiogram.
Angioplasty	A surgical procedure of altering the structure of a vessel by dilating the vessel using a balloon inside the vessel.
Arterial blood gases	Measurement of the amount of oxygen, carbon dioxide, nitrogen in the blood, and a pH reading of the blood. Blood gases are performed in emergency situations and provide valuable evaluation of cardiac failure, hemorrhage, and kidney failure.
Artery graft	A piece of blood vessel that is transplanted from a part of the body to the aorta to repair a defect.
Artificial pacemaker	Electrical device that substitutes for the natural pacemaker of the heart. It controls the beating of the heart by a series of rhythmic electrical impulses. An external pacemaker has the electrodes on the outside of the body. An internal pacemaker will have the electrodes surgically implanted within the chest wall.
Cardiac catheterization	Passage of thin tube (catheter) through an arm vein and the blood vessels leading into the heart. It is done to detect abnormalities, to collect cardiac blood samples, and to determine the pressure within the cardiac area.
Cardiac enzymes	Complex proteins capable of inducing chemical changes within the body. Cardiac enzymes are taken by blood sample to determine the amount of heart disease or damage.
Cardiac magnetic resonance imaging (MRI)	A noninvasive procedure in which images of the heart and blood vessels are captured for examination to determine effects.
Cardiolysis	A surgical procedure to separate adhesions that involves a resection of the ribs and sternum over the pericardium.
Cardiorrhaphy	Surgical suturing of the heart.
Cardioversion	Converting a cardiac arrhythmia (irregular heart rhythm) to a normal sinus rhythm using a cardioverter to give counter shocks to the heart.
Commissurotomy	Surgical incision to change the size of an opening. For example, in mitral valve commissurotomy, a stenosis or narrowing is corrected by cutting away at the adhesions around the mitral opening.
Coronary artery bypass surgery	Open heart surgery in which a shunt is created to permit blood to travel around the constriction in the coronary vessel(s).
Doppler ultrasonography	Measurement of sound waves as they bounce off tissues and organs to produce an image. Can assist in determining heart and blood vessel damage; also called an echocardiogram.

(continued)

Procedure/Test	Description
Electrocardiogram (ECG)	Record of the electrical activity of the heart. Useful in the diagnosis of abnormal cardiac rhythm and heart muscle (myocardium) damage. This procedure is explained fully in Chapter 45.
Electrolytes	Measurement of blood sodium (Na), potassium (K), and chlorides (Cl).
Embolectomy	Surgical removal of an embolus or blood clot from a vessel.
Heart transplantation	Replacement of a diseased or malfunctioning heart with a donor's heart.
Holter Monitor	Portable ECG monitor worn by the patient for a period of a few hours to a few days to assess the heart and pulse activity as the person goes through the activities of daily living. Used to assess a patient who experiences chest pain and unusual heart activity during exercise and normal activities when a cardiogram is inconclusive.
Lipoproteins	Measurement of blood to determine serum cholesterol and triglyceride levels.
Open heart surgery	Surgery that involves the heart, coronary arteries, or the heart valves. The heart is actually entered by the surgeon.
Percutaneous balloon valvuloplasty	Insertion through the skin of a balloon catheter across a narrowed or stenotic heart valve. When the balloon is inflated, the narrowing or constriction is decreased.
Percutaneous transluminal coronary angioplasty (PCTA)	Method for treating localized coronary artery narrowing. A balloon catheter is inserted through the skin into the coronary artery and inflated to dilate the narrow blood vessel.
Phleborrhaphy	Suturing of a vein.
Prothrombin time	Measurement of the time it takes for a sample of blood to coagulate.
Stress testing (Treadmill test)	Method for evaluating cardiovascular fitness. The patient is placed on a treadmill or bicycle and then subjected to steadily increasing levels of work. An ECG and oxygen levels are taken while the patient exercises. The test is stopped if abnormalities occur on the ECG.
Valve replacement	Surgical procedure to excise a diseased heart valve and replace with an artificial valve.
Venography	X-ray of the veins by tracing the venous flow. Also called phlebography.

cholesterol) the less likely you are to have a heart attack. Overall for very high-risk patients, the new goal is to have an LDL below 100 mg/dl. In moderate risk patients, the new goal is an LDL under 130 mg/dl.

Very high risk is defined as those who have just had a heart attack, who have heart disease, diabetes, are regular smokers, and have hypertension. At high risk are those with heart disease, metabolic syndrome, and other multiple risk factors. Moderately high-risk patients are those with multiple risk factors. All at-risk patients should begin therapeutic lifestyle changes (low-fat diet, exercise, stop smoking) regardless of LDL level.

Treatment of Heart Disease

Treatment of heart disease is varied because of the wide number of conditions associated with the cardiovascular system. Three treatments will be examined here. For more information regarding heart disease and treatments, organizations such as the American Heart Association are excellent resources.

- Hypertension or high blood pressure is one of the first symptoms a patient may exhibit. Blood vessels become more rigid and constricted and as a result, blood pushes on the vessel with more force.

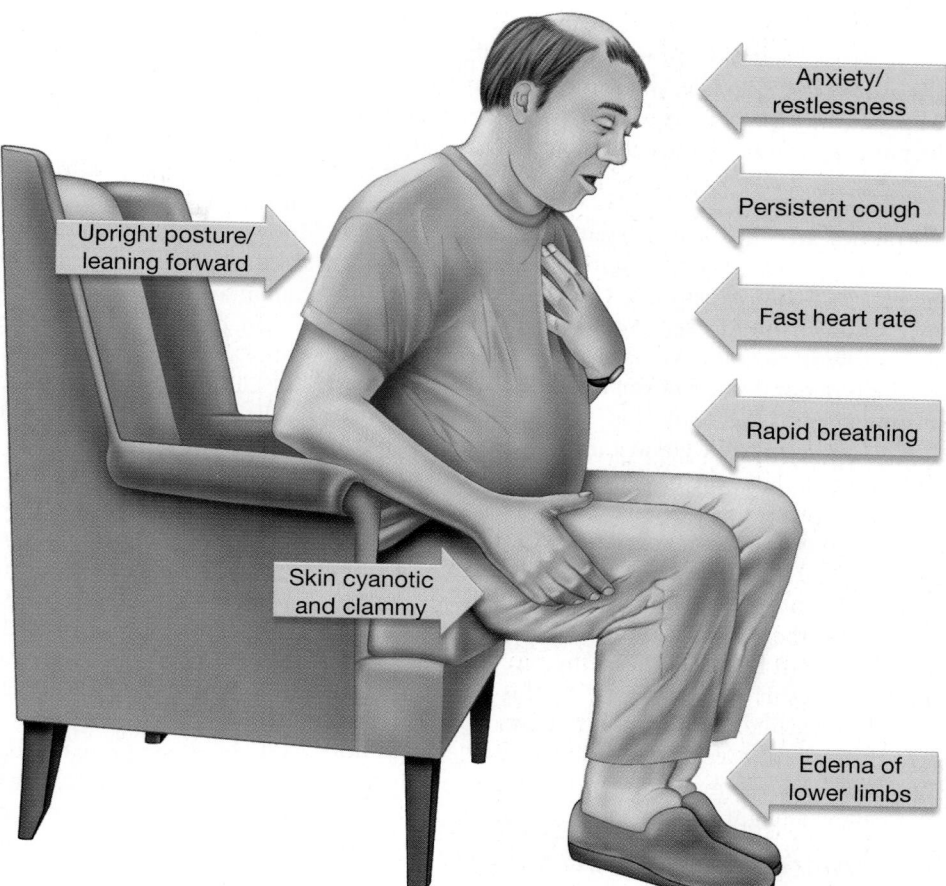

Anxiety/restlessness

Persistent cough

Fast heart rate

Rapid breathing

Upright posture/leaning forward

Skin cyanotic and clammy

Edema of lower limbs

FIGURE 35-5 Examples of symptoms of congestive heart failure (CHF).

Treatment for hypertension includes making life changes to reduce risk factors such as obesity, smoking, and lack of exercise. A variety of medications are available to reduce blood pressure, including diuretics, which help eliminate excess fluid from the body. Cholesterol medications, known as statins, may be prescribed. Blood pressure should be monitored regularly.

- Dysrhythmia is an abnormality of the rhythm or rate of the heartbeat. Dysrhythmia is caused by a disturbance of the electrical system in the heart. Tachycardia is a rapid heartbeat over 100 beats per minute and bradycardia is a slow heart rate under 60 beats per minute. A pacemaker to override the heart's rhythm and provide electrical impulses to regulate rhythm may be necessary. Pacemakers can either be attached externally or implanted internally.

- Coronary artery blockage occurs when plaque and fatty deposits occlude or block one or more of the coronary arteries (arteries that supply the heart muscle with oxygenated blood). There are various methods used to open the coronary vessels including clot-breaking drugs, such as TPA, and balloon angioplasty (Figure 35-6). If these efforts fail, coronary artery bypass surgery using a graft of patient's vein or an artificial vein to bypass the occluded area of the heart muscle may be necessary.

Endocrinology

Endocrinology is the study of the endocrine system. There are two types of glands in the endocrine system, exocrine glands and endocrine glands. Exocrine glands release secretions through a duct or another organ. Endocrine glands are ductless, produce hormones, and

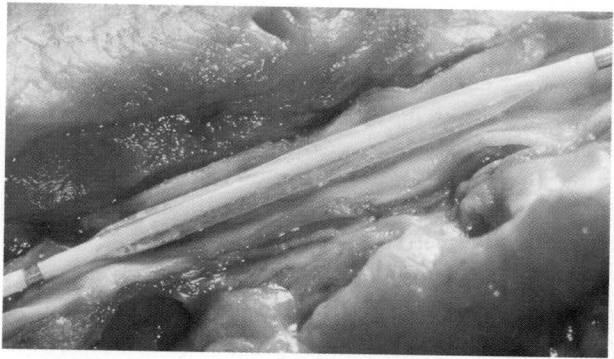

FIGURE 35-6 Balloon angioplasty is used to open coronary vessels.

secrete directly into the blood stream. The endocrine system includes the following organs: two adrenal glands, two ovaries in the female, two sets of parathyroid glands, the pancreas (islets of Langerhans), two testes in the male, the pituitary gland, thymus gland, and thyroid gland.

Hormones

Hormones are chemical messengers produced by the endocrine glands and transported to target tissue by the blood stream. Hormones transfer information and instructions from one set of cells to another. They regulate growth, sexual development, mood, metabolism, and help maintain homeostasis. Each hormone targets specific cells in the body. For example, thyroxin produced by the thyroid gland targets all the cells in the body and regulates the basic metabolic rate of each cell and thus the body as a whole. Hormones are regulated by the nervous system, endocrine control, and a feedback system. The under- or overproduction of even a small amount of hormone can have drastic consequences for the patient. For instance, the underproduction of growth hormone from the pituitary gland in a child can result in dwarfism. In this condition, the body has normal proportions but attains a height of only three to four feet. Overproduction of growth hormone can result in giantism, and the person may grow to a height of eight feet.

Treatments Using Hormones

Many conditions are treated with hormones. For example, diabetes mellitus is treated with insulin, which is now produced synthetically. Steroids, a type of hormone naturally produced in the body, can be used as anti-inflammatory agents to fight disease. Infertility may be treated with estrogens.

Diabetes Mellitus

One of the most common hormonal imbalances the medical assistant will encounter is diabetes mellitus (DM). Approximately 17 million Americans have been diagnosed with DM and nearly 200,000 die each year from the disease. Diabetes mellitus is characterized by hyperglycemia (too much sugar in the blood) and results in a lack of insulin or resistance to the effects of insulin by cells. Without insulin to assist the transportation of glucose into the cells, a patient will experience adverse symptoms, including elevated blood glucose level, excessive thirst (polydipsia), excessive urination (polyuria), rapid weight loss, fatigue, itching, skin infections, and vision problems. If untreated, life-threatening conditions such as stroke, cardiovascular disease, loss of limbs due to infection, blindness to due retinal damage, kidney damage, and diabetic coma can result.

Types of Diabetes Mellitus

Type 1 DM or insulin-dependent diabetes mellitus (IDDM) is characterized by the destruction of the beta cells of the islets of Langerhans in the pancreas and a complete lack of insulin. Type 1 DM has a rapid onset, is believed to be an autoimmune condition triggered by a virus, and occurs most often in children. Scientists believe there maybe a genetic predisposition for this type of DM. Type 1 DM is treated by administration of insulin by injection. Blood glucose levels must be monitored carefully sometimes as many as eight to ten times a day to calculate the amount of insulin needed to maintain normal glucose levels.

In Type 2 DM or noninsulin-dependent diabetes mellitus (NDDM), the insulin that is produced by the islets of Langerhans in the pancreas has little or no effect on cells because of a deficiency of insulin receptors on cell membranes. The majority of diabetes cases fall into this category. Type 2 DM has a slow onset, and risk factors include obesity and family history of diabetes. Control of Type 2 DM may not require insulin injection but may be controlled with medications that enable the insulin to react with cell receptors. Careful food management and moderate exercise are also important for controlling Type 2 DM. The American Diabetes Association noted that Type 2 DM has increased by 33 percent in the past 10 years and investigators relate the increase to the rapidly increasing rate of obesity.

The medical assistant will be taking an active part in educating the patient on diabetes management, performing glucose monitoring, and helping the patient understand and comply with the treatment plan the physician has established (Figure 35-7). The newly diagnosed diabetic patient will have to make life changes to regulate his or her blood sugar to avoid the long-term complications of this devastating disease.

Table 35-5 lists procedures and diagnostic tests relating to the endocrine system. Legal and Ethical Issues discusses more on patient education and the legal responsibilities of the medical assistant.

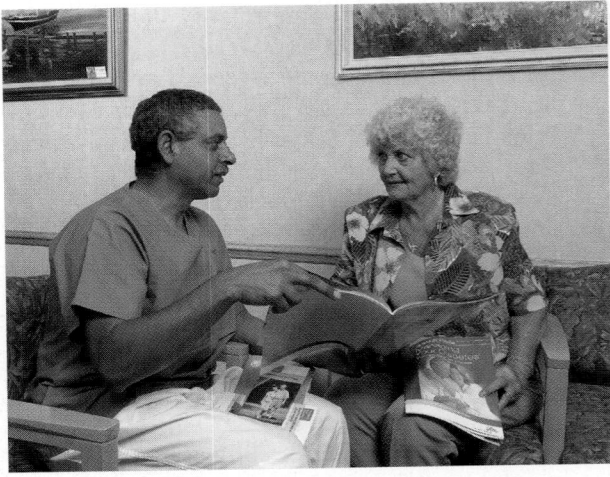

FIGURE 35-7 Using educational materials, a medical assistant discusses lifestyle changes with a diabetic patient.

TABLE 35-5 **Procedures and Diagnostic Tests Relating to the Endocrine System**

Procedure/Test	Description
Basal metabolic rate	Somewhat outdated test to measure the energy used when the body is in a state of rest.
Blood serum test	Blood test to measure the level of substances such as calcium, electrolytes, testosterone, insulin, and glucose. Used to assist in determining the function of various endocrine glands.
Fasting blood sugar	Blood test to measure the amount of glucose circulating throughout the body after fasting for 12 hours.
Glucose tolerance test (GTT)	Test to determine the blood sugar level. A measured dose of glucose is given to a patient either orally or intravenously. Blood samples are then drawn at certain intervals to determine the ability of the patient to utilize glucose. Used for diabetic patients to determine their insulin response to glucose.
Parathryroidectomy	Excision of one or more of the parathyroid glands. This is performed to halt the progress of hyperparathyroidism.
17-hydroxycorticosteroids (17-OHCS)	Test performed on urine to identify adrenocorticosteroid hormones. It is used to determine adrenal cortical function.
17-ketosteroids (17-KS)	Test performed on urine to determine the amount of 17-KS present. 17-KS is the end product of androgens and is secreted from the adrenal glands and testes. It is used in diagnosing adrenal tumors.
Protein bound iodine test (PBI)	Blood test to measure the concentration of thyroxin (T4) circulating in the blood stream. The iodine becomes bound to the protein in the blood and can be measured.
Radioactive iodine uptake test (RAIU)	Test in which radioactive iodine is taken orally or intravenously and the amount of iodine eventually taken into the thyroid gland (uptake) is measured to assist in determining thyroid function.
Radioimmune assay test (RIA)	Test used to measure the levels of hormones in the plasma of the blood.
Serum glucose test	Blood test performed to assist in determining insulin levels and useful for adjusting medication dosage.
Thymectomy	Surgical removal of the thymus gland.
Thyroid echogram	Ultrasound examination of the thyroid that can assist in distinguishing a thyroid nodule from a cyst.
Thyroidectomy	Surgical removal of the thyroid gland. The patient is then placed on replacement hormone (thyroid) therapy.
Thyroid function tests	Blood tests used to measure the levels of T3, T4, and TSH in the blood stream to assist in determining thyroid function.
Thyroparathroidectomy	Surgical removal (excision) of the thyroid gland and parathyroid glands.
Thyroid scan	Test in which a radioactive element is administered that localizes in the thyroid gland. The gland can then be visualized with a scanning device to detect pathology such as tumors.
Total calcium	Blood test to measure the total amount of calcium to assist in detecting parathyroid and bone disorders.
Two-hour postprandial glucose tolerance test	Blood test to assist in evaluating glucose metabolism. The patient fasts over night and then eats a high carbohydrate meal in the morning. A blood sample is then taken two hours after the meal.

Many of the procedures and immunizations discussed in this chapter require written consent either from the patient or legal guardian, if the patient is a child. Careful explanation of the benefits and risks associated with all treatments should be explained by the physician. The medical assistant needs to reinforce the physician's explanation and determine if the patient has understood the explanation.

The patient has a right to privacy and confidentiality during the examination process. Doors should be closed during any examination or procedure and patients, including children, should be draped to protect their modesty. The examination of infants and children carries an additional safety risk since they are unable to protect themselves. The medical assistant must never leave an infant or child unattended.

Gastrointestinal System

The gastrointestinal or digestive system includes the mouth, esophagus, stomach, small and large intestines, and the accessory organs liver, gallbladder, and pancreas. This system stores and digests food, eliminates waste, and utilizes nutrients. Table 35-6 lists procedures and diagnostic tests relating to the digestive system.

The digestive system involves many organs and similar symptoms may be present in a number of disorders and conditions. A patient who sees a gastroenterologist is usually referred by the primary care physician (PCP). Proctology is a subspecialty of gastroenterology. A proctologist treats disorders of the rectum and anus only.

Many of the examinations associated with the digestive system may be uncomfortable and embarrassing for the patient, such as a digital rectal examination or colonoscopy. You must be prepared to provide reassurance to the patient before, during, and after procedures. Patients have the right to privacy and every effort must be made to drape the patient to prevent him or her from being unnecessarily exposed and further embarrassed. When gathering information from patients, listen carefully to their replies. If pain is involved, ask the patient to show you where the pain is located. Pain may be referred (appear somewhere else), and not over the involved organ. For example, gall bladder pain may be in the upper right back, not the abdomen (Figure 35-8). Symptoms such as colic (acute abdominal pain) may be present in a number of conditions. Indigestion is a symptom of gastroesophageal reflux disease (GERD) and also may be present in some patients who are having a heart attack. Many of the procedures associated with the gastrointestinal system involve endoscopy (looking into an opening of the body with a lighted instrument), therefore, proper patient preparation is important to obtain valid results.

Common Disorders of The Digestive System

One of the most commonly encountered GI disorders is gastroesophageal reflux disease (GERD). Approximately

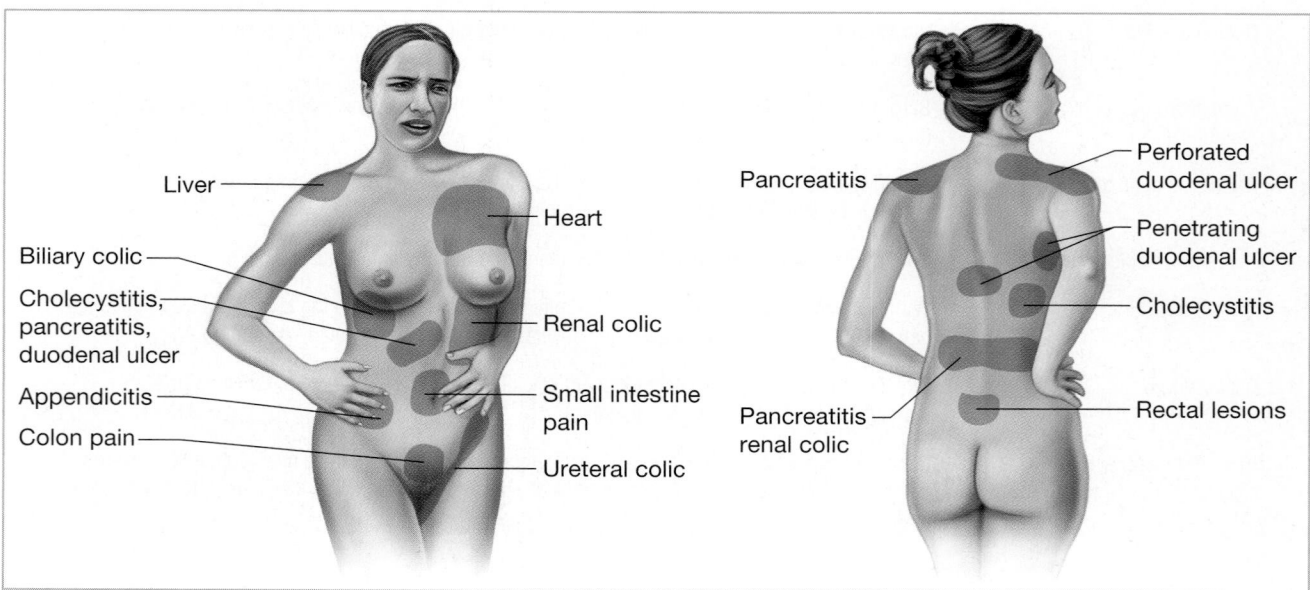

FIGURE 35-8 Examples of sites of referred abdominal pain.

TABLE 35-6   Procedures and Diagnostic Tests Relating to the Digestive System

Procedure/Test	Description
Abdominal ultrasonography	Using ultrasound equipment for producing sound waves to create an image of the abdominal organs.
Air contrast barium enema	Using both barium and air to visualize the colon on x-ray.
Anastomosis	Creating a passage way or opening between two organs or vessels.
Appendectomy	Surgical removal of the appendix.
Barium enema (lower GI)	Radiographic examination of the small intestine, large intestine, or colon in which an enema containing barium is administered to the patient while x-ray pictures are taken.
Barium swallow (upper GI)	A barium mixture swallowed while x-ray pictures are taken of the esophagus, stomach, and duodenum. It is used to visualize the upper GI tract. Also called esophogram.
Colectomy	Surgical removal of the entire colon.
Cholecystectomy	Surgical excise of the gallbladder. Removal of the gallbladder through the laparoscope is a newer procedure with fewer complications than the more invasive abdominal surgery. The laparoscope requires a small incision into the abdominal cavity.
Cholecystogram	Dye given orally to the patient is absorbed and enters the gallbladder, then an x-ray is taken.
Choledocholithotomy	Removal of a gallstone through an incision into the bile duct.
Choledocholithotripsy	Crushing of a gallstone in the common bile duct. Commonly called lithotripsy.
Colonoscopy	A flexible fiberscope passed through the anus, rectum, and colon is used to examine the upper portion of the colon. Polyps and small growths can be removed during the procedure.
Colostomy	Surgical creation of an opening of some portion of the colon through the abdominal wall to the outside surface.
Diverticulectomy	Surgical removal of a diverticulum.
Endoscopic retrograde cholangiopancreatography (ERCP)	Using an endoscope to x-ray the bile and pancreatic ducts.
Esophagoscopy	The esophagus is visualized by passing an instrument down the esophagus. A tissue sample for biopsy may be taken.
Esophagram (barium swallow)	As barium is swallowed the solution is observed traveling from the mouth into the stomach.
Esophagogastrostomy	Surgical creation of an opening between the esophagus and stomach.
Esophagostomy	Surgical creation of an opening into the esophagus.
Exploratory laparotomy	Abdominal operation for the purpose of examining the abdominal organs and tissues for signs of disease or other abnormalities.
Fistulectomy	Excision of a fistula.
Gastrectomy	Surgical removal of part or all of the stomach.

(continued)

Procedure/Test	Description
Gastrointestinal endoscopy	A flexible instrument or scope is passed either through the mouth or anus to facilitate visualization of the GI tract.
Gastric levage	Obtaining a sample of gastric contents by insertion of orogastric tube through the mouth to stomach.
Glossectomy	Complete or partial removal of the tongue.
Hemorrhoidectomy	Surgical excision of hemorrhoids from the anorectal area.
Hepatic lobotomy	Surgical excision of a lobe of the liver.
Ileostomy	Surgical creation of a passage way through the abdominal wall into the ileum. The fecal matter (stool) drains into a bag worn on the abdomen.
Intravenous cholangiogram	A dye is administered to the patient that allows for visualization of the bile vessels.
Intravenous cholecystography	A dye in administered intravenously to the patient that allows for visualization of the gallbladder.
Jejunostomy	Surgical creation of a permanent opening into the jejunum.
Lithotripsy	Crushing of a stone located within the gallbladder.
Liver biopsy	Excision of a small piece of liver tissue for microscopic examination. This is generally used to determine if cancer is present.
Liver scan	A radioactive substance is administered to the patient by IV route. This substance enters liver cells and the organ can then be visualized to detect tumors, abscesses, and other hepatomegaly.
Occult blood	A test performed on feces to determine the presence of invisible amounts of blood. Positive results may indicate gastrointestinal bleeding.
Ova and parasites	A test performed on stool to identify ova and parasites. A positive result indicates protozoa infestation.
Proctoplasty	Plastic surgery of the anus and rectum.
Splenectomy	Surgical removal of the spleen.
Stool culture	A test performed on stool to identify presence of organisms.
Ultrasonography, gallbladder	A test to visualize the gallbladder by using high frequency sound waves. Used to detect gallbladder inflammation biliary obstructions, or gall stones.
Ultrasonsography, liver	A test to visualize liver by using high frequency sound waves. Used to detect hepatic tumors, cysts, abscess, and cirrhosis.
Upper gastrointestinal fiberoscopy	The direct visualization of the gastric mucosa via a flexible fiberscope. Used to detect gastric neoplasm.
Vagotomy	Surgical resection of the vagus nerve in an attempt to decrease the amount of acid secretion into the stomach. Used as a treatment for ulcer patients.

one-third of Americans suffer from this common disorder. GERD is also known as acid reflux or acid indigestion and is caused by stomach acid flowing back up into the esophagus. Normally the sphincter muscle at the juncture of the stomach and esophagus prevents the reflux of acid. If this sphincter muscle is weak, acid reflux may occur. In some patients, the presence of hiatal hernia, eating spicy or greasy foods, and drinking alcohol may cause a local irritation. A hiatal hernia occurs when the upper portion of the stomach protrudes into the chest through the esophageal opening or hiatus of the diaphragm. GERD symptoms include heartburn, burping, and a sour taste in the back of the throat. Persistent acid reflux increases the risk of esophageal cancer. To diagnosis GERD, an upper GI series and barium swallow, and gastroscopy are usually ordered. Treatment of gastroesophageal reflux disease includes making some life changes such as eating small meals six times a day, eating a least two to three hours before bedtime, modifying diet to avoid problem foods, losing weight, and moderating amounts of coffee and alcohol. If those measures fail, then a medication that reduces acid secretions can be ordered or purchased over the counter. Repeated use of antacids is not recommended because they can disrupt body chemistry and cause the stomach to increase acid secretions.

Another common GI disorder is diverticular disease. Diverticula are out-pouching or small sacs found mainly in the lower part of the colon or large intestine and occasionally in other parts of the digestive tract. A diverticulum is a bulging of the inner lining of the intestinal wall through the muscular layers of intestines. Chronic constipation and low fiber diet are thought to be causative factors. Diverticulosis, the presence of diverticula, is found in about half of those over 60 years of age in the United States. Many individuals with diverticula are asymptomatic. Diverticulitis is an inflammation of one or more diverticula causing severe pain, muscle spasm, nausea, and fever. The patient may complain of cramping and tenderness on the left side of the abdomen, small round hard stools, and gas. Untreated diverticulitis may cause narrowing of the intestine, intestinal obstruction and peritonitis, inflammation of the lining of the abdominal cavity, if the diverticula burst.

Diagnosis of diverticular disease depends on patient history, x-ray of the lower GI tract, barium enema, and sigmoidoscopy or colonoscopy. Diverticular disease requires no treatment except to encourage the patient to avoid constipation, and to increase dietary fiber intake. Diverticulitis requires treatment with antibiotics and possibly antispasmodic medication to relieve abdominal pain. In the case of intestinal blockage, hospitalization, and intravenous fluids are necessary. A colectomy, surgical removal of all or part of the colon, may be necessary and possibly a colostomy, creation of an opening of the colon through the adominal wall to allow for passage of stools. Dietary restriction of foods containing seeds, nuts, and corn is recommended by some physicians, while others say it is not necessary to avoid these foods because research has not shown them to be directly linked to diverticular disease.

Sigmoidoscopy

The sigmoidoscopy, also called proctoscopic or proctosigmoidoscopic examination, is an examination of the interior of the sigmoid colon for diagnostic purposes. This is a useful procedure to assist in the detection of cancer of the colon, polyps, ulcerations, and other disorders of the lower intestinal tract.

The sigmoidoscope, a flexible, metal or plastic instrument with a light source and magnification lens, is used for the sigmoidoscopy. The flexible sigmoidoscope, more widely used by physicians, allows the physician to see further into the colon and view the mucous membranes of the intestines. It is more comfortable for the patients as well. For this procedure the patient may be placed in the Sims' position or on a proctoscopic examination table (Figure 35-9).

Preparation for this examination is important. Patients should be told to empty their bowel and bladder before coming in for the procedure. The physician will usually have the patient take a commercially prepared enema two hours before the examination. Patients should be advised to drink plenty of clear liquids and eat sparingly the day before the examination. Some physicians will request the patient to refrain from eating raw fruits and vegetables, grains, and dairy products a few days prior to the examination so the colon

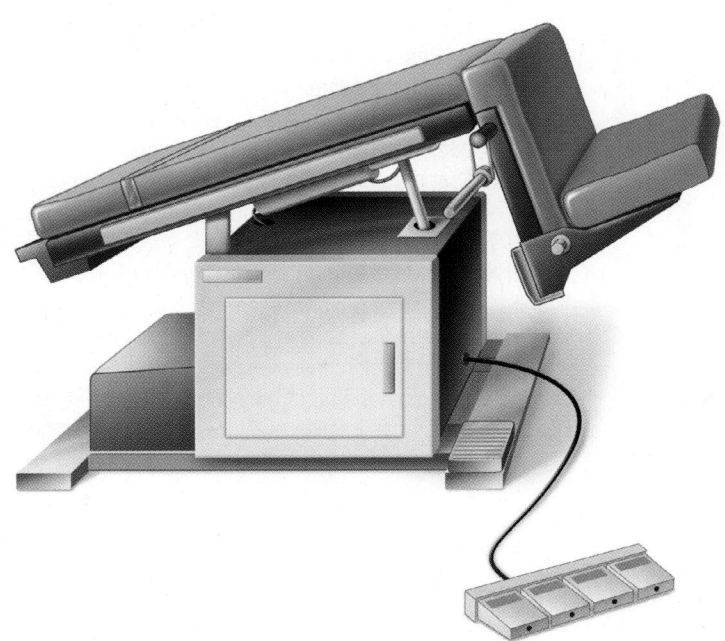

FIGURE 35-9 Proctoscopic examination table.

Assisting with a Sigmoidoscopy

OBJECTIVE: Assist the physician during the sigmoidoscopic examination by positioning the patient, handling all equipment, biopsy material, and providing support for the patient throughout the procedure without error.

Equipment and Supplies

sigmoidoscope with obturator, flexible or inflexible (metal or plastic); anoscope; rectal speculum; insufflator; suction equipment; sterile specimen container with preservative; sterile biopsy forceps; cotton applicators (long); lubricating jelly; basin of warm water; patient drape; gloves; patient gown; small towel or examination table pad; tissue; biohazard waste container

Method

1. Perform hand hygiene.
2. Prepare equipment and supplies. Check all lights and light bulbs in equipment. Prepare a basin of warm water to receive used instruments. Test suction equipment. Place obturator within the sigmoidoscope.
3. Identify patient and explain procedure. Make sure the patient has followed the enema and diet instructions. Check to make sure the consent form has been signed.
4. Ask patient to undress, put on a patient gown, and empty bladder.
5. Assist patient into the Sims', lateral, or knee-chest position or onto the proctology table. **Rationale:** In the knee-chest position, the abdominal contents and organs move forward and away from the pelvic area, which makes it easier to insert the sigmoidoscope.
6. Drape the patient and place a towel or disposable examination pad under the perineal area.
7. Don gloves.
8. Place lubricant on the physician's gloved fingers for a digital examination.
9. Place metal scope in basin of warm water to warm it before insertion into patient.
10. Lubricate the tip of the scope.
11. Attach the inflation bulb (for air inflation during the procedure) and attach the light source. Turn the scope on just before the physician is ready to use it. **Rationale:** The scope tip becomes warm/hot if turned on too soon and may harm the patient.
12. Remind the patient to take deep breaths and relax the abdominal muscles and observe for any undue reactions.
13. Assist the physician by handing instruments and equipment such as suction and cotton tipped applicators, as they are needed. Place used equipment, including suction tubing, into basin of water.
14. Assist with biopsy by holding open specimen containers to receive specimen, while maintaining sterility of container.
15. Clean around patient's anal opening with tissue. Discard in biohazard waste container.
16. Remove gloves and perform hand hygiene.
17. Assist patient to slowly sit up. **Rationale:** Sitting up too quickly from the Sims' position can result in dizziness.
18. Ask patient to dress and provide assistance as needed.
19. Label specimen container with patient's name, address, date, source of specimen, and ID number.
20. Apply gloves and clean equipment, sterilize equipment as needed, clean room.
21. Remove gloves and document procedure. The physician will document the results of the procedure.

Charting Example

2/14/XX	9:00 A.M.

Assisted patient with sigmoidoscopic examination. Biopsy sent to lab. No dizziness or discomfort noted after procedure.

M. King, CMA

will be easier to visualize. It is critical that every attempt is made to ensure the patient follows the instructions for the preparation because an improperly prepared bowel may result in having to reschedule the procedure.

This procedure can be uncomfortable for patients. It is made easier for patients if they are instructed to concentrate on breathing deeply through the mouth while trying to relax the abdominal muscles. Even though the procedure only lasts a few minutes, the patient will need encouragement throughout the procedure. It is helpful to inform patients after the procedure that they might experience flatus (gas) as a result of the air introduced during the procedure.

The physician may take several biopsy samples during the procedure requiring that specimen containers be part of every sigmoidoscopy setup. The patient should sign a consent form for both the procedure and any biopsy of materials. Procedure 35-2 provides the steps for assisting with a sigmoidoscopic examination.

Colonoscopy

Colonoscopy procedures are performed in a hospital outpatient area because an IV sedative is administered prior to the procedure. Colonoscopy allows the physician to examine more of the large intestine than the sigmoidoscopy. American Cancer Society recommends all individuals over the age of 50 have a colonoscopy to screen for cancer.

Lymphatic System

The lymphatic system, which consists of lymph glands, ducts, nodes, tonsils, thymus gland, and spleen, is the basis of the body's defense or immune system. This system protects the body against the invasion of foreign microorganisms. It works in conjunction with the circulatory system to purify the blood and drain fluids throughout the body.

Immunity is the body's ability to defend itself against pathogenic organisms and toxic substances. Immunity is either natural or acquired. Natural immunity is nonspecific and does not require exposure to pathogenic microorganisms. An example of natural immunity is when macrophages (special cells) roam through the body ingesting bacteria and other foreign substances. Acquired immunity develops following exposure to a specific pathogenic microorganism. Immunizations are a type of acquired immunity where a weakened form of the pathogen is given to the patient and specific antibodies to that particular pathogen develop. For example, a child is given the polio vaccine to develop antibodies to the polio virus. The child is then immunized from getting polio.

In some diseases, such as acquired immune deficiency syndrome (AIDS), part of the body's immune system has been destroyed; therefore, the natural ability to fight off infection is lost. AIDS is discussed more fully in Chapter 26. Table 35-7 lists procedures and diagnostic tests related to the lymphatic system.

TABLE 35-7 **Procedures and Diagnostic Tests Relating to the Lymphatic System**

Procedures/Tests	Description
Bone marrow aspiration	Removing a sample of bone marrow by syringe for microscopic examination. Useful for diagnosing diseases such as leukemia. For example, a proliferation (massive increase of white blood cells) could confirm the diagnosis of leukemia.
CT scan (CAT)	Use of computerized tomography to diagnose disorders of the lymphoid organs.
ELISA (enzyme-linked immunosorbent assay)	Blood test for an antibody to the AIDS virus. A positive test means that the person has been exposed to the virus. There may be a false-positive reading and then the Western blot test would be used to verify the results.
Lymphadenectomy	Excision of a lymph node. This is usually done to test for a malignancy.
Lymphangiogram	X-ray taken through the lymph vessels after the injection of dye into the foot. The lymph flow through the chest is traced.
Splenopexy	The artificial fixation of a moveable spleen.
Tonsillectomy	The surgical removal of the tonsils. Usually adenoids are removed at the same time. This procedure is known as T&A.
Western blot	This test is used as a backup for the ELISA blood test to detect the presence of the antibody to HIV (AIDS virus) in the blood.

Musculoskeletal System

The treatment of conditions for the musculoskeletal system (bones and muscles) is called orthopedics, and physicians who diagnose and treat conditions related to the musculoskeletal system are orthopedists. Osteopaths treat the body by realigning the skeletal system to promote healing. They also use conventional medical methods as well. Rheumatologists see patients with joint inflammations and treat patients with autoimmune disorders such as rheumatoid arthritis and lupus. Chiropractors use manual adjustment of the spine to promote healing and maintain homeostasis. A medical assistant's training is comprehensive enough to permit employment in any of the specialties mentioned. Radiology and diagnostic imaging are usually needed to evaluate musculoskeletal conditions (Figure 35-10). Many orthopedists, chiropractors, and osteopaths have x-ray equipment in or associated with their offices. Radiology is discussed in Chapter 44. In some states, medical assistants are not permitted to take x-rays, therefore it is important for you to be familiar with state regulations.

Musculoskeletal System and The Medical Assistant

There are 206 bones in the body and over 600 muscles. Muscles account for approximately 50 percent of body weight. In addition to bones and muscles, the musculoskeletal system includes all the connective tissue, such as tendons, ligaments, cartilage, necessary for proper functioning of this complex system. The functions of the musculoskeletal system are to provide movement, protect internal organs, produce blood cells of all types, and store minerals. See Chapters 21 and 22 for a review of the skeletal and muscular systems. In your career as a medical assistant, regardless of which specialty you work in, you will encounter patients with musculoskeletal conditions.

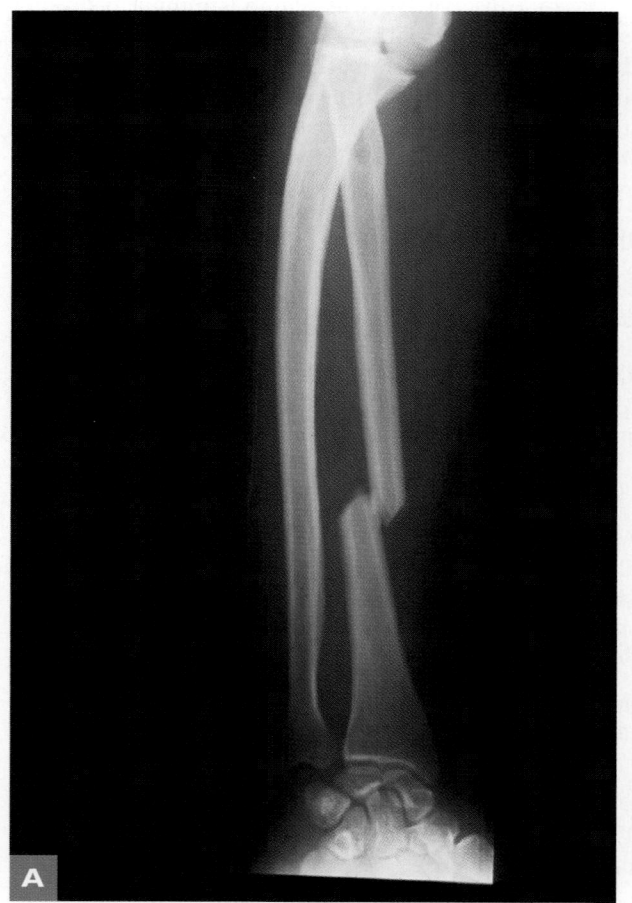
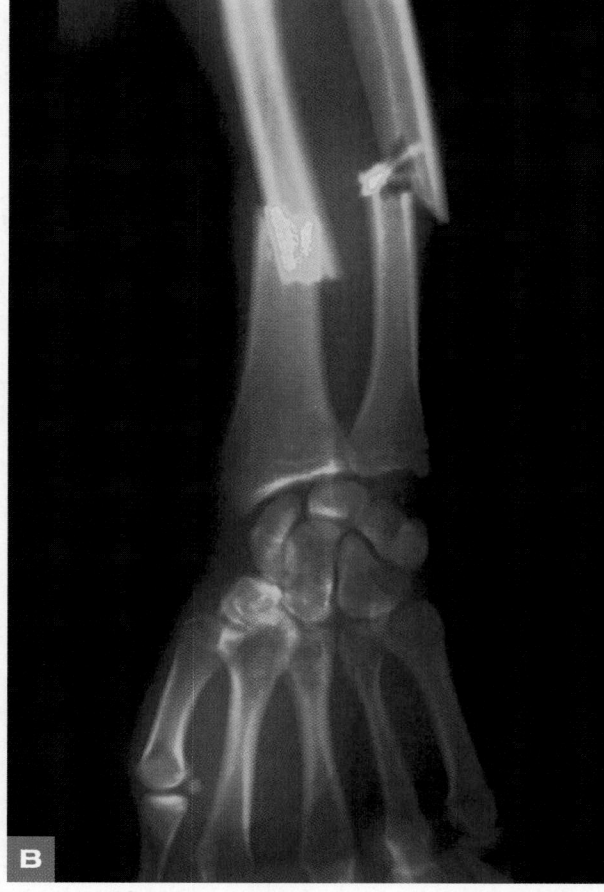

FIGURE 35-10 (A) An x-ray of complete fracture of the radius; (B) An enhanced color x-ray of forearm fractures.

The symptoms a patient may present related to this system are numerous and vary widely. Many of the symptoms patients experience have a great bearing on their quality of life. For example, the young woman suffering from rheumatoid arthritis may be so disabled and in so much pain she cannot work or care for herself. Consider the elderly patient who falls and fractures a hip, requiring a total hip replacement (THR), or the young child who suffers from muscle weakness and lack of motor control due to muscular dystrophy. Lifespan Considerations discusses how aging affects the systems of the body, including the musculoskeletal system.

Your role includes listening carefully to the patient's description of the problem: when did it start, what was done to alleviate the problem, and what are his or her concerns at present. Note carefully the exact location of pain and ask the patient to quantify it on a scale from one to ten. Offer to assist the patient to the examining room and provide a wheelchair, if necessary. Once in the examining room, make any accommodations necessary to ensure that the patient is comfortable, such as providing a blanket for warmth or an extra pillow to support the injured part. When evaluating muscle strength, recall that it should be equal on both sides of the body. For instance, if you ask a patient to squeeze your hands, the amount of pressure the patient exerts with each hand should be equal. Observe the patient's gait and the range of motion of the affected area. All are important clues the physician needs to help make an accurate diagnosis.

Therapeutic modalities, such as application of heat and cold, will be covered in Chapter 46. Table 35-8 lists procedures and diagnostic tests relating to the musculoskeletal system.

Arthritis

Arthritis means inflammation of the joint. There are over 100 types of arthritis affecting more than 40 million Americans. Chances are great that you will encounter patients with this painful and sometimes crippling disorder.

Osteoarthritis, also known as degenerative joint disease (DJD), is a natural consequence of aging. The articular cartilage in weight-bearing joints like the knee, hip, and ankle wears away and the surface becomes rough. The result is a painful, stiff joint. Obesity, trauma, and genetic predisposition increase the risk of osteoarthritis. Treatment involves reducing pain with medication such as nonsteroidal anti-inflammatory drugs (NSAIDs) (for example ibuprophen) and maintaining normal motion.

Nervous System

The study of the nervous system is neurology. A neurologist specializes in treating and diagnosing conditions of the nervous system. A neurosurgeon performs surgical procedures on the nervous system resulting from disease or trauma. A psychiatrist treats mental and neurological conditions that affect behavior.

Patients with nervous system conditions exhibit many different types of symptoms. A neurological examination focuses on the state of consciousness of the patient reflex response, motor response, speech patterns, and patterns of behavior. If as a medical assistant, you notice inappropriate responses, or changes in grooming habits, the physician should be made aware of your observations. Your role in the neurological examination is to have all the necessary equipment set up for the physician including:

- Otoscope
- Ophthalmoscope
- Percussion hammer
- Penlight
- Tuning fork
- Cotton ball
- Pin
- Tongue depressor
- Small vials containing hot and cold liquid, vials with different scents, and vials with different tasting liquids per the physician's order

Provide support and encouragement to patients and assist in positioning them as needed. Many types of tests and procedures may be ordered as follow-ups to the initial examination. Table 35-9 discusses procedures and diagnostic tests relating to the nervous system.

Cerebral Vascular Disease

Cerebral vascular disease is any disease affecting the blood vessels of the brain. Because the brain requires about 20 percent of the body's blood supply, any decrease in blood and oxygen supply has major consequences and causes brain dysfunction. There are many causes of cerebral vascular disease: atherosclerosis, arteriosclerosis, hemorrhage, and thrombus (blood clot). Stroke or cerebral vascular accident (CVA) is any situation that causes an interruption of the blood supply to the brain and is the third leading cause of death in the United States. Risk factors for stroke are similar to those for coronary artery disease, namely hypertension, obesity, high cholesterol, smoking, diabetes, family history, sedentary life style. Regardless of the cause, thrombus,

Lifespan
Considerations

The process of aging affects each system of the body. Keep in mind the impact that aging has on the human body and treat elderly patients in an understanding, respectful manner.

- *Dermatology—The effects of aging are visible to all. The layers of skin thin and wrinkle as collagen and elastin fibers deteriorate. The skin becomes drier because sebaceous glands and sweat glands are less active. Loss of fat in subcutaneous tissue makes the elderly more sensitive to cold.*

- *Musculoskeletal—Bones lose calcium, making them more brittle and susceptible to fractures. Articular cartilage erodes, especially in the weight bearing joints of knees, hips, and small joints in the fingers. Pain and stiffness, particularly on rising in the morning, are part of everyday life. With age, muscles atrophy and are slower to contract. However, regular exercise can delay atrophy and maintain strength.*

- *Nervous—Some forgetfulness is common as is slower problem solving. However, normally memory remains intact. Mental impairment in elderly is more often caused by depression, dementia, medication side effects, and malnutrition. Voluntary movements and reflexes are slower. Recently, studies have found that solving puzzles and studying foreign languages helps to keep the brain active and possibly the neurons from slowing.*

- *Endocrine—Normal aging does not usually lead to acute hormone deficiency. Endocrine secretions do decline with age but are sufficient to function adequately with age.*

- *Cardiovascular—With age, the heart muscle is less efficient, and both heart rate and cardiac output decrease. Atherosclerosis and arteriosclerosis are more common with age and may cause the heart to work harder and blood pressure to elevate. Regular exercise and a diet lower in saturated fats can modify these age-related changes. Vein walls thin and weaken, leading to varicosities and phlebitis, both of which are more common in elderly.*

- *Respiratory—As with other tissues in the body, lung tissue and respiratory muscles lose elasticity. This deterioration leads to decreased ventilation and, depending on the severity of the reduction, a decrease in oxygen available to the heart and body.*

- *Digestive—Less saliva, less sense of taste, loss of teeth, less digestive secretions, and slower peristalsis are consequences of the aging process. There is a greater chance for indigestion, diverticula development, constipation, hemorrhoids, and colon cancer. A decrease in appetite can lead to malnutrition in the elderly.*

- *Urinary—The aging process decreases the number of nephrons in the kidney and in some, the ability to concentrate urine. However, unless other disease factors are present, kidney function remains adequate. The bladder muscles weaken and urinary tract infection risk is greater due to inability to empty the bladder completely.*

- *Reproductive (Female)—The ability to reproduce ends in the female at menopause (45 to 55 years of age). The decreasing amount of estrogen ends ovulation and menstruation, and leads to increase of bone loss, lipidemia, and drying of vaginal tissue.*

  (Male)—Testosterone continues to be produced throughout life in most males. Production of sperm diminishes with age but fertility is still possible. Enlargement of the prostate leading to urination difficulty is fairly common as males age.

---

embolus (thrombus that has moved from its place of origin), or hemorrhage, the resulting condition is referred to as a stroke. When blood is decreased to an area of the brain (ischemia) and is temporary, it is referred to as transient ischemic attack (TIA). A prolonged decrease of blood to an area results in death (necrosis) of the tissue in the vicinity of the incident. In the case of the brain, this often means irreversible damage or death. A TIA is often a warning sign of impending stroke and immediate medical evaluation and possible treatment is important. Since signs of a TIA are temporary, often lasting only a few seconds or minutes to several hours, patients

TABLE 35-8 Procedures and Diagnostic Tests Relating to the Musculoskeletal System

Procedure/Test	Description
Aldolase	A blood serum test to measure ALD enzyme present in skeletal and heart muscle to diagnose Duchenne's muscular dystrophy before symptoms appear.
Antinuclear antibody (ANA)	Antibodies present in a variety of immunologic diseases such as rheumatoid arthritis and systemic lupus.
Amputation	Partial or complete removal of a limb for a variety of reasons, including tumors, gangrene, intractable pain, crushing injury, or uncontrollable infection.
Anterior cruciate ligament reconstruction (ACL)	Replacing a torn ACL with a graft by means of arthroscopy.
Arthrocentesis	Removal of synovial fluid with a needle from a joint space, such as in the knee, for examination.
Arthrodesis	Surgical reconstruction of a joint.
Arthrography	Visualization of a joint by a radiographic study after injection of a contrast medium.
Arthroplasty	Surgical reconstruction of a joint.
Arthroscopic surgery	Use of an arthroscope, a lighted instrument with camera/video capabilities, to facilitate performing surgery on a joint.
Arthrotomy	Surgically cutting into a joint.
Bone graft	Piece of bone taken from the patient that is used to take the place of a removed bone or a bony defect at another site, or to be wedged between bones for fusion of a joint.
Bone scan	Use of scanning equipment to visualize bones. It is especially useful in observing progress of treatment for osteomyelitis and cancer metastases to the bone.
Bunionectomy	Removal of the bursa at the joint of the great toe.
Calcium	A blood serum test to determine levels of calcium. Calcium is essential for muscular contraction, nerve transmission, and blood clotting.
Carpal tunnel release	Surgical cutting of the ligament in the wrist to relieve nerve pressure caused by repetitive motion, for example, typing (carpal tunnel disease).
Computerized axial tomography	Computer-assisted x-ray used to detect tumors and fractures. Also referred to as CT-scan.
Creatine phosphotase (CPK)	A blood serum test to measure the CPK level that is increased in necrosis or atrophy of skeletal muscle, traumatic muscle injury, strenuous exercise, progressive muscular dystrophy, and after heart attack.
C-Reactive Protein (CRP)	Positive result may indicate rheumatoid arthritis, acute inflammatory change, or widespread metastasis.
Electromyography (EMG)	Study and record of the strength of muscle contractions as a result of electrical stimulation. Used in the diagnosis of muscle disorders and to distinguish nerve disorders from muscle disorders.

(continued)

Procedure/Test	Description
Fasciectomy	Surgical removal of the fascia, which is the fibrous membrane covering and supporting muscles.
Goniometry	The measurement of joint movements and angles via a goniometry.
Lactic dehydrogenase (LDH)	A blood serum test to measure the level of LDH enzyme. It is increased in muscular dystrophy, after damage to skeletal muscles, after pulmonary embolism, and during skeletal muscle malignancy.
Laminectomy	Removal of the vertebral posterior arch to correct severe back problems caused by compression of the lamina.
Magnetic resonance imaging (MRI)	Medical imaging that uses radio-frequency radiation as its source of energy. It does not require the injection of contrast medium or exposure to ionizing radiation. The technique is useful for visualizing large blood vessels, the heart, brain, and soft tissues.
Menisectomy	Removal of knee cartilage (meniscus).
Muscle biopsy	Removal of muscle tissue for pathological examination.
Myelography	Study of the spinal column after injecting opaque contrast material.
Phosphorous (P) blood test	Phosphorous level of the blood may be increased in osteoporosis and fracture healing.
Photon absorptiometry	Measurement of bone density using an instrument for the purpose of detecting osteoporosis.
Reduction	Correcting a fracture by realigning the bone fragment. A closed reduction of the fracture is the manipulation of the bone into alignment and the application of a cast or splint to immobilize the part during healing process. Open reduction is the surgical incision at the site of the fracture to perform the bone realignment. This is necessary when there are bone fragments to be removed.
Serum glutamic oxaloacetic transaminase (SGOT)	A blood serum test to measure the level of SGOT enzyme. It is increased in skeletal muscle damage and muscular dystrophy. This test is also called aspartate amino-transferase (AST).
Serum glutamic pyruvic transaminase (SGPT)	A blood serum test to measure the level of SGPT enzyme. It is increased in skeletal muscle damage. This test is also called alanine aminotransferase (ALT).
Serum rheumatoid factor (RF)	An immunoglobulin present in the serum of 50 to 95 percent of adults with rheumatoid arthritis.
Spinal fusion	Surgical immobilization of adjacent vertebrae. This may be done for several reasons, including correction of a herniated disk.
Thermograph	The process of recording heat patterns of the body's surface. Used to investigate the pathophysiology of rheumatoid arthritis.
Total hip replacement (THR)	Surgical replacement of a hip by implanting a prosthetic or artificial joint.
Uric acid blood test	Uric acid is increased in gout, arthritis, multiple myeloma, and rheumatism.

TABLE 35-9 Procedures and Diagnostic Tests Relating to the Nervous System

Procedures/Tests	Description
Babinski's sign	Reflex test developed by John Babinski, a French neurologist, to determine lesions and abnormalities in the nervous system. The Babinski reflex is present or positive when the great toe extends instead of flexes when the lateral sole of the foot is stroked.
Brain scan	Injection of radioactive isotopes into the circulation to determine the function and abnormality of the brain.
Carotid endartectomy	Surgical procedure for removing an obstruction within the carotid artery. It was developed to prevent strokes but is found useful only in severe stenosis with a TIA.
Cerebral angiogram	X-ray of the blood vessels of the brain after the injection of radio opaque dye.
Cerebral spinal fluid shunts	Surgical creation of an artificial opening to allow for the passage of fluid. Used in the treatment of hydrocephalous.
Cordectomy	Removal of part of the spinal cord.
Craniotomy	Surgical incision into the brain through the cranium.
Cryosurgery	Use of extreme cold to produce areas of destruction in the brain. Used to control bleeding and treat brain tumors.
Echoencephalogram	Recording of the ultrasonic echoes of the brain. Useful in determining abnormal patterns of shifting in the brain.
Electromyogram	Written recording of the contraction of muscles as a result of receiving electrical stimulation.
Laminectomy	Removal of a vertebral posterior arch.
Lumbar puncture	Puncture with a needle into the lumbar area (usually the fourth intervertebral space) to withdraw fluid for examination and for the injection of anesthesia.
Nerve block	Method of regional anesthetic to stop the passage of sensory stimulation along a nerve path.
Pneumoencephalography	X-ray examination of the brain following withdrawal of cerebrospinal fluid and injection of air or gas via spinal puncture.
Positron emission tomography (PET)	Use of positive radionucleotides to reconstruct brain sections. Measurement can be taken of oxygen and glucose uptake, cerebral blood flow, and blood volume.
Romberg's sign	Test developed to establish neurological function in which patients are asked to close their eyes and place their feet together. This test for body balance is positive if the patient sways when the eyes are closed.
Spinal puncture	Puncture with a needle into the spinal cavity to withdraw spinal fluid for microscopic analysis.
Sympathectomy	Excision of a portion of the sympathetic nervous system. Could include nerve or ganglion.
Transcutaneous electrical nerve stimulation (TENS)	Application of a mild electrical stimulation to skin electrodes placed over a painful area, causing interference with the transmission of painful stimuli. Can be used in pain management to interfere with the normal pain mechanism.
Trephination	Process of cutting out a piece of bone in the skull to gain entry into the brain to relieve pressure.
Vagotomy	Surgical incision into the vagus nerve. Medication can be administered into the nerve to prevent its function.

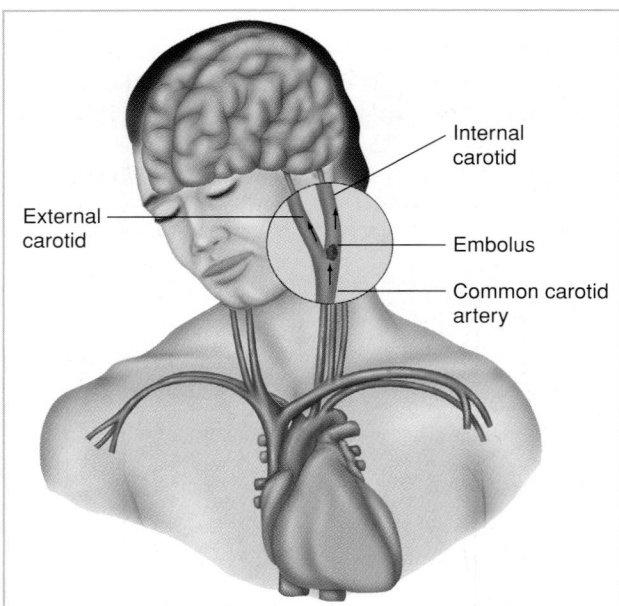

FIGURE 35-11 Embolus traveling to the brain.

and family members often dismiss them as inconsequential. Figure 35-11 depicts an embolus traveling through the carotid artery to the brain.

Recent research recommends that an individual seek medical assistance immediately if there is suspicion of a stroke. Quick intervention with thrombolytic drugs and other medications may restore blood supply and prevent irreversible brain damage. Symptoms of a CVA include sudden severe headache, difficulty in speaking or loss of speech, confusion, one-sided numbness or paralysis, facial droop, memory loss, and blurred vision.

Many patients and family members are unaware that a stroke is in progress and delay seeking help. It is recommended that anyone who suspects they may be having a stroke seek help immediately at a facility prepared to administer clot dissolving medications. Physical, occupational, and speech therapy for CVA patients also should begin as soon as their conditions allow. It is possible for some patients (mainly those under 50) to retrain the many extra neurons in the cerebral cortex that are not in use and recover some functions.

Dementia

Dementia is a condition resulting in progressive loss of memory and intellectual ability. It can occur at any age and is not a normal result of aging. Approximately half of dementia patients suffer from Alzheimer's disease. There are no specific tests to obtain a definitive diagnosis. It is important to rule out possible underlying causes such as low thyroid function, alcohol abuse, depression, certain vitamin deficiencies, brain tumors, and drug interactions. If an underlying cause is found, treatment to correct the problem may be successful and progressive deterioration may cease. However, in most cases, dementia is irreversible. Dementia patients may require supervision to ensure their safety. Behavior problems make this devastating condition, difficult for patients, family members, and health care providers. Dementia results ultimately in the need for 24-hour care, and inevitably death for the patient.

Assisting with Lumbar Puncture

The physician may wish to examine spinal fluid for the presence of red cells, white cells, or pathogenic microorganisms. Examination of cerebral spinal fluid is an important diagnostic tool to assist in determining conditions such as stroke, brain hemorrhage, meningitis, encephalitis polio, and tumors of the brain and spinal cord. Cerebral spinal fluid (CSF) normally is clear, colorless, and sterile, (free of any microorganisms). Three tubes of cerebral spinal fluid are sent to the laboratory for tests. They include a culture for the presence of microorganisms that are found in infectious diseases such as meningitis; cell count, of red cells or white cells that would be present in cases of hemorrhage and infection respectively; and chemical tests for glucose and protein that help to pinpoint the diagnosis. A lumbar puncture is an invasive procedure; therefore, extra care should be taken when handling the CSF tubes and universal precautions should be carefully observed.

During this procedure a needle is inserted into the subarachnoid space of the spinal cord. This is usually performed at the level of the fourth lumbar intervertebral space. A small gauge needle (22) is passed through the dura. When the stylet, or thin probe, is removed from the needle, cerebrospinal fluid (CSF) will escape and can be collected into tubes for microscopic examination. Patients are prone to headaches after this procedure due to leakage of fluid from the spinal spaces. Headaches can be diminished if the patient is instructed to lie perfectly flat for several hours (six to twelve) after the procedure. This procedure is more commonly performed in a clinic setting rather than a medical office to allow the patient to remain flat for the intended time.

Reproductive Systems

The main function of the male and female reproductive systems is to produce offspring to continue the human species. All of the male and female gonads or sexual organs develop from the same embryonic tissue and only begin to differentiate approximately two months after conception. For a review of the reproductive systems, see Chapter 31.

Female Reproductive System

Gynecology is the branch of medicine that deals with disorders and diseases of the female reproductive system. The practice of gynecology is closely related to the medical specialty of obstetrics, which is the branch of medicine concerned with the management of women during pregnancy, childbirth, and the period of time immediately after childbirth, the puerperium. A gynecologist may also be an obstetrician.

An examination of the female reproductive organs will include a breast examination and a pelvic examination to determine the condition of both the external and the internal organs of reproduction. In addition, a Papanicolaou (Pap) test may be performed for the early detection of precancerous or early cancer of the cervix and endometrium of the uterus. Many gynecologists also perform a digital rectal examination as part of a routine pelvic examination. Examination of the female reproductive organs is routine in a busy obstetrics and gynecology (OB/GYN) office.

Assisting the Obstetrics and Gynecology (OB/GYN) Patient

Patients in an obstetrical/gynecology practice will cover a wide age span and present a variety of symptoms and conditions. You may encounter the teenager having her first pelvic examination, the first-time mother, the mother of seven, the premenopausal female, the middle-aged menopausal female, and the aging postmenopausal female. Because they are in distinct life stages, their emotional and physical needs will be different. Hormones play a large part in the stages of development in the female and will have a bearing on the emotional status of your patients as well. One of your tasks is to help identify patients' problems and provide information to the physician. Using your listening skills and being empathetic will provide an environment in which the patient is comfortable enough to convey her feelings and discomforts.

The Breast Examination

The breast examination by the physician precedes the pelvic examination. The patient lies in the supine position for this examination and is generally asked to place her hand behind her head on the side that is being examined first. This allows the physician to examine the lymph nodes under the axilla. The physician palpates the breast using his or her fingertips in a circular fashion around all of the breast tissue to search for lumps, tenderness, or inflammation. In addition, any dimpling or puckering of the skin around the breast and nipple is noted. The nipples are checked for cracking, bleeding, or discharge.

The physician will advise the patient to perform a breast self-examination every month, a week after the menstrual period. Women who have reached menopause should examine their breasts on the same day each month. The American Cancer Society advises a monthly self-examination of both breasts. It is estimated by the American Cancer Society that over a life time one in eight women will develop breast cancer. The medical as-

sistant may have the responsibility of explaining the correct procedure for the breast self-examination. If the woman notes any abnormality during a self-examination, she should call her physician for an appointment and not wait for another month to see if the abnormality disappears. See Procedure 35-3 with Figure 35-12 for the correct way of instructing a woman on how to perform self-examination of the breasts. Figure 35-13 illustrates a medical assistant using a prosthetic teaching breast to instruct a patient on breast self-examination.

The American Cancer Society recommends that:

- Women between the ages of 20 and 39 have a breast examination performed by a physician every three years; a baseline mammogram should be done at the age of 35.

- Women over the age of 40 should have a yearly breast examination by a physician, and a mammogram every one to two years.

- Women over the age of 50 should have a yearly breast examination by a physician and a yearly mammogram.

The Pelvic Examination

The gynecologic examination, or pelvic examination, is included as part of a routine physical examination for the female by some internal medicine and family practice physicians. Other physicians prefer that the patient see a gynecologist for the examination. A pelvic examination alone may be conducted in order to diagnose a problem relating specifically to the female reproductive organ. The patient should be advised not to douche for 24 to 48 hours before the examination. Doing so may wash away cervical cells that are obtained during a Pap smear.

The gynecological examination begins with taking a thorough history from the patient. Questions about the menstrual cycle, past pregnancies, and discomfort during sexual intercourse are important to obtain a picture of the patient's overall health status. You should have knowledge of conditions and diseases affecting this system and a thorough understanding of the signs and symptoms of sexually transmitted diseases (STDs). Sexually transmitted diseases, including their signs, symptoms, and treatments, will be reviewed later in this chapter. Bruises and other signs of physical abuse must be reported. Preparing for Externship discusses more on recognizing the signs of abuse. You should also be familiar with signs and symptoms of drug abuse.

For legal reasons, the medical assistant is usually present to assist with a gynecologic examination. Before beginning the pelvic examination, the physician will listen to the patient's heart and lungs. The pelvic examination begins with an examination of the external genitalia for swelling, redness, or ulcerations. The vaginal speculum is inserted into the vagina to inspect the vagina and cervix for color, lacerations, nodules, or

Instructing a Patient on Breast Self-Examination

OBJECTIVE: Instruct the patient how to do a breast self-examination.

Equipment and Supplies

breast model (if available); pamphlets on breast self-examination

Method

1. Perform hand hygiene.
2. Assemble equipment.
3. Identify patient and explain the necessity for performing the procedure correctly in three different positions each month. Use the breast model to explain the correct application of fingertips.
4. In the shower, Figure 35-12A:
   - Raise right arm. Use the left hand to examine the right breast, then raise left arm and use right hand to examine the left breast.
   - Using the flat fingertips, check breast tissue and underarm tissue gently feeling for any lump or thinkening. Touch every part of the breast when skin is wet.
     Rationale: Hands will move easily over the softened wet skin.
5. Before a mirror:
   - Inspect the breasts for any irregularity in shape while arms are at the side of the body.
   - Look for swelling, dimpling, or puckering of the skin, lumps, or changes in the nipples, such as retracting. Gently squeeze both nipples and look for discharge.
   - Raise the arms overhead and look for size, shape, and contour changes in each breast.
   - With palms resting on hips, flex chest muscles to observe for any obvious differences in breasts, Figure 35-12B.

   Note: the left and right breasts on most females do not match exactly.

6. Lying down:
   - To examine the right breast, place a pillow or folded towel behind the right shoulder and place the right hand behind the head, Figure 35-12C. Examine the right breast with your left hand and the left breast with your right hand.
   - Using your hand with fingers flat, gently press the breast tissue using small circular motions starting at the outermost top of the breast in the 12 o'clock position and spiraling toward the nipple, Figure 35-12D. Cover all the breast tissue feeling for lumps or any abnormal changes in breast tissue. Gently squeeze the nipple of each breast between thumb and index finger to note lumps or discharge.
   - Repeat the procedure for the left breast.
7. With the arm resting on a firm surface, Figure 35-12E, use the same circular motion to examine the underarm area. This is breast tissue too. Repeat procedure for both underarm areas.
8. Report any abnormalities to the physician. This self-examination is not a substitute for periodic examinations by a qualified physician.

Charting Example

2/14/XX	2:00 P.M.

Breast self-exam explained to patient using breast model.

M. King, CMA

---

discharge. The size of the speculum selected will depend on the sexual maturity and physical state of the patient. Vaginal specula may be either metal, and need to be sanitized and sterilized after each use, or disposable and meant for one use only. Warming the speculum in warm water or keeping it warm in a drawer equipped with a heating pad make the examination more comfortable for the patient. Figure 35-15 illustrates the speculum and the manual pelvic examination for females. The patient may need reassurance that the procedure is painless, especially if it is her first gynecologic examination.

Pap Smear

The Pap smear is usually included as part of a pelvic examination. It is a cytological screening test named for a Greek physician, George Papanicolaou. The Pap test is based on the fact that cells are sloughed off the vaginal and cervical mucosa. A thin scrapping of these

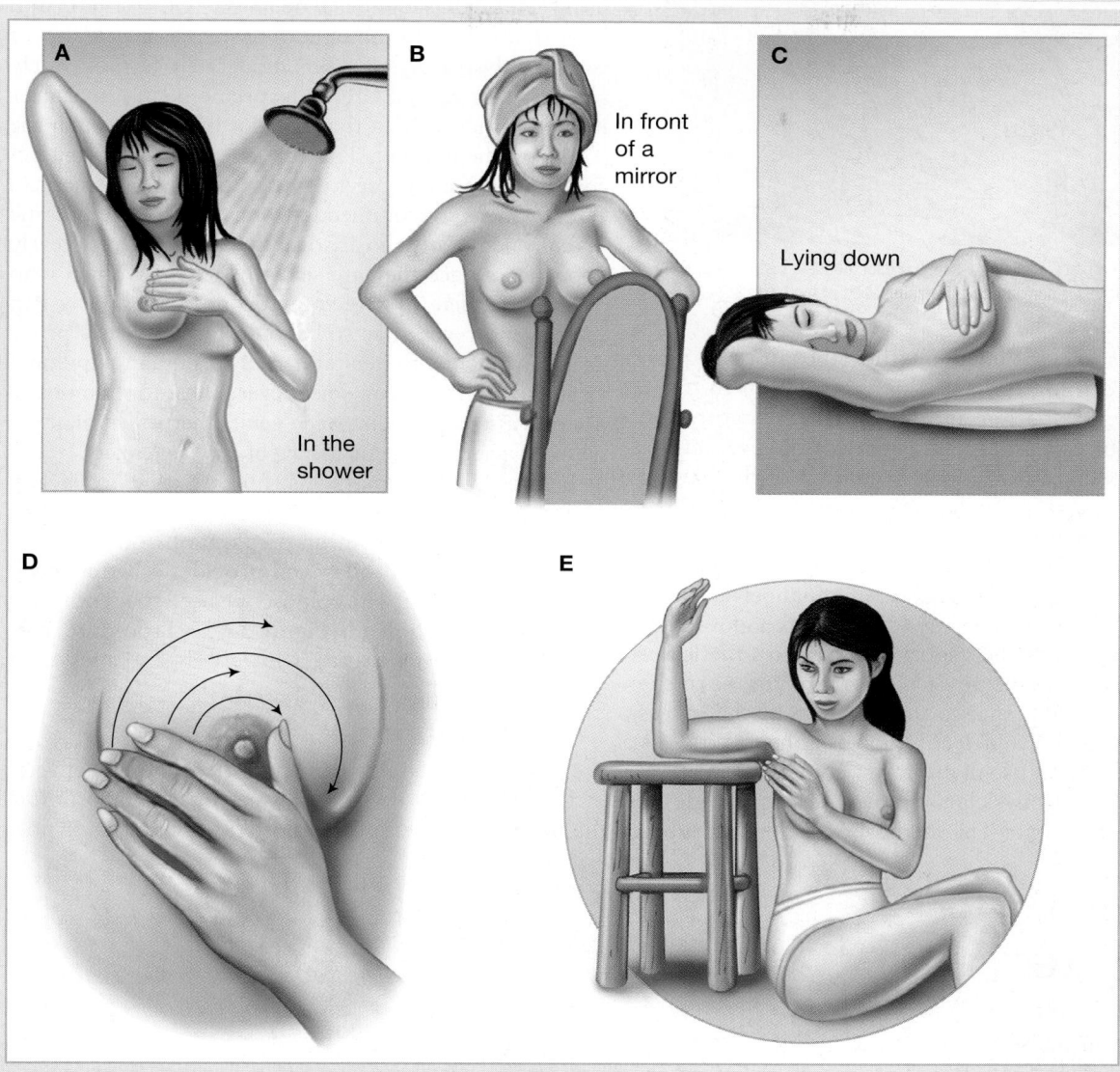

FIGURE 35-12 Demonstrations of correct procedures for breast self-examination.

exfoliated cells is taken from the cervix, vagina, and endocervical canal using a cervical spatula and cervical brush or broom. Presently, two methods of Pap smear collection are used. In the older "dry" method, separate slides are made by the physician, and the medical assistant labels the slides C, V, E, and sprays them with fixative to preserve the cells. The newer more accurate "liquid" method requires the specimen to be collected in a similar fashion, but the plastic vaginal speculum and brush or broom that are used are swirled around several times in a liquid cytology medium in order to suspend and preserve the sample. With either method of collection, the properly labeled specimens are then sent to the laboratory for examination. A cytologist prepares, stains, examines, and evaluates the three slides for evidence of infection, dysplasia (abnormal cells), or cancerous cells. The date of first day of the patient's last menstrual period

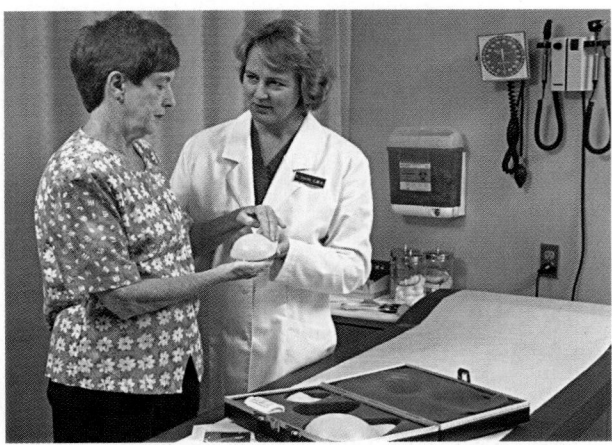
FIGURE 35-13 A medical assistant using a breast model to instruct a patient on proper technique for performing self-examination of the breasts.

(LMP) must be included on the laboratory request form. The cytologist needs this information to make an accurate evaluation and to provide a maturation index (MI) if it is requested as part of the evaluation. An MI provides a hormonal evaluation of the patient that may assist in evaluating causes of infertility, menopausal or postmenopausal bleeding, or amenorrhea (absence of menstrual periods).

After collecting the smears, a bimanual pelvic examination is performed. The physician inserts a gloved, lubricated finger into the vagina and palpates the lower abdomen. Between the physician's two hands, he or she can detect the size, shape, and position of the uterus and ovaries, and also detect lumps or abnormalities. A rectal examination usually follows. To perform a rectal examination the physician removes his or her gloves and dons a new pair. The medical assistant will lubri-

cate one finger, which is then inserted into the rectum to check for hemorrhoids, polyps, or other abnormalities.

Grading Pap Smears

Several methods of grading Pap smears are used. One system provides a grading system for cervical changes, using cervical intraepithelial neoplasia (CIN) criteria of I, II, or III and uses the amount of dysplasia present. CIN I is mildly dysplastic, CIN II is moderately to moderately severe dysplasia, and CIN III is carcinoma in situ (cancer in that particular area that has not broken through the basement membrane). The Pap smear is 95 percent accurate in detecting cervical carcinoma. The American Cancer Society recommends women who have become sexually active, or who are over the age of 18 have yearly Pap smears once they are sexually active. Women who have a complete hysterectomy do not need yearly Pap smears. However, they still should have a yearly pelvic exam. Women with genital herpes or human papilloma virus should have a Pap smear every three to six months. There is a strong link between genital herpes, human papilloma virus and the incidence of cervical cancer.

Figure 35-15 displays instruments used for a Pap smear, and Figure 35-16 illustrates preparing a Pap smear. The thin Pap smear preparation (one layer of cells) is widely used today and provides a better specimen for evaluation. The colposcope used to identify abnormal tissue is shown in Figure 35-17. Procedure 35-4 lists the steps for assisting with a pelvic examination and a Pap test.

Prenatal Care

Prenatal care includes care provided before delivery, including a series of visits and specific tests to promote the health of both mother and fetus. Postnatal or post

Preparing for
Externship

An integral part of your professional development should include an awareness of abuse problems among all ages of patients. Children, women, and the elderly are particularly vulnerable to abuse. Vigilance in your interviewing and observation techniques will help you detect suspicious signs of abuse. Signs of abuse or domestic violence include, bruising, and reluctance on the part of the patient to explain the injury. Elder abuse takes many forms, such as neglect, poor hygiene, poor nutrition, bruises and sores, and being overly concerned about money. Establishing a secure comfortable environment in the office may help abused patients feel at ease to talk about their problems.

Many states mandate that suspicions of abuse be reported. How you go about reporting suspicions and to whom to report should be part of your office policy. Take the initiative and prepare a folder, including the names and numbers of state agencies, women's shelters, and domestic violence hotlines. If there is no clear cut set of standards for you to follow, contact agencies in your state such as the Department of Health, the Department of Aging, and the Department of Children and Family Services. All of these agencies will have printed material and guidelines to help you understand what and how to report your suspicions. Any immediate concerns should be brought to the physician at once. Ignoring the situation helps no one.

partum care covers from the delivery of the infant through the mother's six-week follow-up checkup.

Pregnancy normally lasts forty weeks or nine months. It is divided into three trimesters or stages of approximately three months each. The first trimester includes the period of time from implantation of the embryo in the uterus through the fourteenth week. This is a most critical stage of fetal life because most of the major organ systems develop during this period. It is also the period in which the embryo is most vulnerable to substances that may cause birth defects such as bacterial and viral infections, drugs, alcohol, and other chemical substances. After the eighth week, the embryo is referred to as a fetus. The second trimester begins at the end of the fourteenth week and continues to the end of the sixth month. During this period, refinement of all the organs takes place and fetal movement (quickening) may be felt. The third trimester is the period from the end of the sixth month to birth and is marked by an increase in the size and weight of the fetus. During this stage, the fetus usually assumes a head down position and is said to have reached the age of viability (able to sustain life on its own) at seven months.

First Prenatal Visit

The first prenatal visit usually takes place after the patient has missed her second menstrual period. This visit requires more time than follow-up visits because a full history and prenatal assessment must be done. In addition, a complete physical examination, pelvic examination, including a Pap smear, and cultures (as needed) must be performed. Blood tests are ordered at this visit and it is up to you to reinforce the importance of the patient complying with the physician's orders. Blood tests include CBC, ABO/Rh, serology test for syphilis, and Rubella titer. Usually a complete urine analysis (UA) is ordered as well. These test results provide a baseline to compare with results obtained later in pregnancy.

Prenatal History

Prenatal history includes recording the menstrual history, including the age of onset of menstruation, menstrual interval cycle, duration of period, amount of flow, any menstrual cycle problems, and what type of contraception was used, if any. The past obstetrical history also is a component of the prenatal record. This includes gravida (number of times patient has been pregnant), para (births after 20 weeks of gestation, regardless of whether the infant is born dead or alive), and number of abortions (number of fetuses that did not reach the age of viability). This information should be charted, using

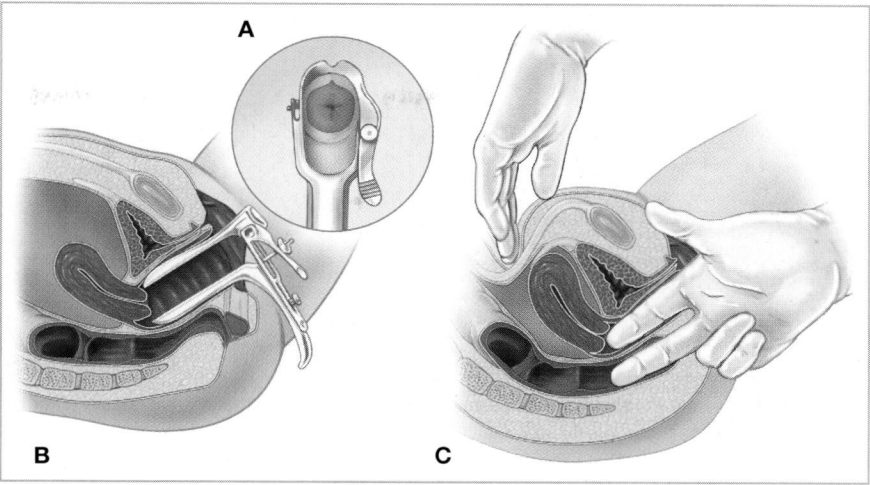

FIGURE 35-14 (A) and (B) Pelvic examination of female using a vaginal speculum; (C) A bimanual examination.

Roman numerals. For example, a woman pregnant for the first time would be gravida I, para 0. A woman pregnant at the current visit, who delivered a single child during her first pregnancy, delivered twins on her second pregnancy, and had one miscarriage would be charted as follows: gravida IV, para III, abs I.

After obtaining the patient's past history, it is important to gather information pertaining to her present pregnancy history. The patient is asked the following question.

- Do you have any preexisting conditions? Heart disease, kidney disease, and diabetes are especially important.

- Do you have any symptoms such as morning sickness, fatigue, headaches, vaginal bleeding, discharge, or breast changes?

- Are you taking any prescriptions, over-the-counter medications, vitamins, or herbal supplements?

- Do you drink, smoke, or use recreational drugs? If so, what and how much?

- Are you employed, married, divorced, or single?

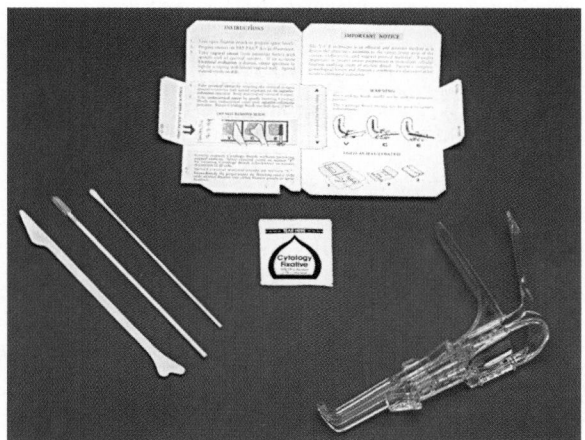

FIGURE 35-15 Instruments needed for a "dry prep" Pap smear.

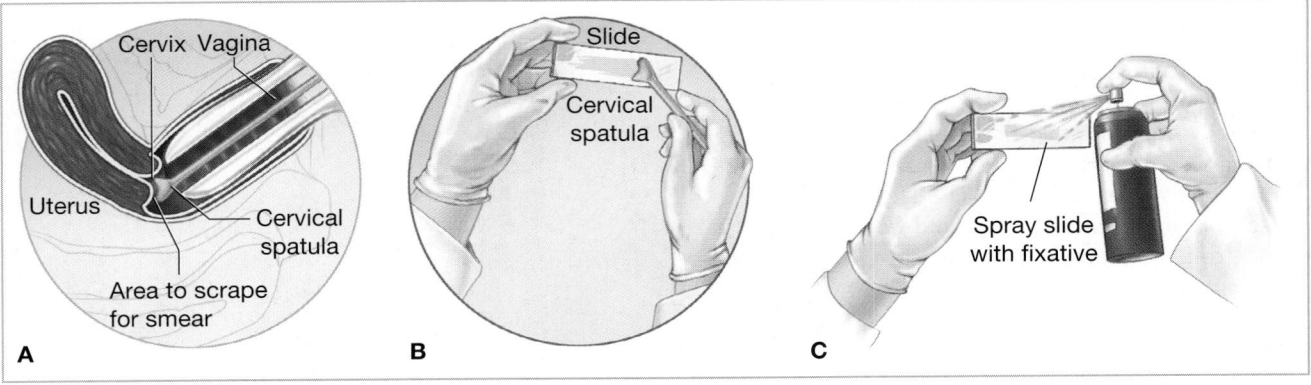

FIGURE 35-16 (A) The female reproductive organs showing location for obtaining a scraping for a Pap smear; (B) Making the Pap smear; and (C) Spraying the Pap smear with fixative.

More often than not, the information most important to the patient during her first prenatal visit is the expected date of delivery. A gestation calculator may be used to predict the estimated date of delivery (EDD). Another method to calculate EDD is to use Nagele's rule, applying the following formula: LMP (last menstrual period) + 7 days − 3 months + 1 year = EDD. For example, if the LMP was June 10, 2004; add 7 days (which = 17); subtract 3 months from June (which = March); add 1 year (which = 2005). The EDD is March 17, 2005.

Prenatal Patient Education

The initial prenatal visit affords an opportunity to provide the patient with information about what to expect at each stage of pregnancy, nutritional guidelines, vitamin and mineral requirements, and substances to be avoided. Pamphlets and brochures should be available in the reception room and examining room. At this visit the physician will order blood tests and other diagnostic procedures, such as an ultrasound, to be completed at a later date. When scheduling procedures and follow-up visits for the patients, reinforce the importance of these visits.

Follow-Up Visits

The patient will return for a follow-up visit every four weeks through the twenty-eighth week, every two weeks up to the thirty-sixth week, and every week until delivery. These return visits offer another opportunity for you take time to educate the patient on the importance of maintaining her follow-up visit schedule. During these visits, you can reinforce proper nutritional guidelines and answer any questions the patient may have. On each subsequent visit you will:

- Set up the examining room
- Obtain a urine specimen from the patient
- Weigh the patient
- Obtain blood pressure
- Ask her to describe any problems
- Chart all information
- Assist the patient onto the examining table, drape her appropriately

The physician will review your results, ask the patient to recline so the fundal height can be measured, check for signs of edema, use a fetoscope for listening to the fetal heart rate, and answer any questions the patient may have.

The fundal height measurement taken on the initial visit is used as a guideline for all subsequent visits. It is the height from the top of the pubic symphysis to the fundus (top of the uterus) using a non-stretchable tape measure. Normally during pregnancy, the uterus enlarges and rises into the abdominal cavity and the fundal height increases each month.

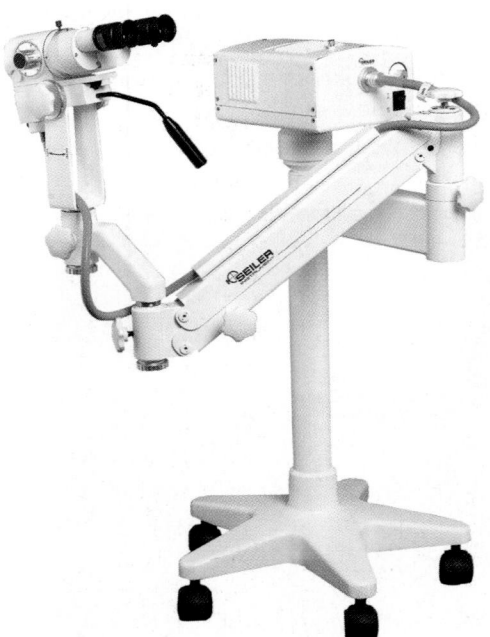

FIGURE 35-17 An example of a colposcope.

PROCEDURE

Assisting with a Pelvic Examination and Pap Test

OBJECTIVE: Set up and assist with a gynecologic examination, including collection of "dry" or "liquid" prep method Pap smear without error.

Equipment and Supplies

vaginal speculum; water-soluble lubricant; cotton-tipped applicator; patient drape; Pap smear materials: Dry Prep—cervical spatula brush, glass slides, fixative spray or liquid slide holder, identification label; Liquid Prep—plastic cervical spatula, broom or brush, cytology transport medium vial, identification label; laboratory request form; cleansing tissue; gloves; container for contaminated vaginal speculum; goose-neck lamp; biohazard waste container

Method

For "dry prep" collection:

1. Perform hand hygiene.
2. Assemble equipment.
3. Label slides, and complete the laboratory form.
4. Identify patient and explain procedure.
5. Direct the patient to the bathroom to empty her bladder.
6. Request patient to remove clothing and put on gown with opening in front and drape patient appropriately.
7. Assist patient into supine position for breast and abdominal examination.
8. Assist and instruct patient to assume dorsal lithotomy position with her buttocks at the edge of the table and feet in the stirrups. Knees should be relaxed and rotated outward. Expose the genitalia by moving the drape away from this area while it still covers the legs.
9. Adjust goose-neck lamp and place physician's stool in proper position at end of examination table.
10. Assist the physician with procedure:
    - Apply gloves.
    - Hand gloves and equipment to physician as needed. Place lubricant onto the speculum as the physician holds it.
    - Hold the microscopic slide as the physician smears slides. Mark slides: E for endocervical, C for cervical, and V for vaginal.
    - Spray fixative from about 6 inches away from the slide.
    - Place the slide into container with label.
11. Hold the receptacle as the physician places the contaminated speculum into it. Set the container into the sink for later cleaning.
12. Apply lubricant to the physician's gloved fingers in preparation for the manual examination.
13. Properly dispose of gloves into hazardous waste container and perform hand hygiene.
14. Assist the patient to sit up by (1) helping her move back on the table, (2) taking her feet out of the stirrups, and (3) helping her to a sitting position.
15. Sanitize and sterilize equipment as needed.
16. Perform hand hygiene.
17. Prepare Pap to be sent to laboratory.

For "liquid prep" collection:

18. Proceed through steps 1–9 above.
19. Open the vial of liquid transport medium and hold for physician to place both plastic spatula and either brush or broom containing speciman in vial.
20. Rinse broom vigorously by pushing to bottom of vial ten times.
21. Use spatula to scrape cells from brush and swirl both in vial to mix before removing.
22. Label vial and dispose of hazardous waste appropiately.

NOTE: The physician will chart the procedure.

The normal fetal heart tone (FHT) is 120–160 beats per minute and can be detected at 10–12 weeks using a Doppler fetal pulse detector. If there is fetal distress indicated by extremely rapid or slow heart rate, fetal stress tests may be ordered to evaluate the condition of the fetus.

The physician will discuss delivery options with the patient. Closer to the date of delivery, the patient will attend classes on prepared childbirth, delivery, and breastfeeding. Classes are usually given at the facility chosen for delivery. Other procedures and diagnostic tests relating to the female reproductive system are described in Table 35-10.

Screening Tests

Additional screening tests are performed during pregnancy to detect abnormalities and to be better prepared for a high-risk newborn. Some of these tests are offered to the mother and she may choose whether or not she wishes have the test performed.

Alpha-fetoprotein (AFP) test is a blood test taken between the fifteenth and eighteenth week of pregnancy to detect certain birth defects or multiple births.

Amniocentesis, performed between the twelfth and sixteenth week of gestation, involves using a fine needle to take a sample of amniotic fluid from the sac around the fetus. The fluid containing fetal cells will be cultured, grown in a laboratory, and screened to detect chromosomal defects such as Down's syndrome. Amniocentesis is also used to assess fetal gender, maturity, and development. Woman over 35 and who have a family history of genetic defects are recommended to have this test.

Glucose tolerance test is performed to test for gestational diabetes. This blood test is performed between 24 and 28 weeks of pregnancy. After fasting, the patient is given a specific dose of glucose and blood is taken one hour later. An elevated test will require an additional, more comprehensive three-hour glucose tolerance test. Women who develop gestational diabetes are at higher risk of developing diabetes later in life. A diet low in fat, moderate in carbohydrates, high in fiber, and regular exercise are recommended. Insulin may be needed if diet and exercise are not sufficient to lower blood sugar. Group B Streptococcus is a common inhabitant of the urinary and reproductive tract and normally does not cause illness. A vaginal culture at 35 to 37 weeks is recommended. One to two percent of infants may be infected, and infection may be life threatening. A patient who tests positive will be treated with antibiotics during labor to prevent fetal infection.

Ultrasound is used to determine the age, growth rate, position of the fetus, and obvious birth defects. It is generally performed at 16 to 20 weeks, and is generally painless. A vaginal ultrasound may be done to examine the fetus more closely.

Delivery

Parturition or birth occurs anytime from week 38 to 42 under normal circumstances. Labor involves three stages and is triggered by the release of the hormone *oxytocin*. The first stage of labor varies in length and ends with complete dilation (widening of the cervix) and effacement (thinning of cervical walls). Stage two, the pushing stage, is the period from complete dilation and effacement through the birth of the fetus. Stage three is the period from the birth of the fetus to the expulsion of the placenta.

Postpartum Visit

During the puerperium, a span of four to six weeks after delivery, the patient's body slowly returns to its prepregnant state. The uterus shrinks or involutes and healing of the birth canal takes place. During this time, the patient experiences vaginal discharge from the lining of the uterus called lochia. This discharge consists of blood, tissue, mucus, and white blood cells. The color of lochia is an indication of healing in the uterus. Normally lochia is bright red until about the fourth day. The discharge then becomes brownish red, by the tenth day, the discharge becomes yellow-white, and disappears altogether after about three weeks. If at any time the discharge becomes bloody or foul smelling, the patient is instructed to call the physician as these may be symptoms of infection and bleeding. Menstruation should resume after about eight weeks in the nonnursing mother and six months in the nursing mother.

During the puerperium, the patient should be encouraged to eat balanced meals, continue taking vitamins, avoid fatigue, and the lifting of heavy objects. A postpartum visit should be scheduled approximately six weeks after delivery. At this time, the overall health status of the patient is evaluated and information about contraceptive methods provided, if desired.

This office visit includes measuring height, weight, vital signs, performing pelvic and breast examination, rectal examination to detect hemorrhoids, and an anemia evaluation (hemoglobin and hematocrit).

Complications During Pregnancy

Placenta previa is a complication in which the placenta develops in the lower portion of the uterus, blocking the opening in the cervix. During labor, the cervix is unable to dilate and efface completely. The result is oxygen deprivation for the fetus and maternal hemorrhage. Both can be life-threatening and an emergency Cesarean section (C-section) may be required. Ultrasound examination can detect the placental placement and a scheduled C-section may avoid an emergency situation. Placenta abruptio is a complication that occurs when the placenta tears away from the uterine wall resulting in hemorrhage and fetal distress. This requires an emergency C-section.

TABLE 35-10   Procedures and Diagnostic Tests Relating to the Female Reproductive System

Procedures/Tests	Description
Abortion	Termination of a pregnancy before the fetus reaches a viable point in development.
Amniocentesis	Puncturing the amniotic sac using a needle and syringe for the purpose of withdrawing amniotic fluid for testing. Can assist in determining fetal maturity, development, and genetic disorders.
Breast examination	Visual inspection and manual examination of the breasts for changes in contour, symmetry, "dimpling" of skin, retraction of the nipples, and for the presence of lumps.
Cauterization	Destruction of tissue using an electric current, a caustic product, a hot iron, or freezing.
Cervical biopsy	Taking a sample of tissue from the cervix to test for the presence of cancer cells.
Cesarean section (C-section)	Surgical delivery of a baby through an incision into the abdominal and uterine walls.
Chorionic villus sampling (CVS)	Procedure that involves the insertion of a catheter into the cervix and into the outer portion of the membranes surrounding the fetus. A sample of the chorionic villi can be examined for the chromosomal abnormalities and biochemical disorders. This procedure can be done 8 weeks into pregnancy.
Colposcopy	Visual examination of the cervix and vagina.
Conization	Surgical removal of a core of cervical tissue or a partial removal of the cervix.
Cryosurgery	Exposing tissue to extreme cold in order to destroy tissues. This procedure is used in treating malignant tumors, to control pain and bleeding.
Culdoscopy	Examination of the female pelvic cavity using an endoscope.
Dilation and curettage (D&C)	Surgical procedure in which the opening of the cervix is dilated and the uterus is scraped or suctioned of its lining and tissue. A D&C is performed after spontaneous abortion and to stop excessive bleeding from other causes.
Doppler ultrasound	Using an instrument placed externally over the uterus to detect the presence of fibroid tumors and to outline the shape of the fetus.
Endometrial biopsy	Taking a sample of tissue from the lining of the uterus to test for abnormalities.
Episiotomy	Surgical incision of the perineum to facilitate the delivery process. Can prevent an irregular tearing of tissue during birth.
Estrogens	Urine or blood serum test to determine the level of estrone, estradiol, and estriol.
Fetal monitoring	Using electronic equipment placed on the mother's abdomen to monitor the fetus' heart and strength of uterine contractions during labor.
Human chorionic gonadotropin (HCG)	Urine or blood serum test to determine the presence of HCG. A positive result may indicate pregnancy.
Hymenectomy	Surgical removal of the hymen.
Hysterectomy	Surgical removal of the uterus.

(continued)

TABLE 35-10 Procedures and Diagnostic Tests Relating to the Female Reproductive System (*continued*)

Procedures/Test	Description
Hysterosalpingography	Taking an x-ray after injecting radio opaque material into the uterus and oviducts.
Hysteroscopy	Inspection of the uterus using a special endoscope instrument.
Intrauterine device (IUD)	Device inserted into the uterus by a physician for the purpose of contraception.
Kegel exercises	Exercises named after A.H. Kegel, an American gynecologist who developed them to strengthen female pelvic muscles. The exercises are useful in treating incontinence and as an aid in childbirth.
Laparoscopy	Examination of the peritoneal cavity, using an instrument called a laparoscope. The instrument is passed through a small incision made by the surgeon into the peritoneal cavity.
Laparotomy	Making a surgical opening into the abdomen.
Mammography	Process of obtaining pictures of the breast by use of x-rays. This procedure is able to locate breast tumors before they grow to 1 cm. It is the most effective means of detecting early breast cancers.
Oophorectomy	Surgical removal of an ovary.
Panhysterectomy	Excision of the entire uterus, including the cervix.
Panhysterosalpingo-oophorectomy	Surgical removal of the entire uterus, cervix, ovaries, and fallopian tubes. Also called a total hysterectomy.
Pap (Papanicolaou)	Test for the early detection of cancer of the cervix named after the developer of the test, George Papanicolaou. A scraping of cells is removed from the cervix for examination under the microscope.
Pelvic examination	Physical examination of the vagina and adjacent organs performed by a physician by placing the fingers of one hand in the vagina. A visual examination is performed using a speculum.
Pelvimetry	Measurement of the pelvis to assist in determining if the birth canal will allow the passage of the fetus for a vaginal delivery.
Pelvic ultrasonography	Use of ultrasound waves to produce an image or photograph of organ or fetus.
Polypectomy	Surgical removal of a polyp.
Pregnanediol	Urine test that determines menstrual disorders or possible abortion.
Pregnancy test	Chemical test on urine that can determine pregnancy during the first weeks of pregnancy. This can be performed in the physician's office or with an at-home test. Also a blood serum test can be performed at an outside laboratory.
Salpingo-oophorectomy	Surgical removal of the fallopian tube and ovary.
Tubal ligation	Surgical tying off of the fallopian tube to prevent conception from taking place. This results in the sterilization of the female.
Wet mount or wet prep	Examination of vaginal discharge for the presence of bacteria and yeast. A vaginal smear is placed on a microscope slide, wet with normal saline, and then viewed under a microscope by the physician.

Hypertension during pregnancy or gestational hypertension occurs in roughly 10 percent of pregnancies. If protein in the urine occurs as well, then preeclampsia exists. Preeclampsia develops in approximately five percent of pregnant women and usually occurs after the twentieth week of pregnancy. Although the cause of preeclampsia is not definitively known, experts believe that the placenta has spasms of the blood vessels that elevate the blood pressure. The blood flow to the placenta can be compromised, and if left untreated, the placenta can be damaged and the fetus will die. The high blood pressure can also affect the brain, kidneys, liver, and lungs. If seizures develop, then the condition is known as eclampsia.

The symptoms of preeclampsia include agitation and confusion, changes in mental status, decreased urine output, headaches, nausea and vomiting, pain in the upper right quadrant, shortness of breath, sudden weight gain, swelling of the face or hands, and visual impairment.

There are no known ways to prevent preeclampsia. All pregnant women should have good prenatal care and should watch their blood pressure closely.

Contraception

It is important for the medical assistant to have an understanding of the various methods of birth control and the effectiveness of each. The patient chooses the most suitable method, based on physical condition, cost, side effects, and effectiveness.

Contraceptive Methods

Contraceptive methods include barrier methods hormonal methods, intrauterine devices, natural family planning, and coitus interruptus or withdrawal of the penis during intercourse.

BARRIER METHODS   Barrier methods include male condoms, female condoms, diaphragms, and cervical caps. All of these methods should be used with a spermicide to enhance protection.

- The male condom is worn over the penis during intercourse and prevents the sperm from entering the vagina. It is inexpensive, easy to use, and available without prescription. The condom provides a measure of protection from sexually transmitted diseases.

- The female condom is a polyurethane sheath that lines the vagina with an inner ring that fits over the cervix and an outer ring that permits entrance of the penis. The sheath is removed after ejaculation.

- The cervical cap is a small flexible device that fits over the cervix. It is obtained by prescription and requires a physician to determine the size needed. It must be in place 30 minutes before intercourse and remain in place for six to eight hours afterwards.

- The diaphragm is a flexible dome of rubber that fits over the cervix and prevents the entry of sperm. An examination and physician's prescription are needed. It can be inserted six hours before intercourse and must be left in place six hours afterwards.

- A contraceptive sponge is a piece of polyurethane foam impregnated with spermicide that blocks the cervical opening. It can be inserted up to 24 hours before intercourse and must remain in place six hours afterwards. The failure rate is high because of the tendency of the sponge to be displaced during intercourse.

HORMONAL METHODS   Hormonal methods of birth control are based on using hormones to change the levels of female hormones in the body to prevent ovulation or implantation of the fertilized ovum. They include birth control pills, hormonal implants, and the morning-after pill. These methods are easy to use and very effective. They must be prescribed by a physician.

- Birth control pills (the "pill"), the most widely used method, contain either a combination of estrogen and progestin or only small amounts of progestin. They are contraindicated—their use is not advised—in women who smoke, are over 35, or who have had a history of blood clots, high blood pressure, breast cancer, liver disease, and advanced diabetes.

- The morning-after pill or a series of pills containing estrogen and progestin inhibit the possibility of implantation and may be used in cases of rape and sexual abuse.

INTRAUTERINE DEVICES   An intrauterine device is a small metal with copper or plastic device with progestin that is placed in the uterus by the physician.

NATURAL FAMILY PLANNING   Natural family planning or the rhythm method is based on avoiding intercourse around the time of ovulation. It relies on if the woman having a relatively normal menstrual cycle and ovulation is quite predictable.

COITUS INTERRUPTUS   Coitus interruptus is the withdrawal of the male's penis before ejaculation in the vagina. It is unreliable because sperm may be released even before a male ejaculates.

Male Reproductive System

The male reproductive system is a combination of reproduction and urinary systems. The major male organs of reproduction are located outside the body in the scrotum and penis. The scrotum (scrotal sac) contains two testes and the seminal ducts. The penis contains the urethra, which carries both urine and sperm to the outside of the

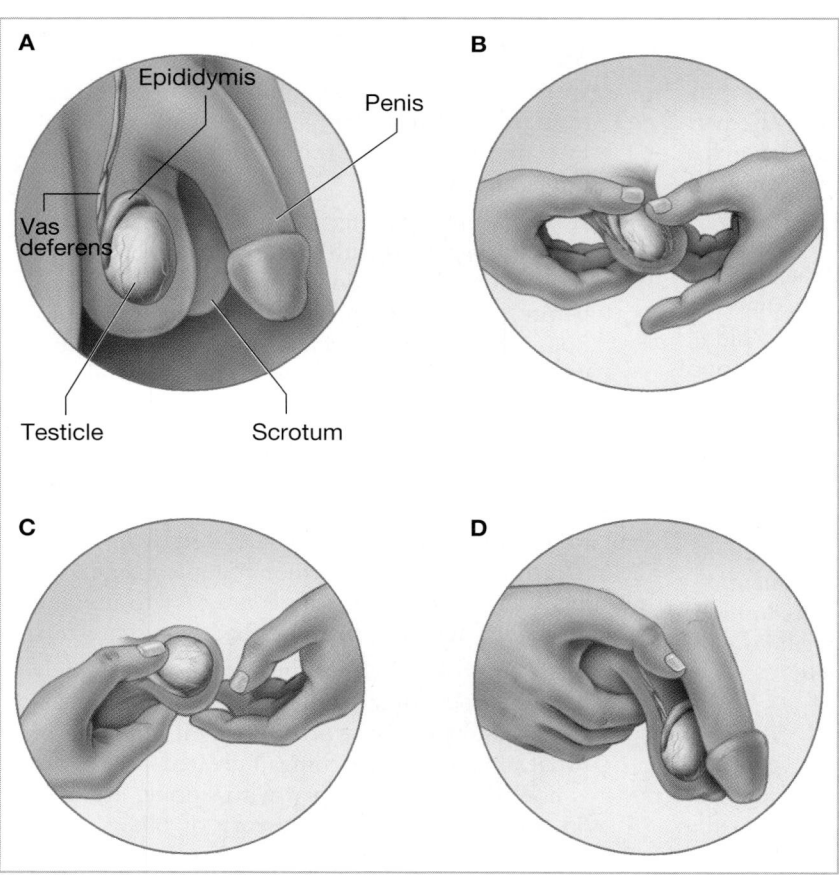

FIGURE 35-18 (A) Male reproductive system; (B) Begin by examining the testicles. Roll the testicle gently between the thumb and fingers applying very slight pressure while attempting to feel any hard, painless lumps; (C) Next examine the cord behind each testicle (the epididymis). This may be tender and is the location of most non-cancerous conditions; (D) Continue the examination by gently feeling the tube that runs up from the epididymis (the vas deferens). The vas deferens is normally a smooth, firm tube.

body. The internal organs of reproduction are the seminal vesicles, ejaculatory duct, and the prostate gland.

The Testicular Examination

Procedures and diagnostic tests relating to the male reproductive system are described in Table 35-11. Figure 35-18 provides an explanation of testicular self-examination for the male patient.

Sexually Transmitted Diseases (STDs)

Sexually transmitted diseases caused by bacteria are generally treated successfully by antibiotics such as penicillin and tetracycline. Although recently, antibiotic resistant strains of organisms that cause gonorrhea and syphilis have developed, making it more difficult to treat these diseases. Viral STDs, such as herpes, genital warts, hepatitis, and HIV, are incurable at this time. Some treatments do exist that reduce the symptoms of these conditions.

Individuals infected with a sexually transmitted disease may not have any symptoms at all. In fact most people who have HIV, for example, have no symptoms. HIV may not produce the symptoms of AIDS until 10 years

or more after infection. Gonorrhea symptoms do not appear in females until two months after exposure. Genital warts may not appear until five months after exposure. Symptoms of the presence of sexually transmitted diseases include sores, discharge, itching, and pain in both males and females. Women may develop pelvic inflammatory disease (PID), which causes abdominal pain, fever, malaise, and severe pain on manipulation of the cervix. Because PID symptoms are similar to those of other abdominal conditions, such as appendicitis, diverticulitis, ectopic pregnancy, and ulcerative colitis, a thorough history and diagnostic tests are necessary. PID can result in blood clots, peritonitis and even death if untreated. In the male, additional symptoms, such as profuse discharge from the penis, swelling and pain in the testicles, and painful urination, may occur. Males frequently will seek help at this point because of the difficulty with urination. See Box 35-1 for information on infertility due to chlamydia infection and treatment of infertility with in vitro fertilization.

Although there are certain examinations and some laboratory procedures that can identify infective organisms and symptoms, for many STDs, there are no completely accurate tests to diagnose patients. Patients may have the disease but test negative until later in the cycle of the disease, as with HIV.

TABLE 35-11 **Procedures and Diagnostic Tests Relating to the Male Reproductive System**

Procedures/Tests	Description
Castration	Excision of the testicles in the male or the ovaries in the female.
Cauterization	Destruction of tissue with an electric current, a caustic agent, hot iron, or by freezing.
Circumcision	Surgical removal of the end of the prepuce or foreskin of the penis. Generally performed on the newborn male at the request of the parents. The primary reason is ease of hygiene. Circumcision is also a ritual practiced in some religions.
Digital rectal examination	Manual examination for an enlarged prostate gland performed by palpating the prostate gland through the rectum wall.
Epididymectomy	Surgical excision of the epididymis.
Erickson sperm separation method	Process of separating the Y-chromosome sperm from the X-chromosome sperm. A sperm sample is taken and placed in a tube of albumin. Those sperm that survive are Y-chromosome sperm, which produce male infants. Females inseminated with these sperm have a 75–80 percent chance of producing a male child.
Fluorescent treponemal antibody absorption	Test performed on blood serum to determine the presence of *Treponema pallidum*, the microorganism that causes syphilis.
Orchidopexy	Surgical fixation to move undescended testes into the scrotum and attaching them to prevent retraction.
Orchiectomy	Surgical removal of the testes.
Paternity test	Test to determine whether a certain male could be the father of a specific child. The test can indicate only who is not the father. Types of tests that may be used are blood type, human leukocyte anitgen (HLA), white blood cell, enzyme, protein, and genetic. The blood type of the child and the alleged father are analyzed for compatibility. For example, a parent with type O blood cannot be the parent of a child with type AB blood. HLA looks at the body's tissue compatibility system, and the white blood cell test looks at chemical markers (antigens) on the surface of the white blood cells. Enzyme and protein tests look at red blood cell enzymes and a new genetic test is being developed that uses molecular and protein biology to look at family-related genetic patterns.
Prostatectomy	Surgical removal of the prostate gland.
Prostate-specific antigen (PSA)	Blood test to screen for prostate cancer. Elevated blood levels of PSA are associated with prostate cancer.
Semen analysis	Procedure used when performing a fertility workup to determine if the male is able to produce sperm. Sperm is collected by the patient after he has abstained from sexual intercourse for a period of 3 to 5 days. Also used to determine if a vasectomy has been successful. After a period of 6 weeks, no further sperm should be present in a sample from the patient.
Sterilization	Process of rendering a male or female sterile or unable to conceive children.
Testosterone toxicology	Test performed on blood serum to identify the level of testosterone. Increased level may indicate benign prostatic hyperplasia. Decreased level may indicate hypogonadism, testicular hypofunction, hypopituitarism, or orchidectomy.
Transurethral resection of the prostate (TURP)	Surgical removal of the prostate gland by inserting a device through the urethra and removing prostate tissue.
Vasectomy	Removal of a segment or all of the vas deferens to prevent sperm from leaving the male body.
Venereal disease research laboratory (VDRL)	Test performed on blood serum to determine the presence of *Treponema pallidum*. Used to detect syphilis.

Infertility and In Vitro Fertilization (IVF)

In vitro fertilization is one method of treating infertility in those who are unable or have a diminished capacity to conceive. There are many causes of infertility and selecting the correct treatment depends on determining whether the cause is functional or a result of infection.

Repeated infections of sexually transmitted diseases, such as chlamydia, often symptomless, may cause scarring and occlusion (blockage) of the fallopian tube. When this happens the ovum released during ovulation is unable to make its way to the uterus through the fallopian tube. Normally conception occurs in the upper one-third of the fallopian tube and the zygote (fertilized ovum) then moves down the tube to implant into the uterus. If the fallopian tube is blocked or scarred, conception and implantation cannot take place. Many women are unaware that they have ever had a chlamydia infection and when they decide it is time to conceive, they find it is impossible.

In vitro fertilization is fertilization outside the body, usually in a petri dish in the laboratory. A woman who wishes to conceive may be given hormones (FSH) to stimulate the release of more than one ovum. The ova are then removed through laparoscopic surgery and put into the petri dish. Sperm, from either the husband or a sperm donor, is added to the petri dish. After fertilization and cleavage (cell division of the zygote) have taken place, the zygote is then placed in the woman's uterus. Since the birth of the "first test tube baby" in 1978, there have been thousands of babies born through in vitro fertilization. It is not always successful however, and it may be necessary to have this procedure repeated several times—each attempt is very costly.

Sexually Transmitted Disease Education

Treating and preventing the spread of STDs depends on education and identification of sexual partners who may have been exposed. The only foolproof means of prevention of sexually transmitted disease is complete abstinence from sexual activity. Agreeing to have a monogamous relationship goes a long way in reducing the chance of being infected. If individuals are going to be sexually active, there are strategies that will reduce the chance of exposure to STDs.

- Use a barrier device (condom) and spermicide during every act of sexual intercourse.

- Limit the number of sexual partners.

- Know your sexual partners well.

- Seek prompt treatment of any suspected STD.

- Complete all cycles of medication and comply with follow-up testing.

- Cooperate in tracing sexual contacts.

Educating patients about sexually transmitted diseases, their causes, symptoms, and treatments is very important. Often the medical assistant is the individual with whom the patient feels most comfortable discussing potentially embarrassing problems. You will need to feel comfortable yourself with the facts about STDs and be able to discuss these issues in an unemotional, nonjudgmental manner. Brochures and pamphlets should be readily available and easily accessed in your office. Patients may feel more comfortable picking up reading material they can review in the privacy of their own home than asking questions in person. Patient Education discusses effective learning aids for educating patients about their diagnoses and treatment plans.

Reporting Sexually Transmitted Disease

In your role as a medical assistant, you should understand the different types of STDs, recognize their symptoms, and comprehend your role in the legal ramifications of reporting sexually transmitted diseases to the proper state and national agencies. For example, in all 50 states, confirmed cases of HIV/AIDS are reportable conditions either by statute or administrative act. Other sexually transmitted diseases, such as gonorrhea and syphilis, are reportable diseases in most states. Legally you need to be aware of your responsibility wherever you are employed. Confidentiality is extremely important when dealing with sensitive information such as testing positive for an STD. Many states require a post-treatment follow-up for certain diseases; therefore, your role in patient compliance is vital. Identifying partners of infected patients is one way to stop the spread of STDs and protect the health of unsuspecting persons. Office policy should spell out clearly your role in these sensitive matters.

Types of Sexually Transmitted Diseases

Chlamydia infections are characterized by urethritis, and in males, epididimytis, and in females, no symptoms initially, then there is the possibility it may lead

Many patients are not ready either physically or emotionally to fully understand their medical diagnosis. The medical assistant will need to be able to clearly explain, in simple language, any terms that are confusing to the patient. All follow-up instructions regarding further treatment, appointments, medications, and mobility need to be explained and documented.

The medical assistant will need to utilize many teaching methods to facilitate the patient's comprehension of his or her diagnosis and treatment plan. Many patients will not be able to understand the medical terminology relating to their illness. Drawing charts for medication dosages, writing instructions for home care and appointment schedules, and asking the patient to repeat what the physician has told them are all effective learning aids.

to pelvic inflammatory disease (PID). Infected females have an increased risk of ectopic pregnancy and sterility. Infants born to infected mothers may develop conjunctivitis or pneumonia. Chlamydial infection can be successfully treated with antibiotics such as tetracycline or erythromycin.

In the male, gonorrhea (GC) is characterized by penile drainage, clear at first, becoming thick and milky, burning, itching, and pain on urination. Females are often asymptomatic, then they develop a yellowish-green discharge. Gonorrhea may possibly lead to PID. Other symptoms that may be experienced by both sexes include sore throat, swollen glands, anal discharge, and fever. Treatment of GC includes large doses of penicillin or tetracycline with follow-up examinations because antibiotic resistant strains of the organisms complicate treatment.

Painful lesions erupting in three to seven days in the genital area is a primary symptom of genital herpes in both male and female. Type I herpes is associated with cold sore lesions. There is no known cure for herpes at present. The lesions are usually self-limiting but reoccur during stressful situations. Recently new treatments have reduced the severity of the reoccurrences.

Human Papilloma virus (HPV) infection refers to a group of viruses that cause this common sexually transmitted disease. Genital warts, or condylomas, are found in clusters on the external organs of both the male and female and internally in the female, in the vagina and cervix. HPV can be discovered by a Pap smear, though the patient may not have visible signs of warts. It may take several months to several years after contact for the person to show signs of infection. Genital warts increase a female's risk of developing cervical cancer.

Trichomoniasis is a protozoal infection caused by the organism *Trichomonas vaginalis*, resulting in an infection of the lower genitourinary tract. Trichomoniasis causes a white or yellow, foamy vaginal discharge with a foul odor in females. The male usually has no symptoms except urethral itching. Diagnosis can be made by obtaining a sample of vaginal secretions and preparing a slide with normal saline. Microscopic examination will reveal the oval Trichomonas parasite with four hairlike flagella whipping across the field. Treatment for both male and female is a course of the antibiotic metronidazole taken orally.

Urinary System

The function of the urinary system is to filter and remove metabolic waste products from the blood, help maintain electrolyte and pH balance, excrete waste from the body in the form of urine, and help regulate red blood cell production and blood pressure. In your role as a medical assistant, it is important for you to comprehend the functions and importance of the urinary system in the overall health of the patient. Symptoms of urinary tract disorders vary as do the age related problems of this intricate system. For example, increased urine production is seen in diabetes, frequency of urination is seen in urinary tract infection, severe pain in episodes of kidney stone movement, swelling and weight gain is seen in congestive heart failure (CHF) and renal dysfunction, decreased urinary output is seen in urinary obstructions (Figure 35-19). The maximum volume of urine the bladder can hold declines with aging, leading to increased frequency of urination and in some individuals, incontinence.

Most people urinate four to six times per day and excrete about 2,000 cc or two quarts of urine per day. Urine specimens are an easily obtainable, noninvasive way to evaluate the homeostatic condition of the body and are among the most frequently ordered tests in the medical office. Collecting, processing, and testing urine specimens will be one of your duties. See Chapter 42. Normally after the patient is greeted and escorted to the examining room, a urine sample may be requested. The patient should be given clear directions on the type of sample required and given an appropriately labeled container. Urine samples are potentially infectious and gloves should be worn when handling patient samples. After the sample is obtained it is tested or stored for later processing. Be sure to follow the processing guidelines to maintain the integrity of the specimen and ensure valid results. Dealing with a variety of patients, some with special needs, you will need to be sensitive to their abilities. Offer assistance as needed and provide for patient privacy. Procedures and diagnostic tests relating to the urinary system are described in Table 35-12.

Prostate Cancer

Prostate cancer is a slow growing malignant tumor of the prostate gland. Prostate cancer may spread to adjacent urinary tract and male reproductive organs, as well as to the lymph nodes and bones. It is the second most common form of cancer in men, with one in eight males affected. Because of its slow rate of growth, prostate cancer can be detected and treated in its early stages with regular medical examinations. The cause of prostate cancer is not known, but age, heredity, and a high fat diet increase the risk of developing it. Symptoms include weak stream of urine, blood in the urine, erectile dysfunction, nocturia (frequency of urination at night), and pelvic pain. The protein specific antigen (PSA) blood test and a digital rectal examination are used to screen for prostate cancer. The PSA test checks for a protein released by the prostate. If levels are elevated, then a biopsy of prostate tissue is done, usually in the office. If the results are positive for cancer cells, then a bone scan is done to detect possible spread of the disease. Treatments for prostate cancer vary from watching and waiting with regular checkups, to surgery, radiation, hormone therapy, and chemotherapy. PSA results of under 4 mg/dl is considered normal. The interpretation of these results and additional testing are needed because a very high result may not mean prostate cancer and very low results may not mean the individual is cancer-free.

Renal Failure

Kidney failure is the inability of the kidneys to adequately filter metabolic waste products from the blood. There are many causes leading to the decline of kidney function and kidney failure is classified as acute or chronic.

Acute Renal Failure

Acute kidney failure has a rapid onset of a few days to a few weeks. It is caused by any condition that decreases blood supply to the kidney, obstructs the flow of urine anywhere in the urinary tract, or by injury within the kidney.

The symptoms vary with the cause and rate of onset and include fluid retention in the hands and feet, dark colored urine, decrease in urinary output, fatigue due to increase in metabolic waste levels in the blood stream, nausea, and pruritis (itchiness). Diagnosis is made based on symptoms and blood tests, such as blood urea nitrogen, creatinine, electrolytes, and diagnostic tests such as CAT scan and ultrasound. Acute renal failure can affect people of any age; however, it is more common in older people. The survival rate is about 60 percent and kidney dialysis and transplants have improved the survival rate greatly.

Chronic Renal Failure

Chronic kidney failure is a slow progressive decline in kidney function over a period of months to several years. Acute kidney failure can become chronic if after treatment, kidneys do not fully recover. Any condition that

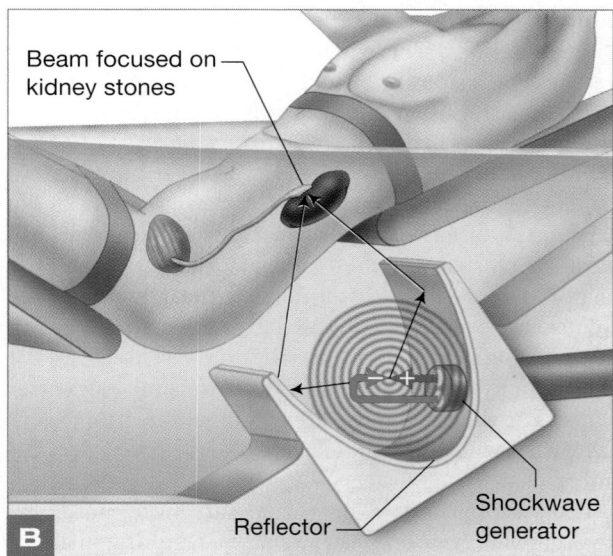

FIGURE 35-19 Extracorporeal shockwave lithotripsy uses acoustic shockwaves created by the shockwave generator to travel through soft tissue to shatter the renal stone into fragments, which then are eliminated in the urine. (A) A shockwave generator that does not require water immersion; (B) An illustration of water immersion lithotripsy procedure.

TABLE 35-12 Procedures and Diagnostic Tests Relating to the Urinary System

Procedures/Tests	Description
Blood urea nitrogen	A blood test to determine the amount of urea that is excreted by the kidneys. Abnormal results indicate urinary tract disease.
Catheterization	The insertion of a sterile tube through the urethra and into the urinary bladder for the purpose of withdrawing urine. This procedure is used to obtain a sterile urine specimen and also to relieve distension when the patient is unable to void on his or her own.
Clean catch specimen (CC)	Urine sample obtained after cleaning off the urinary opening and catching or collecting a sample in midstream (halfway through the urination process) to minimize contamination from the genitalia.
Creatinine	A blood test to determine the amount of creatinine present. Abnormal results indicate kidney disease.
Creatinine clearance	A urine test to determine the glomerular filtration rate (GFR). Abnormal results indicate kidney disease.
Culture, urine	A urine test to determine the presence of microorganisms. Abnormal results indicate urinary tract infection.
Cystography	The process of instilling a contrast material or dye into the bladder by catheter to visualize the urinary bladder.
Cystoscopy	Visual examination of the urinary bladder using an instrument called a *cystoscope*. The patient may receive general anesthesia for this procedure.
Dialysis	The artificial filtration of waste material from the blood. It is used when the kidneys fail to function.
Extracorporeal shockwave lithotripsy (ESWL)	Use of ultrasound waves to break up stones. Process does not require invasive surgery.
Excretory urography	Injection of dye into the bloodstream followed by taking an x-ray to trace the action of the kidney as it excretes dye.
Hemodialysis	Use of an artificial kidney that filters the blood of a person to remove waste products. Use of this technique in patients who have defective kidneys is lifesaving.
Intravenous pyelogram (IVP)	An x-ray examination of the kidneys, ureters, and bladder by injecting radio opaque dye into the circulatory system and tracing its route as it is excreted.
Kidney, ureters, bladder (KUB)	A flat plate x-ray is taken of the abdomen to indicate the size and position of the kidneys, ureters, and bladder.
Lithotripsy	Destroying or crushing kidney stones in the bladder or urethra with a device called a *lithotriptor*.
Meatotomy	Surgical enlargement of the urinary opening.
Peritoneal dialysis	The removal of toxic waste substances from the body by placing warm chemically balanced solutions into the peritoneal cavity. This is used in treating renal failure and in certain types of poisonings.

(continued)

Procedures/Test	Description
Renal biopsy	The removal of tissue from the kidney. Abnormal results may indicate kidney cancer, kidney transplant rejection, and glomerulonephritis.
Renal transplant	Surgical placement of a donor kidney.
Retrograde pyelogram	A diagnostic x-ray in which dye is inserted through the urethra to outline the bladder, ureters, and renal pelvis.
Sound	Metal rod curved at one end with a handle at the other end used to treat stricture or an obstruction in the urethra. A physician will pass the sound up the urethra.
Urinalysis	A laboratory test that consists of the physical, chemical, and microscopic examination of urine.
Urography	The use of contrast medium to provide an x-ray of the urinary tract.
Ultrasonography, kidneys	The use of high frequency sound waves to visualize the kidneys. The sound waves (echoes) are recorded on an oscilloscope and film. Abnormal results may indicate kidney tumors, cysts, abscess, and kidney disease.

can cause acute renal failure can cause chronic kidney failure. The most common causes of chronic failure are diabetes mellitus and hypertension. Other causes include kidney abnormalities, kidney disease (glomerulonephritis), and autoimmune disorders (systemic lupus).

The patient may experience mild symptoms including nocturia and elevated blood urea nitrogen. As the condition progresses, fatigue, lack of mental alertness, anemia, loss of appetite, and shortness of breath affect the patient's quality of life. Diagnosis is based on patient history, symptoms, and blood tests for levels of creatinine and blood urea nitrogen. Chronic renal failure is fatal if not treated. Survival for patients with end-stage renal disease is a few months. Treatments include various medications to adjust blood pressure, regulate electrolyte balance, and counteract anemia, and restriction of pro-

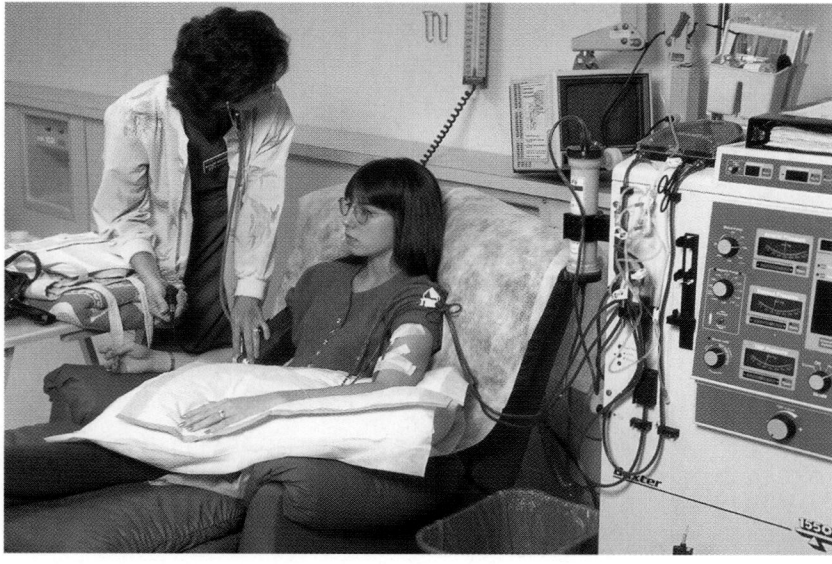

FIGURE 35-20 A patient undergoing hemodialysis in a dialysis unit.

Dialysis

Dialysis is the process of removing waste products and excess fluids from the body. Hemodialysis is the use of an artificial kidney machine to perform the functions of the nephrons of the patient's kidneys. The patient's blood is passed through tiny tubules surrounded by fluid (dialysate), which has the same chemical composition as blood plasma. Waste products and excess fluids pass out of the patient's blood into the fluid of the machine. They are thus eliminated and purified blood is returned to the patient. Hemodialysis needs to be repeated on average three times per week. To achieve this goal, easy access to the patient's bloodstream is necessary. This may be accomplished by a number of means such as creating an arteriovenous fistula or creating a synthetic graft between an artery and vein. Either type of access requires a surgical procedure. Because of the tendency of the blood to clot, heparin is administered during hemodialysis.

Peritoneal dialysis involves the use of the peritoneum, the membrane that lines the abdomen and covers the abdominal organs, to function as a filter for dialysis. The peritoneum has a large surface and rich blood supply making filtration easier. Dialysate is put into the abdominal cavity through a catheter and left for a period of time (hours or overnight) to allow waste and excess fluids to be removed from the blood stream, and then the filtrate is drained out and discarded. Several types of peritoneal dialysis are available, however, each requires varying amounts of time ranging from 10 to 12 hours over night, or every 3 to 4 hours four times a day. A catheter may be placed in the abdominal wall temporarily or permanently as needed. Choosing the type of dialysis depends on many factors such as age, physical condition, type of renal disorder, and lifestyle. Either type of dialysis restricts a patient's life in terms of loss of time, specialized diet, loss of mobility, and loss of independence. In children, renal disease may stunt their growth and cause a feeling of isolation.

tein and calcium in the diet. When these treatments are no longer effective, kidney dialysis or transplant are the alternatives (Figure 35-20). Most patients with advanced kidney failure die within five to ten years even with the improvements of dialysis. Box 35-2 discusses hemodialysis and peritoneal dialysis.

SUMMARY

The topics presented in this chapter represent a variety of medical specialty areas. No physician's practice will include all of them. Since the profession of medical assisting is for the multiskilled individual, he or she is expected to have a general knowledge of medicine.

Much of the clinical role of the medical assistant involves assisting with procedures relating to the body systems including: digestive, musculoskeletal (orthopedics), reproductive, urinary, respiratory, integumentary, endocrine, lymphatic, and cardiovascular. No matter what the task involves, the trademark of a good medical assistant should be careful attention to detail.

Chapter Review

COMPETENCY REVIEW

1. Define and spell the terms to learn for this chapter.
2. Develop a teaching plan for a patient with diabetes mellitus.
3. Develop a brochure instructing female patients how to do a breast self-examination and male patients a testicular self-examination.
4. Describe the setup for a Pap smear. What is the medical assistant's responsibility for assisting with this procedure?

1. A round, raised skin lesion with itching that is a positive sign of reaction to allergic testing is a
   A. nodule
   B. vesicle
   C. papule
   D. wheal
   E. macule

2. Skin, oil glands, hair, and sense organs are part of which system of the body?
   A. cardiovascular system
   B. dermis system
   C. lymphatic system
   D. respiratory system
   E. integumentary system

3. A benign neoplasm that results in enlarged blood vessels is a
   A. melanoma
   B. nevus
   C. keratosis
   D. lipoma
   E. hemangioma

4. A cardiovascular condition that results in death of tissue from lack of blood supply is a(n)
   A. angioma
   B. myocardial infraction
   C. aneurysm
   D. Reynaud's phenomenon
   E. murmur

5. Which conditions would NOT be diagnosed by an examination of CSF?
   A. brain hemarrhage
   B. encephalitis polio
   C. gonnorrhea
   D. meningitis
   E. tumor of the spinal cord

6. What disease results from over production of growth hormone?
   A. myxedema
   B. giantism
   C. Graves' disease
   D. Cushing's syndrome
   E. myasthenia gravis

7. A procedure in which contrast medium is used to visualize the bile ducts is
   A. peritoneoscopy laparoscopy
   B. choledocholithotripsy
   C. intravenous cholangiogram
   D. endoscopic retrograde cholangiopancreatography (ERCP)
   E. cholecystogram

8. An immunoassay test used for detecting an antibody to the AIDS virus is
   A. fluorescein angiography
   B. Romberg test
   C. falling test
   D. ELISA
   E. fungal scraping

9. A musculoskeletal disorder in which a softening of bone occurs that may result from a deficiency in vitamin D is
   A. osteomalacia
   B. osteoporosis
   C. osteoarthritis
   D. scoliosis
   E. talipes

10. The sexually transmitted disease that is caused by a protozoa is
    A. gonorrhea
    B. syphilis
    C. Trichomoniasis
    D. Candidiasis
    E. chlamydia

CRITICAL THINKING

1. What other tests do you think the physician should order based on Brian's results? Why?

2. What implications do these findings have on his work as a laborer?

3. What information about his home environment could be pertinent to the findings?

4. Dr. Thompson speaks to Brian about his smoking and asks you to follow up with information for him. What would you say to Brian to help him understand the dangers of smoking?

ON THE JOB

Shelia Meyer, a medical assistant in Dr. Ryan's large cardiovascular practice, is taking the medical history of Edna Helm, an obese elderly woman with congestive heart disease. Edna states, "I'm always short of breath and I perspire all the time. I guess I'm gaining weight, but the funny thing is that only my legs seem heavier. My heart is pounding when I lie down at night; it even seems to stop sometimes. I've even started to wear red nail polish to hide the funny blue color of my nails."

Edna gives you a copy of her medical history from an out-of-state physician. The medical history indicates that she has had the following conditions, tests, and procedures:

Conditions	Tests	Surgical Procedures
Positive Babinski sign	Holter Monitor testing	Basal cell carcinoma removed in 1992
Allergic rhinitis	Radioimmunoassay test	Sebaceous cyst removed in 1982
Aortic insufficiency	Protein bound iodine test	Meniscectomy in 1978
Ascites	Glucose tolerance test	Rhytidectomy in 1970
Gastritis		
Osteoarthritis		

1. Using correct medical terms, chart Edna's presenting symptoms.
2. Define each of the procedures and conditions listed on her medical record.

INTERNET ACTIVITY

Radiologists are considered allied health professionals. Perform an Internet search and discover their duties, educational requirements, in what types of facilities they are normally employed, employment opportunities, and licensure, certification or registration requirements.

MediaLink More on medical specialties, including interactive resources, can be found on the Student CD-ROM accompanying this textbook.

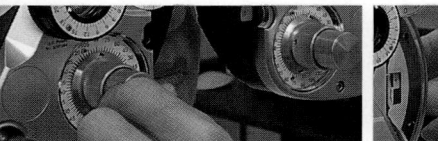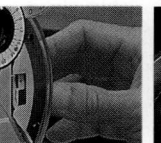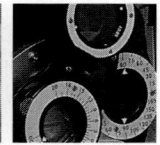

Medical Assistant Role Delineation Chart

HIGHLIGHT indicates material covered in this chapter.

ADMINISTRATIVE

Administrative Procedures

- Perform basic administrative medical assisting functions
- Schedule, coordinate and monitor appointments
- Schedule inpatient/outpatient admissions and procedures
- Understand and apply third-party guidelines
- Obtain reimbursement through accurate claims submission
- Monitor third-party reimbursement
- Understand and adhere to managed care policies and procedures
- *Negotiate managed care contracts*

Practice Finances

- Perform procedural and diagnostic coding
- Apply bookkeeping principles

- Manage accounts receivable
- *Manage accounts payable*
- *Process payroll*
- *Document and maintain accounting and banking records*
- *Develop and maintain fee schedules*
- *Manage renewals of business and professional insurance policies*
- *Manage personnel benefits and maintain records*
- *Perform marketing, financial, and strategic planning*

CLINICAL

Fundamental Principles

- Apply principles of aseptic technique and infection control
- Comply with quality assurance practices
- Screen and follow up patient test results

Diagnostic Orders

- Collect and process specimens
- Perform diagnostic tests

Patient Care

- Adhere to established patient screening procedures
- Obtain patient history and vital signs
- Prepare and maintain examination and treatment areas
- Prepare patient for examinations, procedures and treatments

- Assist with examinations, procedures and treatments
- Prepare and administer medications and immunizations
- Maintain medication and immunization records
- Recognize and respond to emergencies
- Coordinate patient care information with other health care providers
- Initiate IV and administer IV medications with appropriate training and as permitted by state law

GENERAL

Professionalism

- Display a professional manner and image
- Demonstrate initiative and responsibility
- Work as a member of the health care team
- Prioritize and perform multiple tasks
- Adapt to change
- Promote the CMA credential
- Enhance skills through continuing education
- Treat all patients with compassion and empathy
- Promote the practice through positive public relations

Communication Skills

- Recognize and respect cultural diversity
- Adapt communications to individual's ability to understand
- Use professional telephone technique

- Recognize and respond effectively to verbal, nonverbal, and written communications
- Use medical terminology appropriately
- Utilize electronic technology to receive, organize, prioritize and transmit information
- Serve as liaison

Legal Concepts

- Perform within legal and ethical boundaries
- Prepare and maintain medical records
- Document accurately
- Follow employer's established policies dealing with the health care contract
- Implement and maintain federal and state health care legislation and regulations
- Comply with established risk management and safety procedures
- Recognize professional credentialing criteria
- *Develop and maintain personnel, policy and procedure manuals*

Instruction

- Instruct individuals according to their needs
- Explain office policies and procedures
- Teach methods of health promotion and disease prevention
- Locate community resources and disseminate information
- *Develop educational materials*
- *Conduct continuing education activities*

Operational Functions

- Perform inventory of supplies and equipment
- Perform routine maintenance of administrative and clinical equipment
- Apply computer techniques to support office operations
- *Perform personnel management functions*
- *Negotiate leases and prices for equipment and supply contracts*

- *Denotes advanced skills.*

SOURCE: Reprinted by permission of the American Association of Medical Assistants from the AAMA Role Delineation Study: Occupational Analysis of the Medical Assisting Profession.

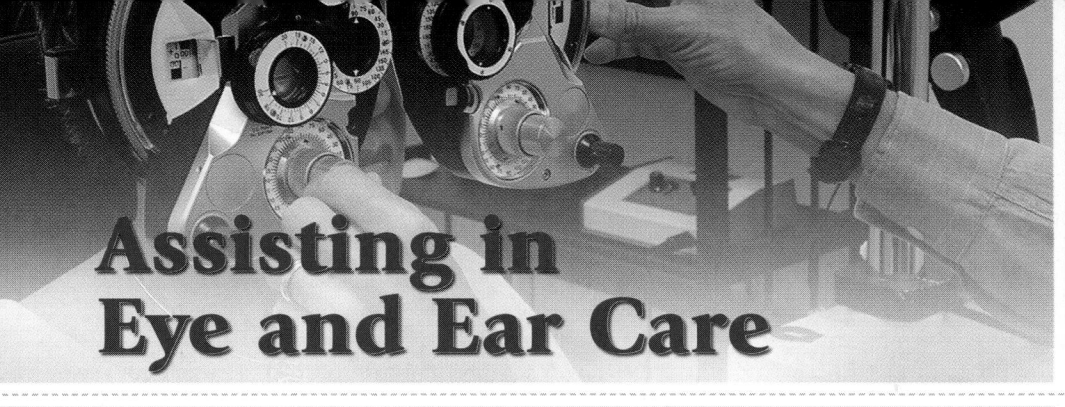

chapter 36

Assisting in Eye and Ear Care

Learning Objectives

After reading this chapter, you should be able to:

- Define the terms to learn in this chapter.
- Explain how vision occurs.
- List and explain five age-related changes in the eye.
- Explain procedures to evaluate distance vision, color blindness, near vision, and contrast sensitivity.
- Explain procedures to irrigate the eye and instill eye medications.
- Name three causes of blindness.

- Explain how hearing occurs.
- Name and explain two types of hearing impairment.
- Explain procedures to irrigate the ear and instill ear medications.
- Explain the procedure to evaluate hearing acuity using an audiometer.
- Explain the procedure for assisting vision impaired patients to prepare for physical examinations.

OUTLINE

The Study of the Eye	708
Irrigation of the Eye	715
Instillation of Eye Medications	715
Patient Safety Guidelines	715
Assisting the Blind Patient	716
The Study of the Ear	717
Hearing Acuity and Assessment	719
Examination of the Nose and Throat	722

Terms to Learn

astigmatism
audiogram
audiometer
cerumen
conduction hearing loss
cornea
electronystagmograph (ENG)
frequencies
hearing acuity
hyperopia

instill
irrigate
Ishihara test
myopia
myringa
ophthalmologist
ophthalmoscope
optician
optometrist
organ of Corti
otology

otorhinolaryngologist (ENT)
otoscope
presbycusis
presbyopia
sensorineural hearing loss
Snellen eye chart
specula
strabismus
tympanum
visual acuity

Case Study

KYLE IS A NINE-YEAR-OLD BOY WHOSE PARENTS are concerned that he is having trouble seeing the blackboard in school. Kyle is shy and will not ask the teacher to change his seat. Kyle's parents both have had glasses since their teens. Dr. Sims asks you to perform a Snellen eye exam. The results are 20/80 OD and 20/60 OS. After Dr. Sims sees the results, he orders a further eye exam that requires eye drops to both eyes to dilate the pupils. Kyle does not want to have this procedure done.

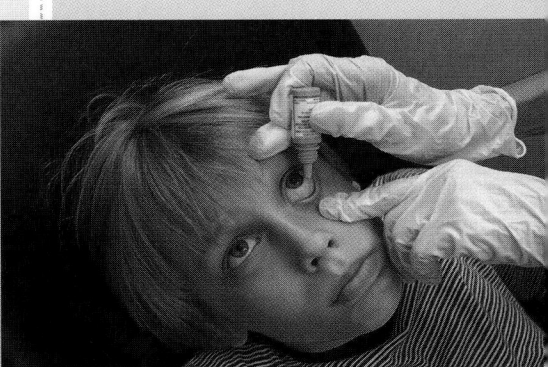

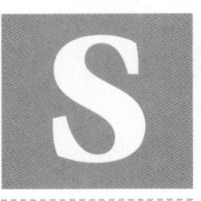Special examinations and procedures relating to specific body systems are commonly performed in the medical office. In this chapter we will consider examinations and procedures relating to the eye and ear. The role of the medical assistant is to assist the physician during special examinations and procedures and to instruct the patient before, during, and after procedures. You will learn the procedures to perform visual and auditory acuity (sharpness) testing, to instill or put in eye and ear medications, and to irrigate or rinse both eyes and ears. Keep in mind you are representing the physician and are important in setting the tone and positive atmosphere in the office. All patients should be treated with respect during all phases of the procedures.

The Study of the Eye

The eye is the organ of sight. The study of the eye is called ophthalmology. An ophthalmologist is a medical doctor who can perform eye examinations and eye surgery, and prescribe medications, eyeglasses, and contact lenses. An optometrist is a doctor of optometry, not a medical doctor, who can perform eye examinations, prescribe medications needed for an eye examination, and write prescriptions for eyeglasses and contact lenses. An optician is a technician who specializes in grinding lenses and preparing eyeglasses and contact lenses. See Chapter 24 to review the structure and function of the eye.

Eye Instruments

There are a number of complex tests used to diagnose and treat vision problems, many of which are done in the office of specialists, such as ophthalmologists or otorhinolaryngologists (ENT), eye, ear, nose, and throat specialists. In primary care and pediatric offices, routine screening examinations for vision problems are performed as part of physical examinations. The otoscope is used to examine the tympanum or myringa for signs of infection and inflammation and will be discussed later in the chapter. *Tympanum* or *myringa* are medical terms for the eardrum. The ophthalmoscope is used to view inner parts of the eye. The physician positions the ophthalmoscope so light penetrates the pupil of the patient's eye and screens for retinal damage and vascular problems. The care and maintenance of the otoscope and the ophthalmoscope is a routine task performed by the medical assistant. These instruments utilize batteries that must be recharged on a regular basis. The tiny bulbs used in both instruments must be replaced occasionally. Most physicians use disposable ear and nasal specula to examine the tympanic membrane and nose. A speculum—singular for the plural, *specula*—is any instrument that holds open an opening of the body to permit inspection. Monitoring supplies for the examining room is a routine task performed by the medical assistant.

Before every eye examination the overall appearance of the eye is evaluated for symptoms such as redness, pus-like discharge, and excessive tearing. In addition, the physician evaluates the status of the patient's pupils. PERRLA in an acronym that stands for Pupils Equal, Round, React to Light and Accommodation and focus on objects at different distances. Normally the pupils of the eyes are the same size and change or accommodate when a beam of light is focused on the eye and is then removed. Injuries to the brain may result in the patient having pupils of unequal size.

Visual Acuity and Refractive Errors

Normal visual acuity, or clearness of vision, is referred to as 20/20 vision, which means the eye should see an object 20 feet away clearly. Errors of refraction occur when the eyeball is either too long, too short, the lens loses its elasticity, or the lens or cornea has an irregular curvature. The cornea is the clear, transparent covering of the eye. Each of these refractive errors will be discussed individually.

Myopia or nearsightedness means that the eye sees near objects well but distant ones appear blurry. This occurs either because the eyeball is too long or because the lens is too thick, and the light rays do not reach the retina. The shape of the eyeball and lens are hereditary. The myopic eye requires a concave lens to correct vision. Hyperopia or farsightedness means that the eyes see distant objects well, but near objects are blurry, and the eyeball is too short or the lens too thin. The hyperopic eye requires a convex lens to correct the visual defect. Presbyopia is farsightedness that occurs with aging. The lens loses its elasticity and glasses are needed for reading. Astigmatism is a refractive disorder where the lenses or cornea are uneven and light is not bent or refracted evenly. Images may be clear in the center of the field and blurry at the outer edges of the visual field. Figure 36-1 shows how lenses correct visual problems.

Strabismus is an eye disorder caused by weakness in the external eye muscles resulting in the eyes looking in different directions. Normally the eyes focus on a subject in coordination or else double vision results. Children with strabismus appear "cross-eyed" and may need to wear a patch over the "good" eye to strengthen the weaker eye. You may need to teach the patient basic eye exercises as part of the treatment plan. It is important that treatment begin at an early age to prevent permanent damage to the eye. If the patch and exercise

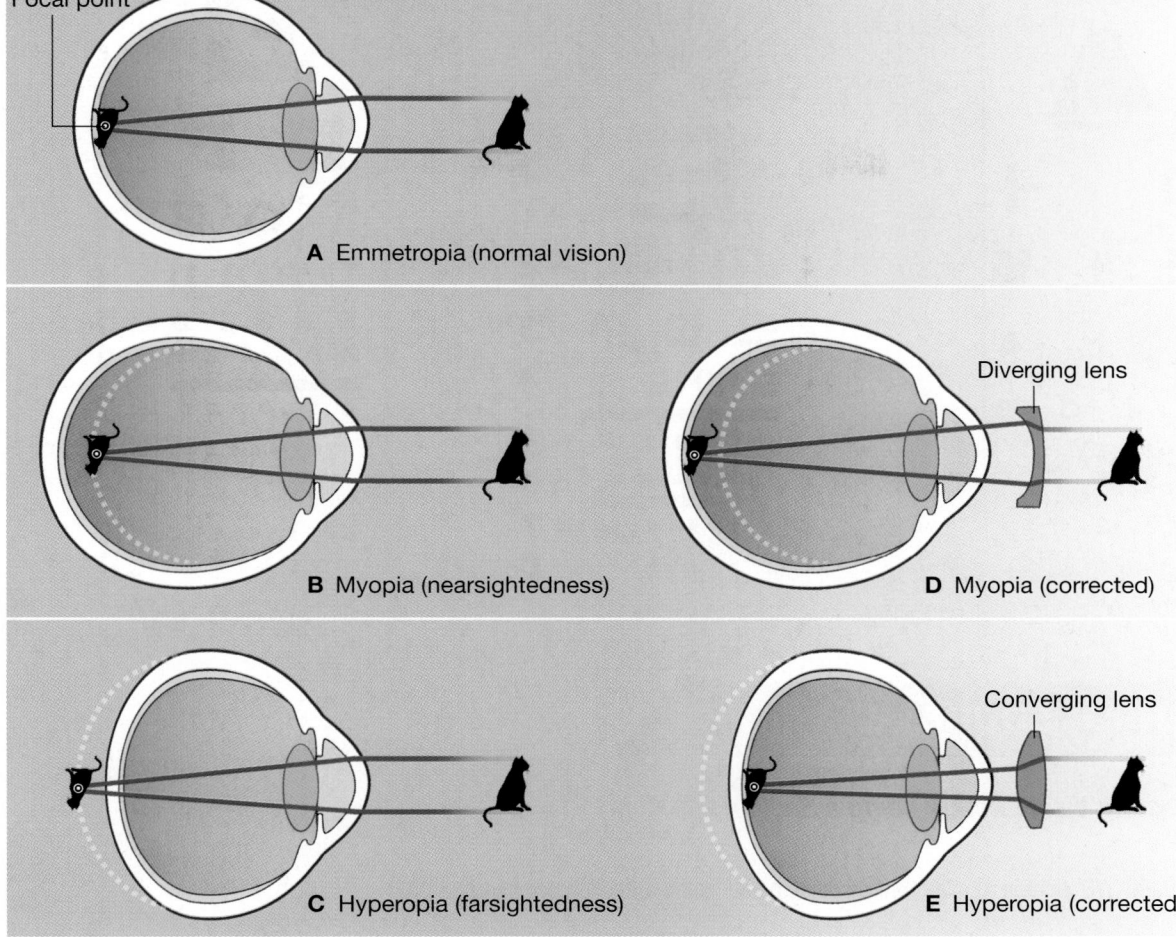

Focal point

A Emmetropia (normal vision)

Diverging lens

B Myopia (nearsightedness)

D Myopia (corrected)

Converging lens

C Hyperopia (farsightedness)

E Hyperopia (corrected)

FIGURE 36-1   How lenses correct visual problems: (A) Emmetropia, (B) Myopia, (C) Hyperopia.

plan are ineffective, surgery on the eye muscle may be necessary.

Assessment of Visual Acuity

As noted previously, visual acuity testing is frequently performed in a variety of medical settings. Performing these tests is usually the task of the medical assistant. Distance acuity testing, near vision acuity testing, and testing for color blindness will be discussed.

Distance Acuity

Distance acuity is measured using the Snellen eye chart for patients who can read and do not have a language barrier. The Snellen charts place the largest symbols on the top line and each line after is of decreasing size. The person with normal vision would be able to read the top line at 200 feet. To the right of each line is a ratio indicating that a person with normal vision could read at decreasing distances of 100, 70, 50, 40, 30, and

20 feet. A result of 20/20 vision means that a person with normal distance acuity could read that line at a distance of 20 feet.

The abbreviation for the right eye is OD (oculus dexter), for the left eye it is OS (oculus sinister), and the abbreviation for both eyes is OU (oculus uterque). These abbreviations should be used when documenting any eye procedure.

For preschool children, or patients who are illiterate or have a language barrier, the Snellen E, the Landolt C, or pictorial charts are used. Figure 36-2 shows different types of Snellen eye charts.

If you are unsure whether or not the patient has the ability to recognize the Snellen eye chart letters, you should verify his or her ability by using a demonstration chart prior to testing. With the Snellen E chart, have the patient demonstrate by pointing his or her finger in the direction the E is pointing prior to testing so as to determine whether or not the patient can follow your directions. When dealing with young children, it may be

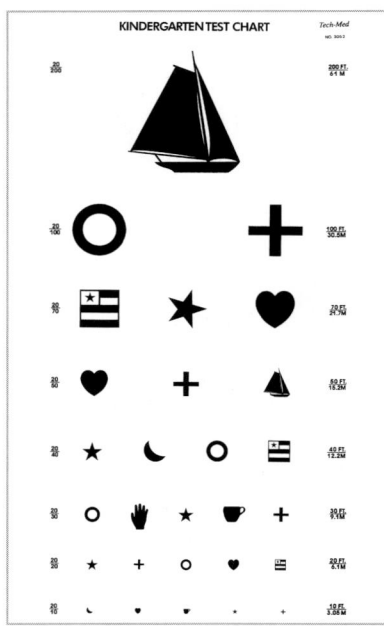 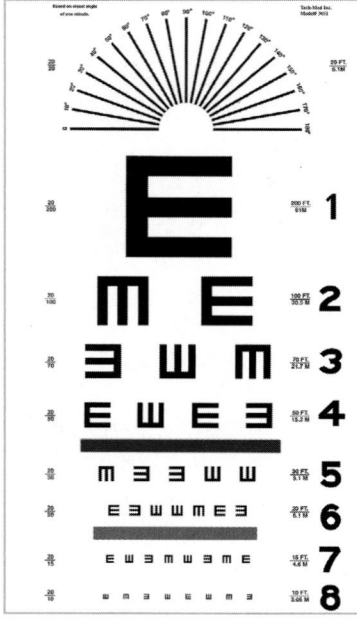 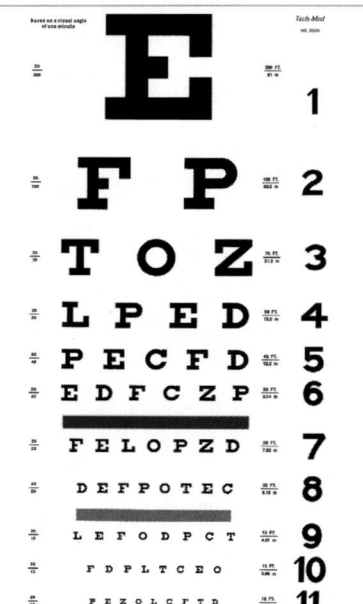

FIGURE 36-2 Different types of Snellen eye charts.

PROCEDURE

Testing Visual Acuity Using a Snellen Eye Chart

OBJECTIVE: Screen a patient for distance acuity using a Snellen eye chart.

Equipment and Supplies

Snellen eye chart placed at a distance of 20 feet; eye shield or occluder; pointer; pen and paper; alcohol and gauze

Method

1. Assemble equipment.
2. Perform hand hygiene and identify patient.
3. Explain procedure.
4. Determine patient's ability to recognize letters. If the patient is unable to read letters use the necessary chart to accommodate patient's abilities.
5. Place patient 20 feet from the chart, either seated or standing, as long as the Snellen eye chart is at eye level.
6. Follow office policy regarding testing with or without corrective lenses.
7. Have patient read the lines with both eyes first at a distance of 20 feet.
8. Following office policy (regarding which eye to test first) have the patient cover the other eye with a cup or occluder.
9. Instruct the patient to keep both eyes open even though one eye is covered.
10. Use pointer and point to letters or appropriate symbols in random order.
11. Record the ratio numbers adjacent to the line the patient can read without error. If there is an error, note it (e.g., OS 20/40 –1 or OS 20/40 –1 with correction—meaning glasses were worn during testing).
12. Repeat the procedure with the other eye and record result, noting any unusual symptoms such as squinting, or blinking excessively.
13. Clean the occluder with gauze and alcohol.
14. Remove gloves and perform hand hygiene.
15. Document results accurately.

Charting Example

2/14/XX	4:00 P.M.	Snellen eye test
OD 20/30	OS 20/30	OU 20/30
		M. King, CMA

Screening for Near Vision Acuity

OBJECTIVE: Screen near vision acuity using the Jaeger system.

Equipment and Supplies
Jaeger near vision acuity chart; gloves; paper and pen

Method
1. Perform hand hygiene.
2. Assemble equipment.
3. Identify patient.
4. Explain procedure.
5. In a well-lighted room, have patient hold the Jaeger card at a distance of 14 to 16 inches.
6. With both eyes open ask the patient to read aloud the smallest paragraph or line possible without error (Figure 36-3).
7. Document results accurately, noting any unusual symptoms such as squinting.

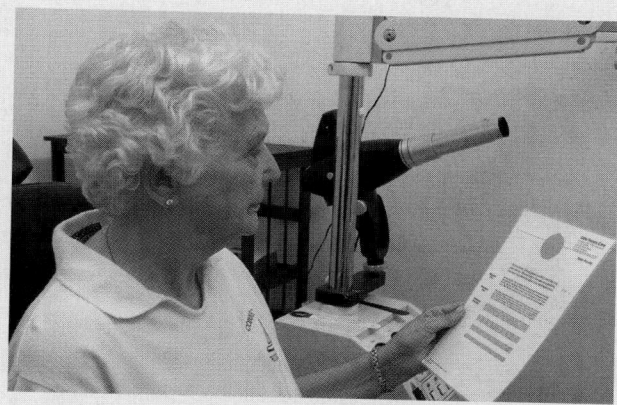

FIGURE 36-3 A patient using a near vision acuity card.

helpful to make a game of it, showing them how to hold their hands to illustrate which direction the E is facing. Following is the procedure for performing a distance acuity test. Procedure 36-1 presents the steps for performing a distance acuity test using the Snellen eye chart.

Near Vision Acuity

Testing for near vision acuity should be done if the patient complains of difficulty reading or performing other close range tasks. It is done to test for hyperopia or presbyopia. The lens of the eye loses its elasticity with age and cannot change from viewing distant objects to close work as readily as before. Close work appears blurry and the individual tends to hold the book or newspaper farther away to make it appear clearer.

Testing for near vision acuity is done by having the patient read a card held at normal reading distance (14 to 16 inches). The card has a series of paragraphs decreasing in size of print with a number above each. The patient's result is the number above the last paragraph he or she can read easily. Office policies differ on whether or not to have patients wear corrective lenses during the test and whether to test each eye individually or both eyes together. As a medical assistant you will follow the policy in your facility.

Procedure 36-2 presents the steps to perform a near vision acuity test.

Color Blindness

Color blindness is the inability to distinguish colors of the spectrum distinctly. Defects in color vision are congenital or inherited, or acquired through disease, or injury. Congenital means the individual was born with the condition. Congenital color blindness is more prevalent in males. It is important to test for color vision defects because changes in color vision may indicate diseases of the retina, optic nerve, or thyroid.

The ability to distinguish colors depends on the cones of the retina, which react to light and permit us to see shades of red, green, and blue. The inability to see any colors is rare and is most likely due to a defect or absence of the cones in the retina. The most common type of color vision defect, which is inherited, is the inability to distinguish red and green. Other types of color blindness prevent patients from distinguishing shades of various colors.

The Ishihara test is printed in either card or booklet form with a single color-dot illustration containing a number, or curved lines and shapes for illiterate patients or children. For instance, a person with normal color vision would be able to see the green number 27 on the red/orange background as in Figure 36-4. The

PROCEDURE

Screening for Color Vision Acuity

OBJECTIVE: Screen a patient for color vision defects.

Equipment and Supplies
Ishihara screening book/cards; paper and pen

Method
1. Perform hand hygiene.
2. Assemble equipment.
3. Identify patient.
4. Explain the procedure.
5. Have patient assume a comfortable position and ask patient to keep both eyes open.
6. In a well-lighted room at a distance of 30 inches, have patient identify the number that is formed by the colored dots on each card or page within three seconds per page or card.
7. If patient is unable to identify the numbers, have the patient trace the number with his or her finger.
8. Score each plate as it is read. If the patient is able to identify the number then record the number seen after the plate number, for example, Plate 1:7. If the patient was unable to identify a number on a plate, record the plate number and mark an X next to it.
9. Note any unusual symptoms.
10. Document the results accurately.

Charting Example

2/14/XX	3:00 P.M.	Ishihara eye normal.
		M. King, CMA

---

patient is shown 14 color plates or pages and must correctly identify 10 to be considered to have color vision within normal limits. The Ishihara booklet or cards should be stored out of direct light to prevent fading of the color plates. Procedure 36-3 presents the steps to perform a screening for color vision acuity using the Ishihara test.

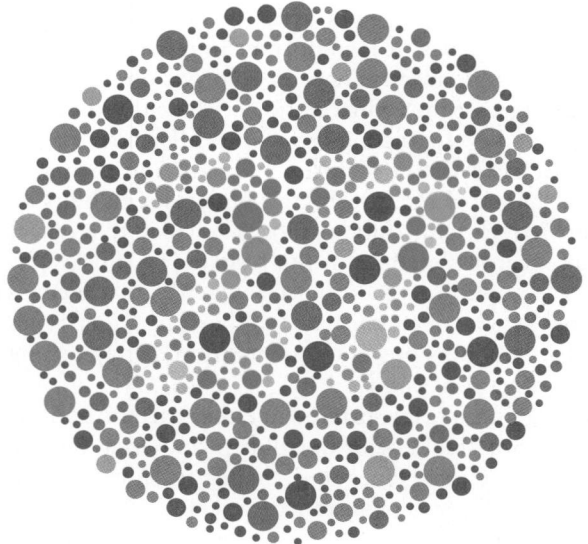

FIGURE 36-4 Color vision chart.

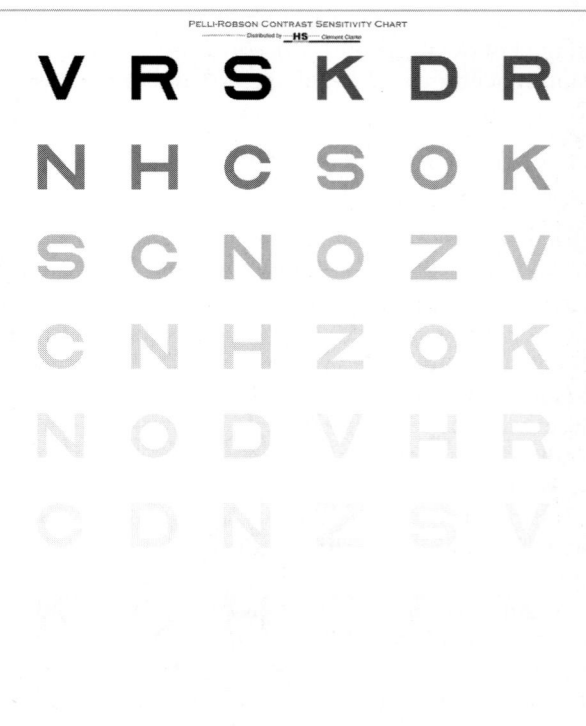

FIGURE 36-5 Pelli-Robson contrast sensitivity chart.

Contrast Sensitivity

Contrast sensitivity measures the patient's ability to distinguish faint differences in shades of grey. There are several new testing procedures or instruments used to test for contrast sensitivity such as the Vistech Consultant system and the Pelli-Robson chart. To perform a procedure for contrast sensitivity, adhere to manufacturer's directions and observe the usual procedural steps for appropriate patient care, such as hand hygiene and correct documentation. It has been determined that contrast sensitivity is affected by most major eye conditions such as macular degeneration, cataracts, glaucoma, and diabetic retinopathy. Figure 36-5 shows a Pelli-Robson chart for testing contrast sensitivity. Figure 36-6 illustrates a patient having a glaucoma test. Table 36-1 lists and explains tests and procedures related to the eye.

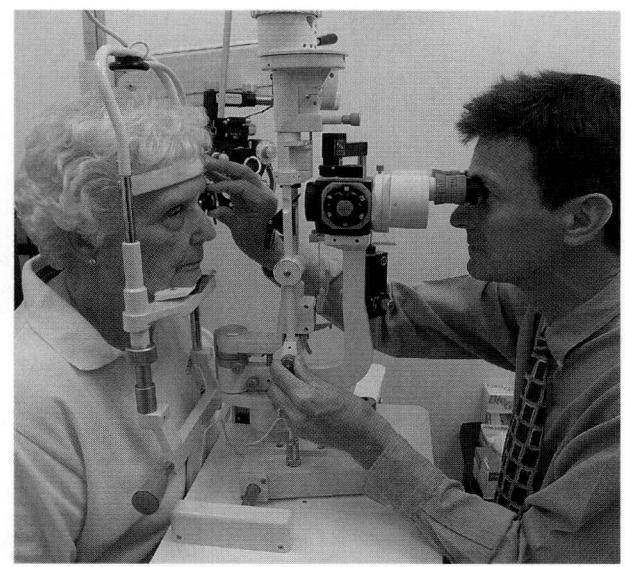

FIGURE 36-6 Patient having a glaucoma test.

TABLE 36-1 Procedures and Diagnostic Tests Relating to the Eye

Test	Description
Corneal transplant	The surgical process of transferring the cornea from donor to a patient.
Electroretinogram	A record of the electrical response of the retina to light stimulation.
Fluorescein angiography	The process of injecting dye (fluorescein) to observe the movement of blood for detecting lesions in the macular area of the retina to determine if there is detachment of the retina.
Gonioscopy	Use of gonioscope to examine the anterior chamber of the eye to determine ocular motility and rotation.
Keratometry	Measurement of the cornea using an instrument called a keratometer.
Keratoplasty	Surgical repair of the cornea.
Laser surgery	Surgical procedure performed with a laser handpiece that transfers light into intense, small beams capable of destroying or fixing tissue in place.
Optomyometer	An instrument used to measure the strength of the muscles of the eye.
Phacoemulsification	The process of using ultrasound to disintegrate a cataract. A needle is inserted through a small incision and the disintegrated cataract is aspirated.
Radial keratotomy	A surgical procedure that may be performed to correct nearsightedness (myopia). Delicate spoke-like incisions are made in the cornea to flatten it, thereby shortening the eyeball so that light reaches the retina. Not all patients have their vision improved and complications could lead to blindness.
Slit-lamp microscopy	The instrument used in ophthalmology for examining the posterior surface of the cornea.

(continued)

TABLE 36-1 **Procedures and Diagnostic Tests Relating to the Eye** (*continued*)

Test	Description
Tonometry	Measurement of intraocular pressure of the eye using a tonometer to check for glaucoma. An air puff tonometer records the cornea's resistance to pressure.
Visual acuity	Measurements of the sharpness of a patient's vision. Usually a Snellen eye chart is used and the patient identifies letters from a distance of 20 feet.
Vitrectomy	A surgical procedure for replacing the contents of the vitreous chamber of the eye.

36-4 PROCEDURE

Irrigation of the Eye

OBJECTIVE: Cleanse or irrigate the eye.

Equipment and Supplies
nonsterile gloves; sterile basin; emesis basin; sterile solution; sterile irrigating syringe; sterile gauze; towel; tissues; pen and patient's chart

Method
1. Identify patient and explain procedure.
2. Assemble equipment.
3. Review physician's order.
4. Check the name, expiration date, and concentration of solution three times.
5. Perform hand hygiene and put on gloves.
6. Ask patient which position he or she would prefer, sitting or lying down.
7. Place towel over patient's shoulder.
8. Open irrigating solution and fill syringe.
9. Ask patient to tilt head to the affected side if seated and hold basin.
10. Open patient's eye using index finger and thumb of nondominant hand.
11. Hold tissue on patient's cheekbone below lower lid and pull down and expose conjunctiva.
12. Hold syringe ½ inch from the eye (Figure 36-7).
13. Gently irrigate from inner to outer canthus, or corner of eye, aiming at the lower conjunctiva.

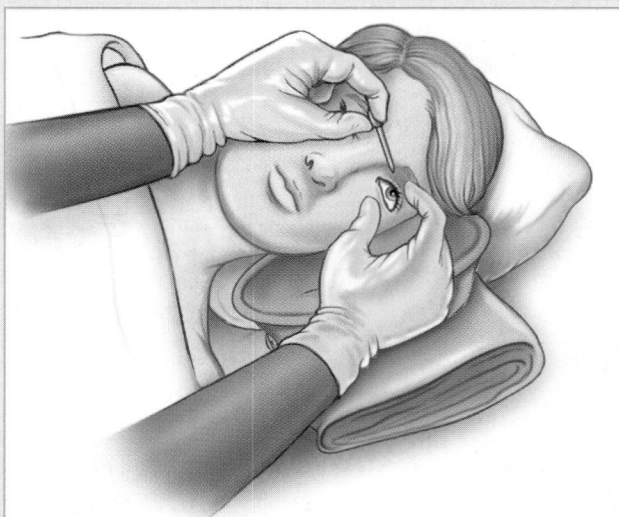

FIGURE 36-7 Irrigation of the eye.

14. Continue irrigating until solution is used up.
15. Dry area around eye with sterile gauze.
16. Dispose of equipment properly.
17. Perform hand hygiene.
18. Document information in patient's chart in appropriate manner.

PROCEDURE

Instilling Eye Medication

OBJECTIVE: Instill eye medication following the physician's orders.

Equipment and Supplies

sterile medication; sterile eyedropper (if needed); tissues; sterile gauze squares; nonsterile gloves; drape or towel

Method

1. Perform hand hygiene.
2. Check physician's orders.
3. Identify patient and explain procedure.
4. Check the type of medication, expiration date, and concentration three times.
5. Ask patient if he or she has any known allergies to the medication.
6. Give patient tissue to blot cheeks.
7. Put on gloves.
8. Position patient with head tilted back and looking up.
9. Pull down lower eye lid exposing the conjunctiva (Figure 36-8).
10. Insert the proper amount of drops to center of conjunctiva or if ointment is used, apply as a thin strip from inner to outer canthus.
11. Do not touch dropper or ointment tube to eye.
12. Ask patient to gently close eye and rotate eyeball.
13. Dry excess medication from inner canthus to outer canthus using sterile gauze.
14. Explain to patient that vision may be blurry.
15. Clean area and dispose of unused medication.
16. Remove gloves and perform hand hygiene.
17. Document procedure appropriately.

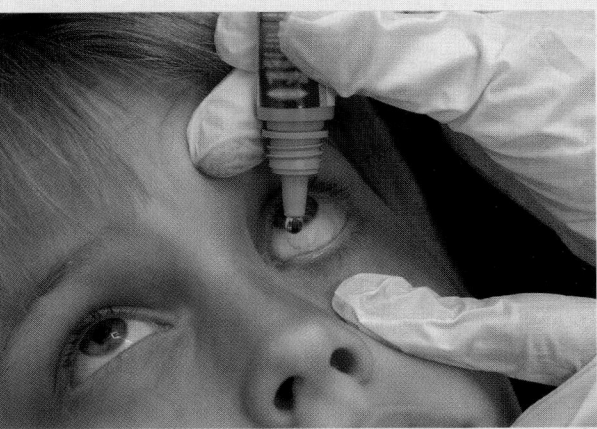

FIGURE 36-8 Instilling eye medication.

Irrigation of the Eye

Irrigation or lavage of the eye is necessary to remove foreign substances or chemicals. Eye irrigation requires the use of sterile technique and equipment. As with any procedure, the medical assistant must first explain the procedure to the patient and answer any questions. Never try to remove a foreign object from the eye using an applicator stick as this may cause corneal abrasions. Procedure 36-4 presents steps for irrigating the eye.

Instillation of Eye Medications

Instilling eye medications may be one of your duties. Only ophthalmic or optic medications can be used in the eye and they must be sterile. It is important that you reinforce the need for sterile medications with your patients. Encourage them to discard eye medications when the prescribed treatment time has been completed. In addition, instruct them that eye medications should never be shared with others or even used in their other eye if treatment is needed. The danger of contamination is great. Procedure 36-5 provides the steps to perform instillation of eye medication. Patient Education discusses more on assisting patients with medications and treatments.

Patient Safety Guidelines

Patients should be made aware of some general safety guidelines to protect their sight. Regular physical examinations on a yearly basis may discover conditions or diseases, such as diabetes or hypertension, that impact their vision. An eye examination every one to two years is important to monitor

The medical assistant acts as the educator and resource person to help the patient achieve the goals set by the physician. You may be required to explain many different topics, including safety issues, medication use, and the need for follow-up visits with specialists. Teaching methods include verbal instructions, demonstration, return demonstration, educational pamphlets, and drawings. Several of these techniques may be necessary, depending on what you are teaching and the patient's educational and motivational levels.

For example, the correct use of optic or otic medication ordered by the physician is very important. The patient must be made to understand that he or she must read the label carefully. You will need to explain that otic medications are for the ear and optic medications are for the eye. It is important to stress this point because the words are easy to confuse. The sterility of these medications is critical. Furthermore, you need to reinforce with the patient or family members the fact that once the course of treatment is concluded, these medications should be discarded. The danger of cross-contamination is great. Patients should be made aware of signs and symptoms related to the eye and ear. They may not connect the symptoms appearing in eyes or ears as being related to other systemic conditions.

changing conditions in the patient's vision. Encourage patients to wear sunglasses to protect eyes from ultraviolet rays, which can damage the cornea. For minor eye problems, tell patients to avoid rubbing and apply cold compresses. Advise patients to wear protective eyewear when using tools or machinery that can cause flying objects. Make patients aware that when chemicals splash in the eye, they should flood the eye for 20 minutes and seek immediate medical attention. Remind patients of the importance of maintaining sterility of optic medications.

Changes in the Aging Eye

The eye ages just like the rest of the body. Because these changes may impair vision, care must be taken to instruct the elderly on safety issues. Their depth perception and difficulty seeing at night make them more vulnerable to falling. Box 36-1 lists some changes that occur in the structure and function of the eye with age.

BOX 36-1

Changes in Structure and Function of the Eye with Age

- Eyelids droop because of decrease in amount of fatty tissue in the lids.
- Tears decrease both in quantity and quality.
- Cornea develops a ring of fat around it.
- Whites of eye may develop brown spots.
- Conjunctiva becomes thinner and drier.
- Irises become smaller and less light enters eye.
- Retinal changes may make vision fuzzy.
- Night vision may be impaired.
- Eyes become more sensitive to glare.
- Depth vision is diminished.
- Floaters or wavy lines or spots may appear in visual field.
- Lenses lose elasticity and impair ability to focus.

Assisting the Blind Patient

Blindness occurs due to accident, birth defect, injury, or disease. Some people are totally blind and have been that way since birth. Their frame of reference to the world depends on descriptions from others. Some individuals can sense light and dark but may not be able to discern anything else. Others have some vision but cannot read. To be declared legally blind a person must see at 20 feet what a normal person would see at 200 feet. Those who have lost their sense of sight need special training and education. Blindness is a devastating impairment, both physically and psychologically. Box 36-2 lists techniques to assist the blind patient, and Guidelines 36-1 provides steps to assist a vision impaired patient prepare for a physical examination.

The Study of the Ear

The study of hearing is known as otology. Physicians who specialize in the ear are known as otologists or otorhinolaryngologists, or ENT (ear, nose, and throat) doctors. Every physical examination includes an examination of the nose and throat as well as the ears. In patients, infections that affect the throat or nose may also affect the ear.

The ear is the organ of hearing and balance. Most parts of the ear are internal and are protected by the temporal bone of the skull. For a review of the structures and function of the ear, see Chapter 24.

Instruments Used in Ear Examinations

The instruments used in the office for ear examinations are the otoscope, tuning fork, and audiometer. The otoscope is a lighted instrument with a small, disposable speculum inserted into the ear canal to examine the tympanic membrane. Figure 36-9 shows a physician performing an ear examination using an otoscope. A healthy eardrum should be pearly gray and concave. An infected eardrum appears reddened, swollen, and bulging. See Box 36-3 for an explanation of ear infections in children.

The tuning fork is a metal, forked-shaped instrument that produces vibrations when struck. The vibrating instrument is then held near the patient's ear or placed on various locations on the head to give a rough hearing assessment. An audiometer

BOX 36-2
Assisting the Blind Patient

- Ask a person how much he or she can see.
- Face the patient when speaking and speak slowly and clearly.
- Identify yourself when you enter a room.
- Explain your reason for being in the room.
- Do not touch the patient unless you ask permission first.
- Identify others in the room, where they are located, and why.
- Describe the room.
- Provide step-by-step directions for procedures as you perform them.
- Offer assistance and respect the patient's answer.
- To assist the patient with walking, walk slightly ahead of him or her and offer your arm. Tell the patient which arm, right or left, you are offering.
- Describe obstacles—for example, steps, doorways.
- Keep hallways examination rooms free of clutter.
- Walk at a normal pace.
- Treat the blind patient with dignity and respect.

36-1 GUIDELINES
Assisting the Vision Impaired Patient to Prepare for Physical Examination

- Call the patient by name and identify yourself.
- Face the patient and speak clearly.
- Ask if the patient needs assistance and offer your arm to him or her.
- Guide the patient to the examining room.
- Explain specifically what you would like the patient to do.
- Again offer your assistance to help the patient disrobe, put on the gown, sit on the examination table, etc.
- Describe what will be happening, how long the procedure will take, and what level of discomfort the patient will experience.
- Ask if the patient would like you to remain in the room with him or her until the physician arrives.

- After the examination is complete, offer your assistance to help the patient get off the examination table, dress, and speak with the physician.
- Ask the patient if he or she has any questions or concerns.
- Relay any concerns to the physician.
- Offer your arm to escort the patient from the examination room.
- Locate his or her coat and belongings for the patient.
- Ask the patient if he or she would like you to arrange for transportation.
- Speak to the patient with respect and empathy.

Otitis Media in Children

Otitis media, middle ear infection or inflammation, is the most frequent ear problem in the pediatric patient, particularly those under six years of age. There are several types of otitis media: acute, recurring, otitis media with effusion (fluid buildup in middle ear), and chronic otitis media.

Because of their age and inability to explain how they feel, it is important to know the symptoms of earaches in children. In an upper respiratory infection, whether viral or bacterial, organisms may spread from the mucous membranes of the nose and throat through the eustachian tube or auditory tube, which connects the nasopharynx and the middle ear. Allergies may also cause fluid buildup in the middle ear. When excess fluid or pus builds up in the middle ear, sound waves cannot be transmitted as easily and there is increased pressure on the tympanic membrane. The eardrum will become reddened and inflamed and bulging or convex. It may even rupture and ear pain can be intense. Signs that an infant or small child has an ear infection are: pulling on ear, redness of external ear, drainage from ear, fever, crying, crankiness, and being unsteady on their feet.

Treatment in the case of infection is usually antibiotics; if allergy related, an antihistamine will be prescribed. An analgesic to reduce fever and discomfort may also be necessary. Children who have frequent ear infections, regardless of the cause, run the risk of hearing impairment due to scarring of the eardrum. Scar tissue renders the tympanic membrane less flexible to incoming sound waves. In addition, chronic ear infections can lead to ossification of the tiny ear bones. The bones become fused together and cannot transmit sound waves effectively leading to a form of conductive loss of hearing.

Surgical treatments for children with reoccurring ear infection are a myringotomy or cutting the eardrum to release pressure and inserting a small plastic tube to permit drainage of the middle ear. After several months to a year, the tubes will fall out unassisted. When tubes are placed in the ear, it is important to restrict water from entering the ear canal. Earplugs should be used for shampooing and swimming.

(Figure 36-10) is an electronic instrument that measures more precisely the frequencies or the number of fluctuations per second of energy in the form of sound waves. The intensity of the sounds patients hear is evaluated as well. A person with normal hearing should hear all frequencies up to 15 decibels under normal conditions. There are many varieties of audiometers in use today. Sales representatives often give inservice demonstrations to staff when an instrument is purchased. A procedure document should be drawn up based on the manufacturer's specifications for audiometer use and should be included in the office

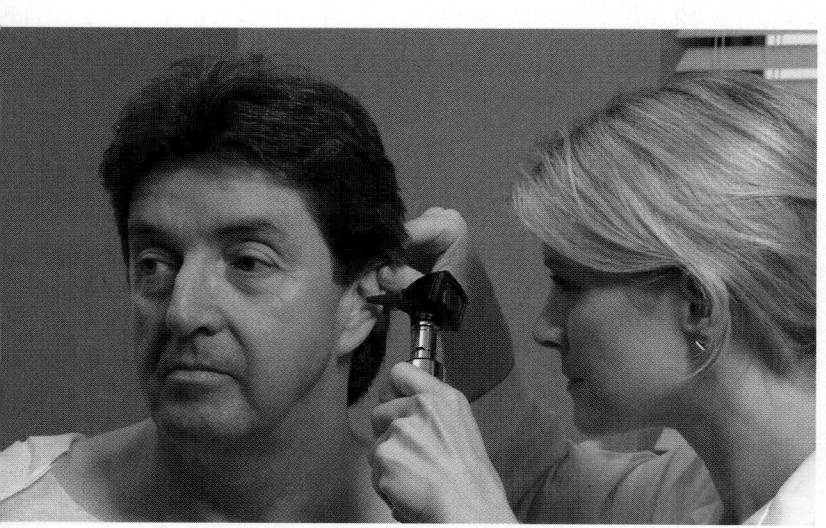

FIGURE 36-9 Examination of the ear using an otoscope.

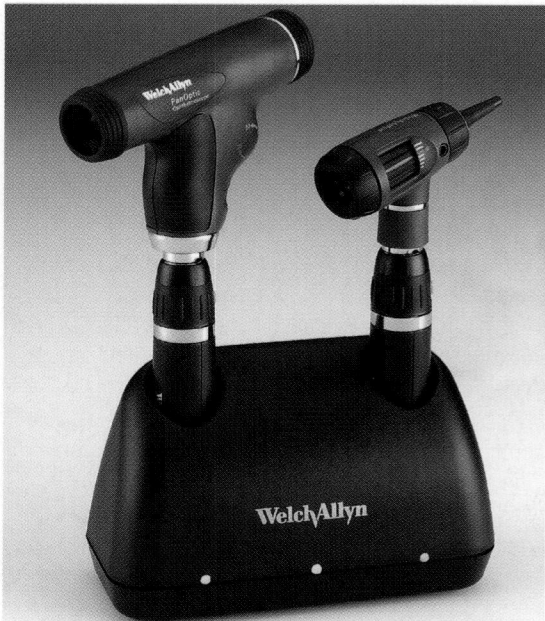

FIGURE 36-10 Audiometer.

Professionalism

Your occupation as a medical assistant often brings you into contact with other allied health professionals. To improve communication with other health care workers, it is important that you understand the duties and training of other members of the allied health team. Ophthalmic assistants work under the supervision of an ophthalmologist and work in offices or clinics. While some ophthalmologists hire medical assistants and train them on the job to perform the functions necessary in their office, others will only hire an ophthalmic assistant (OA). There are specific programs of training for the OA as there are for the medical assistant. The OA must have a high school diploma or equivalency and attend a clinical program approved by a review committee of ophthalmic medical personnel. The student must pass a national examination, which would earn the title of certified ophthalmic assistant (COA). An OA's duties include conducting acuity testing, tonometery, adjusting glasses, assisting during surgical procedures, and administering some eye medications. In addition, the OA may be trained in the use and care of more highly technical instruments. For information on this field, contact the Joint Commission on Allied Health Personnel in Ophthalmology, 2025 Woodlane Drive, St. Paul, MN 55125-2995, (800) 232-3937.

Another health professional you may encounter is the audiologist. An audiologist is an allied health professional who performs diagnostic hearing tests, assesses patient's hearing, fits hearing aids, teaches proper use of the hearing aid, and rehabilitates clients with hearing loss. To become an audiologist one must graduate from an accredited, five-year masters degree program and pass a national certification examination. Audiologists work in hospitals, schools, and private offices. For further information on this profession contact the American Academy of Audiology. Figure 36-11 shows examples of three different kinds of hearing aids.

FIGURE 36-11 (A) Small hearing aid in ear canal, (B) large hearing aid in ear canal, (C) hearing aid attached to glasses. (Jane Schemilt/Science Photo Library/Photo Researchers, Inc.)

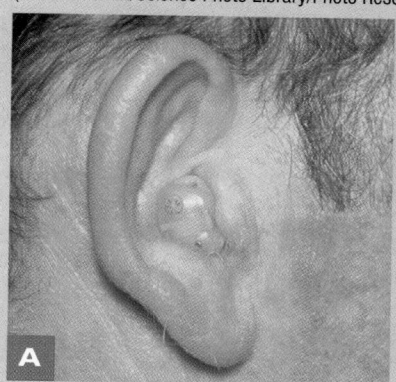 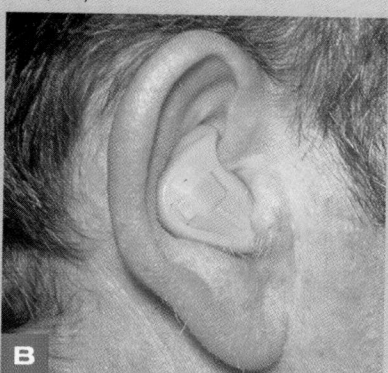 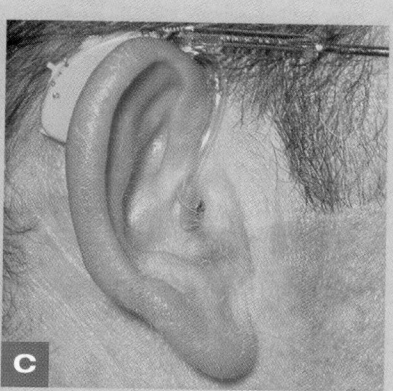

procedure manual. See Professionalism for information on dealing with other allied health professionals.

Hearing Acuity and Assessment

Hearing is essential in the process of learning to talk because speech is based on imitation of sounds and mimicking the way words are used to communicate. As with vision, there are many degrees of hearing loss. Hearing impairments fall into two main categories, sensorineural hearing loss and conduction hearing loss. Sensorineural hearing loss—nerve damage—is due to damage of the organ of Corti, or auditory nerve. The organ of Corti, located in the cochlea (a part of the inner ear), contains hairlike fibers that convert the waves of sound that travel through the ear. The sound waves are then sent to the brain via the auditory nerve. When the sound waves reach the inner ear but are unable to be converted into electrical impulses and sent to the brain, damage is present. Nerve deafness can be hereditary, or may be due to loud noises or viral infections. Conduction hearing loss is due to obstruction of sound waves; thus the sound waves never reach the organ of Corti. Foreign material or excess cerumen (earwax) in the external ear canal, calcification of the bones in the inner ear, infection or fluid buildup in the middle ear, or a combination of these problems may cause conduction hearing loss.

There are a number of tests used to evaluate hearing acuity (sharpness of hearing). The abbreviations AD (aurus dextra) for right ear, AS (aurus sinistra) for left

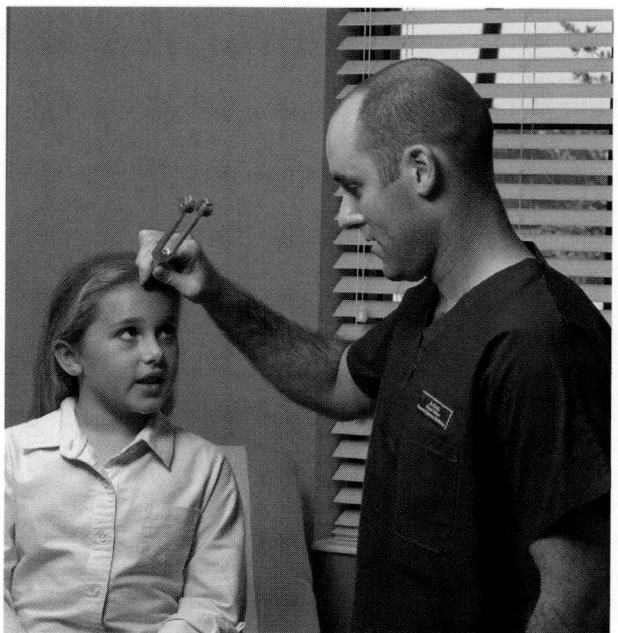

FIGURE 36-12 Testing hearing acuity using tuning fork.

emits sounds of varying frequencies and decibels to which the patient is asked to respond by pushing a button or signaling to the evaluator. The patient wears headphones that block sound in one ear while the technician evaluates the other ear. The decibel levels vary from very high to very low. When the patient indicates his or her ability to hear a sound, a recording or *audiogram* is made. The audiogram, which is a record of patient responses, is then used by the physician to evaluate the patient's hearing. Hearing is considered within normal limits if the patient hears sounds up to 15 decibels, depending on environmental noise. Prolonged exposure to loud noise over 85 decibels can cause temporary or permanent hearing loss. Figure 36-13 illustrates the decibel levels in various locations and associated with various conditions.

A diagnostic test known as tympanometry is used to measure the ability of the myringa or eardrum to move, thereby estimating the pressure in the middle ear. If the middle ear is filled with fluid the tympanic membrane will be more rigid. A printout of the results is produced for the physician to evaluate.

The *electronystagmograph (ENG)* is a special examination that evaluates balance through measurement of the movement of the eyes. ENG is used to evaluate patients with vertigo (a false sense of spinning or motion that can cause dizziness) and other disorders that affect hearing and vision. Electrodes are placed above and

ear, and AU (aurus uterque) for both ears should be used when charting results involving ears. The tuning fork gives a rough evaluation of hearing acuity (Figure 36-12). The audiometer is an electronic device that

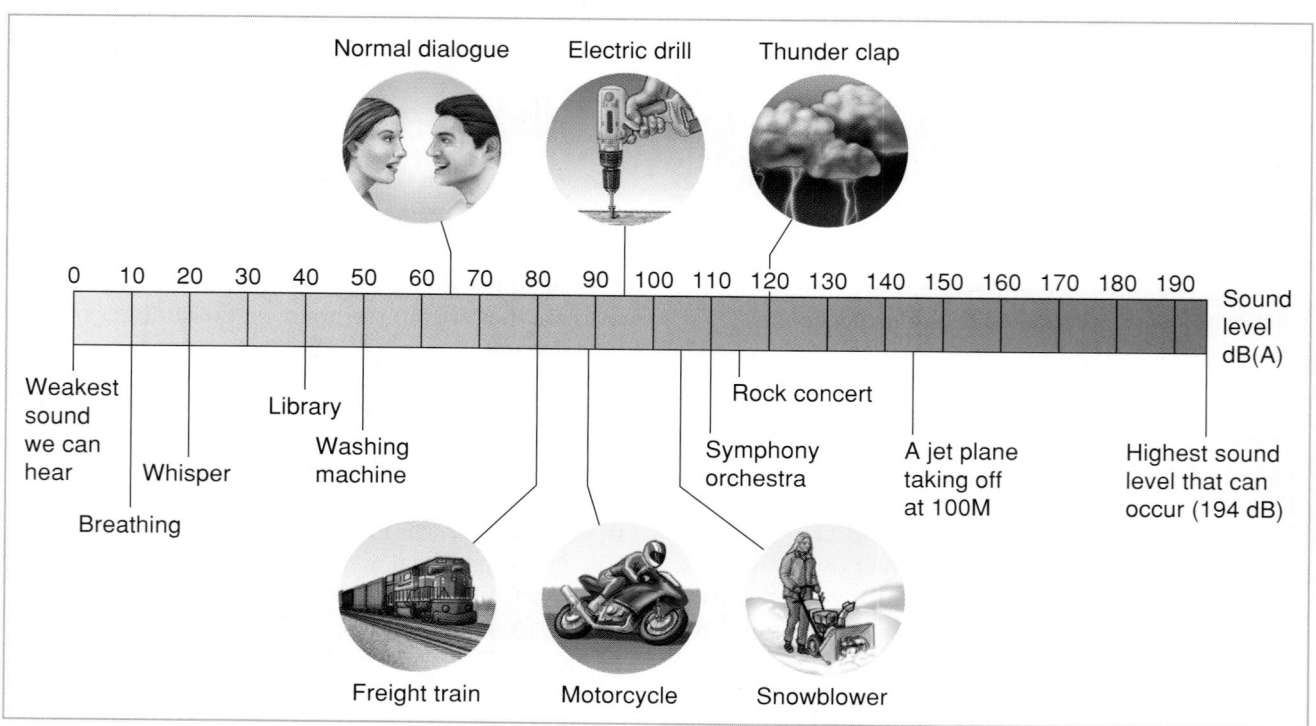

FIGURE 36-13 This illustration shows the decibal levels in various locations and associated with different conditions.

below the eye to record electrical activity. By measuring electrical changes in the electrical field in the eye, an ENG can detect nystagmus (involuntary rapid eye movement) in response to stimuli.

There are several different types of ENG examinations. In the water caloric test, warm or cool water is put into the ear canal so that it touches the tympanic membrane. Air can be used in this procedure instead of water in patients who have a damaged eardrum. A normal response to the stimuli means no nystagmus. If nystagmus does not occur on stimulation, a problem may exist within the ear, nerves associated with the ear, or certain parts of the brain. Legal and Ethical Issues reviews issues that may arise when performing tests and procedures.

Special Needs Patients

It is important to provide for the comfort level of the hearing impaired patient as much as possible in your office setting. Accommodations, such as having available pamphlets in large print and telephones with hearing amplifiers, demonstrate that your care is patient centered. It is important not to lose patience with the patient who is having difficulty hearing your instructions. Remember to face the patient when speaking to him or her and to speak clearly without raising your voice.

Presbycusis is a decline in hearing acuity and is a normal part of aging. You will be encountering many elderly patients in the office. Elderly patients may be reluctant to admit that they are having hearing problems but the family will frequently volunteer the information. Signs like speaking louder, turning up the radio or television, not hearing what is said from another room, are all indications that hearing loss has occurred. As the customer service person in the office, you must handle these situations with delicacy. Your responsibility is to act in the patient's best interest and speak to the physician about your concerns. Other signs of aging are narrowing of the ear canal, dryness of earwax, lessened flexibility of the eardrum, and sclerosis of the ear bones. Lifespan Considerations has more on accomodating patients with special needs.

Ear Safety Guidelines

Remind patients never to put anything in the ear canal. Earwax is a protective substance produced by the body to prevent foreign objects and substances from getting to the eardrum. Digging wax out is dangerous and could cause perforation of the tympanic membrane.

Patients need to understand the connection between repetitive exposure to loud noise and deafness. Young people who listen to loud music on earphones or at concerts are particularly susceptible to this danger. Workers who must engage in duties that require them to be exposed to loud noise should wear protective ear gear.

Legal and Ethical Issues

The medical assistant has an ethical responsibility to use careful, proper technique when performing procedures since an incorrect test result could lead to misdiagnosis and result in serious consequences for the patient and possibly lawsuits for the physician. Proper technique includes following procedures to the letter and documenting completely; it also includes documenting patient results in a timely manner. As a medical assistant, you often will be rushed and pulled in several directions at the same time. Never skip a step like performing hand hygiene to speed up the procedure. Additionally, always properly dispose of hazardous waste material according to OSHA guidelines.

The safety of the patient is your responsibility when he or she is under your care. Patients with diminished visual or hearing capacities will need extra care to avoid accidents and injuries. Always ask hearing or visually impaired patients if they need assistance; offer your arm to ensure their safety, and never allow them to leave immediately after a procedure requiring anesthesia.

Patients who are hearing impaired and cannot use devices such as hearing aids may need other strategies to help increase their awareness of their surroundings at home. Devices such as doorbells that light up when rung, telephone amplifiers, and close-captioned television are accommodations that help the hearing impaired.

Irrigation of the Ear

Irrigation of the ear is necessary to remove impacted earwax or a foreign matter from the ear. Figure 36-14 shows irrigation of the ear. Patients may be apprehensive about the discomfort of the procedure and it is your responsibility to put them at ease as much as possible. Procedure 36-6 outlines steps for irrigating the patient's ear.

Instillation of Ear Medication

Instilling ear medication is a task that you may be asked to perform. You may also be required to instruct a patient how to administer eardrops. You may use the same steps to instruct the patient that you would use performing instillation of medications in the office.

Provide the patient with a printed list of instructions and review the guidelines with them in the office. Ask the patient to demonstrate the steps prior to leaving the office to ensure that he or she understands the procedure. Procedure 36-7 provides the steps to perform instillation of eardrops.

Audiometry

The medical assistant may be asked to perform an audiometer test and may do so if he or she has undergone the proper training. While most audiometers function in similar way, it is important for you to follow the instructions provided by the manufacturer. The physician will interpret the results and inform the patient of the outcome. You are not permitted to release results to a patient unless you have been specifically instructed to by the physician. Procedure 36-8 provides necessary steps to performing an audiometer test on a patient. Table 36-2 lists and explains some of the tests and procedures related to the ear.

Examination of the Nose and Throat

Examination of the nose and throat is part of a physical examination and is considered routine in most offices. The physician will use a nasal speculum to inspect the mucous lining of the nose for signs of irritation and infection. He or she will use a tongue depressor to examine the throat for signs of infection, enlarged tonsils, and abnormalities of the tongue or oral cavity. If signs of infection are present in the throat, a throat culture may be ordered to determine the infecting agent. An appropriate antibiotic will then be ordered for the patient. The most common cause of throat infection is the *Streptococcus* bacteria, Group A. When untreated, this organism can cause secondary infections and possibly serious damage to the kidney, heart, and other organs. Signs and symptoms of nasal problems include nosebleeds or epistaxis, reduced sense of smell, congestion, and allergic rhinitis, which is inflammation of the lining of the nose.

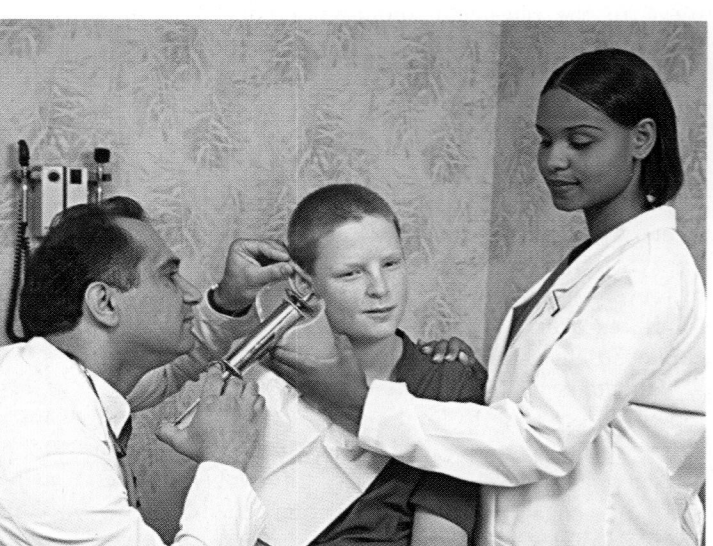

FIGURE 36-14 Ear irrigation.

PROCEDURE

Irrigation of the Ear

OBJECTIVE: Irrigate ear following the physician's orders.

Equipment and Supplies

gloves; ear syringe; sterile basin; emesis basin; warm irrigation solution per physician's order; towels; cotton balls

Method

1. Perform hand hygiene.
2. Assemble equipment.
3. Check irrigating solution three times for name, concentration, and expiration date.
4. Identify patient and explain procedure.
5. Apply gloves.
6. Have patient seated with affected ear tilted slightly downward.
7. Place towel over shoulder and ask patient to hold emesis basin.
8. Clean external ear with moistened cotton ball.
9. Pour warmed solution into sterile basin and fill syringe with 50 cc of solution.
10. For adults, pull the earlobe up and back to straighten the ear canal; for children, pull the earlobe down and back to straighten the ear canal.
11. Expel air from syringe and insert tip into the ear canal; aim stream of flow toward the roof of the canal (Figure 36-15).
12. Repeat until the return from the ear is clear.
13. Remove basin, dry outer ear, and remove towel.
14. Give patient cotton balls to wipe any external drainage.
15. Instruct the patient about home care if needed.
16. Dispose of waste material properly.
17. Perform hand hygiene.
18. Document procedure, noting type of drainage and any patient symptoms such as pain or dizziness.

Charting Example

2/14/XX	11:00 A.M.

Ear irrigation to both ears. Cerumen plug removed from right ear. No pain or dizziness experienced. Patient remained lying on right side for 15 minutes.

M. King, CMA

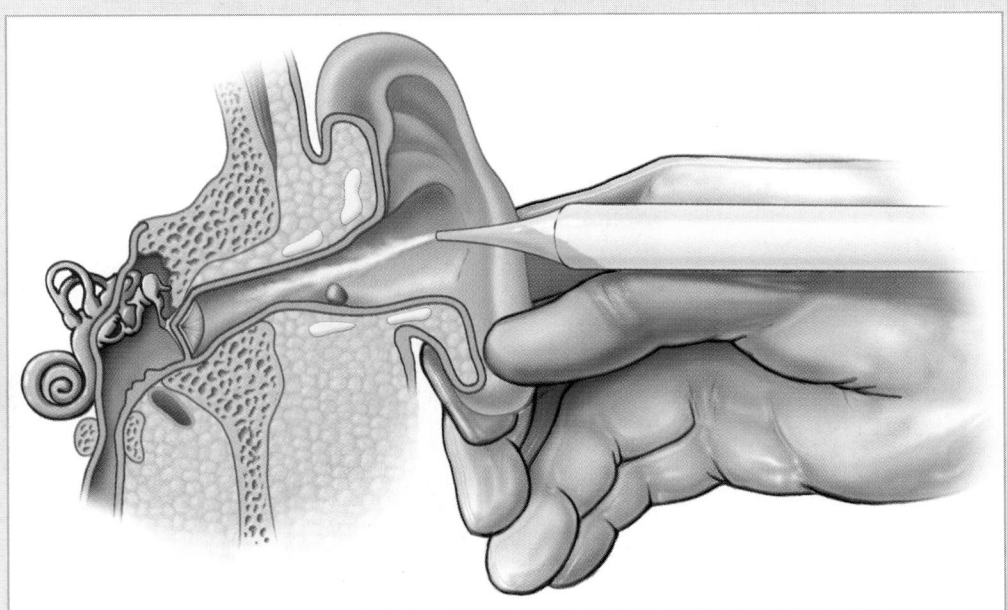

FIGURE 36-15   Irrigating the ear to remove a foreign body.

Instilling Ear Medication

OBJECTIVE: Instill ear medication as ordered by physician.

Equipment and Supplies

otic drops in dropper bottle; cotton balls; disposable gloves

Method

1. Perform hand hygiene.
2. Assemble equipment.
3. Identify patient.
4. Check medication label three times for correct name, expiration date, and concentration.
5. If the medication is cold, warm it by rolling between palms.
6. Have patient tilt head away from the affected ear or lie down with affected ear facing up.
7. Pull earlobe up and back for an adult (Figure 36-16), down and back for a child (Figure 36-17).
8. Place dropper in ear canal without touching sides of canal (Figure 36-18).
9. Instill appropriate number of eardrops along side of canal.
10. Instruct patient to remain in the same position for 3 to 5 minutes.
11. Give instructions for home care if needed.
12. Dispose of equipment and clean area.
13. Perform hand hygiene.
14. Document accurately.

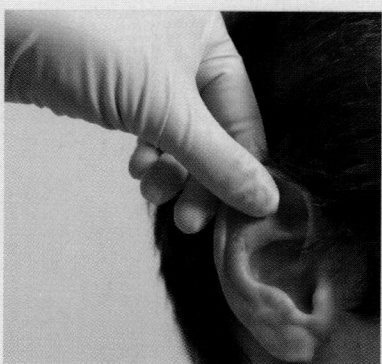

FIGURE 36-16 Straigtening the ear canal of an adult.

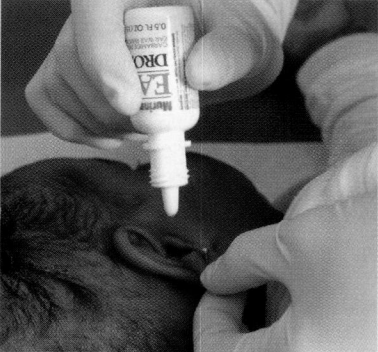

FIGURE 36-17 Straigtening the ear canal of a child.

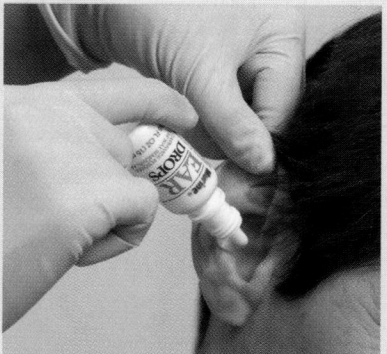

FIGURE 36-18 Instillation of eardrops.

PROCEDURE

Assisting with Audiometry

OBJECTIVE: Perform audiometric test without error.

Equipment and Supplies

audiometer with headphones; quiet room or small, enclosed cubicle

Method

1. Perform hand hygiene.
2. Prepare equipment and room.
3. Test equipment and make sure power is on.
4. Identify patient and explain procedure.
5. Establish signal response patient will give if no automatic button is available; nodding head or holding up a finger are acceptable signals (Figure 36-19).
6. Have patient assume a comfortable position.
7. Place headphones over one of patient's ears.
8. Begin with low frequency and watch patient for indication sound is heard; push button to record if machine does not do it automatically.
9. Gradually increase frequency until test is completed in the first ear.
10. Proceed to the other ear and repeat the entire procedure.
11. Clean equipment following manufacturer's instructions.
12. Perform hand hygiene.
13. Document procedure.

Charting Example

2/14/XX	9:00 A.M.

Audiometry test administered in both ears. Results given to Dr. Williams.

M. King, CMA

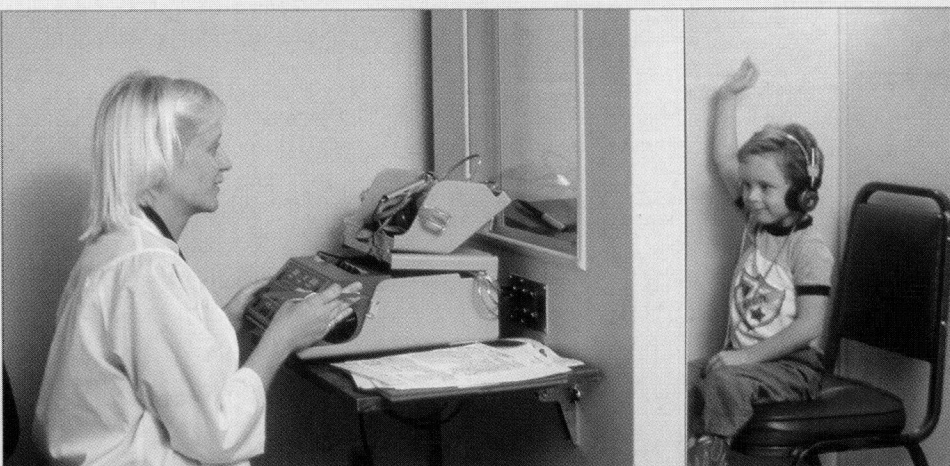

FIGURE 36-19 Hearing test on child.

TABLE 36-2 Procedures and Diagnostic Tests Relating to the Ear

Audiogram	A chart that shows the faintest sounds a patient can hear during audiometry testing.
Audiometric test	A test of hearing ability by determining the lowest and highest intensity and frequencies that a person can distinguish. The patient may sit in a soundproof booth and receive sounds through earphones as the technician decreases and changes the volume and tones.
Electrocochleography	A recording of the electrical activity produced when the cochlea is stimulated.
Electronystagmography	A recording of eye movement in response to specific stimuli, such as sound, water, or air. It is used to determine the presence and location of a lesion in the vestibule of the ear, to help diagnose unilateral hearing loss of unknown origin, and to help identify the cause of vertigo, tinnitus, and dizziness.
Falling test	A test used to observe balance and equilibrium. The patient is observed standing on one foot, then with one foot in front of the other, and then walking forward with eyes open. The same test is conducted with the patient's eyes closed. Swaying and falling with the eyes closed can indicate an ear and equilibrium malfunction.
Mastoid antrotomy	Surgical opening made in the cavity within the mastoid process to alleviate pressure from infection and allow for drainage.
Mastoid x-ray	An x-ray taken of the mastoid bone to determine infection, which can be an extension of a middle ear infection.
Myringoplasty	Surgical reconstruction of the eardrum.
Myringotomy	Surgical puncture of the eardrum with removal of fluid and pus from the middle ear; it is used to eliminate a persistent ear infection and excessive pressure on the tympanic membrane. A tube is placed in the tympanic membrane to allow drainage of the middle ear cavity.
Otoplasty	Corrective surgery to change the size of the external ear or pinna. The surgery can either enlarge or decrease the size of the pinna.
Otoscopy	The use of a lighted instrument to examine the external auditory canal and the middle ear.
Rinne and Weber tuning fork tests	The physician holds a tuning fork, an instrument that produces a constant pitch when it is struck against or near the bones on the side of the head. These tests assess both nerve and bone conduction of sound.
Stapedectomy	Removal of the stapes bone to treat otosclerosis (hardening of the bone). A prosthesis or artificial stapes is implanted.
Tympanometry	Measurement of the movement of the tympanic membrane that can indicate pressure in the middle ear.
Tympanoplasty	Another term for the surgical reconstruction of the eardrum. Also called myringoplasty.

SUMMARY

In this chapter, we have considered signs and symptoms of disorders of the eye and ear. As a multiskilled health care professional, you will be expected to assist with or perform a number of technical functions while you aid the physician. The procedures in this chapter deal with irrigating the eye and ear and instilling medications in the eye and ear. You will be expected to be able to accomplish these independently and without error. In addition, you will be asked to assess both visual and hearing acuity using the procedures provided in this chapter. Dealing with special needs patients, such as children, the elderly, patients with dementia, or those who are illiterate, requires extra skills. Knowing the changes in vision and hearing that occur with age enables you to be more sensitive to these patients.

Educating the patient to perform certain technical skills, such as administering eye and ear medications at home, is an important factor in his or her treatment. As a patient advocate, you can encourage eye and ear safety suggestions. At all times, it is your responsibility to provide the most respectful and empathetic care for the patient.

Chapter Review

COMPETENCY REVIEW

1. Define and spell the terms to learn for this chapter.
2. Develop a teaching plan for a young child with strabismus.
3. What are several precautions the medical assistant should take in the office to assist the hearing impaired elderly patient?
4. Explain how you would remove impacted cerumen from the ear canal of a 40-year-old male.
5. A patient has a visual acuity reading of 20/10 in the left eye. Using this information, answer the following questions:
   A. How far was the patient from the eye chart?
   B. At what distance would a person with normal acuity be able to read this line?
6. Mrs. Evans is 81 years old and has a contrast sensitivity test result below normal. List several conditions that could cause this abnormal result and why it occurs.
7. When measuring visual acuity, explain why you would not permit a patient to do the following:
   A. study the Snellen eye chart.
   B. close his or her eye while testing using Snellen eye chart.
8. A two-year-old child needs to have a myringotomy and tympanoplasty performed because the child has had more than six bouts of otitis media within one year. Explain to the parents what these procedures entail.

PREPARING FOR THE CERTIFICATION EXAM

1. An ophthalmic condition in conjunctiva caused by bacteria is
   A. retinitis pigmentosa
   B. macular degeneration
   C. glaucoma
   D. ectropion
   E. conjunctivitis

2. Ear irrigations are performed
   A. to remove cerumen
   B. to remove a foreign object
   C. to relieve inflammation
   D. as part of a physical exam
   E. answers A, B, and C

3. Myopia is NOT
   A. a refractive error
   B. the same as being nearsighted
   C. means the individual sees things clearly close up
   D. occurs when light rays focus in front of the retina
   E. the same as being farsighted

4. Presbycusis is defined as
   A. loss of hearing in children
   B. loss of hearing associated with aging
   C. loss of eyesight
   D. total loss of hearing
   E. loss of eyesight due to cataract

continued on next page

5. The Snellen eye chart is used to measure
   A. near vision acuity
   B. color acuity
   C. distance acuity
   D. astigmatism
   E. contrast sensitivity

6. To instill eardrops into the ear of a one-year-old child, you would
   A. pull the earlobe up and out to straighten the ear canal
   B. not touch the earlobe because it is painful
   C. pull the earlobe down and back to straighten the ear canal
   D. tell the physician it is too difficult for you
   E. tell the mother to leave the room

7. When performing distance acuity eye examination on someone who is illiterate, you would
   A. let the patient pick the chart he or she would like to use
   B. ask a family member to help the patient read the chart
   C. use a chart that uses pictures instead of letters
   D. first let the patient practice on his or her own
   E. let the patient stand closer to the chart

8. How would you document the results on a patient who had a reading of 20/60 in the right eye and 20/80 in the left eye with one error?
   A. 20/60 OS, 20/80 OU
   B. 20/60 OD, 20/80 OS –1
   C. 20/60 OU, 20/80 AU –1
   D. 20/60 AD, 20/80 AS –1
   E. 20/60 OU, 20/80 OU –1

9. Color blindness is
   A. more prevalent in older women
   B. not important to a patient's health
   C. is hereditary more often in males
   D. sensitivity to distance acuity
   E. a very common problem

10. The most common type of ear infection in children is
   A. otitis externa
   B. otitis media
   C. otitis interna
   D. earlobe inflammation
   E. excess cerumen

CRITICAL THINKING

1. What do Kyle's results of the Snellen examination mean? What would you tell Kyle about his results?

2. What explanations would you use to convince Kyle to let you instill the eyedrops? What would you do if he still resisted?

3. What precautions should you use before using any eye medications, and why?

4. Dr. Sims gives Kyle's parents a prescription for eyeglasses. When they leave the room, he tells you that he isn't going to wear them and look like a "geek" no matter what! How should you handle this?

5. Are you obligated to tell Kyle's parents and Dr. Sims about his feelings?

ON THE JOB

Agnes Jones, the medical assistant in a busy ENT office, is asked to transcribe the following ophthalmology report for the physician.

Reason for consultation: evaluation of progressive loss of vision in right eye.

History of present illness: Patient has noted a gradual deterioration of vision and increasing photophobia over the past year, particularly in the right eye. She states that it feels like there is a film over her right eye. She denies any change of vision in her left eye.

Results of physical examination:

Visual acuity test showed no changes in this patient's long-standing hyperopia. The eye muscles function properly, and there is no evidence of conjunctivitis or nystagmus. The pupils react properly to light. Intraocular pressure is within normal limits (WNL). Ophthalmoscopy after application of mydriatic drops revealed presence of a large, opaque cataract forming in the right eye. There is no evidence of retinopathy, macular degeneration, or keratitis.

1. The results of the physical exam state that the patient's pupils react properly to light. What does this mean? How do pupils react in bright and dim light? Why is this important?
2. This patient wears corrective lenses for which condition?
    A. farsightedness
    B. nearsightedness
    C. abnormal curvature of the cornea
3. The patient history states that Ms. Jones does not have nystagmus or conjunctivitis. Explain these two conditions.

INTERNET ACTIVITY

Lasik surgery is a popular eye procedure. Research it on the Internet. If you were a candidate for this procedure would you have it done? Why, or why not? How will the information you obtain help you in dealing with patients?

MediaLink More on assisting with eye and ear care, including interactive resources, can be found on the Student CD-ROM accompanying this textbook.

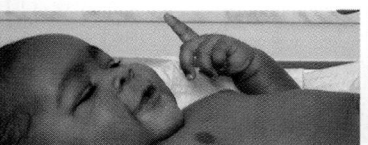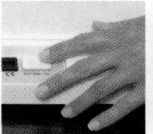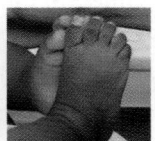

Medical Assistant Role Delineation Chart

HIGHLIGHT indicates material covered in this chapter.

ADMINISTRATIVE

Administrative Procedures

- Perform basic administrative medical assisting functions
- Schedule, coordinate and monitor appointments
- Schedule inpatient/outpatient admissions and procedures
- Understand and apply third-party guidelines
- Obtain reimbursement through accurate claims submission
- Monitor third-party reimbursement
- Understand and adhere to managed care policies and procedures
- *Negotiate managed care contracts*

Practice Finances

- Perform procedural and diagnostic coding
- Apply bookkeeping principles

- Manage accounts receivable
- *Manage accounts payable*
- *Process payroll*
- *Document and maintain accounting and banking records*
- *Develop and maintain fee schedules*
- *Manage renewals of business and professional insurance policies*
- *Manage personnel benefits and maintain records*
- *Perform marketing, financial, and strategic planning*

CLINICAL

Fundamental Principles

- Apply principles of aseptic technique and infection control
- Comply with quality assurance practices
- Screen and follow up patient test results

Diagnostic Orders

- Collect and process specimens
- Perform diagnostic tests

Patient Care

- Adhere to established patient screening procedures
- Obtain patient history and vital signs
- Prepare and maintain examination and treatment areas
- Prepare patient for examinations, procedures and treatments

- Assist with examinations, procedures and treatments
- Prepare and administer medications and immunizations
- Maintain medication and immunization records
- Recognize and respond to emergencies
- Coordinate patient care information with other health care providers
- Initiate IV and administer IV medications with appropriate training and as permitted by state law

GENERAL

Professionalism

- Display a professional manner and image
- Demonstrate initiative and responsibility
- Work as a member of the health care team
- Prioritize and perform multiple tasks
- Adapt to change
- Promote the CMA credential
- Enhance skills through continuing education
- Treat all patients with compassion and empathy
- Promote the practice through positive public relations

Communication Skills

- Recognize and respect cultural diversity
- Adapt communications to individual's ability to understand
- Use professional telephone technique

- Recognize and respond effectively to verbal, nonverbal, and written communications
- Use medical terminology appropriately
- Utilize electronic technology to receive, organize, prioritize and transmit information
- Serve as liaison

Legal Concepts

- Perform within legal and ethical boundaries
- Prepare and maintain medical records
- Document accurately
- Follow employer's established policies dealing with the health care contract
- Implement and maintain federal and state health care legislation and regulations
- Comply with established risk management and safety procedures
- Recognize professional credentialing criteria
- *Develop and maintain personnel, policy and procedure manuals*

Instruction

- Instruct individuals according to their needs
- Explain office policies and procedures
- Teach methods of health promotion and disease prevention
- Locate community resources and disseminate information
- *Develop educational materials*
- *Conduct continuing education activities*

Operational Functions

- Perform inventory of supplies and equipment
- Perform routine maintenance of administrative and clinical equipment
- Apply computer techniques to support office operations
- *Perform personnel management functions*
- *Negotiate leases and prices for equipment and supply contracts*

- *Denotes advanced skills.*

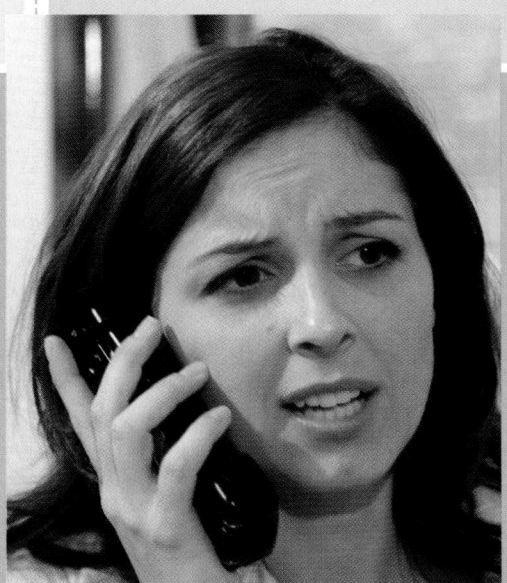

chapter 37

Assisting in Life Span Specialties

Learning Objectives

After reading this chapter, you should be able to:

- Define and spell the terms to learn in the chapter.
- Identify and explain childhood growth and development patterns.
- Accurately measure a child's height, weight, and head circumference accurately.
- Identify five genetic disorders affecting children.
- Correctly apply a pediatric urine device.
- Summarize guidelines for effective communication with the elderly.

- Explain the impact of an aging population on health care in the United States.
- Describe the aging process and its effects on each system of the body.
- Compare and contrast dementia, depression, and confusion in the elderly.
- Identify legal issues of aging patients.
- Identify six safety measures to recommend to caregivers of aging patients.

OUTLINE

Assisting in Pediatrics 732

The Pediatric Office 732

The Pediatric Patient 733

Pediatric Office Visits and Procedures 733

Pediatric Diseases and Disorders 743

Assisting the Elderly 747

Aging Population 747

Facts about the Elderly 749

The Aging Process 750

The Aging Body 750

Legal and Medical Decisions 756

Elder Abuse 758

Safety Guidelines for Children and Elders 758

Terms to Learn

ageism
body mass index (BMI)
cognitive ability
excoriation
failure to thrive (FTT)

febrile seizures
hydrocephalous
microencephaly
orthostatic hypotension

respiratory synctial virus (RSV)
respite care
stridor

Case Study

CONNOR SMITH IS 19-MONTHS OLD and lives with his grandmother, Mildred Graves, who is the primary caregiver. It is 1:00 PM when Mildred calls Dr. Field's office because Connor is sick. She indicates that Connor has had diarrhea twice so far today and "feels warm." She isn't worried yet because the baby is teething and that's what is probably causing his "runs." In case he gets worse in the next 24 hours, she wants to know "what to give him to eat?"

This chapter discusses assisting the population of patients at either end of life, namely, pediatric patients and geriatric patients. Pediatric office visits include well-child visits and sick-child visits. During well-child visits, medical assistants perform measurements such as height, weight, head circumference, vital signs, and record the information on growth charts. Childhood diseases and disorders are examined, including such conditions as croup and upper respiratory infections. Inherited disorders such as cerebral palsy and thalassemia, or conditions such as autism and sudden infant death syndrome (SIDS) are included. Since injuries are the number one cause of death in children, safety issues in the office and at home are discussed with an emphasis on educating caregivers.

The United States has an increasing aging population. It can be expected that a great number of the patients that medical assistants encounter are elderly. Changes in anatomy and physiology impact the quality of life for elders. Encouraging proper nutrition, exercise, and socializing with others can help elders live more productive and fulfilling lives. The role of the medical assistant is to help elders adjust to some of these changes, deal with their major health issues, and be informed about their medications. Dementia and Alzheimer's disease, legal and medical decision issues concerning the elderly, and safety issues affecting both children and the elderly are discussed in this chapter.

Preparing for
Externship

To prepare for your externship and ultimately your future position in health care, it is helpful to gather experience in health care facilities as a volunteer. By volunteering at a children's hospital or long-term-care facility, you would be able to develop a working relationship with these populations. Should you decide to volunteer, utilize some of the suggestions learned in this chapter to help you establish connections with children or elders. With either group of patients, make sure to look beyond the surface of the patient to find the real person inside. Being at ease with elderly or pediatric patients will enable you to be better prepared when you begin your externship. You may even decide that you would like to work solely with either group of patients. In addition, you would be providing much needed assistance and emotional support to these patients.

Assisting in Pediatrics

Pediatrics is the branch of medicine dealing with the care and development of children and the diagnosis and treatment of childhood illnesses. A pediatrician is a medical doctor who specializes in the treatment of newborns, infants, children, and adolescents. Primary care physicians and osteopaths may also care for pediatric patients. Subspecialties of pediatrics include pediatric surgery and oncology. Medical assistants who genuinely like working with children may enjoy employment in pediatrics. Establishing trust and a good rapport with a child goes a long way toward having a more cooperative patient. Many children have a way of sensing those who are comfortable being around them. Some children have had negative experiences and have fears from previous medical experiences. You may gain children's confidence if you: smile when addressing children, speak to them at their level and in simple terms, or take a few moments to interact or play with them. Preparing for Externship discusses some of the benefits of volunteering at health care facilities.

The Pediatric Office

Several factors of prime importance in a pediatric office include telephone triage guidelines, safety of infants and children, and maintaining a healthy environment for these young patients. Filling out the vast numbers of forms encountered in pediatrics (school physical, sports, and health insurance forms) correctly and in a timely fashion is also salient.

Telephone Triage

Telephone triage guidelines for the office staff could be a matter of life and death in the pediatric office. It is important for the physician to establish the guidelines to ensure the truly sick child gets attention quickly and to screen the other calls effectively. Office staff should be well trained in handling calls and triaging appropriately. In some states triaging can only be done by nurses and is beyond the scope of medical assisting practice.

Office Reception Room

The reception room in a pediatric office needs to be bright, welcoming, and interesting. Toys for various age groups should be available. Easy-to-clean plastic toys without tiny pieces are most practical. The reception room is a place for well children to pass the time before their appointment. Sick children should be brought directly into an examination room, if possible, to avoid spreading infection. During office hours, toys should be picked up as needed and put away to prevent falls. Sanitizing toys should be done on a regular basis.

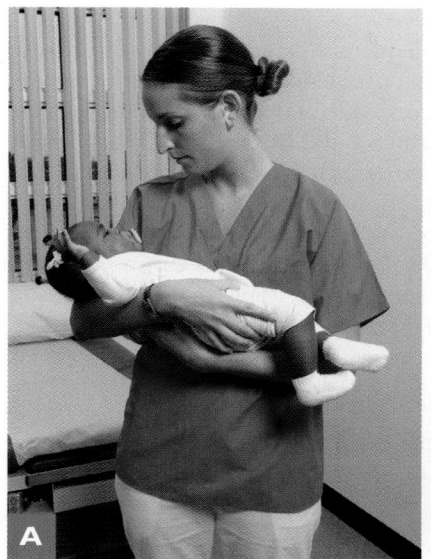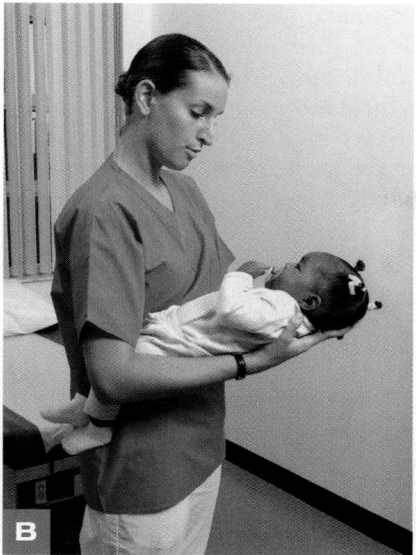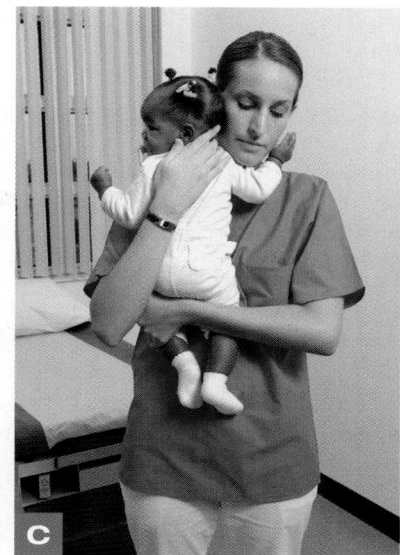

FIGURE 37-1 (A) The cradle hold; (B) The football hold; (C) The shoulder hold.

Patient Safety

Once the child enters your office, his or her safety is your prime concern. No child should be left alone on an examining table, scale, toilet, or other place that could pose a danger. Always place your hand on the infant to protect him or her from falling. When carrying an infant, it is helpful to notice the way the caregiver holds the child. This position is most likely preferred by the infant. Three positions used for carrying an infant, the cradle hold, the football hold, and the shoulder or upright hold, are shown in Figure 37-1. Support the infant's head when using the upright position. At times, it may be necessary to restrict the movements of the infant or small child to perform a procedure or evaluation. A small sheet or receiving blanket may be used to wrap the child in "papoose fashion," binding the arms to his or her sides (Figure 37-2). To restrict movement of the head, hold your hands on either side of the head and avoid sealing off the ears or touching the fontanel (soft spots) on the baby's head.

The Pediatric Patient

Growth and development refer to changes the child makes as he or she matures. Growth patterns provide valuable information on the physical progress of the child. Development refers to the motor, mental, and social progress that the child achieves. The pediatrician looks for markers to detect abnormalities in growth, social, emotional, and intellectual development. The earlier a problem is detected, the better the outcome for the child. Information from each office visit is compared to national standards and charts. Children mature at different rates; however, the stages they pass through are consistent, as are the age ranges. It is important for you to understand the stages of growth and development in your role as health care provider. Table 37-1 is a developmental checklist of the various physical, mental, and social skills children achieve during their first five years.

Pediatric Office Visits and Procedures

Pediatric office visits are divided into well-child visits and sick-child visits. During well-child visits, growth and development are measured, immunizations given, and health information provided. Well-baby visits are scheduled routinely after birth: 1 month, 2 months, 4 months, 6 months, 9 months, 12 months, 15 months, 18 months, 24 months, and then on a yearly basis. Immunizations will be discussed in Chapter 20.

During the sick-child visit, the ill child is brought in for examination to diagnose and recommend treatment for an illness. Most pediatric offices allow time in the daily schedule for sick-child visits.

Newborns through adolescents come in for both well-child and sick-child visits. Allowing for their differences and providing age relevant care is vital. Adolescents especially may be embarrassed to be examined by the physician in front of parents and other staff members. Offer them as much privacy as possible and provide adequate gowns and draping to protect their sense of modesty.

Growth

The average infant weighs about seven pounds at birth. By six months, that weight has doubled and at a year, the child's length has doubled and the weight tripled. The child will not experience a similar growth spurt until he or she reaches puberty. By three years old, the child reaches half his or her adult height. From ages five to ten, the child grows two to three inches and gains three to five pounds yearly. Infants and small children grow from the top down, with the head growing considerably in the first four months. Adult proportions will not be reached until about age 12.

Failure to Thrive (FTT)

Gaining insufficient weight according to the standardized baby growth charts is called failure to thrive (FTT). Children have irregular growth patterns; however, if an infant is considerably under the goal for his or her age, normal development could be affected. Babies whose weight is under three percentile on the growth chart are in the failure to thrive syndrome category. The most frequent cause is inadequate nutrition. For example, new mothers with feeding problems, colicky babies, mothers who used alcohol, or inadequate nutrition during pregnancy may result in a child with FTT. Other causes could be cleft palate, which affects the ability to suck well, and malabsorption disease, which prevents food from being absorbed normally. In addition, insufficient stimulation and lack of nurturing can cause failure to thrive. Social problems such as abuse, poverty, and drug or alcohol dependence can affect the parent's ability to care for and nourish the child.

Measurements

When the child arrives for a well-child visit, the physical examination follows a similar pattern as an adult examination. The physician will examine the patient from head to toe.

Vital Signs

As a medical assistant, it will be your role to obtain temperature, pulse, respirations, and blood pressure measurements. Most pediatricians do not require a blood pressure measurement unless there are cardiovascular or kidney disorders. Some physicians require blood pressure readings on every patient regardless of age. Procedure 37-1 describes steps for measuring pediatric vital signs including temperature (rectal, aural, and axillary methods), apical pulse, respiration, and blood pressure using a pediatric cuff. While all the procedures are similar to performing vital signs on an adult, a blood pressure cuff measuring no wider than two thirds of the child's upper arm must be used. In addition, a pediatric stethoscope has a smaller bell that makes it easier to place over the brachial artery. The blood pressure reading in children is lower than in adults.

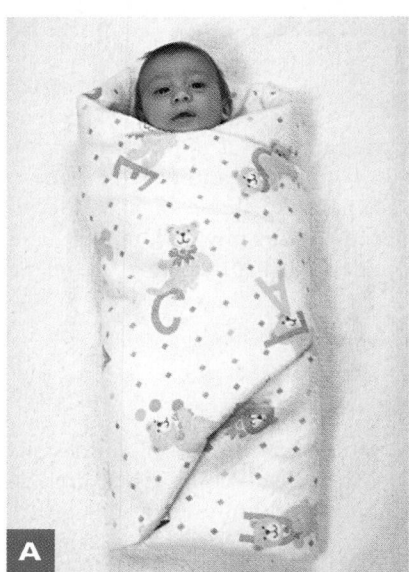

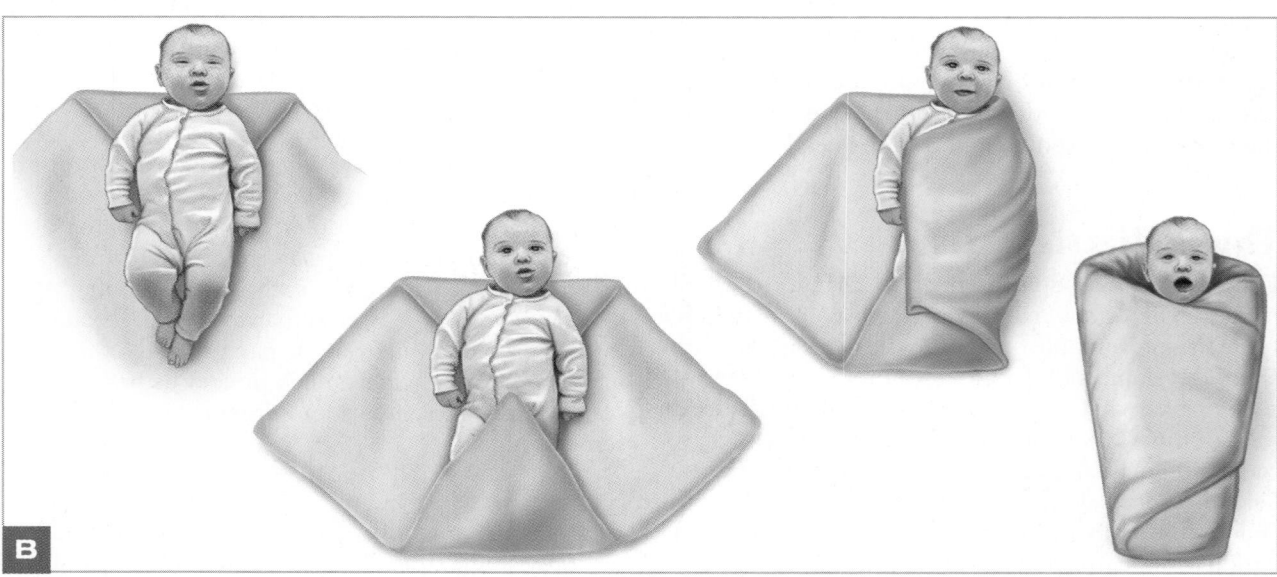

FIGURE 37-2   (A) A baby wrapped for self containment; (B) How to wrap and secure a baby's arms

TABLE 37-1   Developmental Checklist for Young Children Birth to Five Years

Age	Developmental Check
One Month	Able to raise head from surface when lying on tummy; pays attention to someone's face in his or her line of vision; moves arms and legs in energetic manner; likes to be held and rocked.
Two Months	Smiles and coos; rolls partially to the side when lying on back; grunts and sighs; startled by loud sounds.
Three Months	Eyes follow moving object; able to hold head erect; grasps objects when placed in his or her hand; babbles.
Four Months	Holds rattle for an extended period of time; laughs out loud; sits supported for short periods of time; recognizes bottle and familiar faces; rolls from stomach to back.
Five Months	Reaches for and holds objects; stands firmly when held; stretches out arms to be picked up; likes to play peek-a-boo; turns toward sound of a voice.
Six Months	Turns over from back to stomach; turns toward sounds; sits with a little support; persistently reaches for objects out of his or her reach; listens to own voice; crows and squeals; reaches for and grasps objects and brings them to mouth; holds, sucks, bites cookies and begins chewing; says mama or dada to anyone.
Seven Months	Can transfer an object from one hand to the other; can sit for a few minutes alone; pats and smiles at image in mirror; creeps pulling body with arms and leg kicks; is shy at first with strangers.
Eight Months	Can sit steadily for five minutes; crawls on hands and knees; grasps things with thumb and first two fingers; likes to be near parent.
Nine Months	Says mama or dada; responds to own name; can stand for a short time holding on to support; eats with fingers; can pick up small objects.
Ten Months	Able to pull self up at side of crib or playpen; can drink from a cup when it is held.
Eleven Months	Can walk holding onto furniture; can find an object placed under another.
Twelve Months	Waves bye-bye; can walk with one hand held; says two words besides mama and dada; enjoys some solid foods; finger feeds self; likes to have an audience.
Fifteen Months	Walks by self; stops creeping; shows wants by pointing and gesturing; scribbles on paper after shown; begins to use a spoon; cooperates with dressing.
Eighteen Months	Can build a tower with 3 blocks; likes to climb and take things apart; can say 6 words; tries to put on own shoes; drinks from a cup held in both hands; likes to help parent; can throw a ball.
Two Years	Able to run; walks up and down stairs using alternate feet; says at least 50 words; sometimes uses 2 word sentences; points to objects in a book; can undress with help.
Three Years	Can repeat 2 numbers in a row; knows his or her sex; dresses self except for buttoning; can copy a circle; can follow 2 commands of on, under, or behind (stand on the rug); knows most parts of the body; jumps lifting both feet off the ground; can build tower of 9 blocks; can name a color; stays dry during the day and night.
Four Years	Can repeat a simple 6-word sentence; can wash hands and face without help; can copy a cross; can stand on one foot; can catch a tossed ball.
Five Years	Can follow 3 commands; can copy a square; can skip.

Note: If a child is late doing several activities in a time period, seek further evaluation. A child born prematurely will be delayed by the number of months he/she was born early.

Source: Adapted from United Way's Child Development Centers Developmental Checklist 2004.

PROCEDURE

Measuring Pediatric Vital Signs

OBJECTIVE: Perform all steps of the procedures and provide readings with accuracy according to the instructor's guidelines.

Equipment and Supplies

gloves; tympanic thermometer; glass thermometer; electronic thermometer; watch with second hand; stethoscope–pediatric; pediatric blood pressure cuff

Method

1. Gather appropriate equipment.
2. Perform hand hygiene.
3. Identify patient and explain procedures to the parent.
4. Speak reassuringly to child to win his or her trust.
5. Explain to the parent how he or she can assist you in holding an infant.

Obtain temperature with tympanic thermometer as follows:

1. Remove thermometer from base and note that it reads "ready."
2. Attach disposable probe cover to earpiece.
3. Gently pull in a downward direction on outer ear to straighten ear canal of the child.
4. Insert probe into ear canal.
5. Press scan button (Figure 37-3).
6. Observe temperature reading.
7. Gently withdraw the thermometer and eject the probe cover into a bio-hazardous waste container.
8. Record temperature reading using T to denote the tympanic reading.
9. Return thermometer to base.

Obtain temperature reading using axillary method as follows:

1. Take thermometer out of container and rinse with cool water; inspect for defects.
2. Shake down the thermometer to 95°F/ 35°C.
3. Place thermometer in the infant's armpit and hold arm across chest for required time (10 minutes).

4. Read thermometer and record by designating reading with AX to indicate method used.
5. Clean and disinfect thermometer when finished with patient.

Obtain temperature reading rectally by using a glass thermometer as follows (Figure 37-4):

1. Put on gloves.
2. Attach the disposable tip to the top of the probe.
3. Lubricate thermometer to provide easy insertion.
4. Place child on bed in supine or prone position.
5. Insert thermometer ½ inch into rectum and hold in place with hand to prevent expelling.
6. Hold the child securely to restrict movement.

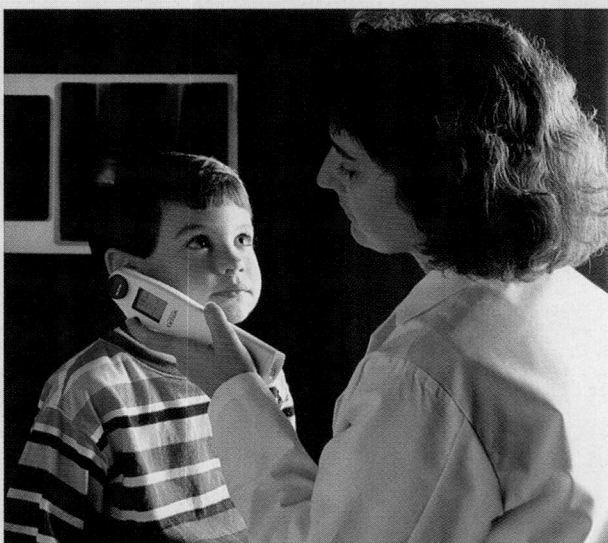

FIGURE 37-3 Tympanic thermometers are particularly helpful when measuring the temperature of a child.

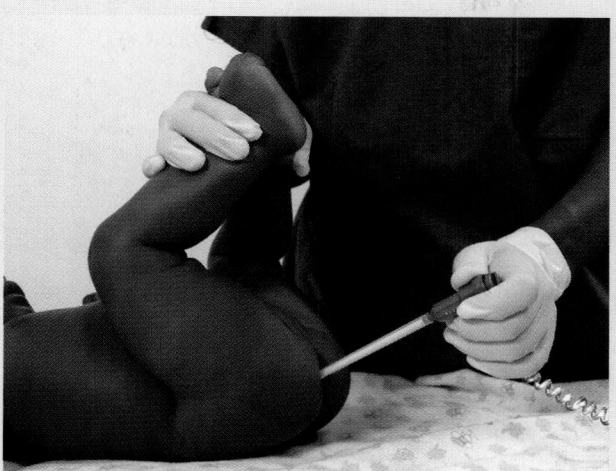

FIGURE 37-4 Obtaining a temperature reading rectally.

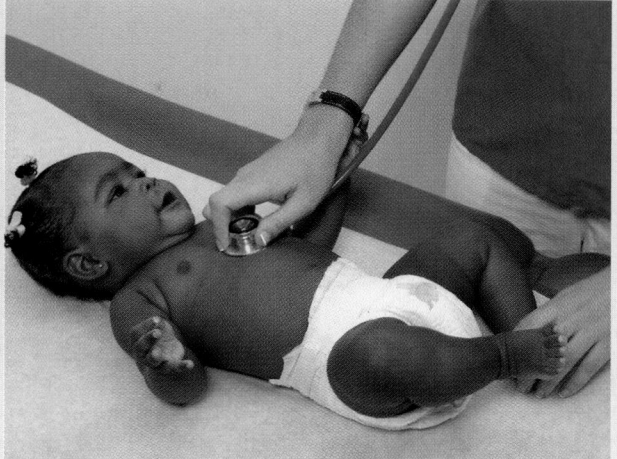

FIGURE 37-5 Measuring the apical pulse of an infant.

7. Leave the thermometer in for the required time (3–5 minutes), according to policy.
8. Remove thermometer, wipe off lubricant, and take the reading.
9. Record reading using R to indicate method used.
10. Clean and disinfect thermometer when finished with patient.

Note: If electronic or digital thermometers are used, follow manufacturer's directions about use and maintenance.

Measure heart rate/pulse by apical measurement as follows:

1. Place the stethoscope on the child's chest at the midpoint between the sternum and the left nipple (Figure 37-5).
2. Listen for the apical beat.
3. Count apical beat for 1 full minute.
4. Record apical pulse using Ap before the pulse to indicate apical reading.

Measure infant respirations for 1 full minute as follows:

1. Place your hand on the child's chest and count the rise and fall of the chest as 1 respiration.
2. Record the results.

Measure the infant's blood pressure using a pediatric cuff and stethoscope as follows:

1. Wrap cuff securely around the upper arm.
2. Feel for the brachial pulse.
3. Place stethoscope earpieces in ears and place diaphragm near pulse.
4. Pump up cuff until pulse in no longer heard.
5. Release valve slowly listening for systolic and diastolic sounds.
6. Record results.

Charting Example

4/10/XX	T 99°F / 37.2°C (T), AP 90, R 20, BP 136/78
	M. King, CMA

TABLE 37-2 **Normal Values from Birth to Adolescents**

Age	Respirations	Pulse	Systolic BP mmHg	Diastolic BP mmHg
Infants	30–60	120–160	74–100	50–70
Toddlers	24–40	90–140	80–112	50–80
Preschoolers	22–34	80–110	82–110	50–78
School Age	18–30	75–100	84–120	54–80
Adolescents	12–16	60–90	100+age	30–40 less than age

Note: Pulse and Respirations are taken for one full minute. The apical pulse is used with a child under two.

In children under five, temperature should be measured with tympanic or axillary thermometers. Chapter 34 covers the information about care and maintenance of all glass (non-mercury), electronic, and tympanic ther-

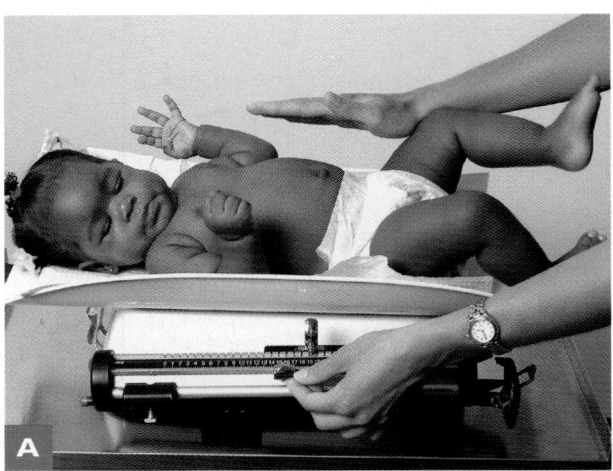

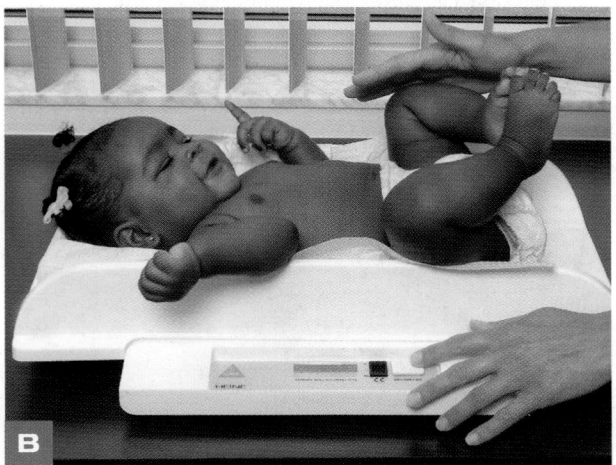

FIGURE 37-6 (A) Balance baby scale; (B) Electronic baby scale.

mometers. The procedures for measuring body temperature in young children are the same as they are in adults. Keeping the child still and calm is the major difference.

To measure an infant's body temperature rectally, place the infant in the supine position and place your non-dominant hand under the baby's bent knees securely. With the other hand, insert the thermometer and hold securely in place to avoid breakage or having the child expel it. If it is an older child, place the child in the prone position, insert the thermometer, and hold securely in place.

In children under two, the apical pulse should be measured by placing the stethoscope on the left side of the chest to the right of the nipple and counting for one full minute. Respirations are easy to count due to the visible rise and fall of the chest in a small child. The younger the child, the higher the respiratory rate will be. Table 37-2 provides the normal pulse, respiration, and blood pressure values for children from birth to adolescents. Normal body temperature is dependent on the method used. The values are as follows:

- Oral 98.6°F / 37°C
- Aural 98.6°F / 37°C
- Axillary 97.6°F / 36.4°C
- Rectal 99.6°F / 37.6°C

Height, Weight, and Head Circumference
Height and weight measurements covered in Chapter 34 should be reviewed if needed. Infants and children are weighed and measured at each office visit. Weighing infants should be done by subtracting the weight of the diaper (Figure 37-6) or by weighing without a diaper. The length of an infant is measured on the examining table until the child can stand reasonably still on the adult scale. Height and weight are measured without shoes. Procedure 37-2 lists the steps for measuring the infant's height and weight.

Measuring the Weight and Height of Infants

OBJECTIVE: Obtain a weight and height that is equal to the instructor's observance, unless otherwise instructed.

Equipment and Supplies

baby scale; patient record; pen; small towel or protector for scale; tape measure

Method

1. Perform hand hygiene.
2. Identify infant by stating the infant's name to the parent. Have the infant remain with parent while the equipment is being prepared.
3. Place a towel or protector on the baby scale.
4. Balance the scale by placing all the weights to the far left side. Turn the bolt at the right edge of the scale until the balance bar pointer is at the middle of the balance bar.
5. Undress infant (or ask parent to undress infant). A clean diaper may be kept in place. Gently lay the infant on the scale. Always keep one hand on the infant until the weights are adjusted. Do not leave the infant unattended at any time.
6. Keeping one hand over the infant's body as a safety precaution, move the large pound weight into the groove closest to the weight estimated for the baby. Then move the smaller ounce weight by tapping it gently until it reaches a point in which the pointer floats in the center of the frame.
7. Keep the weights in place while the infant is moved to the examination table for height measurement.

Continue with Height

8. Holding the tape measure with one hand, place the tape at the top of the side of the infant's head. Stretch the infant out full length as you pull the tape measure down to the bottom of the feet (Figure 37-7). If you are using a table with a measure bar, place the infant's head at one end of the table with the soles of his or her feet

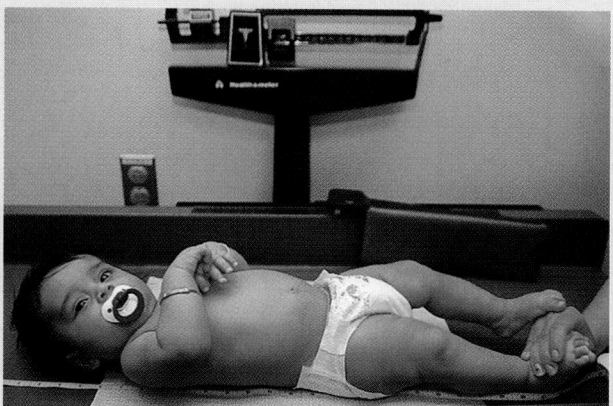

FIGURE 37-7 Measuring an infant from the top of the head to the base of the heels.

touching the footboard. Note: It is preferred to have two people measure the length of an infant. The parent can assist by holding the infant's head still. To measure an active child, make pencil marks on the exam table paper at the top of the child's head and at the bottom of the feet. When the child is removed, measure the area between the marks.

9. Note the height in inches and fractions of an inch and write it on the paper covering the exam table.
10. Ask the parent to hold the infant while the height and weight are charted in the infant's record.
11. Tell the measurements to the parent.
12. Discard paper towel.
13. Perform hand hygiene.

Charting Example

2/14/XX	weight 16 lb. 3 oz., length 30 inches
	M. King, CMA

PROCEDURE

Measuring Infant Head Circumference

OBJECTIVE: Obtain an accurate measurement of infant's or small child's head circumference.

Equipment and Supplies
flexible tape measure (no elasticity); growth chart

Method
1. Perform hand hygiene.
2. Identify the patient.
3. Talk to the infant to gain trust.
4. Explain procedure to the parent or caregiver.
5. Position the infant on examination table or have caregiver hold the infant.
6. Hold the end of tape (0 inches) on the forehead over the patient's eyebrows.
7. Bring the tape around head and over ears to meet in front (Figure 37-8).
8. Take measurement with accuracy to the fraction of an inch or centimeter.
9. Repeat if in any doubt.
10. Document results and record on growth chart.
11. Perform hand hygiene.

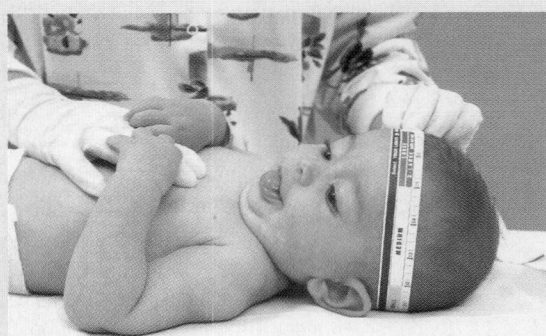

FIGURE 37-8 Measuring the head circumference of an infant.

Charting Example

4/10/XX	Time: 1:35 P.M.

Head circumference 42.5 cm

M. King, CMA

Measurement of the circumference of the head is part of each well-baby office visit until the age of six. Procedure 37-3 provides the steps to measure the circumference of a baby's head. Rapid growth of the head may indicate hydrocephalous, which is excessive fluid around the brain that may lead to brain damage. Head growth that falls below the normal percentile may indicate microencephaly. This condition may be caused by a premature closing of the fontanel, constricting brain growth and leading to mental retardation. Normal head circumference at birth should be between 12.5 to 14.5 inches or 31.75 to 36.83 cm. Generally the head and chest circumferences are equal at about one to two years of age.

Chest circumference measurement is not normally performed at each visit. It may be performed when there is suspicion that over or under development of the heart or lungs or that calcification of the rib cage would constrict the growth of organs. To measure the chest circumference, wrap a measuring tape around the chest at nipple level and read during the resting phase between respirations.

Growth Charts

Every patient has a copy of the National Center for Health Statistics growth chart as part of his or her permanent medical record. Individual growth graphs are available for boys and girls from birth to 36 months and 2 to 20 years. These growth charts are part of the child's permanent record. Pediatricians usually provide a growth booklet for each child so caregivers have a copy of the child's measurements. After the measurements are taken, the medical assistant charts the information in both areas.

Charts also exist for body mass index (BMI) and head circumference. Once measurements are obtained, it is necessary to record them on the patient's chart and in the caregivers' growth booklet.

Hearing and Vision Evaluations

Hearing tests are done in many hospitals at birth as part of special state and federal programs to detect hearing difficulties at an early age. Early detection is important because speech development depends on

Perform a Snellen Eye Exam on a Child

OBJECTIVE: Perform a Snellen eye exam for distance acuity on the child

Equipment and Supplies

Snellen E eye chart and oculator; pencil and paper; mark on floor at a distance of 20 feet from the chart

Method

1. Assemble the equipment.
2. Perform hand hygiene.
3. Identify the patient.
4. Explain the procedure to the patient and parent/caregiver.
5. Ask the child to indicate which way the legs on the E are pointing to make sure child understands the directions.
6. If the child understands, position him or her in front of the Snellen E chart at a distance of 20 feet.
7. Make sure the child is comfortable.
8. Ask the child to hold the oculator over his or her first eye and remind the child to keep both eyes open (Figure 37-9).
9. Point to the Es on the chart and make sure the child is pointing his or her fingers in same direction as the E on the chart. Proceed until you have results from the first eye.
10. Repeat procedure with the other eye.
11. Record results OS, OD, OU.
12. Complement the child and caregiver on how well he or she performed.
13. Perform hand hygiene.
14. Sanitize and replace equipment.

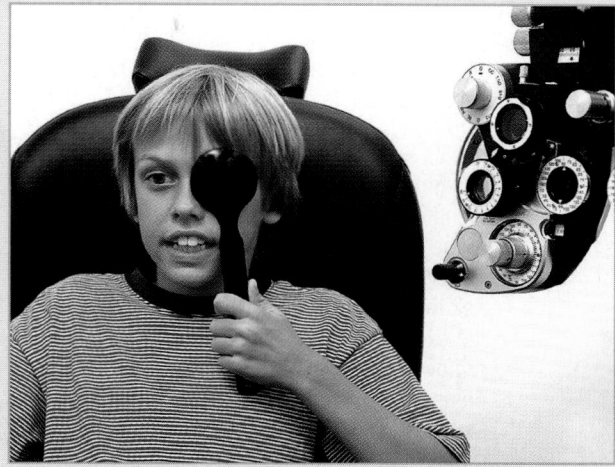

FIGURE 37-9   Testing distance acuity using the Snellen eye exam

Charting Example

4/10/XX	Visual acuity using Snellen E chart
	OD 20/20; OS 20/30; OU 20/20
	M. King, CMA

---

a child's ability to mimic sounds, word selection, and use of words. If the child tests below normal during the first test, it is repeated at about six weeks. Newborns respond to light and older infants are able to follow light. At the yearly examination, visual acuity is measured on children three years and over using Snellen eye chart. Procedure 37-4 lists steps for performing a Snellen visual acuity test on a young child.

Sick-Child Visits

When a caregiver brings in a child who is ill, the infected child should be put immediately in an examination room, if at all possible, to reduce spreading infection among such a vulnerable population in the office recep-

tion room. Based on the patient symptoms, the physician may request a urine sample. If the child is toilet trained and over two to three years old, ask the parents to collect the specimen after providing instruction on cleansing the genital area. The instructions are the same as those for cleansing prior to attaching a urine collection device, which is explained later in the chapter. If the child is too ill or too young, a pediatric urine collection device should be applied as soon as possible to increase the possibility of collecting a sample. When collecting a urine sample, ask the parent or caregiver specific questions to uncover other urinary tract related problems, for example:

- Have there been any changes in amount of urine produced recently?

Applying Pediatric Urine Collection Device

OBJECTIVE: Properly apply a urinary collection device.

Equipment and Supplies

pediatric urine collection bag; laboratory specimen container with label; antiseptic wipes; gloves; bio-hazardous waste container

Method

1. Assemble all equipment.
2. Identify the patient and explain the procedure to the caregiver.
3. Perform hand hygiene and put on gloves.
4. Ask the parent/caregiver to place the child on the examination table in a supine position and remove the diaper.
5. Cleanse genitalia with antiseptic wipes.
   Male: Cleanse the urinary meatus with a circular motion starting at the opening and progressing outward. Repeat with a clean wipe if the child is uncircumcised, retracting the foreskin to clean the meatus. When finished cleaning, replace the foreskin to the normal position.
   Female: Hold the labia open with your non-dominant hand, cleanse the labia from superior to inferior, wiping in one directional motion. Discard the wipe and repeat with a new wipe.
6. Make sure the area is dry. Unfold the collection device and remove the upper portion of paper protecting the adhesive surface. Apply to the mons pubis and press to secure. Continue removing paper and applying to perineum securing the device and making sure it does not stick to the patient's leg (Figure 37-10).
7. Offer water or suggest that the parent try to get the child to drink to increase the likelihood of obtaining a urine specimen.
8. When a sufficient urine sample is collected, remove the bag, wipe down the area that the bag was attached to and re-diaper the infant.
9. Pour the sample into a labeled laboratory container and handle according to routine in your facility.
10. Dispose of all used equipment in a bio-hazardous waste container.
11. Remove gloves and perform hand hygiene.
12. Chart the procedure.

Charting Example

4/10/XX	9:00 A.M. Pedi urine bag attached
	9:25 A.M. No spec obtained
	10:00 A.M. Pt offered H$_2$O. Recheck at 11:00 A.M.

M. King, CMA

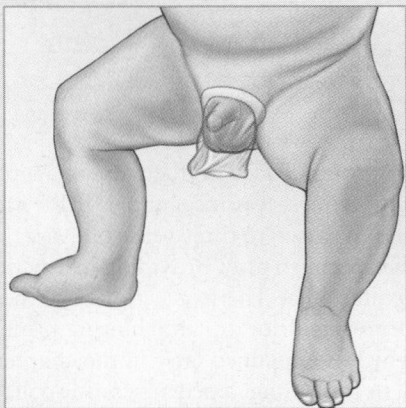 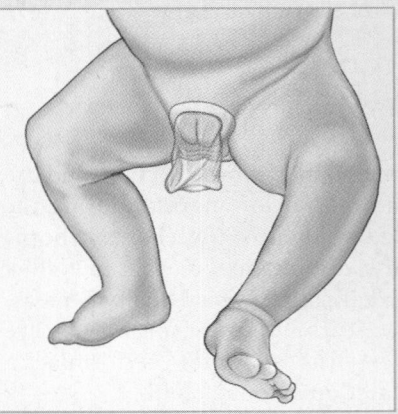

FIGURE 37-10 Applying urine collection device on a male and female infant.

- Does the child complain of burning, itching, or pain during urination? (urinary tract infection, UTI)
- Is there a persistent diaper rash? (diarrhea, change in urine composition)
- Has the child reverted to bed wetting or loss of bladder control? (stress, UTI)
- Is the child in diapers, how many diapers does the child wet each day? (dehydration)

Positive response to any of the above question could indicate urinary tract problems.

After obtaining the patient's temperature, pulse, respiration, height, and weight measurements, a urine collection device should be applied. Procedure 37-5 lists the steps necessary to apply a urine collection device on a child who is unable or unwilling to urinate into a container. In some cases, a child may be catheterized to obtain a specimen. Urine samples reflect the health status of many systems in the body and are an important diagnostic tool. After these procedures are complete, your duty is to remain ready to assist in the examination in whatever manner necessary. Once the visit is completed, be sure to review the physician's instructions with the caregiver and take a few moments to bond with the child. Remember to document any results.

Pediatric Diseases and Disorders

Children experience frequent colds, gastrointestinal upsets, and other fairly routine conditions, which are seen in a pediatric practice. Additional diseases and disorders to those which immunizations are recommended will be covered in Chapter 49.

Upper Respiratory Diseases

The common cold is caused by over 200 varieties of rhinovirus, highly contagious, and usually self-limiting after about a week. In infants and children, there may be low-grade fever, nasal congestion, and coughing. Children during the ages one to two may have six to ten colds a year. It may be necessary to instruct the caregiver on the use of a nasal bulb syringe to remove excess secretions and facilitate nursing or bottle-feeding. Treatment of colds is usually with over-the-counter medications to reduce fever, congestion, and coughs. Secondary infection such as strep throat or otitis media may result from colds.

Strep Throat

Strep throat is caused by group A beta hemolytic streptococcus pyogenes. These highly infectious bacteria may lead to other problems such as scarlet fever and rheumatic fever, which can damage heart valves.

The physician may order a throat culture to confirm that strep is the causative agent. Many pediatrician offices perform these tests on site. Strep throat is treated with antibiotics. Caregivers should be reminded that children must finish the entire prescription to prevent relapse. Most upper respiratory infections are spread easily by droplets from the nose, throat, or contaminated items handled by the infected person. Handwashing is the best defense to ward off colds.

Otitis Media

Otitis media is an infection of the middle ear due to cold, allergies, or other respiratory infections. Fluid builds up and applies pressure to the eardrum, which can cause pain, irritability, and sometimes fever. Treatment of otitis media consists of decongestants, analgesics, and sometimes antibiotics. Repeated infections can lead to damage to the eardrum and loss of hearing. Children with chronic ear infections may require a myringotomy, a tube inserted through the eardrum to permit drainage of fluid.

Croup

Croup is an inflammation of the larynx and trachea, which leads to a distinctive barking cough and hoarseness. There are two types of croup and both begin with a cold. Spasmodic croup begins suddenly at night with the distinct "seal" type of cough and viral croup develops more slowly with swelling, mucous secretions, and noisy breathing called stridor. Antibiotics are not effective against viral illness. Croup is treated at home unless breathing is extremely labored and emergency medical help is needed. Sitting in a steamy bathroom, with the door closed for 15–20 minutes helps restore normal breathing. Afterwards, a cool steam vaporizer or humidifier in the child's room adds moisture to the air and may help breathing. Exposing the child to cool moist night air is also frequently effective.

Bronchiolitis

Bronchiolitis is an inflammation of the bronchioles and is more common in children under two years old. Children who have upper respiratory infections, such as colds, may develop bronchiolitis. Children with asthma and those exposed to second-hand smoke are at a higher risk. Symptoms include cold-like symptoms such as nasal and chest congestion and low-grade fever. Treatments are the same as those used to treat colds. If excessive coughing is present, using a cool steam vaporizer or humidifier may help add moisture to the air and reduce coughing.

Respiratory synctial virus (RSV), which occurs in winter and early spring, is the most common cause of bronchiolitis. It can spread by contact with upper respiratory secretions and may last two weeks. When very young children are affected, they may need hospitalization for intravenous fluids, bronchodilators, and oxygen therapy. Confirmation of RSV is the presence of viral antibodies.

Asthma

Asthma is the most common chronic disease in children, affecting one out of seven children usually before age four. Inflammation and spasms of the bronchi, mucous secretions, and narrowing of the airways make it difficult to exhale and inhale. Symptoms include wheezing, shortness of breath, tightness in the chest, difficulty speaking, and anxiety. The cause for asthma is unknown. However, triggers such as allergies, exposure to pollutants, cigarette smoke, cold viruses, and strenuous exercise may bring on an asthma attack. Children who experience two or more asthma attacks per week should be seen by a specialist. Inhalers or nebulizers may be necessary during attacks. If attacks occur more frequently than twice a week, then daily anti-inflammatory medications will most likely be the treatment. In both cases, an asthma plan should be developed so that the caregiver understands what to do in each stage of an attack culminating in emergency treatment at a hospital if necessary. Bronchodilators are administered either by inhaler or nebulizers. A peak flow meter may be used to measure the capacity of the child's ability to exhale forcefully. If specific allergens are identified, then removing the offending allergens from the child's environment is helpful.

Gastrointestinal Disorders

Diarrhea, nausea and vomiting are common conditions affecting children. Diarrhea is defined as two or more watery stools in 24 hours.

Diarrhea

Diarrhea may be caused by bacterial, viral, and parasitic infections, food allergies, and medications. Infants and children may have diarrhea with no apparent cause. If diarrhea persists for more than two days, the child may need to be seen in the office. Diarrhea in infants and small children can rapidly lead to dehydration. Dehydration can trigger an imbalance of electrolytes causing the child to be lethargic and possibly to hyperventilate. Acidosis and death can occur. The signs of dehydration are vital for you and the caregiver to recognize. They are listed in Box 37-1. In addition to dehydration, diarrhea may cause excoriation, or painful chafing or rawness of the skin in the diaper area. Other symptoms include cramping, weakness, fever, and irritability. Pediatricians often recommend the BRAT diet consisting of bananas, rice/cereal, applesauce and toast. Avoiding diary products is also advised until diarrhea subsides. Foods and dairy products may be reintroduced gradually.

Colic

Colic is severe gastrointestinal pain in infants occurring in both breast-fed and bottle-fed babies. The cause of colic is unknown, although some suspect immaturity of the digestive system. Colic is harmless and usually disappears by four months. Symptoms include intense crying, irritability, fussiness, distended abdomen, and gas. Parents and caregivers feel frustrated, angry, at fault, and exhausted. There is no specific treatment. The trial and error approach to feedings, how to hold the baby, and soothing remedies like rocking and patting the baby's back is the usual treatment. Some babies find relief being held in the football position lying on their bellies along the parent's arm or leg.

Obesity

Obesity is defined as being 20% above the patient's ideal weight with a body mass index (BMI) over 30. Body mass index is a measurement of body weight relative to height and is associated with the amount of body fat. BMI is calculated using the following formula:

$$\text{Body weight in lbs} \times 700 \div \text{height} = \text{value} \div \text{height} = \text{BMI}$$

A BMI of 25 to 27 means a child is overweight. Very few children are obese due to endocrine disorders. Genetic tendencies, family patterns of overeating, poor food choices, and lack of exercise cause children to be obese. Fifty percent of the United States population is considered obese. It is estimated that 30% of children over five are obese. Obesity carries serious consequences to health in the short and long terms and may cause damage to a child's self-esteem. A medical assistant can provide support, encouragement, educational materials, and be a link to community resources for the family dealing with an obese child.

Other Disorders

There are other conditions or disorders that do not fit in any specific category. These will be discussed in the following paragraphs. For a discussion on issues related

---

BOX 37-1
Signs of Dehydration in Infants

- Decrease in urine output—dry diapers
- Weakness and lethargy
- Dry pale skin with loss of elasticity
- Decrease in tear production
- Sunken eyes
- Increased thirst
- Confusion

---

to child abuse, see Legal and Ethical Issues. Patient Education discusses teenage suicide.

Autism

Autism is a nervous system disorder or group of disorders beginning in childhood affecting the child's ability to relate to others. Autism is four times more frequent in males and is noticeable by the age of three. Autism affects 1 in 166 children according to the National Autism Association. The cause is unknown; however, recent research indicates that as many as five to twenty genes may be involved. Other factors implicated as possible causes are exposure to toxic chemicals during pregnancy, pesticides, flame-retardant chemicals, prenatal or postnatal viruses, and exposure to heavy metals like mercury. There is no link between autism and immunizations according to the latest CDC research. Symptoms of autism are varied and may include:

- Failure to make eye contact
- Engaging in repetitive behavior
- Delayed language skills
- Preference for solitary activities
- Upset by changes in routine
- Indifference to people

There is no cure, but recent research indicates that early intervention by specialists can be beneficial. The earlier autism is diagnosed and interventions designed to the child's needs are started, the better the prognosis.

Sudden Infant Death Syndrome

Sudden Infant Death Syndrome (SIDS) is the leading cause of death in children in the first year of life. The highest number of deaths occurs between one and four months. SIDS happens more frequently in winter and is more prevalent in boys. Among the probable causes proposed are immature waking centers in the brain leading to sleep apnea, abnormal regulation of breathing, heart rates, and lack of airway control. Factors that increase the risk of SIDS are low-birth weight, premature birth, family history of SIDS, putting the child to sleep on his or her stomach, births from very young mothers, and exposure to alcohol, drugs, and smoking before birth. Possible prevention techniques include having the infant sleep in a back or side position for at least the first six months, using apnea monitors, and knowledge of infant CPR by the parents. The loss of a child to SIDS is particularly difficult because parents often feel that they were at fault. Support groups and therapy may help devastated parents. The SIDS association has local and national chapters that can provide valuable information and help.

Febrile Seizures

Febrile Seizures are suffered by some children with high fevers following a rapid spike in body temperature.

Legal and Ethical Issues

Child abuse in the United States affects 1 in 20 children each year. Child abuse is defined by the American Medical Association as "emotional, physical, or sexual mistreatment, or neglect of a child." Children are very dependent on the adults who surround them, therefore they are very vulnerable. Caregivers, close family members or friends are usually the abusers and abuse crosses all socioeconomic, racial, religious, and ethnic backgrounds. Physical and psychological abuse can impact brain development, intellectual growth, delay normal growth and social development, and have long-term health problems. Moreover, the psychological effects of abuse last though the abuse is over. Abused children are at increased risk of suffering from low self esteem, depression, emotional highs and lows. As adults, they often are substance abusers and have eating disorders. Sexual abuse is anything of a sexual nature that the child is asked to witness or participate in without consent and yet do not completely understand.

The pediatrician's office is the first step in suspicion of abuse. The physician is asked to evaluate the child's condition and provide treatment. Physicians are required by federal Child Abuse Prevention and Treatment Act to report any suspicions of abuse. You, in turn, are required to report your suspicions immediately to the physician. Your role is to be alert to any suspicious bruises, burns, excessive fractures, changes in behavior, and changes in hygiene, which may indicate abuse. Victims of any type of abuse will require counseling and assistance from a broad spectrum of social service agencies. The effects of abuse cannot be washed away in a short time. In some case, it may takes of years of therapy to resolve the problems caused by child abuse.

Seizures can involve jerking arms and legs, loss of consciousness, and stiffening of the child's body. After a seizure, the child may be sleepy and have a headache. Watching a child have a febrile seizure is alarming for parents; however, there is no lasting effect on the child and these seizures are not associated with epilepsy.

Suicide is the third leading cause of death after accidents and homicides in teenagers and young adults. Educating yourself, parents, and caregivers about the warning signs of suicide could save a life. No one knows exactly what causes someone to commit suicide. There are many factors implicated in suicides; however, others with the same risk factors do not commit suicide. A Center for Disease Control survey found that 28% of high school students had suicidal thoughts and 8.3% had attempted suicide. Girls attempt suicide three times more often than boys. Boys, however, are four times more likely to die in the suicide attempt.

Many people talk about suicide well before they actually make an attempt. This provides a window of opportunity for family, friends, and health care professionals to be alert to their threats and take action to prevent the attempt. Risk factors for teenagers are similar to those of adults including death of a family member, end of a dating relationship, move from familiar school or house, failure at school, substance abuse, and trouble with the law. Most commonly, depression and substance abuse are implicated in suicides. In teenagers, behavior imitation is sometimes a factor. After a publicized suicide of an idol for instance, teenage suicide attempts sometimes increase. As health care professionals, you are in a position to identify those who exhibit any of the following behaviors:

- Decline in hygiene
- Access to firearms and prescription drugs
- Preoccupation with morbid thoughts
- Substance abuse
- Family history of suicide
- Dramatic changes in grades, mood, or contact with friends
- Decrease in appetite and change in sleep patterns
- Previous suicide attempt

Experts say that any suicide attempt must be taken seriously even if it is only a couple of scratches on the wrist or a couple of pills. All suicide attempts should be evaluated in a hospital emergency room for treatment or hospitalization. Crisis hotlines are helpful especially for worried parents and friends. Having information about suicide allows you to be prepared to alert caregivers to suicide risks and inform them to look for certain behavior.

There is no treatment necessary except to reduce the fever. During the seizure, the child should be placed on his or her side in an area free of sharp objects. Do not put anything in the child's mouth nor restrain the child.

Infectious Diseases

A number of other infectious diseases that affect children do not fit previous categories and will be discussed in the following page.

Meningitis

Meningitis or inflammation of membranes surrounding the brain and spinal cord can be caused by viral or bacterial infection. Viral meningitis is more common and is not life threatening; while bacterial meningitis is life threatening and requires immediate medical attention. Usually meningitis results from an infection originating elsewhere in the body and migrating to the brain and spinal cord through the blood stream. Viral meningitis more often affects those under 30 and occurs more frequently in winter. Bacterial meningitis can be caused by several different types of bacteria including streptococcus, staphylococcus, hemophilus influenza, and menigingococcus. Bacterial meningitis can affect all ages, but occurs more frequently in children. Symptoms of the bacterial form of the disease include rapid onset of fever, headache, stiff neck, nausea, and vomiting. Some behavioral changes may occur such as confusion and sleepiness. Evidence of any previous set of symptoms requires immediate medical attention preferably in a hospital. A lumbar puncture is needed to confirm diagnosis and large amounts of antibiotics administered intravenously is the treatment of choice. Complications from the illness include deafness, brain damage, and blindness.

Immunization with HIB vaccine has greatly reduced the number of meningitis cases in the United States. The Advisory Committee on Immunization Practices (ACIP) recommends that children 11–12 years of age, teens entering high school and college freshmen receive the newly licensed (January, 2004) meningococcal vaccine. According to CDC statistics, in the United States, about 2,000 people develop meningococcal disease annually, 10 to 14 percent of those die, and 11 to 19 percent have permanent disabilities. It is recommended that when 11–12 year olds receive their tetanus-diphtheria booster that they receive this new vaccine at the same time.

Fifth's Disease

Fifth's Disease or erythema infectiosum is a mildly contagious viral disease that occurs during spring in children over two years old. It is caused by the parvovirus B19. Symptoms, which last about a week, include reddened cheeks, fever, a rash on arms and legs. If Fifth's disease is contracted during pregnancy, the fetus may suffer damage or die in utero.

Roseola

Roseola is a common early childhood viral infection characterized by a sudden high fever, which can last about four days, followed by a rash of tiny pink spots on the head and trunk. Treatment includes bringing down the child's fever with acetaminophen and sponging the body with lukewarm water.

Hand, Foot, and Mouth Disease

Hand, foot, and mouth disease is another mild viral infection causing blisters to appear in the mouth, on hands, and feet. It commonly occurs in summer and early fall affecting young children in daycare or nursery schools up to four years of age. It is usually caused by the Coxsackie virus and is spread by the fecal-oral route, saliva, or direct contact with blisters. In addition to blistering, symptoms include fever and loss of appetite. Treatments include acetaminophen, rinsing the mouth with warm salty water, and drinking fluids. Handwashing especially after diaper changes, washing toys, and surfaces possibly contaminated by infected children help prevent reinfection.

Inherited or Birth-Related Disorders

In a pediatric practice, genetic defects and birth-related disorders in infants and children will be seen in lesser numbers than infectious diseases or routine upper respiratory and gastrointestinal problems.

Cerebral Palsy

Cerebral palsy is not a single disease with a single cause. It is a group of disorders that appear early in life and impair movement. Acquired cerebral palsy is the result of brain injury at birth or after, or the result of an infection such as meningitis. Congenital cerebral palsy is present at birth and can be caused by infections during pregnancy, jaundice in the newborn, Rh incompatibility, severe oxygen shortage, or head trauma during delivery. Cerebral palsy has a wide array of symptoms including lack of muscle control, muscle weakness, spastic muscles, mental retardation, delayed development, and hearing and vision problems. Diagnosis is by examination and medical history. Physicians look for abnormal muscle tone or "floppy baby" syndrome. There is no cure for cerebral palsy. Patients usually require a team of health care professionals including occupational, physical, and speech therapists to help them achieve their potential.

Thalassemia

Mediterranean anemia or thalassemia is a group of inherited hemoglobin disorders affecting mainly people with ancestors from the Mediterranean area namely, Greece, Italy, North Africa, Spain, and southern Asia. This is a recessive disorder requiring two genes to develop the disease. People with one gene have thalassemia minor or trait. The trait form produces a mild incurable anemia treatable with iron supplements. Thalassemia major is a severe hemolytic anemia. In hemolytic anemia, red blood cells rupture and cannot deliver the required amount of oxygen needed for normal metabolism in the body. Thalassemia major patients require blood transfusions monthly, which cause iron to build up in the body's tissues. Normally, iron is excreted in small amounts daily; however, the body is unable to excrete the excess amount of iron accumulating from the transfusions. These large amounts of iron can deposit in the heart, brain, and liver. With the advances, medications bind with iron to aid excretion and these patients can have longer life expectancies. Blood tests can determine if an individual is a carrier of this gene and prenatal tests can determine if the fetus has thalassemia. For more information on other genetic disorders, see Table 37-3.

Assisting the Elderly

Gerontology, a relatively new area of medical practice, is the study of the process of aging and the effects of aging on people. A geriatrician diagnoses and treats diseases and conditions, such as osteoarthritis, congestive heart failure, arthritis, emphysema, cerebrovascular accident (CVA), and Alzheimer's disease that affect older patients. In general, some of the same conditions that affect a younger population also affect elders. Surprisingly, the elderly have fewer acute illnesses than younger age groups; though when they become acutely ill, they take longer to recover. Chronic illness is the major problem for the older population. Some of the physical problems associated with aging may cause patients to lose their independence; however, many elders remain active and relatively healthy into their late 80s (Figure 37-11).

Aging Population

Every culture treats its elders according to its own traditions (Cultural Considerations). In the United States, our traditions have undergone change, in part, because we are a mobile society and families often are spread across the country. In the early 20th century, grandma

TABLE 37-3 Genetic Disorders

Disorder	Description
Alopecia	Baldness in particular patterns, especially on the head.
Cooley's anemia	A rare form of anemia or a reduction of red blood cells that is found in some people of Mediterranean origin.
Cystic fibrosis	A disorder of the exocrine glands that causes these glands to produce abnormally thick secretions of mucus. The disease affects many organs, including the pancreas and the respiratory system. One reliable diagnostic test in children is the sweat test, which will show elevated sodium and potassium levels. There is presently no known cure for the disease, which can shorten the life span.
Down syndrome	A disorder that produces moderate-to-severe mental retardation and multiple defects. The physical characteristics of a child with this disorder are a sloping forehead, flat nose or absent bridge to the nose, low-set eyes, and a general dwarfed physical growth. The disorder occurs more commonly when the mother is over 40. Also called Trisomy 21.
Duchenne muscular dystrophy	A muscular disorder in which there is progressive wasting away of various muscles, including leg, pelvic, and shoulder muscles. Children with this disorder have difficulty climbing stairs and running. They may eventually be confined to a wheelchair. Other complications relating to the heart and respiratory system can be present. It is caused by a recessive gene and is more common in males. This disorder often results in a shortened life-span.
Hemophilia	A bleeding disorder in which there is a deficiency in one of the factors necessary for blood to clot. There is an abnormal tendency to bleed, and victims of this disorder may require frequent blood transfusions. The female (mother) carries this recessive gene and it is passed on to males. Therefore, it is found almost exclusively in boys.
Huntington's chorea	A rare condition characterized by bizarre involuntary movements called chorea. The patient may have progressive mental and physical disturbances, which generally begin around 40.
Retinitis pigmentosa	Chronic progressive disease that begins in early childhood and is characterized by degeneration of the retina. This can lead to blindness by middle age.
Sickle cell anemia	Severe, chronic, incurable disorder that results in anemia and causes joint pain, chronic weakness, and infections. Occurs more commonly in people of Mediterranean and African heritage. The blood cell in this disease is sickle shaped.
Spina bifida	A congenital disorder that results in a defect in the walls of the spinal column, causing the membranes of the spinal cord to push through to the outside. It may be associated with other defects, such as hydrocephalus, which is an enlarged head as a result of the accumulation of fluid on the brain.
Tay-Sachs disease	A disorder caused by a deficiency of an enzyme, which can result in mental and physical retardation and blindness. It is transferred by a recessive trait and is most commonly found in families of Eastern European Jewish decent. Death generally occurs before the age of 4.

and grandpa had no choice economically except to live with their married children until they died. In 1914, Dr. I. L. Nascher wrote the first geriatric textbook. Fortunately much has changed in the lives of elders since that time. One of the most important improvements in elders' lives was the passage of the Federal Old Age Insurance Law in 1935 under Social Security, which provided elders some financial security. In 1965, in response to an aging population, the Administration on Aging and Older Americans Act, Medicaid, and Medicare were all enacted. As the numbers of older adults continues to increase, there is more attention given to the needs of the elderly in the areas of health care, living conditions, and living a fulfilling old age.

Today's grandmas and grandpas do not want to leave their friends by moving across the country to live with their children. Many are still working into their 70s and are enjoying an active social life through their 80s. Box 37-2 lists some famous older people who were successful in later years. The elderly are no longer lumped into one group of people over 65. Sociologists place the elderly into four distinct age groups.

- Young old: 65–75
- Old: 75–85
- Old-old: 85–100
- Elite old: over 100

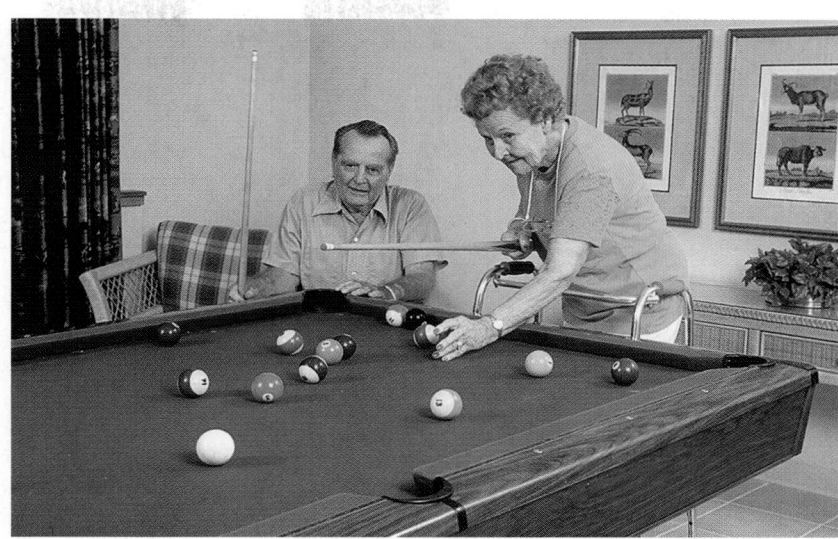

FIGURE 37-11 Older adults can live active lives into their 80s and beyond.

Facts about the Elderly

In the United States currently, people over 65 years of age make up 12% of the total population. This figure is rising and it is estimated that in 2020, the elderly will make up 20% of the population. Life expectancy is increasing as shown in Box 37-3 due to better living condition, medical advances, better nutrition, new medications, and once they reach old age, elders are living longer. Forty percent of the elderly population is over age 85.

Baby boomers are Americans born between 1946 and 1964. The oldest of this group reaches senior citizen status in 2008. The baby boomers have several

Cultural Considerations

People from various ethnic and cultural backgrounds have specific beliefs about aging and the role of elders in the family. As you work with geriatric patients, it is important to remember each person's uniqueness and consider the influences of their ethnic origins on their concept of aging. For example, many African Americans consider the attainment of old age an accomplishment, not something to be looked on with dread. Most elderly African Americans are respected in their families and are less likely to live in long-term-care facilities than white Americans.

Native Americans have close family bonds, elders are respected and viewed as teachers and leaders. They believe that each person has a right to make his or her own health care decisions and may find the probing questions that health care providers need to ask inappropriate.

Many Hispanic Americans view their health status as God's will. Health is a reward for living correctly and taking care of your body, while being ill is a punishment for not living appropriately. Wearing or having medals and crosses in their rooms is an important part of prayer and healing. Older relatives are held in high regard and they view old age in a positive light. The traditions of other ethnic or cultural groups are not odd or weird, they are just different. As health care providers, we should seek to honor the traditions of others and not change them.

Facts that Counteract Aging Assumptions

- Eleanor Roosevelt, wife of Franklin D. Roosevelt, chaired the United Nations Commission on Human Rights from age 62–67 and she wrote her autobiography at 74.
- Frank Lloyd Wright designed the Guggenheim Museum in New York City at age 91.
- Nelson Mandela was inaugurated as president of South Africa at age 75 after 27 years in prison and winning the country's first multiracial election.
- Grandma Moses the famous American painter started her career in art during her 70s.

medical information. Baby boomers have, for the most part, higher incomes than other groups and will require long-term health care facilities to provide amenities. They exercise to keep fit more than previous age groups and will demand workout equipment in long-term-care facilities. A decline in some "traditional" chronic diseases seen in old age may result. On the other hand, they have less leisure time than previous groups, resulting in more stress-related conditions among this group.

The elderly will be using more health care resources in the coming years. Only 5% of the older population is in long-term care at any given time; however, one in four elders will spend some time in a nursing home during his or her last years. It is estimated that most seniors citizens rely on Social Security for 50% of their income. With more people requiring Social Security for longer periods of time, the long-term demands on this beneficial program are obvious.

characteristics that will impact on health care and your role as a provider of health care. They have fewer children than previous generational groups; therefore they will receive less assistance from their children in their old age. They are the best-educated generational group and thus will be more informed, proactive, and involved about their care. They are accustom to high-tech electronics and will have greater access to up-to-date

The Aging Process

The aging process begins at birth and continues until death. It is a not an illness, but a normal part of life that progresses at different rates in each person. There are many theories about the causes of aging. We can identify some factors that impact how we age, such as genetics, lifestyle choices, occupational hazards, poor nutrition, lack of health care, and physical and social environment.

Ageism

Ageism is defined as a prejudice against and incorrect assumptions about an individual because of his or her age. Aging is not easy. Much of our society tends to stereotype the elderly and have many misconceptions, measuring the whole group with one yardstick. It is safe to say that all elders: are not senile, do not retired with lots of money, do not live in nursing homes, do not have all medical expenses covered by Medicare, and are not less productive workers. Many elderly do have contact with family, do enjoy learning new things, have an interest in and are able to have sexual relations. Our goal should be to view the aging adult as an individual and get to know him or her.

Life Expectancy at Birth for Men and Women

Birth Year	Life Expectancy
1920	54.1 years
1930	59.7 years
1940	62.9 years
1950	68.2 years
1960	69.7 years
1970	70.9 years
1980	73.7 years
1990	75.4 years
2000	77.1 years
2010 (projected)	78.5 years

(Adapted from U.S. Department of Commerce [2001]. *Statistical Abstract of the United States* [121st ed. p. 73]. Washington DC: Bureau of the Census.)

The Aging Body

Understanding the effects that the aging process has on the human body as a whole and to each body system will help foster a better awareness of elders' needs to increase respect and empathy for them from health care providers.

Physical Changes

Review Table 37-4 for the physical changes of aging on each system of the body. Important points for the medical assistant to consider relevant to each system follow.

TABLE 37-4 Physical Changes of Aging

Body System	Physical Changes
Integumentary	Hair loses color and becomes thinner; skin dries, becomes less elastic, and wrinkles develop; skin tears easily; skin bruises easily (senile purpura); fingernails and toenails thicken; reduced amount of sweat; increased sensitivity to cold; age spots more common.
Nervous	Problems with balance; temperature regulation off; sensation of pain decreases; deep sleep shortened; more awakening during the night; brain cells lost, but intelligence intact unless pathologic condition present; decreased sensitivity of nerve receptors for heat, cold, pain, and pressure.
Sensory	More difficult to see close objects; night vision may decrease; cataracts (clouding of the lens) more common; peripheral vision and depth perception diminish; hearing diminishes; smell and taste receptors less sensitive.
Musculoskeletal	Less muscle strength; less flexibility; slower movements; arthritis and osteoporosis more common; body is more stooped.
Respiratory	Breathing capacity lessens.
Urinary	Kidneys decrease in size; urine production less efficient; empting bladder completely more difficult; stress incontinence may develop.
Digestive	Primary taste sensations of salt, sweet, and sour decrease; constipation increases; flatulence increases; movement of food through the digestive tract slows.
Cardiovascular	Blood vessels less elastic and more narrowed; heart may not pump as efficiently; decrease in cardiac output and circulation.
Endocrine	Decrease in estrogen and progesterone; hot flashes, nervous feelings; higher levels of parathormone and thyroid stimulating hormone; weight gain; insulin production less efficient; diabetes mellitus more likely.
Reproductive	Females: ovulation and menstruation cease; vaginal walls thinner and drier. Males: scrotum less firm; prostate gland may enlarge.

If during your time with the patient, you notice new problems in the older patient, chart them accordingly and report them to the physician for immediate evaluation. Table 37-5 lists some diseases that usually affect older people.

Integumentary System

Integumentary system changes are visible to the eye. The skin is the first line of defense against infection, temperature change, exposure to sunlight, and perception of pain. Observe the patient as he or she prepares for the examination. Pay particular attention to bruises and signs of infection. Since pain receptors are diminished with age, an elderly person may not even be aware of an injury. Make sure the examining room is the proper temperature and that sufficient coverings are available to make the patient comfortable. Since adhesive bandages may damage the skin during removal, select a type of covering that will cause the least discomfort. Diabetes mellitus is a problem for many elderly and impacts the ability to heal. Examine fingernails and toenails, since the patient may not be able to keep them properly trimmed and may cut too deep leading to infection. Your patient may need to see a podiatrist or have a visiting nurse trim toenails to reduce chance of infection.

Nervous System

The nervous system begins to slow down and reaction times are delayed with age. Cognitive ability (ability to think, reason, and perceive) and dementia will be discussed later in the chapter. Allow extra time for older patients to follow directions and respond to questions. Do not finish sentences for older patients or ignore a patient while talking about the patient to his or her caregivers or family members. Slower responses to

TABLE 37-5 **Diseases That Mainly Affect the Elderly**

Disease/Condition	Explanation
Alzheimer's disease and other dementias	Brain disorders that lead to progressive loss of memory and other intellectual functions.
Aortic aneurysm	Dilation of the wall of the aorta that can rupture and lead to death if left untreated.
Atrophic urethritis and vaginitis	Thinning of the tissue of the urethra and vagina that can lead to burning on urination and painful intercourse.
Decubitus ulcers (bedsores)	Breakdown of skin from prolonged pressure.
Benign prostatic hyperplasia	Enlargement of the prostate gland, which blocks the flow of urine.
Cataracts	Clouding in the lens of the eye, which impacts vision.
Chronic lymphocytic leukemia	A type of leukemia that usually has a long phase with little growth or progression (indolent phase), but has many other characteristic features of cancer.
Diabetes mellitus type 2	A type of diabetes that may not require insulin treatment, usually begins in middle age.
Glaucoma	Elevation of the pressure in one of the chambers of the eye that can decrease vision and lead to blindness, usually begins in middle age.
Hypothyroidism	Thyroid gland is under active and produces too little thyroid hormone, can eventually result in anemia, low body temperature, mental confusion and heart failure.
Osteoarthritis	Degeneration of the cartilage that lines the joints, usually begins in middle age.
Osteoporosis	Loss of calcium from the bones, makes them fragile and leads to fractures.
Parkinson's disease	Slowly progressive degenerative brain disease that leads to tremor, muscle rigidity, difficulty moving, and instability.
Prostate cancer	Cancer of the prostate gland.
Shingles (herpes zoster)	A reawakening of the dormant chicken pox virus that causes skin rash and can lead to prolonged pain.
Stroke	A blockage or bleeding of a blood vessel in the brain that leads to weakness, loss of sensation, difficulty talking, or other neurological problems.
Urinary incontinence	Inability to control urine flow.

changes of balance can make the elderly patient more prone to falls and injuries. Offer your arm to a patient when walking and assist him or her on and off the examination table. Make sure the step stool is secure as your patient gets on and off the examination table.

Sleep cycles are affected by the aging process in the brain. Ask your patients how they are sleeping, how many hours, and if they feel rested. Sometimes, elderly take frequent naps during the day, which can affect their ability to sleep restfully at night.

Sensory Changes

Sensory changes in the eyes, ears, nose, and mouth affect elders' ability to react to the world. Impairment of hearing and eyesight reduces their ability to interact with the environment around them. As an elderly patient prepares for his or her examination, inquire about hearing and sight abilities. Ask if his or her hearing aid is functioning well, whether glasses are helping him or her to see well enough, does the patient still drive, and how does he or she react to the glare of lights at night?

Speak clearly and slowly enough so the patient can understand your message. Sensory information from the nose and mouth declines until about age 80 when approximately half the sense of smell is lost. Taste depends mostly on smell. The elderly may not have much interest in food and therefore may not be taking enough nourishment. Elders often are "tea and toasters." Instead of eating a nutritious meal, they will have tea and toast or crackers periodically during the day. As a result, they feel full, but they are not taking in protein, vitamins, and minerals needed to keep them healthy. Poor oral hygiene and side effects of medications also can affect eating. Engage elder patients in a discussion of favorite foods and what they normally eat each day. Observe their teeth and oral hygiene, ask if they wear dentures and check that the dentures fit properly.

Musculoskeletal System

Musculoskeletal system aging is characterized by a decrease in muscle strength and loss of flexibility. Both of these conditions increase older people's risk of falling and sustaining fractures. You can promote regular exercise perhaps at the local senior center (Figure 37-12) and provide exercise information that the elderly can perform at home while seated to increase upper body strength. Encourage eating proper amounts of dairy products to supply needed calcium. Discuss safety issues at home that can put the elderly patient at risk. Speak to them about how they bathe: do they have grab rails and chairs in the tub area? Encourage them to use the assistive devices that they seem to need—canes, walkers, and bedside commodes (portable toilet). Review safety concerns with caregivers and family members.

Respiratory System

Respiratory system aging is characterized by loss of elasticity in the alveoli and lungs themselves leading to a reduction in exchange of gases. Additionally, as the respiratory muscles become weaker, it becomes more difficult to move air into and out of the lungs. Inactivity in the elderly combined with reduced pulmonary functions make them more prone to pneumonia. Breathing exercises can be taught through videos or written materials helping the elderly to increase the depth of breathing and exercise respiratory muscles. Any activity that will increase their endurance will be beneficial in protecting them from respiratory infections and improving the oxygen supply to all body systems.

Urinary System

Urinary system changes that can occur with aging result in a reduced ability to concentrate urine and slower waste removal by the kidneys. Slower waste removal combined with the number of daily medications taken by most elderly places older patients more at risk for toxic medication overload that can have

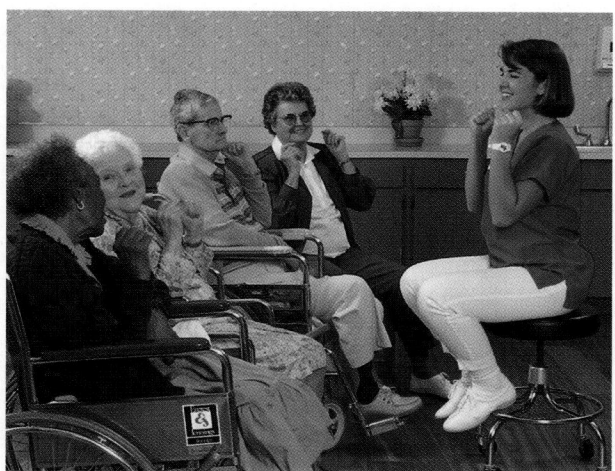

FIGURE 37-12 Exercise is beneficial and provides socialization.

significant impact on their quality of life. Decrease in bladder storage capacity and the inability to empty the bladder provides opportunity for infection. Increased frequency of urination, nocturia, and urgency may all become problems for many elderly. Disruption of sleep may make some patients tired and irritable. Urgency makes them feel reluctant to leave home for fear they may embarrass themselves by not making it to the bathroom in time. Some patients may feel that reducing fluid intake is the way to cope with these problems; however, this can lead to dehydration, electrolyte imbalance, and increased risk of urinary tract infection. Being able to speak to the patient about the consequences of reducing fluids enables the patient to be better informed and possibly make better choices to get through the day. The proper amount of water and other fluids are critical to maintain homeostasis in the body.

Digestive System

Digestive system aging is characterized by slower passage of food leading to less absorption of food, minerals, vitamins, and increased constipation and flatulence. Stressing the importance of proper nutrition including all the food groups is helpful. Provide a brochure with a diagram of appropriate food portion sizes as well as lists of foods in each food group that the patient may bring home. Supplying examples will be helpful for the overweight patient also. Since the liver slows down with age it takes longer for drugs and alcohol to be absorbed, which can cause an increase in the risk of adverse drug interactions.

Cardiovascular System

Cardiovascular changes are age-related and are frequently the cause of disease and disorders in elders. However, lifestyle habits such as smoking, high-fat diet, and lack of exercise also take a toll on the cardiovascular system. Hypertension and decrease in strength of cardiac contractions decreases cardiac output and reduces the oxygen supply needed by the organs of the body. Orthostatic hypotension occurs in some elderly. Orthostatic hypotension is a 20 to 30 mm Hg drop in blood pressure that is associated with dizziness and fainting when changing position from lying down or sitting to standing. Dizziness can increase elders' risk of injury. The medical assistant should help the patient understand why this may happen and suggest that rising more slowly and holding onto something steady may prevent the dizziness.

Endocrine System
Endocrine system aging is characterized by decreasing levels of estrogen, thyroid hypofunction, and insulin resistance. The decrease of estrogen in females ends menstrual cycles, decreases vaginal secretions, and may lead to hot flashes, night sweats, and sleep disturbances. Thyroid hypofunction can lead to overweight, fatigue, and mental confusion, which can be mistaken for dementia. Many elderly develop diabetes mellitus and will need guidance in menu selections and obtaining and testing blood samples. Encourage elders to have blood work done regularly to screen for endocrine dysfunction.

Reproductive System
Reproductive system changes have been discussed in Chapter 31. Since elders are aging more gracefully and in better health than ever before, it follows that the desire for sex in many is present. As medical assistants, you may not be able to imagine older patients being sexually intimate; however, they are. Psychologists say that patterns of sexual interest later in life mirror lifelong patterns. Older patients may find it difficult to discuss anything about sex. If the opportunity presents itself, you must be ready to discuss these issues comfortably and non-judgmentally. Again, written materials for the patient to read at home are important educational tools.

Mental Changes

Mental deterioration is not a normal part of aging. As people age, the risk for mental deterioration increases, as does the risk of age-related disorders. Mental health is the capacity to cope effectively with life changes, manage life's stresses, and achieve a state of emotional balance. It is a fact that brain function slows with aging; however, there are many factors that impact on a patient's mental status. People can bring into old age some of the mental health problems they had in earlier years. To maintain good mental health, individuals need to participate in activities they find interesting and interact socially. The elderly need to be able to feel a sense of self worth and to feel they are of value to society.

Cognitive Ability
Cognitive ability is affected by many factors. Normal aging does not reduce cognitive ability. The psychological

status of the mind is altered by health status, genetics, social factors, educational accomplishment, and physical activity. Normally an individual's personality does not change with age unless there is a pathologic problem.

Memory
There are three types of memory: short term (about 30 seconds or so), long term (what was learned long ago), and sensory (information gained through the senses lasting a few seconds). Aging does not mean a loss of memory or cognitive ability in the elderly. With age, the ability to retrieve information from long-term memory may be slower. Basic intelligence is unchanged throughout the life span, as are the abilities for verbal comprehension, arithmetic operations, and problem solving. Learning is not altered by aging. Working memory, the ability to retain information while using other information, slows with age. The expression, use it or lose it, could apply to the brain as well as other muscles. Keeping the brain active with games, puzzles, and other types of stimulation, help maintain memory retrieval. Activities such as knitting and crocheting are beneficial to stimulate the brain. In addition, physical exercise increases oxygen flow and helps maintain blood supply to the brain. Some may find that the first stages of learning something new may take longer, but once learning has taken place, elders as a group, are able to keep up with others.

Effect of Medications on Mental Abilities
Medications taken for other problems may impair mental abilities if taken in the wrong amount, at the wrong time, or skipped altogether. Older patients take an average of four to five different medications and one to two over-the-counter medications daily. Providing the patient with a pill organizer, a printed list of the medications he or she is taking, and why he or she is taking them, may help decrease incorrect medicating. The caregivers should be provided with these aids if the patient is not competent. Warn the patient about possible food or drug interactions with written and verbal information. When taking a patient history, ask several times about over-the-counter preparations, vitamins, and herbal supplements since the patient may not view these products as "medications."

Confusion
Confusion, a term used by physicians and health care providers to indicate that the person cannot follow a conversation, answer questions appropriately, understand where he or she is, remember important facts, or make appropriate safety judgments. Confusion is not a normal consequence of aging. If confusion is noted in a patient, the cause needs to be determined. As stated previously, it could be from medication reactions, thyroid dysfunction, or pathologic conditions such as

Alzheimer's disease, stroke, brain tumor, or substance overuse or abuse. Pinpointing the exact cause may be difficult and may finally be determined by the process of elimination of other possible causes.

SUNDOWNER SYNDROME   Sundowner syndrome is a type of confusion occurring in some older patients after sundown or at night. It happens more frequently in those with some cognitive impairment. Factors that may increase the incidence of sundowner syndrome are disruption of routine such as hospital admission, unfamiliar surrounding, disturbance in sleep patterns, restraints, or excessive sensory stimulation, such as leaving lights on all night or excessive noise. In the morning, symptoms subside. Surrounding the patient with familiar objects, establishing a routine, controlling room lighting, temperature, and noise level may relieve the problem.

Depression

Depression is defined by the American Medical Association as "an abnormal and persistent mood characterized by sadness, melancholy, slowed mental processes, and changes in eating and sleeping habits." Medical depression is confirmed if the five above symptoms have been present daily for two weeks. Life changes may overwhelm the aging person causing depression that can worsened with some medication interactions. Depression is often overlooked in the elderly or misdiagnosed as crankiness or part of another problem. Sometimes depression can be misdiagnosed as dementia. Maintaining a good rapport with elderly patients so they feel comfortable enough to speak to you is beneficial. You can detect changes in their mental state, making you a better member of the health care team.

Dementia

Dementia is a syndrome marked by progressive loss of memory and other intellectual functions. It can occur at any age, but more frequently it is found in the elderly. Dementia affects about seven percent of people over 65. The onset is usually slow and because changes in behavior are subtle at first, it may be difficult to detect. Dementia is not a normal consequence of aging and is irreversible unless caused by a treatable condition such as electrolyte imbalance or thyroid dysfunction. Half of the people over 100 have no signs of dementia. Dementia is different from normal age-related forgetfulness. An older person may misplace keys or fail to remember a person's name, while a dementia patient forgets that he or she has a car and fails to recognize the individual at all. Approximately half of dementia patients suffer from Alzheimer's disease. Other causes may be:

- Stroke
- Parkinson's disease
- Brain tumor
- AIDS
- Drug and alcohol abuse

DEMENTIA SYMPTOMS   In patients with dementia, symptoms gradually worsen at different rates over a two to ten year period. Patients with vascular dementia progress differently from other dementia patients. After a vascular incident, symptoms tend to worsen and then seem to improve between strokes. In dementia or Alzheimer patients, there is a steady decline with no improvement. The first sign of dementia is usually forgetfulness regarding recent events or places. The individual has difficulty learning new information and may ask repetitive questions. The patient may forget what he or she is doing while in the middle of a task. He or she may forget the correct word for everyday objects, have difficulty with time orientation, and misplace items or put them in an inappropriate place. Often the patient will show a lack of emotion, have mood swings, and demonstrate lack of initiative or disinterest in something he or she previously loved to do such as play golf. As dementia progresses, patients become unable to follow conversations, perform activities of daily living, and eventually become bedridden as the brain shuts down leading to death.

Alzheimer's Disease

Alzheimer's disease (AD) is a progressive disorder of the central nervous system that eventually destroys mental capacities. It occurs more frequently in the elderly. At this time, there is no known cause or cure for this disease. Genetic factors do play a role. Scientists have pinpointed several gene abnormalities linked to the type of AD that seems to run in families.

Alzheimer's disease can have a devastating effect on family members as well as on the patient. One of the first signs of Alzheimer's disease is loss of memory. While there is a normal loss of some memory age (forgetting dates, names, and telephone numbers), the memory loss with Alzheimer's is profound. The patient may not remember where he or she lives and forget who family members are.

SYMPTOMS OF ALZHEIMER'S DISEASE   In the United States, AD affects about 10% of the people over 65 years of age, 20% of those over 75, and 50% of those over 85. It costs billions of dollars each year to care for these patients and the costs will rise as the elderly population increases. Recognizing the symptoms of this and other forms of dementia are necessary for medical assistants so they may be proactive in providing assistance to the patients and caregivers.

Diagnoses of dementia and AD are done by eliminating other potential factors. A patient who is suspected of having dementia should have a complete physical examination, blood profile, a thorough medical and family history, a MRI, and a PET scan. After ruling out possible causes, such as thyroid and medication imbalance, the patient should be given a frequently used mental status examination called Mini Mental Status Exam. This test requires about five to ten minutes and consists of a series of tasks to evaluate recall, writing, and math skills. If the patient scores lower than expected for his or her age, more extensive testing should be ordered. A significant portion of the AD/dementia diagnosis depends on symptoms revealed by the patient and family members or caregivers. The ultimate diagnosis of Alzheimer's disease may only be confirmed by an autopsy with the detection of plaque, dense protein deposits around the brain's nerve cells and tangles, which are twisted protein fibers inside the nerve cells. Initially, dementia patients may try to cover up errors or inabilities and are unwilling to accept that they are having difficulties. Other symptoms include agitation, restlessness, irritability, an inability to care for oneself, incontinence, and inability to communicate. Alzheimer's disease progresses through various stages over a two to ten year period.

TREATMENT   There is no treatment to recover any of the mental functions that have been lost and no way to prevent the loss of more functions in Alzheimer patients. During early stages of dementia, medications, such as Aricept, are purported to slow the progression of the disease. Patients should not drink alcohol, which can worsen the symptoms of AD. Some depressed AD patients may benefit by taking antidepressants in the early stages. Creating a soothing home environment, avoiding criticism, and avoiding constantly correcting errors, helps reduce the stress for AD patients (Figure 37-13). Using community resources for patients and caregivers can help them to deal with the complex circumstances caused by this condition. Support groups can help the caregivers establish contact with others in the same situation.

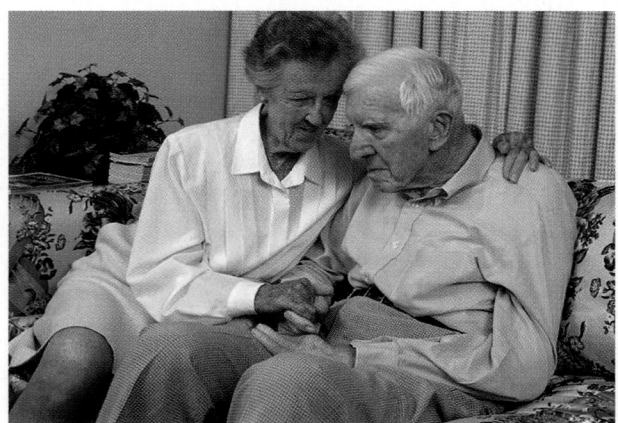

FIGURE 37-13   Familiar objects and a stable environment can reduce some behavioral problems with dementia patients.

Often support groups provide ideas for coping strategies that have worked for others. Helping caregivers locate respite care, which is a temporary interlude of care for the patient to allow the caregiver time for relaxation, can be of great assistance. Many caregivers provide 24-hour care with no outside help for extended periods of time. This often leads to caregiver burnout and in some cases, results in elder abuse. Respite care relief will help caregivers relieve the extraordinary demands of this disease.

Dementia Patient in the Office

In the office, dealing with a dementia patient can be challenging. The patient with Alzheimer's disease must be kept in safe surroundings with someone observing his or her movements. The patient cannot be left alone in a reception or examination room. Having routines and structure in the AD patient's daily life seems to reduce anxiety and stress in the dementia patient. Following a simple routine within the office may be helpful. Always tell the patient what you are going to do and what to expect next, although they may not comprehend your information. Speak to the patient in slow simple terms and be ready to repeat instructions without exasperation. Make eye contact with the patient and use appropriate body language. A warm smile is often reassuring and a simple touch on the arm to guide the patient may encourage him or her to following your instructions. Sometimes using tactics of diversion and distraction such as directing attention to something else works to relieve tension. Keep in mind that the dementia patient cannot control his or her impulses. Allow the patient to "save face" and maintain dignity because no one really knows what is going on in his or her mind. On the other hand, the patient may be uncooperative and the physician will need to decide if the circumstances warrant taking a firm stand with the patient and more extraordinary measures. Procedure 37-6 provides steps for communicating effectively with the elderly.

Legal and Medical Decisions

Families of elders who are progressively declining will ultimately face difficult decisions such as when to take away car keys for safety reasons, when to speak about advanced directives, what to do with a "living will" once it is written, when to take over the decision making, and ultimately if and when to place the patient in a long-term-care facility. It is the professional responsibility of physicians and lawyers to provide guidance to caregivers when making these difficult decisions. However, having an understanding of these difficult decisions, an awareness of where to locate materials to help the caregivers, and acting as a go-between the family and the physician may make things easier for the caregivers.

Communicating Effectively with the Elderly

OBJECTIVE: Communicate effectively with a new elderly patient preparing for a physical examination.

Equipment and Supplies

pen and paper; patient history form; examination table; gown and drapes; other physical examination equipment as needed

Method

1. Welcome the patient in the front office warmly with a smile.
2. Face the patient and speak clearly and directly to him or her.
3. Introduce yourself. Be sincere and polite.
4. Address the patient by Mr., Mrs. or Ms. unless otherwise instructed by the patient.
5. Observe the patient for cues to indicate comprehension of your remarks.
6. If it appears that the patient does not comprehend, paraphrase using other words and simple gestures.
7. Ask the patient to follow you to the examination room.
8. Allow sufficient time for the patient to process information.
9. Observe the patient's overall physical ability to comply with your request.
10. Offer assistance if you think it appears he/she needs it. Allow the patient to do as much for him or herself as possible.
11. Ask the patient to be seated while you begin to gather information for the patient history.
12. Speak respectfully and convey a feeling of warmth and empathy. If the patient's replies to questions become too lengthy, gently interrupt, and bring the patient back to the subject.
13. Never assume the patient is incompetent of understanding you because he or she is old.
14. If answers to some of your questions appear to be inappropriate, do not correct the patient. Gently distract them with another topic and proceed with examination preparations.
15. Save questions pertaining to patient's history that received inappropriate answers to ask caregiver or family member at a later time.
16. Do not leave the patient unattended if they are confused.
17. Do not argue with the patient's view of reality. Remember that relaxed body language, facial expressions, and a caring touch are most important in caring for confused patients.
18. Chart all your findings and impressions.

Charting Example

03/18/XX	Pt appeared confused. Unable to follow
	directions or to undress w/o help. Attitude cheerful.
	M. King, CMA

Informed Consent

Informed consent must be obtained from the patient and a written document to that effect placed in the patient's chart for any procedure other than basic care. In the case of a patient who is too ill, confused, or suffering from dementia, the family may consent to the procedure. Family members may need to be encouraged to obtain the appointment of guardian to grant consent for the incompetent individual. It is the responsibility of the court to grant guardianship. You may provide the family with information about how to proceed with obtaining it and identify a state agency that can assist them. Guardianship invalidates a power of attorney because power of attorney implies competency of the patient.

Advanced Directives

Death and dying issues are dealt with mainly in an inpatient facility. Understanding advanced directives and do not resuscitate (DNR) orders allows you to function more professionally to help patients and caregivers. To review, an advanced directive or living will provides guidelines or directives formulated by the patient that expresses his or her desires about terminal care. In an advanced directive, the individual may state whether or not he or she wants to be resuscitated. The

Professionalism

patients and family members should be aware that they need to spell out what other directives they wish to choose if the patient degrades into a persistent vegetative state. These other directives may indicate if he or she wants medicine withheld, except for pain relief and whether they want feeding and hydration withheld. Patients and families often are under the assumption that when they have a DNR order written it covers all life-sustaining treatments as well. Providing families and patients with information, such as Internet sites to obtain samples of a living will is helpful. In most states, unless the physician writes a specific order restating what the patient has expressed in the advanced directive, a directive is not binding on the staff and facility. Just having a copy of the living will in the bedside table is not enough. Ways to keep current in your field so that you may better assist patients and their families (such as with information regarding DNRs) are discussed in Professionalism.

Elder Abuse

Elder abuse may occur at home from family members or caregivers and in institutions. Elder abuse has many forms including stealing a patient's belongings, inflicting injury and pain, mishandling funds, withholding care such as food, drink, or medication, sexual abuse, threatening a patient, and confining a patient. As a medical assistant, you must be alert to all signs of abuse. All cases of abuse suspected or known must be reported. Organizations such as the National Center of Elder Abuse, American Association of Retired Persons, and state agencies on aging provide information on abuse.

Safety Guidelines for Children and Elders

Since both children and the elderly have to rely on others for care and living accommodations, safety issues are of prime concern. Patients and caregivers should be aware of safety risks and interventions to eliminate or reduce those risks.

Safety of the Elderly

The elderly may be faced with increased risk of injury and may have a reduced capacity to protect themselves. The U.S. Department of Commerce states that the rate of injury per 1,000 in the population is 110.8 for those under 12, 167.5 for those ages 12–21, and 113.8 for those over 65. While the elderly rate of injury is slightly higher than that of young children, it is well below the rate of injury of teens and young adults. The normal aging processes and declining health place the elderly at risk for falling, sustaining fractures, and other injuries. Early identification and correction of health problems helps reduce safety risks. Confusion, disorientation, decreased memory, and poor judgment decrease the ability of the elderly to reduce hazards to their health and safety. Environmental risks in the following areas should be identified and corrected:

Lighting—Provide adequate lighting and reduce glare. Several smaller areas of light are better in a room than one overhead light which produces glare. The elderly's eyes are sensitive to glare.

Electrical cords—Electrical cords should not be in traffic flow areas. Overloaded electrical outlets may cause fire.

Furniture—Furniture for the elderly should be sturdy with good armrests lending support for standing. Rooms stuffed with furniture and bric-a-brac increase a patient's risk of falling.

Rugs—All area rugs should be removed.

Floor wax—Highly polished floors increase the risk of falling.

Bathroom—A small light in the bathroom that is on all the time is helpful. The elderly use the bathroom frequently and can avoid reaching for a switch inside the room. Tub and showers should have non-stick surfaces and grab bars and chairs for support in bathing. Toilets should have grab bars and if the toilet is low a raised seat attachment is needed.

Emergency numbers—emergency numbers should be near each phone including police and fire departments, close relatives, or friends.

Safety of Children

The number one cause of death in children is injury. Injuries cause more deaths than all diseases combined. To reduce risk for children under five, the following suggestions should be followed:

- Smoke detectors on every floor of a house
- Use protective covers over electrical outlets

- Never leave a small child alone in a bathtub or pool even for a few seconds
- Keep side rails up on cribs
- Keep a night light on in halls and bathrooms
- Store dangerous products out of reach
- Post poison control number by the telephone
- Teach all children how to dial 911
- Remove any toys with small parts that could obstruct airways

SUMMARY

The medical assistant should be prepared to function competently with both pediatric and geriatric patients. Medical assistants need to have an understanding of childhood growth and development, the common childhood disorders, uncommon diseases, and genetic disorders. As a medical assistant, you must be able to accurately perform procedures such as obtaining vital signs on children, measuring their height and weight, and assisting with all phases of the sick and well-child examinations.

The geriatric patient may have many chronic problems that will require medical attention. As a medical assistant, comprehending the aging process and how it affects those over 65 is vital to providing good health care. Comprehending facts about the aging United States population and the impact it will have on health care is important. The number of dementia and specifically Alzheimer's patients will be increasing. You must understand the devastating effects of these conditions and be prepared to provide intelligent assistance to the patient and caregivers. After completing this chapter, you can be an understanding, compassionate, competent caregiver to both categories of patients.

Chapter Review

COMPETENCY REVIEW

1. Define and spell the terms to learn in this chapter.
2. The pediatrician has asked you to develop a teaching plan for obese children under 8. What is your plan?
3. Your office has several patients suffering from dementia. Each is in a different stage. You are asked to prepare a summary of the different stages and related behaviors for the next staff meeting to help coworkers better understand these patients.

PREPARING FOR THE CERTIFICATION EXAM

1. A medical doctor who treats and diagnoses the elderly is a(n)
   A. neurologist
   B. pediatrician
   C. geriatrician
   D. gastroenterologist
   E. orthopedist

2. Bacterial meningitis can be caused by
   A. streptococcus
   B. rubeola virus
   C. roseola virus
   D. rubella virus
   E. herpes zoster virus

continued on next page

3. Infants should always be put to sleep on their backs to
   A. prevent SIDS
   B. prevent stomach aches
   C. prevent vomiting
   D. allow for hiccups
   E. allow mother to see if the child is asleep

4. At twelve months of age a child who is developmentally on target is NOT able to
   A. wave bye-bye
   B. stand unassisted
   C. take a few steps
   D. feed self with fingers
   E. drinks from a cup

5. Signs of dementia include all of the following EXCEPT
   A. wandering and pacing
   B. disorientation of time
   C. depression
   D. exhibit interest and spontaneity
   E. exhibit signs of persecution

6. Which of the following is true about elders?
   A. live comfortably on Social Security
   B. have the different emotional needs than younger people
   C. like to live with their children
   D. are not interested in sex
   E. are not less productive workers

7. Signs of aging in the integumentary system do NOT include
   A. thickening of the skin
   B. graying of the hair
   C. easily bruising
   D. dryness of skin
   E. age spots

8. Medical assistants who assist the elderly should NOT exhibit the following characteristics
   A. patience
   B. kindness
   C. empathy
   D. sense of humor
   E. sternness

9. The average weight of a newborn is
   A. 5 pounds
   B. 6 pounds
   C. 7 pounds
   D. 8 pounds
   E. 9 pounds

10. A genetic disorder that causes mild incurable anemia to severe hemolytic anemia is
   A. muscular dystrophy
   B. cystic fibrosis
   C. thalassemia
   D. PKU
   E. sickle cell anemia

CRITICAL THINKING

1. What questions should you ask Grandma Graves? Why?

2. What should you tell her to do in the next 24 hours for Connor? Why?

3. After consulting with the physician, he tells you to have the caregiver bring the child in if the fever is over 101°F and he has two to three more episodes of diarrhea within the 24-hour period. He also recommends the child be given liquids like Pedialyte as often as possible, and Tylenol, not aspirin if Connor's fever elevates. Why are these specific recommendations made?

ON THE JOB

Olive Johnson is a 62-year old practicing lawyer and a patient of Dr. O'Brian. She is coming in today for an annual physical examination. On arrival, she seems cheerful, talkative, and cooperative as usual. After placing her in the examination room, giving her instructions about obtaining a urine sample, and where to have the gown opening, she seems confused and frustrated. She is unable to open the gown properly and mistakes the door to the hallway for the bathroom door. After directing her to the bathroom, you can hear her crying from the other side of the door.

1. How should you handle the situation?
2. What possible conditions could be causing her confusion?
3. How and when should you inform Dr. O'Brian about Olive's behavior?
4. What tests do you think the doctor should order?

INTERNET ACTIVITY

Select your own ethnic group or one in which you are interested (Greek, Irish, Chinese) and do an Internet search for issues related to aging in that group using "_____-elderly."

MediaLink More on assisting in life span specialties, including interactive resources, can be found on the Student CD-ROM accompanying this textbook.

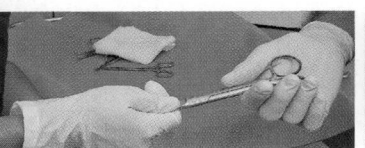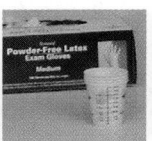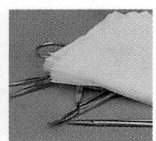

Medical Assistant Role Delineation Chart

HIGHLIGHT indicates material covered in this chapter.

ADMINISTRATIVE

Administrative Procedures

- Perform basic administrative medical assisting functions
- Schedule, coordinate and monitor appointments
- Schedule inpatient/outpatient admissions and procedures
- Understand and apply third-party guidelines
- Obtain reimbursement through accurate claims submission
- Monitor third-party reimbursement
- Understand and adhere to managed care policies and procedures
- *Negotiate managed care contracts*

Practice Finances

- Perform procedural and diagnostic coding
- Apply bookkeeping principles

- Manage accounts receivable
- *Manage accounts payable*
- *Process payroll*
- *Document and maintain accounting and banking records*
- *Develop and maintain fee schedules*
- *Manage renewals of business and professional insurance policies*
- *Manage personnel benefits and maintain records*
- *Perform marketing, financial, and strategic planning*

CLINICAL

Fundamental Principles

- Apply principles of aseptic technique and infection control
- Comply with quality assurance practices
- Screen and follow up patient test results

Diagnostic Orders

- Collect and process specimens
- Perform diagnostic tests

Patient Care

- Adhere to established patient screening procedures
- Obtain patient history and vital signs
- Prepare and maintain examination and treatment areas
- Prepare patient for examinations, procedures and treatments

- Assist with examinations, procedures and treatments
- Prepare and administer medications and immunizations
- Maintain medication and immunization records
- Recognize and respond to emergencies
- Coordinate patient care information with other health care providers
- Initiate IV and administer IV medications with appropriate training and as permitted by state law

GENERAL

Professionalism

- Display a professional manner and image
- Demonstrate initiative and responsibility
- Work as a member of the health care team
- Prioritize and perform multiple tasks
- Adapt to change
- Promote the CMA credential
- Enhance skills through continuing education
- Treat all patients with compassion and empathy
- Promote the practice through positive public relations

Communication Skills

- Recognize and respect cultural diversity
- Adapt communications to individual's ability to understand
- Use professional telephone technique

- Recognize and respond effectively to verbal, nonverbal, and written communications
- Use medical terminology appropriately
- Utilize electronic technology to receive, organize, prioritize and transmit information
- Serve as liaison

Legal Concepts

- Perform within legal and ethical boundaries
- Prepare and maintain medical records
- Document accurately
- Follow employer's established policies dealing with the health care contract
- Implement and maintain federal and state health care legislation and regulations
- Comply with established risk management and safety procedures
- Recognize professional credentialing criteria
- *Develop and maintain personnel, policy and procedure manuals*

Instruction

- Instruct individuals according to their needs
- Explain office policies and procedures
- Teach methods of health promotion and disease prevention
- Locate community resources and disseminate information
- *Develop educational materials*
- *Conduct continuing education activities*

Operational Functions

- Perform inventory of supplies and equipment
- Perform routine maintenance of administrative and clinical equipment
- Apply computer techniques to support office operations
- *Perform personnel management functions*
- *Negotiate leases and prices for equipment and supply contracts*

■ *Denotes advanced skills.*

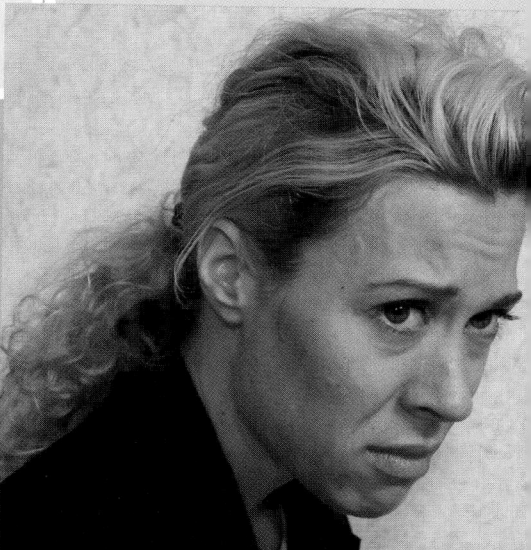

Assisting with Minor Surgery

Learning Objectives

After completing this chapter, you should be able to:

- Define and spell the terms to learn for this chapter.
- Discuss all guidelines for surgical aseptic technique.
- List and differentiate between the types of ambulatory surgery.
- Describe the differences between medical asepsis and surgical asepsis.
- List and describe instruments for cutting, dissecting, grasping, clamping, probing, and dilating.
- Explain the guidelines for handling instruments.
- Give five examples of suture materials, including gauge ranges, with examples of when they may be used.

- Describe the preparation of the patient for minor surgery.
- List equipment and supplies used for preparing the patient's skin for surgery.
- Define informed consent. Discuss the medical assistant's role in the process.
- Describe at least five surgical procedures that can be performed in the physician's office and indicate the responsibility of the medical assistant for each procedure.
- Explain the four types of wounds.
- Describe the stages of healing.
- Discuss postoperative care as it applies to recovery from anesthesia, wound care, and suture removal.

OUTLINE

Ambulatory Surgery	764
Principles of Surgical Asepsis	764
Handling Sterile Instruments	769
Surgical Assisting	779
Preparing the Patient for Minor Surgery	783
Postoperative Patient Care	786
Surgical Procedures Performed in the Medical Office	791

Terms to Learn

ambulatory surgery	eschar	Mayo stand
anesthesia	evisceration	outpatient surgery
biopsy	hyfrecators	scrub assistant
cryosurgery	incision	sterile field
debridement	invasive procedure	surgical scrub
dehiscence		

Case Study

MRS. JONES, A 38-YEAR-OLD FEMALE, has an appointment to have a cyst removed from her right scapula. You have given her information about the procedure, including the fact that there might be some discomfort when she receives the local anesthetic, but the doctor does not believe that sutures will be required. She is very apprehensive about the procedure and has called your office several times this week with more questions. When she arrives for her appointment, she begins to cry as you bring her to the examining room to prepare for her procedure.

This chapter discusses surgical aseptic technique also known as sterile technique. Procedures requiring sterile technique, such as minor surgical procedures, suture insertion and removal, breast biopsy, incision and drainage, removal of growths, and wound treatment, are included. Strict adherence to aseptic technique is necessary when assisting with these procedures. It is important to always remember that an item is either sterile or nonsterile. If there is any doubt about sterility, assume it is nonsterile.

Medical assistants perform many duties related to minor surgery (Figure 38-1). Prior to surgery you will perform administrative duties such as completing insurance forms, obtaining consent forms, and meeting with the patient to answer questions related to the procedure. Upon completion of the procedure, your duties will include providing postoperative instructions such as wound care. Other duties will comprise of setting up the instruments for the procedure, assisting the physician during the procedure, cleaning the examining room after the surgery, sanitizing and disinfecting or autoclaving the instruments used, and restocking supplies as needed.

Ambulatory Surgery

Ambulatory surgery is a method for performing surgical procedures in which the patient is able to walk into and out of the surgical facility on the day of the surgery. This includes outpatient surgery, surgicenter surgery, and office surgery. Since ambulatory surgery is on the increase, the medical assistant is spending more time assisting the physician with surgical procedures.

Ambulatory surgery, with its emphasis on surgical procedures performed outside the hospital setting, has resulted in a cost savings to the consumer and to the insurer. Hospitalization is not required unless there is an unexpected complication. The patient is able to return home after a brief recovery time in the outpatient facility or medical office. The disadvantage to this type of surgery is the short time the health care team has for assessing the patient's postoperative condition. It is important for each outpatient facility to develop a consistent follow-up procedure to track the patient's condition after leaving.

Outpatient Surgery

Outpatient surgery is generally limited to procedures requiring less than 60 minutes to perform. Today, many surgeries are performed in free-standing surgicenters or surgical centers that are part of a hospital complex. Categories of surgeries are as follows:

- Elective—considered medically necessary, but can be performed when the patient wishes (for example, removal of benign growths)

- Emergency—required immediately to save a life (for example, hemorrhage) or prevent further injury or infection

- Optional—may not be medically necessary, but the patient wishes to have it performed (for example, cosmetic surgery and vasectomy)

- Outpatient—does not require an overnight stay in a hospital

- Urgent—to be performed as soon as possible, but is not an immediate or acute emergency (for example, cancer surgery)

Principles of Surgical Asepsis

Surgical asepsis, or sterile technique, is used when sterility of supplies and the immediate environment is required, as in surgical procedures. Sterile technique results in the killing of all microorganisms and spores. It is necessary during any invasive procedure, a procedure in which the body is entered, such as when administering an injection, making a surgical incision, or working with an open wound.

Open tissues provide an excellent reservoir (host) for infection. Infections can delay the healing process, cause permanent harm or death to a patient, and result in additional medical costs. Sterile technique prevents microorganisms from being introduced into the body, thereby decreasing the risk of infection.

Both medical asepsis and surgical asepsis are similar in their overall purpose of decreasing the risk of infection. Medical asepsis is a reduction in the number of microorganisms, such as when you wipe a counter top with disinfectant. Medical asepsis results in a "clean" approach in which materials can be handled with clean hands or nonsterile gloves. Surgical asepsis means a complete absence of microorganisms and spores. Surgical asepsis requires a sterile hand washing or scrub, sterile gloves, and sterile technique when handling materials. A way to remember the difference is to recall,

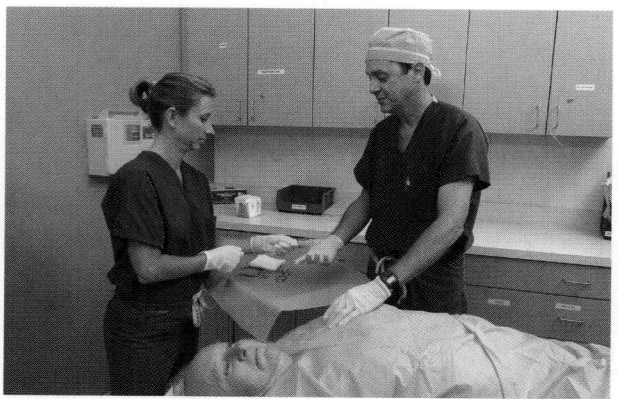

FIGURE 38-1 A medical assistant helps with a dressing change.

"clean for clean" and "sterile for sterile." For example, use clean hands when applying a clean bandage to unbroken skin. Use sterile procedure when handling sterile materials, such as using sterile gloves when touching sterile instruments. See Table 38-1 for a comparison of medical and surgical asepsis.

Guidelines for Surgical Asepsis

When practicing surgical asepsis, follow the guidelines presented here or those used in your office. Guidelines 38-1 provides some rules for surgical asepsis. Refer to this list of key points often as you read through the chapter. They are the ground rules for establishing a sterile field.

The purpose of personal protective equipment (PPE) (also see Chapter 32) is to protect the patient and health care worker from exposure to pathogenic organisms. Remember that nonsterile scrub suits should not be worn home. All personnel should change to street clothes before leaving a medical facility.

TABLE 38-1 Surgical Asepsis versus Medical Asepsis

Surgical Asepsis	Medical Asepsis
Sterile technique used	Clean technique used
Absence of microorganisms	Controls microorganisms
Surgical scrub performed	Basic hand hygiene procedure used
Sterile equipment and supplies required	Clean equipment and supplies
Sterile field	Clean field

38-1   **GUIDELINES**   **Surgical Asepsis**

A sterile item can only touch another sterile item.
- If a sterile item touches a nonsterile item, it is contaminated.
- If a clean item touches a sterile item, it is contaminated.
- A sterile packet that is torn, wet, or punctured is contaminated.
- A sterile packet is contaminated after the date on the packet.
- If unsure of sterility, consider the item contaminated.
- Skin is always considered contaminated. It cannot be sterilized only disinfected.

A sterile item on a sterile field must be within your field of vision and above your waist.
- If you cannot see an item, it is contaminated.
- If items or your hands are below your waist, they are contaminated.
- If you turn your back on a sterile field, it is contaminated.
- If you leave a sterile field unattended, it is contaminated.

Airborne microorganisms contaminate sterile fields.
- Do not place sterile fields in a draft.
- Avoid extra movements near the sterile field.

- Do not talk, cough, sneeze, or laugh over a sterile field.
- Wear a mask if you need to talk during a procedure.
- Do not reach over a sterile field.
- Avoid spills on a sterile field. A wet field is contaminated.

The edges of a sterile field are contaminated.
- If an item touches any part of the one-inch border around the sterile field, it is contaminated.

Sterile gloves must only touch sterile items.
- Do not touch the outside of sterile gloves with bare hands.
- Sterile gloves are contaminated if punctured. Remove and dispose of the item and gloves, rescrub, and reglove.

Sterile packets may be touched on the outside with bare hands.
- Outer wrappings are considered contaminated.
- Open sterile packets away from you to avoid contaminating the packet by touching your clothing.
- Never rewrap an unused sterile packet. The unused items must be re-sanitized, rewrapped, and re-autoclaved.

Be honest if you make an error or suspect you have made an error.
- Remove the contaminated item and correct the error.
- Report contamination to your superior.

PROCEDURE

Surgical Hand Hygiene/Sterile Scrub

OBJECTIVE: Perform surgical scrub on hands and arms using the correct procedure for the appropriate length of time.

Equipment and Supplies

germicidal dispenser soap (not bar soap); sterile scrub brush; sterile towel pack (with 2 to 3 sterile paper or cloth towels); paper towels; sterile gloves (prepackaged); running water (foot pedal preferable); nail file

Method

1. Remove all jewelry. With a nail file, remove any gross dirt from beneath fingernails before scrubbing. Rationale: microorganisms can accumulate in crevices of rings or watches and under fingernails.
2. Assemble equipment.
3. Stand at the sink without allowing your body to touch it. Rationale: Sink is considered contaminated with microorganisms.
4. Remove your lab coat. Roll up your sleeves above elbows. Keep your hands and arms above waist

level at all times. Rationale: All areas below the waist are considered contaminated.
5. Regulate running water temperature to warm, not hot. Rationale: Hot water can cause hands to chap and crack, which can provide a source of cross-infection.
6. Place hands under running water with hands pointed upward. Allow water to run from fingertips to elbows. Rationale: If water ran downward from the unscrubbed arm to the hands, it would contaminate the scrubbed hands.
7. Apply a circle of soap from the dispenser and lather well.
8. Vigorously scrub your hands and wrists with a scrub brush (Figure 38-2A). Wash thoroughly between fingers. Scrub under fingernails. Scrub toward the elbows using 5 minutes on each hand (Figure 38-2B, C).

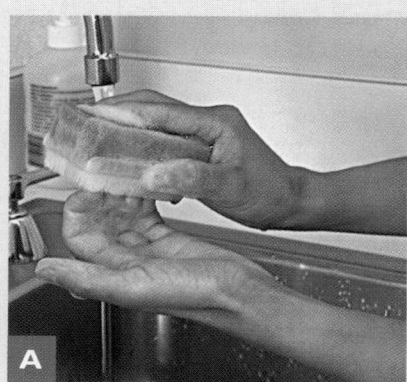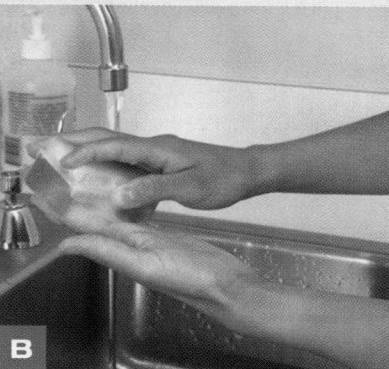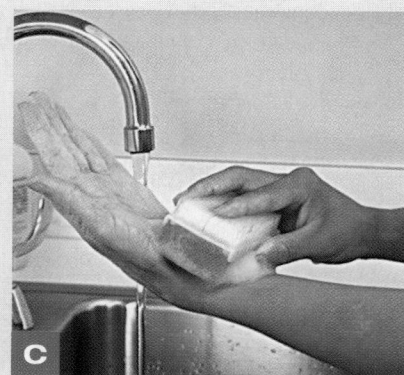

FIGURE 38-2 Sterile scrub hand hygiene.

9. Raise hands, bending at the elbow, and place them under running water to rinse off soap (Figure 38-2D). Allow water to flow from fingertips to elbows (Figure 38-2E).

10. If performing a second lather and scrub is the policy in your facility, use 3 minutes for each hand.

11. Using a sterile towel (if possible), pat hands dry moving from fingertips to wrists, and then to elbows. Hands should still be held above the elbows (Figure 38-2F).

12. Turn off faucet with a fresh towel if foot lever not available (Figure 38-2G). Rationale: The faucet and handles are considered unclean. A towel protects clean hands from contamination.

13. Glove immediately. Keep hands above waist and folded together until the procedure begins.

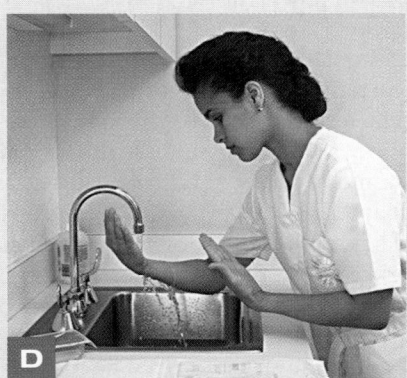
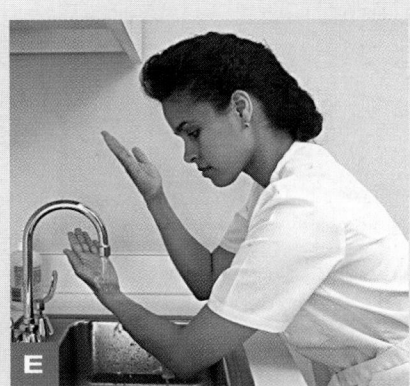
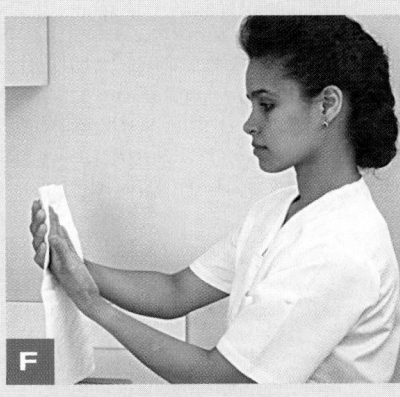
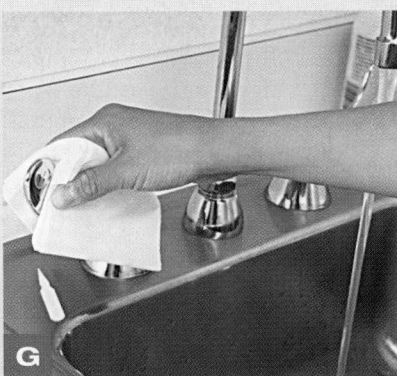

FIGURE 38-2 (*continued*)

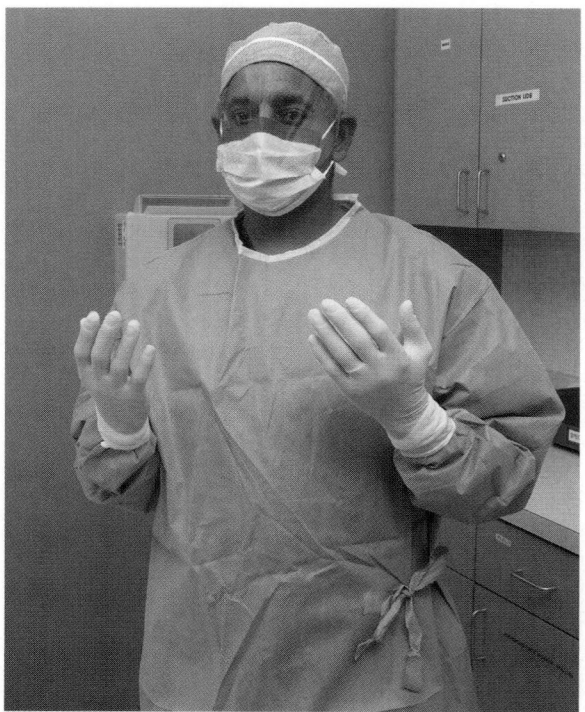

FIGURE 38-3 A medical assistant wearing PPE—gown, face shield, and gloves.

Sterile Scrub and Gloving

In Chapter 32, medical asepsis and hand hygiene were introduced. Performing hand hygiene is the number one way to prevent spreading infection. In this chapter, you will learn the procedure for surgical asepsis or a surgical scrub. A surgical scrub removes microorganisms more effectively than regular hand washing. It is necessary that the hands be as free from microorganisms as possible in the event that sterile gloves are punctured during a procedure. Procedure 38-1 and Figure

38-2 demonstrate the steps and rationale involved in performing surgical hand hygiene. Figure 38-3 shows a medical assistant in personal protective equipment (PPE) including face shield, gown, and gloves preparing to assist with a surgical procedure. Personal protective equipment provides a barrier between infectious or hazardous material and the wearer. Remember if a sterile glove is punctured or if you touch the outside of the glove with your hand it is considered nonsterile and must be replaced after you perform another surgical scrub. Procedure 38-2 and Figure 38-4 lists the steps and rationale for surgical gloving and glove removal.

Sterile Packaging

Sterile packages (packets) are prepared for use in surgery. Each one may contain either a single instrument or piece of equipment or several items packed together. These packets are then autoclaved with sterilization indicators and dated. Sterile packs may be purchased from a medical supply company or packaged by the medical assistant in the office. To prepare sterile packets, you must know the names and uses of instruments routinely used in minor surgery and this will be discussed later in the chapter. Review Chapter 32 for packaging and autoclaving procedures. Sterile packets are used for various procedures. For example, all the instruments needed for a procedure, such as a biopsy, are packaged together in a tray and autoclaved. Procedure 38-3 and Figure 38-5 explain the steps for opening a sterile packet.

When assisting the physician or surgeon with the procedure, the medical assistant will set up the specific tray or instruments before the procedure begins. The packets are set up on a Mayo stand, which is a small portable table with enough room to hold an instrument tray. For some procedures, more than one Mayo stand is used. After the sterile packet is opened,

Professionalism

If as a medical assistant you find assisting with minor surgery fascinating, you may wish to pursue additional training to become a surgical technologist. A surgical technologist, also known as a surgical technician or operating technician, works in an operating room as a member of the surgical team. An operating technician's duties include, but are not limited to the following:

- Set up the operating room
- Set up surgical instruments and supplies
- Prepare the patient for surgery
- Drape the incision site
- Assist physicians and nurses don PPE equipment
- Measure vital signs

- Pass instruments
- Operate suction machines, lights
- Prepare specimens for the laboratory
- Dress patient's wound
- Restock operating room supplies

There are about 130 programs for surgical technologists recognized by Committee on Accreditation of Allied Health Education Programs (CAAHEP). Programs average one to two years in length. After completion of the program, you may take a national certification examination. For further information contact the Association of Surgical Technologists, 7108-C South Alton Way, Englewood, CO 80112.

Handling Sterile Instruments

Surgical instruments have been developed over the past centuries to meet a specific need during an operation such as cutting, suturing, or grasping. In some cases, an instrument developed by a surgeon bears the name of the surgeon, for example Kelly forceps, Halstead mosquito clamp, and the Bozeman uterine forceps.

Instruments Used in Minor Office Surgery

The general classification of instruments is based on their use: cutting, dissecting, grasping, clamping, dilating, probing, visualization, or suturing. There are specific instruments related to individual specialties such as gynecology; urology; orthopedics; ear, nose, and throat; proctology; obstetrics; and neurology. A minor surgical setup will include a standard group of instruments such as scalpel, blades, scissors, hemostat, and suture materials. Instruments are usually made of steel and treated to be rust and heat resistant, stain proof, and durable. It is important to be able to identify common instruments used in your facility. Some physicians

the inside of its wrapper becomes the sterile field (a specific area free of all microorganisms that will be the work area for a surgical procedure). The outer, one-inch border all around the open wrapper is considered contaminated. If the field becomes wet, it is contaminated and a new packet must be opened. The physician may want an additional instrument while performing a procedure; you would open a sterile packet and drop the instrument carefully onto the field. Procedure 38-4 and Figure 38-6 show the steps and rationale for dropping a sterile packet onto a sterile field.

Sterile Transfer

In order to place instruments and supplies onto a sterile field or to move them around on the sterile field, you would need to put on sterile gloves or use transfer forceps. Procedure 38-5 and Figure 38-6 for the steps and rationale for transferring sterile objects using transfer forceps. Remember not to reach across the sterile field or turn your back on the field unless it is covered with a sterile towel.

text continues on page 773

Surgical Gloving

OBJECTIVE: Apply sterile gloves without a break in sterile technique.
NOTE: This procedure follows a surgical hand scrub.

Equipment and Supplies
   double-wrapped sterile glove pack

Method
1. Assemble equipment and check the tape or seal for expiration date and condition of pack.
2. Place the pack on a flat surface at waist height with the cuffed end of the gloves toward you.
3. Open the outside wrapper by touching only the outside of the pack. Leave the opened wrapper in place to provide a sterile work field.
4. Open the inner wrapper without reaching over the pack or touching the inside of the wrapper.

Pull inner wrapper edges to each side without touching the inside of the pack (Figure 38-4A). Rationale: Nonsterile persons or items contaminate a sterile field by reaching across it.

5. Using the thumb and fingers of your left hand (if you are right-handed) pick up the glove on the right side of the pack by grasping the folded inside edge of the cuff (Figure 38-4B). The glove can be dangled slightly off the sterile packing material for easier insertion. Rationale: The folded inside edge of the glove will be placed against the skin and thus will be contaminated. The outer portion of the glove must not be touched by an ungloved hand because it must remain sterile.

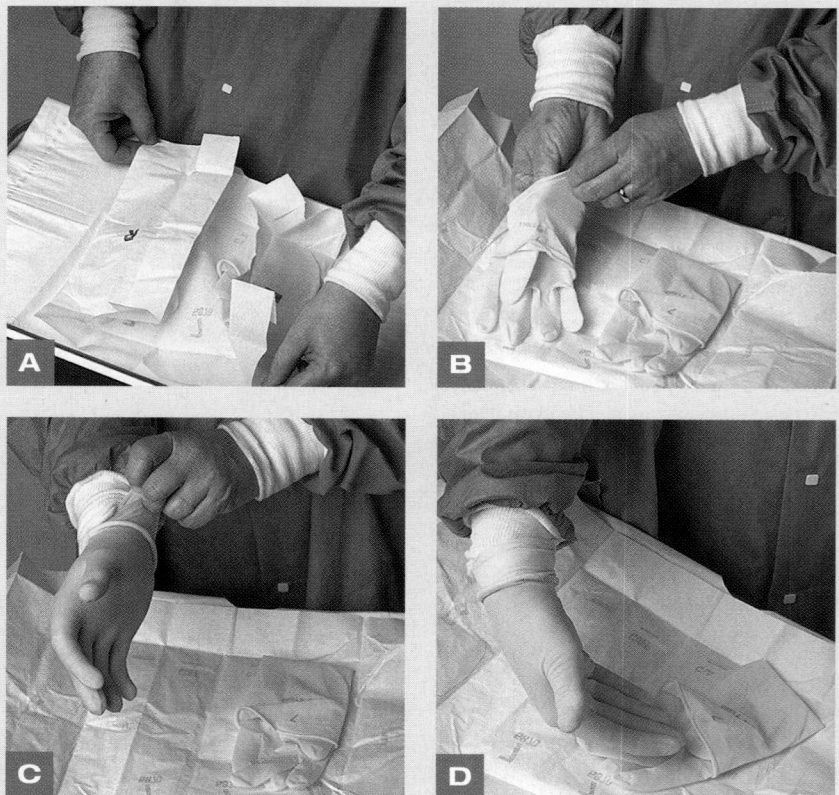

FIGURE 38-4   Sterile gloving and glove removal technique.

6. Pull the glove onto the right hand using only the thumb and fingers of left hand (Figure 38-4C). Do not allow fingers to touch the rest of the glove.
7. Place the fingers of the right-gloved hand under the cuff of the left glove and pull onto the left hand and up over the left wrist (Figure 38-4D). Note: The thumb of the right-gloved hand should not touch the cuff.
8. With the gloved right hand, place your fingers under the cuff of the left glove and pull up over the left wrist (Figure 38-4E). The thumb should not touch the cuff. Rationale: The areas under the cuff are considered sterile. Only gloved fingers can touch this area.
9. After the gloves are in place, the fingers can be adjusted, if necessary, by using the gloved hands (Figure 38-4F).
10. Removing gloves (Figure 38-4G and H): Remove the first glove by grasping the edge of that glove (with fingers of the other gloved hand) and pull the first glove over the hand inside out. Discard the first glove into the proper biohazardous waste container. Remove the other glove by grasping the edge of the cuff with your fingers (from the ungloved hand) and pull the second glove down over the hand, inside out. Discard the gloves appropriately. Rationale: Turning the glove inside out seals in blood and body fluids.

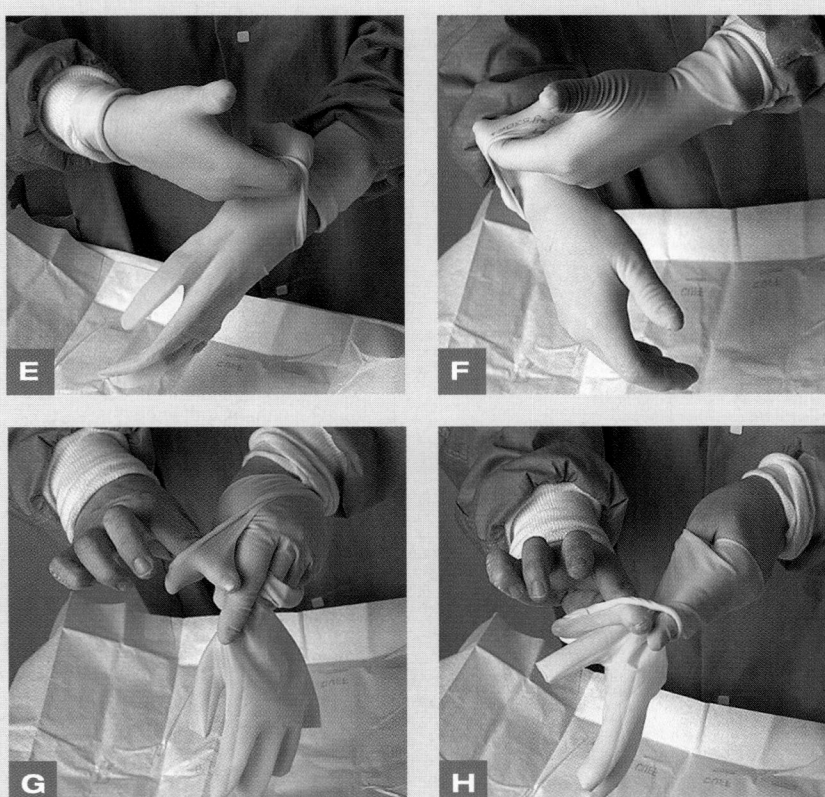

FIGURE 38-4 (*continued*)

PROCEDURE

Opening a Sterile Packet

OBJECTIVE: Open a sterile packet (pack) and use it to set up a sterile field without a break in the sterile technique.

Equipment and Supplies

sterile packet; Mayo stand; waste container; sterile forceps

Method

1. Perform hand hygiene.
2. Assemble equipment. Adjust the Mayo stand to correct height.
3. Place packet on the Mayo stand with the folded edge on top. Position the packet on the stand so that the top flap will fold away from you.
   Rationale: You will not have to reach over the sterile field to open the last flap.
4. Remove the tape or fastener and check the sterilization indicator and date. Discard in a waste container.
5. Pull the corner of the pack that is tucked under and lay this flap away from you. It will hang down over the edge of the Mayo stand (Figure 38-5A and B).
6. With both hands, pull the next two flaps to each side (Figure 38-5C and D). The packet will still be covered with the last layer of the outer wrapper.
7. Grasp the corner of the last flap, without reaching over the sterile field, and open the flap toward your body without touching it (Figure 38-5E and F).
8. The inside of this outer wrapper is now your sterile field. If you need to arrange items within this field, use sterile forceps. If an inner packet needs to be opened with an instrument setup, then someone wearing sterile gloves must open it.

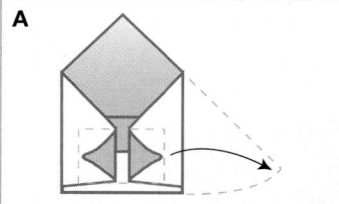
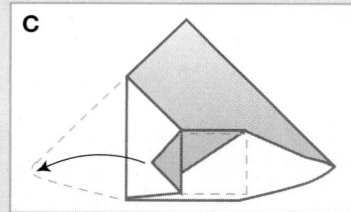
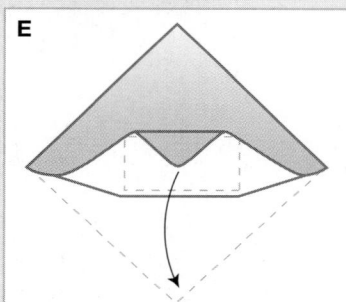
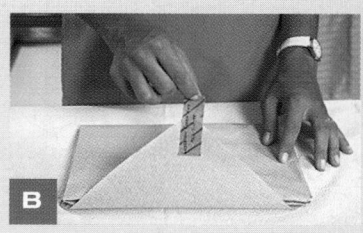
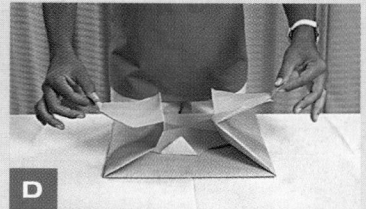
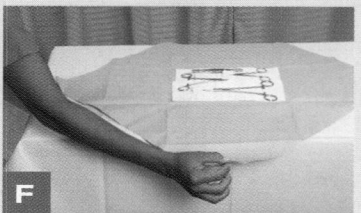

FIGURE 38-5 Opening a sterile packet.

PROCEDURE

Dropping a Sterile Packet onto a Sterile Field

OBJECTIVES: Place (drop) a sterile item onto a sterile field or into a gloved hand without contaminating the packet or the field.

Equipment and Supplies

sterile pack (containing for example: prepackaged items such as a specimen container or needle and syringe in a pull-apart packet)

Method

1. Assemble equipment; check expiration date and sealed condition of packet.
2. Locate the edge on the prepackaged item and pull apart by using the thumb and forefinger of each hand. Do not let your fingers touch the inside of the packet. Rationale: The inside of the packet is sterile and the outside is considered contaminated.
3. Pull the packet apart by securely placing the remaining three fingers of each hand against the outside of the packet on each side. The wrapper edges will be pulled back and away from the sterile item.
4. Holding the item securely about eight to ten inches from the sterile field, gently drop the packet contents inside the sterile field (Figure 38-6). Instead of having you drop the item, the

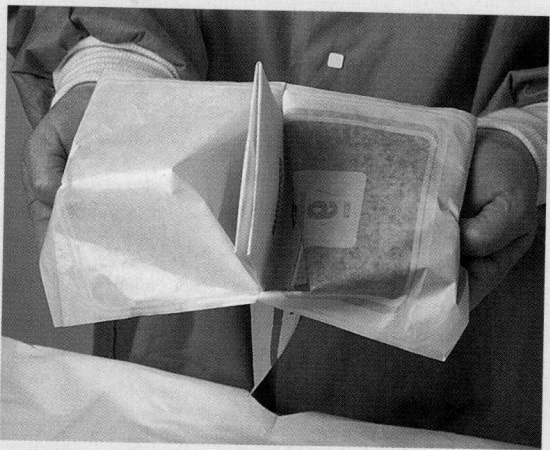

FIGURE 38-6 Dropping sterile supply onto a sterile field.

physician may wish to remove the item directly from the packet by grasping it firmly with his or her gloved hand. Rationale: Nonsterile hands and arms should not be placed over the sterile field.
5. Discard the paper wrapper in a waste container.

---

will use the full name of the instrument, for example Pederson vaginal speculum, and others will just refer to it as a vaginal speculum. The following tips will help you identify instruments.

- Categorize the instrument by its use: to cut, probe, grasp, clamp, retract, dilate
- Examine the types of parts of the instrument and ask yourself the following questions:
  - What type of handles does it have? ring (like scissors), serrated
  - What type of tip does it have? pointed, blunt, teeth, no teeth, serrated
  - What type of closure does it have? spring, box-lock (with a screw), ratchet
  - What type of edges does it have?
  - How long is it? (may indicate what body part it is used for)
  - Whose name does it bear?

Each time you encounter an instrument you are unfamiliar with, answer the above questions to determine its characteristics and remember the name.

Cutting Instruments

Scalpels or knives are used to make incisions, which are surgical cuts into tissue. They are small curved instruments that are made to fit easily into the surgeon's hand. Figure 38-8 illustrates a variety of scalpels and blades. A scalpel blade must be inserted into the scalpel handle. Blades come in various sizes depending on the type of incision and tissue.

Dissecting Instruments

The most common tool for dissecting or cutting tissue is a scissor. For example, scissors are used for debridement (removal of dead tissue around wound edges using sterile technique) or to cut sutures (thread). Scissors have two blades with sharp edges that come together when the handles are drawn together.

PROCEDURE

Transferring Sterile Objects Using Transfer Forceps

OBJECTIVE: Move sterile objects, such as instruments and supplies, within or onto a sterile field or into a gloved hand.

Equipment and Supplies

sterile transfer forceps in a forceps container with a sterilant solution, such as Cidex; Mayo stand with sterile field setup; sterile 4 × 4 gauze package (opened)

Method

1. Grasp forceps handles firmly without separating the tips and remove vertically from the container. Rationale: Open forceps tips could touch the sides of the container which are considered contaminated. Remove vertically to avoid dripping solution onto exposed contaminated portion of forceps.
2. Holding forceps vertically with tips down, gently tap tips together to drop excess solution onto dry sterile 4 × 4 gauze or touch the sterile 4 × 4 gauze to dry the tips.
3. Pick up the sterile item to be transferred by holding transfer forceps vertically with tips down. Do not touch the sterile field. Grasp the article to be transferred firmly at its midsection.
4. Place sterile item within the sterile field (Figure 38-7). Rationale: Remember that the

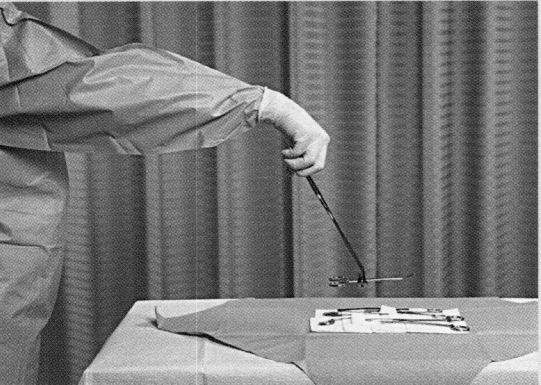

FIGURE 38-7 Proper technique to handle sterile equipment with transfer forceps in a sterile field.

outer one inch of the sterile field is considered contaminated.
5. Place forceps back into container without touching the sides of the container.
6. Clean and sterilize the forceps and container in the autoclave once a week. Change the solution.

The tips of scissors vary greatly to perform a variety of functions. Some scissors have blunt tips that can slide under bandages and dressings to cut without damaging the skin. Metzenbaum scissors are short, curved scissors that are blunt to use on and prevent piercing delicate tissue. Operating scissors or suture scissors are used to cut suture material during surgery. They have a hook on one edge that fits under the suture for ease in suture removal. Dissecting scissors are also called straight or Mayo scissors. Operating scissors are straight or curved with a combination of blades such as sharp/sharp (s/s), blunt/blunt (b/b), and sharp/blunt (s/b); bandage scissors have a blunt tip and a blunt flat edge to allow it to fit easily under a bandage for cutting. Figure 38-9 illustrates a variety of scissors.

Grasping and Clamping Instruments

Forceps are used to grasp tissue or objects (Figure 38-10). One type of forceps is a two-pronged instrument, which has a spring-type handle used to clamp together tightly to prevent slipping. Another type of closure mechanism is called a ratchet closure or clasp. The ratchet clasp allows the forceps to close with differing degrees of tightness. Forceps often have serrations or teeth-like edges that prevent tissue slipping out of the forceps.

TYPES OF FORCEPS   Several different types of widely used forceps are listed below.

- Tissue forceps have teeth and are used to grasp tissue.
- Thumb forceps are two-pronged with serrated tips to hold tissue.
- Splinter forceps are used to grasp foreign bodies.
- Needle holder forceps are used to grasp needles during suturing.
- Hemostats are applied to blood vessels to hold vessels until they can be sutured (Figure 38-11).

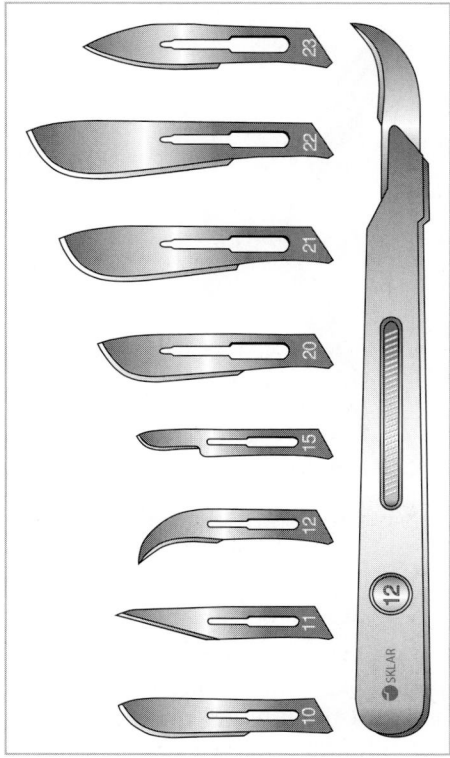

FIGURE 38-8 A variety of scalpels and blades.

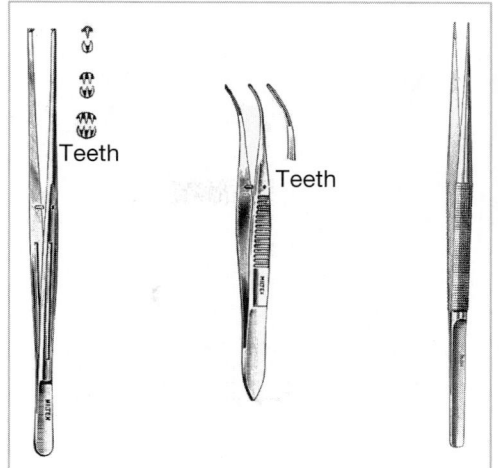

FIGURE 38-10 Types of forceps.

- Sponge forceps are used for holding sponges during surgery.
- Towel clamps are used to hold the edges of sterile drapes together.

Probing and Dilating Instruments

Instruments used to enter body cavities for probing or dilating purposes include:

- Scope—usually lighted, it is inserted into a body cavity or vessel to visualize the internal structures. Figure 38-12 shows different sizes of laryngoscopes that are used to look at a patient's voice

box or larynx. An obturator is placed inside a scope to guide it into a cavity or canal and then removed during visualization of the surgical site. Some obturators have a point used to puncture tissue.

- Speculum—unlighted instrument with movable parts that when inserted into a cavity, such as the vagina, it can be spread apart for ease of visualization and tissue sample removal (Figure 38-13).
- Probe—used to explore wounds and cavities usually with a curved, blunt point to facilitate insertion (Figure 38-14).
- Trocar—used to withdraw fluids from cavities. It consists of a cannula (outer tube), and a sharp stylette that is withdrawn after the trocar is inserted (Figure 38-15).
- Punch—used to remove tissue for examination and biopsy to detect cancerous cells.

Specialized instruments are used for disciplines, such as gynecology and obstetrics (Figure 38-16), urology (Figure 38-17), and orthopedics (Figure 38-18).

Suture Materials and Needles

Suture (thread) materials are used to bring together or approximate a surgical incision or wound until healing takes place. Suture materials are added to the surgical tray setup when they are needed for a procedure. Sutures come either with or without an attached needle. The package label will indicate type, size, and length of the suture material. Suture types include absorbable and non-absorbable.

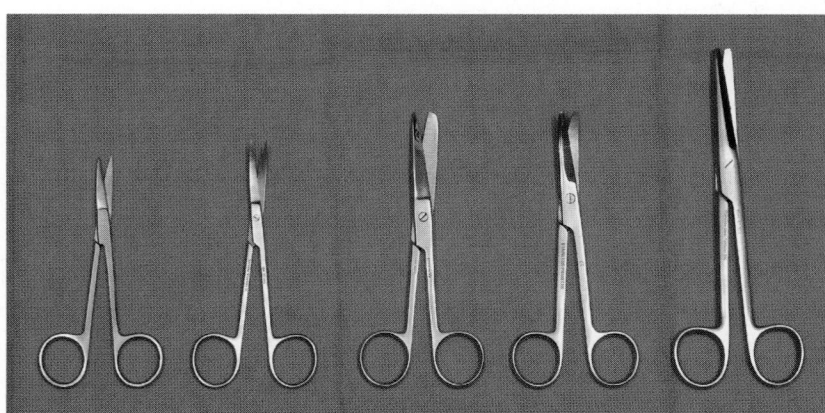

FIGURE 38-9 A variety of types of scissors.

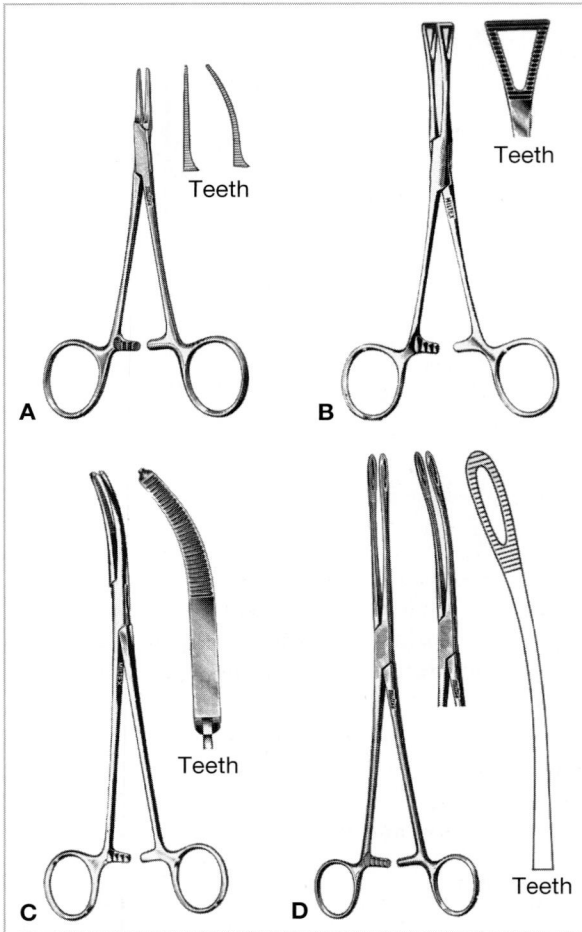

FIGURE 38-11   Hemostats: (A) mosquito forceps; (B) Pennington hemostatic forceps; (C) curved forceps; (D) sponge forceps.

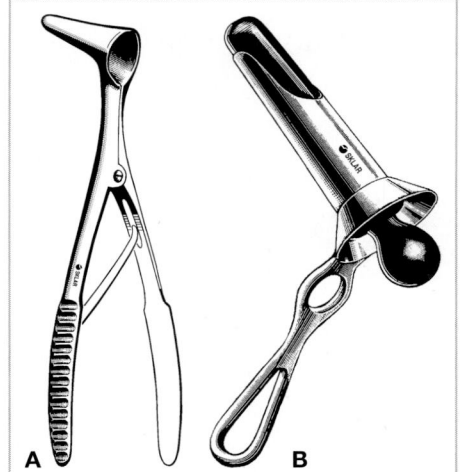

FIGURE 38-13   Speculums: (A) Vienna nasal speculum; (B) Ives-Fanster rectal speculum.

ABSORBABLE SUTURES   Absorbable sutures are digested by tissue enzymes and absorbed by the body tissues. They do not have to be removed. Absorption usually occurs 5 to 20 days after insertion. This type of suture, such as surgical catgut (made from sheep's intestinal lining), is used for internal organs such as the bladder and intestines, subcutaneous tissue, and ligating or tying off blood vessels. They include plain catgut, surgical catgut, and chromic catgut. Plain catgut is used in areas where rapid healing takes place such as highly vascular areas of the lips and tongue. Surgical catgut is used on tissues that are fast healing such as the vaginal area. Chromic catgut has a slower absorption rate and can be used to hold tissue together longer, such as for muscle repair.

NONABSORBABLE SUTURES   Nonabsorbable sutures are used on skin surfaces where they can easily be removed after incisional healing takes place. This type of suture material, such as nylon, cotton, silk, dacron, and stainless steel, is not absorbed by the body. Black silk is the most commonly used nonabsorbable suture.

SUTURE MATERIAL   Suture materials vary and are selected based on how they are used.

- Silk suture, while the most expensive, is also considered the most dependable. An all-purpose suture, it is widely used and easy to tie.

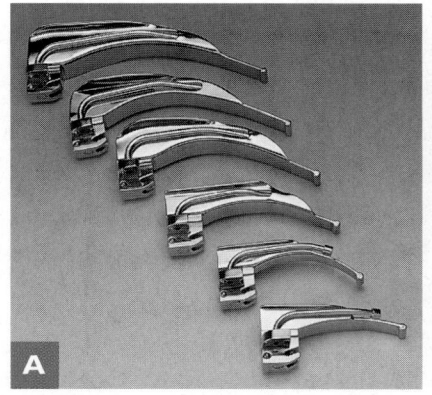

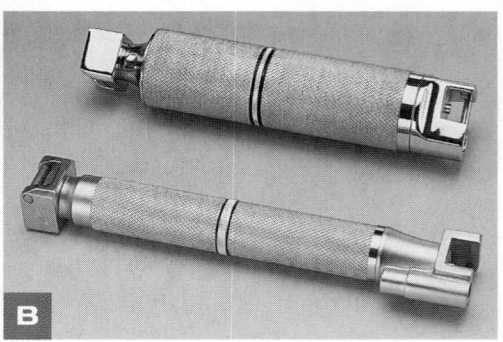

FIGURE 38-12   Laryngoscopes: (A) scopes; (B) handles.

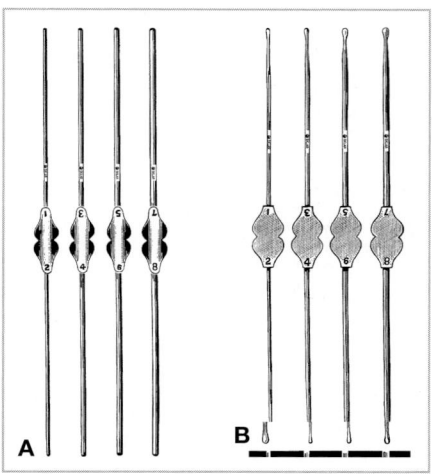

FIGURE 38-14 Lachrymal probes: (A) Bowman; (B) Williams.

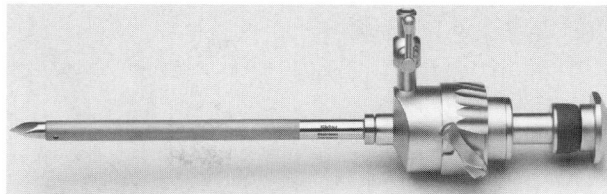

FIGURE 38-15 Trocar.

- Nylon suture has elasticity and strength that makes it ideal for use in joints and for skin closure. The disadvantage is the difficulty in forming a tight knot.
- Polyester suture is the second strongest of all the standard suture material, steel is the strongest. Polyester is used in ophthalmic, cardiovascular, and facial surgery, which all require a strong, un-

breakable suture since a broken suture could result in permanent damage to the patient.

- Steel is used in staples, and is the most widely used suture material in major surgery. It is the strongest of all suture material.
- Cotton suture, with less strength than other suture materials, is no longer widely used.

The size of the suture material, which is measured by the gauge or diameter, is stated in terms of 0s, decreasing in size with the number of zeros. For example, 0 is the thickest and 6-0 (000000) is the smallest. Sizes 2-0 through 6-0 are most commonly used. Delicate tissue, on areas such as the face and neck, would be sutured with 5-0 to 6-0 suture material. These fine sutures would leave less scarring. Heavier sutures, such as 2-0,

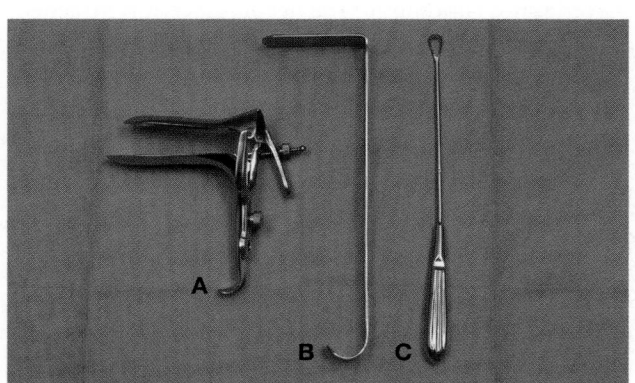

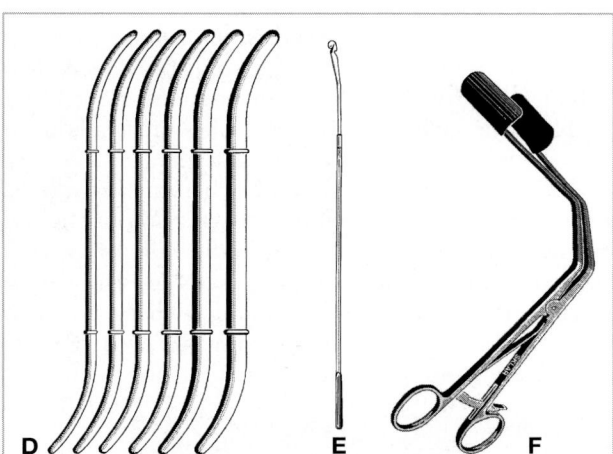

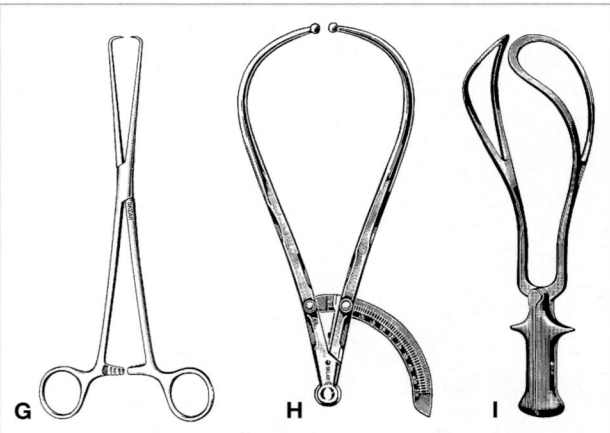

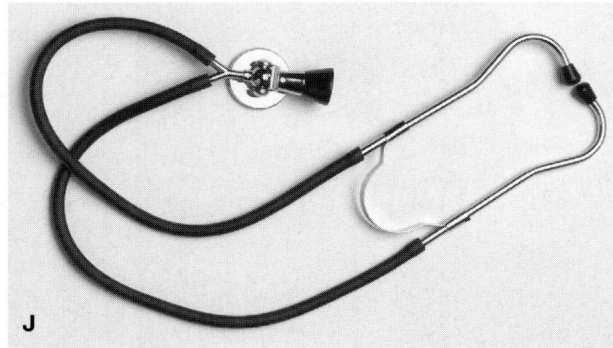

FIGURE 38-16 Gynecological instruments: (A) vaginal speculum; (B) retractor; (C) uterine curette; (D) uterine dilators; (E) IUD extractor forceps; (F) lateral vaginal retractor; (G) Schroeder uterine tenacumlum forceps; (H) Martin pelvimeter; (I) De Lee OB forceps; (J) Bowles obstetrical stethoscope.

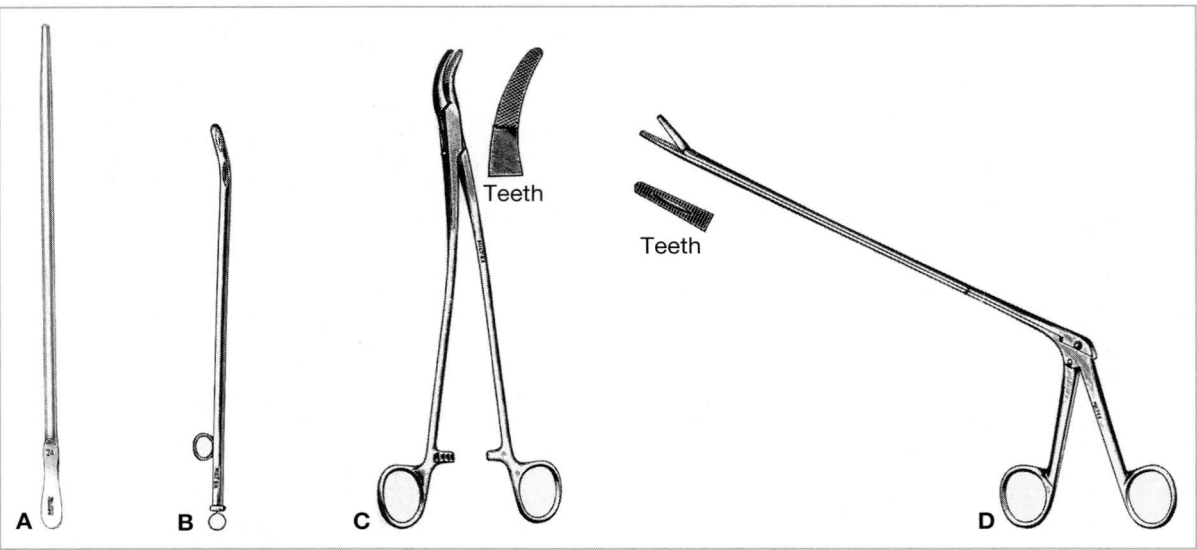

FIGURE 38-17 Urological instruments: (A) sound; (B) female catheter; (C) needle holder; (D) urethral forceps.

would be used for the chest or abdomen. The physician determines the type and gauge of sutures to be used. Table 38-2 summarizes suture uses, sizes, and types. Figure 38-19 illustrates different suture material.

SUTURE NEEDLES Suture needles are available in differing shapes depending on where they are used (Figure 38-20). Needles have either a sharp cutting point used for tissues that provide some resistance, such as skin, or a round non-cutting point used for more flexible tissue such as peritoneum. They are available in three shapes: straight, curved, or swaged.

The straight needle is used when the needle is pushed and pulled through the tissue without the use of a needle holder. This type of needle will have an eye that is threaded with the suture material. The suture material thickness will be double when threaded through the needle since it will enter the eye from one side and come out the other.

Curved needles allow the surgeon to go in and out of a tissue when there is not enough room to maneuver a straight needle. This type of needle requires a needle holder.

A swaged needle and suture materials are combined in one length. This offers the advantage of the suture material not slipping off the needle since it is attached. A swaged needle pack will contain a label indicating the gauge, type of needle point (cutting or noncutting), and type and length of the suture material.

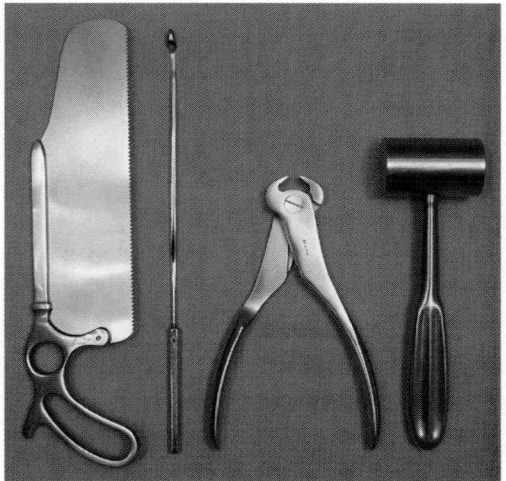

FIGURE 38-18 Orthopedic instruments.

TABLE 38-2 Suture Use, Size, and Type of Material

Use	Gauge	Type of Material
Blood vessels	3-0 to 0 3-0 3-0 to 0	chromic gut cotton silk
Eyelid	6-0 to 4-0 6-0 to 5-0	silk polyester
Skin	6-0 to 2-0 5-0 to 3-0 5-0 to 2-0	nylon polyethylene stainless steel
Fascial	2-0 to 0 2-0 to 0 2-0 to 0	chromic gut silk cotton
Muscle	3-0 to 0 3-0 to 0 3-0 to 0	plain gut chromic gut silk

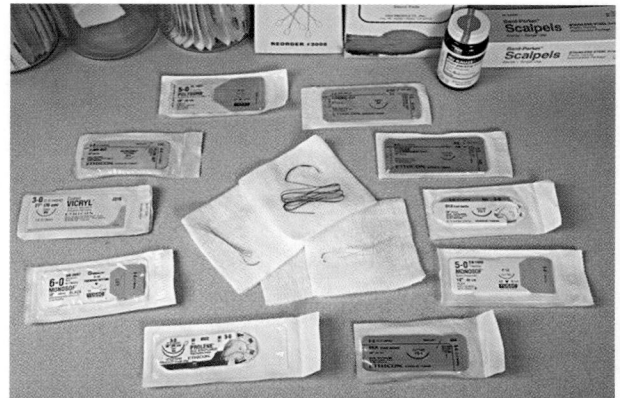

FIGURE 38-19   Types of suture material.

OTHER WOUND CLOSURE MATERIALS   Other materials used for wound closure include sterile tapes, such as Steri-Strips (Figure 38-21) and staples. Sterile tapes are nonallergenic and available in a variety of widths. They are used instead of sutures when not much tension will be applied to a wound such as on a small facial cut. Staples are made of stainless steel and applied with a surgical stapler.

Guidelines for Handling Instruments

Surgical instruments are expensive and may be delicate. They require special care and attention. In some instances, there might not be a duplicate of an instrument. Even slight damage to an instrument can result in malfunction at a critical time during surgery. Guidelines 38-2 provides guidelines for handling instruments.

Surgical Assisting

The medical assistant's role in surgical assisting varies depending on the type of practice and the needs of the physician. For example, an eye surgeon who performs a large number of outpatient cataract operations may employ a full time scrub assistant, scrub technician

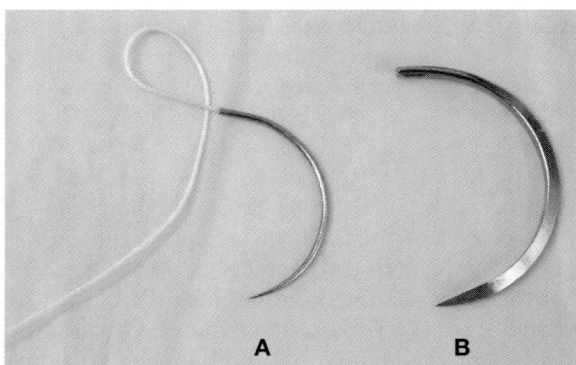

FIGURE 38-20   Surgical needle shapes: (A) taper point; (B) cutting point.

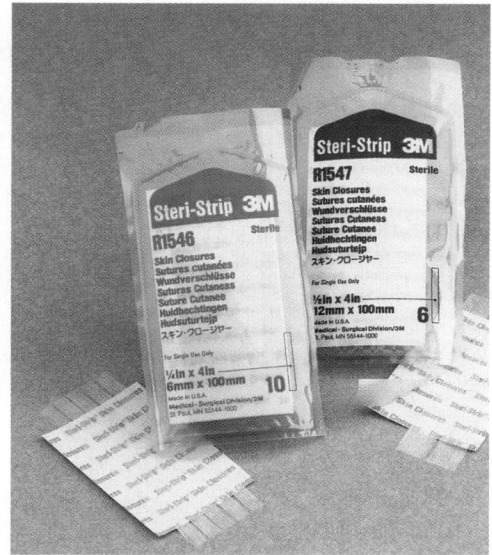

FIGURE 38-21   Steri-Strips from 3M.

(scrub tech), or operating technician (OR tech) who will apply sterile gloves and hand instruments to the surgeon (Professionalism). In this case, the medical assistant might act as the nonsterile assistant, who positions the patient, uses transfer forceps to bring additional supplies as needed, holds the vial of local anesthetic while the surgeon draws up the correct

---

38-2   **GUIDELINES**

Handling Instruments

- Instruments should be rinsed, cleaned, and scrubbed with a brush as soon as possible to prevent hardening of blood and tissue materials.
- Handle carefully. Do not throw instruments into the basin for cleaning.
- Avoid allowing large amounts of instruments to become tangled. They are difficult to separate and could result in damaging your protective gloves.
- Sharp instruments should remain separated from other instruments.
- Delicate instruments, such as those with lenses, should be handled separately.
- Instruments with ratchets should be stored open to maintain their good working condition.
- Check all instruments for defects before sterilizing them. All tips on the instruments should close tightly, scissors should cut evenly, and the cutting edges should be smooth.

- Always be aware of where your hands are because they should never touch a nonsterile area. Immediately re-glove if sterility is broken.
- Arrange the surgical tray for efficiency closing all instruments that were left open during the autoclave process.
- Close all instruments before passing them. Protect the surgeon from injury by handing needles with the point away from the physician, paying close attention to where scalpel blades and scissors' points are in relation to the physician's hands.
- Anticipate the physician's needs by memorizing the types of instruments used in a procedure and the order they are most often used. An index card with a list of the preferences for each procedure is useful for this purpose.
- Do not release your grip on the instrument until you feel the physician take it away. This prevents an instrument from falling to the floor and being damaged. In addition, you may not have a duplicate of that particular instrument on your tray and it will cause a delay in the procedure.

- Place the instrument with a firm "slap" into the physician's extended hand. Since the physician may not look up from the surgical site when his or her hand is extended, do not look away from the instrument until you feel it being taken from you. The handles should be placed into the physician's hands first.
- If asked to provide retraction to open the incision area for better visualization, follow directions from the surgeon regarding the amount of pull needed. Move slowly and deliberately when retracting. Do not make abrupt, forceful moves.
- If sutures are used to close the wound, be prepared to cut the suture material. The physician will pull both ends of the suture material together away from the wound. Cut both ends at the same time $1/8$ to $1/5$ inch above the knot.
- Many requests for assistance will not be verbalized by the physician. It is important to pay attention and anticipate what instruments or assistance will be required next.

dosage into a syringe, and applies dressings. Anyone not in sterile attire and assisting with a procedure can be described as a nonsterile assistant. He or she may also be referred to as a floating assistant, circulating assistant, circulator, or floater.

In many practices, the medical assistant will scrub, apply sterile gloves, and act as the only assistant for the surgeon. A good assistant can help the procedure flow smoothly. The exact surgical tray setup and sequence of passing instruments will vary depending on the procedure and the surgeon's preferences.

A good assistant will anticipate the needs of the physician, use care in handing instruments efficiently, use care that injury does not occur, and account for all materials and instruments used during the procedure. The assistant must maintain an accurate count of absorbent sponges used for cleaning out the wound site during surgery to ensure that all sponges are removed before the patient's wound is closed.

Scrub Assistant

The scrub assistant performs all procedures in sterile protective clothing using sterile technique. His or her responsibilities include arranging the surgical tray to meet the operating physician's preferences, handing instruments, swabbing (sponging) bodily fluids away

from the operative site, retracting the incision area, and cutting suture materials. See Guidelines 38-3 for guidelines of sterile technique for scrub assistants. In order to become competent as a scrub assistant, practice reaching for an instrument with your eyes closed. This is similar to the conditions under which the physician works since he or she does not look up from the operative site when reaching for instruments.

Instruments should be passed to the physician firmly and by the handle first. An instrument should remain in your grasp until you feel confident that the physician has a firm grip on it. Figure 38-22 illustrates a medical assistant using proper technique when passing instruments to the physician. Procedure 38-6 and Figure 38-23 show the steps for transferring sterile solutions onto a sterile field. All of the preceding procedures are vital for you to master in order to properly assist the physician with minor surgery as described in Procedure 38-7.

Floating Assistant

The floating assistant performs nonsterile duties during a surgical procedure and thus "floats" between the operating table, supplies, and equipment. One of the major roles of the float assistant is to monitor the patient by taking vital signs every five to ten minutes. Other duties include providing additional sterile equipment, opening sterile packets, adding sterile equipment to the field, and performing the necessary counts of supplies utilized such as gauze squares. Other guidelines for proper floating technique during surgery are listed in Guidelines 38-4.

Either category of assistant may be responsible for setting up the sterile field prior to surgery following appropriate guidelines. A surgical setup for a typical minor surgical procedure would include:

- Local anesthetic materials
- 3 cc syringe with needle(s)
- Alcohol sponges to cleanse vial top
- Sterile gloves for surgeon
- 4 × 4 and 2 × 2 gauze sponges
- No. 3 scalpel blades and handle, extra scalpel blades (No. 10, 11, and 15)
- Curved iris scissors

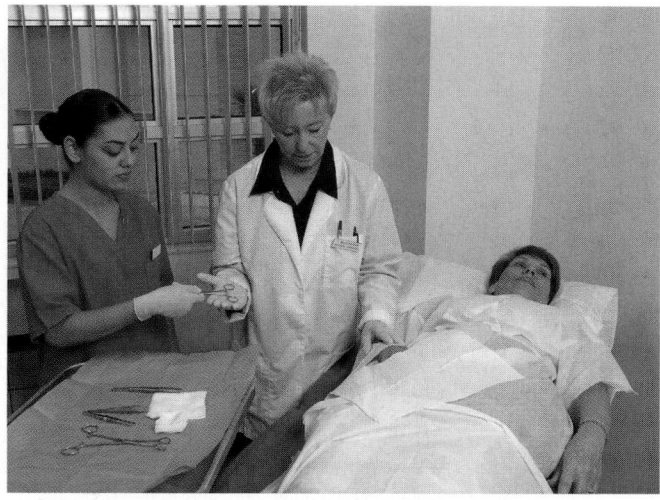

FIGURE 38-22   A medical assistant using the proper technique when passing instruments to the physician.

38-6   **PROCEDURE**

Transferring Sterile Solutions onto a Sterile Field

OBJECTIVE: Pour sterile fluid into a sterile basin on a sterile field without spilling the solution or contaminating the field.

Equipment and Supplies
   sterile saline or other solution as ordered; sterile basin; Mayo stand or side tray; waste container

Method
1. Perform hand hygiene.
2. Assemble all equipment. Check expiration dates on the solution and sterile basin pack.
3. Set up sterile basin on the Mayo tray using inside of wrapper to create a sterile field.
4. Remove cap of the solution and place it on a clean surface with the outer edge down (inside facing up). Avoid touching the inner surface of the cap. Rationale: The inside of the cap is considered sterile.
5. Check the label on the bottle before pouring the solution.
6. Pour a small amount of the liquid into a waste container for discarding. Rationale: This will dislodge any bacteria that may have collected on the edge of the bottle after opening it.

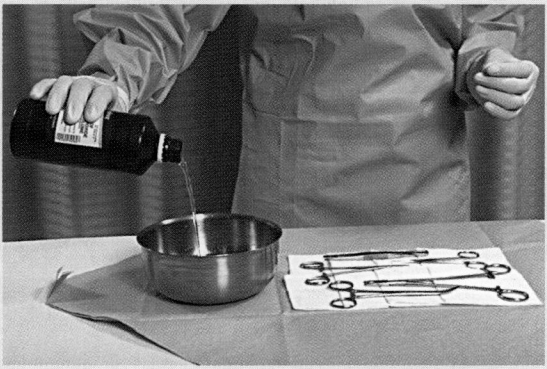

FIGURE 38-23   Pouring sterile solution into a sterile container.

7. Pour the bottle with the label held against the palm (Figure 38-23). Rationale: To protect the label from drips that can destroy the name of the solution.
8. Hold the bottle about six inches above the basin and pour slowly to avoid splashing.
9. Replace the lid immediately after using.

Assisting With Minor Surgery

OBJECTIVE: Prepare all materials and equipment for immediate use in a surgical procedure using sterile technique.

Equipment and Supplies

Mayo stand; side stand; transfer forceps and container; sharps container; waste container/plastic bag; biohazard waste container; anesthetic; alcohol swab; sterile specimen container, depending on type of surgery; sterile pack (2 pairs sterile gloves, towel pack, 4 × 4 sponge pack, patient drape, needle pack, and suture materials); instrument pack(s) including towel clamp pack; syringe pack; 2 sterile basin packs

Method

1. Perform hand hygiene.
2. Open sterile tray packs on Mayo stand and side stand. Use sterile wrapper to create a sterile field. The wrapper will hang over the edges of the tray.
3. Use sterile transfer forceps to move instruments on tray or to place equipment from packets. Materials in peel-away packets should be flipped onto the tray.
4. Open sterile needle and syringe unit and drop gently onto the sterile field. Use care not to reach over the sterile field.
5. Open sterile drape packs and towel clamp packs.
6. Open a set of sterile gloves for the physician.
7. After the tray is ready with all equipment open and arranged, pull the edge of the sterile towel across the tray using sterile transfer forceps. Rationale: The sterile towel will provide a protective covering for the sterile tray until the procedure begins. The medical assistant should not leave the room once the tray is set up (Figure 38-24).
8. When the physician has donned the sterile gloves, remove the sterile towel covering the tray of instruments.

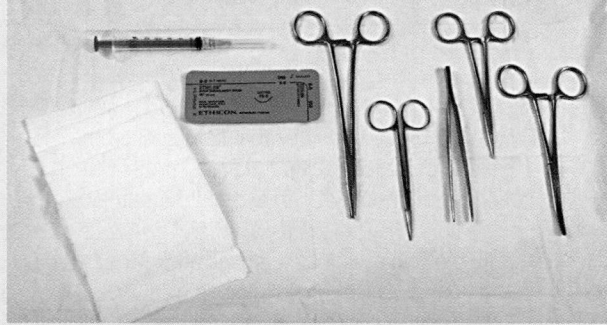

FIGURE 38-24 Sterile instrument setup.

9. Remove the towel by standing to one side and grasp the two distal corners. Lift the towel toward you so that you do not reach over the unprotected sterile field.
10. Cleanse the vial of anesthetic with a sterile alcohol swab and hold it upside down in the palm of your hand with the label facing toward the physician. Hold it steady while the physician draws up the anesthetic.
11. Stand to one side of the patient and assist the physician as requested. Provide additional supplies as needed. Note: If you assist by handing instruments directly to the physician, you must perform a surgical scrub and wear a sterile gown and gloves.
12. Hold all containers for specimens, drainage, or contaminated 4 × 4s. Wear nonsterile gloves to protect yourself from contact with drainage.
13. Collect and place all soiled instruments in a basin out of the patient's view.
14. Place all soiled gauze sponges (4 × 4s) and dressings in a plastic bag. Do not allow wet items to remain on a sterile field.
15. Immediately label all specimens as they are obtained. Close the specimen container tightly.
16. Periodically reassure the patient by quietly asking how he or she is doing. Do not touch the patient with soiled gloves.
17. When the procedure is complete, wash your hands before assisting the patient.
18. Allow the patient to rest and recover from the anesthetic. Periodically, check the patient's vital signs according to your office policy.
19. Provide clear oral and written postoperative instructions for the patient. Make sure the patient is stable before he or she leaves the office.
20. Send specimen(s) to the laboratory with a requisition slip.
21. Clean, sanitize, and sterilize the instruments. Clean and sanitize the room in preparation for the next patient.
22. Perform hand hygiene.

Charting Example

11/8/20XX	9:00 A.M.

The physician will chart the details of the surgical procedure.

- Immediately report any unusual observations about the patient to the operating physician.
- Use care not to touch the physician during any assisting since this will contaminate him or her and cause a delay in the procedure while the physician regloves (and regowns if necessary).
- Provide additional medications such as local anesthetics that are needed during the procedure. When providing medication during the procedure: follow the correct procedure to identify the medication, clean top of the vial/bottle with alcohol, hold vial/bottle upside down so that the physician can insert a sterile needle into the vial without touching the contaminated outer surface, and keep the label in plain view for the physician to read. Hold the vial firmly with both hands at your shoulder height to provide the physician with easy withdrawal. Do not place the vial in front of your face.

Note that the physician will have to use some force when inserting the needle into the vial.
- Since the floating assistant is not sterile, this person must perform all lighting adjustments, patient repositioning, chart notations made during the procedure, requisition forms, and specimen container labeling.
- The floating assistant can place additional sterile materials and instruments onto the sterile field by opening the packet without touching the sterile inside and gently dropping them into sterile field on the Mayo stand. The sterile scrub assistant or physician may remove them from the inside of the packet as the floating assistant holds firmly onto the outside.
- When holding a container to receive a specimen, tilt the container slightly so the physician can place the specimen inside without touching the rim of the container.

- Tissue forceps
- Straight and curved mosquito forceps
- Straight and curved Kelly forceps
- Towel forceps
- Sterile drape towels
- Needle holder with mounted needle and suture materials
- Sterile specimen container with preservative solution

Additional Surgical Supplies

Other surgical supplies may be needed during a procedure. Wound drains such as a rubber Penrose drain may be inserted at the end of a procedure to remove excess fluid. Other packing materials such as sterile petroleum jelly saturated gauze squares or sterilized iodoform gauze strips of varying lengths may also be used to pack wounds. Additional sterile syringes may be necessary to irrigate the wound or extra sterile gauze squares may be needed to absorb blood from a surgical area. In preparation for minor surgery and before the procedure begins, check the supply inventory thoroughly.

Preparing the Patient for Minor Surgery

The medical assistant is often responsible for providing instructions before and after minor surgery. Preoperative and postoperative instructions can be presented in

a variety of formats including one-on-one discussion, videotapes, brochures, pamphlets, and models. These instructions need to be reinforced through a telephone reminder. It is especially important to provide postoperative instructions in a variety of formats since the patient may not be fully alert right after surgery. Family members should be included in these explanations whenever practical.

Patient Instructions

Box 38-1 provides guidelines for preoperative and postoperative instructions. For purposes of efficiency, some preoperative patient preparation can take place before the patient arrives for the procedure. For example, patient education with an explanation of the procedure, preoperative and postoperative instructions, and laboratory testing can take place up to a week before the actual procedure. Preoperative instructions might include an explanation of what laboratory testing is needed and when it is to be done, food and fluid restrictions, directions for special bathing/skin cleansing preparations or cleansing enemas, and restrictions on bedtime sedative use. Postoperatively, patients should have a clear understanding of what to expect during recovery, and how to care for the surgical incision at home.

Informed Consent

The patient must be provided by the physician, an honest, thorough explanation of the surgical procedure, including the benefits and risks. Informed consent is explained

Preoperative and Postoperative Patient Instructions

Preoperative Instructions
- Explain the procedure verbally and provide printed materials.
- Be honest about the level of discomfort expected.
- Advise the patient on the length of the procedure.
- Explain what type of clothing to wear for the procedure.
- Schedule preoperative diagnostic tests—blood, x-ray, etc.
- Describe what at-home preparations the patient will need, such as fasting, and for how long.
- Explain that someone must accompany the patient.

- Inform the patient how long he or she will be out of work.
- Confirm the informed consent form has been signed.
- Answer any questions.
- Measure vital signs.

Postoperative Instructions
- Provide verbal and written instructions of follow-up care.
- Explain when the patient should notify the physician of possible postoperative problems such as fever, bleeding, swelling, or other symptoms.
- Schedule a follow-up visit, if required.

in more detail in Chapter 3. Any invasive procedure with a scalpel, scissors, or other device requires written permission (consent) from the patient. Procedures in which a body cavity is entered for the purposes of visualization, though no incision is made, such as in bronchoscopy, cystoscopy, and colonoscopy also require written consent. The procedure, with all the risks involved, must be explained by the physician. Every attempt must be made to determine if the patient actually understands the explanation given by the physician. The medical assistant can witness the patient's signing the consent form. Legal and Ethical Issues deals with more about signing informed consent forms and other legal concerns.

Positioning and Draping

Before the surgical procedure, ask the patient to remove all clothing and put on a patient gown with the ties at the back, unless otherwise instructed. Have the patient void before assisting him or her onto the operating table and place him or her in the proper position

for the procedure. Every attempt should be made to ensure the patient's comfort since the patient may have to remain in one position for an extended period of time. General guidelines for positioning and draping are discussed in Chapter 33.

Anesthesia

Anesthesia, medication that causes the partial or complete loss of sensation, is used to block the pain of surgery. Anesthesia can also relax muscles, produce amnesia, calm anxiety, and cause sleep. Medical assistants do not administer anesthetics, but they should be familiar with them and their effects.

The two types of anesthetics are general or local (conduction).

General anesthesia

A general anesthetic depresses the central nervous system (CNS) to cause unconsciousness. It is usually administered through inhalation or intravenous injection

Patient Education

Medical assistants play a vital role in minor surgery as we have seen. Protecting the patient from infection by instructing him or her on proper home management of wounds is important. When explaining wound care to patients, it is helpful to explain how to perform wound care and why wound care procedures are important. The basic goal of wound care is to hasten the healing process and reduce scarring. To achieve these goals, it is necessary to protect the wound and surrounding tissues from further

trauma, reduce strain on the tissues adjacent to the wound, protect the wound from excessive movement, and reduce the number of microorganisms in and near the wound. Individuals are more inclined to comply with your requests if they know why the requests are important. Use any opportunities to educate your patients about proper wound care. Encourage them to keep wounds clean and dry, drink extra fluids, get enough rest, and eat properly.

(IV). Inhaled anesthetics are generally in the form of gases or volatile liquids. In many cases, these are administered after a patient has received a sedative or narcotic to relieve pain or a tranquilizer to relieve anxiety. Sedatives and narcotics are usually administered intramuscularly before surgery. In some cases, they are administered by IV immediately before the general anesthetic is given.

Intravenous anesthetics are hypnotic sedatives that produce anesthesia, or sleep, when given in large doses. Sodium pentothal is an example of this type of anesthetic. Precautions to be taken when administering a general anesthetic include:

- Administering the anesthetic only to a patient on an empty stomach to prevent vomiting and possible aspiration of vomitus into lungs resulting in pneumonia.

- Cautioning patients not to drive or engage in other activity that could result in harm from impaired consciousness. General anesthetics can interfere with the patient's alertness for 12 to 24 hours after the surgery.

- Advising patients to avoid alcohol and depressant drugs two to three days before the surgery and one day after the surgery.

Local Anesthesia

Local anesthetics provide a loss of sensation in a particular area of the body without overall loss of consciousness. A local anesthetic is also referred to as a conduction anesthetic. The conduction of pain transmission by way of the nervous system is blocked. Examples of this type of anesthetic are:

- Topical and local infiltration—act on nerve endings
- Nerve block—affects pain transmission along a single nerve
- Regional block, spinal, epidural, or saddle blocks—affect a group of nerves

A local infiltration anesthetic is injected directly into the tissue that will be operated upon. Examples of a local are lidocaine hydrochloride (Xylocaine) and procaine hydrochloride (Novocain). This type of anesthetic is used for such procedures as removal of skin growths, skin suturing, and dental surgery. Local anesthesia takes from 5 to 15 minutes to become effective and lasts from one to three hours. During longer procedures additional injections of anesthetic may have to be administered when the first dosage has worn off.

Epinephrine, a vasoconstrictor that causes superficial blood vessels to narrow, is often added to the local anesthetic when the physician is operating on the face and head. The addition of epinephrine allows for better visualization of the surgical site because it diminishes bleeding. Epinephrine causes local anesthetics to be absorbed by the body more slowly and gives them a longer lasting effect. Clearly mark anesthetics that have been prepared with the addition of epinephrine. Patients with heart problems could have a reaction to epinephrine causing tachycardia or other irregularities.

Nerve blocks are administered by injection into a nerve adjacent to the operative site. This type of anesthetic is used for surgery on hands, fingers, and toes.

Topical anesthetics are local pain control medications that are applied to the skin and produce a numbing effect. These can be applied by drop, spray, or swab. They are commonly used in eye procedures. An example of a spray anesthetic is ethyl chloride, which produces a freezing effect on the skin. Benzocaine (Solarcaine) is another example of a topical anesthetic.

ADMINISTERING ANESTHESIA   Only physicians or anesthesiologists can administer an anesthetic and only they must chart the administration. Either the medical assistant or the physician will draw up the local anesthetic. Using the correct procedure for drawing up medication is discussed in Chapter 49. The medication vial must be correctly identified and then wiped with an alcohol sponge. If the medical assistant draws up the medication, then he or she must present both the syringe and the vial to the physician so that the physician can read the label. The anesthetic will be injected into the patient's prepared skin by the physician before the physician has donned gloves. This syringe is not placed onto the sterile field because it has been contaminated by the medical assistant's ungloved hands.

If the physician prefers to draw up the anesthetic, it can be done using a sterile syringe after he or she has applied gloves. The medical assistant will hold the vial securely while the physician withdraws the anesthetic without contaminating the needle. The outside of the vial cannot be touched by the physician's sterile gloved hand. This syringe can then be placed onto the sterile field.

Some physicians prefer to change the needle after drawing up the local anesthetic. For example, they may draw up the drug using a 21-gauge needle and then administer the solution using a 23-gauge or 25-gauge needle.

Preparation of the Patient's Skin

While skin cannot be sterilized, it can be cleaned using medical aseptic technique. Careful cleansing of the skin before performing a surgical procedure will reduce the number of microorganisms on the skin. This will decrease the chance of carrying infection-producing microorganisms through the skin during the invasive procedure (incision into skin or entrance of a probe).

In some situations, the physician may order the surgical site to be shaved since bacteria can reside in hair. See Procedure 38-8 and Figure 38-25 for skin preparation and shave. Care must be taken to avoid scraping

Preparing the Patient's Skin for Surgical Procedures

OBJECTIVE: Prepare patient's skin for surgical procedure using sterile scrub and shave.

Equipment and Supplies

antiseptic germicidal soap; sterile saline; antiseptic such as betadine; 8 sterile applicators; Mayo tray; waste receptacle (may be included in sterile pack); hazardous waste container; plastic bag for soiled dressings; sterile pack: (sterile gloves, 3 to 4 towel packs, sterile basin pack with 3 basins, patient drape, 4 × 4 gauze sponge pack with 12 to 24 sponges, shave preparation kit)

NOTE: This procedure follows a surgical hand scrub.

Method

1. Perform hand hygiene.
2. Assemble equipment by placing packs on Mayo stand or side tray and opening outer wraps from all packs.
3. Identify the patient and explain the procedure.
4. Have the patient remove appropriate clothing and put on gowning. Ask the patient to void, if necessary.
5. Position and drape the patient to provide exposure of the operative site.
6. Unwrap the basin pack. Pour germicidal soap solution into one basin; sterile saline into the second basin; and antiseptic into the third.
   Rationale: Liquids are poured by holding the outer nonsterile surface of the containers before applying sterile gloves.
7. Wash hands using sterile scrub and apply sterile gloves.
8. Drape the skin with two towels placed three to five inches above and below the surgical site.
9. With a sterile gauze or sponge, apply soapy solution to patient's skin. Use a circular motion starting at the site of proposed incision and move outward (Figure 38-25). Pass over each skin area only once. Place each used sponge into a waste receptacle immediately.
   Note: Some physicians prefer the patient receive a dry shave.
10. Take a fresh sterile gauze or sponge for each cleansing wipe. Repeat this process until the area is completely washed. The last area cleansed will be the outer edges.
11. Rinse using sterile saline on a clean gauze or sponge. Pat dry with a dry gauze only on the area that has been washed. Avoid touching any other skin area.
    Rationale: The surrounding skin is considered contaminated because it has not been washed.

If shaving is ordered, then proceed with the following steps.

1. Apply soap solution to the site area. Remove razor from shave preparation pack. Pull the skin taut and shave the surgical site in the same direction as the hair is growing. Rinse with a

---

or cutting the skin during the shaving process. The physician will order either a wet shave (moistening the skin with soap and water) or dry shave (Figure 38-26). Some physicians feel that shaving the skin presents more risk of skin injury and prefer only to have the patient's skin cleansed carefully.

Postoperative Patient Care

Postoperative care includes monitoring the patient during recovery from anesthesia, wound care, applying dressings, and communicating patient instructions. Patient Education addresses more about instructing patients on home care of wounds.

Recovery from Anesthesia

Topical and other local anesthetics take affect either immediately or within a few minutes. Their effects wear off quickly. The use of large amounts of local anesthetic, beyond normal dosages, is not recommended and may result in an adverse reaction in patients. Some patients are allergic to anesthetics and may slip into anaphylactic shock, which requires emergency treatment (see Chapter 39). An emergency tray or cart including drugs used to counteract shock should always be available in the office. Many facilities require employees to have current CPR certification.

The patient treated with a local anesthetic in his or her mouth or throat should be advised not to eat until

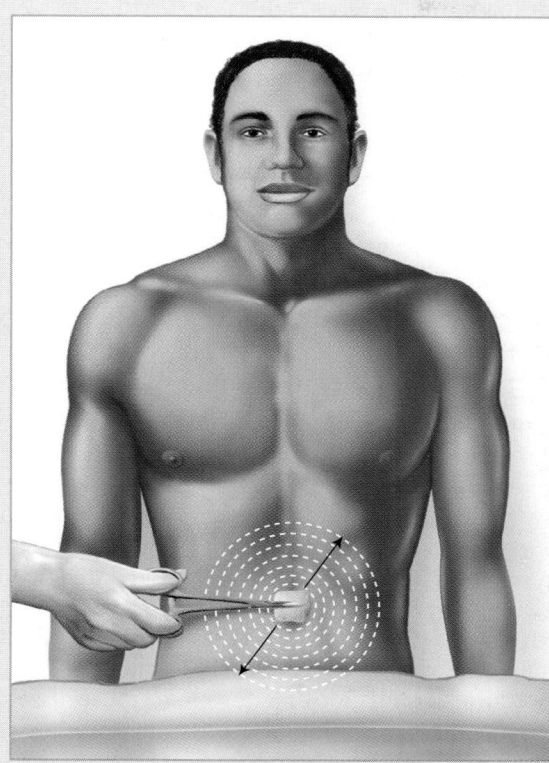

FIGURE 38-25 Preparing the patient's skin at the surgical site.

saline solution using the single-pass, circular motion as before and pat it dry.

Rationale: Shaving against the direction of hair growth can irritate the skin. This skin break-down will allow bacteria to enter.

2. Reapply soap solution to the area and repeat the above process according to your office policy (around five minutes).
3. Pat the entire area dry with the third sterile towel.
4. Apply the antiseptic solution using two cotton applicators together in the same single-pass, circular motion.
5. Cover the prepared surgical site with the remaining sterile towel.
6. Properly dispose of gloves and soiled materials into biohazard container.

To dispose of soiled dressings, use the following steps.

1. Remove gloves.
2. Place one hand into the empty plastic bag.
3. Using the hand covered with the plastic bag, pick up all the soiled materials. With the other hand, pull the outside of the bag over the soiled dressings.
4. Dispose of bag in a hazardous waste container.
5. Perform hand hygiene and document.

Charting Example

3/12/XX	11:00 A.M.

Pt arrived for removal and biopsy of growth on outer aspect of left forearm, Surgical site prepared using betadine. No cuts of lesions noted.

J. Wall, RMA

the effects of the anesthetic wear off to prevent choking on food or burning the mouth. Table 38-3 contains examples of local anesthetics. Patients must be observed carefully after surgery for signs of adverse reaction to the anesthetic, bleeding, and circulatory problems. The patient's vital signs (blood pressure, temperature, pulse, and respiration) should be monitored immediately after surgery and then every 15 minutes for the first hour. Never give fluids to a patient who is not fully alert. This can result in choking. Oral medications for pain, nausea, and vomiting have to be withheld until the patient is fully recovered from anesthesia. Medications may be given by injection until recovery occurs.

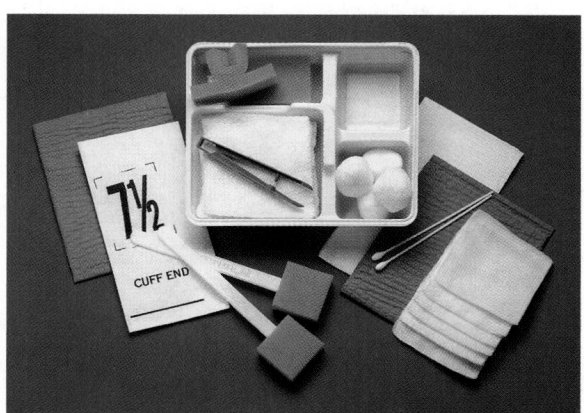

FIGURE 38-26 Dry skin prep tray.

TABLE 38-3 Local Anesthetics

Anesthetic Agent	Use
Benzocaine	Topical use only
Chloroprocaine	Nerve block, epidural
Lidocaine (Xylocaine)	Infiltration or topical
Mepivacaine	Infiltration nerve block
Procaine (Novacaine)	Infiltration; seldom used now
Tetracaine	Infiltration, topical nerve block, spinal

Excessive disorientation and inability to revive within a normal time for recovery should be reported immediately to the physician. The patient should be observed for nausea and vomiting. Medications may be ordered by the physician to counteract nausea and vomiting.

Types of Wounds

The skin acts as a protective barrier and is the body's first line of defense. Any break in the skin, whether from injury or a surgical incision, is referred to as a wound. A surgical procedure requiring an incision through the skin is considered an invasive procedure because a wound is created when the skin is entered. Wounds cause blood vessels to rupture and blood to seep into tissues, which results in skin color changes. Typically, skin coloration will change from erythema in a fresh wound to a greenish yellow color during the healing process, which involves oxidation of blood pigments. There are four types of wound classification:

- Abrasion—outer layers of skin are rubbed away due to scraping; will generally heal without scarring.
- Incision—smooth cut resulting from a surgical scalpel or sharp material, such as razor or glass; may result in excessive bleeding and scarring if deep.
- Laceration—edges are torn in an irregular shape; can cause profuse bleeding and scarring.
- Puncture—made by a sharp, pointed instrument such as a bullet, needle, nail, or splinter; external bleeding is usually minimal, but infection may occur due to penetration with a contaminated object and there may be scarring.

Healing Process

Wounds pass through various stages of healing, including inflammation, as the body starts to fight off potential infection. Inflammation is the body's protective response to trauma and invasion by microorganisms. It is generally localized around the site of trauma or infection. Signs of inflammation are redness or erythema, swelling, warmth, and pain. Wounds go through three phases before healing or restoration of structure and function take place.

- Inflammatory phase—(3 days) blood clot forms to stop bleeding and plug the opening of a wound; eschar or scab forms to keep out microorganisms.
- Proliferating phase—(3 to 21 days) fibrin threads extend across opening of wound and pull edges together; cells multiply to repair the wound.
- Maturation phase—(21 days to 2 years) tissue cells strengthen and tighten the wound closure, form a scar; scar eventually fades and thins.

Wound Complications

Wound complications include (a) infection—signs of inflammation, purulent or pus-like drainage, fever; (b) hemorrhage or bleeding; (c) dehiscence—separation of wound edges; and (d) evisceration—separation of wound edges and protruding of abdominal organs. Uneven or ragged-edged wounds and large wounds take more time to heal. Without proper wound care infection will set in. Infection is the result of wound contamination during or after the injury or surgical procedure. Drainage occurs as fluid and cells escape from the tissues during the inflammatory phase of wound healing. The amount and type of drainage observed on a dressing should be charted. Types of wound drainage are:

- Serous drainage—clear, watery drainage such as the fluid in a blister.
- Sanguineous drainage—bloody (bright red is fresh blood, dark red is older blood), the amount and color of sanguineous drainage is important.
- Serosanguineous drainage—thin watery drainage tinged with blood.
- Purulent drainage—thick pus-like drainage that is green, yellow, or brown.

Cleansing a Wound

A wound must be cleaned before a sterile dressing can be applied. The physician will indicate which of the many products available for wound cleansing he prefers. Warm water and soap are used to remove surface dirt from around the wound area.

To clean a wound using sterile gauze or swab, work from the clean area near the wound outward to less clean areas. This will prevent dragging more microorganisms into the wound. Wipe in one direction and then discard the sterile swab or gauze. Cleanse a linear wound from top to bottom with one stroke per sterile

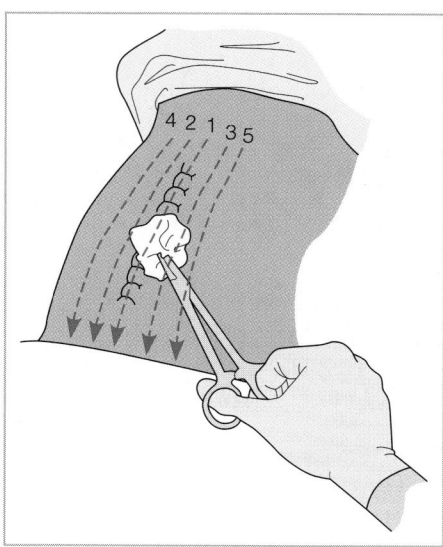

FIGURE 38-27 Cleanse a linear wound by using a new sterile gauze pad for each stroke, begin next to the wound and work from the top to the bottom of the wound area,

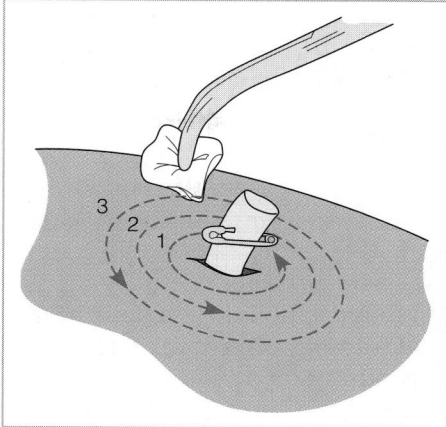

FIGURE 38-28 To cleanse an open wound, begin close to the wound and work outward in full or half circles.

gauze or swab (Figure 38-27). Use a new sterile gauze or swab for each stroke. Work outward from the wound in parallel lines. To cleanse an open wound, such as a pressure ulcer, work in circles, half or full, beginning in the center and work outward (Figure 38-28).

Always clean at least one inch beyond the edge of the dressing to be applied. If no dressing is to be applied, clean two inches beyond the edges of the wound. Use a new gauze pad for each circle.

The size and shape of the dressing needed will depend on the size, location, and amount of drainage from the wound. Sterile 4 × 4 inch gauze pads (called four by fours) are used for most dressings. If there is drainage expected from the wound, a prepared dressing, such as Telfa, may be used to prevent the dressing from sticking to the wound. See Figure 38-29 for an example of a wound closure kit.

Each patient should be asked how long it has been since he or she received a tetanus shot. In the event that the shot was not received within the last ten years, the physician should be informed.

Sutures

A suture is a thread used to sew body tissues together. Sutures used to attach tissues beneath the skin are often made of an absorbable material that disappears in several days. Skin sutures, by contrast, are made of nonabsorbable materials such as silk, cotton, linen, wire, nylon and Dacron (polyester fiber). Silver wire clips or staples are also available. Sutures or staples are inserted by the surgeon at the end of a procedure to hold tissues in alignment during the healing process. The steps necessary to assist with suturing are given in Procedure 38-9. Sutures generally remain in place from five to six days and then have to be removed if they are nonabsorbable. If sutures remain in the body too long, they can cause skin irrita-

tion and infection. The suture acts as a wick to carry bacteria through the skin and into the subcutaneous tissues. Suture removal times differ depending upon the site:

- Facial sutures may be removed after only 24 to 48 hours to prevent scarring.
- Head and neck sutures remain for three to five days.
- Abdominal sutures remain for five to seven days.
- Sutures over weight-bearing joints and large bones may remain seven to ten days.

The medical assistant prepares the patient for suture or staple removal by taking off the dressing, if one is present. Each edge of the dressing is removed by pulling toward the suture line. If the dressing is adhering to the suture line then a small amount of sterile saline or hydrogen peroxide can be used to moisten the dressing to ease removal.

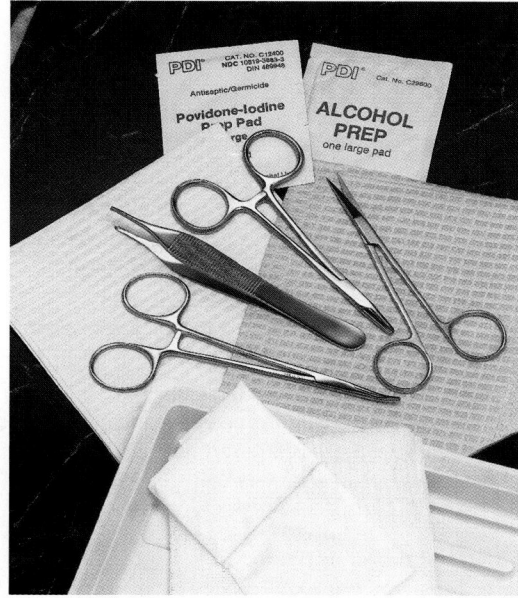

FIGURE 38-29 Wound closure kit.

PROCEDURE

Assisting with Suturing

OBJECTIVE: Assist with suture repair of an incision or laceration using sterile technique.

Equipment and Supplies

Mayo stand; side stand; anesthetic; sterile transfer forceps; sterile saline; waste container/plastic bag; biohazardous waste container; sharps container; sterile gloves (2 pairs); sterile pack(s) (patient drape, towel pack–four towels, 4 × 4 gauze sponge pack); scalpel blades pack (No. 10 and 15); needle and syringe pack; suture and needle pack (according to physician's preference); 2 sterile basins; suture pack–scalpel handle, needle holder, thumb forceps; 2 scissors; 3 hemostats)

Method

1. Use a sterile scrub and gloving procedure.
2. Stand across from the physician.
3. Place two sponges ready for the physician near the wound site. Rationale: The physician will use sponges to clear drainage during the initial inspection of the wound.
4. Assist by using additional sponges to keep wound dry.
5. Pass instruments, such as scissors, to the physician using a firm snap of the handle into his or her hand. Rationale: The instrument should be firmly placed in the physician's hand without letting go until the physician has a firm grasp.
6. The blade is placed into the scalpel using a hemostat.
7. Hand the scalpel to the physician with blade edge down to avoid cutting the physician.
8. Continue to use sponges to keep the wound free of drainage.
9. Pass all instruments to the physician as requested. Try to anticipate the next instruments that the physician may need, such as another hemostat or scissors for cutting suture.
10. Pass the toothed forceps to the physician if laceration edges need to be grasped.
11. Mount the needle into the needle holder and pass as one unit to the physician using care to keep the suture within the sterile field. Pass the needle holder with the needle pointing outward. Hold the suture with the other hand and do not let go of it until the physician sees it.
12. Using the suture scissors, prepare to cut the suture as directed by the physician (usually ⅛ to ¼ inch from the knot).
13. Sponge the closed wound once with a sponge and discard.
14. Repeat this step with each suture.
15. Place all soiled instruments after they are used onto the sterile field if they will be used again or discard others into the instrument basin.
16. When the procedure is complete, remove your gloves and perform hand hygiene before assisting the patient.
17. Allow the patient to rest and recover from the anesthetic. Periodically, check the patient's vital signs according to your office policy.
18. Provide clear oral and written postoperative instructions for the patient. Make sure the patient is stable before he or she leaves the office.
19. Clean, sanitize, and sterilize the instruments. Clean and sanitize the room in preparation for the next patient.
20. Perform hand hygiene.

Remove staples as follows.

1. Perform steps 1 through 10 above.
2. Place the lower tips of a sterile staple remover under the staple.
3. Squeeze the handles together until they are completely closed. Pressing the handles together causes the staple to bend in the middle and pulls the edges of the staple out of the skin. Do not lift the staple remover when squeezing the handles.
4. When both ends of the staple are visible, gently move the staple away from the incision site.
5. Hold the staple remover over a disposable container, release the staple remover handles and release the staple.
6. Perform steps 13 through 21.

Charting Example

The physician will chart the details of the surgical procedure.

In some office practices and in some states, medical assistants are permitted to remove sutures. The procedure should be explained to the patient reminding them that they may feel a pulling sensation. The skin is then thoroughly cleansed with an antiseptic such as alcohol or betadine solution. After opening the sterile suture packet (Figure 38-30) and creating a sterile field with the wrapper, the knot of the suture is gently picked up using a thumb forceps. The suture is then cut with suture scissors below the knot as close to the skin as possible. The suture is removed by pulling the long remaining suture out. Suture material that is outside of the skin should not be pulled through the skin due to the danger of pulling infection-causing microorganisms along with it. Procedure 38-10 and Figure 38-31 provide the steps to remove sutures. Very little of the suture is actually pulled through the skin.

Sterile Dressing

A dressing is the application of a sterile covering over a surgical site or wound using surgical asepsis. A patient who has had an injury or surgical procedure may need to schedule an appointment to remove the old dressing and apply a new sterile dressing. Procedure 38-11 and Figure 38-32 demonstrate the steps for changing a sterile dressing.

Bandaging the Wound

After the wound is dressed, the physician may request you to apply a bandage to hold the dressing in place. Bandages may be gauze, fabric, or elasticized and need not be sterile (Figure 38-33). Bandages are available in various sizes, lengths, and shapes. Some bandages are self-adhering and easier to apply to awkward areas. Elastic bandages are used to support an injured part and reduce swelling. Care must be taken not to bandage too tightly and restrict circulation. Procedure 38-12 and Figure 38-34 show the steps for applying a bandage to patient's forearm.

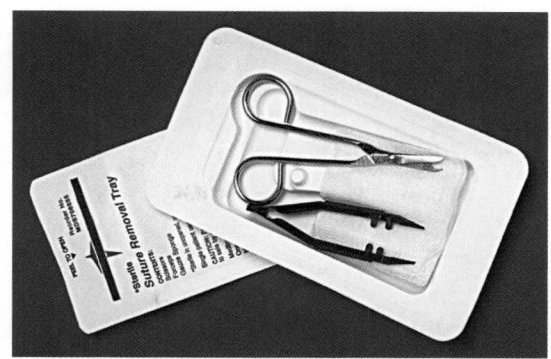

FIGURE 38-30 Disposable suture removal set.

Surgical Procedures Performed in the Medical Office

Many minor surgical procedures can be performed efficiently in the physician's office. This saves the patient the time and expense of having to go into an ambulatory surgical facility or a hospital. The basic surgical setup is the standard setup with the addition of specific instruments for each procedure. Some minor procedures performed in the medical office include biopsy, cautery, colposcopy, cryosurgery, laser surgery, endocervical curettage, endoscopic procedures, suture removal, removal of foreign bodies, incision and drainage, vasectomy, and removal of growths and tumors. Preparing for Externship suggests ways to observe and learn about surgical procedures during your externship.

The medical assistant does not administer these procedures, but must understand them and their effects so that he or she can assist the physician and the patient. A brief description of some procedures follows.

Electrosurgery

Electrocautery, or cautery, is the use of high frequency, alternating electric current to destroy, cut, or

Preparing for Externship

Depending on the type of practice you are assigned to as an extern, you will have opportunities to observe and then later assist with many types of surgical procedures. Showing interest, asking questions at the appropriate time, and volunteering to do tasks that need to be done within your scope of practice, demonstrates initiative and responsibility. If there are quiet times in your office with no assigned tasks, take the opportunity to look through surgical supply catalogues at instruments, types of dressings and bandages, and other supplies to familiarize yourself with the vast array of equipment and supplies available. Each time you assist with or observe a procedure, make an index card including names of instruments, numbers of each instrument, how the physician wishes the packets to be set up, other supplies needed, and types of conditions that the procedure is used to treat. These cards will be valuable to you when you begin your profession as a medical assistant. In some offices, surgical procedures are done so infrequently you may forget what the procedure requires. Your index cards will be a quick reference for you and help you to feel more confident.

Removing Sutures

OBJECTIVE: Remove sutures using proper sterile technique as per the physician's order.

Equipment and Supplies

suture removal pack (suture scissors, sterile gauze squares, thumb forceps, skin antiseptic, sterile gloves, band-aids, biohazardous waste container)

Method

1. Perform hand hygiene.
2. Assemble equipment and check expiration date on pack.
3. Identify the patient.
4. Explain the procedure to the patient and place into a comfortable position.
5. Remove old dressing using proper technique.
6. Perform hand hygiene.
7. Open suture removal pack using proper technique.
8. Apply sterile gloves using proper technique.
9. Cleanse the wound as needed.
10. Place a gauze square next to the wound to put sutures as they are removed.
11. Grasp the knot of the suture with thumb forceps and lift gently (Figure 38-31).
12. Insert the suture scissors and cut suture at skin level. Pull out the suture.
13. Place the cut suture on the gauze and check to see that all sutures have been removed.
14. Repeat these steps until all sutures are removed.
15. Count sutures.
16. Clean wound with antiseptic and allow it to dry.
17. Dress wound as ordered.
18. Properly dispose of equipment and supplies.
19. Remove gloves and perform hand hygiene.
20. Instruct the patient on wound care.
21. Document procedure, including condition of wound, number of sutures or staples removed, and patient instructions on wound care

Charting Example

2/14/XX	11:00 A.M.

Removed sutures and cleansed wound with antiseptic. Wound healing well. Pt. instructed on wound care.

M. King, CMA

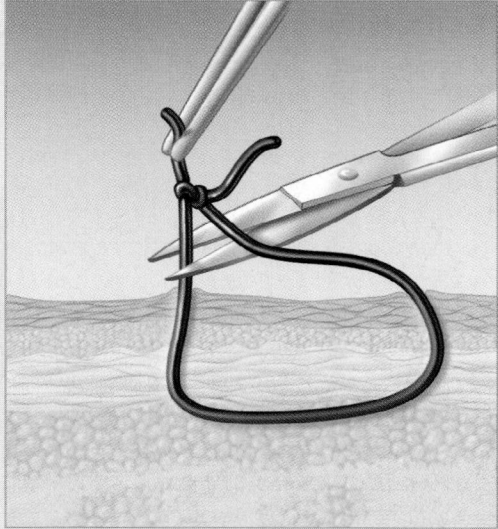
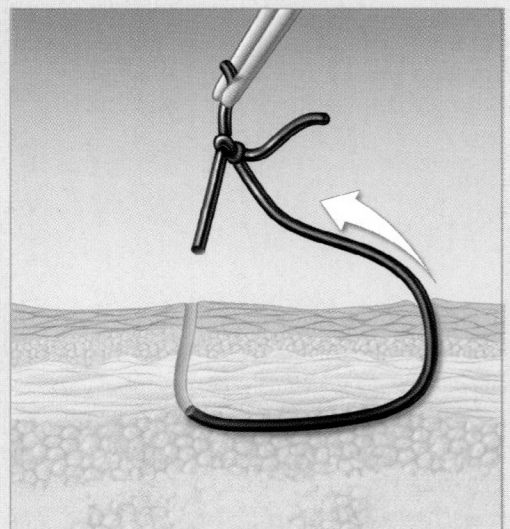

FIGURE 38-31   Removal of sutures.

PROCEDURE

Changing a Sterile Dressing

OBJECTIVE: Change a wound dressing using proper sterile technique.

Equipment and Supplies

disposable gloves; antiseptic solution; solution container; prepackaged dressing pack; thumb forceps; sterile cotton balls; sterile gloves; sterile dressing; adhesive tape; scissors, if necessary for tape; waste container/plastic bag; biohazardous waste container; Mayo stand or side tray;

Method

1. Perform hand hygiene.
2. Assemble equipment using the Mayo stand.
3. Prepare the sterile field applying aseptic technique using prepackaged dressing packet. Employ sterile transfer forceps to place additional sterile items onto the sterile field.
4. Explain the procedure to the patient.
5. Assist the patient into a comfortable position with the area to be dressed resting on a support, such as an examination table.
6. Apply nonsterile gloves.
7. Remove dressing from the wound by loosening tape with gloved hands or forceps and pulling it from both sides toward the wound (Figure 38-32A). Without passing the soiled dressing over the sterile field, place it into the soiled waste bag. Do not allow the dressing to touch the outside or edges of the bag (Figure 38-32B).
8. Inspect the wound for signs of infection and inflammation. Note any discharge by its type, the amount, and its odor (Figure 38-32C).
9. Discard your gloves and contaminated forceps properly. Disposable gloves and forceps are placed in waste container. Reusable forceps are placed in the basin for later cleaning.
10. Open sterile gloves and apply properly.
11. Drop antiseptic onto several cotton balls until they are moist, but not saturated. Clean the wound by using sterile forceps to hold the cotton. Cleanse the wound by moving from the top to the bottom of the wound once. Use a new cotton ball with antiseptic for each wipe. Move from the inside of the wound to the outside edges.
12. Pick up the sterile dressing with gloved hands and place over the wound.
13. Discard your gloves and forceps.
14. Apply adhesive tape to hold the dressing in place. Do not apply too tightly as to restrict circulation. The strips of tape should be long enough to hold the dressing in place. Do not wrap the tape entirely around an extremity or completely cover the dressing.
15. Instruct the patient on dressing care and set a follow-up appointment to see the physician.
16. Chart the procedure, including the date, time, location and condition of the wound, and instructions given to the patient.

Charting Example

2/14/XX	11:00 A.M.

Drsg. change on right anterior forearm. Moderate amt. serous drainage with slight erythema surrounding wound. Incision healing well with edges aligned. Cleansed with betadine. Sterile drsg. applied. Pt. instructed on wound care.

M. King, CMA

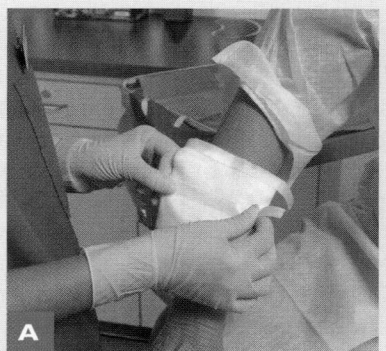 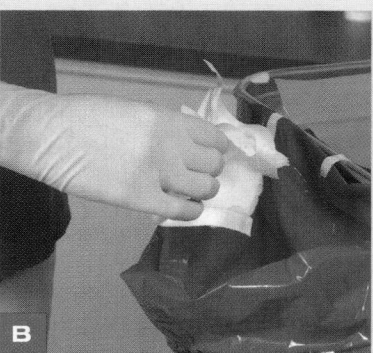 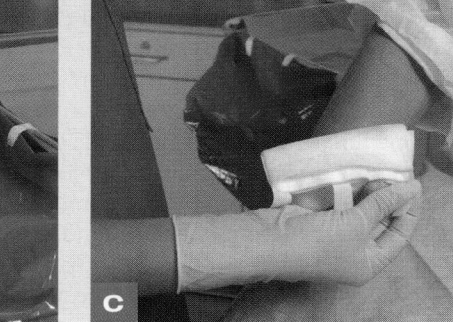

FIGURE 38-32 Wound dressing (A) removal, (B) disposal, and (C) inspection.

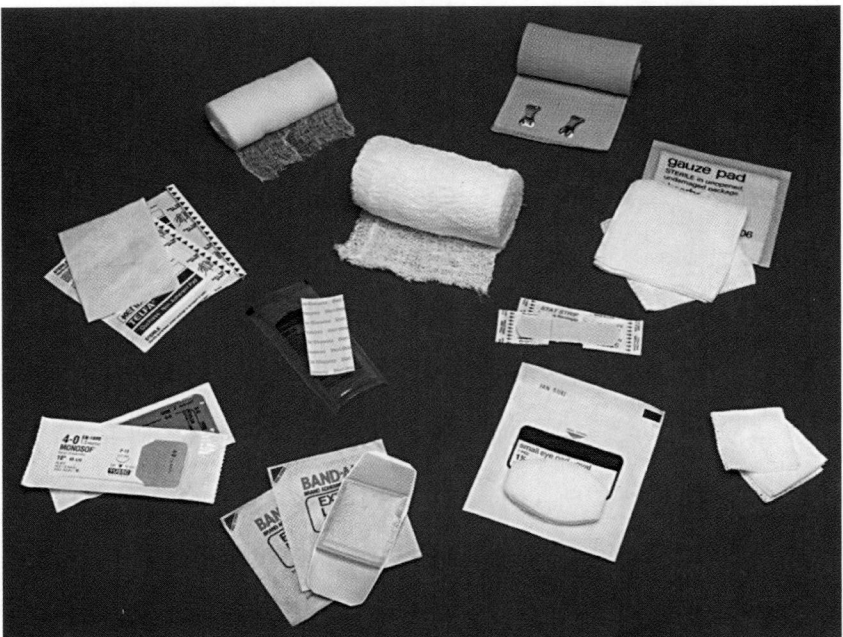

FIGURE 38-33 Various types of bandages.

remove tissue. Electrocautery is also used to coagulate small blood vessels, thereby reducing bleeding and cell loss. See Figure 38-35 for photo of a disposable cautery unit. Four types of currents are used in electrosurgery.

- Electrocoagulation—destroys tissues and controls bleeding by coagulation.

- Electrodessication—destroys tissue by creating a spark gap when the probe is inserted into unwanted tissue.

- Electrofulguration—destroys tissue with a spark emitted from the tip of a probe positioned a short distance away from the unwanted tissue.

- Electrosection—uses electric current to incise and excise the tissue.

Some physicians have miniature electrocautery units called hyfrecators (Figure 38-36). The use of electrocautery is being replaced by the electrosurgical unit (ESU) and the ultrasonic surgical unit (USU).

The ESU is able to provide a more controlled, less damaging form of electric current through the use of a variety of attachments. For example, an incision can be made using ESU with a small electrode blade. The blade cauterizes as it cuts thus minimizing bleeding. Other attachments can be used to coagulate and suction.

The USU uses high-frequency sound waves to break apart calcified or sclerosed tissue that can be removed in small segments. Some models have the ability to suction as they break apart and dissolve body calcifications. In some forms of electrosurgery, a local anesthetic may be administered.

Laser Surgery

The term laser is an acronym for Light Amplification by Stimulated Emission of Radiation. A laser emits an intense beam of light and originally was used to treat diseases of the retina. Today laser surgery is used to treat a wide variety of diseases and conditions including vascular, neurological, orthopedic, and dermatologic problems. Laser surgery has the advantage of promoting quick healing and not destroying surrounding tissue. A medical assistant may need extra training to assist with laser surgery. When a room is to be used for laser surgery, it is important to shut out any stray light rays, post OSHA's laser warning sign, and make sure everyone including the patient is wearing safety goggles. After surgery is complete, the wound should be cleaned with antiseptic and dressed with a sterile dressing.

Colposcopy

Colposcopy is an examination of the vagina and cervix performed using a lighted instrument called a colposcope with the patient in the lithotomy position. The colposcope allows the physician to observe the tissues of this area in great detail through light and magnification. Abnormal areas of tissue or cells can then be removed for biopsy, or microscopic examination of cells for cancer. In some cases, cryosurgery using freezing temperatures to destroy cells is then applied.

Colposcopy is performed:

- When an abnormal tissue development is observed by the physician during a routine pelvic examination.

- When a Papanicoulaou (PAP) smear result is in abnormal range.

- For magnified visualization.

- To obtain a biopsy specimen.

If the physician is unable to visualize the entire cervical canal during the colposcopy, he or she may perform an endocervical curettage (ECC) to scrape endocervical cells from inside the cervical canal. These cells are then sent for further testing to determine any abnormality. Note: Abnormal cell growth can be a sign of a pre-cancerous condition that, if untreated, could lead to the development of cancer.

The patient may experience slight bleeding after this procedure if a biopsy is taken. Provide a perineal pad for the patient with instructions for home care. The patient

PROCEDURE

Applying a Bandage over a Sterile Dressing

OBJECTIVE: Apply a bandage to the forearm.

Equipment and Supplies

nonsterile gloves; bandage material prescribed by physician or office procedures; bandage scissors; tape

Method

1. Identify the patient.
2. Perform hand hygiene.
3. Don nonsterile gloves.
4. Explain the procedure.
5. Hold bandage against the skin with nondominant hand one inch below the dressing.
6. Wrap bandage around wrist two to three times to secure (Figure 38-34A).
7. Wrap forearm from distal (part farthest away from the body) to proximal (closest to the body) with overlapping spiral turns (Figure 38-34B).
8. Check that the bandage is not restricting blood flow.
9. Continue wrapping to at least one inch above the dressing (Figure 38-34C).
10. Wrap two more times to secure bandage and cut.
11. Tape the cut end to the bandage; do not tape the end to the patient's skin.
12. Check again for any blood flow restriction.
13. Remove your gloves.
14. Perform hand hygiene.
15. Explain home care to the patient.
16. Document procedure accurately.

Charting Example

1/18/XX	9:30 A.M.

Applied bandage to sterile dressing. Pt instructed on home care for dressing.

M. King, CMA

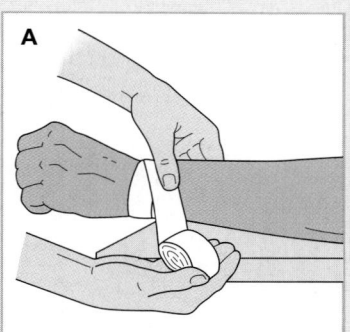
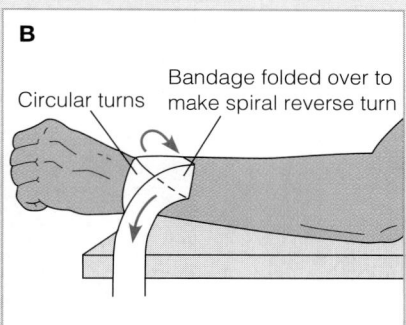
Circular turns — Bandage folded over to make spiral reverse turn
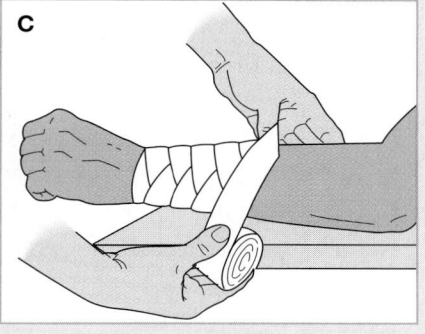

FIGURE 38-34 Bandaging a forearm.

---

should receive instructions to call the physician if there is abnormal pain or bleeding after this procedure.

Endoscopy

An endoscope is an instrument used to look into a hollow organ or body cavity. An endoscope is used to examine the larynx, bladder, colon, sigmoid colon, stomach, abdomen, and some joints. There are attachments utilized with some endoscopes such as light source, suction, monitor, and video recorder. Great care must be taken with these sensitive instruments. In most instances, the patient will need preparation prior to the examination. For example: fasting, taking a laxative, and an enema may be required prior to colonoscopy. Figure 38-37

is an example of flexible colonoscope with monitor and video recorder.

Cryosurgery

Cryosurgery is used to treat cervical erosion and chronic cervicitis. This procedure is also known as cryocautery rooted in the term *cautery*, which refers to a destruction of tissue. With the patient in the lithotomy position, the colposcope is used to magnify the surface of the cervix. Then a probe, capable of reaching freezing temperatures, is placed within the colposcope. The probe produces a freezing effect on tissues to destroy the abnormal cells.

The patient may experience mild cramping and a watery discharge after the procedure. The physician

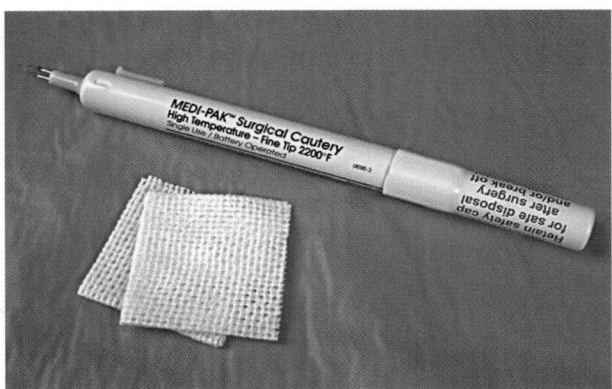

FIGURE 38-35 A disposable cautery unit.

may advise her to take a mild analgesic, such as Tylenol. The patient should be advised against using a tampon which could irritate sensitive tissues for at least a month. Additional instruction should include details on reporting any unusual pain or foul discharge, abstaining from sexual intercourse for one month, and when to return for a follow-up visit. The probe used in cryosurgery needs to be sterilized according to manufacturer's instructions immediately after use.

Endometrial Biopsy (EMB)

An endometrial biopsy (EMB) consists of using a curette or suction tool to remove uterine tissue for testing. EMB is performed for a variety of reasons including:

- To detect precancerous and cancerous conditions of the endometrial lining of the uterus.
- To detect inflammatory conditions.
- To determine if polyps are present.
- To assess abnormal uterine bleeding.
- To assess the effects of hormonal therapy.
- To screen for early detection of endometrial cancer (particularly if risk factors are present).

The American Cancer Society considers women with the following factors to be at high risk for endometrial cancer:

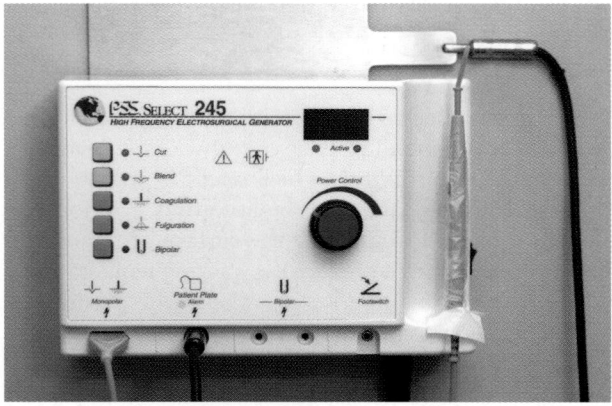

FIGURE 38-36 A hyfrecator, an electrocautery unit.

- Currently on estrogen therapy
- Obesity
- History of failure to ovulate
- History of infertility
- History of abnormal bleeding

An EMB is performed with the patient in the lithotomy position. The physician performs a bimanual examination of the uterus and administers a local anesthetic. A uterine sound is inserted into the uterus after the anesthetic has taken effect. The specimen is taken by means of a curette or with a suction device to aspirate a specimen. The specimen is sent to the laboratory in a container containing a 10 percent formalin preservative solution.

Provide a perineal pad for the patient with instructions for home care. The patient should receive instructions to call the physician if there is abnormal pain or bleeding after this procedure. She may experience mild cramping for which the physician may advise her to take a mild analgesic. She should be advised against using a tampon or douching for at least 72 hours.

Incision and Drainage (I & D)

Incision and drainage is performed to relieve the buildup of purulent (pus) material as a result of infection. The purulent discharge may need to be cultured to determine what microorganism is causing the infection, and thus, what antibiotic would be effective. The procedure is performed using sterile surgical technique. It is important to remember that the purulent material

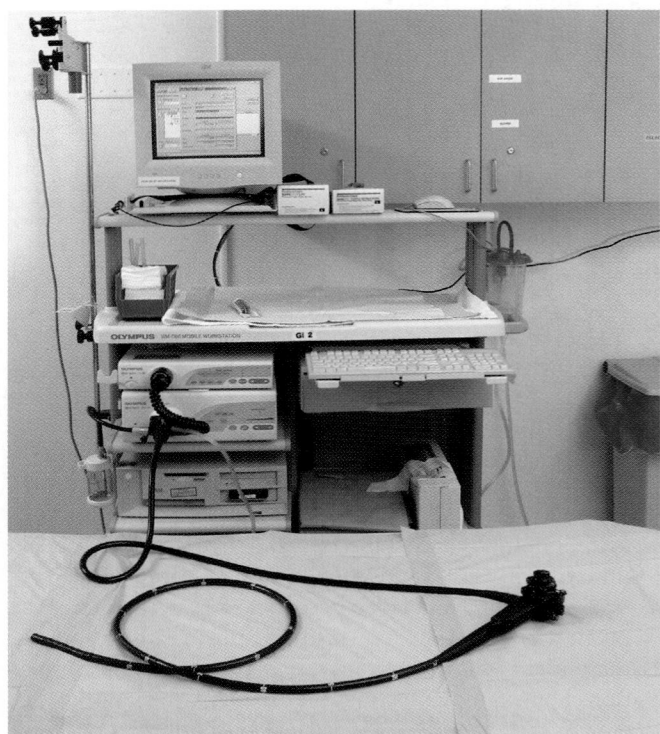

FIGURE 38-37 A flexible colonoscope with monitor and video recorder.

may be highly infectious. All soiled dressings and 4 × 4s should be immediately placed in a plastic waste container and then disposed of properly using OSHA guidelines.

A tray setup for an I & D would include:

- Scalpel handle and blades (No. 11)
- Curved iris scissors
- Tissue forceps
- Kelly hemostat
- Retractor
- Thumb dressing forceps
- 4 × 4 gauze squares

Removal of Foreign Bodies and Growths

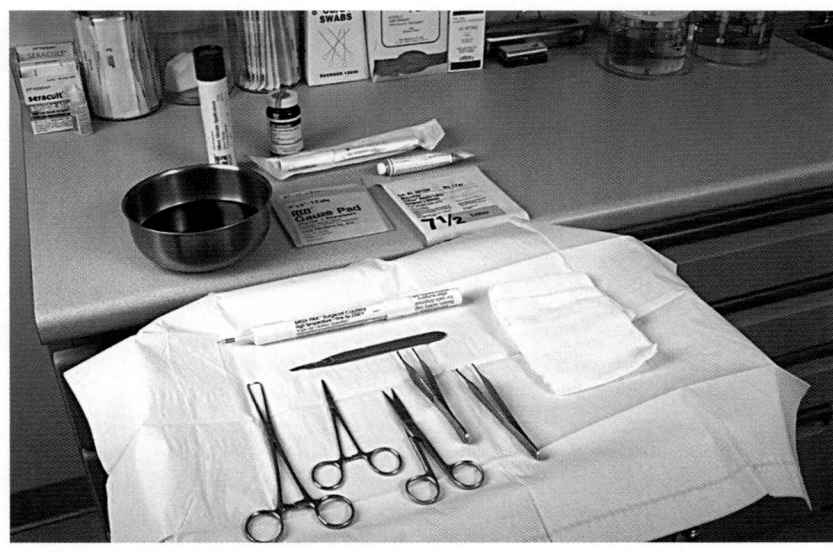

FIGURE 38-38 Surgical tray set up for biopsy procedure.

A foreign body can include a variety of materials from a small splinter or fishhook to a large object, such as an arrow that is imbedded in tissue. Splinter forceps are needed on an instrument tray for foreign body removal.

Growths include tumors, warts, moles, cysts. The most frequent growth removal procedure in the medical office is for cysts, which are enclosed fluid-filled sacs. Some growths will be sent to the laboratory for biopsy testing depending upon the physician's instructions. The removal of a foreign body or neoplasm (new growth) requires a surgical setup that includes:

- Thumb dressing forceps
- Retractor
- Scalpel handle and blades (No. 10 and 15)
- Curved tissue scissors
- Tissue forceps
- Hemostats
- Blunt probe
- Splinter forceps
- Needle holder
- Suture materials and needles
- Sterile 4 × 4 gauze

Figure 38-38 shows a surgical tray for biopsy removal. Figure 38-39 shows a medical assistant holding a specimen container so the physician can place the biopsy specimen into it without touching the rim or outside of the container and the contaminating tissue.

Vasectomy

The vasectomy procedure, tying and cutting of the vas deferens, on the male patient is a surgical procedure that is now commonly performed in the urologist's office. A vasectomy provides a permanent form of birth control for the male. As with any surgical procedure, a consent form needs to be signed and placed in the patient's record

before beginning this irreversible procedure. The patient should be instructed to have someone available to drive the patient home after the procedure. The patient will be uncomfortable for a short period of time (two to three days). He should be given detailed instructions on home care including activity level and sexual intercourse. The instructions may vary somewhat from one urologist to another. A typical vasectomy tray will include:

- Scalpel handle and No. 15 blade
- Dressing forceps
- Towel clamp
- Straight and curved mosquito forceps
- Curved tissue scissors
- Tissue forceps
- Retractor
- Needle holder and suture material
- Suture scissors

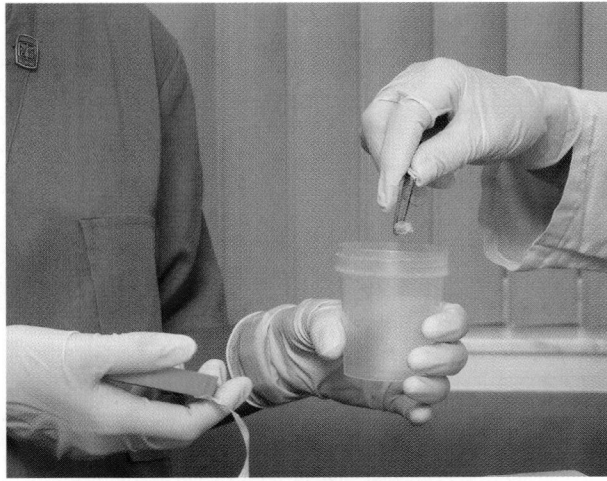

FIGURE 38-39 A medical assistant holds a specimen container to receive a biopsy sample.

SUMMARY

Assisting with surgery includes maintaining aseptic technique, a thorough knowledge of gowning, gloving, surgical hand hygiene, setting up sterile instrument trays and passing equipment to the physician, packaging and surgical setup, and preparing the patient for the procedure. Assisting with surgical procedures carries with it a grave responsibility to maintain absolute sterile technique. The medical assistant incorporates a variety of clinical skills when assisting with a surgical procedure.

Chapter Review

COMPETENCY REVIEW

1. Define and spell the terms to learn for this chapter.
2. Perform hand hygiene using medical aseptic technique; using surgical aseptic technique.
3. Identify by name the pieces of equipment needed for:
   A. suture removal
   B. incision and drainage
   C. suture of a laceration
   D. cervical biopsy
   E. removal of a foreign body
   F. dressing change with a wound culture
   G. endometrial biopsy
4. You have an open sore on your hand. What procedure should you follow when preparing to assist the surgeon?

PREPARING FOR THE CERTIFICATION EXAM

1. Which of the following should NOT touch a sterile field?
   A. 4 × 4s
   B. transfer forceps
   C. gloved hands
   D. sterile specimen container
   E. used instruments

2. The area that is considered sterile on a draped Mayo stand is
   A. within a 2-inch border
   B. outside a 2-inch border
   C. within a 1-inch border
   D. outside a 1-inch border
   E. the entire drape is sterile

3. The portion of a hemostat located near the handle that protects it from slipping once it is closed is the
   A. tooth
   B. ratchet
   C. serrated tip
   D. lock
   E. clamp

4. An instrument used by an obstetrician to measure an expectant mother's pelvis is the
   A. curette
   B. dilator
   C. pelvimeter
   D. speculum
   E. vaginal speculum

5. What is the correct method for shaving a surgical patient during the skin prep?
   A. dry shave going with the grain
   B. wet shave going against the grain
   C. wet shave before preparing the patient's skin
   D. wet shave going with the grain
   E. dry shave after preparing the patient's skin

6. Surgical hand hygiene is performed
   A. for 10 minutes using a clean hand brush
   B. for 10 minutes using a sterile hand brush
   C. by scrubbing for 2 minutes after removing rings
   D. with a brush and disinfectant
   E. using a germicidal soap

continued on next page

7. An example of a small gauge suture used for the skin is
   A. stainless steel 5-0
   B. stainless steel 0
   C. plain gut 3-0
   D. chromic gut 2-0
   E. nylon 2-0

8. When applying sterile gloves
   A. pick up first glove under the cuff and pull over the other hand slowly
   B. hold gloves over the sink while applying since the sink is considered "clean"
   C. place the fingers of the gloved hand under the cuff of the second glove, and then apply
   D. leave the cuffs turned down after applying to catch any spilled fluids
   E. apply gloves before setting up the equipment

9. When transferring sterile solutions to a sterile field
   A. place the cap with outside edge facing up
   B. place the cap with inside facing up
   C. place the cap on the Mayo stand
   D. pour the liquid by stabilizing the bottle on the edge of the basin
   E. discard the liquid remaining in the bottle

10. A typical surgical setup consists of
   A. scalpel, blades, trocar, probe, scope
   B. scalpel, blades, hemostat, probe, scope
   C. scalpel, blades, hemostat, scissors, suture
   D. scalpel, blades, hemostat, scissors, suture, scope
   E. scalpel, blades, scissors, suture, speculum

CRITICAL THINKING

1. How can you help Mrs. Jones feel more comfortable and less apprehensive?

2. Mrs. Jones becomes more upset when she sees you begin to assemble the equipment for the procedure. What is the best way to handle this situation?

3. Should you inform the physician of Mrs. Jones' apprehension and that she is crying?

4. You are the scrub assistant for this procedure. What steps may need to be taken to ensure that Mrs. Jones remains still during the procedure?

5. How would you chart this procedure?

ON THE JOB

Victor Krenz is assisting Dr. Connors with the fifth cataract surgical procedure for the day. The patient is Kathy Wall, a diabetic patient, whose condition has been stable enough for her to undergo a surgical procedure. Victor has performed a six minute surgical scrub on his hands before each of the five procedures. Dr. Connors indicates that he is in a hurry to get back to his office for a heavy afternoon schedule of patients. After both Dr. Connors and Victor are scrubbed, gowned, and ready to begin the operation, Victor feels a slight prick on the tip of his gloved finger as he moves the sterile syringe and needle on the tray. Dr. Connors, who does not notice the accidental needle prick to Victor's glove, states again that he is in a hurry to finish this procedure. Victor knows that if he has to change gloves, it will delay the surgery. He also knows that his hands have had a surgical scrub five times that morning and they are clean.

1. Can Victor justify not changing into new gloves?
2. What could happen to Ms. Wall as a result of Victor's needle prick?
3. How should Victor handle this situation?

INTERNET ACTIVITY

Research the Internet for the newest information about using laser surgery to reduce or remove facial wrinkles. After examining the information, do you think you would elect laser surgery to remove wrinkles? Would you recommend this procedure to others?

MediaLink More on assisting with minor surgery, including interactive resources, can be found in the Student CD-ROM accompanying this textbook.

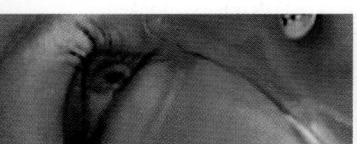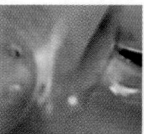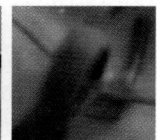

Medical Assistant Role Delineation Chart

HIGHLIGHT indicates material covered in this chapter.

ADMINISTRATIVE

Administrative Procedures

- Perform basic administrative medical assisting functions
- Schedule, coordinate and monitor appointments
- Schedule inpatient/outpatient admissions and procedures
- Understand and apply third-party guidelines
- Obtain reimbursement through accurate claims submission
- Monitor third-party reimbursement
- Understand and adhere to managed care policies and procedures
- *Negotiate managed care contracts*

Practice Finances

- Perform procedural and diagnostic coding
- Apply bookkeeping principles

- Manage accounts receivable
- *Manage accounts payable*
- *Process payroll*
- *Document and maintain accounting and banking records*
- *Develop and maintain fee schedules*
- *Manage renewals of business and professional insurance policies*
- *Manage personnel benefits and maintain records*
- *Perform marketing, financial, and strategic planning*

CLINICAL

Fundamental Principles

- Apply principles of aseptic technique and infection control
- Comply with quality assurance practices
- Screen and follow up patient test results

Diagnostic Orders

- Collect and process specimens
- Perform diagnostic tests

Patient Care

- Adhere to established patient screening procedures
- Obtain patient history and vital signs
- Prepare and maintain examination and treatment areas
- Prepare patient for examinations, procedures and treatments

- Assist with examinations, procedures and treatments
- Prepare and administer medications and immunizations
- Maintain medication and immunization records
- Recognize and respond to emergencies
- Coordinate patient care information with other health care providers
- Initiate IV and administer IV medications with appropriate training and as permitted by state law

GENERAL

Professionalism

- Display a professional manner and image
- Demonstrate initiative and responsibility
- Work as a member of the health care team
- Prioritize and perform multiple tasks
- Adapt to change
- Promote the CMA credential
- Enhance skills through continuing education
- Treat all patients with compassion and empathy
- Promote the practice through positive public relations

Communication Skills

- Recognize and respect cultural diversity
- Adapt communications to individual's ability to understand
- Use professional telephone technique

- Recognize and respond effectively to verbal, nonverbal, and written communications
- Use medical terminology appropriately
- Utilize electronic technology to receive, organize, prioritize and transmit information
- Serve as liaison

Legal Concepts

- Perform within legal and ethical boundaries
- Prepare and maintain medical records
- Document accurately
- Follow employer's established policies dealing with the health care contract
- Implement and maintain federal and state health care legislation and regulations
- Comply with established risk management and safety procedures
- Recognize professional credentialing criteria
- *Develop and maintain personnel, policy and procedure manuals*

Instruction

- Instruct individuals according to their needs
- Explain office policies and procedures
- Teach methods of health promotion and disease prevention
- Locate community resources and disseminate information
- *Develop educational materials*
- *Conduct continuing education activities*

Operational Functions

- Perform inventory of supplies and equipment
- Perform routine maintenance of administrative and clinical equipment
- Apply computer techniques to support office operations
- *Perform personnel management functions*
- *Negotiate leases and prices for equipment and supply contracts*

- *Denotes advanced skills.*

SOURCE: Reprinted by permission of the American Association of Medical Assistants from the AAMA Role Delineation Study: Occupational Analysis of the Medical Assisting Profession.

Assisting with Medical Emergencies

Learning Objectives

After completing this chapter, you should be able to:

- Define and spell the terms to learn for this chapter.

- Explain the primary assessment.

- Discuss the difference between treating complete and incomplete airway obstruction in an adult.

- Describe the differences between first-, second-, and third-degree burns.

- Explain the sequential steps you would take during the first minute after finding a patient seated in an examination room who looks like he's in cardiac arrest.

- List at least 10 things that might cause a patient to seize.

- Discuss the two major kinds of diabetic crises, and explain why you would want to administer sugar for either one.

- Discuss the differences between the four kinds of musculoskeletal injuries.

- Describe the differences in pathophysiology between heat exhaustion and heat stroke.

- Compare and contrast at least five kinds of shock.

OUTLINE

The Emergency Medical
Services System   802

Guidelines for Providing
Emergency Care   802

The Office Emergency
Crash Kit   806

Medical Emergencies   806

Terms to Learn

asphyxia

bandage

chief complaint

dressing

emergency kit
(crash cart)

first responder

heat exhaustion

heat stroke

hyperglycemia

hyperventilation
syndrome

hypoglycemia

hypothermia

immediate history

intubate

past medical history

primary assessment

Rule of Nines

stridor

tidal volume

triage

Case Study

A PATIENT BY THE NAME OF ANNIE HEDLEY just walked into the medical office holding a towel on her head stating "I cut my head open." Bradley Warbington, RMA immediately takes Ms. Hedley to one of the examination rooms.

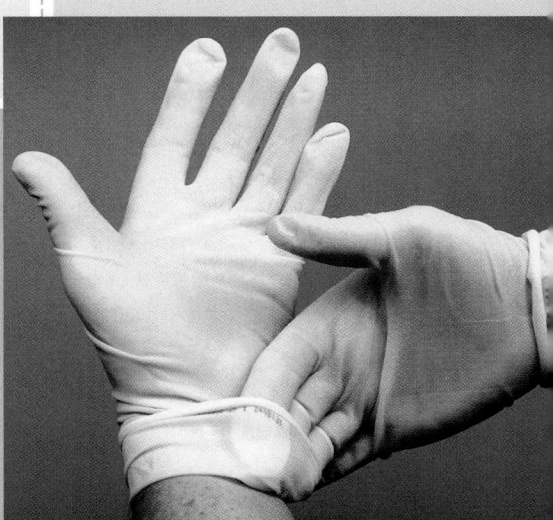

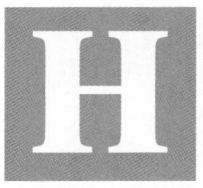ave you ever witnessed the actions of emergency crews at an auto accident scene, or maybe even at a shopping center where someone has had a medical emergency? Maybe you noticed how calm those emergency people were: no running, no shouting, everybody with a job to do . . . almost automatically.

What makes that kind of performance possible under even the worst circumstances is a solid foundation in the basics. The basics include an understanding of what causes most medical emergencies, and knowledge of some basic first steps to take, no matter what is happening around you. A medical assistant who is equipped with that knowledge is prepared to make that first contact with someone who has had a medical emergency. Find out how ill or injured the person is, and what treatment is needed, and make sure the patient gets it. Those are the elements of emergency first aid.

A variety of medical emergencies are presented in this chapter. The physician must be notified immediately regarding all medical office emergencies. In some cases the Emergency Medical Services (EMS) system will need to be notified by calling 911. Medical assistants are cautioned not to perform procedures outside their scope of practice to ensure the patient's safety until additional medical help arrives.

The Emergency Medical Services System

The medical assistant is an important part of a community's EMS system. The medical assistant must exercise good judgment and inform the physician or call 911 immediately if a patient's problems are more serious than he or she can handle. In response, you will quickly obtain the help of people, equipment, and a communication system that are all designed for the kinds of emergencies that the office staff is not equipped to handle.

Typically an EMS system employs first responders—individuals who are trained to recognize medical conditions, initiate basic life support, and access other parts of the system. The first responder would look to the medical assistant as a medical professional for detailed information about the patient's complaint, the immediate and overall history, medications taken and allergies, and the care that has been administered up to the point of their arrival.

After accessing the system, the medical assistant would inform the patient that he or she will be transported to a hospital. The medical assistant would also continue assessing and caring for the patient until the arrival of an ambulance or emergency medical personnel. First responders carry emergency equipment, which

may not be in the medical office, and they can provide the necessary staffing to handle, for example, a cardiac arrest. The emergency crew may also be staffed by one or more paramedics depending on the system.

Paramedics can intubate, which involves inserting a tube into the trachea as and emergency airway, and they can start an IV in seconds. They have ample oxygen supplies and an assortment of emergency medications, and they are licensed to perform other invasive procedures. EMS personnel are accustomed to working with health care professionals. One of them will ask the office staff for all the pertinent patient information and make sure that observations become part of the patient chart. In addition, this communicator will operate the radio system that connects your patient to the receiving hospital.

Specialized Resources

Apart from emergency response teams, the medical assistant will occasionally need to consult with specialists in such areas as poison control, pediatrics, trauma, and burns. Some consults will be under emergency conditions, so make sure the specialists' telephone numbers are displayed prominently near the phones in the office.

Guidelines for Providing Emergency Care

Medical assistants need to be able to handle emergencies in three ways. The most common way is on the telephone, when a patient or patient's relative calls to ask for advice during an emergency outside the office. Another way is when an emergency occurs near the doctor's office and someone brings the patient to the office. The third way is when an emergency occurs in the office.

In some states, triage, or assessing the emergency care needed by patients, is not within the scope of practice of the medical assistant. In these states the medical assistant should not work alone in the medical office (see Legal and Ethical Issues).

In an emergency the medical assistant needs to be able to look at someone, listen to them on the phone, and quickly assess whether they are ill or injured and require emergency care. The medical assistant may ask the physician for advice anytime he or she is in the office, or make the decision to access the EMS by calling 911.

The Primary Assessment

Every patient contact by a medical professional begins with a few simple questions and a basic patient examination called the primary assessment. This assessment is critically important for the medical assistant, whose role it is to organize the process of caring for patients. The key to effective patient assessment is the combination of careful observation with automatic, medically sound routines that are applied in every patient situation. The following steps describe both.

Determine the Patient's Name, Approximate Age, and Gender

Always ask the patient's name first, for two reasons.

1. Identifying the patient enables access to their medical records, and helps you to protect every patient against accidentally receiving the wrong care.

2. All people have names, and all people are supposed to know their names even when not fully alert. The way patients answer to their names (or do not answer) can reveal a lot about how well their mind and body are functioning—and how ill they are.

When you ask patients their names, they must quickly go through an extensive neurological process in order to give a simple appropriate answer. They must be able to:

- Hear you.
- Localize the sound of your voice, using both ears and both eyes.
- Look at you with a symmetrical gaze and focus on you with both eyes.
- Reason that you are a caregiver, and then process the meaning of your words, hopefully in your own language (but maybe not).
- Remember their name, and formulate a meaningful response.
- Answer in coherent speech and with a symmetrical face.

During that brief period of time, you may learn a lot about patients' mental function by observing other things such as facial expressions and body language.

When you ask for a patient's name, ask for the patient's medications at the same time. The labels can provide the date of birth and the correct spelling of the name. The medicine labels can also provide some clues as to the medical history and the name(s) of one or more physicians.

Decide If the Patient Is Ill or Injured

Determine the patient's medical condition early on and reassess it throughout every patient contact. If the patient is really ill, there is no time to ask a lot of questions. A patient's status may change in a matter of seconds. The fastest way to determine if someone is really ill is to look at the person. When a patient looks really ill, that is a good indication that something is wrong. A patient who cannot be aroused or who cannot stay awake deserves serious concern. Does the patient seem too weak to stand up? Does the skin color seem very pale, or perhaps blue? Is the patient very sweaty for no apparent reason (such as hot weather or recent exercise)? Is the patient bleeding uncontrollably, or struggling to breathe?

These are all signs of serious trouble. Stop everything else and alert your physician right away. If the

Legal and Ethical Issues

As a medical assistant, you have three primary legal responsibilities in the face of an emergency. The first is obviously a duty to act within your scope of practice. Even though we all feel a little intimidated by the thought of an emergency, you are a medical professional. As such, in case of an emergency you are accountable to yourself, your employer, and the public for actions that measure up to your degree of medical training.

Once you do receive medical training, your duty to act never really goes away. You will always be expected to act like someone who has had the same kind of training that you have. You will never be able to witness an accident in a public place without some responsibility to do the best you can to help.

Your second legal responsibility is to document the constant emergency readiness of the office you work in. You not only need to check your equipment when you come to work every day or as deemed by your employer (an ethical responsibility), but you need to be able to prove that you did so (a legal responsibility). That means documentation, by means of timed, dated, and signed logs as required in your office. When a piece of equipment fails that you were supposed to check but did not, the failure is at least partially on your shoulders.

Your third legal responsibility, which you share with others in your workplace, is to do all you can to prevent emergencies, for example, correcting things like loose carpet, spills and water leaks, and electrical hazards. Educating patients and their families about their own safety is also part of emergency prevention.

Always stay alert within your scope of practice; know what is beyond your scope; and let your physician know.

physician is not available, contact 911 and anticipate transport to an emergency department.

Determine a Chief Complaint

Another way to find out if someone is really ill, if it is not obvious, is to determine the chief complaint. A patient's chief complaint is the main reason he or she is seeking medical help.

To obtain a chief complaint ask, watch, and listen for it. Try hard to use open-ended questions that leave

One of the best things about being a good caregiver is that people trust you. They believe what you say, and that makes it possible for you to convince them to do or avoid things that will keep them healthy and safe.

There are a thousand little ways to make sure that people's lives are a little healthier without ever preaching to anyone or giving them unqualified medical advice. And you're just the one to do it. The best emergency medicine is preventive care. The medical assistant should be alert to the many opportunities to teach patients healthy habits in order to avoid burns, falls, fractures, and poisoning.

the patient free to choose his or her own words and gestures to describe how he or she feels.

A patient who clutches his chest all the time may be having chest pain. A child who seems to carry, or "cradle," one elbow with the opposite hand may be having some pain in her clavicle or upper extremity. An infant who seems very quiet and who drools a lot may have a sore throat.

A patient whose breathing seems noisy and labored, or who is silent, may have a respiratory obstruction of some kind. It is difficult to talk when it is difficult to breathe. All of these are important findings that may change by the time help arrives. Observations, described in the observer's own words, are very important to an emergency caregiver.

Sometimes the complaint itself is all you need to know. Some specific complaints always warrant prompt attention, including the following:

- Trouble breathing (extremely labored or noisy, shallow, slow or absent)
- Severe or persistent bleeding
- Chest, neck, jaw, or left arm pain that is unrelieved by rest, O_2, or nitrates
- Prolonged or recurrent seizures (especially in the unresponsive patient)
- Extreme weakness (especially if the patient gets dizzy on standing)
- Impending emergency childbirth
- Severe headache, unrelieved by aspirin or acetaminophen
- Palpitations (patient is able to feel heart beating in chest)
- Major trauma (probably not seen in a physician's office)

In addition to this list, never ignore what you think you see, smell, or hear. For instance, skin color and breath or body odors can indicate a variety of medical problems, including poisons, intestinal bleeding, cancer, and diabetes. All of these things can provide crucial hints about a patient's chief complaint.

Obtain the History

There are two kinds of history: the patient's immediate history (or history of the event) and the patient's past medical history (or lifelong history). They are both extremely important.

The immediate history can reveal a lot about the nature of a problem. For instance, a patient who feels "dizzy" upon awakening in the morning with a cold is a lot different than a patient who feels the same way after several episodes of dark-colored, foul-smelling diarrhea. Although both of these patients have the same complaint (dizziness), their histories differ. By itself, the first patient's history suggests an ear infection, whereas the second patient's history points to GI bleeding. Another example would be a caller who describes where his terrible headache is located and then loses consciousness. The data reported in the patient's history would prompt the initial decisions and actions of an entire team of people who would then care for that patient.

The past medical history is the medical story of a person's life, intended to include everything remarkable that has ever happened to the person medically. Sometimes it reveals clues that are essential to a diagnosis. For instance, a person who develops severe shortness of breath along with a simple chest cold might surprise you until you learn from the history that the patient has only one lung.

The best way to gather the past medical history is to use a checklist, whether mental or written. The questions you ask may depend on your employer's standard procedures, but should probably be the same for every patient, regardless of the complaint. Specifically, they might include the following:

- Heart problems? (Heart "attack"?)
- Lung problems? (Does the patient have both lungs?)
- Asthma or allergies
- Kidney problems? (Does the patient have both kidneys?)
- Diabetes? (Does the patient take insulin/has the patient had insulin today and, if so, when?)

- High or low blood pressure? (Which?)
- Seizures?
- Fainting spells?
- Any possibility of pregnancy/OB/GYN history/LMP? (Normal?)
- Previous similar events? (When, treatment, outcome?)

Except for allergies, this list of questions includes all of the conditions that may be fatal to people.

During history taking and throughout all contact with patients and their relatives, listen closely to what people say and watch their eyes. Is somebody extremely concerned about his or her modesty, or does someone feel cold? Is someone expecting bad news about a spouse of 50 years? The answers are part of the history and should be communicated to the physician who will be continuing the care.

The most frightening thing about any emergency is often patients' perceptions of it. Try very hard to anticipate their feelings, and to explain everything in plain language before it happens. Concentrate on their comfort and check up on them every few minutes, just to let them know how important they are.

Gather the Medications

Save the patient's original medicine containers for whomever will continue the care. Make sure you write them down for later reference. Knowing when a patient's medicines were prescribed by observing the date on each label is also helpful. It can reveal how recently the patient was treated by a physician for the medical problem.

If the patient seems confused about his or her medications, the physician needs to be made aware of this. Sometimes the patient just needs help getting organized. The patient who takes a lot of different kinds of medicines may benefit from a daily medication organizer. They come in various configurations, but most consist of rows and columns of small plastic boxes. Sometimes, as is the case with some elderly patients (who often have more than one physician and take too much medicine), the patient's whole list of medications may need to be reevaluated and simplified.

Finally, many medical conditions are caused by interactions among medications or by a patient's reaction to one or more of them.

Determine the Allergies

Most caregivers underestimate the importance of allergies. People can go into anaphylaxis from an allergic reaction. Thousands of patients are violently allergic to some of the medicines that are dispensed every day. Many wear some kind of jewelry as a reminder, in the form of bracelets, wristbands, or necklaces. Usually they are keenly aware of their allergies, but it happens sometimes during a medical crisis that people will either forget about their allergies or become unable to communicate about them. It is good practice to check for warning tags and jewelry during the patient examination, even if a patient denies having any allergies.

Remember, too, that asthma may be induced by an allergy and that people with allergies tend to have more than just one. Be extra suspicious of allergies when a patient's medical history includes asthma—or when, during your questions about medications, the patient reveals a pocket inhaler.

Do a Physical Examination

If a physician is not available, do a comprehensive, quick, basic physical examination when someone looks ill.

When performing a quick physical assessment, start with the things that do not require the use of equipment. After asking permission and before putting on gloves on, gently place the back of one hand or wrist against the skin of the patient's forehead and then on the cheek. Finally, grasp both the patient's hands, perhaps for less than a second. The patient's skin moisture and temperature will be felt, as well as any trembling or shivering that might not be obvious. When people are nervous, their hands get clammy. But when a patient's face gets cold and moist, he or she is more than just nervous.

Look into the patient's eyes for a moment. The pupils should be normal and equal in size. The patient's gaze should appear symmetrical. Use a penlight, if available, to check the pupils of first one eye, then the other.

Observe the patient's overall physical and emotional state. Does the patient seem well nourished, articulate, dressed appropriately, angry or irritable, or abnormally tired? Is the patient coughing or sneezing and can you hear his or her respirations? Does the patient seem to be holding onto a part of the body as though injured, or possibly cradling an aching head in his or her hands? When you walk the patient to the scale, do you notice anything unusual about his or her gait? What is your overall impression of how ill the patient is?

All of the physical observations you have made take only a minute or so but are potentially very important.

Take the Vital Signs

With the patient's permission, take the vital signs. Take the patient's temperature and then count his or her respirations for about 30 seconds. Then spend 30 seconds checking the pulse, and follow that with taking the blood pressure. Record these readings on the chart. If the patient has a potentially serious complaint, or if anything in the vitals or the patient's appearance concerns you, terminate the physical examination and notify the physician immediately. If the physician is unavailable, call 911. Have the patient lie down on the examination table, and make him or her comfortable. Oxygen may need to be administered as ordered by the physician.

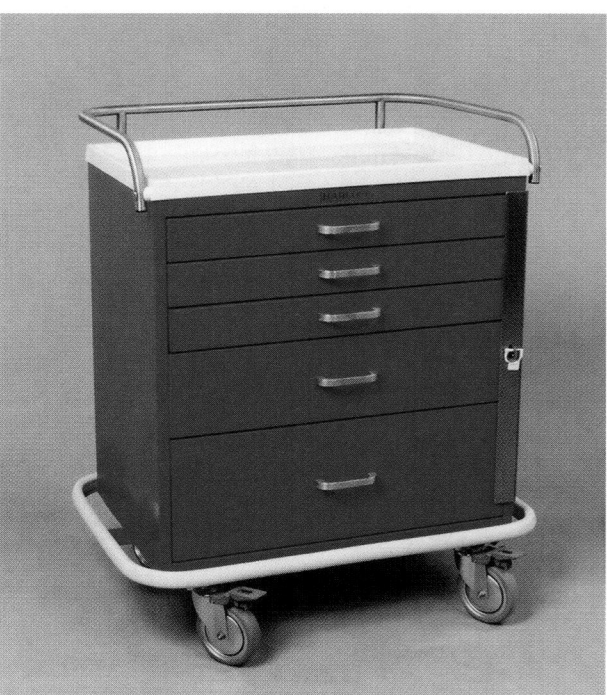

FIGURE 39-1 Crash cart.

The Office Emergency Crash Kit

Every doctor's office has an emergency kit or box (sometimes called a crash cart) that contains all supplies that may be needed during an emergency and which is instantly accessible by anyone in the office (see Figure 39-1). A crash cart resembles a large roll-around tool box with drawers that can be used to store emergency medications, intubation equipment, needles and syringes, assorted small instruments, a resuscitator, a monitor-defibrillator, an oxygen supply, and airways and suction devices. This cart may contain items that are not within the scope of practice for a medical assistant. However, a physician or nurse may use them. In a small office, a crash kit can be brought to the side of any patient within moments of an emergency (also called a "code").

The emergency supplies need to be checked routinely. It is suggested that the cart be restocked after every use and maintained at least once a month on a regular basis, with expiration dates checked, for two reasons. First, emergency medications do not tend to get used often, and they expire. The same is true of the batteries that power the monitor-defibrillator, laryngoscopes, and suction device. When these items do get used, someone who is not currently dealing with the aftermath of an emergency needs to double-check them. Second, being able to use emergency equipment under pressure in an emergency situation requires comfortable, hands-on familiarity with the equipment. When emergencies are infrequent, as in the case of most physicians' offices, familiarity can only come from handling the equipment during frequent maintenance checks. Mock practice sessions can also help medical assistants become more familiar with the equipment and how to respond.

Finally, a crash cart needs to have a physician checklist that names every drug container and every piece of equipment the cart contains. The checklist should provide space for a daily date and signature, and someone in the office should be accountable for maintaining the cart. But everyone who is likely to use the cart needs to check it personally as well, for the sake of their own performance. The physician should decide what equipment and supplies should be stocked in the emergency cart.

Medical Emergencies

The following sections of this chapter present on overview of the descriptions and treatment of medical emergencies that are seen in the medical office. Always remember to check the ABCs when giving emergency care: A = airway (Is the patient's airway open?), B = breathing (Can the patient breathe on his or her own?), and C = circulation (Has something interfered with normal blood flow?)

Airway Obstruction (Foreign Body Airway Obstruction)

Normally, the airway does a good job of protecting itself and keeping itself clean. But airway obstruction can be disastrous. How can the medical assistant help the patient who comes into the office choking on an obstruction? First of all, alert a fellow staff member to notify the physician immediately. The patient exhibits the universal choking sign—both hands to the neck, possible facial reddening or cyanosis, and a look of panic, but no respiratory sounds (see Figure 39-2).

Chances are that if the patient walks into the office with or without help, she does not have a complete

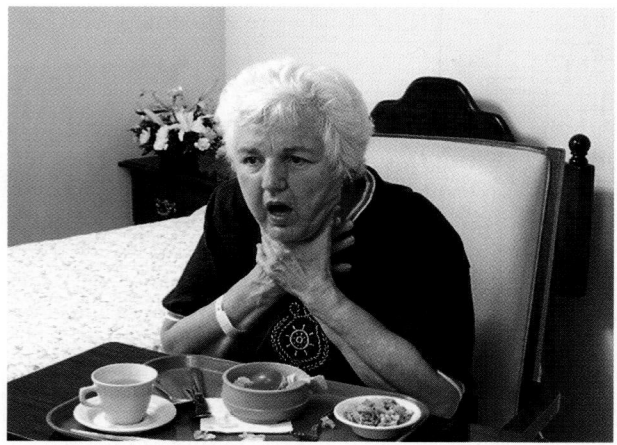

FIGURE 39-2 The universal choking sign.

airway obstruction. As soon as you see the patient, walk up to her calmly, look into her eyes and ask, "Are you choking?" If she can make any breathing sounds at all, do not do anything initially but reassure her. The last thing you want to do is to convert a partial obstruction into complete one.

Heimlich Maneuver

A patient with a complete airway obstruction will be vocally silent. If she nods yes when asked if she is choking, tell her you are about to help her. Walk around behind the patient, encircle her with your arms, locate her navel and the bottom end of her sternum (xiphoid process), and place the thumb side of your closed fist against her abdomen directly between these two points. Grab your fist with your other, free hand, and deliver a firm thrust into the patient's abdomen in an upward direction toward you (Figure 39-3). Keep doing that until the patient coughs up the obstruction or until she loses consciousness.

If the patient does become unconscious after administering one or more abdominal thrusts, ease her to the floor and place her on her back. Call for help and attempt ventilation. If ventilation does not work, grasp the mandible with your thumb and forefinger and pull it forward. Use the index finger of your other hand to sweep the mouth. Do not spend a lot of time at it, but see if you can retrieve an obstruction that may have been freed when the patient lost consciousness.

If you are not able to see and remove the obstruction, kneel beside the patient's thighs and place the heels of your hands (as though you were doing CPR) on the surface of her abdomen midway between her navel and xiphoid. Deliver five firm thrusts into her abdomen, aimed toward her chest. Try once again to ventilate, and keep repeating these steps in sequence as quickly as you can until you can ventilate the patient (see Procedure 39-1).

Variations

There are some patients in whom abdominal thrusts cause injury. They are pregnant women, infants, and very large persons. In those patients, perform chest thrusts instead of abdominal thrusts. If the pregnant patient with a complete airway obstruction is conscious, approach her from behind, encircle her chest with your arms, and place your fist against the middle of her sternum. Seize your fist firmly with your other hand, then deliver a firm thrust backwards. Repeat the maneuver until the obstruction is cleared or she becomes unconscious. Figure 39-4 illustrates a chest thrust to be used on a large person or pregnant woman.

If the patient becomes unconscious, attempt to ventilate. If ventilation does not work, do a jaw lift and finger sweep. It that does not work, kneel beside her

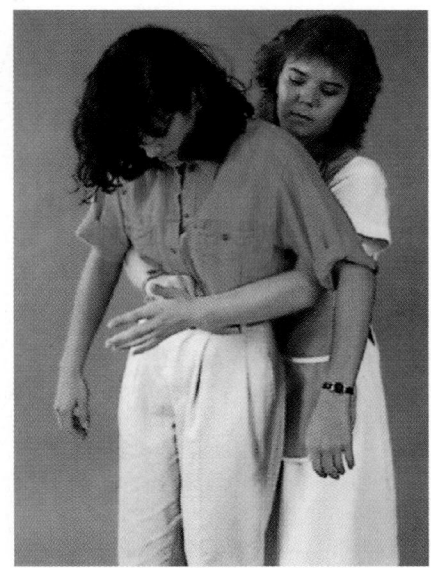

FIGURE 39-3 Heimlich maneuver.

body, as with the abdominal thrust on an unconscious patient, and deliver five chest thrusts to her midsternum (see Figure 39-5). Start all over again, and continue the sequence as quickly as you can until the obstruction is cleared or until the physician or emergency team tells you to stop.

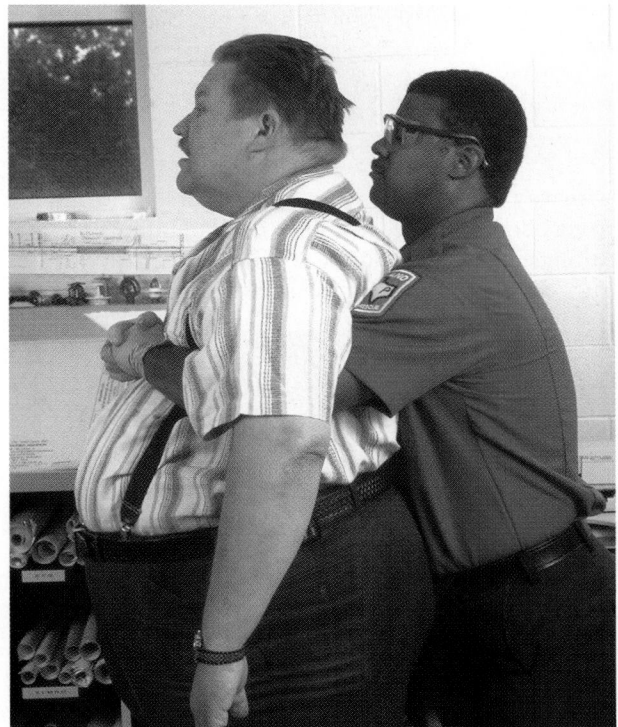

FIGURE 39-4 Chest thrusts are used on very large persons and pregnant women.

Responding to an Obstructed Airway (Conscious Adult, Child, or Infant)

OBJECTIVE: Be able to respond to an obstructed airway.

Equipment and Supplies
disposable gloves, mannequin

Method for a Conscious Adult or Child

1. Ask the choking patient "Are you choking?" If the patient nods his or her head yes or demonstrates the universal sign for choking, ask the patient "Can you speak?" If the patient shakes his or her head no or demonstrates the universal sign for choking, tell the patient your name and ask the patient "Can I help you?"
2. Immediately stand behind the patient.
3. Place your arms around the patient's abdomen.
4. Make a fist with one of your hands. Place your fist with the thumb side toward the abdomen. Your fist should be just above the patient's navel.
5. Place the other, free hand over the fist.
6. Give an upward thrust quickly until the object comes out of the patient's mouth or the patient becomes unconscious.

Method for a Conscious Infant

1. Ask the person with the infant "Is the baby choking?" If person tells you "Yes," tell the person your name and ask the person "Can I help you?"

2. If the infant is not coughing or crying, have the person give you the infant.
3. Place the infant face down on your forearm with your fingers cradling the head, and rest your forearm on your thigh. Keep the child's head dependent. Using the heel of your free hand, deliver five back blows between the child's shoulder blades.
4. Using your forearms to sandwich the child's body, now place the child face up on your opposite forearm and rest that forearm on your thigh on the same side. Place two fingers on the midline of the child's chest just below the nipple line and deliver five quick chest compressions, almost as though you were doing CPR.
5. Repeat back blows and chest compressions in rapid sequence until the object is dislodged. Remove it immediately, but only if you can visualize it in the pharynx. If the infant is still choking, quickly repeat the whole sequence until the obstruction is removed or until the physician or paramedic takes over or the infant becomes unconscious.

Airway obstructions in small children and infants are very common, because children and infants put lots of things into their mouths. A child with an airway obstruction is treated the same as an adult, with one exception. Only remove an obstruction from a child's airway if you can see it. Blind finger sweeps are not recommended.

Any patient who has lost consciousness as a result of an airway obstruction requires x-rays to verify that nothing was aspirated (sucked) into the lungs.

Abdominal Pain

Although a thorough discussion of abdominal pain is beyond the scope of this text, some general concepts are essential to all caregivers. All complaints of abdominal pain should trigger two thoughts: surgery and pregnancy (in females). Because so many abdominal complications can only be resolved by surgery, the patient who complains of abdominal pain should thereafter not ingest anything by mouth (NPO) pending a physician's diagnosis. Second, because of their potentially serious consequences, complications of pregnancy should always be considered a possibility in the female patient who complains of abdominal pain.

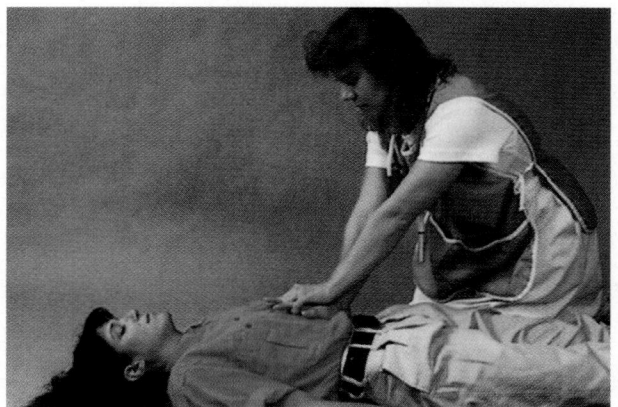

FIGURE 39-5 Chest thrusts are delivered with a firm thrust into the patient's abdomen in an upward movement.

Observe the patient with abdominal pain. Is the patient in shock? Is the skin warm or cool or moist? These signs may indicate a fever, infection, or bleeding. Get a quick set of vitals, including the temperature. Ask the patient if he or she needs to lie down. Ask a few questions that can get you the most important information you need, quickly:

- Has there been vomiting?
- Irregularities of stool or urine?
- Any abnormal discharges (from mouth, rectum, urinary tract)?
- Change in diet?
- Trouble breathing?
- Recent injury?
- Last menstrual period?
- Any possibility of pregnancy?

Not all disorders related to the abdomen are emergencies. But many emergencies related to the abdomen are surgical and, therefore, not performed in the physician's office. Apply high-flow oxygen if ordered by the physician. Keep the patient flat with knees bent to relieve pain. Contact EMS.

Allergic Reactions

The way our bodies respond to substances and pathogens in the environment is supposed to be automatic, unconscious, and trouble free. Except for an occasional bout of poison oak or mosquito attack, that is how life is for most of us. But for some, life is a constant struggle with allergies in the forms of discomfort, fear of environmental substances, and even the reality of sudden death.

Any one of us can discover a severe allergy at any time, but people with severe allergies tend to have many of them rather than just one or two. Fortunately, allergic emergencies are usually easy to recognize and not difficult to treat.

Patients with an allergic reaction usually have red, warm skin. They may have some difficulty breathing, and parts of their body (like the face) may appear so puffy that the family will say that they look like somebody else. The patient may have localized or widespread hives (irregular, white blotchy areas where the skin seems to be raised). If breathing is a problem, wheezing may be heard even without a stethoscope. Usually, but not always, the patient will be able to describe an encounter with a substance to which he has a known allergy (an allergen). If not, and he says he has allergies to other substances, you can surmise that he is having an allergic reaction to an unknown substance.

If the patient's systolic blood pressure is below 100 in addition to the preceding findings, you should probably get the patient to lie down, raise the lower extremities, and treat him for anaphylactic shock.

Treatment for an allergic reaction always begins with the same step: Break contact between the patient and the allergen. If there is no clear identification of the allergen, remove the patient's clothing and do a thorough physical examination. Make sure there is not a stinger somewhere, an ointment or cream, a new kind of hair spray, evidence of a recent injection, or some other substance or object that might be responsible. Find out about recent meals, especially if they included seafood. Consider the recent use of unfamiliar latex contraceptives (male or female). If the patient has a diaphragm in place, it should probably be removed by the patient or by a physician. Do whatever else is necessary to remove anything suspicious. Alert the physician and administer oxygen if ordered. Chances are that no matter how ill the patient appears, he or she will begin to respond within a minute or so to subcutaneous epinephrine (1:1000) (adrenaline). The medical assistant can prepare the epinephrine injection for the physician to administer. Some patients with a history of severe allergic reactions may be given a prescription for an epinephrine auto-injector or kit.

The patient who has been in shock may require transport to a hospital.

Amputation

Amputation of an extremity or body part is such a profound insult that these injuries do not tend to find their

---

Cultural Considerations

Family in some populations is extremely important to the patient. Family members provide not only emotional and physical support but are an essential part of the medical decision-making process. Do not be surprised if your patient brings along the entire family, including parents, grandparents, siblings, aunts, and uncles to discuss an important medical condition. Be prepared for a large crowd and do not get annoyed. Make them as comfortable as possible and consider them part of the healing process.

way into physicians' offices until after they have been cared for in the emergency department (ED) of the nearest hospital. They are fairly easy to care for, since the body normally reacts almost immediately to amputation by shutting down the blood flow to the severed extremity. If amputation does occur nearby and the patient is brought to the physician's office, call EMS and arrange transport to the hospital. Be sure to save the body part in a cooler with ice. (Avoid placing it directly on the ice.)

Asphyxia

Asphyxia or suffocation can occur as a result of almost any mechanical disruption of the organs or structures that enable us to breathe. Some examples include a ruptured lung or diaphragm, blockage of a major pulmonary vessel, crushed rib, or crushed trachea or larynx.

The patient suffering from asphyxia would be blue from the clavicles upward. The neck veins would be very distended, and if conscious the patient may be struggling frantically to breathe but unable to do so. The patient has almost no tidal volume (the volume of air we exchange with each cycle of breathing).

Alert the physician immediately, and contact EMS even if the physician is available. Try to ventilate the patient with 100 percent oxygen as ordered by the physician. Allow the patient to remain in the position of choice. If the patient can be helped at all, it will be by means of an advanced procedure by a physician or a paramedic.

Birth (Emergency)

A pregnant patient may come into the medical office in active labor, which means the birth is imminent. In this case, it is not wise for the patient to then leave the office and make the trip to the hospital for the delivery, particularly if she is unaccompanied or drove the vehicle herself. EMS needs to be called in order to deliver the baby, to provide care to the mother and baby immediately after birth, and to provide transport to the hospital.

Childbirth is a normal process unless the mother is hemorrhaging or the baby is in fetal distress. Fetal distress can be caused by conditions such as a prolapsed umbilical cord or placenta previa, which is blockage of the birth canal by the placenta.

Labor is the actual process of expelling the fetus from the uterus and through the vagina. The length of time of labor varies in women from a few hours to 24 hours or more. A mother who has had several previous births may deliver a baby very quickly. While she will have strong contractions just before birth, there may have been a few or no labor pains or contractions that she was aware of. When a mother who has delivered several babies (multipara) comes into the office in labor, be prepared to conduct an emergency childbirth.

The first stage of labor is referred to as the stage of dilation. During this stage the uterine muscles contract in an attempt to expel the fetus. During this process the fetus presses on the cervix and causes it to dilate or expand. When the cervix is completely dilated at 10 centimeters, the second stage of labor begins. The thinning of the cervix is referred to as effacement. This stage ends with the birth of the baby. Generally the head of the baby appears first. This is referred to as crowning. In some cases, the baby's buttocks will appear first, and this referred to as a breach birth. The last stage of labor is the placenta stage, during which the placenta or afterbirth is delivered. Immediately after childbirth the uterus again begins to contract, causing the placenta to be expelled through the vagina.

Bites and Stings (Venomous and Nonvenomous)

There are three common kinds of bites and a variety of stings that you may expect to see, depending on the area where you work. To some extent, the advanced resources for treating venomous bites and stings will be specialized to meet the needs of your area.

Venomous Bites and Stings

Fortunately, venomous creatures do not always inject venom when they bite. If they do, pain is usually immediate and intense, and swelling follows within minutes to hours. Other variables include:

- The type of creature that bit or stung the patient
- The age and size of the patient
- The location of the site of the sting or bite
- The amount of activity following the bite (less is better)
- The elapsed time since the bite (less is better)

A complete discussion of all kinds of bites or stings is not within the scope of this text, but general descriptions follow.

There is not much to be done for the victims of most venomous bites or stings in the office setting. Most will require the resources of a trauma center and the kind of antivenin that is specific to their injuries. But it is important to recognize the appearances of the injury sites that may not be associated with serious signs or symptoms until 12 to 24 hours or more after envenomation. It is also important to remember that even common insect stings, such as those from bees, may trigger severe allergic reactions, including anaphylactic shock, in some patients. For a bee sting, be careful to scrape the stinger out rather than squeezing it out.

VENOMOUS SNAKEBITE Most venom attacks are not fatal. Small children and elderly adults are most at risk, and so are victims of snakes with fangs that allow the venom to enter the bloodstream directly.

There are two kinds of poisonous snakebites, namely, those from snakes with fangs and those from snakes without fangs. Snakes with fangs (for example, rattlesnakes, copperheads, and cottonmouths) leave distinctive marks from well-developed paired fangs, and the onset of pain and swelling is almost immediate. Be aware that the fang marks may look like abrasions or small cuts instead of puncture wounds. Snakes without fangs (for example, coral snakes) inject their venom during a kind of chewing motion as they bite. Systemic signs—signs indicating that the entire body is affected—may not develop for many hours following these bites.

To help a snakebite patient, contact EMS and apply oxygen if ordered by the physician. The physician may want to start an IV and monitor the patient for signs of an allergic reaction.

VENOMOUS SPIDER BITE With a snakebite, the patient usually knows what bit him, along with where and when it occurred. This is usually not true with spider bites.

Bites by the brown recluse spider are often painless for the first few hours. By the time you see one of these bites, it will have evolved into a small blister surrounded by a painful, reddened area of tissue.

Early recognition and prompt treatment for brown recluse bites by a physician may prevent the development of a large necrotic ulcer (involving the death of tissue). There is no effective first aid, unless the patient is allergic to the venom.

Black widow venom is extremely potent, but fortunately this spider is not particularly aggressive. When it does bite, pain and swelling are immediate and intense, and systemic signs develop over several hours. Fatalities can occur in people who are already in poor health, especially those with high blood pressure. Systemic signs include nausea and vomiting, diaphoresis (sweating), hypertension, and profound painful muscle spasms over large areas of the body adjacent to the bite, followed by a decreased level of consciousness, paralysis, and seizures.

To help a patient who has been bitten by a black widow spider, contact EMS. This patient needs black widow antivenin, and because systemic complications are such a concern, the patient belongs in an emergency department. Apply oxygen if ordered by the physician. The physician may wish to administer an IV. He may also want to administer diazepam to control muscle spasms and seizures. Watch for signs of allergic reaction. Finally, monitor the vital signs, especially blood pressure.

VENOMOUS STINGS (SCORPIONS) Scorpions are found throughout the world. They are reclusive and mostly nocturnal and only a few species have produced human fatalities. The venom of scorpions is neurotoxic and cardiotoxic. Pain at the injection site may progress to numbness, and the patient may exhibit a wide variety of neurological signs, including:

- Hyperactivity, especially in children
- Muscular twitching
- Slurred speech
- Nausea and vomiting
- Excessive salivation
- Convulsions

Contact EMS, because this patient may need antivenin, especially if several neurological signs are obvious. The physician may apply a constricting band above the site and monitor the patient for signs of allergy.

NONVENOMOUS BITES Bites are not all handled in the same way. Important findings include bleeding and whether there appears to be tissue missing. Missing tissue needs to be found quickly, if possible.

The treatment for nonvenomous bites does not vary much by type of bite. But it should be noted that there is probably no nonvenomous bite more disfiguring or more prone to infection than a human one. Human bites are jagged and dirty, and are almost sure to produce scarring and infection. They are also very often associated with other kinds of trauma, both physical and emotional. Most human bite victims are assault victims, and you should inform police when you suspect this.

Bites from squirrels, raccoons, bats, and dogs are also common, and should also result in a police contact, especially if the bite involves a child. In most places, any mammal bite results in mandatory containment of the animal and a rabies examination as soon as possible. Bites by nonvenomous birds or snakes should be treated like any other simple wound.

Severe Bleeding (Hemorrhage)

To the average person, external, visible arterial bleeding is a dramatic and frightening thing. But a smart caregiver knows how easy that is to fix, and how much more worrisome is the prospect of hidden bleeding, deep inside the abdomen, chest, or head. The kinds of findings you need to be most alert for are the signs of hypovolemic shock. They are discussed in the Shock section later in this chapter.

In addition to shock, be alert for other signs of bleeding, system by system. Sometimes the first clues about hidden bleeding come from the nature of the pain associated with it. Headache is an important sign of bleeding inside the head, especially severe, debilitating headache or very sudden onset, with or without other neurological findings. This kind of complaint should be considered a true emergency until ruled out by a neurologist using a CAT scan.

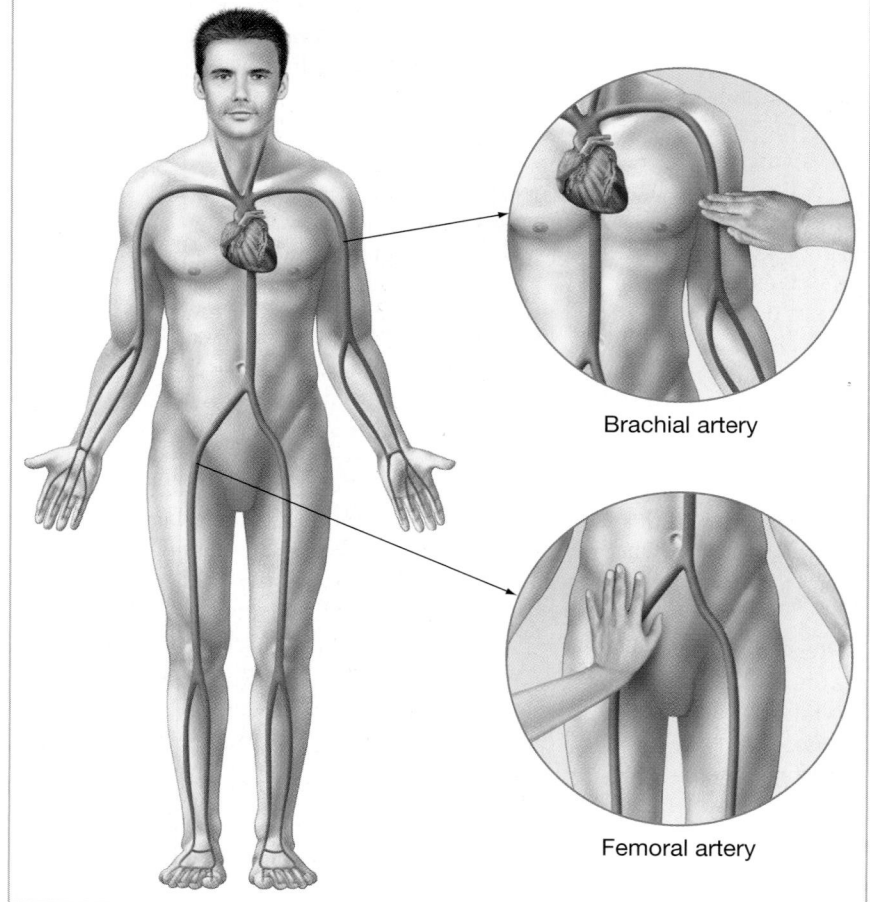

FIGURE 39-6 Pressure points of the body.

Brachial artery

Femoral artery

duced as a by-product of digested blood.

Patients who cough up pink or reddish-colored sputum, or who cough blood as opposed to vomiting it, tend to be bleeding somewhere in the airway. That includes the mouth, the nose, the pharynx, the trachea, and the mainstem bronchi and lungs. Patients whose urine seems bloody may be bleeding somewhere from their kidneys or elsewhere in their genitourinary system.

Fortunately, the body does a good job of controlling its own blood loss. When it fails, the most effective thing to do is also the simplest. Direct pressure with a gloved hand over a bulky compress will stop almost any external bleeding, even arterial bleeding. Do not forget that persistent bleeding is just as important as rapid bleeding. Simple suspicion that a patient may be bleeding internally and treating for shock can be lifesaving.

Pressure Points

There are points on the surface of the body where one can apply pressure (pressure points) in order to stop external bleeding (Figure 39-6). Applying pressure to these points is recommended as a last step to control bleeding because direct local pressure is so much more effective. Unfortunately, this process is uncomfortable for the patient. Never apply pressure directly on the carotid artery. Not only can this cause a stroke, but it also directly stimulates the vagus nerve, which slows the heart rate and can in some cases disrupt cardiac output.

Breathing Emergencies

The respiratory system is a complex network of structures and organs that keeps us alive. In health it keeps itself clean, protects itself against infection and obstructions, and generally makes our breathing so easy that we are not even aware of it. For many people breathing is both laborious and frightening.

There are two kinds of breathing emergencies: those that occur suddenly in healthy people and those that are based on complications of existing disorders. Some may be corrected in the physician's office, and some require emergency hospitalization. Determining which is which can be a challenge even for a well-equipped physician. The most important steps in helping them are the same regardless of their disease process.

Stabbing pain that comes on suddenly, deep in the abdomen or between the shoulder blades, that is unrelieved by anything comes from a dissecting aneurysm of the aorta, which is the body's largest artery. The patient may have a history of high blood pressure. This kind of pain is associated with a spreading bubble between layers of the vessel. If it ruptures, the patient can bleed to death internally within a few minutes. Or, if the bubble is on the inside of the vessel, it can occlude the blood flow to a large area of the body.

Sometimes the biggest clues about the origin and seriousness of bleeding come from the patient's body orifices, or openings. If the bleeding is in the esophagus, bright red undigested blood may be found in the vomit, possibly mixed with brown, predigested blood. The patient who bleeds into the small intestines vomits brown, foul-smelling digested blood. Both of these patients will exhibit a characteristic breath odor of digested blood. The patient who bleeds into his lower GI tract may not vomit at all, but will report dark, tarry, foul-smelling diarrhea. And the patient who bleeds from the rectum discharges red blood rectally. People who are bleeding into their digestive systems tend to have firm, oversized abdomens. That results from the presence of gas pro-

Obstruction of the airway by a foreign body is a common type of emergency, especially among small children and among people who attempt to eat while intoxicated. Airway obstruction is discussed separately earlier in this chapter.

People with respiratory disorders range in severity from the child with a cold to the busy wage earner who comes in with a fever and a cough, to the 70-year-old ex-smoker who is panicky, struggling for her life, and is an ashen gray color. In each case, a caregiver looks at four basic things:

1. What is the patient's overall appearance?
2. What is the degree of effort?
3. What is the respiratory rate?
4. What are the respiratory sounds?

The urgency presented by a patient in this kind of distress can be so desperate that you may feel compelled to treat the patient immediately, thinking you have no time to assess anything. Actually, though, you can take these assessment steps simultaneously as you initiate treatment. Since the physician's actions will depend on a set of accurate vital signs, the process of taking them can benefit the patient a great deal. By convincing the patient that the treatment he or she needs is about to be given, the patient may become less fearful and better able to cooperate in his or her own care.

Observe how the patient is communicating. Communication is our highest mental function, and it is a very reliable indicator of how well we are oxygenating our brains. Is the patient expressing spontaneous humor? If so, chances are the patient is not in grave distress. Is he or she ignoring you and concentrating only on breathing? That is not good, especially if the patient seems very tired. This patient may require intubation and artificial breathing by EMS providers. Between those two extremes are various communication levels. Simple observation during contact will help determine if there is improvement or degeneration (see Table 39-1).

In addition to assessing levels of mental awareness, pay attention to the number of syllables of speech a person uses with each breath. Somebody who spontaneously communicates using 10 to 15 syllables per breath is probably not having much respiratory trouble. But when the patient can utter only one or two syllables per breath, there is a problem.

Finally, remember that respiratory distress can either result from or cause cardiac disorders. These patients need to be monitored and will probably require chest x-rays.

TABLE 39-1 **Communication (Mental Awareness) Levels**

Range	Level	Description
Best	1	Spontaneous expression of humor
	2	Spontaneous speech, even when not being questioned (note syllables per breath)
	3	Intelligible speech in response to questions only (responses are meaningful)
	4	Nonintelligible speech in response to questions (responses are not meaningful)
	5	Obeys commands appropriately, but does not answer questions
	6	Reacts to commands, but does not obey them
	7	Appears awake, but does not answer questions or obey commands
	8	Falls asleep, but verbally arousable
	9	Localizes/avoids noxious stimuli, but never wakes up
	10	Localizes deep pain by trying to push it away
	11	Withdraws from deep pain, but does not localize it
	12	Postures in response to deep pain, but does not withdraw or localize it
Worst	13	Totally unresponsive to any stimuli

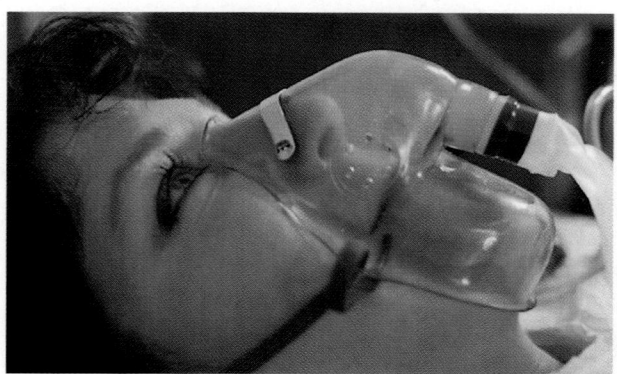

FIGURE 39-7 Application of oxygen.

If the patient has a breathing disorder that can be treated in the office (for instance, asthma or an allergic reaction), efforts to oxygenate can be cut back as status improves. Other patients who have more severe breathing problems, such as emphysema, pneumonia, or congestive heart failure are harder to treat. The physician may be able to ease the distress of these patients somewhat, but these patients will need transport to a hospital with treatment continuing en route. Still other patients such as those with a pulmonary embolus or a lung tumor are in such dire straits that they simply need to get to a hospital right away.

All of these patients need the same kind of basic care. Any patient with difficulty breathing should be considered a potential "code" patient. The cardiac monitor should be connected and a 12-lead ECG should be run. The crash cart should be ready. Figure 39-7 shows an oxygen mask being applied.

When paramedics arrive, inform them in detail about what changes you have seen and in response to what treatment.

Burns

A burn injury occurs when an area of tissue is destroyed by the action of physical heat, chemical activity, high electrical current, or heavy exposure to radiation. The severity of a burn depends on the amount and depth of tissue injury. Survival depends on those factors in addition to the amount of surface area that is destroyed.

Destruction of skin surface is an important consideration because of all of the skin functions that are lost: insulation, regulation of fluids, sensation, and protection from infection. All of these are crucial to life.

The medical assistant may stop the burning and remove any metal jewelry from the burn patient.

Classification of Burns

Burns are classified in two basic ways: by surface area and by depth. The Rule of Nines is a useful tool for estimating surface area (see Figure 39-8). For an adult, each of the following areas represents 9% of the body surface: head and neck, each upper extremity, chest, abdomen, upper back, lower back and buttocks, the front of each lower extremity, and the back of each lower extremity. These make up 99% of the body's surface. The remaining 1% is assigned to the genital region.

In the Rule of Nines, the percentages are modified for infants and young children, whose heads are much larger in relationship to the rest of the body. In addi-

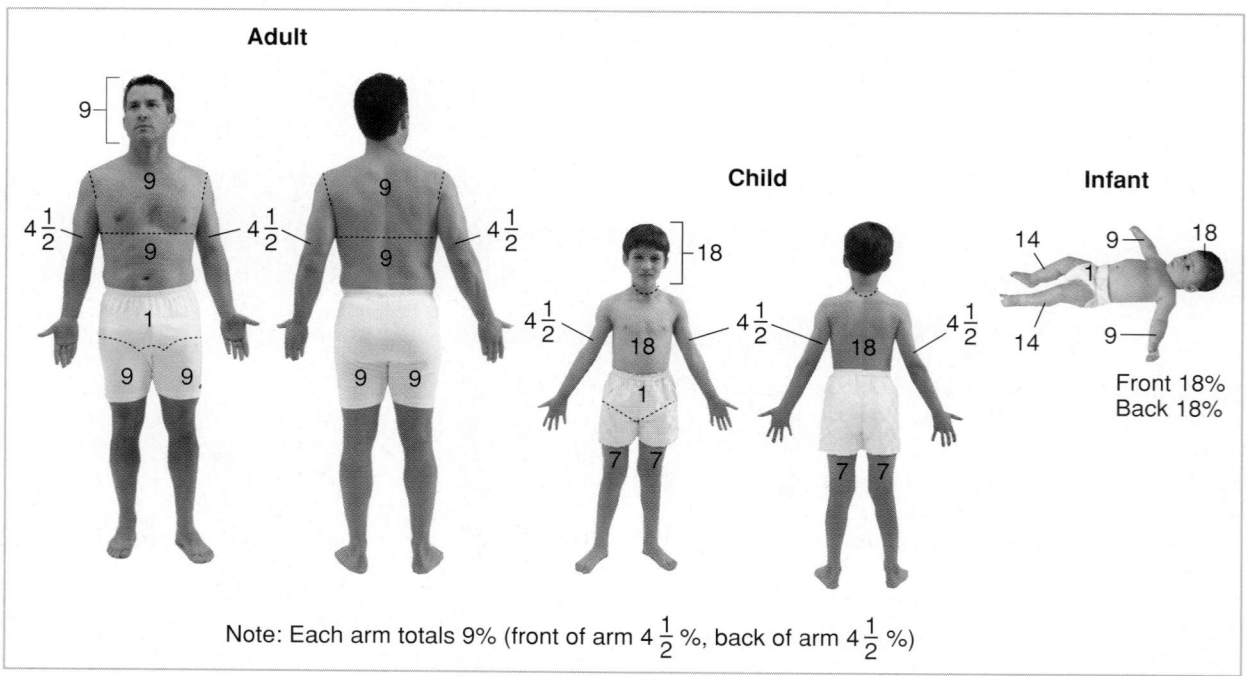

Note: Each arm totals 9% (front of arm $4\frac{1}{2}$%, back of arm $4\frac{1}{2}$%)

FIGURE 39-8 Rule of Nines for burns.

tion, Table 39-2 will give you a basic idea of burn severity by depth.

First- and second-degree burns are extremely painful, even those involving very small areas. Third-degree burns tend not to be painful immediately because, along with the entire dermis, this kind of burn destroys sensory nerve endings. But it also disrupts all of the normal functions of skin, including its self-regenerative properties and its ability to resist infection. Third-degree burns are profound injuries, even if they only involve a small amount of surface area.

Certain special considerations can also help determine the seriousness of a burn:

- The mortality of serious burns is higher for elderly patients and for very young patients.

- The mortality is higher if the patient was burned in a closed area (partly due to the possibility of carbon monoxide poisoning and partly due to the possibility of airway burns).

- Burns of the genitalia are always considered serious, regardless of depth.

- Always consider the possibility of other injuries besides burns, especially in a patient who was burned in an auto or industrial accident.

- Patients with chemical burns should have the area irrigated immediately with large amounts of water. If the burns resulted from an alkali substance, irrigation should be continued for a minimum of 20 minutes. Contact EMS as soon as you encounter such a patient to be sure that if you are dealing with a hazardous substance that cannot be rendered harmless, you have access to the proper resources as early as possible.

- Electrical burns serious enough to leave marks on the body are considered serious burns, because of the probability of internal injuries. (Electrocution by lightning is always considered serious until proven otherwise.)

These factors are all regarded as stand-alone admission criteria by trauma centers in most places. Treatment for first-degree burns involving less than 10 percent of the body surface includes pain relief by means of cool water. That instantly relieves pain, but it is not appropriate for larger surface areas. Damaged skin may not be able to regulate body temperature, so the use of cooling measures over large surface areas can cause hypothermia. Analgesic creams and ointments are appropriate for use on first-degree burns *only if ordered by the physician.*

Cool water can also be used to soothe second-degree burns for small surface areas, as long as there are no broken blisters. Second-degree burns of any size should not be treated with creams or ointments, due to

TABLE 39-2 Classification of Burns

Degree	Characteristics
First	Reddening, swelling of epidermis (like a mild sunburn)
Second	Reddening, swelling of epidermis and outer dermis; blisters noted
Third	Charring of all layers of skin and at least some deeper structures

the risk of breaking blisters and the resulting potential for infection.

Burns of any kind that involve broken skin may need to be debrided (removal of dead or damaged tissue) by a physician. If third-degree burns are present in any amount, the patient warrants treatment at a trauma center. Burns should be dressed with dry sterile dressings, and pain should be managed with injectable analgesics as ordered. If the patient will be transported by paramedics, they will start the IV and administer analgesics via that route if the physician has not already done so.

Upper airway burns constitute a dire emergency and always warrant prompt intubation by the physician or EMS with the largest tube that can be inserted. The epiglottis can swell quickly and make intubation very difficult or impossible at a later time. If the patient sounds even slightly hoarse or complains of difficulty breathing, or if you notice stridor (noisy breathing) in any burn patient, consider the possibility of airway burns and notify the physician right away. Administer oxygen as ordered by the physician.

Large surface-area burns should be dressed with dry sterile sheets, wrapped entirely around the patient's body. These patients benefit most from prompt transport to a trauma center. All burn patients should be monitored for signs of shock, especially in the case of large surface-area involvement.

Cardiac Arrest

Because cardiac arrest is not a frequent occurrence in the physician's office the experience can seem more intimidating than it needs to be.

The patient in cardiac arrest is fairly easy to recognize. The skin color may be normal, but more often it is pale, gray, or slightly blue. Most of all the patient seems inappropriately quiet.

When someone appears unresponsive, call the individual's name if you know it, or ask repeatedly, "Are you OK?" and shake the patient to establish responsiveness.

litigious situation for the physician. When using the AED, it is critical not to touch the patient during the analyzing and delivering shock steps. Figure 39-9

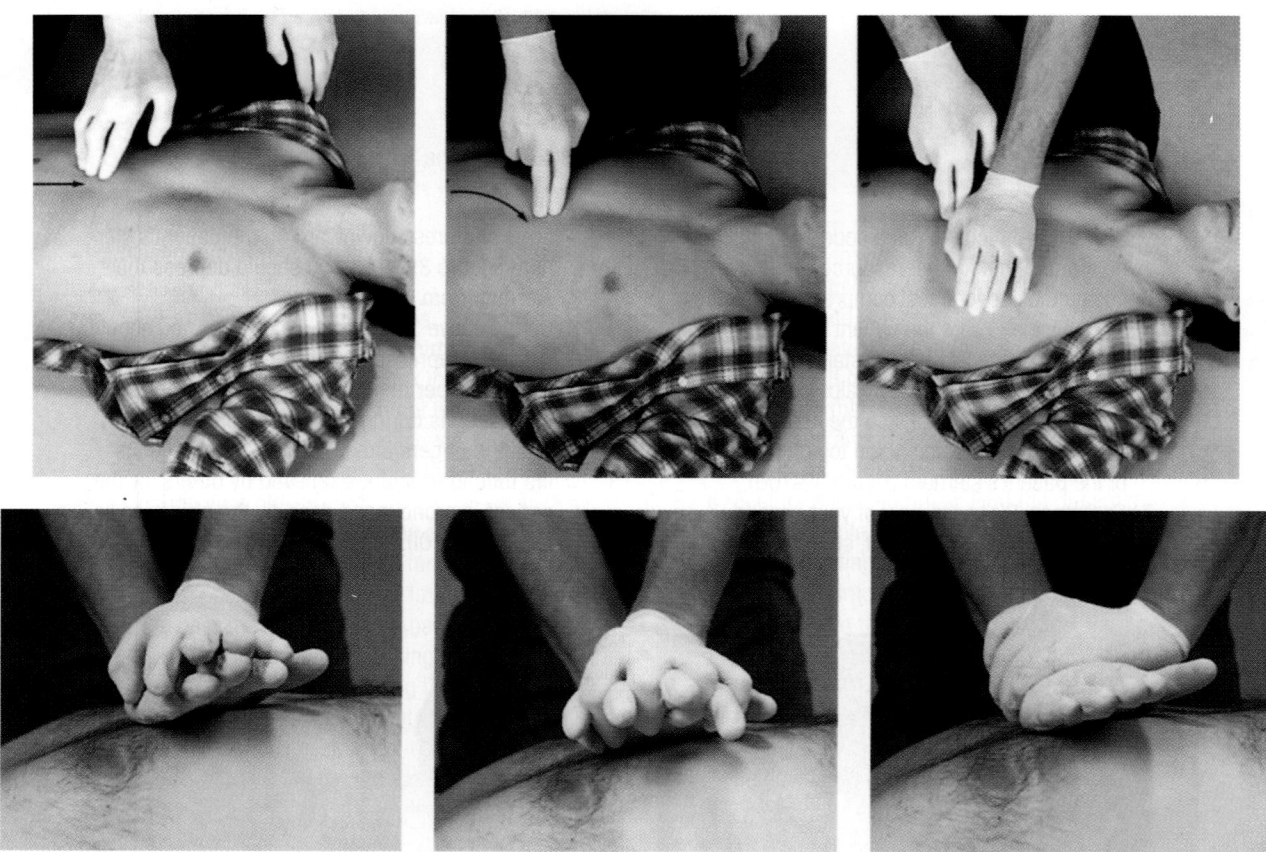

FIGURE 39-11   Location and position of hand during chest compressions.

and do what you can to keep them quiet and comfortable.

Convulsions (Seizures)

Convulsions, or seizures, are produced by disorganized electrical activity in the brain and are characterized by involuntary muscle contractions that may alternate between contraction and relaxation of mus-

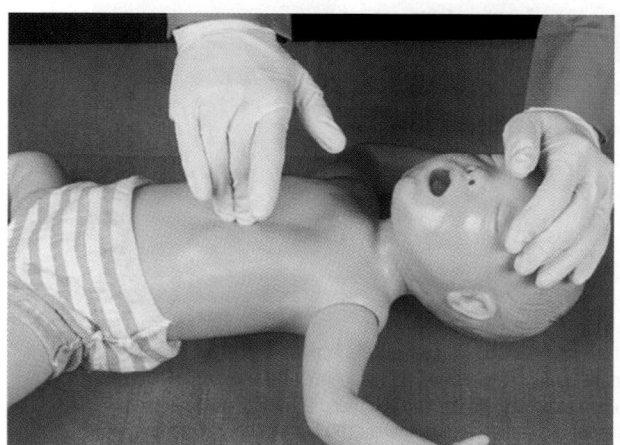

FIGURE 39-12   Infant compressions.

cles (see Table 39-4). In some cases the convulsions are generalized, involving the entire body, or localized and limited to a specific area of the body. Convulsions can result from a number of problems or combinations of problems.

By themselves, convulsions are not life threatening. But the muscle spasms that come with full-body seizures can restrict breathing. Seizure patients may also bite their tongues causing bleeding and swelling, which can obstruct the airway. Finally, seizure patients are sometimes injured when their convulsions cause them to fall.

Once a seizure stops, especially a full-body seizure, it is normal for a patient to remain unconscious for as long as 15 minutes. During that time, most patients cannot control their secretions, for example, urine, the way they would in normal sleep. In addition, whatever caused the first seizure may produce more.

A medical assistant can do two important things for a seizing patient. First, prevent injuries. Keep the patient from falling, and prevent the head from striking anything until the seizure stops. Second, pay close attention to what the patient is experiencing in order to be able to describe it later. Observations will eventually be very important to the patient's neurologist.

Assess the patient's breathing and color, and estimate how long the seizure lasts. Once it stops, reassess breathing. If breathing seems inadequate or absent, the physician may order oxygen. Immediately alert the rest of the staff that you have an emergency in your location, and check for a pulse. If there is no pulse, initiate CPR and contact EMS.

If breathing seems adequate, note the patient's response, apply oxygen as ordered, and place the patient on the left side to allow the secretions to drain. Listen for noise in the airway, and be prepared to assist the patient. Notify your physician. If the physician is not available, contact EMS and anticipate transport. Continue to assess the patient until EMS personnel arrive, and communicate your findings to them.

If the patient's teeth are clenched, *do not* try to force something between them or pry the mouth open. Observe the patient for breathing problems. Once the patient begins to regain consciousness, explain what has happened and make him as comfortable as possible. If there is no history of seizures, the patient will require transport to the ED. He may need extra reassurance, especially if he is incontinent or if this is his first seizure.

Diabetic Crisis

In health, insulin enables body tissues to produce energy from sugar. Several complex mechanisms maintain a constant balance between sugar and insulin in the blood. Diabetes is a disorder that disrupts this balance. It can occur in childhood or in later life. Some forms can be controlled by diet alone; others require treatment with oral or injectable medicines.

Most diabetics routinely monitor their blood sugar levels by means of small handheld computers. Many inject themselves with insulin one or more times per day. But this produces a crude sugar–insulin balance at best, with levels that vary widely.

Diabetics can suffer two kinds of crises: insulin shock, which is a kind of hypoglycemia (too little sugar in the blood), and diabetic coma, a kind of hyperglycemia (too much sugar). Either condition can be fatal eventually, but insulin shock tends to evolve suddenly and can produce death within minutes. Insulin shock results when a diabetic takes his insulin but strays from his diet. It is probably the most common of all metabolic emergencies, and one of the most common true emergencies you will see in the office.

It is also possible for a diabetic to accidentally inject insulin into a small vein, rather than the fatty deposits beneath the skin where it is normally injected. The brain has no tolerance for an absence of sugar or oxygen, because it has no ready reserves to borrow from. When insulin is injected intravenously, its concentration in the blood can climb so quickly that any circulating sugar is absorbed by tissues all over the body

TABLE 39-4   Conditions Causing Seizures

Alcohol	Fever
Airway obstruction/apnea	Head trauma
Brain infection	Hypoglycemia
Brain tumor	Hypovolemia
Cardiac arrest	Hypoxia
Cardiac rhythm disturbance	Metabolic disorder
Cerebral edema	Overdose
Diabetes	Poisoning
Drugs	Respiratory arrest
Electrolyte imbalance	Sepsis
Epilepsy	Stroke

almost immediately, and the brain is confronted by a sudden near absence of sugar. Brain cells can begin to die in minutes.

Unlike insulin shock, diabetic coma occurs when a diabetic either overindulges in sugar or ingests a normal amount of dietary sugar but fails to take her insulin (or other diabetic medication). Look for signs of shock in the absence of trauma, including pale skin, weakness, nausea/vomiting, and inappropriate sweating (which may be profound). The pulse may be normal or elevated, the blood pressure may be normal or low, and the respirations may be rapid and deep. Blood sugar, if you have access to it, may be either very low or very high. If there is no access to a good history, check for the presence of medical jewelry indicating the patient is a diabetic.

The immediate treatment for potential diabetic crisis of either type begins with checking the airway. Can the patient talk? The physician may check for a gag reflex by stimulating the back of the tongue with a tongue blade. If the patient can talk or has a positive gag reflex, the physician will order you to administer a small amount of sugar in any form by mouth. It can be in the form of fruit juice, candy, milk, or anything sweet. If the patient does not have a gag reflex, nothing should be administered by mouth. If the physician is not available, contact EMS immediately.

If the patient is in a diabetic coma, there will be no response to the sugar. If instead the problem is insulin shock, the patient will typically respond within 30 seconds or so. Either way, the patient will eventually need to be evaluated by a physician familiar with the case.

Epistaxis (Nosebleed)

Nontraumatic nosebleed may be messy and embarrassing, but it is usually a benign (non-life-threatening) occurrence caused by picking the nose or by blowing it forcefully. Nosebleed tends to occur most commonly in dry weather or in dusty conditions, and is usually easy to correct.

Bleeding from both nostrils tends to be more serious than bleeding from just one nostril. Nosebleed that occurs after a head injury and does not stop should be considered a serious emergency until proven otherwise. If there is no history of trauma, there are at least three other circumstances that should worry a caregiver about persistent nosebleeds. One is high blood pressure, especially in a patient who has recently changed or stopped taking medicines for high blood pressure. Another is a clotting disorder of some kind, and the third is a patient history of nosebleeds that have caused shock in the past.

Nosebleeds severe enough to cause changes in a patient's vital signs are rare, but they do occur. If the patient's vital signs are normal in the absence of trauma, the patient should be seated upright. If the vital signs are compromised, the patient should lie on the affected side and may need oxygen.

If the blood emerges from both nostrils, its origin is not in the nose but somewhere above it, and it requires the immediate attention of a physician or stat (immediate) transport to an emergency department. A nosebleed that emanates from one nostril is easily treated by a physician. To stop it, the physician will grasp a facial tissue by one corner and twist that corner firmly into a Christmas-tree shape about 4 inches long. Continuing to twist it, the pack is inserted deeply into the patient's affected nostril until the nostril is firmly packed. Then a washcloth is placed over the patient's upper face and the patient is instructed to hold a chemical cold pack against the wash cloth so it fits the bridge of the nose like a saddle.

Bleeding should stop after only a few minutes, at which time the packing can be removed. If bleeding does not stop, electrocautery may be necessary. The physician may be able to perform this treatment in the office, or the patient may require transport to an ED.

If trauma is a possible factor, the physician in the medical office may not attempt to pack the nose or stop bleeding. In this case, contact 911 immediately and anticipate transport to the emergency department. The physician may insert an oral airway if the patient is unresponsive. (Do not use a nasal airway in this kind of patient.) Place the patient on high-flow oxygen by nonrebreather mask and stay with him. Monitor him carefully for changes in status.

Fainting (Syncope)

Many serious disorders cause unresponsiveness. Simple fainting (syncope) occurs often in some people and almost never in others. Fainting or syncope, the sudden loss of consciousness, seems to be caused by a brief interruption in the body's ability to control the brain's circulation. When fainting does occur, it usually does so just after a patient has received an emotional shock of some kind. The patient usually collapses and becomes totally unresponsive, but within a minute, should awaken and return to normal function. Patients seldom become incontinent or have seizures as a result of simple fainting, but may be injured in the course of a fall. Table 39-5 lists some serious disorders that can produce fainting.

There is always a reason for unresponsiveness and determining the reason is important. However, early in your contact with any unconscious patient, your first concern should be to take care of the ABCs (airway, breathing, and circulation). A patient who suddenly becomes unresponsive, may be experiencing arrhythmia such as ventricular fibrillation or ventricular tachycardia.

Make sure that a patient who appears unresponsive really is. Shake and shout at the patient. If there is no response, provide oxygen if the physician orders this. Check the ABCs and call for help. If the patient is breathing well but you cannot wake him, place him on his left side and contact your physician. If your physician is not available, contact EMS. While you await their arrival, try to get a good set of vital signs and if possible obtain a blood sugar reading.

TABLE 39-5 Disorders That Can Result in Fainting

Airway obstruction/apnea	Cerebral Edema	Hypoglycemia	Poisoning
Assault	Diabetes	Hyperglycemia	Respiratory arrest
Brain infection	Drugs or alcohol ingestion	Hypovolemia	Seizure
Brain tumor	Electrolyte imbalance	Hypoxia	Sepsis
Cardiac arrest	Epilepsy	Metabolic disorders	Shock (any kind)
Cardiac rhythm disturbance	Head trauma	Overdose	Stroke

Never leave an unresponsive patient alone for more than a few seconds, and then never on an examination table that is not equipped with railings and/or restraining straps.

Foreign Bodies in Nose, Ear, or Eye

Foreign bodies in the nose and ear are common among children. They seldom present among adults, and they seldom represent serious medical emergencies. The kinds of objects children insert can be tough to extract when doing so depends on the patient's cooperation.

Foreign bodies in the eye are more common in adults. They can produce serious consequences in the absence of competent care.

Nose or Ear

While not common, incidents do occur involving impaled objects in the facial orifices of adults, largely as a result of domestic violence. Among children, it is much more common for small round objects such as BBs, jelly beans, coins, beans, and small objects to find their way into openings. Typically, the result is uncomfortable and the parents bring the child in because the child has become unusually cranky and has been fussing with the affected body part.

Impaled objects of any kind should never be removed by anyone but a physician. Objects impaled in the head should not be removed except at a trauma center.

Eye

Metal or wood splinters are commonly found embedded in the eye and its surrounding membranes. Due to the extreme sensitivity of the area, they are never tolerated for long and are likely to be visible. The sclera of the eye will probably appear reddened and inflamed, and you may be able to see an object with the aid of an examination lamp.

The physician may be able to remove a small splinter by means of vigorous irrigation, as long as the object is not lodged in the cornea. Place the patient on her back or on the affected side, and place several absorbent towels beneath and around the area in which the physician will be working. Using one hand to hold the lids open, the physician will direct a small stream of sterile normal saline (0.9%) from the medial side (inner can thus) of the eye laterally. Even if the object is dislodged, the physician will examine the eye and may prescribe ophthalmic antibiotics in the form of drops to prevent infection.

All ferrous objects (those containing iron) that become lodged in the cornea warrant follow-up by an ophthalmologist as soon as possible (preferably on the same day). They tend to leave particles and/or rusty residues embedded in the cornea that cannot be visualized in the office setting and that must be removed at high magnification. If not removed, these residues can cause corneal ulcers that do not heal.

If the physician is unable to remove the object, patch both eyes. Inform the patient that she will need a ride to an ophthalmologist's office or a trauma center, and help to arrange that. Keep the patient in an examination room with the lights off, to minimize eye movements, and contact EMS.

Fractures (Musculoskeletal Injuries)

All potential fractures are important, because broken bone ends are like broken glass. They can cause severe, permanent soft tissue injuries during movement if mishandled (see Figure 39-13).

The physician's approach to splinting will vary somewhat depending on the physician's specialty. The following are some general principles.

Any patient who describes a forceful mechanism of injury that has produced pain, loss of use, and/or swelling of a body part should be treated for a fracture until the x-rays say otherwise. That treatment may come from the physician, or the physician may decide to stabilize the injury temporarily and refer the patient to an orthopedist. Therefore, the medical assistant may have two roles in the treatment of fractures: to stabilize a patient who has not yet seen a physician, and to splint the patient who has been seen by a physician and is being referred to a specialist.

When a patient comes into the office with a painful disability, pay attention to the history of the injury. How did it happen? How long ago? Does the patient have function and feeling in the injured area and, especially, distal to it? These findings may change later, and they

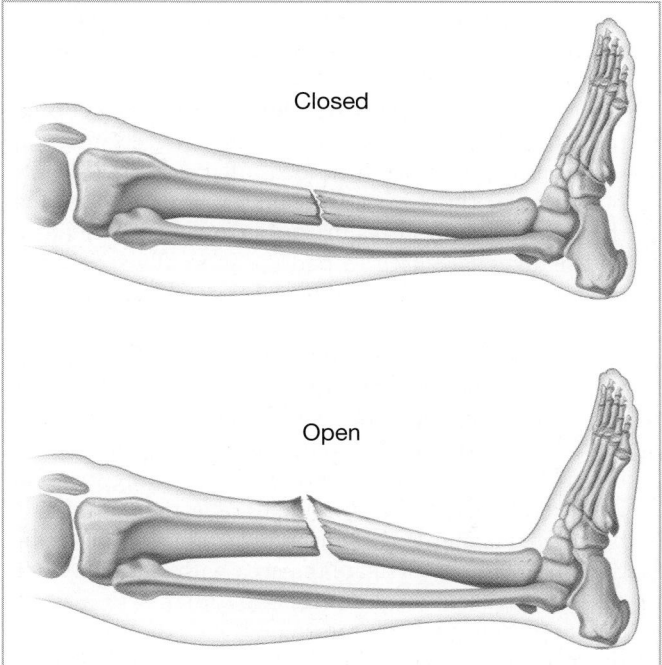

FIGURE 39-13 Types of fractures.

PROCEDURE

Applying an Arm Sling

OBJECTIVE: Apply an arm sling accurately.

Equipment and Supplies
two pieces of triangular-shaped cloth; gauze

Method
1. Perform hand hygiene.
2. Gather supplies.
3. The sling starts with a triangular piece of cloth that is 50 to 60 inches at its base and 36 to 40 inches on each side. Fold it to any width needed.
4. Check distal pulse, sensation, and motor function. Position sling over the chest. The point is toward the injured side and beyond the elbow with the upper end placed over the shoulder.
5. Bring the bottom end up and over the patient's injured arm. Keep the hand elevated above the elbow.
6. Tie the two ends together. Pad the knot with gauze or a small cloth to make sure it does not rest on the patient's neck. Reassess distal pulse and sensation.
7. Secure the point of the sling with a knot or pin to form a pocket for the elbow.
8. Fold another triangular piece of material to form a sling. Tie it around the patient. Be sure it is positioned to support the arm and to maintain elevation.
9. Reassess distal pulse and sensation.

---

are important to the physician. It is possible for swelling to cause permanent nerve damage.

Besides fractures, there are three other major kinds of musculoskeletal injuries: dislocations, sprains, and strains (in decreasing order of severity). Prior to treatment by the physician, they should all be treated as fractures. Musculoskeletal injuries are described in Chapter 22.

Do not waste time with a lot of elaborate splinting prior to the physician's examination. You do not want to obscure any injury from examination, either by the physician or the x-rays. Instead, pay attention to how the patient immobilizes his or her own injury. Pillows and blankets are used to pad the injured area accordingly. Cold compresses minimize swelling. Keep the patient comfortable and still.

Exercise special care to prevent a closed fracture from becoming an open one in which there is protruding bone tissue. Open fractures usually require surgery; closed ones may not. For an open fracture, sterility and moisture are both very important for healing to occur. Be careful to preserve the membrane that covers the bone (periosteum). If there is protruding bone tissue, the physician may irrigate the area with sterile 0.9 percent normal saline solution. Follow that with a sterile dressing that has been moistened with the same solution (not water), and follow that with a sterile occlusive dressing. Keep any loose teeth or bone fragments in

sterile saline, preferably in a sealed sterile container. You can cut the corner out of an IV bag, if one is available, and use that.

The kinds of injuries that need to be stabilized might involve joints or long bones. Do not try to straighten a joint injury. Instead, try to make the splint fit the injury. Then, to prevent movement, stabilize the bone above the injury and the bone below it. Be sure to pad for comfort, because the patient may be wearing the splint for several hours (see Procedure 39-3).

In the case of a long bone injury, the physician will try to stabilize the joint above the injury and the joint below it. You need to contact EMS if the physician is unavailable.

The value of cervical collars has been questioned vigorously in recent years. There is little in the medical literature that supports the use of anything but a few specialized versions of these devices during extrication from certain kinds of major trauma situations. In fact, they may have the effect of raising intracranial pressures. Patients with suspected spinal injuries should be handled by EMS crews, who are specially equipped to handle those circumstances.

Several commercial mobility aids are now available. Physicians should select the specific type and brand they want used in their offices. Staff should then be trained on that specific equipment, because some may be just a little different than the others.

Fractures of the Neck and Back

It is unlikely you will see spinal fractures in the office setting. The reason is that spinal fractures almost always produce too much pain and loss of function to permit travel to a doctor's office. There are, however, two situations when a patient who has spinal fractures might come to the office. One occurs when the patient with a bone disorder suffers a pathologic or disease-related fracture as a result of weakened bones. Pathologic fractures sometimes occur all by themselves, in the absence of external trauma. Cancer and osteoporosis patients are prone to pathologic fractures.

The other kind is a fracture that is so minor it seems stable. The patient with this type of fracture of the neck or back, for instance, might feel very sore or stiff, yet not be incapacitated. These fractures sometimes do not show up in x-rays but may show in an MRI or CT scan.

Treatment for anyone suspected of having a bone injury of the neck or back almost always includes calling EMS. Notify the physician immediately and keep the patient as comfortable as you can without moving him until the EMS arrives.

Eventually, a patient with bony spinal injuries may need to see an orthopedist, and possibly a neurologist. The specialists' jobs are facilitated if a good history is available. Once you've made the patient comfortable and asked her to lie still, determine her motor and sensory status. What happened, and how did she get to your office? Can she feel and move all of her fingers and toes? What are her vital signs? Does she hurt anywhere besides at the site of her injury? Record the times of your observations, including the patient's body position throughout your assessment.

Fractured Jaw

The mandible and nose are probably the weakest structures in the face, and are commonly fractured in fistfights as well as auto accidents in which the driver of a vehicle strikes his face on the steering wheel. They are painful, but only produce a real threat if the mandible is shattered. This is because it is the mandible and its muscular (hyoid) floor that keep the tongue in place.

A fractured mandible would not necessarily be unstable. If it were, the patient would consciously limit his speech and any movements of the mouth and would not permit examination. Oral bleeding might be present. A caregiver should be concerned about the possibility of broken teeth, which could lead to airway obstruction and further lacerations of the oral mucosa. In addition, an impact great enough to shatter the mandible might also produce bony neck injury as well other facial injuries.

An unstable mandible will eventually require surgical repair. A painful mandible in a patient who is con-

trolling his own secretions and in whom there is no bleeding may be left alone, or may be gently immobilized by the physician in the position of function (with the mouth closed) using a conforming bandage (preferably a 5½-inch Kerlix). The patient with this kind of injury will often complain about the teeth not fitting properly, because even the smallest dimensional change inside the mouth can seem very large.

Patients with more serious, less stable injuries should be warned not to swallow their secretions, should be offered a basin to drool or spit into, and should be allowed to choose whatever position permits their secretions to drain. Uncontrollable oral bleeding from such an injury should be left to a physician to treat. If a physician is not available, contact EMS immediately and anticipate transport to an emergency department. As a last resort, it may be prudent to inform the patient that he is bleeding and instruct him as to where he should apply his own pressure dressing.

The physician may apply high-flow oxygenation for any patient with severe bleeding, but it should be loosely applied. If the patient has trouble controlling bleeding and/or secretions, the physician will use suction as necessary. Do not discard the suction reservoir in case it contains tooth fragments that may still be reused many hours later.

Heat and Cold Exposure (Hyperthermia and Hypothermia)

The human body normally controls its internal temperature very effectively, despite extreme variations in its surroundings (by as much as 100°F). But when the body is exposed to a high or low temperature extreme for a long enough time, or when there is a breakdown in the body's internal heat-regulating ability, it can become hyperthermic (overheated) or hypothermic (its temperature can drop unacceptably). Either circumstance causes a systemic breakdown and can eventually result in death if not corrected.

Heat Exhaustion

The hyperthermic patient can suffer a wide assortment of disorders, ranging from a series of warning signs called simple heat exhaustion to a lethal condition called heat stroke. Heat exhaustion occurs when a patient is exposed to a hot environment and does not drink adequate amounts of fluids to maintain a healthy body temperature. Urine output falls, tachycardia, dizziness, nausea and vomiting, headache, muscle cramps and diarrhea result, and the patient may faint when he trying to stand up.

This patient needs fluids and electrolytes, especially sodium. If he can drink and is not vomiting, any "sports drink" (like Gatorade) will resolve his discomfort within an hour. An ECG is important, even if there is a history of working in a hot environment, because

Professionalism

the patient to accept fluids. Then reassess the vitals.

- How was it taken, and was it mixed with anything else? (by mouth, inhaled, etc; with alcohol)

The patient's age and weight are also important findings. All toxic substances act differently in the very old and the very young than they do in healthy adults. A 300-lb male has a much larger liver and bigger kidneys than a 90-lb female. Most toxins are broken down in the liver or the kidneys or in both.

Pay special attention to the affect, or mood, of a person who has ingested a poison. Intentional poisoning always warrants psychiatric support. Consider the possibility of an injection, ingestion, or inhalation any time a patient's mental capacity seems impaired if he does not have an underlying condition such as diabetes.

Finally, pay attention to what the patient's body is doing. Without knowing anything at all about what substances a patient has absorbed, you may notice breath odors that will later disappear. Likewise, there may be odors in the perspiration. If the patient voids

urine or stool, collect specimens. They may provide hints that are important to the poison control center and emergency department where this patient may eventually be seen.

Treating a poisoning patient begins with the poison control center phone number. Although you may be able to administer the first few rounds of treatment to a toxic patient, chances are that even the physician and emergency departments will contact the poison center before doing anything else. The poison center has instant access to the best available information about poisons.

Shock

Circulation is the body's way of perfusing individual cells—supplying them with the nutrients they need and removing their wastes. Shock is the process of cell death that occurs anytime perfusion is not adequate. It can be caused by blood loss, nerve or brain damage, heart disease, a severe allergic reaction, diabetes, sepsis (infection), poisoning, and lung collapse or any major disruption of the pulmonary circulation.

The outward appearance of a shock patient may not vary much by cause, but there are some general differences. Patients with most kinds of shock tend to be very cold to the touch and very pale, almost white. Those with disruption of their respiratory systems are almost always the color of blood that has not been oxygenated in a long time: blue. Almost all shock patients get dizzy (or they may just plain faint) when they stand up after sitting for a while. Almost all become diaphoretic (sweaty). An exception to the notion about pale, cold skin is the patient in anaphylactic (allergic) shock. These patients act just like other shock patients, only their skin color may be bright red.

Another important sign of shock is irritability. A patient who was nice on arrival and who gradually becomes more irritable for no reason as time goes by is getting worse.

Patients in cardiogenic (cardiac) shock do not always follow the rules. They vary a lot, both in appearance and in vital signs. They may remain awake and alert with no detectable pulse or blood pressure until they die. Their heart rates can be slow, normal, or fast. Their skin color may be pale, cyanotic, gray, or even normal to the very end. They often will say that they are going to die.

Treatment does vary between shock patients, because the correct treatment is to support life while correcting the cause of shock. Always reassure the patient, helping him or her to lie down. Contact EMS if directed by your physician and anticipate transport. Consult Table 39-6 for treatment specific to the probable cause of shock, and monitor the patient for changes.

TABLE 39-6	**Treatment for Shock in the Medical Office**
Cause	**Treatment**
Anaphylactic shock	Epinephrine
Cardiogenic shock	IV dopamine, (pacemaker), stat transport to ED
Hemorrhagic shock	Stop bleeding, replace volume, stat transport to ED
Hypovolemic shock	Replace volume
Insulin shock	Sugar, by any means tolerated (IV if patient unconscious)
Neurogenic shock	IV dopamine, stat transport, surgery (not likely to see in the office)
Poisoning	Consult poison center, treat specifically for poison
Respiratory shock	ET intubation, stat transport, surgery
Sepsis	Fluids, IV dopamine, transport to ED

SUMMARY

An understanding of what causes most medical emergencies, a knowledge of some basic first steps to take, and the will to help are essential elements of emergency first aid and of all emergency medicine. Become certified in CPR and recertify yearly as required by the AAMA. Professional-level CPR courses and a basic first aid course like those from the American Red Cross and the American Heart Association provide you with the knowledge needed to work with other health care providers and equipment in the medical office. By keeping current and updated on new emergency office equipment and procedures, you will be prepared in the event of most emergencies that come through the door of your medical office.

Chapter Review

COMPETENCY REVIEW

1. Define and spell the terms to learn for this chapter.
2. Elicit a good primary assessment without wasting time.
3. Respond appropriately to a patient who walks into the office complaining of a severe headache and then immediately goes into full-body seizure in front of you.
4. Correctly perform CPR on an adult.
5. Correctly perform aid for an obstructive airway on infant and adult, unconscious and conscious, victims.
6. Correctly apply an arm sling to a patient.
7. Demonstrate the correct procedure to control bleeding.

PREPARING FOR THE CERTIFICATION EXAMINATION

1. Heat stroke is usually defined by a number of signs, in addition to:
   A. a temperature of 104°F
   B. a rectal temperature of 105°F
   C. any central temperature over 100°F
   D. high blood pressure
   E. low blood pressure

2. Your overall impression about the appearance of a patient in shock is:
   A. not a very important consideration
   B. a very important finding
   C. not affected by your medical experience
   D. totally irrelevant
   E. reassuring

3. The best single question to ask any patient before you ask them anything else is:
   A. what happened
   B. why they came in to the physician's office today
   C. their name
   D. which doctor they want to see
   E. where they work

4. The first thing you need to do when you discover that a patient has arrested is:
   A. call for help
   B. check the airway
   C. contact EMS
   D. drag the patient somewhere where you have some room to work
   E. get the crash cart and charge the defibrillator paddles

5. Patients who have suffered a major amputation are very likely to:
   A. be in a state of shock
   B. have very little blood loss
   C. have no other injuries
   D. be taken to a physician's office
   E. be taken to an urgent care

6. A patient in diabetic coma, if administered sugar:
   A. will usually get worse
   B. will have no response to the sugar
   C. will respond immediately
   D. should not be given insulin
   E. will have a response to sugar

continued on next page

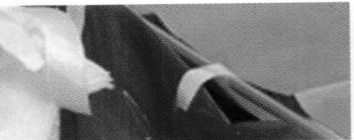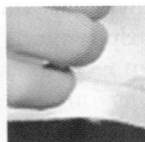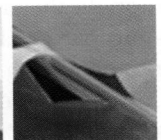

Medical Assistant Role Delineation Chart

HIGHLIGHT indicates material covered in this chapter.

ADMINISTRATIVE

Administrative Procedures

- Perform basic administrative medical assisting functions
- Schedule, coordinate and monitor appointments
- Schedule inpatient/outpatient admissions and procedures
- Understand and apply third-party guidelines
- Obtain reimbursement through accurate claims submission
- Monitor third-party reimbursement
- Understand and adhere to managed care policies and procedures
- *Negotiate managed care contracts*

Practice Finances

- Perform procedural and diagnostic coding
- Apply bookkeeping principles

- Manage accounts receivable
- *Manage accounts payable*
- *Process payroll*
- *Document and maintain accounting and banking records*
- *Develop and maintain fee schedules*
- *Manage renewals of business and professional insurance policies*
- *Manage personnel benefits and maintain records*
- *Perform marketing, financial, and strategic planning*

CLINICAL

Fundamental Principles

- Apply principles of aseptic technique and infection control
- Comply with quality assurance practices
- Screen and follow up patient test results

Diagnostic Orders

- Collect and process specimens
- Perform diagnostic tests

Patient Care

- Adhere to established patient screening procedures
- Obtain patient history and vital signs
- Prepare and maintain examination and treatment areas
- Prepare patient for examinations, procedures and treatments

- Assist with examinations, procedures and treatments
- Prepare and administer medications and immunizations
- Maintain medication and immunization records
- Recognize and respond to emergencies
- Coordinate patient care information with other health care providers
- Initiate IV and administer IV medications with appropriate training and as permitted by state law

GENERAL

Professionalism

- Display a professional manner and image
- Demonstrate initiative and responsibility
- Work as a member of the health care team
- Prioritize and perform multiple tasks
- Adapt to change
- Promote the CMA credential
- Enhance skills through continuing education
- Treat all patients with compassion and empathy
- Promote the practice through positive public relations

Communication Skills

- Recognize and respect cultural diversity
- Adapt communications to individual's ability to understand
- Use professional telephone technique

- Recognize and respond effectively to verbal, nonverbal, and written communications
- Use medical terminology appropriately
- Utilize electronic technology to receive, organize, prioritize and transmit information
- Serve as liaison

Legal Concepts

- Perform within legal and ethical boundaries
- Prepare and maintain medical records
- Document accurately
- Follow employer's established policies dealing with the health care contract
- Implement and maintain federal and state health care legislation and regulations
- Comply with established risk management and safety procedures
- Recognize professional credentialing criteria
- *Develop and maintain personnel, policy and procedure manuals*

Instruction

- Instruct individuals according to their needs
- Explain office policies and procedures
- Teach methods of health promotion and disease prevention
- Locate community resources and disseminate information
- *Develop educational materials*
- *Conduct continuing education activities*

Operational Functions

- Perform inventory of supplies and equipment
- Perform routine maintenance of administrative and clinical equipment
- Apply computer techniques to support office operations
- *Perform personnel management functions*
- *Negotiate leases and prices for equipment and supply contracts*

- *Denotes advanced skills.*

SOURCE: Reprinted by permission of the American Association of Medical Assistants from the AAMA Role Delineation Study: Occupational Analysis of the Medical Assisting Profession.

The Clinical Laboratory

Learning Objectives

After completing this chapter, you should be able to:

- Define and spell the terms to learn for this chapter.
- Explain the role of the clinical laboratory in patient care.
- Identify and explain three types of clinical laboratories and their roles.
- Describe the role of the medical assistant in the physician's office laboratory (POL).
- Summarize OSHA laboratory safety regulations.
- Explain the three CLIA categories of testing.

- Define quality assurance and list at least five components of a QA program.
- Identify several different types of laboratory equipment found in a POL.
- Identify and explain the parts of a microscope.
- Operate and properly care for a microscope.
- Communicate effectively with patients regarding laboratory test preparation and specimen collection.
- List patient information necessary to complete a laboratory request form.

OUTLINE

Role of Clinical Laboratory in Patient Care   836

Laboratory Safety Regulations   837

Laboratory Hazards   838

Quality Assurance   839

Laboratory Equipment   841

Laboratory Measurements and Equipment   842

Clinical Laboratory and Patient Communication   845

Terms to Learn

aliquot	diluent	proficiency testing
analyte	hemolyzed	qualitative test
calibrate	icteric	quantitative test
centrifuge	incubator	reagent
Clinical Laboratory Improvement Amendments (CLIA)	outside laboratory	reference laboratory
	photometer	resolution
compound microscope	physician's office laboratory (POL)	stat
control sample		turn-around time
	pipette	

Case Study

IDA HERMAN IS A 65-YEAR-OLD WOMAN who was seen recently complaining of excessive thirst and frequent urination. Dr. Frank suspects she may be a diabetic, however, her glucose test on the day of her office visit was within normal limits. He ordered a 2-hour postprandial (PP or pc) glucose test, which was performed 3 days later. Ms. Herman is calling the morning after her test to get the results. You put her on hold and check her chart. There is a glucose test report in her chart but it is not dated or initialed.

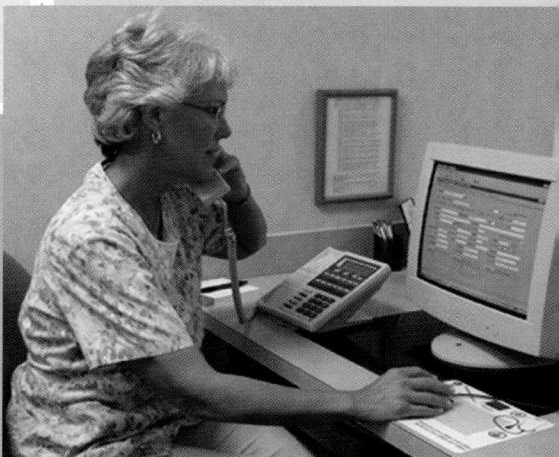

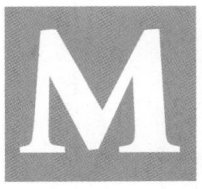**M**ost of us have had laboratory tests performed on samples of blood, urine, or tissue at one time or another. Clinical laboratory tests provide part of the framework on which the physicians base their diagnoses and monitor patients' health.

Role of Clinical Laboratory in Patient Care

Clinical laboratory test results are an essential part of patient care and may be helpful in the following ways:

- To screen for disease
- To confirm a condition suspected by the physician
- To rule out a condition such as pregnancy
- To monitor effectiveness of a treatment such as the use of an anticoagulant medication
- To assess the progress of disease such as cancer

Laboratory data should be used in conjunction with other clinical findings to provide quality care. Relying on laboratory results alone to diagnosis or treat a patient is imprudent.

Clinical laboratories analyze specimens, report results, and provide reference ranges for comparison of the patient results. Tests may be performed manually, using specialized instruments, or automatically. Laboratory tests fall generally into two categories: qualitative or quantitative tests. A qualitative test analyzes for the presence or absence of a substance or analyte in the specimen and may be reported as positive or negative. A quantitative test analyzes a specimen for the presence of a substance and the amount of the substance present. Quantitative tests are usually reported using numerical values or units.

Types of Clinical Laboratories

There are three types of clinical laboratories, which perform tests of varying levels of complexity. They are the outside laboratory, the reference laboratory, and the physician's office laboratory (POL).

Outside Laboratory

The outside laboratory, either a hospital based or independent laboratory, handles specimens collected from many types of facilities and performs tests ranging from simple to very complex. For example, the local hospital in your town may perform Pap tests collected in gynecologists' offices. Or your physician may have a contract with a managed care company that requires her to send all specimens to be tested at a specific laboratory named in their contract.

Reference Laboratory

The reference laboratory may be associated with a specific teaching hospital or medical school or be independently owned. This type of laboratory handles more complex tests than an outside laboratory and those tests that are infrequently requested. Tests performed on a regular basis at a reference lab may provide more accurate results than tests performed a few times a year in an outside laboratory.

Physician's Office Laboratory

A physician's office laboratory (POL) is one in which some of the tests the physician orders are performed in the office. In the POL the doctor has the advantage of receiving the results more rapidly than if tests were done outside of the office. Turn-around time is the length of time it takes for the test to be performed, results generated, sent back for physician review, and added to the patient's chart. Disadvantages to the POL are that in-house testing may require more employees and the purchase of expensive equipment.

Clinical Laboratory Departments

Clinical laboratories are divided into various departments that perform specific categories of tests. The typical clinical laboratory may include departments such as specimen processing, chemistry, special chemistry, hematology, blood bank, microbiology, histology, urinalysis, cytology, serology, parasitology, and toxicology. A physician's office lab performs a narrower range of tests, mainly those related to chemistry, hematology, urinalysis, and microbiology.

Cultural Considerations

Medical assistants must be sensitive to patients from different cultures. Collecting a urine sample may seem routine to you but it may be culturally offensive to the patient. If there is a language barrier, keep directions to patients simple and use pictures to reinforce your directions. At times you may encounter female patients who are not allowed to be examined or to speak to a male physician without their husband or father with them. Allowances must be made for these patients and they should be treated at all times with respect and dignity.

In a physician's office, laboratory medical assistants are usually the caregivers who provide information to the patient regarding preparation for laboratory tests. You must be very clear about the preparation required for a test and never assume that because the patient has had the test before he or she will know what to do. It is always better to give the patient instructions in writing whenever possible.

A period of fasting and/or a special diet may be required prior to a test. The decision to have the patient abstain from medications is made by the doctor who will inform the patient which medications should or should not be taken. It is helpful to testing laboratory personnel to know what medications the patient is taking so they may be alert to possible test interference from certain drugs.

Clinical Laboratory Personnel

As mentioned in Chapter 2, several different categories of health professionals and paraprofessionals may be employed in the clinical laboratory. The director of a clinical lab is usually a pathologist/MD or a clinical laboratory scientist with a doctorate degree. The clinical laboratory scientist (CLS) or medical technologist (MT) supervises and performs laboratory tests. These professionals have a 4-year degree and additional clinical training and have passed a national examination. A medical laboratory technician (MLT) usually has a 2-year degree, additional training, and has passed a national examination. The medical laboratory assistant (MLA), clinical lab assistant (CLA), certified medical assistant (CMA), and registered medical assistant have some specialized training and have passed a certification or registration examination. Other categories of personnel such as phlebotomists who draw blood samples and specimen processors who process and prepare samples may be employed in the laboratory.

Medical Assistant's Role in the Clinical Laboratory

Medical assistants are particularly suited to working in POLs and clinical laboratories because of their cross-training in administrative and clinical areas. All medical assistants are trained in phlebotomy and have basic knowledge of laboratory testing. In addition, their multiskilled abilities help them to perform the many administrative tasks needed in the laboratory field. The patient-oriented training that medical assistants receive helps them be empathetic caregivers.

Laboratory Safety Regulations

Patients are entitled to quality medical care and health care personnel deserve to work in a safe environment. The safety of both patients and personnel must be the central concern of every clinical laboratory regardless of size. The accuracy and validity of test results is crucial to the health of the patient. Chapter 5 in discusses quality assurance and its role in providing quality health care. In the following paragraphs laboratory safety issues and regulations impacting clinical laboratories are discussed.

Several agencies and committees set and review safety guidelines affecting clinical laboratories. They include the Occupational Safety and Health Administration (OSHA), the Centers for Disease Control and Prevention (CDC), the National Committee for Clinical Laboratory Standards (NCCLS), the Environmental Protection Agency (EPA), and the College of American Pathologists (CAP). It is important that medical assistants have a working knowledge of the guidelines and regulations of these agencies and keep up to date on changes in order to provide better health care.

OSHA Regulations (1970)

OSHA was established within the Department of Labor in 1970 by Congress to create safeguards covering nearly every employee in the United States. Two programs of standards under the OSHA umbrella particularly impact the clinical laboratory. They cover exposure to chemical hazards and bloodborne pathogens. Both have been discussed in some detail in Chapter 32, so will only be briefly considered here. OSHA develops specific guidelines governing a particular field and they must be adhered to. If no specific guidelines exist, then the "general duty clause" must be followed, which means that all employers must provide a safe work environment free of hazards that may cause serious injury or death. OSHA also oversees the Universal Precautions guidelines of the CDC. Copies of these general guidelines can be obtained on the Internet.

Clinical Laboratory Improvement Amendments

In 1988 Congress enacted the Clinical Laboratory Improvement Amendments (CLIA) in response to widespread concern over the accuracy of laboratory tests. The government mandates that all laboratories that test human specimens must be regulated to help ensure accurate patient test results. CLIA divides laboratories into the three categories discussed earlier and specifies what types of test may be performed in each and who may perform them. States may have their own laboratory safety requirements, but they must be at least as stringent as the federal government regulations. Information regarding state regulations may be obtained from state health departments. In 1992 CLIA was updated to reflect changes in standards, accrediting programs, fees, and enforcement. Tests are classified as Certificate of Waiver tests, Level I tests, and Level II tests.

Certificate of Waiver Tests

Certificate of Waiver tests (WTs) are the least complex and present the least risk if performed incorrectly. Many of these tests have been approved by the Food and Drug Administration for home use. The early pregnancy detection kit is an example of such a test.

A POL that wishes to perform WTs must apply to perform these tests and is then restricted to performing none of the more complex tests from Level I or Level II and is exempt from complying with CLIA 1988 standards. Quality assurance and quality control methods should be observed. The laboratories that perform WTs may be subject to random inspections and investigation if test results are questioned or there are complaints against the laboratory. A Certificate of Waiver is given to laboratories that perform only low-complexity tests. A POL qualified to perform moderate complexity and waived tests receives a Certificate of Provider-Performed Microscopy (PPM). Box 40-1 lists examples of some CLIA waived tests. A medical assistant employed in a facility with a PPM certificate can perform moderate complexity tests with further training and under the supervision of a laboratory professional or physician.

Level I Tests

Level I Tests are moderately complex and include analysis of specimens in the areas of chemistry, hematology, microbiology, immunohematology, virology, parasitology, and immunology. Any laboratory that wishes to perform Level I testing must be headed by a pathologist/MD or PhD. All personnel must have training past high school. The laboratory must perform proficiency testing and is subject to unannounced inspections. Examples of Level I laboratory tests include a complete blood count (CBC) and cholesterol screenings.

Level II Tests

Level II tests include those that are highly complex; any tests involved in cytology, histopathology, or histocompatibility; and any tests not categorized by Centers for Medicare and Medicaid Services (CMS, formerly HCFA, the Health Care Finance Administration). The laboratories that perform tests in this category must be subject to unannounced inspections, perform proficiency testing, and be headed by an MD or PhD scientist, and tests may only be performed by qualified personnel as specified in the CLIA 1988 standards.

Laboratory Hazards

The laboratory includes biohazards, chemical hazards, and physical hazards; however, most accidents are preventable. Laboratory safety must be the concern of all who are employed in the laboratory field. Medical assistants must be familiar with the following regulations:

- Hazard Communication Standard
- Universal Precautions and Bloodborne Pathogen Standards
- Hazardous Waste Operations
- Needlestick Safety and Prevention Act

Chemical Hazards

Material Safety Data Sheets (MSDS) provide safety information for all in the laboratory environment.

MSDS provide product identification, safety information about proper storage and disposal, potential health hazards, handling precautions, and fire and explosion information. All laboratory personnel have the right to know about hazards pertaining to materials they are using and must receive training appropriate to the materials in use. Each hazardous substance must have a hazardous material label attached to the container that provides a shortened version of the MSDA information. Figure 40-1 is an example of an MSDS label.

Bloodborne Pathogens/Universal Precautions

Biohazards are hazards that have the potential to infect others. As of 1992 OSHAs Occupational Exposure to Bloodborne Pathogen Program must have been in place at all laboratories. In addition the CDC specimen handling precautions known as Standard Precautions (formerly Universal Precautions) must be employed when dealing with any infectious materials. All potentially biohazardous material must be labeled with the biohazard label as shown in Figure 40-2. Chapter 32 includes a list of bloodborne pathogen standards.

Needle-Stick Hazards

OSHA revised the Bloodborne Standards in 2000 to include the following changes. Health care employers must review all new safety devices to lessen the needle-stick risks of their employees, and they must ask for safety input from their employees on an annual basis. A detailed report of all contaminated needle-stick incidences must be kept.

Fire and Safety Hazards

Care must be taken to reduce the chances of fire and electrical accidents by having an awareness of the floor plan and exits and the location of safety devices such as eye washes, showers, and safety blankets.

Hazardous Waste Removal

Hazardous waste includes blood, blood products, body fluids and tissues, cultures, vaccines, sharps, gloves, inoculation loops, and paper contaminated with body fluids. All must be disposed of in proper containers, identified with biohazard labels, and sharps must be placed in puncture-proof, leak-proof containers. Guidelines 40-1 provides a list of laboratory safety guidelines.

Quality Assurance

The most important tasks of the clinical laboratory are to ensure accurate test results and to report them

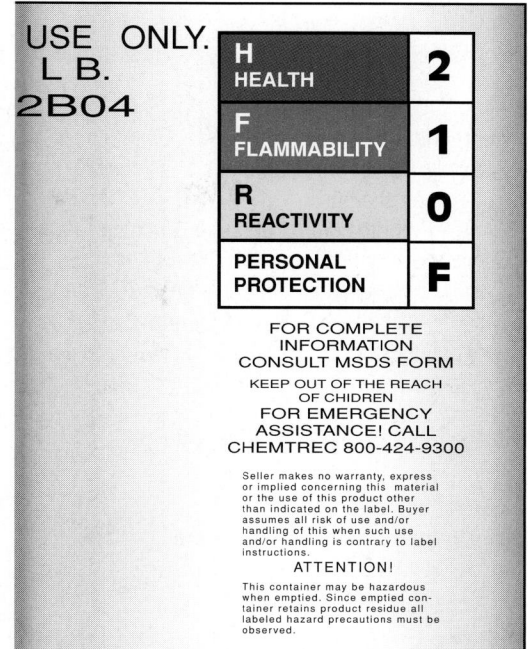

FIGURE 40-1 MSDS labels provide an abridged version of the substance hazards information and must be permanently attached to their containers.

in a timely manner. Each facility must have in place a quality assurance program. A quality assurance program is a written program that includes mechanisms to evaluate laboratory procedures and policies, identify and correct problems, and ensure reliable and prompt reporting of results and testing by competent individuals. (See also Preparing for Externship.)

Quality Assurance in the Laboratory

The CLIA 1992 standards mandate that there must be written policies and procedures for a comprehensive quality assurance program that will "evaluate the

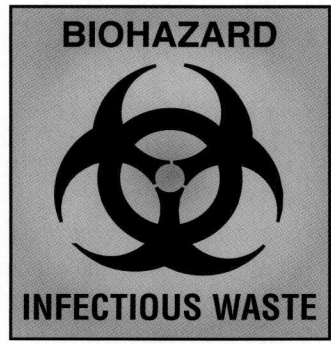

FIGURE 40-2 An orange-red biohazard symbol indicates that bloodborne pathogens maybe present and items should be treated accordingly.

GUIDELINES Laboratory Safety

1. Wear appropriate personal protective equipment (PPE) in the lab only. Do not wear lab coats, masks, and gloves outside of the lab.
2. Avoid hand-to-mouth contact or hands touching the eyes, nose, or ears while in the lab.
   a. No pens, pencils placed in mouth or behind the ears.
   b. No food or drink in lab or lab refrigerator.
   c. Never apply cosmetics such as lipstick or lip balm or handle contact lens while in the lab.
3. Dress appropriately.
   a. Never wear long chains, dangling earrings, or bracelets.
   b. Always tie back hair.
   c. Keep fingernails short, well manicured, with no polish or artificial nails.
4. d. Wear comfortable, sturdy shoes with nonslip soles—no sandals, open-toed shoes, or heels.
4. Do not draw material up through a pipette using suction from the mouth.
5. Do not store caustic material above the eye level.
6. Locate fire extinguishers in the lab and know how to use them.
7. Be sure hands are dry when transferring reagent bottles.
8. Keep first aid manual and supplies available.
9. Avoid inhaling any chemical substance that might cause injury to nasal membranes or lungs.
10. Never use chipped, broken, or cracked glassware.
11. Follow written cleanup policies and procedures for spills.
12. Discard contaminated material in appropriate container.

ongoing and overall quality of the testing process." To this end, the laboratory is required to:

- Evaluate the effectiveness of its policies and procedures
- Identify and correct problems
- Ensure reliable and prompt test results
- Ensure the competence and adequacy of staff
- Take corrective action if errors are found
- Integrate corrective procedures into future policies and procedures
- Document employee training and assess competency yearly after the first year
- Maintain the identity and integrity of patient samples during the entire testing process
- Be subject to inspection every 2 years if performing moderate or high complexity tests

Quality Control

Quality control (QC) programs in clinical laboratories monitor the testing of patient specimens to ensure reliable and consistent results. Patient specimens or samples may be whole blood, serum, plasma, body fluids such as cerebrospinal fluid and urine, feces, tissue, and swabs such as throat, vaginal, or wound.

Control Samples

Control samples are samples similar to the testing specimen required that have been previously tested and that have a known value. Controls are usually purchased from a manufacturer and each batch has an assigned lot number and accompanying value sheet. In addition, information regarding dilution of controls is provided along with information on proper storage.

Reagents

Reagents are substances required for a chemical reaction or which are used to detect the presence of

Preparing for
Externship

In many activities in the medical facility, no one but you knows whether or not you have followed the proper procedure. Whether you wash your hands each and every time you go to a new patient, whether you change gloves as required, whether you perform a test proce-

dure correctly, whether you write down the correct test results, whether you actually perform controls as required are all up to you. Your integrity, honesty, and reliability are on the line every day. Keep in mind the Code of Ethics and the Medical Assistants' Creed, which should be followed to uphold the profession and the quality of health care.

another substance. For example, when a fingerstick blood glucose test is performed, the reagent is on the test strip already and it reacts with the patient's blood drop which is the sample. To determine that the machine and the test strips are working correctly and that medical assistant is performing the tests correctly, control samples with a positive and negative known result should be performed and the results recorded on QC sheets.

Calibration

Some laboratory tests require the medical assistant or whoever is performing the test to calibrate the machine or instrument prior to testing a specimen. To calibrate an instrument, a known standard is used to measure the accuracy of the equipment to be utilized in the test procedure.

Maintenance

All laboratory equipment must be maintained on a regular basis according to manufacturers' instructions. A written record of the maintenance performed must be readily available. In addition, a record of each piece of equipment with model and serial numbers, date of purchase, and manufacturers' inserts should be available when repair is necessary or the laboratory is being inspected.

Documentation

If there is no written record of a test result, a control result, maintenance performed, or temperature recorded, then you have no proof. The end result is the same as if you did not perform the procedure. If it is not written down in the appropriate place, you did not do it.

Proficiency Testing

Proficiency testing is an external quality control program that monitors the accuracy of test systems by comparing your results to results provided by a College of American Pathologists or American Association of Bioanalysts survey program. Unknown samples are sent to your laboratory periodically throughout the year. Under CLIA 1988 standards, laboratories must participate in proficiency testing three times a year, and if any analyte has an unacceptable rating in two of the three testing surveys, suspension of certification or permission to perform that test occurs. The laboratory may not perform that test for patients until appropriate action is taken and two subsequent proficiency tests are within acceptable limits.

Proficiency tests may be performed on whole blood, serum, plasma, or urine, and the samples will have a range of results similar to any group of patients. Some will be high, some normal, and some low.

Laboratory Equipment

Clinical laboratories utilize a wide array of equipment. A POL, however, requires less equipment for clinical laboratory testing than does an outside or reference laboratory. An autoclave, centrifuge, photometer, incubator, microscope, and measuring devices are generally found in most physician's office laboratories.

Autoclave

The autoclave is discussed in Chapter 32. It is used to sterilize equipment or instruments that are used on patients or in certain test procedures.

Centrifuge

The centrifuge is an instrument used to separate specimens into component layers. In the medical office they are used to separate urine so urine sediment can be examined under the microscope (see Chapter 42). A microcentrifuge is used to separate whole blood samples into layers to measure patient hematocrit (see Chapter 43).

Photometer

A photometer is an instrument that measures light intensity. A glucometer is a type of handheld photometer that is used to test glucose levels in patients.

Incubator

An incubator is used to maintain a specific temperature to achieve a specific result. For example, incubators that mimic body temperature are used in POLs to encourage growth of throat and urine cultures. Once the culture has grown sufficiently, identification of the infecting organism can be made (see Chapter 41).

Microscope

Microscopes are frequently used in the medical office to examine urine sediment, vaginal and bacteriological smears, and differential smears, which categorize types of white cells in a sample. This optical instrument magnifies structures unseen by the naked eye for the purpose of counting, naming, or differentiating. Figure 40-3 shows an example of a compound microscope (one that has two sets of lenses, oculars, and objectives). The resolution of a microscope refers to the ability to distinguish clearly between two adjacent but distinct objects. Better microscopes have better resolution.

Parts of the Microscope

The components of a microscope are

1. Eyepiece(s) (monocular or binocular) with magnification printed on them

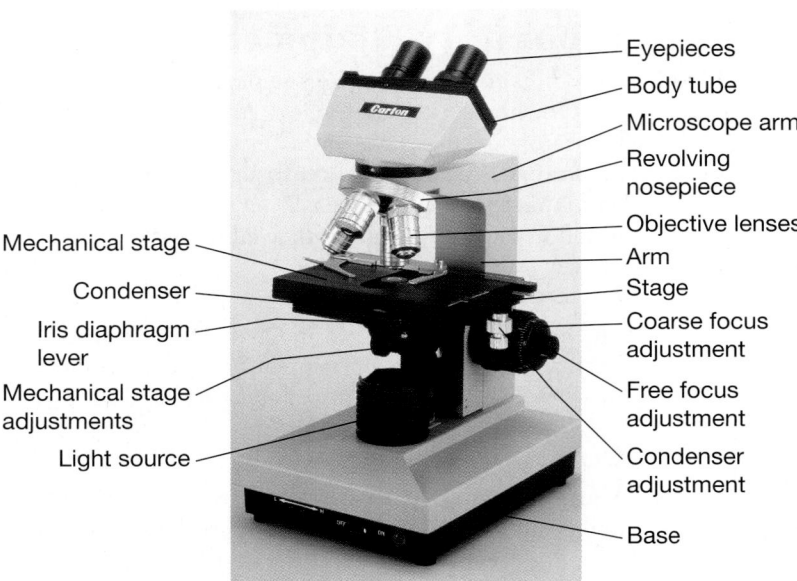

FIGURE 40-3 Binocular microscope with parts labeled.

Labels on figure:
Eyepieces
Body tube
Microscope arm
Revolving nosepiece
Objective lenses
Arm
Stage
Coarse focus adjustment
Free focus adjustment
Condenser adjustment
Base
Mechanical stage
Condenser
Iris diaphragm lever
Mechanical stage adjustments
Light source

of 100 times the size of the sample. Procedure 40-1 list the steps needed to properly use a microscope.

It is important to use the correct lens for the type of microscopic work to be done. For example, the low-power objective, 10×, is used to view epithelial cells, such as skin scrapings; the high dry setting, 40×, is used for urine RBCs (red blood cells), WBCs (white blood cells), or blood RBCs; the oil immersion setting, 100× is for differential blood smears (stained with Wright's stain) or bacteria slides (stained with Gram stain). Microscopic work on the high dry setting is done with a cover glass on the specimen.

Care of the Microscope

Microscopes are delicate instruments that will last for many years if maintained properly. Guidelines 40-2 lists the rules for the proper care and maintenance of the microscope.

Laboratory Measurements and Equipment

The validity of laboratory test results depends on accurate measurements and correct calculations using laboratory equipment. Thermometers are used to measure the temperature of various pieces of laboratory equipment such as refrigerators, freezers, incubators, and water baths, which must be maintained within specific ranges. Each piece of equipment must have its own log of temperature readings with date, time, and the initials of the individual who performed the reading. In addition, medical assistants need to be aware of the laboratory units of measurement that are used to report results. A laboratory result must never be reported without a unit of measurement after it. Metric system units are used most frequently in the laboratory.

Time

To ensure accurate test results, all test procedures must be precisely timed. In tests such as the glucose tolerance test (GTT) specimen collection must be timed precisely in order to provide accurate, meaningful test results. Laboratory time is based on the 24-hour clock or military time to avoid confusion that may result from using the A.M. and P.M. designations of Greenwich Time. The 24-hour clock uses four numbers with noon being expressed as 1200 (twelve hundred

2. Body tube (directional light source)

3. Arm (used in carrying the microscope)

4. Revolving nosepiece (holds objectives and rotates for selection)

5. Objectives (magnification printed on each objective: 10, low-power setting; 40, high dry setting; and 100 or oil immersion setting; (settings are described in the next section)

6. Stage

7. Mechanical stage (movable device that holds slide)

8. Mechanical stage adjustments (two knobs that control vertical/horizontal movement of slide)

9. Coarse and fine adjustment knobs (small knob atop larger knob that adjusts stage up and down for focusing)

10. Condenser (lens system used to increase light for sharper focus)

11. Condenser adjustment knob

12. Light source (illuminator set in base)

13. Iris diaphragm lever

14. Base (holds illuminator, rheostat, and microscope upright and is used while carrying microscope)

Using the Microscope

The magnification of an object is calculated by multiplying the objective magnification by the eyepiece magnification. On low power, magnification would be 10 (the objective) times 10 (the eyepiece) equaling magnification

Using the Microscope

OBJECTIVE: Observe a slide under the microscope using 10×, 40×, and 100× oil immersion and the correct procedure.

Equipment and Supplies

microscope; slide (prepared with specimen to be examined); lens paper/lens cleaner; dust cover for microscope

Note: Follow Standard Precautions and safety guidelines when working with body fluid samples. Use care to avoid splashing or spilling body fluids. Wipe up all spills using guidelines established by OSHA.

Method

1. Make sure the stage is in the down position before starting.
2. Place prepared slide on stage.
3. Turn light on.
4. Rotate nosepiece until 10× objective is directly over the slide.
5. Use the coarse adjustment knob to raise stage until objective is close to slide on stage.
6. Look through eyepiece and adjust coarse focus knob until microscope field is seen. (This will look like a round circle of bright light.)
7. Use fine adjustment knob for clearer image.
8. Open diaphragm. Adjust rheostat to focus if necessary.
9. Raise or lower condenser to alter light refraction. The condenser is usually lowered when using the low-power objective.)
10. Observe.
11. Change objective to 40× and readjust. Use oil on 100× oil immersion.
12. When finished, always lower stage before removing slide.
13. Turn off light.
14. Clean eyepieces and objectives with lens paper and oil immersion lens with lens cleaner.
15. Unplug electrical cord and wrap around base.
16. Cover microscope with dustcover.

hours) and midnight as 2400 (twenty-four hundred) hours). A military time of 4:15 P.M. would be 1615 (sixteen-fifteen hundred hours), which is calculated by adding 4 hours and 15 minutes to 1200. Some workers are required to use 24-hour time clocks to monitor their work arrival and departure times.

Temperature

The two scales used for measuring temperature and necessary calculations for converting Fahrenheit and Celsius were discussed in Chapter 33 and will not be presented here. Table 40-1 lists some temperatures routinely associated with the laboratory environment.

1. Follow cleaning requirements during mandatory daily maintenance.
2. Always use two hands to carry a microscope: one hand to hold the arm of the microscope and one to support the base.
3. Clean oculars, objectives, and stage using only lens paper and lens cleaner.
4. Keep extra light bulbs on hand.
5. Document inspections and repairs in log book.
6. Store with electrical cord wrapped loosely around base.
7. Cover the microscope with a dust cover when it is not in use.

TABLE 40-1 Common Laboratory Temperatures

Laboratory Temperatures	Fahrenheit	Celsius
Freezer	32	0
Autoclave	254	121
Refrigerator	41	5
Incubator	98.6	37
Room	68	20

Laboratory Units of Measurement

The United States uses the English system of measurement in everyday life. The English system uses ounces and pounds for weight; inches, feet, and yards for length; and cups, pints, quarts, and gallons for liquids. In the medical field and throughout most of the world, the metric system is used. The metric system is based on a decimal system combined with various designations—liquid (liter), weight (gram), and length (meter). An apothecary system is also used in pharmacology to measure some medications. These systems and the conversions from one to another will be discussed more fully in Chapter 47.

Most commonly the units used to express laboratory results are the following: millimeter (mm), centimeter (cm), and milligram (mg). The appropriate unit and correct designation must be used when reporting test results. Exact placement of the decimal in a test result is *critical* to the health and safety of the patient. Table 40-2 lists some abbreviations commonly used when reporting patient test results.

TABLE 40-2 Abbreviations Commonly Used in Reporting Laboratory Results

Unit	Abbreviation
Gram	g
Milligram	mg
Liter	L
Milliliter	mL
Microliter	μL
Microgram	μg
Millimoles per liter	mmol/L
Cubic centimeter	cc
Milligrams per deciliter	mg/dL
Pint	pt
Quart	qt
Ounce	oz
Unit	U
Quantity not sufficient	QNS

Measuring Devices

Various measuring and mixing devices are employed in the laboratory. These include beakers, flasks, cylinders, test tubes, and pipettes. They may be made of glass or plastic and be reusable or disposable. Figure 40-4 depicts various types of glassware, and Figure 40-5 depicts pipettes of various types. Beakers and flasks can be used to mix liquids. They are not accurate measuring devices. The graduated cylinder and the volumetric flask are accurate measuring devices.

The graduated pipette is used for measuring and the volumetric pipette is used for transferring liquid from one vessel to another. The graduated pipette is marked with *TD* which means "to deliver," and it will deliver that specific amount. If it is marked with *TC*, "to contain," it must be emptied completely to deliver the exact amount. A serologic pipette has graduations down to the tip and is used to make serum dilutions in the laboratory. The serologic pipette allows for more rapid flow because of its larger opening but is less accurate and should not be used for making reagent dilutions. Micropipettes are used to deliver very small amounts (microliters) of liquid and manufacturers' directions must be carefully followed.

Dilutions

For certain types of tests, dilutions of either the reagent or patient sample may be required. The term *dilution* means parts of the whole volume. For example, if a patient's test result is too high to provide an accurate reading, the test directions may say to repeat the test using a 1 in 10 dilution of the patient's serum in a specific diluent (a liquid such as saline or water). The medical assistant would measure out one part of patient's serum and add it to nine parts of diluent. This is a 1:10 dilution of the sample. You could use 1 mL of serum and 9 mL of diluent or 0.5 mL of serum and 4.5 mL of diluent and the result would be a 1:10 dilution in either case.

Clinical Laboratory and Patient Communication

The medical assistant is often responsible for communicating directly with the patient regarding preparation for specimen collection. Test results are only as good as the specimen provided for analysis. As a result, the medical assistant must make every effort to obtain the appropriate specimen from the patient.

Laboratory Requisition

The laboratory testing process begins with the physician's request for a test. As a medical assistant you will need to complete a requisition that the patient will bring to the laboratory at the time of the test. If the physician

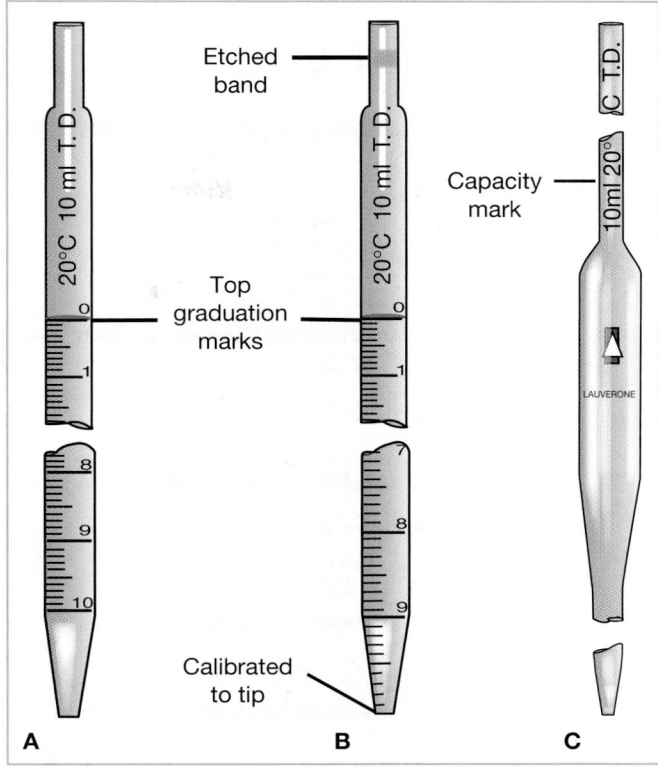

FIGURE 40-5 Types of manual pipettes: (A) graduated; (B) serologic; (C) volumetric.

wants the results immediately for a medical intervention, then the requisition must be labeled stat and processed accordingly. Box 40-2 lists the information necessary to complete a patient request form. Figure 40-6 is an example of a laboratory test requisition. Be sure to use the appropriate laboratory requisition slip since the office may send specimens to several different testing sites.

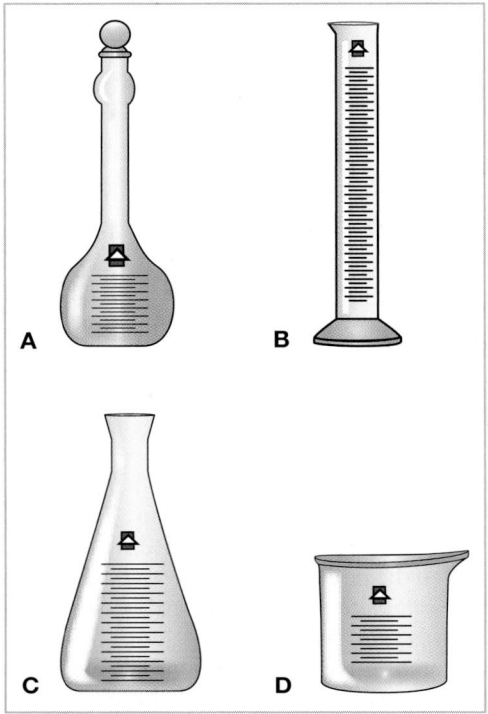

FIGURE 40-4 Laboratory glassware: (A) volumetric flask; (B) graduated cylinder; (C) Erlenmeyer flask; (D) beaker.

BOX 40-2
Laboratory Requisition Information

- Physician's name, address, phone number, account number
- Patient's full name, address, phone number
- Patient's compete insurance information
- Patient's age, date of birth (DOB), and gender
- Source of specimen
- Fasting or nonfasting specimen
- Date and collection time
- Specific tests requested
- Patient's present medications
- Diagnosis if possible
- Stat or regular request

Lab Services

IMPORTANT
Patient instructions
and map on back

PHYSICIAN ORDERS

Patient _____ Last Name _____ First _____ M.I. _____   D.O.B. _____   M ☐ Patient   F ☐ SS# _____ — _____ — _____

Address _____ City _____ Zip _____ Phone # _____

Physician _____

ATTACH COPY OF INSURANCE CARD

Diagnosis/ICD-9 Code _____
(Additional codes on reverse)

Date & Time of Collection: _____
Drawing Facility _____

☐ 789.00 Abdominal Pain ☐ 414.9 Coronary Artery Disease (CAD) ☐ 244.9 Hypothyroidism
☐ 285.9 Anemia (NOS) ☐ 250.0 DM (diabetes mellitus) ☐ 272.4 Hyperlipidemia
☐ 780.7 Fatigue/Malaise ☐ 401.9 Hypertension
☐ 272.0 Hypercholesterolemia ☐ 483.9 URI (upper respiratory infection)

☐ ROUTINE   ☐ PHONE RESULTS TO: # _____
☐ ASAP   ☐ FAX RESULTS TO: # _____
☐ STAT   ☐ COPY TO: _____

HEMATOLOGY	CHEMISTRY	CHEMISTRY	MICROBIOLOGY
☐ 1021 CBC, Automated Diff (incl, Platelet Ct.)	☐ 5550 Alpha Fetoprotein, Prenatal	☐ 5232 HBsAg	Source _____
☐ 1023 Hemoglobin/Hematocrit	☐ 3000 Amylase	☐ 3175 HIV (Consent required)	☐ 7240 Culture, AFB
☐ 1020 Hemogram	☐ 3153 B12/Folate	☐ 3581 Iron & Iron Binding Capacity	☐ 7200 Culture, Blood x _____
☐ 1025 Platelet Count	☐ 3156 Beta HCG, Quantitative	☐ 3195 LH	Draw interval _____
☐ 1150 Pro Time Diagnostic	☐ 3321 Bilirubin, Total	☐ 3590 Magnesium	☐ 7280 Culture, Fungus
☐ 1151 Pro Time, Therapeutic	☐ 3324 Bilirubin, Total/Direct	☐ 3527 Phenobarbital	☐ Culture, Routine
☐ 1155 PTT	☐ 3009 BUN	☐ 3095 Potassium	☐ 7005 Culture, Stool
☐ 1315 Reticulocyte Count	☐ 3159 CEA	☐ 3689 Pregnancy Test	☐ 7010 Culture, Throat
☐ 1310 Sed Rate/ Westergren	☐ 3348 Cholesterol	Serum (HCG, qual)	☐ 7000 Culture, Urine
	☐ 3030 Creatinine, Serum	☐ 3653 Pregnancy Test, Urine	☐ 7300 Gram Stain
URINE	☐ 3509 Digoxin (recommend 12 hrs, after dose)	☐ 3197 Prolactin	☐ 7353 Occult Blood x _____
☐ 1059 Urinalysis	☐ 3515 Dilantin	☐ 3199 PSA	☐ 7365 Ova & Parasites x _____
☐ 1082 Urinalysis w/Culture if indicated	☐ 3168 Ferritin	☐ 3339 SGOT/AST	☐ 7400 Smear & Suspension
Urine-24 Hr _____ Spot _____	☐ 3193 FSH	☐ 3342 SGPT/ALT	(includes Gram Stain/Wet Mount)
Ht. _____ Wt. _____	☐ 3066 ▼ Glucose, Fasting	☐ 3093 Sodium/Potassium, Serum	☐ 7060 Rapid Strep A Screen (_____)
☐ 3033 Creatinine	☐ 3061 Glucose, 1st Post 50 g Glucola	☐ 3510 Tegretol	☐ 7065 Rapid Strep A Screen only
☐ 3036 Creatinine Clearance (also requires blood)	☐ 3075 ▼ Glucose, 2nd Post Glucola	☐ 3551 Theophylline	☐ 7030 Beta Strep Culture
☐ 3095 Protein	☐ 3060 Glucose, 2nd Post Prandial (meal)	☐ 3333 Uric Acid	☐ 5207 GC by DNA Probe
☐ 3096 Sodium/Potassium	☐ 3049 ▼ Glucose Tolerance Oral GTT		☐ 5130 Chlamydia by DNA Probe
☐ Microalbumin 24 Hr _____ Spot _____	☐ 3047 ▼ Glucose Tolerance Gestational GTT		☐ 5555 Chlamydia/GC by DNA Probe
SEROLOGY	☐ 3650 Hemoglobin, A1C		☐ 7375 Wright Stain, Stool
☐ 8020 ANA (Antinuclear Antibody)			
☐ 8040 Mono Spot			
☐ 3494 Rheumatoid Factor			
☐ 8010 RPR			
☐ 5365 Rubella	Additional Tests _____		

PANELS & PROFILES

☐ ✗ **3309 CHEM 12**
Albumin, Alkaline Phosphatase, BUN, Calcium, Cholesterol, Glucose, LDH, Phosphorus, AST, Total Bilirubin, Total Protein, Uric Acid

☐ ▼ **3315 CHEM 20**
Chem 12, Electrolyte Panel, Creatinine, Iron, Gamma GT, ALT, Triglycerides

☐ ▼ **3357 CARDIAC RISK PANEL**
Cholesterol, HDL, LDL, Risk Factors, VLDL Triglycerides

☐ ✗ **3042 CRITICAL CARE PANEL**
BUN, Chloride, CO₂, Glucose, Potassium, Sodium

☐ **3046 ELECTROLYTE PANEL**
Chloride, CO₂, Potassium, Sodium

☐ ▼ **3399 EXECUTIVE PANEL**
Chem 20, Iron, Cardiac Risk Panel CBC, RPR, Thyroid Cascade

☐ **5242 HEPATITIS PANEL, ACUTE**
HAVIgMAb, HBsAg, HBsAb, HBcAb, HCVAb

☐ ▼ **3355 LIPID MONITORING PANEL**
Cholesterol, Triglycerides, HDL, LDL, VLDL, ALT, AST

3112 LIVER PANEL
Alkaline, Phosphatase, AST, Total Bilirubin, Gamma GT, Total Protein, Albumin ALT

☐ ✗ **3083 METABOLIC STATUS PANEL**
BUN, Osmolality (calculated), Chloride, CO₂ Creatinine, Glucose, Potassium, Sodium, BUN/Creatinine, Ratio, Anion Gap

☐ ✗ **3376 PANEL B**
Chem 12, CBC, Electrolyte Panel

☐ ▼ **3382 PANEL D**
Chem 20, CBC, Thyroid Cascade

☐ ✗ **3385 PANEL F**
Chem 12, CBC, Electrolyte Panel, Thyroid Cascade

☐ ▼ **3391 PANEL G**
Chem 20, Cardiac Risk Panel, CBC, Thyroid Cascade

☐ ▼ **3393 PANEL H**
Chem 20, CBC, Cardiac Risk Panel, Rheumatoid Factor, Thyroid Cascade

☐ ▼ **3397 PANEL J**
Chem 20, Cardiac Risk Panel

5351 PRENATAL PANEL
Antibody Screen, ABO/Rh, CBC, Rubella, HBsAg, RPR
☐ 1059 with Urinalysis Routine
☐ 1062 with Urinalysis w/Culture if indicated

☐ ✗ **3102 RENAL PANEL**
Matabolic Status Panel, Calcium, Phosphorus

3188 THYROID CASCADE
TSH, Reflex Testing

▼ – patient **required** to fast for 12-14 hours
✗ – patient recommended to fast 12-14 hours

LAB USE ONLY	
☐ SST	☐ PLASMA
☐ PURPLE	☐ SERUM
☐ YELLOW	☐ SWAB
☐ BLUE	☐ SLIDES
☐ GREEN	☐ DNA PROBE
☐ GREY	☐ B. CULT BTLS
☐ URINE	
☐ BLACK	
☐ OTHER: _____	
RECV. SPECIMEN:	☐ FROZEN
☐ AMBIENT	☐ ON ICE

Special Instructions/Pertinent Clinical Information _____

Physician's Signature _____   Date _____

These orders may be FAXed to: 449-5288   LAB _____   7060-500 (7/96)

FIGURE 40-6 Laboratory requisition slip.

Patient Preparation

Various tests require different types of patient preparation. A fasting specimen means that the patient must not take in any food for a prescribed number of hours prior to collecting the specimen. For most tests the fasting period is at least 8 hours. Postprandial (PP) or *post cibum* (pc) means "after a meal." A fasting blood glucose would be drawn after the patient has abstained from eating for 8 hours at least. Two-hour PP or ac glucose means that the patient eats a prescribed amount of food for a meal and a blood glucose level is drawn exactly 2 hours after completion of the meal. Timing of specimens is important in testing for certain medication levels to assess the highest level of medication in the patient's system (peak) or the low point (trough) and thus to determine the correct dose to be administered.

Specimen Identification

Any specimen obtained from a patient must be labeled clearly with patient's name, date and time of collection, and specimen processing number if required by the testing laboratory. An improperly labeled specimen should not be tested. The patient or office should be called with a request for a new specimen.

Specimen Handling and Preservation

Once the specimen is obtained and labeled, it must be stored according to the directions provided by the testing laboratory's manual. Prior to obtaining the specimen the medical assistant should fill out the requisition, check the laboratory manual for type and amount of specimen needed, type of preservative or anticoagulant required, and how the specimen is to be handled after it is obtained (see Legal and Ethical Issues). For example, some specimens must be mailed to reference laboratories, frozen and in dry ice. Other specimens are to be picked up by a laboratory collection service and must be refrigerated until tested. Preservatives and anticoagulants will be discussed in later chapters.

Patient Results and Records

A patient's test results are reviewed by the physician, who will then make them known to the patient (see also Professionalism). In some circumstances the physician will allow patient results be given to the patient by phone. Release of information must comply with HIPAA guidelines to protect patient confidentiality. After the test results are reviewed by the physician, they must be filed according to office policy in the patient's chart.

SUMMARY

In this chapter the role of the clinical laboratory in health care has been examined. Different types of laboratories, the types of clinical laboratory departments, and categories of laboratory personnel were discussed. OSHA and CLIA guidelines and laboratory safety issues were considered. The medical assistant has an important role in laboratory testing. It is up to the medical assistant to secure the integrity of the specimen and ensure the proper processing, handling, transporting, and recording of test results. Quality assurance and quality control and their roles in ensuring accurate test results were discussed. The microscope, its parts, and how to utilize it in the POL were covered. Other types of equipment such as incubator, glassware, centrifuge, photometer, and the microscope were introduced.

COMPETENCY REVIEW

1. Define and spell the terms to learn for this chapter.
2. Define quality assurance and explain its impact on the clinical laboratory.
3. Explain the role of the clinical laboratory in patient care.
4. Explain the three categories of CLIA testing and give an example of a test that would be performed in each category.
5. Define proficiency testing and how it helps clinical laboratories provide more accurate test results.

PREPARING FOR THE CERTIFICATION EXAM

1. All of the following information should be included on a lab slip EXCEPT:
   A. date specimen is obtained
   B. time specimen is obtained
   C. time specimen is sent to the laboratory
   D. physician's name
   E. patient's name

2. Microscopic slides are placed on what portion of the microscope?
   A. diaphragm
   B. stage
   C. substage
   D. revolving nosepiece
   E. rheostat

3. When working with the microscope, which of the following is correct?
   A. carry the microscope with one hand
   B. the 10× setting is used for oil immersion
   C. the 40× setting is used for a high dry power
   D. lower stage after removing slide
   E. the level of light should remain constant for all examinations

4. Testing in all clinical laboratories is regulated by which of the following federal agencies?
   A. American Association of Blood Banks (AABB)
   B. Medicaid
   C. Medicare
   D. Clinical Laboratory Improvement Amendments of 1988 (CLIA)
   E. College of American Pathologists (CAP)

5. A quantitative test is one that:
   A. tests for presence of substance only
   B. tests for all substances found in sample
   C. tests for the presence and amount of substance in sample
   D. is usually only performed at home
   E. does not require a trained technician

6. An MSDS provides information on:
   A. patients
   B. phlebotomy procedures
   C. sharps disposal containers
   D. bloodborne pathogens
   E. chemicals

7. OSHA requires adherence to what rules when exposed to blood?
   A. Standard Precautions (OSHA)
   B. Federal Drug Administration (FDA)
   C. National Fire Prevention Association (NFPA)
   D. Joint Commission on Accreditation of Healthcare Organizations (JCAHO)
   E. Medicare

8. A control sample is all of the following EXCEPT:
   A. the same as patient sample
   B. tested at the same time test is performed
   C. important to ensure the accuracy of test results
   D. part of a QC program
   E. purchased from manufacturer

9. Certificate of Waiver tests:
   A. are very complex
   B. are simple and may be performed at home
   C. can only be performed by high-level laboratory personnel
   D. are never done in reference laboratories
   E. are not important in health care

10. A pipette:
    A. is a large piece of laboratory equipment
    B. is never used by medical assistants
    C. is used to measure fluids
    D. may be put in mouth
    E. may be used if tip is broken

CRITICAL THINKING

1. What should you tell Mrs. Herman on the telephone?

2. What steps should you take to obtain the results from yesterday's 2-hour PP glucose test?

3. Dr. Frank asks you to find out who did the test but no one in the office seems to know who did it and there is no record in the chart to indicate the test was performed. Identify several errors that are apparent in the handling of this patient's test.

4. How would a QC program in the office help to prevent the problems with this test?

5. If you were the office manager, what would you do to ensure these problems do not occur again?

ON THE JOB

Carmel Lopez has been working in a busy internal medicine office mainly performing clinical procedures. She often performs Certificate of Waiver tests and has helped train new medical assistants to perform them correctly. Carmel observes Rachel not bothering to run the controls that came with a test kit necessary to perform a waived test. Rachel has worked in the office longer than Carmel.

1. Why are controls important when performing a test?
2. What should Carmel do? What should Carmel do if Rachel reacts in a negative way?
3. How would you handle this situation?
4. How might a patient be affected by the actions of Rachel?

INTERNET ACTIVITY

In preparation for an office meeting, your supervisor asks you to research the Clinical Laboratory Improvement Amendments 1988 and 1992 and make a short presentation. Go to http://www.fda.gov/cdrh/clia to prepare for your presentation.

 MediaLink More on clinical laboratories, including interactive resources, can be found on the Student CD-ROM accompanying this textbook.

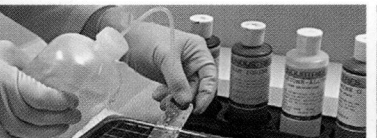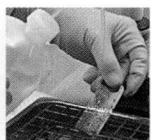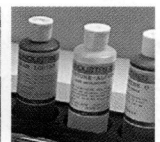

Medical Assistant Role Delineation Chart

HIGHLIGHT indicates material covered in this chapter.

ADMINISTRATIVE

Administrative Procedures

- Perform basic administrative medical assisting functions
- Schedule, coordinate and monitor appointments
- Schedule inpatient/outpatient admissions and procedures
- Understand and apply third-party guidelines
- Obtain reimbursement through accurate claims submission
- Monitor third-party reimbursement
- Understand and adhere to managed care policies and procedures
- *Negotiate managed care contracts*

Practice Finances

- Perform procedural and diagnostic coding
- Apply bookkeeping principles

- Manage accounts receivable
- *Manage accounts payable*
- *Process payroll*
- *Document and maintain accounting and banking records*
- *Develop and maintain fee schedules*
- *Manage renewals of business and professional insurance policies*
- *Manage personnel benefits and maintain records*
- *Perform marketing, financial, and strategic planning*

CLINICAL

Fundamental Principles

- Apply principles of aseptic technique and infection control
- Comply with quality assurance practices
- Screen and follow up patient test results

Diagnostic Orders

- Collect and process specimens
- Perform diagnostic tests

Patient Care

- Adhere to established patient screening procedures
- Obtain patient history and vital signs
- Prepare and maintain examination and treatment areas
- Prepare patient for examinations, procedures and treatments

- Assist with examinations, procedures and treatments
- Prepare and administer medications and immunizations
- Maintain medication and immunization records
- Recognize and respond to emergencies
- Coordinate patient care information with other health care providers
- Initiate IV and administer IV medications with appropriate training and as permitted by state law

GENERAL

Professionalism

- Display a professional manner and image
- Demonstrate initiative and responsibility
- Work as a member of the health care team
- Prioritize and perform multiple tasks
- Adapt to change
- Promote the CMA credential
- Enhance skills through continuing education
- Treat all patients with compassion and empathy
- Promote the practice through positive public relations

Communication Skills

- Recognize and respect cultural diversity
- Adapt communications to individual's ability to understand
- Use professional telephone technique

- Recognize and respond effectively to verbal, nonverbal, and written communications
- Use medical terminology appropriately
- Utilize electronic technology to receive, organize, prioritize and transmit information
- Serve as liaison

Legal Concepts

- Perform within legal and ethical boundaries
- Prepare and maintain medical records
- Document accurately
- Follow employer's established policies dealing with the health care contract
- Implement and maintain federal and state health care legislation and regulations
- Comply with established risk management and safety procedures
- Recognize professional credentialing criteria
- *Develop and maintain personnel, policy and procedure manuals*

Instruction

- Instruct individuals according to their needs
- Explain office policies and procedures
- Teach methods of health promotion and disease prevention
- Locate community resources and disseminate information
- *Develop educational materials*
- *Conduct continuing education activities*

Operational Functions

- Perform inventory of supplies and equipment
- Perform routine maintenance of administrative and clinical equipment
- Apply computer techniques to support office operations
- *Perform personnel management functions*
- *Negotiate leases and prices for equipment and supply contracts*

- *Denotes advanced skills.*

SOURCE: Reprinted by permission of the American Association of Medical Assistants from the AAMA Role Delineation Study: Occupational Analysis of the Medical Assisting Profession.

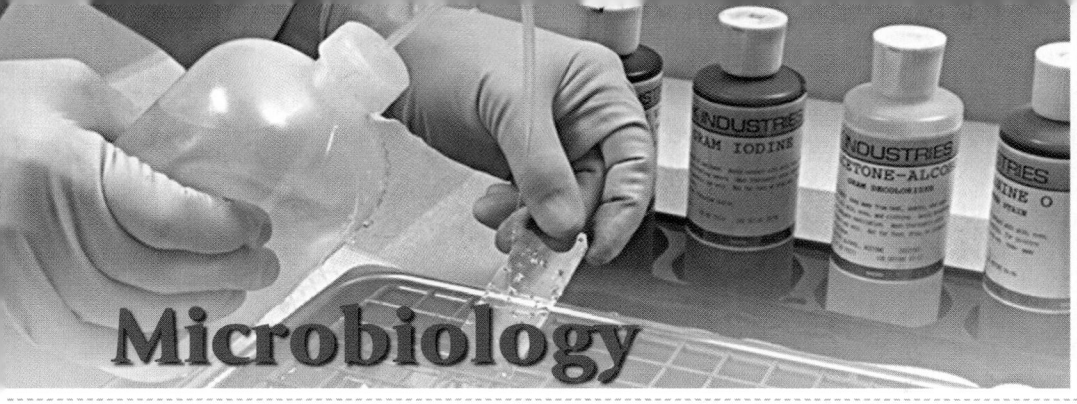

Microbiology

Learning Objectives

After completing this chapter, you should be able to:

- Define and spell the terms to learn for this chapter.

- Define microbiology and its importance in patient care.

- Explain the purpose of obtaining a specimen.

- Explain how microorganisms are classified.

- Explain the differences among bacteria, viruses, protozoa, fungi, and parasites.

- List general guidelines for obtaining specimens.

- Identify a disease caused by each of the five categories of pathogens.

- Identify three different shapes of bacteria and a disease caused by each.

- Describe the different growth media needed for culturing microorganisms.

- Understand how cultures are interpreted.

- Explain the importance of the Gram stain.

- Define sensitivity testing and explain how it is done.

- Describe the basis for serological testing and name three examples performed in a POL.

OUTLINE

Role of the Medical
   Assistant in Microbiology   852

Classifications
   of Microorganisms   853

Types of Microorganisms   854

Specimen Collection
   and Transportation   860

Overview of the Process
   of Diagnosing Infection   862

Microbiology Equipment
   and Procedures   863

Types of Specimens   867

Serology Testing   875

Terms to Learn

acid-fast stain
agar
agglutination
colony
culture media
Culturette
enteritis
eukaryotic
exudates
facultative anaerobe
feces
fixed

inoculated
microbiology
microorganisms
methicillin-resistant
Staphylococcus aureus
(MRSA)
morphology
mycology
necrotizing fascitis
normal flora
organelles
prokaryotic
sequela

serology
smear
spore
sputum
Staphylococcus aureus
(staph)
stool
steatorrhea
streak culture
subcellular
swabs
viable
wet mount

Case Study

A PATIENT ARRIVES AT YOUR OFFICE with a wound on the left forearm. A dressing has been applied by the patient's family, but it is saturated with drainage that appears to contain pus.

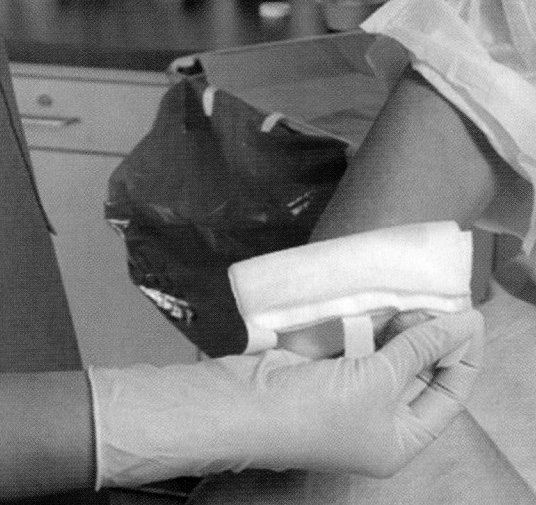

he field of microbiology is the fascinating study of living organisms too small to be seen with the naked eye (microorganisms). Van Leeuwenhoek's invention of the microscope in 1680 allowed mankind to observe for the first time a variety of microbes. Louis Pasteur, the father of microbiology, developed methods for culturing and identifying microbes in the laboratory. Review Chapter 2, for other pertinent historical facts in the field of microbiology.

We are surrounded by microorganisms both on our bodies—in the cavities opening to the outside of our bodies—and in the environment. The microbes that live on the surface of the body and inside the body openings are generally nonpathogenic and are referred to as normal flora. Normal flora are beneficial bacteria that help us resist pathogens. A bacterium that is harmless in one area may be pathogenic in another especially an area that is normally sterile. Sterile areas include body cavities, the bloodstream, bladder, heart, lungs, brain, and other organs.

Bacteria in the environment help us to decompose and recycle waste. This chapter will cover the characteristics of microorganisms and how they are identified and the diseases some pathogens cause. It will also cover the proper collection and transportation of specimens.

Role of the Medical Assistant in Microbiology

The medical assistant is given many responsibilities in the office. These include, but are not limited to:

- Proper use of personal protective equipment (PPE)
- Monitoring equipment for repairs needed
- Performing quality control checks on equipment
- Patient teaching (see Patient Education)
- Confidentiality concerning the patient and test results
- Proper collection and testing of certain specimens

The medical assistant is responsible for instructing patients on the proper collection process for urine, stool, or sputum specimens. It is your responsibility to make the patient as comfortable as possible, particularly when discussing specimens such as stool and urine, which may cause embarrassment.

In some offices, the medical assistant will also test the specimens within CLIA guidelines for waived testing (Chapter 40). If samples are not tested at your facility, you will prepare them for transportation to outside laboratories. No matter what course of action is requested, careful handling of specimens is required for the patient's and medical assistant's safety and to obtain an uncontaminated sample. Safety guidelines, the infectious process cycle, and infection control were discussed in Chapter 32 and will not be repeated here.

Observing HIPAA regulations concerning privacy must always one of your chief concerns. Consider the importance of information you will be handling such as test results for sexually transmitted infections (STIs) and HIV. Information concerning the patient should be given only on a "need-to-know" basis. In other words, the receptionist does not need to know the results of the lab test, but the clinical medical assistant does. Certain information should not be shared, even with coworkers in your facility. Although HIPAA regulations affect everyone in the office, those who have most exposure to patients must be informed of methods of enforcement.

Your efficiency can assist the physician in making a proper diagnosis. The physician and the patient are

Patient Education

The role of the medical assistant in the education of the patient regarding the careful handling of all specimens and testing materials cannot be overemphasized. There is a danger of contamination with microorganisms to everyone coming into contact with the specimen if the patient has not carefully practiced hand hygiene and other infection control measures when obtaining the specimen.

Some patients are reluctant to collect specimens, and the medical assistant can do much to allay their fears by explaining the value of specimen collection. The calm, professional attitude the medical assistant displays while explaining the collection of sputum and stool (feces) may mean the difference between a useful specimen and a contaminated one. An informed patient is more likely to be a compliant patient. Do not overuse medical terminology in the explanation, because your patient may not understand it. As the patient if he or she has any questions. Answer these properly, and if you are unsure of the answer, check with the physician or another worker. Allow the patient to repeat instructions back to you. Always document your teaching.

depending on you to complete the test properly and then to accurately document the results.

Classifications of Microorganisms

Although medical assistants will not be responsible for identifying and naming specific microorganism, it is important to understand how they are classified and named. There are many types of microorganisms and we know already that they are divided by their ability to cause disease into two categories: pathogens and non-pathogens. Most microbes are nonpathogenic (98% to 99%); only 1% to 2% are pathogenic.

Naming Microorganisms

Scientists use a binomial system to name all living organisms—animals, plants, bacteria, fungi, and protozoa. Just as we each have two names—a first name and last name—each organism has two names: the genus (always capitalized) and species (lowercase). For example, the organism that causes strep throat is known as *Streptococcus pyogenes*. Literally it means a chain of round bacteria that produce pus. While you are not expected to learn all the genus and species names, it is important for you to understand the system of nomenclature when receiving laboratory reports over the phone or reading a patient's chart.

Structural Characteristics

The many different types of microorganisms are usually classified by their major structural differences. Differences such as cell structure and the presence or absence of organelles (small structures in the cytoplasm of a cell) are used to classify organisms. Eukaryotic cells have a nucleus and organelles in the cytoplasm. Protozoa, fungi, and parasites are examples of eukaryotic cells. Prokaryotic cells are simpler in structure, without a nucleus or organelles, such as bacteria. Subcellular microorganisms, such as viruses, are those comprised of hereditary material (RNA or DNA) with a protein outer coat.

Retention of Dyes

Bacteria are also characterized by their reactions to certain stains. A stain is a dye used in coloring microorganisms to allow for visibility under a microscope. The Gram stain, named for Jans C. J. Gram, a Danish physician, is a commonly used method of staining bacteria. A gram-positive bacterium retains the violet color of the stain used in the staining of the microorganism. Some of the more common gram-positive bacteria are *Staphylococcus aureus* and *Streptococcus pneumoniae*. Figure 41-1 shows gram-positive streptococci.

A gram-negative bacterium has the pink color of the counterstain used in Gram's method of staining

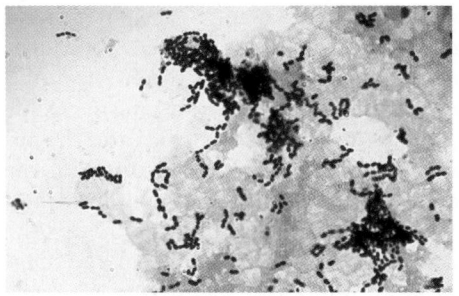

FIGURE 41-1 Gram-positive *Streptococcus pyogenes* bacteria in chains.

microorganisms. A few of the most common gram-negative bacteria are *Escherichia coli, Neisseria gonorrhoeae* and *Salmonella typhi*. Figure 41-2 shows gram-negative *N. gonorrhoeae*. Some organisms do not stain well with Gram stain and require a special stain, such as the acid-fast stain used for the organism that causes tuberculosis.

Use of Oxygen

Bacteria can also be categorized by whether they survive in an oxygen-rich environment (aerobes) or die in the presence of oxygen (anaerobes) or are anaerobes that are flexible and can live with some oxygen (facultative anaerobes). Successful culturing requires an understanding of the oxygen requirements of bacteria. If the ultimate goal is to grow and identify a sample of the organism that is causing disease in a patient, then we must provide proper oxygen, moisture, nutrient, and temperature in the laboratory setting.

Hemolytic Properties

Bacteria are also categorized by their ability to hemolyze (burst) red blood cells in the blood agar. First a word about colonizing microbes for identification. Agar is a gelatin-like substance made from seaweed that is added to culture media to provide nutrition and a semisolid surface on which microbes can grow. The most common types of media are broth and agar. A culture is the propagation of microorganisms or living cells in a special media that enhances their growth. Some types of media contain special dyes or ingredients

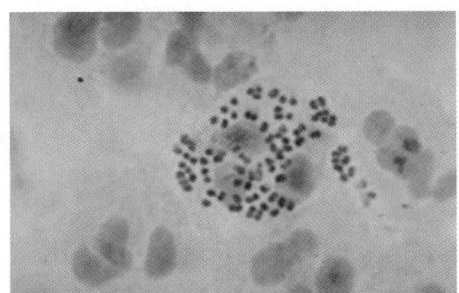

FIGURE 41-2 Gram-negative *N. gonorrhoeae*.

that will enhance the growth of one type of bacteria while retarding growth of others to enable easier identification. The microbiologist observes the culture for a colony (growth of one type of microorganism visible with the naked eye on the surface of media) and the appearance of the colony and examines a sample of the specimen under a microscope for morphology and staining properties. Each bit of information about the nature of the bacteria assists in identification and diagnosis. Hemolysis is an important identifying property of certain microbes. A specimen such as a throat swab is applied to a blood agar plate and incubated for 24 hours. The plate is then held up to the light to enhance reading for hemolysis. No change in color around the colony in known as gamma hemolysis or nonhemolytic (the preferred term). A narrow green-colored zone around a colony is known as alpha hemolysis, and a clear zone around the colony is beta hemolysis. Beta hemolysis indicates that the microorganism in that colony has burst the red blood cells, leaving a clear colorless zone around it. The organism that causes strep throat is beta hemolytic.

Other Identifying Characteristics

Microbes may be either motile or nonmotile. If they are capable of movement, their means of motility is unique to specific categories of microorganisms. They may possess flagella, long whip-like extensions of the cytoplasm, or cilia, fine hair-like extensions. For example, *Trichomonas vaginalis*, the protozoa that is responsible for one type of vaginitis, has four flagella at one end that produce the characteristic circular whip-like movement seen in wet preparations and urine microscopic examinations of infected individuals.

Biochemical analysis, often done on semiautomated analyzers, provides the microbiologist with information to assist in identification of certain pathogens such as enteric organisms.

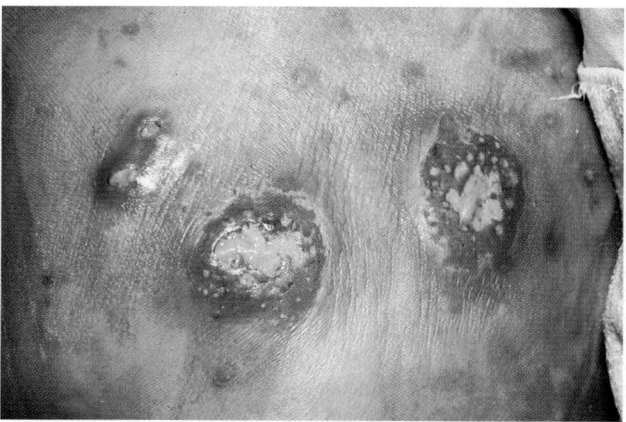

FIGURE 41-3 Carbuncles caused by *S. aureus*.

Types of Microorganisms

Microbes are also divided into groups based on shared special characteristics. Bacteria, viruses, protozoa, fungi, parasites, and other organisms with similar characteristics are discussed next. Table 41-1 provides a list of microorganisms, including descriptions and examples of each.

Bacterium/Bacteria

Bacteria are small, unicellular microorganisms that are capable of rapid reproduction. Their reproductive ability explains how some infections become overwhelming in a short period of time and can be dangerous. As an example, one *Escherichia coli* organism, the most common cause of urinary tract infections (UTIs), reproduces in about 30 minutes. This one *E. coli* cell at the end of a 24-hour period will produce an enormous number of cells capable of creating an infection if they have been introduced into the bladder. Bacteria may be named for their morphology (shape): cocci (spherical), bacilli (rod-shaped), or spirilla (spiral shape). We will consider each group of bacteria classified by their morphology.

Coccus/Cocci

Cocci are round bacteria that are arranged in various configurations. Staphylococci are found in grape-like clusters, streptococci in chains, and diplococci in pairs.

STAPHYLOCOCCI Staphylococci are gram-positive, grape-like clusters of cocci some of which are pathogenic. Nonpathogenic staphylococci are found on our skin and in many of our body orifices, or openings. *Staphylococcus aureus* (*S. aureus*) or Staph is the major pathogen of this genus and may be found as normal flora in the nose and on the skin. It causes infection especially when resistance is lowered by a break in the skin or in the mucous membranes. The skin is the most common site of infection by *S. aureus*. It produces infections such as impetigo in children and is associated with infection of wound sites and surgical incisions. It causes pus-producing abscesses such as boils, carbuncles, and folliculitis. Figure 41-3 shows an example of carbuncles. *S. aureus* is a common cause of nosocomial infections and may also cause pneumonia, meningitis, and septicemia in individuals with reduced resistance. Toxic shock syndrome is also caused by this virulent organism. *S. aureus* produces one type of enteritis (food poisoning) that occurs within in a few hours of eating improperly refrigerated food contaminated with the toxin produced by the bacteria. This toxin causes nausea vomiting, diarrhea, and abdominal cramping. *S. aureus* is coagulase positive, meaning it produces an enzyme that can be used to help differentiate *S. aureus* from other species of this organism.

TABLE 41-1 **Classes of Microorganisms with Descriptions and Examples**

Microorganism	Description	Example
Bacteria	Most numerous of all microorganisms Unicellular Many are pathogenic to humans Identified by shape and appearance	(See cocci, bacilli, and spirilla entries)
■ Cocci	Three types of spherical bacteria	
1. Staphylococci	Form grape-like clusters of pus-producing organisms	Boils, pimples, acne, osteomyelitis
2. Streptococci	Form chains of cells	Rheumatic heart disease, scarlet fever, strep throat
3. Diplococci	Form pairs of cells	Pneumonia, gonorrhea, and meningitis
■ Bacilli	Rod-shaped bacteria	Gram-positive bacilli: tetanus, diphtheria, gas gangrene Gram-negative bacilli: *E. coli* (urinary tract infection), *Bordetella pertussis* (whooping cough)
■ Vibrios		Cholera
■ Spirilla	Spiral-shaped organisms	Syphilis
■ Fungi	Parasitic and some nonparasitic plants and molds Depend on other life forms for their nutrition, such as dead or decaying organic material Reproduction method is budding Yeast is a typical fungus Fungus means "mushroom" in Latin Feed on antibiotics and flourish on antibiotic therapy	*Histoplasma capsulatum* (histoplasmosis), tinea pedis (athlete's foot), candidiasis (yeast infection), and ringworm
Protozoa	One-celled organism Both parasitic and nonparasitic Can move with cilia or false feet Typically 2–200 mm in size	Amebic dysentery, malaria, and *Trichomonas* vaginitis
Rickettsia	Visible under a standard microscope Susceptible to antibiotics Transmitted by insects (ticks, fleas)	Rocky Mountain spotted fever
Virus	Smallest of microorganisms Can only be seen with electron microscope Can only multiply within a living cell (host) Difficult to kill with chemotherapy since they become resistant to the drug Can be destroyed by heat (autoclave sterilization) but generally not by chemical disinfection More viruses than any other category of microbial agents Feed on antibiotics and flourish on antibiotic therapy	Herpes virus, HIV, ARC, AIDS, common cold, influenza virus, smallpox, hepatitis A, hepatitis B, mumps, shingles

Preparing for
Externship

In preparing for your externship, review medical terminology. Physicians use many specialized terms and abbreviations, and you must be familiar with them. If you are working in a specialty area, such as orthopedics, you might hear abbreviations that you would not hear, for example, in obstetrics. When you are assigned an externship site, review disorders, diseases, and abbreviations related to that field.

Today because of increased reliance on treatment with antibiotics to treat low-level infections, "super bugs" are becoming common. This term refers to various microorganisms that are mutating to produce antibiotic-resistant forms. Of particular interest is methicillin-resistant *Staphylococcus aureus* (MRSA). These forms of *S. aureus* produce an enzyme the makes the organism resistant to penicillins and cephalosporins normally used for treatment and renders these antibiotics ineffective. Tests are available to indicate the presence or absence of this enzyme and help determine the most favorable treatment. The problem of antibiotic resistance is a major concern for health care providers and is being experienced worldwide.

STREPTOCOCCI Streptococci are round, gram-positive bacteria arranged in chains some of which are nonpathogenic, others of which are dangerous to humans. Streptococcal organisms are part of the normal flora of the upper respiratory tract and skin. As previously mentioned one classification of streptococcal organisms is based on the type of hemolysis the organisms cause on blood agar plates. In addition, streptococci can be classified serologically with antisera specific for antigens in cell walls that are specific for each group (A–H and K–V). Identification of the specific group of strep organisms is important in epidemiology, the study of outbreaks of infections.

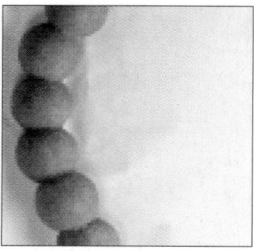

FIGURE 41-4 Streptococci: individual bacteria that have a rounded shape and have clumped together to form a chain.

Group A beta-hemolytic *Streptococcus pyogenes* causes a variety of diseases varying from mild such as strep throat to life threatening such as necrotizing fascitis (severe infection due to destruction of subcutaneous tissue and fascia with a 30% mortality rate). This organism also causes other infections, including pneumonia, tonsillitis, scarlet fever, rheumatic fever, acute glomerulonephritis, and bacterial endocarditis, as well as abscesses, wound infections, and bacteremia. Figure 41-4 shows a model of streptococci. *Streptococcus pneumoniae* (also called *pneumococcus* or *Diplococcus pneumoniae*) frequently are found as normal flora in the throat. However, it is the frequent cause of bacterial pneumonia particularly in the older population, middle ear infections in children, and meningitis in older children and adults.

Commercial kits are available for rapid detection of group A beta-hemolytic strep in the office or laboratory setting. Any negative test should be followed up by a culture that includes bacitracin sensitivity. Sensitivity to the antibiotic bacitracin is a useful tool to separate group A beta-hemolytic strep from other strep organisms. The information about rapid strep tests and the procedure for a throat culture with bacitracin will be covered later in the chapter.

DIPLOCOCCI Diplococci occur in pairs. Some diplococci are gram positive, such as *S. pneumoniae*, which causes bacterial pneumonia. Others such as *N. gonorrhoeae* and *Neisseria meningitidis* are gram negative, the former causing gonorrhea, a sexually transmitted infection, and the latter causing a form of bacterial meningitis and septicemia. Meningococcal meningitis has a high mortality rate and requires immediate treatment. A vaccine for meningococcal meningitis is now available that is recommended for students entering high school or college or for those joining the armed services and other individuals who may be at high risk.

Although these diplocal organisms are pathogenic, many of the diplococci, both gram negative and gram positive, are normally found in areas such as the upper respiratory tract.

Bacillus/Bacilli

Rod-shaped bacilli may be pathogenic or nonpathogenic. Some bacilli are gram positive and others are gram negative. Figure 41-5 illustrates bacilli. Bacilli are responsible for a wide variety of illnesses including gastroenteritis, UTIs, whooping cough, tetanus, botulism, tuberculosis, and pneumonia.

GRAM-NEGATIVE BACILLI Enterobacteriaceae are a large family of gram-negative bacilli found mainly in the intestinal tract; however, many of them will cause infections in other body locations. One type, *Escherichia coli,* is most frequently associated with urinary tract infections (UTIs). Another is the group of Salmonella organisms. Salmonella organisms are a major cause of foodborne illnesses worldwide. They can be classified serologically to differentiate which among the thousands of members of this pathogenic group are causing the outbreak of disease. Most frequently outbreaks of food poisoning are caused either by *Salmonella enteritidis* or *Salmonella typhimurium*. Symptoms of enteric food poisoning include rapid onset, abdominal pain, nausea, diarrhea, and in some children even death. Contaminated food such as raw eggs, chicken, or beef is the usual route of transmission.

Typhoid fever is caused by *S. typhi* and is frequently found in third world countries and natural disaster areas where their is a lack of proper sanitation. Another member of this family of gram-negative bacilli is a group of Shigella organisms that causes bacillary dysentery, characterized by frequent bloody, pus or mucous-containing stools. This bacillary dysentery results from inadequate sanitary conditions.

Another gram-negative bacilli not a member of the previously mentioned family is *Helicobacter pylori*, which was discovered in the early 1980s. This organism is found in about half of the population and causes no symptoms in most individuals. It was discovered that *H. pylori* is the causative agent of peptic ulcers and a risk factor in gastric malignancy in some infected persons. The organism is responsive to a number of antibiotics including tetracycline. The discovery of *H. pylori* led to major breakthroughs in ulcer treatment. Previously it was believed peptic ulcers were due to nerves or increased acid production and treatments were generally ineffective.

GRAM-POSITIVE BACILLI   Gram-positive bacilli may be found in chains or singly, and are spore forming or nonspore forming. A spore is a thick-walled reproductive cell produced by some organisms that is capable of withstanding unfavorable environmental conditions. Notable in this group are *Clostridium botulinum*, which causes botulism, and *Clostridium tetani*, which causes tetanus. Tetanus immunizations are given to protect from the extremely potent neurotoxin produced by *C. tetani*. Tetanus is a disease resulting from a cut or injury associated with contaminated soil such as a rusty farm implement. Botulism is a severe, possibly fatal form of food poisoning caused by the powerful neurotoxin produced by the anaerobe *C. botulinum*. It is associated with improper canning processes and with use as a possible bioterrorism agent.

VIBRIO/VIBRIOS   Vibrios are comma-shaped bacilli. The main pathogen is *Vibrio cholerae* whose enterotoxin causes cholera. Cholera is characterized by profuse watery stools, vomiting, leg cramps, dehydration, and shock. It is caused by ingesting drinking water or eating shellfish from water contaminated with in-

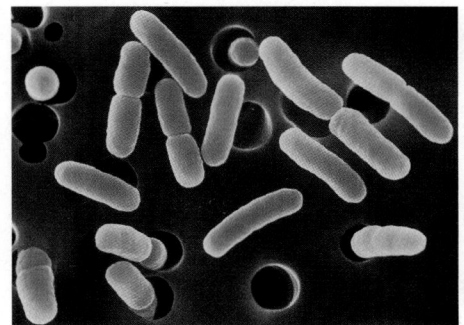

FIGURE 41-5   Bacilli.

fected, urine, feces, or vomitus. Cholera is common in Asiatic countries, and travelers to these areas can be vaccinated for protection; however, they still should boil all drinking water and avoid uncooked foods. Figure 41-6 illustrates a vibrio.

Spirillum/Spirilla

Spirilla, or spirochetes as they are also known, are spiral-shaped or corkscrew-shaped organisms. Technically they are rods that are twisted in various shapes; however, they are classified as a separate category of bacteria. As with other shapes of bacteria some are nonpathogenic and are found in certain areas of the body and others, such as *Treponema pallidum*, cause the sexually transmitted infection syphilis. *Borrelia burgdorferi*, spirillum, was discovered in the mid-1970s to be the causative agent of Lyme disease. Lyme disease is a deer tick-borne disease named after a town in Connecticut that was investigating a cluster of juvenile arthritis cases. Ticks are infected by feeding on deer or rodents, which are natural hosts for the organism. The infected tick then bites a human and transmits the organism. This tick is so tiny that many people are unaware of the bite until the characteristic expanding rash is discovered, followed after a period of time by fever, muscle pain, headache, and fatigue. Immunoassay tests exist to aid in the diagnosis of Lyme disease. Figure 41-7 illustration spirilla.

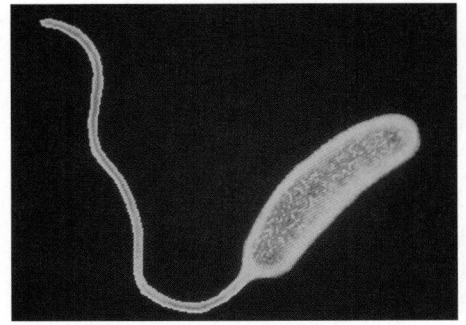

FIGURE 41-6   Vibrio.

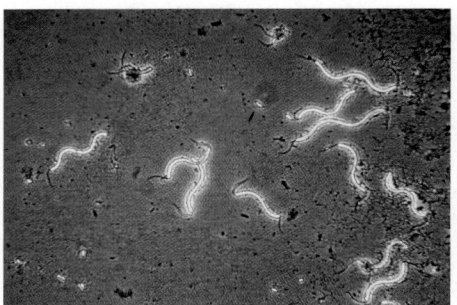

FIGURE 41-7 Spirilla bacteria.

Special Categories of Bacteria

Some types of bacteria do not fall clearly into any of the previously mentioned groups. These are mycobacteria, rickettsia, mycoplasmas, and chlamydia. Mycobacteria have a different type of material in the cell wall and can only be stained with an acid-fast stain. Two members of this genus are fairly well known.

Mycobacterium tuberculosis is the causative agent of tuberculosis and *Mycobacterium leprae*, the cause of leprosy. These organisms do not stain well with a Gram stain. In a positive slide for acid-fast bacilli (AFB), the slender bacilli will appear pink with an acid-fast stain.

Rickettsia, chlamydia, and mycoplasma are very tiny bacteria in the size range of viruses. Rickettsia are bacterial parasites that live in ticks and mites and transmit the disease when they bite humans. Rocky Mountain spotted fever and typhus are both rickettsial diseases. Chlamydia is also an obligate parasite, but it does not live in arthropod hosts. Chlamydia must invade living cells to reproduce. *Chlamydia trachomatis* is an STI that may be a silent inhabitant of the vagina or cause mild burning sensations and discharge. After repeated infections, this organism may cause scarring in the Fallopian tubes making conception difficult. Rickettsia and chlamydia cannot be grown on artificial media. Tissue cultures or serological testing must be done for identification.

Mycoplasma were thought to be viruses at one time but they are very tiny bacteria lacking a rigid cell wall. They cause mycoplasma pneumonia and a type of venereal disease.

Virus/Viruses

Although potent, a virus is the smallest known infectious organism and requires the use of an electron microscope for visualization. A virus, a simpler form of life than a cell, is parasitic, depending on living cells of other organisms for growth. When a virus enters a cell, it may immediately cause a disease, such as influenza. Or it may remain dormant for days or even years. Figure 41-8 shows an example of an influenza virus. For instance, herpes zoster may cause an outbreak of chickenpox within 7 to 14 days of exposure. Yet, HIV can lie dormant for a long period of time, sometimes years, before any symptoms are noted.

Viruses cause many common diseases such as colds, chickenpox, mumps, infectious mononucleosis, and warts. Other illnesses caused by viruses are hepatitis, measles, encephalitis, and herpes. Fortunately, vaccines are available to protect people from diseases such as polio, German measles, measles, hepatitis B, mumps, and chickenpox.

Protozoa

Although single-celled parasites, protozoa are usually larger than bacteria. Most protozoa live in the soil and receive nourishment from dead or decaying organic material. Lack of proper sanitation can lead to rapid spread of infections. Some protozoa are pathogenic and may cause diseases such as *Trichomonas vaginalis* (a type of STI) or malaria transmitted by the bite of an infected *Anopheles* mosquito. The organism inhabits the red blood cells (RBCs) in the affected individual. Figure 41-9 models malaria protozoa.

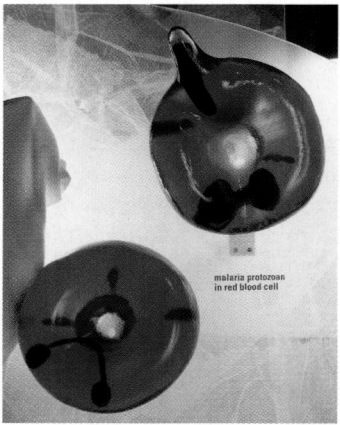

FIGURE 41-9 Model of malaria protozoa in a red blood cell. New parasites are produced, mature in the RBC, then push their way out of the cell.

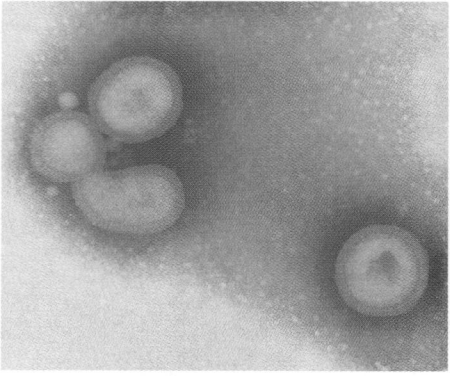

FIGURE 41-8 Influenza virus.

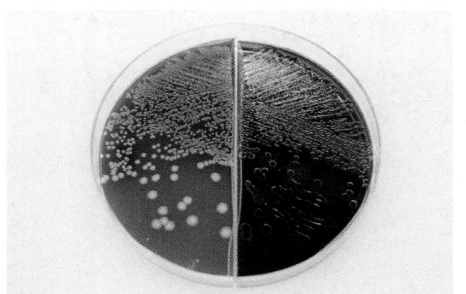

FIGURE 41-10 Mold is growing on red/green agar in a divided Petri dish.

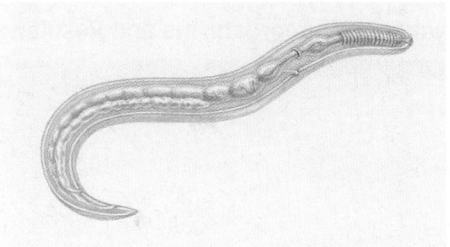

FIGURE 41-11 A female roundworm. Roundworms have long, cylindrical bodies with a tough covering. Eggs laid by the females are excreted in the feces of infected people.

Fungus/Fungi

Fungi are unable to make their own food, so they depend on other life forms. Included in this classification are yeasts and molds. In our environment we encounter fungi in the form of mushrooms and mold in form of penicillin mold on stale bread. Penicillium mold was discovered by Alexander Fleming, and its antibiotic properties changed modern medical treatment. Penicillin is now synthetically produced. Figure 41-10 shows an example of a mold. The study of fungi is known as mycology. Fungi are present in soil, water, and air.

Single-celled fungi that reproduce by budding are known as yeast. Those fungi which produce spores are called molds. Most fungi are not pathogenic and cause few diseases in humans. Of the ones that do, most will produce only superficial infections, such as athlete's foot (tinea pedis) or ringworm. A few do produce life-threatening illnesses when they invade the internal organs of the body.

Candida albicans is the causative agent of moniliasis or candidiasis, a yeast infection, and thrush. Individuals with compromised immune systems or those who have been on long-term antibiotic therapy may develop severe infections. In these cases the normal flora that protect the openings of the body cavities are killed by the antibiotic therapy and allow fungi a fertile environment in which to reproduce. This type of infection is referred to as a "super infection." As anyone who has endured the unpleasantness of athlete's foot knows, it takes a long time and persistence to get rid of a fungal infection. Fungal infections are resistant to antibiotics and must be treated with antifungal agents.

Parasites

As previously noted, a parasite receives nourishment from another organism. As a result of this activity, the host organism becomes diseased. Parasites may be single celled such as chlamydia or multicellular like pinworms.

Some examples of parasites include worms and insects:

• Worms (helminths)—The person may ingest the egg, an immature form of the worm, or it may penetrate the skin. Some of the worms that infect people are flat worms, roundworms, tapeworms, and pinworms. Figure 41-11 shows a female roundworm. Round, flat, and tapeworms inhabit the intestines. Tapeworms, for instance, may grow to be many feet in length. The stool of the patient can be inspected for the presence of ova and mature forms of the worm. The procedure for collecting stool for ova and parasites (O&P) will be covered later in the chapter.

• Insects—Insects may bite, burrow under, or attach to the skin of the human. An example of a disease occurring by attachment of an insect is Lyme disease, caused by a tick-transmitted spirochete. Lyme disease has been documented in many parts of North America and has an incubation period of from 3 to 32 days. Figure 41-12 shows a tick. With early detection and treatment with antibiotics, many patients have complete recovery. Arthritis may be a sequela (long-lasting effect) of Lyme disease. Cardiac conduction abnormalities, aseptic meningitis, and Bell's palsy may also be associated conditions. Scabies and lice infestations are examples parasites. Both are transmitted by direct contact with bedding or clothing and cause severe itching.

Refer to Table 41-2 for some examples of pathogenic microorganisms, their location in the body, and diseases they produce.

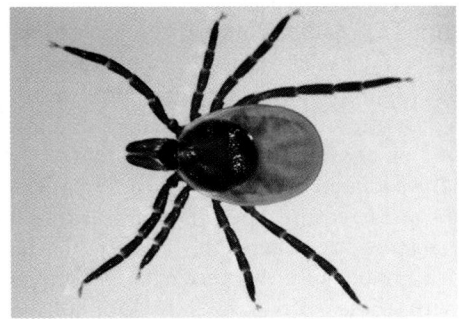

FIGURE 41-12 A deer tick can cause Lyme disease.

TABLE 41-2 **Pathogenic Microorganisms and Resulting Diseases**

Body Location	Pathogen	Disease
Respiratory system	*Streptococcus pyogenes* *Corynebacterium diphtheriae* *Mycobacterium tuberculosis* *Haemophilus influenzae* type B *Streptococcus pneumoniae*	Strep throat, scarlet fever Diphtheria Tuberculosis Influenza Pneumonia
Central nervous system	*Neisseria meningitidis* Polioviruses Rabies virus	Meningitis Poliomyelitis Rabies
Genitourinary system	Herpes simplex viruses 1 and 2 *Candida albicans* (fungus) *Chlamydia trachomatis* *Escherichia coli*	Genital herpes Vaginitis Vaginitis Urinary tract infection
Integumentary system	*Staphylococcus aureus* Varicella zoster virus	Boils, carbuncles Chickenpox Scabies Lice
Gastrointestinal system	Hepatitis A, B, and C viruses *Salmonella enteritidis* *Escherichia coli*	Hepatitis A, B, and C Food poisoning *E. coli* diarrhea
Circulatory system and blood, immune system	*Streptococcus pyogenes* *Staphylococcus aureus* *Plasmodium falciparum, P. vivax, P. malariae, P. ovale* Human immunodeficiency virus Epstein-Barr virus *Borrelia burgdorferi*	Septicemia, endocarditis Malaria HIV/AIDS Infectious mononucleosis Lyme disease
Tissue	*Streptococcus pyogenes*	Necrotizing fascitis

Specimen Collection and Transportation

Specimens for microbiology must be collected according to protocols established by the microbiology department of the laboratory performing the testing. One of the first priorities of quality control (QC) is proper specimen collection. There can be no shortcuts taken in the collection process. Any incorrect steps could result in a contaminated or altered specimen, delayed diagnosis, and postponed or possibly harmful treatment.

The first step in specimen collection is proper patient education. Many tests require special preparation to obtain accurate results for diagnosis. It is up to the medical assistant to make sure the patient understands and complies with these instructions by doing two things: (1) carefully reading and explaining the instruc-

tions, answering any questions the patient might have, and (2) giving written instructions for the patient to follow or refer to at home. Refer to Figure 41-13 for an illustration of a medical assistant explaining a laboratory procedure to a patient. Carefully document any patient teaching and verify that the patient verbalizes understanding of the instructions.

The second important step is to follow the basic guidelines for specimen collection. Guidelines 41-1 provides guidelines for specimen collection. Keep in mind when dealing with microbiological specimens that they are living organisms and must have proper conditions to survive but not to multiply.

Laboratory Request Information

In addition to the specimen label information consisting of patient's name, date and time of collection, type

Professionalism

Maintaining a professional attitude as well as a professional appearance will cause your patients to feel more at ease in your facility. Remember that first impressions often last forever. Your uniform, shoes, hair, and fingernails combine to assist in making that first impression. Your outward appearance can sometimes influence the patient's idea of your competence to perform procedures. So, approach your patient as a competent, professional medical assistant, thus establishing rapport immediately.

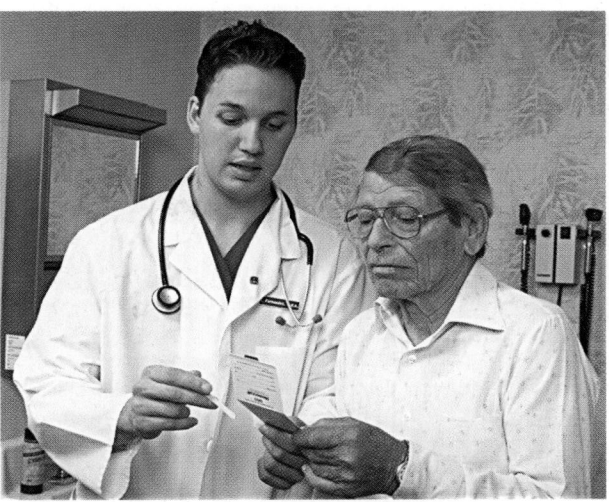

FIGURE 41-13 Medical assistant explains to patient how to use a collection specimen kit.

and source of specimen, doctor's name, and your initials, the following information should be included on the requisition:

- Patient's address
- Identification number
- Age
- Gender
- Insurance information
- More specific information regarding the type and the source of the specimen (nasal swab, left nostril)
- Test requested

- Medication patient is currently receiving
- Diagnosis, if available
- Physician's information (name, address, telephone number)
- Special information or orders

Specimens are rejected by outside laboratories if the label and/or requisition information is incomplete, and for insufficient quantity or packaging of specimens. Tests may have to be repeated and the specimen

---

41-1 GUIDELINES — Specimen Collection

The basic rules for specimen collection are:

1. Confirm the identity of the patient by asking the patient to state his or her name and spell it, if necessary.
2. Screen the patient to determine if pretest preparation was followed.
3. Collect specimen prior to beginning antibiotic treatment.
4. Collect sufficient quantity of material for testing.
5. Use only appropriate collection technique by observing proper cleaning and aseptic procedures to control contamination.
6. Only sterile containers may be used.
7. Select the proper containers for collection that comply with the reference lab's or outside laboratory's requirements.
8. Ensure that the collection container is tightly closed/appropriately sealed to avoid leakage and contamina-

tion of the specimen and any surface the container may come in contact with.

9. Label the specimen accurately at the time of collection with the following information:
   a. Patient's full name
   b. Date
   c. Time of collection
   d. Type of specimen
   e. Antibiotic treatment in use, if any
   f. Your initials
10. Fill out the requisition form for the reference lab and double-check that the information matches the label.
11. Deliver specimen promptly to laboratory and document it. Or maintain proper storage of specimen until delivery can take place or it is transported appropriately. Cerebrospinal fluid always requires immediate delivery.

FIGURE 41-14 Examples of sterile swabs (removed from protective wrappers).

collected again. This means additional delay and discomfort for the patient.

Collection Devices

Sterile swabs are frequently used in collection of specimens. The shafts and the tips of swabs vary in terms of the type of material used. They are wrapped in a sterile wrapper or container to preserve sterility. Figure 41-14 shows examples of sterile swabs of various types. Cotton swabs are used less frequently today because certain microbes are inhibited by the natural ingredients in cotton. Polyester and rayon are used for the tips and wood, plastic or wire for the shaft. Swabs also vary in size of tip and flexibility of the shaft to permit collection in difficult to reach areas. After a swab is collected it is placed in a sterile container which may or may not contain culture media.

Swabs, Culture Tubes, and Other Collection Devices

The Culturette system is a disposable, clear plastic tube that contains a sterile, cotton-tipped applicator swab and a sealed plastic vial of medium (broth containing nourishment for bacteria and a preservative). This system is used to obtain many types of specimens, from sites ranging from the throat, nose, or eyes to wounds

and the genital or urethral areas. It is important that these types of specimens, collected in Culturettes, be transported immediately so that microorganisms remain viable, or capable of living, when they reach the laboratory. Commercially available swab collection and transportation units are used widely. Some of these units contain two sterile swabs, one for culturing and one for preparing the direct smear. A smear is thin layer of microorganisms spread on a glass slide for identification purposes. Figure 41-15 demonstrates a variety of collection devices including a swab and Culturette in the lower left of the photograph.

Specimens such as exudates (wound drainage) may be collected with Culturette units. Collection devices are available for anaerobic cultures also. Sterile containers are available for urine, stool, blood, and cerebrospinal fluid. Fluids drained from body cavities may require larger sterile containers.

Transporting Specimens to an Outside Laboratory

Specimens may be picked up by courier to deliver to a local laboratory testing site. Or the testing site may be located in a distant location requiring special mailing devices and instructions. In addition to moisture and specific nutrition requirements, specimens must be maintained at appropriate temperatures to ensure viability. Temperatures may differ with the type of specimen. The length of time between collection and arrival at the testing site can be crucial. Throat cultures and samples for gonorrhea should never be refrigerated. Always consult the office laboratory manual for complete transporting instructions.

Overview of the Process of Diagnosing Infection

When a patient comes to the office with an apparent infection, exactly what steps are taken to diagnose and begin treatment of the infection? First the patient is examined and the usual procedures are followed including patient identification, vital signs, chief complaint, and present illness. If the infection is one such as chickenpox that can be diagnosed on sight by the physician, further testing will not be necessary. If there is an open infected wound, the site should be measured, described, and charted including information about drainage, odor, and level of patient discomfort.

Next specimens are collected and labeled and prepared safely for

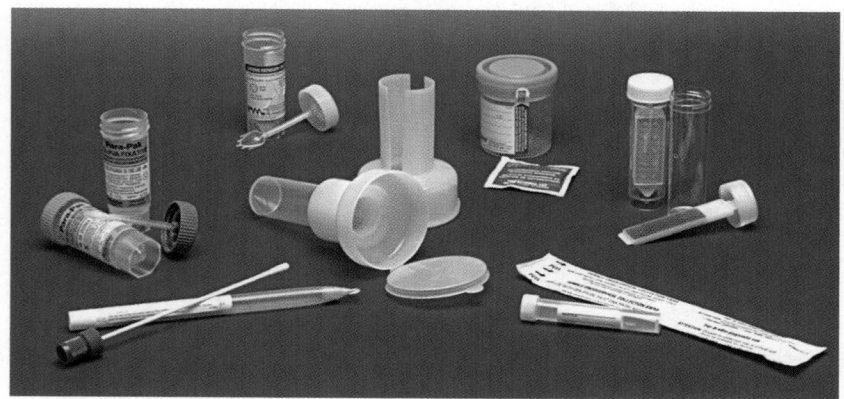

FIGURE 41-15 Examples of specimen collection containers.

transportation to ensure any organisms remain alive and safety issues are observed. A culture of the specimen may be necessary. In this case a swab of the specimen is streaked on appropriate culture medium in such a way to allow individual colonies of microorganisms to develop. This permits easier identification. A second culture plate may be inoculated (microorganisms placed on) heavily to be tested for antibiotic sensitivity. Certain microorganisms are sensitive to specific antibiotics and resistant to others. The culture plates are incubated at 37°C for 24 hours to allow the organisms to grow.

After 24 hours a zone of no growth around an antibiotic disk indicates the organism is sensitive to that drug, and if it is used to treat the patient, it should work in the same way. If the patient is allergic to that particular medication, then the antibiotic with the next largest zone of inhibition is chosen for treatment. If direct examination of the specimen is required then a direct smear is made. This involves placing a thin layer of the specimen material on a slide that is properly labeled, allowed to dry, and then stained. The physician or other qualified personnel will examine it for microorganisms considering their morphology and stain reactions (gram positive or gram negative). In some cases a presumptive diagnosis can be made and treatment determined.

Preparation of a wet mount may be necessary in cases where the organisms, if present, must be kept alive to observe for motility and morphology. A wet mount is a preparation in a liquid that will preserve motility of the microbe. The ultimate goal all of these steps is to select the most favorable treatment that will restore the patient to a healthy condition. A more detailed discussion of the preceding steps follows.

Microbiology Equipment and Procedures

The equipment and supplies necessary in a microbiology laboratory vary with the size and type of facility. A typical physician's office laboratory (POL) will have a microscope, incubator, autoclave, refrigerator, biohazardous waste containers, and a variety of specimen collection devices and containers, all of which have been discussed in previous chapters. Inoculation equipment such as loop, needle, and incineration equipment and culture media are also necessary to process microbiology specimens.

Inoculating Equipment

A loop is a long instrument with a small loop on the end designed to pick up fluids and transfer them to culture media. Specifically calibrated loops for urine cultures are available that allow for the transfer of

1 μL of urine to a culture plate. This precise amount of urine allows for quantitative evaluation of the number of microorganisms to evaluate whether a urinary tract infection is present. A needle is a long straight instrument with a pointed end used to sample individual colonies of microorganisms. Inoculating loops and needles may be purchased in sterile, prewrapped packages or may be made of metal. After a prewrapped sterile loop or needle is used, it is discarded in a biohazard container. A metal loop or needle requires incineration before and after use to ensure sterility. Bunsen burners requiring a natural gas supply or electric incinerators are used.

Culture Media

Once a specimen has been obtained, it must be inoculated onto a medium that will enhance the growth of the microorganism. Media may be solid like a slant (agar in a tube placed in a tilted position to harden), semisolid like agar, or liquid like broth. Media will either inhibit or encourage the growth of

TABLE 41-3 Culture Media and Isolates

Common Culture Media	Isolates
Blood agar	Most bacteria
Chocolate agar	*Neisseria, Haemophilus*
EMB	Gram-negative bacteria
MacConkey agar	Gram-negative bacteria
Thioglycollate broth	Anaerobic microorganisms
GN broth	Fecal microorganisms

certain pathogens and are classified as supportive, selective, differential or enrichment.

- Supportive—used to grow a wide variety of organisms
- Selective—encourages growth of some organisms and restricts growth of others (e.g., vaginal and stool cultures)
- Differential—includes dyes or chemicals that give organisms a different appearance (e.g., differentiate staphylococci)
- Enrichment—contains special organic substances needed to encourage growth of organisms that are fastidious (fussy) (e.g., gonorrhea organisms)

In many POLs, commercial culture units are widely used. For example, units are available for urine that

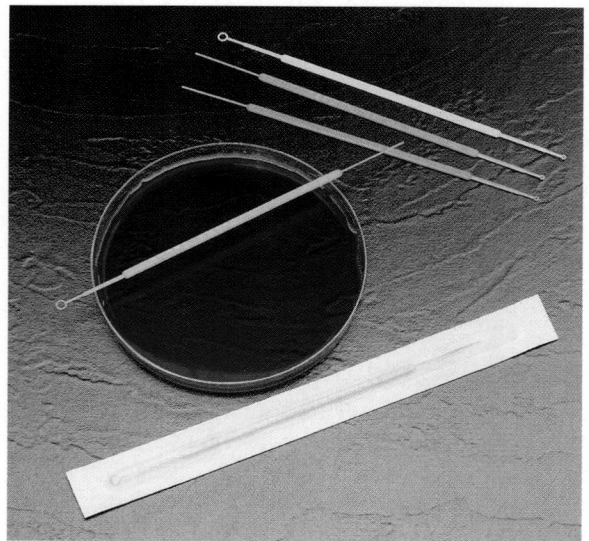

FIGURE 41-16 Blood agar plate and equipment for culture.

make inoculation easy. A paddle with different media on either side is dipped in a clean-catch or catheterized urine sample and replaced in the vial; it is then incubated for 24 hours. Commercial units for blood, vaginal, and throat specimens are also available. All media should be inspected for contamination before use to ensure the integrity of the culturing process.

Inoculating Media

Pathogens are identified by growing cultures, which are the propagation of microorganisms, taken from the specimen. Colonies of bacteria can be grown only on certain media. Pathogens are often identified by the manner in which they grow on a particular medium. An example of this would be streptococci bacteria that cause strep throat. Mucus swabbed from a sore throat inoculated on a medium that contains blood will produce pinpoint-sized colonies that have a transparent ring around each, which is the result of hemolysis or bursting of red blood cells by the streptococci in the surrounding medium. Table 41-3 lists common culture media and microorganisms that can be isolated on each. Figure 41-16 shows a blood agar plate and examples of inoculating needles and loops.

The main goal in growing cultures is to separate pathogenic colonies of organisms from colonies of normal flora. To isolate colonies, the agar must be streaked properly. The specimen is transferred by rubbing the swab across one small area of the agar near the edge. Next, a wire inoculating loop is sterilized in a Bunsen burner flame or electric incinerator, cooled, and used to streak through the area already inoculated and onto an unmarked area of the agar in a zigzag motion. The wire loop is then sterilized again, cooled, and is used to streak through the zigzag area onto the remainder of uninoculated agar with the same technique as before. This is called streaking for isolation (streak culture) and is illustrated in Figure 41-17.

After inoculation, the lid or top of the Petri dish is replaced and the agar plate inverted and placed into an incubator (See Figure 41-18). The inversion of the agar plate allows moisture to collect on the lid of the Petri dish and not on the culture itself. The culture is allowed to grow in the incubator at 37°C for a 24-, 48-, or 72-hour period. Fungi take longer to grow and may need to grow at slightly lower temperatures.

A secondary culture can be obtained by selecting an isolated colony from the initial agar plate and placing it on another media plate using a sterile loop or needle. This provides a pure culture, a colony containing only one single type of organism. Identification of the organism is made by using the pure culture to prepare and stain a slide and by performing various biochemical tests.

Instruments such as Vitek and Autobac use automated technology to facilitate organism identification.

The BAC-T Screen Bacteruria-Pyuria Detection Device is an automated system that immediately determines if significant numbers of bacteria are present in a urine specimen, avoiding the 24- to 48-hour wait for complete growth and identification. Tests such as those mentioned are performed by medical laboratory specialists.

Sensitivity Testing

Once the physician or laboratory specialist identifies the pathogenic organism on the culture, it is necessary to determine which antibiotics will be effective in killing these bacteria. This method of detection is called *sensitivity testing*. A Petri dish with Mueller-Hinton agar and antibiotic disks are used. The Mueller-Hinton agar is inoculated with the pure culture specimen in overlapping strokes and the antibiotic disks are placed in a circle on top of the inoculated agar. The lid of the Petri dish is replaced, inverted, and placed in the incubator for 24 hours. After 24 hours, the organism will have grown all over except around those disks that inhibit its growth. These zones around the disks are measured to determine the susceptibility of the organism to each particular antibiotic disk. After the most effective antibiotic is identified, the patient is started on drug therapy.

Direct Examination

Two methods are used to prepare a specimen for direct examination under the microscope: the direct smear and the wet mount preparation. These methods allow the physician to obtain information quickly in the office and thus start treatment immediately.

Direct Smear

A direct smear may be from a swab of the specimen or from a colony on a culture plate (see Procedure 41-1). The smear from a specimen is made after the culture is inoculated to prevent contamination of the media since slides are not usually sterile. The swab is rolled carefully across the slide so all areas of the swab touch the slide. The slide is labeled by placing the patient's name and specimen type on the frosted end of the slide. The smear air dries; do not wave it in the air, which could spread microorganisms. The slide must be fixed to ensure that the specimen material remains on the slide during the staining process. It is fixed by passing the clear underneath part of the slide through an open flame three to four times or flooding the slide with methanol and letting it dry. These steps must be done prior to any staining procedure.

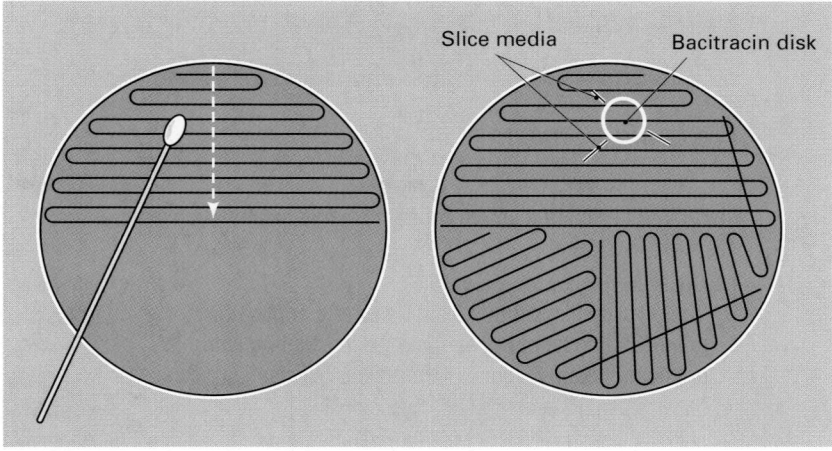

FIGURE 41-17 Culture technique.

Slice media   Bacitracin disk

Wet Mount Preparation

Wet mount preparation involves taking a sample of either a colony or directly from a patient specimen, placing it on a frosted slide, and adding a drop of sterile normal saline and a coverslip. A wet mount preparation such as this allows the physician to observe the motility of the organism and what types of cytoplasmic extensions the organisms have (cilia, flagella). These observations render important identifying information. Refer to Procedure 41-2 for instructions on preparation of a wet mount slide.

Often in the POL a wet mount for fungus is performed using potassium hydroxide (KOH). Fungus is

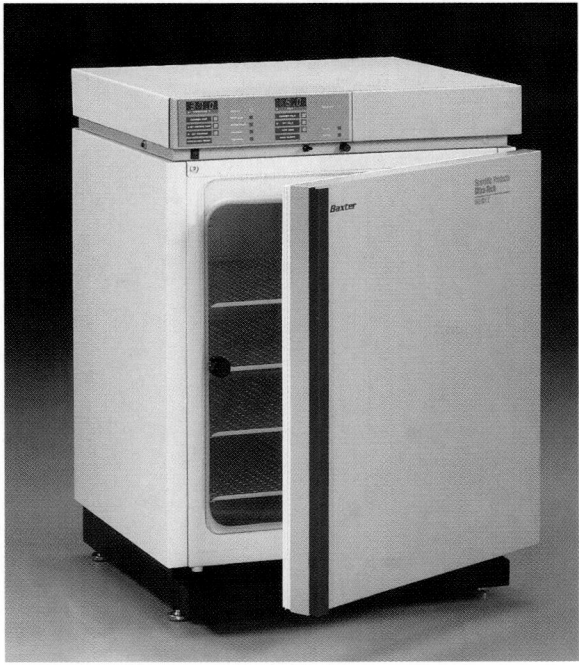

FIGURE 41-18 An incubator for office use.

Preparing a Smear

OBJECTIVE: Prepare a smear for microscopic examination without error.

Equipment and Supplies

frosted slides; specimen from Culturette applicator or inoculating loop; Bunsen burner; inoculating loop (or swab); microscope; oil immersion; gloves; hazardous waste container

Note: Follow Standard Precautions and safety guidelines when working with body fluid samples. Use care to avoid splashing or spilling body fluids. Wipe up all spills using guidelines established by OSHA.

Method

1. Perform hand hygiene and apply gloves.
2. Assemble equipment.
3. Label clean slide with patient's name, date, and type of specimen.
4. Inoculate slide by transferring specimen to slide. This is done by rolling swab over slide, ensuring all areas of swab touch the slide. Or place a drop of sterile saline on slide, and after flaming a needle or loop, pick up material from one type of colony and place in saline and spread gently over two-thirds of the slide.
5. Allow slide to air dry for 20 to 30 minutes.
6. Hold the slide with thumb forceps and pass slide over Bunsen burner flame. This heat "fixes" the specimen to the slide, known as smear fixation. Let the slide cool. Or flood the dry smear with methanol and let dry to fix slide if open flame is not available.
7. Slide is then ready to be stained.

Charting Example

11/16/XX	Direct smear from abscess RT thigh prepared for staining.
	M. King, CMA

---

often difficult to see on direct preparation because keratin from the body, particularly nails, hair, and skin, often obscures the fungal structures. Potassium hydroxide dissolves the keratin, allowing visualization of any fungi present (Figure 41-19). To prepare a KOH mount, a specimen is suspended in one drop of 10% potassium hydroxide and a coverslip is applied. Allow the specimen to sit at room temperature for 30 minutes to dissolve the keratin. The slide will be examined by the physician or laboratory specialist for evidence of fungi in the wet mount.

Staining Specimens

The use of stained smears in microbiology is extensive. The color and shape (morphology) of microorganisms on smears can be observed, for example, in vaginal and nasopharyngeal specimens. The medical assistant should know how to prepare a smear and have a general knowledge of the Gram stain and why it is used. The Gram stain, because several colors are used, will differentiate, or separate, bacteria into two groups: gram positive and gram negative. Different bacteria stain differently, depending on the compounds in their walls. Gram-positive bacteria retain the crystal violet-blue color and gram-negative bacteria retain only the pink safranin color. Thus, gram-positive (violet) bacteria can be distinguished from gram-negative (pink) bacteria. Precautions must be taken in Gram staining in that temperature, age of specimen, or length of incubation could cause a change in gram-positive bacteria.

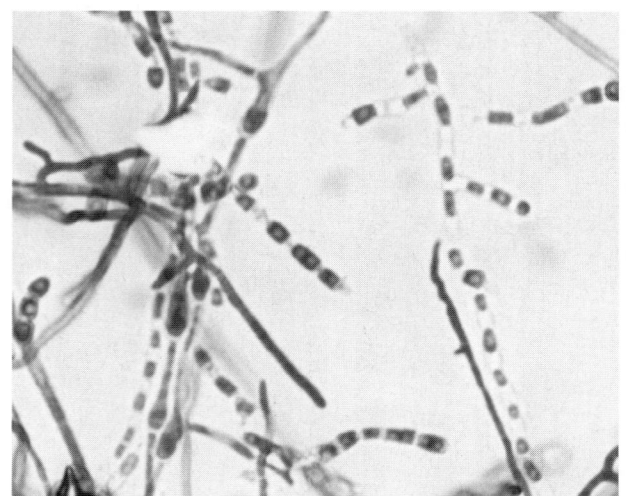

FIGURE 41-19 Example of fungi.

PROCEDURE

Preparing a Wet Mount Slide

OBJECTIVE: Prepare a wet mount slide. For microscopic examination without error.

Equipment and Supplies

clean, dry slide, frosted; coverslip; saline; specimen from a Culturette applicator or swab; paper/pen; microscope; gloves

Note: Follow Standard Precautions and safety guidelines when working with body fluid samples. Use care to avoid splashing or spilling body fluids. Wipe up all spills using guidelines established by OSHA.

Method

1. Perform hand hygiene and apply gloves.
2. Label dry slide with patient's name and date.
3. Inoculate the dry slide by rolling swab containing specimen across surface.
4. Place a drop of saline solution on top of specimen.
5. Place coverslip on top of smeared slide.

Note: The following steps would be performed by a physician or laboratory specialist.

6. Observe immediately under the microscope.
7. Special stains may be used to enhance characteristics.
8. Note on paper what is observed, remove slide, dispose of properly.
9. Remove gloves and wash hands.
10. Chart findings on patient's record.

Charting Example

11/16/XX	Wet mount prepared from vaginal swab for physician to examine.
	M. King, CMA

Gram stains must always be accompanied by culture for microorganism identification.

Procedure 41-3 lists the steps needed to perform a Gram stain correctly. Particular attention must be paid to the timing of the various steps. Crystal violet is poured on a fixed smear for 1 minute. The stain is washed off with water, and iodine is applied for 1 minute. The iodine is washed off and the decolorizer is used to wash for 15 seconds. (Care must be taken not to decolorize too long because it will make the slide difficult to evaluate.) Next safranin is applied to the slide for 30 seconds, followed by washing the slide and wiping off the back side of the slide to remove excess stain and standing it upright to dry. Refer to Figure 41-20 for illustrations of the Gram stain procedure.

The staining properties, shape, and size of the organisms can sometimes be used to identify pathogens in specimen samples. As previously noted, bacilli are rod-shaped cells found singly or in groups. Cocci are round bacteria found singly, in pairs (diplococci), in strings (streptococci), or in clusters (staphylococci). Spirilla, curved or spiral rods, can be arranged singly or in strands. Some bacteria can produce resistant forms called spores under adverse environmental conditions. Spores can lie dormant for thousands of years and, when conditions are right, revert back to active form. This trait makes it difficult to destroy these pathogenic bacteria.

Types of Specimens

Pathogens can be observed in specimens of blood, feces, cerebrospinal fluid, mucus, urine, sputum, wounds, tissue, and other substances from the body. The following paragraphs will discuss these types of specimens and information for obtaining the specimens.

Throat

One of the most frequently requested specimens in a POL is the throat swab or culture. Based on signs and symptoms the patient presents with, such as upper respiratory infection, sore throat, or sinus infection, the physician will order a throat culture to identify the pathogen involved and begin treatment. Confirmation of *Streptococcus pyogenes* is important because of its virulence and possible complications. When performing a throat culture, it is important not to touch the insides of the mouth or the tongue with the swab to avoid contaminating it. A tongue depressor is used to hold the tongue down. The procedure

PROCEDURE

Performing a Gram Stain

OBJECTIVE: Prepare a slide for a Gram stain to differentiate a gram-positive organism from a gram-negative organism.

Equipment and Supplies

Gram-stain kit with decolorizer; culture specimen; slides; Bunsen burner or methanol; staining rack; water wash bottle; water; immersion oil; stopwatch; gloves; slide stand; paper towels; hazardous waste container

Note: Follow Standard Precautions and safety guidelines when working with body fluid samples. Use care to avoid splashing or spilling body fluids. Wipe up all spills using guidelines established by OSHA.

Method

1. Perform hand hygiene and apply gloves.
2. Assemble equipment.
3. Make a smear, label, air dry the smear, and heat or methanol fix.
4. Place slide on staining rack, smear side up.
5. Pour crystal violet solution all over the slide; let stand 1 minute (see Figure 41-20A).
6. Tilt slide to drain excess and rinse with water (see Figure 41-20B).
7. Pour Gram's iodine stain all over the slide; let stand 1 minute (see Figure 41-20C).
8. Tilt slide to drain excess and rinse with water.

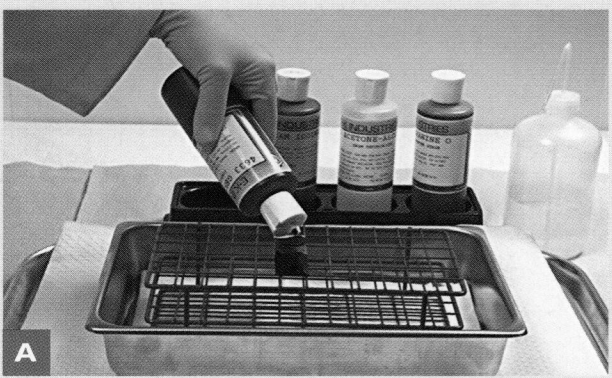

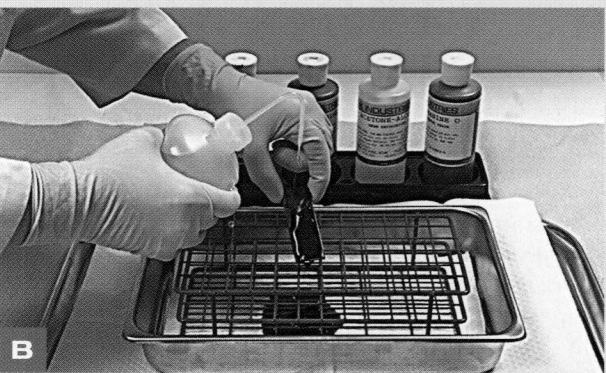

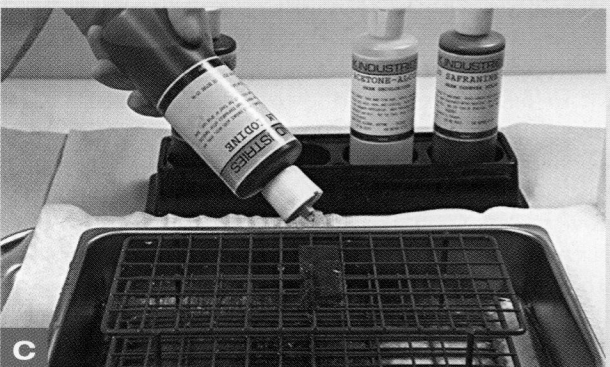

FIGURE 41-20 Gram stain procedure. (A) crystal violet; (B) rinse; (C) iodine.

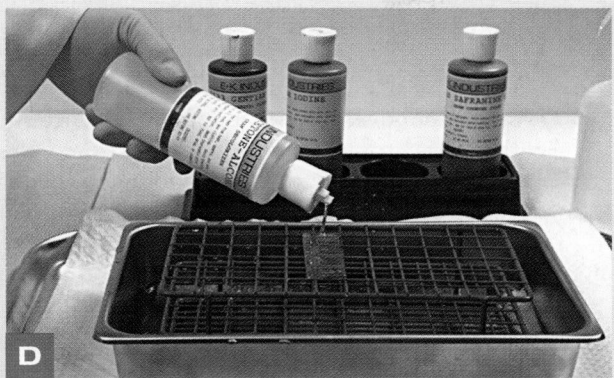

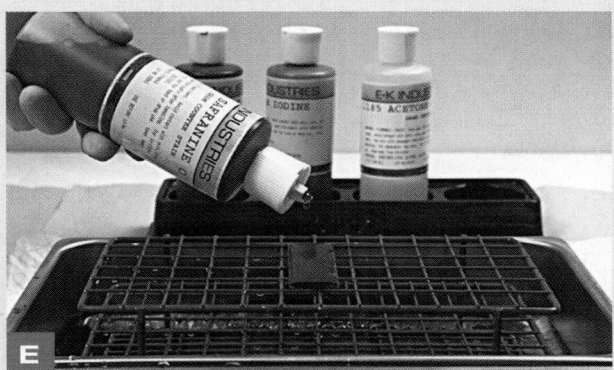

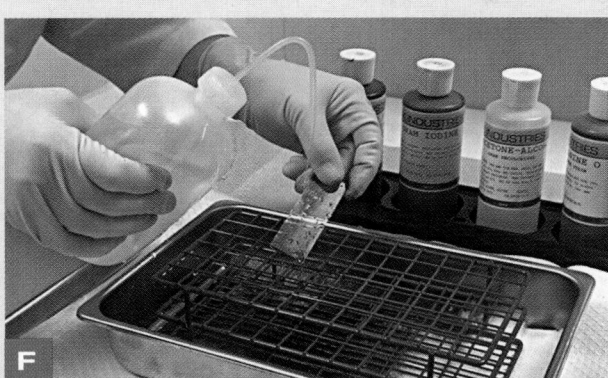

FIGURE 41-20 (*continued*) (D) acetone; (E) safranin; (F) rinse (finish).

9. Gently pour decolorizer with alcohol-acetone all over slide for 15 seconds or until color blue stops running (see Figure 41-20D).
10. Rinse with water.
11. Pour safranin stain all over slide, let stand 30 seconds (see Figure 41-20E).
12. Tilt slide to drain excess and rinse with water. Wipe back of slide (see Figure 41-20F).
13. Stand slide on end on paper towel or in slide drying rack, air dry.

Note: Examination of Gram-stained slide is beyond the scope of practice of the medical assistant. It should be performed by a physician or laboratory specialist.

14. Examine under microscope, using oil immersion lens and oil.

Charting Example

11/16/XX	Gram stain of spec. from abscess of RT thigh prepared for physician to examine.
	M. King, CMA

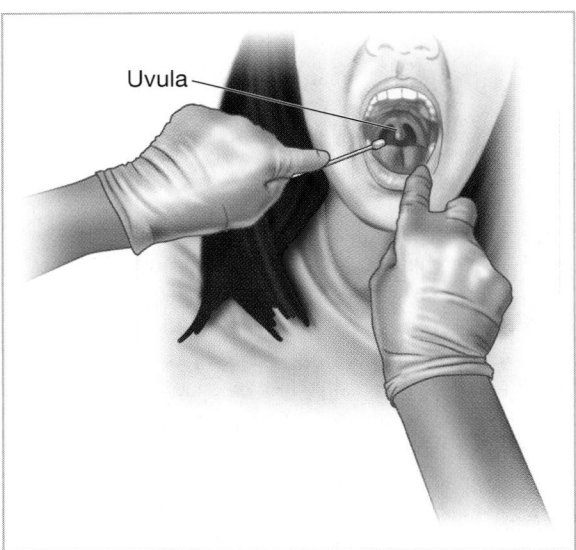

Uvula

FIGURE 41-21 When swabbing for a throat culture, avoid the uvula. Swab on each side in tonsil area.

of swabbing is uncomfortable and should be done quickly, avoiding the uvula because touching it will cause gagging (Figure 41-21). If the patient is a child, the procedure should be done with the child lying down, asking the assistance of the parent or other medical assistant. If the child refuses to open his or her mouth, squeeze the nostrils shut and he or she will open the mouth. Once the swab is removed, place it at once in its plastic covering taking care not to touch the outside of the covering.

If the culture is to be done in house, then it is streaked as mentioned previously. A bacitracin antibiotic disk will be placed on the culture plate in the area with the heaviest inoculation. A zone of no growth around the disk is presumptive evidence that the pathogen is group A beta-hemolytic strep. Other strep organisms are not sensitive to bacitracin. Bacitracin is not used to treat strep throat, only as a differentiating antibiotic. Broad-spectrum antibiotics such as penicillin, ampicillin, and erythromycin are used to treat strep. Procedure 41-4 provides the steps to correctly obtain and culture a throat specimen. If strep is suspected, an antigen antibody test for strep may be ordered. These types of tests will be discussed later in the chapter.

Nasal swabs are sometimes requested and care should be taken to label the swabs "right" and "left" to identify from which nostril the specimen was taken.

41-4 PROCEDURE

Obtaining a Throat Culture

OBJECTIVE: Collect a throat or nasopharyngeal culture without contaminating the specimen.

Equipment and Supplies
Culturette system; laboratory requisition; tongue depressor; gloves; hazardous waste container
Note: Follow Standard Precautions and safety guidelines when working with body fluid samples. Use care to avoid splashing or spilling body fluids. Wipe up all spills using guidelines established by OSHA.

Method
1. Perform hand hygiene.
2. Assemble equipment and Culturette system.
3. Identify patient and explain procedure.
4. Apply gloves.
5. Position patient facing a light source and have the patient open his or her mouth as wide as possible. The gag reflex may be diminished if the patient says "Aaaah."
6. Remove sterile swab from Culturette.
7. Depress tongue, insert swab, and roll it firmly across back of patient's throat or nasopharyn-

geal area where infected. Be careful not to contaminate the swab on the teeth, lips, tongue, or inside of cheeks. Avoid uvula to prevent gagging.
8. Insert swab into plastic vial. Crush the internal vial of transport medium making sure swab is saturated.
9. Place in labeled mailing or transporting envelope and staple shut if necessary. Or if being evaluated in the office laboratory immediately inoculate the culture plate, and apply a bacitracin disk according to office procedure.
10. Wash hands.

Charting Example

2/14/XX	9:00 A.M.

Throat culture obtained. Specimen labeled and sent to outside lab. (Specify name of the lab.)

M. King, CMA

Obtaining a Sputum Specimen for Culture

OBJECTIVE: Collect a sputum specimen without contaminating the specimen.

Equipment and Supplies

sterile labeled sputum container with lid; lab requisition form; gloves; hazardous waste container

Note: Follow Standard Precautions and safety guidelines when working with body fluid samples. Use care to avoid splashing or spilling body fluids. Wipe up all spills using guidelines established by OSHA.

Method

1. Perform hand hygiene and apply gloves.
2. Identify patient.
3. Explain the procedure and give written instructions that the patient can take home, if necessary.
   a. Cough deeply and expel fluid into center of container. A specimen obtained first thing in the morning would be best.
   b. Make sure no other fluids find their way into the cup, such as tears, nasal mucus, or saliva.
   c. Fit lid securely and write the time and date the specimen was obtained.
   d. Bring specimen into doctor's office as soon as possible or place in a refrigerator for no longer than 2 hours.
4. Label envelope with information, staple shut, and transport immediately.
5. Wash hands.

Charting Example

2/14/XX	10:00 A.M.

Sputum specimen collected. Labeled and sent to outside lab. (Specify name of the lab.)

M. King, CMA

Smaller sterile swabs with thinner more flexible shafts are generally used for nasal specimens.

Sputum

To obtain a sputum specimen, which is the mucous substance expelled by coughing or clearing the bronchi, the patient must be carefully instructed to cough deeply, "spitting" the coughed up material into a sterile container. Explain to the patient that this should not be saliva from the mouth. Often it is possible to obtain a "good" sputum specimen if the patient is reminded to try on rising in the morning. The purpose for obtaining a sputum specimen is to isolate and diagnose diseases such as streptococcal pneumonia, influenza, and tuberculosis. Refer to Procedure 41-5 for directions on obtaining a sputum specimen.

Urine

Urinalysis is discussed in Chapter 42; however, obtaining a urine culture is an important procedure in this chapter on microbiology. A urine specimen for culture must be either a catheterized specimen or a clean-catch midstream sample (CCMS). Both methods provide sterile samples. Any other type of urine specimen (one for routine analysis for example) would be contaminated by organisms in the container or on the hands or genitals of the patient. See Procedure 42-1 in the next chapter for collection of a clean-catch midstream urine specimen from both male and female patients.

Procedure 41-6 provides the steps for performing a urine culture from a CCMS sample of urine. In doctor's offices and smaller facilities, self-contained culture units are purchased and used. Many varieties are available and each provides specific procedures and charts to facilitate reading the results. Often urine cultures require a means to provide a quantitative result of the number of microorganisms in the sample. By using selective media and an inoculating loop that is specifically calibrated to deliver 1 µL of urine, quantitative results are possible. Each colony growing on the media represents 1,000 colony-forming organisms per milliliter of urine. One hundred colonies represent 100,000 colony-forming units and indicate the presence of a UTI.

Stool

Stool or feces, waste product from bowel, may be tested for bacterial, parasitic, or protozoal infections, for the presence of occult blood, and for excessive amounts of fat (steatorrhea). The collection of stool specimens

Performing a Urine Culture

OBJECTIVE: Inoculate a urine plate to aid in the identification of a UTI.

Equipment and Supplies

lab requisition form; urine specimen (CCMS) collected in a sterile container; incinerator (electric or Bunsen burner); 1.0 μl loop; agar plates (usually blood, MacConkey, and nutrient); gloves; hazardous waste container

Note: Follow Standard Precautions and safety guidelines when working with body fluid samples. Use care to avoid splashing or spilling body fluids. Wipe up all spills using guidelines established by OSHA.

Method

1. Perform hand hygiene
2. Apply gloves and face protection.
3. With lid on, swirl urine sample to mix.

4. Sterilize loop, remove lid, replacing between inoculating plates.
5. Inoculate each media plate in pattern to allow for isolated colonies (see Figure 41-17).
6. Label bottom of plates.
7. Place media in incubator with agar side up for 24 hours.
8. Results will be interpreted by a physician or laboratory specialist.
9. Document appropriately.
10. Clean area, remove and dispose of gloves, and wash hands.

Charting Example

| 2/14/XX | Urine culture performed. |
| | M. King, CMA |

---

varies with the type of test ordered. Discussing stool sample collection is often embarrassing to both patient and medical assistant; however, correct collection is critical to an accurate result. Fecal specimens must be free of urine or water from the toilet and toilet tissue.

Cultural Considerations

You may have patients who are from a culture where the discussion of bodily functions is taboo. If so, maintaining a professional attitude cannot be stressed enough. The patient may be embarrassed, for example, when discussing stool specimens. Explain the procedure, while attempting to stay away from using any words that would be offensive. If brochures and diagrams are available, these could be helpful. Allow the patient to read these. Allow time for questions from the patient, and answer them truthfully and professionally.

Stool Culture

To detect bacteria or viruses a small amount of feces is needed. The collection containers must be sterile, and aseptic technique must be used in the collection process. Once collected, the stool must be sent immediately to the testing facility. Sterile collection devices are available. Sheets of special paper, coverings for the toilet, and bedpans can be used to collect specimens. Sterile tongue depressors or applicator sticks can be used to transfer a small of amount of stool to a sterile container for transportation to the laboratory or office. In the office a sterile bedpan may be used or sterile pan placed over the bowl of the toilet. Procedure 41-7 provides the steps to collect a stool sample for culture and sensitivity.

Occult Blood

A stool specimen is required to test for occult or hidden blood that may indicate bleeding in the gastrointestinal tract. Often the patient is given the test units to take home and collect the specimen. Directions are provided on each test unit, however, you should review the instructions each time they are given to a patient. Patients are instructed to write their name, date, and doctor's name on label of the unit. Using one of the wooden spatulas provided, they are to collect a small

PROCEDURE

Obtaining Stool Specimen for Culture and Sensitivity

OBJECTIVE: Instruct a patient how to collect a stool sample for culture and sensitivity in a sterile container using correct infection control procedures.

Equipment and Supplies

sterile stool collection container; bedpan or container for collection of stool; tongue depressors; sterile applicator sticks; transportation/mailing container; labels; laboratory request form; gloves; hazardous waste container

Note: Follow Standard Precautions and safety guidelines when working with body fluid samples. Use care to avoid splashing or spilling body fluids. Wipe up all spills using guidelines established by OSHA.

Method

1. Perform hand hygiene.
2. Assemble equipment.
3. Identify patient and explain the procedure, giving written instructions as well. Do not overuse medical terminology, which might cause the patient to misunderstand your instructions.
4. Instruct patient to defecate in container or bedpan. If patient is collecting specimen at home, a sterile container and written instructions with diagrams should be given.
5. Using sterile tongue depressor or applicator stick, take small amount of stool from different parts of the specimen and place in container, making sure no other contaminants are included (toilet paper, urine, etc.).
6. If patient provides the stool specimen in a bedpan or other container, using gloves, proceed as above.
7. Fill out lab request form and wrap around container securing with a rubber band.
8. Place in proper mailing container.
9. Deliver or mail to outside lab facility.

Charting Example

2/14/XX	9:00 A.M.

Stool specimen obtained C&S. Specimen labeled and sent to outside lab. (Specify the name of the lab.)

M. King, CMA

---

amount of stool and place it in one of the circles on the back of the booklet, obtain another sample from a different area of the stool, and place this sample on the other circle. Patients should close the unit and take it or mail it to the doctor's office or the laboratory as requested. Figure 41-22 shows Hemoccult test kits.

For more accurate results patients should be instructed to refrain from vitamin C and red meat for 3 days prior to testing because they may cause false positives. It is important to check the expiration date of any test kit before giving it to the patient.

Stool for Ova and Parasites

The presence of microbial organisms, such as ova and parasites (O&P), may be determined by testing feces or stool. The presence of ova or eggs or other forms of a parasite indicate parasitic infestation. Identification of the parasite aids in selecting the correct treatment.

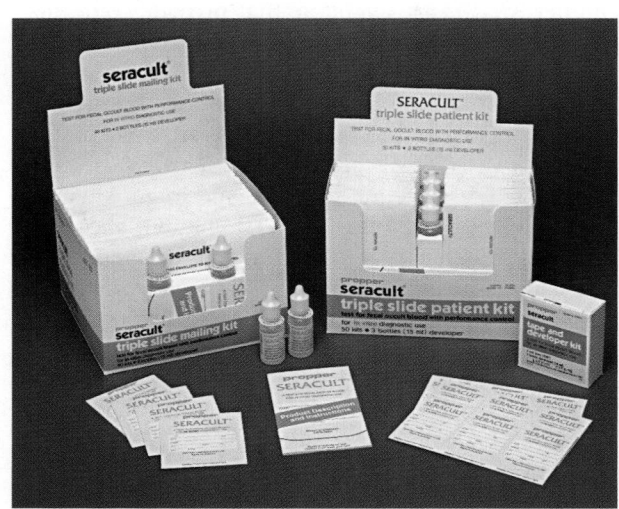

FIGURE 41-22 Examples of Hemoccult test kits.

Obtaining Stool Specimen for Ova and Parasites

OBJECTIVE: Instruct a patient to collect a stool sample for ova and parasites using the correct infection control and procedure. Both fresh and preserved specimens are required.

Equipment and Supplies

Stool collection kit with container for fresh specimen and vials for preserved specimen (formalin and polyvinyl alcohol; bedpan or container for collection of stool; tongue depressors; sterile applicator sticks; mailing container; labels; laboratory request form; gloves; hazardous waste container

Note: Follow Standard Precautions and safety guidelines when working with body fluid samples. Use care to avoid splashing or spilling body fluids. Wipe up all spills using guidelines established by OSHA.

Method

1. Perform hand hygiene.
2. Assemble equipment.
3. Identify patient and explain the procedure, giving written instructions as well. Do not overuse medical terminology, which might cause the patient to misunderstand your instructions.
4. Instruct patient to defecate in container or bedpan, if available. If patient is collecting specimen at home, written instructions including diagrams should be given.
5. When patient returns with the specimen, apply your gloves.
6. Using tongue depressor, take small amount of stool from different parts of the specimen and place in each vial using a new depressor or sterile wooden applicator stick for each vial making sure no other contaminants are included (toilet paper, urine, etc.).
7. Fill out lab request form and wrap around container securing with a rubber band.
8. Place in proper mailing container.
9. Deliver or mail to outside lab facility.

Charting Example

2/14/XX	9:00 A.M.

Stool specimen obtained for O&P. Specimen labeled and sent to outside lab. (Specify the name of the lab.)

M. King, CMA

Commercial kits are available that provide containers for fresh stool specimen and two additional vials for preserved specimens, one containing formalin and the other containing polyvinyl alcohol. The patient should be instructed to mix portions of stool in each vial and seal. If O&P are suspected, three specimen collections will be requested. The specimen is usually obtained in the early morning. The patient should be instructed to defecate into a stool specimen container or by using a bedpan, if available, placed over the toilet. The stool specimen samples should be taken from several different parts of the stool since ova and parasites may be in one portion of the stool and not another. Refer to Procedure 41-8 for collecting a stool specimen for O&P.

One examination for ova and parasites may be performed in the office. The pinworm (*Enterobius vermicularis*) is a common parasite that inhabits the lower gastrointestinal tract with mature pinworms migrating out of the anus at night, causing intense itching. Transmission is by the fecal-oral route or by ingesting eggs with hand-to-mouth transmission. Adult worms male in the colon and the female migrates out of the anus at night to lay eggs. The eggs stick to the anal area, pajamas, and other items of clothing. Collection of a specimen should be done first thing in the morning before a bowel movement or bathing in order to detect ova or worms. Procedure 41-9 provides the steps needed to either perform the collection of a pinworm specimen in the office or to instruct a parent to do so at home. Medications are available for treatment, and reexamination is recommended after a cycle of medication has been completed. In addition, parents and other infected individuals must be told to observe strict personal hygiene including laundering of all bedding and underclothing on a regular basis. It may be necessary

Obtain Stool Specimen for Examination for Pinworms

OBJECTIVE: Collect a rectal swab using cellulose tape for pinworm examination.

Equipment and supplies

glass slide; tongue depressor; gauze or colon balls; microscope; toluene; lab requisition form;

Method

1. Gather equipment and supplies
2. Prepare slide by attaching the sticky side of a piece of cellulose tape to the slide surface and wrapping tape around one end. Leave room to attach small square of paper for labeling at the other end. Do not use Magic tape.
3. Perform hand hygiene and apply gloves.
4. Prepare patient on examination table or parent's lap with anal area exposed.
5. Peel tape off slide by labeled end and wrap around tongue depressor or swab with sticky side out.
6. Press tape to area around anus on both sides.
7. Replace tape on slide sticky side down and smooth with gauze.
8. Label slide with patient's name and date. Fill out lab requisition form.
9. Physician will examine the slide for presence of pinworms or ova. (A drop of toluene may be added before the examination to make ova more visible.)
10. Dispose of all waste, wash hands, and document appropriately.

Charting Example

11/16/XX	Slide prepared for pinworm examination by physician.
	M. King, CMA

to examine other family members and playmates for signs of infection if reinfestation occurs.

Wound Specimens

Sterile swabs are used to obtain a specimen from a wound, abscess, or incision to test for pathogenic microorganisms. The procedure is similar to obtaining a throat culture. Several specimens may be necessary from different locations. Be certain to label each appropriately as to the source. Refer to Procedure 35-1 on obtaining a wound culture and Procedure 38-11 on changing a sterile dressing for the steps needed to also obtain a wound specimen.

Other Types of Specimens

Cerebrospinal fluid (CSF) is always treated as a stat procedure. The procedure to collect CSF is uncomfortable for the patient, and the specimen must be handled with care. Usually three tubes are collected under sterile conditions and sent for testing. The culture and sensitivity test should be performed before chemical and other tests using the second of the three tubes. Tubes one and three are more likely to be contaminated because of the entry and removal processes of collection.

Blood cultures to test for septicemia or bacteremia will be covered in Chapter 43. Commercially available containers containing a broth media are widely used. Blood and CSF under normal conditions are free of any type of microorganisms.

Serology Testing

Serology is the study of the antigen and antibody reactions of the body's immune system. The body's ability to recognize a foreign substance (antigen) and produce an antibody against it is called the immune response. Antibodies are specific for a particular antigen. For example, polio antibody is specific for polio only.

This antigen–antibody reaction is a frequently used testing tool and is used to test for pregnancy, rheumatoid arthritis, mononucleosis, and strep among others. This testing is serologic since it studies or tests the serum component of the blood. These testing kits contain all of the equipment and supplies necessary and assist the medical assistant in ensuring that reagents are fresh and quality control is maintained. The kits standardize testing, thus ensuring accuracy, precision, and quality control. It is absolutely essential to follow exactly the manufacturer's directions.

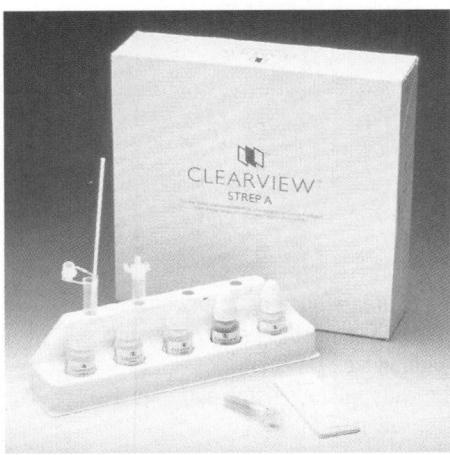

FIGURE 41-23 Strep test kit.

Strep Test

The Group A Strep Screen is a test that is done frequently in POLs. It is especially efficient in the pediatric office because it is self-contained and can be done while the patient waits. This screen is an antigen detection test for group A beta-hemolytic streptococci and follows the general procedure for antigen–antibody agglutination tests, which produce a clumping of cells. One such test, called Q-test STREP, is a commercially prepared diagnostic testing kit that includes detailed instructions and contains reagents as well as controls and quality control suggestions. Figure 41-23 shows an example of a strep test kit.

A variety of other serological test kits are available for infectious mononucleosis, rheumatoid arthritis, and HIV to name a few. The specialty of the physician will determine which tests will be used.

SUMMARY

Microbiology, as practiced by the medical assistant in POLs, is one of the most important aids to diagnosis for the physician. By correct processing and testing of patient specimens, early diagnosis and treatment of disease can take place. The medical assistant plays an important role in the process.

Chapter Review

COMPETENCY REVIEW

1. Define and spell the terms to learn for this chapter.
2. What does it mean to say that a microorganism is nonpathogenic?
3. In what ways are bacteria categorized?
4. If a bacterium is aerobic, what does it require in order to survive?
5. Tinea pedis is an example of which type of microorganism?
6. What is the incubation period for a culture?
7. A specimen is sent to an outside laboratory for culture and sensitivity testing. Your office receives a report that the bacterium is resistant to penicillin. What does that mean?

PREPARING FOR THE CERTIFICATION EXAM

1. Material for a throat culture can include the following areas:
   A. throat
   B. back of tongue
   C. mucus from inside of cheeks
   D. teeth
   E. uvula

2. Material for a sputum specimen is collected from what area?
   A. mouth
   B. throat
   C. lungs and bronchial tubes
   D. pharynx
   E. saliva glands

3. Which of the following would most likely be a source of *Vibrio* bacilli?
   A. whole grains
   B. fruits
   C. vegetables
   D. raw shellfish
   E. well-cooked meat

4. Which of the following is caused by a fungus?
   A. candidiasis
   B. malaria
   C. herpes zoster
   D. gastroenteritis
   E. meningitis

continued on next page

5. When collecting a specimen, which of the following is/are necessary?
   A. selection of proper container for specimen
   B. labeling the specimen
   C. completion of requisition form
   D. avoiding specimen contamination
   E. all of the above

6. When collecting a sputum specimen, which of the following is incorrect?
   A. Explain the procedure or give written instructions if the patient is to obtain the specimen at home.
   B. A specimen obtained first thing in the morning is best.
   C. Patient should "clear the throat" and expectorate this material into the specimen cup prior to coughing deeply.
   D. Patient should cough deeply to obtain the specimen.
   E. Specimen is examined for upper respiratory infection agents.

7. Which is not necessary to perform a Gram stain?
   A. safranin
   B. decolorizer
   C. crystal violet
   D. blood agar
   E. iodine

8. *Staphylococcus aureus* is best described by which of the following?
   A. gram-negative bacilli in chains
   B. gram-positive cocci in chains
   C. gram-positive cocci in grape-like clusters
   D. gram-negative diplococci
   E. acid-fast bacilli

9. The causative agent of scarlet fever and strep throat is:
   A. *Streptococcus pneumoniae*
   B. *Streptococcus pyogenes*
   C. *Neisseria meningitidis*
   D. *Staphylococcus enteritidis*
   E. *Chlamydia trachomatis*

10. The study of the serum portion of blood is known as:
    A. cytology
    B. serology
    C. mycology
    D. parasitology
    E. hematology

CRITICAL THINKING

1. What equipment will you need prior to removing the dressing?
2. The physician orders a culture. How do your obtain the specimen using the Culturette system?
3. What technique would be used for a streak culture?

ON THE JOB

You have been asked to speak to a high school class about the clinical aspects of your job. In particular, they are interested in microbiology because they have just completed a unit on microorganisms in class.

1. What would you tell them about your functions as a medical assistant?
2. What would you say to those who asked if you looked through the microscope and reported your findings?
3. One student asks what type of training one would need to work solely in microbiology in a laboratory setting. How would you answer her?

INTERNET ACTIVITY

Research a type of bacteria, such as the staphylococci that can cause gastroenteritis.

 MediaLink More on microbiology, including interactive resources, can be found on the student CD-ROM accompanying this textbook.

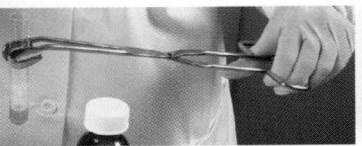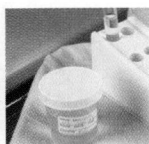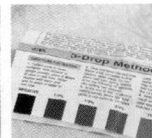

Medical Assistant Role Delineation Chart

HIGHLIGHT indicates material covered in this chapter.

ADMINISTRATIVE

Administrative Procedures

- Perform basic administrative medical assisting functions
- Schedule, coordinate and monitor appointments
- Schedule inpatient/outpatient admissions and procedures
- Understand and apply third-party guidelines
- Obtain reimbursement through accurate claims submission
- Monitor third-party reimbursement
- Understand and adhere to managed care policies and procedures
- *Negotiate managed care contracts*

Practice Finances

- Perform procedural and diagnostic coding
- Apply bookkeeping principles

- Manage accounts receivable
- *Manage accounts payable*
- *Process payroll*
- *Document and maintain accounting and banking records*
- *Develop and maintain fee schedules*
- *Manage renewals of business and professional insurance policies*
- *Manage personnel benefits and maintain records*
- *Perform marketing, financial, and strategic planning*

CLINICAL

Fundamental Principles

- Apply principles of aseptic technique and infection control
- Comply with quality assurance practices
- Screen and follow up patient test results

Diagnostic Orders

- Collect and process specimens
- Perform diagnostic tests

Patient Care

- Adhere to established patient screening procedures
- Obtain patient history and vital signs
- Prepare and maintain examination and treatment areas
- Prepare patient for examinations, procedures and treatments

- Assist with examinations, procedures and treatments
- Prepare and administer medications and immunizations
- Maintain medication and immunization records
- Recognize and respond to emergencies
- Coordinate patient care information with other health care providers
- Initiate IV and administer IV medications with appropriate training and as permitted by state law

GENERAL

Professionalism

- Display a professional manner and image
- Demonstrate initiative and responsibility
- Work as a member of the health care team
- Prioritize and perform multiple tasks
- Adapt to change
- Promote the CMA credential
- Enhance skills through continuing education
- Treat all patients with compassion and empathy
- Promote the practice through positive public relations

Communication Skills

- Recognize and respect cultural diversity
- Adapt communications to individual's ability to understand
- Use professional telephone technique

- Recognize and respond effectively to verbal, nonverbal, and written communications
- Use medical terminology appropriately
- Utilize electronic technology to receive, organize, prioritize and transmit information
- Serve as liaison

Legal Concepts

- Perform within legal and ethical boundaries
- Prepare and maintain medical records
- Document accurately
- Follow employer's established policies dealing with the health care contract
- Implement and maintain federal and state health care legislation and regulations
- Comply with established risk management and safety procedures
- Recognize professional credentialing criteria
- *Develop and maintain personnel, policy and procedure manuals*

Instruction

- Instruct individuals according to their needs
- Explain office policies and procedures
- Teach methods of health promotion and disease prevention
- Locate community resources and disseminate information
- *Develop educational materials*
- *Conduct continuing education activities*

Operational Functions

- Perform inventory of supplies and equipment
- Perform routine maintenance of administrative and clinical equipment
- Apply computer techniques to support office operations
- *Perform personnel management functions*
- *Negotiate leases and prices for equipment and supply contracts*

- *Denotes advanced skills.*

SOURCE: Reprinted by permission of the American Association of Medical Assistants from the AAMA Role Delineation Study: Occupational Analysis of the Medical Assisting Profession.

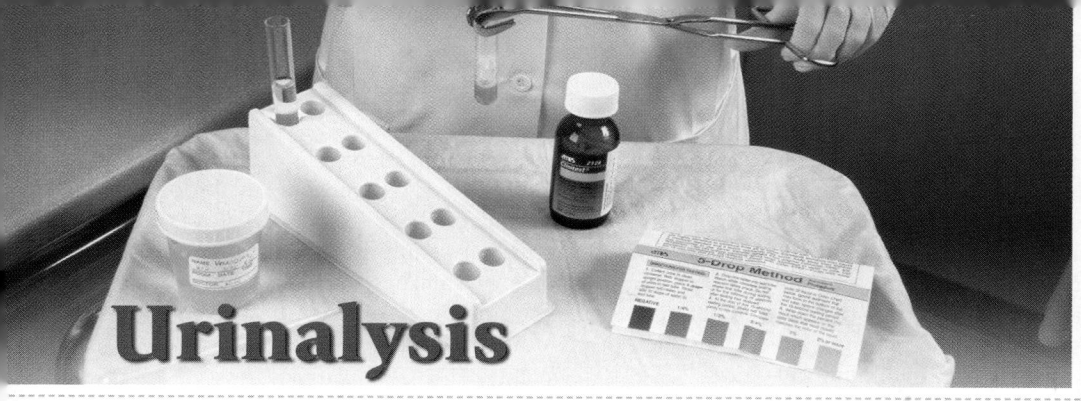

Urinalysis

chapter 42

Learning Objectives

After completing this chapter, you should be able to:

- Define and spell the terms to learn for this chapter.
- List nine types of urine specimens that can be collected.
- Understand the purpose of routine urinalysis.
- Describe the steps for collecting a clean-catch urine specimen.
- Describe the physical components of urine.
- Describe the chemical components of urine.
- State normal values for physical and chemical examination of urine.
- Describe some of the cellular and noncellular elements that might be found during a urine microscopic examination.
- Demonstrate the procedure for measuring specific gravity using a urinometer.
- Demonstrate the procedure for preparing urine for microscopic examination.
- Demonstrate the procedure for glucose testing using tablets.
- Demonstrate a method for pregnancy testing.
- Discuss quality control as it applies to urinalysis.

OUTLINE

Asepsis	880
Collecting the Specimen	880
Routine Urinalysis	884
Urine Pregnancy Testing	894
Quality Control	896

Terms to Learn

amorphous	ketones	renal threshold
anuria	micturate	sediment
bacturia	occult	specific gravity
fetid	oliguria	supernatant
glomerulonephritis	parasites	turbid
glycosuria	polyuria	urinalysis
hematuria	proteinuria	void

Case Study

EDNA HARVEY DROPS OFF A URINE SPECIMEN for routine urinalysis per Dr. Freedman's order. The specimen is properly labeled and you accept the specimen and take it to the laboratory area of the office for testing. On testing the specimen a few minutes later, you discover that the urine smells of ammonia and the chemical strip tests are positive for protein, nitrites, and bacteria. Dr. Friedman noted many bacteria when he performed the microscopic examination.

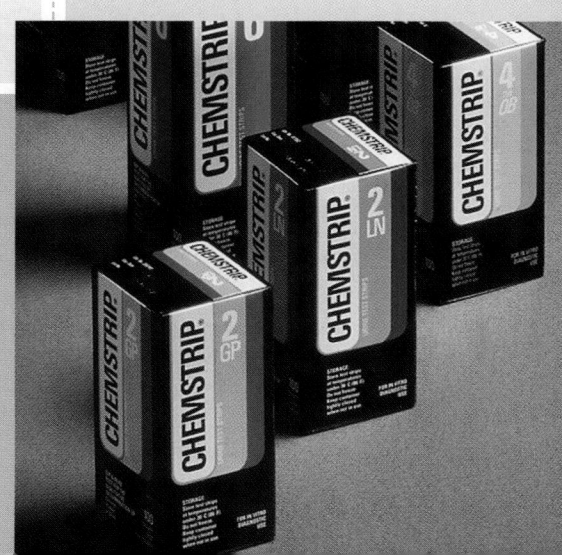

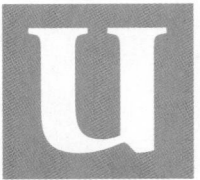 rinalysis refers to the testing of urine for the presence of infection or disease. A routine urine analysis consists of examining the physical, chemical, and microscopic characteristics of urine, and it is one of the most common laboratory tests performed. Urine is readily available, easily collected, and often provides the first clues to illness. Urinalysis provides valuable information about many functions in the body, including kidney functions. The patient needs to be clearly instructed about methods of collection in easily understood terms. Patients do not necessarily comprehend medical terms, therefore words meaning to urinate such as void and micturate may not be understood. Instead words such as "passing water" may need to be used especially with elderly patients.

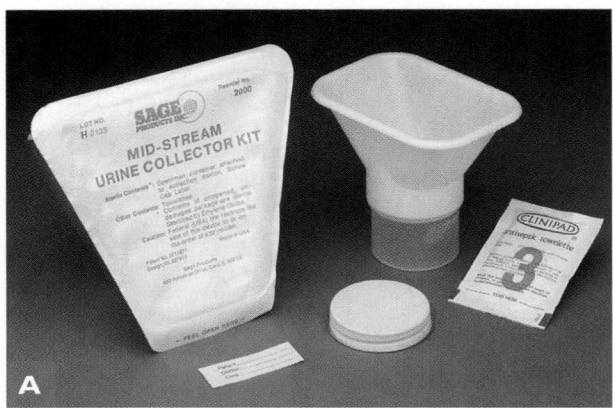

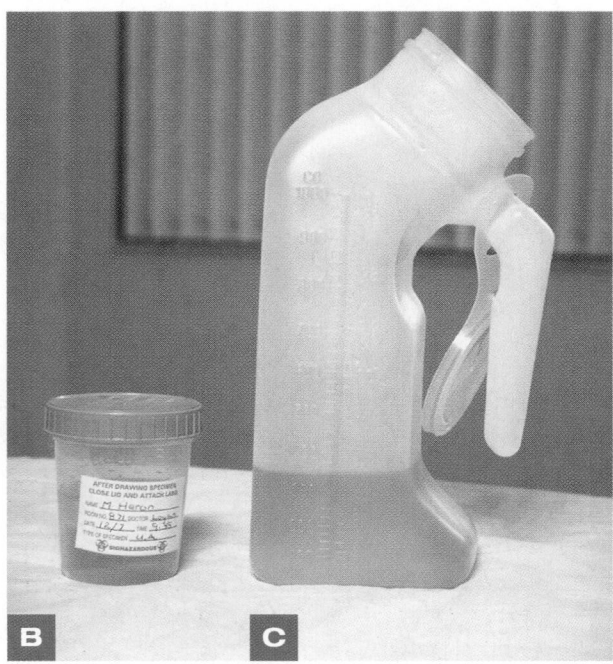

FIGURE 42-1   Various urine specimen containers: (A) midstream clean-catch container; (B) urine collection cup; (C) 24-hour urine container.

Asepsis

Asepsis is very important in urinalysis. Standard Precautions must be followed whenever any blood or body fluids are handled. Wear nonsterile gloves and avoid contaminating any equipment with the urine. If there is any chance of splashes occurring, then a lab coat and goggles should be worn. See Chapter 32 for a thorough discussion of asepsis.

Collecting the Specimen

Urine samples provide valuable indicators of the overall health of the patient. Although urine is readily available in most instances, medical assistants must do their utmost to maintain the integrity of the specimen. A test result is only as reliable and valid as the specimen collected. Anyone who handles specimens must understand how to store and maintain each type of urine specimen collected. In most cases urine samples are refrigerated if testing will not take place within 2 hours. Always consult the office or laboratory manual for further information about specific storage of urine and addition of preservatives for specific tests.

Generally, at least 10 mL of urine is needed for testing depending on the test ordered. Figure 42-1 shows different types of urine collection containers. There are nine types of urine specimens that might be collected:

- Routine (random) sample
- Morning specimen—first voided
- Timed specimen
- Twenty-four-hour specimen
- Two-hour postprandial
- Catheterized specimen (sterile specimen)
- Clean-catch midstream (sterile specimen)
- Pediatric specimen
- Suprapubic specimen

See Patient Education for more information about collecting specimens.

Routine (Random) Sample

A random sample of urine is the most commonly collected type of urine specimen. This specimen is collected in a nonsterile container, and can be collected in the office during the patient's visit or may be brought in from home. It is preferable to provide the patient with urine specimen containers for any sample to be brought in from home to ensure that containers are clean. Random samples are used only for routine screenings, since the composition of urine changes during the day. See Guidelines 42-1 for guidelines for collecting routine urine specimens.

The medical assistant may be the only individual to instruct the patient in the correct method of collecting a urine specimen. It is important to be sure that the patient understands the correct method of collection. Be sure to use terminology that can be easily comprehended by the patient. If the patient is doing an "at home" test, provide written instructions that clearly describe each step of the procedure. Another helpful idea is to place instructions in the lab collection restroom.

When collecting clean-catch specimens, be sure that the patient understands how to clean the labia in the female and the foreskin in the male. Diagrams are helpful both in the laboratory restroom and in the written directions. Patients need a clear explanation of what "midstream" means. When explaining the procedure for samples collected at home, it is important that the patient understands the need for refrigeration for any specimens not brought immediately into the laboratory.

It is especially important to be very professional while giving the instructions. Many patients are sensitive about the subject of elimination, so the medical assistant needs to be sure that the patient's desire for modesty is honored. Be sure to give all instructions for the collection of urine specimens in private, out of hearing distance of other individuals.

Morning Specimen—First Voided

A morning specimen (first void) is the most concentrated urine and is collected immediately on arising in the morning. This specimen is used for tests such as pregnancy testing, urine cultures, and microscopic examinations. The patient is given a specimen container and collects the urine when he or she first arises in the morning. The specimen should be brought to the office for testing within 30 minutes to an hour. If the examination cannot be performed within 2 hours, the sample should be refrigerated, or a preservative added to the container depending on the test procedure to be completed.

Timed Specimen

Timed specimens are necessary for quantitative analysis of substances such as protein, creatinine, or glucose in urine. Urine specimens must be obtained at specific time intervals. The most common timed specimens are 24-hour and 2-hour postprandial specimens.

24-Hour Specimen

It is important to clearly explain to the patient what needs to be done to collect an acceptable 24-hour specimen. Changes occur in urine specimens over time, thus instructions should be given in writing. It should be made clear that when the collection is completed, the specimen should be delivered at once to the laboratory or physician's office. Refrigeration of a specimen slows growth of bacteria and specimen deterioration, but does not stop it. Often preservatives are added by the facility before giving the container to the patient. Some of these may be caustic and containers must be labeled appropriately to prevent injury to the patient and anyone else handling the specimen.

(For more information about labeling specimens, see Legal and Ethical Issues.)

To collect a 24-hour specimen, the patient is given a large, clean, and properly labeled container to take home. Collection begins after he or she voids the first time in the morning. After flushing the first voided urine in the commode, every drop of urine is collected in the container for the next 24 hours, up to and including the first voided specimen on the second morning.

The 24-hour urine test is used to determine the glomerular filtration rate of the kidneys (creatinine clearance), to check specific hormone levels, and to check for other metabolic abnormalities. See Guidelines 42-2 for collecting a 24-hour specimen.

42-1 GUIDELINES

Collecting a Routine Urine Specimen

1. Provide the patient with a nonsterile container that is labeled with the patient's name and date.
2. Ask the patient to use the bathroom and void into a container. Tell the patient to only fill the container two-thirds of the way to avoid spillage.
3. Explain where you want the patient to leave the container of urine. Place a paper towel in the designated area to avoid contamination of the work area.
4. Wearing nonsterile gloves, take the specimen and test the urine immediately if possible.
5. If you are not able to test within 30 minutes, place it in the refrigerator. Note, however, that urine should be at room temperature before testing.

1. Explain why the patient is being asked to save all urine for 24 hours.
2. Give patient large container (one-gallon size) labeled with patient's name, date, time to begin collection, and time to end collection. Note times on laboratory slip also.
3. Include preservative if required by laboratory manual. Label container appropriately if preservative is caustic.
4. Instruct patient to begin at 7 A.M. and void in toilet and flush so bladder is empty at the beginning of the test.
5. Instruct the patient to save every drop of urine voided during the 24-hour period including the first A.M. specimen the following morning.

6. Instruct the patient to urinate into a container with a spout and then pour the specimen into the 24-hour collection container. Caution the patient against spilling any urine.
7. Instruct patient to keep the container with specimen cool in a portable cooler for the duration of the test and during transport of the specimen to the testing facility.
8. Provide detailed instructions on where to take the completed specimen reminding the patient it must be transported immediately after test is completed.
9. Written instructions should be provided after verbal instructions are given at the office.

2-Hour Postprandial Specimen

A 2-hour postprandial urine specimen is collected 2 hours after a meal has been eaten. This test is used as screening for glucose that may be spilled into the urine once the blood levels exceed the renal threshold. Renal threshold is the concentration at which a substance excreted by the kidneys such as glucose begins to appear in the urine. For example, a normal blood glucose level is 70 to 110 mg/DL; if a patient is diabetic once the blood glucose level exceeds 160 to 180 mg/DL the kidneys begin to remove the excess glucose and it will be found in the urine.

Legal and Ethical Issues

The labeling of all specimens *must be accurate and correct. Be sure, prior to giving the patient the specimen container, that the container is labeled with the correct name and date and time of collection. If there is any question regarding the ownership of the specimen—recollect it. Getting the wrong laboratory results could be disastrous for the patient, so it is absolutely imperative that the specimen be correctly labeled.*

Patient confidentiality must always be maintained. Never leave a message stating any lab results when calling a patient's house; instead, ask the patient to call you back.

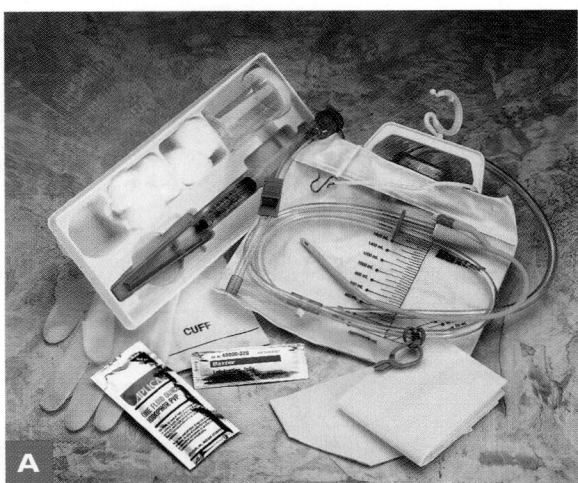

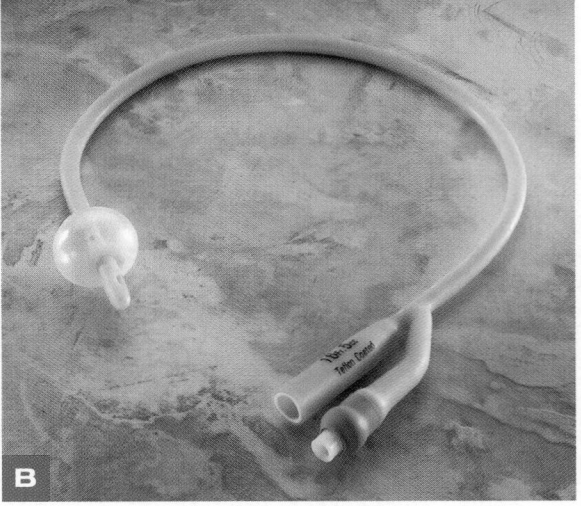

FIGURE 42-2 (A) Foley catheter tray; (B) Foley catheter.

Catheterization Specimen

Catheterization is used to collect a sterile urine specimen, which results in the ideal urine specimen—one that is free of contamination. Typically, a nurse will perform this procedure, but the medical assistant may be called to assist. During catheterization, the urethra and its surrounding tissues will be cleaned and a sterile field will be created. A small, sterile tube will be inserted through the urethra to the bladder and the urine will be collected in the sterile container. Figure 42-2 shows a Foley catheter tray and a catheter.

Catheterization may be performed to test for urine residuals after the patient believes he or she has emptied the bladder, to collect urine from a patient who is unable to void or who is incontinent, to empty the bladder completely before surgery, or to collect sterile urine for diagnostic tests.

Clean-Catch Midstream Specimen

Often it is not practical to collect a catheterized specimen. A clean-catch specimen is a satisfactory alternative. Clean-catch midstream urine samples are used to detect urinary tract infections and other dysfunctions. A clean-catch urine sample maybe cultured for microorganisms and tested to determine what antibiotics, if any, will provide effective treatment for the patient. The patient will need clear instructions to obtain a urine specimen that is free of contamination. Procedure 42-1 provides

---

42-1 PROCEDURE

Collecting a Clean-Catch Midstream Urine Specimen

OBJECTIVE: Instruct both male and female patients to correctly obtain a contaminant-free, clean-catch midstream urine specimen.

Equipment and Supplies
sterile midstream urine container; antiseptic towelettes; written patient instructions

Method
1. Perform hand hygiene.
2. Assemble equipment.
3. Identify and greet patient.
4. Explain procedure to *male* patient as follows:
   - Perform hand hygiene and expose penis. Pull foreskin back if uncircumcised and hold back until specimen has been collected.
   - Cleanse each side of the urethral opening from top to bottom using a separate antiseptic wipe, wiping in one direction only. Cleanse across the top of the urethral opening with a third antiseptic, wiping in one direction only.
   - Void a small amount of urine into toilet. Then void into the container taking care not to touch the insides of the container. Remove container.
   - Continue voiding remainder of urine into toilet.
   - Recap container immediately taking care not to contaminate the inside of the lid.
   - Deliver specimen as instructed.
5. Explain procedure to *female* patient as follows:
   - Perform hand hygiene and remove underwear.

- Expose urinary meatus by pulling apart labia and hold open with nondominant hand.
- Use dominant hand to cleanse around one side of the urinary meatus from front to back with one antiseptic wipe. Use second wipe to cleanse other side in same manner. Using a third wipe, cleanse across the opening of the meatus it self. Continue holding labia apart until procedure is complete
- Begin voiding into the toilet. Place container into position and void into container without touching the inside of the container with fingers.
- Remove container and continue voiding into toilet.
- Wipe in usual manner and cover container with lid, avoiding contaminating the inside of the lid.
- Deliver specimen as instructed.
6. Label specimen container.
7. Perform hand hygiene.
8. Document chart appropriately.

Charting Example

4/23/XX	clean-catch midstream urine specimen collected from patient at 11:00 A.M. Sent to lab for C&S.
	M. King, CMA

---

the steps to follow including instructions for male and female patients to collect sterile midstream clean-catch urine specimens.

Pediatric Specimen

Catheterization or obtaining a midstream clean-catch specimen may not be alternatives in the pediatric patient. Attaching a pediatric urine specimen bag is often the method of choice. This is covered in Chapter 37, Assisting in Life Span Specialties.

Suprapubic Specimen

A suprapubic puncture is performed using a sterile needle and syringe, so the resulting urine specimen is sterile. This procedure is usually performed by a physician and is used for cytology examinations.

Routine Urinalysis

A routine urinalysis will consist of a description of color and appearance of urine. Tests for pH and specific gravity and chemical analyses for glucose, bacteria, protein, and other chemical elements are performed. Lastly, the sediment, the solid material remaining at the bottom of a test tube after centrifugation, is examined. Table 42-1 is a listing of routine urine analysis categories.

Physical Characteristics

Urinalysis begins with an examination of the physical characteristics of urine: appearance, color, odor, quantity, and specific gravity. Evaluating the physical characteristics of urine is covered in Procedure 42-2.

Appearance

When observing a urine specimen, first notice if the specimen is clear or cloudy. If it is cloudy, more specific definitions will include terms such as *slightly cloudy, cloudy with sediment,* or turbid, meaning the urine is opaque and does not allow light to pass through. Turbidity (cloudiness) is caused by a number of factors including bacterial infection, white, red, or epithelial cells, or yeast or vaginal contaminants. Always report exactly what is seen in the sample using appropriate terms. It is also important to remember to observe the

---

TABLE 42-1   Routine Urinalysis Categories

Physical	Chemical	Microscopic
Appearance (clarity/turbidity)	Reaction (pH)	Cells
Color	Protein	Blood (RBCs, WBCs)
Specific gravity	Glucose	Epithelial cells (squamous, transitional, renal)
Odor	Blood	Casts (hyaline, cellular, granular, waxy)
Quantity (24-hour specimen only)	Ketones	Crystals (acid/alkaline)
	Bilirubin	Other: bacteria, spermatozoa, parasites, yeast
	Urobilinogen	Artifacts
	Nitrite	
	Leukocytes	

PROCEDURE

Evaluating the Physical Characteristics of Urine

OBJECTIVE: Evaluate the physical characteristics of urine and properly record the results.

Equipment and Supplies

urine specimen; centrifuge tube; laboratory slip; personal protective equipment as needed

Method

1. Perform hand hygiene and don gloves.
2. Mix urine by carefully swirling, avoiding spills.
3. Label centrifuge tube with patient's name.
4. Assess the color of the specimen and record using appropriate terms: straw, yellow, dark yellow, amber (other colors if noted).
5. Assess clarity and record using appropriate terms: clear, slightly cloudy, cloudy, turbid.
6. Clean area.
7. Remove gloves and perform hand hygiene unless proceeding with complete urinalysis.

Charting Example

4/23/XX	Rand ur. spec. collected. Clear, pale yellow.
	M. King, CMA

---

appearance of the specimen before it begins to cool, because crystals can form during the cooling process, changing the appearance of the sample.

Color

The normal color of urine is called straw—a pale yellow color. However, concentrated urine, along with other variables including medications, vitamins, and some foods, can cause urine colors to range from pale yellow to amber. Occasionally, urine will appear brown or black, indicating a serious illness. Reddish brown color may indicate bleeding, either in the urinary tract or from menstruation. Orange urine may be a result of Pyridium (a medication used to treat bladder spasms). Large quantities of the B vitamins can cause the urine to appear bright yellow. Figure 42-3 shows examples of color variations in urine.

Odor

Normally odor is not usually recorded, but any abnormal aroma should be documented. Individuals testing positive for ketones (from fat metabolism) may have a "fruity" odor to their urine. This can be indicative of uncontrolled diabetes. Fetid or foul odors might indicate infection. Ammonia odors usually result from urine breaking down after a period of time, similar to a diaper with old urine.

Quantity (Volume)

Quantity is measured when timed urine specimens are collected, but not for routine samples. In a 24-hour urine specimen, there should be between 700 and 2,000 mL, with the average being 1,500 mL (3 pints).

This does vary depending on the amount of fluid ingested by the patient. Polyuria (excessive amounts of urine) may indicate disorders such a diabetes or kidney disease. Oliguria (decreased amounts of urine production) can be indicative of dehydration, bleeding, decreased fluid intake, or kidney disease. If renal failure or an obstruction is present, then anuria (the absence of urine) may result. Individuals with these disorders may need to closely monitor their intake and output by recording all fluids ingested and all urine excreted.

Specific Gravity

Specific gravity is the weight of a substance in relation to the weight of the same amount of distilled water. The

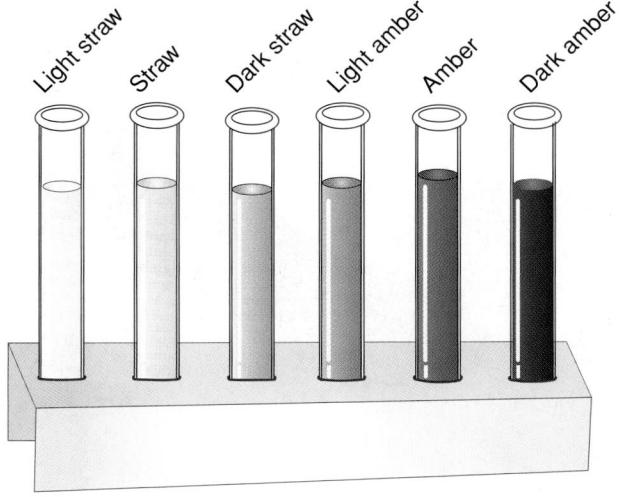

FIGURE 42-3 Color ranges of urine specimens.

concentration of urine changes during the day depending on the amount of fluid intake. Specific gravity is a rough estimate of the amount of substances dissolved in urine. This measurement indicates how well the kidneys can concentrate or dilute urine. Normal specific gravity ranges between 1.010 and 1.030. Readings outside this range may be the first indication that the kidneys are not be working properly. The presence of protein, glucose, or x-ray dyes may increase the specific gravity of urine.

Several methods are used to test urine specific gravity, including the dipstick or reagent strip method, the refractometer method, and in the past the urinometer method. This latter method is used infrequently now. Today most facilities perform the dipstick method; however, information and the procedure are offered for the refractometer method of testing in the event that it is being performed in some areas. Lifespan Considerations provides guidance on how to obtain specimens from older patients.

DIPSTICK The dipstick method is the most commonly used method of measuring specific gravity. This is done by dipping a chemically treated piece of plastic (the dipstick) into the sample of urine and then reading the chemical reaction that takes place on the dipstick Reading the test strip is performed by a chemical analyzer or by visual comparison with results on the side of the test strip bottle.

REFRACTOMETER A refractometer may be used to determine specific gravity. A refractometer uses light, a prism, and a calibrated scale to measure the concentration level of the specimen. Figure 42-4 shows a refractometer. Procedure 42-3 provides the steps necessary to accurately measure the specific gravity of urine using a refractometer.

Chemical Characteristics

Chemical analyses can provide more detailed information about the patient. The most commonly used method is the dipstick, or reagent strip, method. The dipstick has small chemically treated pads that react with specific chemicals in the urine to allow for measurement of specific elements. The color changes caused by the chemical reactions are then compared to charts on the outside of the reagent strip container with the normal and abnormal value of each provided or evaluated by chemical urine analyzers. Dipstick tests are available for pH, protein, glucose, ketones, blood, bilirubin, urobilinogen, nitrite, leukocytes, and specific gravity. These tests provide information about the functioning of the kidneys, liver, and other organs. Examples of boxes of reagent strips measuring from two to nine

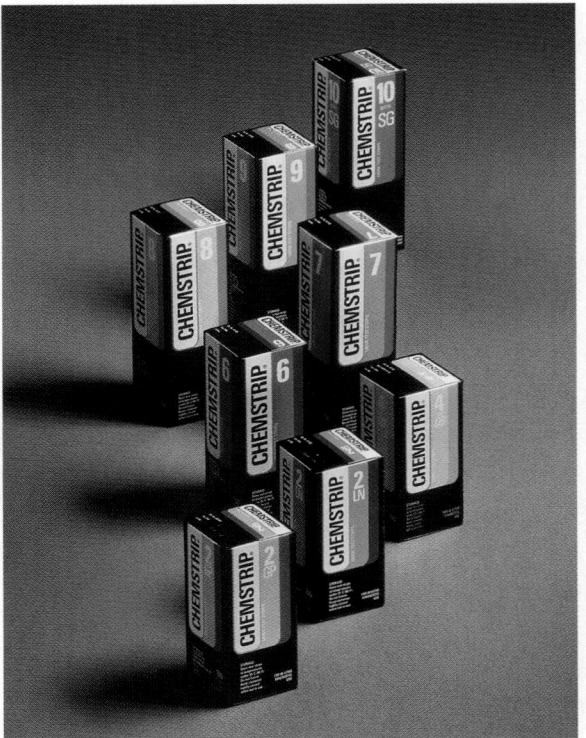

FIGURE 42-5 Ames chemical reagent strips.

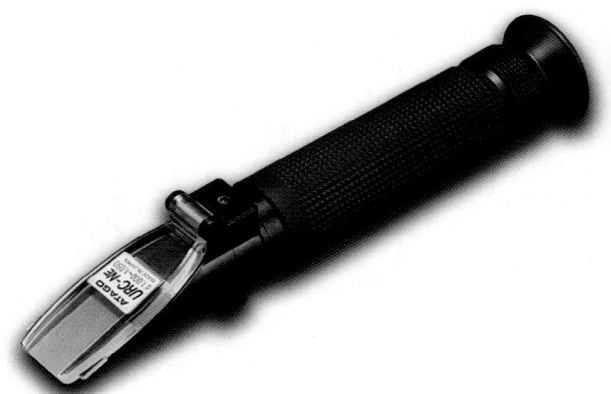

FIGURE 42-4 Portable digital refractometer.

PROCEDURE

Measuring Specific Gravity (SG) with a Refractometer

OBJECTIVE: Perform procedure without error and not more than 0.01 difference from instructor's reading.

Equipment and Supplies

antiseptic cleaner; biohazardous waste container; blood and body fluid protection—lab coat, protective eyewear, nonsterile gloves; distilled water; medicine dropper/pipette; paper, pen/pencil; paper towels; refractometer; urine specimen

Method

1. Perform hand hygiene.
2. Don gloves and protective clothing.
3. Assemble equipment and materials.
4. Before using the refractometer, perform a quality control check by using a sample of distilled water first. The value with distilled water should be 1.000.
   a. Clean the prism and refractometer cover with distilled water. Wipe dry.
   b. Close the cover. Using the medicine dropper or pipette, place a drop of distilled water on the notched area of the cover. If the refractometer does not have an attached cover, place the water directly onto the prism, and then place a cover plate on top of the prism.
   c. Tilt the refractometer to allow light to enter. Read the specific gravity by noting the division line between the light and dark area. This reading should be 1.000. If it is not, retest with fresh distilled water.
5. To test the urine sample, swirl the urine specimen gently to avoid splashing. Using the medicine dropper, remove a small sample and place one to two drops onto the notched area of the cover.
6. Follow instructions in step 4c to read the specific gravity.
7. Record the reading on a piece of paper.
8. Discard the urine appropriately.
9. Remove gloves and protective clothing, and dispose of them properly.
10. Perform hand hygiene.
11. Document findings in patient record.
12. Clean work area and equipment.

Charting Example

4/23/XX	1:00 P.M.	SG 1.012
		M. King, CMA

---

different chemicals in the urine are shown in Figure 42-5. Physicians decide which chemical elements they want to test for based on the patient's status and possible diagnosis. Obstetricians for example usually test for two main elements: glucose and protein. Most physicians test for all of the above-mentioned elements when a patient has an annual physical examination.

Each test has a specific time associated with reading the test, and that information is given on the side of the reagent strip container. The medical assistant must ensure that when a strip has been dipped in a specimen it does not touch the outside of the container when comparing the charts—this would contaminate the outside of the container (Figure 42-6). See Procedure 42-4 for the proper steps to evaluate the presence of certain chemicals in the urine using reagent strips.

Reaction pH

The pH of a solution indicates acidity and alkalinity. The pH is measured on a scale of 0 to 14, with 0 being the most acidic, 14 being the most basic (alkaline), and 7 being neutral (Figure 42-7). Normally, urine is slightly acidic at about 6.0. The ability of the kidneys to dilute and concentrate urine helps maintain the narrow pH range of blood (7.35 to 7.45) necessary for the body to be in homeostasis. Normal kidneys produce urine with pH ranging from 4.6 to 7.9. In urinary tract infections, the pH is typically more alkaline (higher than 7.0) because some bacteria break down urea to ammonia. Urine samples must be examined when fresh to avoid bacteria multiplying and causing inaccurate results. Higher pH is common in fever, phenylketonuria, and diets high in vitamin C. Some causes of low pH include respiratory acidosis, diets high in fruits or vegetables, and administration of some drugs.

Protein

Protein is normally not found in urine of healthy individuals. Urine may contain a small quantity of protein after exposure to the cold, after strenuous muscular

PROCEDURE

Testing Urine with Reagent Strips

OBJECTIVE: Perform chemical testing on urine using chemical reagent strips.

Equipment and Supplies

urine specimen; reagent test strips; timer; paper towel; laboratory slip; pen/pencil; personal protective equipment as needed

Method

1. Perform hand hygiene and don personal protective gear.
2. Check specimen for patient identity, date, and time of collection.
3. Check expiration date on chemical reagent strips.
4. Bring specimen to room temperature and swirl gently to mix.
5. Dip chemical reagent strip in urine, making sure all pads on strip are moistened (Figure 42-6A).
6. Read each pad by comparing to the chart on the side of the bottle appropriately timing each test (Figure 42-6B). (Do not hold test strip against the side of the bottle as contamination will result). Ignore color changes after prescribed time has elapsed.
7. Record results on patient's laboratory slip.
8. Clean work area, remove gloves, and perform hand hygiene.

Charting Example

Note: Normally a urine test slip would be used to record all results of chemical tests. Then when examination is complete and the physician has reviewed it, the test slip would be placed in patient's chart.

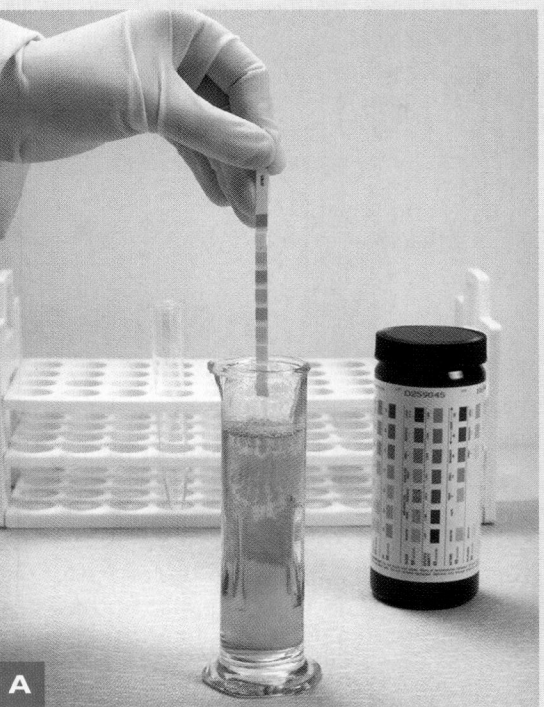

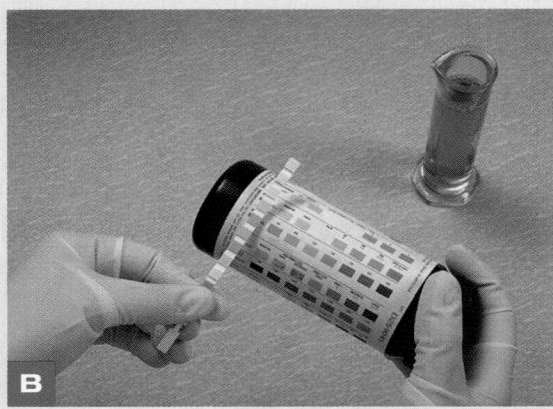

FIGURE 42-6   (A) Dip reagent strip into urine and withdraw; (B) compare color changes on reagent strip to chart on side of container without touching strip to side of container.

activity, or after eating large amounts of protein. However, these are considered physiological responses and not symptoms of disease. The presence of protein (proteinuria) can indicate renal dysfunction, preeclampsia in pregnancy, congestive heart failure, and glomerulonephritis. Glomerulonephritis is a kidney disease involving inflammation and lesions of the glomeruli.

Glucose

Normal urine should not contain glucose. However, after eating a high carbohydrate diet, small quantities of sugar may be present in the urine. This, however, is not a normal condition. If urine levels of glucose do not return to normal fairly quickly, it may be indicative of diabetes, pregnancy, stress, infection, or Cushing's syndrome or it may be caused by the use of some medications. Glycosuria is the name of any abnormal sugar in the urine. Sugar typically spills into the urine when the blood sugar levels exceed the renal threshold for glucose.

Blood

Hematuria (blood in the urine) is abnormal unless it is a contamination from menses. The presence of occult (hidden) blood in urine may indicate anemia, urinary tract infections, kidney stones, or trauma. It is occasionally caused by some medications. Female patients must be asked if menses is present when collection of a urine sample is required. If a patient is menstruating, it should be noted on the laboratory slip.

Ketone

Ketones are by-products of fat metabolism. Normally fats break down into water and carbon dioxide. If fats are burned as a source of energy instead of glucose, ketones will found be in the urine. If this persists long enough, a condition of acidosis may occur resulting in coma and death if untreated. Normally urine is negative for ketones. Elevated ketones are typically seen in conditions such as poorly controlled diabetes, dehydration, starvation, ingestion of large quantities of aspirin, and occasionally after general anesthesia. Ketones tend to evaporate at room temperature, therefore ketone testing must be done immediately or the specimen should be covered and refrigerated.

Bilirubin

Under normal circumstances, bilirubin is not found in the urine. Bilirubin is a product of the breakdown of hemoglobin. Hemoglobin is released from old red blood cells and is converted by the liver into bilirubin and into urobilinogen in the small intestines. The presence of bilirubin in urine may be one of the first signs of liver disease, obstructive biliary disease, or mononucleosis. Large amounts of bilirubin in the urine will cause the urine to turn yellow-brown to dark orange. If a specimen is found to have large quantities of bilirubin, then it should be stored away from light until further testing, because light causes the breakdown of bilirubin.

Urobilinogen

Urobilinogen is a result of red blood cell destruction. It is elevated in any condition causing an increase in bilirubin. It is present in small quantities under normal conditions. If no urobilinogen is present, there may be a bile duct obstruction. However, reagents strips usually are not sensitive enough to detect an absence of urobilinogen.

Nitrites

Measurement of nitrites is a method for detection of bacturia (bacteria in the urine). Thus the presence of

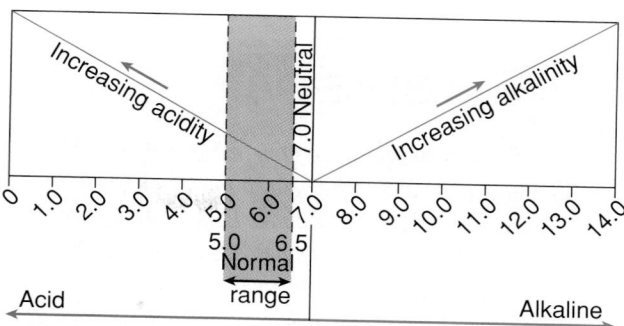

FIGURE 42-7 Urine pH scale.

nitrites often indicates a urinary tract infection. Nitrites are a by-product of chemical breakdown by certain bacteria. Most common urinary tract infections are caused by *Escherichia coli* (*E. coli*), which is typically found in bowel material. Bacteria, when introduced into the urinary meatus, travel up the urethra to the bladder. The bladder is sterile under normal conditions. An infection may result if enough bacteria are present in the bladder. Females should be reminded after voiding or having a bowel movement to wipe from front to back, away from the urinary meatus, to lessen the chance of developing urinary tract infections (UTIs).

False positives for the presence of nitrites can happen if the specimen sits at room temperature too long, because bacteria can begin to multiply at room temperature. Specimens that cannot be immediately tested should be refrigerated.

Leukocytes

Leukocytes are white blood cells and under normal conditions few leukocytes are found in urine. When leukocytes are present in sufficient quantity, they are usually indicative of a UTI. Leukocyte esterase on the reagent strip detects the esterase released by white blood cells. The darker the color on the strip, the greater the number of WBCs. When a positive leukocyte test is found, always check to see if the results correlate with the rest of the patient's report. If there is a positive leukocyte test, then there should be a positive protein test, possibly an elevated pH, and bacteria in the microscopic evaluation.

As mentioned, urine samples provide vital information to the physician treating a patient. Usually when one has an annual physical, all of the preceding tests are performed on the urine specimen. For example, an abnormal urine glucose result may require a follow-up fasting blood sugar or glucose tolerance test to confirm or rule out diabetes mellitus. An abnormal protein result may indicate bladder infection or infection higher in the urinary tract or it may indicate hypertension. Follow-up tests such as a 24-hour urine specimen for protein, x-rays of the kidney, and a clean-catch midstream urine test may be ordered for culture and

Microscopic Examination

Microscopic examination identifies the type and approximate numbers of organisms present in a urine specimen. Microscopic examination helps physicians to determine a disease process. This is not a CLIA waived test. A certificate of provider-performed microscopy (PPM) procedures is issued to a physician's office laboratary (POL) qualified to perform waived tests, moderate complexity tests, and microscopic procedures. If the PPM certificate is not granted, the specimen may be sent to an outside laboratory. In some states, medical assistants may perform microscopic examinations after further training if the facility has a PPM certificate. Medical assistants must be able to properly prepare a urine specimen for microscopic examination and understand the meaning and importance of the results of a urine microscopic examination.

Preparing a Urine Specimen for Microscopic Examination

After performing the necessary physical and chemical analyses, the urine is placed in a centrifuge tube and then into a centrifuge (Figure 42-10). The sediment is the solid material found in urine remaining after the supernatant (liquid portion) is poured off. The sediment may contain organized material such as red blood cells, white blood cells, epithelial cells, casts, bacteria, parasites, yeast, fungi, and spermatozoa. The unorganized sediment consists of all chemical materials, including crystals and amorphous material (material without a shape). A special stain may be used to provide better contrast to the formed elements present. Specimens that are to be examined under the microscope should be fresh. Ideally, they should be collected by the clean-catch method. Procedure 42-6 provides the steps needed to prepare a urine specimen for microscopic examination.

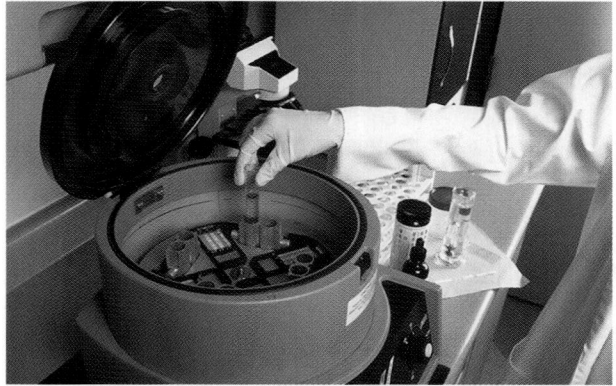

FIGURE 42-10 The centrifuge is used to spin urine specimens in preparation for a microscopic examination.

Reporting and Understanding Urine Microscopic Examinations

As mentioned previously, examining urine sediment under the microscope is not a CLIA waived test and as a medical assistant you should understand CLIA regulations and review your state's regulations regarding these procedures.

To better understand results of a urine microscopic examination, an explanation of the method used to estimate the numbers of formed elements observed is necessary. The meaning of each individual formed element will be discussed in subsequent paragraphs. Once the slide is made and coverslipped, it is examined first under the low-power field (lpf) setting of the microscope (10×) and low light to locate casts, which if present are found near the edges of the coverslip. Ten to fifteen fields are scanned and the number and type of casts or cells is noted. For example, in 10 to 15 fields the examiner sees a range of 0 to 4 hyaline casts. This means that in some fields there were no casts, others one, two, three, or four casts thus the report of 0–4 hyaline casts per lpf. Counting and reporting procedures are the same when using 40×, or the high-power field (hpf) setting. It is preferable to use a numerical range when reporting formed elements. Other elements may be reported using the following words to estimate the amounts:

- Occasional 0–3
- Few 3–6
- Moderate 6–12
- Many 12 or more
- TNTC Too numerous to count

Cells

Cells that may be found in urine are epithelial cells, red blood cells, and white blood cells. The presence of red blood cells, an excessive number of white cells, and certain types of epithelial cells indicate urinary tract conditions or disease.

EPITHELIAL CELLS Epithelial cells are classified as squamous, transitional or bladder, and renal epithelial cells. Squamous epithelial cells line the urinary tract from the external meatus to the bladder. Therefore, a few epithelial cells (0–5/hpf) are to be expected in a urine sample. They also line the vagina and may be considered vaginal contaminants in urine. Finding bladder or renal epithelial cells is an abnormal finding and may indicate the presence of disease in the bladder or kidneys.

RED CELLS One to two red blood cells per hpf is normal; anything more is considered abnormal. The presence of RBCs could represent a bladder infection

PROCEDURE

Preparing a Specimen for a Microscopic Urine Specimen Examination

OBJECTIVE: Perform microscopic examination of urine sediment for casts and cells within a 1% error deviation from instructor's measurements.

Equipment and Supplies

biohazardous waste container; body and body fluid protection—lab coat, goggles, nonsterile gloves; capillary pipette; centrifuge; centrifuge tube; microscope; microscope slide; paper, pen/pencil; Sedi-stain (optional); urine specimen

Note: Medical assistants are not expected to perform a microscopic examination. They may be requested by the physician to prepare the specimen to step 11.

Method

1. Perform hand hygiene.
2. Put on gloves and protective clothing.
3. Assemble equipment and materials.
4. Mix the specimen gently to stir up the sediment that has settled to the bottom.
5. Place 10 mL of urine into the centrifuge tube. Place cap on tube. Place the tube in the centrifuge and balance this with another tube of 10 mL of water on the opposite side of the machine (Figure 42-10).
6. Set centrifuge timer for 5 minutes.
7. After the centrifuge has stopped, remove the tube and pour the supernatant fluid (the clear liquid left on the top of the specimen after centrifuging) off leaving only the sediment. *Alternate method:* Some medical assistants prefer using stain (such as Sedi-stain) to help identify sediment more easily. Place one drop of the commercially prepared stain in the test tube.
8. Mix the sediment by holding the top of the tube and tapping bottom with a finger mixing well to ensure a correct reading.
9. Use a capillary pipette to transfer one drop of sediment to a clean slide.
10. Cover the drop of sediment with a coverslip.
11. Place the slide on the microscope stage.
12. Focus under low power and reduced light for casts and epithelial cells.
13. Carefully examine for anything abnormal paying close attention to the edges, which are where casts are seen if present.
14. Examine 10 to 15 fields using low power. Count the number of casts or other abnormalities seen in each field. If there is nothing in one field, then record zero. Average the count from the 10 to 15 fields for the final result.
15. Use the high-power magnification and adjust for more light reviewing the 10 to 15 fields. Identify casts if present. Count RBCs, WBCs, round, transitional, and squamous epithelial cells. Average the count from the 10 to 15 fields for each formed element seen and record appropriately.
16. Observe for crystals and identify. Observe for bacteria, sperm, yeast, and parasites. Report them as few, moderate, or many.
17. Discard the urine according to OSHA guidelines.
18. Remove gloves and protective clothing, and dispose of them properly.
19. Perform hand hygiene.
20. Document findings in patient record.
21. Clean work area and equipment according to OSHA guidelines.

---

or kidney disorder such as nephritis. Red blood cells are pale, round, have no nucleus (core), and are nongranular. They indicate that bleeding may be taking place somewhere in the urinary system. Acidic urine may cause the red blood cells to rupture and be invisible or mistaken for white blood cells under micro-scopic examination. RBCs may be an indication of menstruation in female patients.

WHITE CELLS White blood cells contain a nucleus and are larger than RBCs with a granular surface. Zero to five white blood cells per hpf would be considered

One member of the clinic or office team will be designated as an OSHA officer. That individual is responsible for ensuring that all OSHA policies are followed, and that all team members are educated appropriately in following those policies. Sharps containers should be provided in any exam room or lab where needles or other sharps are used. Material data safety manuals must be kept up to date, listing all the chemicals used in the facility.

Per OSHA standards, Universal Precautions must be observed at all times. When a medical assistant is in a situation where exposure to blood and body fluids is a possibility, gloves must be worn. If appropriate, a lab coat and goggles and/or face mask should also be utilized.

normal. Large numbers of WBCs may indicate an infection in the urinary system. Further testing would be needed to pinpoint the infection location.

Casts

Casts result from protein formation in the kidney tubules. Different types of casts are classified according to the substances that form them. Casts are counted under the low power of the microscope, but are identified under the high powered magnification. Casts may be identified as hyaline, granular (coarse or finely granular), cellular (WBC, RBC, or epithelial), mixed (containing more than one type of cell), or waxy. Hyaline casts indicate kidney disease. Red blood casts are found in diseases such as glomerulonephritis. Waxy casts are rarely seen and are indicative of severe renal disease.

Bacteria

Bacteria are not normally found in fresh urine. A specimen can become contaminated during collection or with vaginal secretions. Large numbers of bacteria in the urine indicate a urinary tract infection. A specimen with bacteria and white blood cells can be considered a confirmation of UTI. A urine culture may be done to determine the type of bacteria and the correct antibiotic therapy.

Yeast

Yeast may be present in the urine of a female who has a vaginal yeast infection (moniliasis). It can also be present in both males and females with diabetes mellitus.

Parasites

Parasites are organisms that live within other organisms. They may be present in urine as a result of contamination from vaginal or bowel excretions. *Trichomonas vaginalis* is the most frequently found parasite in urine and it causes vaginal infection.

Spermatozoa

Spermatozoa, the male sex cell, can be seen in both male and female urine after sexual intercourse.

Crystals

Crystals can form in the urine either in the kidney, bladder, or in the specimen container on standing. They are found in both acid and alkaline urine. As urine cools solid crystals will precipitate out. The presence of crystals is not usually clinically significant unless found in large numbers. Crystals are identified by their appearance and the pH of the urine in which they are found. In certain metabolic disorders, abnormal crystals such as leucine or tyrosine and cystine may be found. In addition certain drugs such as sulfa drugs may cause the production of crystals.

Contaminants

Many substances can cause contamination of a urine specimen, including clothing fibers, mucous threads, hair, talc, or other body contaminants. There is never a complete guarantee of a contaminant-free specimen, but patient education can help keep the chances of specimen contamination to a minimum. Figure 42-11 identifies different structures that may be found in a urine microscopic examination.

Urine Pregnancy Testing

Pregnancy testing is based on the detection of human chorionic gonadotropin (hCG), which is produced by the placenta and is present in the urine of pregnant women. Levels of hCG may be detectable as early as 10 days after fertilization has taken place. A first morning specimen is preferred for this test because the concentration of the hormone is greatest at that time. The technology of the pregnancy test is fairly complex but the tests themselves are easy to perform. CLIA waived pregnancy tests performed in POLs fall into two categories: agglutination or enzyme immunoassay. The more frequently used enzyme immunoassay (EIA) tests involve the reaction of antigen and antibody and a second antibody attached to an enzyme. Pregnancy tests are produced with built-in controls that are run along with the patient test to provide quality control. Procedure 42-7 lists the steps necessary to perform a urine pregnancy test using the EIA testing method.

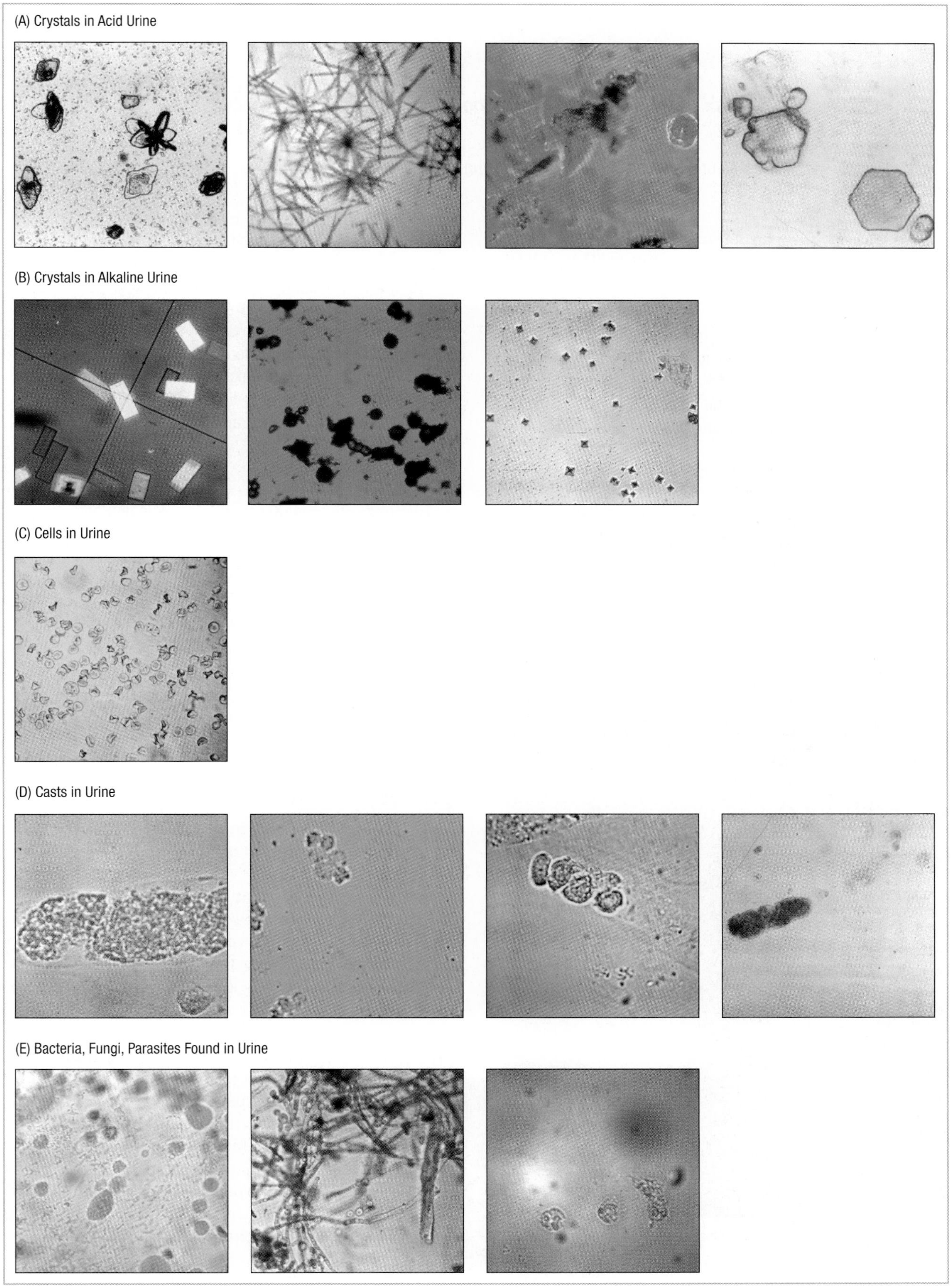

(A) Crystals in Acid Urine

(B) Crystals in Alkaline Urine

(C) Cells in Urine

(D) Casts in Urine

(E) Bacteria, Fungi, Parasites Found in Urine

FIGURE 42-11   Urine sediment chart (Courtesy of Bayer Diagnostic).

Performing a Urine Pregnancy Test Using the Enzyme Immunoassay Method

OBJECTIVE: Perform a urine pregnancy test for hCG using an EIA test and interpret results correctly.

Equipment and Supplies

patient's first A.M. urine specimen; EIA test kit for hCG; timer; gloves; laboratory report

Method

1. Perform hand hygiene and don gloves.
2. Gather supplies and equipment.
3. Allow testing materials and specimen to come to room temperature.
4. Label the test with patient name or ID number.
5. Label one area positive and one negative for controls.
6. Place patient's urine on test chamber following manufacturer's directions.
7. Place positive and negative controls in correct areas.
8. Time the test according to manufacturer's directions.
9. Interpret results correctly.
10. Record results on patient's laboratory slip.
11. Record positive and negative controls in quality control log book according to office policy.
12. Dispose of equipment and perform hand hygiene.

Charting Example

| 10/19/XX | 4:00 P.M. | Preg test pos. |
| | | M. King, CMA |

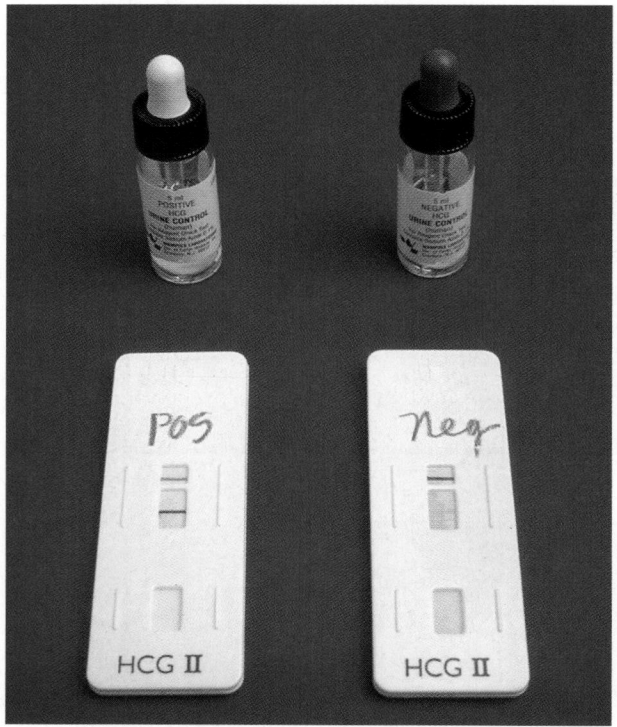

FIGURE 42-12 Urine pregnancy control test—positive and negative.

Figure 42-12 shows positive and negative urine pregnancy control results.

Quality Control

Quality control is a system of ensuring that patients' test results are accurate and reported in a timely manner. Each testing product typically is sold with a quality control testing program. Testing should be done on a regular schedule, following the appropriate protocol and all documentation should be kept in a quality control log. The tests you use for urinary pH, protein, blood, glucose, ketones, bilirubin, nitrite, urobilinogen, and specific gravity should be checked periodically by using solutions that contain a known amount of each of these substances. It is important to precisely follow the directions that are supplied by the manufacturer when using this testing material. Document control results in the quality control log. New employees in your facility should be appropriately trained to perform urine tests and the training documented. All instrumentation associated with urine testing should be cleaned and maintained on a regular basis and documented accordingly.

SUMMARY

Urinalysis is one of the most common laboratory procedures performed by the medical assistant. Because urine is a body fluid, Universal Precautions must be observed, including aseptic technique. Many steps are taken to ensure accurate lab results, including good patient education, proper specimen labeling, and following laboratory procedures exactly.

The three primary components of a urinalysis include the physical (appearance, color, odor, volume, and specific gravity), chemical (pH, protein, glucose, blood, ketones, bilirubin, urobilinogen, nitrate, and leukocytes), and microscopic (cells, casts, bacteria, yeast, parasites, spermatozoa, crystals, and contaminants) examinations. Quality control is the final component of urinalysis.

Chapter Review

COMPETENCY REVIEW

1. Define and spell the terms to learn for this chapter.
2. Explain the procedure for a microscopic examination of urine.
3. Discuss two types of commercial products for doing the chemical analysis of urine specimens.
4. Why do we measure specific gravity?
5. Under what conditions can a urinometer give a false result?
6. What causes a "fruity" odor in urine? In what disease condition is it found?
7. What is the purpose of catheterization?

PREPARING FOR THE CERTIFICATION EXAM

1. When handling a patient's urine, a medical assistant must follow universal handling of fluid precautions, meaning:
   A. aseptic procedures must be followed
   B. gloves and a lab coat must be worn
   C. gloves, lab coat, and goggles must be worn
   D. A and B
   E. A, B, and C

2. Which of the following statements regarding the collection of a routine (random) urine sample is false?
   A. It is collected in a nonsterile container.
   B. It can be collected at any time during the day.
   C. It should remain at room temperature at all times prior to testing.
   D. At least 10 mL of urine should be collected.
   E. The container should be labeled with the date and the patient's name.

3. A 24-hour specimen would be an example of a _____ specimen.
   A. morning
   B. timed
   C. postprandial
   D. clean-catch
   E. clean-catch midstream

4. Fetid, in regards to urine, would refer to the:
   A. odor
   B. color
   C. quantity
   D. turbidity
   E. specific gravity

5. The normal specific gravity of urine, which measures the ability of the kidneys to concentrate urine, ranges from:
   A. 1.000 to 1.005
   B. 1.005 to 1.010
   C. 1.010 to 1.020
   D. 1.010 to 1.030
   E. 1.010 to 1.040

6. Glycosuria, an abnormal condition, is the presence of _____ in the urine:
   A. white blood cells
   B. red blood cells
   C. sugar
   D. bacteria
   E. parasites

continued on next page

7. Which of the following statements is true?
   A. Urine voided by healthy patients is slightly acidic.
   B. Urine voided by healthy patients on a normal diet is slightly alkaline.
   C. A pH greater than 7.0 is common in the presence of a UTI.
   D. A pH lower than 7.0 is common if a patient is consuming large amounts of vitamin C.
   E. An odor of ammonia in urine may indicate infection.

8. The presences of which of the following may signal the onset of liver disease?
   A. leukocytes
   B. erythrocytes
   C. ketones
   D. bilirubin
   E. nitrates

9. Sediment in urine, both organized and unorganized, includes:
   A. casts, cells and crystals
   B. casts, cells, bacteria, parasites, yeast, and fungi
   C. casts, cells, bacteria, parasites, yeast, fungi, and spermatozoa
   D. casts, cells, bacteria, parasites, yeast, fungi, spermatozoa, and crystals
   E. casts, cells, bacterial, parasites, yeast, fungi, spermatozoa, crystals, and amorphous material

10. Which of the following statements is true?
    A. Casts are visualized microscopically under high power.
    B. Cells are visualized microscopically under low power.
    C. Crystals are visualized microscopically under low power.
    D. The findings are charted after averaging what has been seen in five fields.
    E. The findings are charted after averaging what has been seen in 10 fields.

CRITICAL THINKING

1. What conclusions can you make about the urine test?
2. How long may a urine specimen remain at room temperature prior to testing?
3. Why is an ammonia-like odor linked to this specimen?
4. What should you do about the test results?

ON THE JOB

Jose Menendez is an elderly patient of Dr. Juarez, a board-certified urologist. He has a history of recurrent UTIs dating back more than 10 years. When Mr. Menendez becomes symptomatic, he has been instructed to call Dr. Juarez's office and schedule a urinalysis. Dr. Juarez's receptionist has just received a call from Mr. Menendez. He says he knows he is supposed to come in for a urine test, but that he just wants a prescription phoned in to his pharmacy instead. The receptionist asks Emilia, Dr. Juarez's medical assistant, to take the call from Mr. Menendez.

Emilia listens as Mr. Menendez recounts that he is experiencing dysuria—painful, burning urination. She asks him to come in for a urinalysis, explaining that, as per standing orders, a clean-catch midstream specimen needs to be collected. Mr. Menendez repeats to Emilia that he does not want to come in to the office. "Why can't you call in a prescription for Bactrim? That is what I took last time and it helped."

What is your response?

1. Should the responsibility for this call have fallen on Emilia or should the receptionist have either handled the call herself or passed it on to Dr. Juarez?
2. What, if anything, could or should Emilia say to Mr. Menendez to persuade him to come in for the urinalysis?
3. Might the cost of the procedure be a factor in the reason why Mr. Menendez does not want to have a urinalysis, and, if so, what, if anything, can Emilia do or say about the cost?

4. Is it appropriate in this case, given the patient's extensive history, to indeed call in a prescription for Bactrim?
5. If not, how should Emilia handle Mr. Menendez's request for his prescription?
6. If so, what procedure should Emilia follow in order to arrange for a prescription?
7. How should this telephone call be charted?
8. What, if anything, should Dr. Juarez be told about the conversation with Mr. Menendez?

INTERNET ACTIVITY

Use the Internet to research OSHA regulations regarding personal protective equipment.

MediaLink  More on urinalysis, including interactive resources, can be found on the Student CD-ROM accompanying this textbook.

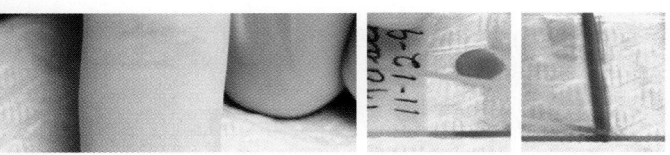

Medical Assistant Role Delineation Chart

HIGHLIGHT indicates material covered in this chapter.

ADMINISTRATIVE

Administrative Procedures

- Perform basic administrative medical assisting functions
- Schedule, coordinate and monitor appointments
- Schedule inpatient/outpatient admissions and procedures
- Understand and apply third-party guidelines
- Obtain reimbursement through accurate claims submission
- Monitor third-party reimbursement
- Understand and adhere to managed care policies and procedures
- *Negotiate managed care contracts*

- Manage accounts receivable
- *Manage accounts payable*
- *Process payroll*
- *Document and maintain accounting and banking records*
- *Develop and maintain fee schedules*
- *Manage renewals of business and professional insurance policies*
- *Manage personnel benefits and maintain records*
- *Perform marketing, financial, and strategic planning*

Practice Finances

- Perform procedural and diagnostic coding
- Apply bookkeeping principles

CLINICAL

Fundamental Principles

- Apply principles of aseptic technique and infection control
- Comply with quality assurance practices
- Screen and follow up patient test results

Diagnostic Orders

- Collect and process specimens
- Perform diagnostic tests

Patient Care

- Adhere to established patient screening procedures
- Obtain patient history and vital signs
- Prepare and maintain examination and treatment areas
- Prepare patient for examinations, procedures and treatments

- Assist with examinations, procedures and treatments
- Prepare and administer medications and immunizations
- Maintain medication and immunization records
- Recognize and respond to emergencies
- Coordinate patient care information with other health care providers
- Initiate IV and administer IV medications with appropriate training and as permitted by state law

GENERAL

Professionalism

- Display a professional manner and image
- Demonstrate initiative and responsibility
- Work as a member of the health care team
- Prioritize and perform multiple tasks
- Adapt to change
- Promote the CMA credential
- Enhance skills through continuing education
- Treat all patients with compassion and empathy
- Promote the practice through positive public relations

Communication Skills

- Recognize and respect cultural diversity
- Adapt communications to individual's ability to understand
- Use professional telephone technique

- Recognize and respond effectively to verbal, nonverbal, and written communications
- Use medical terminology appropriately
- Utilize electronic technology to receive, organize, prioritize and transmit information
- Serve as liaison

Legal Concepts

- Perform within legal and ethical boundaries
- Prepare and maintain medical records
- Document accurately
- Follow employer's established policies dealing with the health care contract
- Implement and maintain federal and state health care legislation and regulations
- Comply with established risk management and safety procedures
- Recognize professional credentialing criteria
- *Develop and maintain personnel, policy and procedure manuals*

Instruction

- Instruct individuals according to their needs
- Explain office policies and procedures
- Teach methods of health promotion and disease prevention
- Locate community resources and disseminate information
- *Develop educational materials*
- *Conduct continuing education activities*

Operational Functions

- Perform inventory of supplies and equipment
- Perform routine maintenance of administrative and clinical equipment
- Apply computer techniques to support office operations
- *Perform personnel management functions*
- *Negotiate leases and prices for equipment and supply contracts*

- *Denotes advanced skills.*

SOURCE: Reprinted by permission of the American Association of Medical Assistants from the AAMA Role Delineation Study: Occupational Analysis of the Medical Assisting Profession.

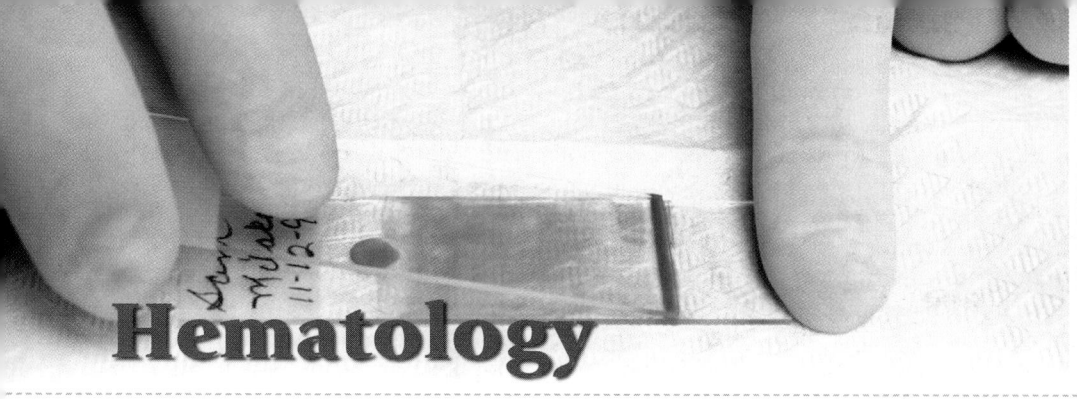

Hematology

Learning Objectives

After completing this chapter, you should be able to:

- Define and spell the terms to learn for this chapter.

- List the components of blood, including the liquid and cellular portions and functions of each.

- Describe how to prepare a patient for collection of a blood specimen

- via venipuncture and capillary puncture methods.

- Discuss how to process a blood specimen for routine testing in a physician's office.

- State the normal values for each of the blood tests discussed.

OUTLINE

The Medical Assistant's Role	902
Blood Formation and Components	902
Function of Blood	903
Blood Specimen Collection	904
Routine Blood Tests	909
Erythrocyte Sedimentation Rate	921
Phenylketonuria	921
Mono Testing	921

Terms to Learn

antecubital space	hematology	heparin
capillaries	hematopoiesis	plasma
electrolytes	hemoglobin	platelets
erythrocyte sedimentation rate (ESR)		

Case Study

MARY O'SHEA, CMA HAS JUST BEEN HIRED AS A MEDICAL ASSISTANT at a physician's office. The first task that Mary has been asked to do is to obtain blood samples from a male patient. The order in the patient's chart indicates that blood samples are to be drawn for the following tests: CBC, serum chemistry tests, and a prothrombin time. What method(s) should Mary use to collect the samples?

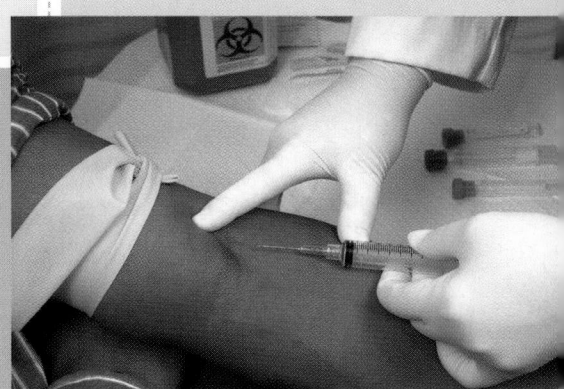

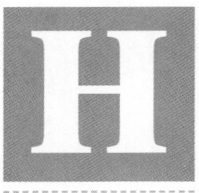**ematology** is the study of blood and the tissues that produce it. Blood and its components are studied to detect pathological conditions and to determine the appropriate course of treatment. Blood analysis is one of the most common diagnostic tests performed in the doctor's office. As a result, the medical assistant must have a thorough understanding of how to collect, handle, package, and analyze a blood specimen correctly.

The Medical Assistant's Role

When the physician orders a blood test, the role of the medical assistant is to collect the specimen. The actual testing of the blood is not commonly done in the medical office but rather is done in an outside laboratory that is contracted with the patient's medical insurance. When a patient's blood is drawn, the medical assistant must ensure that proper specimen labeling has occurred and that the blood is stored correctly until the laboratory courier has arrived for pickup.

Blood Formation and Components

The formation of blood cells is called hematopoiesis. Hematopoiesis begins at the stem cell level during fetal development. Blood is formed with both cellular and liquid components.

Cellular Formation and Components

All blood cells originate from the hematopoietic stem cell, but mature into one of seven individual cells:

1. Red blood cells (erythrocytes)
2. White blood cells (leukocytes)—five types

   A: Granular leukocytes (have granules in their cytoplasm):
   - Neutrophil
   - Eosinophil
   - Basophil

   B: Nongranular leukocytes (do not have granules in their cytoplasm):
   - Lymphocyte
   - Monocyte

3. Platelets (thrombocytes)

Hematopoiesis occurs primarily in the bone marrow of the adult. Lymphocytes, one of the types of white blood cells (WBCs), are produced in the lymph nodes.

Red Blood Cells

Red blood cells (RBCs) are formed in the bone marrow. They are important for the human body because

they contain hemoglobin. Hemoglobin has two functions. The first is to carry oxygen from the lungs to the cells of the body. The second function is to carry carbon dioxide (a waste product) from the body back to the lungs, where it can be expelled with exhalation. When the hemoglobin is carrying oxygen, it is called *oxyhemoglobin*. When it is carrying carbon dioxide, it is called *carboxyhemoglobin*. Arterial blood has a higher concentration of oxygen, explaining its bright red color. Venous blood is darker in color because of the carboxyhemoglobin.

The formation of red blood cells is controlled somewhat by erythropoietin, which is secreted by the kidneys in an adult, and by the liver in a fetus. When the amount of erythropoietin is decreased, red blood cells will not be formed in proper amounts, which may result in certain types of anemia. For instance, patients who are being treated with chemotherapy may develop anemia that then can be treated with an artificial erythropoietin called Procrit that assists in the reproduction of red blood cells. Red blood cells last for about 4 months and are continually being reproduced in the body. The normal RBC range for a male adult is 4.5 to 6 million/mm^3. The normal female RBC range is 4 to 5.5 million/mm^3.

White Blood Cells

White blood cells are also known as leukocytes, which are produced in the bone marrow and are divided into several different types. They originate in the bone marrow from stem cells. White blood cells are larger than red blood cells and their principal function is to defend against infection. The five types of white blood cells are neutrophils, lymphocytes, monocytes, eosinophils, and basophils. The range of WBCs in an adult is 4.5 to 11 thousand/mm^3.

NEUTROPHILS Neutrophils are divided into two categories: segmented neutrophils and nonsegmented neutrophils. Segmented neutrophils have a nucleus that is divided into multiple segments connected by small thin threads. Nonsegmented neutrophils are also called stabs (or bands) and are more immature neutrophils than the segmented ones. The presence of a large number of stabs may indicate the existence of a bacterial infection. Neutrophils are named this because the granules are neutral in color on the laboratory-stained slide. The body reproduces neutrophils on an ongoing basis, and they only survive for a few days. Reproduction is increased when bacterial infection is occurring. Neutrophils combat infection by phagocytosis. Phagocytosis is the process in which the neutrophil surrounds, swallows, and digests the bacteria.

EOSINOPHILS Eosinophils are also assumed to be produced by the bone marrow. Detection of a large number of eosinophils can indicate a parasitic condition or the presence of certain allergic conditions. Eosinophils have granules that produce a red color on the laboratory-stained slide. Eosinophils are called this due to the stain eosin, which is used in the staining of blood smears.

BASOPHILS Like the other white cells, basophils are thought to be produced by the bone marrow, and they produce heparin. Heparin is a substance that prevents clotting. When an individual has a condition that is creating inflammation, heparin may be used to assist in diminishing or preventing the occurrence of clotting. Increased amounts of basophils may be found in patients who have had their spleen removed. Patients who have had excessive exposure to radiation may also have increased basophils.

LYMPHOCYTES Lymphocytes are produced in the bone marrow and in the lymphoid tissue such as the spleen and lymph nodes. The function of lymphocytes is primarily to produce antibodies against foreign substances such as bacteria, viruses, and pollens. Lymphocytes are small and large and can proliferate into B and T cells. B cells may convert into plasma cells, which produce antibodies. T cells can produce helper cells, cytotoxic cells, and suppressor cells. To diagnose an individual with HIV, testing is performed to evaluate the type and amount of T cells present. Lymphocytes do not have granules and are nonsegmented.

MONOCYTES Monocytes are formed in the bone marrow from stem cells. Monocytes assist in phagocytosis. They ingest foreign particles or bacteria that the neutrophils are unable to digest and assist in cleaning up cellular debris that may have been left from the infection. An increase in monocytes is seen in patients who have certain diseases such as tuberculosis, typhoid, and Rocky Mountain spotted fever.

Platelets
Platelets (also called thrombocytes) are the smallest cells found in the blood and are formed in the bone marrow. The main function of platelets is to assist in the clotting of blood. Platelets increase around an area that is bleeding to assist in the formation of clots. The platelets and the injured tissue release thromboplastin. The thromboplastin combines with other elements in the blood to produce thrombin. The thrombin acts on a protein in the blood called fibrinogen, resulting in the formation of fibrin. Fibrin is tiny threads that create a mesh that catches the red cells and other cells to form a clot. There are typically between 150,000 and 400,000 platelets/mm^3.

Understanding the process of normal clotting and absence of normal clotting is important because laboratory tests are designed to determine why clotting is not occurring properly, particularly in patients who are receiving anticlotting drugs such as heparin and Coumadin.

Lifespan Considerations

Drawing blood from an older individual can sometimes be challenging due to the condition of their veins. Patients do not want to have any more needle sticks than necessary. To ensure that a successful needle stick occurs requires both experience and patience. If patients will be returning to the office for blood work at a later time, inform the patient to drink a lot of fluids prior to arrival at the office. Being well hydrated is helpful for finding veins. Use of items such as a small ball placed in the patient's hand to squeeze in order to pump up the veins is also helpful. If the hand must be used for the draw site, place a warm cloth over the area to allow for the vein to rise up. All of these techniques can help in making the first try a success.

Liquid Blood Formation and Components

For the medical assistant to understand how blood is formed requires a thorough comprehension of the cellular and liquid components of blood. The liquid component of blood is called plasma. Plasma is about 55% of the composition of blood and carries cellular elements and other substances. Plasma transports substances in the blood to the different parts of the body. Plasma does contain fibrinogen, which converts to fibrin during the clotting process. Plasma without the fibrinogen is called serum.

Ninety percent of plasma is water, while the other 10% is solid substances, called solutes. These solutes may include the plasma proteins (albumin, globulin, fibrinogen, and prothrombin), electrolytes (sodium, potassium, and chloride), glucose, amino acids, lipids and carbohydrates, metabolic waste products (urea, lactic acid, uric acid), creatinine, respiratory gases (oxygen and carbon dioxide), and miscellaneous substances (hormones, antibodies, enzymes, vitamins, and mineral salts).

Function of Blood

The function of blood is transportation and protection. It carries oxygen and nutrients to the body and removes the waste product carbon dioxide. The blood carries the waste products to the liver, kidneys, and skin for elimination.

Legal and Ethical Issues

It is legal in most states for a medical assistant to perform a venipuncture. Check with the local American Association of Medical Assistants (AAMA) chapter for specifics in your state. When performing basic in-office lab tests, the medical assistant must keep all results confidential. Confidentiality is a moral and ethical obligation for all health care team members.

The heart pumps blood through the body by way of the arteries, veins, and capillaries. The capillaries connect the arteries and veins that pump the blood to and from the heart. When blood flows away from the heart it flows in arteries, and when it returns back to the heart it flows through veins. Arteries have thick walls that allow them to withstand the pressure sustained when the heart is pumping. The blood carried in the arteries contains oxygen. This blood with its high level of oxygen sustains tissue function. As oxygen is being released from the blood, carbon dioxide is being transported to the lungs to be expelled as a waste product.

The blood regulates body temperature. When the body becomes warm, the capillaries dilate and release heat, which in turn cools the body. When the body is cold, the capillaries constrict allowing for less blood flow, which increases the body temperature.

Blood Specimen Collection

Laboratory testing of blood and the collection of all blood and body fluids is strictly regulated by OSHA regulations, and the CDC's Universal Precautions must be followed at all times. CLIA (Clinical Laboratory

---

43-1 PROCEDURE

Quality Control for Collecting a Blood Specimen

OBJECTIVE: Perform quality control procedure while collecting a blood specimen without errors.

Equipment and Supplies

antiseptic cleaner; biohazard waste container; necessary sterile equipment; specimen collection container; disposable alcohol wipe; disposable gloves; appropriate requisition or paperwork required of collection; pen or pencil; patient's chart

Method

1. Review request and verify test ordered.
2. Prepare necessary equipment and work area.
3. Perform hand hygiene and don gloves.
4. Identify the patient and explain the procedure, and make sure he or she understands the procedure.
5. Confirm that patient has followed any pretest preparation requirements.
6. Collect the specimen properly, using the appropriate equipment and technique.
7. Use the appropriate collection container and the right preservatives.
8. Immediately label the specimen with the patient's name, date and time of collection, test's name, and the name of the person collecting the specimen.
9. Follow correct procedures for disposing of hazardous specimen waste and decontaminating work area and equipment according to OSHA guidelines.
10. Remove gloves and dispose in appropriate container. Perform hand hygiene. Dispose of all used needles, etc., in biohazard waste container.
11. Thank the patient and observe for any signs or symptoms of inappropriate response to the procedure.
12. Document the procedure in patient's chart.
13. If the specimen is to be transported to an outside laboratory, prepare it for transport in the proper container, with all the appropriate information according to OSHA guidelines.

Improvement Amendments) sets the standards that all laboratories must adhere to, including training of personnel and testing and transport of specimens (see Chapter 42). It is important when performing specimen collection that the medical assistant follow the regulation guidelines established by these organizations (see Procedure 43-1).

The type and amount of specimen to be acquired is determined by the test to be done. If a very small amount is needed, then the specimen may be obtained by capillary puncture. Larger volumes are collected through venipuncture.

Venipuncture

Three methods of venipuncture are used: the vacuum tube method, the syringe and needle method, and the butterfly method (see also Legal and Ethical Issues).

Methods

The most common method of venipuncture is the vacuum container method because multiple samples can be obtained at the same time, requiring fewer "sticks" for the patient and faster collection for the medical assistant. In using the vacuum container method, it is important to use a large vein, because the vacuum can collapse smaller veins. If the patient has no accessible larger veins, then it is appropriate to use a small needle with a syringe to obtain the specimen. (See Figures 43-1 and 43-2 and Procedure 43-2 for obtaining venous blood with a sterile syringe and needle.)

The butterfly method uses a needle that is attached to 6-to12-inch tubing. The end of the tubing can at-

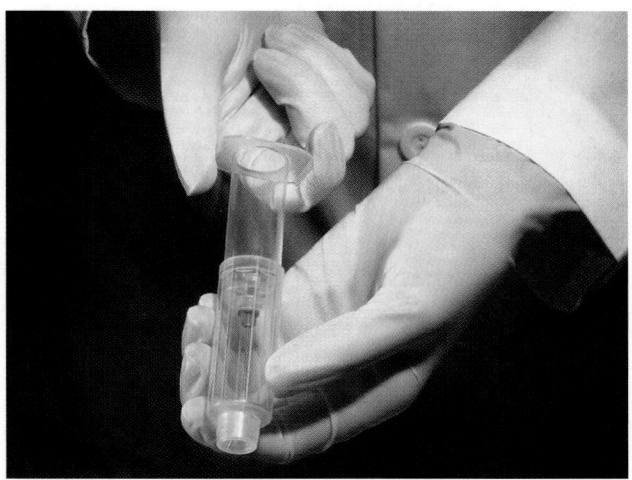
FIGURE 43-2 Vacutainer brand safety lock needle holder.

tach to the syringe or the vacuum container tube holder. The butterfly method is used for small veins that are difficult to draw with the standard vacuum container method or syringe and needle method. It is called the butterfly method because the needle on the end has a winged portion that keeps the needle from turning and anchors the needle into the small vein. The needle used for the butterfly method is a small 21-, 23-, or 25-gauge needle. The drawback to performing the butterfly method is the cost. The needle is more expensive than a standard needle. The butterfly method is not used for the majority of blood draws due to its expense.

Equipment

Figure 43-3 shows the equipment that a medical assistant will need to perform a venipuncture using the

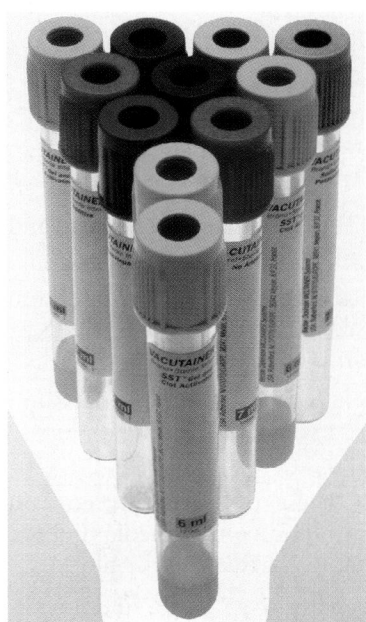
FIGURE 43-1 Vacutainer evacuated specimen tubes with Hemogard closure blood collection tubes.

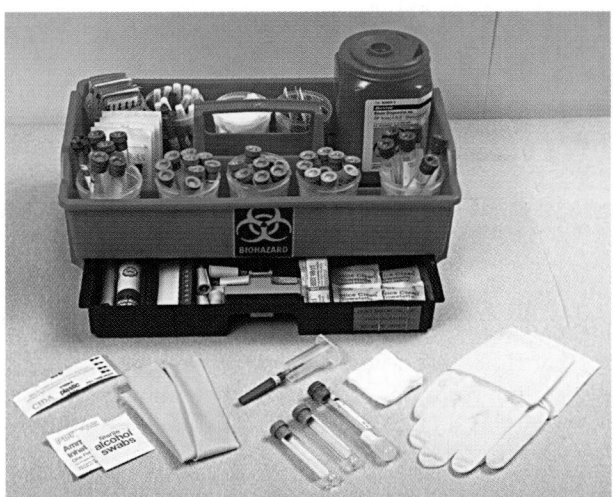
FIGURE 43-3 Venipuncture equipment.

Obtaining Venous Blood with a Sterile Syringe and Needle

OBJECTIVE: Perform a venipuncture using the syringe and needle method.

Equipment and Supplies

sterile 22-gauge needle and 10- to 20-mL syringe; appropriate vacuum specimen tubes for tests ordered; tourniquet; examination gloves; alcohol sponge; cotton balls or dry gauze square; adhesive bandage; patient's record; pen; lab coat; biohazard sharps container

Note: Always identify the patient by his or her arm-band and by asking the patient his or her name.

Method

1. Perform hand hygiene and assemble necessary equipment and supplies.
2. Securely attach the sterile needle to the syringe.
3. Put on examination gloves.
4. Apply a tourniquet 3 to 4 inches above the venipuncture site.
5. Palpate vein and clean the venipuncture site with an alcohol sponge and then dry with a clean gauze.
6. Have the patient make a fist and hold it shut until told to release it.
7. Make sure there is no air in the syringe.
8. Remove the needle guard and insert the needle into the vein.
9. Slowly pull back the syringe plunger until the proper amount of blood has been obtained.
10. Instruct the patient to open his or her fist.
11. Release the tourniquet and withdraw the needle quickly.
12. Fill the appropriate vacuum tubes to the proper level.
13. Apply gentle pressure to the puncture site with a piece of cotton or gauze with the patient's arm slightly raised for a few minutes. This may prevent hematomas from occurring.
14. Apply a bandage to the puncture site.
15. Discard the used needle and syringe into a biohazard sharps container.
16. Remove gloves and discard into appropriate container.
17. Perform hand hygiene.
18. Record procedure in patient's record.
19. Label tubes and send to lab.

---

vacuum container method. All equipment should be assembled and the expiration dates checked prior to attempting to use. Expired tubes should not be used, because they may not have a vacuum. There are various types of tubes, marked by their color. Each tube has a different chemical additive (anticoagulant) to keep the blood from clotting for different types of tests.

- Red top tubes: Contain no anticoagulant and have a sterile interior. A red top tube is typically used for serum chemistry testing.

- Marbled top (either red and gray or black, also called a tiger top) tubes: This is a serum separator tube (SST), which has a gel that separates the serum from the clot after centrifuging. It also contains a clot activator. This tube is commonly used for chemistry testing.

- Lavender/purple top tubes: These tubes contain ethylenediaminetetraacetic acid (EDTA) and are used for testing whole blood or plasma. This tube is used when testing a CBC or glycosylated hemoglobin.

- Green top tubes: These tubes contain heparin and are used for testing whole blood or plasma.

- Light blue top tubes: These tubes contain sodium citrate and are used when testing a PT/INR or PTT (clotting tests).

- Gray top tubes: These tubes contain potassium oxylate and are used when performing a glucose tolerance test.

- Yellow top tubes: These tubes usually contain some type of liquid blood culture media and are used when checking for bacteria in the blood.

Vacuum blood tubes come in 5-, 7-, 10-, and 15-mL sizes. The amount of blood needed for each test differs, so the tube sizes differ accordingly.

When drawing blood by the vacuum container method, it is important to fill the tubes in the recommended order specified by the National Committee for Clinical Laboratory Standards (NCCLS):

- Yellow top tubes: These tubes are filled first to ensure that the collection of blood is sterile.
- Tubes with no additives such as the red top and marble top tubes: These tubes are filled second in order to provide time for the blood to clot.
- Blue top tubes.
- Lavender, green, and gray top tubes: These are the last tubes to be filled.

It is important that all tubes be filled completely as recommended by the individual laboratory where the tubes will be sent for analysis. To avoid hemolysis, do not shake the red top tubes or the marble top tubes. The process of hemolysis is the releasing of the hemoglobin into the plasma of the cells. Shaking the tubes causes the red cells to rupture and release hemoglobin into the plasma or serum.

Sites

The antecubital space is the most commonly used site for venipuncture. This is the space just below the joint in the elbow. This space has four large veins that are easy to access, making this the site of choice. The most common vein used is the median cephalic vein (see Figure 43-4). Depending on a patient's condition, the medical assistant may need to obtain blood using a different site such as the back of the hand or heel of the foot.

Patient Preparation

The blood tests done in a physician's office typically require little preparation (see Patient Education). For some tests, such as a glucose tolerance test, cholesterol, or lipid level test, the patient should fast for 12 to 14 hours prior to the test. Few other tests require fasting. If fasting is required it is important to educate the patient on how many hours to fast prior to the blood draw. If the medical assistant has any question about issues such as fasting in preparation for the blood draw, a good resource is the laboratory to which the specimen is being sent. Testing labs typically have a lab assistant available to address these questions.

At the time of the blood draw, some patients may be anxious. It is important for the medical assistant to communicate clearly what the process involves in order to assist in alleviating the patient's fears (see Cultural Considerations). If the patient is a child, the parent's participation may be helpful in calming the patient.

Being prepared at the time of the blood draw can also help in diminishing patient anxieties. A patient is encouraged when sensing that the medical assistant is competent and knowledgeable in performing the blood

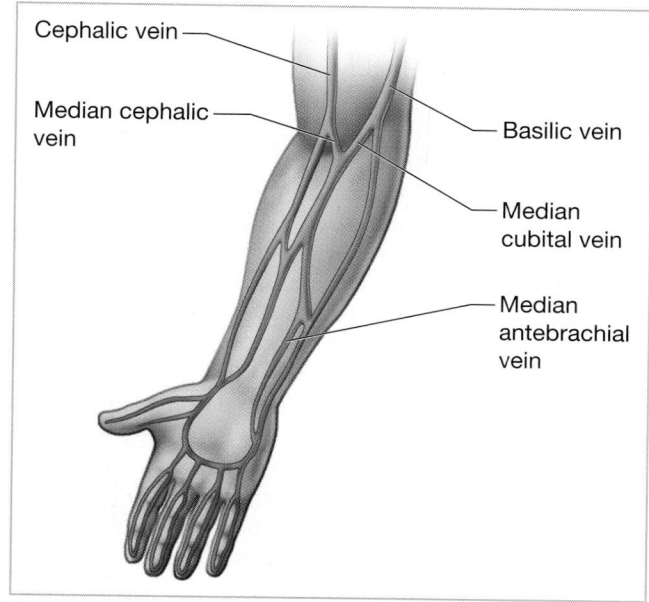

FIGURE 43-4 Anatomy of an arm for venipuncture.

When a test is going to be performed on a patient, it is important that the test be well explained to the patient. By doing so, the medical assistant can help lower the patient's anxieties and fears. Sometimes, depending on the patient's nationality, his or her native tongue may not be English. If this is the case, do not assume that you can explain the procedure clearly by speaking slowly and showing examples. If possible, locate an individual in the office who speaks the patient's native language. A family member may also be present to help. Request permission from the patient to have his or her family member assist in the explanation. Many medical offices now also have on hand various procedures that have been written out in other languages. These are extremely useful.

draw. Competency can be demonstrated by having the appropriate equipment assembled prior to the blood draw and ensuring that the correct blood specimens are drawn correctly. Patients who experience callbacks due to errors such as incorrect specimen handling will lose confidence in the medical assistant and the physician's office.

Unexpected events can happen when performing venipunctures. These include fainting, nausea, excessive anger exhibited by a patient, and uncontrollable bleeding. It is important that the medical assistant remain calm and deal with these situations professionally. When a patient begins to show signs of fainting, it is important to immediately withdraw the needle and request that the patient place his or her head and arms downward. The patient may need to lie down to further ensure his or her safety while recovering. Often in treatment rooms, ammonia is available and can be used to help revive a patient. If a patient does not immediately respond it is important to call another member of the clinical team for assistance.

When a patient becomes nauseous, have him or her breathe deeply through the mouth and provide an emesis basin if necessary. If a patient becomes angry during the procedure, it is important to remain calm and reassuring. If the behavior continues or is disruptive and endangers either the medical assistant or the patient, the procedure should be stopped immediately and the medical assistant should call for assistance in dealing with the situation.

Occasionally, uncontrollable bleeding can occur when the needle is withdrawn. If this occurs it is important to apply pressure to the site. Once pressure has been applied, it is important to call for assistance.

Other complications can make it difficult to perform the procedure or obtain the necessary amount of blood. For example, if a patient has small veins, it is sometimes helpful to apply a hot compress to the area. By doing so the veins may expand and may be easier to access. When veins have a tendency to roll, it is important to place one finger above the area where the needle is to be inserted in order to prevent the vein from moving. An incomplete draw may occur if a patient's vein does not produce enough blood. If this occurs, it will be necessary to obtain blood from a different vein. Some patients present a challenge to the inexperienced phlebotomist. Requesting that a more experienced professional perform the procedure may be necessary.

When drawing blood the medical assistant should wear personal protective equipment such as:

- Gloves
- Goggles and mask
- Gown or lab coat

Although these items are worn to protect the medical assistant from coming in contact with contaminated items, this attire can also promote a professional image that patients desire in their medical assistant.

See Figure 43-5 for an illustration of venipuncture equipment. To perform a venipuncture utilizing the Vacutainer method, review the procedures as outlined in Procedure 43-3.

Capillary Puncture (Manual)

Capillaries are the microscopic blood vessels that are the bridges between arterioles and venules. Oxygen and carbon dioxide are exchanged at the capillary level. Small amounts of blood can easily be obtained from the capillaries in a capillary puncture or "fingerstick" (see Figure 43-7).

Puncture Sites

Figure 43-8 shows the common capillary puncture sites for adults and infants. When performing capillary punctures, the medical assistant should take precautions to avoid using the thumb and index fingers on the hand of adults, because the skin is thicker there than on other fingers. The tissues on the lateral sides of the fingers are less sensitive than that in the middle, but a larger specimen can be obtained from the medial

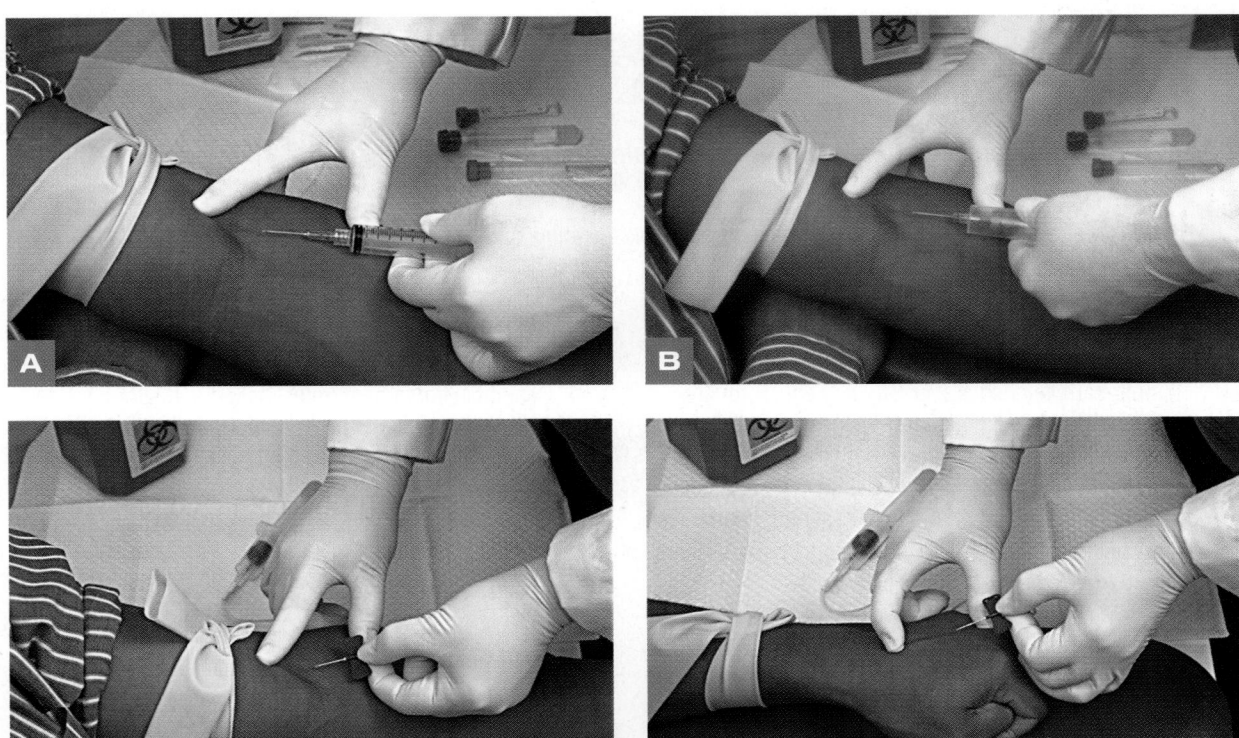

FIGURE 43-5 Demonstrating venipuncture equipment.

portions of the fingers. Earlobes are also a common site for adults. When doing a capillary puncture on infants, their fingers are not large enough to yield a sufficient sample, so the heels may be a better option.

Equipment and Supplies

Figure 43-9 shows the equipment needed for a capillary puncture. Lancets may be either manual or automatic (see Figure 43-10). The primary advantage of the automatic lancet is that the depth of the puncture is controlled by a spring-loaded mechanism, causing less pain to the patient. After a lancet is used, it should immediately be placed in a sharps container to prevent needle sticks. Procedure 43-4 outlines the process for a manual capillary puncture.

Routine Blood Tests

Blood analysis is one vital and routine tool of medicine. The medical assistant performs routine blood tests and procedures in the physician's office. More complex tests are performed by specially trained individuals, either a medical lab technician (MLT) or medical technologist (MT). Figures 43-12 and 43-13 show different hematology analyzing systems.

Physicians frequently order a complete blood count (CBC). A CBC typically consists of a microhematocrit, hemoglobin, WBC count, RBC count, platelet count, and differential white blood cell count (diff).

The medical assistant may be asked to perform a coagulation test. This test is done to determine how well a patient's blood is clotting. It is done on a routine basis with patients who are on blood-thinning medications such as Coumadin. This test is called a *prothrombin time*, more commonly referred to as a *protime*. Prothrombin is a protein in the blood plasma that is then converted to thrombin as part of the clotting process.

Often blood tests ordered for patients are ordered in panels. Common panels include the lipid panel and the liver panel. Included in the lipid panel are such tests as cholesterol, triglycerides, and high-density lipid. A liver panel includes tests such as SGOT and SGPT that can be used in the diagnosis of hepatitis. When performing blood tests, it is always essential that the medical assistant utilize the office lab manual to determine how much blood and the specific blood tube required for each test.

Diabetics monitor their blood sugar by the use of a portable machine such as the One Touch (Figure 43-14) or the Accu-chek. A patient who is diagnosed

text continued on page 914

PROCEDURE

Performing a Venipuncture Using the Vacutainer Method

OBJECTIVE: Perform venipuncture by correctly assembling, locating, and entering vein and withdrawing blood sample.

Equipment and Supplies

biohazard sharps container; Vacutainer tubes; multi-sample needle; 2 or 3 2-inch gauze squares; alcohol pads; examination gloves; Vacutainer sleeve; tourniquet; bandage; cotton balls; adhesive; ink pen; lab coat; patient record; ammonia ampules

Note: Follow Standard Precautions and safety guidelines when working with blood samples. Use care to avoid splashing or spilling blood. Wipe up all spills using guidelines established by OSHA.

Method

1. Perform hand hygiene.
2. Assemble equipment (refer to Figure 43-6A).
3. Identify the patient and explain the procedure. Ensure the patient is either sitting or lying down.
   Rationale: Explaining the procedure helps decrease anxiety. A sitting or lying down position is safer if the patient becomes faint (to prevent falls).

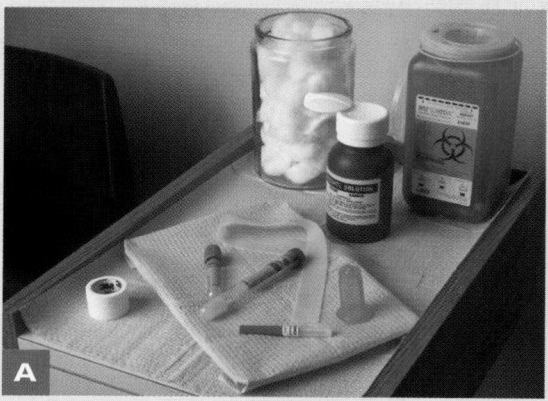
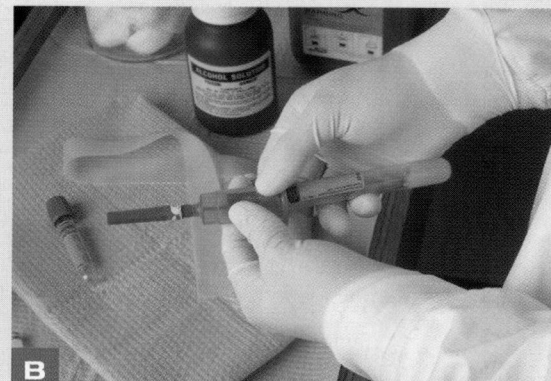
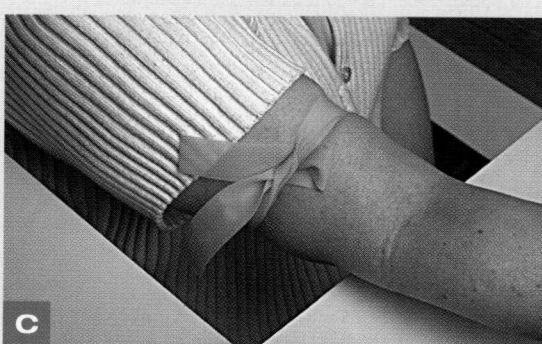
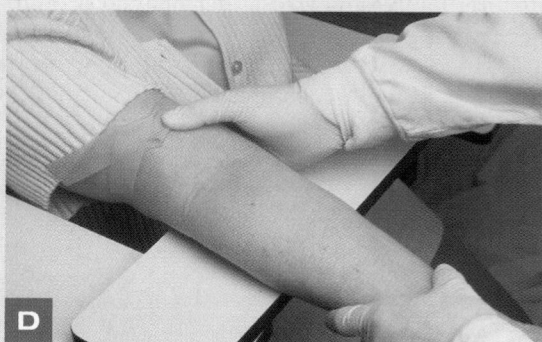

FIGURE 43-6 Venipuncture procedure.

4. Apply examination gloves.
5. Screw the Vacutainer needle into the plastic sleeve (Figure 43-6B). Insert the tube into the other end of the sleeve. The top of the colored stopper should reach the thin guide line on the sleeve. Do not press tube. If the tube exceeds the line, discard the tube; it may not have a vacuum.
6. Apply the rubber tourniquet about 2 inches above the antecubital space (Figure 43-6C). Place the middle of the tourniquet on the posterior (elbow) side of the arm. Crisscross the ends. While holding one end stable, tuck the other end in. This creates a tie that can be quickly released with one hand. In addition, the tourniquet should apply enough tension to engorge the vein with blood.

7. The arm should be in an extended position with the palm facing up (Figure 43-6D). Palpate the vein with your fingertips (Figure 43-6E). If a vein cannot be felt in one arm, try the other.
8. Wipe the site with an alcohol pad in a circular pattern beginning at the insertion site (Figure 43-6F). Let alcohol evaporate. Cleanse your gloved finger with alcohol in case you need to repalpate after site is cleansed.
9. Anchor or "fix" the vein by placing thumb of nondominant hand 2 inches below insertion site and pull skin toward hand (Figure 43-6G). *Rationale:* Veins are superficial and may roll when needle is inserted.
10. While holding onto the tube's sleeve with your dominant hand, insert needle smoothly and

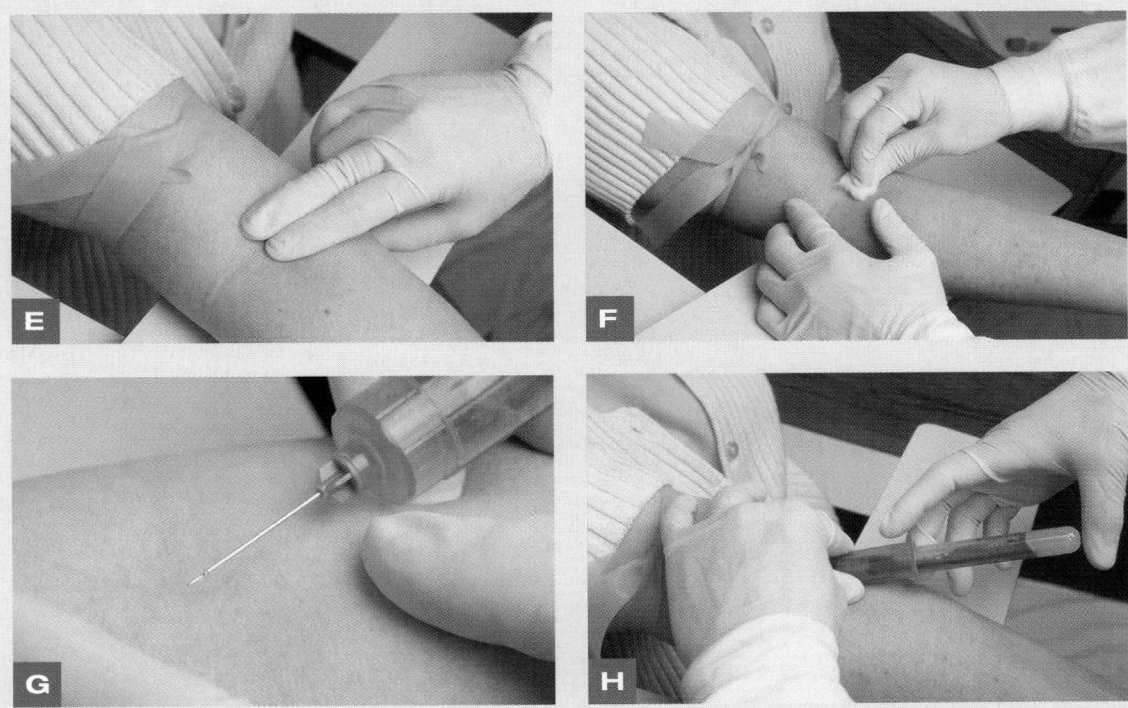

FIGURE 43-6 (*continued*).

Performing a Venipuncture Using the Vacutainer Method

rapidly at a 15-degree angle with the bevel up. The needle only needs to be inserted just past the bevel. If inserted too far, it will puncture both vein walls. Also keep needle in line with the vein.

11. While stabilizing the sleeve, push the tube into the sleeve. Use your thumb to push the tube and hold sleeve with index and middle finger on the flange (Figure 43-6H).
    Rationale: The sleeve must be perfectly stable or needle will damage the fragile vein and will result in a hematoma (bruise).

12. Allow the tube to fill. The vacuum will automatically fill the tube three-quarters full.

13. Remove the tube very carefully without moving the needle and apply a second tube if needed (Figure 43-6I). Gently roll the tube five to six times after removing it from the sleeve to allow the blood to mix with the additive. If both a red and purple tube are needed, collect blood in the red tube that contains no additive first.

14. After removing the last tube, release the tourniquet as soon as blood flow is established or just after the initial tube is full.

15. Remove the needle while covering the site with a gauze square. Immediately have patient apply firm, continuous pressure using a cotton ball or gauze square (Figure 43-6J).
    Rationale: Firm, continuous pressure will decrease chance of hematoma (bruise) formation.

16. Discard needle in sharps container (Figure 43-6K). Never recap needle if sharps container is available.
    Rationale: Recapping a needle is the most common cause of a needle stick. The main dangers from blood due to a needle stick are from hepatitis B and AIDS.

17. Gently invert all tubes collected 8 to 10 times in a figure-eight pattern.
    Rationale: RBCs are fragile and may hemolyze if handled improperly.

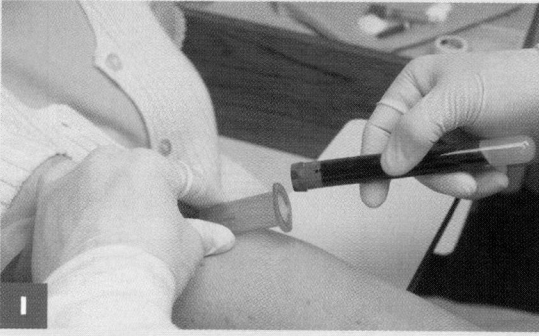
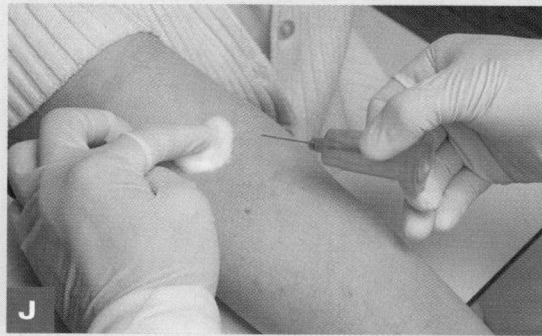

FIGURE 43-6   (*continued*).

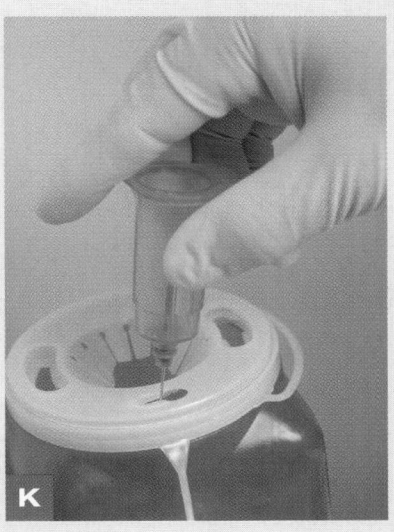

18. Assess the patient. Check the venipuncture site for bleeding, then apply some cotton and a strip of adhesive or a bandage (Figure 43-6L). Ask if the patient is dizzy or lightheaded.
    Rationale: If patient is dizzy or lightheaded, he or she may faint when attempting to stand.
19. Label tubes with patient's name, date, time, ID number, specimen type, tests to be done, and phlebotomist's initials. Fill out laboratory requisition sheet (Figure 43-6M).
20. Remove gloves. Perform hand hygiene.
21. Record procedure on patient's medical record.

Charting Example

2/28/XX	1.00 P.M.

Withdrew 10 mL of blood from L arm, no complications. Sent blood to in-office lab for CBC.

M. King, RMA

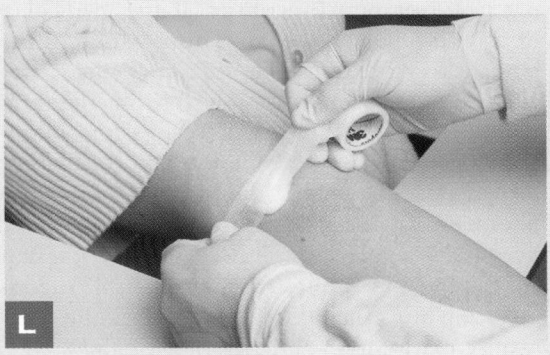

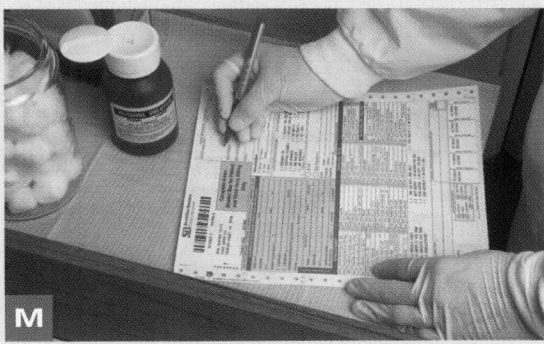

FIGURE 43-6 (*continued*)

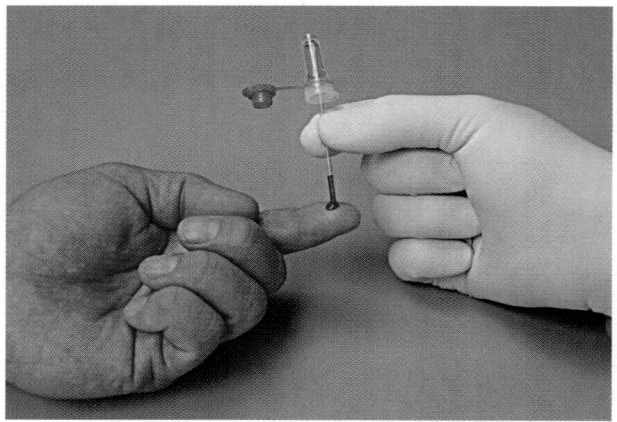

FIGURE 43-7   A fingerstick is useful for obtaining small amounts of blood.

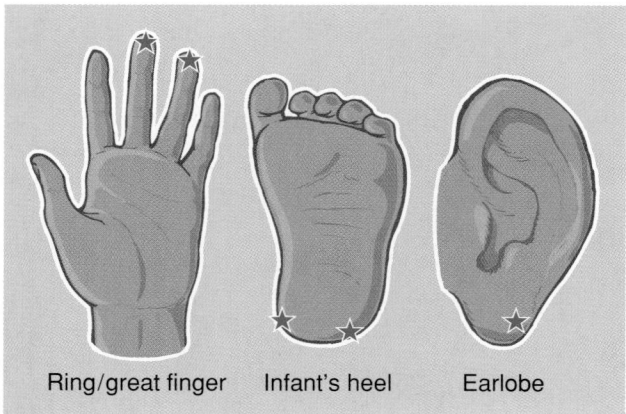

Ring/great finger   Infant's heel   Earlobe

FIGURE 43-8   Capillary puncture sites.

with diabetes may be anxious about performing this test. Proper education of the patient will be helpful in addressing their concerns. A recheck visit or follow-up call to the patient may be necessary to ensure that the patient's comfort level is achieved. This daily test is very critical to address the patient's diabetic condition.

The physician will often order a glycosylated hemoglobin (HbgA1C) to test the long-term control of diabetes. For this test it is critical that the patient be instructed to fast. If the patient fails to fast, the test results will be inaccurate. Concerns expressed by the patient regarding his or her medications should be directed to the physician. The physician will then determine if changes in medication must occur. To screen for blood glucose levels in diabetics, a glucometer may be utilized (see Procedure 43-5).

Other tests that a physician may order on a diabetic patient could include the glucose tolerance test. Although this test was traditionally done in a physician's office, it is now done more often in the outpa-

tient department at a hospital. The patient should be given clear instructions as to the location of the outpatient hospital department. Often hospitals provide maps that are useful to provide to the patient. The patient should be informed that this test requires several hours. This is due in part to the preparation, which involves drinking a solution and several blood draws.

Laboratory results are reported from the lab to the physician's office in a variety of ways including phone calls from the laboratory or by copies of the report being faxed or sent by courier. If the medical assistant receives a call from the laboratory with results, it is important to write down the correct results. Often physicians' offices will have standard forms that are used to record laboratory results. Lab slips for common tests such as urinalysis and common blood panels are often provided. This makes the process of recording the phone information easier. If a lab report does come in by phone it must be followed up with the hard-copy containing the results from the lab. The contents of most lab slips include the patient's name, the written results of the test, and the range values. Table 43-1 provides a list of some commonly performed laboratory tests and the range values.

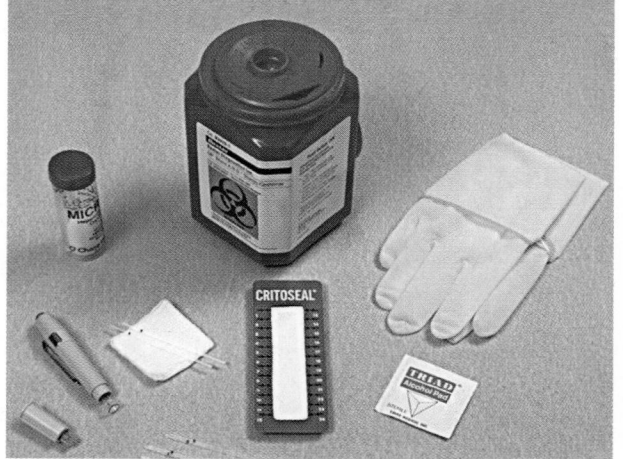

FIGURE 43-9   Capillary puncture equipment.

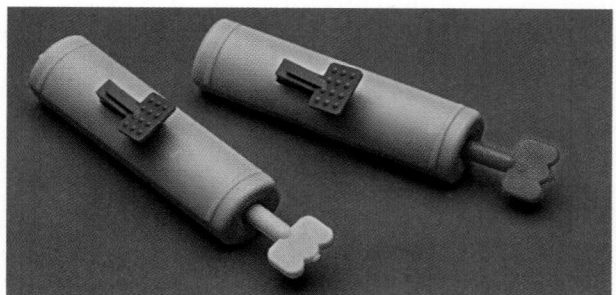

FIGURE 43-10   Spring-activated lancet.

PROCEDURE

Performing a Capillary Puncture (Manual)

OBJECTIVE: Perform a capillary stick using a lancet or spring-loaded lancet following correct aseptic technique and obtaining an adequate sample.

Equipment and Supplies

biohazard sharps container; examination gloves; alcohol pad; 2 × 2 gauze square; lancet or spring-loaded lancet; capillary tubes; sealing clay; ammonia ampules; bandage; lab coat

Note: Follow Standard Precautions and safety guidelines. Use care to avoid splashing or spilling blood. Wipe up all spills using guidelines established by OSHA.

Method

1. Perform hand hygiene.
   Rationale: Hand washing helps prevent the spread of infection.
2. Assemble equipment.
3. Identify the patient and explain the procedure. Have the patient either sitting or lying.
4. Apply examination gloves.
5. Select either the ring or great finger on the nondominant hand. Wipe the site with an alcohol pad. Let alcohol evaporate.
6. Remove plastic protective tip to expose the lancet.
7. Grasp patient's hand and gently squeeze the finger 1 inch below the chosen puncture site.
8. Puncture the site using a quick, jabbing motion across the fingerprints to obtain a full round drop of blood (Figure 43-11A). Do not puncture the direct center of the finger pad since the skin is generally tougher there. Immediately discard lancet in sharps container. (A spring-loaded lancet may also be used.)

9. Wipe away the first drop of blood with a gauze square.
   Rationale: The first drop contains alcohol and tissue fluid and will not provide accurate test results (Figure 43-11B).
10. Obtain the sample using a microhematocrit capillary tube (Figure 43-11C). The finger may be gently massaged to increase blood flow. Seal one end of the capillary tube in clay sealer (Figure 43-11D).
    Rationale: The reason for gently massaging rather than squeezing the finger is to avoid mixing the blood with other tissue fluids that may in turn hemolyze the red blood cells.
11. Apply clean gauze over the site and ask patient to apply firm, continuous pressure until the bleeding stops.
    Rationale: Firm, continuous pressure will decrease hematoma formation.
12. Assess patient and the site. Apply a bandage, if needed. Ask patient if he or she is dizzy or lightheaded.
13. Remove gloves and perform hand hygiene.
14. Record procedure on patient's medical record.

Charting Example

2/28/XX	1:30 P.M.

Performed capillary puncture on L ring finger, no complications.

M. King, RMA

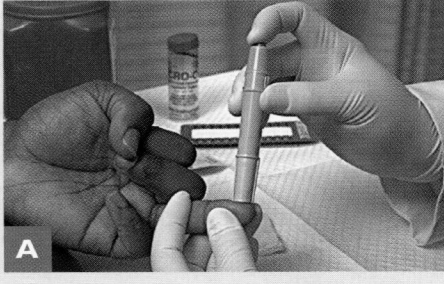
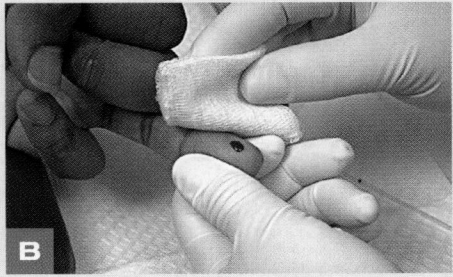
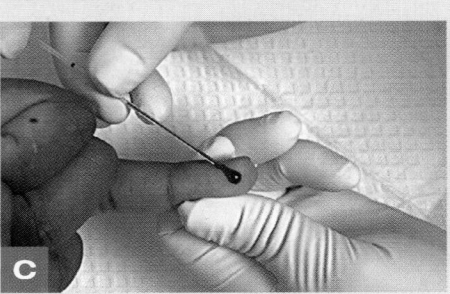
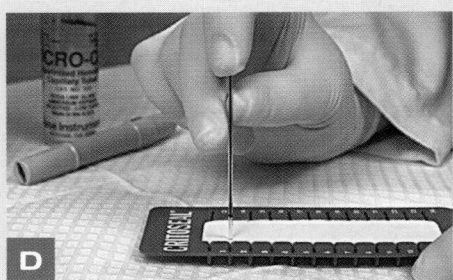

FIGURE 43-11   Capillary puncture procedure.

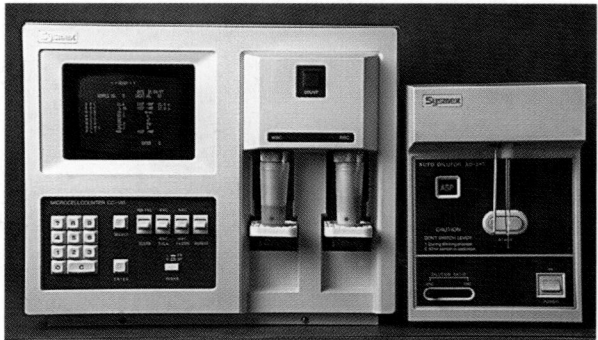

FIGURE 43-12   Whole-blood analyzer.

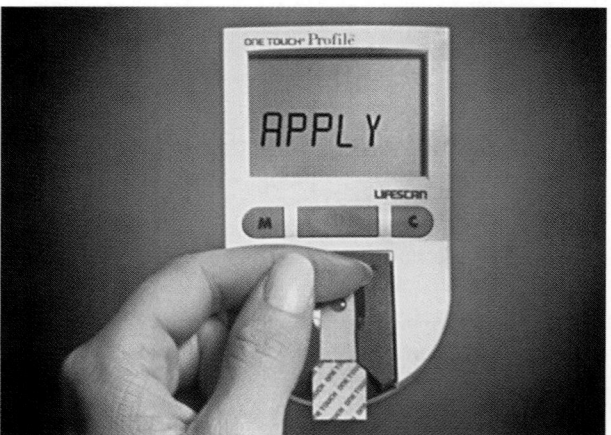

FIGURE 43-14   ONE TOUCH Profile diabetes blood sugar monitoring system.

Microhematocrit Procedure

The microhematocrit (crit) provides the physician with information about the patient's red blood cell volume. A low hematocrit indicates anemia (decrease in the quantity of circulating RBCs) or hemorrhage. An elevated hematocrit indicates dehydration or polycythemia. A normal hematocrit is 40% to 50% in males and 35% to 45% in females.

To perform a microhematocrit, the patient's blood must be drawn using capillary tubes. The patient's finger is cleansed with an alcoholic sponge and then dried with sterile gauze. The patient's finger is then punctured utilizing an automatic lancet or a manual lancet. The first drop of blood is wiped away with dry sterile gauze. The second and subsequent drops are drawn up using a capillary tube that is either tilted horizontally or slightly downward. When the tip of the tube touches the blood, the tube will automatically

draw the blood up by capillary action. The tube should be filled two-thirds to three-quarters of the way full and then sealed on each end. These tubes are then placed in a microhematocrit centrifuge that

TABLE 43-1	**Common Laboratory Tests and Their Normal Values**
Total cholesterol	130–200 mg/dL
Glucose	70–120 mg/dL
Triglycerides	40–150 mg/dL
Creatinine	0.7–1.4 mg/dL
Uric acid	3.5–7.5 mg/dL
BUN	8–20 mg/dL
Sodium	132–142 mEq/L
Potassium	5–5 mEq/L
Chloride	98–106 mEq/L
CO_2	25–32 mEq/L
White blood cell count	5,000–10,000/mm^3
Red blood cell count	$3.5–5.5 \times 10$/mm^3
Hemoglobin	12–16 g/dL
Hematocrit	35.5–49%
Sedimentation rate	0–10 mm/hr
Platelet count	15,000–35,000/mm^3

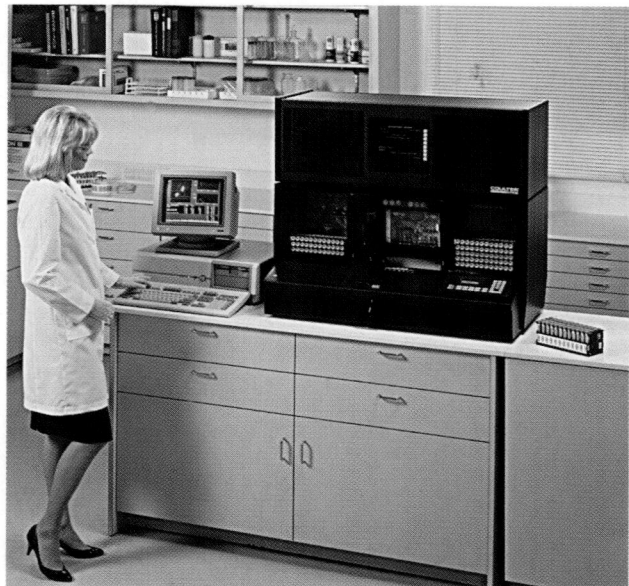

FIGURE 43-13   The COULTER STKS hematology analyzer system.

Screening for Glucose (Blood Sugar) Level

OBJECTIVE: Determine blood glucose level using a glucometer.

Equipment and Supplies

sterile lancet; reagent strips; glucometer; examination gloves; cotton balls; alcohol sponges; gauze squares; watch or clock; pen; lab coat; patient's record

Method

1. Identify the patient and make sure the patient is fasting if required.
2. Assemble the equipment and supplies.
3. Make sure the glucometer has been turned on the required amount of time and has been calibrated for accuracy according to the manufacturer's instructions.
4. Wash hands and put on examination gloves.
5. Perform a capillary blood puncture utilizing a sterile lancet.
6. Remove a plastic reagent strip from the bottle without touching the chemically treated portion.
7. Apply a large drop of blood from the capillary puncture to the chemically treated area so that it is completely covered.

8. Immediately begin timing for the duration specified by the manufacturer.
9. When the duration specified is complete, place the reagent strip into the glucometer and close the door.
10. At this time provide the patient with a dry gauze square to hold over the puncture site after wiping the site with an alcohol sponge.
11. Record the number of mg (milligrams) of glucose per 100 mL (milliliters) as displayed by the instrument.
12. Discard all used equipment and supplies. Remove gloves and wash hands.

Note: Several different types of testing instruments may be used to perform this test. It is critical to follow the manufacturer's instructions for the testing equipment provided.

---

performs cellular separation. For the complete procedure, review Procedure 43-6 and Figure 43-15.

Hemoglobin Determination

Hemoglobin (Hgb) provides the physician with information regarding the amount of hemoglobin present in the sample. A low Hgb may indicate iron-deficiency anemias, while elevated readings are present in patients with polycythemia and in extreme situations, such as burns. Normal values for adult females are 12 to 16 g/dL, and for males 14–18 g/dL.

Hemoglobin can either be measured by an automated blood analyzer or manually by using a hemoglobinometer (see Figures 43-16, 43-17, and 43-18). Typically, the manual method is less accurate and not as reliable as the automated blood analyzer.

Hemoglobin values can be determined utilizing two methods: the specific gravity method or the cyanmethemoglobin method. The specific gravity method is a screening method for blood donors. The cyanmethemoglobin

Preparing for
Externship

For some medical assistants blood draws can be both challenging and rewarding. If you find that performing laboratory tests are not your strength, be sure to work on this area while you are still in school. Ask your instructor to provide extra time in class or outside of class to test your skills. When selecting an externship it will be important to select one that will continue to provide you encouragement and assistance in gaining skills in this area. Communication regarding areas that continue to be challenging will be important so that the right type of help can be provided to you so that your skills can be developed. With some assistance and practice you will become proficient.

Performing a Microhematocrit

OBJECTIVE: Perform a microhematocrit on a capillary blood sample using proper aseptic technique.

Equipment and Supplies

biohazard sharps container; examination gloves; capillary tubes; sealing clay; microhematocrit centrifuge; whole blood; hematocrit card or other reader

Note: Follow Standard Precautions and safety guidelines when working with blood samples. Use care to avoid splashing or spilling blood. Wipe up all spills using guidelines established by OSHA.

Method

1. Perform hand hygiene and apply examination gloves.
2. Assemble equipment as shown in Figure 43-15A.
3. Fill two capillary tubes three-quarters full. The blood specimen can be obtained from a vacuum tube of anticoagulated blood using a plain capillary tube or directly from a fingerstick site using a heparinized capillary tube. Seal one end in the sealing clay.
4. Place capillary tubes in centrifuge with the sealed ends against the rubber gasket (Figure 43-15B). If more than one patient's blood is being tested, mark down the number of the slot the patient's tube is in. Spin for 3 to 5 minutes at 10,000 rpms. (Always check manufacturer's recommendations for proper time and speed.) After centrifuging, the sample will be separated into three layers:
   - Top layer is the plasma.
   - Middle layer, or the buffy coat, is made up of WBCs and platelets.
   - Bottom layer is packed RBCs.
5. Remove tubes immediately after centrifuge stops. *Rationale:* If tubes are not removed immediately, blood may begin to mix together.
6. Determine results. Use the Hct card by placing the sealing clay just below the zero line on both tubes. Then on both tubes match the top of the plasma with the 100 line. Read results on both tubes directly below the buffy coat. Then add those results together and divide by 2.
7. Discard tubes into sharps container.
8. Remove gloves and perform hand hygiene.
9. Record the value as a percentage on the patient's medical record.

Charting Example

| 2/28/XX | 1:45 P.M. | Hct 47%. |

M. King, CMA

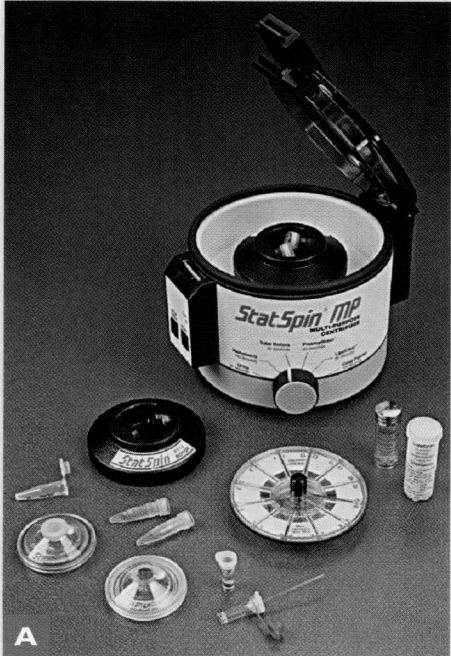

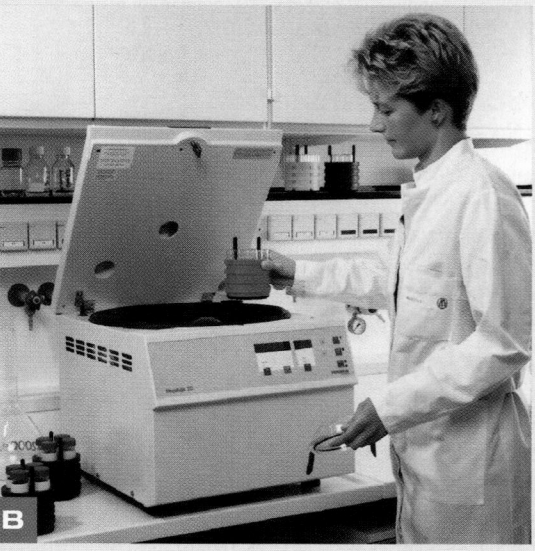

FIGURE 43-15 (A) Centrifuge and supplies; (B) loading a centrifuge.

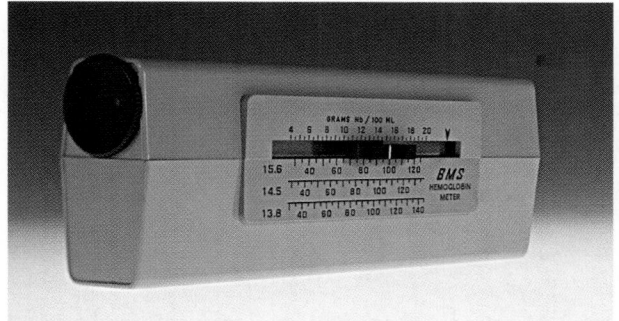

FIGURE 43-16 Hemoglobinometer.

is a more specific and accurate method to give exact hemoglobin levels using hemoglobin analyzers. (See Procedure 43-7 for a hemoglobin determination using the hemoglobinometer.)

White Blood Cell Count

Normal WBC counts range from 4.5 to 11 thousand/mm^3 in adults. An elevated level usually indicates infection (leukocytosis) or, if grossly elevated, may be leukemia. A low level usually indicates a viral infection or auto immunodeficiency.

A WBC count can be performed either manually by the medical assistant using a microscope or by an automated blood analyzer. The manual method of obtaining white blood counts is through the use of a hemacytometer. A hemacytometer is a special slide counting chamber that allows for counting of cells under the microscope. If testing is preformed manually, the medical assistant may use an automated tabulator to assist in counting the various types of cells (see Figure 43-19). Always follow the instructions on the automated analyzer exactly to ensure the validity of the results.

Red Blood Cell Count

Normal RBC volume in an adult female is 4.5 to 5.0 million/mm^3. In the adult male, it is about 5.0 to

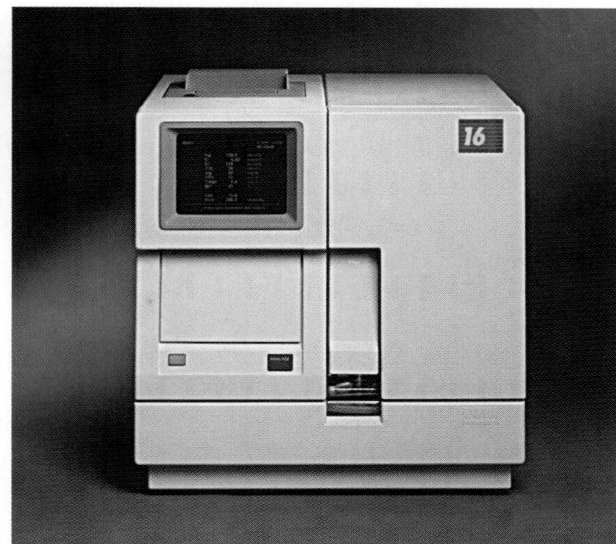

FIGURE 43-17 Nova 16 analyzer.

6.0 million/mm^3. An increase in the number of circulating RBCs may indicate polycythemia, whereas a decrease may indicate anemia.

A manual RBC count is similar to a manual WBC count. Both require small samples of the specimen to be diluted in a special solution. Then the sample is placed on a hemocytometer, which is placed on a microscope used to count the red and white blood cells.

Automated testing for RBCs is more common than manual testing. Always follow the machine's procedure manual exactly. The manual method of counting red blood cells is done with the hemacytometer.

Differential White Blood Cell Count

A differential white blood cell count (diff) determines the percentages of each type of WBC, RBC morphology, and platelet estimation. Performing this test manually is a skill that requires practice to achieve proficiency. The testing is done using a microscope with a bright light

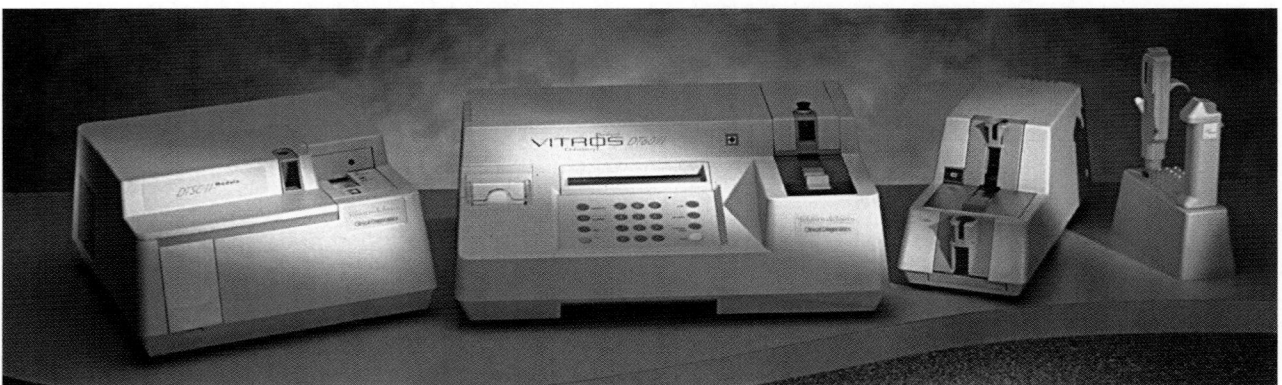

FIGURE 43-18 VITROS DT60II system.

PROCEDURE

Determining Hemoglobin Using the Hemoglobinometer

OBJECTIVE: Perform a blood test to determine hemoglobin levels using the hemoglobinometer.

Equipment and Supplies

hemoglobinometer; glass slide chamber; hemolysis applicator (plastic or wooden); sterile lancet; cotton balls; dry gauze square; alcohol sponges; examination gloves; patient's record; lab coat; biohazard sharps container

Note: Follow Standard Precautions and safety guidelines when working with blood samples. Use care to avoid splashing or spilling blood. Wipe up all spills using guidelines established by OSHA.

Method

1. Perform hand hygiene and put on examination gloves.
2. Gather the necessary equipment and supplies.
3. Using a manual lancet or auto lancet, obtain capillary blood.
4. Pull the glass chamber out of the hemoglobinometer and position the lower part of the slide so that it is slightly offset.
5. Place a large drop of capillary blood onto the slide.
6. Wipe the patient's puncture site with a cotton ball and provide the patient with a dry gauze square to apply mild pressure to the puncture. This should stop further bleeding.
7. Mix blood with hemolysis applicator until the blood becomes clear.
8. Push the glass chamber into the clip and place into the slot on the left side of the hemoglobinometer.
9. Hold the hemoglobinometer in your left hand at eye level while using your left thumb to turn on the light by depressing the bottom button. Look into the instrument to see a split green field.
10. Slide the button on the right side of the meter with your right thumb and index finger while looking into the meter until a matching green field occurs. Leave the sliding scale on the calibrated line where the solid green field appeared.
11. Read the hemoglobin value at the top scale. The results are read as grams of hemoglobin per 100 mL of blood (g/dL).
12. Wash chamber and reusable hemolysis applicator with a detergent solution, rinse, dry, and return to the instrument for the next test.
13. Remove gloves and perform hand hygiene. Discard gloves and nonreusable supplies in appropriate containers.
14. Record the results in the patient's record.

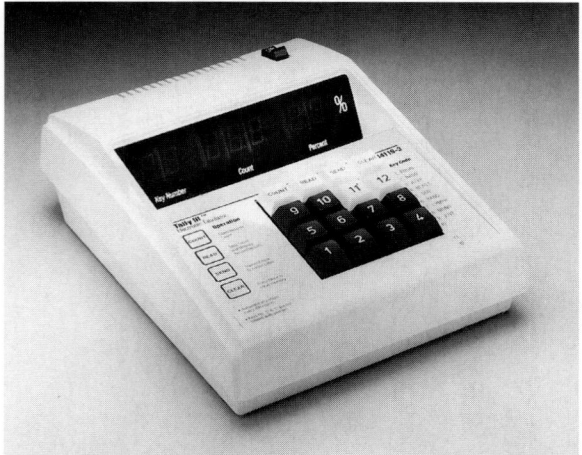

FIGURE 43-19   Electronic tabulator.

and 100× magnification with an oil immersion slide. Focus near the edge of the stained slide where the cells are feathered, and where the cells are one layer thick. This test can also be performed by the automated analyzer (see Procedure 43-8 for slide preparation and also Figures 43-20 and 43-21.)

Red Blood Cells

RBCs are the most numerous, are salmon colored, and appear oval with a slightly pale center. RBCs have no nucleus or granules. RBCs with a nucleus are called reticulocytse (immature RBCs). Normal looking RBCs are recorded as "normal RBC morphology."

Platelets

Platelets are the smallest of the formed blood elements. They are about half the size of a RBC. They stain purple and tend to appear in a clump, although they may also exist singly. They appear if they have a rough outer edge and contain small granules. There are between 200,000 and 300,000 platelets per cubic millimeter of the blood. There are typically between 5 and 20 platelets in one field of view. If this number is counted, then record the platelet count as "adequate platelet estimation."

White Blood Cells

There are five types of white blood cells, each of which has a distinct identifying characteristic when using the Wright's staining method. Count 100 WBCs, then express each of the cell types as a percentage. Normal values for adults are:

- Neutrophils 50–70%
- Eosinophils 1–4%
- Basophils 0–1%
- Lymphocytes 20–35%
- Monocytes 3–8%

Values may differ between manual and automated analyses.

GRANULATED WHITE BLOOD CELLS The neutrophil, or seg, is the most numerous WBC. The neutrophil has small cytoplasmic granules that stain pink or lilac with a multilobed nucleus with small strands connecting each of the lobes, which stain purple. A band neutrophil is an immature neutrophil. It appears similar to the neutrophil except that the nucleus is nonsegmented and curved with a band-like structure. Cytoplasmic granules stain blue to pink.

Eosinophils have segmented nuclei and large, reddish staining granules that are found in the cytoplasm. Basophils are rarely seen in a diff count. This WBC has an S-shaped nucleus and large, irregularly shaped purplish-blue granules that almost entirely cover the nucleus.

ANGRANULOCYTIC WHITE BLOOD CELLS Lymphocytes have a single round or lightly indented nucleus, which almost completely fills the cell. The cytoplasm is clear and stains a pale blue. Lymphocytes are the smallest WBC.

Monocytes are the largest WBC and have a distinct kidney-bean-shaped nucleus. The cytoplasm is abundant and clear, and it stains a grayish blue.

Erythrocyte Sedimentation Rate

The erythrocyte sedimentation rate (ESR) (also called the sed rate) measures the rate at which RBCs settle at the bottom of a tube. Drawing a patient's ESR can be done utilizing either the Wintrobe or Westergren method.

When performing the Wintrobe method, the Wintrobe tube is calibrated in mm/hr. The rate is the height of the RBCs in the bottom of the tube (see Procedure 43-9 and Figure 43-22).

Depending on the type of method used, the normal values may vary. Utilizing the Wintrobe method the normal ESR in an adult female is 0 to 20 mm/hr and in an adult male 0 to 9 mm/hr. Increased values may mean inflammation. An individual's ESR may also be elevated due to a variety of reasons including menstruation, pregnancy, and malignant tumors.

An ESR itself is not diagnostic, but it is used in conjunction with other tests for diagnosis. As an example, when testing for rheumatoid arthritis or fibromyalgia, an ESR may be done in conjunction with the antinuclear antibody test (ANA).

The sed rate is related to the condition of the red blood cells and the amount of fibrinogen in the plasma. When an individual presents with a disease, the surfaces of the membranes of the cells are affected. When a sed rate test is conducted on a patient, the rate at which the RBCs fall indicates the existence of possible conditions.

Phenylketonuria

Phenylketonuria (PKU) is a congenital disease caused by a defect in the metabolism of the amino acid phenylalanine. The unmetabolized protein accumulates in the bloodstream and, if undetected and untreated, will result in mental retardation. The PKU test is always performed on newborns to determine the presence of the unmetabolized protein phenylalanine. The test is typically performed in the hospital but may be performed in the office if not done in the hospital. To perform the PKU test see Procedure 43-10.

Mono Testing

The mono test, which is also known as the mononucleosis spot test, is used to help determine whether a patient has inefectious mononucleosis (see Procedure 43-11). It is frequently ordered along with a CBC (complete blood count). A step test may be ordered with the mono test to determine whether a person's sore throat is due to a streptococcal infection instead of or in addition to mononucleosis.

A mono test is primarily ordered when an adolescent patient has symptoms such as fever, headache, swollen glands, and fatigue that the doctor suspects are due to infectious mononucleosis. The test may be repeated when it is initially negative but suspicion of mono remains high. The physician may order a repeat test in a week or so to see if heterophile antibodies

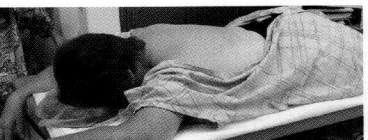 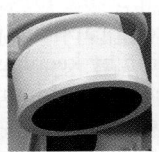 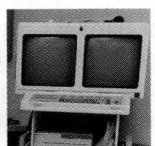

Medical Assistant Role Delineation Chart

HIGHLIGHT indicates material covered in this chapter.

ADMINISTRATIVE

Administrative Procedures

- Perform basic administrative medical assisting functions
- Schedule, coordinate and monitor appointments
- Schedule inpatient/outpatient admissions and procedures
- Understand and apply third-party guidelines
- Obtain reimbursement through accurate claims submission
- Monitor third-party reimbursement
- Understand and adhere to managed care policies and procedures
- *Negotiate managed care contracts*

Practice Finances

- Perform procedural and diagnostic coding
- Apply bookkeeping principles

- Manage accounts receivable
- *Manage accounts payable*
- *Process payroll*
- *Document and maintain accounting and banking records*
- *Develop and maintain fee schedules*
- *Manage renewals of business and professional insurance policies*
- *Manage personnel benefits and maintain records*
- *Perform marketing, financial, and strategic planning*

CLINICAL

Fundamental Principles

- Apply principles of aseptic technique and infection control
- Comply with quality assurance practices
- Screen and follow up patient test results

Diagnostic Orders

- Collect and process specimens
- Perform diagnostic tests

Patient Care

- Adhere to established patient screening procedures
- Obtain patient history and vital signs
- Prepare and maintain examination and treatment areas
- Prepare patient for examinations, procedures and treatments

- Assist with examinations, procedures and treatments
- Prepare and administer medications and immunizations
- Maintain medication and immunization records
- Recognize and respond to emergencies
- Coordinate patient care information with other health care providers
- Initiate IV and administer IV medications with appropriate training and as permitted by state law

GENERAL

Professionalism

- Display a professional manner and image
- Demonstrate initiative and responsibility
- Work as a member of the health care team
- Prioritize and perform multiple tasks
- Adapt to change
- Promote the CMA credential
- Enhance skills through continuing education
- Treat all patients with compassion and empathy
- Promote the practice through positive public relations

Communication Skills

- Recognize and respect cultural diversity
- Adapt communications to individual's ability to understand
- Use professional telephone technique

- Recognize and respond effectively to verbal, nonverbal, and written communications
- Use medical terminology appropriately
- Utilize electronic technology to receive, organize, prioritize and transmit information
- Serve as liaison

Legal Concepts

- Perform within legal and ethical boundaries
- Prepare and maintain medical records
- Document accurately
- Follow employer's established policies dealing with the health care contract
- Implement and maintain federal and state health care legislation and regulations
- Comply with established risk management and safety procedures
- Recognize professional credentialing criteria
- *Develop and maintain personnel, policy and procedure manuals*

Instruction

- Instruct individuals according to their needs
- Explain office policies and procedures
- Teach methods of health promotion and disease prevention
- Locate community resources and disseminate information
- *Develop educational materials*
- *Conduct continuing education activities*

Operational Functions

- Perform inventory of supplies and equipment
- Perform routine maintenance of administrative and clinical equipment
- Apply computer techniques to support office operations
- *Perform personnel management functions*
- *Negotiate leases and prices for equipment and supply contracts*

- *Denotes advanced skills.*

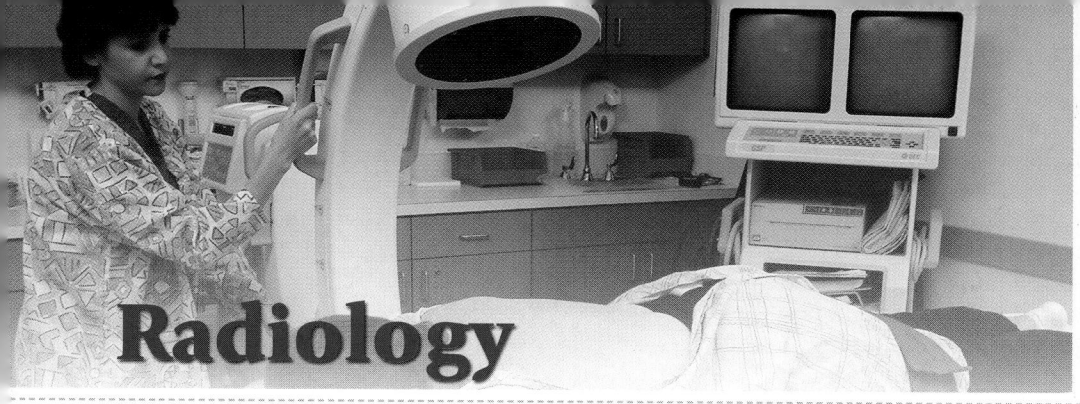

Radiology

chapter
44

Learning Objectives

After completing this chapter, you should be able to:

- Define and spell the terms to learn for this chapter.

- List and explain four basic positions used for taking x-rays.

- Discuss positron emission tomography (PET), computerized tomography (CT), magnetic resonance imaging (MRI) and ultrasound.

- Define and discuss the use for radiology, radiation therapy, and nuclear medicine.

- Describe the process and medical use of fluoroscopy.

- Describe the safety precautions to take for health care workers and patients relating to x-ray procedures.

- List four side effects of radiation therapy.

- List six x-ray procedures that require preparations ahead of time. Describe the preparations.

- Discuss the proper methods for storage of x-ray film and x-rays.

OUTLINE

Radiology	930
Diagnostic Imaging Overview	931
Preparing and Positioning the Patient	932
Diagnostic Imaging Procedures	936
Radiation Therapy	945
Nuclear Medicine	946
Safety Precautions	947
Radiographic Equipment	949
Processing X-ray Film	950
Storage and Records	951
Ownership of Film	951

Terms to Learn

angiography	grid	radiolucent
bucky	nuclear medicine	radiopaque
claustrophobia	rad	rem
collimeter	radioactive	retrograde
cumulative	radiation	transducer
dosimeter	radiograph	x-ray
fluoroscopy	radiologist	
gantry	radiology	

Case Study

IVAN THOMAS, A 17-YEAR OLD MALE PATIENT, has been referred to your diagnostic imaging facility for an IVP. He had a pre-college physical examination and his blood urea nitrogen test (BUN) was slightly elevated. The physician recommended that he have an IVP and told him to report at the assigned time for his procedure. While they explained that an IVP was a type of x-ray, the office staff at his primary physician's office neglected to tell him how to prepare for the test. He does not want to have the procedure in the first place. When he shows up, you begin by asking him some basic questions.

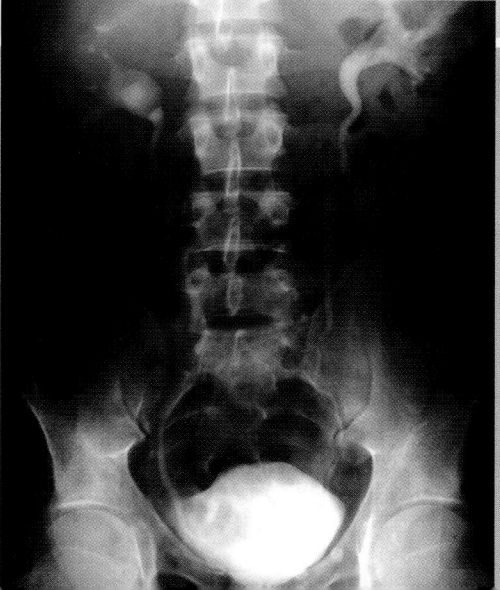

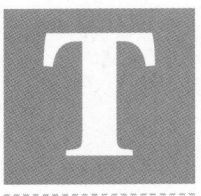he study of radiology includes an understanding of the use of x-rays, diagnostic radiology, radiation therapy, and nuclear medicine. A radiologist is a physician specializing in radiology. A radiographer or radiologic technologist is involved in making diagnostic radiographs or x-rays. His or her duties include positioning patients for radiographic procedures, determining the proper voltage, current, exposure time for each x-ray, adjusting radiographic equipment, developing the film, and assisting the radiologist with special procedures. To become a radiologic technologist requires a two- to four-year college program. The medical assistant in a radiology department will require additional training in order to assist with radiologic procedures. Professionalism discusses further information about requirements. Safety issues and requirements must also be followed when working in and around x-ray equipment.

Radiology

Radiology is the branch of medicine that uses radioactive substances or matter that give off radiation and various techniques for visualizing the internal structures of the body for the diagnosis and treatment of disease.

Professionalism

During your educational program preparing for medical assisting, you have been introduced to the field of radiography. Radiography is a complicated field and to become a radiologic technologist or radiographer takes advanced schooling and training experience. Radiographers perform imaging procedures ordered by physicians; operate several different types of imaging equipment, produce images through the use of ultrasound, magnetic resonance imaging, or radionuclide procedures. "Rad Techs" as they are known in the health care field, have career opportunities in doctors' offices, private imaging facilities, hospitals, and clinics.

To become a radiologic technologist, a student must graduate from a two- or four-year degree program in radiology and pass a national registration examination administered by the American Registry of Radiologic Technologies. Passing this examination earns the candidate the title of Registered Radiologic Technologist (RRT). For more information regarding a career in radiology, contact the American Society of Radiologic Technologists, 15000 Central Avenue SE, Albuquerque, NM 87123, Tel (800) 444-2778.

Radiology uses x-rays, radioactive substances, and other forms of radiant energy such as ultraviolet rays. Radiology can be divided into three specialties: diagnostic radiology, radiation therapy, and nuclear medicine. A discussion of various x-ray, fluoroscopic, and radiologic procedures follows.

Principles of X-rays

X-rays were discovered by Wilhelm Konrad Roentgen in 1895. X-rays are produced in a vacuum tube when electrons, traveling at the speed of light (186,000 miles per second), collide into a target made of specific materials such as tungsten. This collision produces electromagnetic rays that have high energy and very short wavelengths, which are not visible to the human eye. When x-rays are emitted from the tube, they form a cone-shaped x-ray beam. The radiation field is the cross section of the x-ray beam and the point of use (Figure 44-1). The patient is placed between the tube producing the x-ray beam and the film.

The discovery of the x-ray revolutionized the diagnosis of disease. X-rays can penetrate most materials and therefore are useful for making photographic images for diagnostic purposes. They are used in the procedures of radiography and fluoroscopy.

X-ray images or radiographs are produced by projecting x-rays through organs or structures of the body onto photographic film. Some structures such as bones are more radiopaque and allow fewer x-rays to pass through; other softer tissues, such as skin and lungs, are radiolucent permitting greater penetration of x-rays. Thus radiopaque tissue, such as bone, appears light on the film and radiolucent tissue, such as the lungs, leave a shadowy, dark image. X-rays films can then be examined for defects in bones and tissues. In addition, x-rays that penetrate the body are able to change the basic structure of body cells. Thus they have been useful in the diagnosis and treatment of tumors.

Characteristics of X-rays

X-rays have several characteristics that make them useful in the field of medicine. X-rays:

- are able to penetrate substances of different densities to varying degree
- cause ionization of the substances through which they pass (Ionization is the process, which causes the gain or loss of electrons from a neutral atom. Loss of electron = positive charge; gain of electron = negative charge)
- cause fluorescence of certain substances (Internal structures show up dark on a glowing screen as x-rays pass through allowing physicians to visualize structures in motion)
- travel in a straight line so the x-ray beam can be directed at a specific area

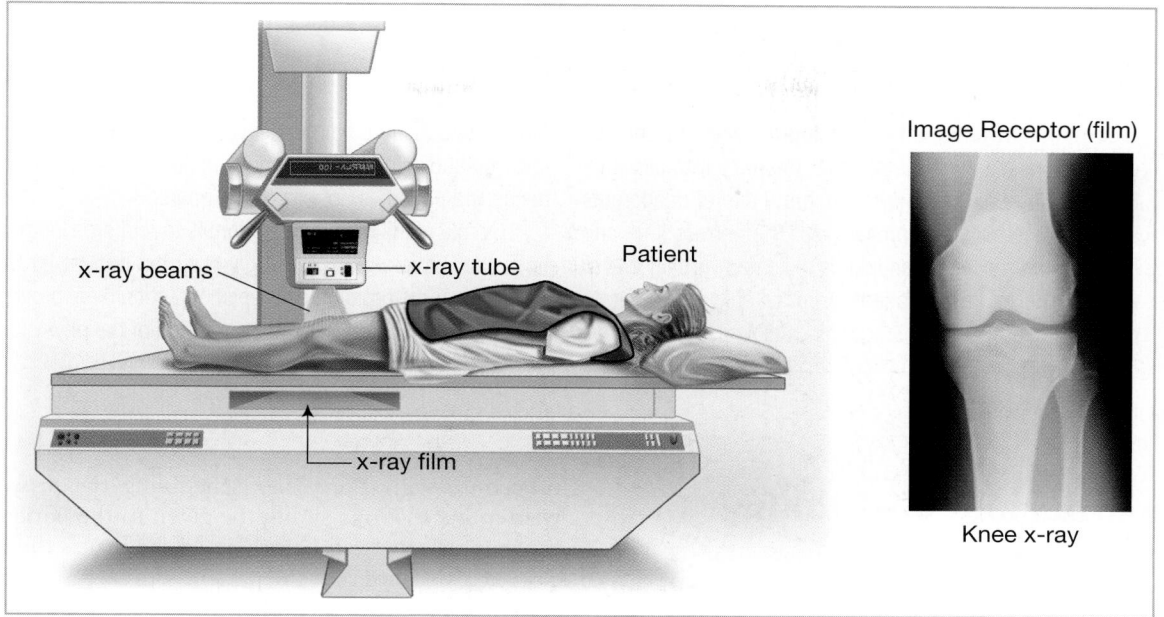

FIGURE 44-1 The patient is placed between the x-ray tube, which emits a cone-shaped x-ray beam, and the film or image receptor. Bones do not allow the x-ray beam to pass through, resulting in an image of the bones on the film.

- can destroy body cells and can be used to kill cancer cells

Since x-rays are invisible and produce no sound or smell, precautions must be taken to protect patients and employees from unnecessary exposure. Safety precautions will be discussed later in the chapter.

Diagnostic Imaging Overview

Diagnostic imaging involves the use of x-rays, ultrasound, radiopharmaceuticals, radiopaque media, and computers to produce images of internal structures and processes. Advances in the field of electronics have made possible noninvasive procedures for visualizing organs and processes that previously required surgical procedures.

The Use of a Contrast Medium

A contrast medium is a radiopaque substance, which does not allow the passage of x-rays, but facilitates radiographic imaging of internal structures that are difficult to visualize on a regular x-ray or fluoroscopic screen. The body structure or organ with the contrast medium, for example the gallbladder, is seen in contrast to adjacent structures.

Contrast media include liquids (barium), powders, air, and gas. They are administered orally, by injection (parenterally), or by enema. The contrast medium acts to convert an organ or structure into an opaque area. In this way, the actual function of that particular organ or structure can be visualized under fluoroscopy or by film.

Barium Sulfate

Barium sulfate and iodine are positive contrast media, which means they have more density and thus can absorb more radiation. Positive contrast media will appear white on x-ray images. This differs from air, a negative contrast medium, which allows more x-rays to pass through. Barium sulfate consists of a chalky compound mixed with water and flavoring to the right consistency for a patient to drink or for a technician to administer as an enema. Barium sulfate is used for fluoroscopic examination of the gastrointestinal tract.

Iodine Contrast Compounds

Iodine compounds used to form radiopaque compounds are employed for thyroid studies, pyelograms, angiograms, and cholecystograms. Iodine compounds should not be used if the patient is allergic to seafood or iodine. In addition, iodine radiopaque compounds interfere with nuclear medicine. Therefore, these two types of studies should not be performed during the same time period.

Negative Contrast

Negative contrast media include air, carbon dioxide, and other gases. These will appear black on x-rays. These media are used to visualize the spinal cord, as in a myelogram, and joints. The introduction of gas and air into the body can result in severe headaches following procedures such as myelograms. Negative contrast studies have largely been replaced with the use of the magnetic resonance imaging (MRI).

Thorough instructions for radiologic procedures include explanations, such as the need for the patient to administer cleansing enemas and to avoid the use of deodorants and powders for some procedures. The correct time and place for the procedure should be indicated verbally and in writing. The informed patient is better able to cooperate during the preparation stage for radiologic procedures.

Clear instructions ultimately save time and money for all involved and help to prevent the need to repeat procedures because a patient is not properly prepared.

The role of the medical assistant is to reinforce instructions that have already been given to the patient by the physician or the radiology therapist. You should not provide advice for the patient without permission of the physician.

Preparing and Positioning the Patient

The role of the medical assistant is to schedule the procedure ordered by the physician, educate the patient about the procedure, explain the preparations needed before hand, and inform him or her how long the entire procedure will take. After scheduling the procedure, written instructions should be given to the patient and thoroughly reviewed before he or she leaves the office. This helps ensure that the patient will be prepared correctly for the procedure when arriving at the appointed time. Patient Education has more information about patient preparation. Once the procedure is concluded,

TABLE 44-1 **X-ray Procedures Requiring Special Preparations**

Procedure	Preparation
Angiogram	No breakfast if morning examination or lunch if afternoon examination.
Barium enema (Lower GI)	Enemas until the bowel return is clear on the evening before the examination, may order rectal suppository in the morning or a cathartic such as 2 oz. of castor oil or citrate of magnesia at 4:00 P.M. the day before the x-ray, clear liquids and jello for dinner, nothing by mouth (NPO) after midnight.
Barium meal (Upper GI)	NPO after midnight.
Bronchogram	NPO.
Cholecystogram (GB series)	Light supper of non fatty food such as fruit and vegetables without butter or oil the evening before the x-ray, gallbladder tablets (prescribed by the physician) are taken with water after supper, NPO except for water until x-ray the following day.
Computerized tomography (CT)	NPO for 4 hours before x-ray if a contrast media is used.
Intravenous cholangiogram	NPO.
Intravenous pyelogram (IVP)	Three Dulcolax tablets or 2 oz. castor oil at 4:00 P.M. the day before the x-ray, eat a light supper, NPO after midnight.
Myelogram	NPO.
Retrograde pyelogram	Enemas or laxatives on the evening before x-ray, NPO for 8 hours before the procedure.
Ultrasound	May require a full bladder or laxatives depending on the type of ultrasound.

it will be your duty to assist the patient, provide post procedure instructions, and inform him or her when to expect the test results. For some x-ray procedures, special patient preparation must be performed before the patient can be examined. These procedures are described in Table 44-1.

For many radiology examinations, the patient will be asked to undress and wear a patient gown. Many of the procedures involve positions and interventions that may be embarrassing to the patient. The medical assistant must make every effort to provide an ample size gown and drape the patient to preserve his or her privacy. Cultural Considerations reviews some cultural factors when preparing patients for procedures. Request that the patient remove all metallic materials such as jewelry, belt buckles, watches, eyeglasses, hairpins, earrings, and hearing aids. In some x-rays of the head, mouth, and neck, the patient may have to remove dentures. Since the patient is not able to wear jewelry during the procedure, a safe container or locker should be provided for personal belongings.

The patient may need assistance getting onto the x-ray table. A footstool should be available if the table is high. X-ray tables do not have side rails. If there is a concern that the patient may become confused, then someone must remain in the room with the patient until the procedure begins. The x-ray technician should be told about the patient's confused state. Children may require special attention and need someone to help them maintain the correct position. Anyone who has to be in the room during an x-ray procedure must follow the strictest safety considerations.

Positioning

Although it is unlikely that you will be positioning a patient for a diagnostic imaging procedure, it will be helpful for you to understand that the patient position relative to the source of x-rays determines the images produced. It may be helpful to review anatomical locations on or in the body presented in Chapter 19.

Preparing for Externship suggests how to have a better understanding when positioning patients. Figure 44-2 illustrates x-ray pathways and the image produced when the patient is placed in a specific position. The position of the patient and the position of the x-ray beam need to be known ahead of time by the technician. The position of the patient is critical for an accurate x-ray. Table 44-2 lists radiology positions and descriptions of each position. Procedure 44-1 lists the steps for a general x-ray examination.

Scheduling Guidelines

The medical assistant often has the responsibility of scheduling the patient and providing instruction for radiologic procedures. If the procedure is performed in a facility other than the medical office, you may have to call to make the appointment. When setting an appointment, have the patient's name, type of insurance with pre-certification or approval number,

Preparing for
Externship

In preparation for your externship, work with a classmate in your laboratory and practice all the positions required for x-rays. You must be completely familiar with all the terms referring to anatomical positions so you are able to correctly instruct the patient to assume those positions. By taking turns as medical assistant and then patient, you will experience first hand how difficult it would be for some patients to readily take the positions as instructed. By putting yourself in the patient's shoes, you will become a more empathetic, understanding health care provider.

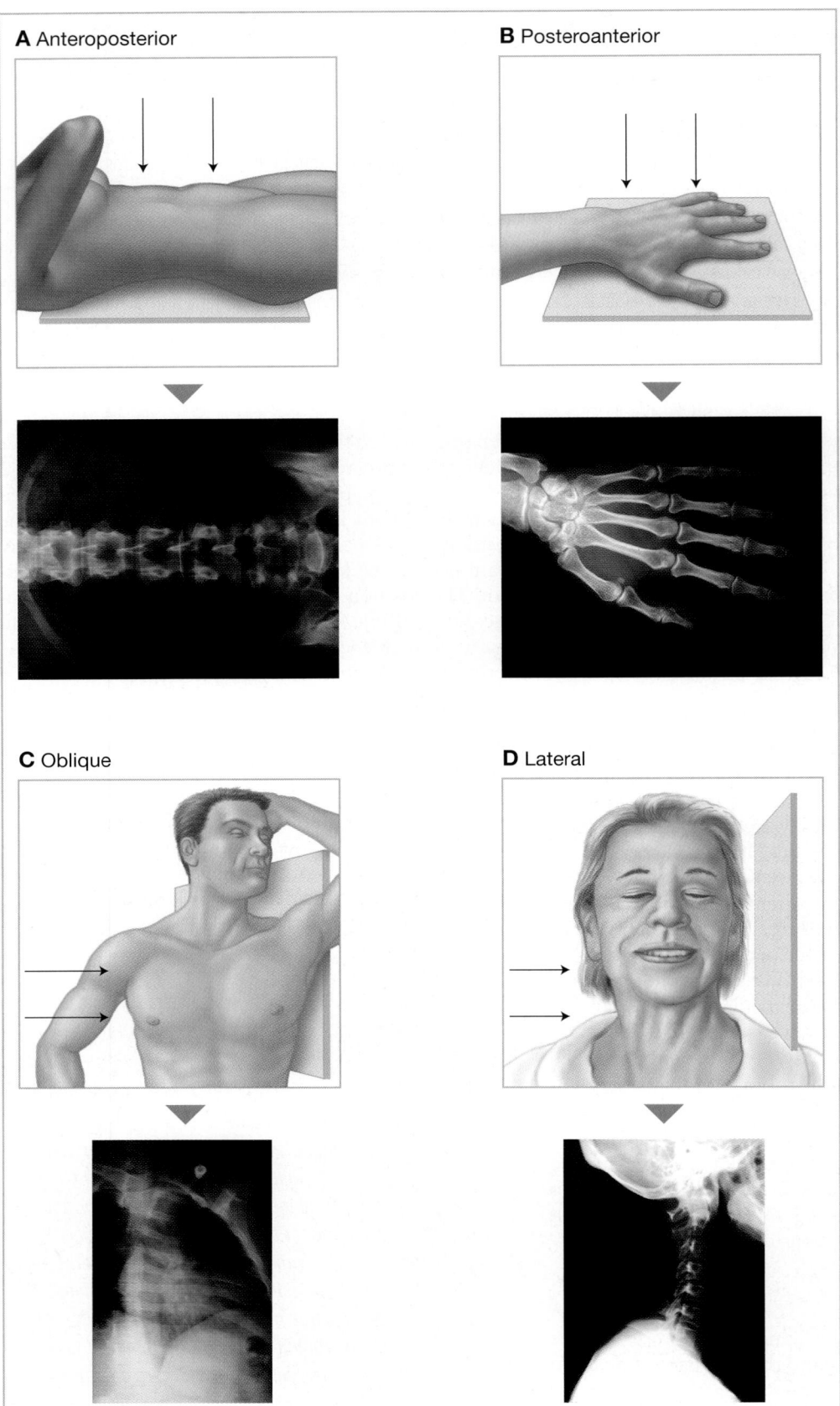

FIGURE 44-2 Examples of the most common x-ray positions and the images they produce.

TABLE 44-2 Radiology Positions

Position	Description
Anterioposterior (AP)	The x-ray beam is directed from front to back. Patient may be standing or supine. The patient's front will face the x-ray equipment and patient's back will be near the film plate.
Posterioanterior (PA)	The x-ray beam is directed from back to front. Patient will be standing upright. Patient's back will face the x-ray equipment and his or her front will be near the film plate.
Oblique	The patient is turned at an angle to the film plate so the x-ray beam can be directed at areas that would be hidden on an AP, PA, or lateral x-ray.
Lateral	The x-ray beam is directed toward one side of the body. In the right lateral (RL) position, the patient's right side is near the film plate and left side is near the x-ray equipment. In a left lateral (LL) position, the patient's left side is near the film plate.
Axial	The x-ray tube is angled to direct a ray along the axis of the body or body part. Cephalad angulation, the x-ray beam is directed at an angle from the feet toward the head. Caudad angulation, the x-ray beam is directed from the head toward the feet.

44-1 PROCEDURE

Procedure for General X-ray Examination

OBJECTIVE: Assist with a radiologic procedure under the supervision of a physician or radiologic technologist.

Equipment and Supplies

order for x-ray examination; dosimeter badge; appropriate x-ray equipment—x-ray film and holder, machine; processing equipment; drape; lead patient shield

Method

1. Check x-ray examination order.
2. Check necessary x-ray equipment as needed.
3. Identify patient.
4. Determine patient compliance with procedure preparation instructions.
5. Explain procedure to patient.
6. Instruct patient to remove all clothing appropriate for procedure.
7. Ask patient to remove all jewelry and metals as needed for procedure.
8. The following steps will most likely be performed by a radiologic technologist:

9. Position and drape the patient correctly.
10. Align the x-ray tube and cassette at correct distance and set controls.
11. Ask patient to hold breath as necessary.
12. Leave room and stand behind lead shield to take x-ray.
13. Ask patient to take comfortable position while x-rays are processed and reviewed.
14. Instruct patient to dress if x-rays are satisfactory.
15. Label the x-rays and place in envelope according to office procedures.
16. Document appropriately.

05/05/XX	7:00 A.M.

Chest x-ray done.

M. King CMA

the referring physician's name, and type of radiologic procedure to be performed. Legal and Ethical Issues has more about assisting with radiologic procedures.

Special dietary restrictions involving radiographic procedures often call for an all-liquid diet on the day before the test. All-liquid diets mean that the patient may have any of the following beverages: coffee, tea, carbonated beverages, clear gelatin desserts, strained fruit juices, bouillon, clear broth, and tomato juice. He or she may not have any dairy products. Remind the patient that NPO means nothing by mouth. It is up to the physician to decide whether the patient should or should not take his or her daily medications.

When multiple procedures need to be scheduled, it is important to consider the sequence of scheduling. Attention to sequencing is important because some procedures, such as those that require the use of contrast medium, may interfere with other tests. In addition, the patient may not be able to tolerate multiple procedures on one day. In general, examinations that do not require the use of contrast medium are performed before those examinations with contrast medium. For example, an abdominal x-ray would be taken before a barium enema. Always check with the facility performing the tests to obtain specific instructions for scheduling. Guidelines 44-1 provides guidelines for sequencing multiple diagnostic procedures.

Some procedures require long waiting periods between filmings because it takes time for the contrast medium to move through portions of the body. This should be carefully explained to the patient in order to schedule his or her time appropriately. The patient may have to allow a full morning for a series of x-ray procedures.

Diagnostic Imaging Procedures

Diagnostic imaging procedures can be divided into invasive and noninvasive procedures or divided into categories based on those that use contrast media and those that do not. The latter classification will be used in this chapter. Table 44-3 identifies the most frequently ordered tests and the conditions they are used to diagnose.

Radiologic Imaging Procedures Requiring Contrast Media

Various radiologic procedures involve the use of contrast media. They are as follows: angiography, arthrography, barium enema (lower GI), barium swallow (upper GI), cholangiography, cholescystography, fluoroscopy, intravenous pyelogram (IVP), myeolography, nuclear medicine studies retrograde pyelogram, and sometimes magnetic resonance imaging (MRI). Contrast media can be administered by mouth, by enema, by injection through intravenous lines or a catheter.

Fluoroscopy

Fluoroscopy is a technique in radiology for visually examining a portion of the body or the function of an

---

44-1   GUIDELINES

Sequencing Multiple Radiographic Procedures

- Schedule all radiographic examinations and tests that do not require contrast media and iodine uptake.
- Radiographic tests of the urinary tract.
- Radiographic tests of the liver and gall bladder.
- Do CT scans of abdomen and pelvis before procedures requiring barium.
- Lower gastrointestinal series (barium enema).
- Upper gastrointestinal series.

Note: CT procedures that require IV contrast media may be done AFTER blood is drawn for iodine uptake series.

TABLE 44-3 **Diagnostic Imaging Procedures and Conditions Diagnosed/Treated**

Test	Conditions Diagnosed/Treated
Angiography Cardiovascular	Status of blood flow, collateral circulation, aneurysm, hemorrhage, vessel malformation
Cerebral	Aneurysm, hemorrhage, evidence of CVA, arteriosclerosis
Gastrointestinal (GI)	Upper gastrointestinal bleeding
Pulmonary	Pulmonary emboli, evaluation of pulmonary circulation in heart conditions prior to surgery
Renal	Abnormalities of blood vessels in urinary system
Arthrography	Joint conditions
Barium enema (lower GI)	Obstructions, ulcers, polyps, diverticulosis, tumor, and motility problems of colon or rectum
Barium swallow (upper GI)	Obstruction ulcers, polyps, diverticulosis, tumors, and motility problems of esophagus, stomach, duodenum and small intestines
Cholangiography and cholecystography	Gallstones, gallbladder, or common bile duct stones or obstructions, ability of gallbladder to concentrate and store dye
Computed tomography (CT)	Aortic and heart aneurysms, disorders of liver and biliary systems, renal and pulmonary tumors, brain abnormalities (tumors, blood clots, CVA, outlines of brain ventricles), GI tract lesions, GI tract disorders (pancreatic cyst, abdominal abscesses, biliary obstruction), breast diseases and disorders, spinal disorders, biopsy guides
Fluoroscopy	Structure, process, and function of organs in motion to detect abnormalities
Intravenous pyleography (IVP), Excretory urography	Urinary system abnormalities, including renal pelvis, ureter, and bladder (kidney stones); abnormal, size, shape, or structure of kidneys, ureter, bladder; space occupying lesions; pyelonephrosis; hydronephrosis; trauma to urinary system
KUB (kidneys, ureters, bladder) radiography	Size, shape, and position of urinary organs; urinary system diseases or disorders; kidney stones
Magnetic resonance imaging (MRI)	Cancerous tissue, arthosclerotic tissue, blood clots, tumors, and deformities, particularly of the heart valves, brain, spine, and joints
Mammography	Breast tumors and lesions
Myelography	Irregularities or compression of spinal cord
Nuclear medicine (radionuclide imaging)	Abnormal function, lesions or disorders of bone, brain, lungs, kidneys, liver, pancreas, thyroid, and spleen
Radiation therapy	Treatment of cancer and some benign tumors or scars
Retrograde pyelogram	Obstruction of ureters, bladder, or urethra
Stereoscopy	Fractures, dense areas that indicate tumor or increase pressure within skull
Thermograph	Breast tumors, breast abscesses, fibrocystic disease
Ultrasound	Abnormalities of gallbladder, liver, spleen, heart kidneys, gonads, blood vessels, lymph system, fetal conditions: (number of fetuses) age, sex, fetal development, position, and deformities
Xeroradiography	Breast cancer, abscesses, lesions, and calcifications

organ using a fluoroscope. This technique allows the radiologist to have immediate images which can be used to assess heart function such as cardiac catheterization. The moving image that is seen on the fluoroscope can then be filmed using a radiograph (x-ray) to obtain a permanent record. Contrast media are often used during fluoroscopic procedures to better visualize organ function and abnormalities. Fluoroscopic procedures include the gastrointestinal series, intravenous pyelogram (IVP), cholecystogram, and myelogram.

GASTROINTESTINAL SERIES   A gastrointestinal (GI) series is a fluoroscopic study of the digestive tract using contrast media to detect abnormalities such as tumors, ulcers, polyps, and diverticulosis. An upper gastrointestinal (upper GI) series is an examination of the esophagus, stomach, duodenum, and small intestine. The patient drinks a barium solution and a fluoroscope outlines the esophagus, stomach, and small intestine as the barium moves through the system. The procedure takes one to two hours and produces little discomfort. The barium may cause

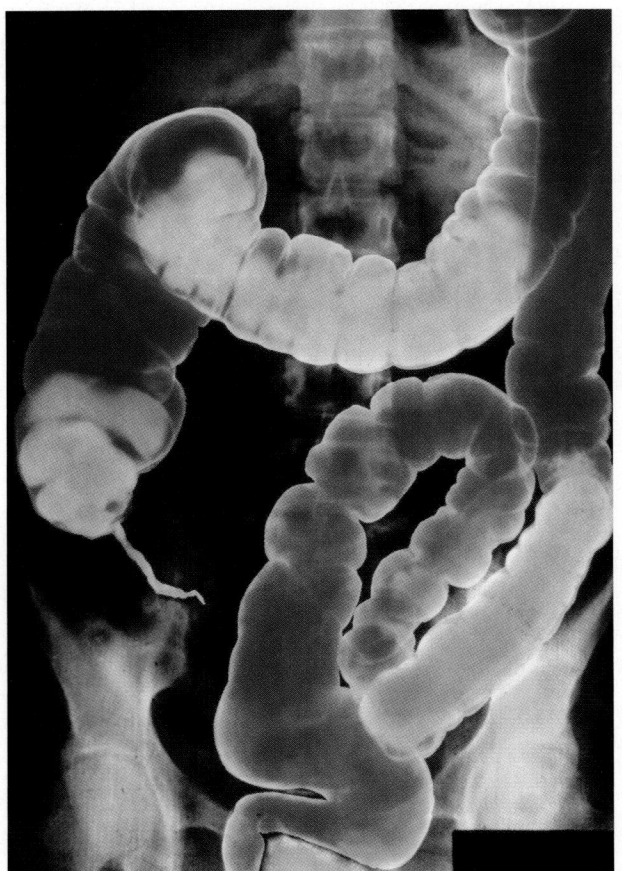

FIGURE 44-3   Radiograph of the colon after a barium enema.

constipation and white stools for several days following the procedure. The patient should also be advised to drink plenty of liquids to help push the barium through his or her system.

A lower gastrointestinal (lower GI) series is the administration of a barium enema, which outlines the colon and rectum on a radiographic picture. The lower GI series is done by giving the patient a barium enema and also air to better illuminate the lower part of the digestive tract. Figure 44-3 shows a radiograph of the lower GI tract after a barium enema. Some patients may have cramping and a feeling of urgency to move their bowels. They should be encouraged to take deep breaths during the procedure to help relax their abdominal muscles. After the procedure is completed, the patient may defecate and more x-rays may be taken of the empty colon. The patient should be encouraged to drink water to help move barium out of his or her system and made aware of the possibility of white stools due to the barium.

The patient should receive written instructions prior to these procedures. In addition, the medical assistant should explain the instructions and the procedure. Careful preparation is necessary for good results on these procedures. If the patient's digestive tract is not properly prepared and cleaned, the procedure may have to be repeated. This results in added expense, time, and patient discomfort. Guidelines are provided for the patient who will undergo upper GI series (Guidelines 44-2) and lower GI series (Guidelines 44-3).

INTRAVENOUS PYELOGRAM (IVP) OR INTRAVENOUS UROGRAM   The intravenous pyelogram, also called a pyelogram, is a radiologic examination of the kidneys, ureters, and bladder. This procedure takes about one to one and half hour and the patient should be screened for iodine sensitivity prior to the procedure. The patient will be instructed to eat a low-residue diet and drink plenty of water the day before the procedure. The patient will be allowed nothing by mouth (NPO) after midnight. A cathartic, such as castor oil or citrate of magnesia, may be ordered along with an enema to be taken the night before the examination.

The patient will need to undress and wear a patient gown for this procedure. A contrast medium containing iodine is injected into the vein (IV). This substance may cause the patient to have a warm, flushed feeling and a metallic taste in the mouth. The patient should be instructed to notify the radiologist if there are any unusual symptoms, such as shortness of breath or itching, that could indicate an allergic reaction to the dye.

The patient is tipped into various positions on the x-ray table, which allows the radiologist to view the dye as it flows through the urinary system. The patient

Upper GI Series

- The patient should not eat or drink after midnight since the stomach must be empty for this procedure. No water should even be swallowed while brushing teeth. The physician may order that no morning medications be taken.
- The patient should be instructed not to smoke since this can stimulate gastric secretions.
- The patient will have to undress and put on a patient gown.
- A barium sulfate drink is prepared for the patient to drink. This may be flavored but will still retain a slightly chalky taste.
- The patient will stand in front of the fluoroscopic screen while drinking the mixture. The radiologist will observe the progress of the barium as the patient drinks.
- The patient is then placed on an x-ray table that will tip into various positions for additional views. Permanent x-rays are taken while the patient will be told to hold his or her breath.
- The procedure may last for several hours during which time the barium will move out of the stomach and into the small intestine.
- The patient may resume normal eating after the examination, but should be reminded to drink water to assist in flushing out the remaining barium, as this may cause constipation. The stool may remain chalky for a couple of days.

Lower GI Series

The colon and rectum need to be free of stool for a clear view of the area on x-ray.

Day before the Examination
- The patient may be instructed to follow a low residue diet for several days before the test. On the morning before the test, he or she will change to an all-liquid diet (such as water and clear soup) because NO solid foods may be taken until after the procedure.
- A cathartic, such as castor oil or citrate of magnesia, may be ordered to be taken at 4:00 P.M. the day before the procedure. Enemas need to be taken until the return fluid is clear.

Day of the Examination
- The patient must undress and wear a patient gown for the procedure. Another cleansing enema may be given before the procedure.
- The patient lies on his or her side on the x-ray table while the technician gives an enema of barium sulfate. The patient is asked to retain or hold the enema within the rectal and colon area.
- The patient is then moved or tipped into different positions on the table while the radiologist observes the flow of barium on the fluoroscope. Periodically radiographs (x-rays) are taken during the procedure.
- The patient is asked to expel the barium into the toilet. Then a final x-ray is taken of the empty bowel.
- The patient may return to a regular diet after this procedure. Whitish stools may be present for one or two days after the procedure. The patient should be encouraged to drink water to flush out the remaining barium with stool.

may be asked to urinate, and then have one final x-ray taken. After the examination, the patient can return to a normal diet. He or she should be encouraged to drink water to flush out the contrast medium through the kidneys.

Retrograde (against the normal flow) pyleography involves inserting a catheter into the urinary tract through the bladder into the ureters. The dye is sent up the tube into the ureters and kidneys and x-rays are taken to evaluate the function of the ureters, bladder, and urethra. The post procedural recommendations are the same as those for the IVP.

CHOLECYSTOGRAM   A cholecystogram is a radiologic examination of the gallbladder using a contrast medium, usually iodine. This procedure is done to detect abnormalities such as the presence of gallstones. Although this procedure has been replaced by ultra-sound in many facilities, it is still ordered when ultrasound scanning fails to provide a definitive diagnosis.

It is important for the patient to understand that there is a significant time involved in preparation the night before and the day of the procedure. The patient is instructed to have a fat-free meal the evening before the procedure and nothing by mouth (NPO) after midnight. The contrast medium, in the form of pills, is taken after dinner. The patient is instructed to take one pill at a time every few minutes with water until the six pills have been ingested. In some facilities, the contrast medium is administered by intravenous (IV) injection. The patient undresses and wears a patient gown for this procedure. An initial x-ray is taken to see if the gallbladder is visible. A study is then conducted using the fluoroscope. Radiographs (x-rays) are taken also. After this portion of the procedure, the patient is asked to eat a fatty meal. This meal stimulates the gallbladder to empty. Another x-ray is taken one hour after the meal. The patient can resume a normal diet after the procedure is complete; however, the patient should be told that diarrhea is an expected side effect of the contrast medium used in this procedure. Patients should be encouraged to drink plenty of fluids to replace the fluids lost as a result of diarrhea.

MYELOGRAPHY Myelography is a fluoroscopic procedure of the spinal cord. A lumbar puncture is done to remove some cerebrospinal fluid (CSF) and instill contrast medium. This procedure produces a myelogram and is used to detect compression of the spinal cord or herniated disks. CT scans and MRIs are more commonly done now; however, a myelogram may be needed if the other procedures do not reveal enough detail. A pneumoencephalograph is performed by injecting air instead of contrast media after some cerebral spinal fluid has been removed. This procedure allows visualization of the cavities of the brain.

Angiography

Angiography is the x-ray visualization of the internal anatomy of blood vessels after a radiopaque material has been injected into the blood vessels. This procedure is used to assist in the diagnosis of many conditions including myocardial infarction (MI or heart attack), cerebrovascular accident (CVA or stroke), renal artery stenosis as a cause of hypertension, clots, stenosis in arteries in the lower extremities and abdomen, aneurysm of the aorta, and pulmonary emboli or clots.

Contrast medium is injected into an artery or vein by way of a catheter and threaded through the vessel until it reaches the correct site. Since iodine is used as the contrast medium, the patient should be tested for allergy to iodine before the procedure begins. The patient is monitored for a few hours after the procedure for any signs of bleeding from the puncture site.

Angiography may be used to study the blood vessels of the brain—cerebral angiography, the kidneys—renal angiography, and the heart—cardiography. This procedure is usually done in the hospital or same day surgical facility and requires the use of local anesthetic. Cardiac catheterization, a form of angiocardiography, is frequently performed to assess the status of the coronary arteries. A catheter is inserted into the femoral artery and fed through the arteries until it reaches the heart. If obstructions are discovered, therapeutic interventions can take place, such as balloon angioplasty or stent insertion, to relieve blockage of coronary arteries. These procedures are costly, carry risks, and are not

usually performed unless other procedures have failed to provide enough information. Facilities that specialize in angiography have patient preparation sheets available. It would be helpful for you to have a copy of each preparation in the office as reference material.

Arthrography

Arthrography is a diagnostic procedure used to produce an arthrogram or image inside a joint. It is performed by a radiologist to help diagnose abnormalities of the joints, tendons, ligaments, and cartilage of the knee, hip, or shoulder. The procedure involves injecting a local anesthetic followed by contrast medium or air or both into the joint. A fluoroscope is used to evaluate the function of the joint. The procedure usually takes about one hour and the patient should be advised to expect some slight discomfort and swelling for a day or two. The patient should be advised to rest the joint during that time.

Radiology Procedures Not Requiring Contrast Media

There are several diagnostic radiologic examinations that do not require the use of a contrast material. Table 44-4 lists several radiology procedures commonly performed with no contrast material. The procedures not requiring contrast media include films of the abdomen, bones, chest, kidneys, ureters, bladder (KUB), and paranasal sinuses.

These examinations or films require that the patient is positioned properly; however, no prior preparation, such as enemas, is required. One of these procedures is the mammogram.

Mammography

Mammography is the radiology examination of the soft tissue of the breast to provide identification of benign and malignant neoplasms (tumors). Breast masses are often as small as one centimeter or less. Women are encouraged to perform monthly breast examinations and check for unknown lumps because finding any mass early increases the cure rate significantly. Contrast medium is not used for this procedure. The patient should be instructed not to use underarm deodorant, talcum powder, body lotion, or perfume prior to the procedure since the clarity of the image could be affected.

The patient stands in front of the x-ray equipment and the technician positions the patient carefully to have all breast tissue examined under x-ray. The patient should be instructed to follow the technician's direction regarding placement of hands, arms, and body position. Patients of childbearing age are given a lead apron to wear during the procedure.

Each breast is alternately compressed by the mammography equipment to spread the tissue for better viewing. The x-rays are directed at angles into the breast tissue. The procedure takes a few seconds for

TABLE 44-4 Radiology Procedures Not Requiring Contrast Material

Type of X-ray	Description and Use
Abdomen	Flat plate or survey of abdomen used for suspected tumors, hematomas, enlarged organs, or abscesses.
Bone	X-ray studies of bones for suspected abnormalities from disease or trauma such as fractures and tumors. Commonly performed spinal x-rays are: Cervical—x-ray of neck area Thoracic—x-ray of the middle back Lumbosacral—x-ray of lower back
Chest	Routine chest x-rays are taken to rule out any abnormality and to pick up hidden disease in the lungs and some cardiac abnormalities (cardiomegaly), the patient assumes the posteroanterior erect position and a lateral position.
Kidneys, Ureters, Bladder	This abdominal x-ray studies the kidneys, ureters, and bladder (KUB), abdominal wall, pelvic bones, and unusual masses.
Paranasal sinuses	X-ray of the sinuses found within the maxillary, frontal, ethmoid, and sphenoid bones for signs of infection, inflammation, and abnormalities.

each view with the entire procedure lasting about a half hour. Some patients may feel discomfort during the procedure due to pressure during the breast compression. For most patients, the discomfort is over as soon as the compression is completed (less than a minute). Occasionally patients will complain of discomfort for several days after a mammogram and the physician may suggest they take an over-the-counter analgesic.

Women over the age of 40 are advised by the American Cancer Society to have a yearly mammogram for early detection of breast cancer. Figure 44-4 shows a woman receiving a mammogram.

If a lump is detected, the patient should follow up immediately with further testing and not wait to see if the lump disappears over time. Many abnormalities detected on mammograms are benign and present no danger to the patient. Figure 44-5 is an example of a normal mammogram. Once a mammogram reveals suspicious tissue, a breast biopsy should be done to confirm the type of mass detected. A new type of biopsy known as stereotactic breast biopsy is less invasive and less painful than previous types of biopsies. This procedure is done with the patient lying face down with the breast compressed between two paddles with the suspicious mass centered in the window of the paddle. A computer determines the precise positioning of the biopsy needle. A small sample of cells is taken and sent for review by a pathologist. After the examination is complete, the physician informs the patient of the pathologist's findings. Figure 44-6 is an example of an abnormal mammogram showing microcalcifications.

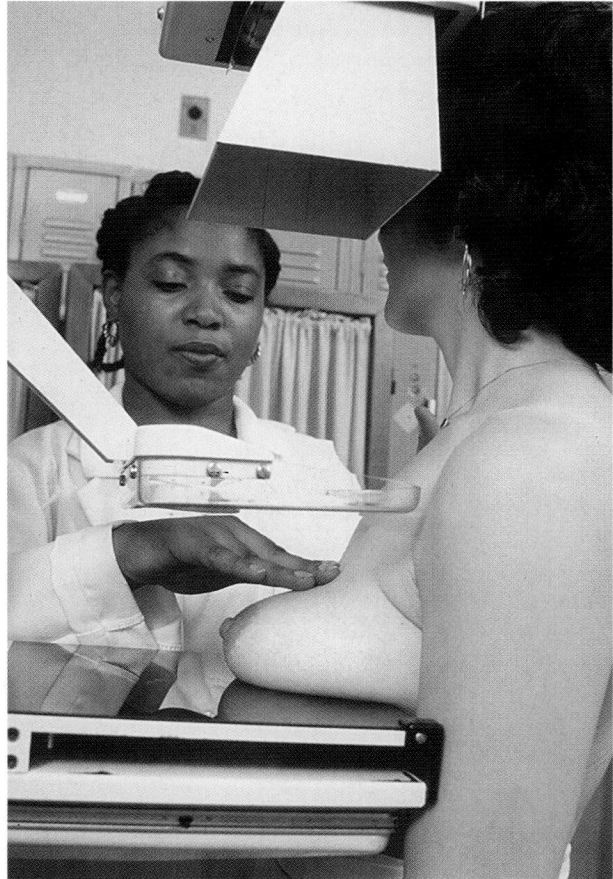

FIGURE 44-4 Compressing the breast between plates provides a better image of breast tissue. Regular mammograms help detect early cancers.

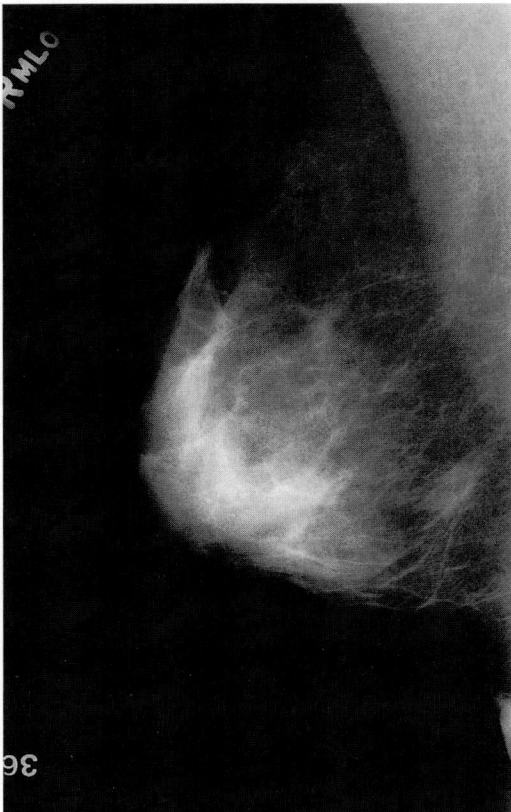

FIGURE 44-5 Normal mammogram.

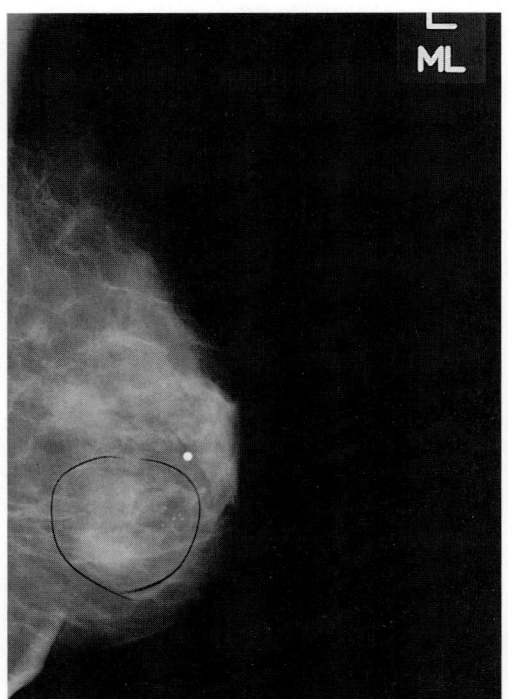

FIGURE 44-6 Mammogram showing microcalcifications.

Kidneys, Ureters, and Bladder (KUB)

A KUB or abdominal flat plate is used to assess the size, shape, and location of the organs of the urinary tract, to detect kidney stones, and diseases of the urinary tract. It is also used to detect the location of an IUD or other foreign object.

Tomography

Tomography, or the sectioning of the body using roetgenography, allows the technician to penetrate dense areas of the body that could not otherwise be visualized. When tomography was first introduced it was considered the most significant advancement in diagnostic medicine since the discovery of the x-ray. Tomography produces tomograms and computed tomography produces CT scans, previously known as CAT scans. Traditional tomography uses a computerized x-ray camera that moves back and forth in an arc over the patient's body producing a series of images. Tomography has the ability to remove, or blur out areas that are not within the plane being examined.

Computed Tomography (CT)

Computed tomography combines radiography with computer analysis of tissue density. In computed tomography scans, the x-ray camera rotates completely around the patient and the computer accumulates cross

sectional slices from each rotation of the camera. The CT scanner consists of a moveable table with a remote control, the circular structure or gantry that houses the x-ray equipment, and an operator console with monitor and computer equipment. Ancillary software and hardware sort, manage, retrieve, and store images.

The patient lies on a narrow table that slides into the scanner. This procedure is painless, noninvasive, and requires no special preparation. In this procedure, a narrow beam of x-ray rotates in a continuous 360-degree motion around the patient to slice the images of the body in cross-sectional angles. The computer then calculates various factors including tissue absorption and displays a printout that determines the density of the tissue. In this way, tissue masses, such as tumors, bone displacement, and fluid accumulation are detected. These images are more detailed than those obtained through conventional x-rays.

CT scan is a valuable diagnostic tool for identifying and discovering space-occupying lesions such as those found in the brain, liver, gallbladder, and spleen. It is especially valuable in evaluating malignant conditions in the lungs and bones. It can eliminate the need for more invasive procedures. Figure 44-7 is a CT of the skull showing multiple facial fractures.

Computerized tomography and magnetic resonance imaging (MRI) have largely replaced the use of tomography except in areas where these two techniques are not available. CT scans are useful when there is conflicting information about the cause of the patient's condition or defining exactly where radiation therapy must be directed for tumor masses. Other uses for CT include: detecting cerebral abnormalities, such as tumors, hematomas (Figure 44-8), childhood cancers, abdominal masses, and surveying difficult to visualize glands, such as the pituitary gland and tissue. The CT scanner is able to scan the entire body in 15 to 20 minutes, which allows one scanner up to about 20 patients to be scanned in one day.

CT Scan Preparation

In many instances, CT scans involve little prior preparation for the patient. For some CT procedures, a contrast medium is used so the patient may be instructed to have NPO for four hours before the procedure. The imposing size of computed tomography equipment may cause considerable apprehension in a new patient. As with any procedure, a thorough explanation when scheduling the scan helps to relieve patient anxiety. Many patients have never seen a CT scanner and having a diagram listing the major parts and their basic functions is helpful.

Instruct the patient to remove all metallic objects and inquire whether or not he or she has a pacemaker or metallic prosthesis. Any metallic objects will interfere with the CT scan. The table may move continuously in a spiral scanning motion or stop and start depending on the area being scanned. The patient should be reassured that he or she will not be in a confined space as with an MRI.

Positron Emission Tomography

Positron Emission Tomography (PET) is a computerized radiographic method that uses radioactive substances to examine the metabolic activity within the body.

For PET scans, the patient is either injected with or inhales a chemical, such as glucose, which carries a radioactive substance. This substance then emits positively charged particles, called positrons that combine with negatively charged electrons found within the body. The rays that are produced are converted into color-coded images that indicate the degree of metabolic activity. PET is used to assist in the treatment of epilepsy, brain tumors, stroke, Alzheimer's disease, blood flow, and metabolism of the heart and blood vessels. This procedure can detect mild early changes in the brain before nerve damage, memory loss, or other symptoms occur. The radioactive elements used in PET are short-lived, which results in minimal radiation exposure for patients.

Magnetic Resonance Imaging (MRI)

One of the newest imaging technologies, magnetic resonance imaging (MRI), has changed the field of radiology. The MRI uses a powerful magnetic field to visualize internal tissues, organs, and structures. The images produced with this technique are excellent. All areas of the body can be scanned using the MRI. There

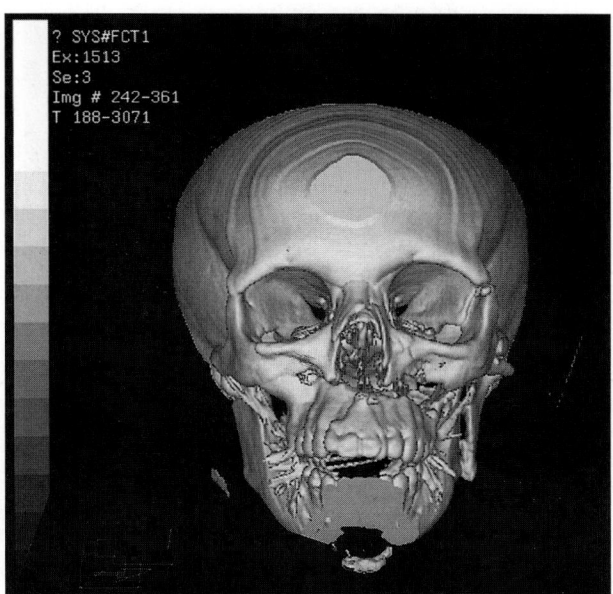

FIGURE 44-7 3-dimensional CT scan of the skull shows multiple facial fractures.

is no ionizing radiation used and the MRI has no known risks. See Figure 44-9 for a color-enhanced MRI image.

The signal or nuclear magnetic resonance produced by the MRI varies with different body tissues. These signals are processed by the computer and form a visual image. An MRI scan can give the viewer a three-dimensional view of tissues or organs of the body in total or as slices. This can be useful for tumor detection.

Explaining the procedure to the patient should include a description of the type of chamber in which the

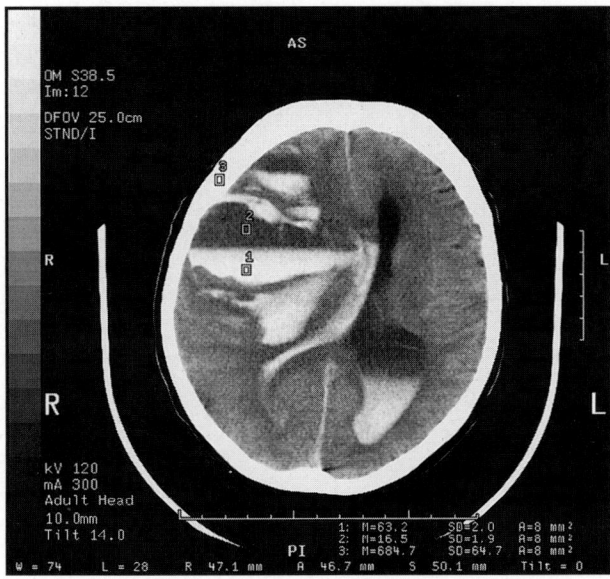

FIGURE 44-8 CT scan of the head shows a massive bleed with a midline shift.

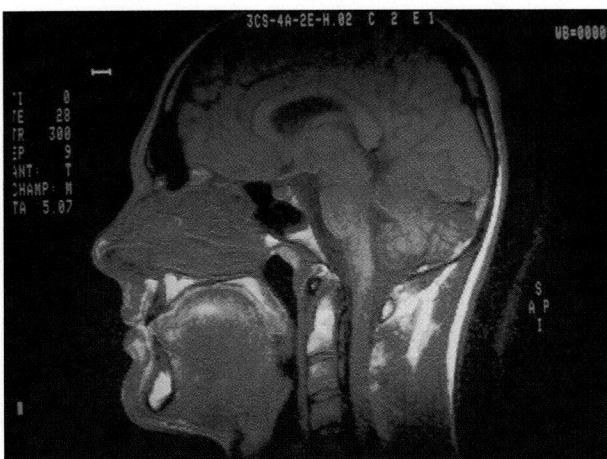

FIGURE 44-9　A color-enhanced MRI image of the skull.

patient will be placed. One type of chamber consists of a large cylindrical electromagnet. The patient is rolled into it on a pallet. The chamber is sealed, which allows the patient's entire body to come into contact with the electromagnetic field. The procedure, while painless, can be upsetting to patients who have claustrophobia, or are afraid of closed in spaces. The space inside a closed MRI machine is only slightly larger than the average patient. The MRI machine makes loud thumping noises intermittently during the procedure. The patient should be made aware of this possibility and be provided with earplugs or earphones to listen to music. In cases of extreme apprehension, the patient may need to be given a medication to promote relaxation. Open MRIs are available for patients who are too large for the enclosed MRI or too apprehensive; however, the

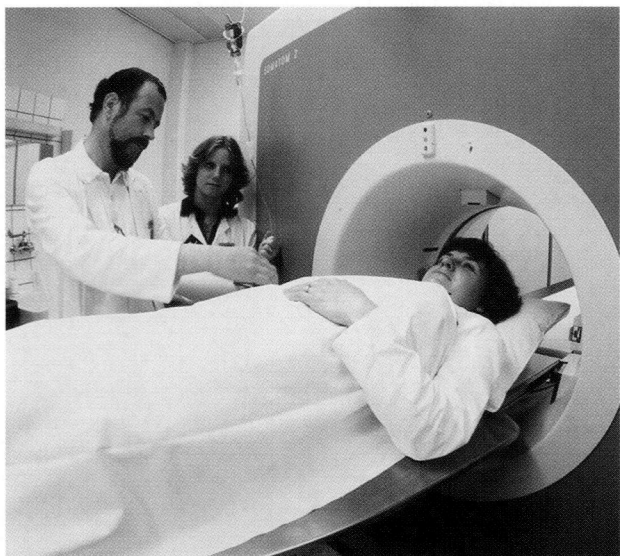

FIGURE 44-10　An open chamber MRI may be more comfortable for the patient, but images may not be as distinct.

images produced may not be as accurate or detailed (Figure 44-10).

There are some limitations to the use of the MRI. It is not possible to view the hard portion of bone matter. For visualizing fractures and other abnormalities, the CT scan and general x-rays are still used. In addition, the strong magnetic field is not appropriate for patients who have pacemakers or metallic clips on blood vessels. The patient should be instructed to:

- Remove all jewelry, eye shadow, and metallic objects, such as watches, belts, hearing aids, and hairpins.
- Identify which devices, if any, have been inserted within his or her body such as pacemakers, dental implants, surgical staples, intrauterine devices, joint or bone pins, prosthesis, metallic clips on blood vessels, or metal fragments, for example from a gunshot. These will all be present on the scan and can interfere with magnetic conduction. In addition, metallic clips on blood vessels can become loosened.
- Leave credit cards or devices, which contain metallic or magnetic code strips outside the MRI chamber.
- Use a patient gown if the patient's clothing has zippers or metal snaps.

The technician is not in the chamber with the patient during the procedure. The patient should be told that the technician will be in constant contact with the patient via a microphone and camera. The patient should be instructed to remain still during the procedure. An MRI scan takes from 20 to 60 minutes depending on the amount of the body to be scanned.

Advancement in MRI technology, called the functional MRI, enables physicians to observe the function of organs. Functional MRIs are able to provide information about nerve activity in the brain and locate areas of the brain activated in memory.

Digital Radiology

Digital radiology is the use of standard fluoroscopy, which is digitized, stored as computer bits, processed, and then converted into an image on a television or video monitor screen. The image is stored on a videotape or digital disc. Digital angiography is used for cardiac and pulmonary arteries and head and neck angiograms.

Ultrasound/Sonography

Ultrasound or sonography is the use of high frequency sound waves to image internal structures. Ultrasound imaging consists of projecting a beam of sound waves into the body. The waves at about 20,000 cycles per second, bounce back as the beam comes into contact with a structure, such as a fetus, which then produces an outline of the internal structure. Ultrasound has valuable medical applications, such as fetal monitoring and detecting abnormalities, such as gallstones, tumors, and heart defects. It is used to scan organs such as the liver, heart, kidneys, thyroid, gonads, and blood vessels. Ultrasound is not used to image the lungs, brain, or skeleton since they are made of or surrounded by bone, which sound waves cannot penetrate.

Ultrasound uses no ionizing radiation and is a painless noninvasive procedure. It has been widely accepted as a safe examination of delicate tissues and the fetus. Fetal ultrasound is commonly performed to detect the presence of multiple pregnancies, fetal and placental positioning, and internal organ development. The use of ultrasound is not recommended simply to determine gender of the fetus.

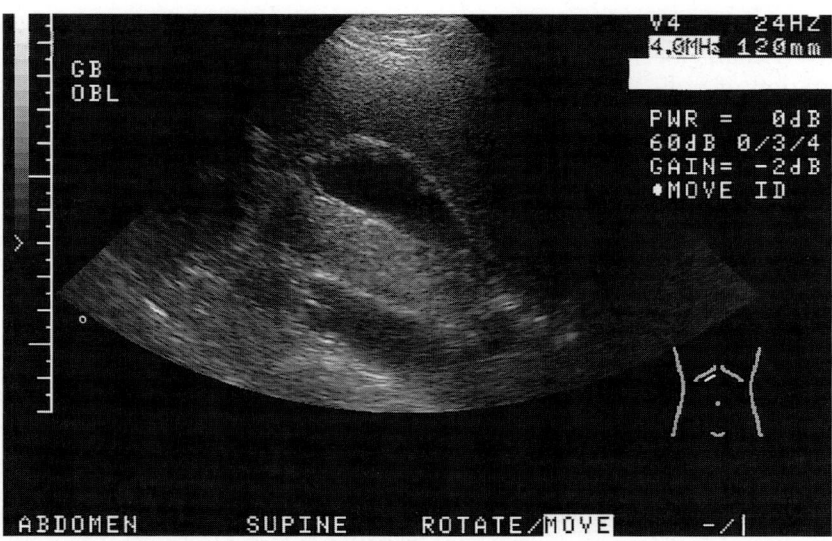

FIGURE 44-11 An ultrasound echogram or sonogram of the abdomen.

Ultrasound Scanning

To perform an ultrasound procedure, a conduction material such as water, special jelly, or oil is used to conduct the sound waves into the body. An instrument called a transducer with a conduction head is then placed on or near the skin. As sound waves pass through the skin, they bounce off the body tissues or fetus and remit an echo reflection of the image back to the instrument. These echoes of the body tissue or fetus are then recorded as a series of dots on an oscilloscope, an instrument that displays a visual picture. The record is called an echogram or a sonogram (Figure 44-11). The patient is often able to view the sonogram on the screen as it occurs. A printout of this visual picture can then be printed for the patient's record and in some cases, a copy of this printout is given to the patient. Usually, it will require some interpretation. The medical assistant should not attempt to explain the results of a sonogram to the patient.

Patient preparation for the ultrasound examination is minimal. The patient should wear loose fitting garments or clothing that is easy to remove since the procedure is performed over bare skin (Figure 44-12). During a fetal ultrasound or pelvic ultrasound, the patient is instructed not to urinate right before the test since a full bladder displaces the intestines and allows for a better view of the uterus. In fact, the patient may be asked to drink a quart or more of water just prior to either of these examinations. For an ultrasound of the gallbladder or liver, the patient may be asked not to eat for several hours before the procedure.

Ultrasound is also used in physical therapy and is discussed in Chapter 46.

Radiation Therapy

Radiation is the use of a radioactive substance in the diagnosis and treatment of disease. When radiation is used to treat cancers or other conditions, it is called radiation therapy. Radiation therapy is the process of administering a particular dosage of radiation to a specific area on the patient's body for the purpose of killing diseased cells. Radiation actually alters the cells so they cannot reproduce and thus eventually die leaving no new cells to develop. Both diseased and normal cells are altered with radiation. Diseased cells are eventually destroyed; however, normal or healthy cells are able to repair themselves and regrow new cells. Radiation therapy is also known as cobalt treatment, x-ray treatment or radiotherapy.

Radiation Rays

In radiation therapy, the radioactive substances used emit three types of rays: alpha, beta, and gamma rays.

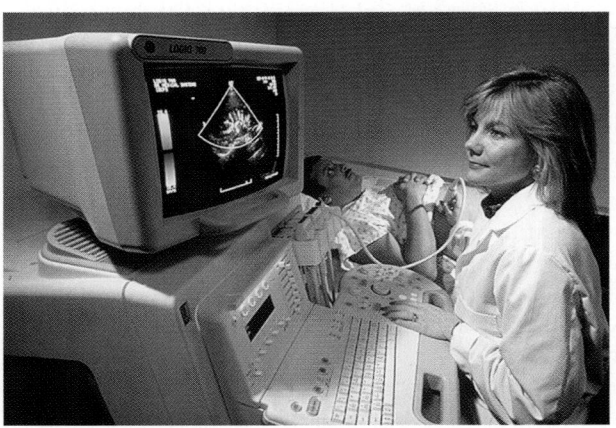

FIGURE 44-12 An ultrasound being performed on a patient.

Alpha rays are the least penetrating rays and are positively charged helium particles released by the disintegration of radioactive material. Beta rays are able to penetrate body tissues a few millimeters and are negatively charged electrons released when atoms of radioactive substances disintegrate. Gamma rays have great penetrating power and are electromagnetic waves emitted by atoms of radioactive elements as they undergo disintegration. Gamma rays can penetrate most body tissue, but are absorbed by lead. These rays are similar to x-rays, but they come from the element's nucleus, while x-rays come from the orbit of the element's atom.

Uses of Radiation Therapy

Radiation therapy is administered after the tumor is well defined in the patient. Tumors are located through the use of CT scan and ultrasound. The boundary of the tumor can be localized by these radiologic procedures. There are a few factors to consider when determining whether or not to use radiation therapy to treat a cancer patient: the tumor must be surrounded by normal tissue that can repair itself after radiation treatment, radiation is used to alleviate symptoms if the cancer has metastasized, and the tumor must be sensitive to radiation.

Patients receive radiation therapy for a variety of types of cancers including: cancer of the ovaries, testes, skin, larynx, and oral cavity. Hodgkin's disease, Wilms' tumor (a type of kidney tumor found in children), and retinoblastoma are also treated with radiation therapy. For some types of malignancies, such as cervical cancer, a combination of radiation and chemotherapy is used. In some cases, when a cure is not probable, radiation may be used to shrink tumors to alleviate pain, relieve pressure, or stop bleeding. In these instances, radiation therapy may improve the patient's quality of life. Certain benign conditions may be treated with radiation such as keloids (abnormal scars), and malformed blood vessels in the brain, which cannot be accessed any other way.

Radiation Therapy Techniques

There are two methods for administering radiation: external radiation therapy (ERT) and internal radiation therapy (IRT).

EXTERNAL RADIATION THERAPY External radiation therapy involves administering calculated doses of radiation from a machine positioned at a specific distance from the site (tumor). A marker or tattoo is placed on the patient at the exact site or port of entry. A computer calculates the dosage required to destroy the largest number of malignant cells while causing the least damage to surrounding cells. It may be necessary to schedule a series of ERT treatments over a period of weeks or months.

INTERNAL RADIATION THERAPY Internal radiation therapy can be administered into the body in two forms: sealed or unsealed radiation therapy. Sealed radiation involves the implantation of sealed containers of radioactive material near the tumor in the body. For example, radium, cesium–137, or cobalt–60 may be sealed in small gold containers or seeds and implanted in or near the tumor site. Unsealed radiation involves introducing a liquid form of radioactive substance into the patient by mouth, blood stream, or instilling into a body cavity. For instance, radioactive iodine–131, phosphorous–32, and gold–198 may be administered in unsealed forms.

Radiation therapy is not usually disfiguring, but may cause side effects in some patients including hair loss, skin changes, nausea, diarrhea, irritation of the mucous membranes in the mouth, throat, bladder, and vagina, and chromosome changes. The symptoms vary in intensity and may last three to six weeks.

Nuclear Medicine

Nuclear medicine, is a branch of medicine that uses radioactive isotopes in the diagnosis and treatment of disease. Isotopes are chemical elements, which may have several forms but identical properties. Radioactive refers to the ability to give off radiation as the result of the disintegration of the nucleus in an atom. Nuclear medicine is also known as radionuclide imaging.

Radioactive isotopes of iodine, cobalt, and other elements are used in nuclear medicine for the treatment of tumors and for nuclear imaging certain parts of the body. Radionuclides, isotopes whose nuclei (central core) are undergoing decay, are administered to the patient intravenously, orally, or instilled into body cavities or organs. The radionuclides then travel to a point within the body that attracts them. For example, iodine is attracted to the thyroid and creates an image or outline of that organ or tumor (abnormality). Radionuclides have a short life, which results in very few side effects for the patient. Radionuclide imaging exposes the patient to lower doses of radiation than some other radiologic procedures.

A concentration of radionuclides is referred to as either "hot" or "cold." If the radionuclide is in an area with an abnormality, it is referred to as "hot." If the radionuclide does not concentrate into a tumor, but is situated in the surrounding area, it is referred to as "cold." Both hot and cold areas can indicate the presence of abnormalities. Scans of different areas of the body require various preparations and varying lengths of time. The patient must be informed of the expected time. For instance, a bone scan takes about an hour (Figure 44-13); however, the patient is given an injection two hours prior to the scan and then must drink a quart of water. Kidney scans last two hours and thyroid uptake may not be completed until two days. After the patient takes the initial capsule, he or she must return 24 and 48 hours after the capsule is taken. The process of studying an area with a concentration of a radioactive substance is called scanning. The technician uses a gamma counter or camera that detects the radiation and converts it into an image or scintigram, which is displayed on a screen. The thyroid, liver, and brain are frequently evaluated using the scanning process.

If a radioisotope is used in a high dose for treatment, then the patients may have symptoms that are similar to those found with radiation. These include: hair loss, nausea, diarrhea, mucous membrane irritation (in the mouth, throat, and bladder), and chromosome changes.

Safety Precautions

Radiation dose is measured in several different units, all of which relate to the amount of energy deposited. The units include the roentgen (R), the gray (Gy), and the sievert (Sv). The sievert and the gray are similar, except that the sievert takes into account the biologic effects of different types of radiation. The biological effect of radiation exposure varies with the type of radiation and its energy. Equal doses of different types of radiation will not always result in the same biological effects. A rad, which stands for radiation absorbed dose, is the unit used to measure the amount of ionizing radiation absorbed during an x-ray procedure. To measure occupational exposure or other exposure that may involve more than one type of radiation, the unit used is the rem, which stands for roentgen equivalent in man. The dosimeter or personal radiation badge containing the occupational exposure dose is reported in rem (Figure 44-14).

Radiation Exposure

People are constantly exposed to low levels of natural ionizing radiation or background radiation from outer space and radon exposure. In addition, people are exposed to ionizing radiation from human made sources such as nuclear weapons testing and radiation from medical testing and treatments. On average, diagnostic imaging emits lower doses of ionizing radiation than occur naturally. Advances in diagnostic imaging have reduced the radiation dose a patient is exposed to during a diagnostic procedure. Excessive exposure to radiation causes tissue damage and side effects.

Overexposure to radiation may result in radiation sickness causing symptoms such as lowered red blood cell and white blood cell count, bone marrow alteration, burns, damage to ovaries and testes, fetal damage (especially during the first three months of pregnancy), and

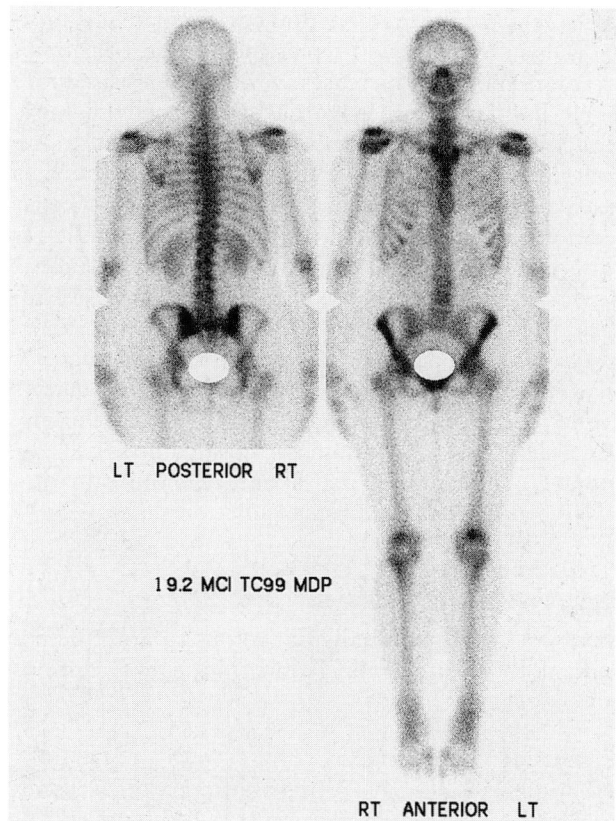

LT POSTERIOR RT

19.2 MCI TC99 MDP

RT ANTERIOR LT

FIGURE 44-13 A nuclear medicine bone scan.

cancer. Radiation sickness from overexposure is usually the result of long-term exposure and is generally delayed. Radiation sickness may result in cancer and premature aging. The severity of radiation sickness depends on the dose of radiation, the type of radiation, duration of exposure, and what areas of body were exposed. Radiation sickness can occur after nuclear reactor accidents.

Cellular Effects of Radiation

At the cellular level, radiation damages the DNA of cells in both malignant and normal cells. Normal cells are better able to repair DNA damage than cancer cells; therefore treatment with radiation kills the

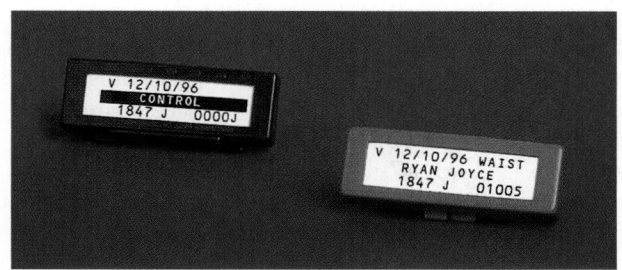

FIGURE 44-14 Dosimeter or personal radiation badge.

cancer cells, while after a period of time, damaged normal cells in the area will repair themselves. Sensitivity to radiation of cells increases with their increased rate of cell division. In other words, cells that divide more frequently, such as hair, mucous membranes of nose, mouth, skin, GI tract, as well as some glands, such as breast and thyroid, are more sensitive. The less specialized a normal cell is, the more affected by radiation it will be. Cells of the bone marrow, germ cells, such as sperm and ovum, fall into this category. Excessive radiation to embryonic cells causes spontaneous abortion, retardation, genetic abnormalities, and increase risk of leukemia and other cancers. The genetic defects can be passed on to future generations. Some cancers, such as leukemias, lymphomas, and squamous cell carcinomas of the mouth and skin, are more radiation sensitive and are treated using radiation therapy.

Patient and Personnel Safety Precautions

Since x-rays are potentially dangerous to both the patient and the health care personnel, special precautions must be taken.

Personnel Precautions

Radiation is discussed in terms of primary and secondary radiation. Primary radiation strikes the patient for either therapeutic reasons or for an x-ray examination. Once the primary beam strikes the patient, it can then become secondary radiation as it bounces off the patient. Secondary radiation is strongest closest to the patient. Lead has been proven to be an effective barrier to an x-ray beam. Lead aprons, shields, and gloves are provided for personnel coming into close contact with x-ray equipment. X-ray technicians do not normally remain next to the patient during the x-ray process. They stand behind a lead shielded divider. X-ray rooms are lined with metal (one-inch thick) as a precaution against x-ray beams escaping from the room. Some facilities have a red flashing light when x-ray equipment is in use to warn others not to enter.

A film badge or dosimeter is worn on the outer clothing of all personnel working with or near radiologic equipment. The badge records the level and intensity of radiation exposure. It is periodically examined to assure the health care worker is not exposed to excessive radiation. Radiation exposure is cumulative, meaning that each exposure to radiation is added to the effect of all previous exposures. All radiographic equipment should be checked on a regular basis to ensure it is in good working condition and to check for radiation leakage. Radioactive diagnostic materials must be stored in a safe environment and amounts of radioactive material closely monitored. Radioactive materials should be stored in lead containers and handled only with forceps never with bare hands. Most facilities have a radiation, safety monitor who specifies the requirements for the facility making sure OSHA guidelines are observed.

Patient Safety Precautions

The guiding principle in the use of radiation is ALARA or as low as reasonably achievable. In other words, the exposure of both patients and workers should always be guided by the idea that it is most prudent to use the lowest amount of exposure to perform the task.

Patient safety requires that a thorough history of the patient be taken. If the patient is female, the 10-day rule about the possibility of pregnancy should apply. An x-ray may be taken only within 10 days of the last menstrual period to avoid taking an x-ray of a female who is unknowingly pregnant. If a patient is unsure about a pregnancy, then a pregnancy test should be performed or the radiographic test postponed until a pregnancy test is completed unless an emergency situation exists. In cases of emergency, the danger of exposure to the embryo or fetus should be explained to the mother.

Patients should be protected from secondary or scatter radiation by the use of a grid during radiographic procedures. Excess scatter may add density to the image and expose the patient unnecessarily. The grid is positioned between the x-ray machine and the patient to absorb radiation scatter before it reaches the film. A Potter–Bucky diaphragm or a bucky is a type of grid that has alternating strips of lead and radiolucent material. Not all secondary radiation is absorbed by a grid, therefore other safety precautions are necessary.

A lead barrier or lead shields should be used by both patients and workers. Patients should be provided with a lead shield for gonads, eyes, breasts, and thyroid whenever appropriate. Employees should use gonad shields, if at the reproductive age (55 or under), whenever the sex organs are going to be exposed to radiation. For a female patient, the gonad shield should be placed with its lowest margin at the level of the pubic symphysis. In the male, the upper edge of the lead shield should be placed one inch below the pubic symphysis.

An implant may present a hazard while the implant is in place. In the patient who is undergoing radiation therapy. The length of time the hazard exists depends on the half-life of the material used. The half-life is the time it takes for ½ of the isotope to decay. Symptoms caused by radiation therapy will generally not begin for several days after the first treatment. This allows time for the patient and family to thoroughly understand what to expect and what steps to take to make the patient more comfortable. The skin is at most risk and frequently results in inflammation similar to sunburn. If the burns are deep enough hair roots are damaged and hair will

TABLE 44-5 Radiation Side Effects, Healing Time, and Interventions

Effect on/in Body	Healing Time	Intervention
Skin 1st to 4th degree burns	7 days to several weeks or months	Assess skin daily; do not use drying substances such as alcohol; avoid lying on area, avoid direct sunlight or direct heat source.
Alopecia	Hair may grow back in several months	Shampoo with mild soap, brush, and comb gently; wear scarves or wigs if hair loss is extensive.
Oral mucosa	Within weeks if irritation not severe	Increase fluid intake; avoid hot, spicy foods and liquids, restrict smoking; suck ice chips, use lip balm, use artificial saliva is necessary.
Intestinal mucosa	Several weeks or months depending on irritation	Check intake/output levels; assess for diarrhea and vomiting; administer antidiarrhetic or antiemetic agents if necessary; encourage intake of potassium rich food; avoid diary products; weigh daily.
Urinary mucosa	Several weeks to months depending on level of irritation	Increase fluid intake, measure urinary output, and urinalysis, administer antibiotics if infection present.
Bone marrow and lymphoid tissue	Depends on dosage and degree of damage	Protect from infection, assess for anemia, watch for bleeding and signs of thrombocytopenia; avoid trauma from injections and IVs.
Eyes	Depends on dosage and degree of damage	Assess for drying, excessive tearing, conjunctivitis, damage to lens, cataract formation; use artificial tears as needed and antibiotic for infection.
Ear	Depends on dosage and degree of damage	Assess for blockage of Eustachian tube and bulging eardrum; protect from falls due to dizziness, assess for hearing loss, administer antibiotic for infection.
Nervous system	Necrosis of brain can develop as late as a year after treatment	Assess for level of cognition, dizziness, slurred speech, weakness, and numbness or tingling in extremities; assess for spinal cord damage, changes in gait, pain; incontinence.

fall out. Radiation side effects, healing time, and patient interventions are summarized in Table 44-5.

Guidelines 44-4 provides a summary of guidelines for safeguarding the safety of health care workers and Guidelines 44-5 provides a summary of guidelines for patients.

Radiographic Equipment

Medical assistants will not be performing the duties of a radiology technician in most cases. However, you may be employed in a facility where x-rays are taken and a basic familiarity with radiographic equipment may be helpful.

The source of the radiation is the x-ray tube and it is located inside a protective covering or housing. The housing protects the x-ray tube and provides places for various attachments that allow the radiographer to move the tube and adjust the size and shape of the x-ray beam. The housing may be attached to the ceiling or mounted on a stand to provide mobility and flexibility of positioning. The x-ray or radiographic table provides support for the patient, but is highly specialized as well. Figure 44-15 illustrates an x-ray machine with x-tube, collimeter (device which controls the size and shape of the x-ray field coming from the tube), table, and bucky tray for film and cassette. Some tables have adjustable heights, tilt into various positions, and float to allow ease in positioning the patient. A grid and bucky slide below the table to prevent excess scatter radiation. The bucky holds a cassette tray, which holds the x-ray film. The grid is placed between the tabletop and the film. The bucky moves the grid during exposure so that it is invisible on the x-ray. The control console is located in the lead-lined booth where the radiographer stands. Here the radiographer determines exposure factors and controls the functions of the procedure. The cassette provides a rigid structure to hold the film and also holds two intensifying screens one in front and one behind the film. These screens are coated with phosphors or fluorescent crystals that emit light when exposed to x-rays. Intensifying screens enable lower doses of radiation to be used on the patient. Radiographic film is very sensitive to light emitted by the intensifying screens. Routine x-ray film is coated with an emulsion on both sides so that the film responds to the intensifying screens on both sides. Films and cassettes come in various sizes and are labeled in inches and centimeters.

Processing X-ray Film

Film development takes place in the darkroom of the facility because exposure to light can ruin the film. Red or orange safe lights in the darkroom are dim, but provide enough light to see where items are located. The darkroom should always be locked when processing film. Both manual and automated processing methods are used. The automated processing method is able to meet quality control standards since the equipment can be tested frequently for accuracy. Automated processing may take about 90 seconds or up to 10 minutes depending on the equipment used. The film is fed into the processor that transports the film through processing chemicals, dries the film, and moves it out of the equipment for the radiologist to view and read.

Storage and Records

X-ray materials for radiologic procedures must be kept in special storage containers that protect the film from damage due to light, heat, chemical fumes, and moisture. In order for film to remain fresh, it should be kept in a dry, cool place within a sealed package. X-ray film should be stored on end to prevent pressure damage from stacking the film. The expiration dates, which are printed on the top end of the package, can be seen clearly when stored on end. X-ray developer is also kept in a cool location that is moisture-free since damage to this fluid can affect the quality of the film. When handling film, it should only be touched with one hand hanging the film vertically to avoid damage. The film packages are only opened in the darkroom of the medical facility because light will destroy the film imaging ability.

All film records are maintained in a record or log book that is kept in the x-ray room. Entered in this record book are the film identification number, patient's name, date, and type of x-rays taken. Each film taken will have an identification number, which is created by placing lead letters or numbers in the film holder or cassette, at the time the x-ray is taken (time of exposure). These numbers will identify the physician's name, date, and patient's name. This data will then be permanently on the film after it is processed.

Films that have been processed should be stored in custom envelopes and filed in specially designed film cabinets. They are usually filed alphabetically. If a chronological numbering system is used based on the identification number of each film, a master log must be maintained. If a film has to be removed from the file cabinet, an insert explaining where the film was sent is filed in place of the film within the file cabinet.

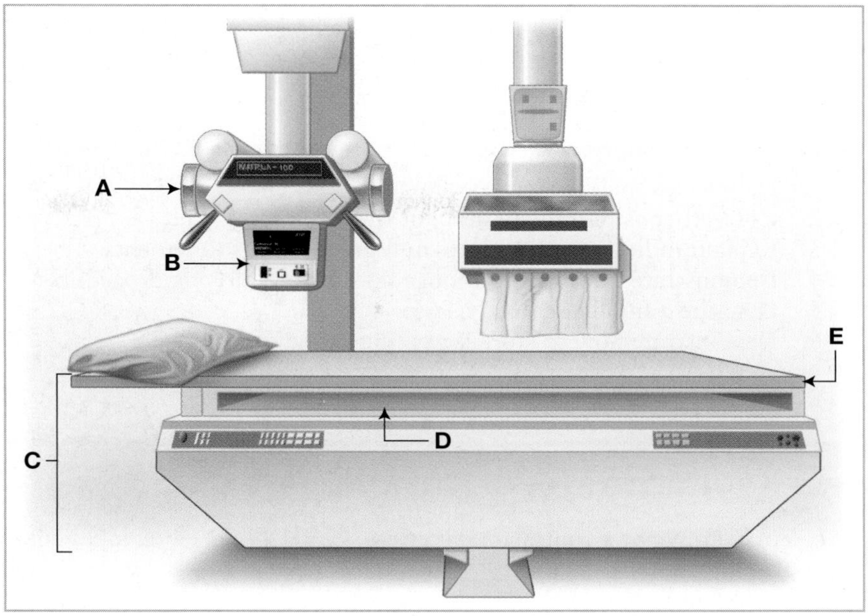

FIGURE 44-15 Generic parts of radiographic equipment: (A) x-ray tube; (B) collimeter; (C) radiographic table; (D) bucky tray for cassette and film; (E) movable table.

Ownership of Film

The medical assistant is frequently called upon to explain the ownership of film to the patient. Although the patient has paid for the film, it is the property of the medical facility or hospital that performed the x-ray. Written reports prepared by the radiologist are sent to other physicians at the request of the patient, but the film generally remains in the original office or hospital. The reason for this is simple: if the film remains in one location, it can always be accessed for future examination and comparison. Once it leaves the originating facility, it can be misplaced and lost.

Physicians are able to loan their films to referring physicians for further examination. The patient has to sign a release of records form for this to take place, but the film must then be returned to the original facility. Since films are a permanent record of the patient at a particular moment, they need to be preserved carefully. It is possible, in some locations, for the patient to obtain a duplicate copy of a film. The patient would have to pay for the copy to be made.

SUMMARY

The use of radiology in medical practice makes it possible to view internal body structures and functions and therefore assist in diagnosis and treatment. These procedures include radiology, radiation therapy, and nuclear medicine. There are inherent risks to the patients, technicians, and the medical assistants in performing these procedures. The use of proper safety precautions can greatly reduce or eliminate these risks altogether.

COMPETENCY REVIEW

Note: These competencies may only be practiced by a medical assistant if permitted by state law.

1. Define and spell the terms to learn for this chapter.
2. Correctly position the patient for the AP, PA, RL, and LL.
3. Explain radiologic procedures and preparations to patients.
4. Demonstrate safety precautions relevant to radiology procedures.
5. Describe a film badge and its use.
6. Demonstrate how to store x-ray film in the office.

PREPARING FOR THE CERTIFICATION EXAM

1. An example of a contrast medium is
   A. lidocaine
   B. epinephrine
   C. sodium chloride
   D. barium oxalate
   E. barium sulfate

2. Which procedure, relating to x-rays, are NOT performed by medical assistants?
   A. instructing the patient
   B. handling x-ray film
   C. positioning the patient
   D. interpreting x-ray film
   E. preparing the patient

3. Secondary radiation is
   A. emitted by the direct x-ray beam
   B. scattered from the patient being x-rayed
   C. emitted through the radiology room walls
   D. the second beam of x-ray
   E. not dangerous

4. An IV pyelogram is an examination of the
   A. gallbladder
   B. small intestine
   C. kidneys, ureters, and bladder
   D. colon
   E. pyloric sphincter of the stomach

5. A patient is scheduled for a cholecystogram. This is an examination of the
   A. gallbladder
   B. small intestine
   C. kidneys, ureters, and bladder
   D. colon
   E. pyloric sphincter of the stomach

6. If a patient notices a white stool after having a lower GI, what advice can be given?
   A. drink plenty of fluid(s)
   B. eat a large meal
   C. take an antacid product
   D. take a laxative
   E. only the physician can give medical advice

7. A radiologic procedure that does NOT require a contrast medium is
   A. IVP
   B. mammogram
   C. LGI
   D. UGI
   E. cholecystogram

8. Symptoms the patient should NOT expect after having radiation treatments are
   A. hair loss
   B. nausea
   C. diarrhea
   D. hemorrhage
   E. irritated throat

9. NPO means
   A. nothing by mouth except water
   B. nothing by mouth after the procedure
   C. only clear fluids
   D. nothing by mouth
   E. nothing except medications

10. A patient who is having a cholecystogram will take the dye
    A. as oral tablets
    B. in enema form
    C. in liquid form
    D. as a barium sulfate drink
    E. no dye is used in this procedure

CRITICAL THINKING

1. What questions would you ask Ivan when he arrives?

2. What preparations for an IVP should Ivan have done?

3. What will you tell Ivan upon realizing that he is not properly prepared?

4. How will you convince Ivan to reschedule his appointment?

5. What will you tell the primary care physician office when the office calls for Ivan's results?

ON THE JOB

Marge Riley, an overweight 50-year old woman with a history of abdominal pain, has been scheduled for a barium enema and a cholecystogram on Monday morning. She states she has board meetings every Monday morning at which breakfast is served and that she will come in for her x-rays after the meeting is over. Marge indicates that she doesn't understand why she needs these procedures.

1. What, if anything, would you tell the patient regarding her need for these procedures?

2. How would you describe these procedures to the patient?

3. What combination of teaching methods would you use to explain the procedures?

4. You are still concerned, after explaining everything to Marge, that she won't follow the instructions. What do you do?

INTERNET ACTIVITY

Search the Internet for information about the history of radiology. When were x-rays first taken? When did physicians first realize that radiographic waves were dangerous?

 MediaLink More on radiology, including interactive resources, can be found on the Student CD-ROM accompanying this textbook.

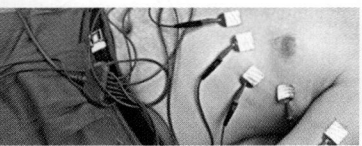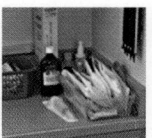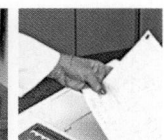

Medical Assistant Role Delineation Chart

HIGHLIGHT indicates material covered in this chapter.

ADMINISTRATIVE

Administrative Procedures

- Perform basic administrative medical assisting functions
- Schedule, coordinate and monitor appointments
- Schedule inpatient/outpatient admissions and procedures
- Understand and apply third-party guidelines
- Obtain reimbursement through accurate claims submission
- Monitor third-party reimbursement
- Understand and adhere to managed care policies and procedures
- *Negotiate managed care contracts*

Practice Finances

- Perform procedural and diagnostic coding
- Apply bookkeeping principles
- Manage accounts receivable
- *Manage accounts payable*
- *Process payroll*
- *Document and maintain accounting and banking records*
- *Develop and maintain fee schedules*
- *Manage renewals of business and professional insurance policies*
- *Manage personnel benefits and maintain records*
- *Perform marketing, financial, and strategic planning*

CLINICAL

Fundamental Principles

- Apply principles of aseptic technique and infection control
- Comply with quality assurance practices
- Screen and follow up patient test results

Diagnostic Orders

- Collect and process specimens
- Perform diagnostic tests

Patient Care

- Adhere to established patient screening procedures
- Obtain patient history and vital signs
- Prepare and maintain examination and treatment areas
- Prepare patient for examinations, procedures and treatments
- Assist with examinations, procedures and treatments
- Prepare and administer medications and immunizations
- Maintain medication and immunization records
- Recognize and respond to emergencies
- Coordinate patient care information with other health care providers
- Initiate IV and administer IV medications with appropriate training and as permitted by state law

GENERAL

Professionalism

- Display a professional manner and image
- Demonstrate initiative and responsibility
- Work as a member of the health care team
- Prioritize and perform multiple tasks
- Adapt to change
- Promote the CMA credential
- Enhance skills through continuing education
- Treat all patients with compassion and empathy
- Promote the practice through positive public relations

Communication Skills

- Recognize and respect cultural diversity
- Adapt communications to individual's ability to understand
- Use professional telephone technique
- Recognize and respond effectively to verbal, nonverbal, and written communications
- Use medical terminology appropriately
- Utilize electronic technology to receive, organize, prioritize and transmit information
- Serve as liaison

Legal Concepts

- Perform within legal and ethical boundaries
- Prepare and maintain medical records
- Document accurately
- Follow employer's established policies dealing with the health care contract
- Implement and maintain federal and state health care legislation and regulations
- Comply with established risk management and safety procedures
- Recognize professional credentialing criteria
- *Develop and maintain personnel, policy and procedure manuals*

Instruction

- Instruct individuals according to their needs
- Explain office policies and procedures
- Teach methods of health promotion and disease prevention
- Locate community resources and disseminate information
- *Develop educational materials*
- *Conduct continuing education activities*

Operational Functions

- Perform inventory of supplies and equipment
- Perform routine maintenance of administrative and clinical equipment
- Apply computer techniques to support office operations
- *Perform personnel management functions*
- *Negotiate leases and prices for equipment and supply contracts*

- *Denotes advanced skills.*

SOURCE: Reprinted by permission of the American Association of Medical Assistants from the AAMA Role Delineation Study: Occupational Analysis of the Medical Assisting Profession.

chapter 45

Electrocardiography and Pulmonary Function

Learning Objectives

After completing this chapter, you should be able to:

- Define and spell the terms to learn for this chapter.

- Maintain and operate electrocardiogram and pulmonary function equipment.

- Identify by name and function the controls on an electrocardiograph machine.

- Name the standard 12 leads and the locations of their sensors.

- State the cause and correction of artifacts.

- Explain forced vital capacity (FVC), forced expiratory volume in 1 second (FEV1), and maximal midexpiratory flow (MMEF).

- Differentiate between obstructive and restrictive pulmonary disease.

OUTLINE

Heart Structure and Function	956
The Electrocardiogram	957
Special Tests	967
Pulmonary Function	970
Pulmonary Function Tests	970
Treatments	975
Pulmonary Diseases	975

Terms to Learn

Einthoven's triangle

electrocardiogram

expiratory reserve volume (ERV)

forced expiratory volume (FEV)

forced vital capacity (FVC)

functional residual capacity (FRC)

heart rate

Holter monitor

inspiratory capacity (IC)

inspiratory reserve volume (IRV)

leads

maximal midexpiratory flow (MMEF)

pacemaker

residual volume (RV)

rhythm

stress test

tidal volume (VT)

total lung capacity (TLC)

vital capacity (VC)

wave

Case Study

MRS. NAGLE HAS JUST ARRIVED AT THE OFFICE for an ECG test and Holter monitor application. She states that prior to getting dressed this morning, she forgot to read the directions she was given and applied talcum powder. After assuring Mrs. Nagle that she can still take the test, you provide her with a patient gown and direct her to remove her clothing including her stockings. You also direct her to remove the talcum powder.

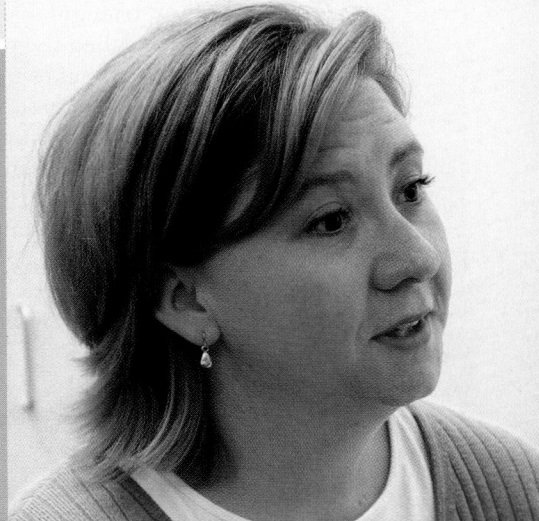

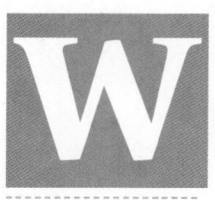ithin the thoracic cavity or chest are the major organs of both respiration and circulation. Because these two systems work very closely together, both are vital for survival, and a problem with one will often lead to a problem with the other. Because many patients suffer with disorders of these two systems, both primary care physicians and specialists monitor and treat these patients. In many clinics, tests associated with these disorders are done by the medical assistant.

All patients visiting a physician should have their heart and lungs assessed, regardless of their chief complaint. A stethoscope is used to evaluate the sounds made as the heart works. These sounds represent the closing of the valves and usually occur closely together followed by a pause, as in "lubb-dubb . . . lubb-dubb." The first sound, the "lubb," is called the S_1 and is the first sound of the pattern, representing the closing of the tricuspid and bicuspid (mitral) valves. The second sound, the S_2, results from the closing of the aortic and pulmonary valves. The physician will document normal heart sounds, along with any rubs, murmurs or gallops, or other abnormal heart sounds that are present, in the medical record.

When more specific cardiac information is needed, an electrocardiogram (ECG) is performed. The electrocardiogram is a tracing, or recording, of electrical activity as it moves through the heart. The ECG represents only the electrical activity of the heart, and not the actual mechanical performance. The physician orders this painless, noninvasive test when the heart sounds are unusual, the rhythm is irregular, or the patient has any heart-related complaints or has a condition that might affect the heart or be due to the heart. A recording will also be made to serve as a reference with which to compare future recordings in evaluating any changes. This may be called a baseline electrocardiogram, not to be confused with the baseline in the recording itself.

Heart Structure and Function

Located between the lungs behind the sternum, the heart is a hollow triangular organ enclosed within a double-walled sac called the pericardium. The middle layer or myocardium makes up most of the heart wall and is composed of interconnected muscle and fibrous tissue. The endocardium lines the upper chambers, or atria, and lower chamber, or ventricles, of the heart.

Blood circulates throughout the body and returns from the general circulation by way of the superior and inferior venae cavae, to the right atrium, moving in one direction through the heart. When the right atrium is full, the atrium contracts and blood is pumped into the right ventricle through the tricuspid valve. Upon filling, blood is pumped by contraction of the right ventricle through the semilunar valves into the pulmonary artery going to the lungs. There, blood is oxygenated and returned to the left atrium through the four pulmonary veins. When that chamber is full, it contracts and blood is squeezed into the left ventricle through the mitral (bicuspid) valve. In the left ventricle, blood will enter the aortic semilunar valve and move into all parts of the body except the lungs. Blood travels to all parts of the body via the aorta and then goes into all other arteries.

Heart valves act as gates to prevent the backward flow of blood. They open and shut in response to the changing pressure brought about by cardiac contraction and relaxation. The contraction and relaxation of the chambers occurs in sequence because electrical impulses move smoothly along the electrical conduction system of the heart.

This conduction system involves the movement of charged particles or ions during different phases. Minerals (sodium, potassium, and calcium) are responsible for smooth contractions and consistent rhythm. At rest, the cells of the heart are polarized; that is, they are charged with energy (negative inside the cell and positive outside). As the cells are stimulated to contract, the mineral particles move like a wave, and charge within the cells changes to positive inside and negative outside. The cells are depolarized and contraction occurs. The cells then return to a resting state, called repolarization, as their electrical charge returns to the original negative inside and positive outside.

The four major components of this conduction system are the sinoatrial (SA) node, atrioventricular (AV) node, the bundle of His with the right and left bundle branches, and the Purkinje fibers. The heartbeat is controlled by rhythmic impulses that arise in the SA node and move through the conduction system. The SA node, located in the right atrium, is made of modified myocardial cells and acts like a battery. It is known as the pacemaker of the heart because it establishes the pace. It may accelerate or slow the heart rate, beats per minute, under the influence of the autonomic nervous system.

The conduction system carries the impulse from the SA node and spreads it through the atria. This process is called atria depolarization. The impulses reach the AV node (also made of modified myocardial cells) where they are momentarily delayed. During this delay, the atria rest and recover. This is known as atrial recovery, atrial rest, or atrial repolarization. The impulse passes from the AV node down the bundle of His as it divides into two bundle branches, carrying the impulse along both sides of the interventricular septum. The bundle branches spread to form a network, the Purkinje system,

THE CHILD

ECGs are rarely performed on children except in cardiac offices, in cases of emergencies, or before some sports physicals. Lead placement is exactly the same as in an adult, but sometimes placing the leads can be a challenge due to the smaller available space for them.

Children need extra time and coaching for pulmonary function tests (PFTs). Take the time to explain to them that they will need to blow "really hard" until you tell them to stop, and then they will need to take a big breath back through the tube. It may take a couple of practice runs the first time this procedure is performed for them to perform the test accurately, which will, of course, change the validity of the results. PFTs are never performed on a child who is unable to cooperate with the testing.

Since it is critically important to have cooperation for both the ECG and the PFTs, parents may need to help persuade the child to cooperate. If the child is frightened, the test may not be accurate.

THE OLDER ADULT

The positioning of ECG leads on the older adult is the same as that for other adults. However, sometimes making the leads truly accurate can be a challenge secondary to a loss of elasticity in the skin. The use of towels may be required to hold the leads in place after they are positioned—just fold the towel several times and place it on top of the leads so the weight holds them in place. Older adults also have fragile skin. Be very careful not to rip off the electrodes from the skin, but instead hold traction on the skin and work the electrode off carefully. It may take a few minutes of being careful, but the patient will be grateful for the consideration.

When doing PFTs, explain the procedure clearly to them. They may not be able to perform multiple efforts, so each must be a valid try. Watch their technique and offer constructive hints if needed to help improve the validity of each effort. Be very supportive to them and coach the patient throughout the procedure.

that distributes the impulse to all parts of the ventricular muscle, resulting in ventricular contraction and or ventricular depolarization. Ventricular depolarization follows atrial repolarization, and is followed by a period of ventricular recovery known as ventricular repolarization or rest. There is a brief pause, and the cycle begins again. Atrial and ventricular depolarization plus atrial and ventricular repolarization comprise the cardiac cycle, one pulse and one heartbeat.

A unique property of cardiac muscle is that all conductive tissue has the potential to serve in the role of pacemaker; that is, any area can set the cardiac rate if the SA node fails. Under abnormal circumstances, such as when damage has occurred, other areas may assume the role of the pacemaker. Slower rhythms will be generated by the AV node (40 to 60 beats per minute), by the bundle of His (less than 40 beats per minute), and by the Purkinje system. But normally the SA node generates the controlling impulses at a resting rate of 60 to 80 beats per minute.

The Electrocardiogram

The electrical charges created by the cardiac conduction system can be sensed throughout the body. Electrodes placed in specific areas of the skin can detect those electrical charges and then transmit them to a computer for amplification of the signal to be recorded on paper for physician assessment. If no energy is sensed, then the equipment records a flat line, or isoelectric line. When the equipment senses an electrical charge, this will be recorded as either an upward or a downward deflection on the read-out. Movement away from the baseline is called a deflection or wave. The waves or deflections may go up (positive) or down (negative) from the baseline and represent amplitude or voltage. The strength or voltage of the electrical impulse will determine the size of the deflection. Large voltages will cause larger deflections, whereas small voltages will create smaller deflections. The deflections from the heart are labeled P, Q, R, S, and T. (Sometimes a small U wave follows the T wave. This is considered normal and is most probably due to a potassium deficiency.) A normal cardiac cycle is one series of PQRST waves. The P represents atrial depolarization (change in electrical activity), the QRS complex represents ventricular depolarization, and the T is repolarization (a return to the resting electrical state).

On an ECG, the horizontal axis (line) represents time; a slower heart rate will have more space between the PQRST complexes. On a patient with a faster heart rate, the cardiac cycles will be closer together. When a heart skips a beat, there is a long flat line between PQRSTs. Additionally, the amount of space between

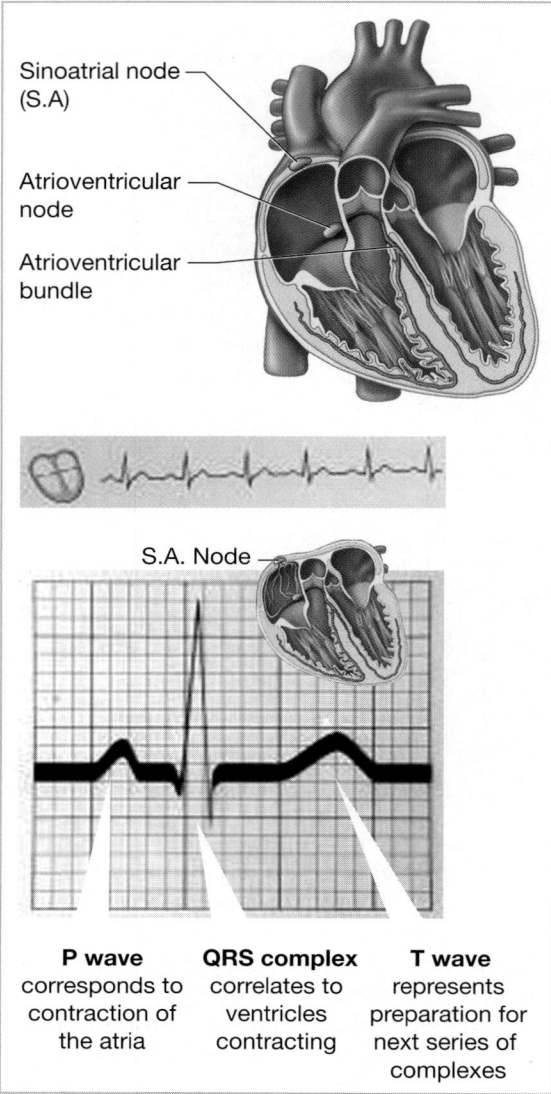

Sinoatrial node
(S.A)

Atrioventricular
node

Atrioventricular
bundle

S.A. Node

P wave
corresponds to
contraction of
the atria

QRS complex
correlates to
ventricles
contracting

T wave
represents
preparation for
next series of
complexes

FIGURE 45-1 The heart and an electrocardiogram tracing.

the P wave and the QRS complex indicates the time required for the conduction system to carry the impulse from the SA node to the Purkinje fibers.

Recordings are made from a variety of perspectives or angles known as leads. Each lead will record from a specific combination of sensors. When completed, the 12-lead ECG produces a three-dimensional record of cardiac impulses. The pattern of deflections will appear quite different on each lead. The pattern of deflections recorded, voltage or amplitude and time, assist the physician in evaluating the status of the patient's heart.

In some instances, it may be necessary to enlarge or shrink the recording. Under ordinary circumstances, a recording is made in sensitivity 1, which represents a 10-mm deflection per 1 millivolt (mV) of electricity. The size is doubled in sensitivity (2) or halved in sensitivity (½).

Lifespan Considerations has pointers on assisting children and adults during an ECG test.

Time and the Cardiac Cycle

The P wave represents the impulse that originated in the SA node and spread through the atria, called atrial depolarization. When the P wave is present in normal size and shape, then the stimulus causing the heart to beat originated in the SA node.

Normally, the P-R interval (time from the beginning of P to the beginning of QRS) is between 0.12 and 0.20 seconds (three to five small boxes on the ECG graph paper). A deviation from these times could represent an abnormality in the electrical system of the heart or in the structure of the heart that impacts the electrical system. This interval represents the time it takes for the impulse to cross the atria and the AV node and reach the ventricles. A P-R interval that is too short means the impulse has reached the ventricles through a shorter than normal pathway. If the interval is too long, a conduction delay in the AV node might be assumed.

The QRS complex represents the time necessary for the impulse to travel through the bundle of His, the bundle branches, and the Purkinje fibers to complete ventricular activation or contraction, known as ventricular depolarization. This usually takes less than 0.12 second (three small ECG boxes).

The ST segment and the T wave represent repolarization of the ventricles. The ST segment is normally flat (on the isoelectric line or baseline) or is only slightly elevated. The T wave represents a part of recovery of the ventricles after contraction. The QRS complex and the T wave typically point in the same direction, and T waves that are opposite in direction from the QRS may indicate a problem in the heart or its electrical system. While the medical assistant should not try to interpret the electrocardiogram, understanding what is normal in the cardiac cycle is helpful. Figure 45-1 shows the heart and an electrocardiogram tracing.

If the patient has an implanted automatic pacemaker, spikes will appear on the ECG with each cardiac cycle. These spikes should be rhythmically spaced on the ECG if the pacemaker is programmed for a certain rate. In fact, even when a patient is dead, the pacemaker spike will be recorded if an ECG is done—but, unfortunately, the heart muscle will not respond to the electrical stimulus. Some pacemakers are fixed rate or continuous. Some fire only when needed (on demand). Some are rate responsive to physiological changes. The atrial-paced pacemaker will show a spike with the P wave. Pacemakers that spike with the QRS wave are ventricular paced. Notify the physician if the implanted pacemaker is visible on the surface of the skin. Figure 45-2 shows an electrocardiogram tracing with a pacemaker firing.

ECG Machines

Many types of ECG machines are in use, but all should be calibrated to align with the international standard. This means that the paper in all machines moves at

As a medical professional, the medical assistant needs to look at his or her "job" as a career instead of "just a job." This means being interested in seeing what else there is to learn so that each task performed can be done better. Keeping up with current trends is very important, since the medical assistant needs to reinforce the information that the physician is teaching to the patients. Reading journals and listening to lectures are easy ways to keep up.

Although you have been taught to do an ECG correctly, you may notice other health care professionals incorrectly placing leads. You must still check for landmarks and lead placement, even if other, more seasoned employees have adopted sloppy and unprofessional habits.

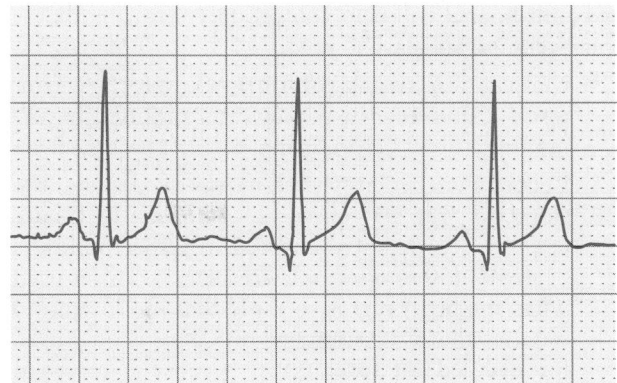

FIGURE 45-2   Electrocardiogram tracing with pacemaker spike.

the same speed of 25 mm/second and, given the same amount of electrical energy, the recording stylus will move the same distance (1 mV of electricity input will cause the stylus to deflect 10 mm), thus giving uniform recordings worldwide. Standardization is a means of verifying that each machine deflects 10 mm in response to 1 mV of electricity in sensitivity.

Older models are manual, meaning you must tell the machine what to do. You may record from arms and legs in fairly rapid succession, but you must move the chest sensor and record from each lead, then move the sensor again.

Newer models of electrocardiographs are computerized. Computerized models have automatic features so you may only need to push a button. All 10 sensors are placed on the patient at the beginning of the procedure and the computer switches from lead to lead in rapid succession. Before operating the machine, the medical assistant will enter data into the computerized electrocardiograph. Data usually include the patient's name, date of birth, diagnoses, height, weight, age, blood pressure, medications taken, and pertinent information to the ECG. The medical assistant may ask the patient these questions while placing the data in the computer, which helps the patient to relax a bit before beginning the procedure. The operator may override the automated machines if there is a need for manual controls. For example, the physician may have just ordered one rhythm strip of lead II, rather than a complete 12-lead ECG. Many computerized models can

record from more than one lead at once, to save time. Each is recorded in a separate channel or pathway for the signal and, typically, these machines record three channels at once. Other machines have a built-in interpretive feature (see Figure 45-3) and will print out a statement as to the status of the heart. Others can connect directly via fax with a regional office that will carry out the interpretation function and fax results to your office.

Although computerized electrocardiographs save considerable time in mounting ECGs, care should still be taken to ensure that a clear ECG is made before disconnecting the sensors. Computerized electrocardiographs should still be monitored for artifacts, or errors.

It is your responsibility to produce a clear and accurate tracing from each patient, so you must be familiar with the machines in your office. Read the manufacturer's instructions for the machine before using. Knowledge of

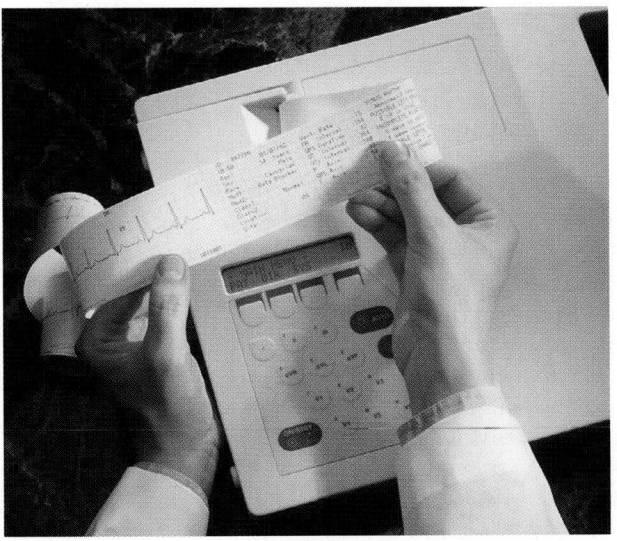

FIGURE 45-3   Single-channel electrocardiograph with interpretation of results.

the control panel will help you produce a tracing that is clear, accurate, and easy to read.

- Main power switch (off/on): Allow for a warm-up of 2 minutes (or whatever is specified by the manufacturer) before using.
- Record switch: This switch moves the paper at the standard "run 25" speed (25 mm/sec). ECGs are usually recorded at this speed. Another option is "run 50" (50 mm/sec or twice as fast). This is used when the heart rate is so rapid that interpretation requires that it be stretched out. This is only used for detailed interpretations, because it tends to waste paper and can be more difficult to read.
- Lead selector: This determines from which sensors the machine will record:
  - Standard (limb) leads: Record from two sensors placed on all extremities.
  - Augmented leads: Record from the midpoint between two limb sensors to a third limb sensor.
  - Chest leads (also called precordial leads): Record from various positions on the thorax.
- Standard adjustment screw: Increases or decreases the size of the deflection in response to 1 mV of electricity.
- Sensitivity control: Allows the operator to increase or decrease the recording size in order to enlarge or shrink the deflections to fit on the paper. When changing from the international standard of sensitivity 1 to sensitivity of ½ or 2, the operator needs to include a standard for the interpreter information.
- Standard button: Allows verification of calibration to the international standard.
- Stylus control: Centers the recording in the middle of the page or the center of each channel by moving the stylus.
- Stylus heat control: Increases or decreases heat and adjusts for the sharpest tracing.
- Marker: Indicates, by a code, which lead is being recorded.

Electrocardiogram Paper

On an ECG machine using thermal paper, a heated stylus melts the light-colored coating and reveals the black base of this special electrocardiogram paper. The stylus temperature is adjustable with a screwdriver; if it becomes too hot, a hole will be burned in the paper. If it is not hot enough, insufficient coating is removed and the line revealed is very faint. The paper is also pressure sensitive and must be handled carefully. If this paper is exposed to light for long periods, the markings will fade with time.

Many newer machines use ink in the stylus and provide a longer lasting printout. Be sure to read the man-ufacturer's instructions carefully when changing the ink cartridges in the pens.

"Time" markers, referred to as 3-second markers, are printed on all electrocardiogram paper. Look for them at the top of single-channel paper and between channels in multichannel paper. The time markers are small squares with a light line and larger squares with a darker line. The small squares are 1 mm by 1 mm square and represent 0.1 mV of voltage in the height and .04 second time in the width. The larger squares are 5 mm by 5 mm square and represent 0.5 mV of voltage in the height and 0.20 second time in the width. Thus, the paper records both time (horizontally) and voltage (vertically).

Heart Rate

Heart rate is the same as beats per minute. It is possible to estimate the heart rate from an electrocardiogram. Some offices have a protocol that states you should record some additional cycles if the heart rate is above or below certain numbers. Many cardiologists also expect you to perform an exact calculation of the heart rate before you place the recording in the patient record or on the doctor's desk. We next discuss two methods for estimation of the heart rate and one for exact calculation.

Note the 3-second markers that are printed by the manufacturer on the paper. To estimate the cardiac rate (beats per minute) from the tracing use the *6-second method*. Begin at one 3-second marker and go to the right for two additional markers, a total of 6 seconds. Count the number of QRS complexes between the first and third markers and add a zero. This is your estimated ventricular rate per minute. A similar atrial estimate can be made by counting the P waves between these markers. This estimate is accurate even if the rhythm is irregular (arrhythmia).

The heart rate can also be estimated by locating a QRS complex close to a 5-mm line, the darker line on the paper. Move to the next deflection at the right or the left, counting how many 5-mm lines intersect the tracing before the next QRS complex. Count off at each 5-mm line, beginning at the deflection near the 5-mm line and saying "zero, 300, 150, 100, 75, 60, 50." Stop counting when you reach the next QRS complex. This *count-off method* is an estimate of the ventricular rate. This estimate is accurate only for the complexes where it was done.

To obtain on exact calculation of the heart rate, recall that the paper moves at a standard speed of 25 mm/second, so it will move at 1500 mm/minute (25 mm × 60 seconds = 1500). An exact calculation of ventricular heart rate is achieved by counting the millimeter boxes between two QRS complexes and dividing that number into 1500. For instance, if there are 20 mm between two QRS complexes, 1500 divided by 20 equals 75 beats per minute. An exact calculation of atrial heart rate is achieved by counting the millimeter boxes between two P waves and by dividing that number into 1500. These calculations are accurate only for the complexes where they were done.

Rhythm is the regularity of the occurrence of heartbeats. Ventricular rhythm is determined by measuring the distance between QRS complexes. There should be a fairly consistent space between complexes. Atrial rhythm is determined by measuring the distance between P waves. There should be a fairly consistent space between waves. Again, train yourself to look at the rhythm while you are recording. Some offices have protocols about what extra tracings to record in the event the rhythm appears irregular to you.

Sensor Placement

The ECG machine records the cardiac cycle through sensors placed on the patient's bare skin. Sensors are placed over the fleshy part of the inner aspect of both lower legs, and either both upper arms or both forearms, avoiding the bony prominences. These locations are abbreviated LA for left arm, RA for right arm, LL for left leg, and RL for right leg. The RL sensor serves as an electrical reference point and is not actually used in the recording. If you have a patient on whom you cannot place one extremity sensor as planned, you must place the sensors on both extremities symmetrically. For example, a patient in a cast up to the knee requires that both sensors be placed above the knee. If a hand and forearm are amputated, both arm sensors are placed on the upper arm. The chest sensor, abbreviated with V, is used in six locations, with a number following the V, as in V1, V2, and so forth. Placement of chest sensors must be anatomically correct. Figure 45-4 show a 12-lead ECG.

By recording from different combinations of sensors, the electrical activity of the heart is seen from different angles. A lead selector switch or lead indicator selects the combination of sensors for that lead. One sensor is used for chest (unipolar) leads. A combination may be two sensors, as with standard limb (bipolar) leads, or three sensors, as with augmented limb leads.

With many sensors and many views possible, you will need to indicate on the tracing from which lead you are recording. An international marking system has been devised using dashes and dots. Some machines automatically mark the code just above the cardiac tracing. Others require manual marking with the international code. Table 45-1 lists limb, augmented, and chest leads indicating proper placement and marking codes.

It is beneficial to memorize the sensors used in the limb and augmented leads. Then, if you have difficulty getting a clear recording from one lead, you do not have to look at all the sensors, only those involved. Some find it easier to remember all the leads

and the sensors being recorded (see Table 45-1) or by picturing Einthoven's triangle which is a pictorial guide to leads. (See Figure 45-5.)

Patient Preparation

A well-informed patient is more cooperative and less anxious. Explain the equipment and procedure as well as what you will expect the patient to do. The surroundings should be pleasant and the table wide enough for adequate support. Patients will need to be bare to the waist so privacy should be provided for disrobing. Offer female patients a gown, to be worn with the opening at the front. In addition, you will need access to bare skin on the lower legs. Patients may have to remove socks or stockings. Roll long pant legs out of the way. Position the patient comfortably supine with a pillow under the head, and another under the knees, if needed, to eliminate back strain. If the patient cannot tolerate lying down, use the semi-Fowler's position instead and note that the ECG was done in that position. Jewelry usually does not interfere with sensor placement. Prepare the skin where the sensors will be applied. Any area that has been treated with talcum powder or skin lotion must be rubbed with alcohol to remove the residue to facilitate the adherence of the leads. Some shower gels leave sufficient moisturizer as a residue that can interfere with sensor contact. Such residue must be removed with alcohol. Then the electrolyte sensors may be applied.

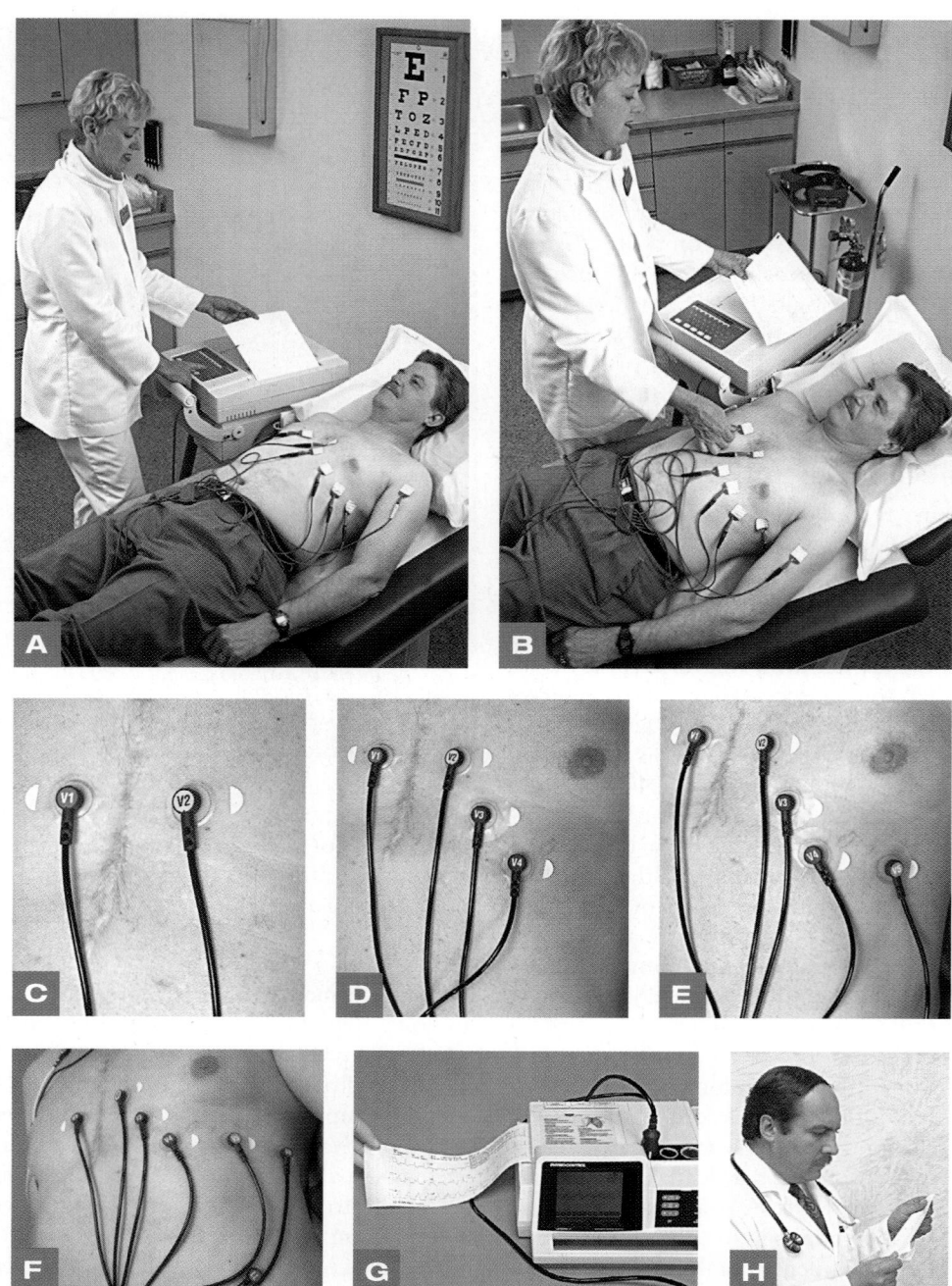

FIGURE 45-4 (A–H) Sensors of a 12-lead ECG.

Preparations

If you are to obtain a clear recording of the patient's cardiac cycle, you will need a machine, calibrated and in good working order with a good supply of paper. You may also need a screwdriver for adjustment of stylus temperature and the standard control screw. You will also need the sensors to place on the skin and a supply of electrolyte or conduction cream, gel, or pads to improve the contact between the skin and electrodes. The sensors may be metal plates that attach with rubber straps or they may be small suction cups called Welch electrodes. These will need to be cleaned between patients to prevent the accumulation of electrolyte. Adhesive disposable sensors that contain electrolyte are also available.

To begin, assemble the necessary supplies, plug the machine into a properly grounded outlet, allow it to warm up, and verify that the machine is operational and in compliance with the international standard.

TABLE 45-1   Sensor (Lead Placement and Marking Codes)

Leads	Placement	Abbreviation	Marking Code
Limb Leads			
Lead I	Right arm to left arm	RA-LA	•
Lead II	Right arm to left leg	RA-LL	••
Lead III	Left arm to left leg	LA-LL	•••
Augmented Leads			
aVR	RA-midpoint (LA-LL)	(LA-LL) RA	-
aVL	LA-midpoint (RA-LL)	(RA-LL) LA	--
aVF	LL-midpoint (RA-LA)	(RA-LA) LL	---
Chest Leads			
V1	4th intercostal space, right sternal border		—•
V2	4th intercostal space, left sternal border		—••
V3	Midway between V2 and V4		—•••
V4	5th intercostal space, midclavicular left		—••••
V5	Left anterior axillary fold, horizontal to V4		—•••••
V6	Left midaxillary, horizontal to V4 and V5		—••••••

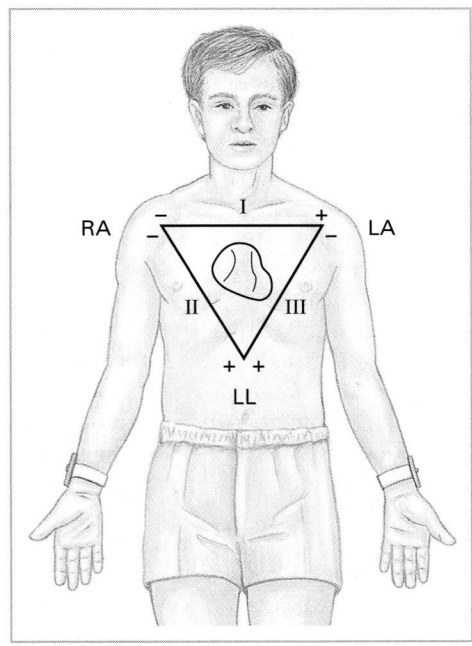

FIGURE 45-5 Einthoven's triangle.

Using manual controls, run the machine at the "run 25" setting and push the standard button briefly to release 1 mV of electricity. Stop the machine and count the small boxes covered by the deflection of the stylus. The 1 mV of electricity should have caused a positive deflection of 10 mm. If not, adjust the standard screw with a screwdriver until the deflection is precisely 10 mm, or call your service representative.

Identify, interview, and instruct the patient. Following skin preparation, the electrolyte and sensors may be applied. Electrolyte comes in many forms, including gel, lotion, and paste. Each office selects one that is compatible with the type of sensors they are using and their machines. The most recent development is a disposable gummy sensor-containing electrolyte. It requires that small alligator clamps be added to the sensor wires. These clip onto the edge of the sensor.

The procedure to attach the sensors will vary slightly, depending on the machine you are using. Some sensors are secured with a rubber strap. One electrolyte-saturated pad is placed on the skin and the sensor plate strapped over it. The limb sensors are attached

Patients with pulmonary diseases may need some educational materials on breathing exercises, a breathing program, a moderate exercise program, the avoidance of inhaled irritants, and the use of an inhaler. As you work in these areas, you will pick up some interesting tips from other patients that you can pass along.

Many patients need dietary guidance especially regarding the reduction of salt and cholesterol, and some will need information about weight loss and moderate exercise programs. However, do not give out materials or educational information without the specific direction of the physician.

and the first six leads are recorded, one at a time. Then the one chest sensor is moved from position to position as each lead is recorded. Newer machines use a small amount of electrolyte lotion and Welch electrodes. Electrolyte and all sensors are placed on the skin at once. All 12 leads are run in rapid succession because the computerized machines can switch from one lead to another quickly.

The placement of chest sensors must be precise. It is possible to complete this task without unnecessary exposure for female patients. The landmarks you will need to palpate or view are the sternum, the fourth intercostal space, both clavicles, and the left axilla. Stand on the left side of the patient and expose the sternum. Locate the right clavicle and the space immediately inferior to it. This is a supracostal space; that is, it is above the first rib and does not count as an intercostal space. Proceed toward the feet at the right edge of the sternum and, using the tips of your fingers, palpate the first rib and first intercostal space, second rib and intercostal space, and so forth until you feel the fourth intercostal space. This space at the right sternal margin is the location of V1. Lead V2 is placed at the same level on the left side of the sternum. Next, you will need to locate V4 to find V3. From the middle of the left clavicle, draw an imaginary line toward the feet, stopping one intercostal space below the level of V2. This is V4 (5th intercostal space, midclavicular left). Lift a female patient's gown up from the hemline in respect of patient privacy. Lead V4 must be at the base of the breast and, in some patients, under the breast. In males, it should be at about nipple level. Now you can locate V3 midway between V2 and V4. It is on a rib. V5 is at a point where two imaginary lines intersect. Continue to work under the patient's gown. Draw a line from the front of the left axillary fold toward the feet, parallel to the table on which the patient is lying. Draw another line toward the table from V4. Where these lines intersect is V5. Lead V6 is placed at the midaxilla, in line with V4 and V5. You will need to practice locating the landmarks and sensor sites on different body sizes and shapes. Remember to keep your female patients covered. You might need to delicately move pendulous breasts to place the sensors beneath them. Figure 45-6 shows the correct placement of leads. Procedure 45-1 shows the procedure for performing an ECG.

Arrange the patient cable to follow body contours, avoiding coils. Connect the patient cable and begin to record by performing a standard. For manual machines, select the STD lead, "run 25," and push the standard button. Stop the machine and count the boxes included in the deflection. You should get a reading of 10 mm. If you get more or less, adjust the standard control as needed with a screwdriver. Then use the lead selector knob and select the leads in sequence, running a 6-inch strip, marking the lead code, if necessary. The length of the tracing you will need depends on how your office mounts single-channel cardiograms. Have information about your mounting format before you begin to record. Adjust the stylus to the center of the paper. For automatic machines, depress "auto-run" and adjust the stylus to the center of each channel. Record the tracing, using problem-solving skills. When the cardiogram is completed, remove the sensors and wipe the electrolyte from the patient's skin. Dismiss the patient. Clean the machine. Mount the electrocardiogram, if necessary, and transfer the patient information. Sign or initial your work.

Making Adjustments

A satisfactory tracing is one that is accurate, readable, clear, travels down the center of the page, and has a baseline that is consistently horizontal. If the baseline begins to drift upward or downward, use the position control knob to return it to the center of the page. Observe whether the tracing remains within the graph portion of the paper. If the deflections are so large that they exceed the upper and lower limits of the graph, you will have to reduce the sensitivity from 1 to ½. This will make the tracing half as large, and you will need to include a standard to let the interpreter know what you have done. One millivolt of electricity will cause a deflection of 5 mm in sensitivity ½. However, if the tracing in sensitivity 1 is so tiny that it is not readable, increase the size by

Recording a 12-Lead Electrocardiograph

OBJECTIVE: Perform an ECG without assistance.

Equipment and Supplies

ECG machine with sensors, patient cable, power cord; ECG paper; electrolyte, if needed; alcohol; screwdriver, for adjustments, if needed; patient gown, if needed

Method

1. Perform hand hygiene.
2. Assemble necessary supplies.
3. Attach and plug in the power cord.
4. Verify that the machine is operational and positioned properly.
5. Identify, interview, and instruct the patient on the procedure.
6. Offer female patients gowns to be worn with the opening down the front.
7. Position the patient flat on the table with a pillow under the head and one under the knees if needed.
8. Prepare the electrode sites and attach the electrodes. Limb electrodes should be applied over the fleshy part of the inner aspects of the lower legs and forearms. Chest leads should be applied as illustrated in Figure 45-6.
9. Connect the patient cable.
10. Instruct the patient to relax, breathe normally, and refrain from speaking.
11. Standardize the machine.
12. Adjust the stylus to the center of the paper or the center of each channel.
13. Record. For automatic machines, depress AUTO-RUN; for manual machines select the leads in sequence and use RUN 25. Use your problem-solving skills if you encounter artifacts.
14. Mark the leads, if necessary.
15. Remove the sensors; wipe electrolyte from the patient's skin, if used.
16. Politely dismiss the patient, aiding the patient in getting up and dressed, if necessary.
17. Perform hand hygiene.
18. Clean the machine, straps, and sensors according to manufacturer's instructions.
19. Mount the ECG if necessary and transfer patient information.
20. Chart the procedure in the patient's record. Sign or initial your work.

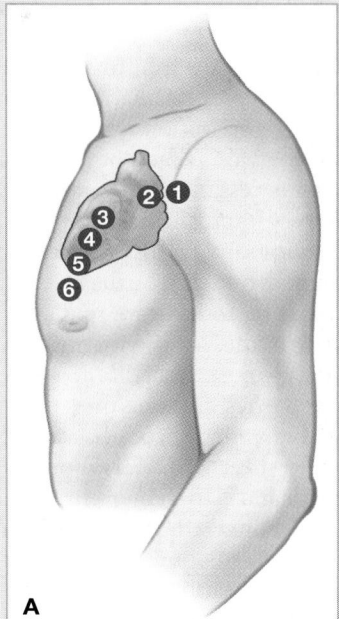

A

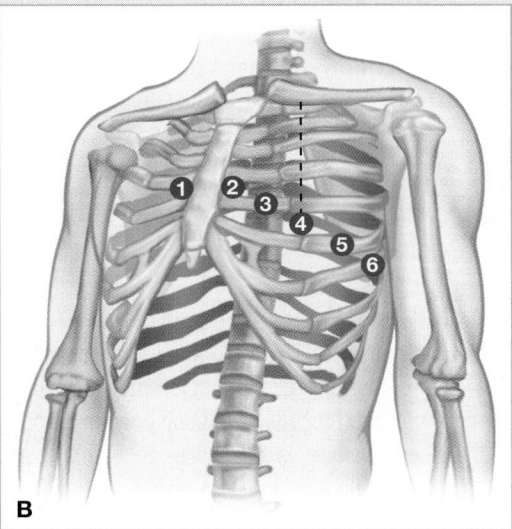

B

FIGURE 45-6 Placement of chest leads.

Charting Example

3/11/XX	2:10 P.M.

12-lead ECG performed and given to MD to read.

W. Short, CMA

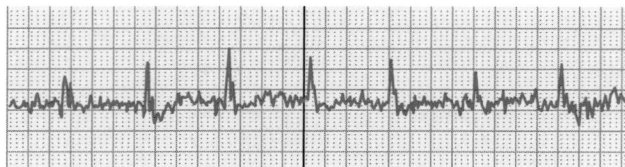

FIGURE 45-7 Somatic tremor.

changing the sensitivity from 1 to 2. Again, place a standard on the page to let the physician know that you have made a change. One millivolt of electricity will cause a deflection of 20 mm in sensitivity 2.

Because the paper moves through the machine at the rate of 25 mm/second, an option available in recording is to move the paper twice as fast, or at 50 mm/second. This would only be necessary if the cardiac cycles were compacted by a very rapid heart rate. In this case, a better quality cardiogram would be produced if the cycles were stretched out. If you have to change the speed, mark the tracing to indicate that you did so. In machines that mark the lead with an international code, the code marks are stretched out; the dots appear as dashes, and the dashes are long ones.

Multichannel machines produce an ECG very quickly, on a single sheet of paper about 8 inches by 11 inches. You will have to center three baselines. A sensitivity or speed change affects all three channels.

Knowledge of the leads and their sensor locations will help the medical assistant to trace back to the source any irregular or erratic markings, known as artifacts. You can also perform other troubleshooting techniques during the recording process. Failure to make the necessary corrections will result in an unsat-

Cultural Considerations

Be very careful to protect the privacy of your patient while doing an ECG, making sure the door to the exam room is closed and that it remains closed during the entire procedure. Expose only as much of the chest wall as is necessary to attach the leads and then be sure to use a drape or sheet to carefully cover the chest before starting the test. Some cultures forbid a male professional to do this procedure on a female so be very respectful of these cultural habits. Even a male patient should have his chest covered during the test, unless he verbalizes other wishes. If possible, a female medical assistant should do the ECG on a female patient.

isfactory or no tracing. The physician will not be able to read and interpret such a recording.

Artifacts

Occasionally, the sensors will detect electrical activity from a source other than the heart. These deflections or artifacts impair accurate interpretation of the tracing. The medical assistant needs to find the cause of the artifact and correct it. The different causes of artifacts and how to correct them include the following:

1. Somatic tremor. A tense muscle or a muscle contraction, even one that you cannot see, is called somatic tremor. It may result from patient discomfort, tension, chills, and talking or moving. Calm and reassure the patient. Suggest that the patient relax, breathe normally, and not talk. If necessary, place the patient's hands palm-side down under the hips. This is especially helpful if the patient is not relaxed on the narrow table. This position is also best for patients with a tremor disorder. They will display the smallest number of artifacts in this position. (See Figure 45-7.)

2. Wandering baseline and baseline shift. This artifact is caused by poor sensor contact with the skin, such as when sensors are dirty or applied too tightly or too loosely, when lotion or talcum prevents good contact with the skin, or when the patient cable slips toward the floor, pulling on the lead wires. You need to readjust, reapply, or clean the sensors, and place the patient cable securely on the table. You may need to clean the skin with alcohol or cut chest hair. (See Figure 45-8.)

3. AC (alternating current) interference. Electrical current in wires and equipment may be picked up by the patient's body and the recording machine. This appears in the recording as small regular spikes or static, and is due to improper grounding, nearby electrical equipment in use, or twisted and coiled lead wires. Ground the machine properly. Unplug other electrical equipment in the area. Move the machine to the patient's feet and away from walls containing cables. You may have to wait until a procedure in an adjacent room, such as an x-ray, is completed. (See Figure 45-9.)

4. Erratic stylus. Loose or broken lead wires cause the stylus to thrash erratically, and go off the page. Repair the wires, replace them, or call for service on the equipment.

Mounting an Electrocardiogram

Machines that record one lead at a time produce a tracing that is 6 or 12 feet long. To have a document that will fit into the patient record, use a mounting device. Manufacturers make heavy paper folders with pockets or self-stick areas labeled for each of the leads. Many different forms are available. Knowing the form you will use for mounting will help avoid the waste in obtaining a longer tracing than you need. Select the best part of the recording for that lead. It must have a straight baseline and no artifacts. Cut and trim it, and place it in the appropriate area of the folder. Double-check your work to make certain you have read the international code for leads correctly. Repeat the process until all 12 leads have been properly mounted. Employer preference will determine where to place the standardization. Machines that record from three leads at once do not require mounting. The final product fits nicely into a patient record.

What Is Normal?

A normal sinus rhythm means that each heartbeat has three distinct waves: a P wave, a T wave, and between the two, a QRS complex where the Q is a downward deflection, the R is an upward deflection, and the S is a downward deflection following an R. The beats come at regular intervals, indicating the impulse originates in the SA node. Within the lead being recorded, each cardiac cycle appears the same as previous cycles.

Abnormalities

Occasionally a tracing will reveal an abnormality caused by cardiac pathology in the patient. An observant medical assistant will recognize the more common abnormalities and draw them to the attention of the physician or follow office protocol, which often calls for an additional recording in a particular lead. Table 45-2 lists some cardiac pathology that can be visualized by ECGs.

Special Tests

Some ECG-related diagnostic procedures are performed regularly in the primary care office or in cardiology. The two discussed next involve recording additional lengths of tracings, and may be part of written office protocol for cardiograms.

In the first one, a rhythm strip will be run in lead II for 20 seconds on the physician's request or, in some instances, if the medical assistant sees anything that appears abnormal on the tracing. This is not cut and mounted, but carefully folded and given to the physician for interpretation.

In the second one, an inspiration strip is run on lead II for 10 seconds with the patient holding his or her breath. This is of greatest value when, as the patient breathes, your tracing shows wandering baseline. This will eliminate any respiratory impact on the tracing.

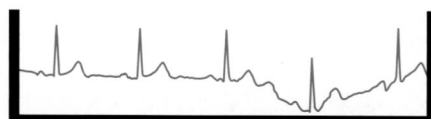

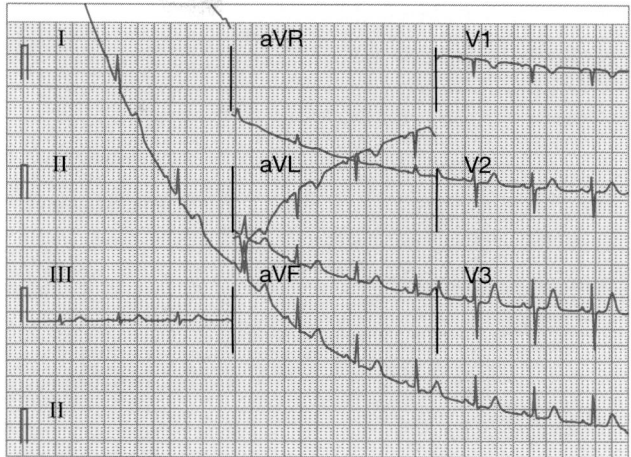

FIGURE 45-8   Wandering baseline.

Exercise Tolerance Testing

A stress test or treadmill is an evaluation of the heart's response during moderate exercise following a 12-lead electrocardiogram. This may be used to evaluate patients with a high risk for developing heart disease or known to have early heart disease, and for patients about to begin a strenuous exercise program. This test is also done on patients who have cardiac complaints when exercising and as an evaluation of their rehabilitation following cardiac surgery.

The patient should be given instructions before the scheduled test day to wear comfortable exercise or

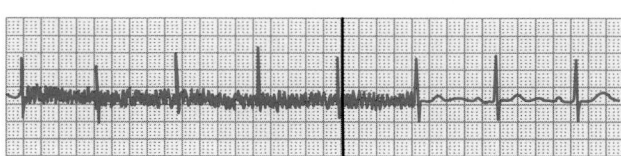

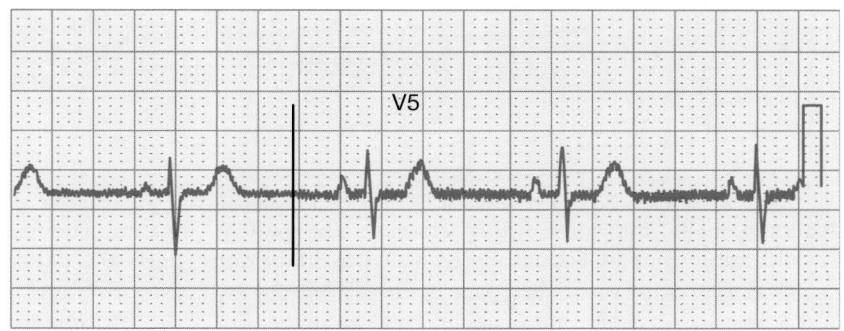

FIGURE 45-9   AC (alternating current) interference.

TABLE 45-2 Abnormalities Caused by Cardiac Pathology

Abnormality	Description
Sinus tachycardia	There are more than 100 beats per minute; cycles are normal.
Sinus bradycardia	There are fewer than 60 beats per minutes; cycles are normal.
Sinus arrhythmia	Normally seen in children and young adults; all aspects of the ECG are normal except the irregularity. The space between QRS complexes is not equal. The heart rate increases on inspiration and decreases on expiration.
Premature atrial contractions (PACs)	A P wave occurs earlier than expected, usually from a source outside the sinus node. Therefore, P waves are distorted.
Paroxysmal atrial tachycardia (PAT)	There is a common arrhythmia, usually seen in young adults with normal hearts. There are no visible P waves because they are hidden by the T wave of the previous cycle. The atrial rate is between 140–250/minute. In many ways it looks on the ECG like repeated PACs.
Atrial flutter	This rapid fluttering of the upper chambers looks on the ECG like the pattern of teeth on a saw. The atrial rate is 250–350/minute. Not all of the impulses are conducted through the AV node because they are coming too fast. There is some "blockage" at the AV node. This is one type of heart block.
Atrial fibrillation	There are as many 350 irregular P waves and 130–150 irregular QRS complexes per minute.
AV heart block	The node is diseased and does not conduct the impulse well. There are three types: First degree, where the PR interval is prolonged; second degree, where some waves do not pass through to the ventricles; and third degree or complete AV block, where the atria and ventricles beat independently.
Premature ventricular contractions (PVCs)	The wide QRS complexes occur without preceding P waves. They may be caused by electrolyte imbalance, stress, smoking, alcohol or toxic reactions to drugs and in a majority of patients who have had a heart attack.
Ventricular tachycardia	Three or more consecutive PVCs. Usually originating below the SA node, the complexes are wide and bizarre in appearance.
Ventricular fibrillation	The waves are irregular and rounded, the contractions uncoordinated. Death may occur in as little as 4 minutes.
Myocardial infarction (MI)	There are broad and deep Q waves. *Old injury:* The ST segment is usually depressed below the baseline. *New injury:* The ST segment is usually elevated above the baseline. Angina pectoris is the name for the syndrome of pain and oppression in the anterior chest due to heart tissue being deprived of oxygen. If this pain lasts 20–30 minutes, suspect a myocardial infarction in which the heart tissue is actually dying.

walking shoes and loose-fitting clothes. The patient should know that ECGs will be recorded as he or she walks at a carefully prescribed pace in the presence of the physician. Increases in rate or incline will be made, but the patient should not feel discomfort or shortness of breath. The medical assistant prepares the patient, connects the patient to the recording devices (ECG, heart rate, BP), and frequently checks blood pressure during the test. The sensors are all placed on the torso. The precordial sensors (V1–V6) are placed as for the regular

PROCEDURE

Treadmill Stress Test

OBJECTIVE: Apply monitors, instruct the patient, monitor, and record ECG, BP, and heart rate periodically and make adjustments to the treadmill as requested.

Equipment and Supplies

treadmill; sensors; blood pressure monitor

Method

1. Assemble necessary supplies.
2. Plug in the power cord and turn on the machine.
3. Verify that the treadmill is operational.
4. Identify, interview, and instruct the patient. Offer female patients a gown, to be worn to open down the front.
5. Perform a baseline ECG (see Procedure 45-1).
6. Disconnect the patient cable from the ECG machine.
7. Attach a sphygmomanometer to the patient's arm.
8. Permit the patient to walk about the room or on the slow-moving treadmill to see what it feels like.
9. Connect the patient to all recording devices.
10. Check with the physician to determine the pace and incline of the treadmill.
11. Record BP, ECG, and heart and respiratory rate periodically as you observe the patient's face for redness, difficulty breathing, chest pain, and so forth.
12. When the test is completed, clean the patient's skin and assist with dressing as needed.
13. Organize the documentation into the patient record.

Charting Example

3/11/XX	3:10 P.M.

Stress test performed. Patient observed for 15 minutes after test. Patient tolerated the procedure well.

M. Shapiro, CMA

ECG, but the arm and leg sensors are put at the midclavicular line on the top of the torso and on the midclavicular line on the abdomen. The physician evaluates the effect of exercise on the heart rate, blood pressure, and the electrocardiogram. The physician may order the test to be stopped if the patient has trouble breathing or complains of chest pain. Thallium is sometimes injected into the patient's vein before a stress test for better understanding of blood flow. Procedure 45-2 describes how to perform a stress test.

Because there is always the risk of cardiac arrest, the medical assistant becomes responsible for maintaining emergency equipment that might be needed and having it in the room at the time of the test. Oxygen equipment, a defibrillator, an airway, intravenous solutions, and medications should be periodically checked and replaced, if outdated or not functioning. Figure 45-10 shows the patient being closely observed during a stress test. Always be sure a physician is present when a stress test is done.

Holter Monitor

The Holter monitor records cardiac activity while the patient is ambulatory for at least a 24-hour period. Holter monitoring is performed when the ECG is not conclusive or the cardiac irregularity was not captured on the tracing. A small tape recorder and a patient diary are used to

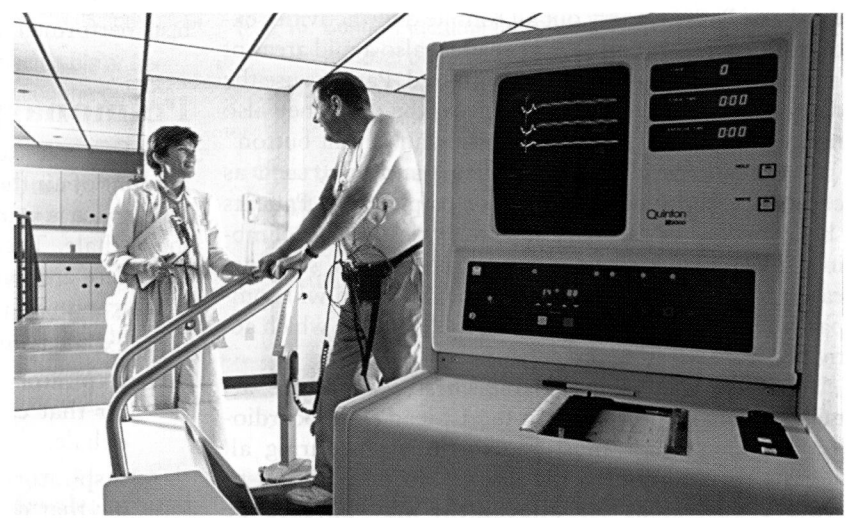

FIGURE 45-10 The patient must be observed very closely during a stress test.

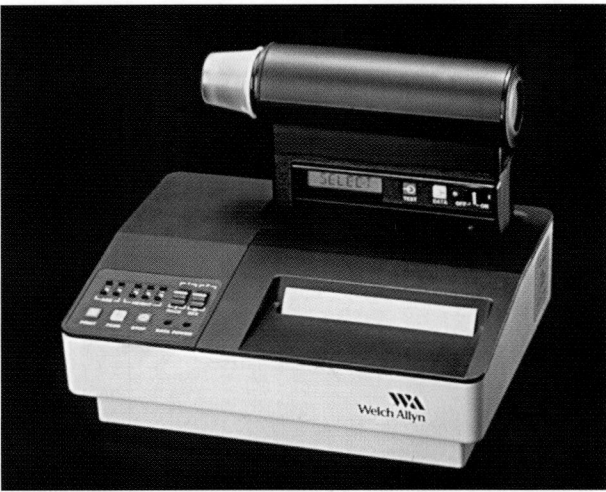

FIGURE 45-13 One type of spirometer.

- Inspiratory capacity (IC): the amount of air that can be inhaled after normal expiration.
- Functional residual capacity (FRC): the amount of air remaining in the lungs after a normal expiration.

Total lung capacity and functional residual capacity will increase in obstructive lung disease (those diseases that obstruct the flow of air out of the lungs and generally slow expiratory rate and increase residual volume). Patients with asthma have a decreased ability of the lungs to deflate during expiration. In restrictive lung disease the volumes are decreased because expansion of the lungs is prevented, thereby diminishing total lung capacity, vital capacity, and inspiratory capacity.

These tests are performed by a respiratory care specialist, usually in a hospital setting, as ordered by the pulmonologist. The capacities are included here because, in working with the specialist and pulmonary patients, you encounter the terms and volumes. Sometimes, however, spirometry testing is done in an occupational medicine office, allergy specialist's office, or pulmonologist's office. It is helpful to know what they describe. To continue monitoring the effects of respiratory disease, an evaluation can be carried out by the medical assistant in an office or clinic.

Volume Capacity Spirometry

A diagnostic spirometer is employed to evaluate the patient's ability to ventilate during a maximum forced exhale. This device measures and records the volume exhaled and the time required completing it. This air movement is recorded on special paper with vertical second marks and horizontal liter marks in one of three ways:

- Forced vital capacity (FVC): amount of air exhaled after maximum inspiration or one of the two timed FVCs.

- Forced expiratory volume (FEV) in 1 second (FEV1): amount of air exhaled during the first second of FVC maneuver
- Maximal midexpiratory flow (MMEF) is the average flow rate during middle half of FVC.

Figure 45-13 shows one type of spirometer.

Patient Preparation

The patient must have accurate instructions and reassurance with questions answered. Generally, preparation begins when the patient schedules the appointment. Patients should eat lightly and not smoke prior to the test, and should avoid using analgesics or bronchodilators for 24 hours prior to the test, if the physician so orders.

Patient preparation for spirometry testing is important and must be thorough. When the procedure is scheduled, a brochure explaining the test should be provided to the patient. Instruct the patient to refrain from smoking for 6 hours and to not use bronchodilators or nebulizers for 6 hours prior to the test.

On arrival, again explain the test, the steps involved, and determine if there are reasons the test should not be performed such as flu, cold, or allergy. Weigh and measure the patient, and measure and record vital signs. The height and weight are necessary for calculations after the test. Demonstrate and explain in simple terms what you would like the patient to do. If the patient has ill-fitting dentures ask him or her to remove them, because lips must be sealed tightly around the mouthpiece. Have the patient loosen any tight clothing, ties, girdles, bras, or belts that could impede the test. The patient should be encouraged to sit because light-headedness may cause dizziness. The patient's feet should be flat on the floor, legs uncrossed, and head and chin slightly elevated for the entire procedure. This proper upright position must be maintained during a spirometry test. If the patient prefers a standing versus sitting position, that is acceptable because it makes no difference with the results, the choice depends on patient comfort.

The test should be repeated three times successfully and the best two maneuvers should be used to calculate the pulmonary function. Results are considered normal if the patient's best result is 80% of pretest calculated values. The effectiveness of bronchodilator medication can be evaluated if the results are abnormal. The patient may be given a bronchodilator and then retested to determine the effectiveness of the medication.

Spirometric measurements depend on patient effort, which, in turn, depends on the coaching of the medical assistant. Generally, three good measurements are performed and the best is considered for evaluation. Patients usually need some practice with wrapping their lips around the disposable mouthpiece and forcibly exhaling.

Spirometry Procedure

Pulmonary function tests (PFTs) to evaluate lung volume and lung capacity are performed mainly in a pulmonary function laboratory. One noninvasive PFT, spirometry, is regularly performed in the office setting. Spirometry assesses lung function, by measuring how much air can be held in the lungs and how much and how quickly air can be exhaled. There are many types of spirometers on the market. Some are mechanical, others are computerized. All spirometers consist of a mouthpiece and tubing connected to a recording device. The patient is asked to inhale as deeply as possible and then exhale as forcefully, and as completely as possible, while measurements are being taken. Several different measurements can be made from a spirometer test.

See Table 45-3 for a list of lung capacity tests and definitions. Spirometry results reflect the elasticity of the lungs, their ability to ventilate, and the strength of the respiratory muscles. These tests are good screening tools for pulmonary function and help the physician determine impaired function due to narrowing or obstruction in conditions such as emphysema, asthma, bronchitis, and diseases that cause muscle weakness such as myasthenia gravis. Spirometry tests can be used to evaluate the effectiveness of a specific dose of medication. To obtain an accurate result, the patient must inhale deeply and then exhale as forcefully as possible for as long as possible. Your role will be to act as cheerleader and coach to induce the patient to give a peak performance.

Procedure 45-4 lists the steps necessary to determine a patient's forced vital capacity using a spirometer.

A variety of spirometers are available in the marketplace, but they must meet minimum standards for acceptable performance. When using automated computerized machines, the spirometry procedure is complicated by the necessity of dealing with the computer program. You must enter patient data into the computer, such as

age, height, weight, vital signs, and medication, depending on the machine and the computer program used. The machine usually makes predictions about what the graphic representation should look like.

There are changes anticipated with lung disease. Note that in obstructive disease, more time is required for a complete exhale, and in a restrictive pattern, maximum exhale is reached quickly but the volume is small. With the test results, the patient's pulmonary measurement is compared to the predicted values for the patient's height, weight, age, race, and sex by the physician who takes into account the patient's clinical status at the same time. Clinical status refers to the patient's

TABLE 45-3 Pulmonary Function Tests

Lung Function	Definition
Total volume (TV)	Amount of air inspired and expired in a normal respiration
Vital capacity (VC)	Maximum amount of air that can be expired after a maximum inspiration
Inspiratory capacity (IC)	Maximum amount of air that can be inspired after a normal expiration
Expiratory reserve volume (ERV)	Maximum volume of air left that can be exhaled after normal expiration
Residual volume ((RV)	Volume of air left in lungs after forced expiration
Functional residual volume (FVR)	Amount of air left in the lungs after normal expiration
Forced vital capacity (FVC)	Amount of air that can be forcefully exhaled from a maximum inhalation
Maximal volume ventilation (MVV)	Maximum volume that patient can breathe in and out in 1 minute

PROCEDURE

Performing a Spirometer Test to Measure Forced Vital Capacity

OBJECTIVE: Perform a forced vital capacity test.

Equipment and Supplies

functioning spirometry machine; nose clip; patient mouthpiece; disinfectant; biohazardous waste container; paper and pencil; scale for height and weight; sphygmomanometer and blood pressure cuff

Method

1. Perform hand hygiene.
2. Assemble all equipment.
3. Calibrate spirometer as necessary, according to manufacturer's instructions.
4. Identify patient.
5. Question patient about preparing for test by not smoking and not using bronchodilators for the preceding 6 hours.
6. Inquire about general health at present.
7. Explain and demonstrate procedure to patient.
8. Weigh and measure patient and record.
9. Measure patient's vital signs and record.
10. Explain the proper positioning and loosen any tight clothing.
11. Start machine and enter needed data.
12. Review procedure with patient. Be sure that patient knows to breathe forcibly several times into spirometer.
13. Apply nose clip.
14. Have the patient take a big breath in.
15. Have the patient place the mouthpiece in his or her mouth and seal his or her lips around the mouthpiece.
16. Push the start button at the same time as you give the instructions to the patient.
17. Encourage the patient to blast breath out as hard, fast, and long as possible.
18. Make recommendations to improve outcome, if necessary.
19. Obtain second set of maneuvers.
20. Obtain third set of maneuvers.
21. Continue until you have three acceptable outcomes. You may obtain up to eight attempts, if needed, to obtain three good trials. Some computerized machines will select the best attempt and print it.
22. Remove nose clip and ask patient to remain until physician reviews results.
23. Give physician trial information.
24. Record results in patient's chart.
25. Clean tubing and dispose of mouthpieces, using Standard Precautions.

Charting Example

3/12/XX	8:30 A.M.

Spirometry performed with 3 good results submitted to MD.

K. Christianson, CMA

---

physical condition at the time of the test. A fever, asthma attack, poor night's sleep, scoliosis, or any of a number of other variables could affect the pulmonary function results. A prediction indicator result of 85% to 100% would indicate no impairment; 75% to 85% would be slight impairment, and so on. Procedure 45-4 describes how to perform spirometry tests.

Peak Flow Meter

Peak flow meters measure the patient's ability to move air into and out of the lungs. Keeping a record of peak flow either daily or when attacks occur helps the physician establish effective treatments and prepare a treatment plan.

It may be your responsibility to teach the patient and family members how to use a peak flow meter correctly. Specifically, it measures the fastest rate at which the patient exhales after taking a maximum breath (peak expiratory flow rate). Instruct the patient to put the mouth around the mouthpiece and blow forcibly into the meter, which will measure the peak expiratory flow rate. The patient should keep a diary of the flow rates to see if medication is helping or the disease is getting worse.

A patient may use a flow meter at home to monitor breathing. This information will assist the physician with determining the most effective medication regimen. On a "good" day, the patient blows as hard as possible into the device to establish a goal or baseline against which to compare other expiratory attempts.

Oximeter

For patients suffering from cardiac and pulmonary disorders it may be necessary to determine the oxygen content of the blood. An electronic device called an oximeter, which can be clipped on the bridge of the nose, the forehead, earlobe, or to the tip of a finger, determines the oxygen concentration in arterial blood. This equipment allows for the measurement of blood oxygenation and can determine whether treatments are effective or not. A pulse oximeter is illustrated in Figure 45-14.

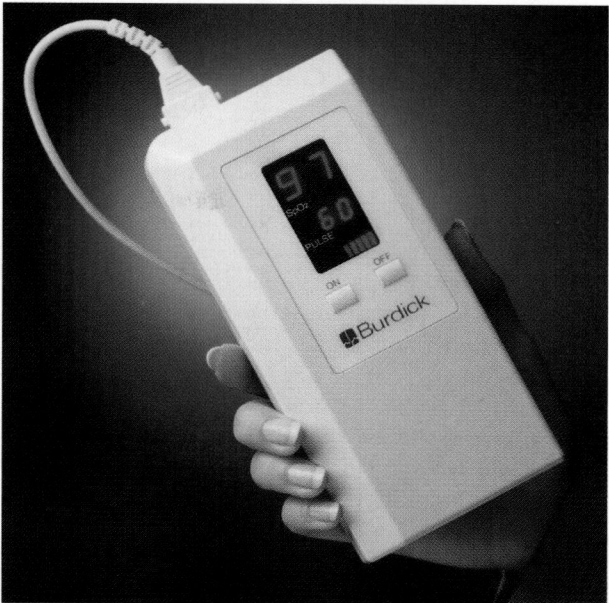

FIGURE 45-14 Burdick 100 pulse oximeter.

Treatments

After a basic test, some patients are asked to breathe an aerosolized bronchodilator, and the physician evaluates the value of the drug in causing an increase in capacity. The graphic test results become part of the patient's permanent record.

Nebulizers and inhalers are used to treat asthma and other respiratory conditions. Nebulizers deliver medication directly to deeper areas in the lungs. Inhalers are used to deliver a measured amount of medication directly into the respiratory tract to dilate the airways.

Nebulizers

The small-volume nebulizer is sometimes used to treat breathing difficulties. If a handheld nebulizer is used, a small amount of aerosolized liquid medication mixture is placed in a chamber. Then the patient is asked to put the nebulizer in the mouth and breathe deeply for 8 to 10 minutes. A high-pressure gas stream of either air or oxygen passing through a small opening actually creates the aerosol. The aerosol is then delivered into the patient through either a mouthpiece or a mask. The procedure for a nebulizer is to first note the patient's baseline data (auscultation, vital signs, oximeter reading, and peak expiratory flow rate). Then assemble the handheld nebulizer and select a mouthpiece or a mask for delivery. Using a mask can decrease the amount of drug that reaches the lungs by about 1% or 2% because of deposition on the face. The mask should be used only when the patient is unable to take the treatment with a mouthpiece.

Measure the proper dosage of drug and diluent into the nebulizer. Set the gas flow to the nebulizer at 6 to 8 L/min. Position the patient in a semi-Fowler's position. Implement the therapy and encourage the patient to breathe slowly through the mouth. Instruct the patient to deeply inspire periodically and to hold a breath for about 4 to 10 seconds. When no aerosol is flowing, discontinue treatment. Monitor and evaluate the patient's response to the treatment.

Encourage the patient to cough well, quantifying the amount and describing the type of sputum if the cough is productive. Monitor the patient's pulse, breath sounds, peak expiratory flow rates, and blood oxygenation. Disassemble and store the equipment properly. Record the data in the patient's chart.

Inhalers

One type of inhaler, a metered-dose inhaler (MDI), holds about 200 doses of the prescribed medication in a pressurized container with an attached mouthpiece. Patient teaching is very important because MDIs are frequently misused, resulting in inadequate treatment. As with instructions on how to properly use nebulizers, demonstrate for the patient first and then ask him or her to repeat the demonstration for you. Written backup material is provided to the patient as well.

The patient should put the mouth over the mouthpiece of the inhaler and inhale when the medication container is pressed into the inhaler. A puff of medication will be dispensed. After the dose is dispensed, remove the medication and clean the plastic inhaler with soap and water.

Pulmonary Diseases

The medical assistant usually performs pulmonary function tests in the office for chronic obstructive problems, such as asthma (spasms of the bronchial tubes or swelling of the mucous membranes), chronic bronchitis (inflammation of the bronchial mucous membranes), cystic fibrosis (faulty exocrine glands secrete too much mucus, which obstructs the lungs), or emphysema (permanent enlargement of air spaces beyond the terminal bronchioles). These obstructive pulmonary diseases tend to be chronic and worsen over time if treatment is not effective. As the lungs are unable to expand or are restricted from expanding, the pulmonary function tests will show altered TLC, IC, and VC. As a medical assistant, you may find yourself doing many pulmonary function tests on the same patient to assess whether the drug treatments are effective.

SUMMARY

The use of electrocardiography and spirometry for the early diagnosis and treatment of heart and lung disease has contributed to the lengthened life expectancy of many patients and has improved their quality of life. ECGs are usually performed while lying down. Sometimes ECGs are done in combination with stressful exercise to see the effect on the heart. The patient may be monitored for 24 hours with a Holter monitor to see which activities stress the heart. The medical assistant may also be asked to perform pulmonary function tests (spirometer, oximeter, and peak flow meter) to assess patient breathing function, or may be asked to give patient treatments with nebulizers or inhalers. Pulmonary function tests are not usually done when the problem is an upper respiratory one. The oximeter can be used in an acute event to determine blood oxygenation, and spirometers can be used to determine pulmonary response to medications and treatments. Accuracy in carrying out your duties during these tests will provide the physician with the best possible data to make that diagnosis and institute the correct treatment.

Chapter Review

COMPETENCY REVIEW

1. Define and spell the terms to learn for this chapter.
2. Describe how to maintain and operate electrocardiograph equipment and pulmonary function equipment.
3. Identify by name and location of their sensors the standard 12 leads on an electrocardiograph machine.
4. Name and describe four ECG artifacts.
5. Explain the differences between *obstructive* and *restrictive* pulmonary disease.
6. Explain the purpose of pulmonary function tests.

PREPARING FOR THE CERTIFICATION EXAM

1. Which of the following is the amount of air that can be forcibly inspired after a normal inhalation?
   A. tidal volume
   B. expiratory reserve
   C. inspiratory reserve
   D. total lung capacity
   E. residual volume

2. When performing an ECG on a patient with a right lower leg cast, the leg sensors are placed:
   A. on the left leg
   B. on both upper legs
   C. on both upper arms
   D. on the bottom of the feet
   E. they are eliminated.

3. An electrocardiogram is a:
   A. recording of the voltage with respect to time
   B. recording of the mechanical action of the heart
   C. technique for making recordings of heart activity
   D. machine used to make cardiac tracings.
   E. recording of the size of the heart.

4. Normally, a complete ECG consists of _____ sensors and _____ leads.
   A. 10, 10
   B. 8, 10
   C. 6, 12
   D. 12, 10
   E. 10, 12

5. The Purkinje fibers are located on or in the:
   A. right atrium
   B. left atrium
   C. apex
   D. ventricles
   E. septum between the atria

6. The portion of the ECG that relates to ventricular depolarization is the:
   A. P wave
   B. QRS complex
   C. T wave
   D. U wave
   E. P-R interval

continued on next page

7. The patient uses which of the following at home to measure respiratory function?
   A. peak flow meter
   B. spirometer
   C. oximeter
   D. inhaler
   E. nebulizer

8. The little "spark" that begins or starts the heartbeat originates in the:
   A. Purkinje fibers
   B. vagus nerve
   C. SA node
   D. AV node

9. The correct order of stimulation in the electrical conduction system of the heart is:
   A. AV node, SA node, bundle of HIS, bundle branches, Purkinje network
   B. SA node, AV node, bundle of His, bundle branches, Purkinje network
   C. Bundle of His, AV node, SA node, bundle branches, Purkinje network
   D. Purkinje network, Purkinje fibers, SA node, AV node
   E. Bundle of His, SA node, AV node, bundle branches, and Purkinje network

10. Sensors placed at the 5th intercostal space, midclavicular line are:
    A. V1   D. V4
    B. V2   E. V5
    C. V3

CRITICAL THINKING

1. State the patient explanation and preparation you would give for a patient having his or her first cardiogram.
2. During the procedure, Mrs. Nagle asked why you used the "cold paste" and why she had to remove her stockings and the talcum powder. How would you answer Mrs. Nagle's questions?
2. Explain to Mrs. Nagle what an ambulatory monitor does and what she will be expected to do.
3. Why does she need to have a 12-lead cardiogram first?

ON THE JOB

Bonny Glidewell, CMA, works in a cardiologist's office. She passes out a questionnaire to all her patients about their lifestyle habits (exercise, eating, smoking, etc.) in order to create patient teaching brochures.

1. Which questions should she ask to determine which behaviors are the most prevalent in this practice?
2. What would you expect to be the usual diet of a person with coronary artery disease?
3. What instructions might she give on how to stop smoking?
4. Construct a brochure to give to patients to help them change their diets.
5. Create a patient teaching brochure on the importance of exercise.

INTERNET ACTIVITY

Go to www.americanheart.org and www.lungusa.org and create two brochures to teach patients about heart and lung health.

MediaLink More on electrocardiography and pulmonary function, including interactive resources, can be found on the Student CD-ROM accompanying this textbook.

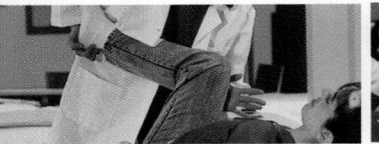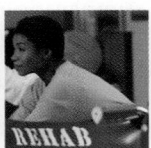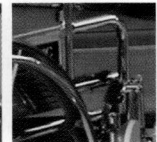

Medical Assistant Role Delineation Chart

HIGHLIGHT indicates material covered in this chapter.

ADMINISTRATIVE

Administrative Procedures

- Perform basic administrative medical assisting functions
- Schedule, coordinate and monitor appointments
- Schedule inpatient/outpatient admissions and procedures
- Understand and apply third-party guidelines
- Obtain reimbursement through accurate claims submission
- Monitor third-party reimbursement
- Understand and adhere to managed care policies and procedures
- *Negotiate managed care contracts*

Practice Finances

- Perform procedural and diagnostic coding
- Apply bookkeeping principles

- Manage accounts receivable
- *Manage accounts payable*
- *Process payroll*
- *Document and maintain accounting and banking records*
- *Develop and maintain fee schedules*
- *Manage renewals of business and professional insurance policies*
- *Manage personnel benefits and maintain records*
- *Perform marketing, financial, and strategic planning*

CLINICAL

Fundamental Principles

- Apply principles of aseptic technique and infection control
- Comply with quality assurance practices
- Screen and follow up patient test results

Diagnostic Orders

- Collect and process specimens
- Perform diagnostic tests

Patient Care

- Adhere to established patient screening procedures
- Obtain patient history and vital signs
- Prepare and maintain examination and treatment areas
- Prepare patient for examinations, procedures and treatments

- Assist with examinations, procedures and treatments
- Prepare and administer medications and immunizations
- Maintain medication and immunization records
- Recognize and respond to emergencies
- Coordinate patient care information with other health care providers
- Initiate IV and administer IV medications with appropriate training and as permitted by state law

GENERAL

Professionalism

- Display a professional manner and image
- Demonstrate initiative and responsibility
- Work as a member of the health care team
- Prioritize and perform multiple tasks
- Adapt to change
- Promote the CMA credential
- Enhance skills through continuing education
- Treat all patients with compassion and empathy
- Promote the practice through positive public relations

Communication Skills

- Recognize and respect cultural diversity
- Adapt communications to individual's ability to understand
- Use professional telephone technique

- Recognize and respond effectively to verbal, nonverbal, and written communications
- Use medical terminology appropriately
- Utilize electronic technology to receive, organize, prioritize and transmit information
- Serve as liaison

Legal Concepts

- Perform within legal and ethical boundaries
- Prepare and maintain medical records
- Document accurately
- Follow employer's established policies dealing with the health care contract
- Implement and maintain federal and state health care legislation and regulations
- Comply with established risk management and safety procedures
- Recognize professional credentialing criteria
- *Develop and maintain personnel, policy and procedure manuals*

Instruction

- Instruct individuals according to their needs
- Explain office policies and procedures
- Teach methods of health promotion and disease prevention
- Locate community resources and disseminate information
- *Develop educational materials*
- *Conduct continuing education activities*

Operational Functions

- Perform inventory of supplies and equipment
- Perform routine maintenance of administrative and clinical equipment
- Apply computer techniques to support office operations
- *Perform personnel management functions*
- *Negotiate leases and prices for equipment and supply contracts*

- *Denotes advanced skills.*

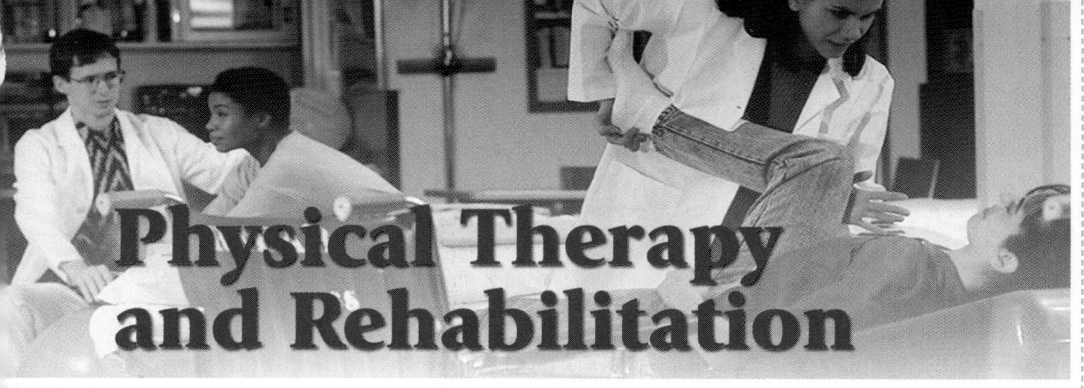

Physical Therapy and Rehabilitation

Learning Objectives

After completing this chapter, you should be able to:

- Define and spell the terms to learn for this chapter.
- Differentiate between a physiatrist and a physical therapist.
- Describe ten modalities used in physical therapy.
- Discuss ten range of motion exercises.
- Describe the difference between ultraviolet radiation, diathermy, and ultrasound.
- List and discuss three applications of heat and cold therapy and their uses.

- State the physiologic reactions to the applications of heat and cold. State any contraindications.
- Differentiate between electromyography, evoked potential studies, and somatosensory evoked potentials.
- Describe the two-point, three-point, and four-point gait in crutch walking.
- Describe proper body mechanics.
- List and discuss five pieces of adaptive equipment used in rehabilitation.
- Describe AROM and PROM.

OUTLINE

Therapeutic Team	980
Rehabilitation	982
Patient Assessment	983
Conditions Requiring Physical Therapy	983
Physical Therapy Methods	983
Adaptive Equipment and Devices	996
Diagnostic Testing	1007

Terms to Learn

ambulation	massage	prosthetist
atrophy	modalities	range of motion
contracture	orthotist	rehabilitation
diathermy	physiatrist	suppuration
erythema	physiatry	
gait	prosthesis	

Case Study

SHIRLEY JONES IS A CMA IN DR. LITTLE'S BUSY ORTHOPEDICS PRACTICE. One of Dr. Little's patients, Devon Washington, has been using crutches for the past four weeks due to a fractured left femur. When Devon comes in for his weekly checkup appointment, he mentions to Shirley that it hurts under his arms when he uses the crutches. He also says that his hands are always cold and numb now. Shirley relays this information to Dr. Little. After examining and observing the patient, Dr. Little comes to the conclusion that Devon is not using his crutches properly. She asks Shirley to give crutch walking instructions to Devon in the office and in writing.

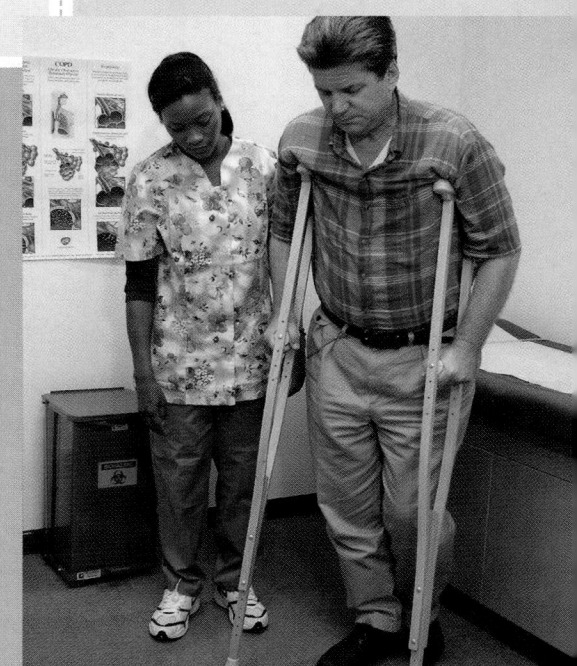

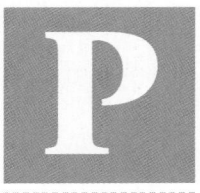**P**hysical medicine, the branch of medicine called physiatry, is the therapeutic use of physical agents for the diagnosis, treatment, management, and prevention of diseases and debilitating illnesses. A physiatrist is a medical doctor or osteopath who must complete four years of residency training and obtain licensure in the state where he or she practices.

The treatments that are prescribed by a physiatrist, sports medicine specialist, or a physician usually are carried out by a physical therapist. Physical therapists are licensed professionals who teach patients the correct use of equipment and body mechanics to prevent further injury or disability. Means and methods used in physical therapy consist of rehabilitation, restoration, and the prevention of disabilities. A physical therapist uses a variety of treatments including heat, cold, massage, exercise, traction, and at times a combination of modalities (an application of any therapeutic agent). Figure 46-1 shows a physical therapist assisting a patient on parallel bars.

Therapeutic Team

Rehabilitation is the process of bringing the patient back as close as possible to his or her normal physical condition after injury or disease. Restorative care is care provided to attain and maintain function and independence.

Patients in need of rehabilitation or physical therapy often require the skilled services of many members of the health care team. This therapeutic team includes the physical therapist (PT), physical therapy assistant (PTA), occupational therapist (OT), occupational therapy assistant (OTA), recreation specialist, exercise physiologist or sports medicine therapist, massage therapist, and prosthetist or orthotist. A prosthetist specializes in designing, preparing, and fitting prosthetic devices such as artificial limbs. An orthotist designs and fits supportive devices such as braces and splints (See Professionalism). Table 46-1 lists several professionals that make up the therapeutic team and the educational requirements for each level of the profession. Members of the therapeutic team may work in hospitals, rehabilitation centers, nursing homes, private physical therapy and occupational therapy practices, schools, sports medicine facilities, and home health agencies. Medical assistants need to have a thorough understanding of the different therapeutic team members and their roles in rehabilitation. In your role as a medical assistant, you may schedule appointments for patients and at times assist with patient treatments.

Role of the Physical Therapist (PT)

A physical therapist receives special training in assisting patients through the use of exercises and equipment to regain body motion and strength (Figure 46-2). The physical therapist is skilled at using special

FIGURE 46-1 Physical therapist helping the patient on parallel bars.

Professionalism

Among the interesting careers mentioned in this chapter are those of the prosthetist and orthotist. A prosthetist designs and fits artificial limbs and an orthotist designs and fits braces, surgical supports, and other appliances. Orthotics and prosthetics are designed to allow the patient to reach his or her potential.

The orthotist applies knowledge, compassion, and biomechanical principles to aid patients in achieving a positive outcome. Orthotic care can range from arch supports for flat feet, to knee supports, to acute fracture care. Orthotists have close ties to the rehabilitation community. They are employed in private clinics, device manufacturing companies, rehabilitation centers, and government agencies. To become an orthotist requires a two-year degree and two years of supervised training.

TABLE 46-1 Careers in Physical Medicine

Career	Education/Experience
Physiatrist (MD or DO)	Medical school graduate, 4-year residency in physical medicine and rehabilitation, state licensure.
Physical Therapist (PT)	Master's degree, licensure required in all states.
Physical Therapy Assistants (PTA)	2-year accredited program or associate degree plus internship, licensure required in some states.
Occupational Therapist (OT)	Bachelor or master degree and internship, licensure required in all states, certification from American Occupational Therapy Association.
Occupational Therapy Assistant (OTA)	1- to 2-year certificate program or associate's degree and internship, licensure or certification required by most states.
Massage Therapist	3-month to 1-year accredited massage therapy program, certification, registration or licensure required in most states.
Recreational Therapist (TR) or Certified Therapeutic Recreation Specialist (CTRS)	Usually a bachelor's degree plus internship, licensure and certification required in a few states, can be certified by National Council for Therapeutic Recreation Certification or registration by Association for Rehabilitation Therapy.
Recreational Therapy Assistants (Activity Director)	1- to 2-year certificate program or associate degree, can be certified by National Council for Therapeutic Recreation (NCTRC).
Sports Medicine (Athletic Trainer, ATS)	Bachelor or master degree, licensure required in some states, can be certified by National Athletic Trainers Association.
Prosthetist/Orthotist	2 years of college and 2 years of supervised training, national certification available, ABC, BOC.

equipment for strengthening muscles, and measuring, fitting, and using assistive devices such as crutches, walkers, and canes.

Role of the Occupational Therapist (OT)

An occupational therapist is a vital member of the rehabilitative team. The occupational therapist is focused on increasing the patient's ability to function within his or her own environment. The occupational therapist assists the patient to relearn and acquire activities of daily living (ADLs) by addressing the following areas:

- Mobilization—activities include assisting patients to maintain balance, reach, grasp, move, and turn while sitting.
- Teaching activities of daily living—include bathing, dressing, feeding,

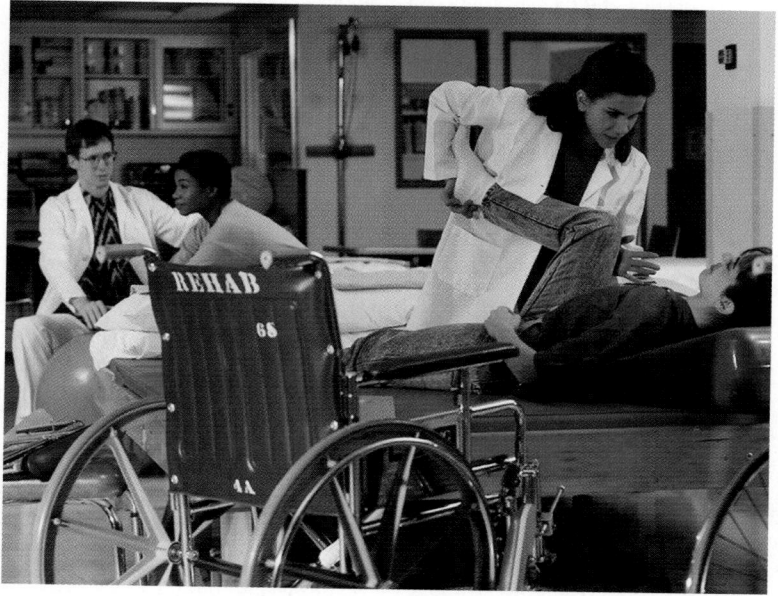

FIGURE 46-2 Physical therapist exercising the patient's leg in a physical therapy department.

grooming, household chores, and leisure activities.

- Coordination, strength, and activity tolerance—includes teaching the patient techniques for using all physical resources without tiring quickly and conserving strength.

To illustrate, a patient recovering from a traumatic injury: will be treated by physicians and nurses, referred to a physiatrist for therapeutic rehabilitation, and given a care plan implementing the doctor's prescription by a physical therapist and occupational therapist who utilize various modalities to try to bring the patient back to pre-trauma levels of function. Since many recoveries involve long-term treatments, the patient may see a recreational therapist to design activities to engage the patient's interest and to boost morale. A physical therapy assistant or occupational therapy assistant will carry out care plans designed and ordered by the professionals.

Role of Medical Assistant

Although as a medical assistant you would need more training and education to perform many of these duties, carrying out orders for treatments such as heat or cold compresses and exercise may be within your scope of practice. A medical assistant may not recommend a course of treatment to any patient. You may, however, need to instruct the patient how to appropriately use heat or cold applications at home and demonstrate the use of assistive devices such as canes and crutches. If in doubt whether or not a specific task is within your scope of practice, obtain information from local, state, or national medical assisting organizations.

Rehabilitation

Rehabilitation is the process of assisting a patient to regain a state of health and the highest level of function possible. Injury, illness, and conditions such as multiple sclerosis cause patients to lose mobility and self-esteem.

The rehabilitation process is a holistic approach to every aspect of the patient's well being, not just the present disease or injury. Goals are set for each patient by professionals on the case and suited to the individual patient's needs. In addition, each patient may have his or her own rehabilitation goal. For some, it may be to return to work, others to be able to care for themselves and live independently. The patient is assisted to resume activities of daily living, such as feeding, toileting, and providing as much of his or her own care as possible. Cultural Considerations discusses additional factors that may affect the patient's course of rehabilitation.

Rehabilitation after a long illness or a debilitating disease causing muscle loss and atrophy requires patience from everyone involved: the patient, family members, and caregivers. Special attention should be paid to the psychological problems, such as depression and anger, that can occur from a feeling of loss of control over one's life. Rehabilitation programs are useful for the following conditions and diseases:

- Surgery (such as hip and knee replacements)
- Trauma, such as broken bones, can result in long periods of inactivity and muscle weakness
- Catastrophic illness such as stroke
- Disease conditions resulting in muscle atrophy or disuse, such as multiple sclerosis, muscular dystrophy, cerebral palsy

A formal rehabilitation program begins as soon as the acute phase of an illness or disease has passed. Short-term and long-term goal setting takes place based on the physician's orders and the patient's willingness to cooperate.

A short-term goal would include objectives such as learning crutch walking and range of motion exercises. Long-term goals aim at independence, and the patient acquiring a feeling of confidence. In this chapter, we are dealing mainly with physical aspects of rehabilitation.

Cultural Considerations

As you pursue your medical assisting career, you will encounter patients with a variety of health care beliefs. Some beliefs may be contrary to those held by traditional medical practitioners in the United States. Alternative treatments may be the patient's course of action, although the physician may not believe that the treatment is compatible with conventional medicine. The patient should be encouraged to reveal any alternative medical treatments he or she is pursuing, because they may affect the conventional treatments prescribed by the physician. If the patient exhibits an interest in alternative therapies, encourage him or her to view them as complementary to those recommended by the physician. Examples of alternative therapies are biofeedback, homeopathy, naturopathy, craniosacral therapy, and acupuncture. It would be helpful for you to have a basic understanding of some of these alternative treatments to be an informed professional.

Patient Assessment

Prior to actually prescribing rehabilitation treatments, the physician must assess the patient's ability to perform certain functions. The physiatrist will inspect and palpate the patient's limbs and joints to evaluate muscle strength and flexibility. Range of motion, the amount of movement in a particular joint, will be evaluated and is discussed later in this chapter. The physiatrist will evaluate the patient's gait, the way a person walks, for clues to specific problems. Posture is also evaluated because the lack of symmetry may indicate scoliosis or curvature of the spine resulting in uneven muscle development. Figure 46-3 illustrates the abnormal types of curvature of the spine. Kyphosis is a thoracic curvature that becomes exaggerated and produces a "hump back" appearance. Lordosis is an abnormal anterior curvature and is sometimes referred to as "swayback."

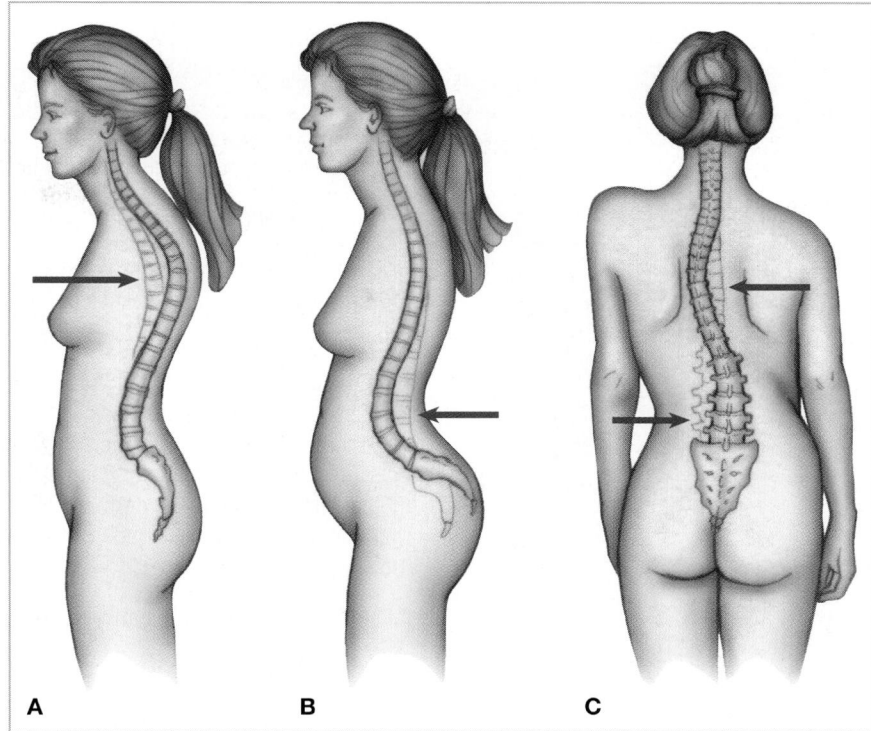

FIGURE 46-3   Three abnormal curvatures of the spine: (A) kyphosis; (B) lordosis; (C) scoliosis.

In scoliosis, there is an abnormal lateral curvature of the spine. Scoliosis can occur in individuals sometimes during adolescence or periods of rapid growth. Treatment of any abnormal curvature may include physical therapy exercises, surgery, a body cast, or a brace depending on the severity.

As a medical assistant, you will assist the physician with these examinations. Once the evaluation is completed, the physician will recommend prescriptions for specific treatments.

Conditions Requiring Physical Therapy

Disease, injury, birth defects, surgery, and amputation all can result in loss of function. Often, the loss of function involves more areas of the body than the specific part affected. For instance, a patient who loses his or her lower leg as a result of diabetes has difficulty with ambulation (the act of walking) and other activities of daily living. The loss of the leg forces the patient to use different muscles groups that may become sore when walking with crutches or a prosthesis. Box 46-1 lists common health problems that require rehabilitation. Table 46-2 lists conditions that may necessitate physical therapy and the services of a physical medicine specialist. Patients requiring physical therapy may be inpatients, outpatients, nursing home residents, home health patients, and those in special facilities such as veterans' hospitals.

Physical Therapy Methods

Methods used in physical therapy include massage, exercise, heat and cold applications, electricity, ultraviolet radiation, ultrasonic diathermy, hydrotherapy, and hot paraffin. These treatment methods are used to

---

BOX 46-1
Common Health Problems Requiring Rehabilitation

- Alcoholism
- Amputation
- Brain tumor
- Cerebral palsy
- Chronic obstructive pulmonary disease
- Traumatic brain injury (TBI)
- Myocardial infarction (MI)
- Spinal cord injury or tumor
- Cerebral vascular accident (Stroke)
- Substance abuse
- Mental illness

TABLE 46-2 Conditions Treated by Physical Therapy

Disorder/Pathology	Description
Amputation	Removal of an extremity due to injury or disease.
Arthritis	Inflammation of a joint that usually occurs with pain and swelling.
Back Pain	Pain along and radiating from the spinal column area resulting from back strain, muscular weakness, and disease or pathology of the spinal cord, such as slipped disc.
Burn	Damage to the skin from 1st-, 2nd-, or 3rd-degree burns resulting in strictures, decreased mobility, and stiffness. 1st-degree: Damage to superficial layer of skin or outer layer of epidermis with no scarring but resulting in erythema; 2nd-degree: Damage extending through the epidermis and into the dermis causing vesicles and scarring; 3rd-degree: Damage to full thickness (epidermis and dermis) and into underlying layers of the skin with scarring.
Bursitis	Inflammation of the bursa between bony prominences and muscles or tendons.
Cardiovascular disease	Diseases of the circulatory and cardiac systems.
Cerebral palsy	Nonprogressive paralysis due to defects in the brain or birth trauma.
Cerebrovascular accident (CVA)	Hemorrhage or clotting in the brain that can result in unconsciousness or paralysis (stroke).
Fracture	Broken bone.
Multiple sclerosis	Inflammatory disease of the central nervous system, generally strikes adults between ages of 20–40 and causes progressive weakness and numbness.
Muscular dystrophy	Wasting disease of the muscles.
Neck trauma	Damage to neck muscles and nerves as the result of trauma or injury (such as whiplash from a car accident).
Osteoporosis	Disease that results in a reduction of bone mass that frequently occurs in post-menopausal women; can result in back pain and fractures.
Paraplegia	Paralysis of the lower portion of the body.
Parkinson's disease	Chronic nerve disease with fine tremors, slow gait, muscular weakness, and rigidity.
Poliomyelitis	Acute viral disease that causes an inflammation of the gray matter of the spinal cord, resulting in paralysis in some cases; it has been brought under partial control through vaccinations.
Quadriplegia	Paralysis of all four extremities of the body.
Rheumatoid arthritis	Form of arthritis with inflammation of the joints, swelling, stiffness, and pain.
Sprain	Pain and disability caused by trauma to a joint; a ligament may be torn in a severe sprain.
Strain	Trauma to a muscle from excessive stretching or pulling.

improve circulation, strengthen muscles, relieve pain, and assist the patient in learning to perform all activities of daily living.

Massage

Massage is kneading or applying pressure by hands to a part of the patient's body to promote muscle relaxation, improve blood circulation, and reduce tension. Massage can consist of the simple act of rubbing an injection site to stimulate absorption and reduce pain. It can incorporate techniques, such as kneading, rolling, stroking, and tapping the skin, that are performed by persons skilled in the art of massage.

Massage is considered a form of passive exercise that is usually applied by someone other than the patient. Terminology related to massage follows:

- Effleurage—light stroking movement that may be performed in a circular pattern.
- Friction—rubbing or deep stroking that produces an increase in circulation and mild heat within the tissues.
- Petrissage—kneading or a rolling method of massage that requires pressing the muscles.
- Tapotement—light tapping or percussion that is performed with the sides of the hands in a cupping position to relieve congestion.

In addition, massage can help restore mobility, decrease swelling, relax muscle spasms, and reduce pain. Physical therapists often incorporate massage in their treatment plans.

Massage therapy is a holistic approach to promoting health that is increasingly valued as a valid form of heath care. Massage therapists require special training and are licensed in many states. They may perform massage in individual private practices and in the hospital setting. There are several types or categories of massage practiced by massage therapists. Traditional or Swedish massage, which is most commonly used in the United States, includes stimulating blood circulation through the soft tissues. Deep tissue massage is used to release chronic patterns of tension or pain by applying massage and pressure at deeper levels. Trigger point massage concentrates finger pressure directly to individual muscles to release "trigger points" or knots in the muscles. Reiki involves channeling the body's energy and spirit through gentle touch and massage.

Exercise Therapy

Being active is an important part of maintaining physical and mental well-being. Inactivity affects every system of the body and the lack of activity can complicate any physical or mental condition. Any person who has exercised regularly and then suspended the exercise activity for a period knows how quickly muscles lose vigor. Atrophy, decrease or wasting away of muscle tissue, occurs rapidly in an inactive patient. Contractures may result increasing the original disability. A contracture is the fixed position of a joint due to muscle shortening and lack of exercise.

Exercise programs are conducted to maintain or regain fitness through planned activity of muscles and joints. Effective exercise programs can help increase or establish lost muscle tone, improve circulation, relieve stress, correct poor posture and body alignment, and increase endurance.

Regular exercise programs, at least three times a week for 20 to 30 minute periods, are recommended for normal adults. Recent research indicates that daily exercise for 30 minutes is actually needed to maintain health. A patient with known medical problems should have a medical consultation with his or her physician to evaluate the medical condition and recommend appropriate exercise.

Types of Exercise

A well-rounded exercise program should involve different types of exercises. In addition to an aerobic exercise program, it is considered beneficial to perform 30 minutes of strength training twice a week to promote healthy bones and improve the ratio of fat to muscle. Various types of exercise are:

- Aerobics—strengthens the cardiopulmonary system.
- Isotonic—maintains uniform (unchanging) tension or tones the muscles upon stimulation.
- Isometric—involves contractions with muscles fixed in place so that the tension occurs without noticeable movement.
- Stretching—results in muscle elongation.

Range of Motion

Patients who have suffered from a temporary or permanent loss of mobility will need instruction on range of motion (ROM) exercises. These exercises can help to maintain muscle tone and flexibility. The medical assistant may need to demonstrate range of motion exercises for the patient's family members if the patient is unable to perform the exercises alone.

Range of motion is the degree of movement in a specific joint without causing pain and is measured with a special type of protractor called a goniometer. During the patient assessment, the physician lines up the two arms of the goniometer with the bones on either side of the joint being measured. Figure 46-4 is an example of a goniometer measuring the range of motion at the patient's elbow. The degree of movement is read from the scale on the hinged arm of the goniometer. Both active and passive movement is measured.

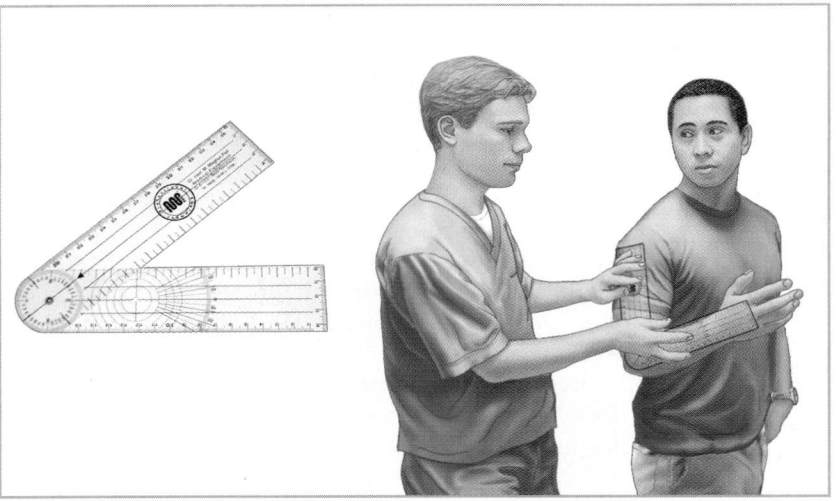

FIGURE 46-4 A goniometer is used to measure range of motion of the patient's arm.

Based on the ability of the patient, the physician may order one of the following types of range of motion exercises:

- Active range of motion (AROM)—The patient is able to move all limbs through the entire range of motion unassisted.

- Passive range of motion (PROM)—The patient must have someone else move his or her limbs through the range of motion exercises because he or she is unable to do it.

- Active assist range of motion (AAROM)—The patient participates to a limited extent in range of

motion exercises, but will require assistance.

Before beginning range of motion exercises, guidelines listed in Guidelines 46-1 should be explained to the patient. The patient and the patient's family should be given printed range of motion instructions and precautions to take home with them.

Range of Motion Exercises

Range of motion (ROM) exercises are used to develop and strengthen muscles and joints. Figure 46-5 illustrates the types of body movements used in range of motion assessment. Terminology used when discussing movement produced by muscles in range of motion exercises is listed in Table 46-3. Most terminology relating to muscle movement is in pairs with opposite meanings. For example, abduction means movement of a body part away from the body and adduction means movement toward the body. Figure 46-6 illustrates range of motion exercises performed on a patient's wrist.

Application of Heat and Cold

Heat and cold are used to treat conditions resulting from trauma and infection. Heat and cold, when used therapeutically, are applied for short periods of time (usually 15–30 minutes). Circulation can be impaired if either hot or cold applications remain on a body part for an extended period of time. Tissue damage may result if hot and cold applications are not monitored closely. Lifespan Considerations discusses factors that affect hot and cold applications.

The medical assistant may have the responsibility to teach the patient the use of heat and cold applications for therapeutic purposes. In some cases, the medical assistant will apply these devices in the office setting (Patient Education).

Heat Applications

Heat is often used to hasten the healing process. The application of heat to a body part causes dilation of blood vessels and allows more blood to circulate to injured tissues. A condition of erythema, or redness of the skin, is caused when the capillaries become congested with blood. This increased circulation assists in providing the body with oxygen and nutrients necessary for repair and healing. Tissue metabolism increases and healing can occur.

Heat can also assist in relieving pain and muscle spasms. In addition, heat can be used to soften hard crusts of exudate produced by damaged body tissues. Exudate is an accumulation of fluid, pus, or serum in tissue that may become hard and crusty.

| **46-1** | **GUIDELINES** |

Performing Range of Motion (ROM) Exercises

- Each exercise should be performed three times unless otherwise ordered by the physician.
- A logical sequence of exercises should be followed so that every muscle and joint receives some movement. In general, ROM exercises begin with the head and move down the body.
- The patient should attempt to do as much as he or she is able to without assistance.
- Never force any part of the body beyond normal range. Do not exercise to the point of pain.
- Exercise should not be performed if a joint is reddened or swollen.
- Limbs should be supported at the joints when exercising.

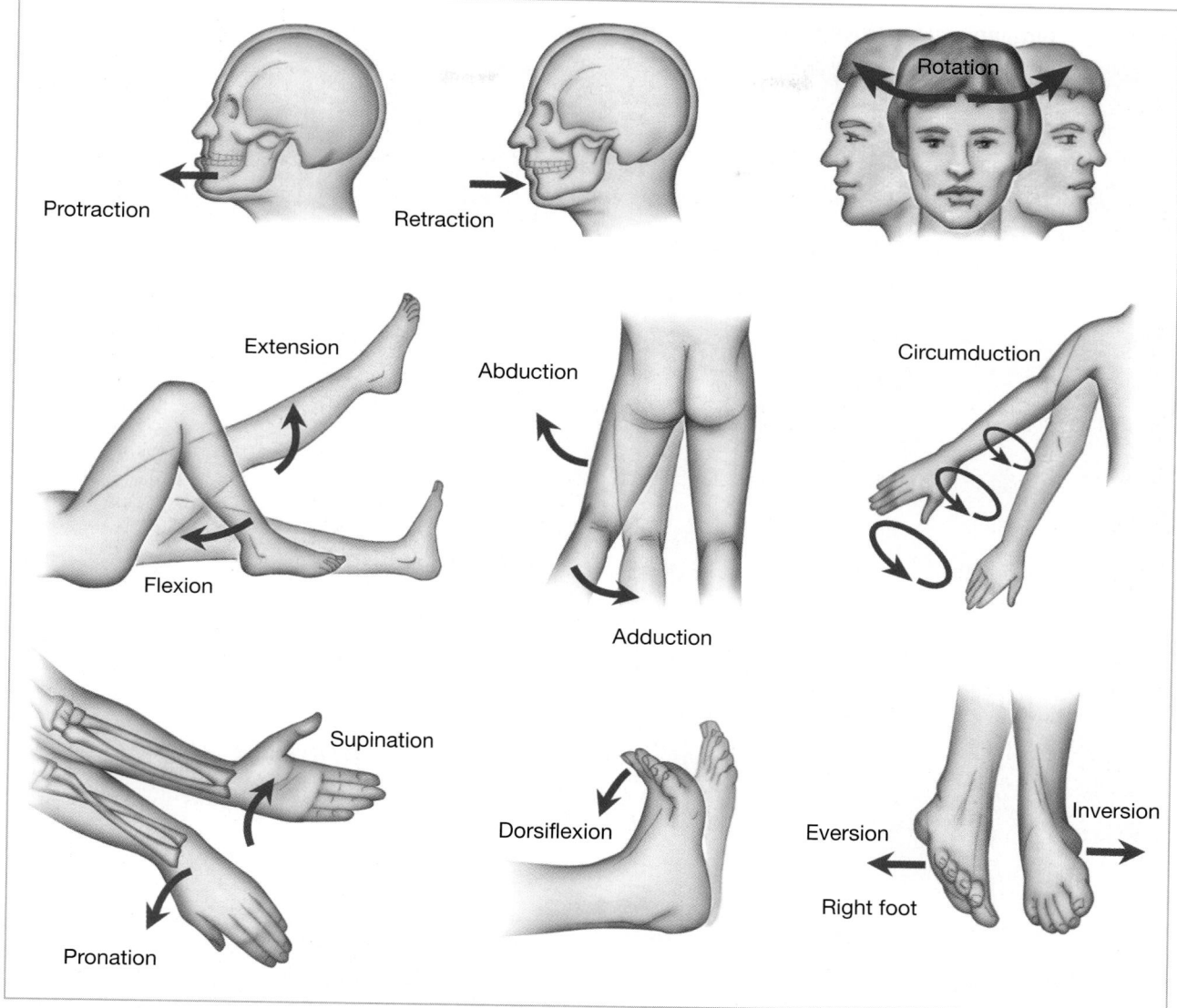

FIGURE 46-5 Types of body movements used in range of motion assessment.

The application of heat, in particular moist heat, can hasten suppuration, a process to relieve the internal buildup of pus formation. Heat application can take the form of either moist or dry applications to produce a dilation of blood vessels in the skin.

MOIST HEAT Moist heat application uses heated water that actually touches the skin, such as in a tub or with a wet compress (pad). Examples of moist heat applications include warm to hot compresses, Sitz baths, tub baths, warm soaks, heat hydrotherapy or whirlpool bath, and paraffin treatment.

Hot compresses, often containing a medicated solution, are applied to hasten healing or cleanse open wounds. Any soft, absorbent cloth, such as a washcloth, small towel, disposable woven towels, or gauze squares, can be used as a hot compress. Procedure 46-1 provides the steps for applying a hot compress. The compress may be kept warm by placing a hot water bottle on top of the compress or re-warming the compress. Applying a hot compress to an open wound requires the use of sterile procedures.

Hot soaks involve having the patient put the affected part of the body into a container of water with or without medication for 15 minutes. The water temperature should be no more than 110°F / 44°C. Procedure 46-2 provides steps for a hot soak application.

A hot pack is a canvas bag of varying sizes filled with a heat retaining gel. Hot packs are commercially available and are used to treat larger areas of the body. The packs are placed in hot water and heated, then wrapped in a towel and applied to the affected area.

TABLE 46-3 Terminology for Movement Produced by Muscles

Term	Description
Abduction	Movement away from the midline of the body.
Adduction	Movement toward the midline of the body.
Circumduction	Movement in a circular direction from a central point.
Dorsiflexion	Backward bending (as of a hand or foot).
Eversion	Turning outward.
Extension	Movement that brings a limb into or toward a straight condition.
Flexion	The act of bending.
Hyperextension	Extreme or abnormal extension or stretching.
Inversion	Turning inward.
Opposition	Ability to move the thumb into contact with other fingers.
Plantar flexion	Bend the sole of foot, point toes downward.
Pronation	Turn downward or backward with the hand or foot, to lie in a prone position is to face downward.
Rotation	The process of turning.
Supination	To turn the palm or hand anteriorly, to turn the foot inward and upward, to lie in a supine position is to face upward.

Lifespan
Consideration

The physician will take into consideration the patient's age, location of treatment, and general condition when ordering hot or cold modalities. Using hot and cold modalities require special consideration when treating pediatric or geriatric clients. All patients must be cautioned to test all warm applications before applying them at home to avoid burning the skin. The skin of elderly patients is especially conducive to burning because their nerve endings lose some sensitivity during the aging process. Some drugs also affect the older person's sensitivity to pain. Confused and dementia patients may not recognize pain; therefore, you must watch for changes in behavior such as restlessness that may signal pain.

Parents must be reminded to carefully test all warm applications on themselves before placing it on an infant or child. Infants and children have fragile skin and are at risk for burns. When undergoing hot or cold treatments, young children should not be left unattended.

Other points to remember: thin skinned areas, such as the back and chest that are normally covered with clothing, are more sensitive to hot and cold treatments and areas with broken skin are more sensitive to tissue damage. Cover all hot or cold applications with a towel or covering before applying directly to the patient's skin. Electrical equipment, such as heating pads, should not come into contact with water. Recognize the signs of complications from hot or cold treatments such as blisters, excessive redness or bluish discoloration, pale skin, and shivering. Always provide for patient privacy through appropriate draping and screening.

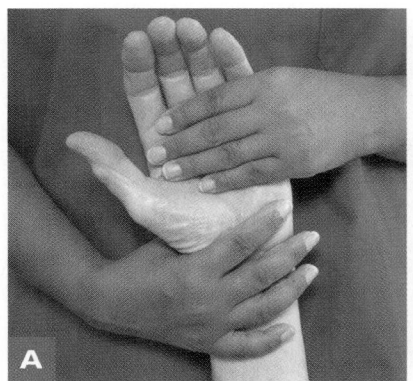
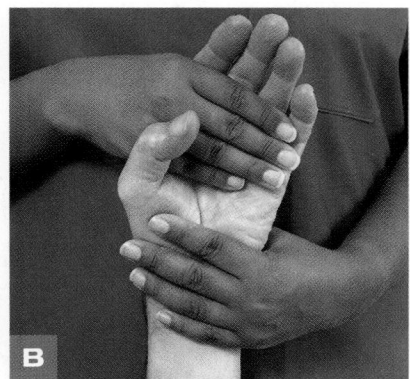
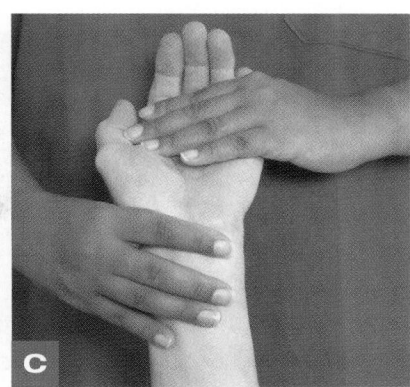
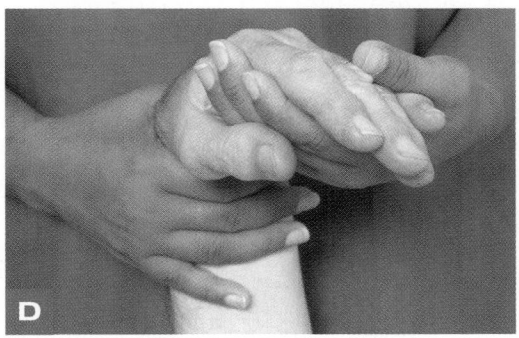

FIGURE 46-6 Range of motion exercises on a patient's wrist. (A) Radial deviation; (B) Ulnar deviation; (C) Extension; (D) Flexion.

These packs have the advantage of retaining heat longer than hot compresses.

Heat hydrotherapy is the use of warm water as a therapeutic or healing treatment. This can be done in bathtubs, swimming pools, and whirlpools. The whirlpool bath, with continuous jets of hot water reaching the body surfaces, promotes circulation and flexibility of muscles and joints. Arthritis patients are encouraged to participate in exercises in a warm pool to maintain flexibility and reduce pain.

Hot paraffin as a form of heat treatment involves placing the extremities into hot wax to relax the muscles and promote healing. The temperature of the paraffin or wax has to be controlled carefully to prevent burning. Paraffin treatments are usually performed by licensed physical therapists using standard paraffin bath equipment. This therapy is useful for patients with rheumatoid arthritis to relieve the pain and stiffness in joints. The hand or limb is inserted into hot melted paraffin that has been heated to 126°F / 54°C. The hand or limb is left in the hot paraffin for about 15 to 30 minutes until there is a thick coating. The relief after this treatment is longer lasting than in some other forms of moist heat treatment. Note: there is a danger of burns if the temperature of the paraffin is not carefully monitored.

DRY HEAT A dry application is a heat application without water, such as with a heating pad. Dry heat, which does not produce moisture, includes infrared radiation (heat lamps), electric heating pads, hot water bottles, chemical hot packs, and aquathermia or aquamatic pads. Figure 46-9 is an example of an aquamatic K-pad, which is an electric, water-filled pad used for dry heat. Another heating pad is a flat electrical pad that provides localized heat by regulating a dial. The physician should specify the temperature required for the treatment (low, medium, high). Patients should be reminded not to lie on heating pads to avoid burns. Procedure 46-3 lists the application steps for a heating pad.

Patient Education

The medical assistant plays an important role in educating the patient with physical therapy needs. In many cases, the medical assistant is the only person providing instructions regarding commonly ordered procedures relating to the application of heat and cold. A team approach, which includes all members of the health care team, patient, and family, is the ideal structure for patient education when handling physical disabilities.

PROCEDURE

Applying a Hot Compress

OBJECTIVE: Perform a hot compress application and document procedure without error.

Equipment and Supplies

soaking solution (or water) as ordered by physician; basin; bath thermometer; absorbent cloths such as washcloths or gauze squares; waterproof cover such as plastic wrap

Method

1. Perform hand hygiene.
2. Assemble the equipment. If an open wound is present, use sterile equipment and Standard Precautions.
3. Identify and explain the procedure to the patient.
4. Fill the basin half full of water or medicated solution prepared according to the directions of the physician.
5. Request the patient to remove any necessary clothing because compresses are performed on bare skin. Assist the patient if necessary.
6. Check the temperature of the solution with a bath thermometer. The temperature range for an adult is between 105° and 110°F (41° and 44°C).
7. Position the patient into a comfortable well-supported position.
8. Place the cloths in the basin of hot water or solution. Wring out one cloth until it is wet but not dripping.
9. Gradually place the compress on the patient's body part (Figure 46-7). Ask the patient to tell you how the temperature feels.
10. Frequently test the temperature of the solution. Replace the water as it cools with more warm water.
11. Time the procedure according to the physician's order (15–30 minutes). Check the patient periodically for any signs of change in redness, swelling, or pain.

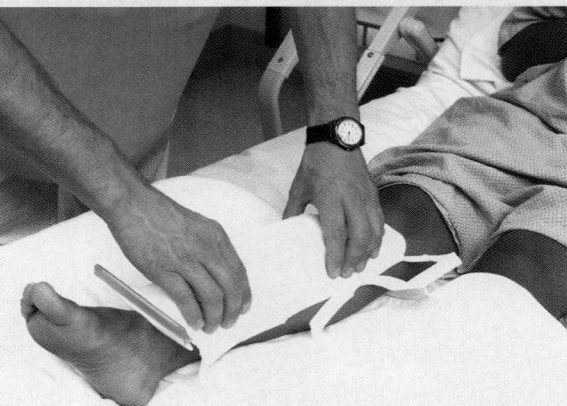

FIGURE 46-7 Applying a hot compress to the patient's leg.

12. Gently dry the affected body part.
13. Instruct the patient on any further care such as continued warm compresses at home.
14. Place towels in the laundry. If an open wound is present, then handle the linens according to Standard Precautions.
15. Clean all of the equipment.
16. Perform hand hygiene and return the equipment.
17. Document the procedure in patient's record.

Charting Example

6/14/XX	3:00 P.M.

Hot compress at 105°F applied to right shin for 20 minutes. Skin with some redness after application. Pt. states there is pain relief. Instructed on application of hot compresses at home.

M. King, CMA

PROCEDURE

Application of Hot Soak

OBJECTIVE: Perform a hot soak application and document procedure without error.

Equipment and Supplies

soaking solution or water as ordered by physician; basin or tub; pitcher; bath thermometer; towels

Method

1. Perform hand hygiene.
2. Assemble the equipment. If an open wound is present, use sterile equipment and Standard Precautions.
3. Identify and explain the procedure to the patient.
4. Fill the basin or tub half full of water or medicated solution prepared according to directions of the physician.
5. Request the patient to remove any obstructing clothing because soaks are applied to the bare skin. Assist the patient if necessary.
6. Check the temperature of the solution with a bath thermometer. The temperature range for an adult is between 105° and 110°F (41° and 44°C).
7. Position the patient into a comfortable well-supported position.
8. Pad the side of the basin or tub with a towel to prevent the patient's body from rubbing on the edge.
9. Gradually place the patient's body part (Figure 46-8) into the solution. Ask the patient to tell you how the temperature feels.
10. Frequently test the temperature of the solution. Using a pitcher, remove part of the liquid every 5 minutes and replace with hot water. Pour the hot water at the edge of the basin or tub and protect the patient by placing your hand between the patient's body part and the hot water as it is poured. Swirl the water while pouring to mix the hot and cool fluid together.
11. Time the procedure according to the physician's order (15–30 minutes). Check the patient periodically for any signs of change in redness, swelling, or pain.
12. Gently dry the affected body part.
13. Instruct the patient on any after care such as further warm soaks at home.
14. Place the towels in the laundry. If an open wound is present, then handle the linens according to Standard Precautions.

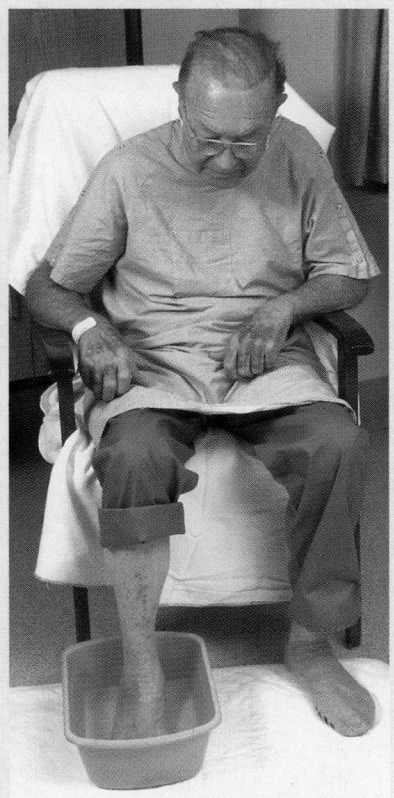

FIGURE 46-8 Place a basin in position for the patient to easily dip his or her foot in water for a hot soak.

15. Clean all of the equipment.
16. Perform hand hygiene and return the equipment.
17. Document the procedure in the patient's record.

Charting Example

1/15/XX	1:00 P.M.

Hot water soak at 105°F applied to right foot for 30 minutes. Skin slightly pink to some redness after application. Pt. states there is pain relief. Instructed on application of hot water soaks at home.

M. King, CMA

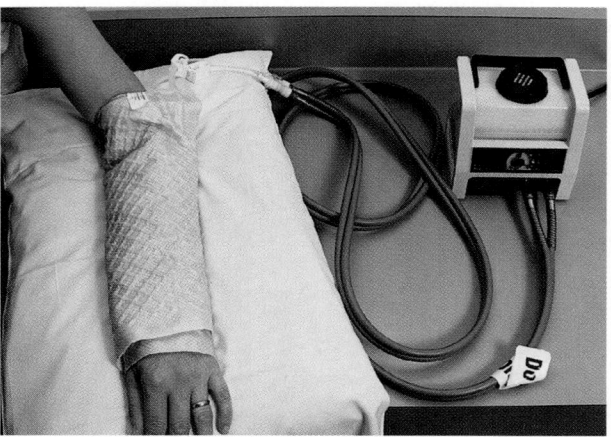

FIGURE 46-9 Aquamatic pad and heating unit provide dry heat treatment to a patient's arm.

Heat lamps use infrared bulbs to produce heat. Since the rays from the lamp penetrate the surface of the skin three to five millimeters, it is essential that the lamp be placed two to four feet away from the patient to avoid burning the skin. Treatments usually last about 20 minutes and must be carefully monitored.

Ultraviolet lamps are used to treat conditions such as psoriasis or wound infections and will be covered later in the chapter.

A hot water bottle is flat, flexible and easy to use. The temperature of the water should not exceed 125°F / 54°C. For the elderly and children under two, the temperature should not exceed 115°F / 46°C. The water bottle should be filled partially and the remaining air expelled. An overly full bottle is less flexible and harder to conform to the affected body part.

46-3 PROCEDURE

Application of a Heating Pad

OBJECTIVE: Perform a heating pad application and document procedure without error.

Equipment and Supplies
heating pad with protective covering or pillowcase

Note: Perform a preliminary check of the heating pad to determine that the wires are in good condition without bending.

Method
1. Perform hand hygiene.
2. Assemble and test the equipment.
3. Identify and instruct the patient concerning the procedure. The patient should be cautioned against using pins, bending the heating elements within the pad, or lying on the heating pad. Rationale: Pins should never be used in a heating pad either to secure a pad to its cover or to attach the pad to the patient's clothing. Pins can puncture the heating pad elements and cause an electrical shock. Lying on the pad may cause too much heat to accumulate in that area and burn the patient.
4. Place the heating pad in a protective covering or pillowcase.
5. Connect the heating pad to an electric plug. Set the temperature selector at the setting ordered by the physician (low or medium).
6. Place the heating pad over the patient's affected area. Ask the patient to tell you how it feels. Rationale: The pad should be warm, but not uncomfortable or too hot.
7. Instruct the patient regarding the proper temperature setting. Tell him or her not to change the setting. Rationale: Some patients, such as the elderly, have poor circulation and may not feel the heat of the pad.
8. Leave the heating pad in place for the amount of time ordered by the physician (15–20 minutes). Check the patient periodically for any signs of change in redness, swelling, or pain.
9. Remove the heating pad when procedure is complete. Instruct the patient on any after care such as further heat treatments at home.
10. Place the protective covering in laundry.
11. Perform hand hygiene and return all of the equipment.
12. Document the procedure in the patient's record.

Charting Example

1/12/XX	9:00 A.M.

Heating pad on medium setting applied to left elbow for 20 minutes. Erythema noted over application site. Pt. states there is pain relief and increased mobility in elbow joint. Instructed on application of heating pad at home.

M. King, CMA

Chemical hot pack is a disposable pack that becomes hot when slapped or kneaded. To use these convenient hot packs, the manufacturer's directions should be followed.

Cold Applications

Cold applications result in constriction of blood vessels, which is the opposite effect of warm applications. Constriction of blood vessels is very useful to prevent or reduce swelling, such as in the case of a sprain. Since the blood flow is actually slowed, the amount of body fluids carried into an injured part, such as a leg, is reduced. Additional benefits of cold applications may include the reduction of pain and control of bleeding due to the slowing of blood circulation.

Cryotherapy is using cold for therapeutic purposes. Cold applications can be applied to a body part, such as an ice bag after a tooth extraction. In addition, cold applications can be placed on the entire body to reduce an elevated body temperature. Cold applications consist of cold compresses, soaks, ice packs, and hypothermia blankets. Procedure 46-4 lists the steps for applying cold compress. Ice in a bag or container (ice pack) is used to treat localized conditions. Procedure 46-5 provides the steps for application of an ice bag. A bag of frozen vegetables, such as peas, makes an effective temporary ice bag.

Chemical cold packs are self-contained packets containing a small amount of water in an inner bag, which when released into a chemical contained in the outer bag, causes a chemical reaction that makes the bag cold. This pack can be used as an alternative to an ice pack. Procedure 46-6 lists the steps for applying a cold chemical pack.

Wet cold applications, such as cold compresses, may be used to treat pain and fever. A washcloth or similar cloth is moistened with ice water and applied to an area.

Patient safety and comfort are a concern when using either warm or cold applications.

Ultraviolet Radiation

Ultraviolet radiation uses rays from natural sources, such as the sun, and artificial sources, such as sun lamps, for healing purposes. Ultraviolet rays stimulate the growth of new epithelial cells and are capable of

---

46-4 PROCEDURE

Application of Cold Compress

OBJECTIVE: Perform a cold compress application and document procedure without error.

Equipment and Supplies
water; absorbent cloths or gauze squares; waterproof cover or plastic wrap; basin; ice

Method
1. Perform hand hygiene.
2. Assemble the equipment. If an open wound is present, use sterile equipment and Standard Precautions.
3. Identify and instruct the patient concerning the procedure.
4. Fill the basin half full of cold water. Add ice cubes and compresses.
5. Wring out the compress until it is wet but not dripping. Gently place the compress on the patient's affected body part. Wrap the compress in a plastic or waterproof covering to prevent dripping.
6. Check the compress every three to five minutes and replace with another cold compress. Add more ice as the water becomes warm.
7. Leave the compress in place for the time specified by the physician (usually 15–20 minutes).
8. Gently dry the affected body part.
9. Place the linens in the proper container. Clean all of the equipment.
10. Perform hand hygiene and return the equipment.
11. Document procedure in the patient's record.

Charting Example

| 10/23/XX | 10:00 A.M. |

Cold compresses applied to right ankle for 20 minutes. Swelling decreased after treatment. Erythema noted over application site. Instructed on application of cold compress at home.

M. King, CMA

Application of Ice Bag

OBJECTIVE: Perform an ice bag application and document procedure without error.

Equipment and Supplies

ice bag with a protective cover (or small hand towel); ice chips or crushed ice

Method

1. Perform hand hygiene.
2. Assemble and test the equipment.
3. Identify and instruct the patient concerning the procedure.
4. Fill the ice bag ½ to ⅔ full of ice. Expel air by squeezing the empty half of ice bag. Replace the cap. (Figure 46-10)
5. Dry the bag and place into a protective covering or small hand towel.
6. Place the ice bag over the patient's affected body part. Ask the patient how the ice bag feels.
7. Refill the bag with ice as needed.
8. Leave the ice bag in place for the time specified by the physician (usually 15–20 minutes).
9. Clean the equipment. Allow the bag to air dry.
10. Perform hand hygiene and return the equipment.
11. Document the procedure in the patient's record.

Charting Example

2/14/XX	2:00 P.M.

Ice bag applied to contusion on right forehead. Swelling reduced after 20 minutes. Erythema noted in treatment area. Instructed on application of ice bag at home.

M. King, CMA

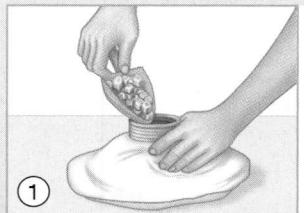 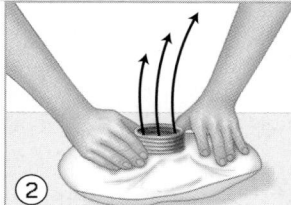 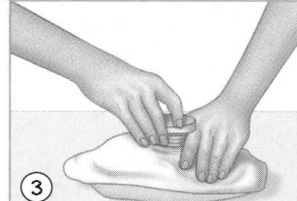 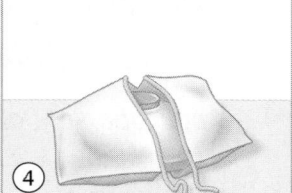

FIGURE 46-10 Preparing an ice bag.

---

killing bacteria. These rays are used therapeutically for the treatment of disorders such as psoriasis. Disorders caused by bacteria, such as acne and pressure sores, are treated effectively with this therapy. The goal of the treatment is to produce a small redness on the skin to stimulate circulation and kill bacteria.

Ultraviolet ray lamp treatment must be carefully controlled since the lamps can cause severe sunburn and even second and third degree burns. Both the timing of the exposure and the distance of the lamp from the patient must be carefully controlled. A patient can receive a second-degree burn after one to two minutes of exposure to a lamp set at 30 inches from the patient. Since a patient does not feel this type of burn occurring, he or she cannot warn the operator to stop treatment.

Treatment is ordered by the second, such as a 20-second lamp treatment placed at least 30 inches from the patient and directed only on the area to be treated. Eye protection, in the form of dark goggles, should be worn by both the patient and medical assistant to protect the eyes from ultraviolet ray exposure.

The patient should never be left unattended during this procedure. If you have to leave the room during the treatment, turn off the lamp until you return. There is a great danger of severe burns if the timing is not exact.

Diathermy

Diathermy is the therapeutic use of high-frequency currency that induces an electrical field within a por-

Application of Cold Chemical Pack

OBJECTIVE: Perform a cold chemical pack application and document procedure without error.

Equipment and Supplies

cold chemical pack; soft cloth

Method

1. Perform hand hygiene.
2. Assemble the equipment (Figure 46-11).
3. Identify and instruct the patient concerning the procedure.
4. Shake the bag to allow crystals to fall to the bottom. Squeeze the pack until the inner bag ruptures. Shake the bag to mix contents. The bag should become cold immediately and remain cold for about 30 minutes.
5. Place the bag inside a soft cloth.
6. Place the cloth-protected bag over the patient's affected body part.
7. Check the patient every three to five minutes.
8. Leave the cold pack in place for the time specified by the physician (usually 15–20 minutes).
9. Discard the ice pack in a proper waste container after use.
10. Perform hand hygiene.
11. Document the procedure in the patient's record.

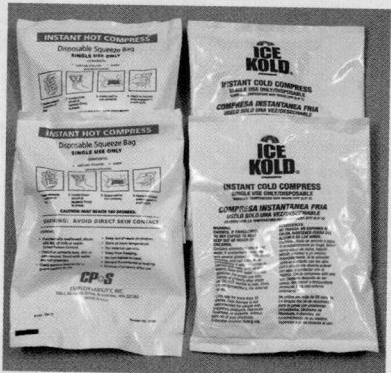

FIGURE 46-11 Examples of disposable hot and cold packs before activation.

Charting Example

7/31/XX	2:00 P.M.

Cold pack applied to left cheek over molar area for 20 minutes. Swelling decreased after treatment. Instructed on application of cold chemical pack at home.

M. King, CMA

---

tion of the body. This electrical field generates heat in various parts of the body and increases blood flow to aid in healing. Diathermy is useful in treating muscular disorders and treatments of tendonitis, arthritis, and bursitis.

The diathermy machine placement must be carefully controlled according to the manufacturer's instructions. Some machines are placed one inch from the patient's skin and may have a built-in spacer to assist with exact placement. Others have applicators with pads that require a towel to be placed between the applicator pad and the patient. Due to the danger of burns inherent in diathermy treatment, it has been replaced in many facilities with ultrasound, which is safer.

Ultrasound

Ultrasound is sound energy from high-frequency sound waves penetrating deep through tissue layers. It works on the same premise as sonar used in oceanography. Ultrasound waves vibrate at the rate of one million times per second, which cannot be heard by the human ear, but produce a mechanical and a heating effect. The mechanical effect or vibration works on connective tissues such as ligaments and tendons. The heat effect works on all body tissues; however, ultrasound treatments should be used carefully near bony tissues to avoid causing injury from concentration of waves. Ultrasound treatments usually are applied for ten minutes or less, as ordered by the physician. The patient may require several ultrasound treatments to receive the benefit.

Ultrasound is used effectively to treat pain, relax muscle spasms, stimulate circulation in patients with vascular disorders, relax tendons and ligaments, and break up calcium deposits and scars. Ultrasound treatments are used in conjunction with other treatments, such as medications, to relieve back spasms.

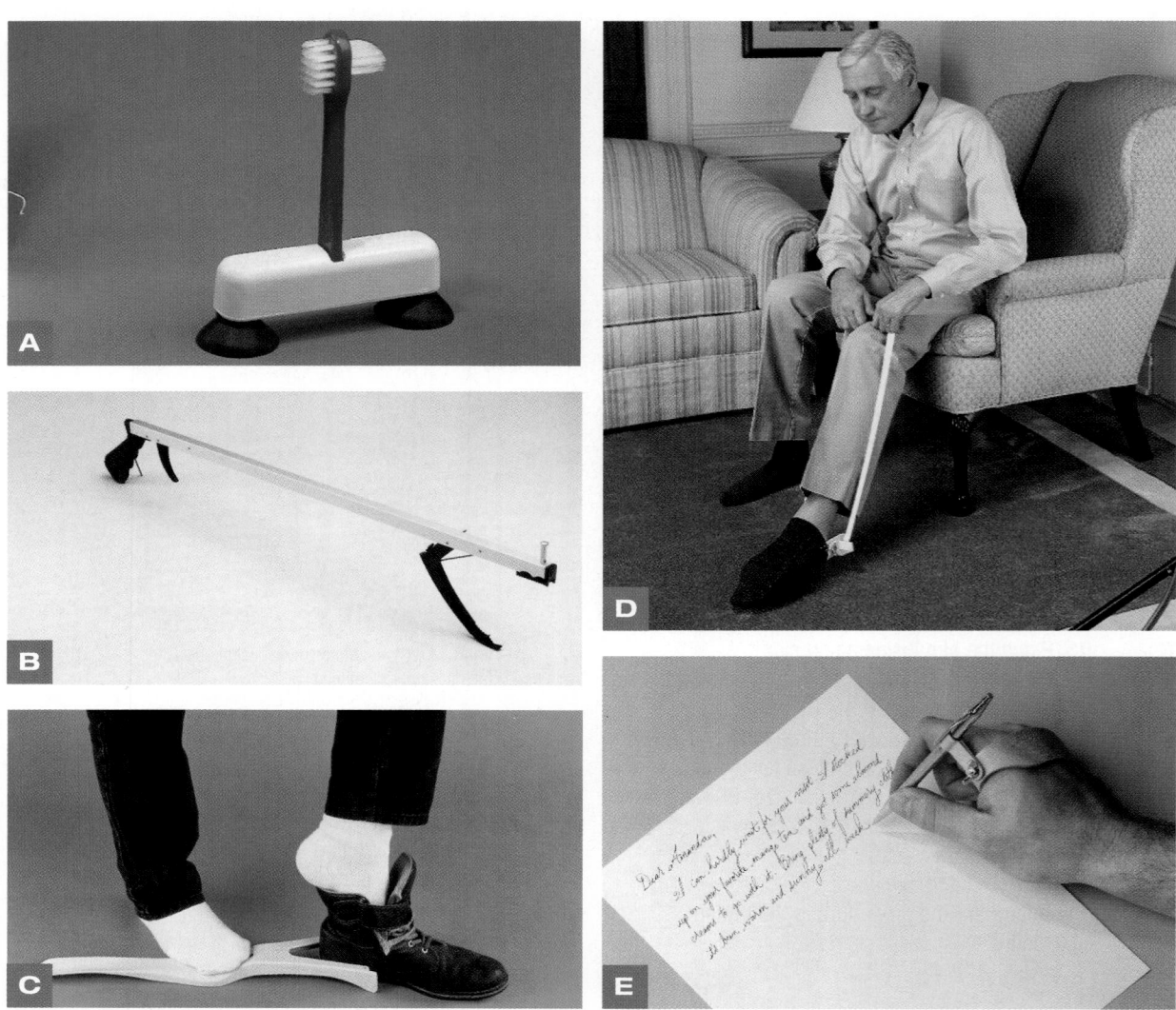

FIGURE 46-12 There are many types of adaptive devices: (A) a toothbrush; (B) a reaching stick; (C) a shoe holder; (D) a stocking helper; (E) a writing aid.

Ultrasound is administered via a machine with an applicator head attachment that can be placed directly on the skin. The ultrasound applicator head contains quartz crystal that vibrates rapidly when an electric current passes through it. Since these waves do not travel through air, they must be kept in contact with the skin. A conducting medium, such as a special gel or mineral oil, must be placed on the skin to conduct the ultrasound into the body. The ultrasound operator applies the ultrasound head to the patient's skin using a steady up and down motion. The operator must keep the ultrasound head in continuous motion over the body part since tissue damage can occur if it is held in one place for a prolonged period of time. Patients should be asked if they have any implants, such as a hip or joint replacement, since the ultrasound could loosen the implant.

Adaptive Equipment and Devices

Equipment used to assist recovery from physical disorders or disabilities includes adaptive equipment, such as wheelchairs, walkers, canes, crutches, and special furniture, such as shower chairs and geriatric chairs. Mobility aids or mobility assistive devices are designed to enable the patient to ambulate. Other devices, including braces, casts, traction, prostheses, splints, and slings, are used by the physical therapist to manipulate the patient's damaged bones and tissues. Adaptive equipment also includes a variety of utensils, such as eating utensils molded to fit the patient's hand and dishes with a wide edge to prevent spilling. Figure 46-12 illustrates adaptive equipment,

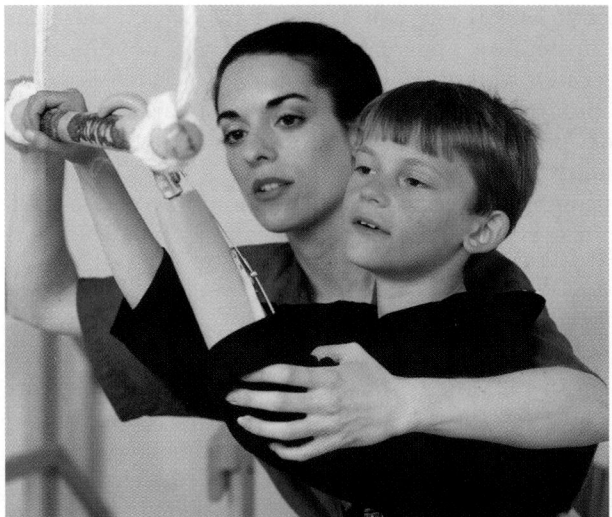
FIGURE 46-13 Therapist assisting an amputee patient to regain mobility and strength after amputation.

Legal and Ethical Issues

Many of the procedures described in this chapter are beyond the scope of practice for a medical assistant beginning his or her first job. Additional training and practice is required before teaching a patient to use crutches, for instance. In some states, only a licensed physical therapist is able to perform many of the procedures discussed. The medical assistant must remember that with many procedures, he or she is "assisting" another licensed person, such as the physician, nurse, or physical therapist. Always check with your local or state medical association regarding the laws in your state if there is any doubt. The patient's safety must always be placed first.

including a toothbrush, a reaching stick, shoe holder, a stocking helper, and writing aid.

Special furniture, such as shower chairs made from aluminum or plastic, allows the patient to sit while taking a shower. The geriatric chair, a wheeled chair that reclines with an attached tray for meals, is useful for patients who can feed themselves but may not be able to sit securely in a regular chair.

Adaptive devices are prescribed by the physician; however, the physical therapist may provide the initial instruction on the use of the device. Figure 46-13 illustrates a physical therapist assisting a patient to regain mobility and strength after amputation. In a general practice setting, the medical assistant will assist the physician with these devices and will provide continuing education and support for the patient when he or she is seen in the physician's office. Legal and Ethical Issues discusses issues regarding a medical assistant's scope of practice.

Crutches

Crutches allow the patient to walk without placing weight on the healing leg part. Weight is transferred to the arms and hands. Crutches are made from metal or wood and should have a rubber tip at the end to prevent slipping on a smooth floor surface. The three most common types of crutches (Figure 46-14) are:

- Axillary crutch—a tall crutch with shoulder rest and handgrip that reaches from the ground to under the axilla. These crutches are commonly used for a patient that has suffered a fractured leg.

- Lofstrand (forearm crutch)—a single aluminum tube with an arm cuff that fits snugly around the patient's forearm and uses a handgrip for weight bearing. This crutch allows the patient to release the handgrip to use the hand while still having the crutch held in place by the arm cuff for support. People with cerebral palsy and paraplegia often choose to use this type of crutch.

- Canadian or elbow crutch is a variation of the Lofstrand crutch that extends further up the arm.

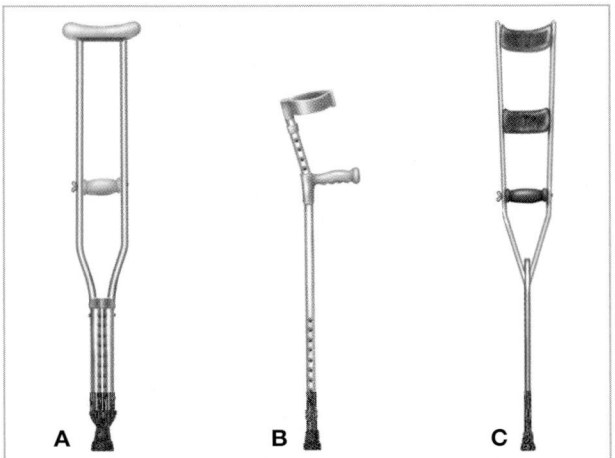
FIGURE 46-14 Three types of crutches: (A) Axillary crutch; (B) Lofstrand or forearm crutch; (C) Canadian or elbow crutch.

Measuring for Axillary Crutches

Axillary crutch measurement has to be taken carefully to prevent pressure damage to the axillae. If the crutch is too long it may cause pressure on the brachial plexus (nerve running under the axilla and down the arm). The patient may develop a condition known as crutch palsy, resulting in muscle weakness in the arm, wrist, and hand. Crutches that are too short can result in the patient having to bend forward while walking. Back pain, nerve damage, and injury to the axilla and palms of the hands can occur if the crutches are improperly fitted. The steps for measuring axillary crutches follow:

1. Have the patient wear walking shoes and stand straight.

2. Place the crutch tips four to six inches to the side and four to six inches in front of each foot.

3. Adjust the crutch, using the bolts and nuts at the sides of the crutch, so that the axillary crutch bars are three-finger-widths below the axilla. Measure this by inserting your own fingers between the patient's axilla and the crutch bar.

4. Next adjust the handgrips so the patient can flex his or her elbows at a 30-degree angle when the crutch is in place and the patient's hands are on the hand bars.

Instructions in both writing and an actual demonstration should be provided to the patient that will be using crutches. To teach the patient how to properly use crutches, have him or her start in the tripod position. Figure 46-15 illustrates the correct position of the crutches and patient's feet. Teaching the patient how to use crutches and proper crutch walking gaits is one of the responsibilities of the medical assistant.

Crutch Walking Gaits

The type of crutch gait or walk that the patient will use depends on the amount of weight bearing the pa-tient's leg or legs will support, his or her muscular coordination, age, and overall physical condition. In a crutch walking gait, each foot and crutch is called a point. For example, a two-point gait consists of two points from the total of four points (two legs and two crutches) that are in contact with the ground during each step. The patient should be encouraged to use a slow gait. Common gaits include the four-point, three-point, two-point, swing-to, and swing-through gaits.

The physician determines the type of crutch necessary for the patient and may fit the crutch for the patient in the office. You may be asked to demonstrate the use of crutches and the appropriate gait required by the patient's condition. The patient should be reminded to use a slow pace in crowded areas or when feeling tired. Using crutches requires a great deal of energy and different muscle groups than the patient is accustomed to using.

FOUR-POINT GAIT   The four-point gait is a slow and steady gait and is used when a patient can bear weight on both legs. This is considered the safest of all gaits since the patient always has three points of support in contact with the ground at all times. This gait is also used for patients who may have muscular weakness and some lack of coordination (Figure 46-16).

To use this gait, first the right crutch is moved forward, followed by the left foot, then the left crutch, and then the right foot. This is repeated over and over. The patient must be able to move each leg separately to use this gait.

THREE-POINT GAIT   The three-point gait is used when one leg is stronger than the other or when there is no weight bearing on one leg. The patient must have good muscle coordination and arm strength. To use this gait, the patient must be able to support his or her full weight on one leg. Have the patient move both crutches and the affected leg forward and then move the unaffected leg forward while weight is balanced on both crutches (Figure 46-17). This gait requires good coordination and muscle strength. This gait is used by patients with musculoskeletal disorders (for example, fractures), recent leg surgery, or amputees without a prosthesis.

TWO-POINT GAIT   The two-point gait is faster moving than the four-point gait and is used by the patient that can bear some weight on both feet and have good balance. Two-point gait occurs when a crutch and the opposite foot are moved forward at the same time. For example, the left crutch and the right leg move together (Figure 46-18).

SWING GAITS   Swing gaits are used by patients with severe leg disabilities such as deformities or paralysis.

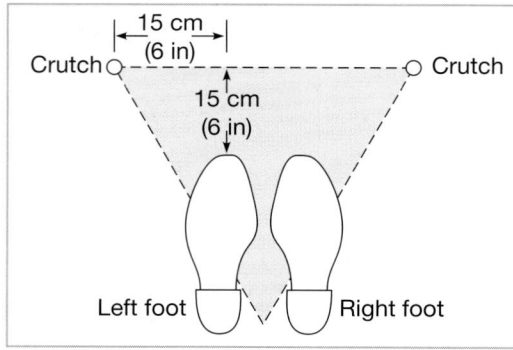

FIGURE 46-15   The correct beginning position for the patient's feet and crutches (Tripod position).

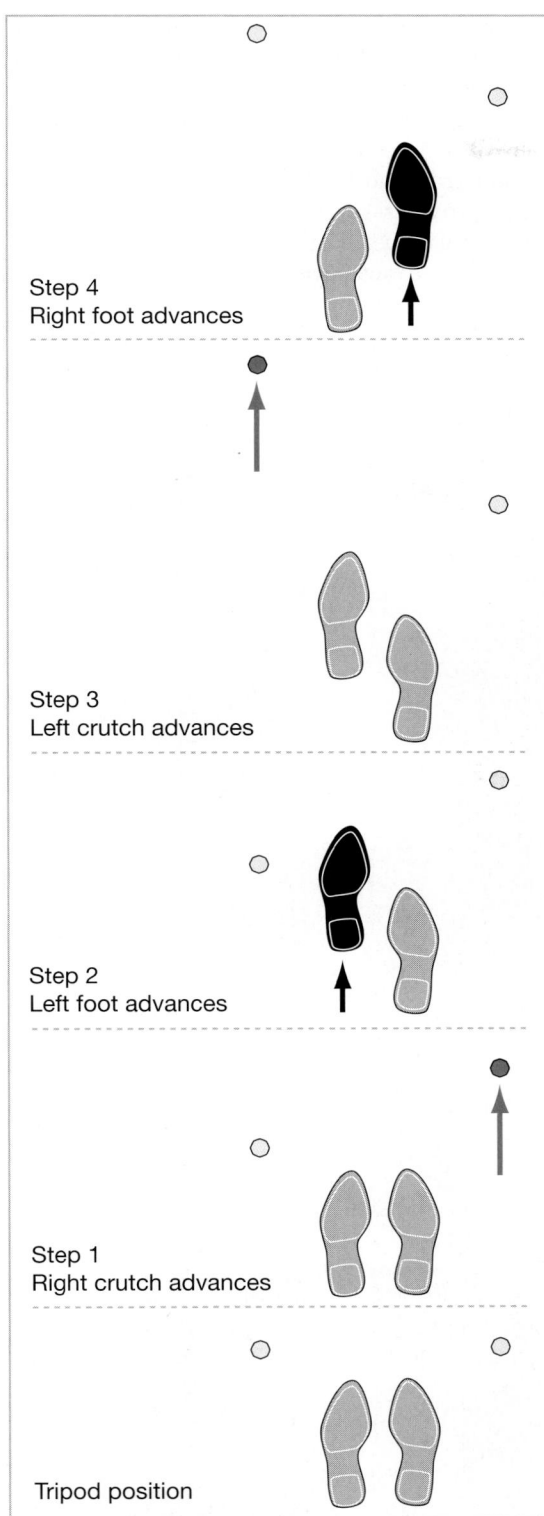

Step 4
Right foot advances

Step 3
Left crutch advances

Step 2
Left foot advances

Step 1
Right crutch advances

Tripod position

FIGURE 46-16 Four-point gait.

They may use either of the two swing gaits: swing-to or swing-through gait.

To use the swing-to gait, the patient moves the crutches forward, lifts his or her body, and then swings the legs up to the same point. Good muscular control is needed for this gait since the patient may lose his or her balance and fall forward with this gait (Figure 46-19).

To use the swing-through gait, the patient moves the crutches forward, as in the swing-to gait, and then swings the legs past the crutches. This provides a good base of support. It is a gait that allows for fast movement. Both the swing-to and swing-through gaits are used by paraplegic patients who are using the forearm type of crutches or by patients with a generalized leg weakness.

Sitting with Crutches

The patient using crutches should be instructed on how to manipulate the crutches and support his or her legs to sit down.

1. The patient should face forward and then back into a straight-back chair with arm rests until the back of his or her legs touch the chair seat.

2. The crutches should be placed in the hand on the strong side of the body, opposite the weak leg.

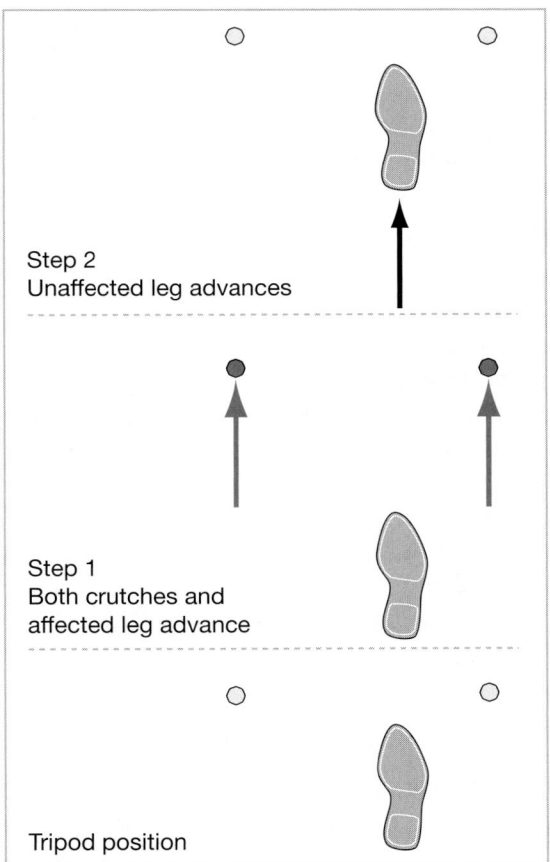

Step 2
Unaffected leg advances

Step 1
Both crutches and
affected leg advance

Tripod position

FIGURE 46-17 Three-point gait.

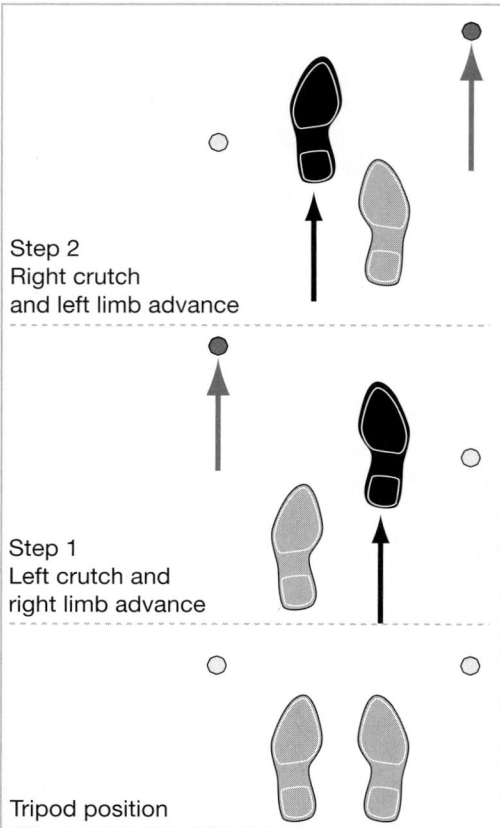

FIGURE 46-18 Two-point gait.

Step 2
Right crutch
and left limb advance

Step 1
Left crutch and
right limb advance

Tripod position

3. The patient should grasp the chair arm with the other hand and lower him or herself gently into the chair.

Standing with Crutches

The patient should be instructed to follow four steps when moving from a sitting to a standing position with the use of crutches.

1. The patient should place the crutches in the hand on the strong side of the body to use as support.
2. The patient should move or slide his or her body forward in the chair.
3. The patient should grasp the chair arm with the free hand on the affected side.
4. The patient should push up to a standing position.

Procedure 46-7 provides the steps for teaching or reinforcing instructions on the correct use of crutches.

Canes

Canes are used by patients that have muscle or bone weakness on one-side or need assistance with balance. Two common types of canes are the standard cane and the four-point (quad) cane shown in Figure 46-22. Sev-

eral types of wooden and aluminum canes are available. The aluminum canes are adjustable for height using nuts and wing bolts. The wooden canes have to be purchased to size or cut to the correct length. All canes should have a rubber tip on the end to prevent slipping. A standard cane has a curved neck for ease of gripping. It provides support for patients who need only slight assistance. The tripod (three-point) and quad (four-point) canes have a wide base with three or

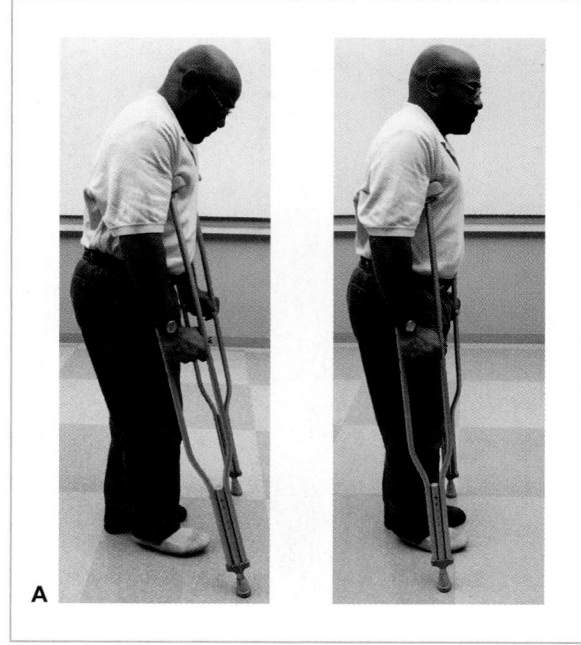

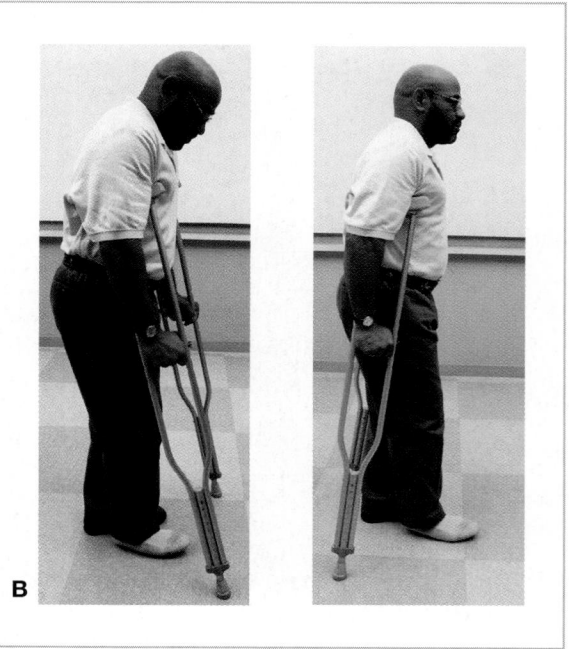

FIGURE 46-19 Swing gaits: (A) swing-to gait; (B) Swing-through gait.

Instructing a Patient to Use Crutches Correctly

OBJECTIVE: Teach a patient how to use crutches correctly.

Equipment and Supplies
crutches; gait belt

Method
1. Assemble the equipment requested by the physician's order.
2. Check the crutches to determine that they are in good working condition.
3. Perform hand hygiene.
4. Identify the patient and explain the procedure.
5. Check to see if the patient is wearing sturdy, non-skid shoes.
6. Demonstrate the correct position.
7. Demonstrate the gait requested by the physician.
8. Have the patient stand against a wall or near a chair for support.
9. Adjust crutch length to appropriate height. The distance between the top of the crutch and the axilla should be three finger widths (Figure 46-20).
10. Instruct the patient to keep his or her head up, stand straight with abdomen in and feet straight with a slight (5 degree) bend at the knee joint. Remind the patient to look ahead and not down while walking with crutches. This will prevent the patient from bending forward.
11. Explain to the patient that the weight should be supported by hands not underarms. The patient should practice standing to maintain balance and place weight on the palms of the hands at the hand bars, and not on the axilla. Instruct the patient not to rest body weight on the axillary bars for more than one or two minutes to prevent injury to the brachial plexus.
12. Instruct the patient to assume basic crutch stance or tripod to provide a firm base of support. The basic crutch stance is the tripod to provide a firm base of support. Feet are slightly

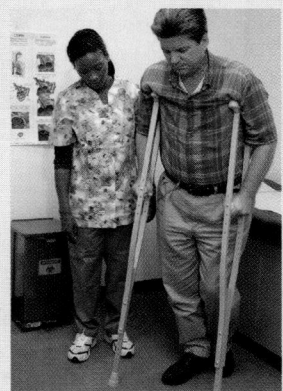

FIGURE 46-21 The medical assistant instructs the patient how to walk with crutches.

apart, and the tips of the crutches are four to six inches in front of and four to six inches to the side of the toes. An imaginary line drawn from the two crutch points to an area behind the center of the feet will form a triangle (tripod).
13. Instruct the patient to take small steps and swing through when first learning to use crutches. The crutches should only move about 12 inches forward with each step to prevent the crutches from slipping. Have the patient move slowly at first (Figure 46-21).
14. Have the patient practice his or her gait.
15. Remind the patient to report any numbness or tingling in arms. The shoulders and hand bars can be padded for extra comfort with either sponge rubber or a soft cloth. The patient should then remeasure and adjust the crutches for the correct length,
16. Crutches should always be moved forward and to the side so the feet can swing through.
17. Remind the patient to periodically check the nuts and wing bolts to maintain tightness and to check the rubber tips frequently for cracks. They can easily be replaced.
18. Make corrections on the patient's use of crutches as needed.
19. Chart appropriately.

Charting Example

9/30/XX	2:00 P.M.

Instructed how to use crutches. Adjusted crutches to fit. Pt practiced for 20 minutes.

M. King, CMA

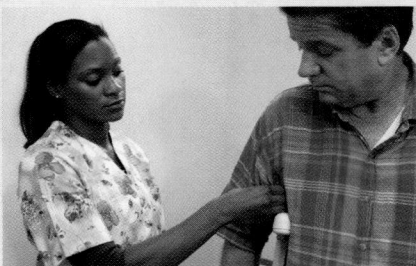

FIGURE 46-20 The medical assistant measures and adjusts the crutch length for the patient.

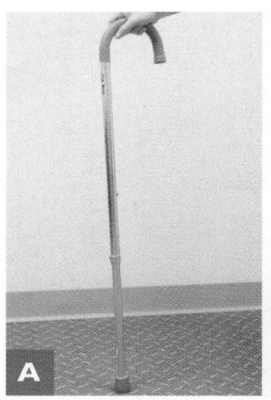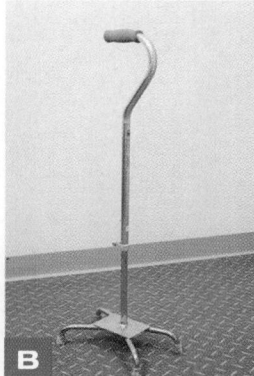

FIGURE 46-22 Two types of canes.

four points to provide steadier support. The neck is bent with a T-shaped handle.

A physical therapist determines the most suitable cane for the patient. To determine the correct cane height, the patient should stand tall so that the handgrip of the cane is level with the hip joint and the elbow is flexed at an angle of 25–30 degrees. Also the handle must be suitable for the patient's hand size. Procedure 46-8 lists the steps for teaching a patient the correct use of a cane.

Walkers

Walkers are assistive devices made of aluminum that provide a base of support for patients who need help with balance and walking. To aid with mobility, many geriatric patients use walkers. The walker should be adjusted to the patient's height and reach just below the patient's waistline (Figure 46-23).

A stationary walker must be picked up by the patient, moved forward, and then used as a base of support while the patient walks into it. This requires strong arm muscle development.

A walker with wheels can be used by patients that have good coordination and balance. This type of walker can be dangerous because it might move too quickly, causing the patient to lose his or her balance and fall. Some walkers with wheels have a stop and release bar that the patient presses to unlock the wheels; if the patient lets go of the bar the wheels lock, thus preventing the walker from moving away from the patient. Procedure 46-9 is presented to help teach or reinforce a patient's use of a walker.

Wheelchairs

Wheelchairs are hand manipulated or power-driven. Many patients operate their own wheelchairs, however, not all patients are able to (nor should they) operate their own wheelchairs (Figure 46-24). For example, an individual paralyzed on one side and the blind or frail patient may not be able to operate his or her own wheelchair and will need assistance.

Wheelchair Transfer

Always think of moving a patient as the process of transferring him or her from one place to another. In many cases, the patient is familiar with the techniques necessary for the transfer and will be able to assist the medical assistant.

A patient, who is paralyzed on one side of the body (hemiplegia) or who has a general weakness, can be moved from a wheelchair by pivoting the patient so that he or she can use the stronger leg to assist you. Explain to the patient that this transfer technique is used to prevent injury to the patient and to the individual

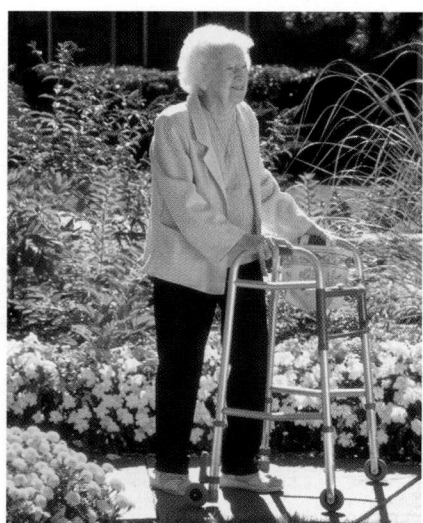

FIGURE 46-23 Walkers help the patient ambulate safely.

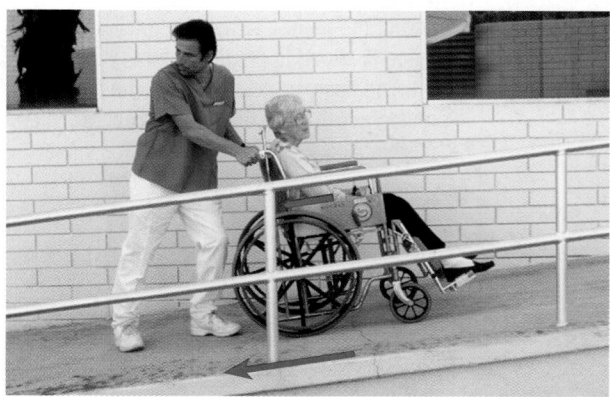

FIGURE 46-24 Wheelchairs are moved down ramps backwards.

Instructing a Patient to Use a Cane or Single Crutch Correctly

OBJECTIVE: Instruct a patient on the correct use of a cane.

Equipment and Supplies
cane suited to the patient's needs; gait belt

Method
1. Assemble the equipment according to the physician's order.
2. Check the cane height and condition of the cane tip.
3. Identify the patient.
4. Perform hand hygiene and explain the procedure.
5. Check to see if the patient is wearing sturdy, non-skid shoes.
6. Demonstrate the correct position.
7. Demonstrate the gait.
8. Instruct the patient to hold the cane (or single crutch) on the opposite side of the injury or affected limb. As the affected leg moves forward, the cane (or crutch) on the opposite side will move forward to provide support.
9. Place the cane (or single crutch) six inches in front of and slightly to one side of the unaffected side. Make sure the cane tip is firmly on the floor and the weight is supported on the strong leg and the cane. The patient's elbow should be slightly flexed during weight bearing.

10. Have the patient look straight ahead, not down at his or her feet.
11. Have the patient move the cane (or single crutch) forward 6 to 12 inches and bring the affected leg forward until it is even with the cane. The weight should be placed on the strong foot and leg.
12. Instruct the patient to move the strong leg forward past the cane and weaker leg. As the unaffected foot moves forward, the weight is shifted to the weak or affected foot and the cane. Thus the cane will provide support for weight bearing on the weaker leg.
13. Have the patient repeat the walking pattern and evaluate his or her balance and endurance using small steps.
14. Document the procedure correctly.

Charting Example

3/3/XX	1:00 P.M.

Instructed on proper use of walking with a cane. Cane height and condition good. Pt balance and gait good. Pt practiced for 10 minutes.

M. King, CMA

---

assisting with the transfer. Procedure 46-10 lists the steps to successfully transfer a patient from a wheelchair to a chair or examination table. Figure 46-26 is an example of moving a patient from a bed to a wheelchair. Figure 46-27 illustrates how to protect a falling patient.

Braces

A brace is one type of orthotic used to support weakened body parts, to correct deformities, and prevent joint movement. Braces may be made out of metal, plastic, or leather and are customized to the patient's needs and anatomy. To wear this type of assistive leg device, the brace is placed in the patient's shoe, the patient's foot is inserted, and a hook-and-loop strap is used to hold the brace in place. Any orthotic positioned over a bony point must be padded to avoid skin breakdown. Prolonged use of a brace may weaken muscles.

Casts

Regardless of the type of specialty office that employs you, in your career as a medical assistant, you will encounter patients with casts. Casts are made of plaster, plastic, or fiberglass and are used to hold a bone in place after reduction of a fracture. Casts are applied over a stockinette to protect the skin. Fiberglass and plastic casts dry quickly, while a plaster of paris cast may take up to 48 hours to dry. Proper cast care and patient assessment are important to avoid further damage to the part of body already affected.

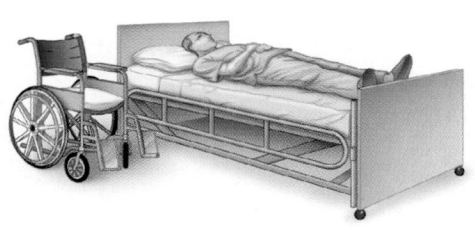

A Position the chair with the back even with the head of the bed.

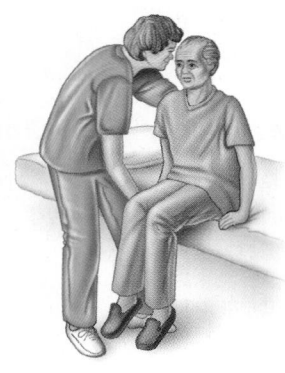

B Assist the patient to dangle.

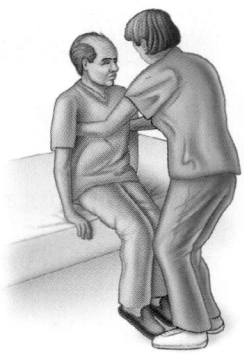

C Brace your knees against the patient's knees and block his or her feet with your feet.

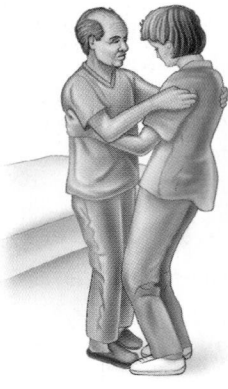

D Bring the patient to a standing position.

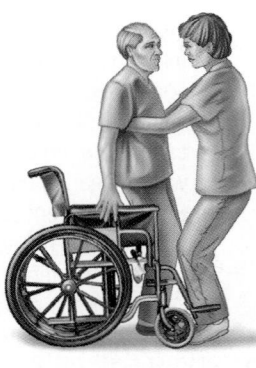

E Ask the patient to grasp the chair as you support him or her.

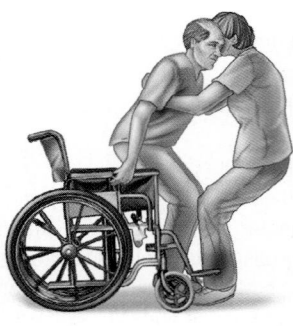

F Bend your knees as you lower the patient to the chair.

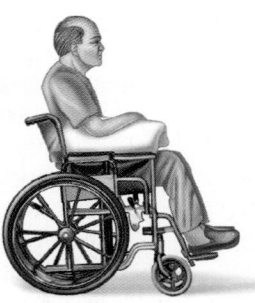

G Use pillows as needed to position the patient in correct body alignment.

FIGURE 46-26 Assisting the patient to transfer from the bed or examining table to a wheelchair.

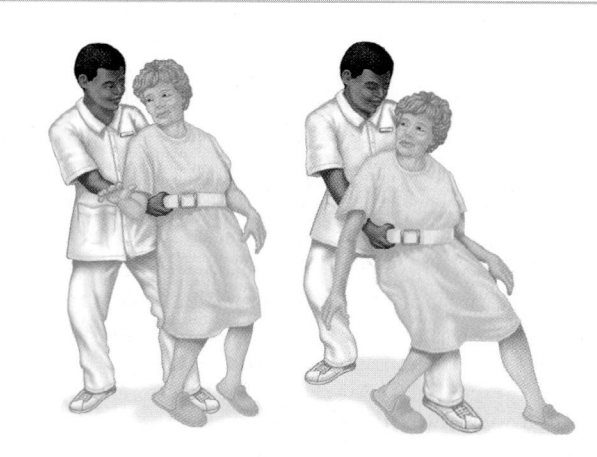

A If the patient begins to fall, pull him or her close to your body with the gait/transfer belt.

B Ease the patient to the floor by letting him or her slide down your leg.

FIGURE 46-27 Assisting a falling patient.

Cast Care

Casts are applied for the purpose of immobilizing a broken bone or muscle strain and sprain. A cast may be applied after a surgical procedure on a limb to immobilize the area until healing takes place. Casts are made from a variety of pliable materials that the physician will mold to fit the body part. A cast can be considered to be a form of nonflexible bandage. Casts are generally applied using a wet plaster-type material around a stockinette liner and cotton padding over the limb. As the cast dries, it becomes hard. Newer synthetic fiberglass materials are being used to form casts that are lighter in weight than a plaster cast. The medical assistant should use caution when handling fiberglass materials by wearing protective glasses or eye shield.

The medical assistant may be asked to assist the physician in applying the cast. It may be necessary to hold the limb at the joint areas as the cast is being applied. Remember to handle a damaged limb gently.

After the cast has been applied, it must be left uncovered during the drying process. The limb may need

PROCEDURE

Teaching a Patient to Correctly Use a Walker

OBJECTIVE: Teach a patient to correctly use a walker.

Equipment and Supplies
walker suited to patient's needs; gait belt

Method
1. Assemble the equipment according to the physician's order.
2. Check the condition of the walker.
3. Perform hand hygiene.
4. Identify the patient and explain the procedure.
5. Check to see if the patient is wearing sturdy, non-skid shoes.
6. Demonstrate the correct stance and gait with the walker.
7. Assist the patient into the walker.
8. Evaluate the walker for proper height and fit. (The top of the walker should reach the patient's hipbone and the patient's hands should be on the handgrip with his or her elbow flexed at a 30-degree angle).
9. Instruct the patient to distribute his or her weight evenly between the walker and both legs.
10. Instruct the patient to move the walker six to eight inches ahead with all four legs of the walker hitting the floor at the same time.
11. Instruct the patient to bring his or her weaker foot into the walker.
12. Instruct the patient to bring the stronger foot forward even with the weaker foot.
13. Have the patient continue walking with the walker while you evaluate his or her balance and endurance.
14. Document appropriately.

Note: The walker is not be used by the patient as a transfer device. Remind the patient to grasp the walker after he or she is in a standing position and not to use the walker to pull up from a sitting position.

Charting Example

5/31/XX	11:00 A.M.

Instructed on proper use of walker. Evaluated walker height to fit. Pt practiced for 15 minutes.

M. King, CMA

---

to be supported on a pillow at this time. The patient should be cautioned against moving around until the cast is dry. The cast may become warm or even hot during the drying process. This is normal.

The patient's limb should not become hot or cold once the cast has been applied. Check the edges of the cast and report any changes to the physician (Figure 46-28). The medical assistant should make frequent checks of the patient's circulation. The patient should be instructed to call the physician if any of the following problems are observed:

- Circulation restricted by the cast.
- Pain as a result of the cast pinching the skin.
- Excessive itching under the cast.
- Numbness or tingling of the fingers or toes.

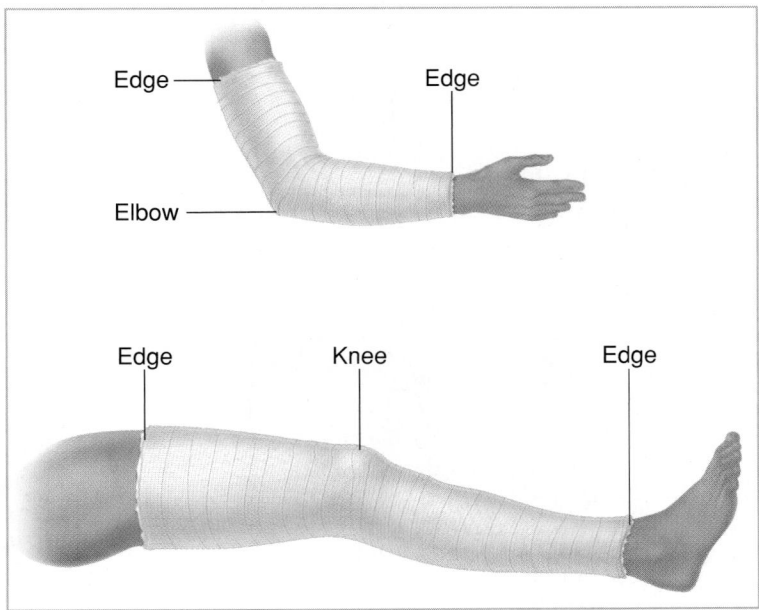

FIGURE 46-28 Check the edges of a cast and report any changes.

Wheelchair Transfer to Chair or Examination Table

OBJECTIVE: Move the patient from a wheelchair to a chair or examination table without error.

Equipment and Supplies

chair or examination table; gait belt, if needed; step stool, if needed

Method

1. Perform hand hygiene.
2. Identify the patient and introduce yourself.
3. Explain what you are going to do before you start. Discuss what the patient will do to assist you.
4. Place the wheelchair at a 45-degree angle to the chair or examination table. This provides a shorter distance to pivot the patient from the wheelchair.
5. Put the wheelchair brakes into the lock position on both sides. The patient's legs should be moved off the pedals by supporting the ankle and lower leg. Gently place the patient's feet on the floor and have the patient shift forward in the chair, if possible. Move the foot pedals up and out of the way so the patient has a clear path to move forward.
6. Make sure the examination table or chair is stable before attempting the transfer.
7. Position yourself near the patient's nonparalyzed side so you can provide support and the patient can use his or her stronger limb. You will move the patient toward the stronger side. Do not refer to the patient's "good" or "bad" side.

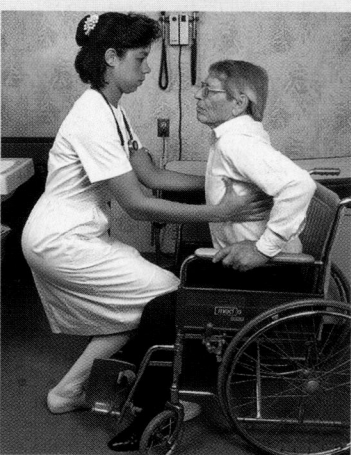

FIGURE 46-25 A medical assistant helps the patient out of the wheelchair.

8. Place one of your feet forward to establish a firm base of support for your body. Move down toward the patient while keeping your back straight.
9. Have the patient place his or her hands on the arm supports of the wheelchair. Then, ask the patient to lean forward and push up as you assist the patient to a standing position, on the count of three (Figure 46-25).
10. Position yourself so that the patient's paralyzed leg is between your knees. Support the paralyzed leg with your knees, if necessary, so the leg will not slip as the patient stands.
11. Place your hands under the patient's armpits and help the patient to stand. Use the muscles in your legs to push your body upward. Do not bend over and use back muscles. Note: a "gait belt" can be placed around a heavier patient's waist for lifting.
12. Allow the patient to stand for a few moments before attempting to move into the chair or onto the examination table.
13. Assist the patient to pivot (turn) toward the non-paralyzed side by pivoting your own body as you hold the patient under his or her armpits. Do not twist your body. Turn it as a unit.
14. Gently lower the patient into a chair by bending your knees and keeping your back straight.
15. If the patient must move up onto an examination table and can assist you, then support the weak side as the patient places his or her stronger leg onto the step stool. Pivot the patient around so he or she can then sit on the edge of the table. Encourage the patient to move back on the table to eliminate the danger of falling.
16. If the patient is unable to assist you, then ask for another assistant to hold one side of the patient as you support the other side. Count aloud "one," "two," "three," and then lift the patient together. Do not attempt to lift—by yourself—a patient who is unable to help you.
17. When assisting the patient into a supine position, support the paralyzed leg gently onto the table.
18. Never leave a physically challenged (disabled) patient unattended.

- Discolored toes or fingers.
- Swelling of the limb around the edge of the cast.
- Discoloration soaking through the cast.
- Loosely fitting cast.
- Foul odor coming from the cast.

The physician should advise the patient on the amount of weight and movement that can be safely applied to the cast. Remind the patient that nothing should be put on the edges of the cast. The cast should not get wet. The patient may be able to tie a strong plastic bag around the cast in order to take a shower.

Traction

Traction is a method of pulling or stretching in two directions used to immobilize fractures, correct deformities, and reduce compression of the vertebrae or other musculoskeletal conditions. Skeletal traction, which is performed on inpatients, is applied by the physician to the patient's bone by inserting a pin or wire through the bone. Skin traction is done by the physical therapist by attaching bandages and strips of material to the skin. Weights are then attached to the material and tension is applied to reduce painful muscle spasm. This type of traction can be set up in a patient's home.

Prosthesis

Removal of a limb or part of a limb surgically is known as amputation. Amputations are performed as the result of trauma, disease, such as gangrene, bone tumors, severe bone infection, and workplace accidents. Major psychological adjustment is needed to help the patient deal with his or her appearance and limitations on independence. A prosthesis is an artificial replacement of a missing body part.

Immediate fitting of a prosthesis involves fitting the patient immediately after the limb is removed, sometimes before leaving the operating room. The benefit of immediate fitting is that the patient is able to begin ambulation the next day. The decision to select a specific type of fitting rests with the physician and must include an assessment of the patient's overall condition, age, and willingness to learn to use the new limb. Many recent improvements in prostheses result in a limb that closely resembles the original and functions efficiently. Prosthetic devices are custom made for the patient and adjustments may be necessary to ensure a comfortable fit for the patient. In the delayed fitting of a prosthesis, stump conditioning is needed and involves shrinking and shaping the stump before a prosthesis can be fitted. Amputees may feel a phantom pain, which although is normal, the cause is unknown. The patient may experience pain in the amputated limb for a short time or, in some cases, for years.

Diagnostic Testing

To determine the presence or full extent of a disabling disease, the physician may order evaluative or diagnostic testing. This may include an examination of the following:

- Muscle strength
- Muscle coordination
- Mobility of joints
- Neuromuscular function
- Circulation and sensory function

Neuromuscular evaluation may include tests, such as electromyography (EMG), nerve conduction studies (NCS), and evoked studies, such as brainstem auditory evoked response (BAER) and somatosensory evoked potentials (SEP), to pick up abnormalities, such as diseases of the peripheral nerves, muscles, and spinal cord.

Electromyography (EMG)

Electromyography (EMG) consists of using an electromyograph to test the electrical activity of muscles. EMG is most often performed when a patient complains of muscle weakness or numbness. The electromyograph consists of electrodes, an oscilloscope to visually produce the waves of muscle activity, an amplifier, loudspeaker, an electrical stimulator, and a camera. The patient may receive sedation before this test is conducted since there can be a painful stimulation from the electric current. The EMG consists of inserting a fine-gauge needle electrode through the skin and into a muscle and then sending a small amount of electric current into the muscle. This procedure permits the physician to examine individual parts of muscles. Abnormal results are found in conditions such as amyotrophic lateral sclerosis (ALS), muscular dystrophy, and peripheral nerve damage.

The electrical activity of the muscle recorded on a graph paper or on film is known as an electromyogram (EMG). This permanent record is then evaluated to determine the adequacy of muscle activity.

A surface electromyogram (SEMG) involves less discomfort for the patient, but the results are less conclusive. In this test, electrodes are attached to the surface of the body to detect electrical activity.

Electrical Stimulation

Electrical stimulation with low-voltage current is helpful to stimulate nerves that supply muscles. An electrical current is applied using disposable gel electrodes. This is a passive means to stimulate muscles when a patient cannot exercise due to injury or disease. This type of stimulation is used to avoid atrophy of muscle tissue.

Transcutaneous electric nerve stimulation (TENS) is another way of using electric stimulation in physical medicine. A TENS unit is attached to the patient in the affected area and a controlled dose of current is sent to the muscle to help control intractable pain when medication has not been effective. TENS units may be used at home.

Evoked Potential Studies

Responses within the brain to external stimuli such as light, sound, and touch are called an evoked potential study. These tests are considered noninvasive since no equipment or needle is inserted into the body. Two types of evoked potential studies are described below.

- Brainstem auditory evoked response (BAER) is used to assess the auditory nerve pathways. This is useful in diagnosing auditory tumors and lesions.
- Somatosensory evoked peripheral nerves (SEP) are used for diagnosing nerve function defects in peripheral nerves, for example, in the legs.

SUMMARY

Physical therapy involves the use of physical measures, equipment, and body movement to promote mobility, circulation, restore normal function, and relieve pain. The medical assistant, working under the supervision of a physician, is able to teach the patient about proper body mechanics, exercise, and the application of various therapeutic devices such as heat and cold applications. In some cases, the medical assistant will apply these devices.

- -

Chapter Review

COMPETENCY REVIEW

1. Define and spell the terms to learn for this chapter.
2. Instruct a partner on the two-point, three-point, and four-point crutch walking gaits.
3. Create patient education materials for the application of hot and cold applications.
4. Using a partner, demonstrate PROM. Demonstrate AROM yourself.
5. Demonstrate the proper method for wheelchair transfer.
6. Talk to a local physical therapist about a typical day in his or her practice.
7. Describe the following testing methods: electromyography (EMG), nerve conduction studies (NCS), evoked potential studies (EPS), and brainstem auditory evoked response (BAER).

PREPARING FOR THE CERTIFICATION EXAM

1. A licensed professional who teaches a patient the correct use of equipment and body mechanics to prevent further injury or disability is referred to as a/an
   A. speech therapist
   B. occupational therapist
   C. physical therapist
   D. psychotherapist
   E. respiratory therapist

2. Which is a moist heat application?
   A. hypothermia blanket
   B. aquamatic K-pad
   C. warm-water bottle
   D. heat lamp
   E. Sitz bath

3. The electrical activity of a muscle is recorded by using which test?
   A. somatosensory evoked potentials (SEP)
   B. electromyography (EMG)
   C. evoked potential studies (EPS)
   D. brainstem auditory evoked response (BAER)
   E. active range of motion (AROM)

4. Rehabilitative programs are useful for treating all of the following EXCEPT
   A. catastrophic illness, for example stroke
   B. trauma
   C. acute illness
   D. diseases resulting in muscle atrophy
   E. chronic illness

continued on next page

5. The process which provides a medicinal or healthful effect is called
   A. suppuration
   B. erythema
   C. therapeutic
   D. contraindicated
   E. supination

6. When applying hot compresses, the correct maximum temperature is
   A. 90° F
   B. 115° F
   C. 120° F
   D. 105° F
   E. 125° F

7. Movement that bends a body part backward is known as
   A. inversion
   B. supination
   C. pronation
   D. dorsiflexion
   E. rotation

8. When the patient faces downward, this is called
   A. inversion
   B. supination
   C. pronation
   D. dorsiflexion
   E. rotation

9. Range of motion exercise performed without assistance from another person is
   A. AROM
   B. PROM
   C. active resistive
   D. ROME
   E. BAER

10. The crutch-walking gait used when a patient is able to bear weight on both legs is
    A. two-point
    B. three-point
    C. four-point
    D. swing-to
    E. swing-through

CRITICAL THINKING

1. What would you do first in working with Devon?
2. What instructions should Shirley give Devon?
3. What signs and symptoms relating to problems with crutch walking must Devon report?

ON THE JOB

Jenny Watmore, a medical assistant working in Dr. Cory's orthopedic practice, has been asked to assist Mr. Ivy from the wheelchair onto the examination table. Mr. Ivy, who is 70 years old, is weakened on the left side of his body from the cerebrovascular accident (CVA). He weighs 200 pounds and is reluctant to provide much help to Jenny when she has to transfer him from the wheelchair to the examination table.

1. How can Jenny get Mr. Ivy to help her assist him?
2. Describe the body mechanics that Jenny should use to assist Mr. Ivy.
3. What patient education does Mr. Ivy need?
4. What documentation should Jenny provide on Mr. Ivy's record?

INTERNET ACTIVITY

Select one of the professions listed in Table 46-1. Do an Internet search to discover the duties, the average salary range, where these professionals are usually employed, and the long-term job opportunities of the profession you selected.

MediaLink  More on physical therapy and rehabilitation, including interactive sources, can be found on the Student CD-ROM accompanying this textbook.

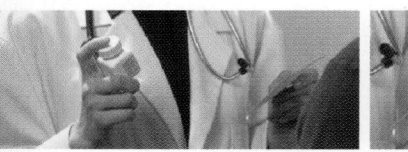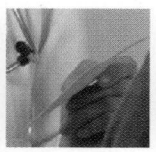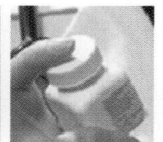

Medical Assistant Role Delineation Chart

HIGHLIGHT indicates material covered in this chapter.

ADMINISTRATIVE

Administrative Procedures

- Perform basic administrative medical assisting functions
- Schedule, coordinate and monitor appointments
- Schedule inpatient/outpatient admissions and procedures
- Understand and apply third-party guidelines
- Obtain reimbursement through accurate claims submission
- Monitor third-party reimbursement
- Understand and adhere to managed care policies and procedures
- *Negotiate managed care contracts*

Practice Finances

- Perform procedural and diagnostic coding
- Apply bookkeeping principles

- Manage accounts receivable
- *Manage accounts payable*
- *Process payroll*
- *Document and maintain accounting and banking records*
- *Develop and maintain fee schedules*
- *Manage renewals of business and professional insurance policies*
- *Manage personnel benefits and maintain records*
- *Perform marketing, financial, and strategic planning*

CLINICAL

Fundamental Principles

- Apply principles of aseptic technique and infection control
- Comply with quality assurance practices
- Screen and follow up patient test results

Diagnostic Orders

- Collect and process specimens
- Perform diagnostic tests

Patient Care

- Adhere to established patient screening procedures
- Obtain patient history and vital signs
- Prepare and maintain examination and treatment areas
- Prepare patient for examinations, procedures and treatments

- Assist with examinations, procedures and treatments
- Prepare and administer medications and immunizations
- Maintain medication and immunization records
- Recognize and respond to emergencies
- Coordinate patient care information with other health care providers
- Initiate IV and administer IV medications with appropriate training and as permitted by state law

GENERAL

Professionalism

- Display a professional manner and image
- Demonstrate initiative and responsibility
- Work as a member of the health care team
- Prioritize and perform multiple tasks
- Adapt to change
- Promote the CMA credential
- Enhance skills through continuing education
- Treat all patients with compassion and empathy
- Promote the practice through positive public relations

Communication Skills

- Recognize and respect cultural diversity
- Adapt communications to individual's ability to understand
- Use professional telephone technique

- Recognize and respond effectively to verbal, nonverbal, and written communications
- Use medical terminology appropriately
- Utilize electronic technology to receive, organize, prioritize and transmit information
- Serve as liaison

Legal Concepts

- Perform within legal and ethical boundaries
- Prepare and maintain medical records
- Document accurately
- Follow employer's established policies dealing with the health care contract
- Implement and maintain federal and state health care legislation and regulations
- Comply with established risk management and safety procedures
- Recognize professional credentialing criteria
- *Develop and maintain personnel, policy and procedure manuals*

Instruction

- Instruct individuals according to their needs
- Explain office policies and procedures
- Teach methods of health promotion and disease prevention
- Locate community resources and disseminate information
- *Develop educational materials*
- *Conduct continuing education activities*

Operational Functions

- Perform inventory of supplies and equipment
- Perform routine maintenance of administrative and clinical equipment
- Apply computer techniques to support office operations
- *Perform personnel management functions*
- *Negotiate leases and prices for equipment and supply contracts*

- *Denotes advanced skills.*

SOURCE: Reprinted by permission of the American Association of Medical Assistants from the AAMA Role Delineation Study: Occupational Analysis of the Medical Assisting Profession.

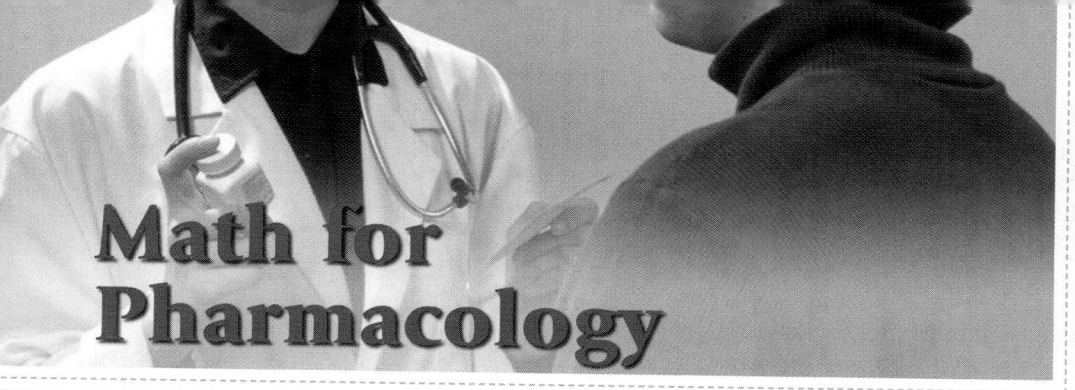

Math for Pharmacology

Learning Objectives

After completing this chapter, you should be able to:

- Define and spell the terms to learn for this chapter.
- State the differences between the apothecary and metric systems.
- Convert dosages between the apothecary and metric systems given the conversion formula.
- Correctly calculate medication dosages using the mathematical conversions.
- State four rules for calculating pediatric dosages.

OUTLINE

Weights and Measures	1012
Drug Calculations	1013
Calculating Dosages	1017
Rules for Conversion	1017
Calculating Pediatric Dosages	1018

Terms to Learn

apothecary system	Fried's law	West's nomogram
body surface area (BSA)	metric system	Young's rule
Clark's rule		

Case Study

MRS. HANOVER, AN ELDERLY LADY, AGED 85, has come to Dr. Horsley's office due to lower back pain that she has been experiencing for a month. Dr. Horsley orders a bone scan, which reveals that Mrs. Hanover, is suffering from osteoporosis. Due to Mrs. Hanover's condition Dr. Horsley prescribes calcium with vitamin D tablets 100,000 USP units 1 every 6 hours for 14 days. The calcium with vitamin D tablet is available in either 8,000 USP units/mL drops or 50,000 USP unit tablets. How would Sue, the medical assistant, calculate how many tablets Mrs. Hanover should take every 6 hours?

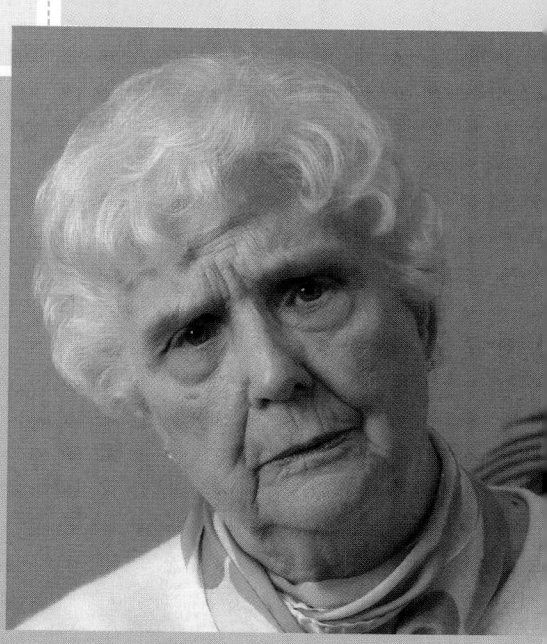

Weights and Measure

Two separate sets of weights and measures are used to calculate medication doses, the apothecary system and the metric system. Generally, most physicians and facilities have moved to the metric system, but the medical assistant must be familiar with both systems, because occasionally medications do appear in the apothecary system. Another aspect to remember is that common household measurements, such as teaspoon and tablespoon do appear, although they are not formal medication measurement units. Most commonly, the household measurements are used in patient education.

The Apothecary System

The apothecary system is considered to be the oldest system of measurement. Dry weight equivalent is 1 grain = 1 gram of wheat. The basic units of measure are the grain (gr). The gram (g), the dram (dr, ʒ), the ounce (oz, ℥), and the pound (lb). Fluid measurements are the minims (m), fluid dram (fl dr, flʒ), fluid ounce (fl oz fl℥), pint (pt), quart (qt), and gallon (gal). Some common household measurements such as the ounce, pint, quart, and gallon are based on the apothecary system.

Roman numerals are used when numbering in the apothecary system. For example, 3 grains would be gr iii. Fractions are also used. Three-fourths of a grain would be gr ¾. The unit of measure in the apothecary system is placed before the actual number.

To accurately write an apothecary notation the following rules should be adhered to:

1. The unit or abbreviation comes before the amount.

    Example: qt iii, rather than iii qt

2. Use lowercase roman numerals to express whole numbers 1 through 10, 15, 20, and 30.

3. Use Arabic numbers for other quantities.

    Example: qt i (one quart), gr 12 (twelve grains), and gr xx (twenty grains)

4. Use fractions to designate amounts less than 1.

    Example: gr ½, NOT 0.50 gr

5. The symbol *ss* is used to designate the fraction ½.

    Example: pt iiiss (three and one-half pints)

When interpreting a drug order or reading a drug label, it is helpful to know the common roman numerals and their Arabic equivalents (see Table 47-1).

The Metric System

The metric system is the most commonly used conversion system for dosage calculations. Metric conversions are simply accomplished by multiplying or dividing by 1000. Multiplying by 1000 would be the same as

TABLE 47-1 Arabic Numbers, Roman Numerals, and Apothecary Notations

Arabic Number	Roman Numeral	Apothecary Notation	Arabic Number	Roman Numeral	Apothecary Notation
1	I	i, ī	8	VIII	viii, v̄iii
2	II	ii, īi	9	IX	ix, īx
3	III	iii, īii	10	X	x, x̄
4	IV	iv, īv	15	XV	xv, x̄v
5	V	v, v̄	20	XX	xx, x̄x
6	VI	vi, v̄i	25	XXV	xxv, x̄xv
7	VII	vii, v̄ii	30	XXX	xxx, x̄xx

moving the decimal point three places to the right. Dividing by 1000 would mean that the decimal point moves three places to the left. For further explanation, review the following example:

Convert: 3.5 g to mg

Equivalent: 1 g = 1000 mg. Conversion factor is 1000.

Multiply by 1000: 3.5 g = 3.5 × 1000 = 3500 mg

Or move the decimal point three places to the right: 3.5 g = 3.500 = 3500 mg

The common units of measure are the liter (volume), the gram (weight), and the meter (length). Table 47-2 lists common abbreviations for weights and measures (see Guidelines 47-1 for conversion within the metric system).

In the metric system, the dosage is written as a decimal number first with the unit of measurement following (2.5 mg). Equivalents are demonstrated in Table 47-3. Common household measures are discussed in Table 47-4, and the comparisons of the three systems for liquid measurements are in Table 47-5.

Drug Calculations

Stock medications are frequently kept in offices for use in the office. However, the stock medications may be a different dosage than the physician's order. Therefore, it is important to understand basic drug calculations to ensure that the correct dose of medication is given. Sometimes, a conversion chart is given, but it is important to double-check and ensure that the dose is correct.

Many factors are involved in calculating the correct dose of a drug, including the patient's age, weight, and current state of health. Another important factor to note is the other medications that the patient is currently taking, because they may strengthen or weaken the new drug.

TABLE 47-2 Common Abbreviations for Weights and Measures

Apothecary System		Metric System	
Symbol/Abbreviations	**Meaning**	**Symbol/Abbreviations Weights**	**Meaning**
gtt drop	drop	mg	milligram
℔ min	minim	gm	gram
dr, ℨ	dram	**Symbol/Abbreviation Volume**	**Meaning**
fl dr, flℨ	fluid dram	l	Liter
oz, ℥	ounce	mL	milliliter
fl oz, fl℥	fluid ounce	cc	cubic centimeter
O pt	pint		
C gal	gallon		
gr	grain		

TABLE 47-3 **Commonly Used Equivalents for the Apothecary and Metric System**

Measure Apothecary	Equivalent Metric	Measure Apothecary	Equivalent Metric
1 gr	65 mg or 0.065 g	**Liquid Measure**	
5 gr	325 mg or 0.33 g	1 fl dr	4 mL
10 gr	650 mg or 0.67 g	2 fl dr	8 mL
15 or 16 gr	1 g	2.5 fl dr	10 mL
15 or 16 m	1.00 mL or cc	4 fl dr	15 mL
1 dram	4 mL	1 fl oz	30 mL
1 oz	30 cc, 30 mL, 8 tsp, 8 drams, 2 tbsp	3.5 fl oz	100 mL
1 lb	450 g	7 fl oz	200 mL
1 lb	0.4536 kg	1 pt	500 mL
1 minim (m)	0.06 mL	1 qt	1000 mL
4 m	0.25 mL	60 gtts	4 mL

The first step in the drug calculation is to ensure that the system of weights and measures in the prescription is the same as in the container of stock medication. If they are different, the first step will be to use Table 47-3 and Table 47-5 to covert them to the same system.

Two methods of drug calculations are explained in this chapter: the ratio method and the formula method. It is important to understand both and then apply the method that seems easiest for you.

Review of Math Principles

A basic review of math principles is necessary to understand drug calculations. See Table 47-6 for examples of mathematical equivalents to review the relationship

---

47-1 **GUIDELINES**

Conversion within the Metric System

1. No change is required to change milliliters into cubic centimeters because they are equal to each other.
2. To change grams to milligrams, multiply grams by 1000 or move the decimal point three places to the RIGHT.
3. To change milligrams to grams, divide milligrams by 1000 or move the decimal point three places to the LEFT.
4. To convert liters to milliliters, multiply liters by 1000 or move the decimal point three places to the RIGHT.
5. To convert milliliters to liters, divide milliliters by 1000 or move the decimal point three places to the LEFT.

TABLE 47-4 **Common Household Measures**

Measure	Equivalent
60 gtts (drops)	1 teaspoon (tsp)
3 tsp	1 tablespoon (T)
2 T	1 oz
4 oz	1 small juice glass
8 oz	1 cup or glass
16 T or 8 oz	1 cup
2 cups	1 pint (pt)
2 pints	1 quart (qt)
4 quarts	1 gallon

TABLE 47-5 Comparison of Household/Apothecary/Metric Liquid Measurements

Household	Apothecary	Metric
1 drop	1 minim (♏)	0.06 mL
1 tsp	1 fl dr (fl℈)	4–5 mL
1 T	4 fl dr (fl℈)	15–16 mL
2 T	1 fl oz (fl℥)	30–32 mL
1 cup or glass	8 fl oz (fl℥)	250 mL
2 cups or glasses	16 fl oz, 1 pt	500 mL
4 cups or glasses	1 qt	1000 mL = approximately 1 liter

between fractions, ratios, percentages, and decimals. For example, ½ is the same as 0.5 and the ratio of 1:2. A ratio and a decimal are different ways of expressing the fraction ½.

Ratios are one method of calculating drug dosages. The medical assistant would compare the amount of drug ordered to the amount on hand.

To determine a percentage in the fraction, divided the numerator (top number) by the denominator (bottom number). The decimal point is then moved to spaces to the right, creating the percentage. For example:

$$½ = 1 ÷ 2 = 0.50$$

$$0.50 = 50.0\% \text{ or } 50\%$$

When there are two ratios to compare, then you have a proportion. A proportion resulting from the fraction ½ or ratio could be 10/20 = ½ or 10:20::1:2. The proportion is read as 10 divided by 20 equals 1 divided by 2, or ten is to twenty as one is to two. Even though the numbers are bigger (10 instead of 1), the proportion is exactly the same—the first number is half the size of the second. If you know three of the four numbers for the two ratios, you can solve for the fourth by using mathematical principles. The symbol x is used for the unknown quantity. For example $10/20 = 1/x$.

To find the unknown quantity, cross multiply. This means to multiply the top number on the left side of the = sign by the bottom number on the right side, and the bottom number on the left is multiplied by the top number on the right. Then, divide both sides by the number with the x: $10x ÷ 10 = 1x$ or x and $20 ÷ 10 = 2$.

TABLE 47-6 Example of Mathematical Equivalents

Fraction	Ratio	Percent	Decimal
1/4	1:4	25%	0.25
1/2	1:2	50%	0.50
2/3	2:3	66%	0.66
3/4	3:4	75%	0.75
7/8	7:8	88%	0.88
1/100	1:100	1%	0.01
1/200	1:200	0.5%	0.005
1/1000	1:100	0.1%	0.001

by each other and the means (the two inner numbers—20 and 1) to solve for x: the (unknown)

$$10:20::1:x$$
$$10 \times x = 20 \times 1$$
$$10x = 20$$
$$x = 20 \div 10$$
$$x = 2$$

To prove this answer is correct, multiply the extremes and multiply the means. If the answer is correct, they will be equal.

$$So\ldots 10:20::1:2$$
$$10 \times 2 = 20 \times 1$$
$$20 = 20\text{—so the answer is correct}$$

Problem: There is a physician order to give 80 mg of Lasix (furosemide). The supply on hand states that there is 40 mg/mL.

There are 40 mg in 1 mL of Lasix. (This is the strength of the medicine.) The question is asking how many mL of Lasix are required to get 80 mg.

$$80\,\text{mg}:x\,\text{mL}::40\,\text{mg}:1\,\text{mL}$$
$$80 \times 1 = 40 \times x$$
$$80 = 40x$$
$$x = 2\,\text{mL}$$

So—2 mL of Lasix are required to get 80 mg.

This means that $x = 2$.

$$\frac{10}{20} = \frac{1}{x} = 10 \times x = 20 \times 1$$
$$10x = 20$$
$$\frac{10x}{10} = \frac{20}{10}$$
$$1x = 2$$
$$x = 2$$

Another method is to convert $10/20 = 1/x$ into the ratio we saw earlier of $10:20::1:x$. Then, multiply the extremes (the two outer numbers—the 10 and the x)

Calculating Dosages

It is possible to calculate dosages easily using a formula. To determine the amount of the drug needed, set up the following formula:

Calculation formula:

$$\frac{\text{Available strength}}{\text{Ordered strength}} = \frac{\text{available amount}}{\text{amount to give}}$$

Available strength is the strength of the drug in stock. The available amount is the amount of drug in the container. The ordered strength is the physician's order, and the amount to give is the unknown quantity (the x).

For example, the physician order is to give 500 mg of a drug, and there is a vial which contains 1000 mg/mL.

Calculation formula:

$$\frac{\text{Available strength}}{\text{Ordered strength}} = \frac{\text{available amount}}{\text{amount to give}}$$

Strength of the drug in the vial $= 1000$ mg/mL

Available amount $= 1$ mL

Ordered strength $= 500$ mg

Amount to give $= x$

$$\frac{1000 \text{ mg}}{500 \text{ mg}} = \frac{1 \text{ mL}}{x}$$

$$1000 \times x = 500 \times 1$$

$$1000x = 500$$

$$\frac{1000x}{1000} = \frac{500}{1000}$$

$$1x = 5/10 = \text{½ mL} = 0.5 \text{ mL}$$

You would fill the syringe with 0.5 mL of liquid to give you the physician's order of 500 mg of medication. To solve a problem using other forms of medications, such as tablets, use the same formula:

Physician's order: Give 10 grains of medication.

Available: Tablets containing 2.5 grains each

Calculation formula:

$$\frac{\text{Available strength}}{\text{Ordered strength}} = \frac{\text{available amount}}{\text{amount to give}}$$

$$2.5 \text{ gr} = 1 \text{ tablet}$$

$$10 \text{ gr } x \text{ (number of tablets)}$$

$$2.5 \times x = 10 \times 1$$

$$2.5x = 10$$

$$\frac{2.5x}{2.5} = \frac{10}{2.5}$$

$$1x = 4 \text{ tablets}$$

Cultural Considerations

It is important to be aware of the responses of patients to the prescriptions written by the physician. Some individuals may not take the medications prescribed by the physician for cultural or religious reasons. For example, certain religions such as Scientology and Jehovah's Witness have specific beliefs that oppose the use of medications for the treatment of medical diseases and psychological disorders. Understanding why the patient may not want to take the medication is important so that the physician might change the plan of care to meet not only the medical needs of the patient, but to also respect the patient's cultural preferences.

Another formula that is frequently used is $D/H \times Q$, where

$D =$ desired or ordered dose

$H =$ supply on hand or available supply

$Q =$ quantity available

Problem: The physician ordered penicillin 250 mg. The bottle from the supply cabinet is labeled "Penicillin 500 mg per mL."

Solution: Set up the formula

$$\frac{\text{Desired}}{\text{Hand}} \times \text{Quantity}$$

The physician's order is placed in the Desired (D) space and the supply you have on hand is placed in the Hand (H) space. The quantity per mL is placed in the Quantity (Q) space:

$$\frac{D}{H} \times Q = \frac{250}{500} \times 1$$

Divide 250 by 500 $\times \dfrac{1}{1} = 0.5$ mL

The answer is 0.5 mL or ½ mL.

Rules for Conversion

When converting from one system to another, it is important to remember that the equivalents may be only approximate, especially when using conversion tables such as the one in Table 47-7. This table, however, should be learned, because the conversions are very

TABLE 47-7 **Conversion List**

Apothecary	Metric
15 or 16 minims (m)	1 mL or 1 cc
1 fluid dr	4 mL or cc
1 fluid oz	30 mL or cc
1 quart	1000 mL or cc
1/60 grain	1 milligram (mg)
1 grain	0.065 gram
15 grains	1 gram
2.2 pounds	1 kilogram

47-2 **GUIDELINES**

Conversion

1. To change grains to grams, divide by 15.
2. To change ounces to cubic centimeters (cc) or milliliters (mL), multiply by 30.
3. To change grains to milligrams (mg), multiply by 60. (Use this rule only when you have less than 1 grain.)
4. To change kilograms to pounds, multiply by 2.2.
5. To change cubic centimeters (cc) or milliliters (mL), to ounces, divide by 30.
6. To change drams to milliliters (mL), multiply by 4.
7. To change cubic centimeters (cc) or milliliters (mL) to minims, multiply by 15 or 16.
8. To change minims to cubic centimeters (cc) or milliliters (mL), divide by 15 or 16.
9. To convert drams to grams, multiply by 4.

helpful when converting from one measuring system to another (see Guidelines 47-2).

Calculating Pediatric Dosages

Pediatric medications and their dosages are different than those for adults. Sometimes, those medications used for adults must be calculated for use in children. It is imperative that the calculations be exact when administering medications to a child. Oftentimes, the physician takes the responsibility for this task, but the medical assistant may be asked to assist or to double-check the dosage.

There are several rules or "laws" for the calculations of medications for pediatrics, including Clark's rule, Fried's law, Young's law, West's nomogram, and the body by weight method. Each of these approaches is named for the individual who developed the rule.

Clark's Rule

Clark's rule is based on the weight of the child. This is the most common law used in the calculation of drug dosage for children, especially since the weight of different children at the same age can vary significantly. The formula for Clark's rule is

$$\text{Pediatric dose} = \frac{\text{child's weight in pounds}}{150 \text{ pounds}} \times \text{adult dose}$$

This rule is followed by dividing the child's weight by 150 pounds and then multiplying that number by the adult dose.

> *Practice:* Penicillin is ordered for a child weighing 35 pounds. The average dose for an adult is 360 mg. How many mg will the child receive?
>
> $$35/150 \times 360 \text{ mg} = 83.9 \text{ mg}$$

To convert the mg into milliliters use the $D/H \times Q$ formula.

Fried's Law

Fried's law is applied to children under the age of 1 year. Fried's assumption is that a 12½-year-old child could take an adult dose, and a fraction of that is taken to figure dosages on a young child. The formula:

$$\text{Pediatric dose} = \frac{\text{child's age in months}}{150 \text{ months}} \times \text{adult dose}$$

This formula uses 150 months in the denominator as the equivalent for 12½ years.

Young's Rule

Young's rule is used for children who are over 1 year of age. The formula used for Young's rule is:

Pediatric dose =

$$\frac{\text{child's age in years}}{\text{child's age in years} + 12} \times \text{adult dose}$$

To use this formula, divide the child's age in years by the same number plus 12. Multiply this number by the adult dose to determine the correct pediatric dosage.

West's Nomogram

The two methods most commonly used for calculating pediatric dosages are body weight (such as mg/kg), and body surface area (BSA). The West's nomogram is the preferred method for sick and underweight children. It can be used for both infants and children. The chart is frequently found in pediatric offices, medical textbooks, and dictionaries.

West's nomogram is the preferred method of pediatric calculation particular for oncology and critical care patients because it is based on the calculation of the body surface area of the child. The body surface area (BSA) is based on a calculation of the child's height and weight, and is expressed as m². The chart has three columns (see Figure 47-1). To calculate the child's BSA, a straight line is drawn from the patient's height in inches or centimeters across the columns to the patient's weight in kilograms or pounds. The straight line will intersect on the BSA column. This

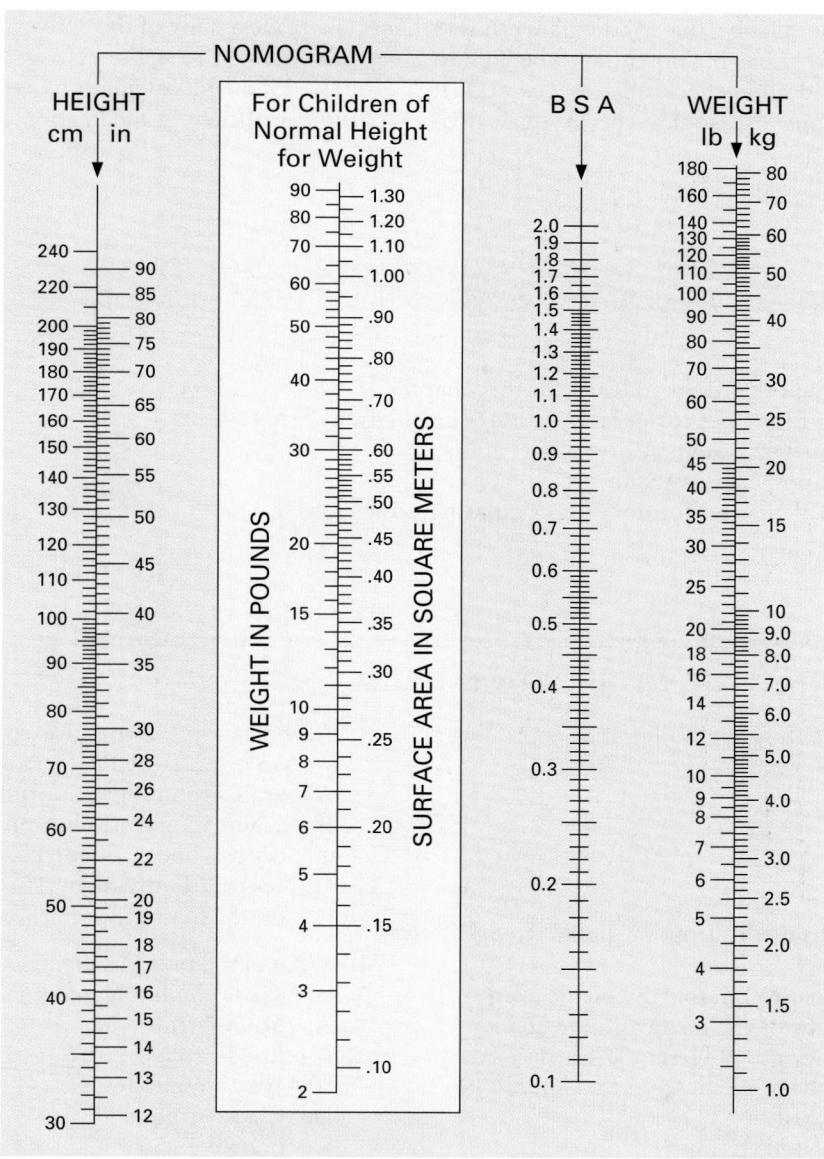

FIGURE 47-1 Nomogram chart.

point will give the BSA average. Once a BSA average is calculated, it is applied to the following formula:

$$\text{Pediatric dose} = \frac{\text{BSA of child}}{1.73 \text{ square meters}} \times \text{adult dose}$$

1.73 meters is the standard adult BSA.

Body Weight Method

The body weight method is the other method that is commonly seen in pediatric situations. Medication dosages are often ordered by the body weight method. The body weight method uses calculations based on the patient's weight in kilograms. This requires converting the patient's weight into kilograms. The following provides an example of how this is achieved.

Example: Convert 77 lb to kg

Approximate equivalent: 1 kg = 2.2 lb.

Conversion factor is 2.2

77 lb = 77 divided by 2.2 = 35 kg

Once the child's weight has been converted into kilograms the correct dosage can be calculated. This is done by calculating the safe drug dosage in mg/kg (as recommended by a reputable drug reference) and then multiplying that amount by the child's weight in kg.

SUMMARY

The medical assistant must be able to calculate dosages correctly since any error has the potential to be fatal to the patient. Always double-check all dosages and, if possible, have someone else double-check your calculations. Have a copy of the conversion factors in an accessible location to make conversions quickly and accurately. Frequent calculations will keep the medical assistant proficient at medication calculations.

- -

Chapter Review

COMPETENCY REVIEW

1. Define and spell the terms to learn for this chapter.
2. What are the four rules for pediatric dosage calculations?
3. What is the metric system?
4. What is the apothecary system?
5. What is the calculation formula for calculating dosages?

PREPARING FOR THE CERTIFICATION EXAM

1. In liquid measures, one fluid ounce is equal to:
   A. 1 mL
   B. 10 mL
   C. 30 mL
   D. 100 cc
   E. 30 cc

2. With regard to medication, available strength refers to:
   A. what actually contains the medication
   B. the potency of the medication in stock
   C. the potency the physician has ordered
   D. the amount of medication that should be administered
   E. the calculated strength

3. According to the rules for converting from one system of measurement to another, to change:
   A. grains to milligrams, multiply by 60
   B. grains to grams, multiply by 15
   C. ccs to ounces, divide by 50
   D. ccs to mL, divide by 15
   E. drams to grams, multiply by 2

4. What is the preferred method of most physicians for calculating pediatric dosages?
   A. Young's rule
   B. Fried's rule
   C. West's nomogram
   D. Clark's rule
   E. body weight

continued on next page

5. Tablets and capsules are measured in metric units of:
   A. grains
   B. millimeters
   C. cubic centimeters
   D. ounces
   E. grams

6. Sometimes the available dosage of a medication on hand is not that same as that which the physician has ordered. The medical assistant must determine how much of the medication should be used. In the equation used for this calculation, the needed dosage is indicated by:
   A. the numerator
   B. the denominator
   C. a whole number
   D. both the numerator and the denominator
   E. numbers less than 10

7. Which of the following choices is NOT a formula used to calculate a dosage of a medication?
   A. West's nomogram
   B. Clark's rule
   C. Young's rule
   D. Fried's law
   E. Blalock-Taussig procedure

8. Which of the two following measurements are equal to each other?
   A. milligrams to grams
   B. liters to milliliters
   C. milliliters to grams
   D. milliliters to cubic centimeters
   E. milliliters to liters

9. When converting a larger unit to a smaller unit, you:
   A. divide
   B. multiply
   C. subtract
   D. add
   E. measure

10. Which of the following formulas is used to calculate a pediatric dose based on the child's weight in ponds?
   A. Young's rule
   B. Clark's rule
   C. Fried's law
   D. West's nomogram
   E. body weight

CRITICAL THINKING

1. How many tablets should Sue instruct Mrs. Hanover to take every 6 hours?
2. How did Sue calculate the dosage?
3. How many tablets should Mrs. Hanover take if instructed to take the medication qid?

ON THE JOB

In the past Mrs. Kennedy has been prescribed Protonix 20 mg a day. Cindy, the medical assistant at Dr. Jones's office, has just spoken to the patient. Mrs. Kennedy tells Cindy that her abdominal pain has increased. After Cindy speaks with the physician on call, the physician increases the dosage to 40 mg once a day. The physician indicates that the patient should take the medication for 2 weeks to see if any further relief can be achieved. Mrs. Kennedy will be stopping by the office to pick up some samples this afternoon. How will Cindy instruct Mrs. Kennedy and document in the patient chart the change in dose?

INTERNET ACTIVITY

Do an Internet search for medical assistant pharmacology.

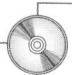 **MediaLink** More on pharmacology, including interactive resources, can be found on the Student CD-ROM accompanying this textbook.

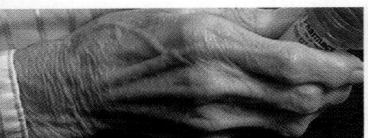 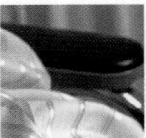 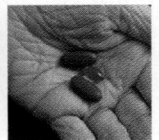

Medical Assistant Role Delineation Chart

HIGHLIGHT indicates material covered in this chapter.

ADMINISTRATIVE

Administrative Procedures

- Perform basic administrative medical assisting functions
- Schedule, coordinate and monitor appointments
- Schedule inpatient/outpatient admissions and procedures
- Understand and apply third-party guidelines
- Obtain reimbursement through accurate claims submission
- Monitor third-party reimbursement
- Understand and adhere to managed care policies and procedures
- *Negotiate managed care contracts*

Practice Finances

- Perform procedural and diagnostic coding
- Apply bookkeeping principles

- Manage accounts receivable
- *Manage accounts payable*
- *Process payroll*
- *Document and maintain accounting and banking records*
- *Develop and maintain fee schedules*
- *Manage renewals of business and professional insurance policies*
- *Manage personnel benefits and maintain records*
- *Perform marketing, financial, and strategic planning*

CLINICAL

Fundamental Principles

- Apply principles of aseptic technique and infection control
- Comply with quality assurance practices
- Screen and follow up patient test results

Diagnostic Orders

- Collect and process specimens
- Perform diagnostic tests

Patient Care

- Adhere to established patient screening procedures
- Obtain patient history and vital signs
- Prepare and maintain examination and treatment areas
- Prepare patient for examinations, procedures and treatments

- Assist with examinations, procedures and treatments
- Prepare and administer medications and immunizations
- Maintain medication and immunization records
- Recognize and respond to emergencies
- Coordinate patient care information with other health care providers
- Initiate IV and administer IV medications with appropriate training and as permitted by state law

GENERAL

Professionalism

- Display a professional manner and image
- Demonstrate initiative and responsibility
- Work as a member of the health care team
- Prioritize and perform multiple tasks
- Adapt to change
- Promote the CMA credential
- Enhance skills through continuing education
- Treat all patients with compassion and empathy
- Promote the practice through positive public relations

Communication Skills

- Recognize and respect cultural diversity
- Adapt communications to individual's ability to understand
- Use professional telephone technique

- Recognize and respond effectively to verbal, nonverbal, and written communications
- Use medical terminology appropriately
- Utilize electronic technology to receive, organize, prioritize and transmit information
- Serve as liaison

Legal Concepts

- Perform within legal and ethical boundaries
- Prepare and maintain medical records
- Document accurately
- Follow employer's established policies dealing with the health care contract
- Implement and maintain federal and state health care legislation and regulations
- Comply with established risk management and safety procedures
- Recognize professional credentialing criteria
- *Develop and maintain personnel, policy and procedure manuals*

Instruction

- Instruct individuals according to their needs
- Explain office policies and procedures
- Teach methods of health promotion and disease prevention
- Locate community resources and disseminate information
- *Develop educational materials*
- *Conduct continuing education activities*

Operational Functions

- Perform inventory of supplies and equipment
- Perform routine maintenance of administrative and clinical equipment
- Apply computer techniques to support office operations
- *Perform personnel management functions*
- *Negotiate leases and prices for equipment and supply contracts*

- *Denotes advanced skills.*

SOURCE: Reprinted by permission of the American Association of Medical Assistants from the AAMA Role Delineation Study: Occupational Analysis of the Medical Assisting Profession.

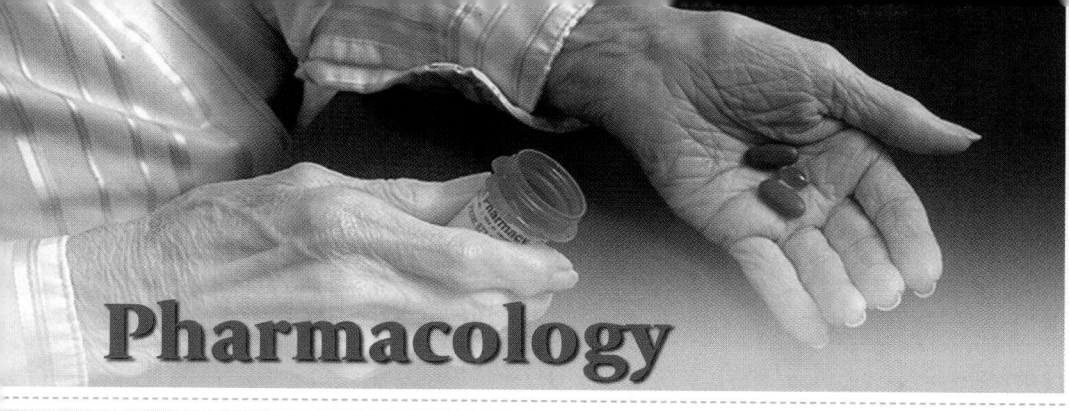

Pharmacology

Learning Objectives

After completing this chapter, you should be able to:

- Define and spell the terms to learn for this chapter.
- Differentiate between the legal (generic) and commercial (trade) and chemical names for a drug.
- Describe the precautions to be observed when administering drugs.
- Describe the drug reference resources that should be accessible in all physician offices.
- List the "ten rights" to medicine administration.
- List the five schedules of the Controlled Substances Act.
- Explain the conditions under which a medical assistant may administer medications.
- Cite the information that must be charted when administering a medication.

Terms to Learn

bioequivalent	generic name	pharmacology
brand name	habituation	prophylactically
broad spectrum	idiosyncratic	side effects
contraindicated	lethal	synthetic
Drug Enforcement Administration (DEA)	pharmacists	toxic

OUTLINE

Drug Names	1024
Regulation and Standards	1024
References	1024
Legal Classification of Drugs	1025
Drug Abuse	1028
General Classes of Drugs	1029
Routes and Methods of Drug Administration	1033
Frequently Administered Drugs	1036
Side Effects of Medications	1037
Drug Interactions	1037
Drug Use During Pregnancy	1038
Reading and Writing a Prescription	1038
Abbreviations Used in Pharmacology	1041

Case Study

SUSAN KREMSKI, CMA, WORKS at Dr. Jones's internal medicine practice. She is responsible for refilling medications that are called in on the prescription refill line at the office. Susan always pulls the patient's chart and documents the medication name, amount to be refilled, if there are to be any additional refills, and the physician's name. She also records the pharmacy phone number and initials and dates the entry.

She has received a call from the pharmacy for a refill for Joe Thomas, for a pain medication. Susan pulls Mr. Thomas's chart and notices that he is calling a week early for his refill. How should Susan handle this request?

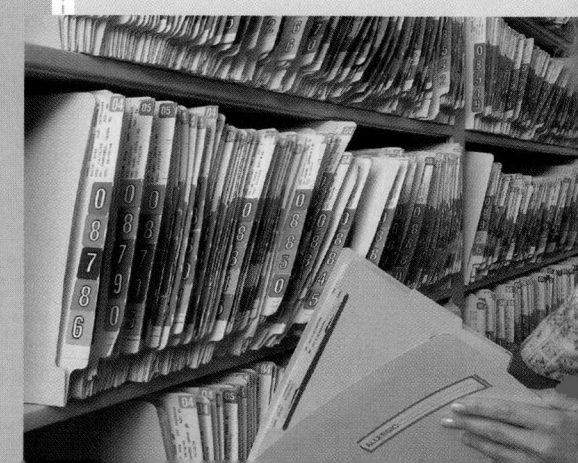

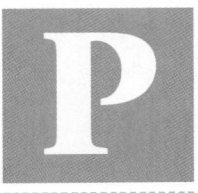**P**harmacology is the study of drugs and their origins, characteristics, and effects. Drugs come from many different sources, including plants, animals, minerals, and synthetics. Some drugs, such as vitamins, are found naturally in the foods we eat. Medications, such as penicillin and other antibiotics, come from molds, which are a form of plant life. The vast majority of drugs used in medicine today are synthetic, created in a laboratory by artificial means.

Drugs, such as antibiotics or antihypertensives, are given to either help improve or eradicate a condition that a patient already has. If drugs are given prophylactically, they are being used to prevent the onset of a condition. Drugs that are given to control infections or to kill cancer cells are called chemotherapy drugs.

The role of the medical assistant is to assist the physician in the treatment of patients. The physician is responsible for prescribing medication for patients. The medical assistant is often required to administer the medication. This requires the medical assistant to develop skills in reading medication orders, properly administering medications, and other aspects of pharmacology.

Drug Names

Three names are used to describe drugs: the generic name (equivalent to what is sometimes called the "official" or nonproprietary" name of a drug), the brand name, and the chemical name. The generic name is the single identifying name, is typically noted in lowercase letters, and is considered the legal name for the drug. Generic drugs are required by Food and Drug Administration (FDA) law to have the same effectiveness, safety, active ingredients, quality, strength, purity, and stability as brand name drugs. Examples of generic names include acetaminophen, ibuprofen, and tetracycline.

The brand name, which is typically noted in uppercase letters, is the name given to a drug by a specific manufacturer. This is also called the proprietary name. This name is often the most familiar name for a specific drug. The company that holds the patent for the drug can manufacture and produce that drug, under that brand name, for 20 years from the date of the patent. Other companies may manufacture the same drug, but must use their own brand name. Advil and Motrin are brand names for the generic durg ibuprofen.

Generic drugs are typically priced lower than drugs with the brand names, and generally are bioequivalent having the same strength and action. It is the active ingredients in generic drugs that are required to be bioequivalent. However, generic drugs are not as closely monitored as the brand name drugs, so their effectiveness may or may not actually be equal. If a physician believes that a specific drug is more effective than a generic version, then the named brand is more likely to be ordered.

The chemical name is the chemical formula typically used by manufacturers and pharmacists. Pharmacists are specially trained and licensed professionals who specialize in the preparation and dispensation of drugs.

Regulation and Standards

The FDA is the specific department within the federal Department of Health and Human Services responsible for the testing, approving, labeling, and enforcing laws about the sales and distribution of drugs. The Federal Food, Drug, and Cosmetic Act of 1938 stipulates the actual control of drugs. This law was enacted to ensure the safety of food, drugs, and cosmetics that are sold within U.S. borders. The Controlled Substances Act of 1970 regulates the manufacture and distribution of drugs that are capable of causing dependencies. The Drug Enforcement Administration (DEA) is the agency of the federal government responsible for enforcing drug control.

All physicians are required to register with the DEA in order to prescribe, dispense, or administer controlled substances.

References

The most common drug resource available is the *Physicians' Desk Reference,* also known as the PDR. The pink section in the PDR is an alphabetical listing of generic and brand names. The blue section in the PDR contains an alphabetical listing by category or classification of generic and brand names. The white section contains current information regarding pharmaceutical manufacturers. The gray section provides product identification and color photos of tablets and capsules. This text is reprinted annually and is a relatively easy-to-read reference published by a private company and purchased by medical offices and hospitals. The *Hospital Formulary* also contains up-to-date information about drugs and their usage. It is published by the American Hospital Formulary Service and is used extensively by pharmacists. Another book that is helpful is the *United States Pharmacopeia–National Formulary* (USP–NF). This book lists all of the official (generic) drugs that are authorized for use in the United States.

Many online references are available, including Web MD and Medline, but the medical assistant must be sure to use recognized, reliable resources when searching the Internet for medical information. Because it is impossible for anyone to remember all of the available medications, it is important for the medical assistant to practice using the available medical references and not rely on memory to ensure that patients receive the correct drug. Many names sound alike, and accuracy in prescribing the correct drug for the correct condition is imperative.

Legal Classification of Drugs

Drugs are classified based on the need for a prescription and their addictive potential. It is important that the medical assistant be able to distinguish between prescription and nonprescription drugs, and also to stay current on the status of drugs because some do change status from prescription to nonprescription.

Prescription Drugs

Physicians are responsible for prescribing medications; however, specially licensed professionals such as physician assistants and advanced practice nurses (such as nurse practitioners and clinical nurse specialists) can also write prescriptions. A prescription is a written explanation to a pharmacist detailing the name of the medication, the dose, the route, and the times of administration. Physicians can also give the prescription verbally to a pharmacist. Examples of prescription drugs include antibiotics, antihypertensives, and pain medications. These drugs must be labeled with the words "Caution: Federal Law prohibits dispensing without prescription."

Nonprescription Drugs

Nonprescription drugs are also known as over-the-counter (OTC) drugs. OTC drugs are found in a variety of stores. Examples include aspirin, antidiarrhea medications, and cold medications.

OTC medications are regulated by the FDA. OTC medications are not without dangers, and patients should be educated to read labels and follow the label's directions (see Patient Education). If taken incorrectly, some OTC drugs can be unsafe since they may react negatively with a prescription drug the pa-

tient is taking. Antacids should not be taken with some antibiotics. Aspirin should not be taken with Coumadin (an anticlotting medication), because of the potential for uncontrolled bleeding. Individuals with stomach ulcers should not take aspirin or ibuprofen because of the risk of bleeding. If there are questions about how to take OTC medications, patients should ask their pharmacists for guidance. Patients should always let their physicians know about all OTC medications they are taking so that there are no complications.

Controlled Substances

Certain drugs are controlled if they have a potential for addiction or abuse. The DEA enforces the control of

TABLE 48-1 Schedule for Controlled Substances

Level	Description	Comment
Schedule I	Highest potential for addiction and abuse. Not accepted for medical use. Examples: marijuana, heroin, and LSD	Not prescribed drugs.
Schedule II	High potential for addiction and abuse. Accepted for medical use in the United States. Examples: codeine, cocaine, morphine, opium, and secobarbital	A DEA-licensed physician must complete the required triplicate prescription forms entirely written in his or her own handwriting. The prescription must be filled within 7 days and it may not be refilled. In an emergency, the physician may order a limited amount of the drug by telephone. These drugs must be stored under lock and key if they are kept on the office premises. The law requires that a dispensing record of these drugs be kept on file for 2 years.
Schedule III	Moderate to low potential for addiction and abuse. Examples: butabarbital, anabolic steroids, and APC with codeine	A DEA number is not required to write a prescription for these drugs, but the physician must hand write the order. Five refills are allowed during a 6-month period and must be indicated on the prescription form. Only the physician can give telephone orders to the pharmacist for these drugs.
Schedule IV	Lower potential for addiction and abuse than Schedule III drugs. Examples: chloral hydrate, phenobarbital, and diazepam	A medical assistant may write the prescription order for the physician, but it must be signed by the physician. Five refills are allowed over a 6-month period of time.
Schedule V	Low potential for addiction and abuse. Examples: low-strength codeine combined with other drugs to form cough suppressant	Inventory records must be maintained on these drugs.

these medications. A drug that has the potential for abuse must be placed on the controlled substances list, according to the Federal Controlled Substances Act (CSA). The CSA has set forth guidelines for controlled substances and divided them into five categories sections according to their potentially addictive level of abuse. See Table 48-1 for examples of these schedules. Controlled substances (also known as narcotics) **must always be kept under lock and key, and strict control must be maintained.** A narcotic log should be used to track all narcotics, including the inventory in stock, who administers a narcotic, how much was given, and the date and name of the patient receiving the drug. Most facilities do not allow medical assistants to administer narcotics.

All controlled substances must be labeled according to CSA specifications, showing the drug's assigned schedule. The schedule identification number is written inside a capital letter C, which stands for controlled substance (see Figure 48-1).

Medical offices have an inventory of a variety of medications in stock including samples from pharmaceutical companies. Commonly stocked injectable drugs are listed on Table 48-2. The medication inventory is

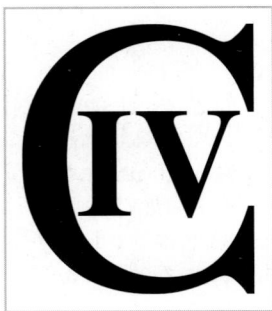

FIGURE 48-1 Controlled substance label.

TABLE 48-2 **Injectable Drugs Commonly in Stock in the Medical Office**

Name Generic	Trade Name	Route	Usage
Amitriptyline HCL	Elavil	IM	Depression
Brompheniramine maleate	Dimetane	IM/SC	Allergy
Chlorpromazine HCL	Thorazine	IM	Psychosis
Diazepam	Valium	IM	Anxiety
Dimenhydrinate	Dramamine	IM	Nausea/vomiting
Diphenhydramine	Benadryl	IM	Allergic reaction
Diphtheria, tetanus toxoid	Same name	IM	Immunization active vaccine
Furosemide	Lasix	IM	Edema
Gentamicin sulfate	Garamycin	IM	Infection
Heparin sodium	Same name	SC	Prevent clotting
Hydromorphone HCL	Dilaudid	SC/IM	Severe pain
Lidocaine HCL 1%, 2%	Xylocaine	SC	Anesthetic for minor surgery
Prochlorperazine	Compazine	IM	Psychosis
Promethazine HCL	Phenergan	IM	Nausea/vomiting
Sodium chloride with benzyl alcohol 0.9%	Sodium Chloride Bacteriostatic		Diluent for injection
Tetanus and diphtheria toxoids	Same name	IM	Immunization (active vaccine)
Tetanus antitoxin	Same name	IM	Prevention (passive vaccine)
Tetanus immune globulin	Hyper-Tet	IM	Prevention (passive vaccine)
Tetanus toxoid	Same name	IM	Immunization (active vaccine)
Tuberculin protein derivative	Tine test	ID	Tuberculin testing
Water for injection	Same name		Diluent for injection
Emergency Drugs			
Bretylium tosylate	Bretylol	IV	Arrhythmia
Epinephrine		IV SC	Cardiac arrest Allergic reaction
Norepinephrine	Levophed	IV	Hypotension
Sodium bicarbonate		IV	Acidosis
Electrolytes/Ringer's 1000 mL		IV	Dehydration

ID, intradermal; IM, intramuscular; SC, subcutaneous; IV, intravenous

Note: Only physician and nurse may administer intravenous medications.

usually the responsibility of the medical assistant (see Legal and Ethical Issues). A log book is used and contains a complete list of all medications on site including sample products. Included in the log book is the name of each medication, quantity on hand, and expiration dates. Typically a separate section in the log book is used to indicate when a medication is dispensed to a patient. When distributing a medication to a patient, the patient's name is entered into this section of the log book and the quantity, date and time of distribution, and medical assistant's initials are noted. Once a month it is important for the medical assistant to review the inventory to ensure that a sufficient supply of all drugs is available and that no medication has expired.

Physicians are required to register with the DEA in order to prescribe, dispense, or administer controlled substances. A special Form, DEA 224, must be completed and submitted to the DEA. Renewal is required every 3 years, using Form 224a.

The expiration dates of all narcotics in stock should be checked regularly, and two staff members should document the destruction of any outdated narcotics. When disposing of expired medications, follow office policy. The signatures of both individuals should be documented on the narcotic log stating that the medications have been destroyed.

Some common controlled substances are:

- Anabolic steroids
- Butabarbital
- Chloral hydrate
- Cocaine
- Codeine
- Diazepam
- Heroin
- LSD
- Marijuana
- Morphine
- Opium
- Phenobarbital
- Secobarbital
- Tylenol with codeine.

Drug Abuse

Although the use of drugs is an important element for treating diseases and conditions, any drug can be abused. Both OTC medications and prescription drugs can be misused. Examples of these drugs include pain medications, sleeping aids, and cold medications. Drug abuse can occur with patients at any age and can lead to dependency or toxicity.

Drug abuse and drug dependency are defined separately. Drug abuse is defined as the use of a drug improperly or wrongly. An individual with drug dependency is one who relies on the medication or uses the medication for psychological support. Individuals who become physically dependent are those who continuously use a substance to function or to avoid physical pain. For physical dependency to occur, the abused substance produces changes in the nervous system that the body begins to rely on. Once the substance is removed, the individual experiences withdrawal symptoms. Depending on the level of addiction, withdrawal symptoms will be mild to severe.

Medical assistants need to be aware of the potential for drug abuse and drug dependency in patients. If the medical assistant suspects a patient to be abusing drugs, the following steps may be taken:

1. Notify the physician. It is not up to the medical assistant to confront the patient.

TABLE 48-3   Drug Types That Are Commonly Abused

Sedatives	Dalmane	Restoril	Seconal
Antianxiety	Valium	Xanax	Librium
Antidepressants	Prozac	Elavil	Tofranil
Pain medications	Demerol	Vicodin	Percocet
Illegal drugs	Heroin	Marijuana	Cocaine

2. Check local pharmacies to see if the patient is obtaining medications from multiple pharmacies.

3. Patients who are frequently calling for refills should be told that another refill will require an office visit.

Items that are important to keep secure in the office include syringes, needles, and prescription pads. Never leave blank prescription pads laying out in examination rooms. Prescription pads should always be stored in secure locations.

Any dispensing of a controlled substance from the office must be documented in the patient's chart and also in the narcotic log. Table 48-3 lists drug types that are commonly abused.

General Classes of Drugs

The classification of drugs is based on their action in the body. Table 48-4 presents a comprehensive list of drug classifications with descriptions of the use or function

TABLE 48-4   Drug Classification Names and Descriptions of Use

Name	Use
Adrenergic	Increases the rate and strength of the heart muscle. Acts as a vasoconstrictor, dilates bronchi, dilates pupils and relaxes muscular walls. Used to treat asthma, bronchitis, and allergies.
Adrenergic blocking agent	Increases peripheral circulation, decreases blood pressure and vasodilation. Used to treat hypertension.
Analgesic	Relieves pain without the loss of consciousness. These may be either narcotic or non-narcotic. Narcotic drugs are derived from the opium poppy and act on the brain to cause pain relief and drowsiness.
Anesthetic	Produces a lack of feeling that may have a local or general effect depending on the type of administration.
Antacid	Neutralizes acid in the stomach.
Antianxiety	Relieves or reduces anxiety and muscle tension. These are used to treat panic disorders, anxiety, and insomnia.
Antiarrhythmic	Controls cardiac arrhythmias by altering nerve impulses within the heart.
Antibiotic	Destroys or prohibits the growth of microorganisms. These are used to treat bacterial infections. They have not been found to be effective in treating viral infections. Antibiotics must be taken regularly for a specified time period to be effective.

(continued)

Name	Use
Anticoagulant	Prevents or delays blood clotting. Also referred to as blood thinners. These may be administered by intravenous injection, such as with the drug heparin. Oral drugs, such as warfarin, cannot be taken along with aspirin since the interaction between the two medications could cause internal bleeding.
Anticonvulsant	Prevents or relieves convulsions. Drugs such as phenobarbital reduce excessive stimulation in the brain to control seizures and other symptoms of epilepsy.
Antidepressant	Prevents or relieves the symptoms of depression. These drugs are also used in the prevention of migraine headaches.
Antidiabetic	Drugs that control diabetes by regulating the level of glucose in the blood and the metabolism of carbohydrates and fat.
Antidiarrheal	Prevents or relieves diarrhea.
Antidote	Counteracts the effects of poisons.
Antiemetic	Controls nausea and vomiting. These generally act on the vomiting center in the brain.
Antifungal	Kills fungus.
Antihelminthic	Kills parasitic worms.
Antihistamine	Counteracts histamine and controls allergic reactions.
Antihypertensive	Prevents or controls high blood pressure. Some of these drugs act to block nerve impulses that cause arteries to constrict and thus increase the blood pressure. Other drugs slow the heart rate and decrease its force of contraction. Still others may reduce the amount of the hormone aldosterone in the blood that is causing the blood pressure to rise.
Anti-inflammatory	Counteracts inflammation.
Antineoplastic	Kills normal and abnormal cancerous cells by interfering with cell reproduction.
Antipruritic	Relieves itching.
Antipyretic	Reduces fever.
Antiseptic	Prevents the growth of microorganisms.
Antitussive	Controls or relieves coughing. Codeine is an ingredient in many prescription cough medicines. It acts on the brain to control coughing.
Astringent	A substance that has a constricting or binding effect by coagulating proteins on a cell's surface. This may be used to stop hemorrhage.
Bronchodilator	Dilates or opens the bronchi (airways in the lungs) to improve breathing.
Cardiogenic	Strengthens the heart muscle.
Cathartic	Causes bowel movements to occur. These drugs may have a strong purging action and can become habit forming.
Contraceptive	Used to prevent conception.

(*continued*)

TABLE 48-4 Drug Classification Names and Descriptions of Use (*continued*)

Name	Use
Decongestant	Reduces nasal congestion and swelling.
Diuretic	Increases the excretion of urine, which promotes the loss of water and salt from the body. This can assist in lowering blood pressure; therefore, these drugs are used to treat hypertension. Potassium in the body may be depleted with continued use of diuretics. Potassium-rich foods, such as bananas, kiwi, and orange juice, along with medications for potassium deficiency, can help correct this deficiency.
Emetic	Induces vomiting
Estrogen	A hormone used to replace estrogen lost during menopause. Estrogen is responsible for the development of secondary sexual characteristics and is produced by the ovaries.
Expectorant	Assists in the removal of secretions from the bronchopulmonary membranes.
Hemostatic	Controls bleeding.
Hypnotic	Produces sleep or hypnosis.
Hypoglycemic	Lowers blood glucose level.
Immunosuppressive	Suppresses the body's natural immune response to an antigen. This is used to control autoimmune diseases such as multiple sclerosis and rheumatoid arthritis.
Laxative	Used to promote normal bowel function.
Miotic	Constricts the pupils of the eye.
Muscle relaxant	Produces the relaxation of skeletal muscle.
Mydriatic	Dilates the pupils of the eye.
Narcotic	Produces sleep or stupor. In moderate doses this drug will depress the central nervous system and relieve pain. In excessive doses it will cause stupor, coma, and even death. Can become habit forming (addictive).
Purgative	Stimulates bowel movements.
Psychedelic	Drugs such as lysergic acid diethylamide (LSD) that can produce visual hallucinations.
Sedative	Produces relaxation without causing sleep.
Stimulant	Speeds up the heart and respiratory system. Used to increase alertness.
Tranquilizer	Used to reduce mental anxiety and tensions.
Vaccine	Given to promote resistance (immunity) to infectious diseases.
Vasodilator	Produces a relaxation of blood vessels to lower blood pressure.
Vasopressor	Produces the contraction of muscles in the capillaries and arteries, which elevates the blood pressure.
Vitamin	Organic substances found naturally in foods that are essential for normal metabolism. Most have been produced synthetically to be taken in pill form.

TABLE 48-5   Classification of Drugs by Type or Usage with Examples

Type/Usage	Example Brand Name (Generic Name)	Type/Usage	Example Brand Name (Generic Name)
Adrenergic	Isuprel (isoproterenol) Sudafed (pseudoephedrine hydrochloride HCL)	Tetracyclines	Acnromycin (tetracycline HCL) Declomycin (demeclocycline) Terramycin (oxytetracycline) Vibramycin (doxycycline hyclate)
Adrenergic blocking agent	Aldomet (methyldopa) Inderal (propranolol HCL)	Anticholinergic	Atropine (atropine sulfate) Banthine (methantheline bromide) Donnatal (belladonna)
Analgesic	Acetylsalicylic acid, or aspirin Advil (ibuprofen) Darvon (propoxyphene HCL) Dilaudid (hydromorphone HCL) Demerol (meperidine HCL) Talwin (pentazocine HCL) Tylenol (acetaminophen)	Anticoagulant	Coumadin (warfarin sodium)
		Anticonvulsant	Dilantin (phenytoin sodium) Phenobarbital (phenobarbital)
		Antidepressant	Elavil (amitriptyline HCL)
Anesthetic	Carbocaine (mepivacaine HCL) Novocain (procaine HCL) Nupercaine (dibucaine HCL) Xylocaine (lidocaine HCL)	Antidiabetic	Insulin and oral medications: Precose and Metformin
Antacid	Milk of Magnesia (magnesia magma) Mylanta (aluminum hydroxide) Maalox (aluminum hydroxide)	Antidiarrheal	Kaopectate (kaolin and pectin mixture) Lomotil (diphenoxylate)
Antianxiety	Valium (diazepam)	Antiemetics	Atarax (hydroxyzine HCL) Compazine (prochlorperazine) Dramamine (dimenhydrinate) Phenergan (promethazine HCL)
Antiarrhythmic	Digoxin (digoxin) Norpace (disopyramide) Pronestyl (procainamide HCL)		
Antibiotic Aminoglycosides	Garamycin (gentamicin sulfate) Kantrex (kanamycin) Mycifradin Sulfate (neomycin sulfate) Nebcin (tobramycin sulfate) Neobiotic (neomycin sulfate)	Antifungal	Mycostatin (nystatin)
		Antihelminthics	Vermox (mebendazole)
		Antihistamine	Adrenalin (epinephrine) Benadryl (diphenhydramine) Chlor-Trimeton (chlorphen-iramine maleate) Dimetane (brompheniramine maleate)
Cephalosporins	Ancef (cefazolin sodium) Anspor (cephradine) Ceclor (cefaclor) Duricef (cefadroxil) Keflex (cephalexin) Keflin (cephalothin sodium)	Antihypertensives	Aldomet (methyldopa) Catapres (clonidine HCL) Lopressor (metoprolol tartrate) Minipress (prazosin HCL)
Penicillins	Amoxil (amoxicillin) Bicillin (penicillin G potassium) Duracillin (penicillin G procaine) Polycillin (ampicillin)	Anti-inflammatory	Aspirin (acetylsalicylic acid) Indocin (indomethacin) Motrin (naproxen) Nalfon (fenoprofen calcium) Naprosyn (naproxen)

(continued)

TABLE 48-5 Classification of Drugs by Type or Usage with Examples *(continued)*

Type/Usage	Example Brand Name (Generic Name)	Type/Usage	Example Brand Name (Generic Name)
Antineoplastic	Cytoxan (cyclophosphamide) Fluorouracil (5FU) Adriamycin (doxorubicin HCL)	Hormone	Testosterone Premarin, estrogen
Antipruritic	Calamine lotion (calamine) Hydrocortone (hydrocortisone sodium phosphate)	Hypnotic	Seconal (secobarbital)
		Hypoglycemic	Precose (oral) Metformin (oral)
Antipyretic	Advil (ibuprofen) Aspirin (acetylsalicylic acid) Tylenol (acetaminophen)	Laxative	Dulcolax (bisacodyl)
		Muscle relaxant	Valium (diazepam) Robaxin (methocarbamol)
Antiseptic	Cidex (glutaraldehyde) pHisoHex (hexachlorophene)	Narcotic	Demerol (meperidine HCL) Percodan
Antitussive	Codeine (codeine phosphate)	Psychedelic	LSD (lysergic acid diethylamide)
Bronchodilator	Alupent (metaproterenol sulfate) Brethine (terbutaline sulfate) Isuprel (isoproterenol HCL) Theolair (theophylline)	Purgative	Ex-Lax (phenolphthalein)
		Sedative and hypnotic	Amytal (amobarbital) Butisol (butabarbital sodium) Nembutal Sodium (phenobarbital) Seconal Sodium (secobarbital sodium) Valium (diazepam)
Contraceptive	Ortho-Novum 10/11-21 (estrogen with progestogen) Enovid-E 21 (estrogen with progestogen)	Stimulant	Dexedrine (dextroamphetamine sulfate)
Decongestant	Neo-Synephrine (phenylephrine HCL) Sudafed (pseudoephedrine HCL)	Tranquilizer	Haldol (haloperidol)
		Vasodilator	Isordil (isosorbide dinitrate) Nitro-bid (nitroglycerin) Nitrostat (nitroglycerin)
Diuretic	Diuril (chlorothiazide) Hygroton (chlorthalidone) Lasix (furosemide)	Vasopressor	Levophed (norepinephrine)
Emetic	Ipecac syrup	Vitamin	Vitamin A Vitamin C Vitamin D Vitamin E Vitamin K
Estrogen	Estrace (estrogen)		
Expectorant	Robitussin (Guaifenesin)		

for each classification. Table 48-5 presents a similar list with examples of specific drugs for the classification.

Routes and Methods of Drug Administration

The route of administration is the method by which the drug is introduced into the body (see Figure 48-2).

The most common routes of drug administration are as Follows:

- Oral. This is any method of drug given by mouth. In most patients, this is the easiest method of drug administration. However, because of the effects of stomach acids and gastric juices, some of the chemical compounds are destroyed in the stomach. Some medications, such as

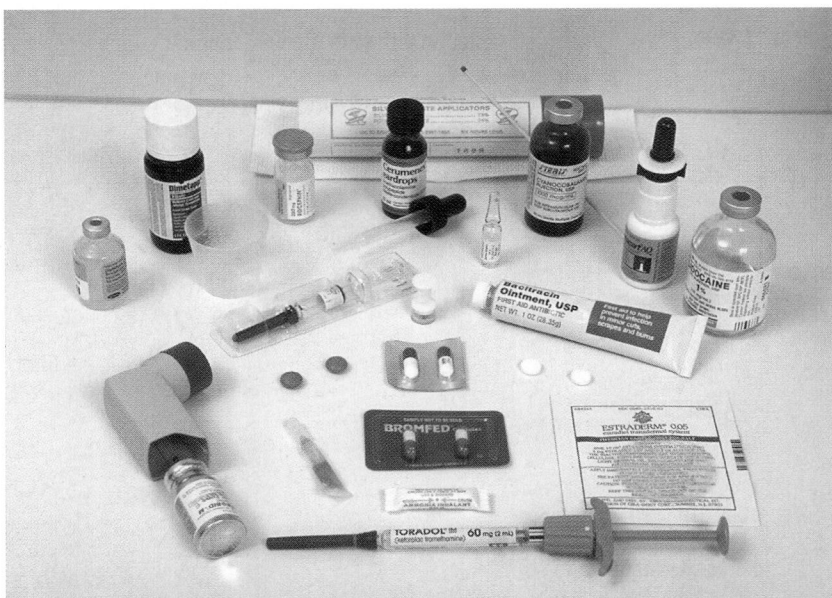

FIGURE 48-2 Different types of medication require different routes of administration.

aspirin, also can have a corrosive action on the stomach.

- Sublingual. Sublingual drugs are held under the tongue where they are absorbed through the tissues and into the bloodstream for distribution to the body. Nitroglycerin is commonly administered this way when it is used for treating heart pains called angina.
- Parenteral. Parenteral administration of medication is given through the skin for absorption through skin tissues, muscle tissue, or in the blood. This usually requires the skin to be punctured by a needle with a syringe attached to administer the

medication. Table 48-6 lists the methods of parenteral administration, and a description of each method.

Most drugs must be given by specific routes to be effective. It is important to be sure that the patient understands the directions for medication administration because the right route must be followed for the medication to be effective. Table 48-7 lists numerous forms in which medications are prepared and the nonparenteral routes through which they are administered.

Sometimes a drug can be administered by a variety of routes. For example, the female hormone estrogen can be administered orally in the form of a pill or topically

TABLE 48-6	**Methods for Parenteral Administration of Drugs**
Method	**Description**
Intradermal	A very shallow injection just within the top layer of skin. This is a method commonly used in skin testing for allergies and tuberculosis.
Subcutaneous (SC)	An injection under the skin and fat layers. The middle of the upper, outer arm is usually used.
Intramuscular (IM)	An injection directly into the muscle of the buttocks or upper arm (deltoid). This method is used when there is a large amount of medication or it is irritating.
Intravenous (IV)	An injection into the veins. This route can be set up so that there is a continuous administration of medication, usually after a major surgery or during a major procedure.
Intrathecal	Injection into the meninges space surrounding the brain and spinal cord.
Intracavity	Injection into a body cavity such as the peritoneal or chest cavity.

TABLE 48-7 **Nonparenteral Methods for Administering Drugs**

Method	Description
Rectal	The drug is introduced directly into the rectal cavity in the form of suppositories or solution. Drugs may have to be administered by this route if the patient is unable to take them by mouth due to nausea, vomiting, or surgery of the mouth.
Oral	Drugs that are taken by mouth and swallowed by the patient.
Inhalation	This category of drugs includes those that are inhaled directly into the nose and mouth. Aerosol sprays are administered by this route.
Topical	These drugs are applied directly to the skin or mucous membranes. They are distributed in ointment, cream, or lotion form. These drugs are used to treat skin infections and eruptions. Transdermal patches are also used; examples include Nicotrol, Estraderm, and Nicoderm.
Vaginal	Vaginal tablets and suppositories are used to treat vaginal yeast infections and other irritations.
Eyedrops	Drugs placed into the eye to control eye pressure in glaucoma. Used during eye examinations to dilate the pupil of the eye for better examination of the interior of the eye. Also used to treat infections.
Eardrops	Drugs placed directly into the ear canal for the purpose of relieving pain or treating infection.
Sublingual or buccal tablets	Drugs, such as nitroglycerin for anginal pain, which are placed under the lip or between the cheek and gum.

in the form of a skin patch. Table 48-8 lists various forms in which medicines are prepared and routes through which they are administered. Before you administer medication to a patient, you should always follow a checklist:

- Be sure that you have the correct patient.

- Check and recheck that you have the correct medication as ordered.
- Check that you are giving the correct dose.
- Make sure you are using the correct route.
- Make sure that the medication has not expired.

TABLE 48-8 **Routes of Drug Administration**

Form	Route	Form	Route
Aerosol	Inhalation	Pills	Oral
Caplets	Oral	Powders	Topical
Capsules	Oral	Skin patch	Topical
Elixir	Oral	Spansules	Oral
Liniment	Topical	Spray	Oral, topical
Lotion	Topical	Suppository	Rectal, vaginal
Lozenges	Oral	Syrup	Oral
Ointment	Topical	Tablet	Oral

TABLE 48-9 The 50 Most Frequently Administered Drugs

Brand Name	Type	Brand Name	Type
1. Amoxil	Antibiotic	25. Theo-Dur	Bronchodilator
2. Lanoxin	Cardiotonic	26. Lopressor	Beta-blocker
3. Zantac	Antiulcer	27. Lasix	Diuretic
4. Xanax	Tranquilizer	28. Voltaren	Nonsteroidal anti-inflammatory
5. Premarin	Hormone (estrogen)	29. Darvocet-N	Analgesic (narcotic)
6. Cardizem	Cardiotonic	30. Dilantin	Anticonvulsant
7. Ceclor	Antibiotic	31. Monistat	Antibiotic (antifungal)
8. Synthroid	Hormone (thyroid)	32. Augmentin	Antibiotic (penicillin)
9. Seldane	Antihistamine	33. Micronase	Oral hypoglycemic agent
10. Tenormin	Beta-blocker	34. Feldene	Nonsteroidal anti-inflammatory
11. Vasotec	Antihypertensive	35. Micro-K	Potassium supplement
12. Tagamet	Antiulcer	36. Provera	Hormone (progestin)
13. Naprosyn nonsteroidal	Anti-inflammatory	37. Motrin	Nonsteroidal anti-inflammatory
14. Capoten	Antihypertensive	38. Mevacor	Cholesterol lowering
15. Ortho-Novum 7/7/7	Synthetic hormone	39. Triphasil	Synthetic hormone
16. Dyazide	Diuretic	40. Prozac	Antidepressant
17. Ortho-Novum	Synthetic hormone	41. Lo/Ovral	Synthetic hormone
18. Proventil	Bronchodilator	42. Valium	Tranquilizer
19. Tylenol with codeine	Analgesic (narcotic)	43. Retin-A	Antiacne
20. Procardia	Calcium channel blocker	44. Cipro	Antibiotic
21. Calan	Calcium channel blocker	45. E-Mycin	Antibiotic
22. Ventolin	Bronchodilator	46. Maxzide	Diuretic
23. Inderal	Beta-blocker	47. Coumadin	Anticoagulant
24. Halcion	Sedative	48. Carafate	Antiulcer
		49. Timoptic	Beta-blocker
		50. Slow-K	Potassium supplement

Frequently Administered Drugs

Pharmaceutical companies are constantly developing, testing, and releasing new drugs. As a result, broad-spectrum antibiotics are frequently prescribed. These antibiotics are effective against a large range of microorganisms, making the treatment of specific illnesses easier. Table 48-9 lists 50 of the most commonly prescribed drugs.

Side Effects of Medications

Drugs not only affect the symptom for which they are taken, they also affect other functions. These other, sometimes undesirable, effects are called side effects. Occasionally, side effects can be lethal, which means they may cause death. Because of this, it is important that side effects be noted and taken seriously. Sometimes, side effects are specific to the individual (idiosyncratic). Food interactions can cause side effects. Other effects can be caused by allergic reactions.

Examples of specific side effects to drugs include the following:

1. Anaphylactic shock: This is a life-threatening reaction to a drug, food, or insect bite. Symptoms can include respiratory distress, edema (swelling) in the mouth and throat, convulsions, and unconsciousness. If untreated, death can result.

2. Drug tolerance is a decrease in the effectiveness of a drug as the body gets used to having the drug in the system. It will take a larger dose of the drug to achieve the same result. This is common when a patient is repeatedly prescribed the same antibiotic, or in patients who require a specific drug, such as a pain control medication, over a long period of time. The dose cannot always be increased, as some drugs can become toxic (harmful)with excessive amounts.

3. Habituation is dependence on a drug. Habituation can develop with a variety of drugs, including narcotics and laxatives.

Unexpected side effects can range from rashes to drowsiness, coughing, runny nose, constipation, dizziness, headache, nausea, or vomiting. Patients should be instructed to call the physician if any of these symptoms occur. The physician may adjust the medication dose, or completely change the prescription to another drug that may not have the same side effects.

Drug Interactions

Many factors contribute to how a patient reacts to medication. A patient can be given a medication and have a completely different reaction one time versus another. Factors that contribute to a patient's reaction to a medication include the patient's age, weight, method of administration, allergies, intolerance, and tolerance.

Patient's Age

Geriatric and pediatric patients specifically are more susceptible to the affects of medications and will usually require lower doses (see Figure 48-3 and Lifespan Considerations). Due to this fact, when a physician prescribes a medication for this population the medical assistant should review the order to ensure that the correct dosage has been ordered.

Patient's Weight

A patient's weight is an important factor to consider when calculating the medication dosage. There is a direct correlation between the patient's weight and medication level. A patient's body weight, will determine the dosage the physician prescribes. If the medication level is too low for the body weight, the patient will not benefit as much from the medication. At the same time, if the medication level is too high for the patient's body weight, the patient could become ill or even have an overdose reaction.

Method of Administration

The method of administration affects the rate at which the body absorbs the medication. Physicians choose the method of administration depending on the response desired. For instance, for a more immediate response the physician would more than likely order an injectable medication. To offer relief over a sustained period of time, a time-released oral medication may be used.

Allergies

An allergy to a medication can occur at any time. A patient may have an immediate allergic reaction or may develop one over time. An allergic reaction can manifest itself in ways such as hives and shortness of breath. This can be moderate to severe. Patients should be educated in what to do if an allergic reaction occurs. Patients who experience an allergic reaction should be told to call the office immediately or if severe go to the nearest emergency room. If a patient has an allergy to any medication, this should be documented in the

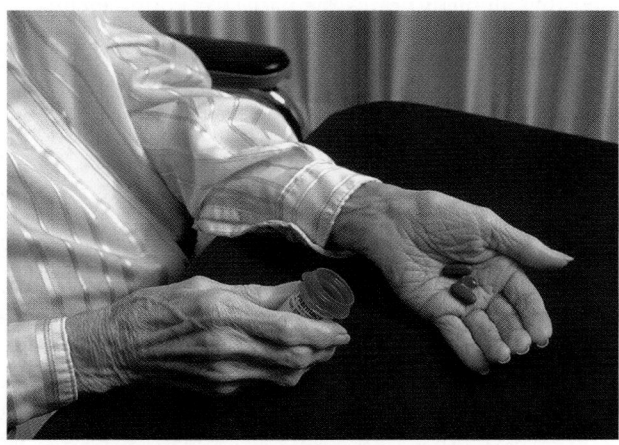

FIGURE 48-3 Older adults may need special assistance with medications.

patient's chart and on an allergy sticker that is placed on the outside of the chart.

Intolerance and Tolerance

Some patients may experience an intolerance to a medication. As with allergies, any intolerances to medication should also be documented in the patient's chart. Vomiting, diarrhea, or abdominal cramping can be indications of intolerance. If an intolerance to a medication is experienced, the patient should alert the physician who may then adjust the dosage or change the prescription as needed.

If a patient takes a medication for an extended period of time the patient may develop a tolerance to that medication. If this occurs, the physician may need to change medications or increase the dosage to obtain the desired result.

The medical assistant needs to get a complete history regarding all medications the patient is taking including herbal and OTC medications. These medications should be documented in the patient's record. This information is then used by the physician to determine the appropriate treatment for the patient.

Drug Use During Pregnancy

Caution should be used when a pregnant woman decides to take a drug. Very few drugs are considered safe for use during pregnancy. Women who are pregnant should consult with their doctors prior to taking any medication. Even OTC medications can have harmful effects on a pregnant woman or her fetus. Prior to prescribing a drug for any female, the date of her last menstrual cycle should be ascertained to ensure that she is not pregnant.

Drug Use and the Breast-Feeding Mother

A lot of medications taken by a breast-feeding mother could appear in breast milk, which would then be swallowed by the nursing infant. There are a few medications that a breast-feeding mother can take, but it is very important that the prescribing physician be aware that the mother is breast-feeding. Several medications, however, are contraindicated. This means the medications are so dangerous for the infant that the mother must stop breast-feeding while she is taking them. These contraindicated medications include:

- Tetracyclines
- Chloramphenicol
- Sulfonamides
- Oral anticoagulants
- Iodine-containing drugs
- Antineoplastics.

Reading and Writing a Prescription

Reading and writing a prescription is fairly easy, with some understanding of the symbols used in writing those prescriptions. The main parts of a prescription follow:

1. The superscription contains the patient's name, address, age, and date on the top line. The symbol ℞

from the Latin term *recipe,* meaning "take thou" is usually preprinted on the prescription form.

2. The inscription gives the name of the medication, actual ingredients, and dosage.
3. The subscription tells the pharmacist how to mix the drug and how much to provide the patient.
4. The signa (Sig.), which means "mark" is the instructions on how the medication should be taken by the patient.
5. The physician's name, address, telephone number, and DEA number. Generally, all but the DEA number are preprinted on the prescription pad.
6. The number of times the prescription may be refilled (usually no more than six times).
7. The prescription may have a DAW (dispense as written) option.

It is important to be sure that each of the main parts of the prescription is filled out completely.

Figure 48-4 shows an example of a prescription. In this example, the physician has ordered the medication Estrace, which is a form of the hormone estrogen. The prescription tells the pharmacist to give 100 tablets, and orders a 1 mg dosage, which is to be taken once a day (1 q am). The instruction to the pharmacist is to refill the prescription three times and not to substitute with another generic medication.

Sometimes, a prescription is written for prn refills, meaning that the prescription can be refilled as needed. The physician will fill in the name, address, age of the patient, and date. The physician must also sign his or her name at the bottom of the prescription. A blank prescription form cannot be handed to a patient.

When the pharmacist fills the prescription, the patient instructions will be placed on the label as instructed by the physician, along with special instructions for taking the medication (such as "take with meals") that can help make sure that the medication is as effective as possible. The pharmacist will also include a package insert with each medication that contains information regarding possible side effects and contraindications. If there are any side effects the patient needs to report these to the physician.

Some prescriptions can be filled by telephone. At such times, the patient's record should be pulled for the physician and the refill order or new medications prescribed should be documented. Usually there is a medication refill form in the chart. The medical assistant should list what the physician has ordered to be filled: the medication, the name of the medication, and the strength and dose of the medication. The medical assistant should also document the name of the pharmacy, the pharmacy phone number, and the time of the call.

Beth Williams, MD
Windy City Clinic
123 Michigan Avenue
Chicago, IL 60000
Telephone (200) 555-9876

Name Jane Doe Age 56

Address

Date 2/14/xx

Rx Estrace 1 mg

Sig. 1 q AM
Disp. # 100

Substitution Permissible ______ M.D.

"Prescriber must hand-write "Brand Necessary" or "Brand Medically Necessary" in the space below in order for a brand name product to be dispensed."
Brand Necessary

B Williams M.D.

Refill 0 1 2 (3) 4 5 6

FIGURE 48-4 Sample prescription.

Only physicians are permitted to sign prescriptions. However, the medical assistant in some cases may complete the prescription form, which the physician then checks for accuracy and signs. See Guidelines 48-1 for the Administration of Medication. (See also Preparing for Externship.)

Preparing for Externship

To prepare for an externship, *the medical assistant needs to be familiar with the various medications appropriate for the specialty in which he or she will be working. It is essential that the medical assistant know how to read and write prescriptions, and ensure that the dosages transcribed are correct. Correct use of abbreviations is mandatory.*

The "ten rights" of medication administration are a cornerstone of the practice of the medical assistant, because they ensure that the directions given by the physician are followed correctly. It is always helpful to be very comfortable with several versions of drug reference guides to ensure quick research when the situation warrants.

1. Medications/drugs can only be administered to a patient under the supervision of a licensed physician. To do otherwise is considered "practicing medicine without a license." The medication order must be written and signed on the patient's medical record by the physician.

2. The medical assistant acts as the liaison or intermediary between the physician and the patient. Some of the duties include ordering, storing, rotating, and checking expiration dates on medications.

3. Medications must be checked three times before administration. The "three befores" are:
   - Before medication is removed from the medication cabinet
   - Before medication is poured, drawn up into a syringe or placed onto a medication cup
   - Before medication is returned to the cabinet.

4. Medications cannot be returned to the container once they have been removed. If they are not administered, they must be discarded.

5. Remember the "ten rights" for administering medications (Figure 48-5). The "ten rights" are:
   - Right patient
   - Right medication
   - Right dosage
   - Right route
   - Right time
   - Right documentation
   - Right client education
   - Right to refuse
   - Right assessment
   - Right evaluation.

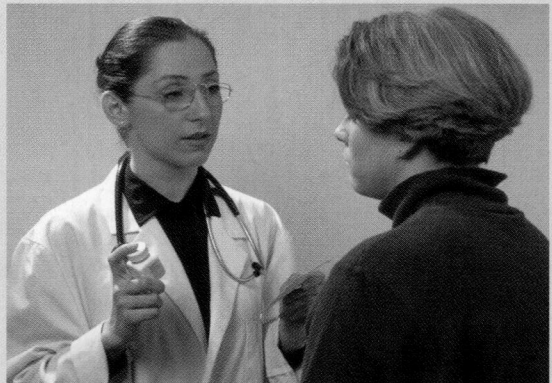

FIGURE 48-5 Remember the "ten rights" when administering medications.

6. Keep a record of all allergies on the patient's medical record. Often these allergies are noted on the front of the medical record as well as within the medical record.

7. The documentation on the patient's medical record must include the following:
   a. Name of the medication
   b. Dosage
   c. Route of administration
   d. Site of administration
   e. Signature of the person administering the medication along with initials designating the person's status, for example, CMA or RMA

8. All narcotics must be documented in a record maintained for that purpose. This is referred to as "logging a narcotic." Every narcotic must be accounted for.

9. Be careful that you administer the medication by the correct route. Methods of administration include:
   a. Oral (by mouth)
   b. Sublingual (under the tongue)
   c. Buccal (in the cheek)
   d. Rectal (inserted into the anal cavity)
   e. Vaginal (inserted into vaginal canal)
   f. Parenteral (by injection)
   g. Topical (applied to the skin)
   h. Inhalation (by breathing the medication)
   Medical assistants do not administer medications by the following routes:
   a. Intrathecal (into the meninges space)
   b. Intracavity (into a body cavity)
   c. Intravenous (IV) (into a vein)

10. Medication labels should be clean and readable. If they become soiled, unreadable, or fall off the container they must be discarded.

11. If you are not familiar with a particular medication, you must look it up in the PDR. Never violate this rule.

12. Know the side effects for the medication you are administering.

13. Always advise the patient to take the complete number of dosages ordered in the prescription. This is especially important when using antibiotics.

14. Advise the patient to only use medication for the member of the family or person for whom it was prescribed.

Abbreviations Used in Pharmacology

Medical abbreviations are used in pharmacology but due to the risk of possible errors taking place in the misreading of information, many physicians are choosing to not use abbreviations in prescription writing and chart documentation. Table 48-10 lists the most commonly used abbreviations. The medical assistant must be very careful to ensure that the abbreviations used are appropriate, correct, and clear, because it is easy to mistake one abbreviation for another. Always use approved abbreviations—never create your own abbreviations.

TABLE 48-10 **Commonly Used Pharmacology Abbreviations**

Abbreviation	Meaning	Abbreviation	Meaning
@	At	DC, disc	Discontinue
a	Before	d/c, disc	Discontinue
aa	Of each	dil	Dilute
ac	Before meals	disp	Dispense
AD	Right ear	dr	Dram
ad lib	As desired	dtd#	Give this number
alt dieb	Alternate days	Dx	Diagnosis
alt hor	Alternate hours	elix	Elixir
alt noc	Alternate nights	emul	Emulsion
am, AM	Morning	et	And
amt	Amount	ext	Extract/external
ante	Before	Fe	Iron
aq	Aqueous (water)	fl	Fluid
AS	Left ear	G	Gauge
AU	Both ears	g	Gram
Ba	Barium	gal	Gallon
bid	Twice a day	gr	Grain
C	100	gt	One drop
c̄	With	gtt	Two or more drops
cap(s)	Capsule(s)	H	Hour/hypodermic
cc	Cubic centimeter	hs	Hour of sleep
d	Day	IM	Intramuscular

(continued)

TABLE 48-10 **Commonly Used Pharmacology Abbreviations** (*continued*)

Abbreviation	Meaning	Abbreviation	Meaning
inj	Injection	qod	Every other day
IV	Intravenous	R	Right
K	Potassium	Rx	Take
kg	Kilogram	s or s̄	Without
L	Liter	SC	Subcutaneous
liq	Liquid	Sig.	Label as follows/directions
M ft	Make	sl	Under the tongue
mcg	Microgram	SOB	Shortness of breath
mg	Milligram	sol	Solution
mitt#	Give this number	ss or ¯s¯s	One-half
mL	Milliliter	stat	At once/immediately
mm	Millimeter	Subc, SubQ	Subcutaneous
noct	Night	subling	Sublingual
non rep	Do not repeat	suppos	Suppository
NPO	Nothing by mouth	susp	Suspension
NS	Normal saline	syr	Syrup
PR	Per rectum	T, tbsp	Tablespoon
pt	Pint	tab	Tablet
pulv	Powder	tid	Three times a day
q	Every	tinc, tr	Tincture
q2h	Every 2 hours	top	Apply topically
qam	Every morning	tsp	Teaspoon
qd	Once a day/every day	u	Unit
qh	Every hour	ung	Ointment
qhs	Every night	UT	Under the tongue
qid	Four times a day	ut dict UD	As directed
qm	Every morning	wt	Weight

SUMMARY

The medical assistant works directly under the supervision and the license of the physician. No matter what kind of medical practice the medical assistant is working in, it is always important to follow all federal, state, and local regulations regarding the administration, dispensing, and inventorying of all medications.

You must remember that you are always ethically and legally responsible for all of your actions. You must consider all aspects of administering a medication and follow your checklist. Never administer a medication with which you are unfamiliar and always get clear instructions from the physician.

Chapter Review

COMPETENCY REVIEW

1. Define and spell the terms to learn for this chapter.
2. Name the governmental agency that enforces drug sales and distribution.
3. Name the federal act that controls the use of drugs causing dependency.
4. List the "ten rights" of drug administration.
5. Discuss the "three befores" that must take place before drug administration.
6. Describe what you would do when a patient indicates a drug allergy.
7. Define "logging a narcotic."
8. List the information that must be charted when administering a medication.
9. List the functions of the following medications: diuretic, sedative, anesthetic.
10. A drug may be known by three different names. What are they?

PREPARING FOR THE CERTIFICATION EXAM

1. The chemical name for the OTC medication Aleve is:
   A. acetaminophen
   B. naproxen sodium
   C. Naprosyn
   D. Tylenol
   E. Aldomet

2. According to the Drug Enforcement Administration, controlled substances:
   A. can be addictive
   B. may have the potential for abuse by a patient
   C. must be kept under lock and key
   D. (the dispensation of) must be recorded in a narcotics log
   E. all of the above

3. An example of a Schedule IV drug is:
   A. Xanax
   B. morphine
   C. vicodin
   D. MS Contin
   E. Tylenol with codeine

4. Capoten, which is an ACE inhibitor, is classified as an:
   A. antibiotic
   B. anti-inflammatory
   C. antipruritic
   D. antihypertensive
   E. antipyretic

5. Which of the following is a method for the administration of a drug by means of an injection under the skin and fat layers?
   A. intradermal
   B. intramuscular
   C. subcutaneous
   D. intravenous
   E. intrathecal

6. A nonparenteral method of administering drugs would be:
   A. inhalation
   B. topical
   C. vaginal
   D. buccal
   E. all of the above

continued on next page

7. The "ten rights" a medical assistant must observe when administering medications include the right medication, the right documentation, and:
   A. time
   B. route
   C. dosage
   D. patient
   E. all of the above

8. Which, if any, of the following routes of administration is not used by a medical assistant?
   A. ID
   B. IV
   C. IM
   D. Z-track IM
   E. SC

9. Which part of a prescription precedes the instructions that should be given to the patient?
   A. Sig.
   B. ℞
   C. superscription
   D. inscription
   E. subscription

10. A common abbreviation, used in pharmacology that means "as needed" is
    A. aa
    B. ac
    C. prn
    D. ante
    E. NS

CRITICAL THINKING

1. What should Susan do to respond to this medication refill request?
2. Should Susan report this request for a refill to Dr. Jones?
3. After talking with the patient, Dr. Jones has approved the request for a refill. What is Susan's next step?

ON THE JOB

Dr. Waring is in solo practice. When she is on vacation, she arranges for Dr. Dumphey to cover her patients. Dr. Dumphey's medical assistant, Theresa, has just received a call from a patient of Dr. Waring's. The patient is an elderly woman, with multiple medical problems, who is possibly having a reaction to a medication that Dr. Waring prescribed 2 days ago for bronchitis. Her symptoms include nausea, upset stomach, dizziness, headache, rash on her chest, and extreme exhaustion. Theresa senses that the patient may be exhibiting some disorientation to time and place because it is difficult to elicit consistent responses from her regarding her medications.

The patient is reporting to Theresa that the newest medication she has been taking is Biaxin. The other medications she takes includes Prinivil, Cardizem CD, Premarin, Prilosec, Robaxin, Zocor, Ambien, Prozac, Fosamax, Seldane, and aspirin. The patient does not know the dosage of any of these medications, but is willing to "open up her bag of medicine" and read each prescription label to Theresa. What should Theresa do?

What is your response?

1. Does Theresa have an obligation, as Dr. Dumphey's medical assistant, to handle this situation with this patient or should Dr. Waring simply be notified?
2. Is this an emergency situation or potential emergency situation and, if so, what should Theresa do immediately?
3. Because the patient seems disoriented, should Theresa even trust what the patient is reporting?
4. Should Theresa have the patient read the label of each of her medications?

INTERNET ACTIVITY

To further understand the elements of the *Physicians' Desk Reference,* go online and type PDR in the search area.

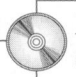

MediaLink More on pharmacology, including interactive resources, can be found on the Student CD-ROM accompanying this textbook.

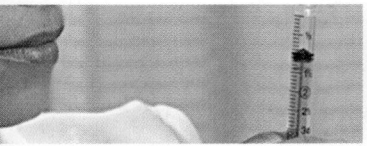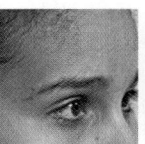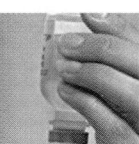

Medical Assistant Role Delineation Chart

HIGHLIGHT indicates material covered in this chapter.

ADMINISTRATIVE

Administrative Procedures

- Perform basic administrative medical assisting functions
- Schedule, coordinate and monitor appointments
- Schedule inpatient/outpatient admissions and procedures
- Understand and apply third-party guidelines
- Obtain reimbursement through accurate claims submission
- Monitor third-party reimbursement
- Understand and adhere to managed care policies and procedures
- *Negotiate managed care contracts*

Practice Finances

- Perform procedural and diagnostic coding
- Apply bookkeeping principles

- Manage accounts receivable
- *Manage accounts payable*
- *Process payroll*
- *Document and maintain accounting and banking records*
- *Develop and maintain fee schedules*
- *Manage renewals of business and professional insurance policies*
- *Manage personnel benefits and maintain records*
- *Perform marketing, financial, and strategic planning*

CLINICAL

Fundamental Principles

- Apply principles of aseptic technique and infection control
- Comply with quality assurance practices
- Screen and follow up patient test results

Diagnostic Orders

- Collect and process specimens
- Perform diagnostic tests

Patient Care

- Adhere to established patient screening procedures
- Obtain patient history and vital signs
- Prepare and maintain examination and treatment areas
- Prepare patient for examinations, procedures and treatments

- Assist with examinations, procedures and treatments
- Prepare and administer medications and immunizations
- Maintain medication and immunization records
- Recognize and respond to emergencies
- Coordinate patient care information with other health care providers
- Initiate IV and administer IV medications with appropriate training and as permitted by state law

GENERAL

Professionalism

- Display a professional manner and image
- Demonstrate initiative and responsibility
- Work as a member of the health care team
- Prioritize and perform multiple tasks
- Adapt to change
- Promote the CMA credential
- Enhance skills through continuing education
- Treat all patients with compassion and empathy
- Promote the practice through positive public relations

Communication Skills

- Recognize and respect cultural diversity
- Adapt communications to individual's ability to understand
- Use professional telephone technique

- Recognize and respond effectively to verbal, nonverbal, and written communications
- Use medical terminology appropriately
- Utilize electronic technology to receive, organize, prioritize and transmit information
- Serve as liaison

Legal Concepts

- Perform within legal and ethical boundaries
- Prepare and maintain medical records
- Document accurately
- Follow employer's established policies dealing with the health care contract
- Implement and maintain federal and state health care legislation and regulations
- Comply with established risk management and safety procedures
- Recognize professional credentialing criteria
- *Develop and maintain personnel, policy and procedure manuals*

Instruction

- Instruct individuals according to their needs
- Explain office policies and procedures
- Teach methods of health promotion and disease prevention
- Locate community resources and disseminate information
- *Develop educational materials*
- *Conduct continuing education activities*

Operational Functions

- Perform inventory of supplies and equipment
- Perform routine maintenance of administrative and clinical equipment
- Apply computer techniques to support office operations
- *Perform personnel management functions*
- *Negotiate leases and prices for equipment and supply contracts*

- *Denotes advanced skills.*

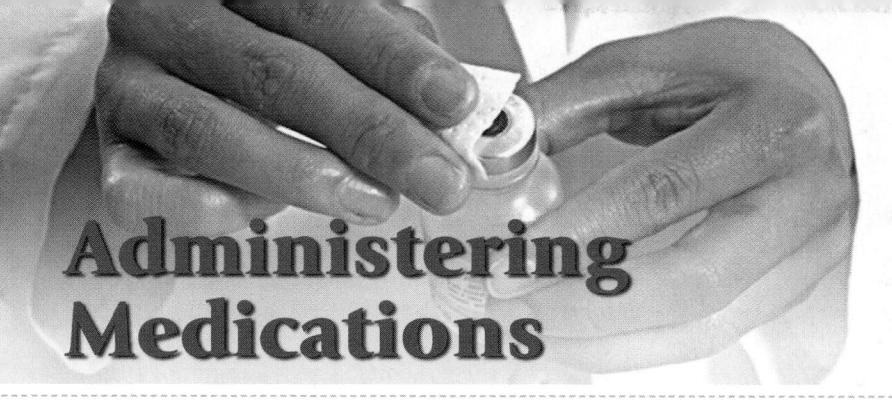

Administering Medications

Learning Objectives

After completing this chapter, you should be able to:

- Define and spell the terms to learn for this chapter.
- Describe the OSHA standards relating to needle sticks.
- Correctly describe the procedure for the administration of oral medications.
- Correctly describe the procedure for the administration of parenteral medications.

- List the standard needle lengths and gauges.
- List and define the four sites for intramuscular injections.
- State the rationale for using the Z-track injection method.
- State the name of 10 drugs commonly found in the medical office.
- List the precautions used when administering an injection to an infant or small child.

OUTLINE

Administration Procedures: OSHA Standards	1048
Medication Administration	1048
Equipment Used for Medication Administration	1053
Sites for Intramuscular Injections	1057
Sites for Subcutaneous Injection	1061
Intradermal Injection	1066
Tuberculin Skin Test	1067
Intravenous Therapy	1071
Immunizations	1072
Reconstituting a Powdered Medication for Administration	1076
Charting Medications	1077

Terms to Learn

ampules

deltoid muscle

diphtheria

dorsogluteal site

hepatitis A

hepatitis B

Hib disease

immunizations

inactivated polio vaccine (IPV)

inhalation medications

intradermal injection

intramuscular (IM) injections

liquid medications

measles, mumps, and rubella (MMR) vaccine

oral medication

oral polio vaccine (OPV)

parenteral medication administration

pertussis

pneumococcal vaccine

polio vaccine

prefilled cartridge injection systems

rectus femoris

subcutaneous injection

tetanus

vaccines

varicella

vastus lateralis muscle

ventrogluteal site

Z-track method

Case Study

LATOYA IS A MEDICAL ASSISTANT in Dr. Reed's office. Dr. Reed is a board-certified pediatrician licensed to practice medicine in the state of Illinois.

A patient, a 4-year-old boy, has been brought in by his baby-sitter for an emergency appointment because of severe nausea and vomiting. He weighs about 30 pounds. Dr. Reed is concerned that the child might be dehydrated.

Dr. Reed, upon examination of the child, orders 2.5 mg of Compazine, rectally, stat. He asks Latoya to administer the medication. The child is upset and crying and appears very fearful of Latoya. Latoya is concerned about being able to administer the medication to the child given his behavior.

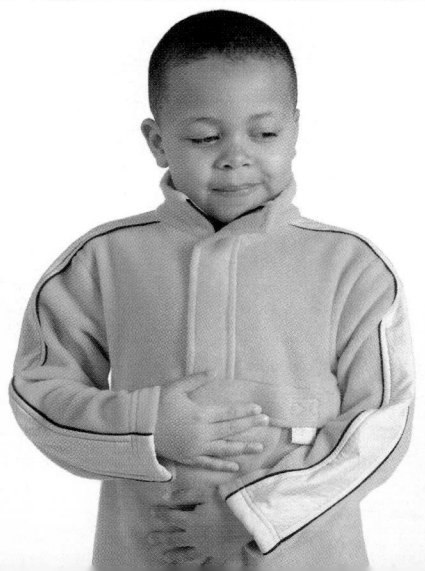

One of the most important functions of the medical assistant is administering medications. Pharmacology and drug therapy use the skills of physicians, pharmacists, nurses, and medication assistants. The medical assistant's specific role is administering the correct medication at the correct dose, time, and route.

Administration Procedures: OSHA Standards

The Occupational Safety and Health Administration (OSHA) has established very specific guidelines regarding the disposal of contaminated needles and syringes. The bloodborne pathogens standard has provisions for follow-up procedures for health care workers who are exposed to a needle stick from a contaminated needle.

If a medical assistant is accidentally stuck with a contaminated needle, the physician should be notified immediately. Specific concerns are exposure to hepatitis B virus (HBV) and human immunodeficiency virus (HIV), which can cause acquired immunodeficiency syndrome (AIDS). There is a much greater chance of developing HBV than of developing HIV/AIDS from a contaminated needle stick.

Immediate reporting of needle sticks is important to ensure that testing and prophylactic treatment can be appropriately initiated. The employer is responsible for providing free medical evaluation and treatment for exposure to contaminated sharps or needles while at work. Investigation of the incident is a second reason for early reporting, because the employer should begin to seek reasons for the incident. Additional training may be necessary in order to prevent other injuries in the office.

According to the law, all medical offices must have a puncture-proof, rigid, locked container labeled with an international biohazard sticker for the disposal of sharps. Smaller biohazard sharps containers may be placed in all of the patient exam rooms. When these smaller containers are two-thirds to three-quarters full they should be closed and placed in a large biohazard container that is in a central location in the office (see Figure 49-1). When the large container is two-thirds to three-quarters full, it should be replaced and disposed of using a waste removal service contracted to incinerate or autoclave the contents. The waste removal service will give the office a document of destruction, which should be kept and filed at the office.

Any time a medical assistant has the potential to come in contact with *any* body fluids—such as saliva, blood, or other substances—Standard Precautions must be observed and followed. Careful hand hygiene must follow the removal of gloves after such contact. For more on biohazadous waste disposal see Chapter 32.

Medication Administration

Medications may be administered orally, topically, by inhalation, vaginally, rectally, or by injection. Specific procedures must be followed when the medical assistant is ordered to administer a medication. The first step is always to check the order, making sure that you can clearly read the order and that you completely understand what is being ordered. Be sure to review the "three befores" and the "ten rights" discussed in Chapter 48 before proceeding with this chapter (see Legal and Ethical Issues). The second step is to ensure that the patient does not have an allergy to the ordered medicine. Then, check the order again, and check the "ten rights". Although this may sound like duplicated effort, this is where mistakes are very often caught and giving an incorrect medication can be deadly. Medical assistants do not administer medications by intravenous fluids nor do they administer chemotherapy drugs or narcotics (see Figure 49-2).

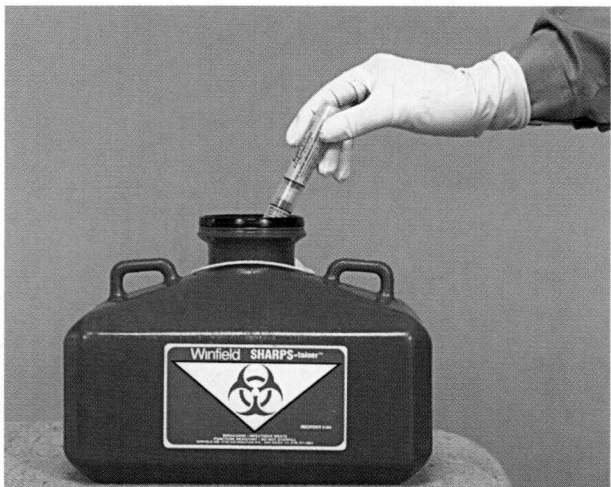

FIGURE 49-1 Biohazard sharps container.

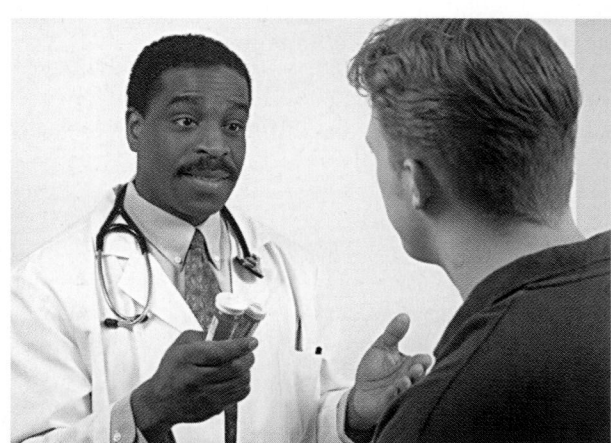

FIGURE 49-2 Provide patient instruction as needed.

Topical Medications

Topical drugs for dermal application and mucosal application come in various forms. For skin conditions that require treatment, topical drug forms include:

- Creams and ointments
- Lotions
- Skin patches.

Topical medications that are applied to mucosal membranes include:

- Eyedrops, eardrops, and nose drops
- Eye ointments
- Vaginal creams
- Rectal and vaginal suppositories
- Sterile douche solutions
- Sublingual or buccal tablets.

As with the administration of any medication, it is important for the medical assistant to wear gloves. When administering ointment to an area, the area should first be cleaned. Once the area has been wiped clean, the ointment should be applied in a thin layer using either a cotton swab or a tongue depressor.

If a patient needs to receive a liquid medication such as a lotion or suspension, the bottle should be shaken well and then applied as directed. When administering a liquid medication that is to be sprayed, caution should be taken to ensure that both the patient and the drug administrator not inhale the spray. In some instances when a topical drug is applied, the area must then be covered with a sterile gauze in order to keep the area clean. When reapplying ointment to an area, the old remaining ointment should be removed prior to applying a new layer of ointment. (See Procedure 49-1 for instruction on administering a rectal or vaginal suppository and Procedure 49-2 for administering sublingual or buccal medication).

Oral Medication Administration

Oral medication administration is giving medication that is administered through the gastrointestinal system. These medications can be pills, syrups, or other liquids. These are medications that are swallowed, enter the body through tissues of the gastrointestinal system, and are then rapidly absorbed in the body. There are a variety of different types of liquid medications including suspensions, emulsions, elixirs, syrups, and solutions. Equipment used for the dispensing of liquid medication includes calibrated cups, spoons, and droppers. As with any medication, it is important to educate the patient on the proper measurement of these medications. Many liquid medications are prescribed for the pediatric patient due to the ease of administration. (See Procedure 49-3 for instructions on administering oral medications).

Inhalation Medication Administration

Inhalation medications are used for dispensing oral medication into the respiratory tract. The equipment used for this route is a metered-dose inhaler (nebulizer) (see Figure 49-3). When a patient requires this type of medication,

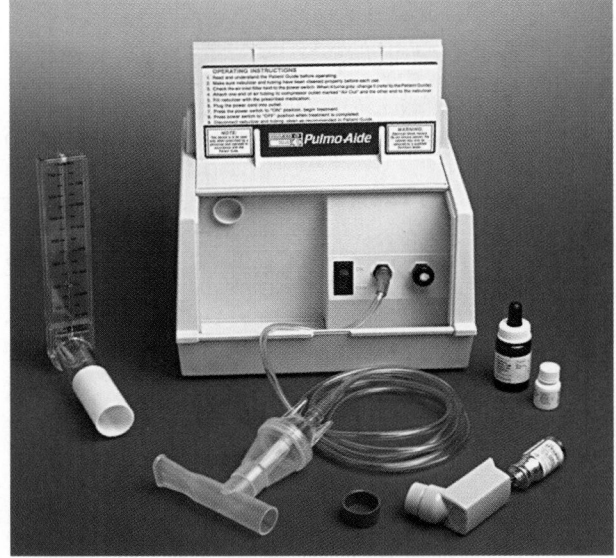

FIGURE 49-3 A metered dose inhaler with a medication inhaler.

Administering (Inserting) a Rectal or Vaginal Suppository

OBJECTIVE: Insert a suppository without error as ordered by the physician.

Equipment and Supplies

medication order signed by physician; lubricant; water; biohazard waste container; patient instructions; vaginal suppository or cream and supplies; sterile gloves; sanitary napkin; rectal suppository and supplies; nonsterile gloves; 4 × 4 gauze square; pen

Method

1. Assemble equipment.
2. Perform hand hygiene.
3. Select the correct medication using the "three befores." If you are not familiar with the medication, look it up in a reference book, read the package insert, and/or consult the physician.
4. Always double-check the label to make sure the strength is correct since medications are manufactured with different strengths.
5. Correctly calculate the dosage in writing. Double-check your calculations with someone else.
6. Check the dosage again against the medication order.
7. Replace the cap on the medication bottle and return the bottle to the storage shelf or refrigerator after reading the label again.
8. Identify the patient both by stating his or her name and examining any printed identification, such as a wrist name band or medical record. Ask the patient if he or she has any allergies.
9. Give patient a gown or sheet. Have the patient remove all clothing from the waist down.
10A. *Rectal suppository:* Have the patient lie on left side, if possible, with top leg bent. Drape a sheet over the patient. Put on nonsterile gloves. Open the suppository wrapper and place suppository on a gauze square. Moisten the suppository with a small amount of lubricant or water. With one hand separate the buttocks. Pick up the suppository with the other hand. Ask the patient to breathe slowly as you insert the suppository from 1 to 1½ inches through the rectal sphincter. Hold the but-

tocks together and instruct the patient not to bear down or push out the suppository. Wipe the anal area with the gauze and discard gauze into a biohazard waste container. Have the patient remain in the side position for around 20 minutes until the suppository melts.

10B. *Vaginal suppository:* Have the patient assume the dorsal recumbent position with legs apart. Drape the patient. Open the sterile glove pack on a flat surface leaving the gloves in place. Use the inside of the glove wrapper as a sterile field. Peel open the suppository container and drop the suppository onto the inside of the glove wrapper. If an applicator is provided, drop it onto the sterile surface also. Glove using sterile technique. With one gloved hand, separate the labia minora and hold it in place. Using the other hand, insert the suppository one finger length into the vagina. If an applicator is used, place the suppository into the applicator and insert it in a downward direction. Instruct the patient to remain in this position for at least 10 minutes for the suppository to dissolve. Place applicator into the glove wrapper. Remove one glove by pulling inside out from the cuff. With the remaining gloved hand, roll the contaminated wrapper and contents. Hold these waste items as you remove the remaining glove over them. Dispose of all materials into a biohazard waste container. Give the patient a sanitary napkin.
11. Remain with the patient until the medication has dissolved.
12. Provide the patient with written follow-up instructions if further medication is to be taken.
13. Chart the medication administration on the patient's record noting the time, medication name, dosage, injection site, route, and your name.

Charting Example

2/26/XX	9:00 A.M.	Dulcolax 15 mg. Rectal supp.
		M. King, CMA

Administering Sublingual or Buccal Medication

OBJECTIVE: Administer a medication to a patient under the tongue or between the cheek and gum.

Equipment and Supplies

medication order signed by physician on the patient's medical record; oral medication; paper cup or receptacle for medication; patient instruction sheet; biohazard waste container; pen

Method

1. Assemble equipment.
2. Perform hand hygiene.
3. Select the correct medication using the "three befores." If you are not familiar with the medication look it up in a reference book, read the package insert, and/or consult the physician.
4. Always double-check the label to make sure the strength is correct since medications are manufactured with different strengths.
5. Correctly calculate the dosage in writing. Double-check your calculations.
6. Place a medicine cup/container on a flat surface.
7. Shake the tablet ordered into the bottle cap and then into a medication container.
8. Check the dosage again against the medication order.
9. Replace the cap on the medication bottle and return the bottle to the storage shelf after reading the label again.
10. Identify the patient both by stating his or her name and examining any printed identification, such as a wrist name band or medical record. Ask the patient if he or she has any allergies.
11A. *Sublingual medication:* Have the patient place the tablet under the tongue. Instruct the patient not to swallow until the tablet has dissolved.
11B. *Buccal medication:* Have the patient place the tablet between the cheek and gum area. Instruct the patient not to swallow until the tablet is dissolved.
12. Tell the patient not to take fluids until the tablet is dissolved.
13. Remain with the patient until the medication has dissolved.
14. Provide the patient with written follow-up instructions if further medication is to be taken.
15. Chart the medication administration on the correct patient's record noting the time, medication name, dosage, route, and your name. After giving the medication to the patient, it is best to have the patient wait in the office for 30 minutes.

Charting Example

2/14/XX	9:00 A.M. Nitroglycerin tab 1 (gr. 1/100), subling., P = 60

N. Young, RMA

Patient Education

The physician is the first individual to discuss medications with a patient. The medical assistant should reinforce the physician's teaching and clarify any questions that the patient may have. Be sure that all explanations include the dosage and frequency of medication administration. If the patient is unclear about the purpose or the dosage of the medication, he or she may not take the medication as directed. Expected results and side effects should also be carefully explained to the patient. The pharmacy may include medication inserts for the patient, but reinforcement can help improve patient understanding and compliance. Be sure that the patient understands the dosing, especially if the medication is in liquid form. He or she may not understand properly measuring the dose in the metric or apothecary system. The education sessions should be documented in the patient's chart.

Special emphasis should be placed on instructing the patient to take the medication for the length of time that the medicine is prescribed. For example, antibiotics should be taken for the entire length of time or they will be ineffective and the infection may reoccur. Other medications are designed to be taken indefinitely, and should only be stopped on the advice of a physician.

Administering Oral Medications

OBJECTIVE: Administer oral medication.

Equipment and Supplies

medication order signed by physician; oral medication; calibrated paper cup or receptacle for medication; water in glass; patient instruction sheet; biohazard waste container; pen

Method

1. Assemble equipment.
2. Perform hand hygiene.
3. Select the correct medication using the "three befores." If you are not familiar with the medication, look it up in a reference book, read the package insert, and/or consult the physician.
4. Always double-check the label to make sure the strength is correct since medications are manufactured with different strengths.
5. Correctly calculate the dosage in writing. Double-check your calculations with someone else.
6. Place a medicine cup/container on a flat surface.
7. Gently shake the medication if it is in liquid form.
8. Hold the bottle so that the label is in the palm of your hand to prevent damaging the label with liquid medication.
9. Recheck the label again.
10. Remove the cap from the medicine container and place it upside down on a clean surface. This will keep the inside of the cap clean, which can then be replaced on the bottle.
11A. *Liquid medication:* Hold the calibrated medicine cup at eye level and pour the medication into the cup stopping at the correct dosage line. Pour the medication away from the label side of the bottle.

If too much medication is poured into the calibrated cup, do not return it to the bottle. Discard it into a sink.

11B. *Tablet or capsule medication:* Shake out the correct number of tablets or pills into the bottle cap. Then place them in the medicine cup. If you accidentally pour out an extra tablet, do not return it to the medication bottle. Discard it.

12. Check the medication again to make sure the dosage is the same as the medication order.
13. Replace the cap on the medication bottle and return the bottle to the storage shelf.
14. Take the prepared medication and a glass of water to the patient.
15. Identify the patient both by stating his or her name and examining any printed identification such as a wrist name band or medical record. Ask the patient if he or she has any allergies.
16. Remain with the patient until the medication has been swallowed.
17. Provide the patient with written follow-up instructions if further medication is to be taken.
18. Chart the medication administration on the correct patient's record noting the time, medication name, dosage, route (oral procedure), and your name. After giving the medication to the patient, it is best to have the patient wait in the office for 30 minutes.

Charting Example

2/14/XX	1:00 P.M.	ASA, 500 mg, po.
		N. Young, RMA

---

the patient may receive the treatment in the office and/or be sent home with the metered-dose inhaler (MDI). It is the responsibility of the medical assistant to ensure that the patient is trained in the use of the MDI. (See also Patient Education). The patient must clearly understand the use of this equipment prior to taking it home. See Chapter 45 for more information on nebulizers.

Parenteral Medication Administration

Parenteral medication administration means administering a medication through injection. These routes include intramuscular, intravenous, subdermal, and intradermal injections. Medication that is given by injection enters the bloodstream more rapidly than medications given by other methods. Parenteral administration allows medication to be targeted to a particular area of the body. For example, a local anesthetic is injected into a specific area on the body. The injection site then becomes numb, allowing the physician to suture the area with no discomfort to the patient.

Injections

Injections are classified by the tissue into which the medication is injected. The most common injections done by medical assistants are intramuscular and intradermal. Intramuscular (IM) injections are given in the muscles, usually the deltoid or the gluteus medius muscles in adults or the vastus lateralis (in the thigh) or

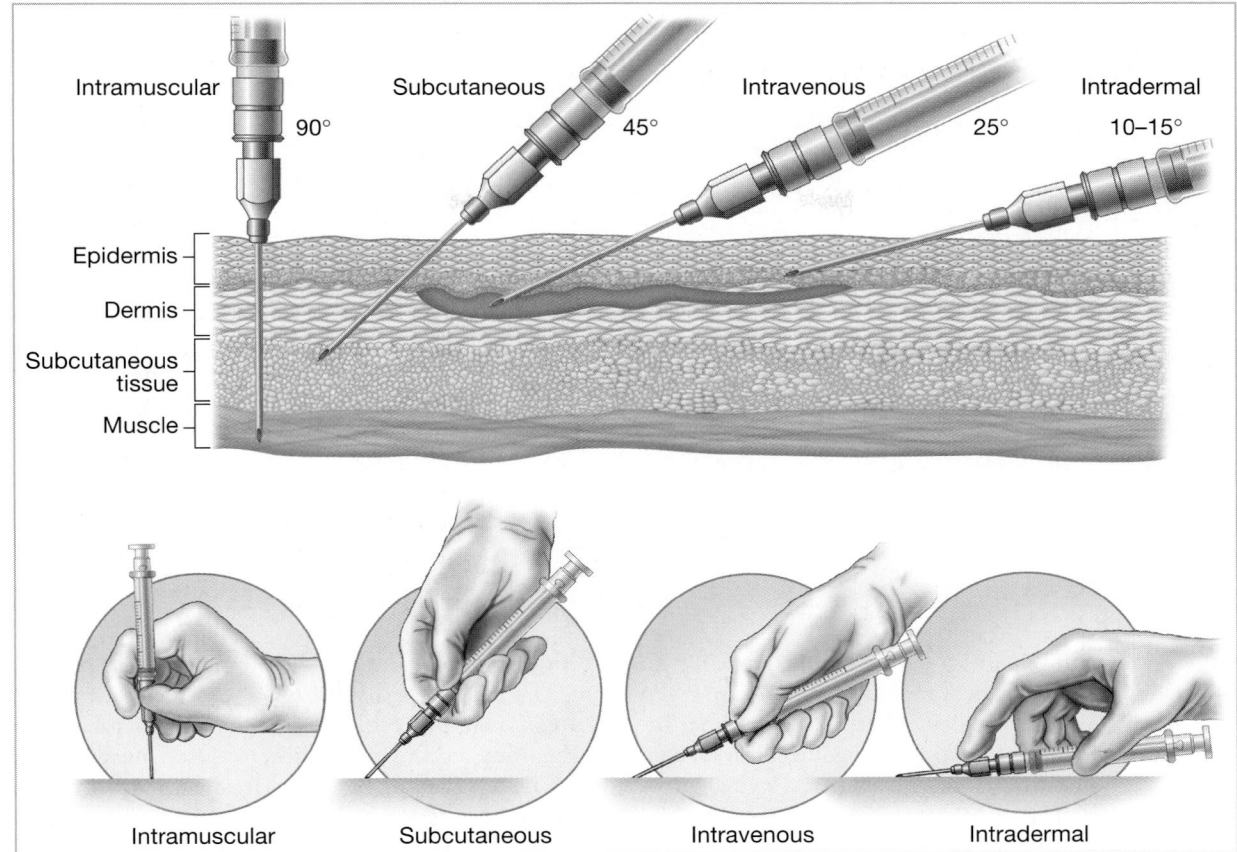

FIGURE 49-4 Angle of needle insertion for four types of injections.

the rectus femoris (middle region of the thigh) muscles in pediatric patients (see also Lifespan Considerations). Syringes are used with disposable needles to give injections (see Figures 49-4 and 49-5).

Equipment Used for Medication Administration

The type of equipment used depends on the type of medication and method of administration. For instance, when an oral medication is being administered, use of a calibrated cup or spoon would be required. Equipment used for injectable medications includes syringes and needles. Medications administrated through inhalants require the use of a metered-dose inhaler. It is important for the medical assistant to be familiar with the various types of equipment used for medication administration.

Syringes

Syringes come in a variety of sizes (see Figure 49-6). The smallest syringe is called a tuberculin syringe, and the measurements are calibrated in 1/100 of a milliliter. Tuberculin syringes are used with 27- or 28-gauge needles and are used to do tuberculosis (PPD) testing and allergy testing, for which all of the injections are done intradermally (in the skin).

Another type of syringe is the insulin syringe. Units are used for insulin administration, done with a small needle and injected directly under the skin (subcutaneous injections). These injections are typically done in the arms, abdomen, or thighs. A 25- or 26-gauge syringe is used for insulin administration.

Larger syringes are calibrated in 2-, 3-, 5-, and 10-mL segments and larger, up to 60 mL. The most commonly used size is the 3-mL syringe, because it is the most accurate with small doses of medication. Most injected doses of medication are less than what the 3-mL syringe can hold. The viscosity of the medication being given also determines the gauge of the needle.

Needles are categorized according to size—both length and gauge (how large the barrel of the needle is). The larger the size of the needle, the smaller the gauge. The largest needles available are 14 to 18 gauge, and are only used in trauma care. IV lines are typically placed with 18-, 20- or 22-gauge needles. This is not a medical assistant responsibility. Intramuscular injections are

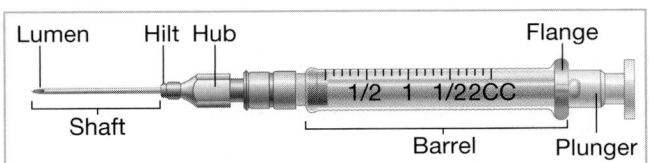

FIGURE 49-5 A hypodermic needle.

THE CHILD

When giving injections to pediatric patients, it is important to make sure that the patients understand that they are going to be given an injection, and it will hurt for a moment. Never lie to pediatric patients, but instead give them a brief statement such as "I am going to give you some medicine with a shot, and it might hurt for just a minute, but then we will put a bandage on it." Be sure that all pediatric dosage calculations are double-checked. A slight dosage miscalculation can create significant problems in a pediatric patient.

Never give medications to a pediatric patient without permission from the parent or guardian. Explain why the medication is being given, and be sure that they are comfortable with the physician's explanation and have given their consent.

THE OLDER ADULT

Elderly patients typically take more medications than do younger patients. Always get a complete medication history. Include questions about over-the-counter medications. If an elderly patient has difficulty swallowing, be sure that the physician is aware of this so that smaller pills or alternate forms of medication can be prescribed.

Elderly patients often have thinner skin and smaller muscles. So when giving them injections, use a smaller needle and use care to not tear the skin or damage the muscle. Adhesive tape may tear their skin, so use gentle pressure on the site, then consider using paper tape if a bandage is needed.

---

usually given with 24- or 25-gauge needles, usually ⅝-inch to 3 inches long. Subcutaneous injections are given with 25- to 26-gauge needles, whereas intradermal injections are given with 27- to 28-gauge needles. Needle length is very important and varies from ⅜ inch to 4 inches in length. The needle length will depend on the route used and the area of body to be injected.

Syringes and needles are disposable. There is a puncture-proof sheath or cover on the needle. It is im-portant to check that the sheath (cover) is in place any time the medical assistant is changing the needle on a syringe. This prevents needle sticks. Never handle an unsheathed needle. Any dirty or used needle should never be handled or recapped (resheathed). If a needle needs to be recapped, put the sheath on a counter and "scoop" the cap with the needle—but *never* touch the needle. After capping the needle, be sure to clean the area with a disinfectant. All needles and syringes

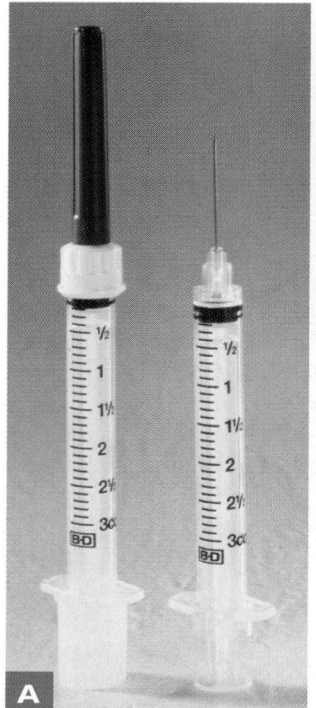
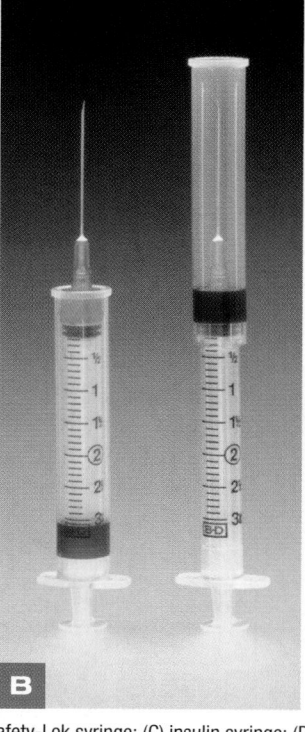
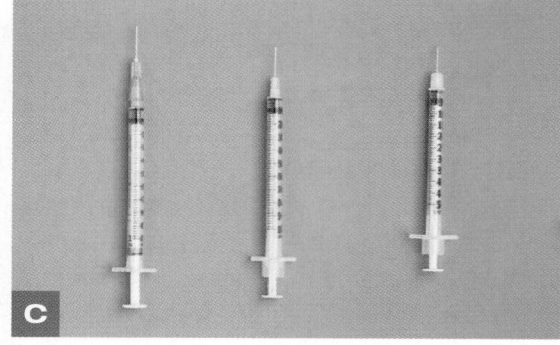
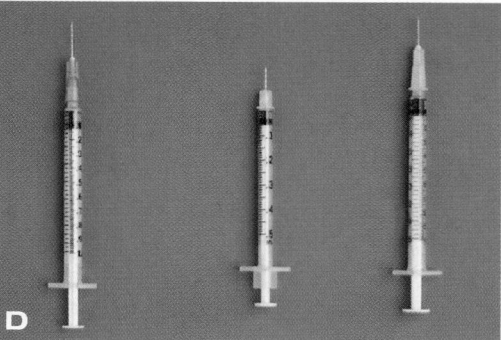

FIGURE 49-6 (A) Med-Saver syringe; (B) Safety-Lok syringe; (C) insulin syringe; (D) tuberculin syringes.

should be placed in a red sharps container, needle down as soon as they are used.

As OSHA standards become stricter, more facilities will adapt to using safety needles, where a protective cover can quickly and safely be engaged to protect the user from exposure to a contaminated needle. It is a good idea to practice engaging the safety mechanism on a clean needle to prevent accidents with contaminated ones. Sharps containers are used for disposal of safety needles. No needle should be disposed in any receptacle except for a sharps container.

Medications for injection are provided in several formats. The most common form for injectable medication is single-dose or multiple-dose vials. These are glass vials with rubber stoppers to protect the medications inside. The needle is inserted through the rubber stopper and the correct amount of medication is drawn out. Single-dose vials are meant to be used, as the name implies, one time. Multiple-dose vials are used multiple times, cleaning the stopper with rubbing alcohol prior to each use.

Ampules are small, sealed glass bottles containing a single dose of medication. There is a small indentation in the neck of the ampule where the tip is broken off to open the container. It is important to use an alcohol pad or cotton pad to hold the vial to prevent glass cuts when opening ampules (see Procedure 49-4 and Figure 49-7).

49-4	**PROCEDURE**

Using an Ampule

OBJECTIVE: Open and withdraw medication from an ampule.

Equipment and Supplies
ampule containing medication; soap; alcohol sponge; needle; syringe; biohazard waste container; pen

Method
1. Do not open the ampule until you are ready to withdraw the fluid.

   Note: Always follow the "three befores" when checking medications against the medication order.
2. Perform hand hygiene.
3. Snap your thumb and middle finger gently against the tip of the ampule to move all the medication away from the neck and into the bottom of the ampule (Figure 49-7A).
4. Clean the neck of the ampule using an alcohol swab.

5. Use gauze between the ampule and thumbs when breaking the ampule. Using one hand to hold the bottom of the vial, snap the top off with the other hand using a gauze square to prevent a cut when the glass neck breaks (Figure 49-7B).
6. If the top of the ampule does not snap off easily, you may have to use a file to create a cut or "score" the ampule at the neck. The glass ampule should then break easily at this point (Figure 49-7C).
7. Insert a needle (attached to a syringe) into the ampule and withdraw the fluid without touching the sides of the ampule.
8. Withdraw all the medication from the ampule. It may be necessary to tip the ampule slightly to withdraw all of the fluid.
9. Discard the broken ampule into a biohazard waste container.

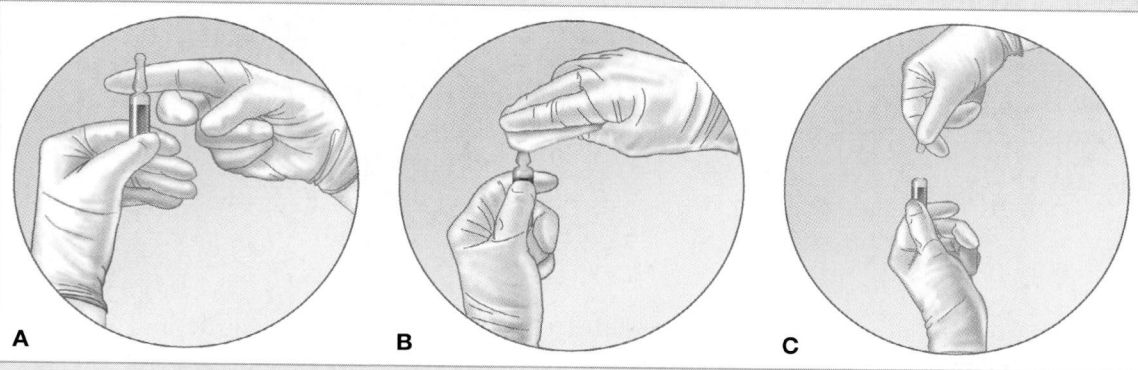

A	B	C

FIGURE 49-7 Breaking a glass ampule containing medication.

PROCEDURE

Withdrawing Medication from a Single-Dose or Multiple-Dose Vial

OBJECTIVE: Withdraw medication from a single-dose and a multiple-dose vial.

Equipment and Supplies

disposable gloves; biohazard waste container; biohazard sharps container; soap; needle; syringe; alcohol sponge; medication vial; pen

Method

1. Check the medication using the "three befores" technique before beginning. Compare the medication vial (bottle) against the physician's order (Figure 49-8A).
2. Select the correct syringe and needle depending on the type of medication and location for the injection site.
3. Perform hand hygiene.
4. Roll the medication vial between your hands to mix any medication that has settled on the bottom.
5. Wipe the rubber stopper with an alcohol sponge firmly in a circular motion. Then set the vial on a clean surface while you prepare the syringe (Figure 49-8B).

6. Remove the protective cap from the needle on the syringe. Maintain the sterility of the inner surface of the protective cap since it will be needed to cover the needle again after you have filled the syringe. Figures 49-8C through 49-8E show the steps involved in filling a syringe.
7. Withdraw the syringe plunger and allow air to enter the syringe in an amount equal to the amount of medication to be withdrawn. Because the vials are vacuum sealed, this will allow for easier withdrawal of fluid.
8. Turning the vial upside down at eye level and using care not to touch the rubber stopper, insert the needle into the rubber stopper and inject the air into the vial. Be extremely cautious concerning contamination as you enter the multiple-dose bottle.
   Rationale: There is an increased danger of contamination since the multiple-dose vial

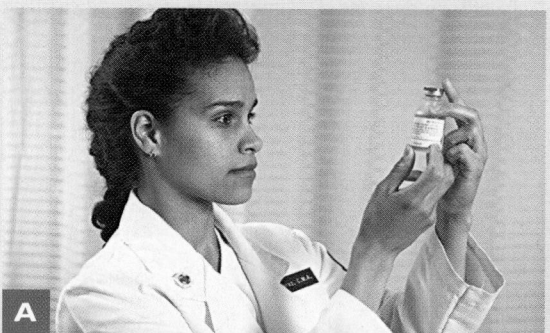
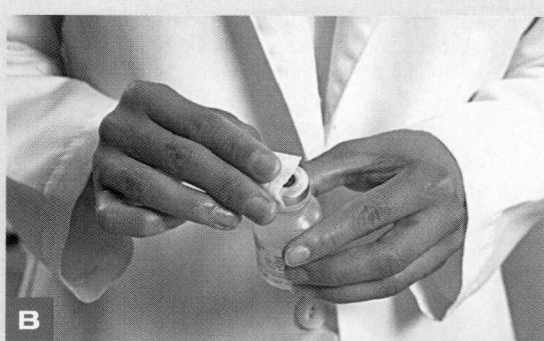

FIGURE 49-8   (A) Read the label on the medication bottle. (B) Clean the top of the bottle.

Prefilled cartridge injection systems are prefilled, single-dose cartridges that fit with a special cartridge holder. This system is convenient in that medications do not have to be drawn up prior to injections. The cartridge holders are sturdy and long lasting. (See Procedure 49-5 for instructions on withdrawing medication from a single-dose or multiple-dose vial and Figure 49-8.)

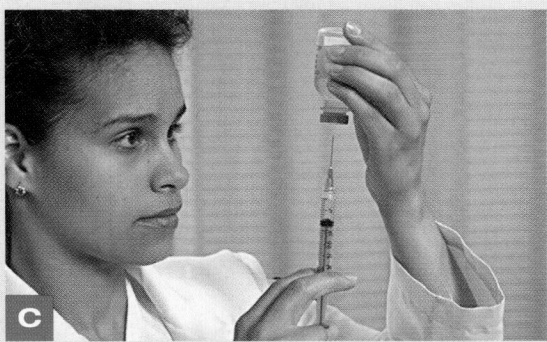

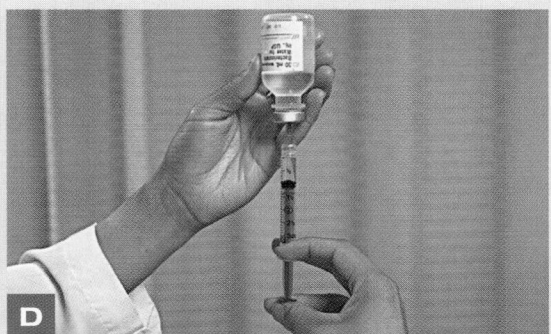

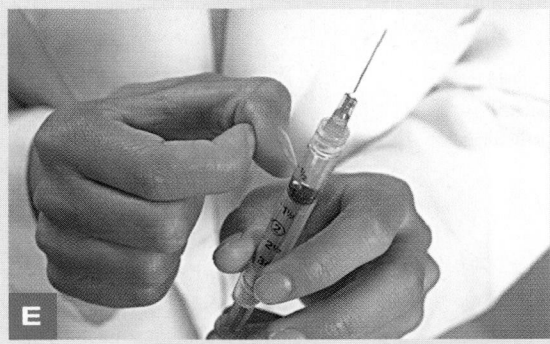

FIGURE 49-8 (*continued*) (C) Invert bottle and inject the same amount of air into the bottle as amount of medication to be withdrawn. (D) Keeping the bottle inverted, draw the correct amount of medication into the syringe. (E) Remove the needle from the bottle and expel the air or tap out the air bubbles.

may be entered more than once by several people.

9. Keeping the upside-down vial at eye level, slowly withdraw the correct amount of fluid medication.
   Rationale: Rapid withdrawal of fluid may cause air bubbles to form in the syringe.

10. While the needle is still in the vial, check to make sure that the dosage is accurate. Any air bubbles in the syringe will give you an inaccurate dose since they take up the space needed for medication. To remove air bubbles, flick your fingers against the side of the syringe until the air bubbles go back into the tip of the syringe. Expel these bubbles back into the vial and withdraw more medication until the dosage is accurate.

11. Remove needle from vial.

12. If you have accidentally withdrawn too much fluid, discard the excess fluid by shooting it into a sink or waste receptacle. Never return medications to the vial or bottle from which they came.

13. Check the medication vial after you have withdrawn the dosage to make sure you are correct. This is the last step of the "three befores" for checking medications. Also, check to see if the multiple-dose vial needs to be refrigerated after opening.

Sites for Intramuscular Injections

IM injections are given in one of four sites. These sites or muscles are the deltoid, vastus lateralis, dorsogluteal, and the ventrogluteal muscles (see Figure 49-9).

Deltoid Muscle

The deltoid muscle is located on the upper outer surface of the upper arm. This site of small muscle mass works well for small-volume injections, but not for

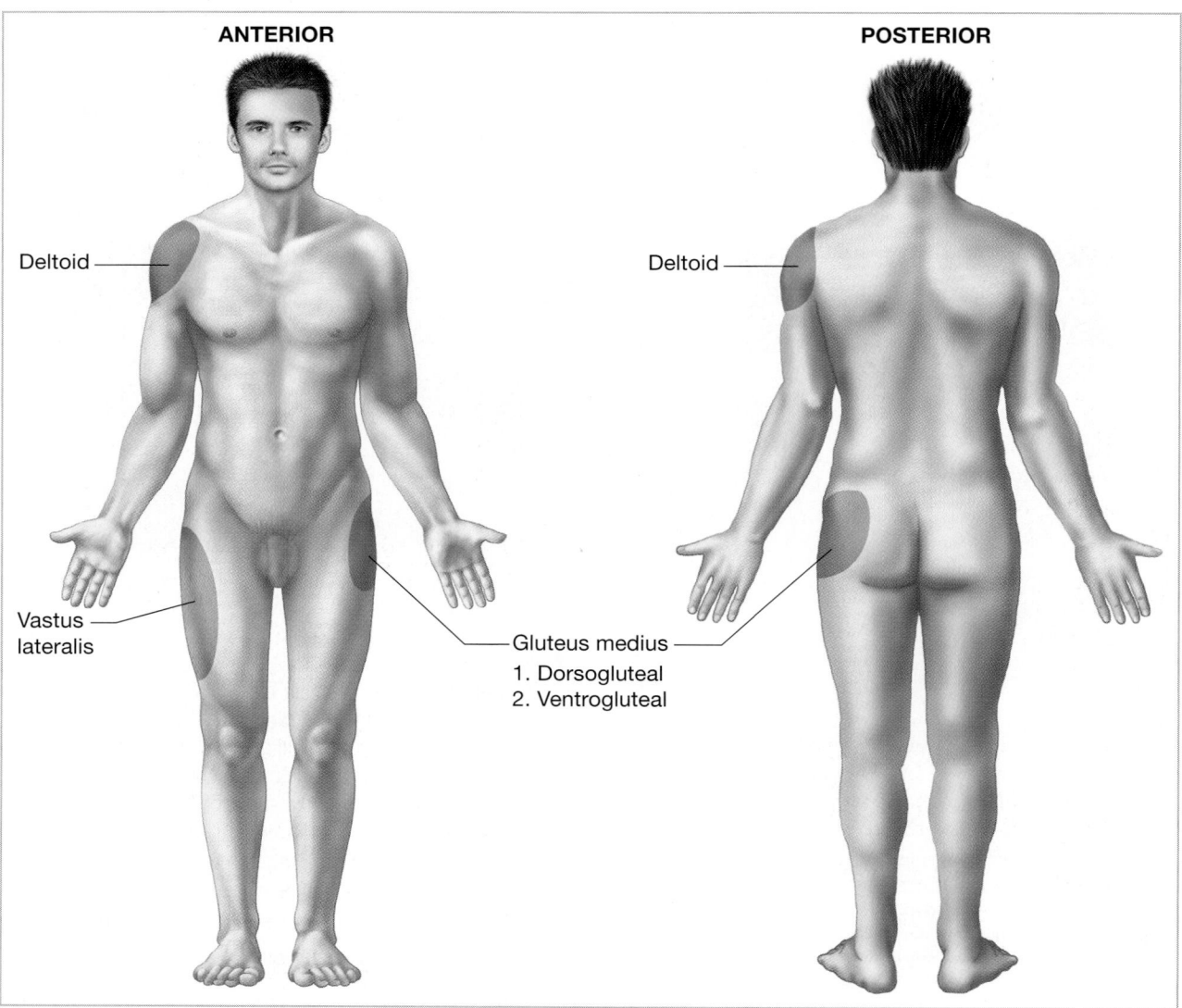

ANTERIOR

Deltoid

Vastus
lateralis

POSTERIOR

Deltoid

Gluteus medius
1. Dorsogluteal
2. Ventrogluteal

FIGURE 49-9 Sites for intramuscular injections.

large ones. Common injections in this site include tetanus boosters in adults. This site should never be used in infants or small children because the size of the muscle is too small.

The deltoid muscle is found by measuring two finger widths below the acromion process of the shoulder. Never give injections in the back of an arm, because there are large blood vessels and nerves in this area.

Use a 23-gauge, 1-inch needle to give injections in the arm. For individuals with small arms, a 25-gauge, ⅝-inch needle is more appropriate.

Vastus Lateralis Muscle

The vastus lateralis muscle is on the outer portion of the upper thigh and is part of the quadriceps. This site is considered the safest site for IM injections, especially in children or small individuals, because there are few major blood vessels in this area. The vastus lateralis muscle lies below the greater trochanter of the femur and within the upper lateral quadrant of

the thigh. This muscle is the well developed in the infant and is recommended by the American Academy of Pediatrics as the preferred injection site for infants and children.

In the adult, the vastus lateralis extends from the middle of the anterior (front) thigh to the middle of the lateral thigh. Typically, it is one handbreadth below the greater trochanter (hip bone), and extends to one handbreadth above the knee. The patient may be either sitting or lying down (supine) for an injection in this muscle.

Dorsogluteal (Gluteus Medius) Muscle

The dorsogluteal site is most commonly used for large-volume, deep IM injections or irritating viscous (thick) medications. Antibiotics are often an IM injection. There is a danger of damage to the sciatic nerve in this area, so this is not the first choice of a site for injections. Landmarks must be carefully observed to ensure proper placement of the injection in this site.

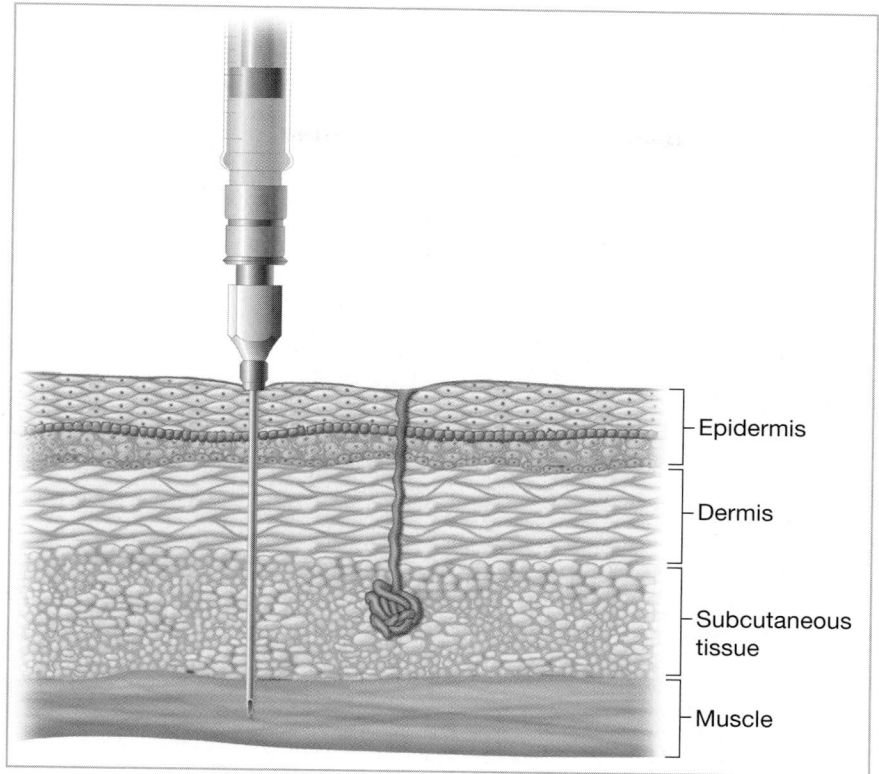

FIGURE 49-10 Needle position for an intramuscular injection.

To give this injection, the patient should be asked to lie prone and point the toes inward. This causes the gluteal muscles to relax. Draw an imaginary line from the greater trochanter of the femur to the posterior superior iliac spine. Give the injection above and lateral to this line. See Figure 49-10 for an illustration of the placement. Another method is to divide the buttocks in four equal parts, and give the injection in the upper outer quadrant (see Figure 49-11).

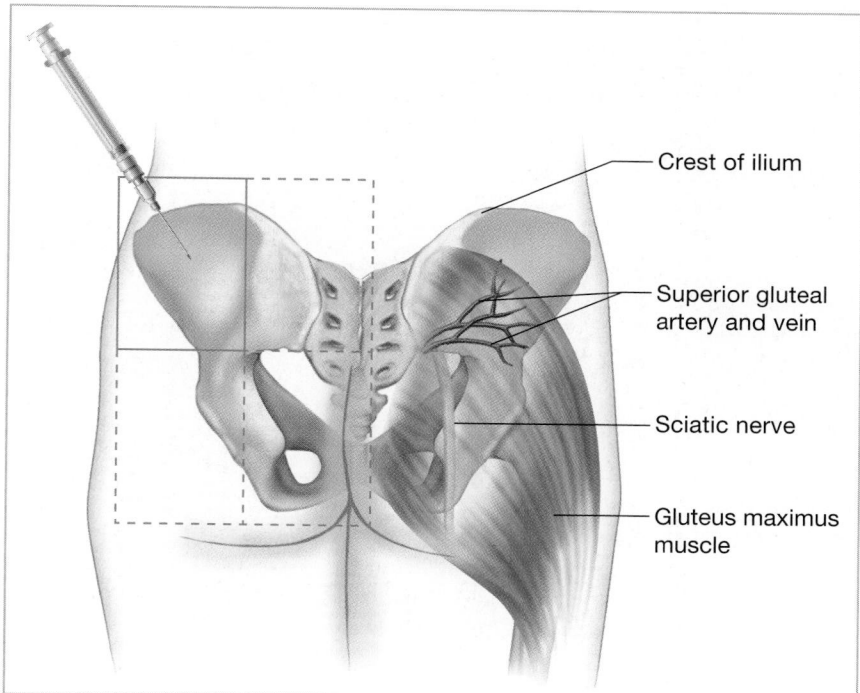

FIGURE 49-11 Injecting the upper outer quadrant of the buttocks.

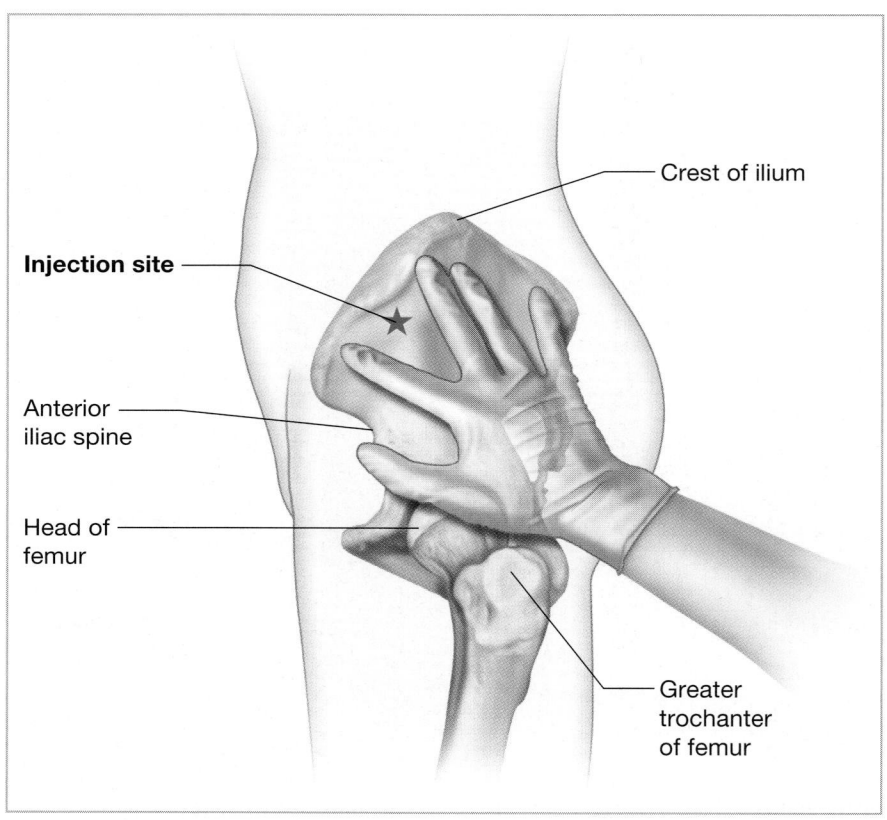

Crest of ilium

Injection site

Anterior
iliac spine

Head of
femur

Greater
trochanter
of femur

FIGURE 49-12 Injecting the ventrogluteal muscle.

TABLE 49-1 **Insulin Types and Duration of Action**

Insulin Name	Type	Common Name	Action Onset	Action Peak	Action Duration
Crystalline	Rapid action	Regular	1 hour	2–4 hours	6–8 hours
Semilente	Rapid	Regular	1 hour	4–10 hours	12–16 hours
Humulin-R	Rapid	—	15 min	1 hour	6–8 hours
Isophane	Intermediate	NPH	2–4 hours	6–15 hours	24–48 hours
Insulin zinc suspension	Intermediate	Lente	2–4 hours	6–15 hours	24–48 hours
Humulin-N	Intermediate	—	1 hour	4 hours	24 hours
Protamine zinc	Slow action	PZI	3–6 hours	12–20 hours	24–36 hours
Ultralente	Slow	PZI	8 hours	12–24 hours	36+ hours

Ventrogluteal (Gluteus Medius) Muscle

The ventrogluteal site is considered safer than the dorsogluteal muscle because there are no major nerves or blood vessels in this muscle. This site is considered safe for infants, children, and adults (see Figure 49-12).

To give an IM injection in the patient's left ventrogluteal muscle, place the palm of the right hand on the greater trochanter and the index finger on the superior iliac crest. Stretch the index finger as far as possible along the iliac crest and then spread the middle finger away from your index finger. The injection is made in the space between the index and middle finger. Always remember to use the hand opposite the side of the planned injection on the patient, for example, your left hand and the patient's right gluteus medius when using this method to determine the injection location. Intramuscular injections are always given at a 90-degree angle.

Sites for Subcutaneous Injection

The subcutaneous injection is given just under the skin in the fat (adipose) tissue. This method is used for small doses of nonirritating medications such as immunizations, insulin, and analgesics. The deltoid area is frequently used for these injections, but other areas include the upper back or (when the patient does self-injection) the abdomen and thighs. Table 49-1 lists insulin types and duration of action. See Figure 49-13 for an illustration of the sites for subcutaneous injections.

The subcutaneous injection is given at a 45-degree angle to the skin surface, unless the injection is heparin or insulin, in which case a 90-degree angle is used (see Figure 49-14). For patients who self-inject (e.g., patients administering insulin), the site of injection must be rotated. The patient must be taught to keep his or her own rotation chart to ensure that they

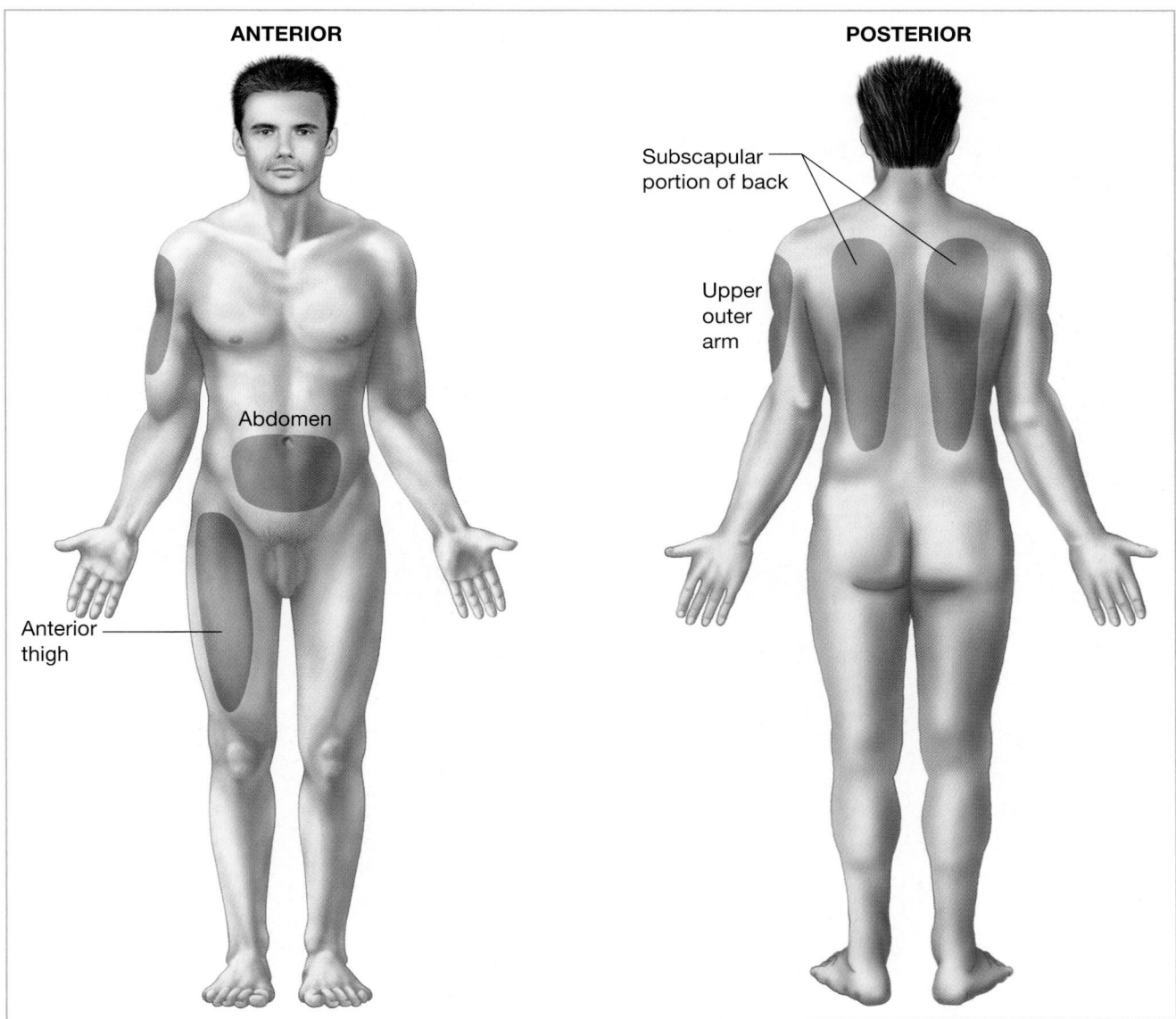

ANTERIOR

Abdomen

Anterior thigh

POSTERIOR

Subscapular portion of back

Upper outer arm

FIGURE 49-13 Sites for subcutaneous injection.

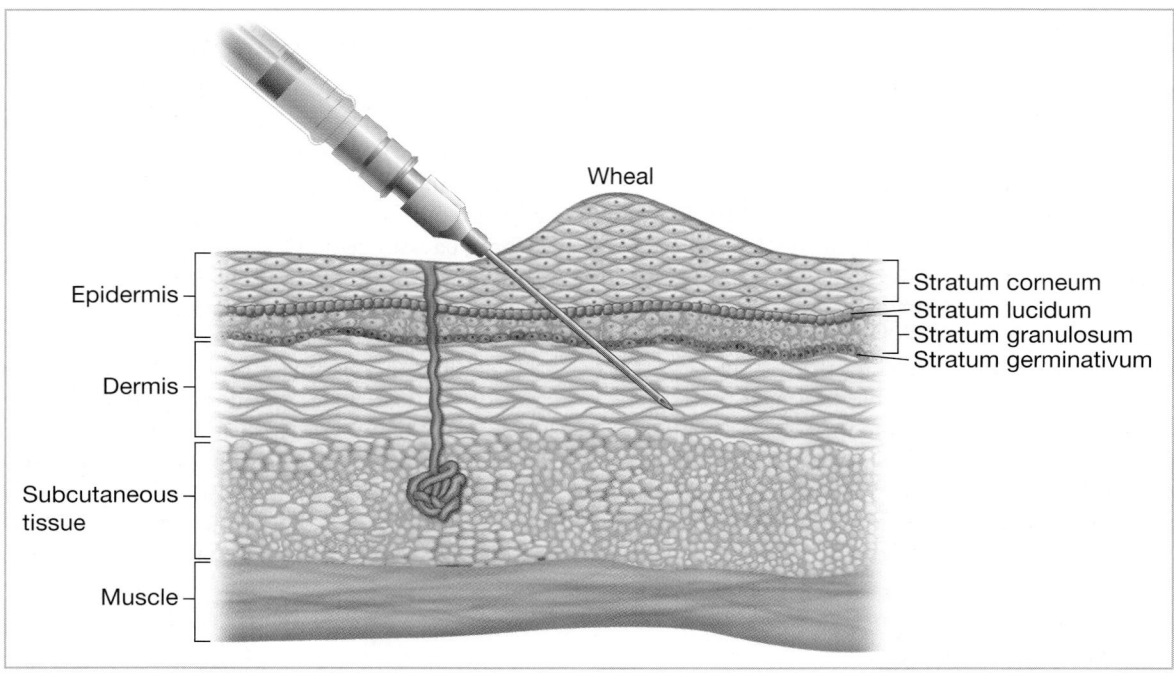

FIGURE 49-14   Needle position during subcutaneous injections.

are protecting their skin. See Figure 49-15 for an example of rotation sites. Patients receiving allergy injections should remain in the office after their injection per the office protocol, usually 20 or 30 minutes *to ensure that the patient is not having any type of allergic reaction.* (See Procedure 49-6 and Figures 49-16 and 49-17 for instructions on administering parenteral injections).

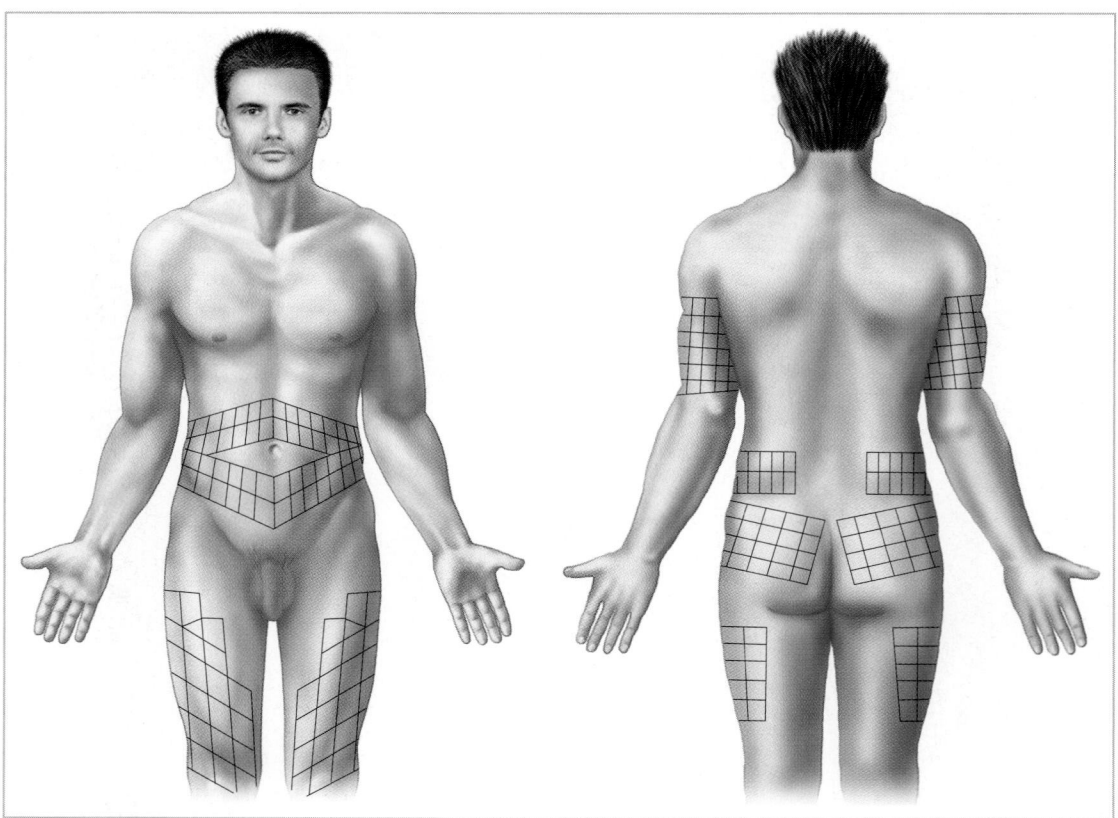

FIGURE 49-15   Rotation sites for administering insulin.

text continues on page 1066

PROCEDURE

Administering Parenteral Subcutaneous (SC) or Intramuscular (IM) Injections

OBJECTIVE: Administer subcutaneous and intramuscular injections without error.

Equipment and Supplies

medication order signed by physician; vial of medication; nonsterile gloves; alcohol sponges; biohazard sharps container; biohazard waste container; *subcutaneous injection:* 25-gauge, ⅝-inch needle for small arm; 23-gauge, 1-inch needle for average arm; disposable 3-mL syringe; *intramuscular injection:* 22-gauge, 1½-inch needle; disposable 3-mL syringe; pen

Method

1. Perform hand hygiene.
2. Apply nonsterile gloves and follow universal blood and body fluid precautions.
3. Select the correct medication using the "three befores."
   Note: Always double-check the label to make sure the strength is correct since medications are manufactured with different strengths, for example, 250 mg/mL and 500 mg/mL.
4. Gently roll the medication between your hands to mix any medication that may have settled. Refrigerated medication can be rolled between your hands to warm it slightly.
5. Prepare the syringe using the correct technique. Carefully carry the covered needle and syringe to the patient.
6. Identify the patient both by stating his or her name and examining any printed identification, such as a wrist name band or medical record. Ask the patient if he or she has any allergies.

7. Position the patient depending on the site you are using.
8. Using a circular motion clean the patient's skin with an alcohol sponge. Wipe the skin with a sweeping motion from the center of the area outward.
   Rationale: This prevents recontamination of the injection site by the alcohol sponge. Figure 49-16 illustrate the sites for administering an injection.
9. Once again check the medication dosage against the patient's order to determine if this is the correct time to administer the dose (one of the "ten rights").
10. Remove the protective covering from the needle using care not to touch the needle. If you accidentally touch the needle, excuse yourself to the patient, then return to the preparation area and change the needle on the syringe. If you are using a self-contained syringe and needle unit that does not come apart, discard the entire syringe with the medication and start the process over again.
    Rationale: A contaminated needle can cause a severe infection in an already ill patient. Remember: The patient's safety is your first priority.
11. When you are prepared to administer the injection, place a new alcohol sponge or a cotton ball between two fingers of your nondominant hand so that you can easily grasp it when you are through with the injection.

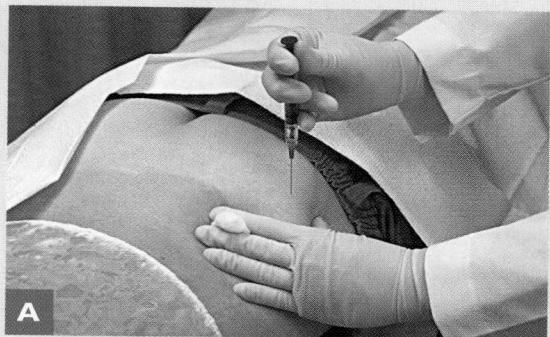
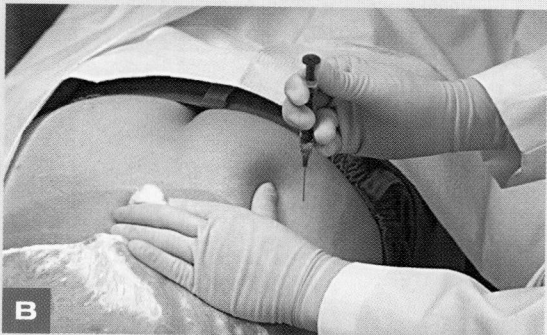

FIGURE 49-16   (A–F) Sites for administering medication.

continued on next page

PROCEDURE (continued)

Administering Parenteral Subcutaneous (SC) or Intramuscular (IM) Injections

12. Firmly grasp the syringe in your dominant hand similar to the way a pencil is held.

13A. *To administer a subcutaneous injection:* With your nondominant hand, pick up the skin at the injection site and form a small mass of tissue. *Rationale:* This will aid in the needle entering only the subcutaneous tissue.

13B. *To administer an intramuscular injection:* With your nondominant hand stretch the skin tightly where you will insert the needle. *Rationale:* Pulling the skin taut allows the needle to enter the skin more easily. (If the patient is thin or a child, you would pinch the muscle into a bundle and squeeze as the

needle is inserted. In this way you would avoid going deeper than the muscle and touching a bone.)

14. Grasping the syringe in a dart-like fashion, insert the entire needle with one swift movement.

15A. *For subcutaneous injection:* Insert into the subcutaneous tissue at a 45-degree angle.

15B. *For intramuscular injection:* Insert needle directly into the muscle at a 90-degree angle. *Rationale:* The selection of the correct size needle is important since you will be inserting the entire needle into the patient.

16. Do not move the needle once you have inserted it. If the needle is pushed in further, contami-

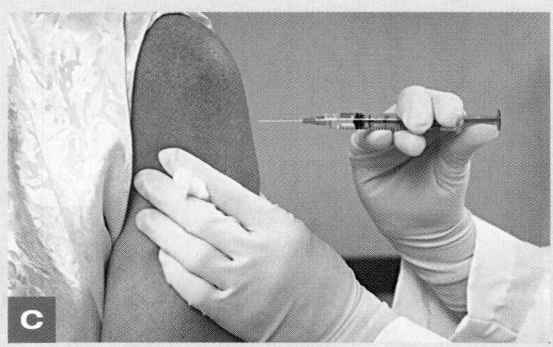
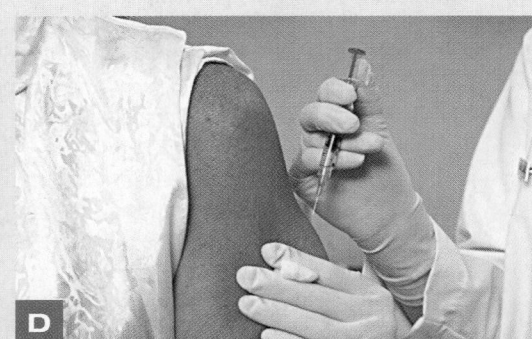
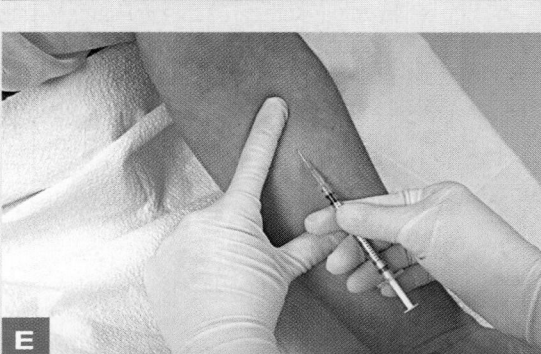
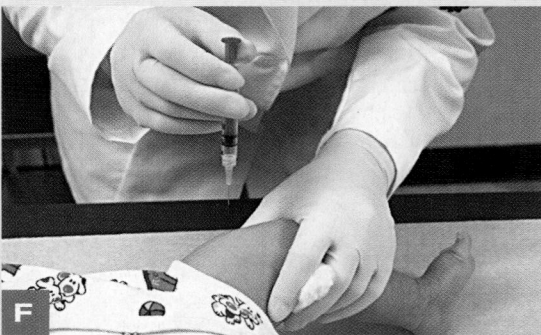

FIGURE 49-16 *(continued).*

nants are carried into the skin from the exposed needle.

17. Aspirate to determine if you have entered a blood vessel. To do this pull back slightly on the plunger with the hand holding the syringe while holding the needle steady in the muscle. If blood appears in the hub area of the syringe, it means that you are in a blood vessel. You will then have to withdraw the needle using correct technique and discard the syringe containing the blood and medication. Begin the procedure again with step 1 and fresh supplies.

    Rationale: You may not administer subcutaneous or intramuscular injection intravenously into a blood vessel.

18. If you do not see a return of blood in the syringe when you aspirate, slowly inject the medication without moving the needle. Do not move the needle until you have completed injecting all the medication. See Figure 49-17 for illustrations of intramuscular injection.

    Note: Insert and withdraw the needle quickly to minimize pain but administer the medication slowly.

19. Taking the alcohol sponge (or cotton ball) from between the last two fingers of your nondominant hand, place it over the area containing the needle. Withdraw the needle at the same angle you used for insertion using care not to stick yourself with the needle.

20. With one hand place the sponge firmly over the injection site. With the other hand discard the needle in a biohazard sharps container.

21. You may gently massage the injection site to assist absorption and ease pain for the patient.

22. Make sure the patient is safe before leaving him or her unattended. Observe the patient for any untoward effect of the medication for at least 15 minutes.

23. Correctly dispose of all materials.

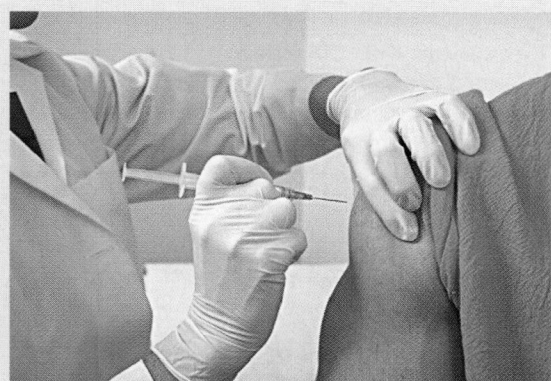

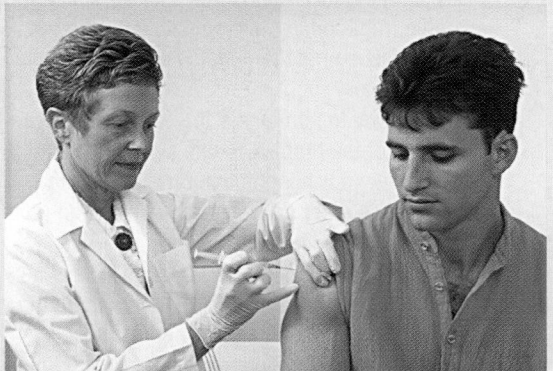

FIGURE 49-17 Intramuscular injections.

24. Remove gloves into a biohazard bag and wash your hands.

25. Chart the medication administration on the patient's record noting the time, medication name, dosage, injection site, route, lot number on the immunizations, and your name.

Charting Example

2/14/XX	1:30 P.M.	Penicillin G. procaine, 600,000 unit	IM Right gluteus.
			M. King, CMA

Administering of a Z-Track Injection

OBJECTIVE: Administer a Z-track injection using proper technique.

Equipment and Supplies
alcohol sponges; biohazard sharps container; biohazard waste container; disposable gloves; medication order signed by the physician; pen; sterile needle and syringe; medication vial

Method
Follow steps 1 through 15 of Procedure 49-6 for administration of an intramuscular injection.

16. After withdrawing the medication from the vial, change to a fresh needle. This will eliminate any irritating medication that may be within the needle from coming into contact with the patient's tissue until the needle is placed into the muscle layer.

17. When ready to administer the medication, pull the skin of the buttock to one side and hold it in place with your nondominant hand. You may wish to use a dry gauze sponge if the skin is slippery (Figure 49-18B).

18. With your dominant hand and using a dart-like grip on the syringe, insert the needle up to the hub quickly into the gluteus medius muscle. Do not move the needle once it is place (Figure 49-18C).

19. While still maintaining a firm hold on the taut skin with your nondominant hand, pull back on the plunger of the syringe to check for a blood return with the fingers of the hand holding the syringe. To do this simply move your fingers up the syringe, while keeping the needle steady within the patient's buttocks, until your thumb and index finger reach the top of the plunger. If blood appears in the hub of the syringe, then using correct technique, withdraw the syringe, discard, and begin with step 1 again.

20. If there is no return of blood, then very slowly inject the medication into the muscle.

21. Wait several seconds after injecting the medication before you withdraw the needle. Cover the area with the alcohol sponge and withdraw the needle at the same angle of insertion. Wait at least 10 seconds before releasing the skin being held by the nondominant hand (Figure 49-18D and E).

22. Do not massage the area. Observe the patient for at least 15 minutes for any untoward reaction. You may advise the patient to walk around to assist in the absorption process of the medication.

23. Correctly dispose of all materials.

24. Remove gloves and wash your hands.

25. Chart the medication administration on the patient's record noting the time, medication name, dosage, injection site, route, and your name.

Charting Example

2/14/XX	3:30 P.M.	Iron dextran, 50 mg Z-track into left gluteus. No C/O pain.
		N. Young, RMA

Z-Track Method

The Z-track method is used when a medication is irritating to the subcutaneous tissues or the medication may discolor the skin. When giving a medication using the Z-track method, you need to pull the skin to the side prior to inserting the needle. The pulling of the skin displaces the tissue; then you inject the medication, release the skin, and the medication will not be able to seep back to the skin's surface. (See Procedure 49-7 and Figure 49-18 on Z-track injections.)

Intradermal Injection

The intradermal injection is commonly used for allergy skin testing in which a minute amount of material is

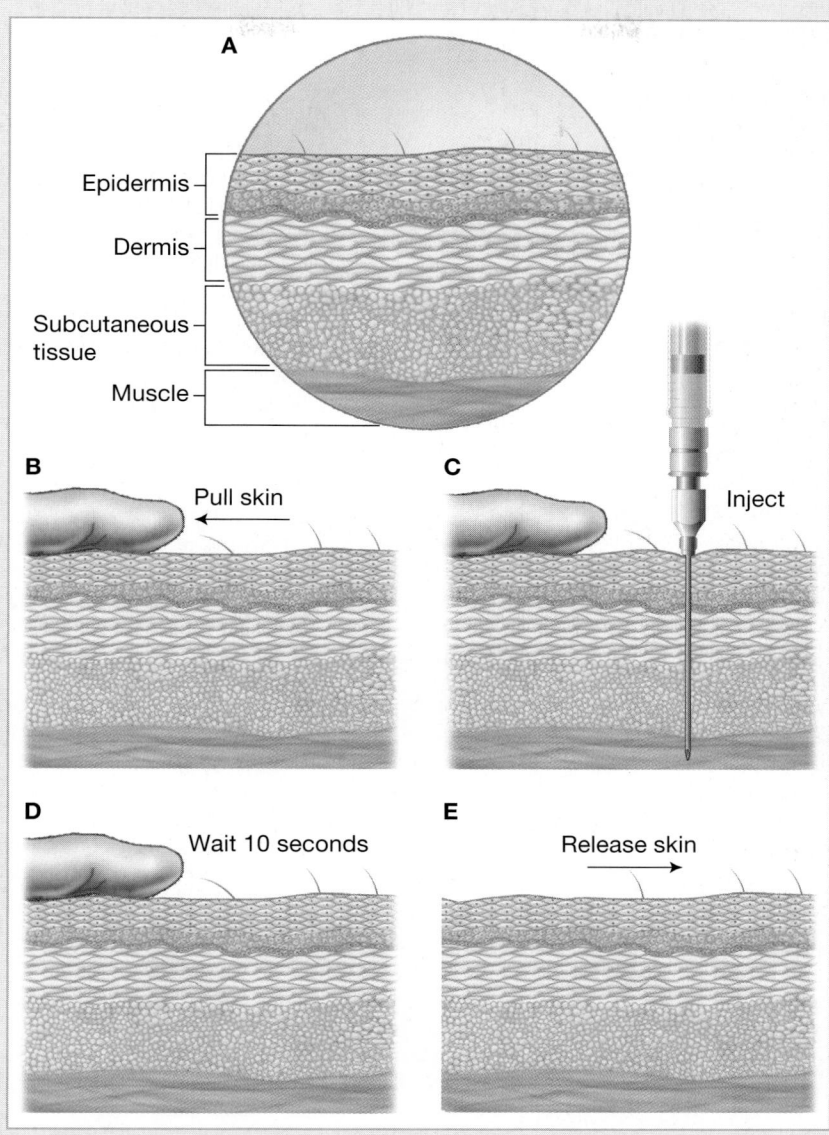

A

Epidermis –
Dermis –
Subcutaneous tissue –
Muscle –

B   Pull skin

C   Inject

D   Wait 10 seconds

E   Release skin

FIGURE 49-18   An example of the Z-track method of injection.

injected within the top layer of skin to determine a patient's sensitivity. Because just the top level of skin is entered, a small "wheal" or bubble that contains the injection fluid appears on the skin. Do not rub the area after giving the injection. (See Procedure 49-8 and Figures 49-19 and 49-20 for administration of an intradermal injection.)

Tuberculin Skin Test

A tuberculin skin test is done to see if a patient has ever had tuberculosis. A small amount of TB protein (antigens) is injected under the top layer of skin on the patient's inner forearm. If the person has ever been exposed to the TB bacteria, the skin will react to the

PROCEDURE

Administering an Intradermal Injection

OBJECTIVE: Administer an intradermal injection.

Equipment and Supplies

disposable gloves; hazardous waste container; alcohol sponges; sterile needle; sterile syringe; vial of medication; medication order signed by physician; pen

Method

I. Preparation

1. Perform hand hygiene.
2. Apply nonsterile gloves and follow universal blood and body fluid precautions.
3. Select the correct medication using the "three befores." Always double-check the label to make sure the strength is correct since medications are manufactured with different strengths, for example, 1:10, 1:100, or 1:1000 dilutions.
4. Gently roll the medication between your hands to mix any medication that may have settled. Refrigerated medication can be rolled between your hands to warm it slightly.
5. Prepare the syringe using the correct technique. Carefully carry the covered needle and syringe to the patient.
6. Identify the patient both by stating his or her name and examining any printed identification such as a wrist name band or medical record.
7. Select the proper site (center of forearm, upper chest or upper back). See Figure 49-19 for intradermal skin injection sites.

8. Using a circular motion, clean the patient's skin with an alcohol sponge. Wipe the skin with a sweeping motion from the center of the area outward. This prevents recontamination of the injection site by the alcohol sponge.
9. Allow time for the antiseptic on the sponge to dry to reduce the possibility of it reacting with the medication.
10. Once again check the medication dosage against the patient's order to determine if this is the correct time to administer the dose (one of the "ten rights").
11. Remove the protective covering from the needle using care not to touch the needle. If you accidentally touch the needle, then excuse yourself to the patient. Return to your preparation area and change the needle on the syringe. If you are using a self-contained syringe and needle unit that does not come apart, you will have to discard the entire syringe with the medication and start the process over again. (Remember: The patient's safety is your first priority. A contaminated needle can cause a severe infection in an already ill patient.)

II. Injection

12. Hold the syringe between the first two fingers and thumb of your dominant hand with the palm down and the bevel of the needle up. Figures 49-20A–F illustrate the steps used to administer an intradermal skin test.

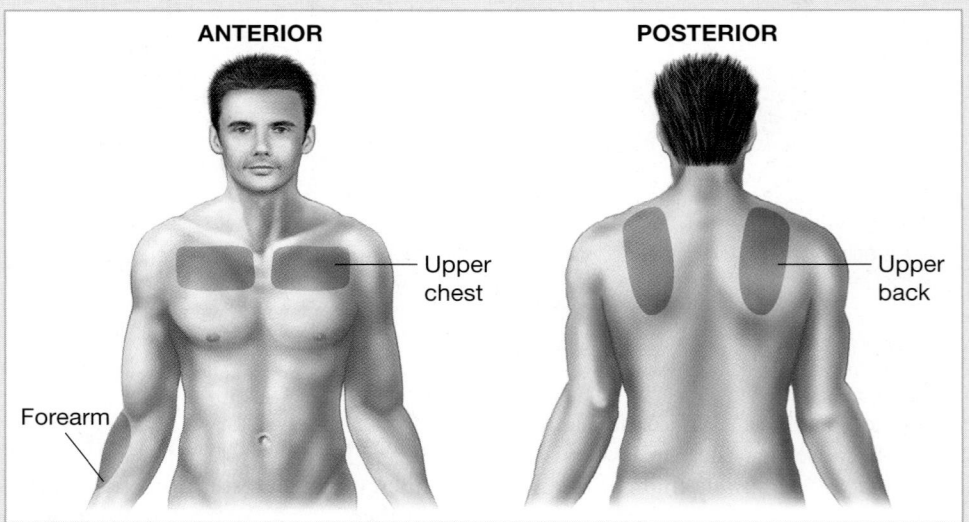

ANTERIOR   **POSTERIOR**

— Upper chest

— Upper back

Forearm

FIGURE 49-19 Intradermal skin injection sites.

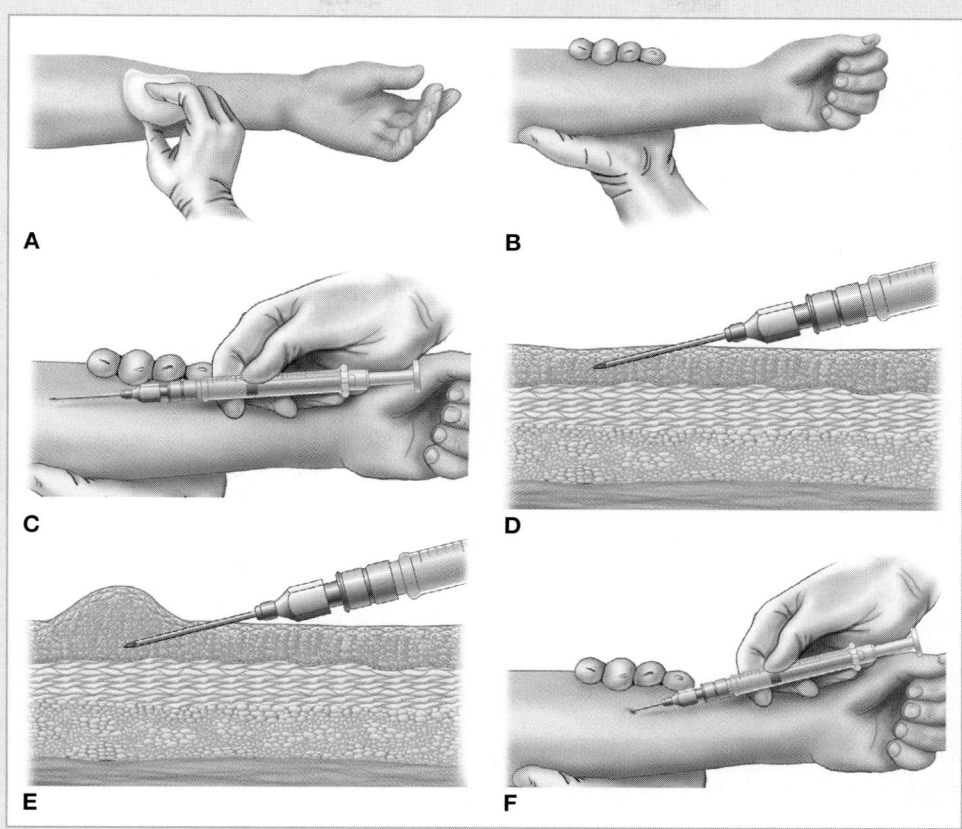

FIGURE 49-20 (A–F) Administering an intradermal skin test.

13. Hold the skin taut with the fingers of your nondominant hand. If you are using the center of the forearm, then place the nondominant hand under the patient's arm and pull the skin taut. This will allow the needle to slip into the skin more easily.

14. Using a 15-degree angle, insert the needle through the skin to about ⅛ inch. The bevel of the needle will be facing upward and covered with skin. The needle will still show through the skin. Do not aspirate.

15. Slowly inject the medication beneath the surface of the skin. A small elevation of skin (wheal) will occur where you have injected the medication.

16. Quickly withdraw the needle. With the other hand discard the needle into the biohazard sharps container.

III. Patient Follow-Up

17. Do not massage the area.

18. Make sure the patient is safe before leaving him or her unattended. Observe the patient for any untoward effect, such as an allergic reaction to the medication, for at least 20 to 30 minutes. Tell the patient not to rub the area.

19. Correctly dispose of all materials.

20. Remove gloves and wash your hands.

21. Chart the medication administration on the patient's record noting the time, medication name, dosage, injection site, route, appearance of the intradermal site after injection, and your name.

Charting Example

2/14/XX	10:00 A.M.	Mantoux (PPD) tuberculin test, 0.10 mLID

Right anterior forearm. Instructed to return on 2/16 to have test read.

M. King, CMA

antigens by developing a firm red bump at the site within 2 days. The test cannot tell if the infection is active or inactive (latent).

The PPD (purified protein derivative) skin test uses a measured amount of TB antigens in a shot that is put under the top layer of skin on the patient's forearm. A Mantoux test is a good test for a TB infection. It is often used when symptoms, screening, or testing, such as a chest x-ray, show that a person may have TB.

Before administering a tuberculin skin test, the medical assistant should ask the patient the following questions:

1. Have you experienced recent symptoms of TB, such as cough, night sweats, or weight loss for no reason?
2. Have you had a positive tuberculin skin test in the past?
3. Have you had TB in the past?
4. Have you experienced risk factors for TB, such as contact with a person or a health care worker with TB, or have you resided in a country where TB is common?
5. Have you recently been given a TB vaccination and, if so, were the results positive?
6. Have you been treated with medicines, such as corticosteroids, that may affect the immune system?
7. Have you been infected with the HIV virus?
8. Do you have a skin rash that may make it hard to read the skin test?

To perform a tuberculin skin test (see also Procedure 49-9), ask the patient to sit down and turn the inner side of his or her forearm up. The skin where the test is done should be cleansed and allowed to dry. Using a tuberculin syringe, a small injection of the TB antigen (PPD) is put under the top layer of skin. The fluid makes

PROCEDURE 49-9

Performing a Tuberculin Skin Test

OBJECTIVE: Perform a tuberculin skin test.

Equipment and Supplies
antiseptic cleaner; biohazard waste container; disposable tuberculin syringe with 26- or 27-gauge needle; disposable alcohol wipe; disposable gloves; PPD antigen; cotton balls

Method
1. Perform hand hygiene.
2. Apply gloves.
3. Assemble equipment and supplies.
4. Using the forearm, inject 0.1mL (5 Tuberculin Units) PPD antigen intradermally, keeping the bevel facing upward.
5. If a wheal of 6 to 10 mm is not produced, another test should be performed immediately on the same arm at a site at least 5 cm (2 inches) from the original site.
6. After administering the test, advise the patient not to rub or scratch the test site.
7. Using a cotton ball, gently dab the area lightly and wipe off any drops of blood that may occur. Do not put a bandage on the test site.
8. Inform the patient to return to the office in 2 to 3 days to read the test.
9. Document the test site in the patient's chart.
10. Discard the syringe/needle in the biohazard waste container.
11. Remove gloves and dispose of them correctly.
12. Clean work area and equipment according to OSHA guidelines.

a little bump (wheal) under the skin. A circle may be drawn around the test area with a pen. Do not cover the site with a bandage. Tell the patient that some redness at the skin site is expected and that the site may itch, but that it is important that it not be scratched, because scratching may cause redness or swelling that would make the test difficult to read. Instruct the patient to return to the office within 2 to 3 days after the test to have the skin test checked.

Test Results

Redness alone at the skin test site is a negative reaction. A firm bump is a positive reaction to the skin test. The size of the firm bump (not the red area) should be measured 2 to 3 days after the test to determine the result.

Although the medical assistant is responsible for reporting abnormal results (or positive results in the case of a TB skin test) to the physician, "interpreting" such tests as being positive or negative is *not* within the scope of practice for the medical assistant and, as such, never should be done. The medical assistant is only allowed to report the findings of "positive" or "negative."

Intravenous Therapy

Intravenous therapy is a process that involves administering fluids and solutions directly into a patient's vein. It can only be prescribed by a physician as either a continuous infusion or as a drip from a bottle or bag or as a single injection.

Continuous infusion means that the fluid must be running into the vein continuously. If the drip of the solution stops, the vein may form a small clot of blood. In this case the IV will have to be restarted. To prevent the patient from undergoing this procedure twice, it is wise to report any cessation of dripping immediately.

When the patient receives a single dosage via the intravenous route on a regular basis, a small needle with a port (opening), called a heparin lock, may be inserted into the patient's wrist area. This is sealed with a cap, and then taped in place. Each time the patient receives the medication, the cap is removed from the port and tubing inserted. Medication is administered through this tubing. In some cases the port opening contains a rubber/plastic stopper and a needle can be placed into the port for direct administration of the drug.

If a patient comes into the physician's office with an IV port in place, the medical assistant should be alert to changes at the IV site and report them to the physician at once. The following should be reported: redness, swelling, heat, bleeding, and loss of feeling at the site of the infusion.

Although medical assistants are not licensed to start intravenous infusions, in many states where they are certified and have had advanced training, they may be permitted to prepare the intravenous (IV) tray for administration of the IV fluids. These fluids may include blood and blood by-products, hydrating solutions that may be needed for hydrating the body or to prevent dehydration, isotonic solutions that are used to replace cellular fluids lost through blood loss, and maintenance solutions, which are used to replace electrolytes that may have been lost through diarrhea and vomiting.

Preparing the IV Tray

The most important point about setting up the IV tray is that the medical assistant must have been trained and possess the knowledge necessary to complete such a task (see Procedure 49-10). This involves understanding some of the possible side effects that intravenous therapy can cause, such as infections at the site of the needle; phlebitis, which is inflammation of the vein; and the most common side effect, infusion. An infusion occurs when the tip of the IV catheter withdraws from the vein or pokes through the vein into surrounding tissue, or when the vein's wall becomes permeable and leaks fluid. Infusion is frequently encountered with peripheral IVs, and almost always requires replacement of the IV at a different location. Other possible reactions that may occur during intravenous therapy include blood or drainage from the area of insertion, redness, pain or swelling in the area, blood backing up into the tubing, and the needle or tube coming loose or being removed by the patient.

Prior to preparing the IV tray, the medical assistant should make sure he or she carefully reads the facility's requirements for this procedure. Instructions for this procedure are frequently located in the office or hospital procedure manual. Once this has been completed, it is important to make sure that you check the doctor's order as to what IV fluid solution is required. When checking the order, remember to check for the following: It is the right patient, the right solution, the right drug, the right technique, and the right route. Also, make sure that the solution is properly labeled with the patient's name, the date and time of administration, and the name of the doctor who has ordered it. Once you have determined that you have the right solution, you will have to prepare the IV administration set. Most facilities have disposable IV administration sets that are ready for use. After you have completed setting up the IV administration set, along with your other supplies, they should all be placed on a separate IV or Mayo tray. Make sure you position the items in the order of their usage. Finally, after you have completed the tray setup, you should notify the health care member who is going to start the IV that the tray is ready for the patient.

Your role as a certified medical assistant is to assist the person starting the IV. This often includes not only

Preparing an Intravenous (IV) Tray

OBJECTIVE: Prepare an IV tray.

Equipment and Supplies

absorbent disposable sheet; alcohol prep pads; betadine swabs; disposable tourniquet; IV setup: IV tubing with attached filter; IV catheter; bag of IV fluid labeled with type and patient's name, date, time; paper tape; syringe; port cap; disposable gloves; gauze (2 × 2 or 4 × 4); IV setup tray; IV pole with pump

Method

1. Perform hand hygiene.
2. Apply gloves.
3. Prepare IV fluid administration set:
   - Inspect fluid bag to make sure it contains desired fluid, that fluid is clear, and that the bag is free from any leaks and has not expired.
   - Select correct administration set (either mini or macro drip) and uncoil the tubing, being careful that the ends of the tubing do not become contaminated.
   - Close flow regulator to the fluid bag.
   - Remove protective covering from the port of the fluid bag and the protective covering from the spike of the administration set.
   - Insert the spike of the administration set into the port of the fluid bag with a quick twisting motion, being careful not to puncture yourself.
   - While holding the fluid bag higher than the drip chamber of the administration set, squeeze the drip chamber once or twice in order to start the flow of the fluid. Fill the chamber to the marker line. If the chamber is overfilled, quickly lower the bag below the level of the drip chamber and squeeze some of the fluid back into the fluid bag.
   - Open the flow regulator and allow the fluid to flush all the air from the tubing. A trash can or the wrapper the fluid came in can be used for the overflow of fluid.
   - Turn off the flow and place the sterile cap back on the end of the administration set (if you had to remove it). Then place this end nearby so it can be easily reached by the person ready to connect it to the IV catheter in the patient's arm.
4. Place absorbent disposable sheet on tray.
5. Assemble equipment and supplies on tray in order of use.
6. If using an IV pole or pump, hang IV solution (bag) on the pole; do not set it up or calculate drops in the pump; this will be done by the person starting the IV.
7. Notify appropriate personnel (RN, LVN, physician) that IV tray setup is ready for administration.
8. Wash hands.
9. Document procedure.
10. Clean work area and equipment according to OSHA guidelines.

---

set up the IV tray, but also frequently involves being available to provide the patient with reassurance during the procedure. It also includes making sure that after the procedure has been completed, the patient and the area have been cleaned and that the equipment and supplies have been properly disposed. Most facilities only require that you document the procedure for setting the tray up. Documentation of the actual IV is done only by the person who has started the intravenous infusion.

The medical assistant will come into contact with patients who have intravenous therapy. These include patients in a clinic setting, homebound patients, or patients who receive chemotherapy on an outpatient basis.

Immunizations

Immunizations or vaccines are given to humans in order to decrease the susceptibility to disease. By becoming immunized the human body can resist the invasion of germs that can cause one to develop a disease. If an individual's immune system is compromised, then the individual is more at risk of becoming sick.

Antibodies are protein substances and are produced by lymphocytes in the spleen, lymph nodes and tissue, and the bone marrow. Antibodies react in response to antigens or foreign substances. The human body naturally produces antibodies. This process occurs when an individual develops an illness such as the measles.

During the process of being ill with the measles, the body begins to develop antibodies to fight off the disease. After the individual has recovered from the measles, the individual is less likely to contract the same strain of measles due to the fact that the body has developed antibodies to fight off this disease. When this occurs the individual is said to have developed immunity, or a resistance, to the disease.

Immunity can be either genetic or acquired. Antibodies are not involved when genetic immunity occurs. Acquired immunity, however, does involve the development of antibodies. This type of immunity may be either natural or artificial and may be acquired either through an active or passive means.

Artificial active immunity is the result of receiving vaccinations with inactive (dead) or attenuated (weakened) organisms. Through the delivery of immunizations and vaccines, an individual's body can be prepared to fight off a disease. For instance, the flu vaccine is given each year right before the flu season begins. Individuals who are more susceptible to contracting the flu, such as elderly adults, receive the flu vaccine. By receiving the flu vaccine, individuals are establishing an immunity in their bodies to the flu and are increasing their chances of being able to fight of the disease. Each year the Centers for Disease Control and Prevention (CDC) recommends that certain individuals receive the influenza vaccination. These individuals usually include:

- Persons aged ≥65 years with comorbid conditions
- Residents of long-term care facilities
- Persons aged 2–64 years with comorbid conditions
- Persons aged ≥65 years without comorbid conditions
- Children aged 6–23 months
- Pregnant women
- Health care personnel who provide direct patient care
- Household contacts and out-of-home caregivers of children aged <6 months.

Immunizations or vaccines are produced by taking a dead infectious agent of a disease and injecting it into the human body. Typically this creates no harm to the patient. Sometimes, an immunization or vaccine can cause an individual to experience some mild symptoms of the disease or to develop fever-like symptoms at the site of injection. For example, some children after receiving the diphtheria, tetanus, and pertussis vaccine (DTaP) will experience some redness and swelling where the injection was given. A fever may also be a temporary symptom. To learn more about the immune system refer to Chapter 26.

Childhood and Adolescent Immunizations

An annual recommended childhood and adolescent immunization schedule is issued each year by the American Academy of Pediatrics, the Advisory Committee on Immunization Practices of the CDC, and the American Academy of Family Physicians. The schedule indicates the recommended ages for routine administration of childhood vaccines (see Figure 49-21).

Hepatitis B Vaccine

Hepatitis B is caused by the hepatitis B virus (HBV) and is transmitted by contaminated serum in blood transfusions or through the use of contaminated needles or instruments. Hepatitis B is a form of viral hepatitis, is highly contagious, and can be fatal. By immunizing children the potential of this disease becoming an epidemic is minimized.

It is recommended that soon after birth all infants be given the first dose of hepatitis B. Only infants whose mother's hepatitis B surface antigen (HBsAg) is negative may be given the first dose by age 2 months. A child should receive a total of four doses of the vaccine. The last dose should not be given to the infant before age 24 weeks. When delivering the hepatitis B vaccine, special attention should be paid to the CDC's vaccination requirements for infants born to HBsAg-positive mothers or infants born to mothers whose HBsAg status is unknown.

Diphtheria Vaccine

The vaccine for diphtheria is given to children in five separate doses. The fifth dose is given between the age of 4 and 6 years. Diphtheria is an acute infectious disease. Transmission of diphtheria is by direct and indirect contact and is diagnosed by obtaining a throat culture. Individuals with diphtheria typically experience symptoms such as headache, fever, and sore throat. Diphtheria is treatable but can be quite serious.

Pertussis Vaccine

Pertussis, also known as whooping cough, is a respiratory disease that is most common in children under the age of 4 years. It is known as whooping cough due to one of the symptoms being a violent cough with a whooping sound. Pertussis is caused by bacteria and is transmitted by direct and indirect contact. Once a child is immunized with the pertussis vaccine the child is no longer susceptible to contracting this disease.

Tetanus Vaccine

Tetanus is a disease of the nervous system and is caused by a bacterium that enters the body through a break in the skin. Individuals with tetanus may experience fever, elevated blood pressure, and severe muscle spasms. Tetanus is not contagious and rarely occurs in individuals living in the United States. Occurrence of

Recommended Childhood and Adolescent Immunization Schedule

UNITED STATES • 2005

Vaccine ▼ / Age ►	Birth	1 month	2 months	4 months	6 months	12 months	15 months	18 months	24 months	4–6 years	11–12 years	13–18 years
Hepatitis B[1]	HepB #1	HepB #2			HepB #3					HepB Series		
Diphtheria, Tetanus, Pertussis[2]			DTaP	DTaP	DTaP		DTaP			DTaP	Td	Td
Haemophilus influenzae type b[3]			Hib	Hib	Hib	Hib						
Inactivated Poliovirus			IPV	IPV		IPV				IPV		
Measles, Mumps, Rubella[4]						MMR #1				MMR #2	MMR #2	
Varicella[5]						Varicella					Varicella	
Pneumococcal[6]			PCV	PCV	PCV	PCV				PCV	PPV	
Influenza[7]					Influenza (Yearly)					Influenza (Yearly)		
Hepatitis A[8]										Hepatitis A Series		

Vaccines below red line are for selected populations

This schedule indicates the recommended ages for routine administration of currently licensed childhood vaccines, as of December 1, 2004, for children through age 18 years. Any dose not given at the recommended age should be given at any subsequent visit when indicated and feasible.

 Indicates age groups that warrant special effort to administer those vaccines not previously given. Additional vaccines may be licensed and recommended during the year. Licensed combination vaccines may be used whenever any components of the combination are indicated and the vaccine's other components are not contraindicated. Providers should consult the manufacturers' package inserts for detailed recommendations. Clinically significant adverse events that follow immunization should be reported to the Vaccine Adverse Event Reporting System (VAERS). Guidance about how to obtain and complete a VAERS form can be found on the Internet: **www.vaers.org** or by calling **800-822-7967**.

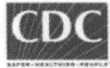

Range of recommended ages
Preadolescent assessment
Only if mother HBsAg(−)
Catch-up immunization

The Childhood and Adolescent Immunization Schedule is approved by:
Advisory Committee on Immunization Practices www.cdc.gov/nip/acip
American Academy of Pediatrics www.aap.org
American Academy of Family Physicians www.aafp.org

DEPARTMENT OF HEALTH AND HUMAN SERVICES
CENTERS FOR DISEASE CONTROL AND PREVENTION

CDC

Footnotes
Recommended Childhood and Adolescent Immunization Schedule
UNITED STATES • 2005

1. **Hepatitis B(HepB) vaccine.** All infants should receive the first dose of hepatitis B vaccine soon after birth and before hospital discharge; the first dose may also be given by age 2 months if the infant's mother is hepatitis B surface antigen (HBsAg) negative. Only monovalent HepB can be used for the birth dose. Monovalent or combination vaccine containing HepB may be used to complete the series. Four doses of vaccine may be administered when a birth dose is given. The second dose should be given at least 4 weeks after the first dose, except for combination vaccines which cannot be administered before age 6 weeks. The third dose should be given at least 16 weeks after the first dose and at least 8 weeks after the second dose. The first dose in the vaccination series (third or fourth dose) should not be administered before age 24 weeks.

   Infants born to HBsAg-positive mothers should receive HepB and 0.5 mL of Hepatitis B Immune Globulin (BHIG) within 12 hours of birth at separate sites. The second dose is recommended at age 1–2 months. The last dose in the immunization series should not be administered before age 24 weeks. These infants should be tested for BHsAg and antibody to HBsAg (anti-HBs) at age 9–15 months.

   Infants born to mothers whose HBsAg status is unknown should receive the first dose of the HepB series within 12 hours of birth. Maternal blood should be drawn as soon as possible to determine the mother's HBsAg status; if the HBsAg test is positive, the infant should receive HBIG as soon as possible (no later than age 1 week). The second dose is recommended at age 1–2 months. The last dose in the immunization series should not be administered before age 24 weeks.

2. **Diphtheria and tetanus toxoids and acellular pertussis (DTaP) vaccine.** The fourth dose of DTaP may be administered as early as age 12 months, provided 6 months have elapsed since the third dose and the child is unlikely to return at age 15–18 months. The final dose in the series should be given at age ≥4 years. **Tetanus and diphtheria toxoids (Td)** is recommended at age 11–12 years if at least 5 years have elapsed since the last dose of tetanus and diphtheria toxoid-containing vaccine. Subsequent routine Td boosters are recommended every 10 years.

3. *Haemophilus influenzae* **type b (Hib) conjugate vaccine.** Three Hib conjugate vaccines are licensed for infant use. If PRP-OMP (PedvaxHIB or ComVax [Merck] is administered at ages 2 and 4 months, a dose at age 6 months is not required. DTaP/Hib combination products should not be used for primary immunization in infants at ages 2, 4 or 6 months but can be used as boosters following any Hib vaccine. The final dose in the series should be given at age ≥12 months.

4. **Measles, mumps, and rubella vaccine (MMR).** The second dose of MMR is recommended routinely at age 4–6 years but may be administered during any visit, provided at least 4 weeks have elapsed since the first dose and both doses are administered beginning at or after age 12 months. Those who have not previously received the second dose should complete the schedule by the visit at age 11–12 years.

5. **Varicella vaccine.** Varicella vaccine is recommended at any visit at or after age 12 months for susceptible children (i.e., those who lack a reliable history of chickenpox). Susceptible persons aged ≥13 years should receive 2 doses, given at least 4 weeks apart.

6. **Pneumococcal vaccine.** The heptavalent **pneumococcal conjugate vaccine (PCV)** is recommended for all children aged 2–23 months. It is also recommended for certain children aged 24–59 months. The final dose in the series should be given at age ≥12 months. **Pneumococcal polysaccharide vaccine (PPV)** is recommended in addition to PCV for certain high-risk groups. See *MMWR* 2000;49(RR-9):1–35.

7. **Influenza vaccine.** Influenza vaccine is recommended annually for children aged ≥6 months with certain risk factors (including but not limited to asthma, cardiac disease, sickle cell disease, HIV, and diabetes), healthcare workers, and other persons (including household members) in close contact with persons in groups at high risk (see *MMWR* 2004;53[RR-6]:1–40) and can be administered to all others wishing to obtain immunity. In addition, healthy children aged 6–23 months and close contacts of healthy children aged 0–23 months are recommended to receive influenza vaccine, because children in this age group are at substantially increased risk for influenza-related hospitalizations. For healthy persons aged 5–49 years, the intranasally administered live, attenuated influenza vaccine (LAIV) is an acceptable alternative to the intramuscular trivalent inactivated influenza vaccine (TIV). See *MMWR* 2004;53(RR-6):1–40. Children receiving TIV should be administered a dosage appropriate for their age (0.25 mL if 6–35 months or 0.5 mL if ≥3 years). Children aged ≤8 years who are receiving influenza vaccine for the first time should receive 2 doses (separated by at least 4 weeks for TIV and at least 6 weeks for LAIV).

8. **Hepatitis A vaccine.** Hepatitis A vaccine is recommended for children and adolescents in selected states and regions and for certain high-risk groups; consult your local public health authority. Children and adolescents in these states, regions, and high-risk groups who have not been immunized against hepatitis A can begin the hepatitis A immunization series during any visit. The 2 doses in the series should be administered at least 6 months apart. See *MMWR* 1999;48(RR-12):1–37.

FIGURE 49-21 Recommended childhood and adolescent immunization schedule.

death with tetanus is low but can occur in people over the age of 60.

DTaP VACCINE When children receive a vaccine for tetanus it is usually given in a combination vaccine of diphtheria, tetanus, and pertussis also known as the DTaP vaccine. Five DTaP shorts are required to fully protect a child. The last booster is given between the age of 4 and 6 years. If a child has a reaction to the first dose of DTaP, the child will then, depending on age, be given the Td vaccine or the DT vaccine. The Td vaccine does not contain pertussis vaccine and contains less diphtheria toxoid than what is contained in the DTaP vaccine. The DT vaccine, which contains diphtheria and tetanus toxoids but no pertussis, may be given to children who have a reaction to their first dose of the DTaP vaccine. The Td vaccine is given to children 7 years and older, and the DT vaccine is given to children under the age of 7.

Haemophilus Influenzae Type B (Hib) Conjugate Vaccine

Although the Hib disease is not well known, a recent statistic from the CDC indicated that 1 out of every 200 children in the United States under the age of 5 contracts Hib. Meningitis, which is a result of Hib, affects about 12,000 children a year. Hib is caused by a bacterium and is spread through the air and enters the lungs or bloodstream. The Hib vaccine became available in 1985 and since then the cases of Hib disease have decreased dramatically.

Measles, Mumps, and Rubella Vaccine (MMR)

The measles, mumps, and rubella (MMR) vaccine is given to children to protect them from developing measles, mumps, and rubella. Once a child is given the one-time shot of MMR the child is protected for life. The MMR is given in two doses. If necessary the vaccines for measles, mumps, and rubella can also be given separately.

Due to the MMR vaccine very few children contract these diseases. A virus causes measles, and prior to development of the measles vaccine almost all children came down with the measles. Measles is extremely serious and can result in brain damage, deafness, or death. Mumps was also a very common childhood disease prior to the development of the vaccine. Mumps is not as serious a disease as the measles, but could result in some undesired side effects including meningitis, encephalitis, and deafness. Rubella, also known as German measles or 3-day measles, is typically a mild disease that affects an individual for about 24 hours. Rubella is caused by a virus and is spread through close contact. Rubella can strike adults and unborn children. Unborn babies can be infected if the woman gets rubella early in the pregnancy. If a pregnant woman does have rubella, there is a high probably that the in-

fant will be born with birth defects. Since the development of the rubella vaccine, only several hundred cases are reported each year.

Varicella Vaccine

Varicella, or chickenpox, is probably one of the most common childhood diseases. Chickenpox, named this due to the blisters that look like chickpeas, is caused by a virus and is spread through the air. Chickenpox, although an uncomfortable disease, is usually not serious. The varicella vaccine became licensed in the United States in 1995 and since then the number of varicella cases has significantly diminished. Although the vaccine has not eradicated the disease, it has dramatically lowered the percentage of individuals infected by this disease.

Pneumococcal Vaccine

The pneumococcal vaccine, until very recently, was not licensed for children under the age of 2. Typically older adults have received this vaccine to protect them from contracting the streptococcus pneumonia bacteria. According to the CDC, this bacteria kills more people in the United States each year than any other vaccine-preventable disease. By obtaining the vaccine, individuals are protected against the seven strains of the pneumococcal bacterium. The pneumococcal bacteria are spread through the air. Winter and early spring are the most common seasons when pneumococcal infections occur.

Hepatitis A Vaccine

Hepatitis A, which is caused by a virus, is the most common type of hepatitis in the United States. Hepatitis A affects the liver but does not cause long-term effects. It is spread through personal contact or by eating contaminated food or drinking contaminated water. The vaccine is given to children 2 years old or older to prevent the risk of contracting hepatitis A. It is recommended that children who live in Alaska, Arizona, and Oregon should receive the vaccine. Individuals who travel to other countries are also encouraged to obtain this vaccine.

Professionalism

There will be regular visits from pharmaceutical representatives in any medical office. These professionals have two goals: to educate the physician about the pharmaceuticals their company sells, and to convince the physician to prescribe their medications. This proves to be a double-edged sword. It is important that the reps, at some point, be able to present their information to the physician because new research is important to the physician, but there must be set rules so that the physician does not get overrun by the reps and cannot see patients. It may fall to the medical assistant to acquire information on the medications for the physician. Always treat pharmaceutical representatives as professionals, but be sure to explain the policies of the office regarding visits by representatives. The medical assistant can offer to take information for the physician, and check the supply of samples. However, the physician must sign for any medication samples left at the office.

Poliovirus

Since 1955 the polio vaccine has been available, resulting in the disappearance of the disease in the United States. Polio though is still common in some parts of the world. A polio epidemic could appear in the United States due to individuals bringing in the disease from another country. Due to this fact, it is important that children even in the United States be immunized. Polio is caused by a virus and is spread through contact with the feces of an infected person. Although paralysis is not a result for all individuals who contract polio, it is an event that does affect some children.

There are two types of polio vaccines: inactivated polio vaccine (IPV) and live oral polio vaccine (OPV). For many years children received the polio vaccine orally (OPV) rather than by injection (IPV). Due to the fact that the oral polio vaccine was found in rare situations to cause polio in children, it is now recommended that all children receive the polio vaccine by injection.

Adult and Other Immunizations

In addition to the influenza vaccination, adults 65 years of age and older should receive the pneumococcal polysaccharide vaccine (PPV).

Adults and children who travel abroad must also be aware of additional vaccines or immunizations that must be obtained prior to travel. The CDC recommends certain vaccinations and preventive medications for travel. The recommendations are divided by the region of travel. For instance, if one were to travel to South Asia, vaccine and medication recommendations would include hepatitis A, hepatitis B, malaria, and typhoid.

Reconstituting a Powdered Medication for Administration

Some medications are supplied in a powdered or dry form. To be injected, these powdered medications

---

49-11 **PROCEDURE**

Reconstituting a Powdered Medication for Administration

OBJECTIVE: Reconstitute a powdered medication.

Equipment and Supplies
alcohol swab; disposable gloves; medication label; medication order signed by physician; pen; sterile needle; sharps container; vial of medication

Method
1. Remove the top from the powder medication and the top from the diluent, then wipe both tops with an alcohol swab.
2. Insert a sterile needle through the rubber stopper on the vial of diluent.
3. Withdraw the appropriate amount of diluent and add to the powder medication.
4. Remove needle from vial and discard in sharps container.
5. To ensure that the medication is mixed well, roll the vial between the palm of your hand.
6. Label the mixed vial with strength of medication prepared, time and date, your initials, and expiration date.
7. Administer the medication to the patient as directed.

must be reconstituted with a diluent, usually sterile water. Once the diluent is added to the powder and mixed well, the appropriate dose is drawn up and administered to the patient. To reconstitute a powdered medication, see Procedure 49-11.

Charting Medications

Parenteral medications are charted using the same documentation as for oral medications: name of medication, dosage, route, date, site, and signature of person administering the medication. It is also necessary to document that you have provided instructions to the patient regarding follow-up care. Examples of charting follow:

9/10/XX	9:00 A.M.	nitroglycerin, 1 tab, sublingually.

Written instructions given to pt. Precautions explained. Told to call progress in to office at 1:00 P.M. today.

M. Richards, CMA

1/19/XX	11:00 A.M.	Monistat-3, 200 mg. Vaginal. PT.

Given written instructions for follow-up care.

M. Richards, CMA

10/10/XX	1:00 P.M.	Mantoux test, 0.01 mL.

Tuberculin Purified Protein Derivative, L forearm, subq., small wheal noted. Pt. instructed not to rub or cover the area and to return for reading in 48 hours.

M. Richards, CMA

SUMMARY

Administering a medication is one of the medical assistant's most important duties and responsibilities. When administering medications the medical assistant is expected to be knowledgeable about the medication and its side effects. Medications come in many forms including oral, parenteral, and inhalants. Medications are always given under the supervision of the physician. The physician must be physically present within the facility at the time that the medical assistant dispenses the medication.

When administering medications the medical assistant must always observe the "three befores" and the "ten rights." Although errors rarely occur, if an error does occur notice must be given immediately to a supervisor so that the situation can be handled quickly for the safety and well-being of the patient.

Chapter Review

COMPETENCY REVIEW

1. Define and spell the terms to learn for this chapter.
2. What are the ten rights of drug administration?
3. What would you do if you see a small amount of blood appear in the plunger of a syringe as you withdraw the plunger?
4. What is the process for giving an oral medication?

PREPARING FOR THE CERTIFICATION EXAM

1. When administering oral or sublingual medication
   A. assemble all of the equipment and use aseptic technique
   B. select the correct medication using the "three befores"
   C. double-check the label on the medication
   D. A and B
   E. all of the above

2. When giving parenteral medication, a smaller gauge needle is used for which type of injection?
   A. intramuscular
   B. Z-track
   C. subcutaneous
   D. intradermal
   E. intravenous

continued on next page

3. Because the entire needle, up to the hub, must go into the patient, what length needle should be used for an intradermal injection?
   A. ⅜ inch
   B. ⅘ inch
   C. ⅝ inch
   D. ⅚ inch
   E. 1 inch

4. Which site, because there are fewer major blood vessels, is considered the safest for an intramuscular injection?
   A. vastus lateralis
   B. deltoid
   C. dorsogluteal
   D. ventrogluteal
   E. gluteus medius

5. Which of the following is NOT a common site for intradermal injections?
   A. forearm
   B. anterior chest
   C. upper back
   D. abdomen
   E. all of the above

6. Which of the following is NOT a common site for subcutaneous injections?
   A. upper outer arm
   B. subscapular portion
   C. anterior thigh
   D. abdomen of back
   E. anterior chest

7. Which is the preferred location for intramuscular injections on a toddler?
   A. deltoid
   B. vastus lateralis
   C. gluteus medius
   D. gluteus maximus
   E. biceps

8. The Z-track method is only used for injections into the:
   A. deltoid
   B. gluteus medius
   C. vastus lateralis
   D. dorsogluteal
   E. adipose tissue

9. A tuberculosis test has to be read within how many hours after being administered?
   A. 12 hours
   B. 24 hours
   C. 48 hours
   D. 36 hours
   E. 16 hours

10. A subcutaneous injection is usually given at what degree of angle?
    A. 15 degrees
    B. 90 degrees
    C. 45 degrees
    D. 10 degrees
    E. 30 degrees

CRITICAL THINKING

1. How should Latoya proceed in order to follow Dr. Reed's instructions?
2. Since the boy's baby-sitter has brought him to the office and is in charge of his care, must Latoya still obtain parental permission before administering the Compazine?
3. Because the child is extremely anxious and upset, should Latoya ask another medical assistant to help administer the medication or might this further alarm the child?
4. Does the prescribed dosage of Compazine seem like the proper one given the child's age and weight?

ON THE JOB

Mrs. Conners comes into Dr. Tyler's office to be seen for a sore throat and fever. The examination reveals that Mrs. Conners has tonsillitis. Dr. Tyler writes an order in the patient's chart for an injection of antibiotic to be given today. The patient is also given a prescription for an oral antibiotic to be taken for the next 10 days.

Joe, the medical assistant, while administering the injection to Mrs. Conners, accidentally punctures his finger with the dirty needle.

What is your response?

1. What should Joe do?
2. Is an incident report necessary?
3. If an incident report is filed, where should it be placed?

INTERNET ACTIVITY

Choose three common drugs and perform searches to get information about them. Select nationally recognized websites that you know you can access again when seeking information for patients.

 MediaLink More on administering medications, including interactive resources, can be found on the Student CD-ROM accompanying this textbook.

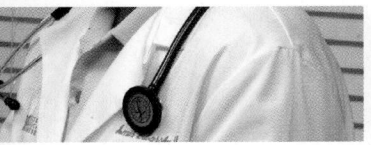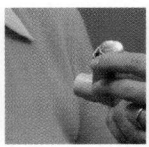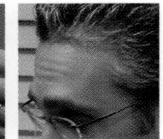

Medical Assistant Role Delineation Chart

HIGHLIGHT indicates material covered in this chapter.

ADMINISTRATIVE

Administrative Procedures

- Perform basic administrative medical assisting functions
- Schedule, coordinate and monitor appointments
- Schedule inpatient/outpatient admissions and procedures
- Understand and apply third-party guidelines
- Obtain reimbursement through accurate claims submission
- Monitor third-party reimbursement
- Understand and adhere to managed care policies and procedures
- *Negotiate managed care contracts*

Practice Finances

- Perform procedural and diagnostic coding
- Apply bookkeeping principles

- Manage accounts receivable
- *Manage accounts payable*
- *Process payroll*
- *Document and maintain accounting and banking records*
- *Develop and maintain fee schedules*
- *Manage renewals of business and professional insurance policies*
- *Manage personnel benefits and maintain records*
- *Perform marketing, financial, and strategic planning*

CLINICAL

Fundamental Principles

- Apply principles of aseptic technique and infection control
- Comply with quality assurance practices
- Screen and follow up patient test results

Diagnostic Orders

- Collect and process specimens
- Perform diagnostic tests

Patient Care

- Adhere to established patient screening procedures
- Obtain patient history and vital signs
- Prepare and maintain examination and treatment areas
- Prepare patient for examinations, procedures and treatments

- Assist with examinations, procedures and treatments
- Prepare and administer medications and immunizations
- Maintain medication and immunization records
- Recognize and respond to emergencies
- Coordinate patient care information with other health care providers
- Initiate IV and administer IV medications with appropriate training and as permitted by state law

GENERAL

Professionalism

- Display a professional manner and image
- Demonstrate initiative and responsibility
- Work as a member of the health care team
- Prioritize and perform multiple tasks
- Adapt to change
- Promote the CMA credential
- Enhance skills through continuing education
- Treat all patients with compassion and empathy
- Promote the practice through positive public relations

Communication Skills

- Recognize and respect cultural diversity
- Adapt communications to individual's ability to understand
- Use professional telephone technique

- Recognize and respond effectively to verbal, nonverbal, and written communications
- Use medical terminology appropriately
- Utilize electronic technology to receive, organize, prioritize and transmit information
- Serve as liaison

Legal Concepts

- Perform within legal and ethical boundaries
- Prepare and maintain medical records
- Document accurately
- Follow employer's established policies dealing with the health care contract
- Implement and maintain federal and state health care legislation and regulations
- Comply with established risk management and safety procedures
- Recognize professional credentialing criteria
- *Develop and maintain personnel, policy and procedure manuals*

Instruction

- Instruct individuals according to their needs
- Explain office policies and procedures
- Teach methods of health promotion and disease prevention
- Locate community resources and disseminate information
- *Develop educational materials*
- *Conduct continuing education activities*

Operational Functions

- Perform inventory of supplies and equipment
- Perform routine maintenance of administrative and clinical equipment
- Apply computer techniques to support office operations
- *Perform personnel management functions*
- *Negotiate leases and prices for equipment and supply contracts*

- *Denotes advanced skills.*

SOURCE: Reprinted by permission of the American Association of Medical Assistants from the AAMA Role Delineation Study: Occupational Analysis of the Medical Assisting Profession.

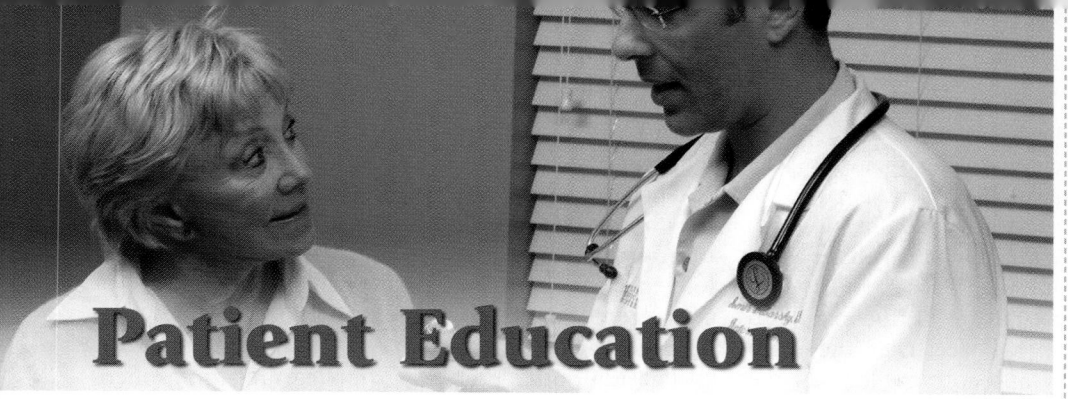

Patient Education

Learning Objectives

After completing this chapter, you should be able to:

- Define and spell the terms to learn for this chapter.
- List and describe five methods that help adults learn.
- State 15 teaching methods and strategies to use for patient education.
- Discuss 12 tips for clear writing.
- Describe the four changes that take place as people age.
- Describe the process used when developing a teaching plan.
- Discuss some of the reasons for noncompliance with patient education.

- Describe how you would adapt education for culturally based needs.
- Discuss how you would adapt education for patients with hearing impairments, patients who don't see well, or those who do not speak English.
- Create a public relations brochure for the office.
- Discuss cast application, care, and removal.

OUTLINE

Patient Education   1082

Developing a Teaching
Plan   1089

Teaching Patients
with Disabilities   1089

Handling Noncompliance   1091

Teaching about Cast
Care   1091

Terms to Learn

dexterity   learning outcomes   noncompliance

Case Study

MR. ALBERT YOUNG IS A 70-YEAR-OLD MAN with a history of colon cancer. Dr. Luo has asked that a teaching plan be developed for him regarding his colostomy care. Of special interest is that Mr. Young's wife (also a patient of Dr. Luo's) is recovering from a stroke and has had frequent *E. coli* infections of a leg wound. Dr. Luo is concerned that Mr. Young has been contaminating his wife's leg wound with the *E. coli* when changing her dressing.

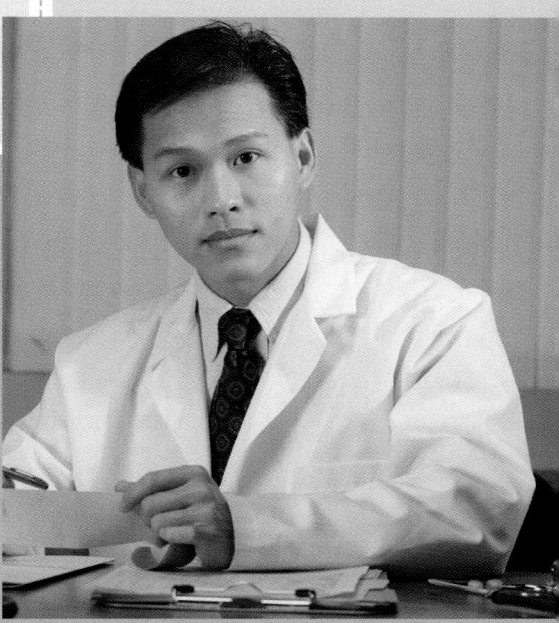

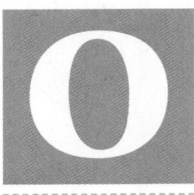ne of the rights patients have is to receive instructions on how they can manage their own health needs. The medical assistant is often the person of choice to provide patient education. Patients become familiar with the medical assistant who escorts them into the exam room, is often present during the examination process, and whom they will see when the exam is complete. This familiarity and comfort level of the patient assists in the learning process.

Patient Education

Most of the patients you will be teaching will be adults. If children need instruction, their parents should be present so they can reinforce the teaching, although communication needs to be adapted to the learner's level of comprehension. Most patient education concepts apply to both the child and adult learner. Some specific learning concepts, however, relate to the adult based on language skills, previous experience, and motivation.

How Adults Learn

Adult learning is an active process and adults prefer to participate actively. Therefore, activities and techniques that call for participation, such as role-playing, will achieve more learning faster than those that do not. For example, a lecture is not as useful as role-playing for patient learning.

Learning must be self-directed for adults. Therefore, the clearer and more relevant the statement of desired learning outcomes, the more learning that will take place. Learning outcomes are the goals of the patient education. They are what the patient should achieve as a result of the teaching. In health care settings, the patient must be taught the advantages of healthy lifestyles and how to achieve their goals. Practical application of learning is desired by most adult learners. Any learning that is applied immediately by the patient is retained longer. For instructions on creating a community resource brochure and a public relations brochure see Procedures 50-1 and 50-2.

The adult often prefers a group learning atmosphere because of the mutual support a group setting offers. In order for learning to be effective, it must be reinforced. This can be done either through the group or by the teacher. Weight loss centers have used this technique effectively by announcing successful weight loss to others in a group meeting.

Learning new material is facilitated when it is reinforced by material that is already known. For instance, when instructing a new colostomy patient on the necessity for meticulous hand washing before and after handling the colostomy material, it is important to build on the patient's previous knowledge of hand washing.

Motivational incentives for adult learners are better health, improved appearance, pride of accomplishment, self-confidence, and praise from others. In addition to frequent praise, the adult learner learns more rapidly when he or she is made aware of progress. The time an adult spends on learning is related to many factors, including:

- Number of years spent in school
- Reading level
- Use of vocabulary
- Satisfaction with previous attempts to learn
- Health status of family member

50-1 PROCEDURE

Creating a Community Resource Brochure

OBJECTIVE: Create a brochure that educates a patient about available community resources.

Equipment and Supplies
computer, printer, pen, phone book, newspaper, stapler

Method
1. Identify one community resource that is available to help patients with disease prevention or health promotion, by using a phone book, newspaper, or website.
2. Create a brochure for distribution to patients that includes the name, location, phone number, and services offered by the resource.
3. Distribute brochures in the office waiting room.

Creating a Public Relations Brochure

OBJECTIVE: Promote the office by creating a brochure for distribution to current and potential patients.

Equipment and Supplies
computer, pen, stapler

Method
1. Gather the necessary data and create a brochure to advertise your office. Be sure to include the following:
   - Office name (e.g., Virginia Adult and Pediatric Allergy Clinic)
   - Type of practice (e.g., dermatology)
   - Office hours

- Office address
- Names and information about physicians
- Insurance plans accepted
- Payment expectations (e.g., copayments are expected before visit begins; all methods of payment are acceptable except cash)
- Emergency management procedures (e.g. after hours, contact the answering service at 703-555-1234)

2. Have the brochure printed and distribute it to patients.

Teaching Methods and Strategy

A combination of teaching techniques should be used for patient education rather than just one. For example, when instructing a newly diagnosed diabetic patient, a combination of brief lecture, models of anatomical sites for injections, demonstration of the injection procedure, use of printed handouts, diagrams of injection site rotation, and videos might all be used at different points in the educational process.

Using language and communication skills that are not suited to the learner creates roadblocks to effective patient learning (see Legal and Ethical Issues). Some roadblocks to effective patient learning are:

- Ordering, commanding, and directing the patient to learn
- Warning or threatening

Legal and Ethical Issues

You need to be able to communicate with your patients, especially in order to get truly informed consent about certain procedures. A responsible office will hire a medical assistant or physician with good foreign language skills or a medical interpreter to ensure patient understanding and compliance.

- Moralizing or preaching ("ought to do," "should do")
- Judging
- Criticizing
- Name calling, stereotyping, labeling
- Sarcasm
- Anxiety
- Culturally inappropriate treatment plans
- Speaking loudly to a blind person
- Age-inappropriate speech

Culture influences learning and can affect readiness, values, feelings of inclusion, what aspect of learning the patients choose, and how they apply it in their own homes (see also Cultural Considerations and Professionalism). Use of personal space, distances maintained, facial expressions, body movements, gestures, and expressions can be misinterpreted in certain cultures and need to be considered when educating a patient. Based on the developmental stage of the child, patient education should be modified to reach that child. A good example would be the importance of teaching a child with asthma to use a nebulizer properly. The approach would need significant modification from the approach used to teach an adult.

Attitudes and illness have a powerful impact on learning readiness. Women and higher educated people have an increased interest in learning, whereas men or less traditionally educated adults are marginalized learners for reasons of race, ethnicity, or class. They may distrust education due to previous negative

Tips for Clear Writing

1. Begin the material with a short introduction to state the purpose and to orient the reader.
2. Use titles and headings that clearly define the topics.
3. Use boldface, italics, or underlining to emphasize important words and ideas.
4. Use a summary paragraph to end a section or recap a point.
5. Use one important idea per paragraph.
6. Start each paragraph with a strong topic sentence.
7. Vary the length of sentences.
8. Use frequent examples to clarify ideas with which the reader may not have had experience.
9. Use active rather than passive voice.
10. Avoid polysyllabic words whenever possible. Use shorter words.
11. Avoid using a specialized vocabulary such as medical terminology.
12. Avoid abbreviations except when commonly understood.

experiences. In addition, illness affects an individual in different ways; fatigue and pain can be obstacles to learning. It is important to create a learning environment that encourages patient readiness. Consider rescheduling the session if the patient is not feeling well at the time.

Table 50-1 describes several teaching methods that can be used effectively for adults and children. As mentioned earlier, a combination of methods may prove useful. Box 50-1 provides and extensive list of tips on how to prepare printed material that is easy for patients to read. Guidelines 50-1 provides additional means for

50-1 GUIDELINES   Effective Health Instruction

1. Always address the patient by name. Do not use the patient's first name unless you have asked permission to do so.
2. Be well organized. Have all materials, models, and brochures together so that you will not have to leave the patient during the education process.
3. Have either a verbal or written order from the physician for teaching medical procedures, such as self-injection.
4. Assume the patient can learn. Do not equate intelligence level with educational level. Avoid talking down to patients.
5. Write or print instructions large enough to be clearly read by the patient.
6. Do not overwhelm the patient with technicalities. The patient does not have to know everything you know.
7. Do not use medical abbreviations when discussing medical procedures or conditions with patients.
8. Define necessary medical terms for patients using simple explanations. Never use "street language" to discuss bodily functions. However, you may have to adapt some medical terms, such as urination, to more common terms or expressions, for example "passing water," if the patient does not understand.
9. Correct patient errors in the learning process without harsh judgment. Reemphasize the correct information.
10. Avoid teaching by performing the procedure over and over for the patient. Give a demonstration of a procedure, such as drawing up insulin for the diabetic patient. Then, allow the patient to immediately practice. If the technique is not perfect, reinforce learning by having the patient perform the procedure again.
11. Establish a quiet, unhurried, nonthreatening atmosphere for patient education. It should not be conducted in a waiting room or hallway.
12. Remember that if a patient is facing you as you demonstrate a procedure, such as bathing a baby or giving CPR, the patient's hands will be reversed when performing the procedure. Whenever possible, have the learner stand next to you during a one-on-one demonstration.
13. Avoid criticism. Always stress the positive with comments, such as "You're doing fine. Let's try it one more time."

TABLE 50-1 Patient Teaching Methods

Method	Description	Advantage	Disadvantage	Usefulness
Lecture	Formal report or instructions delivered to the patient with little interaction between teacher and learner	Efficient No limit to number of learners	No interaction to handle individual learner confusion May be boring for learner	Patients who need general knowledge (new mothers) Large groups (smoking cessation, weight reduction)
Role-play	Short play in which the learner participates in "playing out" the story	Learner sees how others might do something Learner involvement	Time consuming Learner must be willing to "play" the role	Patients with chronic diseases (hypertension, diabetes) Patients learning new interactions (how to direct home health aide) Handling unusual situations that cannot be demonstrated, such as calling 911 in an emergency
Case problems	Applies information to real situations	Believable Concrete rather than abstract	Significant facts may be missing Effectiveness depends on teacher	Patients who must apply new knowledge (patient with angina, new mothers, diabetes)
Demonstration/ return demonstration	Showing patients how to do something and then immediately having them do the same procedure	Presents standards for performance both visual and oral Allows learner to know it can be done	May be difficult to see Limited to small group Patients may be nervous	Patients who need to understand cause and effect Patients who must learn new skills (colostomy care, diabetic injections, baby care, CPR)
Contracting	Setting up goals with clear behaviors and responsibilities for the patient	Requires learner involvement Promotes learner's strengths Identifies acceptable goals	Requires learner decision making May be threatening Time consuming	Patients with chronic disease Well patients who wish to change health habits
Use of significant other	Teaching a close relative/friend the same information the patient receives	Provides learner support and reinforcement Learning continues at home	Other person must be willing to help Other person may be a negative influence Other person may foster dependence	Elderly patients and those with disabilities Patients whose compliance is in question

(*continued*)

TABLE 50-1   Patient Teaching Methods *(continued)*

Method	Description	Advantage	Disadvantage	Usefulness
Past experiences	Building learning on what has been learned in the past rather than creating a new set of knowledge	Identifies potential problems Makes the patient more comfortable	Depends on ability to recall Requires insight	Patients who are anxious or overwhelmed Patients who must change behavior (take medication, use proper diet, exercise)
Group teaching	Bringing together patients who have common learning needs	Efficient and economical Participants support each other Participants are actively involved	Group may digress Some cultures discourage open discussion Transportation may be a problem Difficult for all to agree on a time	Patients and families with common learning needs (weight reduction, smoking cessation)
Programmed instruction	Printed instructions that force the learner to understand one concept before going on to the next Every correct response builds toward the next question; can be computer assisted	Active learner participation Individual pacing Encourages independence Provides immediate feedback	May be impersonal and boring Patient must be literate Lack of personal involvement between patient and teacher Patient must be self-motivated	Self-motivated learners Accommodates lower reading level
Simulations (games)	To create a pretend scenario for learning purposes	Involves the patient in the learning process Nonthreatening Allows patients to see knowledge previously learned	Some patients dislike competition Some patients do not like games Some patients have difficulty following directions or with abstract ideas	Adults and children with acute problems (cast care), chronic problems (asthma) or health promotion issues (dental care, weight control)
Tests of knowledge	Short questions that relate to the patient's knowledge of the subject	Evaluates patient's knowledge at that moment Gives patient a feeling of accomplishment Raises patient's consciousness of what they were unaware of	May make patients anxious Time consuming May embarrass patients with lack of knowledge	Adults and children who must apply knowledge (diabetic patient, postsurgical patient with a dressing change)

(continued)

TABLE 50-1 **Patient Teaching Methods** (*continued*)

Method	Description	Advantage	Disadvantage	Usefulness
Printed handouts	Brochures or instruction sheets printed for the main purpose of imparting knowledge to the patient	Promotes consistency Gives visual reinforcement	Must be accompanied by verbal teaching Difficult to create since they require clarity and simplicity	Well patients (health maintenance literature) Patients who must remember difficult information (presurgical instructions, medication information)
Diagrams	Picture models of concepts	Offers visual reinforcement Attracts attention of the patient Shows proportions and relationships	Must be accurate May require artistic skill to produce	Preschoolers People with limited reading or vocabulary levels
Models	A miniature (usually) representation of an object produced in a substance, such as clay or plaster	Encourages patient participation Offers direct application of skill	May be expensive	School-age children Adults practicing a skill (CPR, breast self-exam, bathing a child)
Film	A video, slide presentation, or moving picture	Recreates real-life situations Effective for patients with limited reading skills	Too fast for the elderly adult May be expensive Takes time to set up and run	Groups of patients Health maintenance material (nutrition, preventive dentistry) Video in waiting room

improving instruction. Also see Procedure 50-3 for instructing patients according to their health maintenance and promotion needs.

Teaching the Older Adult

Older adult patients' abilities, motivations, and social circumstances differ from those of younger patients. Their intellectual capacity does not diminish; it merely changes. Some changes that take place as a person ages include slower processing of new material, decreased short-term memory, decreased dexterity (ability to use their hands), and increased anxiety over new situations (see also Lifespan Considerations).

One type of intellectual ability is based on the intelligence absorbed during life, for example, vocabulary, arithmetic, and the ability to reflect on and evaluate past experience. This type of intelligence can increase with age. Therefore, the older person is able to learn quickly if the learning requires information acquired in the past. When teaching the older adult, it is wise to explore past experiences using concrete examples, such as "Tell me how you calculate the amount of food you eat on your diabetic diet."

Slowed Processing Time

Older patients need more time to think through and absorb new information; therefore, the medical assistant should break down information into small units. When teaching from a list of things, take time to explain each item on the list. For example, when the instructions state "Call your doctor for the following reasons: temperature over 99 degrees, drainage from the incision, inability to take the medication, or pain," each of these reasons should be explained separately. These explanations should be accompanied by a description of the relationship of each item to the patient's problem. It is also helpful to give written instructions so the patient can process the instructions more slowly later.

Decreased Short-Term Memory

The older adult patient can remember easily things that happened in the past but may have difficulty remembering new information that was acquired yesterday. Learning then becomes very frustrating for them. The medical assistant should work with the patient to devise methods to reinforce instruction or prod the memory. The new information should be linked to a well-known past experience when possible. Always attempt to reinforce old ways of doing things rather than introducing new behavior. For example, when teaching the signs and symptoms of an infection to an older diabetic patient, ask the patient to recall the symptoms experienced in the past with an infected wound or cut.

Decreased Dexterity

Due to arthritis and other physical changes, some elderly patients are not able to do the same things they could when they were younger. Advising an overweight elderly patient who uses a cane and is on a reduction diet to get more exercise by walking for 1 hour a day may not be appropriate. Some procedures requiring small muscle dexterity such as flossing teeth and opening medication bottles are almost impossible for the elderly person with arthritis. Adaptive equipment may have to be advised for these patients (see Chapter 46).

Increased Anxiety about New Situations

The medical assistant must give the elderly patient a feeling of confidence. This can alleviate some of the anxiety that may surface during a new learning situation. When patients see that they are able to manage the situation, they will relax and learning will take place.

Teaching methods to use with the older adult range from using handouts with large print to utilizing video and audiovisual displays. Slow-moving slides are preferable to a fast video or movie since the slide can be stopped to reinforce learning. Role-playing can be useful as long as the patient's energy level can be maintained. Family members should be included in the teaching process whenever possible. The elderly person is accustomed to being in control and may not wish to learn anything new if he or she does not see the advantage of doing so.

Instructing Patients According to Their Needs for Health Maintenance and Promotion

OBJECTIVE: Instruct a deaf individual to prepare for outpatient surgery by creating a brochure on steps to minimize infection postoperatively.

Equipment and Supplies

computer, printer, pen, stapler

Method

1. Create postoperative instructions for the deaf patient, including information about activities, medications, dressing changes, diet, and follow-up care. Create a copy for the client and one for the chart.
2. Face the patient so your lips can be easily read.
3. Greet the patient, using the patient's name.
4. Discuss the contents of the postoperative instructions with the patient.
5. Obtain feedback to show understanding from patient.
6. Give copy of information to patient.
7. Have patient sign one copy of the brochure and keep one copy for the patient chart.
8. Document the education.

Charting Example

Instructed patient on postoperative instructions as highlighted in attached brochure. February 20, 20XX

Emily Blodgett, CMA

Developing a Teaching Plan

An effective teaching plan for both the adult and child learner must include desired outcomes. A teaching plan that the medical assistant develops for a condition, such as hypertension (high blood pressure), can be used with some adaptations for all patients with hypertension. Box 50-2 illustrates a sample teaching plan.

Teaching Patients with Disabilities

Because of differences in the learning readiness and processing capabilities of older adults and also of special needs patients such as those with developmental delays, hearing impairments, and visual impairments, or non-English-speaking patients, the medical assistant needs to carefully prepare any brochures or materials given to patients.

Patient education should be adapted to the patient. Many patients will have special needs. Patients who have hearing impairments, visual impairments, are developmentally delayed or mentally retarded, or who do not speak English pose special challenges.

Patients who have hearing impairments frequently read lips. Face the patient and speak slowly. Be sure that you do not stand with your back to the window because such positioning will throw shadows over your mouth. Remove barriers or face masks when speaking to clients with hearing impairments. You may need to hire an interpreter for the deaf. Get a microphone to boost your voice volume and give specific written instructions to clients with hearing impairments.

Patients who have visual impairments may not be able to understand written instructions unless the type is very large—and some will not be able to read at all. The medical assistant may need to make audiotaped instructions of information that is usually written. Be sure to clear clutter from the office that might impede the patient and hold the patient's hand to lead him or her to examinations and procedures.

Patients who have developmental delays or mental retardation may have trouble understanding instructions. The medical assistant may need to instruct the caregiver instead or give the patient simplified, pictorial directions.

Patients who are illiterate or do not understand English pose special challenges. Ask the patient when an appointment is made if he or she would like an interpreter for patient care. Sometimes the patient prefers to bring a relative who speaks English. Be sure to get patient permission to discuss health information with relatives. Send written instructions home with the patient. If a large percentage of patients in the office speak a certain language other than English, it may help to construct brochures in other languages. Consider culture and diet compliance along with patient likes and dislikes for compliance.

BOX 50-2

Sample Teaching Plan for Hypertension

Content

I. Basic anatomy and physiology of the heart and blood vessels
II. What is hypertension?
III. Symptoms of hypertension
IV. Risk factors related to hypertension
V. Situations that might precipitate hypertension
VI. Home treatment for hypertension
VII. Handling medications
VIII. Reasons to contact the physician
IX. Follow-up
X. Community resources/support groups

Learning Objectives

I. The patient describes the anatomy and physiology of the heart muscle and blood vessels in simple terms.
   a. The heart muscle is a strong hollow organ that acts as a pump. It pumps blood throughout the body and lungs.
   b. Blood vessels throughout the body carry oxygen to the tissues and cells.
   c. When the blood vessels become narrowed or do not function properly, the heart may have to work harder. Eventually, pressure within the vessels will rise.
II. The patient states in simple terms the definition and causes of hypertension.
   a. Hypertension is an elevation in blood pressure in which the systolic pressure is 140 mmHg or above and the diastolic pressure is 90 mmHg or above.
   b. An elevated blood pressure reading is a signal that there is a problem which could affect the heart action or even cause a stroke.
   c. Hypertension (high blood pressure) may be caused by a buildup of fatty substances (cholesterol) on the lining of the blood vessels that feed the heart.
III. The patient states the most common symptoms of hypertension.
   a. This is generally a "silent" disease, which means there are few or no symptoms.
   b. The patient may feel very well.
   c. The best indicator is an elevated blood pressure reading on several occasions.
   d. May have headaches or dizziness.
   e. Patient's symptoms are _____.
IV. The patient defines risk factors and describes controllable and uncontrollable risk factors.
   a. Risk factors are habits or characteristics that increase the probability of developing a narrowing of the blood vessels.
   b. Controllable factors are
     1. Obesity (20% over the average weight for the age, sex, and height)
     2. Cigarette smoking

     3. Increased amount of fatty substances in the blood
     4. Stress
     5. Lack of exercise
     6. Diet
   c. Uncontrollable factors are
     1. Family history
     2. Diabetes
     3. Patients over the age of 50
   d. Patient's risk factors are
   Controllable _____
   _____
   Uncontrollable _____
   _____
V. Patient states situations that may precipitate hypertension.
   a. Diet heavy in fats and salt
   b. Stress
   c. Smoking
   d. Family history
   e. Age
   f. Lack of exercise
   g. Patient's hypertension may be precipitated by the following:
   _____
   _____
VI. The patient states the home treatment of hypertension.
   a. Monitor blood pressure with home equipment. Record blood pressure readings.
   b. Take medications on a regular basis at the same time every day.
   c. Adjust diet by eliminating salt and fat and reducing calorie intake.
   d. Use stress reduction techniques.
   e. Exercise moderately.
VII. The patient states how to handle medications.
   a. Patient must call physician for a prescription renewal every 3 months.
   b. Patient must have a supply of medication on hand when traveling.
   c. Patient must come in to have blood pressure checked by physician every 2 weeks.
VIII. The patient states reasons to contact the physician or go to the emergency room.
   a. Dizziness or fainting.
   b. Blood pressure reading of 160/98 or higher.
IX. The patient provides the following:
   Physician #: _____
   Emergency Room #: _____
X. The patient provides a list of community resources/support groups for hypertension.

If the patient and/or significant others are unable to complete some or all of this teaching plan, document evaluation in progress notes on chart.

Handling Noncompliance

Noncompliance, that is, not following a physician's orders, can seriously jeopardize a patient's health and recovery. For instance, a patient with hypertension who fails to take prescribed medication can develop uncontrolled hypertension and have a stroke or heart attack. In addition, health care costs escalate with noncompliance.

Several groups of patients, including those who have had heart bypasses or hemodialysis, have been followed up to determine their compliance level. In both situations, the compliance levels were around 50%. Lack of compliance may be indicated by failure to (1) take medication as ordered, (2) return for follow-up appointments, (3) practice dietary changes, and (4) follow an exercise program. On the other hand, patients with cystic fibrosis, a serious disease causing respiratory problems and failure, were found to be more than 80% compliant with their medication regimen. This compliance was attributed to the possibility that these patients and their families perceived the consequences for failure to take cystic fibrosis medications to be very serious.

Noncompliance with instructions is a problem for all age groups, but children have the least problem as long as their parents are compliant and assist them. Patients who have formed a positive relationship with their health care provider, physician, and other staff, such as the medical assistant, have been found to be more compliant. To help form this positive relationship with the physician, you may choose to create a public relations brochure. See Procedure 50-3 for instructions.

One of the best methods to encourage patient compliance is to convey to the patients the knowledge they need to make educated decisions about their health care. For instance, the cystic fibrosis patients just mentioned were more compliant after realizing the seriousness of their disease.

In addition to having greater knowledge, the patient must also want to comply. The medical assistant can reinforce learning, and reduce noncompliance, by working out a follow-up plan with regular evaluation of progress. This plan should include an objective stating what the patient should be able to do along with a date indicating when the objective should be accomplished. Table 50-2 is an example of a patient education follow-up plan.

Teaching about Cast Care

An example of a case when the medical assistant might need to educate a patient is about cast care. If a patient has had a cast placed on an injured extremity, the patient will leave the office needing to know how to care for the cast.

Putting on a Cast

Casts are applied for the purpose of immobilizing a broken bone or muscle strain and sprain. A cast may be applied after a surgical procedure on a limb to immobilize the area until healing takes place.

The medical assistant may be asked to lay out the instruments required for putting on a cast. Equipment includes the cast material (bandage roll or tape), container of warm water, stockinette, Webril (sheer wadding) padding rolls, bandage scissors, rubber gloves, and sponge rubber (for padding).

Casts are made from a variety of pliable materials that the physician will mold to fit the body part. A cast

TABLE 50-2   Patient Education Follow-Up Plan

Objective	Performance	Date Needed
Self-administer insulin injections with 100% accuracy	1. Understand types of insulin	2/14/XXXX
	2. Practice drawing up insulin × 3	2/14/XXXX
	3. Practice injection on anatomical model × 3	2/16/XXXX
	4. Demonstration on patient by instructor using saline	2/18/XXXX
	5. Return demonstration using saline	2/18/XXXX
	6. Injection of insulin	2/18/XXXX
	7. Follow-up to check technique	3/1/XXXX

Preparing for Externship

can be considered a form of nonflexible bandage. Casts are generally applied using a plaster-type material, which is applied wet around a stockinette liner with cotton padding over the limb. The medical assistant will wet a bandage roll impregnated with calcium sulfate and mold it to the injured body part. As the cast dries, it becomes hard. Newer fiberglass materials are being used to form casts since they are lighter in weight than a plaster cast. They are formed by using tapes with either a polyester-cotton combination, fiberglass, or plastic resin imbedded in the tape. The medical assistant should wear protective glasses or an eye shield when handling fiberglass materials.

Air casts are a type of inflatable immobilizer that use air to apply firm pressure to the wounded limb. They are used primarily for postcast pressure or sprains.

External fixation devices are sometimes used to create appropriate pressure without using casting material. The skin around the fixation pins must be cleaned.

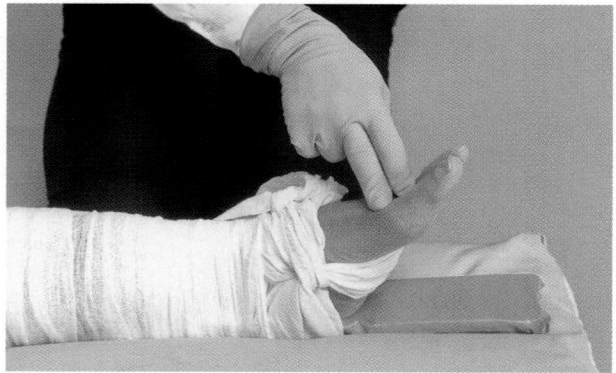

FIGURE 50-1 Checking distal pulses.

The type of casting material is a physician preference and also depends on the body part to which a cast is being applied.

The medical assistant may be asked to assist the physician in applying the cast. It may be necessary to hold the limb at the joint areas as the cast is being applied. Remember to handle a damaged limb gently.

After the cast has been applied, it must be left uncovered during the drying process. The limb may need to be supported on a pillow at this time. The patient should be cautioned against moving around until the cast is dry. The cast may feel warm or even hot during the drying process. Reassure the patient that this normal.

The patient's limb should not become hot or cold once the cast has been applied. Frequent checks of the patient's circulation will alert the medical assistant to any change in the patient's circulation. The patient should be instructed to call the physician if any of the following problems are observed:

- Circulation restricted by the cast
- Pain as a result of the cast pinching the skin
- Excessive itching under the cast
- Numbness or tingling of fingers or toes
- Discolored toes or fingers
- Swelling of the limb around the edge of the cast
- Discoloration soaking through the cast
- Loosely fitting cast
- Foul odor coming from the cast

The physician should advise the patient on the amount of weight and movement that can be applied to the cast. Remind the patient that nothing should be put into the edges of the cast. The cast should not get wet. The patient may be able to tie a strong plastic bag around the cast in order to take a shower.

The patient is an excellent source of information about what is happening under the cast. The injury that caused the fracture leads to swelling, which can create pressure under the cast. Also remember that when the cast dries and hardens, it may constrict blood flow. Always check distal pulses and notify the physician if any abnormality is noted. The physician may need to remove and replace the cast. Figure 50-1 shows how to check circulation distal to the immobilized area.

Some types of casts are:

- Short arm cast (SAC)—extends from the finger to just below the elbow. Used for a fracture or dislocation of the wrist or forearm.
- Long arm cast (LAC)—extends from the fingers to the axilla, with a bend at the elbow. Used for a fracture of the upper arm.
- Long and short leg casts—extend from the thigh to the toes (LLC) or from below the knee to the toes (SLC). They usually include an embedded walking heel.

There are several types of fractures, or breaks. They are termed simple, or closed, when the bone is broken but the skin is not. Compound, or open, fractures occur when both the bone and the skin are broken. A Colles fracture is at the lower end of the radius. A Potts fracture is at the lower part of the fibula and the malleolus of the tibia. These are the most common fractures because we tend to guard our fall with our legs and wrists. A greenstick fracture is bent on only one side and fractured on the other. These are particularly common in children. An oblique fracture runs obliquely to the axis of the bone. Transverse fractures are at a right angle to the axis of the bone. An impacted fracture happens when fractured bone fragments are forced into another bone. A comminuted fracture is a fracture that broke into tiny fragments.

Patient Education

The medical assistant should instruct the patient on how to care for the cast before allowing the patient to leave the office. Educational topics include:

- Clean the cast with a damp cloth.
- Do not cut or trim the cast. If the edge seems sharp, apply masking tape to the sharp edge or use a nail file to trim it down.
- Elevate the extremity with the cast on it to reduce swelling and pain.
- Observe the fingers and toes for color changes, temperature changes, pain, tingling, or decreased sensation.
- Allow the cast material to dry by exposing it to the air and keeping it uncovered, even during the night. If you apply pressure to the cast before it is dry, you can damage the tissue underneath.
- Do not try to scratch under the cast by putting objects into the cast. This will result in broken skin that can lead to infection.
- When decorating a cast, use only water-soluble paints or marking pens. Otherwise the cast will not be able to breathe.
- Call the physician's office if you smell a bad odor coming from the cast, lose sensation or blood flow beyond the cast, feel a burning sensation, or notice blood coming from the cast.

Figure 50-2 shows a cast boot given to a patient with a leg cast before leaving the office. After being sure that the patient understands the importance of cast care, the medical assistant must document the teaching in the patient chart.

Removing a Cast

The medical assistant may need to assist the physician with removing a cast. Equipment needed includes a cast cutter, cast spreader, bandage scissors, bag for disposing

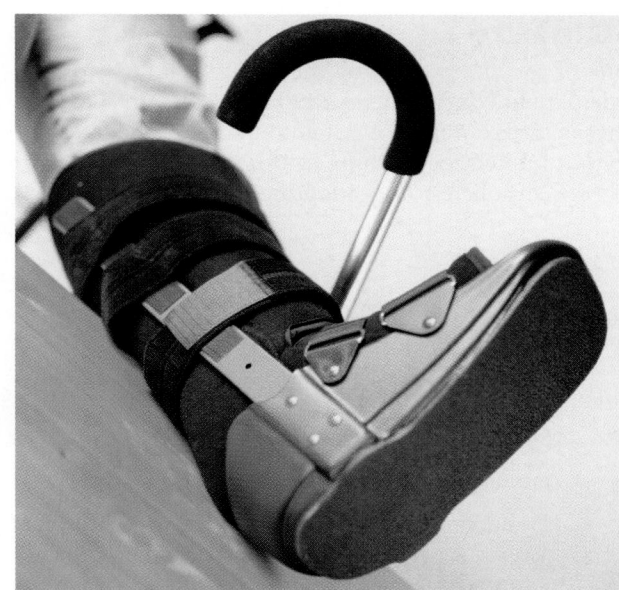

FIGURE 50-2 Cast boot.

of cast materials, and a drape. After washing hands and draping the patient, the medical assistant will need to explain the process to the patient. The cutter vibrates and does not spin. The patient may feel some pressure and warmth. The patient may be shocked to see that the skin under the cast has become white and the muscle tone has decreased, and may need some reassurance that physical therapy will improve the function and appearance of the limb. The medical assistant should stand near the physician and hand the necessary equipment as requested. After the cast is removed, the medical assistant should apply written instructions for postcast care, clean the equipment, wash hands, and document the procedure in the patient chart. Figure 50-3 shows the instruments used for cast removal: cast cutter, cast splitter, and bandage scissors.

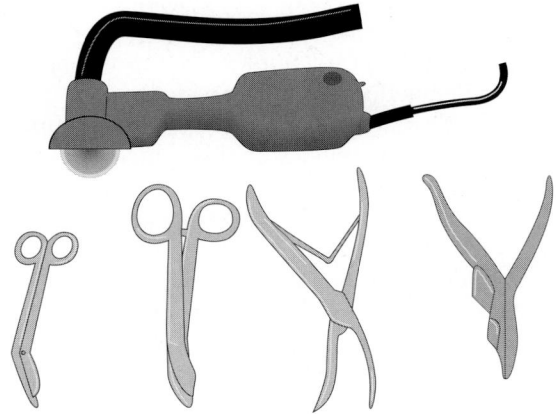

FIGURE 50-3 Cast removal equipment.

SUMMARY

One of the vital tasks of a medical assistant is to provide patient education, as needed, and as directed by a physician. Examples of patient education include, but are not limited to, teaching health promotion, describing office policies, and adapting education to special needs. In addition, the medical assistant often plays a critical role in handling noncompliant patients (for example, a diabetic patient who will not adhere to the prescribed diet). Again, patient education is the most effective means of resolving such a situation.

Chapter Review

COMPETENCY REVIEW

1. Define and spell the terms to learn for this chapter.
2. Create a patient brochure describing a typical medical office. Be sure to include office location, times when patients are seen, contact numbers, physicians, type of practice, and insurance information.
3. Develop a teaching plan for health promotion.
4. Create a community resource brochure. For example, information about support groups, such as a Lions Club or the Red Cross.

PREPARING FOR THE CERTIFICATION EXAM

1. The most effective combination of teaching methods for the older adult is
   A. lecture, printed materials, models
   B. lecture, return demonstration, programmed instruction
   C. role-play, group teaching, return demonstration
   D. video, test of knowledge, group teaching
   E. all of the above

2. When writing instructional booklets to teach diabetics nutritional planning, which of the following statements is TRUE?
   A. Use of medical terminology is fine as long as detailed definitions are provided.
   B. Sprinkle material with medical abbreviations so the patient will know this is medical education.
   C. Combine several ideas into one grouping in order to save space.
   D. Avoid using too many examples.
   E. Show diagrams of injection rotation sites.

3. Which of the following is a potential legal dilemma for the CMA?
   A. The patient asks for information regarding an alternative treatment for breast cancer.
   B. The patient asks for a list of the foods that her baby, who has diarrhea, can eat.
   C. The patient is discharged after day surgery for a hernia repair with only an instructional pamphlet.
   D. The patient states that he or she won't follow the instructions, so none are given.
   E. All of the above.

4. Which of the following should not be included in an office brochure?
   A. office hours
   B. office location
   C. insurance plans accepted
   D. physician's home telephone number
   E. emergency phone numbers and after-hours plan

continued on next page

5. Which of the following is the most therapeutic statement during patient education?
   A. Let me show you a video about your disease.
   B. Tell me what you already know about your disease.
   C. This is what you ought to do.
   D. I will show you how to do this.
   E. Take this pop quiz on your disease when you go home.

6. Which of the following is NOT true about cast care?
   A. Use water-soluble pens to decorate.
   B. Do not allow it to get wet.
   C. Use a ruler to scratch under the cast.
   D. Check distal pulses and color of feet or hands frequently.
   E. Report any odor coming from the cast.

CRITICAL THINKING

1. Describe, in detail, the teaching plan you would develop for Mr. Young.
2. Should there be one or two teaching plans regarding Mr. Young and his wife's care? Why?
3. What should the very first issue discussed with Mr. Young when teaching him about his wife's and his own care?
4. An older patient from Egypt comes in with her son. She speaks no English, but her son is willing and able to interpret for you. Discuss how you would adapt education to her culturally based needs.
5. One of your adult patients is mentally retarded and only reads on a first-grade reading level. How would you adapt your patient education techniques to his special needs?

ON THE JOB

Mary Ruth, a CMA, works in a dialysis clinic. Most of her patients have diabetes mellitus, an endocrine disorder that can destroy the kidneys and leave the patient dependent on dialysis. The patients are usually on the dialysis machine for several hours 3 days per week. This gives Mary Ruth a chance to do a lot of patient teaching.

1. Is it appropriate for the CMA to do patient teaching?
2. What would be the best way for Mary Ruth to teach her patients?
3. If the patient has diabetic retinopathy, what would be the best way to teach this patient?
4. If the patient is old and claims to be "set in my ways," what would be good strategies for teaching the patient about healthy lifestyles?
5. Should family members be involved in the teaching plan? If so, how?
6. Describe a possible teaching plan for diabetic patients.

INTERNET ACTIVITY

Choose a topic that interests you to create an instructional and a community resource brochure. Do an Internet search to gather information. For example go to www.nlm.nih.gov/medlineplus and research heart disease. Then create a patient teaching brochure.

 MediaLink More on patient education, including interactive resources, can be found on the Student CD-ROM accompanying this textbook.

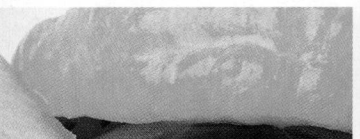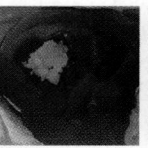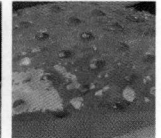

Medical Assistant Role Delineation Chart

HIGHLIGHT indicates material covered in this chapter.

ADMINISTRATIVE

Administrative Procedures

- Perform basic administrative medical assisting functions
- Schedule, coordinate and monitor appointments
- Schedule inpatient/outpatient admissions and procedures
- Understand and apply third-party guidelines
- Obtain reimbursement through accurate claims submission
- Monitor third-party reimbursement
- Understand and adhere to managed care policies and procedures
- *Negotiate managed care contracts*

Practice Finances

- Perform procedural and diagnostic coding
- Apply bookkeeping principles

- Manage accounts receivable
- *Manage accounts payable*
- *Process payroll*
- *Document and maintain accounting and banking records*
- *Develop and maintain fee schedules*
- *Manage renewals of business and professional insurance policies*
- *Manage personnel benefits and maintain records*
- *Perform marketing, financial, and strategic planning*

CLINICAL

Fundamental Principles

- Apply principles of aseptic technique and infection control
- Comply with quality assurance practices
- Screen and follow up patient test results

Diagnostic Orders

- Collect and process specimens
- Perform diagnostic tests

Patient Care

- Adhere to established patient screening procedures
- Obtain patient history and vital signs
- Prepare and maintain examination and treatment areas
- Prepare patient for examinations, procedures and treatments

- Assist with examinations, procedures and treatments
- Prepare and administer medications and immunizations
- Maintain medication and immunization records
- Recognize and respond to emergencies
- Coordinate patient care information with other health care providers
- Initiate IV and administer IV medications with appropriate training and as permitted by state law

GENERAL

Professionalism

- Display a professional manner and image
- Demonstrate initiative and responsibility
- Work as a member of the health care team
- Prioritize and perform multiple tasks
- Adapt to change
- Promote the CMA credential
- Enhance skills through continuing education
- Treat all patients with compassion and empathy
- Promote the practice through positive public relations

Communication Skills

- Recognize and respect cultural diversity
- Adapt communications to individual's ability to understand
- Use professional telephone technique

- Recognize and respond effectively to verbal, nonverbal, and written communications
- Use medical terminology appropriately
- Utilize electronic technology to receive, organize, prioritize and transmit information
- Serve as liaison

Legal Concepts

- Perform within legal and ethical boundaries
- Prepare and maintain medical records
- Document accurately
- Follow employer's established policies dealing with the health care contract
- Implement and maintain federal and state health care legislation and regulations
- Comply with established risk management and safety procedures
- Recognize professional credentialing criteria
- *Develop and maintain personnel, policy and procedure manuals*

Instruction

- Instruct individuals according to their needs
- Explain office policies and procedures
- Teach methods of health promotion and disease prevention
- Locate community resources and disseminate information
- *Develop educational materials*
- *Conduct continuing education activities*

Operational Functions

- Perform inventory of supplies and equipment
- Perform routine maintenance of administrative and clinical equipment
- Apply computer techniques to support office operations
- *Perform personnel management functions*
- *Negotiate leases and prices for equipment and supply contracts*

Denotes advanced skills.

SOURCE: Reprinted by permission of the American Association of Medical Assistants from the AAMA Role Delineation Study: Occupational Analysis of the Medical Assisting Profession.

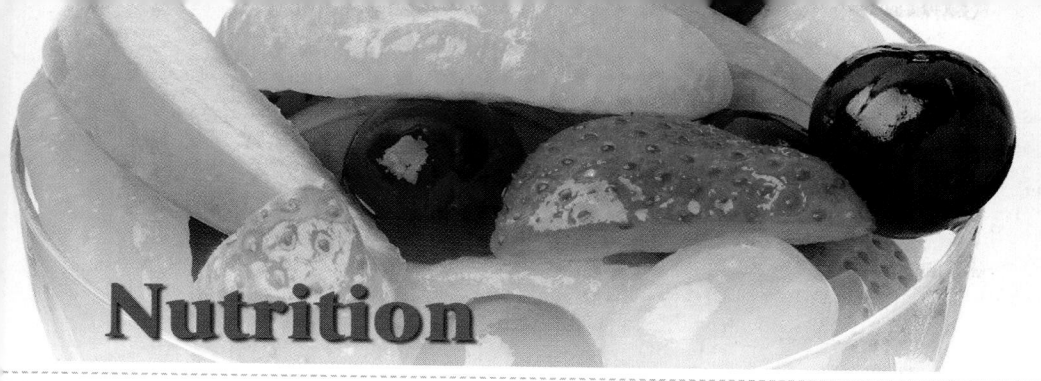

Nutrition

Learning Objectives

After completing this chapter, you should be able to:

- Define and spell the terms to learn for this chapter.
- Define metabolism.
- List and describe six types of nutrients.
- Discuss the difference between saturated and unsaturated fats.
- Discuss the difference between LDL and HDL in cholesterol.
- Describe the food guide pyramid and state its importance for patient education.

- Discuss calories as the term relates to proteins, carbohydrates, and fats.
- State the formula for determining the percentage of calories in a food that are supplied by fat.
- List and discuss six important dietary guidelines.
- State 12 diet modifications and why the physician might order them.

OUTLINE

Nutrition	1098
Stress Management	1116
Time Management	1116

Terms to Learn

BRAT	hydrogenation	nutrient(s)
cholesterol	metabolism	polysaccharides
digestion	monosaccharides	

Case Study

MARY DRAHMS JUST FOUND OUT SHE IS PREGNANT. Her husband Walt states that she eats all the time, mostly at fast-food restaurants. She states she is eating for two now. He is concerned that she may gain too much weight during the pregnancy and have complications because of overeating. Dr. Franklin insists that all his patients receive nutritional counseling during pregnancy.

The medical assistant is responsible for instructing the patient, and sometimes family members, in correct dietary adjustments for her condition.

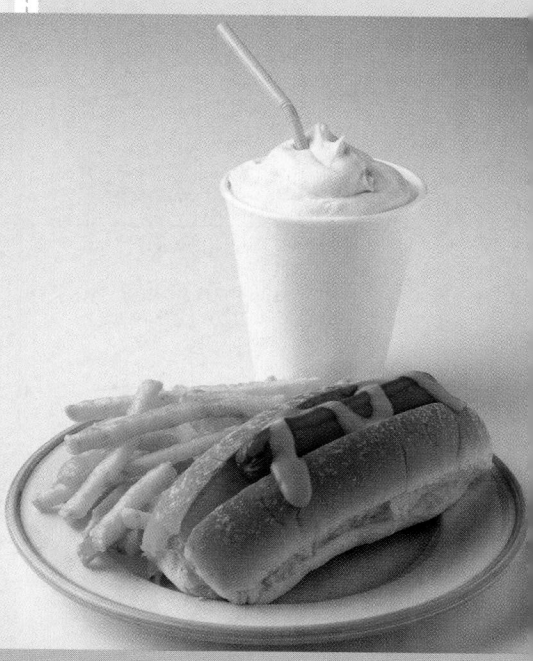

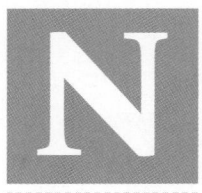

Nutrition includes all of the processes involved in using foods for growth, repair, and maintenance of the body. The nutrition process includes ingestion, digestion, absorption, and metabolism. Some nutrients are capable of being stored in the body and can be used when the food intake is insufficient. Other nutrients such as vitamin C are not stored and need to be continually replenished.

Nutrition

Interest in nutrition has been around for a long time. Debilitating diseases such as scurvy, rickets, and beriberi were found to be caused by deficiencies in the diet. Scurvy was discovered to be a disease of sailors and others who did not receive fresh fruits and vegetables for long periods of time. When sailors began to take lemons and limes along on their sea voyages, the symptoms of scurvy (hemorrhages, anemia, weakness, sallow complexion) disappeared. A lack of vitamin C was the culprit. Rickets, caused by a deficiency of vitamin D, produced bowed legs in young babies and children until this vitamin was added to milk to fortify it. Beriberi, more commonly found in rice-growing regions, caused neurological and cardiovascular abnormalities until thiamin was added to the diet of patients.

The cures for these diseases resulted from research into what people were eating. The study of nutrition is

NUTRIENT CLASS	BODILY FUNCTIONS	FOOD SOURCES
CARBOHYDRATES	Provides work energy for body activities, and heat energy for maintenance of body temperature.	Cereal grains and their products (bread, breakfast cereals, macaroni products), potatoes, sugar, syrups, fruits, milk, vegetables, nuts.
PROTEINS	Build and renew body tissues; regulate body functions and supply energy. Complete proteins; maintain life and provide growth. Incomplete proteins; maintain life but do not provide for growth.	Complete proteins: Derived from animal foods—meat, milk, eggs, fish, cheese, poultry. Incomplete proteins: Derived from vegetable foods—soybeans, dry beans, peas, some nuts and whole grain products.
FATS	Give work energy for body activities and heat energy for maintenance of body temperature. Carrier of vitamins A and D, provide fatty acids necessary for growth and maintenance of body tissues.	Some foods are chiefly fat, such as lard, vegetable fats and oils, and butter. Many other foods contain smaller proportions of fats—nuts, meats, fish, poultry, cream, whole milk.
MINERALS Calcium	Builds and renews bones, teeth, and other tissues; regulates the activity of the muscles, heart, nerves; and controls the clotting of blood.	Milk and milk products except butter; most dark green vegetables; canned salmon.
PHOSPHORUS	Associated with calcium in some functions needed to build and renew bones and teeth. Influences the oxidation of foods in the body cells; important in nerve tissue.	Widely distributed in foods; especially cheese, oat cereals, whole wheat products, dry beans and peas, meat, fish, poultry, nuts.

FIGURE 51-1 A balanced diet begins with eating foods from the basic food groups.

performed by nutritionists and dietitians. Nutritionists provide information on foods and nutrition. Dietitians promote good health through proper diet and the use of diet in the treatment of disease.

It has been said that the typical American diet contains too much fat, too many calories, too much cholesterol, too much salt, not enough fiber, and insufficient complex carbohydrates. Nutritionists believe that many Americans receive more than 40% of their daily calories from fats. The best diet is a well-balanced eating plan with the correct proportion of the major nutrients (see Figure 51-1). A well-nourished person is better able to ward off infection, remain more alert, and may even be able to live longer (see Patient Education).

Digestion

Digestion is the actual process the body undergoes when it converts food into chemical substances that can be absorbed into the blood and used by the body tissues and organs. The actual digestive process is accomplished by physically breaking down, diluting, and dissolving food substances. In the process they are also chemically split into simpler compounds. For example, proteins are broken down into amino acids; carbohydrates are broken down into monosaccharides (simple sugars); and fats are absorbed as fatty acids and glycerol (glycerin).

Actual digestion takes place in the alimentary canal, also referred to as the digestive system or the

NUTRIENT CLASS	BODILY FUNCTIONS	FOOD SOURCES
MINERALS (continued) Iron 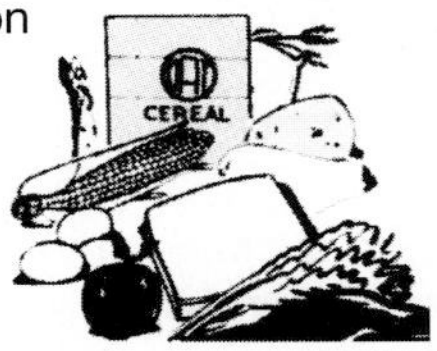	Builds and renews hemoglobin, the red pigment in blood which carries oxygen from the lungs to the cells.	Eggs, meat, especially liver and kidney; deep-yellow and dark green vegetables; potatoes, dried fruits, whole-grain products; enriched flour, bread, breakfast cereals.
Iodine 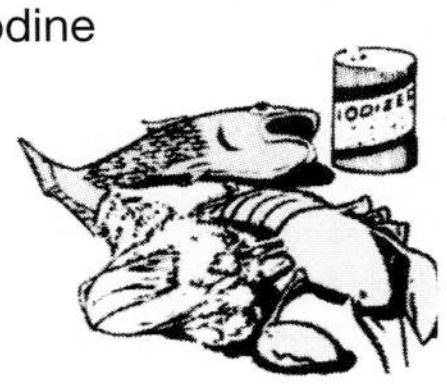	Enables the thyroid gland to perform its function of controlling the rate at which foods are oxidized in the cells.	Fish (obtained from the sea), some plant-foods grown in soils containing iodine; table salt fortified with iodine (iodized).
VITAMINS A 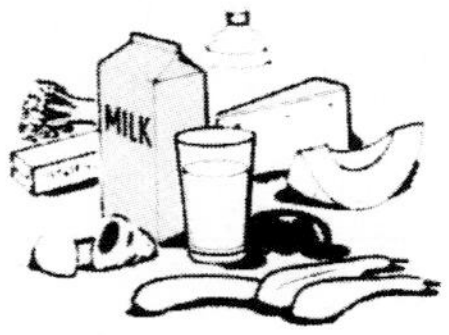	Necessary for normal functioning of the eyes, prevents night blindness. Ensures a healthy condition of the skin, hair, and mucous membranes. Maintains a state of resistance to infections of the eyes, mouth, and respiratory tract.	One form of vitamin A is yellow and one form is colorless. Apricots, cantaloupe, milk, cheese, eggs, meat organs, (especially liver and kidney), fortified margarine, butter fish-liver oils, dark green and deep yellow vegetables.
B Complex B$_1$ (Thiamine) 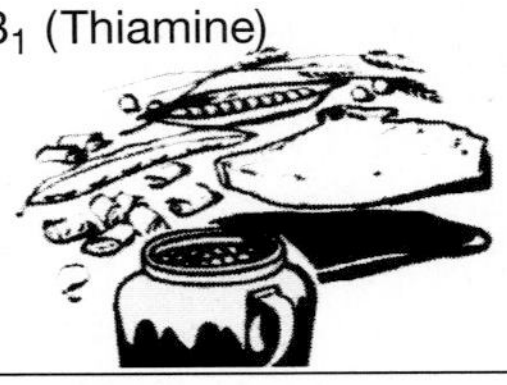	Maintains a healthy condition of the nerves. Fosters a good appetite. Helps the body cells use carbohydrates.	Whole grain and enriched grain products; meats (especially pork, liver and kidney). Dry beans and peas.
B$_2$ (Riboflavin) 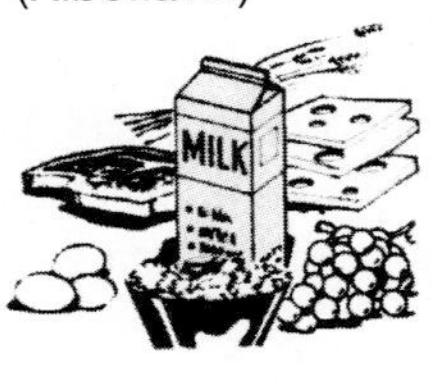	Keeps the skin, mouth, and eyes in a healthy condition. Acts with other nutrients to form enzymes and control oxidation in cells.	Milk, cheese, eggs, meat (especially liver and kidney), whole grain and enriched grain products, dark green vegetables.

FIGURE 51-1 Continued.

NUTRIENT CLASS	BODILY FUNCTIONS	FOOD SOURCES
VITAMINS (continued) Niacin 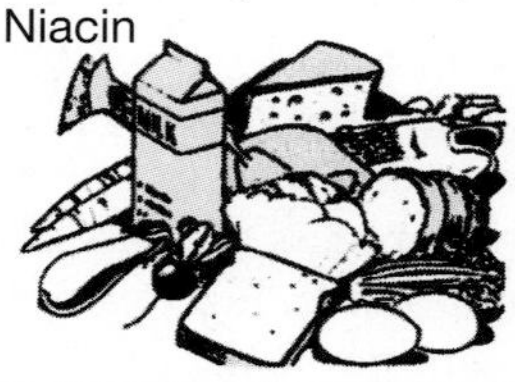	Influences the oxidation of carbohydrates and proteins in the body cells.	Liver, meat, fish, poultry, eggs, peanuts; dark green vegetables, whole grain and enriched cereal products.
B_{12} 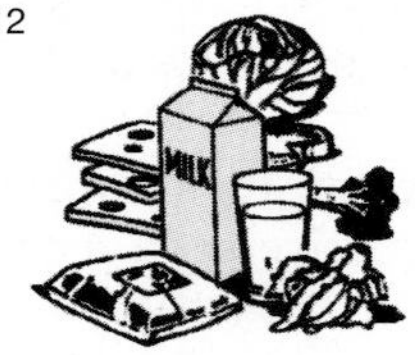	Regulates specific processes in digestion. Helps maintain normal functions of muscles, nerves, heart, blood—general body metabolism.	Liver, other organ meats, cheese, eggs, milk, leafy green vegetables.
C (Ascorbic Acid) 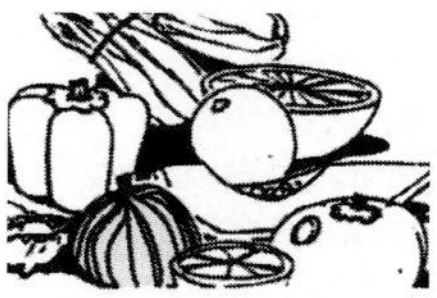	Acts as a cement between body cells, and helps them work together to carry out their special functions. Maintains a sound condition of bones, teeth, and gums. Not stored in the body.	Fresh, raw citrus fruits and vegetables—oranges, grapefruit, cantaloupe, strawberries, tomatoes, raw onions, cabbage, green and sweet red peppers, dark green vegetables.
D 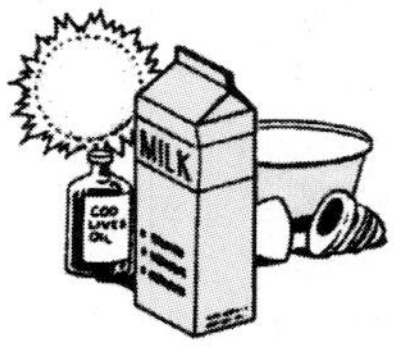	Enables the growing body to use calcium and phosphorus in a normal way to build bones and teeth.	Provided by vitamin D fortification of certain foods, such as milk and margarine. Also fish-liver oils and eggs. Sunshine is also a source of vitamin D.
WATER 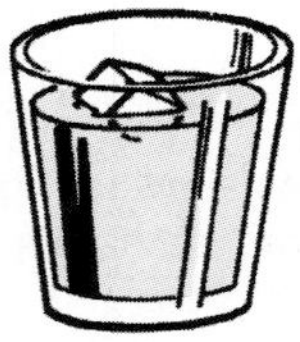	Regulates body processes. Aids in regulating body temperature. Carries nutrients to body cells and carries waste products away from them. Helps to lubricate joints. Water has no food value, although most water contains mineral elements. More immediately necessary to life than food—second only to oxygen.	Drinking water, and other beverages; all foods except those made up of a single nutrient, as sugar and some fats. Milk, milk drinks, soups, vegetables, fruit juices. Ice cream, watermelon, strawberries, lettuce, tomatoes, cereals, other dry products.

FIGURE 51-1 Continued.

gastrointestinal (GI) tract. Figure 51-2 illustrates the digestive system. Accessory organs including the salivary glands, liver, gallbladder, and pancreas provide essential enzymes for digestion through their secretions. Water, minerals, some vitamins, and some of the carbohydrates in fruit are absorbable as soon as they are ingested.

The average adult stomach holds about 1½ quarts of food and liquid. The stomach will reach a peak in

Patient Education

Perhaps the most important patient education the medical assistant can give is about healthy lifestyles. Poor diet contributes to many diseases, such as diabetes, heart disease, stroke, and gout. The physician should ask about nutritional habits at annual checkups, but if your physician is too pressed for time, you might prepare some brochures to educate patients about a healthy diet. Be sure that you know what comprises a healthy diet before creating the brochures and have your office manager or physician approve them.

the digestive process 2 hours after a meal and may take 3 to 5 hours to empty into the small intestine. It may take 20 minutes for the brain to register that food has entered the system. The digestion process is influenced by emotions as well as the enzyme and chemical actions of the digestive system. A quiet, calm atmosphere at mealtime can enhance the digestive process.

Metabolism

Metabolism is the sum of all physical and chemical changes that take place within the human body. Metabolism is the process of changing food, air, water, and other materials into substances absorbed into the body through the blood and respiratory system. Specific enzymes that are required to maintain metabolism are amino acids, carbohydrates, vitamins, and essential trace minerals.

Approximately 23% of all energy released by nutrients is used by the body to carry on its normal functions, such as respiration, digestion, reproduction, muscular movement, circulation, and cellular regrowth. The remaining 75% of the energy becomes heat. Eating and drinking the wrong foods can negatively affect metabolism.

Classification of Nutrients

Nutrients are the organic and inorganic chemical substances found in foods that supply the body with necessary elements for metabolism. Certain nutrients (carbohydrates, fats, and proteins) provide energy; other nutrients (water, electrolytes, minerals, and vitamins) are essential to the metabolic process (see Professionalism).

There are six main classifications of nutrients, and more than 50 nutrients are required for the human body to function properly. These nutrients must be consumed in the diet on a daily basis. The six classifications of nutrients are as follows:

1. Carbohydrates   4. Water
2. Protein   5. Vitamins
3. Fats   6. Minerals

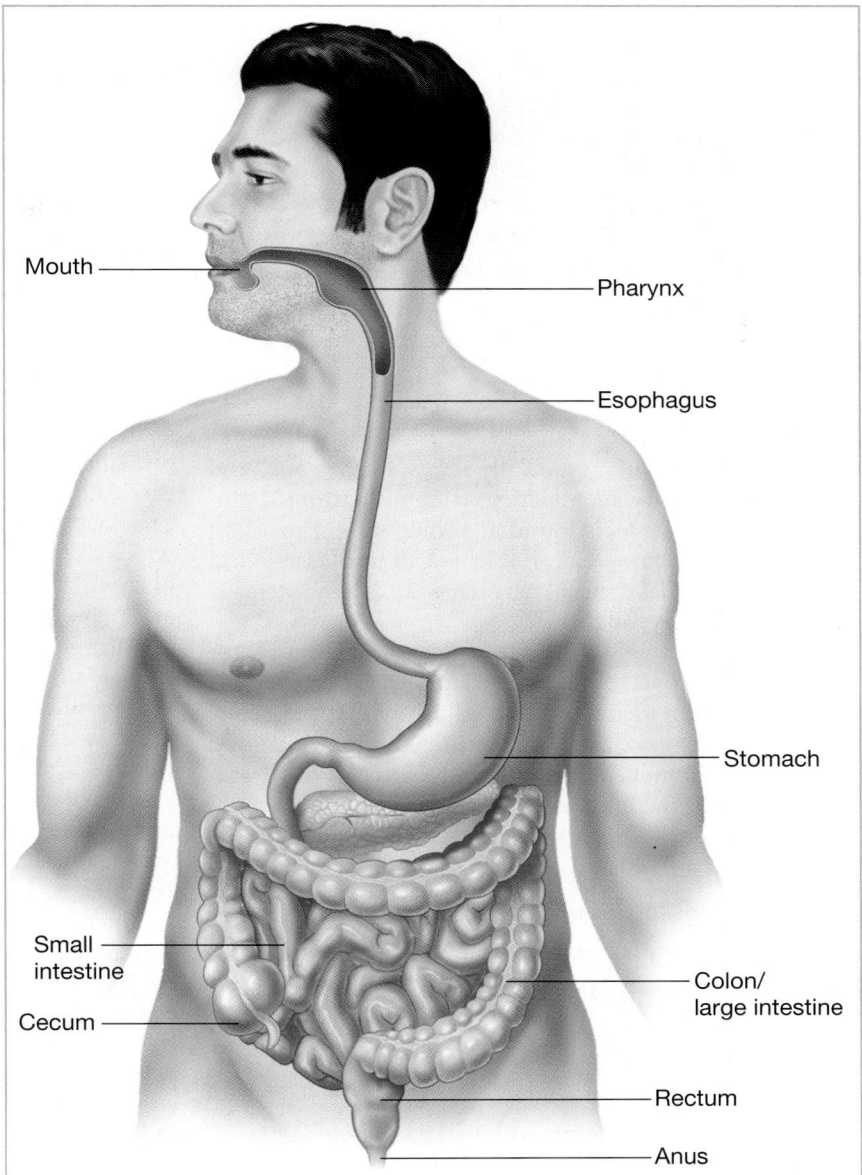

FIGURE 51-2   The digestive system.

Carbohydrates

The main source of energy from foods is from carbohydrates. Carbohydrates are the sugars (simple carbohydrates), starches (complex carbohydrates), and fiber (cellulose) that are found mainly in plants. They are stored in the body as glycogen in virtually all tissues but mainly in the liver and muscles. They form an important source of reserved energy in the body.

Sugars include simple sugars (monosaccharides of glucose, galactose, and fructose) and complex sugars (disaccharide of sucrose, lactose or milk sugar, and maltose). Starches are polysaccharides, which are reduced to glucose during the digestive process and transported into the blood. Most sugars are produced

Professionalism

naturally by plants, especially fruits, sugar cane, and sugar beets. However, lactose, a combination of glucose and galactose, is found in animal milk. Processed or refined sugars (e.g., table sugar, molasses, and corn syrup) have been extracted and concentrated from natural resources.

Carbohydrates provide 4 calories of energy for every gram of carbohydrate. Complex carbohydrates are considered ideal foods for a healthy diet since they are generally low in fat, high in fiber, and are a good source for vitamins and minerals. Excess carbohydrates are stored in the body as fat.

Sources of simple carbohydrates (simple sugars) are:

- Refined table sugar, honey, jelly, syrup, candy
- Natural sugar in fruits and vegetables

Sources of complex carbohydrates (starches) are:

- Vegetables (yams, potatoes, broccoli, carrots, peas, beans)
- Citrus fruits (oranges, grapefruit, lemons, limes)
- Whole grains, cereals, and pastas

Nutritionists recommend that only 10% of the body's calorie requirements should come from refined sugar. Complex carbohydrates should provide 50% to 60% of the daily calorie requirements.

Protein

Proteins are called the "building blocks" of the body because they form the base of every living cell. A protein is linked together, much like a chain, with 20 amino acids. Eleven of the amino acids can be produced by the body. However 9 of the amino acids, referred to as essential amino acids, must be obtained from the diet.

The nine essential amino acids are only found in complete proteins, which include proteins from animal sources, such as meat, cheese, eggs, fish, and milk. Incomplete proteins, which cannot supply the body with all of the essential amino acids, include vegetable proteins, such as peas, beans, and wheat. Fortunately, various combinations of the incomplete proteins can supply the essential amino acids, for example, legumes and rice. It is recommended that 12% to 15% of the daily calories consumed come from proteins.

Proteins are necessary for:

- Producing energy (4 calories of energy for every gram of protein consumed)
- Promoting growth and repair of tissues
- Providing the framework for bones, muscles, and blood

Fats

Fats, also called lipids, are fatty acids that can be chemically classified as saturated or unsaturated. Fats do not dissolve in water. Some fat is necessary in the diet since the fat-soluble vitamins A, D, E, and K are all carried into the blood system by way of fats. There are also two critical fatty acids, linoleic and linolenic, which are "essential" to the diet. Fat is a major source of energy for the body. Fat can be found in both animal and plant food products. When eaten moderately, fat is important for proper growth, development, and maintenance of good health. Fat provides taste, consistency, and stability and helps you feel full. Parents should be aware that fats are an especially important source of calories and nutrients for infants and toddlers (up to 2 years of age), who have the highest energy needs per unit of body weight of any age group.

Saturated fat is produced by animal sources, such as meat, eggs, lard, and dairy products and certain oil-producing plants such as coconuts and palms. Many commercially prepared cakes, cookies, and nondairy creamers contain hidden saturated fat. Saturated fat has many negative effects on the body including raising the level of blood cholesterol. It is recommended that no more than 10% of the daily calorie intake should come from saturated fat. Fat reduction can also reduce the risk of disease, for example, certain types of cancer, heart disease, and stroke.

Unsaturated fats are of two types: polyunsaturated fat and monounsaturated fat. Polyunsaturated fat is found in vegetable oils and fish oils (omega-3 fatty acids). Unsaturated fat is normally liquid at room temperature but can be converted into a solid fat through the process of hydrogenation. Hydrogenation turns liquid unsaturated fat into margarine by adding hydrogen.

Monounsaturated fat is considered to be a more desirable type of unsaturated fat since it has the ability to lower cholesterol levels and LDLs. Monounsaturated fats include canola oil, olive oil, and peanut oil. Fats, in moderation, are beneficial for the body. These fats:

- Are a concentrated source of energy (9 calories of energy for every gram of fat consumed)
- Aid in the transportation of soluble fat vitamins A, D, E, and K

TABLE 51-1 Food Label for Snack Crackers

Nutrition Facts			% Daily Value*
Serving size: 16 crackers (29 g)		Total fat 6 g	9%
Servings per container: about 4		Trans fat 2 g	18%
Amount per serving		Polyunsaturated fat 0.5 g	
Calories	140	Monounsaturated fat 2.5 g	
Calories from fat	50	Cholesterol 0 mg	0%
		Sodium 170 mg	7%
		Total carbohydrate 19 g	6%
		Dietary fiber 2 g	
		Protein 2 g	
		Vitamin A	0%
		Vitamin C	0%
		Calcium	2%
		Iron	4%

*Percent Daily Values are based on a 2,000-calorie diet. Your daily values may be higher or lower depending on your calorie needs.

	Calories	2,000	2,500
Total fat	Less than	65 g	80 g
Sat fat	Less than	20 g	25 g
Cholesterol	Less than	300 mg	300 mg
Sodium	Less than	2,400 mg	2,400 mg
Total carbohydrate		300 mg	375 g
Dietary fiber		25 g	30 g

- Serve as a source of energy
- Provide some taste to foods
- Satisfy appetite
- Provide lubrication for skin and internal tissues
- Are stored for future energy use

Unfortunately, many Americans are eating more fat in their diet than they need. Many foods contain hidden fat. Fat content is indicated on many foods. However, food labeling can be confusing and misleading. A high-fiber muffin may actually contain polyunsaturated fat, eggs, sugar, and very little fiber. See Table 51-1 for an example of food labeling components mandated by the Department of Health and Human Services and the U.S. Department of Agriculture.

TRANS **FATS** Beginning in 2006, all labels must identify the *trans* fats in food. Basically, trans fat is made when manufacturers add hydrogen to vegetable oil. Hydrogenation increases the shelf life and flavor stability of foods containing these fats.

Trans fat is frequently found in vegetable shortenings, some margarines, snack foods, and other foods made with or fried in partially hydrogenated oils. Unlike other fats, the majority of trans fat is formed when food manufacturers turn liquid oils into solid fats such as shortening and hard margarine. A small amount of trans fat is found naturally, primarily in dairy products, some meat, and other animal-based foods.

While unsaturated fats (monounsaturated and polyunsaturated) are beneficial when consumed in moderation, saturated and trans fats are not. Saturated fat and trans fat raise LDL cholesterol levels in the blood. Dietary cholesterol also contributes to heart disease.

Therefore, it is advisable to choose foods low in saturated fat, trans fat, and cholesterol as part of a healthful diet.

When comparing foods, look at the Nutrition Facts panel on the label, and choose the food with the lower amounts of saturated fat, trans fat, and cholesterol. Health experts recommend that you keep your intake of saturated fat, trans fat, and cholesterol as low as possible while consuming a nutritionally adequate diet. However, these experts recognize that eliminating these three components entirely from your diet is not practical because they are unavoidable in ordinary diets. See Table 51-2 for trans fat information.

TABLE 51-2 Total Fat, Saturated Fat, Trans Fat, and Cholesterol Content Per Serving[a]

Product	Common Serving Size	Total Fat (g)	Sat. Fat (g)	% DV for Sat. Fat	Trans Fat (g)	Combined Sat. & Trans Fat (g)	Cholesterol (mg)	% DV for Cholesterol
French fried potatoes[b] (fast food)	Medium (147 g)	27	7	35%	8	15	0	0%
Butter[c]	1 Tbsp	11	7	35%	0	7	30	10%
Margarine, stick[d]	1 Tbsp	11	2	10%	3	5	0	0%
Margarine, tub[d]	1 Tbsp	7	1	5%	0.5	1.5	0	0%
Mayonnaise[e] (soybean oil)	1 Tbsp	11	1.5	8%	0	1.5	5	2%
Shortening[b]	1 Tbsp	13	3.5	18%	4	7.5	0	0%
Potato chips[b]	Small bag (42.5 g)	11	2	10%	3	5	0	0%
Milk, whole[b]	1 cup	7	4.5	23%	0	4.5	35	12%
Milk, skim[d]	1 cup	0	0	0%	0	0	5	2%
Doughnut[b]	1	18	4.5	23%	5	9.5	25	8%
Cookies[b] (cream filled)	3 (30 g)	6	1	5%	2	3	0	0%
Candy bar[b]	1 (40 g)	10	4	20%	3	7	<5	1%
Cake, pound[b]	1 slice (80 g)	16	3.5	18%	4.5	8	0	0%

[a]Nutrient values rounded based on FDA's nutrition labeling regulations.
[b]1995 USDA Composition Data.
[c]Butter values from FDA Table of *Trans* Values, 1/30/95.
[d]Values derived from 2002 USDA National Nutrient Database for Standard Reference, Release 15.

[e]Prerelease values derived from 2003 USDA National Nutrient Database for Standard Reference, Release 16.

Source: www.fda.gov.

Water

Water is a vital nutrient that is necessary for survival. The human body can survive for several weeks without food, but cannot live more than a few days without water. Water is an inorganic nutrient with no caloric value. Approximately two-thirds of the body is water.

The average human body is composed of between 50% and 60% water. The male body has more water than the female due to the greater muscle mass of the male, which can hold more water. The female body, on the other hand, contains a greater percentage of fat than the male body. Fat does not hold as much water as muscle tissue does.

There are a variety of sources for water in the body. Water is found in most fruits and vegetables, ingested as a liquid beverage, or occurs naturally as a result of metabolism. The function of water in the body is described in Box 51-1.

The recommended daily amount of water to be ingested is six to eight glasses. Because water occurs in many foods, such as fruits, vegetables, meats, crackers, and even desserts, most people ingest enough water on a daily basis. Water intake is kept in balance with fluid output through the skin, lungs, urine, and feces. Individuals vary in their requirements for water depending on:

- Age
- Body size
- Exercise
- Climate
- Pregnancy
- Illness
- Metabolic rate
- Diet

Vitamins

Vitamins are organic substances that are essential for metabolism, growth, and development of the body. They are not sources of energy but they are required for health. There are a variety of conditions that increase the need for vitamins above the usual recommended dose. These include pregnancy, lactation, excessive use of alcohol, and some illnesses.

In general, most of the vitamins cannot be formed in the body with the exception of vitamin A, which is formed from carotene. Vitamin D is formed by the action of ultraviolet light on the skin (sunlight) and vitamin K by bacteria of the intestines.

Vitamins are generally identified by their alphabetic letter. The two main classifications of vitamins are fat soluble (A, D, E, and K) and water soluble (B and C). These classifications are important in patients who have diseases that interfere with the digestion of fat, such as in celiac disease, since they will eventually develop a deficiency in the fat-soluble vitamins. The human body cannot manufacture vitamin C, therefore it must be taken in foods, citrus fruits, or as a supplement.

BOX 51-1

Function of Water in the Body

Water is used by the body to:

- Carry oxygen and nutrients to cells.
- Regulate body temperature.
- Prevent dehydration.
- Replace water lost through perspiration, respiration, urination, and defecation.
- Remove waste products from cells.
- Protect organs and tissues.

Sources for water-soluble vitamins are:

- Vitamin B_1: liver, eggs, pork, wheat germ, yeast-enriched cereals, nuts
- Vitamin B_2: milk, liver, egg whites, yeast, wheat germ, almonds
- Vitamin B_6: wheat bran, molasses, liver, soybeans, bananas, raisins
- Vitamin B_{12}: beef, liver, milk, shellfish, cheese
- Niacin: liver, poultry, enriched cereals, tuna, peanuts
- Biotin: egg yolks, legumes, meat
- Folacin: legumes, green leafy vegetables
- Pantothenic acid: legumes, grains
- Vitamin C: citrus fruits, raw vegetables, strawberries

Sources of fat-soluble vitamins are:

- Vitamin A: green and yellow vegetables, animal foods, egg yolks, cheese
- Vitamin D: milk, butter, margarine, sardines, fish liver oils, sunlight
- Vitamin E: wheat germ, corn oil, soybeans
- Vitamin K: green leafy vegetables, liver, cabbage, cauliflower

Vitamins can be destroyed in foods through improper storage and prolonged cooking. They do provide essential organic substances. See Table 51-3 for a further description of individual vitamins.

Minerals

Minerals are inorganic elements that are of neither animal nor plant origin. They are found throughout the body but mainly in bones and teeth, and they compose 5% of the body. The two classifications of minerals are macrominerals (major minerals) and microminerals

TABLE 51-3 **Vitamins and Minerals**

Vitamins/ Nutrient	Source	Functional Deficiency	Toxicity	Recommended Dietary Allowances (RDA)[a]
Vitamin A (carotene): necessary for formation and maintenance of skin, mucous membranes, teeth and hair, and normal vision	Egg yolk, fish-liver oils, liver, green leafy or yellow vegetables, yellow and orange fruits, dairy products	Night blindness, fatigue, scaly skin	Headache, skin peeling, bone thickening, liver and spleen enlargement	5000 IU/day
Vitamin B_1 (thiamine): carbohydrate metabolism, nerve cell function, heart muscle function	Dried yeast, whole grains, meat (liver and pork), nuts, enriched cereals, potatoes, legumes	Beriberi, fatigue, mental confusion		1.5 mg/day
Vitamin B_2 (riboflavin): releases energy during protein metabolism	Milk, cheese, eggs, liver, enriched cereals, almonds	Anemia, dermatosis, skin cracks		1.2 mg/day
Vitamin B_6 (group): nitrogen and protein metabolism, assists in building body tissue	Dried yeast, liver, whole grain cereals, fish, legumes, bananas, avocados	Anemia, seborrheic dermatitis, nervous system disorders, convulsions, skin cracks	Nerve damage	2 mg/day
Vitamin B_{12} (cyanocobalamin): nervous system function, fat and protein metabolism	Milk products, seafood, meat, liver, cheese	Pernicious anemia, fatigue, nervousness		6 mcg/day
Niacin (nicotinic acid): carbohydrate, fat, and protein metabolism	Dried yeast, fish, liver, meat, legumes, enriched cereals, eggs, peanuts, and poultry	Pellagra, dermatosis, glossitis, CNS dysfunction, fatigue		20 mg/day
Vitamin C (ascorbic acid): needed to build bones, muscles, blood vessels, and connective tissue; aids in iron absorption	Citrus fruits, tomatoes, broccoli, potatoes, cabbage, green peppers, berries, and strawberries	Scurvy, loose teeth, hemorrhoids, gingivitis, fatigue	Nausea and diarrhea	60 mg/day
Vitamin D: necessary for calcium and phosphorous absorption, bone and tooth development and maintenance; helps maintain nervous system and heart muscle action	Fortified milk, butter, margarine, eggs, fish-liver oils, liver, sunlight	Rickets, tetany, loss of bone calcium	Diarrhea, weight loss, renal failure	400 IU/day

(*continued*)

TABLE 51-3 Vitamins and Minerals (*continued*)

Vitamins/ Nutrient	Source	Functional Deficiency	Toxicity	Recommended Dietary Allowances (RDA)[a]
Vitamin E: protects blood cell membranes, body tissues and fatty acids from destruction	Vegetable oil, wheat germ, margarine, egg yolks, leafy vegetables, legumes, cereals	Anemia, nerve damage, RBC hemolysis, muscle damage		30 IU/day
Vitamin K: normal blood coagulation, prothrombin formation	Leafy vegetables, liver, pork, vegetable oils, fruit, dairy	Hemorrhage in newborn and in person taking blood thinner		No RDA for Vitamin A
Biotin: metabolism of protein, carbohydrates, and fats	Yeast, liver, kidney, egg yolks, nuts, legumes, cauliflower	Dermatitis, glossitis		0.5 mg/day
Folic acid: RBC production	Dried legumes, green leafy vegetables, organ meats	Anemia, GI disorders, mouth cracks		0.4 mg/day
Pantothenic acid: aids in energy release from carbohydrates and fats	Whole grains, meats, vegetables, fruits, legumes	Muscle cramps, fatigue, vomiting		10 mg/day
Calcium: bone and tooth formation, muscle contractility, blood coagulation, myocardial conduction, neuromuscular function	Milk and milk products, meat, fish, eggs, beans, cereals, fruits, vegetables, tofu, fortified orange juice	Hypocalcemia, tetany, neuromuscular excitability, osteoporosis	Hypercalcemia, kidney stones, renal failure	800 mg/day
Chromium: part of glucose tolerance factor (CTF)	Brewer's yeast and widely distributed in other foods	Impaired glucose tolerance in malnourished children and diabetics		No RDA
Cobalt: part of vitamin B_{12} molecule	Green leafy vegetables	Anemia in children		20 mg/day
Copper: enzyme component	Oysters, organ meats, nuts, dried legumes, whole grain cereals	Anemia in malnourished children		0.3 mg/kg per day
Fluorine: bone and tooth formation	Coffee, tea, fluoridated water	Dental caries	Mottling and pitting of permanent teeth	No RDA

(*continued*)

TABLE 51-3 **Vitamins and Minerals** (*continued*)

Vitamins/ Nutrient	Source	Functional Deficiency	Toxicity	Recommended Dietary Allowances (RDA)[a]
Iodine: thyroxine (T_4) and triiodothyronine (T_3) formation, necessary for energy formation	Seafood, iodized salt, dairy products	Goiter, cretinism	Myxedema	150 mcg/day
Iron: hemoglobin, enzymes	Soybean flour, kidney, beef, liver, beans, peaches	Anemia		30 mg/day
Magnesium: bone and tooth formation, nerve conduction, muscle contractility, enzyme activity	Green leafy vegetables, cereals, nuts, wheat bran, grains, seafood, chocolate	Neuromuscular irritability, weakness	Hypotension, respiratory failure, cardiac disturbances	280 mg/day
Phosphorus: bone and tooth formation, acid–base formation	Milk, cheese, meat, fish, poultry, cereals, nuts, legumes	Irritability, weakness, blood cell disorders		300 mg/day
Potassium: muscle activity, nerve transmission, intracellular acid–base balance, water retention	Milk, bananas, kiwi, raisins, vegetables	Hypokalemia, paralysis, cardiac arrhythmia (irregular heartbeat)	Hyperkalemia, paralysis, cardiac arrhythmia	2000 mg/day
Sodium: maintain acid–base balance, muscle contractility, nerve transmission	Meat (beef, pork), cheese sardines, olives, potato chips, table salt	Hyponatremia, muscle cramping	Hypernatremia, coma, confusion, high blood pressure	500 mg/day
Zinc: growth, wound healing component of insulin and enzyme	Vegetables	Growth retardation		30 mg/day

[a]IU, international units; mg, milligrams; meg, micrograms.

(trace minerals). The macrominerals include calcium, magnesium, phosphorus, sodium, potassium, chlorine, and sulfur. Macrominerals are required in greater amounts than the trace minerals iron, iodine, copper, manganese, cobalt, fluorine, zinc, selenium, chromium, nickel, tin, and vanadium. Minerals are found in the following sources:

- Vegetables and fruits for calcium, iron, phosphorus, copper, and iodine
- Milk and leafy vegetables for calcium
- Balanced diet

Minerals do not supply calories or energy. See Table 51-3 for more information on minerals.

Cholesterol

There is currently much controversy surrounding cholesterol. Cholesterol is a fat-like material that is normally found in the body. It is essential for the function of body systems, such as the nervous system, formation of cell membranes, and many hormones.

Cholesterol is found in only two sources: the human body and in animal sources. Cholesterol does not come from plants. Animal sources of cholesterol provide saturated fat, which may contribute to elevated blood cholesterol in humans.

Cholesterol moves into and out of the body cells within compounds called lipoproteins. These lipoproteins are classified into either high-density lipoproteins

(HDLs) or low-density lipoproteins (LDLs). HDLs are the "good cholesterol" and LDLs are the "bad cholesterol." LDLs are bad since they carry most (60% to 70%) of the cholesterol into the bloodstream. This cholesterol is deposited into blood vessels and can lead to a narrowing of the blood vessels, which leads to heart disease and stroke. HDLs are good because they only contain 20% to 30% of the blood cholesterol and carry cholesterol away from the arteries. It is believed that the higher the HDL level in the blood, the lower the risk for cardiovascular disease.

An increase in cholesterol level has been tied to an increased risk for heart disease: heart attack and stroke. Evidence indicates that unsaturated fats (olive oil and canola oil) may help to lower the amount of cholesterol in the blood. It is important to examine food labels for the amounts of both cholesterol and saturated fat. Many foods contain no cholesterol but have a large amount of saturated fat, which can lead to cholesterol buildup in the body.

Balanced Diet

The key to a balanced diet is eating a variety of foods in the correct amount. Eating food as recommended in the food guide pyramid published by the U.S. Department of Health and Human Services will be adequate for good health. The size of portions and numbers of servings will depend on the age, size, and exercise level of the individual. See Figure 51-1 for an illustration of the basic nutrient classifications.

Food Guide Pyramid

A revised food guide pyramid was introduced in 2005 by the U.S. Department of Agriculture to replace the old "basic four" food groups from 1946 and the 1992 update. Figure 51-3 illustrates the new food guide pyramid. A healthy diet should include a wide variety of foods. Patients can better understand the entire nutritional process if they see the food pyramid (see also Cultural Considerations). Many doctors' offices display a large poster of the pyramid on the wall.

The new food pyramid customizes a regimen according to age, activity, and gender. If patients want a customized food pyramid, they can go to the website to customize an education plan for them. The site addresses appropriate physical activity and describes the six food groups: grains, vegetables, fruits, milk, meat and beans, and fats and oils. The customized pyramid describes an ideal amount for the person to eat daily, with lists of healthy foods in each category. The site promotes fresh, rather than processed foods. It also suggests the use of healthy oils rather than solid fats. The pyramid suggests the user choose lean or low-fat meat and poultry and foods rich in omega-3 fatty acids. It also describes discretionary calories,

such as wine and sweetened cereals, which should be minimized. Sweets, while pleasant to taste, are rarely nutritious.

Recommended Dietary Allowances (RDAs)

The Food and Nutrition Board of the National Academy of Sciences has created standards of recommendations for the amount of protein, vitamins, and minerals that Americans should try to eat and the body weights they should try to maintain for good nutrition. These standards periodically change as the weight ranges and protein needs are reviewed. The charts can be ordered through the National Academy Press, Washington, DC.

Calories

The intake of food is measured in terms of the energy that it produces. A calorie is a measurement of a unit of heat that provides energy. The definition of a calorie is the amount of heat (energy) required to raise the temperature of 1 kg of water 1 degree Celsius ($1°C$).

All food (except water) generates energy in the body. Daily calorie requirements of individuals will vary based on a variety of factors including gender, age, weight, and activity level. Men generally need more calories than women; the young need more calories than older adults; heavier people require more calories to maintain their weight; and active people require more calories because they tend to burn calories faster than individuals who are inactive. Women require more calories during periods of pregnancy and lactation.

Anatomy of MyPyramid

One size doesn't fit all
USDA's new MyPyramid symbolizes a personalized approach to healthy eating and physical activity. The symbol has been designed to be simple. It has been developed to remind consumers to make healthy food choices and to be active every day. The different parts of the symbol are described below.

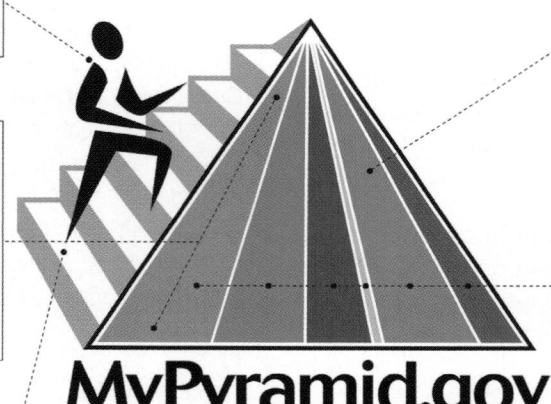

Activity
Activity is represented by the steps and the person climbing them, as a reminder of the importance of daily physical activity.

Moderation
Moderation is represented by the narrowing of each food group from bottom to top. The wider base stands for foods with little or no solid fats or added sugars. These should be selected more often. The narrower top area stands for foods containing more added sugars and solid fats. The more active you are, the more of these foods can fit into your diet.

Personalization
Personalization is shown by the person on the steps, the slogan, and the URL. Find the kinds and amounts of food to eat each day at MyPyramid.gov.

Proportionality
Proportionality is shown by the different widths of the food group bands. The widths suggest how much food a person should choose from each group. The widths are just a general guide, not exact proportions. Check the Web site for how much is right for you.

Variety
Variety is symbolized by the 6 color bands representing the 5 food groups of the Pyramid and oils. This illustrates that foods from all groups are needed each day for good health.

Gradual Improvement
Gradual improvement is encouraged by the slogan. It suggests that individuals can benefit from taking small steps to improve their diet and lifestyle each day.

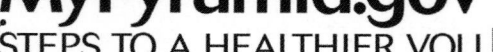

U.S. Department of Agriculture
Center for Nutrition Policy and Promotion
April 2005 CNPP-16

USDA is an equal opportunity provider and employer.

GRAINS VEGETABLES FRUITS OILS MILK MEAT & BEANS

FIGURE 51-3 The 2005 food guide pyramid.

When more calories are taken in than are consumed, they are stored as fat. Overall body weight will increase when this happens on a consistent basis. When fewer calories are taken in than are needed, stored calories are used and the body weight will decrease.

Calories come from the proteins, carbohydrates, and fats in food. To determine the amount of energy generated by the food eaten, use the following figures:

- Protein: 4 calories of energy per gram
- Carbohydrate: 4 calories of energy per gram
- Fat: 9 calories of energy per gram

Note: These figures are just for the protein, carbohydrate, and fat content of foods and not the total weight, including fluid, of the food.

Determining the Number of Calories in Food

Using a cookie that contains 1 g of protein, 4 g of carbohydrates, and 4 g of fat, calculate the total number of calories.

1. 1 g protein (4 calories per gram) — 4 calories
2. 4 g of carbohydrates (4 calories per gram) — 16 calories
3. 4 g of fat (9 calories per gram) — 36 calories

Total calories-56 calories per cookie.

Determining the Percentage of Calories Supplied by Fat

Use this formula when you want to determine the percentage of calories in a food supplied by fat:

1. Fat calories: grams of fat $\times$ 9.
2. Place result of calculation 1 over total calories.

Using the previous example of a cookie containing 56 calories, determine the percentage of calories supplied from fat:

1. $4 \times 9 = 36$ fat calories
2. $36/56 = 0.642 = 64.2\%$

Therefore, 64.2% of the calories in this cookie are supplied by fat.

Dietary Guidelines

Under normal disease-free conditions, the average person should observe the following dietary guidelines:

1. Eat a wide variety of foods to acquire the necessary vitamins and minerals.
2. Choose a diet that is low in fat, saturated fat, and cholesterol.
3. Eat a diet that is rich in vegetables, fruits, and whole grains.
4. Limit intake of salt. Try not to add salt to food.
5. Use sugar in moderation.
6. Use alcohol in moderation. Do not use alcohol at all during pregnancy.

Dietary Modifications

The normal (regular) diet can be modified to adjust to specific patient conditions, such as pregnancy, recovery from surgery, gastrointestinal upset, allergies, dental work, and disease conditions such as diabetes mellitus. A modified diet for health reasons is called a therapeutic diet. Diets can be modified based on calorie content, level of spice and salt content, bulk, nutrients, consistency, and intervals between meals.

Therapeutic diets need to be carefully explained to patients. In some cases, the physician will refer the patient to a registered dietitian (RD) who can discuss all aspects of a therapeutic diet with the patient.

The medical assistant will often provide dietary education for patients in the medical office (see Legal and Ethical Issues). Since lifestyle changes must be made to comply with some of the diets, the patient must be motivated to make the required changes. All of the principles of adult education need to be considered when teaching patients about dietary changes. For example, when a woman is pregnant, it is more important for her to eat good-quality food (high in folic acid and calcium) than to increase the quantity of food. In fact, a pregnant or lactating woman should increase her caloric diet by only 500 calories per day.

Clear Liquid Diet

A clear liquid diet contains no solid food or milk products. A clear liquid diet is frequently required before certain laboratory tests, examinations, or surgery. It may also be prescribed for a patient suffering from gastrointestinal problems. A clear liquid diet is frequently the first diet a patient is placed on after having surgery and a general anesthetic. Patients must not remain on a clear liquid diet for an extended period of time because it has little nutritional value.

Foods included on a clear diet are:

- Clear soup and broth
- Plain gelatin

- Black coffee
- Tea
- Carbonated beverages

Full Liquid Diet

A full liquid diet is often prescribed for patients who are unable to chew and/or digest solid food. This may be due to gastrointestinal problems, infections, or oral surgery. This diet is also prescribed as the next diet step for patients who have been on a clear liquid diet.

Foods recommended on a full liquid diet are:

- All liquids allowed on a clear diet
- Fruit and vegetable juices
- Strained fruit
- Soup (creamed or strained)
- Milk and milkshakes
- Ice cream

As with the clear liquid diet, a full liquid diet is not to be used for extended periods of time.

Mechanical Soft Diet

The mechanical soft diet is recommended for patients who have dental problems, such as a lack of teeth, or who have difficulty swallowing. This diet is often recommended when patients are recovering from surgery.

Foods included on this diet are:

- All soups
- All liquids
- Cooked vegetables
- Canned fruit
- Ground meat and vegetables
- Tender fish and poultry

Bland Diet

A bland diet contains no seasonings or fibers that are irritating. This diet is prescribed for patients who have gastrointestinal problems and allergies. Foods that are gas forming (such as cabbage), contain caffeine or spices, or are high in fiber are eliminated.

Foods included in a bland diet are:

- Mildly flavored foods
- Low-fiber foods
- Milk products
- Cooked fruit
- Noncitrus juices

BRAT Diet

Children suffering from uncontrolled gastrointestinal upsets can become dehydrated more easily than adults due to the depletion of body fluids. Physicians often recommend foods on the BRAT diet since they are easily digested and do not cause further upsets.

BRAT stands for:

Bananas

Rice

Applesauce

Toast

This combination of foods is prescribed for small children who suffer from vomiting, nausea, and diarrhea. Children should be seen by the physician if symptoms continue.

High-Protein Diet

A high-protein diet is recommended for patients recovering from bone injuries. This diet can aid in healing. Protein foods such as meat, dairy products, and legumes need to be eaten along with a variety of fruits and vegetables for a balanced diet. Often a high-protein drink is included for the patient.

Diabetic Diet

A therapeutic diet designed for diabetic patients must consider several factors including:

1. Type of insulin therapy the patient receives
2. Severity of the diabetes
3. Activity and exercise level
4. Ability for activity
5. Calories necessary to maintain the patient's weight

A food exchange system is often used for diabetic patients. This allows for variety in their diet since the patient is able to select foods they prefer. Foods are grouped into the same six categories discussed in the food pyramid: breads, fruits, vegetables, meat, milk, and fat.

Each food plan must be prescribed for the individual patient. All diabetic diets should be given to the patient in writing. The medical assistant will be asked to reinforce the eating plan with the patient.

High-Residue/Fiber Diet

The high-fiber diet is used to treat patients with existing problems as well as to provide prevention for heart disease. New research is demonstrating that a diet high in fiber is effective in preventing colon cancer.

Dietary fiber is thought to provide protection against diabetes, breast and colon cancer, gallbladder disease, constipation, irritable bowel syndrome, hemorrhoids, and diverticulosis. Fiber may also reduce the level of cholesterol within the blood, thereby protecting against heart disease. The recommended daily intake of fiber is between 20 and 30 grams. Dietary fiber is not found in animal products or dairy products.

Fiber sources are:

- Raw fruits and vegetables
- Whole-grain breads and cereals
- Legumes

Low-Residue Diet

A low-residue diet is also called a low-fiber diet. This diet is useful for a variety of patients including those with colitis, diarrhea, indigestion, or a colostomy.

Some low-residue foods are:

- Cooked vegetables and stewed fruit
- Bananas are the only raw fruit allowed
- Lean beef, lamb, chicken, and turkey
- Cooked cereal
- Eggs
- Soups, all except creamed soups

Foods not allowed on a low-residue diet are:

- Fried food
- Milk or milk products
- Seasonings

Low-Fat/Low-Cholesterol Diet

The average American diet contains between 30 and 50 grams of fat per day. A low-fat diet is aimed at keeping the fat content between 20 and 30 grams of fat per day. This diet is recommended for patients who have an intolerance to fat, for example, patients with gallbladder, pancreatic, and/or liver disease. A low-fat diet has been found to reduce the risk of colon, breast, and prostate cancer, heart disease, and obesity.

Foods recommended on a low-fat/low-cholesterol diet are:

- Fruits and vegetables
- Skim milk
- Whole-grain breads and cereals
- Only desserts such as angel food cake, graham crackers, and no-fat wafers

Foods not allowed on a low-fat/low-cholesterol diet are:

- All fried foods
- Visible fat
- Butter and margarine

Low-Sodium/Low-Salt Diet

Therapeutic diets vary in the amount of salt restrictions. Restrictions vary from mild to moderate and severe. Diets are restricted in salt for patients with hypertension and heart or kidney disease. Salt restriction is also recommended for patients on weight reduction diets since an excess of salt/sodium in the diet promotes water retention.

Mild sodium-restricted diets allow between 3,000 and 5,000 mg of sodium per day. Many foods, especially processed foods, contain salt. A mild sodium-restricted diet (2,000 to 3,000 mg) would result in an allowance of 1/2 teaspoon of table salt per day and a very limited amount of foods containing salt.

A moderate salt-restricted diet allows 1,500 to 2,000 mg of sodium per day. This diet allows 1/2 teaspoon of table salt, but all processed and canned foods containing salt are prohibited. No salt is allowed in food preparation. This is the most frequently prescribed level of salt restriction.

A severe salt-restricted diet of 500 mg per day would limit all table salt use, cooking salt, and include only salt-free products in the diet. This diet is difficult to maintain using purchased foods. Patients are recommended to increase the use of fresh fruits and vegetables and to read labels carefully when on severe salt-restricted diets.

Calorie Content Diet

Weight reduction diets are often prescribed for patients whose health is affected by excess weight. Gaining excess body fat can lead to serious health problems, such as high blood pressure, heart disease, and diabetes.

A 1,200-calorie diet using a balance of the five food groups and low-fat foods will result in weight loss. For a healthy diet patients are recommended to eat at least four choices from the grains group; five meat or bean choices; two vegetable choices; two fruit choices; two milk choices; and not more than three fat choices. These choices add up to 1,200 calories. Examples of these foods are listed in Box 51-2.

Patients are encouraged to keep a food diary of all they eat in a day. This helps patients to become more aware of the unhealthy eating they might be doing and to substitute healthy foods for unhealthy ones. Table 51-4 illustrates a sample food diary format.

Healthy Food Choices

Healthy food choices include eating less fat, eating more high-fiber foods, using less salt, and eating less sugar.

BOX 51-2
Basic Food Group Choices for a 1,200-Calorie Eating Plan

Grains

Each of these equals one grain choice (80 calories) and contains 1 gram of fat. For weight reduction, limit to four to six choices a day.

½ cup pasta or barley

⅓ cup rice

1 slice bread or 1 roll

4–6 crackers

½ English muffin, bagel, hamburger/hot dog bun

½ cup cooked cereal

¾ cup dry, unsweetened cereal

3 cups popcorn, unbuttered, not cooked in oil

Vegetables

Each of these equals one vegetable choice (25 calories). Two or more servings are recommended per day.

½ cup cooked vegetables

1 cup raw vegetables

½ cup tomato/vegetable juice

Meat and Beans

Each of these equals one meat choice (75 calories). Five to six servings are recommended per day.

1 oz. cooked poultry, fish, or meat

¼ cup salmon or tuna, water packed

1 tablespoon peanut butter

1 egg (limit to 3 per week)

Each of these equals two meat choices (150 calories). Fat content varies for meat but should be limited to a total of 18 fat grams for meat per day.

1 small chicken leg or thigh

½ cup cottage cheese or tuna

Each of these equals three meat choices (225 calories):

1 small hamburger

1 small pork chop

½ chicken breast

1 medium fish filet

Cooked meat about the size of a deck of cards

Milk

Each of these equals one milk choice (75 calories). Two servings per day are recommended.

¼ cup cottage cheese

1 oz. low-fat cheese, such as mozzarella or ricotta

Fruit

Each of these equals one fruit choice (60 calories). Two servings a day are recommended.

1 fresh medium fruit

1 cup berries or melon

½ cup fruit juice

½ cup canned fruit in juice without sugar

¼ cup dried fruit

Oil

Each of these equals one fat choice (45 calories and 5 grams of fat each). Fat should be limited to three servings per day.

1 teaspoon margarine, oil, mayonnaise

2 teaspoons diet margarine or diet mayonnaise

1 tablespoon salad dressing

2 tablespoons reduced-calorie salad dressing

Do not assume similar products are the same. Be sure to check the Nutrition Facts panel on food lables because even similar foods can vary in calories, ingredients, nutrients, and the size and number of servings in a package. Even if you continue to buy the same brand of a product, check the Nutrition Facts panel frequently because ingredients can change at any time.

Eat Less Fat

- Eat smaller servings of meat. Eat poultry and fish more often. Choose lean cuts of red meat.

- Prepare all meats by roasting, broiling, or baking. Trim off all visible fat. Be careful of added sauces or gravy.

- Remove skin from all poultry.

- Avoid all fried foods. Avoid adding fat during cooking.

- Eat fewer high-fat foods such as cold cuts, bacon, sausage, hot dogs, butter, margarine, salad dressing, nuts, lard, and solid shortening.

- Drink skim or low-fat milk.

- Eat less ice cream, cheese, sour cream, whole milk, cream, and other high-fat dairy products.

Eat More High-Fiber Foods

- Choose dried beans, peas, and lentils more often.

- Eat whole grain breads, cereals, crackers.

TABLE 51-4 Food Diary

Calories Each Day: _____		
Meal Time:	Meal Time:	Meal Time:
_____	_____	_____
_____	_____	_____
_____	_____	_____
_____	_____	_____
_____	_____	_____
_____	_____	_____
_____	_____	_____
Snack Time:	Snack Time:	Snack Time:
_____	_____	_____
_____	_____	_____

- Eat more vegetables, raw and cooked.
- Eat whole fruit in place of fruit juice.
- Try high-fiber foods such as oat bran, barley, brown rice, bulgur, and wild rice.

Use Less Salt

- Reduce the amount of salt you use in cooking.
- Try not to put salt on food at the table.
- Eat fewer high-salt foods such as canned soups, ham, hot dogs, pickles, sauerkraut, and foods that taste salty.
- Eat fewer convenience and fast foods.

Eat Less Sugar

- Avoid adding table sugar, syrup, honey, jam, jelly, candy, sweet rolls, fruit canned in syrup, regular gelatin, desserts, pie, cake with icing, and other sweets.
- Avoid regular soft drinks. One 12-ounce can has nine teaspoons of sugar!
- Choose fresh fruit or fruit canned in natural juice or water.
- If desired, use sweeteners that do not have calories, such as saccharin or aspartame, instead of sugar.
- Avoid heavily processed foods

- Food choices that include hydrogenated fats used to preserve food are not as good as fresh foods.

Food Supplements

Physicians prescribe protein-vitamin-mineral food supplements when patients are debilitated due to disease processes, such as AIDS, or they are unable to tolerate a normal diet. In some cases, the liquid supplement may have to be given via a tube feeding until the patient is strong enough to drink the supplement. Supplements to the diet should only be used under the direction of a physician.

Exercise

Exercise and physical activity should be included as part of the patient's health plan. Activity helps to metabolize the fat in the diet so that it does not become stored in the body. Almost any patient can exercise, after being cleared by the physician. Exercises in a pool can even be enjoyed by patients with arthritis. Walking is a good exercise and can be done with little extra equipment beyond a good pair of walking shoes. Some patients, however, will exercise more if they have made a monetary commitment to a gym or health club. Patients can lose weight by making simple modifications to their lifestyle, such as taking the stairs instead of an elevator, or by parking farther away from the entrance of their workplace. Even small changes can help with weight loss. It is important to match the exercise with the interests and finances of the patient. If you select an exercise program that is impossible for the patient to comply with, you set the patient up for failure. It is better to keep an exercise program simple and reasonable for the patient.

Alcohol

Alcohol is not considered a food product, but it does contain calories and lowers the rate at which calories are burned. Some studies have shown the value of moderate consumption of red wine, but excessive alcohol intake is associated with problems such as alcoholism, auto accidents, and family and work disruptions. Pregnant women are advised to exclude alcohol during pregnancy because of the potential for birth defects such as fetal alcohol syndrome.

Stress Management

It is important to decrease stress in the medical office as much as possible. Sick patients can wear down the patience of the staff and leave the medical assistant feeling frustrated. It is important to realize that patients rarely intend to stress the medical assistant— but it is part of the job to deal with people under stress. Therefore, the employees at a medical office may also feel stressed.

One of the best ways to reduce stress in the medical office is to practice stress management. Some forms of stress management are:

Aromatherapy—Some smells, such as lavender, have been shown to decrease stress.

Biofeedback—Wearing biofeedback dots, rings, or patches shows the wearer if stress has constricted blood flow to that area. Knowing that a person is stressed is the first step in changing the behaviors that lead to stress.

Deep breathing—Breathing deeply can relax your body, especially muscles and heart.

Distraction—Some people find hobbies or vacations distracting from stress.

Exercise—Mild exercise has been shown to decrease stress in most individuals

Guided imagery—Taking a few minutes to imagine being in some restful place can cause your body to relax in response to that stimulus.

Hypnosis—Learning to think more deeply without inhibitions can help people regain control of stress.

Humor—Laughing at one's self or the bizarre predicaments of life can decrease stress.

Meditation/prayer—Numerous studies have shown that focusing on reflection or prayer can relax the body.

Music—Restful music that you enjoy has been shown to decrease stress.

Relaxation—Even in the office, a few minutes of concentrating on relaxing muscle groups (perhaps in the break room) can be rejuvenating.

Slow breath counting—Counting slow breaths can distract and relax the brain.

Water therapy—Some people find a bath can soothe them and help relieve stress.

Stress can also be caused by pain. If stress results from pain, these techniques are recommended:

Heat—Applying heat to different parts of the body can distract the brain from pain. Many people enjoy a hot bath for example.

Cold—Applying cold to different parts of the body can distract the brain from pain. Applying a cold pack to the head, for example, can ease a headache.

Pressure—Applying pressure to certain pressure points can reduce pain. Headache pain, for example, can be reduced by massaging the temples.

Usually stress management can only be used for a few minutes at the office, but the medical assistant should plan activities during free time to decrease stress. Sometimes talking to other health professionals about the stress can help the medical assistant to find new ways to reduce stress.

Time Management

One of the greatest attributes of an effective office manager is the ability to effectively manage time. If the manager is organized, the office is usually organized. Time management requires the ability to prioritize what the important tasks are and to complete them on schedule. This is quite different from doing every task as it comes along. The office manager generally has little control over the tasks presented. The control is in how the tasks are handled and delegated.

One of the main responsibilities of the office manager/medical assistant is to manage all the peripheral office functions so that the physician is free to concentrate on practicing medicine. It is possible for the physician to gain an hour each day to devote to administrative and/or patient-related tasks that only he or she can do, because tasks such as opening the daily mail, restocking the medical bag, searching for the drug sample to give to a patient, and dealing with pharmaceutical and other sales representatives are handled by the office manager or medical assistant.

TABLE 51-5   To Do List

Priority	To Do
2	Order paper supplies.
1	Arrange Dr. Christianson's air transportation to medical convention next month.
2	Prepare performance appraisal for Emily Jane Doro.
3	Reorganize storeroom.
1	Type convention speech.
1	Place ad for medical assistant.
3	Ask Ruthy to remove old magazines from reception area.
1	Call for Pap test report on Mrs. Glidewell.
2	Block out schedule for next quarter.
3	Ask Belinda to take down Christmas decorations.
1	Prepare agenda for Thursday's staff meeting.

Before establishing a time management system, it is important to define the office goals with the physician. Physician's goals vary from complex to simple and from long term to short term. These goals may include collecting all payments at the time of service delivery, reorganizing or computerizing billing, limiting the practice, adding a partner or new service, writing a textbook, or plans for early retirement.

After the goals have been established, priorities can be set. The office manager/medical assistant can establish a priority list of the goals. A priority list is a composite of all the tasks that need to be accomplished to actualize each goal. These can be placed on a To Do list, as they come to the office manager's attention. Each item is as-signed a priority designation of 1, 2, or 3 depending on how critical the item is to complete the task. For example, ordering supplies that are running out is given a number 1, while rearranging a linen cupboard or a file drawer might be assigned a 3. Number 1 priority items must be done first and number 3 last. It is often tempting to do the easier tasks first since they take less time and show an immediate accomplishment. Good use of time management would determine that the inventory order should be placed immediately, and the number 3 priority items could be delegated to someone else or completed later, if necessary. It is a good idea to date a To Do list and to cross off items as they are accomplished. Table 51-5 shows an example of a To Do List.

SUMMARY

One of the vital tasks of a medical assistant is to provide patient dietary education, as needed, and as directed by a physician. An example would be nutritional planning for a diabetic patient. The medical assistant often plays a critical role in handling noncompliant patients, such as a diabetic patient who will not adhere to the prescribed diet. Dietary education should be individualized to the patient and the specific disease or condition the patient has. No one diet works for all, but diet is an important component of health and should be considered with all patients. Stress management for patients, employees, and the medical assistant is also important. Medical careers create stress in the practitioners, so it is important to know how to reduce stress. Time management is critical for the office to operate well. Urgent tasks are not necessarily important tasks. A To Do List can help the medical assistant to list and prioritize tasks.

Chapter Review

COMPETENCY REVIEW

1. Define and spell the terms to learn for this chapter.
2. Design a patient teaching chart based on the food guide pyramid to illustrate the five classifications of nutrients.
3. Develop a sample menu for 3 days based on the food guide pyramid.
4. Determine the number of calories in a piece of pie that has 1 g of protein, 8 g of carbohydrates, and 9 g of fat.
5. Take a food label from a package of cereal and list the number of calories, total fat, cholesterol, sodium, total carbohydrates, dietary fiber, sugars, protein, and vitamins.
6. Write a 1-day food plan for the following therapeutic diets: full liquid, mechanical soft, high fiber, moderate salt restrictive, and 1,200 calorie.
7. Maintain a weekly diary of your intake of food. Analyze each food group intake.

PREPARING FOR THE CERTIFICATION EXAM

1. _____ is an example of a water-soluble vitamin.
   A. vitamin A
   B. vitamin B
   C. vitamin D
   D. vitamin E
   E. vitamin K

2. The recommended percentage of foods from proteins in the daily diet is:
   A. 5%
   B. 8%
   C. 12%
   D. 30%
   E. 50%

3. A BRAT diet has been ordered for Abilene Collis, who is 2 years old. What foods will be included on that diet?
   A. apple juice
   B. milk
   C. strained meats
   D. bananas and rice
   E. vegetables

4. When restricting food on a 1,200-calorie diet that is being adapted for a diabetic patient using food exchange lists, what needs to be remembered?
   A. Alcohol is forbidden for all diabetics.
   B. Exercise increases the need for insulin.
   C. Twelve hundred calories may be too much for a diabetic patient.
   D. Water should be restricted with diabetics.
   E. Consider all elements of the food guide pyramid when developing a diet.

5. An example of a complex carbohydrate is:
   A. jelly
   B. table sugar
   C. meat
   D. syrup
   E. honey

6. Which of the following statements about cholesterol is TRUE?
   A. All cholesterol is bad.
   B. Good cholesterol is low-density lipoproteins (LDL).
   C. There is no evidence that high cholesterol intake is linked to disease.
   D. Cholesterol is an essential element normally found in the body.
   E. The information "cholesterol 0 mg" on a food label means that there is no fat present.

7. Which of the following is not a stress management technique?
   A. music
   B. guided imagery
   C. meditation
   D. vigorous exercise
   E. deep breathing

8. Which statement about carbohydrates is NOT TRUE?
   A. They are the body's main source of energy.
   B. They provide 4 calories of energy for every gram of carbohydrate.
   C. They include the nine essential amino acids.
   D. They include sugar, syrup, and jam.
   E. They include wheat germ, pasta, and sweet potatoes.

continued on next page

9. Goals for time management in the office for the office manager might include all of the following EXCEPT:
   A. computerizing billing
   B. scheduling physician travel
   C. orienting new employees
   D. selecting gifts for the physician's wife
   E. creating presentations for the physician

10. Which percentage of the human body is water?
    A. 5–10
    B. 20–29
    C. 40–49
    D. 50–59
    E. 75–80

CRITICAL THINKING

1. What general information would you give Mrs. Drahms?
2. What foods would you recommend for Mrs. Drahms?
3. How will Dr. Franklin measure her weight gain during pregnancy?
4. What foods should Mrs. Drahms avoid?
5. If her husband asks if they can eat out in fancy restaurants, what would you answer?

ON THE JOB

Gladys Pierce is a 70-year-old patient of Dr. Court Franklin. She is more than 100 pounds overweight and a newly diagnosed type 2 diabetic. She is concerned that she may lose her eyesight and feeling in her arms and legs if she does not get her diabetes under control. She may also have strokes and even a lethal heart attack. Dr. Franklin asks Dan Tyler, CMA, to create a diet for Ms. Pierce.

1. What general instructions would you give Ms. Pierce?
2. What foods would be good dietary choices?
3. Which foods would be poor choices for her?
4. How should Ms. Pierce prepare foods to decrease fat calories?
5. Would processed foods be a good choice for Ms. Pierce or not?

INTERNET ACTIVITY

Visit the website www.supersizeme.com or view the video *Supersize Me* and comment on the man's dietary habits.

Visit the website www.mypyramid.gov and create a dietary regimen suited to your age, gender, and activity level.

MediaLink More on nutrition, including interactive resources, can be found on the Student CD-ROM accompanying this textbook.

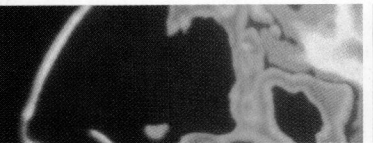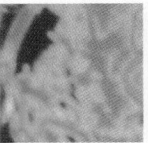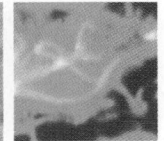

Medical Assistant Role Delineation Chart

HIGHLIGHT indicates material covered in this chapter.

ADMINISTRATIVE

Administrative Procedures

- Perform basic administrative medical assisting functions
- Schedule, coordinate and monitor appointments
- Schedule inpatient/outpatient admissions and procedures
- Understand and apply third-party guidelines
- Obtain reimbursement through accurate claims submission
- Monitor third-party reimbursement
- Understand and adhere to managed care policies and procedures
- *Negotiate managed care contracts*

Practice Finances

- Perform procedural and diagnostic coding
- Apply bookkeeping principles

- Manage accounts receivable
- *Manage accounts payable*
- *Process payroll*
- *Document and maintain accounting and banking records*
- *Develop and maintain fee schedules*
- *Manage renewals of business and professional insurance policies*
- *Manage personnel benefits and maintain records*
- *Perform marketing, financial, and strategic planning*

CLINICAL

Fundamental Principles

- Apply principles of aseptic technique and infection control
- Comply with quality assurance practices
- Screen and follow up patient test results

Diagnostic Orders

- Collect and process specimens
- Perform diagnostic tests

Patient Care

- Adhere to established patient screening procedures
- Obtain patient history and vital signs
- Prepare and maintain examination and treatment areas
- Prepare patient for examinations, procedures and treatments

- Assist with examinations, procedures and treatments
- Prepare and administer medications and immunizations
- Maintain medication and immunization records
- Recognize and respond to emergencies
- Coordinate patient care information with other health care providers
- Initiate IV and administer IV medications with appropriate training and as permitted by state law

GENERAL

Professionalism

- Display a professional manner and image
- Demonstrate initiative and responsibility
- Work as a member of the health care team
- Prioritize and perform multiple tasks
- Adapt to change
- Promote the CMA credential
- Enhance skills through continuing education
- Treat all patients with compassion and empathy
- Promote the practice through positive public relations

Communication Skills

- Recognize and respect cultural diversity
- Adapt communications to individual's ability to understand
- Use professional telephone technique

- Recognize and respond effectively to verbal, nonverbal, and written communications
- Use medical terminology appropriately
- Utilize electronic technology to receive, organize, prioritize and transmit information
- Serve as liaison

Legal Concepts

- Perform within legal and ethical boundaries
- Prepare and maintain medical records
- Document accurately
- Follow employer's established policies dealing with the health care contract
- Implement and maintain federal and state health care legislation and regulations
- Comply with established risk management and safety procedures
- Recognize professional credentialing criteria
- *Develop and maintain personnel, policy and procedure manuals*

Instruction

- Instruct individuals according to their needs
- Explain office policies and procedures
- Teach methods of health promotion and disease prevention
- Locate community resources and disseminate information
- *Develop educational materials*
- *Conduct continuing education activities*

Operational Functions

- Perform inventory of supplies and equipment
- Perform routine maintenance of administrative and clinical equipment
- Apply computer techniques to support office operations
- *Perform personnel management functions*
- *Negotiate leases and prices for equipment and supply contracts*

- *Denotes advanced skills.*

SOURCE: Reprinted by permission of the American Association of Medical Assistants from the AAMA Role Delineation Study: Occupational Analysis of the Medical Assisting Profession.

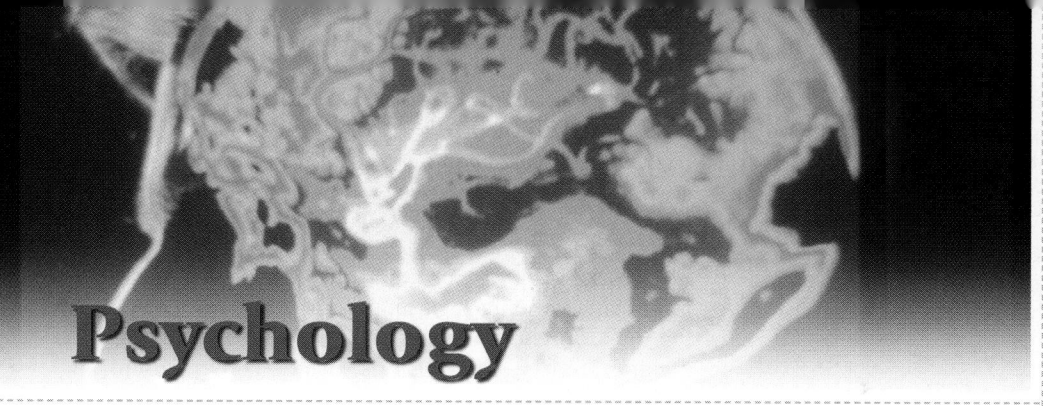

Psychology

Learning Objectives

After reading this chapter, you should be able to:

- Define and spell the terms to learn for this chapter.

- List 11 major diagnostic categories of mental disorders.

- State the difference between neurosis and psychosis.

- Explain psychotherapy, psychopharmacology, and electroconvulsive therapy.

- Discuss Maslow's hierarchy of needs.

- Discuss heredity and cultural and environmental influences on behavior.

- Discuss interpersonal skills and human behavior.

- Explain how to communicate with a patient who is frightened, angry, or depressed.

- Explain motivation.

- Describe eight ways to cope with stress.

- Describe the five stages of grief.

OUTLINE

Psychology	1122
Psychological Disorders	1122
Treatments	1124
Developmental Stages of the Life Cycle	1125
The Mind–Body Connection	1126
Maslow's Hierarchy of Needs	1126
Heredity and Environmental and Cultural Influences on Behavior	1127
Interpersonal Skills and Human Behavior	1128
Emotions	1129
Motivation	1130
Stress	1130
Assisting the Patient with Terminal Illness	1135

Terms to Learn

adolescence
adulthood
bias
bipolar disorder
childhood
electroconvulsive therapy (ECT)
hierarchy of needs
infancy
motivation

neuroses
personality disorders
prejudice
prenatal period
psychiatrist
psychiatry
psychologist
psychology
psychopharmacology

psychoses
psychotherapy
schizophrenia
stereotyping
stress
stressor
terminal illness
Type A behavior
Type B behavior

Case Study

HOLLY SUTTER, CMA, is obtaining a patient history from Christine Smith who just turned 40 years old yesterday. During the interview, Christine starts to cry. She made the following statements: "I wish my life were different," "I can't sleep at night," "It takes all I can do to get up in the morning to go to work," and "Some days I just don't want to be around anyone."

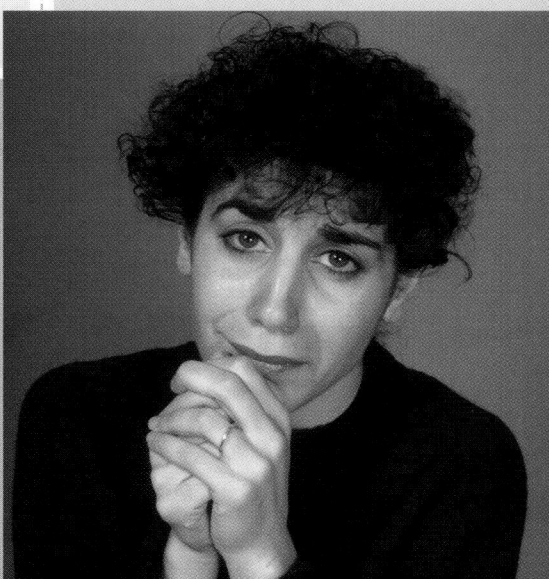

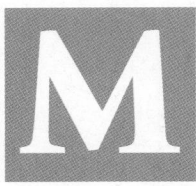any patients who come into the physician's office or clinic will have physical or emotional problems that are not the main reason for their appointment. The medical assistant must be able to care for the entire person in a holistic fashion.

Psychology

Psychology is the science of behavior and the human thought process. This behavioral science is primarily concerned with human beings acting alone or in groups. A psychologist is one who is trained in the methods of psychological analysis, therapy, and research.

There is a distinction between normal and abnormal behavior when studying psychology. Abnormal psychology is the study of behavior that deviates from the normal. This includes psychoneuroses, psychoses, psychosomatic disorders, personality and sociopathic disorders, and disturbances occurring as a result of intoxication, brain damage, and brain disease.

All social interactions, such as might occur in the communication process, pose some problems for some people. These problems are not necessarily abnormal. One means of judging if behavior is abnormal is to compare one person's behavior against others in the community. If a person's behavior interferes with the activities of daily living, it is often considered abnormal.

Psychological Disorders

Psychiatry is the branch of medicine that deals with the diagnosis, treatment, and prevention of mental disorders. A psychiatrist is a physician specializing in the care of patients with emotional disorders. A psychiatrist can prescribe drugs for the treatment of mental disorders.

Many people will have some type of mental disorder during their life. This is considered normal. A continual state of emotional disorder that disrupts life is considered abnormal. Mental disorders are defined as any behavior or emotional state that causes an individual great suffering or worry, is self-defeating or self-destructive, or disrupts the person's day-to-day relationships. The legal definition of a mental disorder is "impaired judgment and lack of self-control." George Albee, a past president of the American Psychological Association, stated, "Appendicitis, a brain tumor, and chickenpox are the same everywhere, regardless of culture or class; mental conditions, it seems, are not."

The guide for terminology and classifications relating to psychiatric disorders is the *Diagnostic and Statistical Manual of Mental Disorders*, Fourth Edition, Text Revision (DSM-IV-TR), which is published by the American Psychiatric Association. Major diagnostic categories of mental disorders in the DSM-IV-TR are described in Table 52-1.

Mental diseases can be divided into three major categories: neuroses, psychoses, and personality disorders.

Neuroses

Neuroses are mild emotional disturbances that impair judgment. Patients suffering from neuroses are able to tell the difference between fantasy and reality. Neuroses include anxiety, compulsions, hysteria, hypochondria, and obsessions.

- Anxiety is a vague feeling of apprehension, worry, uneasiness, or dread. A certain amount of anxiety is normal.
- Compulsions consist of a repetitive act that is performed by the patient to relieve fear connected with an obsession.
- Hysteria is a lack of control over emotions that may result in an outburst, amnesia, or symptoms such as sleepwalking.
- Hypochondria is an abnormal concern about one's health with the false belief of suffering from a disease despite being assured otherwise by the physician.
- Obsession is a neurotic mental state in which a patient has an uncontrollable desire to dwell on an idea or emotion. The patient is usually aware of the obsession and tries to resist the thoughts.

Psychoses

Psychoses are severe mental disorders that interfere with patients' perceptions of reality and their ability to cope with the demands of daily living.

- Delusion is a persistent, strongly held, false belief that is most likely wrong. It is seen in persons with a psychosis who cannot separate delusion from reality. The most serious delusions are those that cause the patient to harm themselves or others.
- Depression is a mental disorder marked by an altered mood. The symptoms may include agitation, loss of energy, feelings of worthlessness, self-reproach, diminished ability to concentrate, and recurrent thoughts of death.
- Hallucination is a false perception that has no relation to reality. It may be visual, auditory, and sometimes even olfactory. The patient's judgment may be impaired and he or she will not be able to distinguish between the real and the imaginary.
- Manic-depressive state is a mental disorder characterized by mood swings between excessive excitement and depression. This is also referred to as bipolar disorder.
- Schizophrenia is a psychotic disorder marked by a variety of symptoms, including delusions,

TABLE 52-1 Major Diagnostic Categories of Mental Disorders

Category	Example
Anxiety disorder	Phobias, panic attack, compulsive rituals
Cognitive disorder	Delirium, dementia, amnesia (resulting from brain damage, or the effects of toxic substances or drugs), degenerative disorders such as Alzheimer's
Disorder diagnosed in infancy and childhood	Mental retardation, attention deficit disorders such as hyperactivity or inability to concentrate, and developmental problems
Dissociative disorder	Dissociative amnesia in which important events cannot be remembered after a traumatic event, and dissociative identity disorder (multiple personality disorder) in which two or more personalities or identities are present in one person
Impulse control disorder	Inability to resist an impulse to perform some act that is harmful to the individual or others such as pathological gambling, stealing (kleptomania), setting fires (pyromania), or having violent rages
Personality disorder	Inflexible behavior patterns that cause distress or the inability to function; these include paranoid, narcissistic, and antisocial disorders
Mood disorder	Major depression, bipolar disorder (manic depression), chronic depressive mood
Schizophrenia and other psychotic disorders	Characterized by delusions, hallucinations, and severe disturbances in thinking and emotion
Sexual and gender identity disorder	Transsexualism (wanting to be the other gender), sexual performance (lack of orgasm, premature ejaculation, or lack of sexual desire), or unusual or bizarre sexual acts
Disorder with physical symptoms and no organic cause	Paralysis, heart palpitation, dizziness; also referred to as hypochondriasis
Substance-related disorder	From excessive use of or withdrawal from alcohol, amphetamines, caffeine, cocaine, hallucinogens, nicotine, opiates, and other drugs

hallucinations, disorganized and incoherent speech, severe emotional abnormalities, and a withdrawal into an inner world.

- Psychopathic behavior occurs when an individual is unconcerned about others to the point of being completely antisocial. These individuals may lack a conscience and are often manipulative.

Personality Disorders

Personality disorders include antisocial reactions, paranoia, and narcissistic behavior.

- Antisocial reactions are characterized by socially negative actions such as stealing, lying, manipulating others, violence, a lack of social emotions (guilt, shame, empathy), and impulsive behavior. This is also referred to as sociopathic behavior. (See also Professionalism.)

- Narcissistic behavior refers to abnormal self-love and self-admiration.

- Paranoia occurs when a patient demonstrates intense feelings of persecution and jealousy. It is also characterized by other symptoms of schizophrenia such as delusions.

Professionalism

When you encounter an angry patient remain calm. A medical assistant should never get angry with the patient, use curse words, or raise their voice at the patient. If you feel you are losing control of the situation, it is appropriate to ask another staff member for assistance so you can maintain your professionalism.

With some mental disorders, particularly severe depression, the patient may become so distraught as to threaten or attempt suicide. Often the suicidal person does not really want to die, but just wishes to escape an intolerable situation.

Treatments

Treatments for mental disorders are varied and include psychotherapy, psychopharmacology, and electroconvulsive therapy.

Psychotherapy

Psychotherapy is a method for treating mental disorders by mental rather than physical means. This includes psychoanalysis, humanistic therapies, and family and group therapy (see Figure 52-1).

- Psychoanalysis is a method of obtaining a detailed account of the past and present emotional and mental experiences from the patient in order to determine the source of the problem and eliminate the effects. It is a system developed by Sigmund Freud that encourages the patient to discuss repressed, painful, or hidden experiences with the hope of eliminating or minimizing the current problem.

- Humanistic therapies are also called "client-centered" or "nondirective therapy." The therapist does not delve into the patient's past when using these methods. The patient is helped to feel better by building self-esteem and a feeling that he or she is respected.

- Family and group therapy is solution focused. The therapist places minimal emphasis on the patient's past history and places a strong emphasis on having the patient state his or her goals and then finding a way to achieve them.

Psychopharmacology

Psychopharmacology relates to the study of the effects of drugs on the mind and brain and particularly the use

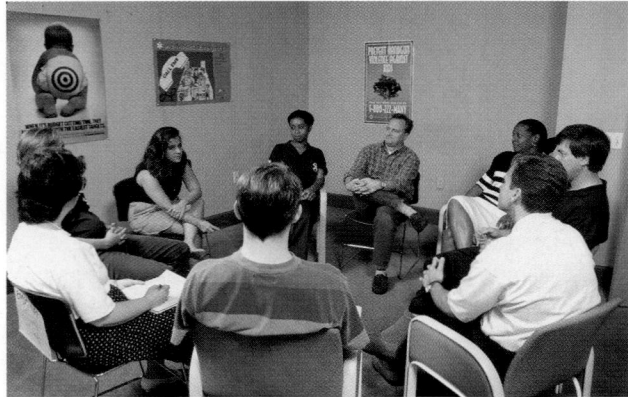

FIGURE 52-1 A group therapy session.

of drugs in treating mental disorders. The brain is a large soft mass of nerve tissue contained within the cranium. It is the cranial portion of the central nervous system. The mind is the integration of and organization of functions of the brain resulting in the ability to perceive surroundings, to have emotions, imagination, memory, and will, and to process information in an intelligent manner. The quality and quantity of the functions of the mind vary with experience and development. The main classes of drugs for the treatment of mental disorders are antipsychotic drugs, antidepressant drugs, "minor" tranquilizers, and lithium.

- Antipsychotic drugs are the major tranquilizers, which include chlorpromazine (Thorazine), haloperidol (Haldol), clozapine (Clozaril), and risperidone (Risperdal). These drugs have transformed the treatment of patients with psychoses and schizophrenia. These medications reduce the patient's agitation and panic and shorten the schizophrenic episode. One of the side effects of these drugs is involuntary muscle movements, which develop in approximately one-fourth of all adults who take the drugs.

- Antidepressant drugs are classified as stimulants and alter the patient's mood by affecting levels of neurotransmitters in the brain. Antidepressants, such as monoamine oxidase (MAO) inhibitors, are nonaddictive, but they can produce unpleasant side effects such as dry mouth, weight gain, blurred vision, and nausea.

- "Minor" tranquilizers include Valium and Xanax. These are also classified as depressants and are prescribed for anxiety. However, they are the least effective in treating emotional disorders. Patients may develop a problem with tolerance after taking these drugs for an extended period of time. (They begin to need larger and larger doses.) In general, antidepressants are preferred to tranquilizers for treating mood disorders.

- Lithium, from the salt lithium carbonate, is a special category of drug. It is used successfully to calm patients who suffer from bipolar disorder (depression alternating with manic excitement). The patient on lithium needs to be carefully monitored because too much of this drug is toxic and too little is ineffective.

Electroconvulsive Therapy

Electroconvulsive therapy (ECT) is a procedure occasionally used for cases of prolonged major depression (see Figure 52-2). This is a controversial treatment in which an electrode is placed on one or both sides of the patient's head, and brief electric current is turned on causing a convulsive seizure. A low level of voltage is used in modern ECT and the patient is administered a

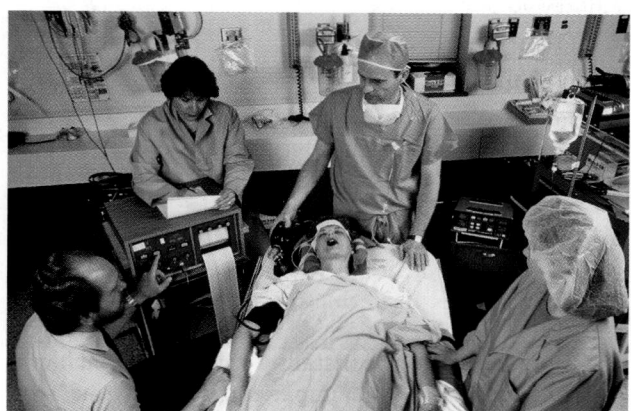

FIGURE 52-2 Electroconvulsive therapy.

muscle relaxant and an anesthesia prior to administration of the current. This helps to prevent violent muscle contractions. Advocates of this treatment state that it is a more effective way to treat severe depression than the use of drugs. It is not effective with disorders other than depression, such as schizophrenia and alcoholism.

Developmental Stages of the Life Cycle

When you are caring for patients it will be important for you to understand the developmental stages of life cycles so that you can take better care of your patients. There are five main developmental periods: prenatal, infancy, childhood, adolescence, and adulthood. Within each developmental period are subdivisions.

Prenatal Period

The first developmental period of child development is the prenatal period, which covers the process from conception until birth. Throughout this period the structures of the body as well as the organs are formed. At this time development is influenced by the environment and heredity.

Infancy

The second subdivision of child development is infancy. This period of vast changes occurs from childbirth until toddlerhood (see Figure 52-3). During this time an infant gains motor ability along with coordination. The infant will also develop language and sensory skills. During this period, the infant will express basic emotions and feelings, develop trust or mistrust, and become attached to caregivers.

Childhood

Childhood is the last subdivision of child development (see Figure 52-4). Ages 3 to 5 are considered early childhood. During children's preschool years, their linguistic, physical, and cognitive capabilities will grow rapidly. The concept of self begins to develop as well as socialization. Ages 6 to 11 are considered middle childhood. During middle childhood, children start to know their world, think logically, and make major advances in reading and writing. Moral and psychosocial development progress rapidly. Achievement is very important to the child during this stage.

Adolescence

Adolescence occurs between childhood and adulthood. Ages 12 to 14 are considered early adolescence. During this time, the beginning of formal operational thinking and sexual maturation take place. Early adolescents want more independence from their parents and they start to form companionships with their friends. Late adolescence occurs from ages 15 to 19. The psychosocial task of positive identity is formed. Late adolescents

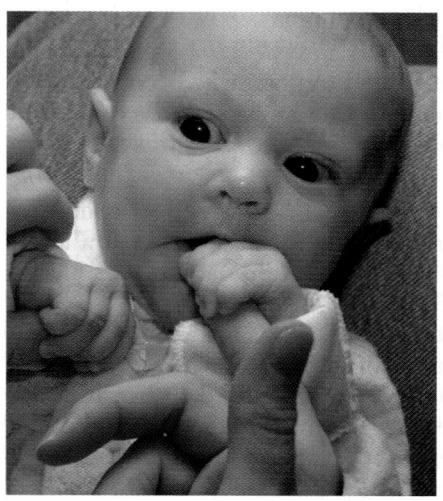

FIGURE 52-3 Infancy.

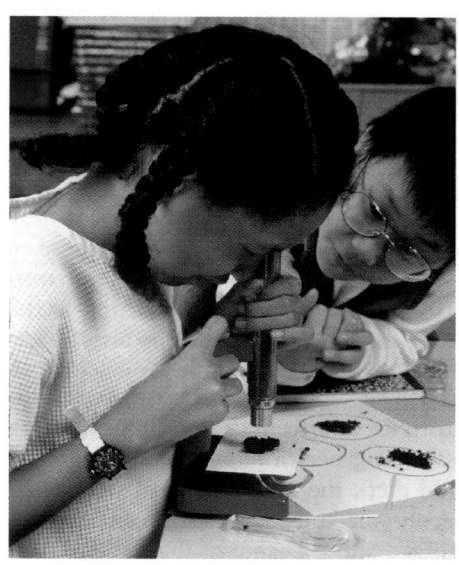

FIGURE 52-4 Childhood.

neip you relate to how that patient might be feeling, and hopefully it will help you display more patience with the patient. Learning about the different cultures in your area will help you be more comfortable around a person from that culture as well as be able to communicate more effectively with him or her.

When you are talking to a patient from another country, use simple and common words. Avoid using

the language? When you encounter a patient who speaks very little English, you will need to be calm, respectful and considerate. As you are talking with the patient use simple words. Avoid using medical terms and never use slang. Try to make the patient feel as comfortable as possible.

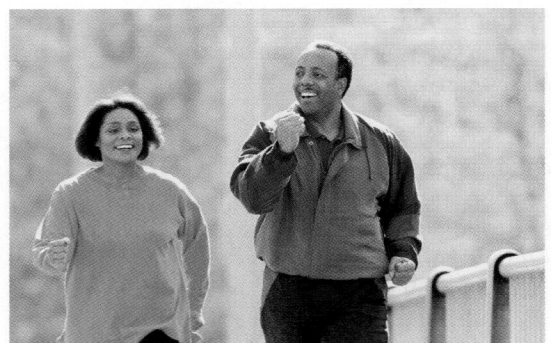

Many patients with a major illness go through a period of depression. The disease may cause emotional changes. In turn worry about the disease may cause unhealthy habits such as an increase in smoking or drinking. Patients who have a physical illness such as heart disease, diabetes, or AIDS may become additionally stressed when confronted with the loss of income or a job.

In addition psychologists believe some individual personality types may cause a person to become ill. The Type A behavior pattern individual is considered

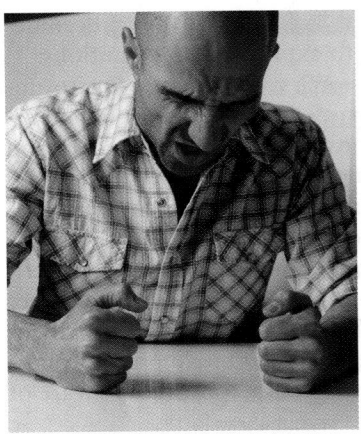

FIGURE 52-8 Emotion—anger.

You are working in the front office when a patient comes to the front reception window and starts screaming, yelling, and cursing at you. How else could you recognize this patient was angry? What should you do?

If a person is angry, he or she may have a reddish color to the face and ears, eyes may be slightly squinted, and fists may be clenched (see Figure 52-8). These are just some of the signs that a person is angry. Once you recognize a person is angry, remain calm yourself. As long as the patient is not being aggressive, allow him or her to communicate the anger. First, let the patient know that you understand he or she is angry. You should then inquire about what is making the patient angry so you can solve the issue. During the conversation make sure you are empathic so the patient knows you are concerned about his or her issue.

Holly Sutter, CMA, is taking a patient's vital signs when the patient tells her, "I failed all my courses last quarter and if I fail anymore courses I'm going to be kicked out of school." During the conversation the patient starts crying and tells Holly, "I'm having trouble sleeping and I am tired of trying so hard in my courses and not succeeding" (see Figure 52-9).

During the conversation with the patient, Holly should be empathic and caring. After Holly allows the patient to express his feelings, she should immediately tell the doctor about the conversation as well as the above statement the patient made. It is also important for Holly to document the situation in the patient's medical record. See Procedure 52-2 to role-play a situation in which a patient is frightened, angry, and depressed.

Motivation

When was the last time you were motivated to complete a task or a goal? What was the task or goal you wanted to accomplish? What motivated you to complete that task or goal?

Motivation is the stimulus that drives us to act. It forms and guides our goal-directed behavior. As a medical assistant there will be many tasks for you to complete every day. Knowing the task or goals you want to accomplish is the first step. Next you need to determine what is motivating you to complete that task or goal. Some people are motivated to complete a task or goal because it challenges them. People also like the rewards or praise they receive from completing the task or goal. There are many types of motivators. Medical assistants who are motivated to accomplish tasks or goals on a regular basis will be successful in their careers.

Stress

Everyone experiences stress at one time or another. Stress is the body's reaction to the world around it. Stress can be emotional, intellectual, or physical. It can also be spiritual, economical, or social. Depending on

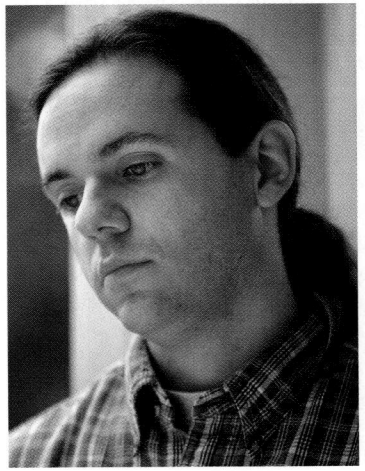

FIGURE 52-9 Emotion—depression.

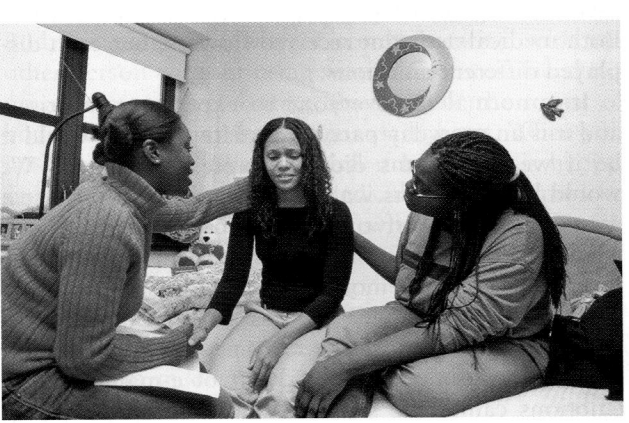

FIGURE 52-10 Signs of stress.

PROCEDURE

Role-Playing a Situation When a Patient Is Frightened, Angry, and Depressed

OBJECTIVE: Learn how to deal with a patient who is frightened, angry, or depressed.

Equipment and Supplies
pen; medical record

Method
1. Choose a classmate.
2. Select a quiet part of the classroom to conduct the procedure.
3. Determine who will be the medical assistant and who will be the patient.
4. Have the student pretending to be the patient express the emotions of being frightened, angry, and depressed.
5. Once you recognize one of these emotions, remain calm.
6. If the patient is not displaying destructive behaviors, allow the patient to express his or her feelings without being interrupted.
7. Let the patient know that you understand.
8. Inquire about the issue so you can solve the issue.
9. During the conversation make sure you are empathic so the patient knows you are concerned about his or her issue.
10. Notify the physician of the conversation.
11. Document the conversation in the medical record.

---

the level of stress, it can be energizing, motivating, or exhausting. Medical research has shown that a certain amount of stress is not a bad thing. The body's reaction to stress determines if it is good stress or bad stress (distress). It has also been implicated in various illnesses (see Figure 52-10 and Patient Education).

A stressor is a real or imaginary event that causes stress. Certain major life events such as the death of a loved one, divorce, an unexpected move away from family and friends, unemployment, illness, getting married, delivering a baby, studying for an examination, or purchasing a new car can trigger stress. Each of these life events or others may be positive or negative. For a life event to be stressful, it doesn't always have to be a negative event.

Symptoms of stress vary from person to person. It is important for you to know what is normal for you and your body. Box 52-1 lists symptoms of stress.

Defense Mechanisms

Defense mechanisms operate at a subconscious level to manage anxiety by denying, misinterpreting, or distorting reality. They often hinder self-awareness by preventing people from being sensitive to anxiety. Defense mechanisms can be helpful in dealing with anxiety; however, consistent use of certain defenses leads to the development of either good or self-destructive behavior patterns. For example, the basic human need to be loved and cared for by another person can result in a variety of behaviors when the fear of losing love produces anxiety. One person may be driven to constantly look for love and affirmation by engaging in frequent one-night sexual encounters. Another person may seek and develop a warm, intimate relationship. A third person may be so frightened of not finding love and so fearful of rejection that he or she avoids relationships to decrease the anxiety. The management of defense mechanisms

Patient Education

The medical assistant may see the patient in the office or handle a question about stress over the telephone. At this time the medical assistant can reinforce healthy habits for coping with stress.

TABLE 52-2 **Defense Mechanisms** (*continued*)

Defense Mechanism	Example(s)	Use/Purpose
Rationalization Justification of certain behaviors by faulty logic and ascription of motives that are socially acceptable but did not in fact inspire the behavior.	A mother spanks her toddler too hard and says it was all right because he couldn't feel it through the diapers anyway.	Helps a person cope with the inability to meet goals or certain standards.
Reaction Formation A mechanism that causes people to act exactly opposite to the way they feel.	An executive resents his bosses for calling in a consulting firm to make recommendations for change in his department but verbalizes complete support of the idea and is exceedingly polite and cooperative.	Aids in reinforcing repression by allowing feelings to be acted out in a more acceptable way.
Regression Resorting to an earlier, more comfortable level of functioning that is characteristically less demanding and responsible.	An adult throws a temper tantrum when he does not get his own way. A critically ill client allows the nurse to bathe and feed him.	Allows a person to return to a point in development when nurturing and dependency were needed and accepted with comfort.
Repression An unconscious mechanism by which threatening thoughts, feelings, and desires are kept from becoming conscious; the repressed material is denied entry into consciousness.	A teenager, seeing his best friend killed in a car accident, becomes amnesic about the circumstances surrounding the accident.	Protects a person from a traumatic experience until he or she has the resources to cope.
Sublimation Displacement of energy associated with more primitive sexual or aggressive drives into socially acceptable activities.	A person with excessive, primitive sexual drives invests psychic energy into a well-defined religious value system.	Protects a person from behaving in irrational, impulsive ways.
Substitution The replacement of a highly valued, unacceptable, or unavailable object by a less valuable, acceptable, or available object.	A woman wants to marry a man exactly like her dead father and settles for someone who looks a little bit like him.	Helps a person achieve goals and minimizes frustration and disappointment.
Undoing An action or words designed to cancel some disapproved thoughts, impulses, or acts in which the person relieves guilt by making reparation.	A father spanks his child and the next evening brings home a present for him. A teacher writes an exam that is far too easy, then constructs a grading curve that makes it difficult to earn a high grade.	Allows a person to appease guilty feelings and atone for mistakes.

situation does occur, you will need to remain calm and focus on the situation. You will be able to handle the situation using the best abilities you possess.

As a medical assistant, you will be taking care of patients who are sick everyday. This can be emotionally, mentally, and/or physically draining. Anytime your stress level is too high and you have trouble coping, you must seek support from a close friend or family member. If a close friend or family member is not able to help you, seek help from a professional.

Develop a Patient Teaching Handout about Stress

OBJECTIVE: Develop an appropriate teaching tool about stress.

Equipment and Supplies
computer; word processor; printer; pen, paper

Method
1. Decide what information should be included on the patient teaching handout.
2. Develop an outline of the information you plan to include of the patient teaching handout.
3. Using a word processing program, develop a patient teaching handout.
4. Make sure your patient teaching includes at a minimum the definition, causes, and ways to cope with stress.
5. Proofread your patient teaching handout on the computer screen.
6. Make any necessary corrections to the patient teaching handout.
7. Print your patient teaching handout.
8. Proofread the hard copy of your patient teaching handout.
9. Make any necessary corrections to the patient teaching handout.
10. Turn in the patient teaching handout to your instructor.

Encountering a patient who is experiencing stress provides an opportunity for patient teaching. After allowing the patient to discuss the stress and stressors, assess the patient's knowledge of the topic of stress. Doing so will establish a starting point for educating the patient. Next, determine the appropriate reading, language, and educational level of the patient so that you can select and prepare materials to use to teach the patient about stress. Some of the educational materials that are used in a medical office include videos, patient teaching handouts (see Procedure 52-3), and booklets. After you gather all of your equipment and supplies, you will be ready to provide the patient with information about stress. When you have completed the patient teaching you will need to document it in the patient's medical record.

Assisting the Patient with Terminal Illness

The medical assistant will come into contact with patients who have a terminal illness. A terminal illness is one that is expected to end in death. This includes conditions and diseases such as cancer, AIDS, progressive heart disease, amyotrophic lateral sclerosis (Lou Gehrig's disease), cystic fibrosis, and multiple sclerosis.

In cases where the dying process is slow for the patient, the medical assistant may have the opportunity to be with the patient on several occasions during office visits. While there is always hope of recovery or finding a cure through research for a disease such as AIDS, it is wise to listen to the patient express his or her fears and concerns rather than to offer false hope for recovery.

Death is a natural process that everyone must face. People have various ways of coping with their own death based on a variety of influences including culture, religion, personal experience, and age.

Culture

People learn what their own culture expects of them at a very early age by observing family and friends as they handle life events such as births and deaths. In some cultures death is considered a normal end to the life process and is therefore accepted with peace. In other cultures death may be feared.

The terminally ill patient and family may have already established a very personal approach or method for handling death and dying. The medical assistant may also have a strong cultural attitude toward death.

Religion

Religious beliefs play an important role in how patients handle death and dying. Some patients will have a strong belief in an afterlife. Other patients will follow no particular religious belief. In both cases, the patients' death and dying process can be meaningful and peaceful.

It is considered unacceptable for the medical assistant to attempt to convert the patient to the medical assistant's religious faith. Professionalism mandates that the medical assistant and other staff members recognize and support the patient's right to embrace his or her own religious beliefs.

TABLE 52-3 **Five Stages of Grief**

Denial	A refusal to believe that dying is taking place. In this stage the patient (or family member) may need time to adjust to the reality of approaching death. This stage cannot be hurried.
Anger	At this stage, the patient may be angry at everyone and may express this intense anger at God, family, and even health care professionals. The patient may take this anger out on the person closest to him or her. Usually this is a family member. In reality, the patient is angry about dying.
Bargaining	The third stage of grief involves attempting to gain time by making promises in return. The patient may bargain with God. The patient may also indicate a need to talk at this stage.
Depression	This stage is marked with a deep sadness over the loss of health, independence, and eventually life. There is an additional sadness of leaving loved ones behind. The grieving patient may become withdrawn.
Acceptance	At the acceptance stage there is a sense of peace and calm. The patient may make comments such as "I have no regrets. I'm ready to die." It is better to let the patient talk and not make denial statements such as "Don't talk like that. You're not going to die.

Personal Experience

The past experiences of the patient and the medical assistant will mold how they approach the topic of death. If the patient has been closely involved with the care of someone who has died a painful death, the patient may fear the same kind of death for himself or herself. These patients will need to be able to discuss their fears. In the same manner, if the medical assistant has had past experiences with the death of friends or relatives, it may be easier to assist the patient.

Age

The elderly usually have less fear of death than younger people. In some cases an elderly person may not feel well, have failing eyesight, hearing, and memory, and may look upon death with relief. If the patient wishes to discuss his or her approaching death, the medical assistant should be ready to listen.

The Stages of Grief

Doctor Elizabeth Kubler-Ross devoted much of her life to the study of the dying process and working with dying patients. She divided the dying process into five stages that she believes all persons go through (Table 52-3). It is helpful to understand these stages when attempting to help the dying patient.

According to Kubler-Ross, all those involved with the dying process may go through the five stages. This would include the patient, family members, and caregivers (such as the medical assistant). The five stages are denial, anger, bargaining, depression, and acceptance. The stages may overlap and may not be experienced by everyone in the stated order, but all are present in the dying person, according to Kubler-Ross.

As the time of death approaches, some of the earlier stages may be repeated. For example, patients who cannot care for themselves may become angry. The critical point to remember when assisting a patient who is dying is that the grieving period is a normal part of the dying process.

Hospice care, which is physical and emotional care provided to the dying person, is a growing movement throughout the United States. The medical assistant should be acquainted with this option of care delivery for the terminally ill.

SUMMARY

Some physical conditions and disabilities cause patients discomfort, but are not the presenting problem when they arrive in the physician's office. The medical assistant must remain flexible and be able to handle all unusual situations. It is vital that all health care workers keep up with literature that relates to their field. The medical assistant will want to read his or her association journal to remain current in the field.

COMPETENCY REVIEW

1. Define and spell the terms to learn for this chapter.
2. Describe how you use the eight health habits to cope with stress.
3. Explain the difference between Type A and Type B behaviors.
4. Explain neuroses, psychoses, and personality disturbances.
5. Discuss the three treatments for mental disorders.
6. Explain how you would communicate with a frightened, angry, and depressed patient.

PREPARING FOR THE CERTIFICATION EXAM

1. A mental disorder that is characterized by delusions and hallucinations is:
   A. cognitive disorder
   B. dissociative disorder
   C. anxiety disorder
   D. personality disorder
   E. schizophrenia

2. An emotional disorder that impairs a person's judgment and concept of reality is:
   A. psychosis
   B. neuroses
   C. delusion
   D. manic-depression
   E. depression

3. During electroconvulsive therapy the patient will receive:
   A. a high level of voltage
   B. a low level of voltage
   C. a muscle relaxant
   D. anesthesia
   E. B, C, and D

4. Which of the following is not considered an antipsychotic drug?
   A. Thorazine
   B. Prozac
   C. Risperidone
   D. Clozaril
   E. Haldol

5. _____ relates to the study of the effects of drugs on the mind and particularly the use of drugs in treating mental disorders.
   A. Psychopharmacology
   B. ECT
   C. Psychotherapy
   D. Pharmacology
   E. Neuroses

6. _____ is a lack of control over emotions, which may result in an outburst, amnesia, or symptoms such as sleepwalking.
   A. Anxiety
   B. Compulsion
   C. Hypochondria
   D. Hysteria
   E. Obsession

7. The _____ behavior pattern individual is someone who is constantly struggling to achieve, is irritable, hostile, and impatient with anyone who gets in the way, and has a sense of time urgency.
   A. Type X
   B. Type Z
   C. Type B
   D. Type M
   E. Type A

8. In Maslow's hierarchy of needs, which level is safety needs level, which includes physical safety as well as security relating to employment?
   A. Level I
   B. Level II
   C. Level III
   D. Level IV
   E. Level V

continued on next page

9. Personality disorders include which of the following?
   A. antisocial reactions
   B. paranoia
   C. narcissistic behavior
   D. A, B, and C
   E. none of the above

10. The guide for terminology and classifications relating to psychiatric disorders is the:
    A. DMS-IV
    B. DMS-IV-TR
    C. DSM-IV
    D. DSM-IV-TR
    E. SDM-IV

CRITICAL THINKING

1. What should Holly do with the information she obtained from Ms. Smith?
2. Should Holly call 911 immediately to have Ms. Smith admitted to a psychiatric hospital?
3. Should Holly notify Ms. Smith's friend who is in the waiting room about her statements?

ON THE JOB

Amy Freeman is a new medical assistant who has recently graduated and passed the CMA examination. During her education she studied ways to cope with stress. Renee Baker, a full-time student and a young mother of two small children, has an appointment to see Dr. Williams. Ms. Baker tells Amy that she is angry at her husband for not being more supportive and angry at herself for not doing that well in school. Because Ms. Baker has opened up to Amy about her feelings, Amy wants to try to help her. Amy decides to provide Ms. Baker with patient teaching about stress management.

1. What information should Amy give about stress management?
2. How would Amy document the patient teaching she gave Ms. Baker?
3. Does Amy have a responsibility to inform the physician of Ms. Baker's situation?

INTERNET ACTIVITY

Visit the www.ctherapy.com/feelings_home.asp website and answer the following questions:

1. What is the purpose of the poster?
2. How would seeing this poster help you understand a patient?
3. What type of professionals would utilize this poster?

MediaLink  More on psychology, including interactive resources, can be found on the Student CD-ROM accompanying this textbook.

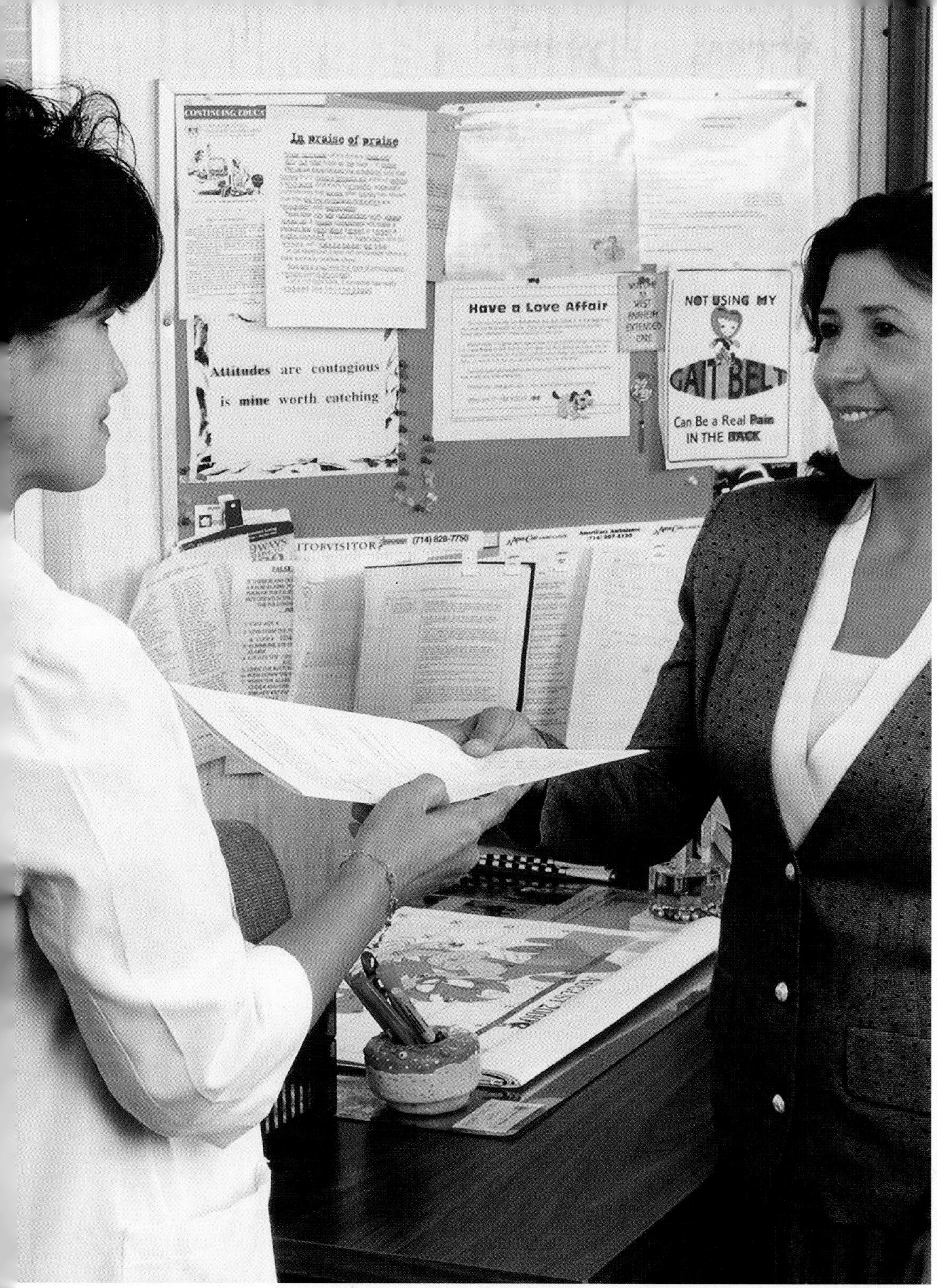

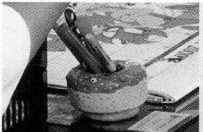
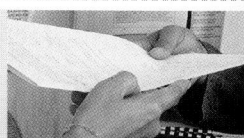

Unit Five

Career Assistance

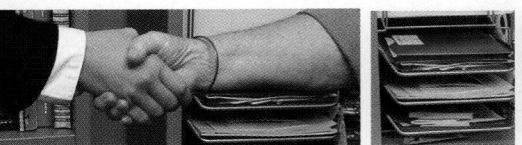

Medical Assistant Role Delineation Chart

HIGHLIGHT indicates material covered in this chapter.

ADMINISTRATIVE

Administrative Procedures

- Perform basic administrative medical assisting functions
- Schedule, coordinate and monitor appointments
- Schedule inpatient/outpatient admissions and procedures
- Understand and apply third-party guidelines
- Obtain reimbursement through accurate claims submission
- Monitor third-party reimbursement
- Understand and adhere to managed care policies and procedures
- *Negotiate managed care contracts*

Practice Finances

- Perform procedural and diagnostic coding
- Apply bookkeeping principles

- Manage accounts receivable
- *Manage accounts payable*
- *Process payroll*
- *Document and maintain accounting and banking records*
- *Develop and maintain fee schedules*
- *Manage renewals of business and professional insurance policies*
- *Manage personnel benefits and maintain records*
- *Perform marketing, financial, and strategic planning*

CLINICAL

Fundamental Principles

- Apply principles of aseptic technique and infection control
- Comply with quality assurance practices
- Screen and follow up patient test results

Diagnostic Orders

- Collect and process specimens
- Perform diagnostic tests

Patient Care

- Adhere to established patient screening procedures
- Obtain patient history and vital signs
- Prepare and maintain examination and treatment areas
- Prepare patient for examinations, procedures and treatments

- Assist with examinations, procedures and treatments
- Prepare and administer medications and immunizations
- Maintain medication and immunization records
- Recognize and respond to emergencies
- Coordinate patient care information with other health care providers
- Initiate IV and administer IV medications with appropriate training and as permitted by state law

GENERAL

Professionalism

- Display a professional manner and image
- Demonstrate initiative and responsibility
- Work as a member of the health care team
- Prioritize and perform multiple tasks
- Adapt to change
- Promote the CMA credential
- Enhance skills through continuing education
- Treat all patients with compassion and empathy
- Promote the practice through positive public relations

Communication Skills

- Recognize and respect cultural diversity
- Adapt communications to individual's ability to understand
- Use professional telephone technique

- Recognize and respond effectively to verbal, nonverbal, and written communications
- Use medical terminology appropriately
- Utilize electronic technology to receive, organize, prioritize and transmit information
- Serve as liaison

Legal Concepts

- Perform within legal and ethical boundaries
- Prepare and maintain medical records
- Document accurately
- Follow employer's established policies dealing with the health care contract
- Implement and maintain federal and state health care legislation and regulations
- Comply with established risk management and safety procedures
- Recognize professional credentialing criteria
- *Develop and maintain personnel, policy and procedure manuals*

Instruction

- Instruct individuals according to their needs
- Explain office policies and procedures
- Teach methods of health promotion and disease prevention
- Locate community resources and disseminate information
- *Develop educational materials*
- *Conduct continuing education activities*

Operational Functions

- Perform inventory of supplies and equipment
- Perform routine maintenance of administrative and clinical equipment
- Apply computer techniques to support office operations
- *Perform personnel management functions*
- *Negotiate leases and prices for equipment and supply contracts*

- *Denotes advanced skills.*

SOURCE: Reprinted by permission of the American Association of Medical Assistants from the AAMA Role Delineation Study: Occupational Analysis of the Medical Assisting Profession.

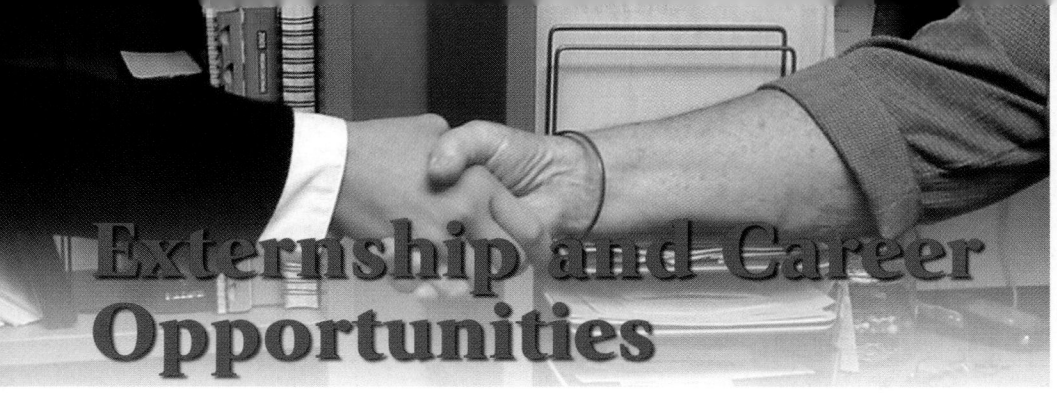

Externship and Career Opportunities

Learning Objectives

After completing this chapter, you should be able to:

- Define and spell the terms to learn for this chapter.
- Discuss three advantages of an externship experience.
- Complete your own personal assessment.
- Develop your own résumé.
- State the purpose of a cover letter.
- Write a letter in response to a classified advertisement from your local newspaper.
- Discuss the steps used in preparing for an interview.
- Develop a follow-up letter to send following an interview.
- Describe an employer's expectations.

OUTLINE

What Is an Externship?   1142

Preparing for the
    Certification
    Examination   1145

The Job Search   1146

The Résumé   1148

The Cover Letter   1151

The Interview   1151

Follow-Up after
    the Interview   1156

What Does the Employer
    Want?   1156

Terms to Learn

application	externship	proofread
blind ad	personal assessment	résumé
certification examination	preceptor	
cover letter	professional reference	

Case Study

ELIZABETH OBERMARK, A MEDICAL ASSISTING STUDENT at one of the local colleges, will be starting her externship today at Dr. Baldwin's office. Elizabeth arrived 25 minutes late to the externship site. She told Melba, the office manager, that she woke up late and then could not find the office. She also told Melba she will need to leave today at noon because she is going out of town to visit a sick friend.

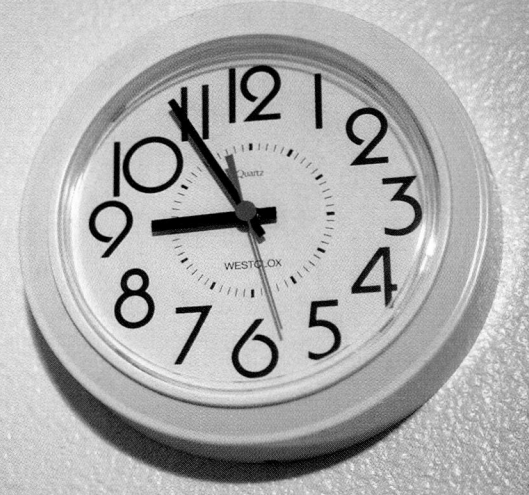

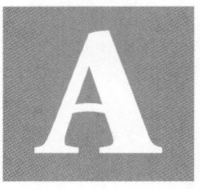

All indications are that job opportunities for medical assistants are expanding at a rapid rate. The U.S. Department of Labor has projected medical assisting to be one of the fastest growing occupations. This demand for health personnel means that a well-prepared medical assistant will have a secure future.

One of the best means to facilitate the transition between the classroom and the medical setting is through the externship experience. This experience can be a time of great challenge and learning since the student is able to gain experience while under supervision. To receive the most benefit from the experience, careful preparation needs to take place. The externship experience is also one of the most exciting components of a medical assisting program.

As the student's formal educational experience in school draws to a close, he or she will prepare for the certification examination offered by the American Association of Medical Assistants (AAMA) or American Medical Technologists (AMT). Most hiring physicians look for this certification. This credential, along with graduation from an accredited program, indicates that entry-level skills have been accomplished.

During this final stage of training, the student will also begin the search for employment. This chapter discusses skills that are useful to both the externship and job searching.

What Is an Externship?

An externship refers to a situation in which one leaves the confines of the classroom and works, without payment, in a health care setting using the newly acquired medical assisting skills under the supervi-

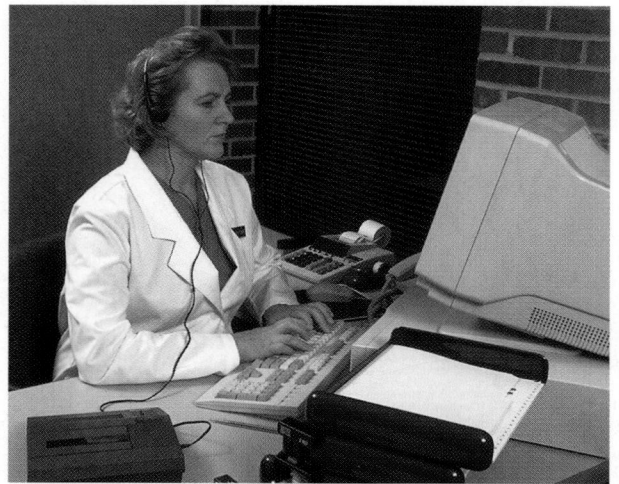

FIGURE 53-1 Medical assistant performing transcription work.

Preparing for
Externship

Physicians expect all of their medical assisting externs to have outstanding clinical and administrative skills. However, the physicians and their staff realize that you are inexperienced and they are generally patient while you are learning. The one area in which physicians and office managers are extremely critical is regarding punctuality. If you are even a minute late for an interview, starting the day, or returning from a break, it will not be overlooked. Because many externships eventually result in full-time jobs, it is important to establish an unbroken rule that you will NEVER be late. The night before starting at your externship site, you should double-check the setting on your alarm clock. Make sure you get up early enough to eat a good breakfast. Prepare all your paperwork to take to the externship site the day before. Don't forget to make sure that your uniform is pressed.

sion of someone at the site. An externship offers the student an opportunity to get on-the-job experience. There is as wide a range of externships as there are medical facilities. An externship can be as short as 4 weeks or as long as one semester of school. Schools that are accredited by the Council on Accreditation of Allied Health Education Programs (CAAHEP) in conjunction with the AAMA require an externship of a minimum of 160 hours. The externship experience should provide the medical assistant with ample experience in both administrative and clinical skills.

Your school and you will work together to select the right externship for you based on your skills, needs, and residence location (Figure 53-1). Ideally, the externship experience is carefully monitored by the clinical instructor/externship coordinator so that problems can be addressed if any arise (see also Preparing for Externship.)

The Externship Experience

Students generally find the externship experience to be the most rewarding part of their school experience. You will have the opportunity to see how a physician's office, ambulatory care setting, or clinic operates on a day-to-day basis (Figure 53-2). In addition you will be exposed to a variety of different personalities in the work setting. Other advantages of the externship include gaining additional experience using your skills such as phlebotomy, taking ECGs and vital signs, conducting urinalysis and hematology testing, using the computer, interviewing patients, performing billing and insurance procedures, and scheduling patients. You will gain experience in budgeting your time and balancing your workday, school day, and your home life.

Your performance and behavior will be carefully observed by your supervisor at the externship site. Some of the areas that will be evaluated are these:

- Administrative and clinical skills and techniques
- Caring attitude
- Empathy for patients
- Enthusiasm
- Ethical standards
- Grooming/dress
- Initiative
- Integrity
- Interpersonal skills with patients and coworkers
- Language skills
- Poise under pressure
- Professionalism
- Punctuality/dependability

Student's Responsibilities

The student has an overall responsibility to prepare well in advance of the interview for the externship. This preparation includes a review of skills, updating the résumé, and planning on how to project a professional appearance.

Each externship site is somewhat unique and may have additional requirements. The externship may require the medical assistant to carry malpractice insurance. Documentation of a recent physical exam and immunizations including hepatitis and tetanus may also be required. A tuberculosis (TB) test is required if you are working near patients. Because some of the immunizations, particularly hepatitis, require several months to complete it is wise to begin this process 8 to 9 months before your expected externship. It is the student's responsibility to make sure that necessary physical examinations, paperwork, and immunizations are completed on a timely basis.

You are being given a great responsibility and opportunity by being allowed to gain experience at the

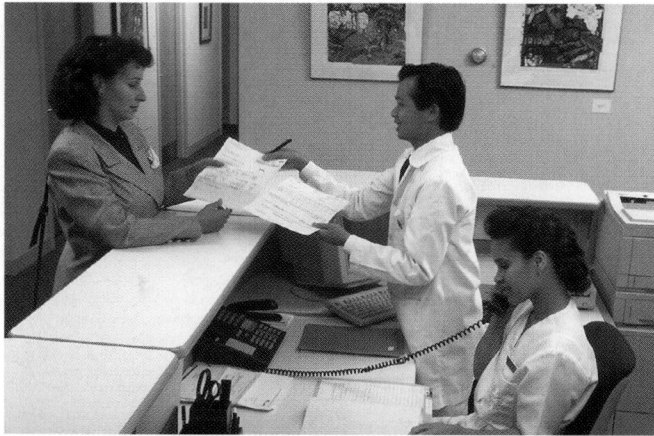

FIGURE 53-2   Medical assistant working in a front office area of a medical office.

externship site (see also Professionalism). The physician or facility providing an externship expects candidates to be extremely cautious regarding ethical and legal concerns. Errors can result in malpractice claims against the physician with whom you are working. If an error occurs, it should be reported immediately to the supervisor without alarming the patient. In many cases when errors are handled immediately, they can be corrected. If you cover up an error or mistake, it could result in immediate dismissal. Regular interviews with the office manager provide opportunities for the medical assistant student to discuss issues that may need clarification (Figure 53-3).

Issues of confidentiality and patient privacy are of great concern to the physician and staff in all facilities. Discussion of information regarding any patient or the physician's practice with anyone outside of that facility is never allowed.

You will receive supervision from your on-the-job supervisor and your externship coordinator. Be sure to ask questions. The externship experience is meant to be a learning experience. If you find that you are not

Professionalism

Remember that as a member of the health care team, you are always under observation. It is not a good idea to use the casual language that one might use at home. And always remember to smile!

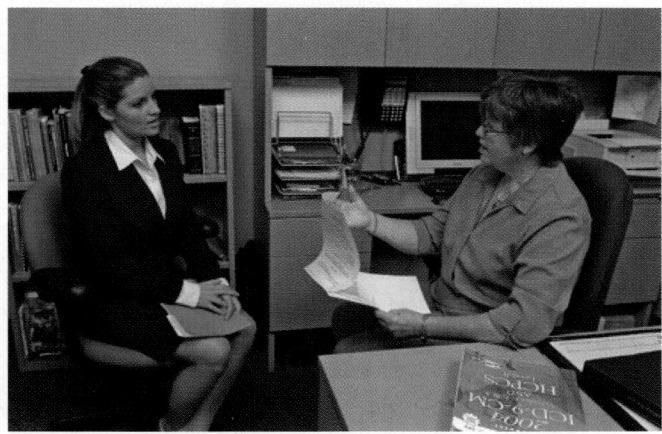

FIGURE 53-3   Medical assistant during an interview with the office manager.

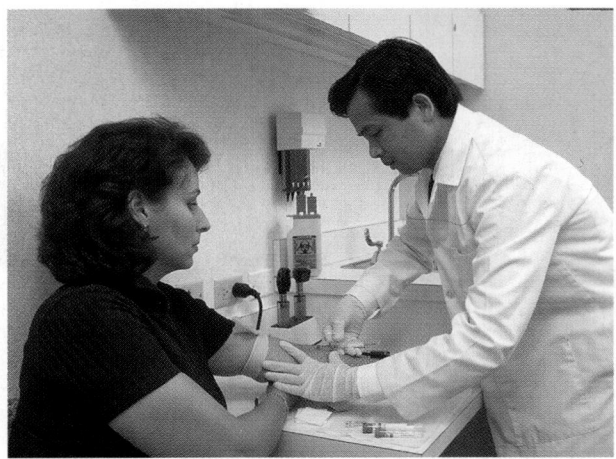

FIGURE 53-4 Drawing blood is one of the procedures the medical assistant may perform in the medical office.

vious student's good performance in that externship. Remember, the behavior and work performance of the medical assistant during the externship is a direct reflection on the school that prepared him or her.

Finding the Right Site

Most schools have an externship coordinator who screens and selects health care sites that are appropriate for training. The screening process requires the coordinator to conduct an interview with the physician or office manager at the site to ensure that the student will benefit from appropriate experiences and receive supervision on site. Often the school has an affiliation agreement with the externship site that is kept on file at the school. Ideally, the externship site will have a former graduate of your program in their employ who can identify what skills and situations are needed.

Generally, it is not a good idea for students to select externship sites without the assistance from the school or the externship coordinator in particular. The school has the responsibility to require that the students are well supervised (Figure 53-4).

receiving the experience you require, bring this to the attention of your clinical supervisor.

Many students are able to take advantage of excellent externship opportunities simply because of a pre-

Areas Evaluated	Ratings*				
Makes effective use of time	1	2	3	4	N/A
Able to work well with others	1	2	3	4	N/A
Accepts suggestions/criticisms willingly	1	2	3	4	N/A
Expresses concern for patients	1	2	3	4	N/A
Protects confidentiality of physician and patients	1	2	3	4	N/A
Always on time for work	1	2	3	4	N/A
Willingly works until the job is completed	1	2	3	4	N/A
Able to work independently	1	2	3	4	N/A
Demonstrates skill as appropriate	1	2	3	4	N/A
Does not perform skills beyond scope of training, education, and personal capability	1	2	3	4	N/A
Practices principles of aseptic technique	1	2	3	4	N/A
Projects a positive attitude	1	2	3	4	N/A
Recognizes emergencies	1	2	3	4	N/A
Dresses appropriately	1	2	3	4	N/A
Practices good hygiene	1	2	3	4	N/A

TABLE 53-1 **Sample Student Externship Form**

*Ratings: 1 = excellent, 2 = good, 3 = average, 4 = needs improvement, N/A = not applicable.

The Preceptor Role

The medical assistant at an externship site always works under the supervision of the physician. However, the physician may designate another member of the health care team as a supervisor for the student.

This person performs in the role of a preceptor. A preceptor provides additional instruction and guidance for a student by observing the performance of particular skills. The preceptor will also provide a formal written evaluation for the student, usually at the midpoint and final point. Table 53-1 lists several areas that are included on a typical evaluation form.

The preceptor is looking for continual improvement in skills as the student gains confidence. The student should make every attempt to establish a rapport, or comfortable work relationship, with the preceptor.

Externship Site Evaluation

At the end of the externship experience, the student will be asked to provide an evaluation of the site. This evaluation may include the following types of questions:

- Was the overall externship experience positive or negative? Explain.
- Was the supervisor or preceptor approachable and available to answer questions?
- What, in your opinion, could be improved about this externship site/experience?
- Should this externship site be offered to other students?

TABLE 53-2 Major Areas Tested on the CMA Examination

Category	Topics Covered
General	Medical terminology
	Anatomy and physiology
	Behavioral science; psychology
	Medical law and ethics
Administrative	Oral and written communication
	Records management
	Insurance and coding
	Computers and office machines
	Bookkeeping, collections, and credit
Clinical	Examination room techniques
	Laboratory procedures
	Pharmacology and medication administration
	Emergency procedures
	Specimen collection

Preparing for the Certification Examination

The certification examination to become a certified medical assistant is offered by the AAMA three times a year (January, June, and October). The examination is given at numerous locations throughout the United States. It is a 4-hour examination. The examination is only available to medical assistants who have completed a CAAHEP-accredited program in medical assisting. The certified medical assistant (CMA) examination is a comprehensive test that includes questions relating to general transdisciplinary knowledge, administrative knowledge, and clinical knowledge. Table 53-2 describes the areas covered under each category.

The certification examination to become a registered medical assistant (RMA) is given as a computer-based test (CBT) or paper-and-pencil test at various times throughout the year. Eligibility to take this examination is either based on 5 years of work experience or a combined training and work program.

Preparation for a certification examination begins as soon as the student begins a training program. All of the subject matter taught in a program is interrelated and forms the basis of the student's knowledge. All class notes and information acquired during the training program should be maintained in an organized fashion so that preparation for the examination can be efficient. A variety of examination preparation courses are offered. In addition, several excellent review books provide the student with sample test questions. These review books should be purchased well before the actual date of the examination. The study questions are generally related to the three major categories covered on the examination: general, administrative, and clinical. Students should time themselves while answering these sample test questions since the actual examination is timed.

See Volume I, Chapter 1, for a further discussion of the credentialing agencies.

The Job Search

Many offices that offer externship opportunities do not have a full-time position available. Do not think it is a reflection of your work if you are not offered a position at the end of your externship. If your externship experience did not lead to a permanent position, then you need to begin the job search in earnest. In some cases, a facility will not want to hire you as a medical assistant until you become credentialed after taking the required examination. However, some facilities will interview you for a permanent position with the understanding that you must pass the certification exam.

Any job search should begin with careful planning. You will need to prepare a list of information sources for identifying job opportunities, update your résumé, rehearse interviewing, and plan your professional attire for the interview process. Six reasons are cited as the most common job search mistakes:

1. Having no clear plan
2. Failing to inform others of your job search
3. Spending too much time answering classified ads
4. Looking for the perfect job
5. Limiting yourself to one field
6. Giving up the search too soon

There are several areas to pursue in your search for job opportunities, some of which are listed in Table 53-3.

Personal Assessment

Before moving ahead with your job search, it is a good idea to perform a personal assessment or evaluation of your own strengths and weaknesses. While it is not a good idea to point out any weaknesses to potential employers, you must be cautious to avoid taking on tasks for which you are not qualified (see Patient Education). Employers often ask about weaknesses. State one and indicate what you are doing about it. This shows you are not aware of limitations, but lets the employer know you are serious about improving yourself. By performing a personal assessment, you can determine in what fields you might enjoy working, which areas require more skill development, and for which positions you are qualified (Figure 53-5).

TABLE 53-3 Sources for Job Opportunities

Internet	Use various Web sites such as monster.com, careerbuilder.com, or jobs.com.
Classified ads	Use local and out-of-town newspapers, professional journals, and trade magazines. Use the local public library's access to national newspapers.
Employment agencies	Place your name with the agency and career consultants.
Health care facilities in your area	Contact hospitals, veteran's facilities, extended-care facilities, and ambulatory case sites.
Local medical society	Obtain a listing of physicians who are looking for help or a listing of all the medical practice offices in your area.
Parents, friends	Network within your own friends and relatives. Make sure they know you are looking for employment.
Personal physician	Your own physician may network for you and call his or her colleagues.
Publications	American Association of Medical Assistants and other local professional publications.
Professional	Use both state and local chapters of your own professional association and other allied health groups.
School placement service	One of the best sources since they know your training and skills well. In many cases the prospective employer will call the schools looking for new employees.
State employment office	After completing the required application forms, your name will be on file for available positions.

Patients are not always clear regarding distinctions among the various health care workers' credentials and responsibilities. During your externship, you may have to clarify that you are a student working under the direction of your supervisor. Doing so protects you from being expected to perform procedures done by health care workers who are certified and/or licensed at levels beyond your credentials. Always wear the insignia of your school and a name pin that designates your status.

You can ask your instructors for guidance and observations on your appearance, attitude, and skills. Although it is never easy to accept criticism, a well-intentioned comment from someone you know about the need to clean your uniforms, eliminate jewelry, change to a more professional hairstyle, or brush up on particular skills may help you obtain the job you are seeking.

You may wish to practice your interview skills with your instructors or in front of a mirror. Use every opportunity to speak up in class to further develop your communication skills. Work on smiling at every opportunity.

Conducting a Job Search

After planning and performing a self-assessment, it is time to gather the equipment and supplies to be successful at your job search. At home, at the school you are attending, or at most local libraries you can access a computer and printer to develop and print your cover letter, résumé, and follow-up letter. If the computer has access to the Internet you can look on various Web sites for jobs that are posted. Searching the Internet has become a very popular way to look for a job. There is no more waiting for a workplace human resource department to open or getting there before it closes. You are able to access the workplace Web site at your convenience to search for job information.

Many Web sites are available on the Internet that can help you with your job search. These Web sites may focus on résumé writing, job applications, interviewing, job postings, and more. Some currently popular Web sites are www.monster.com, www.careerbuilder.com, and www.hotjobs.com. Once you are at one of these Web sites, you will be able to search for a job by category, city/state/zip code/location, and key word. If you want to work for a particular medical office, using any Internet search engine on the Internet, key in the name of the medical office, the city, and the state to see if the office has a Web site available. If you already know the Web address for the medical office, key it in to the address bar of your Web browser. Remember, not all medical offices have Web sites.

Your local library or school library should also have classified ads, various publications, and newsletters to use as sources to find a job. If your school has a placement office, it is one of the best places to receive help with your job search. Most school placement offices have a job posting board and will review your résumé, conduct a mock interview, and help as well as encourage you to find a job.

Being organized is a must while searching for a job. A job search organizer or folder is a wonderful place to keep a copy of your cover letter, résumé, follow-up letter, and applications. It can also be used to keep handy business cards, job advertisements, your contact log, and phone numbers. Having all of this information in one place will help you stay organized and keep you focused during your job search. It will also prevent any of the items just listed from getting lost or misplaced.

A contact log is a great reference for information about the offices or people you have contacted about a job search. Keep the names, addresses, telephone numbers, and e-mail addresses of the people you have contacted in your log.

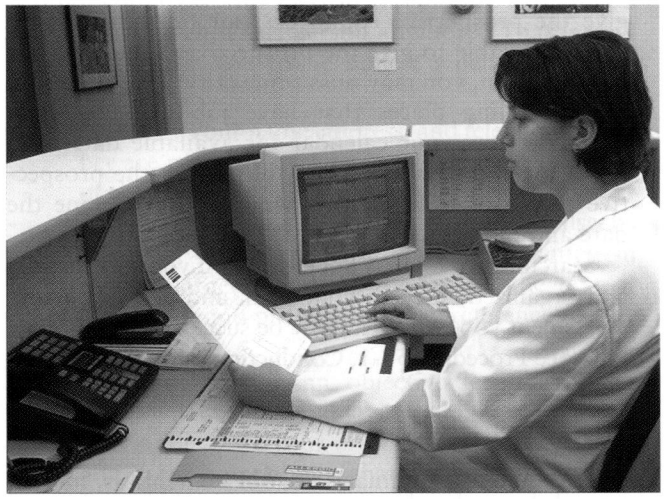

FIGURE 53-5 Medical assistants who perform billing must know and use the proper codes to assure third-party payments by insurance companies.

UNIT 5 *Career Assistance* 1149

have standard questions which may include "Tell me why you went into medical assisting?" or "Why do you want to work here?" You should practice responses to these questions before you go to the interview (Figure 53-8).

Another resource for obtaining information about the interview process is the Internet. If you type the word "interviewing" into an Internet search engine, you will find numerous Web sites that contain information about interviewing such as preparation, questions asked, questions for you to ask, practice interviews, tips, and much more. The information from some of the Web sites you visit will provide a wealth of knowledge that will help you be successful during the interview process.

Many schools have a placement office or career services office to assist you as you are attending school and/or after you graduate. It is important for you to get to know the staff and to understand the services available. Getting to know the staff will help you become more comfortable when you are seeking assistance from them.

Many placement offices offer these services:

- Help you develop a cover letter, résumé, and follow-up letter.

- Review your cover letter, résumé, and follow-up letter.

- Conduct a mock interview.

- Provide you with current job listings.

- Provide career counseling.

- Help you with your job search.

- Host job fairs for you to attend on campus.

- Conduct workshops and seminars about interviewing, cover letters, résumés, and follow-up letters.

Ralph Taylor
222 East Main St.
Chicago, IL 60601
(312) 555-1212

May 20, 20XX

James Stark, M.D.
1450 N. Devonshire
Chicago, IL 60611

Dear Dr. Stark:

This letter is in response to your recent advertisement in the May 19, 20XX, Chicago Sun News for a certified medical assistant.

I believe that my qualifications are a good match for your position. During my medical assisting program at Central State College in Hometown, Illinois, I maintained a 3.6 GPA on a 4.0 scale.

My medical assisting program at Central State College was completed in December 20XX. I passed the American Association of Medical Assistants' certification examination January 27, 20XX. Currently I am completing an associate degree program at CSC and plan to graduate in June 20XX.

The enclosed résumé includes my experience as a part-time nursing assistant for Dr. Jane Young in her family practice office.

I look forward to meeting you to discuss your position needs and my qualifications.

Thank you for your consideration.

Sincerely,

Ralph Taylor

Ralph Taylor, C.M.A.

FIGURE 53-7   An example of a cover letter sent in response to a classified ad.

Preparing for Tough Interview Questions

In addition to the standard questions, there may be some difficult questions such as "We all have our strengths and weaknesses. Tell me one of your weaknesses." It is always a good idea to highlight your strengths. Therefore, to answer a tough question, select a strength. For instance, you might make the following response to the question about your weakness, "I am a perfectionist and may sometimes hold myself to a very high standard that is almost unobtainable" or "I care very deeply about people and must work to empathize with them rather than sympathize."

The interviewer may ask you questions regarding any "gaps" in the chronology. Answer all questions honestly using simple statements, such as "I did not work during that year because I was caring for an elderly relative" or "It has been six months since I finished school. I did not seek employment because I was studying for the CMA examination." It is not necessary to provide lengthy explanations for termination from a position. Be especially careful not to criticize the institution or individual who terminated you.

Preparing a Cover Letter

OBJECTIVE: Prepare a cover letter.

Equipment and Supplies
computer; printer; pen; paper; dictionary; thesaurus; telephone book

Method
1. Gather equipment and supplies.
2. Using Figure 53-7 as an example, prepare a cover letter using a word processing program.
3. Proofread your cover letter.
4. Have a close family member or friend proofread your cover letter.
5. Make any corrections to errors found on the cover letter.
6. Using good-quality, white or off-white paper, print your cover letter.
7. Turn your cover letter in to your instructor.

Some of the questions that could be asked during an interview include:

- What is one of your strengths?
- What is one of your weaknesses?
- What has been your favorite job? Why?
- What goal or goals do you want to accomplish in the next year?
- What goals do you want to accomplish in the next five years?
- Why would you want to work for this medical office?
- Tell me why I should hire you?
- How do you qualify for this position?
- What has been one of your best accomplishments?
- How did you handle a difficult situation at one of your past jobs?

Be prepared to answer the difficult questions with great poise and professionalism. You will have only about 20 minutes to convince your potential employer that you should be the applicant hired. Be absolutely honest about your achievements. However, don't be afraid to talk positively about yourself. There is no one else present at the interview who knows you as well as you do. Guidelines 53-1 lists some guidelines for successful interviewing.

During the interview you should also have questions for the interviewer about the medical office, the position, and the staff. This will give you a clear understanding of the possible place of employment and will help you decide if you want to be employed at that particular medical office.

Here are some questions you might want to ask the interviewer:

- Why is this position open?
- How many patients are seen in the office per day?
- What are the working hours for this position?
- How long is the probationary period?
- When are evaluations conducted?
- How long is the orientation or training period?
- Why do you enjoy working here?

To get a clearer understanding of the medical office, you should also ask for a copy of the job description for the position. If the interviewer hasn't already given you a tour, you should ask to meet the rest of the

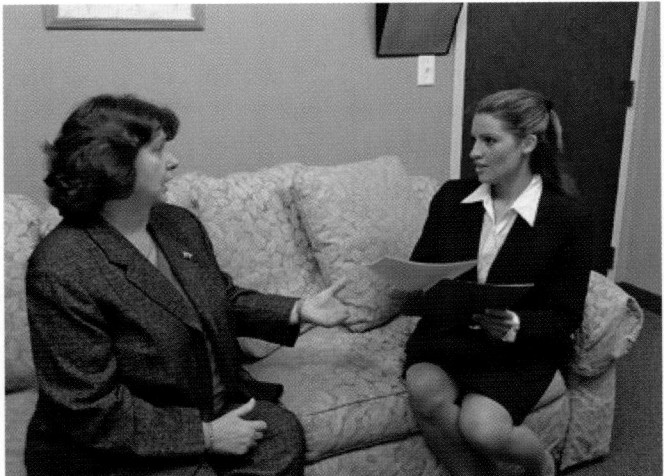

FIGURE 53-8 The job interview.

1. Learn all you can about the organization. Interviewers are impressed by candidates who indicate knowledge of their facility or organization.

2. Have a specific job in mind when you interview so that you project the impression of self-assurance.

3. Know your qualifications for each specific job area/task requirement. Rehearse or review possible responses several times before going to the interview. You can role-play with a friend or relative to build your confidence.

4. Prepare responses to possible "difficult questions" you might be asked or to the request to tell the interviewer something about yourself.

5. Be prepared to discuss where you want to be in 5 years.

6. Carry extra copies of your résumé.

7. Arrive 5 to 10 minutes before your scheduled appointment. You may wish to wait outside the facility if you arrive too early.

8. Dress conservatively to project a professional well-groomed appearance. Generally, a uniform is not required for an interview.

9. Never ask for permission to smoke during an interview. Do not eat anything during an interview unless the interview takes place during a meal. Chewing gum is never acceptable during the interview.

10. Be alert and prompt in giving answers to the interviewer's questions. Do not offer information that is not requested. Keep answers concise.

11. Ask questions about the position and the organization. It is generally not a good idea to inquire about benefits on the first interview.

12. Bring your Social Security number, a pen, driver's license number, extra résumés, and the names of three references with their telephone numbers.

staff and tour the medical office. This will help you decide if you would fit in with the other staff at the medical office.

Professionalism at the Interview

The day of the interview you will be judged immediately by your appearance. You should present a conservative, well-groomed professional appearance. Wear little or no jewelry and avoid showy hairstyles, heavy perfume, bright nail polish, and bright clothing. Of course, this is the same appearance that you will want to present on the job.

Women should wear a suit or dress. Men should wear a suit, a plain shirt, and tie. The colors of the attire you will be wearing during the interview should never stand out or be bright. Your attire should be dark blue or black. Your attire should never have any bizarre patterns, designs, or textures. Low-cut shirts and tight-fitting garments are unacceptable and unprofessional for a job interview. Before you leave for the interview, look at yourself in the mirror. Is the garment you are wearing wrinkled? If so, press it. Never go to an interview with your garment wrinkled. Make sure there is no lint on your garment. Make sure your shoes are clean and polished. Now ask yourself, "Would I want to hire that person in the mirror?" If you are still in a medical assisting program, you may wish to wear a clean pressed uniform with your school insignia.

No one should accompany you to an interview. Introduce yourself to the receptionist and wait quietly in the reception room until you are called for the interview. Be very courteous to all office staff. Many physicians will have their entire office team assist in selecting new employees.

Greet the person interviewing you with a firm handshake. Now is an excellent time to give the interviewer a copy of your résumé and reference list. Even if the interviewer already has a copy of your résumé, it is acceptable to give him or her another copy. Interviewers will generally take a few minutes to ask casual questions that will allow you to relax. Be prepared for questions such as "Tell me about yourself." Have good eye contact with interviewer and answer all questions in a sincere and friendly manner. Never give answers to the interviewer that are misleading or dishonest.

Questions relating to age, ethnic origin, place of birth, marital status, and number of children are prohibited by law. Most interviewers are aware of this law and will not ask these questions. You do not have to answer them if they are asked.

Salary and benefits are not generally discussed in the first interview. If you are called back for a second interview or with a job offer, the topic of salary and benefits can be discussed at that time. Remember to be pleasant when the interview is over. The interviewer will usually indicate the end of the interview by standing up and shaking your hand as you leave (Figure 53-9).

Every interview experience is an opportunity for personal growth. If you are not hired on the first or second interview, do not become discouraged. Reassess your interviewing skills. Ask your instructor or friend to critique your skills to see how you might improve. Immediately send out more cover letters and résumés until you are hired. According to interviewers, the 10 most common mistakes made in interviews are:

1. Poor eye contact
2. Use of slang or improper grammar
3. Inappropriate dress or poor grooming
4. Lack of enthusiasm
5. Poor posture
6. Smoking or chewing gum
7. Talking too much or projecting an overconfident attitude
8. Arriving late
9. Speaking critically of previous employers
10. Inability to ask questions about the organization

Complete Procedure 53-4, Role-Playing an Interview.

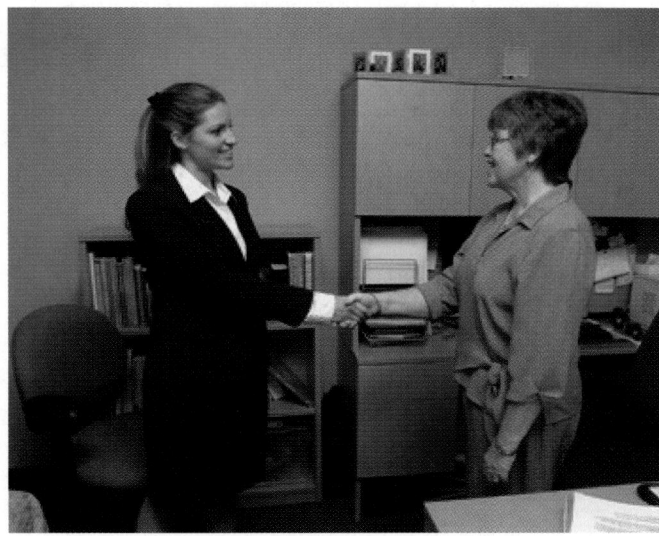

FIGURE 53-9   Medical assistant shaking hands with the interviewer at the close of the interview.

The Application

If you have had work experience, there should be no "gaps" on your application or résumé from the time you began to work. You may have stopped working

---

53-4	**PROCEDURE**

Role-Playing an Interview

OBJECTIVE: Successfully role-play a job interview.

Equipment and Supplies
none

Method

1. Determine five questions that may be asked during an interview.
2. Choose a classmate.
3. Select a quiet part of the classroom to conduct the interview.
4. Determine who will be the interviewer and who will be the interviewee.
5. The interviewer will begin the interview process by giving the interviewee a general idea about the medical office and the employees that work there.
6. The interviewer will ask the interviewee the five questions he or she selected in step 1.
7. The interviewer will gather information about the interviewee's past work experience.

8. The interviewer will gather information about the interviewee's educational experience.
9. The interviewee will answer the interviewer questions.
10. The interviewee will ask the interviewer questions about the medical office and the position.
11. The interviewer will answer the interviewee's questions.
12. Each student should play the part of the interviewer and interviewee.
13. Now have the students discuss the 10 most common mistakes made in an interview. Did either student display any of these mistakes?
14. Each student will assess their interviewing skills.
15. Each student will discuss the appropriate attire to wear to an interview.
16. Each student will discuss the successful interviewing guidelines from their textbook.

Legal and Ethical Issues

***You are responsible for providing** complete and accurate information on application forms. Be sure all the facts surrounding your education and work experience are absolutely accurate. It is especially important to be honest about your skill level. Do not promise to perform procedures or tasks for which you are not trained. Lying on an application or a résumé is considered cause for termination. In some instances there may even be cause for prosecution.*

temporarily to complete your education. The employer will then expect the dates of employment and schooling to run consecutively. "Gaps" with no apparent work or schooling indicated should be clarified. If you were unemployed for a period of time, the potential employer will want to know why.

An application is usually completed at the time of the interview. Therefore, bring along a folder containing all of your documentation such as:

- Social Security number
- Updated résumé and an extra copy for the interviewer
- List of three references with their addresses and telephone numbers
- A chronological list of all your work experience
- Driver's license number and/or photo ID

The neatness of your handwriting and printing will be demonstrated on your application. Be careful to print if that is requested. Questions relating to age, ethnic origin, place of birth, and number of children are prohibited by law. However, some offices and institutions may still have these questions on their application forms. You do not have to answer these questions. Simply leave the questions blank. Applications are discussed further in Legal and Ethical Issues.

Follow-Up after the Interview

Immediately following the interview, on the same day if possible, send a letter thanking the interviewer for his or her time. This is a good opportunity to again express your interest in the position. Be meticulous about proofreading your letter for mistakes. It may be your final professional contact with the interviewer before the decision to hire is made.

You may wish to call the office a few days later to ask about the progress made on filling the position. If you are offered a position and decide not to accept it, you would use the same courtesy when turning down an offer as you use when accepting one. See Figure 53-10 for a sample of a follow-up letter, and Procedure 53-5, Preparing a Follow-Up Letter.

If you are offered a position that you wish to accept, then a letter of acceptance is sent within 5 days of the offer. Accept the offer graciously, clearly stating the position you are accepting, and express your thanks.

Ralph Taylor
222 E. Main St.
Chicago, IL 60601
(312) 555-1212

May 30, 20XX

James Stark, M.D.
1450 N. Devonshire
Chicago, IL 60611

Dear Dr. Stark:

Thank you for giving me the opportunity to discuss the medical assisting position that you are seeking to fill in your office. I believe that my skills would be a good match with your needs.

I enjoyed meeting you and your staff today, and I would be very interested in working for you.

Thank you for considering my application. I look forward to hearing from you.

Sincerely,

Ralph Taylor

Ralph Taylor, C.M.A.

FIGURE 53-10 An example of a follow-up letter following an interview.

What Does the Employer Want?

Employers are looking for a variety of skills from their employees.

PROCEDURE

Preparing a Follow-Up Letter

OBJECTIVE: Prepare an interview follow-up letter.

Equipment and Supplies
computer; printer; pen; paper; dictionary; thesaurus; telephone book

Method
1. Using Figure 53-10 as an example, prepare a follow-up letter.
2. Proofread your follow-up letter.
3. Have a close family member or friend proofread your follow-up letter.
4. Make any corrections to errors found on the follow-up letter.
5. Using good-quality, white or off-white paper, print your follow-up letter.
6. Turn in your follow-up letter to your instructor.

To be successful as a medical assistant, you must master six basic skills:

1. Reading. As a medical assistant you will be reading medical records, orders, instructions, memos, correspondence, resources, references, and much more. You will also read a variety of professional journals to keep your skills current.

2. Listening. A large amount of your time as a medical assistant will be spent listening to patients. You will also use your listening skills during meetings, telephone conversations, and conversing with other staff members. Good listening skills are critical for every medical assistant.

3. Speaking. As a medical assistant you will spend a lot of time speaking to patients and other staff members. When you are speaking with others you will need to speak clearly and use appropriate terms.

4. Writing. Documentation in a medical office is a must. It demonstrates that care or treatment has been done. This could be critical if a physician is called to court for a lawsuit. A medical assistant needs to make sure all documentation is complete, accurate, and spelled correctly.

5. Problem solving. Your problem-solving skills will help the medical office and your duties be more efficient. Employers want their employees to be able to take care of changes and think of new ways to improve situations.

6. Teamwork. A medical office must work as a team for it to run efficiently. As a medical assistant you will share knowledge and responsibilities with other staff members. Good-quality patient care results when all members of the team working together.

Depending on the employer, they will look for a wide range of values and skills in an employee. Not every employer will want the same values or skills. Some of the values and skills employers look for are as follows:

1. Initiative. When the medical assistant takes on a task without being told to do so, this is initiative. Starting a task on your own will show your employer that you are problem solving and using your critical thinking skills.

2. Enthusiasm. A medical assistant's enthusiasm can be expressed verbally or nonverbally. When you are enthusiastic you enjoy what you are doing as well and are passionate about it. Enthusiasm is a positive quality for all medical assistants to acquire.

3. Honesty. For the patients, physician, and other staff members to trust you, you will need to be honest at all times. If you have made a mistake, admit it and learn from it.

4. Dependability. When a medical assistant is late, leaves early, or misses work, this means the office must reassign staff and possibly work understaffed for that time period. This causes more work for everyone. The physician and other staff members depend on you to be there at the scheduled time.

5. Flexibility. Most medical offices are very busy and emergencies do occur. As a medical assistant you will need to be flexible with the changes that can occur daily or even minute to minute in the medical office. This also means that you will need to multitask throughout the workday.

6. Administrative skills. Part of your job duties may include administrative procedures. Take special care to make sure each one is performed correctly.

7. Clinical skills. Part of your job duties may include clinical procedures. It is critical for a medical assistant to perform clinical skills with total accuracy.

You will not be perfect at all of these skills, but you can develop each and every one of them with time, practice, and commitment. The more values and skills you have as a medical assistant, the more employable you will be. Just ask yourself, what would you want in an employee? This will help lead you to the values and skills you need to develop.

SUMMARY

One of the most valuable components of a medical assisting program is the externship because it provides an opportunity to practice skills that have been learned in school, under the direct supervision of the externship coordinator. This important stage of the training provides the student an opportunity to gain insight into strengths and weaknesses, allowing students to work on or correct weaknesses before accepting employment.

The job interview process requires the medical assistant to be honest and sincere about capabilities and the desire to work diligently. A fulfilling career demands careful planning, the ability to arrive on time, and the ability to work diligently for an employer while always keeping the patient's needs in mind.

Chapter Review

COMPETENCY REVIEW

1. Define and spell the terms to learn for this chapter.
2. Describe three areas of student responsibility concerning the externship.
3. List and discuss three externship opportunities in your area that you would like to pursue.
4. List and discuss six areas that your externship supervisor will be evaluating.
5. Write a résumé or update an existing résumé.
6. Select an advertisement for a medical assistant position from your local newspaper's classified section. Write a cover letter in response to that advertisement.
7. Write a follow-up letter after receiving an interview for the position mentioned in Question 6.
8. What are three questions that you would ask a potential employer during an interview?
9. How would you respond to the questions "What is your major strength?" and "What is your major weakness?"

PREPARING FOR THE CERTIFICATION EXAM

1. Working without payment in a health care setting as part of a medical assisting program is called:
   A. a clinical rotation
   B. an in-service
   C. an externship
   D. an internship
   E. a practicum

2. In accordance with the AAMA guidelines regarding externship, a minimum of how many hours must be successfully completed by a medical assistant?
   A. 80
   B. 100
   C. 120
   D. 140
   E. 160

continued on next page

3. Some of the areas that are not evaluated during externship training include:
   A. clinical skills
   B. administrative skills
   C. grooming
   D. enthusiasm
   E. grades received in school

4. Which of the following is not a guideline to successful interviewing?
   A. Carry one extra copy of your résumé.
   B. Dress conservatively.
   C. Be alert.
   D. Arrive 5 minutes early.
   E. Do not chew gum.

5. Which of the following is NOT considered a job hunting mistake?
   A. failing to network with others and tell them that you are looking
   B. looking for the perfect job
   C. limiting yourself to one field
   D. not having a clear plan
   E. spending very little time answering classified ads

6. The process by which a medical assistant self-evaluates one's strengths and weaknesses is referred to in the chapter as:
   A. ego identification
   B. personal assessment
   C. skill evaluation
   D. self-reflection
   E. self-assessment

7. What information is placed at the very top of a résumé?
   A. name
   B. name and address
   C. name, address, and telephone number
   D. name, address, telephone number, and Social Security number
   E. name, address, telephone number, and date of birth

8. A statement from someone who has either worked with you or known you for a long time is called a:
   A. professional statement
   B. professional reference
   C. professional letter
   D. professional resources
   E. professional testimonial

9. The name of the type of correspondence that is intended as a courtesy to introduce yourself is called a:
   A. cover letter
   B. follow-up letter
   C. résumé
   D. interview letter
   E. calling card

10. Which of the following is NOT considered one of the more common mistakes made in an interview?
    A. shaking hands
    B. being critical of a previous employer
    C. not asking questions about the potential employer's organization
    D. being extremely talkative
    E. using very familiar language such as "yep" instead of "yes"

CRITICAL THINKING

1. What could Elizabeth have done to be on time to the externship site?

2. Do you think Melba should terminate Elizabeth from this externship site?

3. Should Elizabeth have scheduled to leave at noon on her first day of her externship experience?

ON THE JOB

Stacy is the lead medical assistant in an ophthalmology practice of 10 physicians. The eye clinic sees patients, literally, from all over the world. Several of the physicians are premier in their specific area of ophthalmology, such as Dr. Keeler, who specializes in retinal diseases.

Today Stacy is going to interview a potential new employee, Sarah Banks. Sarah is currently finishing a CAAHEP-approved medical assisting program at a local college and is searching for full-time employment. She has some on-the-job experience dating back to when she was an after-school receptionist for a general practitioner, but that was more than 10 years ago.

The clinic tends to hire medical assistants who are certified, experienced, and very capable of dealing with patients from different age groups, races, and origins. However, Sarah is being considered for the position because, first of all, her father is a personal friend of Dr. Keeler's and, secondly, medical assistants, because of the high demand, are difficult to find. What should Stacy do to prepare for the interview with Sarah?

What is your response?

1. Considering that the practice is limited to ophthalmology, would any special requirements be warranted in a medical assistant who was going to work in this area?
2. Considering that the clinic's patient population is mixed by age and race, would any special requirements in a medical assistant be warranted in this case?
3. Is it proper procedure for Sarah to be applying for this position given that she has not yet completed her medical assisting program?
4. Should Stacy, given the circumstances, invest a lot of time in interviewing Sarah? Why or why not?
5. Should the rather dated on-the-job experience be factored into Stacy's decision to hire Sarah or not?
6. If Stacy decides not to hire Sarah, does Stacy need to personally contact the reference and thank him anyway, given that he is a friend of Dr. Keeler's?

INTERNET ACTIVITY

Using any Internet search engine, type the words "dressing for an interview." Go to one or more of the resulting Web sites to answer the following questions:

1. Would a person be ready for an interview if he or she had an eyebrow piercing?
2. Should a person chew gum during an interview?
3. What are appropriate colors for dresses or suits?

MediaLink  More on externship and career opportunities, including interactive resources, can be found on the Student CD-ROM accompanying this textbook.

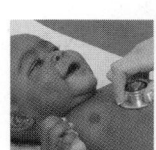

a	ampere; anode; anterior; aqua; area; artery	AKA	above-knee amputation	Ba	barium
AB, Ab	abortion; abnormal; antibody	alk phos	alkaline phosphatase	BAC	blood alcohol concentration
ABC	aspiration biopsy cytology	ALD	aldolase	BaE	barium enema
ABG	arterial blood gases	ALL	acute lymphocytic leukemia	baso	basophil
ABLB	alternate binaural loudness balance	ALS	amyotropic lateral sclerosis	BBB	bundle branch block (L for left; R for right)
ABO	blood group	ALT	argon laser trabeculoplasty; alanine aminotransferase	BBT	basal body temperature
ABR	auditory brainstem response	AMA	American Medical Association	BC	bone conduction
AC	air conduction; anticoagulant	AMD	age-related macular degeneration	BE	barium enema
a.c.	before meals	AMI	acute myocardial infarction	BG, bG	blood glucose; blood sugar
ACAT	automated computerized axial tomography	AML	acute myelogenous leukemia	b.i.d.	twice a day
Acc.	accommodation	Angio	angiogram	BIN, bin	twice a night
ACG	angiocardiography	ANS	autonomic nervous system	BK	below knee
Ach	acetylcholine	A&P	auscultation and percussion; anatomy and physiology	BKA	below-knee amputation
ACL	anterior cruciate ligament			BM	bowel movement
ACLS	advanced cardiac life support	AP, AP view	anterior-posterior; anteroposterior view	BMD	bone mineral density (test)
ACR	American College of Rheumatology	APB	atrial premature beat	BMR	basal metabolic rate
ACS	American Cancer Society	APTT	activated partial thromboplastin time	BNO	bladder neck obstruction
ACTH	adrenocorticoptropic hormone	ARC	AIDS-related complex	BP	blood pressure
AD	right ear (O) (auris dexter); Alzheimer's Disease; advance directive	ARD	acute respiratory disease	BPH	benign prostatic hypertrophy
		ARDS	acute respiratory distress syndrome	Broncho	bronchoscopy
		ARF	acute respiratory failure; acute renal failure	BRP	bathroom privileges
ADA	American Diabetes Association	ARMD	age-related macular degeneration	BS	breath sounds; bowel sounds; blood sugar
ad lib	as desired; freely	AROM	active range of motion	BSE	breast self-examination
adeno-CA	adenocarcinoma	AS	aortic stenosis; arteriosclerosis; left ear (X)	BSI	body systems isolation
ADH	antidiuretic hormone			BSP	bromsulphalein
ADHD	attention-deficit hyperactivity disorder	ASCVD	arteriosclerotic cardiovascular disease	BT	bleeding time
ADL	activities of daily living	As, Ast, astigm	astigmatism	BUN	blood urea nitrogen
ADP	adenosine diphosphate			BX, bx	biopsy
AE	above the elbow	Ascus	atypical squamous cells of undetermined significance	c̄	with (cum)
AF	atrial fibrillation			C1, C2, etc.	first cervical vertebra, second cervical vertebra, etc.
AFB	acid-fast bacillus (TB organism)	ASD	atrial septal defect		
AFP	alpha-fetoprotein	ASH	asymmetrical septal hypertrophy	C&S	culture and sensitivity
A/G	albumin/globulin ratio	ASHD	arteriosclerotic heart disease	CA	cancer; carcinoembryonic antigen
Ag	antigen			Ca	calcium; cancer
AGN	acute glomerulonephritis	ASL	American Sign Language	CABG	coronary artery bypass graft
AH	abdominal hysterectomy	Astigm.	astigmatism		
AHF	antihemophilic factor VIII	AST	aspartate aminotransferase	CAD	coronary artery disease
AHG	antihemophillic globulin factor VIII	ATN	acute tubular necrosis	CAM	complementary and alternative medicines
AI	aortic insufficiency; artificial insemination	ATP	adenosine triphosphate	cap	capsule
		AU	both ears (auris unitas)	CAPD	continuous ambulatory peritoneal dialysis
AIDS	acquired immune deficiency syndrome	AV, A-V	atrioventricular; arteriovenous	CAT, CT	computerized axial tomography
AIH	artificial insemination homologous	AVMs	arteriovenous malformations	cath	catheterization
AK	above knee	AVR	aortic valve replacement	CBC	complete blood count
				CBD	common bile duct
				CBS	chronic brain syndrome
				cc	cubic centimeter
				CC	clean-catch urine specimen; cardiac catheterization; chief complaint

CCU — coronary care unit; cardiac care unit
CD4 — protein on T-cell helper lymphocyte
CDC — Centers for Disease Control and Prevention
CDH — congenital dislocation of the hip
CEA — carcinoembryonic antigen
CF — cystic fibrosis
CGL — chronic granulocytic leukemia
c.gl. — correction with glasses
CGN — chronic glomerulonephritis
CHD — congestive heart disease
chemo — chemotherapy
CHF — congestive heart failure
CHO — carbohydrate
chol — cholesterol
Ci — curie
Cib — food (cibus)
CIC — coronary intensive care
CIN — cervical intraepithelial neoplasia
CIS — carcinoma in situ
CK — creatine kinase
CL, Cl — chloride
CLL — chronic lymphocytic leukemia
cm — centimeter
CMG — cystometrogram
CML — chronic myelogenous leukemia
CMP — cardiomyopathy
CNS — central nervous system
c/o — complains of
CO — cardiac output
CO_2 — carbon dioxide
COLD — chronic obstructive lung disease
COPD — chronic obstructive pulmonary disease
CP — cerebral palsy; chest pain
CPD — cephalopelvic disproportion
CPK — creatine phosphokinase
CPM — continuous passive motion
CPR — cardiopulmonary resuscitation
CPS — cycles per second
CR — computerized radiography
CRF — chronic renal failure
CS, C-section — cesarean section
C&S — culture and sensitivity
C-section — cesarean section (surgical delivery)
CSF — cerebrospinal fluid
C-spine — cervical spine film
CT — computed tomography
CTA — clear to auscultation
CTS — carpal tunnel syndrome
CUC — chronic ulcerative colitis
CV — cardiovascular
CVA — cerebrovascular accident
CVD — cardiovascular disease
CVP — central venous pressure
CVS — chorionic villus sampling

CWP — childbirth without pain
Cx — cervix
CXR — chest x-ray
cyl. — cylindrical lens
cysto — cystoscopic exam
/d — per day
D — diopter (lens strength)
dB, db — decibel
DBS — deep brain stimulation
D/C — discontinue
D&C — dilatation and curettage
D&E — dilation and evacuation
dc — discontinue
DC — discharge
DCIS — ductal carcinoma in situ
DDS — Doctor of Dental Surgery; dorsal cord stimulation
decub — decubitus
Derm — dermatology
DES — diethylstilbestrol
DHT — dihydrotestosterone
DI — diabetes insipidus; diagnostic imaging
diff — differential
dil — dilute; diluted
DJD — degenerative joint disease
DM — diabetes mellitus
DNA — deoxyribonucleic acid
DNR — do not resuscitate
DO — doctor of osteopathy
DOA — dead on arrival
DOB — date of birth
DOE — dyspnea upon exertion
DPT — diphtheria, pertussis, tetanus injection
DRE — digital rectal examination
DRGs — diagnostic related groups
DSA — digital subtraction angiography
DTaP — diphtheria, tetanus and pertussis (vaccine)
DTR — deep tendon reflex
DT's — delerium tremens
DUB — dysfunctional uterine bleeding
DVA — distance visual acuity
DVT — deep vein thrombosis
Dx — diagnosis
EBV — Epstein-Barr virus
ECC — endocervical curettage
ECCE — extracapsular cataract extraction
ECF — extracellular fluid; extended care facility
ECG; EKG — electrocardiogram
ECHO — echocardiogram
E. coli — Escherichia coli
ECSL — extracorporeal shockwave lithotriptor
ECT — electroconvulsive therapy
ED — erectile dysfunction
EDC — estimated date of confinement
EEG — electroencephalogram
EENT — eyes, ears, nose, throat
EGD — esophagogastroduoden-oscopy

ELISA — enzyme-linked immunosorbent assay
EM — emmetropia (normal vision)
EMG — electromyography
ENG — electronystagmography
ENT — ear, nose, and throat
EOM — extraocular movement
eosin, eos — eosinophil
ERCP — endoscopic retrograde cholangiopancreatography
ERT — estrogen replacement therapy; external radiation therapy
ERV — expiratory reserve volume
ESR, SR — erythrocyte sedimentation rate
ESL, ESWL — extracorporeal shock-wave lithotripsy
ESR, SR, sed rate — erythrocyte sedimentation rate; sedimentation rate
ESRD — end-stage renal disease
EST — electroshock therapy
ET — endotracheal; endotracheal
ETF — eustachian tube function
F — Fahrenheit
FACP — Fellow, American College of Physicians
FACS — Fellow, American College of Surgeons
FBS — fasting blood sugar
FDA — Food and Drug Administration
FEF — forced expiratory flow
FEKG — fetal electrocardiogram
FEV — forced expiratory volume
FH — family history
FHR — fetal heart rate
FHS — fetal heart sound
FHT — fetal heart tone
FMS — fibromyalgia syndrome
FROM — full range of motion
FS — frozen section
FSH — follicle-stimulating hormone
FTA-ABS — fluorescent treponemal antibody absorption
FTND — full-term normal delivery
5-FU — 5-fluorouracil
FUO — fever of undetermined origin
FVC — forced vital capacity
FX, fx — fracture
g — gram
Ga — gallium
GB — gallbladder
GC — gonorrhea
GCSF — granulocyte colony-stimulating factor
GERD — gastroesophageal reflux disease
GGT — gamma-glutamyl transferase
GH — growth hormone
GI — gastrointestinal

GIFT	gamete intrafallopian transfer
GnRF	gonadotropin-releasing factor
GOT	glutamic oxaloacetic transaminase
Gpi	globus pallidus
GPT	glutamic pyruvic transaminase
gr	grain
grav I	first pregnancy
GSW	gunshot wound
gtt	drops (guttae)
GTT	glucose tolerance test
GU	genitourinary
gyn, gyne	gynecology
h	hour
H	hypodermic; hydrogen
H&L	heart & lungs
HAA	hepatitis-associated antigen
HAV	hepatitis A virus
HBIG	hepatitis B immune globulin
HBOT	hyperbaric oxygen therapy
HBP	high blood pressure
HBV	hepatitis B virus
HCG	human chorionic gonadotropin
HCl	hydrochloric acid
HCO$_3$	bicarbonate
HCT, Hct, crit	hematocrit
HCV	hepatitis C virus
HD	hemodialysis; Hodgkin's disease
HDL	high-density lipoproteins
HDN	hemolytic disease of the newborn
HDS	herniated disk syndrome
HEENT	head, eyes, ears, nose and throat
HF	heart failure
Hg	mercury
HgB, Hb, Hgb, HGB	hemoglobin
HGH	human growth hormone
HIV	human immunodeficiency virus (causes AIDS)
HLA	human leukocyte antigen
HMD	hyaline membrane disease
HNP	herniated nucleus pulposa (herniated disk)
H$_2$O	water
Hpd	hematoporphyrin derivative
H. pylori	Heliocobacter pylori
HPV	human papillomavirus
HRT	hormone replacement therapy
h.s.	at bedtime
HSG	hysterosalpingography
HSO	hysterosalpingoophrectomy
HSV	herpes simplex virus
HSV-2	herpes simplex virus-2
Ht	height
HT	hypermetropia (hyperopia)
HTLV	human T-cell leukemia-lymphoma virus
HTN	hypertension
Hx	history
hypo	hypodermic
Hz	Hertz
IBD	inflammatory bowel syndrome
IBS	irritable bowel syndrome
IC	intracardiac; interstitial cystitis
ICCE	intracapsular cataract cryoextraction
ICF	intracellular fluid
ICP	intracranial pressure
ICSH	interstitial cell-stimulating hormone
ICU	intensive care unit
ID	intradermal
I&D	incision and drainage
IDDM	insulin-dependent diabetes mellitus
Ig	immunoglobins (IgA, IgD, IgE, IgG, IgM)
IH	infectious hepatitis
IHSS	idiopathic hypertropic subaortic stenosis
IL-2	interleukin-2
IM	intramuscular
inj	injection
I&O	intake and output
IOL	intraocular pressure
IOP	intraocular pressure
IPD	intermittent peritoneal dialysis
IPPB	intermittent positive pressure breathing
IQ	intelligence quotient
IR	interventional radiologist
IRDS	infant respiratory distress syndrome
IRT	internal radiation therapy
IRV	inspiratory reserve volume
IS	intercostal space
ITP	idiopathic thrombocytopenia purpura
IU	international unit
IUD	intrauterine device
IUGR	intrauterine growth rate; intrauterine growth retardation
IV	intravenous
IVC	intravenous cholangiogram; inferior vena cava; intraventricular catheter
IVCD	intraventricular conduction delay
IVF	in vitro fertilization
IVP	intravenous pyelogram
IVS	interventricular septum
IVU	intravenous urogram
J	joule
JNC	Joint National Committee
JVP	jugular venous pulse
K	potassium
KB	knee bearing
KD	knee disarticulation
kg	kilogram
KS	Kaposi's sarcoma
KUB	kidneys, ureters, bladder
kV	kilovolt
kW	kilowatt
L, l	liter
L1, L2, etc.	first lumbar vertebra, second lumbar vertebra, etc.
LA	left atrium
L&A	light and accommodation
lab	laboratory
LAC	laceration; long arm cast
LAK	lymphokine-activated killer (cells)
LAT, lat	lateral
lb	pound
LB	large bowel
LBBB	left bundle branch block
LBW	low birth weight
LCIS	lobular carcinoma in situ
LD	lactate dehydrogenase
LDH	lactic dehydrogenase
LDL	low-density lipoproteins
LE	left eye; lupus erythematosus; lower extremity
LEDs	light-emitting diodes
LES	lower esophageal sphincter
LGI	lower gastrointestinal series
LH	luteinizing hormone
LH-RH	luteinizing hormone-releasing hormone
LIF	left iliac fossa
liq	liquid; fluid
L K & S	liver, kidney, and spleen
ll	left lateral
LLC	long leg cast
LLE	left lower extremity
LLL	left lower lobe
LLQ	left lower quadrant
LMP	last menstrual period
LOM	limitation of motion
LP	lumbar puncture
LPE	laser peripheral iridotomy
LPF	low-power field
LRQ	lower right quadrant
L, lt	left
LTH	lactogenic hormone
LUE	left upper extremity
LUL	left upper lobe
LUQ	left upper quadrant
LV	left ventricle
LVAD	left ventricular assist device
lymph	lymphocyte
M	molar; thousand; muscle
m	male; meter; minim
mA	milliampere
mAs	milliampere second
MBC	minimal breathing capacity
MCH	mean corpuscular hemoglobin
MCHC	mean corpuscular hemoglobin concentration
mCi	millicurie
MCV	mean corpuscular volume
MD	medical doctor; muscular dystrophy

| mEq | milliequivalent | NPUAP | National Pressure Ulcer | Pe tube | polyethylene tube placed in |

VMA	vanillylmandelic acid	WNL	within normal limits	XRT	radiation therapy
VP	vasopressin	WPW	Wolff-Parkinson-White syndrome	XT	exotropia
VPB	ventricular premature beat			XX	female sex chromosomes
		wt	weight	XY	male sex chromosomes
VS	vital signs	w/v	weight by volume		
VSD	ventricular septal defect			YAG	yttrium-aluminum-garnet (laser)
VT	ventricular tachycardia	x	multiplied by		
		XM	cross match for blood (type and cross match)	YOB	year of birth
WBC	white blood cell			yr	year
WDWN	well developed, well nourished	XP	xeroderma pigmentosum		
		XR	x-ray	z	atomic number

CHARTING ABBREVIATIONS AND SYMBOLS

aa	of each	FHT	fetal heart tones	qm	every morning (quaque mane)
ac	before meals (ante cibum)	GB	gallbladder		
AD	right ear (auris dextra)	GI	gastrointestinal	qn	every night (quaque nocte)
ADL	activities of daily living	GU	genitourinary	R	right; respiration
ad lib	as desired	h, hr	hour	RBC	red blood cell; red blood (cell) count
adm	admission	hpf	high power field		
AE	above elbow	hs	hour of sleep; bedtime (hora somni)	Rh	Rhesus blood factor (Rh + or Rh −)
AJ	ankle jerk				
AK	above knee	hypo	hypodermic injection	RLQ	right lower quadrant
alt dieb	every other day	ICU	intensive care unit	R/O	rule out
alt hor	every other hour	IM	intramuscular	ROM	range of motion
alt noc	every other night	I&O	intake and output	RUQ	right upper quadrant
AM, am	before noon (ante meridiem); morning	IU	international unit	SC, sc, subq	subcutaneous
		IV	intravenous	SOB	shortness of breath
AMA	against medical advice	L	left	SOS	if necessary (si opus sit)
AMB	ambulate; ambulatory	L&A	light and accommodation	stat	immediately
ant	anterior	LAT	lateral	Sx	signs, symptoms
AP	anteroposterior	L&W	living and well	T, temp	temperature
A-P	anterior-posterior	LLQ	left lower quadrant	tabs	tablets
approx	approximately	LMP	last menstrual period	TC&DB	turn, cough, deep breathe
AQ, aq	water	LOA	left occipitoanterior	tid	three times a day
ASAP	as soon as possible	LPF	low power field (10x)	tinct	tincture
AS or LE	left ear (auris sinistra)	LUQ	left upper quadrant	TPN	total parenteral nutrition
AV	atrioventricular	MTD	right ear drum (membrana tympani dexter)	trans	transverse
BE	below elbow			ULQ	upper left quadrant
bid	twice a day	MTS	left ear drum (membrana tympani sinister)	ung	ointment
bin	twice a night			URQ	upper right quadrant
BK	below knee	neg	negative	VS	vital signs
BM	bowel movement	NG	nasogastric	WBC	white blood cell; white blood (cell) count
BMR	basal metabolic rate	NPO	nothing by mouth		
BRP	bathroom privileges	NS	normal saline	WM, BM	white male, black male
C	Centigrade, Celsius or calorie (kilocalorie)	OD	right eye (oculus dexter)	WF, BF	white female, black female
		OP	outpatient		
caps	capsules	OR	operating room	×	times, power
CBR	complete bed rest	OS or OL	left eye (oculus sinister, oculus laevus)	−	negative
CC	chief complaint; clean catch (urine)			+	positive
		OU	each eye (oculus uterque)	F	female
CCU	cardiac (coronary) care unit	P	pulse	M	male
		PA	posteroanterior	+/−	positive or negative
c/o	complains of	pc	after meals (post cibum)	*	birth
cont	continue	PI	present illness	†	death
dc	discontinue	po	by mouth (per os)	%	percent
DC	discharge from hospital	PO	postoperative	#	number; pound
DNA	does not apply	PM, pm	afternoon or evening (post meridiem)	&	and
DNR	do not resuscitate			<	less than
DNS	did not show	prn	as necessary, as required, when necessary	=	equal
Dr	doctor			>	greater than
D/W	dextrose in water	q	every (quaque)	?	question
Dx	diagnosis	qd	every day (quaque die)	@	at
EOM	extraocular movement	qh	every hour (quaque hora)	^	increase
ER	emergency room	q2h	every 2 hours	™	trade mark
Ex	examination	q4h	every 4 hours	©	copyright
F	Fahrenheit	qid	four times a day (quarter in die)	®	registered
FHS	fetal heart sounds			¶	paragraph

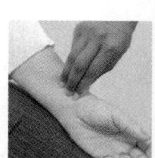

APPENDIX II:
Glossary of Word Parts

PREFIXES

a	no, not, without, lack of, apart	end	within, inner	neo	new
ab	away from	endo	within, inner	nulli	none
ad	toward, near	ep	upon, over, above		
ambi	both	epi	upon, over, above	olig	little, scanty
an	no, not, without, lack of	eso	inward	oligo	little, scanty
ana	up	eu	good, normal		
ant	against	ex	out, away from	pan	all
ante	before	exo	out, away from	par	around, beside
anti	against	extra	outside, beyond	para	beside, alongside, abnormal
apo	separation			per	through
astro	star-shaped	hemi	half	peri	around
auto	self	heter	different	poly	many, much, excessive
		hetero	different	post	after, behind
bi	two, double	homo	similar, same	pre	before
bin	twice	homeo	similar, same, likeness, constant	primi	first
brachy	short			pro	before
brady	slow	hydr	water	proto	first
		hydro	water	pseudo	false
cac	bad	hyp	below, deficient	pyro	fire
cata	down	hyper	above, beyond, excessive		
centi	a hundred	hypo	below, under, deficient	quadri	four
chromo	color			quint	five
circum	around	in	in, into, not		
con	with, together	infra	below	re	back
contra	against	infer	below	retro	backward
		inter	between		
de	down, away from	intra	within	semi	half
deca	ten	ir (in)	into	sub	below, under, beneath
di (a)	through, between			supra	above, beyond
dia	through, between	macro	large	super	above, beyond
dif	apart, free from, separate	mal	bad	sym	together
dipl	double	mega	large, great	syn	together, with
di (s)	two, apart	meso	middle		
dis	apart	meta	beyond, over, between, change	tachy	fast
dys	bad, difficult, painful			tetra	four
		micro	small	trans	across
ec	out, outside, outer	milli	one-thousandth	tri	three
ecto	out, outside, outer	mon (o)	one		
em	in	mono	one	ultra	beyond
en	within	multi	many, much	uni	one

WORD ROOTS/COMBINING FORMS

abdomin	abdomen	aden	gland	alveol	small, hollow air sac
abort	to miscarry	aden/o	gland	ambyl	dull
absorpt	to suck in	adhes	stuck to	ambul	to walk
acanth	a thorn	adip	fat	amni/o	lamb
acetabul	vinegar cup	agglutinat	clumping	ampere	ampere
acid	acid	agon	agony	amputat	to cut though
acoust	hearing	agor/a	market place	amyl	starch
acr	extremity, point	albin	white	anastom	opening
acr/o	extremity, point	albumin	protein	andr	man
act	acting	alimentat	nourishment	andr/o	man
actin	ray	all	other	ang	vessel

ang/i	vessel	cartil	gristle	cost	rib
angin	to choke, quinsy	castr	to prune	cost/o	rib
angi/o	vessel	caud	tail	cox	hip
anis/o	unequal	caus	heat	cran/i	skull
ankyl	stiffening, crooked	cavit	cavity	crani/o	skull
an/o	anus	cavit	cavity	creat	flesh
anter/i	toward the front	celi	abdomen, belly	creatin	flesh, creatine
anthrac	coal	cellul	little cell	crine	to secrete
aort	aorta	centr	center	crin/o	to secrete
aort/o	aorta	centr/i	center	crur	leg
append	appendix	cephal	head	cry/o	cold
arachn	spider	cept	receive	crypt	hidden
arche	beginning	cerebell	little brain	cubit	elbow, to lie
arter	artery	cerebell/o	little brain	culd/o	cul-de-sac
arter/i	artery	cerebr/o	cerebrum	curie	curie
arteri/o	artery	cervic	cervix, neck	cutane	skin
arthr	joint	cheil	lip	cyan	dark blue
arthr/o	joint	chem/o	chemical	cycl	ciliary body
artific/i	not natural	chlor/o	green	cycl/o	ciliary body
aspirat	to draw in	chol	gall, bile	cyst	bladder, sac
atel	imperfect	chole	gall, bile	cyst/o	bladder, sac
atel/o	imperfect	chol/e	gall, bile	cyt	cell
ather	fatty substance, porridge	choledoch/o	common bile duct	cyth	cell
ather/o	fatty substance, porridge	chondr	cartilage	cyt/o	cell
atri	atrium	chondr/o	cartilage		
atri/o	atrium	chord	cord	dacry	tear
aud/i	to hear	chori/o	chorion	dactyl	finger or toe
audi/o	to hear	choroid	choroid	dactyl/o	finger or toe
auditor	hearing	choroid/o	choroid	defecat	to remove dregs
aur	ear	chromat	color	dem	people
aur/i	ear	chrom/o	color	dendr/o	tree
auscultat	listen to	chym	juice	dent	tooth
aut	self	cine	motion	dent/i	tooth
axill	armpit	cinemat/o	motion	derm	skin
		circulat	circular	derm/a	skin
bacter/i	bacteria	cirrh	orange-yellow	dermat	skin
balan	glans penis	cirrh/o	orange-yellow	dermat/o	skin
bartholin	Bartholin's glands	cis	to cut	derm/o	skin
bas/o	base	claudicat	to limp	dextr/o	to the right
bil	bile, gall	clavicul	little key	diast	to expand
bil/i	bile, gall	cleid/o	clavicle	didym	testis
bi/o	life	coagul	to clot	digit	finger or toe
blast/o	germ cell	coagulat	to clot	dilat	to widen
blephar	eyelid	coccyg/e	tailbone	disk	a disk
blephar/o	eyelid	coccyg/o	tail bone	dist	away from the point of
bol	to cast, throw	cochle/o	land snail		origin
brach/i	arm	coit	a coming together	diverticul	diverticula
bronch	bronchi	col	colon	dors	backward
bronch/i	bronchi	coll/a	glue	dors/i	backward
bronchiol	bronchiole	collis	neck	duct	to lead
bronch/o	bronchi	col/o	colon	duoden	duodenum
bucc	cheek	colon	colon	dur	dura, hard
burs	a pouch	colon/o	colon	dur/o	dura, hard
		colp/o	vagina	dwarf	small
calc	lime, calcium	concuss	shaken violently	dynam	power
calc/i	calcium	condyle	knuckle		
calcan/e	heel bone	con/i	dust	ech/o	echo
cancer	crab	conjunctiv	to join together	ectop	displaced
capn	smoke	connect	to bind together	eg/o	I, self
capsul	a little box	constipat	to press together	ejaculat	to throw out
carcin	cancer	continence	to hold	electr/o	electricity
carcin/o	cancer	cor	pupil	eme	to vomit
card	heart	coriat	corium	embol	to cast, to throw
card/i	heart	corne	cornea	emulsificat	disintergrate
cardi/o	heart	corpor	body	encephal	brain
carp	wrist	corpor/e	body	encephal/o	brain
carp/o	wrist	cortic	cortex	enchyma	to pour
		cortis	cortex		

enter	intestine	gon/o	genitals	lacrim	tear
enucleat	to remove the kernel of	granul/o	little grain, granular	lamin	lamina, thin plate
eosin/o	rose-colored	gravida	pregnant	lamp (s)	to shine
episi/o	vulva, pudenda	gryp	curve	lapar/o	flank, abdomen
equ/i	equal	gynec/o	female	laryng	larynx
erget	work			laryng/e	larynx
erg/o	work	halat	breathe	laryng/o	larynx
eructat	a breaking out	hallux	great (big) toe	later	side
erysi	red	hem	blood	laxat	to loosen
erythr/o	red	hemat	blood	lei/o	smooth
esophag/e	esophagus	hemat/o	blood	lemma	rind, sheath, husk
esophag/o	esophagus	hem/o	blood	lent	lens
esthesi/o	feeling	hemorrh	vein liable to bleed	lept	seizure
estr/o	mad desire	hepat	liver	letharg	drowsiness
eti/o	cause	hepat/o	liver	leuk	white
eunia	a bed	herni/o	hernia	leuk/o	white
excret	sifted out	hidr	sweat	levat	lifter
		hirsut	hairy	libr/i	balance
f(erat)	to bear	hist/o	tissue	lingu	tongue
fasc	a band (fascia)	hol/o	whole	lip	fat
fasci/o	a band (fascia)	horizont	horizon	lipid	fat
femor	femur	humer	humerus	lip/o	fat
fenestrat	window	hydr	water	lith	stone
fibr	fibrous tissue, fiber	hymen	hymen	lith/o	stone
fibrillat	fibrils (small fibers)	hypn	sleep	lob	lobe
fibrin/o	fiber	hyster	womb, uterus	lob/o	lobe
fibr/o	fiber	hyster/o	womb, uterus	lobul	small lobe
fibul	fibula			locat	to place
filtrat	to strain through	icter	jaundice	log	study
fixat	fastened	ile	ileum	log/o	word
flex	to bend	ile/o	ileum	lopec	fox mange
fluor/o	fluorescence	ili	ilium	lord	bending
foc	focus	ili/o	ilium	lucent	to shine
follicul	little bag	illus	foot	lumb	loin
format	a shaping	immun/o	safe, immunity	lumb/o	loin
fungat	mushroom, fungus	infarct	infarct (necrosis of an area)	lump	lump
fus	to pour	infect	infection	lun	moon
		infer/i	below	lymph	lymph, clear fluid
galact/o	milk	inguin	groin	lymph/o	lymph, clear fluid
ganglion	knot	insul	insulin		
gastr	stomach	insulin/o	insulin	malign	bad kind
gastr/o	stomach	integument	covering	mamm/o	breast
gen	formation, produce	intern	within	mandibul	lower jawbone
gene	formation, produce	ionizat	ion (going)	man/o	thin
genet	formation, produce	ion/o	ion	mast	breast
genital	belonging to birth	iont/o	ion	masticat	to chew
gen/o	kind	irid	iris	mast/o	breast
ger	old age	irid/o	iris	maxill	jawbone
gest	to carry	isch	to hold back	maxilla	jaw
gester	to bear	ischi	ischium	maxim	greatest
gigant	giant	is/o	equal	meat	passage
gingiv	gums			meat/o	passage
glandul	little acorn	jaund	yellow	med	middle
gli	glue			medi	toward the middle
gli/o	glue	kal	potassium	medull	marrow
glob	globe	kary/o	cell's nucleus	medull/o	marrow
globin	globule	kel	tumor	melan	black
globul	globe	kerat	cornea	melan/o	black
glomerul	glomerulus, little ball	kerat/o	horn, cornea	men	month
glomerul/o	glomerulus, little ball	keton	ketone	mening	membrane (meninges)
gloss/o	tongue	kil/o	a thousand	mening/i	membrane
gluc/o	sweet, sugar	kinet	motion	mening/o	membrane
glyc	sweet, sugar	kyph	a hump	menise	crescent
glyc/o	glucose, sweet, sugar			men/o	month
glycos	sweet, sugar	labi	lip	ment	mind
gonad	seed	labyrinth	maze	mes	middle
goni/o	angle	labyrinth/o	maze	mes/o	middle

mester	month	orth	straight	physi/o	nature
metr	to measure, womb, uterus	orth/o	straight	pil/o	hair
metr/i	womb, uterus	oscill	to swing	pine	pine cone
micturit	to urinate	oscill/o	to swing	pineal	pineal body
miliar	millet (tiny)	oste	bone	pin/o	to drink
minim	least	oste/o	bone	pituitar	phlegm
mi/o	less, smaller	ot	ear	plak	plate
mit	thread	ot/o	ear	plasma	a thing formed, plasma
mitr	mitral valve	ovar	ovary	plast	a developing
mnes	memory	ovul	ovary	pleur	pleura
mucos	mucus	ovulat	ovary	pleura	pleura
mucus	mucus	ox	oxygen	pleur/o	pleura
muscul	muscle	ox/i	oxygen	plicat	to fold
muscul/o	muscle	oxy	sour, sharp, acid	pneum/o	lung, air
muta	to change			pneumon	lung
mutat	to change	pachy	thick	poiet	formation
my	muscle	pancreat	pancreas	poli/o	gray
myc	fungus	paque	dark	pollex	thumb
myc/o	fungus	palat/o	palate	por	a passage
mydriat	dilation, widen	palliat	cloaked	porphyr	purple
myel	bone marrow, spinal cord	pallid/o	globus, pallidus	poster/i	behind, toward the back
myel/o	marrow	palm	palm		
my/o	muscle	palpitat	throbbing	prand/i	meal
my/os	muscle	papill	papilla	presby	old
myring	drum membrane	para	to bear	press	to press
myring/o	drum membrane	paralyt	to disable, paralysis	proct	anus, rectum
myx	mucus	partum	labor	proct/o	anus, rectum
		parturit	in labor	prolif	fruitful
narc/o	numbness	patell	kneecap, patella	prophylact	guarding
nas/o	nose	path	disease	prostat	prostate
nat	birth	path/o	disease	prosth/e	an addition
nat/o	birth	pause	cessation	prot/e	first
necr	death	pector	chest	proxim	near the point of origin
necr/o	death	pectorat	breast	prurit	itching
nephr	kidney	ped	foot, child	psych	mind
nephr/o	kidney	ped/i	foot, child	psych/o	mind
neur	nerve	pedicul	a louse	pudend	external genitals
neur/i	nerve	pelv/i	pelvis	pulm/o	lung
neur/o	nerve	pen	penis	pulmon	lung
neutr/o	neither	penile	penis	pulmonar	lung
nid	nest	pept	to digest	pupill	pupil
noct	night	perine	perineum	purpur	purple
nom	law	periton/e	peritoneum	py	pus
norm	rule	phac	lens	pyel	renal pelvis
nucl	nucleus	phac/o	lens	pyel/o	renal pelvis
nucle	kernel, nucleus	phag	to eat, engulf	pylor	pylorus, gate keeper
nyctal	blind	phag/o	to eat, engulf	py/o	pus
nystagm	to nod	phak	lentil, lens	pyret	fever
		phalang/e	closely knit row	pyr/o	heat, fire
occlus	to shut up	pharyng/o	pharynx		
ocul	eye	pharyng	pharynx	rach	spine
odont	tooth	phas	speech	rachi	spine
olecran	elbow	phen/o	to show	radi	radius
onc/o	tumor	phe/o	dusky	rad/i	radiating out from a center
onych	nail	phim	a muzzle		
onych/o	nail	phleb	vein	radiat	radiant
o/o	ovum, egg	phleb/o	vein	radic/o	spinal nerve root
oophor	ovary	phon	voice	radicul	spinal nerve root
ophthalm	eye	phone	voice	radi/o	ray
ophthalm/o	eye	phon/o	sound	rect/o	rectum
opt	eye	phor	carrying	relaxat	to loosen
opt/o	eye	phos	light	remiss	remit
or	mouth	phot/o	light	ren	kidney
orch	testicle	phragm	partition	ren/o	kidney
orchid	testicle	phragmat/o	partition	respirat	breathing
orchid/o	testicle	phras	speech	reticul/o	net
organ	organ	physic	nature	retin	retina

retin/o	retina	stern	sternum	trop	turning
rhabd/o	rod	stern/o	sternum	troph	a turning
rheumat	discharge	sterol	solid (fat)	tubercul	a little swelling
rheumat/o	discharge	steth	chest	tuss	cough
rhin/o	nose	steth/o	chest	tympan	ear drum
rhonch	snore	stigmat	point	tympan/o	drum
rhytid/o	wrinkle	stom	mouth		
roent	roentgen	stomat	mouth	uln	ulna, elbow
rotat	to turn	strabism	a squinting	uln/o	ulna, elbow
rrhyth	rhythm	strict	to draw, to bind	umbilic	navel
rrhythm	rhythm	superfic/i	near the surface	ungu	nail
rube/o	red	super/i	upper	ur	urine
		suppress	suppress	ure	urinate
sacr	sacrum	surrog	substituted	urea	urea
salping	tube, fallopian tube	sympath	sympathy	uret	urine
salping/o	tube, fallopian tube	synov	joint fluid	ureter	ureter
salpinx	tube, fallopian tube	syst	contraction	ureter/o	ureter
sarc	flesh	system	a composite whole	urethr	urethra
sarc/o	flesh	systol	contraction	urethr/o	urethra
scapul	shoulder blade			urin	urine
scler	hardening	tel	end, distant	urinat	urine
scler/o	hardening, sclera	tele	distant	urin/o	urine
scoli	curvature	tempor	temples	ur/o	urine
scoli/o	curvature	tend/o	tendon	uter	uterus
scop	to examine	tendin	tendon	uter/o	uterus
seb/o	oil	ten/o	tendon	uve	uvea
secund	second	tenon	tendon		
semin	seed	tenos	tendon	vagin	vagina
seminat	seed	tens	tension	vag/o	vagus, wandering
senile	old	tentori	tentorium, tent	varic/o	twisted vein
senil	old	terat	monster	vas	vessel
sept	putrefaction	testicul	testicle	vascul	small vessel
septic	putrefying	test/o	testicle	vas/o	vessel
ser (a)	whey	thalass	sea	vector	a carrier
ser/o	whey, serum	thel/i	nipple	ven	vein
sert	to gain	therm	hot, heat	venere	sexual intercourse
sexu	sex	therm/o	hot, heat	ven/i	vein
sial	saliva	thorac	chest	ven/o	vein
sial/o	salivary	thorac/o	chest	ventilat	to air
sider/o	iron	thorax	chest	ventr	near or on the belly side of the body
sigmoid	sigmoid	thromb	clot		
sigmoid/o	sigmoid	thromb/o	clot	ventricul	ventricle
sin/o	a curve	thym	thymus, mind, emotion	ventricul/o	little belly
sinus	a hollow curve	thyr	thyroid, shield	vermi	worm
situ	place	thyr/o	thyroid, shield	vers	turning
som	body	thyrox	thyroid, shield	vertebr	vertebra
somat	body	tibi	tibia	vertebr/o	vertebra
somat/o	body	tinnit	a jingling	vesic	bladder
somn	sleep	toc	birth	vesicul	vesicle
son	sound	tom/o	to cut	vir	virus (poison)
son/o	sound	ton	tone, tension	viril	masculine
spadias	a rent, an opening	ton/o	tone	viscer	body organs
spastic	convulsive	tonsill	tonsil, almond	volt	volt
sperm	seed (sperm)	topic	place	volunt	will
spermi	seed (sperm)	top/o	place	volvul	to roll
spermat	seed (sperm)	tors	twisted	vuls	to pull
spermat/o	seed (sperm)	tort/i	twisted		
sphygm/o	pulse	tox	poison	watt	watt
spin	spine, a thorn	toxic	poison		
spir/o	breath	trach/e	trachea	xanth/o	yellow
splen/o	spleen	trache/o	trachea	xen	foreign material
spondyl	vertebra	tract	to draw	xer	dry
spondyl/o	vertebra	trephinat	a bore	xer/o	dry
staped	stirrup	trich	hair	xiph	sword
steat	fat	trich/o	hair		
sten	narrowing	trigon	trigone	zo/o	animal
ster	solid	trism	grating	zoon	life

-able	capable	-grade	a step	-penia	lack of, deficiency
-ac	pertaining to	-graft	pencil, grafting knife	-pepsia	to digest
-ad	pertaining to	-gram	a weight, mark, record	-pexy	surgical fixation
-age	related to	-graph	to write, record	-phagia	to eat
-al	pertaining to	-graphy	recording	-phasia	to speak
-algesia	pain			-pheresis	removal
-algia	pain	-hexia	condition	-phil	attraction
-ant	forming			-philia	attraction
-ar	pertaining to	-ia	condition	-phobia	fear
-ary	pertaining to	-iasis	condition	-phoresis	to carry
-ase	enzyme	-ic	pertaining to	-phragm	a fence
-asthenia	weakness	-ide	having a particular	-phraxis	to obstruct
-ate	use, action		quality	-phylaxis	protection
-ate (d)	use, action	-in	chemical, pertaining to	-physis	growth
		-ine	pertaining to	-plakia	plate
-betes	to go	-ing	quality of	-plasia	formation, produce
-blast	immature cell, germ cell	-ion	process	-plasm	a thing formed, plasma
-body	body	-ism	condition	-plasty	surgical repair
		-ist	one who specializes, agent	-plegia	stroke, paralysis
-cele	hernia, tumor, swelling	-itis	inflammation	-pnea	breathing
-centesis	surgical puncture	-ity	condition	-poiesis	formation
-ceps	head	-ive	nature of, quality of	-praxia	action
-cide	to kill			-ptosis	prolapse, drooping
-clasia	a breaking	-kinesia	motion	-ptysis	to spit, spitting
-clave	a key	-kinesis	motion	-puncture	to pierce
-cle	small				
-clysis	injection	-lalia	to talk	-rrhage	to burst forth, bursting forth
-cope	strike	-lemma	a sheath, rind	-rrhagia	to burst forth, bursting forth
-crit	to separate	-lepsy	seizure	-rrhaphy	suture
-culture	cultivation	-lexia	diction	-rrhea	flow, discharge
-cusis	hearing	-liter	liter	-rrhexis	rupture
-cuspid	point	-lith	stone		
-cyesis	pregnancy	-logy	study of	-scope	instrument
-cyst	bladder	-lymph	clear fluid	-scopy	to view, examine
-cyte	cell	-lysis	destruction, to separate	-sepsis	decay
				-sis	condition
-derma	skin	-malacia	softening	-some	body
-dermis	skin	-mania	madness	-spasm	tension, spasm, contraction
-desis	binding	-megaly	enlargement, large	-stalsis	contraction
-dipsia	thirst	-meter	instrument to measure	-stasis	control, stopping
-drome	a course	-metry	measurement	-staxis	dripping, trickling
-dynia	pain	-mnesia	memory	-sthenia	strength
		-morph	form, shape	-stomy	new opening
-ectasia	dilatation			-systole	contraction
-ectasis	dilatation, distention	-noia	mind		
-ectasy	dilation			-taxia	order
-ectomy	surgical excision	-oid	resemble	-therapy	treatment
-edema	swelling	-ole	opening	-thermy	heat
-emesis	vomiting	-oma	tumor	-tic	pertaining to
-emia	blood condition	-omion	shoulder	-tome	instrument to cut
-er	relating to, one who	-on	pertaining to	-tomy	incision
-ergy	work	-one	hormone	-tone	tension
-esthesia	feeling	-opia	eye, vision	-tripsy	crushing
		-opsia	eye, vision	-troph (y)	nourishment, development
-form	shape	-opsy	to view	-trophy	nourishment, development
-fuge	to flee	-or	one who, a doer	-type	type
		-ory	like, resemble		
-gen	formation, produce	-orexia	appetite	-um	tissue
-genes	produce	-ose	like	-ure	process
-genesis	formation, produce	-osis	condition	-uria	urine
-genic	formation, produce	-ous	pertaining to	-us	pertaining to
-glia	glue				
-globin	protein	-paresis	weakness	-y	condition, pertaining to,
-gnosis	knowledge	-pathy	disease		process

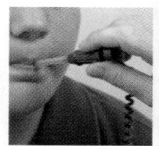

Glossary

Number in parentheses ( ) indicates chapter.

abduction Movement of a body part away from the midline. (21)

accounting The system of reporting the financial results of a business through analysis, statement, or summary about financial matters. (13)

accounts payable The amounts owed to others for equipment and services that have not yet been paid. (14)

accounts receivable Accounts of money owed. (13, 14)

accreditation The process in which an institution (school) voluntarily completes an extensive self-study after which an accrediting association visits the school to verify the self-study statements. (1)

acid-fast stain Special stain used to make visible under the microscope the organism that causes tuberculosis. (41)

acne vulgaris A common skin condition that occurs when oil and dead skin cells clog the skin's pores; usually called simply acne. (20)

acquired immune deficiency syndrome (AIDS) A series of illnesses that occur as a result of infection by the human immunodeficiency virus (HIV), which causes the immune system to break down. (2)

acromegaly A hormonal disorder that results when the pituitary gland produces excess growth hormone, most commonly affecting middle-aged adults and potentially resulting in serious illness and premature death. (30)

active immunity The introduction of immunity by infection or with a vaccine. (26)

active listening Paying attention to a speaker completely, concentrating on the verbal message, observing for nonverbal cues, and offering a response. (4)

active record A record of a patient who has been seen in the past few years and are currently being treated, usually from one to five years. (12)

active transport The process in cells that requires energy to transport materials to, from, and within the cell. Active transport mechanisms include phagocytosis and pinocytosis. (19)

active voice The subject of the sentence performs the action. (10)

acute condition An illness or injury that a patient suddenly experiences and requires treatment but may not be life threatening. (8)

acute pain The pain associated with trauma or surgery that is to be expected and that lasts through the recovery from the condition. (33)

acute renal failure A condition that occurs when something, such as a blockage, toxins, or a sudden loss of blood flow, causes a change in the filtering function of the kidneys. (29)

Addison's disease A condition in which the cortex of the adrenal gland is damaged, decreasing the production of adrenocortical hormones, usually resulting from an autoimmune disorder but also caused by infection, cancer, or hemorrhage into the glands. (30)

adduction The movement of a body part toward the midline. (21)

adolescence The growth step leading from childhood to adulthood. Early adolescence comprises ages 12 to 14 and late adolescence ages 15 to 19. (52)

adulthood Age designation divided roughly into early (20s and 30s), middle (40s and 50s), and late (from 60 to death). (52)

aerobic Requiring oxygen to live. (32)

afebrile The absence of a fever. (33)

agar A gelatin-like substance made from seaweed that is added to culture media to provide nutrition and a semi-solid surface for microbes to grow on. (41)

age analysis The procedure for determining how long an account has been past due, and then instituting the necessary collection procedures. (13)

ageism A prejudice against and incorrect assumptions about an individual because of his or her age. (37)

agglutination The clumping of cells. (41)

aggressive The practice of imposing a point of view on others or trying to manipulate others. (4)

aliquot A small portion of the original specimen. (40)

allergen A substance that enters the body through inhalation, swallowing, contact with the skin, or injection and causes an abnormal response. (35)

alopecia Baldness or loss of hair. (20, 34)

alphabetic filing The most common system for filing records in a physician's office, based on placing files in an A to Z order. (12)

Alzheimer's disease A progressive, degenerative disease of the brain characterized by loss of memory and other cognitive functions. (23)

amblyopia Also called "lazy eye." A disorder in children caused by the eye muscles being weaker in one eye. (24)

ambulation The act of walking. (46)

ambulatory surgery A situation in which a patient is able to walk into and out of the surgical facility the day of the surgery, which includes outpatient surgery, surgicenter surgery, and office surgery. (38)

American Association of Medical Assistants (AAMA) The professional association for medical assistants that oversees program accreditation, graduate certification, and provides a forum for issues of concern to the physician. (1)

American Banker's Association (ABA) number A bank number printed on a check that originates and identifies the bank and location of the bank from which a check is written. (14)

Americans with Disabilities Act (ADA) Legislation to protect the rights of the disabled regarding access to employment, public buildings, transportation, housing, schools, and health care facilities. (9)

American Medical Technologists (AMT) A professional association that provides oversight for the registration and testing of medical technologists. This association, in cooperation with the AMT Institute for Education (AMTIE) has developed a continuing education (CE) program and recording system. (1)

amorphous Without a shape. (42)

amphiarthrotic joint An articulation, or joint, that permits very slight movement. (21)

amplify To make louder. (34)

ampules Small, sealed glass bottles containing a single dose of medication, opened by breaking off the tip at a small indentation in the neck. (49)

amyotrophic lateral sclerosis (ALS) Also called motor neuron disease, Lou Gehrig's disease. A disease of unknown cause that breaks down the nerve cells from the brain to the spinal cord (upper motor neurons) and from the spinal cord to the peripheral nerves (lower motor neurons), which control muscle movement. (23)

anaerobic Not requiring oxygen to live. (32)

analyte The substance sought in the analysis of a specimen. (40)

anaphylactic shock A life-threatening allergic reaction whose symptoms include acute respiratory distress, edema, hypotension, rash, tachycardia, pale cool skin, convulsions, and cyanosis. (35)

anatomical position Term used to describe relationships of the parts of the body. In this position, the body is assumed to be standing, with the feet together, the arms to the side, and the head and eyes and palms of the hands facing forward. (19)

anatomy The study of the structure of an organism. (19)

anemia A condition in which there are insufficient levels of hemoglobin in the red blood cells, caused by decreased healthy red cell production by the bone marrow, increased erythrocyte destruction, or blood loss from heavy menstrual periods or internal bleeding. (25)

anesthesia Medication that causes the partial or complete loss of sensation, used to block the pain of surgery. (2, 38)

aneurysm An abnormal widening or ballooning of a portion of an artery, related to weakness in the wall of the blood vessel. (25)

angina The condition caused by the narrowing of the coronary arteries and subsequent reduction of blood flow to the heart. (35)

angiography The x-ray visualization of the internal anatomy of blood vessels after a radiopaque material has been injected into them, used to assist in the diagnosis of conditions such as myocardial infarction (MI or heart attack), cerebrovascular accident (CVA or stroke), renal artery stenosis as a cause of hypertension, clots, stenosis in arteries in the lower extremities and abdomen, aneurysm of the aorta, and pulmonary emboli or clots. (44)

angioplasty A surgical vessel repair procedure frequently used to reopen blocked coronary arteries. (25)

answering service A telephone response service that can be in effect to relieve staff at designated times. (6)

antagonist A muscle that counteracts, or opposes, the action of another muscle. (22)

antecubital space The most common site for venipuncture, just below the joint in the elbow, where four large veins are accessible, the most commonly used being the median cephalic vein. (43)

anthrax A deadly infectious disease caused by Bacillus anthracisis. Humans contract the disease from infected animal hair, hides, or waste. (2)

anthropometry The science of size, proportion, weight, and height. (33)

antibodies Protein substances produced by lymphocytes in the spleen, lymph tissue and nodes, and bone marrow that reacts to antigens (foreign substances). (26, 32)

antigen A foreign substance that invades the body. (26)

anuria The absence of urine, which may indicate that an obstruction is present or renal failure. (42)

apical The heart rate counted at the apex of the heart. (33)

apnea Lack of breathing. (33)

aponeurosis A wide, thin, sheetlike tendon, made up of fibrous connective tissue, that typically attaches muscles to other muscles. (22)

apothecary system Considered to be the oldest system of measurement. The dry weight equivalent is 1 grain = 1 gram of wheat, and the basic units of measure are the grain (gr), gram (g), dram (dr), ounce (oz), and pound (lb). Fluid measurements are the minims (mn), fluid dram (fl dr), fluid ounce (fl oz), pint (pt), quart (qt), and gallon (gal). The system uses roman numerals and fractions and writes them following the unit of measure. (47)

appendicitis An inflammation of the appendix caused by a blockage of the inside of the appendix, the lumen, which leads to increased pressure, impaired blood flow, and potentially gangrene and rupture. (28)

appendicular skeleton One of the two divisions of the skeletal system, consisting of the 126 bones, including the extremities, that are not part of the axial skeleton. (21)

application A form usually completed at the time of a job interview that includes personal information and a list of previous work experiences. (53)

archive The storage of items, such as files or records for future reference or back up, usually placed in a storage container or facility and kept for a determined number of years. (8)

arrhythmia An irregular heartbeat caused by a disturbance of normal electrical activity of the heart. The two types are tachycardia or fast heart rate, and bradycardia, or slow heart rate. (25)

arteriosclerosis Also called hardening of the arteries. A thickening and loss of elasticity of the arteries, occurring over many years during which the arteries develop areas that become hard and brittle due to deposits of calcium. (25)

arthritis Inflammation of one or more joints caused by various disease processes. (21)

articulation Also called a joint. The place where two bones connect, with the positioning of the bones determining the type of movement the joint performs. (21)

ascites Fluid in the abdomen. (29)

aseptic Germ free. (32)

asphyxia Suffocation. (39)

assertive The practice of making a point in a positive manner by standing firm, making decisions based on principles or values, and trusting ones own ideas or instincts in the situation. (4)

assessment An evaluation to determine a patient's medical problem. (4)

assignment of benefits A patient's written authorization giving the insurance company the right to pay the provider of services directly for billed charges. (13, 16)

asthma A chronic inflammatory condition typically caused when allergens or other irritating substances cause swelling in the lining of the trachea and bronchial tubes, which causes the creation of mucus, which can cause coughing or a sense of struggling to breathe. (27)

astigmatism A disorder in which the lenses or cornea of the eye are uneven, resulting in light not being bent or refracted evenly and causing some parts of images to be clear while others are blurry. (24, 36)

asymptomatic Without symptoms. (33)

atherosclerosis Narrowing of the vessel lumen of the arteries due to a buildup of fatty material and plaque, thus slowing or stopping the flow of blood, which can lead to cell death in the area supplied by the vessel. It is the leading cause of congestive heart disease. (25, 35)

atmospheric pressure The pressure of the air around us, measured as 760 mmHg at sea level, lower at higher altitudes. (27)

atom The smallest chemical unit of matter. (19)

atria The two upper receiving chambers of the heart. (25)

atrioventricular node Also called the AV node. One of the three areas of specialized neuromuscular tissue that initiate the heartbeat, it is located beneath the endocardium of the right atrium and is a "gatekeeper," responsible for transmitting impulses from the sinoatrial node to the inferior portions of the heart. (25)

atrophy A loss of muscle mass and strength that occurs with the disuse of muscles over time. (22, 46)

attitude Opinion that develops from one's value system. (4)

audiogram A record of a patient's responses to varied levels of sound, used to evaluate the person's hearing. (36)

audiology The study of hearing disorders. (24)

audiometer An electronic instrument that measures the frequency, or the number of fluctuations per second, of energy transferred in the form of sound waves. (36)

audit Examination of all financial statements for accuracy. (14)

auditory By hearing. (4)

auscultation Listening to sounds within the body. (34)

automated assistance program An automated telephone system that allows for separating callers to the appropriate people through a series of questions. (6)

axial skeleton One of the two divisions of the skeletal system, consisting of 80 bones from the axis of the body, including the skull and vertebral system. (21)

B lymphocytes White blood cells created and matured in the bone marrow that seek out invading organisms and send T lymphocytes to destroy them. (26)

bacteria Microorganisms that are capable of causing disease. (2)

bactericidal Causing the destruction of disease-producing bacteria. (32)

bacturia The presence of bacteria in urine, often indicating a urinary tract infection and detected by testing for nitrites, a by-product of the chemical breakdown of certain bacteria. (42)

bandage A strip of binding material used to hold a dressing in place. (39)

bandwidth The number of bits processed in a computer at one time to represent and address. (11)

behavior The actions others see. (4)

Bell's palsy A weakness or paralysis of the muscles that control expression on one side of the face. (23)

benefit period The period of time that payments for Medicare inpatient hospital benefits are available. (15, 16)

benign Noncancerous. (35)

benign prostatic hyperplasia (BPH) Also called benign prostatic hypertrophy. An enlargement of the prostate gland, usually occurring in men older than 50, which compresses the urethra, restricting the normal flow of urine. (31)

bias An unfair preference or dislike of something that prevents an impartial opinion of someone or something; when a person favors a certain belief or attitude. (4, 52)

bicuspid valve Also called the mitral valve. Valve through which the blood leaves the left atrium of the heart. (25)

bimanual Two-handed, deep palpation. (34)

bioequivalent The active ingredients in generic drugs being as effective as those in brand name drugs. (48)

biohazard Biological substances, such as medical waste and samples of a virus or bacterium, that pose a threat to human beings and are potentially infectious. (5)

biopsy Microscopic examination of cells for cancer. (38)

bipolar disorder Also called manic-depressive state. A mental disorder characterized by mood swings between excessive excitement and depression. (52)

blind ad An advertisement that does not identify the institution or facility that placed the ad. (53)

block A style or format of letter writing that is spaced with all lines, from the date through the signature line, flush with the left margin. There is a space separating each paragraph and between inside address, salutation, body, and close. (10)

bloodborne pathogens Disease-producing organisms transmitted via the blood. (32)

body mass index (BMI) A measurement of body weight relative to height used to calculate the amount of body fat. (37)

body mechanics Coordination of body alignment, balance, and movement. (5)

body surface area (BSA) A measurement used to establish drug dosage for children, calculated from height and weight and expressed in meters squared (m^2). (47)

bookkeeping The process of managing the accounts for a business, which is a continual process and should be done on a daily basis. (13)

bounding pulse An increased volume or force in the pulse. (33)

bradycardia An abnormally slow heart rate, fewer than 60 beats per minute, which may be regular or irregular. (25)

brand name Also called proprietary name. The name given by a manufacturer to a specific product. (48)

BRAT A selection of foods—bananas, rice, applesauce, and toast—prescribed for small children suffering from vomiting and diarrhea because they can become dehydrated easily. (51)

breach of confidentiality Failure to keep something confidential. When patient information is released to others without authorization from the patient. (16)

breach of contract The failure by either party in a valid contract to comply with the terms of the agreement. (3)

breast cancer The types are infiltrating ductal, the most common, in which the cancer arises in the tiny ducts that run from the milk glands to the nipple; infiltrating lobular, which develops in the lobules; and inflammatory. (31)

broad spectrum Antibiotics effective against a large range of microorganisms. (48)

bronchitis Respiratory system disorder in which the mucous membranes in the bronchial passages become inflamed, resulting in mucus, coughing, and breathlessness. (27)

bucky A type of barrier having alternating strips of lead and radiolucent material that is positioned between an x-ray machine and a patient to absorb radiation scatter before it reaches the film. (44)

bundle of His Also called the atrioventricular (AV) bundle. One of the three areas of specialized neuromuscular tissue that initiate the heartbeat, it extends from the AV node into the intraventricular septum, where it branches off, sending a branch to each ventricle. (25)

bursitis Inflammation of the bursa, a small sac of fluid that cushions and lubricates an area where joint-related tissues, including bones, tendons, ligaments, muscles, and skin, rub against one another. (21)

cadaver A dead human body used to study the human anatomy. (2)

caduceus The recognized symbol for medicine depicts a healing staff with two snakes coiled around the staff. (2)

calibrate To measure the accuracy of equipment against a known standard. (40)

caller ID A telephone function that allows the telephone owners to know who is calling each time the telephone rings. (6)

canceled check A deposited check that has been processed and paid out to creditors by the bank. (14)

cancellous (spongy) bone The reticular tissue that makes up most of the volume of a long bone and that includes the red bone marrow, which manufactures most of the red blood cells found in the body. (21)

capillaries The microscopic blood vessels that are the bridges between arterioles and venules, where oxygen and carbon dioxide are exchanged. (43)

capital equipment Items that require a large dollar amount to purchase (generally more than $500) and have a relatively long life. (9)

carcinoma *in situ* Cancer in a particular structure that has not spread outside the structure. (35)

cardiac muscle A type of involuntary muscle found in the heart, roughly quadrangular in shape, cross striated, and having a single central nucleus. (22)

cardiomegaly An enlarged heart. (30)

cash disbursement Payments made to creditors. (14)

cataract A clouding over the eye's lens that prevents light from entering through it. (24)

cavities Spaces within the body. (19)

cell A basic unit of life that contains the internal organs, or viscera. Comprised of cell membrane, which protects it and regulates the movement of water, nutrients, and wastes; a central nucleus, which contains the cell's DNA (deoxyribonucleic acid) and RNA (ribonucleic acid); and organelles, small structures that help carry out the day-to-day operations of the cell. (19)

cell membrane The membrane that protects the cell from the outside environment and regulates the movement of water, nutrients, and wastes into and out of cells. (19)

cellulitis An acute, spreading bacterial infection below the surface of the skin characterized by redness,

warmth, swelling, and pain. It can also cause fever, chills, and enlarged lymph nodes. (20)

central processing unit (CPU) The brain of the computer or main memory that executes the specific set of instructions. (11)

centrifuge An instrument used to separate specimens into component layers for separate examination under the microscope. (40)

cerebrospinal fluid The fluid produced by the choroid plexus in the ventricles of the brain that fills the spinal canal and the subarachnoid space that surround the brain, cushioning the brain and spinal cord and nourishing them with oxygen and glucose. (23, 35)

certification The issuance by an official body or professional organization of a certificate and credentials to one who has met the educational and experience standards of that organization. (1, 2)

certification examination The four-hour test required for a student to become certified as a medical assistant, offered by the American Association of Medical Assistants (AAMA) three times a year at numerous locations throughout the United States. (53)

Certified Medical Assistant (CMA) A multiskilled health care professional who assists providers in an allied health care setting and who has met the standards of the AAMA by achieving a satisfactory test result and is validated every five years, either by earning continuing education units (CEUs) or through reexamination. (1)

cerumen Ear wax. (36)

cervical cancer Cancer of the cervix. The two main types are squamous cell (epidermoid) and adenocarcinoma. (31)

cervicitis An inflammation of the cervix, most often caused by infection with sexually transmitted infections (STIs). (31)

character The sum of the values, attitudes, and behaviors a person exhibits. (4)

chemotherapy Cancer treatment using drugs. (26)

chief complaint The primary symptom that causes a patient to seek medical treatment. (39)

childhood The third subdivision of child development, with early childhood comprising ages 3 to 5 and middle childhood ages 6 to 11. (52)

cholesterol A fat-like material essential for the function of body systems, such as the nervous system,

formation of cell membranes, and many hormones. (51)

chronic fatigue syndrome (CFS) Immune system disorder of unknown origin. (26)

chronic obstructive pulmonary disease (COPD) Respiratory system condition comprising primarily two diseases, chronic bronchitis and emphysema, in which the flow of air through the airways and out of the lungs is obstructed. (27)

chronic pain Long-term pain, persisting for more than six months and interfering with functions of life. (33)

chronic renal failure A gradual and progressive loss of kidney function, typically as a result of another disease. (29)

chronological Organized according to time. (34)

cilia Hairlike projections in the nose that increase the surface area of a cell, increasing its ability to trap dust, pollen, and other foreign matter to prevent it from entering the nasal cavity. (19, 27)

circumcision Surgical removal of the foreskin of the penis, performed for religious, cultural, or medical reasons. (31)

circumduction The process of moving a body part in a circular motion. (21)

cirrhosis A potentially life-threatening condition that occurs when the liver is damaged, usually after years of inflammation, by scarring, or fibrosis, that replaces healthy tissue and prevents the liver from working normally. (28)

claim A written and documented request for reimbursement for an eligible expense to the insurance company in a correct and timely manner. (15)

clarity In reference to your speaking voice, the quality or state of being understandable. (6)

Clark's rule The most common formula used to calculate drug dosage for children, based on weight: Divide the child's weight by 150 pounds and then multiply the result by the adult dose. (47)

claustrophobia Fear of being in an enclosed space. (44)

clinical diagnosis Also called working diagnosis. A preliminary presumptive diagnosis made by the physician based on the health history and physical examination. (33)

Clinical Laboratory Improvement Amendments (CLIA) Federal law regulating all laboratories that test human specimens to help ensure accurate test results, specifying three categories of tests and authorizing and certifying those who perform them. (40)

clock speed The measurement of how many instructions per second the computer's processor can execute and is represented in MHz. (11)

closed-ended question Question that can be answered with a yes or a no reply. (4)

closed-panel HMO A clinic that is owned by the HMO and the physicians are employees of the HMO. (15)

closed record A record of a patient who has actively terminated his or her contact with the physician. The files are kept in storage for legal reasons. (12)

cognitive ability The ability to perceive, think, and reason. (37)

colic Acute abdominal pain. (35)

colitis Inflammation of the large intestine caused by many different disease processes, including infections, primary inflammatory disorders (ulcerative colitis, Crohn's colitis, lymphocytic and collagenous colitis), lack of blood flow (ischemic colitis), and history of radiation to the large bowel. (28)

collating Collecting into one file all records, test results, and information pertaining to a patient who is scheduled to be seen by the physician. It also refers to organizing the sub-group information (for example, laboratory and x-ray results) in records for the day's appointments as well as when filing. (7)

colleague A fellow member of a profession. (18)

collimeter The device that controls the size and shape of the radiation field coming from the tube in an x-ray machine. (44)

colony The growth of one type of microorganism, visible to the naked eye, on the surface of a medium. (41)

colorectal cancer Collective term for colon cancer, affecting the large intestine, and rectal cancer, affecting the last eight to 10 inches of the colon. (28)

common cold An infection of the upper respiratory tract caused by any one of a number of viruses and differing from other viral infections by its lack of high fever or significant fatigue. (27)

compact bone The dense, hard layer of bone tissue in a long bone. (21)

complement A group of proteins activated by antibodies that assist in destroying bacteria, viruses, and infected cells. (26)

compound microscope A microscope that has two sets of lenses, ocular and objective. (40)

computer A programmable machine, or system of hardware that responds to a specific set of instructions and performs a list of instructions in programmed language called software. (11)

condescending Behavior that adopts a superior attitude and acting as though one is better than someone else. (4)

conduction hearing loss Hearing loss due to obstruction of sound waves, caused by foreign material or excess cerumen (ear wax) in the external ear canal, calcification of the bones in the inner ear, infection, or fluid buildup in the middle ear. (36)

conference call Three or more parties at different locations from each other may speak with one another on the telephone at the same time. (6)

confidentiality Safeguarding a patient's confidences, particularly information in the medical record regarding family history, past or current diseases or illnesses, test results, and medications is vital to the patient and health care professional relationship. (1)

congestive heart failure (CHF) Also called simply heart failure. A condition in which the heart cannot pump enough blood to the other organs, which can result from such conditions as coronary artery disease, past heart attack, hypertension, heart valve disease due to past rheumatic fever or other cause, primary diseases of the heart muscle itself, heart defects present at birth, and any infection of the heart valves or heart muscle, such as endocarditis or myocarditis. (25)

conjunctivitis Also called pinkeye. An inflammation of the conjunctiva, the tissue that lines the inside of the eyelid, frequently caused by a virus, bacteria, or other irritating substance. (24)

constipation A condition in which stools are difficult to pass, involving straining, a feeling of not completely emptying the bowels, and hard or pellet-like stools. (28)

contact dermatitis An allergic reaction of the skin caused by irritating substances coming in contact with it, often resulting in red, irritated skin and occasionally in vesicles and rash. (20)

continuing education units (CEUs) Credit awarded for additional course work beyond certification, a unit of training or education is granted for

each clock hour. The American Association of Medical Assistants requires 60 CEUs over a 5-year period to maintain certification. (1)

contracture The fixed position of a joint due to muscle shortening and lack of exercise. (46)

contraindicated To be strictly avoided because of the potential for a dangerous interaction. (48)

contributory negligence The patient's contribution to the injury, which if proven, would release the physician as the direct cause. (3)

control sample A sample similar to the test specimen that has been tested previously and has a known value. (40)

co-payment (copay) A designated amount of money that is required by a patient/member of some medical insurance plans to pay for medical services or medication, usually at the time of service. (7)

cornea The lens of the eye. (36)

corneal abrasion A lesion or abrasion on the cornea as the result of an injury or infection. (24)

coronary heart disease (CHD) Also called coronary artery disease (CAD). Condition resulting from a narrowing of the coronary arteries that supply blood to the heart, which can lead to a higher risk of heart attack and, potentially, sudden death. (25)

cortex In the kidney, the outer layer, in which the arteries, veins, convoluted tubules, and glomerular capsules are found. (29). In the lymph node, that portion populated mainly by lymphocytes. (26)

cover letter A letter introducing an applicant to an employer, stating the purpose of the correspondence, the position being sought, and the applicant's match to the stated requirements. (53)

credit An addition of funds to an account. (14)

Crohn's disease Also called inflammatory bowel disease (IBD). A chronic inflammatory disease of the intestines that primarily causes ulcerations in the lining of the small and large intestines but can affect the digestive system anywhere from the mouth to the anus. (28)

crossover claim A patient claim that is eligible for both Medicare and Medicaid. It is also called Medi/Medi. (15)

cryosurgery Also called cryocautery. A procedure in which a probe is used to freeze tissue to destroy abnormal cells, used to treat cervical erosion and chronic cervicitis. (38)

culture The values, beliefs, attitudes, views, and customs shared by a group of people and passed on through the generations. (4)

culture media Media, typically broth or agar, for the propagation of microorganisms or living cells to enhance their growth, potentially while retarding the growth of other organisms and potentially containing special dye to enable easier identification. (41)

Culturette A disposable, clear plastic tube that contains a sterile cotton-tipped applicator swab and a sealed plastic vial of medium (broth containing nourishment for bacteria and a preservative), used to obtain many types of specimens. (41)

cumulative The case in which the effects of any individual event are added to the effects of all previous events, as happens in exposure to radiation. (44)

Current Procedural Terminology (CPT) A manual that provides procedure and service codes. (17)

Cushing's disease A rare disorder than develops when too much cortisol is released by ACTH as a result of stimulation of the pituitary. (30)

cyanosis A condition in which a patient does not take in enough oxygen during inhalation, resulting in an increase in carbon dioxide (CO_2) in the blood and a bluish tint to the skin and nail beds. (27, 33)

cycle time The length of time the average patient spends in the medical office. (8, 9)

cystic fibrosis (CF) A chronic and progressive respiratory system disorder, usually diagnosed in childhood, in which the mucus becomes thick, dry, and sticky, causing it to build up and clog passages in many organs but primarily in the lungs and pancreas. (27)

cystitis An inflammation of the bladder that usually occurs when bacteria infect the lower urinary tract. Most cases are caused by *Escherichia coli*, a bacterium found in the lower gastrointestinal system. (29)

cytokinesis The separation of the cytoplasm into two parts. (19)

cytoplasm The substance that fills a cell. (19)

debit A charge against an account. (14)

debridement Removal of dead tissue around the edges of a wound. (38)

decubitus ulcer Also called pressure sores or bedsores. Area of skin and tissue that breaks down when constant pressure is maintained on it. (20)

deductible A sum of money that must be paid by the patient before the insurance plan pays benefits for services rendered. (15)

defamation of character A scandalous statement about someone that can injure the person's reputation. Defamation can result even when the statement is true. (3)

defensive behavior A reaction to a perceived threat that is usually unconscious. (4)

dehiscence The separation of wound edges. (38)

deltoid muscle The muscle on the outer surface of the upper arm used for small-volume injections in adults. (49)

demographic Information or data relating to descriptive information such as age, gender, ethnic background, education, and Social Security number. (7)

deposit Money (cash and check payments) placed into a bank account. (14)

dermis One of the two layers that compose the skin. (20)

desensitizing injection A process in which minute amounts of an allergen are injected into a patient's system over an extended period of time to allow the patient to develop a tolerance for the allergen. (35)

dexterity Ability to use one's hands accurately. (50)

diabetes mellitus A condition in which the body is unable to produce enough insulin to properly control blood sugar levels by converting sugar and starches into energy. The three types are type 1, also known as juvenile diabetes and as insulin-dependent diabetes mellitus (IDDM); type 2, also known as adult-onset and as non–insulin-dependent diabetes mellitus (NIDDM); and gestational diabetes, which occurs during pregnancy. (30)

diagnosis The determination of the cause and nature of a disease. (33)

Diagnostic Related Groups (DRGs) A Medicare hospital payment system, which classifies each Medicare patient according to his or her illness. (2)

dialysis A filter other than the kidneys to remove toxins and maintain water balance. The two types are hemodialysis, which uses a machine that cleans the blood outside the body, and peritoneal dialysis, which is done through the tissues of the abdomen, with a dialysis fluid instilled in the stomach, left for a period while the membranes in the abdomen filter toxins, and then removed. (29)

diaphoresis Excessive sweating. (35)

diaphragm A dome-shaped respiratory muscle that divides the ventral cavity into two parts. (19)

diaphysis The shaft of a long bone. (21)

diarrhea An increase in the frequency of bowel movements or a decrease in the form of stool. The two types are acute, which lasts a few days to a week, and chronic, defined usually as lasting more than three weeks. (28)

diarthrotic joint An articulation, or joint, that allows for free movement in a variety of directions. (21)

diastolic blood pressure Pressure recorded in an artery when the left ventricle relaxes. In standard notation it is recorded below the systolic pressure. (25)

diathermy The therapeutic use of a high-frequency current to induce an electrical field within a portion of the body, generating heat and increasing blood flow to aid in healing, used to treat muscular disorders and tendonitis, arthritis, and bursitis. (46)

differential diagnosis The determination of which of several diseases is the cause of a problem. (33)

digestion The process by which the body dissolves food substances by chemically splitting them into simpler compounds that can be absorbed into the blood and used by the body tissues and organs. (51)

diluent Liquid in which something is diluted. (40)

diphtheria An acute infectious disease that is transmitted by direct and indirect contact and is diagnosed by analyzing a throat culture. (49)

discretion The ability to make decisions responsibly, is tactful in communicating with others, and is able to be fair and be familiar with policies and regulations. (1)

discriminatory Prejudicial. (18)

dislocation A disconnection of the bones that meet at a joint, usually caused by a sudden impact, such that the bones are no longer in their normal positions. (21)

diverticulitis Inflammation of a small pouch or sac in the wall of the colon, generally caused by stool lodging in the diverticula, that can lead to swelling or rupture. (28)

diverticulosis The condition of having diverticula, or small outpouchings, in the large intestine, most typically in the sigmoid colon, a condition that increases with age because of the weakening of the colon walls. (28)

DNA (deoxyribonucleic acid) The genetic code that coordinates protein synthesis. (19)

dorsiflexion The process of bending a body part backward. (21)

dorsogluteal site The gluteus medius muscle in the upper outer quadrant of the buttocks, used for large volume, deep intramuscular (IM) injections or for irritating viscous (thick) medications. (49)

dosimeter A radiation badge that contains a measure of an individual's occupational exposure to ionizing radiation, reported in rems. (44)

double booking Scheduling two patients to be seen during the same time slot without allowing for any additional time in the schedule. (8)

dressing A sterile covering placed directly over a wound to absorb blood and other body fluids, prevent contamination, and protect the wound from further trauma. (39)

Drug Enforcement Administration (DEA) The agency of the federal government responsible for enforcing drug control. (48)

dwarfism A condition characterized by shorter than normal skeletal growth, resulting from more than 300 recognized conditions, with achondroplasia being the most common type of short-limb dwarfism. (30)

dysmenorrhea The presence of abdominal cramps during menstruation. The two types are primary, in which there is no underlying gynecological abnormality, and secondary, in which there is such an abnormality. (31)

dysplasia Abnormal cells found in a cell specimen. (35)

dyspnea Difficulty breathing. (25, 35)

eczema Also called atopic dermatitis. A chronic skin condition characterized by scaling, itching rashes and caused by an allergic-type reaction on the skin. (20)

Einthoven's triangle A pictorial guide to the locations for attaching the leads to a patient for an electrocardiogram. (45)

electrocardiogram A painless, noninvasive test used to evaluate the electrical activity generated by the heart at rest and during activity. The test creates a recording, called a tracing, of electrical activity as it moves through the heart. (45)

electroconvulsive therapy (ECT) A controversial procedure occasionally used for cases of prolonged major depression, in which an electrode is placed on one or both sides of a patient's head and a low-voltage current is turned on briefly, causing a convulsive seizure. (52)

electrolyte Medical/scientific term for salts, specifically an ion that is electri-cally charged and moves to either a negative (cathode) or positive (anode) electrode. Sodium, potassium, and chloride are electrolytes. (19, 43)

electronic medical record (EMR) Electronic medical documentation relating to the patient. (12)

electronystagmograph (ENG) An instrument that measures the movement of the eyes, using electrodes placed above and below the eye to record electrical activity. (36)

embezzlement The taking of funds by a breach of trust. (14)

embolus A thrombus that has moved from its place of origin. (35)

emergency kit (crash cart) A large roll-around toolbox instantly accessible by anyone in the office and containing all of the supplies that may be needed during an emergency. (39)

empathy The ability to be sensitive to or understand the feelings of another individual and identify with what he or she is experiencing without necessarily experiencing the same thing; to have some insight or understanding of the pain or distress a patient is feeling and act in a kindly way that expresses sensitivity to the patient's feelings. (1, 4)

emphysema A progressive respiratory system disease in which the tissues necessary to support the physical shape and function of the lung are destroyed, primarily causing shortness of breath. (27)

encephalitis An inflammation in the brain, most often caused by viral infections. (23)

endocardium The inner lining of the heart wall. (25)

endometriosis A condition in which the endometrium, the tissue lining the uterus, travels outside the uterus into the pelvis or abdominal cavity. (31)

endomysium The connective tissue covering that surrounds an individual muscle cell. (22)

endosteum The tough connective tissue membrane lining the medullary canal and containing the bone marrow in a long bone. (21)

enteritis Food poisoning. (41)

enunciation In reference to your speaking voice, the clear articulation and pronouncement of words. (6)

eosinophil A granular white blood cell that captures invading microorganisms and antibody–antigen reactions through phagocytosis (engulfing or eating). (35)

epidermis One of the two layers that compose the skin. (20)

epididymitis An inflammation or infection of the epididymis, the long coiled tube attached to the upper part of each testicle, where mature sperm are stored before ejaculation. (31)

epilepsy A common neurological disorder in which the nervous system produces intense, abnormal bursts of electrical activity in the brain, which can lead to seizures that temporarily interfere with muscle control, movement, speech, vision, or awareness. (23)

epimysium A thin connective tissue covering muscles. (22)

epiphysis The ends of a developing long bone. (21)

episiotomy An incision in the perineum, the external region between the vulva and the anus, during labor to prevent its tearing during delivery. (31)

erectile dysfunction (ED) The inability to achieve or maintain an erection sufficient for sexual intercourse, resulting from insufficient blood supply, from the smooth muscle failing to relax, or from the penis not retaining the blood that flows into it. (31)

ergonomics Scientific information and data regarding human body mechanics used to design objects and overall environments for human use. (5)

erythema Redness of the skin. (46)

erythrocyte sedimentation rate (ESR) Also called the "sed" rate. The rate at which red blood cells settle to the bottom of a test tube, typically done utilizing either the Winthrobe or Westergren method. (43)

erythrocytes Also called red blood cells. Biconcave cells produced in the red bone marrow that are small enough to pass through capillaries. (25)

eschar The scab that forms on a wound to keep out microorganisms. (38)

established patient Any patient who has been previously seen by the physician and has an existing medical record/chart in the physician's practice. (8)

ethnicity A classification of people based on national origin. (4)

ethnocentric Belief that one's own cultural background is better than any other. (4)

eukaryotic Cells having a nucleus and organelles in the cytoplasm, for example, protozoa, fungi, and parasites. (41)

eupnea Normal breathing. (33)

Evaluation and Management (E/M) A classification of services in the CPT manual that includes codes for office visits, consultations, the physician's component for emergency services, inpatient hospital care, and so forth. (17)

eversion The process of turning the body outward. (21)

evisceration The separation of wound edges and protrusion of abdominal organs. (38)

exclusive provider organization (EPO) A managed care system that allows the patient to only select from a defined panel of providers, who are reimbursed on a modified fee-for-service method. (15)

excoriation Chafing or rawness of the skin. (37)

exophthalmos A condition produced by hyperthyroidism in which the eyeball protrudes beyond its normal protective orbit because of swelling in the tissues behind. (30)

expiratory reserve volume (ERV) The volume of air that can be forcibly exhaled after a normal exhale. (45)

extension The process of straightening a flexed limb. (21)

externship A situation in which a student works, during the final stage of his or her training, without pay in a health care setting under the supervision of someone at the site. (1, 53)

exudates Drainage from a wound. (41)

facsimile (fax) An electronically transmitted document containing print text and graphic information. (7)

facultative anaerobe An anaerobe that can survive in the presence of some oxygen. (41)

failure to thrive (FTT) Infant weight gain that is insufficient according to standardized baby growth charts. (37)

fascia The connective tissue structure covering the skeletal muscles and separating them from one another. (22)

fascicles Sections into which a muscle is divided. (22)

febrile Having a body temperature above 100.4°F (38°C), a fever, at which point the body is producing greater heat than it is losing. (33)

febrile seizures Seizures suffered by some children with high fevers following a rapid spike in body temperature, potentially involving jerking of arms and legs, loss of consciousness, and stiffening of the body. (37)

feces Also called stool. The waste product from the bowel. (41)

fee schedule A list of the amount to be paid by an insurance company for each procedure or service, determined by a claims administrator and applied to claims subject to the fee schedule of a provider's managed care contract. (15)

feedback Any response to a communication. (4)

fetid Foul smelling. (42)

fibrocystic breast disease Also called mammary dysplasia, benign breast disease, and diffuse cystic mastopathy. A condition that involves common, benign changes in the tissues of the breast. (31)

fibromyalgia A musculoskeletal pain and fatigue disorder with no known cause but with evidence pointing to a genetic predisposition to a neuromuscular/neuroendocrine abnormality that disturbs the usual sensory perception, especially of pain signals. (22)

first responder An individual trained to recognize medical conditions, initiate basic life support, and access other parts of the system. (39)

fixed Having ensured that a specimen material will remain on the slide during the staining process, accomplished by passing the slide through an open flame a few times or by flooding the slide with methanol and letting it dry. (41)

flatus Gas in the colon. (35)

flexion The process of bending (or curving) the spine. (21)

floppy disk A small flexible, magnetic disk in a rigid plastic case that stores data from and retrieves data from a computer. (11)

fluoroscopy A technique in radiology for visually examining a portion of the body or the function of an organ using a fluoroscope, which produces a moving image that can be filmed using a radiograph (x-ray) to obtain a permanent record. (44)

folliculitis An inflammation or infection of hair follicles that most often appears in areas that become irritated by shaving or the rubbing of clothes or where follicles and pores are blocked by oils and dirt. (20)

forced expiratory volume (FEV) The volume of air exhaled during the first second of a forced vital capacity maneuver. (45)

forced vital capacity (FVC) The amount of air exhaled after maximum inspiration. (45)

frequencies The numbers of fluctuations per second of energy in the form of sound waves. (36)

Fried's law A formula used to calculate drug dosage for children a year old and younger: Divide the child's age in months by 150 months (representing a child 12.5 years old) and then multiply the result by the adult dose. (47)

functional residual capacity (FRC) The volume of air remaining in the lungs after a normal expiration. (45)

fundus The top of the uterus. (35)

gait An individual's particular way of walking. (46)

gantry The circular structure that houses the x-ray equipment in a computed tomography (CT) scanner. (44)

gastroesophageal reflux disease (GERD) Condition in which the muscle at the superior portion of the stomach (the cardiac sphincter) does not close tightly or relaxes inappropriately, allowing for a "backwash" of gastric fluids and stomach contents into the esophagus and the throat. (28)

gender bias Indicating either male or female role by the language or image used. (10)

generic name Also called official name or nonproprietary name. The single identifying name of a drug, considered to be the legal name and typically denoted in lower case letters. (48)

genetics The study of the make up of animals or plants. (19)

germinal centers The primary resting places for B lymphocytes. (26)

gestational diabetes A condition in which the body is unable to produce enough insulin to properly control blood sugar levels by converting sugar and starches into energy, occurring during pregnancy and typically disappearing afterward but occasionally precipitating ongoing type 2 diabetes. (30)

gigantism A condition in which excessive growth hormone is secreted during childhood, before the closure of the bone growth plates, which causes overgrowth of the long bones, muscles, and organs, usually caused by a pituitary gland tumor. (30)

glaucoma A condition caused by an increase in the amount of pressure in the eye, leading to an excessive amount of aqueous humor, can lead to damage of the optic nerve and eventual blindness. The two basic types are open-angled glaucoma, in which pressure builds up very slowly, and acute-angle closure glaucoma, considered to be much more serious, in which the space between the iris and the cornea decreases, causing a greater degree of pressure to build. (24)

glomerulonephritis Also called glomerular disease. A condition involving inflammation and lesions of the glomeruli that hampers the kidneys' ability to remove waste and excess fluids and can lead to kidney failure. (29, 42)

glycosuria Sugar in the urine. (42)

goiter An enlarged thyroid gland, most commonly caused by Hashimoto's thyroiditis, an autoimmune inflammation. (30, 34)

gonads Sexual organs. (35)

goniometer A special type of protractor used to measure the range of motion possible in a specific joint without causing pain. (34)

gout A disease caused by the formation of crystals in a joint, leading to inflammation. It most commonly seen in men older than 40 and most frequently affects the great toe. (21)

Graves' disease An autoimmune disorder in which the antibodies produced by the immune system stimulate the thyroid to produce too much thyroxine, the most common cause of hyperthyroidism. (30)

grid A barrier positioned between an x-ray machine and a patient to absorb radiation scatter before it reaches the film. (44)

grievance Complaint. (18)

gross annual wage An individual's yearly work earnings before taxes and any withholdings are taken out. (14)

ground fault circuit interrupter (GFCI) An outlet designed to protect people from severe or fatal electric shocks. (5)

group practice Physicians who participate in a practice with other physicians to share the workload and expenses. (1)

guardian ad litem An adult who will act in the court on behalf of a minor. (Latin) (3)

habituation Dependence on a drug. (48)

Hashimoto's thyroiditis An autoimmune inflammation of the thyroid that causes hypothyroidism and goiter. (30)

hay fever Also called seasonal allergic rhinitis or pollinosis. A seasonal allergy that causes inflammation of the mucous membranes of the nose and eyes. (27)

headache Headache categories differentiated by the International Headache Society (IHS) are migraine, tension, cluster, and posttraumatic. (23)

Health Insurance Portability and Accountability Act (HIPAA) A federal act designed to improve portability and continuity of health insurance coverage. (4)

health maintenance organization (HMO) A managed care plan in which a range of health care services are made available to plan members for a predetermined fee (the capitation rate) per member, by a limited group of providers (such as physicians and hospitals). (15)

hearing acuity Sharpness of hearing. (36)

hearing loss The two most common types are conductive, a temporary condition that may develop when sound waves have no way of being conducted through the ear, and sensorineural, which occurs when neural structures of the ear become damaged, eventually leading to deafness. (24)

heart murmur A condition in which a damaged or diseased valve allows blood to escape and move backward through the valve. (25)

heart rate The controlled, rhythmic pulses of the heart, measured in beats per minute. (45)

heat exhaustion A condition that occurs when a person is exposed to a hot environment and does not drink adequate amounts of fluids to maintain a healthy body temperature, causing urine output to fall and leading to tachycardia, dizziness, nausea and vomiting, headache, muscle cramps and diarrhea, and fainting. (39)

heat stroke A condition caused by sufficient overheating (higher than 105° F centrally) long enough to cause failure of the temperature control center in the medulla of the brain, causing red, hot skin, shock, low blood pressure, and potentially disorientation or seizure. (39)

hematology The study of blood, its components, and the tissues that produce it to detect pathological conditions. (43)

hematopoiesis The formation of blood cells, which originate from the hematopoietic stem cell and mature into one of seven cell types: red blood cells (erythrocytes), five types of white blood cells (leukocytes), and platelets (thrombocytes). (43)

hematuria Blood in the urine. (42)

hemoglobin The substance in red blood cells whose function is to carry oxygen (oxyhemoglobin) from the lungs to the body cells and to carry the waste carbon dioxide (carboxyhemoglobin) from the body cells back to the lungs, where it can be expelled with exhalation. (43)

hemolyze Cause the red blood cells to burst. (40)

hemoptysis The coughing up of blood. (27)

hemorrhoids A dilated vein in the walls of the anus and sometimes around the rectum, usually caused by untreated constipation but occasionally associated with chronic diarrhea. (28)

hemostasis The stoppage of bleeding as a result of the smooth muscle at the site of a break causing the vessel wall to contract, creating a spasm that reduces the amount of blood loss and initiates the attachment of platelets to the broken area and to each other there, which forms a plug. (25)

heparin A substance that prevents blood from clotting. (43)

hepatitis A A disease caused by the hepatitis A virus that is transmitted through personal contact or by contaminated food or water and that affects the liver but does not cause long-term effects. (49)

hepatitis B A disease caused by the hepatitis B virus (HBV) that is transmitted by contaminated serum in blood transfusions or through the use of contaminated needles or instruments. (49)

hernia An abnormal protrusion of an organ, or part of an organ, through the wall of the body cavity where it is located, the most common types of abdominal hernias being hiatal and inguinal hernias. (28)

herpes simplex An infection that primarily affects the mouth or the genital area. The two different strains are Herpes simplex virus type 1 (HSV-1), the more common, which usually is acquired in childhood and is associated with infections of the lips, mouth, and face, and Herpes simplex virus 2 (HSV-2), which is sexually transmitted. (20)

herpes zoster Also called shingles. An infection caused by the varicella zoster virus that causes a painful rash. The virus first causes chickenpox and then lies dormant in the nerves, but with the potential to reactivate as shingles. (20)

hiatal hernia A condition in which the upper portion of the stomach protrudes into the chest cavity through a weakened or enlarged esophageal hiatus, an opening in the diaphragm normally large enough to accommodate only the esophagus. (28)

Hib disease A disease caused by a bacterium that enters the body through the lungs or bloodstream and that can result in meningitis. (49)

hierarchy A ranked order. (4)

hierarchy of needs The five levels of need identified by Abraham Maslow: I, physiological needs such as food, water, and shelter; II, safety needs, which includes such things as job security; III, social needs, which includes having a sense of belonging to a group; IV, self-esteem; and V, self-actualization, which occurs when an individual achieves all he or she is capable of. (52)

hilum The notch in the concave border of each kidney, the entrance for the renal artery and vein, nerves, lymphatic vessels, and the opening for the ureters. (29)

hirsutism Excessive hair growth. (34)

histamine The substance that produces the symptoms of allergies. (35)

holistic Viewing the overall situation such as the human body as a whole organism. (4)

Holter monitor A small tape recorder, accompanied by a patient diary, used to detect infrequent heart irregularities, recording cardiac activity while the patient is ambulatory for at least 24 hours and able to record continuously or only when the patient presses a button at the onset of symptoms. (45)

homeostasis The result of an organism's systems working together to maintain balance or equilibrium by adjusting for constant changes. (19)

homophones Words in the English language that have similar pronunciations but very different meanings and spellings. (10)

hordeolum Also called a sty. An inflamed gland of the eyelid, often caused by a bacterial infection, that appears as a pus-filled swelling near the roots of the eyelash. (24)

hospice A facility that provides an interdisciplinary program of care and supportive services for terminally ill patients and their families. (2, 4)

hydrocele A painless buildup of watery fluid around one or both testicles that causes the scrotum or groin area to swell. (31)

hydrocephalous Excessive fluid around the brain that can lead to brain damage. (37)

hydrogenation A process that turns liquid unsaturated fat into solid fat by adding hydrogen. (51)

hyfrecators A miniature electrocautery unit. (38)

hyperglycemia Too much sugar in the blood. (39)

hyperopia Also called farsightedness. A condition in which the eye can see distant objects well but near objects are blurry, caused either by the eyeball being too short or the lens too thin. (24, 36)

hypersensitivity An abnormal response of acute sensitivity to an allergen. (35)

hypertension Also called high blood pressure. Condition in which blood pressure is consistently higher than 140/90, which can lead to kidney failure, stroke, heart attack, peripheral artery disease, and eye damage. (25)

hyperthyroidism A condition in which the thyroid produces excess amounts of hormones, potentially leading to exophthalmos, palpitations, atrial fibrillation, enlargement of the heart, and congestive heart failure. (30)

hyperventilation syndrome A condition in which strong emotional triggers stimulate sudden changes in blood chemistry that produce extreme air hunger, diaphoresis, paresthesias, and emotional distress. (39)

hypoglycemia Too little sugar in the blood. (39)

hypotension Also called low blood pressure. Condition in which blood pressure is consistently lower than 90/60, which can cause inadequate blood flow to the heart, brain, and other vital organs. (25)

hypothermia A body temperature lower than 95° F (39)

hypothyroidism A condition in which the thyroid produces inadequate amounts of hormones, which can lead to an enlarged thyroid gland, a goiter, from the constant stimulation. (30)

hysterectomy A surgical procedure to remove a woman's uterus. The types are complete (total), in which the cervix, fallopian tubes, and ovaries are removed; partial (subtotal), in which the upper part of the uterus is removed but the cervix is not; and radical, in which the uterus, cervix, upper part of the vagina, and supporting tissues are removed. (31)

icteric Having a bilious yellow-green color. (40)

idiosyncratic Specific to an individual. (48)

immediate history The history of the current medical complaint. (39)

immune response A series of immune system attacks on organisms and substances that invade the body systems and cause disease. (26)

immune system The tissues, organs, and physiologic processes used by the body to identify abnormal cells and foreign substances and defend against those that might be harmful, including bacteria, microbes, viruses, toxins, and parasites. (26)

immunity A resistance to disease. The two types are genetic, which does not involve the production of antibodies, and acquired, which does. (32)

immunizations Also called vaccines. The injection of inactive (dead) or attenuated (weakened) disease agents into the human body to establish resistance to the diseases they cause. (49)

immunology The study of immunity or the resistance to or protection from disease. (2)

impacted cerumen Hardened ear wax that obstructs the auditory canal and can lead to hearing loss or tinnitus. (24)

impetigo A contagious skin infection, found most commonly in children, caused by bacteria that form round, crusted, oozing spots, typically around the nose and mouth. (20)

inactive record A medical record of a patient who has not been seen by the physician within the time period determined by office policy. The patient has not received a formal notification that the physician has terminated care. These files are maintained but generally kept in a separate storage file cabinet. They may return when a medical problem develops. (12)

inactivated polio vaccine (IPV) A vaccine to protect individuals against polio, which is caused by a virus and spread through contact with feces of an infected person and can result in paralysis. (49)

incident report A formal written description of any unusual occurrence or accident in the medical setting. (5)

incision A surgical cut into tissue. (38)

incontinence The involuntary and unpredictable flow of urine. The three types are stress, the most common, which happens when sneezing, laughing, or the like; urge, which occurs when the bladder contracts without warning; and overflow, which happens when a blockage prohibits normal emptying and the bladder simply overflows. (29)

incubation The period from exposure to a pathogen to the point at which the disease symptoms develop. (32)

incubator A container in which a specific temperature is maintained to achieve a specific result. (40)

infancy The second subdivision of child development, covering the time from birth to becoming a toddler. (52)

infectious mononucleosis Also called simply mono and "the kissing disease." A viral infection caused by the Epstein-Barr virus (EBV), part of the herpes family, characterized by an increase in white blood cells that contain a single nucleus and commonly found in young adults. (26)

inflection In reference to your speaking voice, the pitch in your voice and the way words and phrases are uttered. (6)

influenza Also called flu. An illness caused by infection of the respiratory tract by viruses. (27)

informed consent Permission or approval given by a patient who is informed by the physician about the possible consequences of both having and not having certain procedures and treatment. (3)

inguinal hernia A condition in which tissue or part of the intestine push through a weak spot in the abdominal wall in the groin area, causing a bulge in the groin or scrotum. (28)

inhalation medications Medications administered through the respiratory tract, using a metered-dose inhaler (nebulizer). (49)

inoculated Exposed to microorganisms. (41)

insertion In locations at which skeletal muscles attach, the attachment point on the bone that moves. (22)

inspection Visual examination. (34)

inspiratory capacity (IC) The volume of air that can be inhaled after normal expiration. (45)

inspiratory reserve volume (IRV) The volume of air that can be forcibly inspired after a normal inhale. (45)

instill To put in eye or ear medication. (36)

insulin-dependent diabetes mellitus (IDDM) Also known as type 1 diabetes, juvenile diabetes. A condition in which the body is unable to produce enough insulin to properly control its blood sugar level by converting sugar and starches into energy, typically diagnosed in children. (30)

integrated delivery system (IDS) An organization of provider sites, such as ambulatory centers, clinics, or hospitals, with a contracted relationship that offer services to subscribers. (15)

integrity Adherence to a code of values, honesty, dependability, and dedicated to high standards. To do what is expected, when it is expected, for the simple reason that it is expected. (1)

International Classification of Diseases, Ninth Revision Clinical Modification (ICD-9-CM) The accurate diagnostic numeric and alphanumeric code listing for patient diagnoses and identification on the medical insurance claim forms used for the insurance billing process. (17)

International Classification of Diseases, Tenth Revision (ICD-10) Diagnosis codes that contain increased specificity and include newly discovered or diagnosed diseases. (17)

Internet A computer network made up of thousands of interfacing networks worldwide. (11)

Internet service provider (ISP) A commercial service that provides access to the Internet. (11)

interstitial cystitis (IC) An inflammation of the bladder wall, the cause of which is unknown. (29)

intractable pain Pain that is overwhelming, difficult to relieve, and all consuming. (33)

intradermal injection The injection of a minute amount of material into the top layer of skin to determine a patient's sensitivity, typically used for allergy testing and characterized by the appearance on the skin of a small wheal, or bubble, containing the injected fluid. (49)

intramuscular (IM) injections The injection of medication into a muscle, including the deltoid, vastus lateralis, and dorsogluteal and ventrogluteal muscles. (49)

intubate To insert a tube into the trachea as an emergency airway. (39)

invasive procedure A procedure in which the body is entered, such as when administering an injection, making a surgical incision, or working with an open wound. (38)

inventory A detailed master list that maintains all of the physical assets or capital equipment in an office. (9)

inversion The process of turning the body inward. (21)

irrigate To rinse the eye or ear. (36)

irritable bowel syndrome (IBS) A common intestinal condition characterized by abdominal pain and cramps, diarrhea or constipation or both, gas, bloating, nausea, and other symptoms. (28)

ischemia Reduced blood supply. (35)

Ishihara test A series of illustrations comprised of colored dots that is used to test a person's color vision. (36)

ketones By-products of fat metabolism found in urine. (42)

kidney stones Also called renal calculi. Deposits of mineral salts in the kidney, usually benign there, that can pass into the ureter, slowing down or blocking urine flow and irritating the ureter, causing bleeding. (29)

kidneys Paired, bean-shaped organs located at the back of the abdominal cavity and lying on either side of the spinal column in the flank area, against the muscles of the back. (29)

kilobyte (K or Kb) The measurement of a computer's memory or storage. Each kilobyte is 1,000 bytes (or characters) of information. (11)

kinesthetic Involving movement. (4)

laryngeal mirror A small mirror attached to a long handle used to examine the larynx. (34)

leads The sensors attached to a patient for recording an electrocardiogram. (45)

learning outcomes The goals of education; that is, what a person should achieve as a result of the learning. (50)

ledger card A record of the charges, adjustments, payments, and current balance for the patient. (13)

Legionnaire's disease A type of pneumonia or lung infection caused by the *Legionella* germ. (27)

lethal Able to cause death. (48)

leukemia A malignant cancer of the bone marrow and blood, affecting the white blood cells. The two types are lymphocytic, affecting the lymphoid cells, and myeloid, or myelogenous, affecting the myeloid cells, and the disease can be acute or chronic. (25)

leukocytes Also called white blood cells. Larger blood cells that fight infection and thus contribute to homeostasis. (25, 26)

licensure Granting of a license and authorization to practice one's profession. (2)

lipolysis The destruction of fats. (30)

liquid medications Medications administered in suspensions, emulsions, elixirs, syrups, and solutions using calibrated cups, spoons, and droppers. (49)

lithotripsy Procedure that involves passing shock waves through the body to break down kidney stones. The two types are extracorporeal shockwave and percutaneous ultrasonic. (29)

living will A document that allows patients to request that life-sustaining treatments and nutritional support not be used to prolong their life. This document gives patients the legal right to direct the type of care they wish to receive when their death is imminent and provides protection for physicians and hospitals when they follow the patient's wishes. (3)

lochia The lining of the uterus. (35)

lung cancer Types include adenocarcinoma, the most common type, bronchoalveolar cell carcinoma, squamous cell carcinoma, and carcinoid lung cancer. (27)

lymph A clear fluid that travels through the body's arteries, circulating

and minerals, and more than 50 nutrients are required for the body to function properly. (51)

objective symptoms Complaints that are felt by a patient and are apparent to observers or measurable. (33)

objective Relating to something measurable. (34)

occult Hidden, indicating that although not visible, there is, for instance, blood in a urine sample. (42)

Occupational Safety and Hazard Administration (OSHA) A governmental agency responsible for the safety of all employees of companies operating in the United States. (5)

office flow The organization of an office environment that lends itself easily to teamwork, time management, organized and efficient office equipment usage, and patient flow. (9)

oliguria Decreased amount of urine production, which may indicate decreased fluid intake, dehydration, bleeding, kidney disease, an obstruction, or renal failure. (42)

oncogenes The genes controlling cell growth and multiplication that are transformed into cancer cells by cancer-causing agents. (26)

open-ended question A question that requires more than a yes or no response. (4)

open-panel HMO A health care provider that is not employed by the HMO and does not belong to a medical group owned or managed by the HMO. (15)

ophthalmologist A medical doctor who can perform eye examinations and eye surgery and prescribe medications, eyeglasses, and contact lenses. (36)

ophthalmoscope Instrument used to examine the inner parts of the eye. (36)

opportunistic infections Infections that take advantage of an immune system already suppressed, such as by stress, poor nutrition, or HIV infection. (32)

optician A technician who specializes in grinding lenses and preparing eyeglasses and contact lenses. (36)

optometrist A doctor of optometry, not a medical doctor, who can perform eye examinations and prescribe medications associated with the eye examination, eyeglasses, and contact lenses. (36)

oral cancer Cancer of the mouth, usually starting in the flat squamous cells that line it. (28)

oral medication Medication administered through the gastrointestinal

system using pills, syrups, or other liquids. (49)

oral polio vaccine (OPV) A vaccine taken orally to protect individuals against polio, which is caused by a virus and spread through contact with the feces of an infected person and can result in paralysis. (49)

organ of Corti Organ located in the cochlea (a part of the inner ear) containing hair-like fibers that convert sound waves for transmission to the brain along the auditory nerve. (36)

organelles Small structures that help carry out the day-to-day operations of a cell. (19, 41)

organs Groups of tissues that serve a common purpose or function. (19)

origin In locations at which skeletal muscles attach, the attachment point on the bone that is more fixed or still. (22)

orthostatic hypotension A 20 to 30 mmHg drop in blood pressure associated with dizziness and fainting when changing position from lying down or sitting to standing. (37)

orthotist Someone who specializes in designing and fitting supportive devices such as braces and splints. (46)

osteoarthritis The most common type of arthritis, resulting from years of wear and tear on joints and occurring most frequently in the hips, knees, and finger joints. (21)

osteopath A medical professional who places great emphasis on the relationship between the musculoskeletal systems and the organs of the body. The skill of manipulation therapy is learned in schools of osteopathy. (2)

osteoporosis The loss of bone density and the thinning of bone tissue, a condition seen most commonly in older adults, especially postmenopausal women, and in individuals who do not consume enough calcium. (21)

otitis media Inflammation of the middle ear caused by viral or bacterial infections. (24)

otology The study of hearing. (36)

otorhinolaryngologist (ENT) An eye, ear, nose, and throat specialist. (36)

otosclerosis A condition in which the tissue surrounding the bone of the stapes grows abnormally around it, preventing it from transmitting sound vibrations to the inner ear and resulting in profound hearing loss. (24)

otoscope Instrument used to examine the eardrum. (36)

outpatient surgery Generally describes procedures requiring less than an hour to perform, often in freestanding surgicenters or surgical centers that are part of a hospital complex. (38)

outside laboratory A laboratory, either hospital based or independent, that handles specimens collected from many types of facilities and performs tests ranging from simple to very complex. (40)

ovarian cancer The three main types are epithelial cell cancer, the most common, which starts in the outer covering of the ovary; germ cell tumors, which start in the egg cells within the ovary and generally occur in younger women and even children; and stromal tumors, which start in the cells that form the structural framework of the ovary. (31)

ovarian cyst Sac filled with a fluid or semisolid material that develops on or within the ovary, typically not disease related and disappearing on its own, when the grown follicle fails to rupture and release an egg and instead of being reabsorbed forms a cyst. (31)

overbooking Scheduling more than one patient in the same time slot. Also referred to as double or triple booking. (7)

ovulation The process of producing an ovum and releasing it into the pelvic cavity and the fallopian tube. (31)

oximetry The process of measuring the oxygen saturation of arterial blood. (33)

oxygen debt The inability of the body to absorb enough oxygen to supply the energy required to sustain a high level of activity, resulting in its utilizing the anaerobic energy system and in the buildup of lactic acid in the muscles. (22)

oxygen saturation The relative amounts of deoxygenated (venous) blood versus oxygenated hemoglobin in arterial blood. (33)

pacemaker The sinoatrial (SA) node, located in the right atrium and made of modified myocardial cells, which acts like a battery, establishing the heart rate. (45)

palpation Using the hands to feel the skin and accessible underlying organs. (34)

palpatory method The feeling of the radial pulse while the blood pressure cuff is deflating, used to determine systolic pressure. (33)

pancreatic cancer The two types are adenocarcinoma, the more common, which arises from the exocrine glands, and neuroendocrine carcinoma, or islet cell tumor, which is rare. (28)

pandemic An outbreak of a disease that infects many people in different countries at the same time such as the bubonic plague. (2)

paraplegia Paralysis from approximately the waist down. (23)

parasites Organisms that live within other organisms. (42)

parenteral medication administration The administration of a medication through injection, including intramuscular, intravenous, subdermal, and intradermal injection. (49)

Parkinson's disease A progressive disorder caused by degeneration of the nerve cells in the parts of the brain that control movement, resulting in a shortage of the neurotransmitter dopamine, which impairs movement. (23)

participating provider A physician or medical facility that will accept the insurance company's allowed amount as payment in full (less patient co-payments) for services rendered. (16)

parturition Birth. (35)

passive listening Simply listening to someone without having to reply such as when listening as a member of an audience. (4)

passive transport Process in cells that does not require energy to transport materials to, from, and within the cell. Passive transport mechanisms include diffusion, osmosis, and filtration. (19)

passive voice The subject of a sentence receives the action. (10)

past medical history A person's lifelong medical history. (39)

pasteurization The process during which substances, such as milk and cheese, are heated to a certain temperature to eliminate bacteria. (2)

patellar Relating to the kneecap bone. (34)

pathogens Disease-producing microorganisms. (32)

pathophysiology The study of diseases or disorders caused by a malfunction or by aging. (19)

payee A person or company named as the receiving party to whom the amount on a check is payable. (14)

payer A person signing a check to release money. (14)

pediculosis An infestation of the hairy parts of the body or clothing with the eggs, larvae, or adults of lice. (20)

pelvic inflammatory disease (PID) An infection of the upper genital area

that occurs when disease-carrying organisms migrate upward from the urethra and cervix, potentially affecting the uterus, ovaries, and fallopian tubes and potentially leading to scarring and infertility or to tubal pregnancy. (31)

peptic ulcer disease (PUD) A condition in which a disruption occurs in the lining of the esophagus, stomach, or duodenum. (28)

percussion Using the fingertips to tap the body lightly but sharply to gain information about the positions and sizes of underlying body parts. (34)

pericardium The outer lining of the heart wall. (25)

perimysium Connective tissue responsible for dividing a muscle into sections. (22)

perineum The external region between the vulva and the anus, composed of muscle covered with skin. (31)

periosteum The membrane that forms the covering of long bones, except at their articular surfaces. (21)

permeable Capable of allowing substances to pass through. (32)

personal assessment Evaluation of one's own strengths and weaknesses. (53)

personality disorders Disorders include antisocial reactions, also called sociopathic behavior, characterized by impulsive behavior, socially negative actions, and a lack of social emotions (guilt, shame, and empathy); paranoia, characterized by intense feelings of persecution and jealousy; and narcissistic behavior, which refers to abnormal self-love and self-admiration. (52)

pertussis Also called whooping cough. A respiratory disease most common in children younger than 4 years, caused by bacteria and transmitted by direct and indirect contact and known as whooping cough because one of the symptoms is a violent cough with a whooping sound. (49)

phagocytes Several types of white blood cells that attack invading organisms, the most common being **neutrophils**, which primarily attack bacteria. (26)

phagocytosis The process by which leukocytes (white blood cells) actively fight pathogenic microorganisms. (32)

phantom pain A sensation felt in a missing body part after it has been removed. (33)

pharmacists Specially trained and licensed professionals who specialize in the preparation and dispensation of drugs. (48)

pharmacology The study of drugs, their origins, characteristics, and effects. (48)

photometer An instrument that measures light intensity. (40)

physiatrist A medical doctor or osteopath who specializes in physical medicine. (46)

physiatry The branch of medicine encompassing physical medicine, involving the therapeutic use of physical agents for the diagnosis, treatment, management, and prevention of diseases and debilitating illnesses. (46)

physician's office laboratory (POL) A laboratory in the office suite in which some simple tests are performed. (40)

physiology The study of the function of an organism. (19)

pipette An instrument used for measuring or for transferring liquid from one vessel to another. (40)

pitch In reference to your speaking voice, the loudness of your voice. (6)

plasma The liquid component of blood, accounting for about 55% of its composition and composed of 90% water and 10% solids (solutes), that transports substances throughout the body. (43)

platelets Also called thrombocytes. The smallest cells in blood, formed in the bone marrow, whose main function is to assist in the clotting of blood. (25, 43)

pleurisy Also called pleuritis. An inflammation of the pleura, the membrane surrounding the lungs, generally stemming from an existing respiratory infection, disease, or injury. (27)

pneumococcal vaccine A vaccine to protect individuals against the *Streptococcus pneumoniae* bacteria, which are spread through the air. (49)

pneumonia An inflammation of the lungs, caused by bacteria, viruses, fungi, or chemical irritants, often following influenza in the elderly and debilitated and with the most common bacterial cause in the United States being *Streptococcus pneumoniae* (pneumococcus pneumonia). (27)

point-of-service plan (POS) A flexible health care plan that allows patients to choose using the panel of providers within the HMO network or to utilize the services of non-HMO providers. (15)

polio vaccine A vaccine to protect individuals against polio, which is caused by a virus and spread through contact with feces of an infected person and can result in paralysis. (49)

polycystic kidney disease (PKD) A disorder in which clusters of cysts, noncancerous sacs of water-like fluid, develop, primarily within the kidneys. (29)

polysaccharides Starches (complex carbohydrates) that are broken down into glucose during the digestive process. (51)

polyuria Excessive amount of urine production, which may indicate disorders such as diabetes or kidney disease. (42)

portal of entry Means of entry, including the respiratory, urinary, and reproductive tracts, skin, mucous membranes, and blood, into a new host from the reservoir host in a chain of infection. (32)

portal of exit Means of exit, including the respiratory, intestinal, urinary, and reproductive tracts and open wounds, of pathogens from the reservoir host who is the beginning of a chain of infection. (32)

post Enter amounts onto a record. (13)

practice of medicine Diagnosing and prescribing treatment or medication. (3)

preauthorization Prior approval from a health care plan administrator to receive reimbursement for surgery and other procedures to be performed. (15, 16)

preceptor A supervisor who provides additional instruction and guidance for a student in an externship and provides a formal written evaluation of the student. (53)

preferred provider organization (PPO) A health care plan that stipulates that the patient must use a medical provider (physician or hospital) who is under contract with the insurer for an agreed-on fee. (15)

prefilled cartridge injection systems Prefilled single-dose cartridges that fit into a special holder for the administration of medications. (49)

prejudice A preformed and unfavorable belief or attitude toward a certain culture or group with little or no information about the culture or group. (4, 52)

premenstrual syndrome (PMS) A condition affecting women who menstruate that may include such symptoms as constipation, diarrhea, nausea, anorexia, appetite cravings, headache, backache, muscular aches, edema, insomnia, clumsiness, malaise, irritability, indecisiveness, mental confusion, and depression. (31)

premium A monthly fee paid by the insured for specific medical insurance coverage. (15)

prenatal period The first subdivision of child development, covering the process from conception to birth. (52)

prepaid plan A group of physicians or other health care providers who have a contractual agreement to provide services to subscribers on a negotiated fee-for-service or capitated basis (also called managed care plan). (15)

presbycusis Hearing loss from the gradual deterioration of the sensory receptors located in the cochlea, seen most frequently in older adults and caused by such factors as long exposures to loud noises, infection, injury, and in some cases side effects caused by certain medications; usually occurs with aging. (24, 36)

presbyopia A disorder that causes the loss of elasticity in the eye's lens as a result of aging; usually occurs with aging (24, 36)

primary assessment The questions asked and examinations conducted at initial contact with a patient: Determine the patient's name, approximate age, and gender, decide if the patient is ill or injured, determine the chief complaint, obtain immediate and past medical histories, identify medications currently being taken, do a physical examination, and take the vital signs. (39)

primary care physician (PCP) A physician who is part of a managed care plan that provides all primary health care services to members of the plan. Generally an internist, family practitioner, gynecologist, or pediatrician is a primary care physician. (15)

prime mover A muscle that is the primary actor in a given movement, that is, the muscle that produces the movement in muscle contraction. (22)

principal diagnosis A diagnosis of a particular condition that a patient sought care for on a particular date. It is used when performing coding in the hospital setting and when a final diagnosis was unable to be determined without further patient follow-up. (17)

printer A device to output information from a computer onto paper or a hardcopy. (11)

probationary period A trial period to observe a new employee at work and to determine if the new employee is suited to the position for which he or she was hired. (18)

problem-oriented medical record (POMR) The charting of medical records based on a patient's problem. (12, 34)

procedural coding The process of transferring a narrative description of procedures into numbers. (17)

professional courtesy (PC) A consideration of service offered by a physician to other physicians, family members, and indigent patients. Conditions must fall within federal guidelines, and be recorded in the patient's record. (13)

professional reference A statement from someone who has worked with you or known you for a period of time attesting to your skills and personal integrity. (53)

proficiency testing An external quality control program that monitors the accuracy of laboratories by having them test samples whose constituents are already known. (40)

prognosis The prediction of the course of a disease and the recovery rate. (33)

prokaryotic Cells lacking a nucleus or organelles, such as bacteria. (41)

pronation The process of lying prone, or face downward; the process of turning the hand so that the palm points downward. (21)

proofread To review a document for errors. (53)

proofreading Reviewing and checking a written document or material for errors in content and typing. (10)

prophylactically Preventing the onset of a condition. (48)

prostate cancer A malignant tumor that grows in the prostate gland. (31)

prosthesis An artificial replacement of a missing body part. (46)

prosthetist Someone who specializes in designing, preparing, and fitting prosthetic devices such as artificial limbs. (46)

proteinuria The presence of protein in the urine, which can indicate renal dysfunction, preeclampsia in pregnancy, congestive heart failure, and glomerulonephritis, a kidney disease. (42)

protraction The process of moving a body part forward. (21)

proximate cause Natural continuous sequence of events, without any intervening cause, which produces an injury. In a legal case of negligence, the defendant's acts (or failure to act) that directly cause an injury. (3)

psoriasis A common skin condition characterized by frequent episodes of redness, itching, and thick, dry scales that result from the accelerated movement of new skin from the lower layers of the skin to the top, causing a buildup of dead skin cells. (20)

psychiatrist A physician specializing in the care of patients with emotional disorders. (52)

psychiatry The branch of medicine that deals with the diagnosis, treatment, and prevention of mental disorders. (52)

psychologist Someone trained in the methods of psychological analysis, therapy, and research. (52)

psychology The science of behavior and the human thought process. (52)

psychopharmacology The study of the effects of drugs on the mind and brain and particularly of the use of drugs in treating mental disorders. (52)

psychoses Severe mental disorders that interfere with a patient's perception of reality and ability to cope with the demands of daily living. (52)

psychotherapy A method for treating mental disorders by mental rather than physical means, including psychoanalysis, humanistic therapies, and family and group therapy. (52)

puerperium The period immediately following childbirth. (35)

pulmonary edema A condition in which fluid accumulates in the lungs, usually caused by failure of the heart's left ventricle but also caused by lung problems such as pneumonia, an excess of intravenous fluids, some types of kidney disease, bad burns, liver disease, nutritional problems, and Hodgkin's disease. (27)

pulmonary embolism (PE) A blood clot in the lung, usually originating in smaller vessels in the leg, pelvis, arms, or heart and traveling to the lung, where it ultimately becomes wedged in a vessel too small to allow it to pass, causing that portion of the lung to die due to lack of oxygen. (27)

pulse deficit The difference between the radial pulse and the apical pulse. (33)

pulse pressure The difference between the systolic blood pressure reading, measured at the highest pressure, as the heart is contracting, and the diastolic pressure, measured at the lowest pressure, when the heart is relaxed (the ventricle is at rest). (33)

Purkinje fibers Specialized conductive fibers located within the walls of the ventricles, responsible for relay-

ing cardiac impulses to the cells of the ventricles, which allow the ventricles to contract. The Purkinje system includes the bundle of His and the peripheral fibers. (25)

pyelonephritis An infection of the kidney and renal pelvis caused by bacteria, usually *E. coli*, entering the kidneys from the bladder. (29)

pyloric stenosis A condition in which a baby's pylorus (the connection between the stomach and the duodenum) gradually swells and thickens, which interferes with food entering the intestine. (28)

pyrexia Also called fever. A body temperature above 100.4°F (38°C), at which point the body is producing greater heat than it is losing. (33)

quadriplegia Paralysis from approximately the shoulders down. (23)

qualitative test The analysis of a specimen for the presence or absence of a substance, usually reported as positive or negative. (40)

quality assurance (QA) Gathering and evaluating information about services provided as well as the results achieved and comparing this information with an accepted standard. (5)

quantitative test The analysis of a specimen for the presence of a substance and the amount of it present, usually reported in numerical values or units. (40)

queue A waiting line. (6)

rad The unit of measurement that describes the amount of ionizing radiation absorbed during an x-ray procedure. (44)

radiating pain Pain that spreads out from an originating area. (33)

radiation The use of a radioactive substance for diagnostic radiology, radiation therapy, or nuclear medicine. (44)

radiation therapy Cancer treatment that uses high-energy waves, such as x-rays, to damage and destroy cancer cells. (26)

radioactive Able to emit radiation as the result of the disintegration of the nucleus in an atom. (44)

radiograph An image produced by projecting x-rays through internal structures of the body onto photographic film. (44)

radiologist A physician specializing in radiology. (44)

radiology The branch of medicine that uses radioactive substances, such as x-rays and ultraviolet rays, to visualize the internal structures of the body for diagnostic radiology, radiation therapy, or nuclear medicine. (44)

radiolucent Permitting greater penetration of x-rays. (44)

radiopaque Permitting fewer x-rays to penetrate. (44)

random-access memory (RAM) The highest amount of memory measured in the number of kilobytes that a computer can hold all at once. (11)

range of motion (ROM) The degree of movement possible in a specific joint without causing pain, measured with a goniometer. (46)

rapport An environment of cooperation. (4)

read-only memory (ROM) Storage of information that is not actively being used by the computer at that moment. (11)

reagent A substance required in a chemical reaction or used to detect the presence of another substance. (40)

real time Refers to automatically placing the appointment, patient needs, and information within the appropriate areas of a computer appointment program versus a manual system. (8)

reasonable person standard Exercising the ordinary standard of care and the type of care that a "reasonable" person would use in a similar circumstance. (3)

receptionist The staff employee in an office who greets and assists incoming patients and performs duties that make the office run smoothly and efficiently; often a medical assistant. (7)

reconciliation The agreement of the figures on the bank statement with the records maintained in the medical office and the adjustment of banking records. (14)

rectus femoris A muscle in the middle region of the thigh into which medication is injected, used most often for pediatric patients. (49)

redundant Repetition of the same statement over again. (10)

reference laboratory A laboratory that handles more complex tests and those tests that are infrequently requested in other laboratories. (40)

referral Paperwork for the insurance company that is required from the primary care physician to send a patient to see a medical specialist for treatment. (6, 15)

referred pain Pain that is felt somewhere other than at the source. (33, 35)

reflex hammer Also called a percussion hammer. Hammer having a hard rubber, triangular head, used for testing reflexes. (34)

Registered Medical Assistant (RMA) A medical assistant who meets the eligibility requirements and who can prove his or her competency to perform entry-level skills through written examination. The RMA is awarded to candidates who pass the AMT certification examination. A multiskilled health care professional assists providers in an allied health setting. (1)

registration A health care professional on record as part of an organization or association in a specific health care field that administers examinations and maintains a list of qualified individuals. (2)

rehabilitation The process of returning a patient as close as possible to the person's normal physical condition after injury or disease. (46)

rem Abbreviation for roentgen equivalent in man. The unit of measure that describes exposure to ionizing radiation that may involve more than one type of radiation. (44)

renal calculi Also called kidney stones. Deposits of mineral salts in the kidney, usually benign there, that can pass into the ureter, slowing down or blocking urine flow and irritating the ureter, causing bleeding. (29)

renal pelvis A sac-like area of the kidney for collecting urine. (29)

renal threshold The concentration in the blood at which a substance such as glucose excreted by the kidneys begins to appear in the urine. (42)

res ipsa loquitur A doctrine meaning, "the thing speaks for itself," applies to the law of negligence. It refers to the breach (neglect) of duty that is so obvious that it does not need further explanation or "it speaks for itself." (Latin) (3)

reservoir Host who is the source of a pathogen, beginning of a chain of infection. (32)

residual volume (RV) The volume of air left in the lungs at the end of an exhale (around 1200 ml). (45)

resolution The ability of a microscope to distinguish clearly between adjacent but distinct objects. (40)

respiratory syncytial virus (RSV) The most common cause of bronchiolitis, spread by contact with upper respiratory secretions, occurring winter and early spring, and lasting up to two weeks. (37)

respite care A temporary interlude of care for a patient to allow the caregiver time for relaxation. (37)

respondeat superior A Latin term meaning "Let the master answer." It refers to the employer or physician who is liable for the negligent actions of anyone working for him or her. In some states, both the physician and the employee may be liable. (3)

résumé A summary of a person's credentials, including employment history, experience, training, and education. (53)

retinal detachment Separation of the retina from the underlying choroids layer. (24)

retraction The process of moving a body part backward. (21)

retrograde Against the normal flow. (44)

rheumatoid arthritis An immune system disorder in which the body's defenses attack the tissue in the joints, leading to inflammation, degeneration of the articular cartilage, and deformation of the joints. (21, 26)

RhoGAM Drug administered to a pregnant woman to inhibit the production of antibodies against the Rh antigen. (25)

rhythm The regularity of the occurrence of heartbeats, with ventricular rhythm determined by measuring the distance between QRS complexes and atrial rhythm by measuring the distance between P waves. (45)

ribosome An important cellular organelle that participates in protein synthesis. (19)

risk management Planning and implementing strategies for reducing the physician's risk of lawsuit in the medical setting. (4)

RNA (ribonucleic acid) A single chain of chemical bases important for protein synthesis. The two types of RNA molecules are mRNA and tRNA. (19)

rosacea A chronic and potentially life-disruptive disorder, primarily of the facial skin and often characterized by flare-ups and remissions. (20)

rotation The process of moving a body part around a central axis. (21)

Rule of Nines Tool for estimating the surface area of a burn. (39)

sanitization The inhibition or inactivation of pathogens by means of scrubbing and washing items. (32)

scabies A contagious disorder of the skin caused by very small, wingless insects or mites called the human itch mite or scabies itch mite. (20)

scheduling system A system that facilitates the coordination of appropriate time segments for staff, patients, and the practice's available equipment to provide efficient services. (8)

schizophrenia A psychotic disorder marked by a variety of symptoms, including delusions, hallucinations, disorganized and incoherent speech, severe emotional abnormalities, and withdrawal into an inner world. (52)

sciatica Pain along the large sciatic nerve that runs from the lower back down the back of each leg, usually caused by pressure on the sciatic nerve from a herniated disc. (23)

scoliosis Curvature of the spine. (34)

scrub assistant A surgical assistant whose responsibilities include arranging the operating physician's surgical tray, handing instruments, swabbing (sponging) bodily fluids away from the operative site, retracting the incision area, and cutting suture materials, all performed in sterile protective clothing using sterile technique. (38)

sebaceous glands Glands in the skin that produce sebum, an oil that acts to protect the body from dehydration and the possible absorption of harmful substances. (20)

sediment The solid portion of a urine sample after it has been separated by a centrifuge, which may contain organized material, such as red blood cells, white blood cells, epithelial cells, casts, bacteria, parasites, yeast, fungi, and spermatozoa, or unorganized material, consisting of all chemical materials, including crystals and amorphous material (material without a shape). (42)

seizure A temporary interference with muscle control, movement, speech, vision, or awareness. (23)

selective permeability The attribute of a cell membrane that allows certain substances to enter the cell while preventing other substances from doing so. (19)

self-referral A health insurance enrollee chooses to see an out-of-network provider without authorization. (15)

seniority A status gained by being the individual who worked for an employer for the longest amount of time. (18)

sensorineural hearing loss Hearing loss due to damage to the organ of Corti or the auditory nerve. (36)

sequela A long-lasting effect. (41)

serology The study of antigen–antibody reactions of the body's immune system. (41)

severe acute respiratory syndrome (SARS) A newly identified respiratory illness caused by a previously unknown virus, denoted SARS-CoV, of the coronavirus family, whose members often cause mild to moderate upper respiratory illness, such as the common cold. (27)

sexually transmitted infection (STI) Also called venereal disease. An infection transmitted through exchange of semen, blood, and other body fluids or by direct contact with the affected area of another person, caused by such organisms as chlamydia, human papillomavirus (HPV), genital herpes, gonorrhea, syphilis, and human immunovirus (HIV) and potentially resulting in birth defects, blindness, bone deformities, brain damage, cancer, heart disease, infertility and other abnormalities of the reproductive system, mental retardation, or death. (31)

side effects Reactions, sometimes undesirable or lethal, other than those sought from a drug. (48)

signee The person who signs a check or document. (14)

sinoatrial node Also called SA node, "pacemaker." One of the three areas of specialized neuromuscular tissue that initiate the heartbeat, it is located in the upper wall of the right atrium, just below the opening of the superior vena cava, and discharges the electrical impulses that cause contractions of the atria, thus initiating the heartbeat. (25)

sinusitis An infection or inflammation of the mucous membranes that line the inside of the nose and sinuses, causing them to swell and thus block the drainage of fluid from the sinuses into the nose and throat. (27)

skeletal muscle Type of voluntary muscle found in the locomotive system that controls movement by being attached to bones in the body, made up of cylindrical fibers of striated cells with the nucleus of each cell tending to be toward the edge of the cell. (22)

smear A thin layer of microorganisms spread on a glass slide. (41)

smooth muscle Type of involuntary muscle found throughout the body, composed of elongated, spindle-shaped cells with the nucleus centrally located and without striations. (22)

Snellen eye chart A chart used to measure the distance acuity of a person's vision. (36)

SOAP A charting method comprising subjective and objective information, assessment, and plan of care. (34)

software A set or sets of programmed language that gives instructions for a computer to process and perform. (11)

solo practice A physician who practices alone. (1)

solvent A company or practice capable of paying its bills and salaries. (18)

source-oriented medical record (SOMR) A charting method in which information is organized into different sections and is placed in the medical record in reverse chronological order. Tabs are used to label the source, such as laboratory, x-ray, consultation, and special study. (12, 34)

specific gravity The weight of a substance in relation to the weight of the same amount of distilled water. (42)

specific time The time allocated on the schedule to each patient depending on the purpose of the office visit or the type of examination or testing that is to be done. (8)

speculum Plural **specula**. An instrument that holds open the entrance to a body cavity to permit inspection. (34, 36)

spina bifida The most frequently occurring, permanently disabling birth defect, resulting from the failure of the spine to close properly during the first month of pregnancy. (23)

spore A thick-walled reproductive cell produced by some organisms, notably *Clostridium botulinum,* which causes botulism, and *Clostridium tetani,* which causes tetanus, that is capable of withstanding unfavorable environmental conditions. (41)

sprain A stretching or tearing injury to a ligament. (22)

sputum The mucous substance expelled by coughing or clearing the bronchi. (41)

squamous cell carcinoma A malignant tumor that affects the middle layer of the skin. (20)

standard of care The level of knowledge, skill, and care a medical practitioner must provide to all patients for the same care that would commonly be provided by other similar medical care professionals under the same circumstances in the same locality. (3)

***Staphylococcus aureus* (staph)** The major pathogen of its genus, found as normal flora in the nose and on the skin, which causes infection especially when resistance is lowered by a break in the skin or in the mucous membranes, manifesting as gram-positive, grape-like clusters of cocci and as impetigo in children and associated with infection of wound sites and surgical incisions. (41)

stat Immediately. (40)

statute of limitations The maximum period of time during which a patient can take legal actions. (3, 13)

steatorrhea Excessive amounts of fat in the feces. (41)

stem cell An undifferentiated cell that can give rise to other cells of the same type or from which specialized cells can develop. (2)

stereotyping Forming negative beliefs concerning specific characteristics of a group that are applied unfairly to an entire population. (4, 52)

sterile field A specific area free of all microorganisms that will be the work area for a surgical procedure. (38)

sterilization The destruction of all microorganisms, both pathogenic and nonpathogenic, using techniques such as heat (steam or dry), chemicals, high-velocity electron bombardment, or ultraviolet light radiation. (32)

stomach ulcers Also called peptic ulcers, gastric ulcers. A condition in which the lining of the stomach or upper part of the small intestine (duodenum) is damaged and the sensitive tissue underneath is exposed to stomach acid. (28)

stool Also called feces. The waste product from the bowel. (41)

stop-payment order An order issued by the payer, to suspend payment on a check not allowing the bank to disburse the funds. (14)

strabismus Also called crossed eyes. An eye disorder caused by weakness in the external eye muscles, resulting in the eyes looking in different directions. (24, 36)

strain A stretching or tearing injury to a muscle or a tendon. (22)

streak culture A culture in which the specimen is transferred to the culture medium by rubbing the swab across one small area of the agar near the edge, followed by "streaking" through that area onto an unmarked area in a zigzag motion using a sterilized wire inoculating loop, which is done to promote separation of pathogenic colonies from those of normal flora. (41)

stress The body's reaction to the world around it, which can be emotional, intellectual, or physical. (52)

stress test A test to evaluate the response of a patient's heart during moderate exercise on a treadmill, administered following a 12-lead electrocardiogram. (45)

stressor A real or imagined event that causes stress. (52)

stridor Noisy breathing. (37, 39)

stroke Also called cerebrovascular accident (CVA). Result of a clot or hemorrhage in the brain blocking the blood supply and causing brain cells to die from a lack of oxygen. (23)

subcellular Relating to microorganisms comprised of hereditary material (RNA or DNA) with a protein outer coat, such as viruses. (41)

subcutaneous injection Injection given just under the skin in the fat (adipose) tissue, used for small doses of nonirritating medications, frequently in the deltoid muscle but also in the upper back, abdomen, or thigh. (49)

subjective Relating to something believed rather than measured. (34)

subjective, objective, assessment, and plan (SOAP) A system used for charting medical records. (12)

subjective symptoms Complaints that are felt by a patient but are not apparent to observers or measurable. (33)

subscriber The person, also known as a member, who holds an insurance policy (that may include family members) providing medical coverage in return for a fixed monthly fee. (13, 15)

sudoriferous glands Also called sweat glands. Glands that occur in nearly all regions of the skin but are most numerous in the palms and soles. The two types of sweat glands are the apocrine glands and eccrine glands. (20)

superbill (charge/encounter slip) The document generated by the medical office of services for billing and insurance processing and used as a charge slip, statement, and insurance reporting form. (13, 16)

supernatant The liquid portion of a urine sample after it has been separated by a centrifuge. (42)

supination The process of lying supine, or face upward; the process of turning the palm or foot upward. (21)

suppuration The discharge of pus. (46)

surgical asepsis The techniques practiced to maintain a sterile environment in order to prevent microorganisms from entering a body, including sanitization, disinfection, and sterilization. (32)

surgical scheduler The person in the surgery department who sets up and maintains the schedule for surgery and procedures. (8)

surgical scrub An intense and thorough hand hygiene to remove microorganisms before surgery. (38)

susceptible host In a chain of infection, a host who is unable to fight off the pathogen. (32)

swabs Tool used in the collection of specimens. (41)

sweat glands Also called sudoriferous glands. Glands that occur in nearly all regions of the skin but are most numerous in the palms and soles. The two types of sweat glands are the apocrine glands and eccrine glands. (20)

symbol Icon or sign used in the CPT manual to distinguish changes or instructions to be used when coding. (17)

sympathy Feeling sorry or pity for a patient. (4)

synarthrotic joint An articulation, or joint, that produces no movement. (21)

synergist A muscle that acts with another muscle to produce movement. (22)

synthetic Created in a laboratory by artificial means. (48)

system A group of organs that work together to perform a specific function. (19)

systemic lupus erythematosus (SLE) System-wide immune system disorder in which the body produces abnormal antibodies that attack its own tissues rather than foreign organisms. Lupus refers to a type of skin rash and erythematosus means red. (26)

systolic blood pressure Pressure recorded in an artery when the left ventricle contracts. In standard notation it is recorded above the diastolic pressure. (25)

T lymphocytes White blood cells created in the bone marrow and matured in the thymus gland that destroy invading organisms identified by the B lymphocytes. (26)

tachycardia An abnormally fast heartbeat of more than 100 beats per minute. The rhythm may be regular or irregular and may not allow the ventricle of the heart to fill properly, causing a lack of oxygen to the brain and body. (25)

tax withholding Money or amount of salary that is withheld from an employee's payroll check by the employer for the purposes of paying governmental taxes. (14)

telephone triage The telephone screening process for determining the order in which to take patients' calls according to the seriousness of their condition. (6)

Telnet (Telnet Protocol) Facilitates login to a computer host to execute commands. (11)

tendonitis Inflammation and irritation of the tendon, caused by microscopic tearing. (22)

tendons The connective tissue that attaches muscles to bones. (22)

terminal digit filing A medical filing system based on the last digits of the ID number, which evenly distributes files within the entire filing system eliminating the need for frequent reshifting of files. (12)

terminal illness Illness that is expected to lead to death. (52)

tetanus Also called lockjaw. A disease of the nervous system that results from the bacteria *Clostridium tetani* entering through a break in the skin and releasing a toxin that affects the motor nerves, causes fever, and elevates blood pressure. It is characterized by severe, painful muscle spasms. Often fatal. (22, 49)

thesaurus A reference book that provides synonyms or similar meaning words. (10)

third-party check A check written by a party unknown to you. (14)

third-party payer A person or party other than the patient, such as an insurance company, who assumes responsibility for paying the patient's bill. (13)

thready pulse Barely perceptible volume or force in the pulse. (33)

thrombophlebitis Condition that occurs when a blood clot causes inflammation in one or more veins, typically those in the lower extremities. The two types are superficial, in which the affected vein is near the surface of the skin, and deep vein, in which the affected vein lies deep within a muscle. (25)

thrombus A blood clot. (35)

tickler file A small file box organized into the dates that a reminder postcard should be mailed. (8)

tidal volume (VT) The volume of air exchanged with each cycle of breathing (about 500 mL). (39, 45)

time patterns Matrixing off time within an appointment schedule for catch-up time or nonscheduled appointments. (8)

tinnitus A symptom associated with many forms of hearing loss, caused by loud noises, medicines, and health problems, such as allergies, tumors, and problems arising from the cardiovascular system, with severe cases causing the individual difficulty hearing, working, or even sleeping. (24)

tissue A grouping of cells that performs a specialized function. There are four types of tissues in the body: epithelial, connective, muscle, and nerve. (19)

tongue depressor A thin, flat, disposable wooden blade used to press down the tongue to observe the mouth and throat. (34)

total lung capacity (TLC) The volume of the lungs at peak inspiration, equal to the sum of the tidal, expiratory reserve, inspiratory reserve, and residual volumes. (45)

toxic Harmful to the body. (48)

trabeculae Inward-pointing structures that subdivide lymph nodes into different compartments. (26)

transducer An instrument used in ultrasound scanning that has a conduction head that directs sound waves into a body and registers their echoes to visualize internal structures of the body, producing a sonogram, or echogram. (44)

triage The process of sorting or grouping patients according to the seriousness of their condition. (8, 39)

tricuspid valve The heart valve from the right atrium to the right ventricle. (25)

Truth in Lending Act Formerly the Consumer Protection Act of 1968. A federal law affecting credit that was enacted to protect the consumer. (13)

tuberculosis (TB) A contagious disease caused by the bacillus *Mycobacterium tuberculosis,* which can grow anywhere in the body but is most commonly found in the lungs, producing granular tumors in the infected tissues. (27)

tuning fork A metal instrument with two prongs extending from the handle that makes a humming sound when struck, used to test a patient's hearing ability. (34)

turbid Opaque; not allowing light to pass through. (42)

turgor The resistance of the skin when grasped between the fingers. (34)

turn-around time The length of time it takes to perform a test, generate the results, and return them for physician review and addition to the chart. (40)

tympanum The eardrum. (36)

Type A behavior A behavior pattern in which the individual is constantly struggling to achieve, is irritable, hostile, and impatient with anyone who gets in the way, and has a sense of time urgency, believed by some psychologists to be more prone to some diseases such as cancer and heart disease. (52)

Type B behavior A behavior pattern in which the individual is relatively calm. (52)

universal serial bus (USB) A small portable storage device that can hold up to 4Gs of data, also known as jump drive, thumb drive, or flash drive. (11)

ureters Tubes that carry newly formed urine from each kidney down to the bladder, made up of an inner coat of mucous membrane, a middle coat of smooth muscle, and an outer layer of fibrous tissue. (29)

urethra The musculomembranous tube extending from the bladder to the urinary meatus, the external opening of the urinary system. (29)

urethritis Inflammation of the urethra. (31)

urinalysis The testing of urine for the presence of infection or disease, including examining its physical, chemical, and microscopic characteristics, describing its color and appearance, testing it for pH, specific gravity, glucose, bacteria, protein, or chemical elements, and examining the sediment. (42)

urinary bladder The muscular sac, located in the pelvic cavity, that serves as a reservoir for urine and whose wall consists of an inner layer of epithelium, a layer of smooth muscle, an outer layer of longitudinal muscle, and a fibrous layer. (29)

urinary meatus The external opening of the urinary system. (29)

Usenet (Network News Transfer Protocol or NNTP) Distributes Usenet news articles derived from topical discussions on newsgroups. (11)

usual, customary, and reasonable (UCR) The fee charged for medical services that is determined by the physician or the practice's partners as a result of taking into consideration the time and services involved as well as the prevailing rate fee in the community. (13)

uterine cancer Also called endometrial cancer, adenocarcinoma. Cancer that starts in the cells of the lining of the uterus and usually develops in the glandular tissue of the endometrium. (31)

uterine fibroids Benign tumors made up of muscle cells and other tissues that grow within the wall of the uterus, manifesting as a single growth or a cluster. (31)

vaccines Also called immunizations. The injection of inactive (dead) or attenuated (weakened) disease agents into the human body to establish resistance to the diseases they cause. (49)

vaginal speculum An instrument used to hold open the walls of the vagina. (34)

vaginitis An inflammation of the vagina usually caused by a change in the normal balance of vaginal bacteria or by an infection, with the most common types being bacterial, yeast infections, trichomoniasis, and atrophic vaginitis. (31)

value A set of standards a person uses to measure the worth or importance of someone or something. (4)

varicella Also called chicken pox. One of the most common childhood diseases, caused by a virus and spread through the air, which is named for the blisters that arise and that look like chickpeas. (49)

vastus lateralis muscle The muscle on the outer portion of the upper thigh, being part of the quadriceps and lying below the greater trochanter of the femur and within the upper lateral quadrant of the thigh, into which medication is injected, especially in children and small individuals. (49)

vendor Supplier of office supplies and equipment. (9)

venom Poison. (35)

ventricles The two lower pumping chambers of the heart. (25)

ventrogluteal site The gluteus medius muscle injection site, considered to be safer than the dorsogluteal site because of the absence of major nerves or blood vessels there. (49)

verbal communication A wide range of words and sounds or tone of voice that a person uses to convey vastly different meanings. (4)

viable Capable of living. (41)

visual By seeing. (4)

visual acuity Also called 20/20 vision. Normal, clear vision. (36)

vital capacity (VC) The volume of air that can be exhaled following forced inspiration, which includes maximum expiration. (45)

vital signs The pulse, blood pressure, body temperature, and rate, rhythm, and depth of respirations. (33)

voice messaging system A system for messages (voice mail) to be left or recorded when the medical assistant is unavailable to answer the telephone. (6)

void To urinate. (42)

warrant A statement issued to indicate that a debt should be paid, but not actually a negotiable check. (14)

warranty A guarantee in writing from the manufacturer that the product will perform correctly under normal conditions of use. (9)

wart A type of infection caused by viruses in the human papillomavirus (HPV) family that can grow on all parts of the body, including on the skin, inside the mouth, on the genitals, and in the rectal area. (20)

wave On an electrocardiogram printout, deflections away from the baseline,

Akinesia, 418
Albee, George, 1122
Albinism, 356
Albumin, 445
Alcohol, 1116
Aldosterone, 525
Aliquot, 847
Allergens, 465, 660
Allergic reactions, 809, 1037–1038, 1062
Allergies, 465–466, 660–661. *See also* Allergic reactions
   common types of, 660t
   conditions related to, 660
   determining, 805
   to medications, 1037–1038
   to scents, 131
   symptoms of, 660
   tests for, 661–662
Allergy and immunology, 27
Alopecia, 367–368, 367f, 646
Alphabetic filing system, 213–216
   key to, 215
   procedure for filing record in, 216
   rules for, 214t
Alpha-fetoprotein (AFP) test, 692
Alpha-Z system (Smead Manufacturing
   Company), 217, 218t
Alternative therapies, 982
Alveoli, 474, 476–477
   with capillaries, 477f
Alzheimer's disease, 415, 755
   symptoms of, 755–756
   treatment, 756
Amblyopia, 426
Ambulation, 983
Ambulatory surgery, 764
American Academy of Audiology, 719
American Academy of Family Physicians, 1073
American Academy of Pediatrics, 1058, 1073
American Association of Bioanalysts, 841
American Association of Medical Assistants
   (AAMA), 4, 9–10, 1142
   Code of Ethics, 57, 59
   Creed of, 57
   DACUM philosophy (1979), 7
   Role Delineation Study (1997), 7
American Association of Retired Persons, 758
American Banker's Association (ABA), 249
American Board of Medical Specialties (ABMS), 23
American Board of Radiology, 29
American Cancer Society, 135, 685, 941
American College of Rheumatology (ACR), 399
American Diabetes Association, 135, 530–531, 670
American Heart Association, 135, 450, 666, 668
American Hospital Association, 58, 87
American Hospital Formulary Service, 1024
American Medical Association (AMA), 106
   definition of child abuse used by, 745
   depression, defined by, 755
   essential of quality care, 106
   ethical behavior, according to, 57
   handling of unethical behavior by, 57
   Principles of Medical Ethics, 57, 58
American Medical Technologists (AMT), 10, 1142
American Occupational Therapy Association (AOTA), 35

American Psychiatric Association, 1122
American Psychological Association, 1122
American Red Cross, 21
American Registry of Radiologic Technologies, 930
American Society of Clinical Pathologists (ASCP), 37
American Society of Radiologic Technologists, 930
Americans with Disabilities Act (ADA), 160, 633
Ames Color File System, 217
Amniocentesis, 356, 692
Amphiarthrotic joints, 380
Ampules, 1055
   procedure for using, 1055
Amputation, 809–810, 1007
AMT Institute for Education (AMTIE), 10
Amyotrophic lateral sclerosis (ALS), 415
Anaerobes, 853
Anal canal, 494
Analyte, 836
Anaphylactic shock, 660, 661, 1037
Anatomical position, 350, 350f
Anatomy, 342
Androgenetic alopecia, 368
Androgens, 526
Androsterone, 526
Anemia, 444, 747
   causes of, 454
   treatments for, 455
   types of, 454–455
Aneroid sphygmomanometer, 621f, 622
Anesthesia, 20, 784–785
   administering, 785
   general, 784–785
   local, 785, 788t
   recovery from, 786–788
Anesthesiology, 27
Anesthetics, 19
Aneurysms, 455
Angina, 451–452, 666
Angiography, 940
Angioplasty, 452
Answering service, 124
   checking, before opening office, 132
Antagonist, 397
Antecubital space, 907
Anthrax, 19
Anthropometry, 593
Antibiotic resistance, 856
Antibiotics, 859, 1024
   broad-spectrum, 1036
   problem of resistance to, 856
Antibodies, 450, 565, 1072–1073. *See also*
   Autoantibodies; Immunoglobulins
   antigens versus, 464–465
Antidiuretic hormone (ADH), 524
Antigen–antibody reaction, 565, 660
   used as testing tool, 875
Antigens, 446, 565, 660. *See also* Blood types
   versus antibodies, 464–465
   development of, 463
Antrectomy, 505
Anuria, 885
Aorta, 437
   aneurysms of, 455
Apical heart rate, 611–612

Aplastic anemia, 455
Apnea, 613
Apocrine glands, 364f
Aponeurosis, 396
Apothecary notation
  accurately writing, 1012
  Arabic numbers, Roman numerals, and, 1012t
  commonly used equivalents for, 1014t
  comparison of household/metric liquid measurements, 1015t
  conversion list, 1018t
Apothecary system, 1012
Appendicitis, 495, 497
Appendicular skeleton, 378, 383, 384f
Appendix, 449, 494, 495
Application form, 1155–1156
  providing complete and accurate information on, 1156
Application programs, computer, 197
Appointment books, 147–148
  archiving, 148
Appointment cards, 150–151
Appointment scheduling, 144–155
  advance booking, 150–151
  appointment books, 147–148
  appointment cards, 150–151
  building free time block into, 152–153
  double booking patients, 145
  for established patients, 154–155
  exceptions, 151–153
  follow-up, 151
  by grouping procedures, 145
  for hospital admission, 151
    patient information to be supplied when setting up, 152t
  inpatient surgical procedures, 153
  legal and ethical issues related to, 148
  methods, comparison of, 146t
  missed appointments and delays, 149–150
  modified wave scheduling, 145
  for new patients, 154
  for nonpatients, 155
  open office hours system, 145
  outpatient procedures, 151, 153
  patient no-shows, 138, 150
  patient referrals, 151
  patient scheduling process, 148–151
  procedure for, 150
  scheduling surgery, 151
  specified time scheduling, 144
  systems, 146–148
  telephone and e-mail, 153–154
  time estimates for specific office procedures, 149t
  wave scheduling, 145
Aqueduct of Sylvius (cerebral aqueduct), 410
Arabic numbers, 1012
Arachnoid, 409
Archives, 148
Aromatherapy, 1116
Arraignment, 52
Arrhythmia, 452–453, 610, 827
Arteries, 440
  "hardening" of, 451
  system of, 441f
Arteriosclerosis, 451

Arthography, 940
Arthritis, 384–385, 679
Articulation, 380–381. See also Joints
Artificial active immunity, 565, 1073
Artificial breeding, 355
Artificial passive immunity, 565
Ascites, 517
Asepsis
  history of, 562
  importance in urinalysis of, 880
  medical, 570–571
  surgical, 574–580, 582
Aseptic techniques
  causing break in chain of infection, 570–571
  maintaining, 569
  need to adhere to, 562
  practicing good, 575
  surgical. See Surgical asepsis
Asphyxia, 810
Assertive behavior, 75
  comparison of aggressive and, 75t
  guidelines, 76
  techniques, 75–76
Assessment, patient, 72
Assignment of benefits, 291
  form, 231
Assisted-living facility, 33
Associate practice, 27
Association of Surgical Technologists, 768
Associative neurons, 407
Asthma, 479, 744
Astigmatism, 426, 708
Atherosclerosis, 419, 451, 666
Atmospheric pressure, 478
Atoms, 342
ATP (adenosine triphosphate), 396
Atria, 436, 956
Atrioventricular bundle, 438, 439
Atrioventricular node, 438, 956
Atrophy, 399, 985
Attention deficit hyperactivity disorder (ADHD), 356
Attitudes, 66
  conveying positive, 71
Audiograms, 81, 720
Audiologists, 81, 719
Audiology, 430
Audiometer, 717–719, 718f, 720
Audiometric testing, 81
Audiometry, 722
  assisting with, 725
Auditory canal (auditory meatus), 428
Auditory learners, 68
Audits, 265
Auricle (pinna), 428
Ausculatory gap, 618
Auscultation, 639
Authoritarian leaders, 322
Autism, 745
Autoantibodies, 469
Autoclave, 578–580, 579f, 841
  drying process after use of, 580
Autoclaving, 579–580
  procedure for wrapping instruments for, 581

Autoimmune diseases, 462, 528
Automated assistance program, 122–123
Automated external defibrillator, 816, 816f
Autonomic nerves, 411
Autonomic nervous system (ANS), 414–415
Autopsies, 19
Axial plane (transverse plane), 350
Axial skeleton, 378, 381–383, 381f
Axons, 407
    neuron with two converging, 407f
AZT, 22

B

Baby boomers, 749–750
Bacilli, 856
    gram-negative, 856–857
    gram-positive, 857
    vibrios, 857
Bacteria, 17, 19, 563, 854, 856–858
    ability of, to hemolyze, 853
    aerobic and anaerobic, 563
    antigens and, 463
    causing cellulitis, 368
    cells that fight off, 464
    conditions required for growth of, 563t
    dye retention and, 853
    special categories of, 858
    in urine, 894
    use of oxygen to categorize, 853
Bacteriology, 19–20, 563
BAC-T Screen Bacteruria-Pyuria Detection Device, 865
Bacturia, 889
Balance, 236
Bandages, 791, 828
    procedure for applying, over sterile dressings, 795
    types of, 794f
Bandwidth, 195
Bank drafts, 251
Banking
    accepting cash, 257
    bill paying, 254–255
    cash disbursement, 258
    checks, 249–254
    deposits, 256–257
    function of, 248
    hold on accounts, 258
    legal and ethical issues related to, 260
    online, 248
    procedures, saving documentation relating to, 259–260
    statements, 258–259
    types of bank accounts, 248
Bankruptcy, 234
Bank statements
    credits and debits on, 258
    procedure for reconciling, 259
    reconciliation of, 258–259
Barium sulfate, 931
Barnard, Christian, 22
Barrett's esophagitis, 501
Barton, Clara, 21
Basal cell carcinomas, 364
Basal metabolic rate (BMR), 524
Basal metabolism, 626

Basophils, 903
Bathrooms, medical office, 163
Battery, 49
B-cell lymphocytes, 463
Bedsores, 662
Behavior, 66
    assertive versus aggressive, 75
    defensive, 77
    exhibiting negative, 68
    heredity and environmental and cultural
        influences on, 1127
    interpersonal skills and human, 1128–1129
    patterns, dealing with wide scope of, 83
Bell, Charles, 415
Bell's palsy, 415
Benefit period, 270, 286
Benign prostatic hyperplasia (BPH), 554–555, 555f
Better Business Bureau, 235
Bias, 79–80, 1127
Bicuspid valve, 437
Bile, 494, 495
Bilirubin, 889
Billing, 229–231
    computerized, 230–231
    credit policy, 231–232
    ledger cards, 229–230
    manual, 230
    methods, 229
    period: frequency, 231
    superbill/encounter form, 229
    third-party payers and minors, 231
Bill paying, 254–255
Bioequivalency, 1024
Biofeedback, 982, 1116
Biohazards, 1048. *See also* Hazardous medical waste
    definition of, 98
Biomedical equipment technician, 38
Biopsy, 547, 663, 794
    breast, 941
    endometrial, 796
Bioterrorism, 585–586, 857
Bipolar disorder, 1122
Birth defects, 356
Births, reports of, 53t
Bites
    nonvenomous, 811
    venomous, 810–811
Black death, 17
Black plague, 17
Blackwell, Elizabeth, 21
Bladder, 512
Bland diet, 1112
Bleeding
    from both nostrils, 822
    controlling, 827, 828
        procedure for, 829
    severe, 811–812
Blind ad, 1151
Blindness, 82, 716
Block letter style format, 180–181, 182f
Blood, 442–443
    circulation of, through heart, 618f
    composition of, 443–445
    defenses in, 445

delivery of oxygen to, 474
flow through heart, 436–437, 437f
formation and components
  cellular, 902–903
  liquid, 903
formed elements of, 445f
function of, 903–904
functions of, 445–446
occult
  in stool, 872–873
  in urine, 889
regulation of body temperature by, 445–446
specimen collection, procedure for quality control for, 904
study of. *See* Hematology
transportation, 445
volume, regulation of, 510
Bloodborne pathogens, 569
Bloodborne Pathogens Standard, 100–101, 838, 839, 1048
Blood clots, 484
Blood pressure, 440–442
average normal readings for, 619t
causes of error in measurements of, 623
equipment for measuring, 620–622
factors affecting, 619–620
high and low, 458
importance of measurement of, 616
measuring, 622
new guidelines for, 619, 619t
physiological factors affecting, 620t
physiology of, 616–617
procedure for measuring, 625
readings, 617
  causes of error in, 626t
  terms related to abnormal, 621t
urinary system and, 510–511
variations, causes of, 620t
Blood types, 446–449
cross-reactions and, 446f
type A, 446
type AB, 447
type B, 447
type O, 447
Blood vessels, 439–440
Blue Cross/Blue Shield, 274
claim forms, 286
B lymphocytes, 464
Body fat measurement, 626–627
Body fluids, 566
Body language, 70, 72
using positive, 75
Body lice, 371
Body mass index (BMI), 627, 740
formula for calculating, 744
Body mechanics, 102
principles of proper, 103t–104t
Body, of letter, 179
Body surface area (BSA), 1019–1020
Body temperature, 596
axillary
  assessing, 606
  procedure for measuring, 609
factors affecting, 597t
normal values, 598–599
  and terms for, 596–598

physiology of, 596
selecting method for measuring, 599t
sites for measuring, 598–599
  aural, 598
  axillary, 598
  oral, 598
  rectal, 598–599
Bone marrow, 449
effect of aging on, 462
formation of blood cells in, 443
lymphocytes in, 464
malignant cancer of, 455. *See also* Leukemia
Bones
classification of, 378–380, 379f
functions of, 379
of lower extremities, 383, 384f
markings of, 380, 380t
structure of long, 380
of upper extremities, 383, 384f
Bookkeeping
double-entry, 237–238
guidelines for manual, 235
patient accounts, 236
single-entry, 237
Bookkeeping systems, 237–243
double-entry bookkeeping, 237–238
pegboard system, 238–243
single-entry bookkeeping, 237
Botulism, 857
Bounding pulse, 610
Bowman's capsule, 511, 512
Braces, 1003
Bradycardia, 452, 606, 669
Bradykinesia, 418
Bradypnea, 613
Brain, 409–411
brainstem, 411
cerebrum, 409
cortex and ventricles of, 409–410
diencephalon, 410–411
effect of aging on, 408
lateral view of, 410f
pituitary gland and relation to, 523f
relationship of 12 cranial nerves to specific
  regions of, 412f
tracts in, 408
Brain scans (CT scans), 416
Brainstem, 409, 410, 411
Brainstem auditory evoked response (BAER), 1008
Brand name drugs, 1024
Brand names, 1024
BRAT diet, 1112
Breach of confidentiality, 295
Breach of contract, 45–46
Breast cancer, 544, 546–547, 685
Breasts, 541
biopsy of, 941
examination of, 685
  demonstrations of correct procedures for self-, 687f
  procedure for instructing patient on self-, 686
Breathing, 476, 613
bubbling, 616
Cheyne-Stokes, 616
deep, for relaxation, 1116

Breathing (*continued*)
emergencies, 812–814
exercises, 753
providing educational materials on, 964
mechanism of, 478
nervous system and, 613
pressure measurements related to, 478
rate of, in children, 613–614
respiratory quality, 616
respiratory volumes and capacities, 478–479
rhythm, 615
sounds, 616
Brochures
creating community resource, 1082
creating public relations, 1083
developing, before externship, 1113
Bronchi, 476–477
Bronchioles, 474, 476
Bronchiolitis, 743
Bronchitis, 479–480
Bubbling breathing, 616
Bubonic plague, 17
Bucky, 948
Bulbourethral glands, 544
Bundle of His, 438, 439, 956
Bureaucratic leaders, 322
Burnout, 68
Burns, 373–374, 814
classification of, 814–815, 815t
considerations for determining seriousness of, 815
Rule of Nines, 373–374, 373f, 814–815, 814f
Bursitis, 385
Business letters
body of, 179
closing of, 179
copy notation, 179
date, 178
enclosure notation, 179
guidelines for using courtesy titles, 179
headings, 178
inside address, 178
procedure for composing, 180
reference initials, 179
salutation, 179
standard components of, 178–179

C

Cadavers, 17
Caduceus, 16, 17f
Calcitonin, 524
Calibration, 841
Calorie content diet, 1113
Calories, 1109–1110
in food, determining number of, 1110
supplied by fat, determining percentage of, 1110
Cancellous bone, 380
Cancer, 467
breast, 544, 546–547, 685
causes and treatment of, 467
cervical, 547
colon, 498
endometrial, 552–553, 796
and immune system, 467

lung, 483
oral, 502–503
ovarian, 549
pancreatic, 503–504
prostate, 556, 700
skin, 364–365
uterine, 552–553
Canes, 1000, 1002
procedure for instructing patient on use of, 1003
Canthus, 424
Capillaries, 440, 444f, 476, 908
alveoli with, 477f
Capillary puncture (manual), 908
equipment and supplies, 909
procedure for performing, 915
sites, 908–909
Capital equipment, 163
Capitalization, rules for, 177
Carbohydrates, 1101–1102
Carbon dioxide
exhalation of, 474
removal of, 474
transfer, 477f
Carcinogens, 467
Carcinoma in situ, 688
Cardiac arrest, 815–815
Cardiac cycle, 439, 956–957
phases of, 439
time and, 958
Cardiac muscles, 396, 438
Cardiology, 27, 663
Cardiomegaly, 533
Cardiopulmonary resuscitation (CPR), 137–138, 452, 816
procedure for administering adult, 818–819
rates and ratios: adult versus pediatric, 817t
Cardiovascular disease. *See also* Heart disease
symptoms of, 664
Cardiovascular system, 663–664, 666, 668–669. *See also* Circulatory system
disorders of, 456t–457t
effect of aging on, 680, 753–754
procedures and diagnostic tests relating to, 667t–668t
Carditis, 453
Career opportunities
in health care field, 33–34. *See also specific positions*
for medical assistants, 10–11
medical transcription, 222, 223
for orthotists, 980
in physical medicine, 981t
for prosthetists, 980
Carpal tunnel syndrome, 386–387
Cash disbursement, 258
Cashier's checks, 251
Casts, 894, 1003
care of, 1004–1005, 1093
checking edges of, 1005f
problems caused by, 1092
putting on, 1091–1093
removing, 1093
types of, 1092
Cataracts, 426
Catheterization, 883
cardiac, 940
CAT scans. *See* CT scans

Cauda equine, 411
Cautery, 791
Cavities, 351, 353, 353f
CDC. *See* Centers for Disease Control and Prevention (CDC)
CD-ROM, 196
Cecum, 494
Cell membrane, 345
Cell phones, 118
Cells, 344–347
    cancer, 467. *See also* Cancer
    cell membrane, 345
    chemistry and, 354–355
    cytoplasm, 345–346
    eukaryotic, 853
    of islets of Langerhans, 525
    in lungs, 477
    major parts of, and structures inside, 345f
    muscle fibers, 394. *See also* Muscles; Muscular system
    nucleus, 345, 346
    phagocytic, 463. *See also* Macrophages
    prokaryotic, 853
    that may be found in urine, 892–894
    types of blood, 442
Cellulitis, 368, 368f, 662
Celsius (C) scale, 599
Centers for Disease Control and Prevention (CDC), 550–551, 837
    influenza vaccination recommendations of, 1073
    isolation guidelines issued by, 565–566
    purpose of, 38
    Standard Precautions, 566, 1048
    Universal Precautions, 101, 220
Centers for Medicare and Medicaid Services (CMS), 229, 838
    Web site, 311
Central lymphoid tissue, 462
Central nervous system (CNS), 408–411, 409f
    nerves in, 407
Central processing unit (CPU), 195
Centrifuge, 841
Centrioles, 346
Cerebellum, 411
Cerebral aqueduct, 410
Cerebral hemispheres, 409
Cerebral palsy, 747
Cerebrospinal fluid, 411, 684, 875
    removal of some, for myelogram, 940
Cerebrovascular accident (CVA), 419, 455, 668, 679–680, 816–817
    symptoms of, 684
Cerebrovascular disease, 679–680, 684
Cerebrum, 409
    lobes of, 409
Certificate of Waiver tests (WTs), 838
Certification, 9
    for health care professionals, 33
    medical assistants and, 55
Certified checks, 251
Certified laboratory scientist (CLS), 37
Certified medical assistant (CMA), 9, 837
Certified medical assistant (CMA) examination
    major areas tested on, 1145t
    preparing for, 1145

Certified medical technologist (CMT), 37
Certified nursing assistant (CNA), 34–35
Certified ophthalmic assistant (COA), 719
Certified registered nurse anesthesiologist (CRNA), 27
Certified respiratory therapy technician (CRTT), 35
Cerumen, 430, 719
Cervical cancer, 547
Cervicitis, 547–54
Cervix, 538
Cesarean section (C-section), 695
CHAMPVA (Civilian Health and Medical Program of the Veterans Administration), 270, 275
Character, 66
Charge slips, 135–136, 229
Charting
    guidelines, 655
    medications, 1077
    six Cs of, 594
    SOAP, 208, 209f, 651–653, 654t
Checks, 249–254
    ABA number on, 249
    accepting, 252–253
    advantages of, 249
    canceled, 258
    completing check stubs, 253
    correctly written, 252f
    endorsement of, 253, 254f
    errors in writing, 252
    mailing, 253
    MICR on, 249–250
    payroll, 261
    procedure for posting non-sufficient funds, 255
    procedure for preparing, 250
    returned, 254
    third-party, 252
    types of, 249, 251
    write-it-once system, 250–252
    writing, 250
    written by agents, 253
Chemical hazards, 98, 838–839
Chemical waste, 99
Chemotherapy, 19–20, 467, 483, 547, 556, 663
Chest pain, 817, 820
Cheyne-Stokes breathing, 616
Chickenpox, 1075
Chief complaint, 592
    determining, 803–804
    warranting prompt attention, 804
Child abuse, 745
    reports of, 53t
Child Abuse Prevention and Treatment Act, 745
Childbirth, 692
    dangers of 19th century, 19
    emergency, 810
Childhood, 1125
Children. *See also* Minors
    abuse of, 53f, 745
    additional assistance for, 632
    administering medications to, 1038
    bones in, 379
    calculating pediatric dosages, 1018–1020
    careful calculations regarding medication dosing for, 1016
    circulatory system development in, 438

Children (*continued*)
consideration of, in medical offices, 161
CPR techniques for, 816
dehydration in, 513, 744
developmental checklist for, birth to five years, 735t
digestive system and, 495
dosage of medication prescribed for, 1013
drinking bottles, proper angle for, 429
ECGs and PFTs for, 957
endocrine system in, 526
failure to thrive (FTT), 734
gaining confidence of, 732
gastrointestinal disorders affecting, 744
giving injections to, 1054
growth charts for, 740
growth of, 733–734
hearing and vision evaluations for, 740–741
hot or cold modalities for, 988
immune response in, 462
infectious diseases affecting, 746–747
inherited or birth-related disorders, 747
lawsuits on behalf of, 48
measuring weight of, 738
muscular development in, 395
needing help during x-ray procedures, 933
nervous system in, 408
normal values from birth to adolescence, 738t
otitis media, 718
otitis media in, 429
pediatric diseases and disorders, 743–747. *See also
specific diseases and disorders*
prescriptions to be kept at school for, 480
procedure for performing Snellen eye chart exam on, 741
procedure for responding to obstructed airway in, 808
rate of breathing in, 613–614
in reception area, 137
reproductive system in, 540
requiring additional accommodations, 722
respiratory system in, 477
safety of, 759
skin conditions in, 365
taking vital signs of, 734, 738
toys and books for, in reception area, 162
Chime, 493
Chiropractors, 24, 678
Cholecystogram, 939–940
Cholelithiasis, 494
Cholera, 19, 857
Cholesterol, 450, 1108–1109
Choroid plexus, 411
Choroids, 424
Christian Scientists, 51
Chromosomes, 346
Chronic fatigue syndrome (CFS), 468
Chronic obstructive pulmonary disease (COPD), 479,
615–616
Chronic pain, 624
Chronic renal failure, 517, 700, 702–703
Chronological record, 651
Cilia
in bronchial tubes, 477
in cells, 346
in lungs, 477
in nose, 474

Circulatory system, 435–458. *See also* Cardiovascular
system; Lymphatic system
blood, 442–446
blood vessels, 439–440
common disorders associated with, 450–458. *See also
specific disorders*
lymphatic system, 449–450
overview of, 436
pulmonary and systemic circulation, 442, 444f
Circumcision, 543
Circumduction, 381
Cirrhosis, 497–498
Civil law, 44–46
contract law, 45–46
tort law, 44–45
Civil War, United States, 21
Claims
clean, 290
denied, 290
dirty, 290
Electronic Media Claims (EMC), 289
forms, 290
invalid, 290
paper, 289
processing, 290–291, 294–295
security, 295
status of insurance, 290
types of submission for, 289
Clarification, 74–75
Clark's rule, 1018
Claustrophobia, 944
Clear liquid diet, 1111
Cleft palate, 356
Clinical area, of medical office, 160
Clinical diagnosis, 590
Clinical laboratories
departments in, 836
equipment, 841–841
maintenance of, 841
measurements and, 842–845
guidelines for safety in, 840
hazards, 838
measuring devices employed in, 844–845
medical assistant's role in, 837
and patient communication, 845–847
personnel, 837
quality assurance in, 839–840
quality control programs in, 840–841
request information, 860–862
requisitions, 845
information on, 845
sample slip for, 846f
role of, in patient care, 836
safety regulations, 837–838
temperatures associated with environment in, 843, 844t
time in, 842–843
types of, 836
units of measurement, 844
Clinical laboratory assistant (CLA), 837
Clinical Laboratory Improvement Act (CLIA), 109
Clinical Laboratory Improvement Amendments
(CLIA), 109
categories and explanation under, 109t
enactment of, 838

proficiency testing, under standards of, 841
  waived tests, 838
Clinical laboratory scientist (CLS), 37, 837
Clinical laboratory technician (CLT), 37
Clitoris, 541
Clock speed, 195
Cloning, 22
Closed-ended questions, 73
Closed fracture, 387, 824
Closed records, 213
Closing, in correspondence, 179
Clots, 444
Cluster headaches, 417
CMS-1500, 277, 286, 290
  completed, 293f
  example of, 288f
  procedure for completing, 291–292
  requirement of use of, for Medicare billing, 300
Coagulation, 444, 445
  defined, 446
Cobalt treatment. See Radiation therapy
Cocci, 854, 856
Cochlea, 428, 429f
Code of Ethics (AAMA), 57, 59
Code of Hammurabi, 16, 56
Codes of ethics, 54
Cognitive ability, 751–752, 754
Coitus interruptus, 695
Cold, 1122
  applications, 993
  compress, procedure for application of, 993
  to distract brain from pain, 1116
  procedure for application of cold chemical pack, 995
  procedure for application of ice bag, 994
Colic, 672, 744
Colitis, 498
Collating records, 132, 133
  procedure for, 133
Collect calls, 123
Collections, 46, 232–235
  aging accounts receivable, 233
  bankruptcy, 234
  claims against estates, 234–235
  credit policy and, 231–232
  delinquent accounts, 233
  guidelines for, 232
  laws governing, 47t
  letters, 234
  making, guidelines for, 233
  process, 232–233
  regulations pertaining to, 233–234
  special problems, 234
  statute of limitations, 235
  techniques, 233
  telephone, 234
  using agency for, 235
College of American Pathologists (CAP), 837, 841
Colles's fracture, 388
Collimeter, 950
Colon, 494f
  with diverticulosis, 500f
Colon cancer, 498
Colonoscopy, 677
Colony, 854

Color blindness, 711–712
Color-coded filing systems, 217–218
  Alpha-Z alphabetic, 218t
  numerical, 218t
Color deficiency, 356
Colorectal cancers, 498
Colposcopy, 794
Comminuted fracture, 388
Commission on Accreditation of Allied Health Education
  Programs (CAAHEP), 5, 9, 10, 768, 1142
Common cold, 481, 743
Communication
  barriers to, 76–77
  channels of, 69, 69f
    information richness, 69t
  clinical laboratory and patient, 845–847
  directive, techniques, 73–75, 74t
  effective, 590–591
  importance of, 66
  as indicator of oxygenation in brain, 813
  between insurance companies and medical care
    providers, 277
  intraoffice, 84–85
  as key to managing efficient office, 322
  levels, 813t
  messages conveying impatience, 70
  nonverbal, 72, 1128
  with other health care workers, improving, 719
  patient, 1083
  patient education and, 89–90
  procedure for effective, with the elderly, 757
  process, 68
  by sign language, 81
  in special circumstances, 80–84
  with superiors, 87
  techniques, 72–75
  verbal, 70–71, 1128
  written, 172–181, 188–189, 1128–1129
Communications clerk, 38
Compact bone, 380
Complement, 464
Complete decongestive therapy (CDT), 469
Compliance plans, 311–312
Compliance, wellness and, 90
Compound fracture, 387
Compound microscope, 841
  with parts labeled, 842f
Compression fracture, 388
Computed tomography (CT). See CT scans
Computerized systems, for accounting, 243
Computers
  billing on, 230–231
  CD-ROM, 196
  components of, 194–198, 196t
  drives, 196
  and ergonomics, 202
  hardware, software, and storage components, 195t
  keyboard, 196–197
  in medicine, use of, 194
  memory, 195
  monitor, 195
  mouse, 197
  patient information stored on, 231
  for payroll duties, 261

Computers (*continued*)
  printers, 197
  removable disk drive, 196
  security for, 198–199
  selecting, 199
  software, 176t, 194, 197
  terms frequently used for, 200t
  types of, 194
Condescension, avoiding, 77, 84
Conduction hearing loss, 719
Conductive hearing loss, 430
Conference calls, 123
  placing, 124
Confidentiality, 8, 59–60, 87–89
  according to Medical Patients Rights Act, 59
  appointment book and, 147–148
  HIPAA rules pertaining to, 59, 198, 202. *See also* Health Insurance Portability and Accountability Act (HIPAA)
  importance of, to office manager, 328
  and the law, 49
  legal and ethical issues for, 222
  medical assistants and, 55
  minors and, 51
  as moral and ethical obligation, 904
  of patient information, safeguarding, 590
  regarding financial information of patients, 231
  when using fax transmissions, 52
Conflict resolution, 85
  steps in, 86
Confusion, 754–755
Congenital disorders, 356
Congestive heart failure (CHF), 452, 666
Conjunctiva, 425
Conjunctivitis, 426
Connective tissue, 347
Consent forms, 49, 211–212
  needed for billing, 229
Consideration, defined, 45
Constipation, 495, 498–499
Consultation report, 212
Contact dermatitis, 368
Contact lenses, 708
Contact Precautions, 568
Contaminants, in urine, 894
Continuing education units (CEUs), 9
Continuous infusion, 1071
Contraception, 695
Contraceptive methods, 695
  barrier methods, 695
  coitus interruptus, 695
  hormonal methods, 695
  intrauterine devices, 695
  natural family planning, 695
Contract law, 44, 45–46
Contracts, 45, 166
  premature termination of physician-patient, 46
  termination of, 46
Contracture, 985
Contrast medium, 931
  radiologic imaging procedures requiring, 936, 938–940
Contrast sensitivity, 713
Contributory negligence, 45
Controlled drugs, 54
  storage of, 54

Controlled substances, 54, 1025–1026, 1028.
  See also Narcotics
  common, 1028
  schedule for, 1026t
Controlled Substances Act (1970), 54, 1024, 1026
Control samples, 840
Conversion
  list, 1018t
  within metric system, guidelines for, 1014
  rules for, 1017–1018
Convolutions, in brain, 409
Convulsions, 820–821
Co-payments, 131, 135, 229, 274
COPD. *See* Chronic obstructive pulmonary disease (COPD)
Coping mechanisms, 77, 80
Copy notation, in correspondence, 179
Cornea, 424, 708
  lesions or abrasions to, 427
Corneal abrasion, 427
Coronal plane (frontal plane), 350
Coronary artery blockage, 669
Coronary artery bypass graft (CABG), 452
Coronary artery disease (CAD), 450, 666
Coronary heart disease (CHD), 450–451
Coronary occlusion, 451
Coronary thrombosis, 451
Coronavirus, 484
Corpus callosum, 408, 409
Cortex
  adrenal, 525–526
  of brain, 409–410
  of kidney, 511
  of lymph node, 463
Corticosterone, 525
Corticotropin-releasing factor (CRF), 522
Cortisol, 523, 525
Court testimony, 52
  pointers for, 52
Cover letter, 1151
  example of, 1152f
  procedure for preparing, 1153
Cowper's glands, 544
Crab lice, 371
Crackles, 616
Cranial cavity, 353
Cranial nerves, 411–414
  12 pairs of, 413t
Craniosacral therapy, 982
Crash cart, 806, 806f
Credit, 236
Credit policy, 231–232
Creed of the American Association of Medical Assistants (AAMA), 57
Cretinism, 524
Crimean War, 21
Criminal law, 44
Critical thinking, 85
  elements of, 86
Crohn's disease, 499
Crossover claims, 275, 286
Cross-referencing, of files, 218
Croup, 743
Crust, 663f

Crutches, 997
  crutch and walking gaits, 998–999
  instructing patient to use single crutch correctly, 1003
  measuring for axillary, 998
  procedure for instructing patient on correct use of, 1001
  sitting with, 999–1000
  standing with, 1000
Cryosurgery, 795–796
Cryotherapy, 663
Crystals, in urine, 894
CT scans, 942–943
  preparation for, 943
Cultural considerations, 78–79
  addressing issues of diabetes, 530
  alternative medical treatments and, 982
  assumptions regarding curative measures, 547
  attitudes toward tobacco smoking, 481
  beliefs about aging and family role of elders, 749
  creating patient education materials, 1088
  dietary habits, 449, 1109
  discussion of bodily functions, 872
  during examinations, 634
  explaining community resources to diverse client population, 26
  explaining tests to patients, 908
  eye contact and, 134
  family participation in medical situations, 809
  having understanding of instructions when taking medications, 1025
  HIV-positive patients, 584
  modesty requirements, 516
  noting patient's cultural and ethnic background, 211
  pain and, 626
  patient's rights and need for modesty, 369
  patients who speak little English, 1127
  personal beliefs influenced by, 8
  procedures requiring disrobing and, 933
  protecting privacy while doing ECG, 966
  psychological implications of some immune system diseases and, 465
  religious practices, 51
  respecting individuality, in communication, 79
  responses of patients to prescriptions, 1017
  risk factors for osteoporosis, 389
  role of diet, and disorders of digestive system, 503
  role of, regarding exercise and holistic health, 399
  sensitivities to discussing specimens related to elimination, 884
  stereotypes about neurological diseases, 418
  terminal illness and, 1135
  urine samples and, 836
  use of interpreters, 354
  variation of viewpoints on drug administration, 1070
  when fielding calls in medical office, 121
Culture
  defined, 853
  inoculating, 863
  procedure for obtaining sputum specimen for, 871
  procedure for performing urine, 872
  stool, 872
  streak, 864
Culture media, 853, 863–864
  classifications of, 864
  and isolates, 864t

Culturette system, 862
Curie, Marie, 20
Curie, Pierre, 20
Current Procedural Terminology (CPT) manual, 243, 305, 307f
  codes for Evaluation and Management (E/M), 307
  examples of sections and codes, 308t
  getting to know, 305, 307
  medical coding, 308
  modifier page from, 309f
  organization of, 307
  symbols, 308
  use of modifiers in, 308
Cushing's disease, 530, 531f
Customer service, 335
Cyanosis, 483, 615
  caused by allergic reactions, 661
Cycle billing, 231
Cycle time, 144, 161
Cystic fibrosis (CF), 356, 481–482
Cystitis, 513–514
Cysts, 516
Cytokinesis, 346, 347
Cytologist, 687, 688
Cytoplasm, 345–346
Cytoplasmic streaming, 345–346
Cytosol. *See* Cytoplasm

D

Damages, 45
Database, in POMR, 651
Date, in correspondence, 178
Day sheets, 238
  balancing, 241, 242t
  sections, 239t
Deafness, 430
Death. *See also* Terminal illness
  dealing with, 82
  reports of, 53t
DeBakey, Michael, 22
Debit, 236
Debridement, 773
Decibels, 720
Deciduous teeth, 491, 492f
  eruption of, 493
Decision making, patient, 89
Decubitus ulcers, 368–369, 662
  four stages of, 369
Deductibles, Medicare, 274
Deductions, 229
Defamation of character, 48–49
  libel, 49
  slander, 49
Defendants, 45
Defense mechanisms, 1131–1132, 1133t–1134t
Defensive behaviors, 77
Defibrillation, 452
Degenerative joint disease (DJD), 679
Dehiscence, 788
Dehydration
  in elderly, 753
  in infants, signs of, 744
Delinquent accounts, 233

Deltoid muscle, 1057–1058
Delusion, 1122
Dementia, 684
    accommodating patients suffering from, 722
    patient in the office, 756
    symptoms of, 755
    treatment, 756
Democratic leaders, 322
Demographic information, 135
Dendrites, 407
Dental hygienists, 36
Dental insurance, 276
Department of Health and Human Services (HHS), 220
Deposition, 52
Deposits, 256–257
    completing deposit slips, 257
    making, 257
    procedure for preparing deposit slip, 256
    to savings accounts, 257
Depression, 755, 1122
Dereliction of, 45
Dermatology, 27–28, 662. See also Integumentary
        system; Skin
    common skin disorders, 662
    dermatological neoplasms, 662–663, 664t
Dermis, 363
    touch originating in, 431
Desensitizing injections, 661
Diabetes, 517
Diabetes mellitus, 526, 530–531, 670
    in elderly, 754
    and impact of ability to heal, 751
    types of, 670
Diabetic coma, 821
Diabetic diet, 1112
Diagnosis, 590
    of disease, importance of x-rays to, 930
    facilitating comprehension of patient's, 699
Diagnosis and treatment plan, 212
Diagnosis-related groups (DRGs), 26, 280
Diagnostic and Statistical Manual of Mental Disorders
    (DSM-IV-TSR), 1122
Diagnostic imaging, 678, 931
    procedures, 936–945. See also specific procedures
        and conditions diagnosed/treated, 937t
Diagnostic imaging technicians, 37
Diagnostic tests, 645, 646t
    evaluations performed by, 1007
    relating to cardiovascular system, 667t–668t
    relating to digestive system, 673t–674t
    relating to endocrine system, 671t
    relating to female reproductive system, 693t–694t
    relating to integumentary system, 665t
    relating to lymphatic system, 677t
    relating to male reproductive system, 697t
    relating to musculoskeletal system, 681t–682t
    relating to nervous system, 683t
    relating to the ear, 726
    relating to the eye, 713t–714t
    relating to urinary system, 701t–702t
Dialysis, 517–518, 703
Diaphoresis, 664
Diaphragm, 351, 474, 612
Diaphysis, 380

Diarrhea, 499, 744
Diarthrotic joints, 380
Diastolic blood pressure, 442, 526
Diathermy, 994–995
Diencephalon, 409, 410–411
Dietary guidelines, 1111
    modifications of, 1111–1113
Dieticians, 35–36
Dietitians, 1099
Differential diagnosis, 590
Differential white blood cell count, 919, 921
Diffusion, 355
Digestion, 490, 1099–1101
    accessory organs of, 494–495
    elimination of waste products of, 494
    organs of, 490f
    in small intestine, 493
Digestive system, 489–505, 490f, 672–677, 1101f.
        See also Gastrointestinal system
    common disorders associated with, 495–505. See also
        specific disorders
    disorders and pathology of, 496t–497t
    effect of aging on, 680, 753
    main functions of, 490
    organs of, 491–494
    procedures and diagnostic tests relating to, 673t–674t
Digital radiology, 944
Dilation, 810
Diluent, 845
Dilutions, 845
Diphtheria, 20, 1073
Diplococci, 856
Direct cause, 45
Direct Distance Dialing (DDD), 123
Disabilities, 716, 717, 721, 1002–1003, 1004, 1006
    teaching patients with, 1089
Disability insurance, 275–276
Disaster plans, 96–97
Disasters
    guidelines for handling, 97
    in medical offices, 96–97
Discharge summary, 212
Discipline, 329–330
Discretion, of medical assistants, 8
Diseases. See also Illness
    autoimmune. See Autoimmune diseases
    caused by contaminated food and water, 19
    caused by microorganisms, 19
    and conditions making use of rehabilitation, 982
    genetic, 399–400. See also Genetic disorders
    genetics, heredity, and, 356–358
    importance of x-rays to diagnosis of, 930
    from infected animal hair, hides, or waste, 19
    pathogenic microorganisms and resulting, 860t
    pulmonary, 975–976
    related to poor nutrition, 1098, 1100
    reportable communicable, 53t
    that mainly affect elderly, 752t
    upper respiratory system, 743–744
Disinfection, 19, 575–577
Dislocations, 388–389
Distance acuity, 709, 711
    procedure for checking child's, 741

Disturbances, managing, 137
Diverticular disease, 675
Diverticulitis, 500, 675
Diverticulosis, 500, 675
DNA (deoxyribonucleic acid), 345, 346
  fingerprinting, 355–356
DNA testing, 23
Doctor of osteopathy (DO), 24
Documentation, 841
  correct, 593
  of failed appointments, 138
  importance of appropriate, 89
  incidents needing certified letter, 46
  legal importance of, 52, 346, 617
  medical assistants and, 55
  of patient medical information, 651–654
Domestic violence, 688
Donning, 578
Do not resuscitate (DNR) orders, 757–758
Dopamine, 526
Dorsal cavity, 351
Dorsal recumbent position, 642f, 644
Dorsiflexion, 381
Dorsogluteal muscle, 1058–1059
Dosimeter, 947
Dot matrix printers, 197
Double booking, 145
Down syndrome (trisomy 21), 356
Drapes, 641, 643, 784
Draping, 784
Dressing, 827–828
Drives, computer, 196
Droplet Precautions, 568
Drug abuse, 1028–1029
  defined, 1028
  reports of, 53t
  steps to be taken for suspicion of, 1028–1029
  types of drugs associated with, 1029t
Drug administration. *See also* Medication administration
  nonparenteral methods for, 1035t
  oral method, 1033–1034
  parenteral, 1034–1035
    methods for, 1034t
  routes of, 1035t
    methods and, 1033–1035
  sublingual, 1034
Drug dependency, 1028–1029
Drug Enforcement Administration (DEA), 53, 54, 1024
Drug regulations, 53–54
  medical assistants and, 55
Drugs. *See also* Medications
  breast-feeding mothers and, 1038
  calculations for, 1013–1016
  chemotherapy, 1024
  classification of
    names and descriptions, 1029t–1031t
    by type or usage with examples, 1032t–1033t
  coding use of, 303
  controlled, 54
  fifty most frequently administered, 1036t
  given prophylactically, 1024
  injectable, commonly in stock in medical offices, 1027t
  interactions and, 1037–1038
  legal classification of, 1025–1026, 1028

names of, 1024
  pregnancy and, 1038
  regulation and standards for, 1024
  resource references for, 1024–1025
  sublingual, 1034
  synthetic, 1024
  for treatment of mental disorders, 1124
  types of, commonly abused, 1029t
Drug samples, 167
DTaP vaccine, 1075
Ductus deferens, 544
Duodenum, 493, 527
Durable power of attorney (DPOA), 52
Dura mater, 409
Duty, 45
Dwarfism, 526, 531–532
Dying process, 82
Dysmenorrhea, 548
Dysplasia, 364, 687
Dysplastic nevi, 364
Dyspnea, 453, 664
Dysrhythmia, 610, 669
Dysuria, 514

E

Ear
  anatomy of, 428
  effect of aging on, 752
  examinations, instruments used in, 717–719
  external ear, 428
  foreign bodies in, 823
  hearing evaluations for children, 740–741
  inner ear, 428, 429
  irrigation of, 721
    procedure for, 723
  medication, instilling, 721–722
    procedure for, 724
  middle ear, 428
  otitis media, 718
  procedures and diagnostic tests relating to, 726
  safety issues, 721
  and sense of hearing, 428
  wax in, 430
Eardrum, 428, 720
Earwax, 719, 721. *See also* Cerumen
Echogram, 945
E codes, 303
  example of, 304f
ECT. *See* Electronic claims transmission (ECT)
Eczema, 369
Edema, 450, 452, 664
Editing, 181, 183
Efferent neurons, 407
Ehrlich, Paul, 19–20
Einthoven's triangle, 961
Elderly. *See also* Aging; Older Adults
  abuse of, 758
    reports of, 53t
  administering medications to, 1038
  assisting, 747
  diseases that mainly affect, 752t
  distinct age groups of, 749
  dosage of medication prescribed for, 1013
  facts about, 749–750

Elderly (*continued*)
    legal and medical decisions pertaining to, 756–758
    procedure for communicating effectively with, 757
    safety of, 758–759
    sensory changes in, 752–753
Elective surgery, 764
Electrical safety, 97
Electrocardiogram (ECG), 956, 957–958
    abnormalities revealed by, 967
    artifacts and, 966
    control panel, 960
    deflection or wave on, 957
    estimating heart rate from, 960–961
    machines, 958–960
        lead placement and marking codes, 963t
        preparations for operating, 962–964
        sensor placement, 961, 962f
    making adjustments, 964, 966
    mounting, 966–967
    normal, 967
    paper, 960
    patient preparation for, 961
    -related diagnostic procedures, 967
    tracing, heart and, 958f
    twelve-lead, sensors of, 962f
Electrocautery, 791, 822
Electroconvulsive therapy (ECT), 1124–1125
Electroencephalogram (EEG), 416
Electroencephalograph technician, 36
Electroencephalography (EEG), 36
Electrolytes, 355, 511, 903
Electromyogram (EMG), 1007
Electromyography (EMG), 1007
Electronic claims transmission (ECT), 201
Electronic data exchange (EDI) information system, 288
Electronic mail. *See* E-mail
Electronic Media Claims (EMC)
    advantages of, 289–290
Electronic medical records (EMR), 208
Electronic medical records (EMRs), 654
    advantages, 654
    disadvantages, 654
Electronic or digital thermometers, 601, 605–606
    procedure for measuring oral temperature using, 607
Electronic signatures, 201–202
Electrons, 342
Electronystagmograph (ENG), 720–721
Electrosurgery, 791
Elimination, 490. *See also* Urinary system
ELISA (enzyme-linked immunosorbent assay), 584
E-mail, 187–188, 201
    different forms of, 188
    to schedule appointments, 153–154
Emancipated minors, 51
Embezzlement, 257
Embolism, 455
Embolus, 680
    traveling to brain, 684f
Emergencies. *See also* Medical emergencies
    breathing, 812–814
    conditions for potential patient, 152
    examples of medical, 154t
    handling telephone, 125
        questions to ask when, 125

    legal responsibilities in face of, 803
    in medical offices, 130
Emergency kit, 806. *See also* Crash cart
Emergency medical services system, 802
Emergency medical technicians (EMTs), 36
Emergency medicine, 28
Emergency surgery, 764
Emotions, 1129–1130
Empathy, 81
    definition of, 71
    of medical assistants, 8
Emphysema, 480–481
Employee handbook, 331–332
Employees. *See also* Team
    difficult, 86
    discipline and probation for, 329–330
    dismissal of, 330
    issues or benefits information for, 332
    maintaining records of, 318
    motivation of, 321–322
    need for identification of, to patients, 335
    orientation and training of, 326
    performance evaluation forms, 330f
    probationary period for new, 326
    protecting confidentiality of, 328
    providing performance feedback to, 328–329
    types of reviews for, 329
Employee safety, 98
    OSHA requirements for, 100–101, 220
Employer, loyalty to, 87
Employer's Quarterly Federal Tax Return (Form 941), 262
Employers, values and skills desired by, 1156–1158
EMS system. *See* Emergency medical services system
Encephalitis, 415–416
Enclosure notation, in correspondence, 179
Endocarditis, 453
Endocardium, 436
Endocrine glands, 669–670
Endocrine system, 521–534, 669–670
    common disorders associated with, 527–533. *See also specific disorders*
    disorders of, 529t–530t
    effect of aging on, 680, 754
    function of, 522
    homeostasis and, 522
    organs of, 670
    primary glands of, 522, 522f. *See also specific glands*
    procedures and diagnostic tests relating to, 671t
Endocrinology, 669–670
Endometrial biopsy (EMB), 796
Endometrial cancer, 552–553, 796
Endometriosis, 548
Endomysium, 396
Endoplasmic reticulum, 346
Endorsements, check, 253, 254f
Endoscopy, 794–795
Endosteum, 380
English system of measurement, 844
Enteritis, 854
Envelopes
    entering ZIP codes on, 185
    folding letters and inserting into, 183–184
    formats, 185
    stationery and, 183t

Environment, customer-friendly, 76
Eosinophils, 660, 902–903
Epidemics, 17
Epidemiology, 856
Epidermis, 362–363
Epididymitis, 555
Epididymus, 542, 544
Epiglottis, 476
Epilepsy, 416
Epimysium, 396
Epinephrine, 523, 526, 809
Epiphyseal fracture, 388
Epiphysis, 380
Episiotomy, 541
Epistaxis, 722, 821–822
Epithelial tissue, 347
Epstein-Barr virus (EBV), 468
Equal Credit Opportunity Act (1975), 47t
Equipment, 163–165
    to assist recovery from physical disorders or disabilities,
        996–1007
    for capillary puncture, 909
    defects, reporting, 166
    inoculating, 863
    laboratory, 841–842
        maintenance of, 841
    life and safety, 166
    for measuring blood pressure, 620–622
    medical transcription, 164
    neurological examination, 679
    purchasing, 165
    radiographic, 949–950
    records, maintaining, 165–166
    used for medication administration, 1053–1056
    used for physical examinations, 634–635, 636f, 641t
    usually found in examining rooms, 635
    venipuncture, 905–907, 905f
    warranties for, 165
Erectile dysfunction, 555
Ergonomics, 102, 202
    in medical offices, 105
Erosion, 663f
Errors, handling accidental, 54
Erysipelas, 662
Erythrocytes, 444. See also Red blood cells
Erythrocyte sedimentation rate (ESR), 921
    test using the Wintrobe method, procedure for
        performing, 924
Eschar, 788
Esophagus, 493
Established patients, 154–155
Estates, claims against, 234–235
Estrogen, 526, 527, 540, 541
Ether, 20
Ethical standards, 56–57
Ethics. See also Legal and ethical issues
    codes of, 54, 57, 59
    definition of, 56
    ethical issues and personal choice, 60
    medical, 56–57
    scientific discoveries and ethical issues, 60–61
Ethnocentricity, 80
Eukaryotic cells, 853
Eupnea, 613

Eustachian tube, 429
Evaluation and Management (E/M), 307
    levels of, 307–308
    understanding, 307
Evaluations
    effective use of performance, 328–329
    giving regular, 328
Eversion, 381
Evisceration, 788
Evoked potential studies, 1008
Examination rooms
    children and, 137
    equipment and supplies, typical, 637t
    escorting patients to, 136–137
    features of, 633
    furnishings for, 162–163
    patient comfort, 634
    preparing, 632
    privacy and, 634
    procedure for cleaning, 633
    safety, 633
    typical, 163
Exclusive provider organizations (EPOs), 273
Exercise
    to decrease stress, 1116
    massage, as form of passive, 985
    as part of patient's health plan, 1115–1116
    range of motion, 985, 986
        guidelines for performing, 986
    therapy, 985
    tolerance testing, 967–969
    types of, 985
Exercise physiologist, 980
Exhalation, 478, 612
Exocrine glands, 669
Exophthalmos, 532, 532f
Expert witness, 52
Expiration, 478f, 612. See also Inhalation
Expiratory reserve volume, 970
Exposure Control Plan, 100–101
Extended-care facility (ECF), 33
Extension, 381
External ear, 428, 428f
External radiation therapy, 946
Externship
    appointment scheduling, 144
    areas to be evaluated during, 1143
    asking questions, 388
    awareness of abuse problems, 688
    being an example to patients, 1092
    being respectful and polite, 368
    defining problem and remedy, 401
    description of, 1142
    developing "library" of medication information, 1075
    drawing blood, 917
    evaluating strengths, 482
    exhibiting integrity during, 23
    experience, 1142–1143
    finding right site for, 1144
    focusing on patients, 516
    following proper procedure, 840
    form, sample student, 1144t
    gaining front office skills, 249
    in gynecology, obstetrical, or urological practice, 553

Externship (*continued*)
  helpful courses for, 236
  importance of clear writing, 356
  keeping up with current trends, 959
  knowledge of first aid procedures and certification in
    CPR, 816
  knowledge of OSHA regulations and Universal
    Precautions, 100
  learning about cultures in your community, 1151
  observing and assisting with surgical procedures, 794
  patient communication, 498
  patient presentations in neurological practices, 418
  pharmacology experience, 1018
  planning commute time appropriately, 649
  practicing good asepsis techniques, 575
  practicing positions required for x-rays, 933
  preceptor role during, 1145
  professional attire, 454
  protecting computer password, 198
  relating to teammates, 469
  requirement of, 5
  reviewing medical terminology, 856
  reviewing OSHA requirements and procedures, 890
  review of local standard of care laws, 47
  site
    evaluation, 1145
    finding out cultures that may be encountered at, 1132
  student's responsibilities during, 1143–1144
  "ten rights" of medication administration, 1039
  thinking ahead, 426
  as time of challenge and learning, 1142
  treating patients with equal respect, 528
  volunteering in health care facilities, 732
  working with insurance process, 280
Exudates, 862
Eye
  anatomy of, 424–425
  assisting blind patients, 716
  changes in structure and function of, with age, 716
  common disorders associated with, 425–427. *See also*
    specific disorders
  effect of aging on, 752
  eyeball and anatomical structures, 424f
  foreign bodies in, 823
  guidelines for assisting vision impaired patient to prepare
    for physical examination, 717
  instruments, 708
  irrigation of, 715
    procedure for, 714
  medication, instilling, 715
    procedure for, 715
  procedures and diagnostic tests relating to, 713t–714t
  and sense of vision, 424
  study of, 708
  vision evaluations for children, 740–741
Eyeglasses, 708

F

Facsimile (fax) machines, 132, 188–189. *See also* Fax
  transmissions
Facultative anaerobes, 853
Fahrenheit/Celsius conversions, 599, 599f
  formulas for, 600t

Fahrenheit (F) scale, 599
Failure to thrive (FTT), 734
Fainting, 822–823
  disorders that can result in, 822t
Fair Credit Reporting Act (1971), 47t
Fair Debt Collection Practices Act (1978), 47t, 233–234
Fair-employment practice (FEP) laws, 325
Fallopian tubes, 538–539
False ribs, 383
Falx cerebri, 409
Family and medical history, 211
Family practitioners, 28
Farsightedness, 426, 708
Fascia, 394, 396
Fascicles, 396
Fats, 1102–1104
  total fat, saturated fat, trans fat, and cholesterol content
    per serving, 1104t
Fax transmissions. *See also* Facsimile (fax) machines
  confidentiality and, 52
  of medical records, 132
Febrile seizures, 745–746
Federal Bureau of Records, 21
Federal Food, Drug, and Cosmetic Act of 1938, 1024
Federal Old Age Insurance Law, 749
Federal Register, 281
Federal Unemployment Tax Act (FUTA), 262, 264
Federation Licensing Examination (FLEX), 24–25
Feedback, 74
  positive, 90
Fees
  professional, 228–229
  questions regarding, 119
  usual, customary, and reasonable, 228
Fee schedules, 271, 280
Felony, 44
Female-pattern hair loss, 368
Female reproductive system, 538–542, 538f, 684–695
  common disorders associated with, 544–554. *See also*
    specific disorders
  disorders and pathology of, 545t–546t
  effect of aging on, 680
  function of, 538
  procedures and diagnostic tests relating to, 693t–694t
Fetal alcohol syndrome, 1116
Fetal heart tone (FHT), 692
Fever, 597
Fibrinogen, 445
Fibrocystic breast disease, 548–549, 549f
Fibroids, 553
Fibromyalgia, 399
Fibrosis, 497
Fifth's Disease, 747
"Fight or flight" syndrome, 526
File folders, 213
Files, locating missing, 219
  guidelines for, 219
File Transfer Protocol (FTP), 201
Filing
  alphabetic system, 214–219
  locating missing files, 219
    guidelines for, 219
  rules for, 214–219
  tickler files, 219

Filing systems, 212–213
  active records, 212
  alphabetic, 214–216
  closed records, 213
  color-coded, 217–218
  cross-referencing in, 218
  file storage, 213
    divider guides, 215
    file folders, 213
  inactive records, 213
  numerical, 215–217
  subject matter, 216
Filtration, 355, 512
Financial management, 318
Fire safety, 97
  RACE plan, 98f
First responders, 802
Fissure, 409, 663f
Flatus, 677
Fleming, Alexander, 20, 859
Flexion, 381
Floating assistants, 780–781, 783
  guidelines for, during surgery, 783
Floppy disk, 196
Flu, 482
Fluoroscopy, 936, 938–940
Follicle-stimulating hormone, 523, 540–541
Folliculitis, 369
Follow-up care, 212
Follow-up letter
  example of, following interview, 1156f
  procedure for preparing, 1157
Food and Drug Administration (FDA), 53, 838
  generic drugs and, 1024
  regulation of OTC medications by, 1025
Food guide pyramid, 1109, 1110f
Food supplements, 1115
Forced expiratory volume, 972
Forced vital capacity, 972
  procedure for performing spirometer test
    to measure, 974
Forceps, types of, 774–775, 775f
Foreign bodies, removal of, 797
Foreign body airway obstruction, 806–808. See also
  Airway obstruction
Foreskin, 543
Form letters, 179–180, 180f
Fowler's position, 642f, 644
Fractures, 387–388, 823–824
  of jaw, 825
  of neck and back, 825
  types of, 823f
  various types of, 388f
Fragile X syndrome, 357
Franklin, Benjamin, 18
FRAXA syndrome, 357
Frequencies, 718, 720
Freud, Sigmund, 20
Fried's law, 1018
Frontal lobe, 409, 410
Frostbite, 826–827
Full liquid diet, 1111
Functional MRIs, 944
Functional residual capacity, 972

Fundus, 690
Fungi, 563, 859

G

Galen, 17
Galileo, 17
Gallbladder, 494
Gallstones, 494
Gastrin, 527
Gastroenterologist, 672
Gastroenterology, 672
Gastroesophageal reflux disease (GERD),
  500–501, 672, 675
Gastrointestinal mucosa, 527
Gastrointestinal series, 938. See also Lower GI series;
  Upper GI series
Gastrointestinal system, 672–677. See also Digestive
  system
General anesthesia, 784–785
General hospitals, 31
Generic drugs, 1024
Generic names, 1024
Genes, 346
Genetic disorders, 356–358, 481, 747, 748t
Genetic engineering, 355
Genetic fingerprinting, 355–356
Genetic immunity, 565
Genetics, 355
  hair color and, 363
  heredity, and disease, 356–358
Genital herpes, 370, 699
Geriatrician, 747
Geriatrics, 28
Germinal centers, 463
Germs, 562. See also Microorganisms
  multiplication of, 563
Gerontology, 747
Gestational diabetes, 531
Gestational hypertension, 695
Gigantism, 526, 532. See also Acromegaly
GI series, 938, 939
Glands
  of endocrine system, 522–527. See also specific glands
  primary, of endocrine system, 522f
Glasgow seven-point scale, 366–367
Glaucoma, 426
Glomerular disease, 514–515
Glomerular excretion, 512
Glomerulonephritis, 514–515, 888, 894
Glomerulus, 511
Gloves, removing, 577f
Gloving, 768
  procedure for surgical, 770–771
Glucose tolerance test, 692
Glycosuria, 889
Goals, setting, 89–90
Goiter, 533, 533f, 647
Golgi apparatus, 346
Gonadotropin, 524
Gonadotropin-releasing hormone (GTRH), 522
Goniometer, 639, 985
Gonorrhea, 699
Good Samaritan laws, 48

Gossip, negative aspects of, 85
Gout, 389
Graafian follicle, 540, 542
   rupture of, 541
   stages of development, 539f
Gram, Jans C. J., 853
Grammar, 177
Gram stain, 853, 866
   procedure for performing, 868–869
Granulated white blood cells, 921
Granulocytes, 444
Graves' disease, 532
Gray (Gy), 947
Gray matter, 408, 411
Greenstick fracture, 388
Grid, 948
Grief, 1136
   five stages of, 82, 1136t
Grievance process, 332
Gross annual wage, 260
Ground fault circuit interrupter (GFCI), 97
Group A Strep Screen, 876
Group practice, 10, 27
Group practice without walls (GPWW), 273
Growth hormone (GH), 523, 526
   excess production of, 527–528
Growth hormone-releasing factor (GHRF), 522
Growths, 797. See also specific growths
   removal of, 797
Guardian ad litem, 48
Guided imagery, 1116
Gynecologic examination, 685–688
Gynecologist, 685
Gynecology, 29, 684–685
   patient, assisting, 685
Gyri, 409

H

Habituation, 1037
Hair follicles, 363
   inflammation or infection of, 369
Hallucination, 1122
Hammurabi, 16
Hand, foot, and mouth disease, 747
Hand washing, 571
   alcohol-based rubs, 571, 574
   importance of, 562
   procedure, 572–573
   technique, 572f–573f
Harvey, William, 17
Hashimoto's thyroiditis, 533
HAV, 582
Hay fever, 482
Hazard Communication Standard, 838
Hazardous medical waste, 99, 570, 1048
   major types of, 99–100
   removal, 839
Hazardous Waste Operations, 838
Hazards
   chemical, 838–839
   fire and safety, 839
   needle-stick, 839, 1048
HAZCOM binders, 98, 102

HBV, 582–583
HDL cholesterol, 450
Headaches, 416–417
Heading, in business letters, 178
Head lice, 371
Health care
   career opportunities, 10–11, 33–34
   costs and payments, 25–26
   cultural traditions in, 79t
   lawsuits related to, 46. See also Law
   religious beliefs about birth, death, and, 83t
   setting, creating customer-friendly environment in, 76
Healthcare Common Procedure Coding System
       (HCPCS), 305
   Level II sections, 306f
Health care institutions, 30–33
   hospice, 33
   hospitals, 30–32
   nursing homes, 32–33
Health care professions, 33–38
   career titles and educational levels, 34t
   certification for, 33
   licensure for, 33
Health information technology, 37
Health insurance
   availability of, 270
   benefits, types of, 276
   Blue Cross/Blue Shield, 274
   cards, 135
      front and back, 273f
   claims. See Claims
   commercial plans, 273
   cost containment, 280
   disability insurance, 275–276
   exclusions, 277
   fee schedules, 280
   government programs, 274–275
   indemnity schedules, 277
   managed care organizations (MCOs), 270–273
   Medicaid, 275
   Medicare, 274–275
   military benefits, 275
   payment of benefits, 276–277
   procedure for applying managed care policies and
       procedures, 280
   procedure for applying third-party guidelines, 279
   procedure for performing billing and collection, 278
   provider preauthorization and precertification, 277–278
   purpose of, 270
   understanding details of, 271
   verification of benefits, 279
   workers' compensation, 275–276
Health insurance claim forms
   Blue Cross/Blue Shield, 286
   example of, 287f, 288f
   managed care, 286
   Medicaid, 286
   Medicare, 286
   military benefits, 286
   rejection of, 295–296
      preventing, 296
   tracking, 295–296
   types of, 286, 289
   workers' compensation, 289

Health Insurance Portability and Accountability Act
   (HIPAA), 59, 76, 220, 444, 590, 852
   coding of services required in, 300
   confidentiality standards
      applying to electronic transmissions, 202
      for computerized records, 198
   guidelines for medical office records area, 161
   inventory requirements, 167
   Privacy Rule, 87–88
Health Maintenance Organization Act of 1973, 271
Health maintenance organizations (HMOs), 26, 271–272
   components of, 272
   models, 272
Health, mind-body connection and, 67–68
Health Plan Employer Data and Information Set (HEDIS),
   108
Hearing acuity, 719
   decline in, 721
   tests used to evaluate, 719–721
Hearing aids, 752
Hearing impaired patients, 81, 721
   procedure for assisting, 81
Hearing loss, 430. *See also* Hearing acuity
Heart, 436–439
   blood flow through, 436–437, 437f
   cardiac cycle, 439
   chambers, interior view of, 437f
   circulation in, 439f
   circulation of blood through, 618f
   conduction system of, 438–439, 440f
   and elctrocardiogram tracing, 958f
   linings of, 437f
   location of, 436f
   pathology, abnormalities caused by, 968t
   physiology of, 437–438
   sounds, 439, 956
   structure and function, 956–957
   valves of, 438f
   vascular system of, 438
Heart attack, 438, 450, 827
   symptoms of, 451–452
Heart disease. *See also* Cardiovascular disease
   risk factors associated with, 666, 668
   treatment of, 668–669
Heart murmur, 437, 439
Heart rate, 956
   estimating, from ECG, 960–961
Heat
   applications, 986–987
   to distract brain from pain, 1116
   dry, 989, 992–993
   moist, 987, 989
   procedure for application of a heating pad, 992
   procedure for applying a hot compress, 990
   procedure for applying hot soak, 991
   uses of, for conditions caused by trauma and infection,
      986
Heat exhaustion, 825–826
Heat stroke, 826
Height
   indications provided by, 593–594
   measuring, 594
   procedure for measuring, 595
      infants', 739

Heimlich maneuver, 807, 807f
   variations on, 807–808
Hematocrit, 443
Hematology, 28, 902
Hematopoiesis, 443, 462, 902
Hematuria, 889
Hemiplegia, 1002
Hemochromatosis, 357
Hemodialysis, 517–518, 703
Hemoglobin, 444, 454, 902
   determining, 917, 919
      procedure for, using hemoglobinometer, 920
Hemoglobin S disease, 455. *See also* Sickle cell anemia
Hemolysis, 847, 853–854
Hemolytic anemias, 454
Hemophilia, 357
Hemoptysis, 485
Hemorrhage, 455, 680, 811–812
Hemorrhoids, 501
Hemostasis, 446
Heparin, 903
Hepatitis A, 582
   vaccine, 1075
Hepatitis B, 220, 582–583, 1048
   vaccine, 1073
Hepatitis C, 583
Hepatitis D, 583
Hepatitis E, 583
Herbal supplements, 754
Heredity
   defined, 356
   genetics, disease, and, 356–358
Hernia, 501–502
Herpes, 699
Herpes simplex, 370
   symptoms of, 370
Herpes zoster, 370
Herpetic whitlow, 370
Hiatal hernia, 501
Hib disease, 1075
Hierarchy of needs, 66–67, 1126–1127, 1127f
High blood pressure, 455, 516, 668–669
High-protein diet, 1112
High-residue/fiber diet, 1112
Hilum, 511
HIPAA. *See* Health Insurance Portability and
   Accountability Act (HIPAA)
Hippocrates, 16, 17, 56
Hippocratic Oath, 17, 18, 56
Hirsutism, 646
Histamine, 660
HIV/AIDS, 221, 1048
Holter monitor, 969–970
   procedure for applying, 971
Homeopathy, 982
Homeostasis, 342, 753
   contribution of white blood cells to, 444
   maintenance of, 522
Homophones, common, 175t
Hordeolums, 427
Horizontal recumbent position, 642f, 643–644
Hormones, 522–523, 670
   adrenal cortex, 525–526
   adrenal medulla, 526

Hormones (*continued*)
   defined, 522
   gastrointestinal mucosal, 527
   gonadotropic, production of, 540
   pancreatic, 525
   parathyroid gland, 524
   pineal gland, 524
   pituitary gland, 523–524
   placental, 527
   produced by ovaries, 527
   release of, 540
   of testes, 527
   thymus gland, 527
   thyroid gland, 524
   treatments using, 670
Hormone therapy, 556
Hospice care, 33, 82, 1136
Hospital Formulary, 1024
Hospitals, 30–32
   categories of, 31
   scheduling for admission to, 151
      patient information to be supplied when, 152t
Housekeeping, medical office, 163
Housekeeping safety, 101–102, 163
   OSHA procedures for, 102
HSV-1 (herpes simplex virus type 1), 370
HSV-2 (herpes simplex virus type 2), 370
Human body
   anatomical locations and positions, 350–354
   anatomical planes of, 350, 352f
   basic building blocks of, 344f. *See also* Cells
   cavities and abdominal regions, 351, 353
   defense of. *See* Immune system
   directional anatomical terms, 350, 351f
   function of water in, 1105
   impact of aging on, 680, 750
   infection control system of, 564–565
   landmarks, 354t
   levels of organization in, 342–347, 343f
   organs and systems, 347
   organ systems of, with major functions, 349f
   pressure points, 812, 812f
   primary pulse points of, 442f
   types of movements in, 381f
   types of tissue in, 348f
Human genome project, 22–23
Human immunodeficiency virus (HIV), 22, 547,
   1048
   and AIDS, 583–584
   infection, stages of, 583–584
   people at highest risk for, 584
Human papillomavirus (HPV), 373, 547, 699
Humor, as stress reliever, 1116
Hunter, John, 17, 18
Hydrocele, 556
Hydrocephalus, 419, 740
Hydrogenation, 1103
Hyperglycemia, 821
Hyperopia, 426, 708, 711
Hypersensitivity, 660
Hypertension, 455, 458, 668–669, 753–754
   chronic renal failure and, 517
   during pregnancy, 695
   sample teaching plan for, 1090

symptoms of, 616
   treatment for, 669
HyperText Transfer Protocol (HTTP), 201
Hyperthermia, 597
Hyperthyroidism, 524, 532
Hyperventilation, 615
Hyperventilation syndrome, 827
Hypnosis, 1116
Hypoglycemia, 821
Hypotension, 458
   caused by allergic reactions, 661
   symptoms of, 616
Hypothalamus, 410–411
   hormones of, 522–523
Hypothermia, 597–598, 826
Hypothyroidism, 524, 532–533, 533f
Hypoventilation, 615
Hysterectomy, 548, 553

I

ICD-9-CM (International Classification of Diseases, Ninth
   Clinical Modification)
   abbreviations, symbols, and other conventions, 303
   coding
      procedure for, 305
      steps in, 302–303
   E-code section of, 304f
   formats and conventions of, 302
   publishing of, 300
   special codes in, 303
   understanding, 300, 302
ICD-10 (International Classification of Diseases, Tenth
   Revision), 303
Ileum, 493
Illness. *See also* Diseases
   differing cultural views regarding, 78
   link between stress and, 67–68, 1126
   poor diet and, 1098, 1100
Immediate history, 804
Immune response, 462, 464
   cancer and, 467
   inappropriate, excessive, or lacking, 465
Immune system, 449, 461–470. *See also* Immunity;
   Tonsils
   in AIDS patients, 584
   anatomy of, 462–464
   and body's defense, 464–465
   cancer and, 467
   common disorders associated with, 465–469, 466t
   structures central to, 462–464
Immunity, 464–465, 565, 677, 1073
   acquired, 566t
   types of, 464
Immunizations, 464, 677, 746, 1072–1073
   adult and other, 1076
   childhood and adolescent, 1073, 1075–1076
      schedule recommended for, 1074f
   for health care employees, 220
Immunoglobulins, 464–465
Immunology, 19–20, 27
   advances in, 20–21
Impacted cerumen, 430
Impetigo, 370–371, 371f

Inactivated polio vaccine, 1076
Inactive records, 213
Incident reports, 104–105, 219–220
    example of typical, 105f
Incision and drainage (I & D), 796–797
Incisions, 773
Incontinence, 513, 515
Incubation, 584
Incubator, 841
Incus (anvil), 428
Individual practice association (IPA), 272
Infancy, 1125
Infants
    assessing vital signs of, 598
    CPR techniques for, 816
    measuring weight of, 738
        procedure for, 739
    procedure for measuring head circumference of, 740
    procedure for measuring height of, 739
    procedure for responding to obstructed airway in, 808
    signs of dehydration in, 744
    signs of ear infection in, 718
Infection control system, 564–565
    blood system, 565. See also Circulatory system
    lymphatic system, 565. See also Lymphatic system
    OSHA and, 569
    physical and chemical barriers, 570–582
    prevention, 564–565
Infections
    chain of, 564f
    factors needed for occurrence of, 563–564
    fungal, 859
    mechanisms promoting spread of, 564
    natural barriers to, 564–565
    nosocomial, 563
    opportunistic, 584
    overview of process of diagnosing, 862–863
    stages of the process of, 564t
    susceptibility to new, 562
    yeast, 859
Infectious mononucleosis, 468
    symptoms of, 921
    test for, 921, 924
Infectious waste, 100. See also Hazardous medical
        waste
    disposal of, 570
Infertility, 698
Inflammation, 565
Inflammatory bowel disease (IBD), 499
Inflammatory process, 565
    acute, 566t
Influenza, 482
Informed consent, 49–51, 757
    definition of, 49
    document, sample of, 50f
    exceptions to doctrine of, 50
    forms, 211–212
    medical assistants and, 55–56
    for surgical procedures, 769
Infundibulum, 411
Inguinal hernia, 501–502, 502f
Inhalation, 478, 612, 615
Inhalation medications, 1049, 1052
Inhalers, 975

Injections, 1052–1053
    angle of need insertion for four types of, 1053f
    Z-track method of, 1067f
Injuries, reportable, 53t
Ink-jet printers, 197
Innate immunity, 465
Inner ear, 428
    common disorders associated with, 429–430
Inoculating
    culture, 863
    equipment, 863
    media, 864–865
Input devices, computer, 195
Insects, 859
Insertion, 397
Inside address, in correspondence, 178
Inspection, 638
Inspiration, 478, 478f, 612. See also Inhalation
Inspiratory capacity, 972
Inspiratory reserve volume, 970
Instant message format, 188
Instilling
    ear medication, 721–722
        procedure for, 724
    eye medication, 715
        procedure for, 715
Instruments
    cutting, 773
    dissecting, 773–774
    grasping and clamping, 774–775
    guidelines for handling, 779
    gynecological, 777f
    handling sterile, 769
    orthopedic, 778f
    probing and dilating, 775
    tips to help with identification of, 773
    urological, 778f
    used in minor office surgery, 769, 773
Insula, 409
Insulin, 525, 531, 534, 541, 821
    types and duration of action, 1060t
Insulin-dependent diabetes mellitus (IDDM), 531, 670
Insulin shock, 821
Insurance. See also Health insurance
    accounts receivable, 236
    billing, 229
    claims. See Claims
    long-term care, 276
    major medical, 276
    malpractice, 48
Insurance cards, 135
Insurance coding, 300. See also ICD-9-CM (International
        Classification of Diseases, Ninth Clinical Modification)
    code linkage, 312
    compliance, 312
    history of, 300
    procedure coding, 303
    procedure for assigning a CPT code, 310
Insurance fraud, 308
    Medicare definition of, 308, 311
    prevention and detection, compliance guidance for,
        311–312
    reporting suspected, 312
    tips, 311

Integrated delivery system (IDS), 273
Integrated provider organization (IPO), 273
Integrity, of medical assistants, 7–8, 23
Integumentary system, 361–374. *See also* Dermatology;
  Skin
  accessory structures in, 362
  common disorders associated with, 364–374. *See also*
    specific disorders
  effect of aging on, 680, 751
  functions of, 362
  overview of, 362
  procedures and diagnostic tests relating to, 665t
Intentional torts, 44t, 45
Intermediate-care facility (ICF), 32–33
Intermittent pulse, 610
Internal medicine, 28
Internal radiation therapy, 946
Internal Revenue Service, 262
International Classification of Diseases (ICD), 243, 300.
  See also ICD-10; ICD-9-CM
International Headache Society (IHS), 417
International health and medical insurance, 276
International List of Causes of Death, 300
Internet, 199
  advertising staff positions on, 324–325
  building medical practice Web site on, 335
  obtaining information about interview process on,
    1152
  services on, 201
  Web sites, as help in job search, 1147
Internet service provider (ISP), 201
Interneurons, 407
Internists, 27, 28
Interoffice memoranda, 181
Interpersonal dynamics, 66–68
Interstitial cystitis (IC), 514
Interventricular foramina, 410
Interview, 1151–1152
  follow-up after, 1156
  guidelines for successful, 1154
  procedure for role-playing an, 1155
  professionalism at, 1154–1155
  questions, preparing for tough, 1152–1154
  ten most common mistakes made during, 1155
Interview process, 325–326
Intractable pain, 624
Intradermal injections, 1053f
  procedure for administering, 1068–1069
Intradermal test, 661
Intramuscular injections, 1052–1053, 1053f
  needle position for, 1059f
  procedure for administering, 1063–1065
  sites for, 1057–1059, 1058f, 1061
Intrapleural pressure, 478
Intrapulmonic pressure, 478
Intrauterine device, 695
Intravenous injections, 1053f
Intravenous pyelogram (IVP), 938–939
Intravenous therapy, 1071
  preparing IV tray for, 1071–1072
  side effects of, 1071
Intravenous urogram, 938–939
Intubation, 802
Invasive procedures, 764

Inventory
  equipment, record of, 166t
  list of sample drugs, maintaining, 167
  order form, sample, 167f
  supply control, 166–167
Inversion, 381
In vitro fertilization (IVF), 698
Iodine compounds, 931
Iris, 424
Iron deficiency anemia, 454
Irrigation
  of the ear, 721
    procedure for, 723
  of the eye, 715
    procedure for, 714
Irritable bowel syndrome (IBS), 502
Ischemia, 455, 680
Ishihara test, 647, 711–712, 712f
Islets of Langerhans, 525
Isolation gown, removing, 576f
Isotopes, 946
IV tray
  preparing, 1071–1072
    procedure for, 1072

J

Jack-knife position, 643f, 645
Jaeger reading card, 647
Janssen, Zacharias, 17
Jehovah's Witnesses, 51
Jejunum, 493, 527
Jenner, Edward, 18
Job applicants
  checking references of, 326
  hiring of, 326
  interview process for, 325–326
  learning important information about, 325
  prohibitions against asking discriminatory questions of,
    325
  testing thinking abilities of, 326
Job search, 1146
  conducting, 1147–1148
    procedure for, 1148
  mistakes, 1146
  performing personal assessment before, 1146–1147
  sources for job opportunities, 1146t
Joint Commission on Allied Health Personnel in
  Ophthalmology, 719
Joint Commission on the Accreditation of Health Care
  Organizations (JCAHO), 31, 220
Joint Review Committee for Ophthalmic Medical
  Personnel, 5
Joints, 380
  movement and, 380–381
  typical, 380f
Juvenile diabetes, 531

K

Kaposi's sarcoma, 584
Keratin, 362, 363
Ketones, 889
Keyboard, computer, 196–197
  ergonomics and, 202
Kidney failure. *See* Renal failure

Kidneys, 511
    external structure of, 511
    internal structure of, 511
    nephrons of, 511
    transplants of, 518
    waste products of, 511
Kidney stones, 515–516
    types of, 515f
Kidneys, ureters, and bladder (KUB), 942
Kinesthetic learners, 68
Klinefelter's syndrome, 357
Knee-chest position, 642f, 644
Knives, 773
Koch, Robert, 19
Korotkoff, Nicolai, 617
Korotkoff sounds, 441, 617–619
    five phases of, 618t
Kubler-Ross, Elisabeth, 82, 1136
Kyphosis, 384, 385f, 983

L

Labia majora, 541
Labia minora, 541
Labor, 692, 810
Laboratory technicians, 37
Laboratory tests, 645, 646t
    common, and their normal values, 916t
Lacrimal apparatus, 425
Lactic acid, buildup of, 396
Lactogenic hormone, 524
Laennec, Rene, 18
Landmark terms, human body, 354f
Laptop computers, 194
Large intestine, 494, 494f
Laryngeal mirrors, 635
Larynx, 476
Laser printers, 197
Laser surgery, 426, 427, 791, 794
Lasik procedure, 426
Lateral recumbent position, 642f, 644
Law. See also Minors
    civil law, 44–45
    classification of, 44–46
    confidentiality and, 49
    criminal law, 44
    governing collections, 47t
    vaccines required by, 53t
LDL cholesterol, 450
Leading questions, 74
Learning
    adult, 1082
    outcomes, 1082
    roadblocks to effective patient, 1087
    styles, 68
Ledger cards, 229–230, 238, 240, 240f
Leeuwenhoek, Anton van, 17, 852
Legal and ethical issues
    accuracy in labeling of specimens, 882
    assisting another licensed person, 997
    calling in prescriptions, 1016
    caution regarding offering false hopes to patients, 1128
    checking patient's past medical history, 387
    child abuse, 745

communicating with patients, 1083
computerized data, 199
confidentiality regarding patient testing, 863
confidentiality standards, 444
dealing with insurance, 276, 295
dealing with reproductive issues, 547
digestive disorders and lifestyle, 500
documentation and, 346
driving and neurological disorders, 416
employer responsibilities according to OSHA
    guidelines, 100
federal coding regulations, 312
financial information regarding patients, 232
guidelines for giving medication, 1049
immunodeficiency disorders, emotional lifestyle and, 467
informed consent, 769
laws regarding diabetes and driving public
    transportation vehicles, 530
legal responsibilities in face of emergency, 803
maintaining aseptic technique, 569
for medical assistants, 6
medical records confidentiality, 222
monitoring of dated material, 172
for office managers, 328
overseeing physician re-registrations and renewals, 25
patient communication and, 77
patient drug abuse concerns, 1028
patient noncompliance, 1111
patient privacy, 512
patient safety during office visits, 138
performing banking procedures, 260
performing venipuncture, 904
physical examinations, 638
prescriptions to be kept at school, 480
providing appropriate explanation of necessary
    procedures, 961
providing complete and accurate information on
    application forms, 1156
relating to scheduling process, 148
removal of clothing and, 372
reporting of equipment defects, 166
requirement of written consent, 672
responsibility to use careful, proper technique, 721
specimens with medicolegal implications, 847
understanding of ethical standards, 56
using proper technique for procedures and measuring
    vital signs, 617
visual difficulties and driving, 427
when speaking with patients over telephone, 117
written orders and written consent, 936
Legal terminology, understanding, 319
Legionellosis, 482
Legionnaire's disease, 482
Lenses, 424
    and correction of visual problems, 709f
    grinding of, 708
Lesions, 662
    caused by genital herpes, 699
    corneal, 427
    tumors of skin, 364
Letter writing, 172–181
    active versus passive voice, 174, 174t
    avoiding personal pronoun I, 174
    business letters, 178–179

Letter writing (*continued*)
  capitalization rules, 177
  for collections, 234
  composition, 174
  error correction in office correspondence, 177–178
  form letters, 179–180
  gender bias, removing, 173
  inflated phrases versus concise terms, 174t
  letter styles, 180–181
  parts of speech, 177
  plurals, 176–177
  repetition and redundancy in, 174
  requesting payment, 172
  sentence and paragraph length, 173
  spelling, 176t
  technical terminology, 172–173
  two-page letters, 179
  use of numbers in, 177, 177t
  word choice, 172
Leukemia, 455
Leukocytes, 442, 444, 445f, 464, 889, 902
  defenses performed by, 445
Level II tests, 838
Level I tests, 838
Liability, preventing, 54–56
Libel, 49
Licensed practical nurse (LPN), 35, 87
Licensed vocational nurse (LVN), 35
Licensure, 24–25
  endorsement, 25
  examination for, 24–25
  for health care professionals, 33
  medical assistants and, 55
  reciprocity, 25
  revocation, 44
  suspension or revocation, 25
Life cycle
  adolescence, 1125–1126
  adulthood, 1126
  childhood, 1125
  developmental stages of, 1125–1126
  infancy, 1125
  prenatal period, 1125
Lifespan considerations, 9
  administering medications to pediatric patients, 1038
  appropriate appearance, 132
  assistance for children, adolescents, and older adults, 632
  bones and, 379
  careful calculations regarding medication dosing for elderly, 1016
  checks written by agents, 253
  child proof and kid friendly medical offices, 161
  circulatory system, 438
  computer preparedness for older employees, 230
  computers and computer terminology, 201
  confusion associated with filing claims, 294
  dealing with elderly patients, 71, 105f
  dealing with infants, 598
  digestive system, 495
  drawing blood from older individuals, 903
  easing patient waiting time, 155
  ECGs and PFTs, 957
  effect of aging on senses, 425

  endocrine system, 526
  fast food, 1112
  giving injections, 1054
  hot or cold modalities for pediatric or geriatric clients, 988
  immune system, 462
  impact of aging on human body, 680
  keeping instructions to the point, 1088
  kidneys, 513
  Medicare patients, 275
  movement and exercise, 395
  nervous system, 408
  obtaining urine specimen from older adult, 886
  participating in minor surgery procedures and providing follow-up care, 769
  patients requiring additional accommodations, 722
  reproductive system, 540
  skin and, 365
  superbill questions, 300
  when handling pediatric cases, 121
Life stages, 66–67, 67t. *See also* Life cycle
Limited checks, 251
Lipids. *See* Fats
Lipoatrophy, 399
Lipodystrophy, 399
Lipolysis, 523
Lipoproteins, 450, 1108–1109
Listening, 1129
Listening skills, 72–73
  active listening, 72
  guidelines for, 73
  passive listening, 72
  procedure for effective, 73
Lister, Joseph, 562
Lithotomy position, 642f, 644
Lithotripsy, 516
Litigation
  appropriate documentation, to avoid, 89
  avoiding, 54
  use of medical records in, 52
Liver, 494–495
  substances manufactured by, 495
Living will, 51, 756, 757
Lobes, 409
Local anesthesia, 785
  agents and use, 788t
Lochia, 692
Long bones, 380
  features found in, 380f
Long, Crawford, 20
Long distance calls, 123
  being aware of time zones when placing, 123
  conference calls, 123
  making, 123
Longitudinal fissure, 409
Long-term care institutions, 32–33, 756
  assisted-living facility, 33
  extended-care facility (ECF), 33
  intermediate-care facility (ICF), 32–33
  skilled nursing facility (SNF), 32
Long-term care insurance, 276
Loop of Henle, 511
Lordosis, 384, 385f, 983
Lou Gehrig's disease, 415

Low blood pressure, 458
Lower GI series, 938
  guidelines for, 939
Lower respiratory system, 474
Low-fat/low-cholesterol diet, 1113
Low-residue diet, 1113
Low-sodium/low-salt diet, 1113
Loyalty, to employer, 87
Lumbar puncture
  assisting with, 684
  confirming meningitis diagnosis with, 746
  myelography and, 940
Lumpectomy, 547
Lung cancer, 483
Lungs, 477
  cells in, 477
  roles of, 477
Luteinizing hormone, 524, 541
Lyme disease, 857, 859
Lymph, 449–450
Lymphatic system, 449–450, 449f, 677. *See also*
    Circulatory system
  central lymphoid tissue, 462
  components of, 449, 463f
  function of, 449
  peripheral, 462–464
  primary responsibility of, 462
  procedures and diagnostic tests relating to, 677t
  spleen, 450
  thymus gland, 450
  tissue fluid, lymph, and lymph nodes, 449–450
Lymphedema, 468
Lymph nodes, 449, 463
  functions of, 463
  structure of, 450f
Lymphocytes, 450, 464, 903
Lysosomes, 345, 346

M

Macrophages, 463
Macular degeneration, 426–427
Macule, 663f
Magnetic Ink Character Recognition (MICR), 249–250
Magnetic resonance imaging (MRI), 942, 943–944
  claustrophobia related to, 944
Mail
  certificate of mailing, 186
  certified, 186
  classifications of, 185–187, 186t
  handling tips, 187
  insurance, 186
  postal money orders, 187
  procedure for opening daily, 188
  recall, 187
  registered, 187
  returned, 187
  size requirements for, 187
  special delivery, 186
  special handling, 186
  special postal services, 186–187
  stationery and envelopes, 183t
  tracing lost, 187
  ZIP codes, 185

Main memory, computer, 195
Major medical insurance, 276
Male-pattern baldness, 368
Male reproductive system, 542–544, 542f, 695–696
  common disorders associated with, 554–556. *See also*
    specific disorders
  disorders of, 554t
  effect of aging on, 680
  external organs, 542–543
  internal organs, 543–544
  procedures and diagnostic tests relating to, 697t
Malignant melanoma, 364, 366–367
Malleus (hammer), 428
Malpractice, 48. *See also* Negligence
Malpractice insurance, 48
Mammary glands, 541
Mammogram, 940–941
  normal, 942f
  showing microcalcifications, 942f
Mammography, 940–941
Managed care
  advantages and disadvantages of, 271
  claim forms, 286
  exclusive provider organizations (EPOs), 273
  health maintenance organizations (HMOs), 271–272
  managed care organizations (MCOs), 270–273
  preferred provider organizations (PPOs), 272–273
  systems, history of, 271
Managed care organizations (MCOs), 270–273
Management service organization (MSO), 273
Manic-depressive state, 1122–1123
Manipulation, 639
Manual decongestive therapy (MDT), 469
Marker X syndrome, 357
Marketing
  assessing target market, 334
  customer service, 335
  free, and public relations, 335
  medical practices, 333–335
  Web sites, 335
Martin-Bell syndrome, 357
Maslow, Abraham, 66–67, 1126–1127
Massage, 985
Massage therapist, 980
  categories of massage practiced by, 985
Massage therapy, 985
Mass storage devices, computer, 194
Mastectomy, 547
Material Safety Data Sheet (MSDS), 98
  example of, 99f
Material Safety Data Sheets (MSDS), 838–839
Math
  equivalents, example of, 1015t
  for pharmacology, 1011–1020
  principles, review of, 1014–1016
Matrix, forming, 148–149
Mature minor, 51
Maximal midexpiratory flow, 972
Mayo tray, 1072
M code, 303
Measles, mumps, and rubella (MMR) vaccine, 1075
Meatuses, 475
Mechanical safety, 98
Mechanical soft diet, 1111–1112

Media
  culture, 863–864
  inoculating, 864–865
Mediastinum, 477
Medicaid, 32, 275, 749
  claim forms, 286
Medical asepsis, 570–571, 764–765
  versus surgical asepsis, 765
Medical assistants. *See also* Medical assisting
  administrative responsibilities, 6
  assisting with medical meetings and speaking
      engagements, 332–333
  certification, 55
  characteristics of good, 7–9
  clinical responsibilities, 7
  collection of blood specimens by, 902
  confidentiality/privacy and, 55
  cultural considerations for. *See* Cultural considerations
  documentation, 55
  drug regulations, 55
  education and training for, 4–5
  externship requirement for, 5. *See also* Externship
  informed consent and, 55–56
  job opportunities, 10–11
      in health care departments and specialties, 11t
      in inpatient and ambulatory settings, 11t
  knowledge of entire medical office necessary for, 161
  legal and ethical issues for. *See* Legal and ethical issues
  letter writing by. *See* Letter writing
  liability prevention role of, 54–56
  licensing, 55
  office management, 55
  principles of medical ethics, 57
  proofreading of correspondence by, 172
  quality assurance role of, 108
  and regulations needing familiarity with, 838
  responsibilities of, 5, 7
  role of, 5–7
      in clinical laboratories, 837
      in microbiology, 852–853
      in physical medicine, 982
      as receptionist. *See* Patient reception
  safety and, 56
  scope of practice issues dealt with by, 86–87
  six basic skills necessary for success as, 1157–1158
  standard of care for, 58
Medical assisting. *See also* Medical assistants
  accreditation for programs in, 5
  definition of, 4
  history of, 4
  as one of fastest growing occupations, 1142
  professional organizations, 9–10. *See also specific
      organizations*
Medical care, quality, 105–106
  defined by AMA, 106
Medical diagnosis, 590
Medical emergencies. *See also* Emergencies
  abdominal pain, 808–809
  airway obstruction, 806–808
  allergic reactions, 809
  amputation, 809–810
  asphyxia, 810
  birth, 810
  bites and stings, 810–8111

  burns, 814–815
  cardiac arrest, 815–815
  cardiopulmonary resuscitation, 816
  chest pain, 817, 820
  convulsions, 820–821
  diabetic crisis, 821
  foreign bodies in nose, ear, or eye, 823
  fractures, 823–824
  guidelines for providing care during, 802–806
  heart attack, 827
  heat and cold exposure, 825–827
  hyperventilation, 827
  open wounds, 827–829
  poisoning, 829–830
  primary assessment, 802–805
  in reception area, 130, 137–138
  severe bleeding, 811–812
  shock, 830
  specialists' telephone numbers for, 802
  stroke, 816–817
Medical ethics, 56–57
  AMA Principles of, 57
  ethical standards and behavior, 56–57
Medical history, 591–593
  areas to be included in, 592
  assessment of body systems, 593
  chief complaint, 592
  family, 592–593
  kinds of, 804
  personal questions for, 593
  present illness, 592
  procedure for interviewing new patient to obtain, 652
  sample of patient's, 591f
  sheet to list patient problems, example of, 653f
  sheet used to record review of systems, example of, 647f
  social or personal history, 593
  standard information for, 591
Medical insurance claims. *See* Claims; Health insurance
  claim forms
Medical laboratories, 37
Medical laboratory assistant (MLA), 837
Medical laboratory technician (MLT), 37, 837
Medical offices
  accounts payable expenditures in, 236–237
  administrative responsibilities, 6
  bathrooms, 163
  care and maintenance of equipment in, 131
  categories of files in, 212–213
  closing, 138, 139
  compliance plans, 311–312
  creating sense of affiliation to, 321–322
  defining goals of, with physician, 331
  documentation needed by, 46
  equipment, 163–165
  ergonomics in, 105, 202
  examination rooms, 136–137, 162–163
  facilities planning, 160
  housekeeping procedures, 163
  importance of procedures manual to, 332
  injectable drugs commonly in stock in, 1027t
  layout, 160–161
  lost and found, 130–131
  maintaining solvency of, 318
  managing clinical aspect of, 318

medical meetings and speaking engagements, 332–333
no-show patients, 138, 150
office flow, 161
opening, 132
  procedure for, 133
petty cash, 260
posting of payment policies, 228
procedure and policy manual, 86
reception area, 130, 137–138, 161–162
recurring monthly expenses of, 255
reference materials, 183
security, 102, 104–105
supplies, 166–167
surgical procedures performed in, 791–797. *See also specific procedures*
telephones in. *See* Medical office telephones
typical layout, 161f
uses of computers in. *See also* Computers
Medical office telephones, 114–125
  answering, 114–115
  business telephone systems, 115–116
    making calls, 115
    things to avoid when placing callers on hold, 116
    transferring calls, 116
    using hold function, 115–116
  and cultural considerations, 121
  handling difficult calls, 122
  handling emergency calls, 125
  long distance calls, 123–124
  making reminder calls and doing callbacks, 118
  message taking, 116–118
    caller ID, 117
    call forwarding, 117
    privacy manager, 117
    procedure for, 117
    speakerphones and headsets, 117–118
    voice messaging system, 116
  pagers and cell phones, 118
  prescription refill requests, 121
    taking message for, 122
  for scheduling appointments, 153–154
  screening calls, 118
  telephone techniques, 114–118
  telephone triage, 121–122
  typical incoming calls, 119–121
    from nonpatients, 120–121
    from patients, 119–120
  using answering service, 124
  using telephone directory, 122–123
Medical Patients Rights Act, 59
Medical practice acts, 24–25
  licensure, 24–25
  registration, 25
  suspension or revocation of medical licenses, 25
Medical practices, 10
  marketing and customer service, 333–335
  types of, 26–27
    associate practice, 27
    group practice, 10, 27
    partnership, 27
    professional corporation, 27
    sole proprietorship, 27
    solo practice, 10, 26–27

  use of professional advertising service by, 333
  ways to promote, 335
Medical practitioners, 23–24
  medical privileges of, 32
  title of doctor, 23
    designations and initials for, 24t
    others with, 23–24
Medical privileges, 32
Medical records, 208
  access to, 221
  collating, 132
    procedure for, 133
  computerized, 198–199
  consultation report, 212
  diagnosis and treatment plan, 212
  discharge summary, 212
  disclosure without consent, 221
  electronic and computerized, 210
  electronic signatures, 201–202
  family and medical history, 211
  fax transmission of, 132
  guidelines for recording information in, 593
  HIPAA guidelines for area containing, 161
  informed consent forms, 211–212
  as legal documents, 209
  operative report, 212
  ownership of, 222–223
  pathology report, 212
  patient correspondence and follow-up care, 212
  patient registration form, 211
  physical examination results, 211
  procedure for adding or changing items on, 210
  procedure to organize patient, 213
  professionalism when handling, 291
  radiology report, 212
  from referred physicians or hospital visits, 211
  reflecting all services and care in, 311
  release form for, 221f
  releasing, 221
  retention and destruction of, 223
  specially protected medical information, 221
  storing, 221
  test results, 211
  transcription of, 222
  types of, 208–210
  types of forms and reports, 210–212
  use of, in litigation, 52
  x-rays, 951
Medical records technician, 37
Medical social workers, 36–37
Medical specialties, 27–29
Medical technologist (MT), 37, 837
Medical terminology. *See also* Abbreviations
  common misspellings of, 176t
  and corresponding synonyms, 173t
  for movement produced by muscles, 988t
  patients and use of, 77
  reviewing, for externship preparation, 856
  skills, need for excellent, 646
  use of correct, 172–173
Medical transcription, 38, 222
  career opportunities, 223
  equipment, 164
  sound-alike words, 221

Medical transcriptionists, 222
  physically challenged, 164
Medicare, 32, 274–275, 749
  billing, use of CMS-1500 for, 300
  claim forms, 286
  coding and reimbursement, 300
  coverage in hospice setting, 33
  definition of insurance fraud, 308, 311
  taxes, 262
Medicare Catastrophic Coverage Act, 300
Medication administration, 1048–1053. *See also* Drug
      administration
  equipment used for, 1053–1056
  guidelines for, 1040
  inhalation, 1049, 1052
  method of, and absorption by body, 1037
  oral, 1049
  parenteral, 1052–1053
  procedures: OSHA standards, 1048
  "ten rights" of, 1039
  topical, 1049
Medications. *See also* Drugs
  age and effects of, 1037
  allergies to, 1037–1038
  calculating dosages, 1017
    body weight method, 1020
    pediatric, 1018–1020
  charting, 1077
  contraindicated for breast-feeding mothers, 1038
  effect of, on mental abilities, 754
  gathering, 805
  for injection, formats for, 1055
  liquid, 1049
  method of administration, 1037
  older patients and, 754
  patient's weight and, 1037
  preparing, 55
  procedure for administering oral, 1052
  procedure for administering sublingual or buccal, 1051
  reconstituting powdered, for administration, 1076–1077
    procedure for, 1076
  religious beliefs opposing use of, 1017
  side effects of, 1037
    idiosyncratic, 1037
    lethal, 1037
  tolerance and intolerance to, 1038
Medicine
  during the 18th century, 17–18
  during the 19th century, 18–20
  during the 20th century, 20–21
  computer use in, 194
  contributions of ancient civilizations to, 16
  early, 16–18
  firsts in, 22
  frontiers of, 22–23
  health care costs and payments, 25–26
  history of early, 16–23
  medical and surgical specialties, 27–30
  medical practice acts, 24–25
  medical practitioners, 23–24
  modern, and the future, 21–23
  remedies used in early, 16
  types of medical practices, 26
  women in, 21

Meditation/prayer, 1116
Mediterranean anemia, 747
MedLearn, 229
Medline, 1024
Medulla
  adrenal, 526
  of kidney, 511
  of lymph node, 463
Medulla oblongata, 411, 613
Medullary canal, 380
Megahertz (MHz), 195
Meiosis
  differences between mitosis and, 347
  stages of, 347
Melanocyte-stimulating hormone, 524
Melanocyte-stimulating releasing factor (MRF), 523
Melanoma, 366–367. *See also* Malignant melanoma
  changes in a mole, ABCDEs of, 366t
Melatonin, 524
Memory, 754
Memos, 181
Menarche, 541
Ménierè, Prosper, 430
Ménierè's disease, 429–430
Meninges, 409
Meningitis, 417, 746
Menopause, 526, 540, 541
Menstrual cycle, 541–542
Mensuration, 639
Mental awareness
  levels of, 813t
    assessing, 813
Mental disorders
  defined, 1122
  treatments for, 1124–1125
Mental health, 754
Mentally/emotionally impaired patients, 82–84
Mercury sphygmomanometer, 621f, 622
Metabolism, 524, 626, 1101
Metastasis, 366, 467
  common sites of breast cancer, 546
Methicillin-resistant *Staphylococcus aureus* (MRSA), 856
Metric system, 842, 844, 1012–1013
  commonly used equivalents for, 1014t
  comparison of household/apothecary liquid
      measurements, 1015t
  conversion list, 1018t
  guidelines for conversion within, 1014
MG. *See* Myasthenia gravis
Microbes, 562–564, 853. *See also* Microorganisms
  motility or nonmotility of, 854
Microbiology
  equipment and procedures, 863–867
  field of, 852
  role of medical assistant in, 852–853
Microencephaly, 740
Microfiche, 208
Microfilm, 208
Microhematocrit, 916–917
  procedure for performing, 918
Microorganisms, 17, 562–564, 852, 853–859
  classes of, with descriptions and examples, 855t
  classifications of, 853
  diseases caused by, 19

growth of, 563
hemolytic properties of, 853–854
naming, 853
other identifying characteristics of, 854
pathogenic, and resulting diseases, 860t
sciences for study of, 563
structural characteristics of, 853
subcellular, 853
transmission of, 563–564
types of, 854–859
viability of, 862
Microprocessors, 195
Microscope, 841
care of, 842
guidelines for maintenance and, 843
parts of, 841–842, 842f
resolution of, 841
using, 842
Microscopic examination, of urine specimens, 892–894
preparing specimen for, 892
procedure for, 893
reporting and understanding, 892
Micturation, 880
Middle digit filing system, 216
Middle ear, 428
common disorders associated with, 428–429
Middle ear infection, 718
Migraine headaches, 417
Military benefits, 275
claim forms, 286
Minerals, 1105, 1106t–1108t, 1108
Mini Mental Status Exam, 756
Minors. *See also* Children
billing, 231
emancipated, 51
lawsuits on behalf of, 48
legal implications when treating, 51
mature, 51
rights of, 51
Minor surgery
additional surgical supplies, 783
anesthesia, 784–785
informed consent, 783–784
instruments used in, 769, 773
patient instructions for, 783
positioning and draping, 784
postoperative patient care, 786–789, 791
preoperative and postoperative patient instructions, 784
preparation of patient's skin, 785–786
preparing patient for, 783
procedure for assisting with, 782
procedures, participating in, 769
Misdemeanor, 44
Mistakes, admitting and correcting, 54
Mitochondria, 345, 346
Mitosis
cell division and, 346–347
differences between meiosis and, 347
stages of, 346f
Mitral valve, 437
Modified block style format, 181, 182f
with indented paragraphs, 182f
Modified wave scheduling, 145
Molecules, 342, 344

Moles, 364
changes in, 365, 366–367, 366t
Money orders, 251
Monitor, computer, 195
ergonomics and, 202
Monocytes, 903
Mononucleosis, 463. *See also* Infectious mononucleosis
Mononucleosis spot test, 921, 924
Monosaccharides, 1099
Mono test, 921, 924
procedure for performing, 925
Mons pubis, 541
Morbidity rates, 20
Morphology, 854
Motivation, 1130
Mouse, computer, 197
Mouth, 491
Mucosum, 363
Multicultural issues, 77–80
bias, prejudice, and stereotyping, 79–80
culture, 78–79
language, 77–78
Multiple sclerosis, 417
Muscle cramps, 399
Muscles. *See also* Muscular system
abdominal, 398
of the arm, wrist, hand, and fingers, 398
atrophy of, 985
cardiac, 396, 438
composition of, 396
energy production for, 396
in eye, 425
fatigue of, oxygen debt and, 396
functions of, 394–395
of the head, 397
of the leg, ankle, and foot, 398
pain and cramps of, 399
of the pectoral girdle, 398
respiratory, 398
skeletal, 394f, 396
smooth, 395–396
terminology for movement produced by muscles, 988t
Muscular dystrophy, 357, 399–400
Muscular system, 393–402. *See also* Muscles;
Musculoskeletal system
common disorders associated with, 398–402. *See also specific disorders*
types of muscle tissue, 395–396
Musculoskeletal system, 678–679
effect of aging on, 680, 753
injuries to, 823–824
and the medical assistant, 678–679
procedures and diagnostic tests relating to, 681t–682t
Music, as stress reliever, 1116
Mutations, 356
Myasthenia gravis (MG), 400
Mycobacteria, 858
Mycology, 563, 859
Myelin sheath, 407
Myelography, 940
Myocardial infarction (MI), 438, 666, 827
symptoms of, 451–452
treatment for, 452
Myocarditis, 453

Myocardium, 347, 436
Myomectomy, 553
Myopia, 426, 708
Myringa, 708, 720
Myringotomy, 718, 743
Myxedema, 524, 533, 533f

N

Nails, 363, 364f
Name pins/tags, receptionist, 131
Narcotics. *See also* Controlled substances
   checking expiration dates of, 1028
   keeping accurate log of, 1028
   maintaining strict control of, 1026
Nares, 475
Nasal mucosa, 475
Nascher, I. L., 749
National Academy of Sciences, 1109
National Archives and Records Administration
   (NARA), 281
National Autism Association, 745
National Board of Respiratory Therapy, 35
National Center for Health Statistics growth chart, 740
National Center of Elder Abuse, 758
National Certification Agency for Medical Laboratory
   Personnel, 37
National Childhood Vaccine Injury Act (1960), 53t
National Cholesterol Education Program, 668
National Committee for Clinical Laboratory Standards
   (NCCLS), 837
National Committee for Quality Assurance (NCQA), 108
National Council Licensure Examination (NCLEX), 35
National Federation of Licensed Practical Nurses, 35
National Health Care Skills Standards (NHCSS), 34
National Institutes of Health, 555
National Pressure Ulcer Advisory Panel, 369
Natural active immunity, 565
Natural family planning, 695
Natural immunity, 677
Natural passive immunity, 565
Natural selection, 355
Naturopathy, 982
Nearsightedness, 426, 708
Near vision acuity, 711
   procedure for screening for, 711
Nebulizers, 975
Necrotizing fasciitis, 856
Needles
   disposable, 1054
   suture, 778f
Needle-stick hazards, 839, 1048
Needlestick Safety and Prevention Act, 838
Negative contrast media, 931
Neglect of duty, 45
Negligence. *See also* Malpractice
   four Ds of, 45
   res ipsa loquitur, 48
Negotiable instruments, 249
Neoplasms, 662–663. *See also* Tumors
   benign, 662, 664t
   malignant, 662–663, 664t
Nephrologists, 29
Nephrology, 28

Nephrons, 511
   structure of, 512f
Nerve cells, 347. *See also* Neurons
Nerve damage, 719
Nerve fibers, 407–408
Nerve(s), 362
   autonomic, 411
   components of, 408
   cranial, 411–414, 413t
   impulses and synapses, 408
   spinal, 414
   types of, 407
Nerve tissue, 347
Nervous system, 405–419, 406f, 679–680, 684. *See also*
   Central nervous system (CNS); Peripheral nervous
   system (PNS)
   breathing and, 613
   common disorders associated with, 415–419. *See also*
      specific disorders
   effect of aging on, 680, 751–752
   functions of, 407
   homeostasis and, 522
   nerve fibers, nerves, and tracts, 407–408
   neurons, 407
   procedures and diagnostic tests relating to, 683t
   use of electrical impulses in, 407
Neuralgia, 417–418
Neuroglia, 407
Neurohypophysis, 524
Neurologist, 679
Neurology, 28, 679
Neurons, 347
   types of, 407
Neuroses, 1122
Neurosurgeon, 679
Neurotransmitters, 408, 524
   in cerebrospinal fluid, 411
Neutrons, 342
Neutrophils, 464, 902
Nightingale, Florence, 21
Nitrites, 889
Nodule, 663f
Non–insulin-dependent diabetes mellitus (NIDDM), 531, 670
Nonabsorbable sutures, 776
Noncompliance
   handling, 1091
   legal and ethical issues regarding patient, 1111
Non-English speaking patients, 77–78
   disadvantages of, 84
Non-mercury glass thermometers, 600
   cleaning and storing, 601
      procedure for, 605
   procedure for measuring oral temperatures using,
      602–603
   procedure for measuring rectal temperatures using, 604
   sheaths for, 600–601
Nonparticipating providers, 294
Nonprescription drugs, 1025
Nonsteroidal anti-inflammatory drugs (NSAIDs), 679
Nonverbal communication, 70, 72, 1128
   use of, with non-English speaking patients, 77–78
Norepinephrine, 523, 526
Normal flora, 852, 854
   isolating colonies of, 864

Norton, William, 20
Nose, 474–475
    effect of aging on, 752
    examination of, 722
    foreign bodies in, 823
Nosebleed, 821–822
No-shows, 138, 150
Nosocomial infections, 563
Nuclear medicine, 28, 946–947
Nucleolus, 346
Nucleus, 345, 346
Numbers, in correspondence, 177, 177t
Numerical filing system, 215–217
    middle digit filing, 216
    serial numbering, 216
    straight numerical filing, 215
    terminal digit filing, 216
    unit numbering, 216
Nurses, 34–35
Nursing homes, 32–33
Nutrients
    classification of, 1101–1105, 1108
    defined, 1101
Nutrition, 1098–1099
    balanced diet, 1098f–1100f, 1109–1111
    diseases related to poor, 1098, 1100
    healthy food choices, 1113–1115
Nutritionists, 1099
Nystagmus, 721

O

Obesity, 744
Objective symptoms, 592
Obstetrician, 685
Obstetrics, 29, 685
    patient, assisting, 685
Occipital lobe, 409, 410
Occult blood
    in stool, 872–873
    in urine, 889
Occupational Safety and Health Administration
        (OSHA), 220, 837
    authority and responsibilities of, 96
    Bloodborne Pathogens Standard, 100–101,
        838, 839, 1048
    Exposure Control Plan, 100–101
    exposure control program of, 569
    guidelines for using personal protective equipment and
        clothing, 101
    Hazardous Communications section regarding chemical
        hazards, 98
    housekeeping procedures, 102
    Occupational Exposure to Bloodborne Pathogen
        Program, 839
    regulations (1970), 837
Occupational therapist (OT), 35, 980
    role of, 981–982
Occupational therapy assistant (OTA), 980
Office flow, 161
Office for Civil Rights (OCR), 220
Office management, 38
    clinical office management, 318
    communication, 319

    creating team atmosphere, 323–324
    employee records, 318
    facility and equipment management, 318
    financial management, 318
    legal concepts, 319
    medical assistants and, 55
    personnel responsibilities, 318
    scheduling, 318
    systems approach to, 318–319
Office managers, 38. See also Personnel management
    alerting physician to patient no-shows, 138
    effective use of performance evaluation by, 328–329
    establishment of priority list by, 331
    general duties, 319–322
    hiring of new staff members by, 324
    importance of time management for, 330–331
    as integral part of team, 323
    leadership styles, 322–323
    monthly planning, 320
    motivation of employees by, 321–322
    orientation and training methods of effective, 326
    responsibilities to employee and physician/
        employer, 319t
    skills observed in good, 319
    staff meetings, 320
    use of personnel policy manual by, 331–332
Office procedures manual, 332
    contents of, 333t
    functions of, 332
Office security, 102, 104–105
Older adults. See also Elderly
    additional assistance for, 632
    bones in, 379
    careful calculations regarding medication
        dosing for, 1016
    changes related to mobility in, 395
    circulatory changes in, 438
    decreased short-term memory in, 1088
    dehydration in, 513
    dexterity decrease in, 1088
    digestive system and, 495
    drawing blood from, 903
    ECGs and PFTs for, 957
    endocrine system in, 526
    giving injections to, 1054
    hot or cold modalities for, 988
    increased anxiety about new situations found in, 1088
    intellectual performance in, 408
    lymphatic tissue in, 462
    obtaining urine specimen from, 886
    reproductive system changes, 540
    respiratory rates of, 477
    sense organs and, 425
    skin and hair in, 365
    slowed processing time of, 1087
    teaching, 1087–1088
Oliguria, 885
Once-a-month billing, 231
Oncogenes, 467
Oncology, 28, 663
Online banking, 248
Open-angle glaucoma, 426
Open-ended questions, 73
Open fracture, 387, 824

Open-panel HMO, 272
Operating technician, 768
Operative report, 212
Ophthalmic assistant (OA), 719
Ophthalmologist, 708
Ophthalmology, 29, 708
Ophthalmoscope, 635, 708
Opportunistic infections, 584
Optical Character Recognition (OCR), 185
Optician, 708
Optional surgery, 764
Optometrist, 708
Oral cancer, 502–503
Oral cavity, 491f. *See also* Mouth
Oral medication administration, 1049
  procedure for, 1052
Oral polio vaccine, 1076
Organ donations, 52
Organelles, 345, 853
Organ of Corti, 428, 719
Organs, 347. *See also* Skin
  of digestive system, 491–494
  formation of special sense, 425. *See also* Special senses
  of respiratory system, 474–477
  of urinary system, 511–512
Organ transplants, 22, 52
Origin, 397
Orthopedics, 29, 678
Orthostatic hypotension, 754
Orthotist, 980
  career as, 980
Osmosis, 355
Osteoarthritis, 385, 679
  X-ray showing, 387f
Osteopaths, 24, 678, 732, 980
Osteoporosis, 389, 526, 532
Otitis externa, 429
Otitis media, 429, 718, 743
Otorhinolaryngologist, 708
Otorhinolaryngology, 29
Otosclerosis, 429
Otoscope, 635, 649, 708, 717, 718f
Outpatient surgery, 764
Output devices, computer, 195
Outside laboratories, 836
Ova and parasites (O&P), 859
  procedure for obtaining stool specimen for, 874
  testing stool for presence of, 873–875
Ovarian cancer, 549
Ovarian cysts, 549–550
Ovaries, 527, 539–541
  functions of, 540
    structure and, 527f
Overbooking, 136
Overflow incontinence, 515
Overlay programs, computer, 197
Over-the-counter drugs, 754, 1025
Oviducts, 538–539
Ovulation, 541
Oximeters, 616, 975
Oximetry, 616
Oxygen. *See also* Oxygen delivery; Respiratory system
  application of, 814f
  bacteria categorization pertaining to, 853

carried by hemoglobin, 902
  monitoring, 816
Oxygen debt, 396
Oxygen delivery, 476–477
  for all parts of body, 474
  lungs and, 474
Oxygen saturation, 616
  procedure for measuring, using pulse oximeter, 617
Oxytocin, 524, 692

P

Pacemaker, of heart, 438, 956
  other areas assuming role of, 957
  spike, ECG tracing with, 959f
Pacemakers, implanted, 669
  atrial-paced, 958
  automatic, 958
  MRIs and, 944
Pagers, 118
Pain, 623–624, 672
  examples of sites of referred abdominal, 672f
  stress caused by, 1116
  threshold, 624
  tolerance, 626
  types of, 624
Palate, 491
Palm pilots, 194
Palpation, 638
Palpebral fissure, 424
Pancreas, 495, 525
Pancreatic cancer, 503–504
Pandemic, 17
Papanicolaou, George, 686
Papanicolaou (Pap) test. *See* Pap test
Paper claims, 289
Papillary layer, of dermis, 363
Pap smear, 686–688. *See also* Pap test
  grading, 688
Pap test, 547, 645, 685. *See also* Pap smear
  procedure for assisting with, 691
Papule, 663f
Paramedics, 36
Paraplegia, 418
Parasites, 859
  in urine, 894
Parasympathetic nervous system, 414–415
  summary of effects of, 414t
Parathormone (PTH), 524
Parathyroid glands, 524, 525f
Parenteral medication administration, 1052–1053
Parietal lobe, 409
Parkinson's disease, 418
Participating providers, 294
Partnership, 27
Parts of speech, 177, 178t
Parturition, 692
Passive immunity, 465, 565
Passive listening, 72
Passive transport, 354–355
Passive voice, 174
Password, computer, 198
Pasteurization, 19, 562
Pasteur, Louis, 19, 562, 852

Past medical history, 592, 804–805
Patch test, 661–662
Pathogens, 445, 562f, 563
  bloodborne, 569
  spread of, 562
Pathologist, 663
Pathology, 29
Pathology report, 212
Pathophysiology, 342
Patient care technician (PCT), 34–35
Patient correspondence, 212
Patient education, 1081–1094
  about physician's specialty and credentials, 24
  clarifying position as student, 1147
  clarity regarding patient test preparation, 837
  communication and, 89–90
  compliance when taking medications, 469
  computer technology, 198
  dietary instructions, 503
  dosage of medication prescribed, 1013
  explaining wound care, 784
  facilitating patient's comprehension of diagnosis and
    treatment plan, 699
  fasting requirements for routine blood tests, 907
  follow-up plan, 1091t
  giving explanations about medications, 1051
  healthy lifestyles and, 1100
  helping achieve goals set by physician, 716
  helping patient cope with stress, 1131
  how adults learn, 1082
  important sites for, 135
  instructing on correct use of equipment, 601
  instruction on correct method of collecting urine
    specimen, 881
  instructions for radiologic procedures, 932
  introduction of caregivers, 335
  maintaining bone health and preventing bone loss, 383
  medical language and, 350
  medication for endocrine disorders, 534
  and medications for neurological disorders, 416
  office banking practices, 252
  ownership of medical records, 222–223
  patients with pulmonary diseases, 964
  physical therapy needs, 989
  presentation techniques for, 90
  printed materials used in medical office, 173
  promoting healthy attitude toward exercise and
    nutrition, 399
  proper angle for child drinking bottle, 429
  proper hygiene and urinary system, 515
  pulmonary diseases and, 480
  regarding role of medical assistants, 4
  relating to legal issues, 54
  safety precautions, 102
  signs and symptoms of heart attack, 448
  skin care, 365
  stressing proper hand hygiene, 569
  suicide, 746
  teaching about cast care, 1091–1093. See also Casts
  teaching about lifestyle changes, 549
  teaching about new medications, 1025
  teaching preventive care, 804
  understanding health insurance details, 271, 290
  understanding policy regarding financial matters, 228

  using telephone system for, 123
  videotapes for, 162
Patient identification system, 215–216
Patient information booklets, 333
  as educational tool, 335
  procedure for developing, 334
Patient/physician relationship, 49
  informed consent, 49–51
  patient rights, 49
  Patient Self-Determination Act, 51–52
  physician rights, 49
  rights of minors, 51
  standard of care, 47
Patient reception, 129–139
  charge slips, 135–136
  closing the office, 138
    procedure for, 139
  duties of receptionist, 130–131
  escorting patient to examination room, 136–137
  greeting patients upon arrival, 134
  managing disturbances, 137
  no-shows, 138
  opening the office, 132
  reception area, 130
  signing-in, 134–135
  time consideration for patients, 136
Patient registration form, 135, 211, 229–230
  example of, 136f
  information needed on, 230
Patients. See also Lifespan considerations
  advising, 89
  angry, 80
  anxious, 81
  assessment of, 72
  assisting blind, 716
    techniques for, 717
  consideration for time of, 136
  as consumers, 85
  dealing with elderly, 105f
  decision making of, 89
  double booking, 145
  draping, 641, 643
  escorting, to examination room, 136–137
  established, scheduling appointments for, 154–155
  financial information regarding, 232
  greeting, 76, 134
  hearing impaired, 81, 721
  information to request from, with telephone calls, 120
  interviewing, 590–591
  legal and ethical issues of telephone conversations
    with, 117
  medical office environment for, 160
  mentally/emotionally impaired, 82–84
  new, scheduling appointments for, 154
  non-English speaking, 77–78, 84
  no-show, 138, 150
  orientation of, 162
  pediatric, 733
  positioning, 643–645
  potential "code," 814
  preparation for tests of, 846
  preparing, for physical examinations, 640–641,
    643–645
  referrals for, 151, 278–279

Patients (*continued*)
    responsibilities for care and treatment of, 7
    rights of, 49
    signing-in, 134–135
    with special needs, 81–82
    telephone dealings with difficult, 122
    terminally ill, 82
    typical incoming calls from, 119–120
    visually impaired, 82
Patient's Bill of Rights, 58, 60, 87, 88t, 590
Patient Self-Determination Act, 44, 51–52
    durable power of attorney (DPOA), 52
    living will, 51
    Uniform Anatomical Gift Act, 52
Payroll, 260–265
    annual tax returns, 265
    deposit requirements, 262
    Federal Unemployment Tax Act (FUTA), 262, 264
    income tax withholding, 261–262
    Medicare taxes, 262
    methods for calculating checks for, 261
    procedure for generating medical office, 262
    Social Security taxes, 262
    state disability insurance, 265
    state unemployment tax, 265
Peak flow meters, 974–975
Pediatricians, 27, 29
Pediatric office, 732
    patient safety, 733
    procedure for measuring pediatric vital signs, 736–737
    reception room, 732
    sick-child visits, 733, 741, 743
    telephone triage, 732
    visits and procedures, 733–743
    well-child visits, 733
Pediatrics, 29
    assisting in, 732
    subspecialties of, 732
Pediculosis, 371, 371f
Peer Review Organization (PRO), 280
Pegboard system, 238–243, 239f, 250, 261
    adjustments, 240–241
    components of, 238, 240
    day sheets, 238
    ledger cards, 238, 240
    locating errors in, 243
    procedure for, 241
    receipt forms, 240
    using, 240
Pelli-Robson chart, 712f, 713
Pelvic cavity, 351
Pelvic examination, 685–688, 689f
    bimanual, 688
    procedure for assisting with, 691
Pelvic inflammatory disease (PID), 550, 696, 699
Pelvis, 383
    male and female, 385f
Penicillin, 20, 859, 1024
Penis, 542–543
    functions of, 543
Peptic ulcer disease (PUD), 504–505
Percussion, 638–639
Percussion hammer, 635
Percutaneous ultrasonic lithotripsy, 516

Pericarditis, 453
Pericardium, 436
Perimysium, 396
Perineum, 541
Periosteum, 380
Peripheral lymphatic system, 462–464
Peripheral nervous system (PNS), 411–412
    nerves in, 407
Peristalsis, 493
Peritoneal dialysis, 518, 703
Permanent teeth, 491, 492f
    eruption of, 493
Permeability, 579–580
Permissive leaders, 322
Pernicious anemia, 454
PERRLA (pupils equal, round, react to light and
    accommodation), 708
Persistent generalized lymphadenopathy, 584
Personal assessment, 1146–1147
Personal digital assistants (PDAs), 194
Personality, 66
Personality disorders, 1123–1124
Personal protective equipment (PPE), 98, 768f, 840, 852
    and clothing, 101t
    purpose of, 765
    wearing, when drawing blood, 908
Personnel management
    advertising positions, 324–325
    hiring procedures: selecting right staff members,
        324–332
    interview process, 325–326
    orientation and training, 326
    responsibilities, 318
Personnel policy manual, 331–332
Perspiration, 362
Pertussis, 1073
PET scans, 943
Petty cash, 260
pH, 884, 887
Phagocytes, 464
Phagocytosis, 445, 660
Phantom pain, 624
Pharmacists, 36, 1024
Pharmacology
    abbreviations, commonly used, 1041t–1042t
    defined, 1024
    experience during externship, 1018
    math for, 1011–1020
Pharmacy, 36
Pharynx, 475–476, 493
    separation of oral cavity from, 491
Phenylketonuria (PKU), 357, 921
    test, procedure for performing, 925
Phlebotomists, 37
Photometer, 841
Physiatrists, 980
Physical examination results, 211
Physical examinations
    adult, 639–640
    assisting physician with, 640–641, 643–645
    body part, method of examination, and equipment used
        during general, 641t
    during emergencies, 805
    equipment and supplies used for, 634–635

examination of nose and throat, 722
  guidelines for assisting vision impaired patient to
    prepare for, 717
  legal considerations regarding, 638
  methods used by physician during, 635, 638–639
  patient preparation for, 640–641, 643–645
  positions for conducting, 642f–643f
  procedure for assisting with complete, 648
  procedure for preparing new patient for, 652
  rooms for, 632–634
  sequence of procedures during, 645–647, 649, 651t
Physical medicine, 29, 980
  application of heat and cold, 986–987, 989–993
  careers in, 981t
Physical therapist (PT), 35, 980
  role of, 980–981
Physical therapy
  adaptive equipment and devices, 996–1007, 996f
  combination of modalities used in, 980
  conditions requiring, 983, 985
  conditions treated by, 994t
  methods, 983, 985–987, 989, 992–996
    means and, used in, 980
  needs, educating patient regarding, 989
Physical therapy assistant (PTA), 980
Physician/employee relationship, 46
  respondeat superior, 46–47
Physician-hospital organization (PHO), 273
Physicians, 26
  behind schedule, 145. See also Appointment scheduling
  codes of ethics for, 56
  defining office goals with, 331
  malpractice insurance, 48
  overseeing re-registrations and renewals for, 25
  patient education regarding specialty and
    credentials of, 24
  professional courtesy offered by, 244
  protecting, from charge of abandonment, 46
  public duties of, 53t
  rights of, 49
  types of practices engaged in by. See Medical
    practices
Physician's assistant (PA), 35
Physician's Desk Reference (PDR), 183
Physicians' Desk Reference (PDR), 1024
Physician's office laboratories (POLs), 836
Physiology, 342
Pia mater, 409
Pineal gland, 524
Pink eye. See Conjunctivitis
Pinna (auricle), 428
Pinwheel, 635
Pinworms, 874
  procedure for obtaining stool specimen for
    examination for, 874
Pipettes, 844
Pituitary gland, 411, 523–524
  anterior lobe, 523–524
  posterior lobe, 524
  and relation to brain, 523f
PKU. See Phenylketonuria (PKU)
Placement offices, 1152
Placenta, 527
Placenta abruptio, 695

Plaintiffs, 45
Plan, in POMR, 651
  sample, 652
Plasma, 442, 443, 445, 903
Platelets, 442, 444, 903, 920–921
Pleura, 477
Pleural space, 477
Pleurisy, 483
Pleuritis, 483
Plurals, forming, 176–177, 177t
Pneumococcal vaccine, 1075
Pneumocystis carinii pneumonia (PCP), 584
Pneumonia, 483
Point-of-service plan (POS), 272–273
Poisoning, 829–830
Poles, 409
Policy and procedure manual, 86
Polio, 21
Poliovirus, 1076
Pollinosis, 482
Polycystic kidney disease (PKD), 516
Polydipsia, 531, 670
Polyphagia, 531
Polypharmacy, 1016, 1038
Polysachharides, 1101
Polyuria, 531, 670, 885
POMR, 208. See also Problem-oriented medical
    record (POMR)
  approach, four sections to, 208–209
Pons, 411
Portal of entry, 563
Portal of exit, 563
Positioning, 784
Positive contrast media, 931
Positron Emission Tomography (PET), 943
Postage meters, 165
Postal money orders, 187
Posting
  correcting errors in, 241
  proof of, 242
Post-traumatic headaches, 417
Post-traumatic stress disorder, 1132
Potter–Bucky diaphragm, 948
Pott's fracture, 388
Power, 322
  types of, 323
Practice of medicine, 44
Preauthorization, 275, 277–278
Precertification, 277–278
Preeclampsia, 695
Preferred Provider Health Care Act, 271
Preferred provider organizations (PPOs),
    271, 272–273
Prefilled cartridge injection systems, 1056
Pregnancy, 689. See also Prenatal care
  complications during, 692, 695
  dietary considerations during, 1111
  drug use during, 1038
  excluding alcohol during, 1116
  history, information pertaining to present, 689
  screening tests performed during, 692
  testing, urine, 894
Prehypertension, 458
Prejudice, 66, 79–80, 1127

Premenstrual syndrome (PMS), 550
  multisystem effects of, 551f
  symptoms of, 551–552
Premiums, 270, 272
Prenatal care, 688–690, 692
  delivery, 692
  first prenatal visit, 689
  follow-up visits, 690–692
  patient education, 690
  postpartum visit, 692
  prenatal history, 689
  screening tests, 692
Prenatal period, 1125
Prepaid plans, 271
Prepuce, 543
Presbycusis, 430, 721
Presbyopia, 426, 708, 711
Prescription
  reading and writing, 1038–1039
  sample, 1039f
Prescription blanks, 54
Prescription drugs, 1025
Present illness, 592
Presenting problem, 592
Pressure points, 812, 812f
Primary assessment, 802
  deciding if patient is ill or injured, 803
  determining allergies, 805
  determining chief complaint, 803–804
  determining patient's name, approximate age, and
    gender, 803
  doing physical examination, 805
  gathering medications, 805
  obtaining history, 804–805
  taking vital signs, 805
Primary care medicine, 28. *See also* Family practitioners
Primary care physicians, 271, 272, 732
Primary medicine, 28. *See also* Internists
Primary radiation, 948
Prime mover, 397
Principal diagnosis, 303
Principles of Medical Ethics (AMA), 57, 58
Printers, 197
Privacy, 852
  in examination rooms, 634
  medical assistants and, 55, 444
  patient, 512
  protecting, while doing ECG, 966
  when taking body measurements, 594
Probation, 330
Probationary period, 326
Probing questions, 73
Problem list, in POMR, 651
  sample, 652
Problem-oriented medical record (POMR), 651–653. *See
  also* POMR
Problem solving, 85
  steps for, 86
Procedure coding, 303
Procedures
  administering (inserting) rectal or vaginal
    suppository, 1050
  administering intradermal injection, 1068–1069
  administering oral medications, 1052

  administering parenteral subcutaneous or intramuscular
    injections, 1063–1065
  administering sublingual or buccal medication, 1051
  application of a heating pad, 992
  application of cold chemical pack, 995
  application of cold compress, 993
  application of hot soak, 991
  application of ice bag, 994
  applying a Holter monitor, 971
  applying a hot compress, 990
  applying an arm sling, 824
  applying bandage over sterile dressing, 795
  applying pediatric urine collection device, 742
  assisting with a sigmoidoscopy, 676
  assisting with audiometry, 725
  assisting with complete physical examinations, 648
  assisting with minor surgery, 782
  assisting with pelvic examination and Pap test, 691
  assisting with suturing, 790
  changing a sterile dressing, 793
  cleaning and storing non-mercury glass
    thermometers, 605
  cleaning examination rooms, 633
  collecting clean-catch midstream urine specimen, 883
  communicating effectively with the elderly, 757
  conducting a job search, 1148
  controlling bleeding, 829
  creating community resource brochure, 1082
  creating public relations brochure, 1083
  determining hemoglobin using hemoglobinometer, 920
  developing patient teaching handout about stress, 1135
  disposal of infectious wastes and substances, 570
  evaluating physical characteristics of urine, 885
  focusing dietary teaching on patient's needs, 1102
  general x-ray examination, 935
  instilling ear medication, 724
  instilling eye medication, 715
  instructing patient on breast self-examination, 686
  instructing patients according to their needs for health
    maintenance and promotion, 1089
  instructing patient to use cane or single crutch
    correctly, 1003
  instructing patient to use crutches correctly, 1001
  for interviewing new patient to obtain medical history
    and prepare for physical examination, 652
  irrigation of the ear, 723
  irrigation of the eye, 714
  measuring adult weight and height, 595
  measuring apical-radial pulse (two-person), 614
  measuring axillary temperature, 609
  measuring blood pressure, 625
  measuring infant head circumference, 740
  measuring oral temperatures
    using electronic or digital thermometer, 607
    using non-mercury glass thermometer, 602–603
  measuring oxygen saturation using pulse oximeter, 617
  measuring pediatric vital signs, 736–737
  measuring radial pulse rate, 612
  measuring rectal temperatures using non-mercury glass
    thermometer, 604
  measuring respirations, 615
  measuring specific gravity with refractometer, 887
  measuring systolic blood pressure using palpatory
    method, 624

measuring temperatures using aural (tympanic membrane) thermometer, 608
measuring weight and height of infants, 739
obtaining sputum specimen for culture, 871
obtaining stool specimen for culture and sensitivity, 873
obtaining stool specimen for examination for pinworms, 875
obtaining stool specimen for ova and parasites, 874
obtaining throat culture, 870
obtaining venous blood with sterile syringe and needle, 906
opening a sterile packet, 772
performing a Gram stain, 868–869
performing a mono test, 925
performing a PKU test, 925
performing a urine culture, 872
performing capillary puncture (manual), 915
performing erythrocyte sedimentation rate test using the Wintrobe method, 924
performing microhematocrit, 918
performing Snellen eye exam on children, 741
performing tuberculin skin test, 1070
performing venipuncture using Vacutainer method, 910–913
preparing a cover letter, 1153
preparing a follow-up letter, 1157
preparing a smear, 866
preparing a wet mount slide, 867
preparing patient's skin for surgical procedures, 786–787
preparing résumé, 1150
preparing slides, 922–923
preparing specimen for microscopic urine specimen examination, 893
quality control for collecting a blood specimen, 904
reconstituting a powdered medication for administration, 1076
recording a twelve-lead electrocardiograph, 965
relating to cardiovascular system, 667t–668t
relating to digestive system, 673t–674t
relating to endocrine system, 671t
relating to female reproductive system, 693t–694t
relating to integumentary system, 665t
relating to lymphatic system, 677t
relating to male reproductive system, 697t
relating to musculoskeletal system, 681t–682t
relating to nervous system, 683t
relating to the ear, 726
relating to the eye, 713t–714t
relating to urinary system, 701t–702t
removing sutures, 792
responding to an obstructed airway (conscious adult, child, or infant), 808
role-playing an interview, 1155
role-playing a situation in which patient is from another culture, 1128
role-playing a situation when patient is scared, angry, and depressed, 1131
sanitizing instruments, 578
screening for color vision acuity, 712
screening for glucose (blood sugar) level, 917
screening for near vision acuity, 711
surgical gloving, 770–771
surgical hand hygiene/sterile scrub, 766–767
taking a wound culture, 666
teaching a patient to correctly use a walker, 1005
testing for sugar in urine using tablets, 890
testing urine with reagent strips, 888
testing visual acuity using Snellen eye chart, 710
transferring sterile objects using transfer forceps, 774
transferring sterile solutions on sterile field, 781
treadmill stress test, 969
using an ampule, 1055
wheelchair transfer to chair or examination table, 1006
withdrawing medication from a single-dose or multiple-dose vial, 1056–1057
wrapping instruments for autoclaving, 581
Proctologic position, 643f, 645
Proctologist, 672
Proctology, 672
Professional corporation, 27
Professional courtesy (PC), 244
Professional fees, 228–229
Professionalism, 8, 9
addressing patients, 499
addressing physicians, 464
addressing topic of money owed, 254
appearance, 442
appearance and grooming of receptionists, 131
avoiding casual language in workplace, 1143
becoming a lifelong learner, 758
becoming a surgical technologist, 768
careers as prosthetist and orthotist, 980
components of, 550
continued updating of skills, 826
continuing education requirements, 34
courtesy and manners, 373
differences in lifestyles and cultures, 1088
dress code requirements, 1012
encountering angry patients, 1123
excessive jewelry, 571
field of radiography, 930
filing system, 213
health insurance procedures, 273f
importance of test results, 847
improving communication with other health care workers, 719
at interviews, 1154–1155
knowledge of entire medical office, 161
listening to unhappy patients, 396
maintaining certification or registration, 973
maintaining demeanor of, 105
maintaining positive attitude, 531
making good first impression, 861
mark of, 381
neurologic patients and, 415
of office manager, 320
OSHA officers, 894
patient information stored on computers or disks, 231
patient records, 291
reflecting services and care in medical record, 311
setting boundaries with patients, 517
setting good example, 72
sharing e-mails and Web sites, 201
taking messages, 357
teamwork, 483
telling the truth, 54
visits from pharmaceutical representatives, 1076
when physician gets behind schedule, 145, 427

Professional liability, 46–49
   defamation of character, 48–49
   determination of, 46
   Good Samaritan Laws, 48
   malpractice, 48
   respondeat superior, 46–47
   standard of care, 47
   statute of limitations, 48
Professional references, 1151
Professional Standards Review Organization (PSRO), 280
Proficiency testing, 841
Progesterone, 527, 541
Prognosis, 590
Progress notes, 209
   in POMR, 651
      sample, 652–653
Prokaryotic cells, 853
Prolactin, 541
Prolactin-releasing factor (PRF), 523, 524
Pronation, 381
Prone position, 642f, 644
Proofreading
   guidelines for, 181
   importance of, 181
   proofreader's marks, 181, 184f
Prostate cancer, 556, 700
Prostate gland, 544
Prosthesis, 1007
Prosthetist, 980
   career as, 980
Protected health information (PHI), 88
Protective clothing, 574
Protein, 1102
Protein specific antigen (PSA) blood test, 700
Protein synthesis, 346
Proteinuria, 888
Protons, 342
Protozoa, 563, 858
Protozoology, 563
Proximate cause, 45
Psoriasis, 371–372, 662
Psychiatrist, 679, 1122
Psychiatry, 20, 29, 1122
Psychological disorders, 1122–1124
   neuroses, 1122
   psychoses, 1122–1123
Psychologist, 1122
Psychology, 82–83
Psychopathic behavior, 1123
Psychopharmacology, 1124
Psychoses, 1122–1123
Psychotherapy, 1124
Puberty, 540, 541, 544
Public Health Service Act, 106
Puerperal sepsis, 19
Puerperium, 685, 692
Pulmonary circulation, 442
Pulmonary edema, 483–484
Pulmonary embolism, 453, 484
Pulmonary function, 970
   calculating pulmonary capacity, 971–972
   diseases related to, 975–976
   treatments pertaining to, 975

Pulmonary function tests (PFTs), 957, 970–975, 973t
   locations for performing, 972–973
   peak flow meter, 974–975
   spirometry, 972–974
   using oximeter, 975
   volume tests, 970–971
Pulmonologist, 970
Pulse, 606
   bounding, 610
   characteristics of, 606, 610
   deficit, 611
   intermittent, 610
   nine sites for measuring, 611f
   oximeter, 616
   pressure, 442
   procedure for measuring apical-radial
      (two-person), 614
   rates, 440
      average, by age, 610t
      defined, 606
      factors influencing, 606, 610t
      measuring radial, 612
   sites, 611–612
      location of common, 611t
   thready, 610
Pulse deficit, 611
Pulse pressure, 617
Pupil, 424
Purchase agreements, 166
Purkinje fibers, 439, 956
Pustule, 663f
Pyelogram, 938–939
Pyelonephritis, 516–517
Pyloric sphincter, 493
Pyloric stenosis, 505
Pyloroplasty, 505
Pyrexia, 597. *See also* Body temperature

Q

Quadriplegia, 418
Qualitative tests, 836
Quality assurance programs (QAPs), 106–107
   implementing, 108, 219
Quality assurance (QA), 106–109, 839–840
   Clinical Laboratory Improvement Amendment
      (CLIA), 109
   definition of, 106
   Health Plan Employer Data and Information Set
      (HEDIS), 108
   incident reports, 219–220
   issues reviewed by QA committee in physician's office, 106
   Joint Commission on the Accreditation of Health Care
      Organizations (JCAHO), 220
   measure to assure, 220–221
   medical assistant's role in, 108
   Occupational Safety and Hazard Administration
      (OSHA), 220
   quality assurance programs (QAPs), 106–107
   Quality Improvement Programs (QIPs), 106
   for quality medical care, 219–221
Quality control, 840–841, 896
   procedure for collecting blood specimen, 904
   specimen collection and, 860

Quality Improvement Programs (QIPs), 106
Quantitative tests, 836
Questions
  to ask before administering tuberculin skin test, 1070
  to ask when gathering past medical history, 804–805
  for patients with abdominal pain, 809
  preparing for tough interview, 1152–1154

R

Rabies, 19
Rad, 947
Radial keratotomy (RK), 426
Radiating pain, 624
Radiation, 945
  cellular effects of, 947–948
  cumulative effects of exposure to, 948
  exposure, 947
  rays, 945–946
  safety precautions, 947–949
    guidelines for maintaining, 950
    patient, 948–949
    personnel, 948
  side effects, healing time, and interventions, 949t
Radiation sickness, 947
Radiation therapy, 467, 483, 547, 663, 945
  techniques, 946
  uses of, 946
Radiculopathy, 419
Radioactive isotopes, 946
Radioactive substances, 945–946
Radioactive waste, 99
Radioallergosorbent test (RAST), 662
Radiographers, 930
Radiographic equipment, 949–950
Radiographs, 930
Radioisotopes, 947
Radiologic procedures
  children and, 933
  guidelines for sequencing multiple, 936
  not requiring contrast media, 940–942, 941t
  patient preparation for, 932–933
  positioning, 933
  requiring contrast media, 936, 938–940
  scheduling guidelines for, 933, 935
Radiologic technologists, 36, 930
Radiologists, 29, 930
Radiology, 678
  defined, 930
  positions, 935t
Radiology report, 212
Radionuclides, 946
Radiotherapy, 663. *See* Radiation therapy
Radium, 20
Rales, 616
Random-access memory (RAM), 195
Range of motion, 985–986
  exercises, 985, 986
    guidelines for performing, 986
    on a patient's wrist, 989f
Rapport, work group, 85
RAST test, 662
Reabsorption, 512
Readings, 617

Read-only memory (ROM), 195
Reagents, 840–841
Reagent strips, 888
Real time, 147
Reasonable person standard, 45
Receipt forms, 240
Reception area, 130
  children in, 137
  components of, 161–162
  medical emergencies in, 137–138
Receptionists
  care and maintenance of office equipment, 131
  duties of, 130–131
  handling of incoming money by, 131
  and lost and found, 130–131
  personal characteristics and physical appearance, 131
  professionalism of, 131
Receptors
  in dermis, 431, 431f
  types of sensory, 408
Recommended dietary allowances (RDAs), 1109
Records. *See* Medical records
Recreation specialist, 980
Rectum, 494
Red blood cell count, 919
Red blood cells, 442, 444, 902, 920
Reed, Walter, 20
Reference initials, in correspondence, 179
Reference laboratories, 836
Referrals, 151, 278–279
  authorization for, 279
Referred pain, 624, 672
Reflecting, 74
Reflex hammer, 635
Reflux esophagitis, 500–501
Refractive errors, 425–426
Refractometer, 886, 887
Registered dietitian (RD), 1111
Registered medical assistant (RMA), 10
Registered medical records administrator, 37
Registered nurse (RN), 35, 87
Registered radiologic technologist (RRT), 930
Registered respiratory therapist (RRT), 35
Rehabilitation
  common health problems requiring, 983
  conditions and diseases benefiting from, 982
  patient assessment prior to prescribing, 983
  process as holistic approach, 982
  therapeutic team, 980–982
Rehabilitative medicine, 29. *See also* Rehabilitation
Relaxation, as stress reliever, 1116
Rem, 947
Removable disk drive, computer, 196
Renal calculi, 515–516
Renal corpuscle, 511
Renal failure, 517–518, 700, 702–703
Renal pelvis, 511
  infection of, 516–517
Renal threshold, 882
Reproductive system, 537–556, 684–696
  effect of aging on, 754
  female, 538–542, 544–554, 684–695
  male, 542–544, 554–556, 695–696

Requisition, laboratory
    completion of, 845
    information for inclusion on, 845, 846f, 861
    sample slip, 846f
Research hospitals, 31
Research, medical, 52
Reservoir host, 563
Residual volume, 971
Res ipsa loquitur, 48
Resource-Based Relative Value Scale (RBRVS), 274, 277
Respiration, 474, 612
    characteristics of, 613
    depth of, 615–616
    physiology of, 612–613
    procedure for measuring, 615
    rate of, 613–614
Respiratory cycle, 612
Respiratory rate, 613–614
    ranges of various age groups, 614t
    situations causing changes in, 615t
Respiratory synctial virus (RSV), 743–744
Respiratory system, 473–485, 474f. *See also* Breathing
    common disorders associated with, 479–485. *See also
        specific disorders*
    effect of aging on, 680, 753
    exchange of gases in, 474
    organs of, 474–477
    primary function of, 474
Respiratory therapist (RT), 35
Respite care, 756
Respondeat superior, 46–47
Restating, 74
Résumés, 1148–1149
    formats for, 1148
    importance of proofreading, 1149
    information to include on, 1149–1151
    items not included on, 1150–1151
    procedure for preparing, 1150
    references and, 1151
    using chronological format, example of, 1149f
Reticular formation, 411
Reticular layer, of dermis, 363
Retina, 424, 711
    disorders affecting, 426–427
Retinal detachment, 426–427
Retraction, 381
Retrograde pyelography, 939
Review of systems (ROS), 593, 635, 645, 650t
    components of, 646–647, 649
    medical history sheet used to record, 647f
Reviews
    orientation or training, 329
    poor performance, 329
    routine performance, 329
    salary, 329
    topics of, for front office personnel, 329
Rheumatoid arthritis, 385, 469
    hand deformities associated with, 387f
Rheumatologists, 29, 678
Rh factor, 447–449
    pregnancy and, 448f
Rhinovirus, 481, 743
RhoGAM, 449

Rhonchi, 616
Rhythm
    breathing, 615
    heart, 961
    normal sinus, 967
Rhythm method, 695
Rib cage, 382, 383f
Ribosomes, 345, 346
Ribs, 382–383
Risk management, 89
RNA (ribonucleic acid), 345
    two types of, 346
Robotics, 22
Roentgenography, 942
Roentgen (R), 947
Roentgen, Wilhelm Konrad, 20, 930
Roget's International Thesaurus, 183
Role-playing
    situation in which patient is from another culture, 1128
    situation when patient is scared, angry, and
        depressed, 1131
Roman numerals, 1012
Rosacea, 372
Roseola, 747
Rotation, 381
Routine blood tests, 909, 914, 916–917, 919, 921
    fasting requirements for, 907
Rule of discovery, 48
Rule of Nines, 373–374, 373f, 814–815, 814f

S

Sabin, Albert, 20–21
Safety issues
    assisting patients to avoid, 640
    chemical hazards, 98
    children and, 759
    in clinical laboratories, 837–838
        guidelines, 840
    disaster plans, 96–97
    elderly and, 758–759
    electrical safety, 97
    employee safety, 98
    examination rooms and, 633
    fire safety, 97
    general safety measures, 96–98
        guidelines for, 96
    guidelines for ear, 721
    hazardous medical waste, 99–100
    housekeeping safety, 101–102
    incident reports, 104–105
    mechanical safety, 98
    medical assistants and, 56
    office security, 102, 104–105
    patient guidelines to protect sight, 715–716
    patient protection during office visits, 138
    pediatric office, 733
    proper body mechanics, 102
    regarding radiation, 947–949
Sagittal plane (median plane), 350
Saliva, 491
Salivary glands, 494
Salk, Jonas, 20–21

Salmonella, 857
Salutation, in correspondence, 179
Sanitization, 575
    of instruments, procedure for, 578
SARS-CoV, 484
Scabies, 372, 372f
Scale, 663f
Scalpels, 773, 775f
Schedule drugs, regulation of sale and use of, 53–54
Schedule I drugs, 54
Schedule V drugs, 54
Scheduling systems, 146–148
    computerized, 146–147
    manual, 147–148
Schizophrenia, 1122–1123
Schwann cells, 407
Sciatica, 418–419
Sclera, 424
Scleroderma, 662
Scoliosis, 383, 385f, 649, 983
Scorpion stings, 811
Scratch test, 661
Scrotum, 542
Scrub assistants, 779, 780
    guidelines: sterile techniques for, 780
Seasonal allergic rhinitis, 482
Sebaceous glands, 363–364
Sebum, 363
Secondary radiation, 948
Secondary sex characteristics, 540, 544
Secretin, 527
Sediment, 884
Sed rate, 921
Seizure disorders, 416
Seizures, 820–821
Selective permeability, 345
Self-awareness, 66
Self-referral, 273
Semen, 544
Semi-Fowler's position, 642f, 644
Seminal fluid, 544
Semi-simplified letter style format, 181
Semmelweiss, Ignaz, 19, 562
Seniority, promotions based on, 320
Sensitive issues, discussing, 76
Sensitivity testing, 865
Sensorineural hearing loss, 430, 719
Sensory ganglia, 413
Sensory receptors, 362, 408
Septum, 436
Sequela, 859
Serial numbering filing system, 216
Serology, 875
Serotonin, 524
Serum, 903
Serum hepatitis, 582–583
Severe acute respiratory syndrome (SARS), 484
Sexual abuse, 745
Sexually transmitted diseases (STDs), 696. *See also* Sexually transmitted infections (STIs)
    educating patients about, 698
    reporting, 698
    types of, 698–699

Sexually transmitted infections (STIs), 550–552, 552f. *See also* Sexually transmitted diseases (STDs)
Sharps, 1048
    containers for, 1055
Sheath, 407
Shelf-life, of autoclaved packages, 582
Shingles, 370
Shock, 830
    treatment for, in medical office, 830t
Shock wave lithotripsy, 516
Shunting, 419
Sick-child visits, 733, 741, 743
Sickle cell anemia, 357, 454
Sievert (Sv), 947
Sigmoidoscopy, 675, 677
    procedure for assisting with, 676
Sign language, 81
Simple fracture, 387
Simplified letter style format, 181, 182f
Sims' position, 642f, 644
Single-entry bookkeeping, 237
Sinoatrial node, 438–439, 956
Sinuses, 475, 484
Sinusitis, 484–485
Sitting position, 643f, 645
Skeletal muscles, 396
    anterior and posterior view, 394f
    attachments to, 397
    major, 397
    structure of, 396–397
Skeletal muscle tissue, 347
Skeletal system, 377–389
    common disorders associated with, 383–389. *See also specific disorders*
    disorders of, 386t
    divisions of, 378. *See also* Appendicular skeleton; Axial skeleton
    human skeleton, 378f
Skilled nursing facility (SNF), 32
Skin. *See also* Dermatology; Integumentary system
    accessory structures of, 363–364
    care, importance of, 366
    disorders, common, 662
    layers of, 362–363
    lesions, 662
    in older adults, 365
    preparation of patient's, for minor surgery, 785–786
    procedure for preparing patient's, for surgical procedures, 786–787
    protection given by, 362
    secretion and, 362
    sensory receptors in, 362, 431f
    signs as objective evidence of illness or disorder, 663f
    as temperature regulator, 362
Skin cancer, 364. *See also* Malignant melanoma
    signs and symptoms of, 364
    three major types of, 364
    treatment for, 364–365
Skin-fold fat measurement, 626
Slander, 49
SLE. *See* Systemic lupus erythematosus
Slides, procedure for preparing, 922–923
Small intestine, 493, 493f

Smallpox, 18
Smears, 862
    direct, 865
    procedure for preparing, 866
Smegma, 543
Smell, sense of, 430–431. *See also* Nose
Smoking
    change in attitude toward, 481
    chronic bronchitis and, 480
    and COPD, 479
    emphysema and, 480
    lung cancer and, 483
Smooth muscles, 395–396
Smooth muscle tissue, 347
Snakebites, venomous, 810–811
Snellen eye chart, 647, 709, 711
    procedure for testing visual acuity using, 710
    using, for children, 741
SOAP charting method, 208, 209f, 651–653, 654t
Social Security Act of 1972, 280
Social Security taxes, 262
Social work, 36–37
Software, 194, 197
    accounting, 243
    for billing, 230–231
    for payroll duties, 261
    programs, 176t
Sole proprietorship, 27
Solid waste, 99
Solo practice, 10, 26–27
Somatic nervous system, 411–412
Somatosensory evoked peripheral nerves (SEP), 1008
Somatotrophic hormone, 523
Sonogram, 945
Sonography, 944–945
Source-oriented medical record (SOMR), 208, 653–654
Special senses, 423–432
    hearing, 428–430
    smell, 430–431
    taste, 430–431
    touch, 431–432
    vision, 424–427
Specialty hospitals, 31
Specific gravity, 885–886
    dipstick method of measuring, 886
    use of refractometer to determine, 886
        procedure for, 887
Specific time slots, 144
Specimens
    blood. *See* Blood
    collection of
        devices for, 862
        guidelines for, 861
        stool, 871–872
        transportation and, 860–862
        urine, 880–884
    handling and preservation of, 846–847
    icteric, 847
    identification of, 846
    other types of, 875
    preparing, for direct examination, 865–866
    problems encountered with, 847
    procedure for obtaining sputum, 871
    proving chain of custody regarding, 847

sending, to outside laboratory, 862
    staining, 866–867
    stool, 873–875
    throat, 867, 870–871
    types of, 867, 870–875
    urine. *See* Urine samples
    wound, 875
Speculum, 635, 708
    nasal, 722
    used in ear canal, 717
    vaginal, 645, 686
Spermatic cord, 544
Spermatozoa, 543, 543f, 894
    in urine, 894
Sphygmomanometer, 441, 620, 621f, 635
    aneroid, 621f, 622
    components of, 621–622
    mercury, 621f, 622
Spider bites, venomous, 811
Spina bifida, 358, 419
Spinal cord, 381–382, 408, 411
    adult, 414
    lesions, results of, 418
Spinal nerves, 414
Spine. *See also* Skeletal system
    abnormal curvatures of, 383–384, 385f
Spiral fracture, 388
Spirilla, 857
Spirochetes, 857
Spirometry tests, 972
    patient preparation for, 972
    procedure for, 972–974
    procedure for performing, to measure forced vital
        capacity, 974
    uses of, 973
Spleen, 449, 450, 450f, 463
Spongy bone, 380
Spores, 857
Sports medicine therapist, 980
Sprains, 400–401
Sputum, 871
    for culture, procedure for obtaining, 871
Squamous cell carcinoma, 365–366, 502
    symptoms, 366
    treatment for, 366
Staff arrangements, 85–87
Staff meetings, 320
    establishing regularly scheduled, 86
    procedures, 321
    sample agenda for, 321
Stains, 853
Standard of care, 47
    for medical assistants, 58
Standard operating procedure (SOP), detailing, 332
Standard Precautions, 566, 839, 1048. *See also* Universal
        Precautions
    equipment and situations, 568t
    summary of, 567
    using, while measuring vital signs, 596
"Standards for Privacy of Individually Identifiable Health
        Information," 220
Standard style letter format, 181
Stapes (stirrup), 428
Staph, 854

Staphylococci, 854, 856
Staphylococcus aureus, 854
Stat, 845
    procedures, 875
Statute of limitations, 48
    regarding collections, 235
Steatorrhea, 871
Stereotactic breast biopsy, 941
Stereotyping, 79–80, 1127
Sterile dressing, 791
    procedure for applying bandage over, 795
    procedure for changing, 793
Sterile field, 769
    contamination of, 765
    procedure for dropping sterile packet onto, 773
    procedure for transferring sterile solutions
        onto, 781
Sterile packet
    procedure for dropping, onto sterile field, 773
    procedure for opening, 772
Sterile scrub, 764
    and gloving, 768
    procedure for, 766–767
Sterile technique, 764
    guidelines for scrub assistants, 780
Sterile transfer, 769
Sterilization, 577–578
    indicators, 580, 583
    methods used for, 578–580
    time requirements, 580t
Stertorous sounds, 616
Stethoscopes, 18, 620, 622, 635, 956
    components of, 623t
Stings, 810–811
Stomach, 493
Stomach ulcers, 505
Stool
    culture, 872
    specimen for culture and sensitivity, procedure for
        obtaining, 873
    specimen for examination for pinworms, procedure for
        obtaining, 875
    specimen for ova and parasites, procedure for
        obtaining, 874
    testing, 871–872
        for occult blood, 872–873
        for ova and parasites, 873–875
Stop-payment order, 254
Strabismus, 426, 708–709
Straight numerical filing system, 215
Strains, 401
Stratum corneum, 362
Stratum germinativum, 363
Stratum granulosum, 362
Stratum lucidum, 362
Streak culture, 864
Strep throat, 743, 864
    test for, 876
Streptococci, 856
Stress, 1130–1131
    coping with, 1132, 1134–1135
    developing patient teaching handout about, 1135
    guidelines for managing, 68
    helping patients cope with, 1131

link between illness and, 67–68, 1126
    symptoms of, 1132
Stress incontinence, 515
Stress management, 1116
Stressors, 1131
Stress test, 967–969
    procedure for treadmill, 969
Striated muscles, 396
Stridor, 616, 743
Stroke, 419, 455, 679, 816–817
    in progress, symptoms of, 684
    risk factors for, 680
Student health insurance, 276
Sty, 427
Subcutaneous injections, 1053f
    needle position during, 1062f
    procedure for administering parenteral, 1063–1065
    sites for, 1061–1062, 1066
Subjective, objective, assessment, and plan (SOAP)
    charting. *See* SOAP charting method
Subjective symptoms, 592
Subpoena, 52
Subpoena duces tecum, 52
Subscribers, 270, 272
Sudden Infant Death Syndrome (SIDS), 745
Sudoriferous glands, 364f
Suicide, 746
Sulcus, 409
Sundowner syndrome, 755
Superbill, 229, 230f, 294
    codes on, 300
    example of, 301f
    helping patients understand diagnosis on, 300
    uses of, 300
Supination, 381
Supine position, 642f, 643–644
Supplies, 166
    for capillary puncture, 909
    drug samples, 167
    expendable office, 167t
    found in examination rooms, 635
    inventory of, 166–167
    order system, 167
    used for health examination, 636f
    used for physical examinations, 634–635
Suppositories, procedure for administering, 1050
Suppuration, 987
Surface electromyogram (SEMG), 1007
Surfactant, 477
Surgeons, 30
Surgery. *See also* Minor surgery
    ambulatory, 764
    antiseptic system in, 19
    aseptic technique in, 562
    cardiovascular, 31t
    categories of, 764
    changes in practice of, 19
    colorectal, 31t
    cosmetic, 31t
    definition of, 30
    hand, 31t
    neurosurgery, 31t
    oral, 31t
    orthopedic, 31t

Surgery (*continued*)
  outpatient, 764
  scheduling, 151
    information needed for, 152
  specialties in, 30
  thoracic, 31t
  use of robotics in, 22
Surgical asepsis, 574–580, 582, 764–765, 768–769
  guidelines for, 765
  versus medical asepsis, 765
  principles of, 764–769
Surgical assisting, 779–781, 783
Surgical insurance, 276
Surgical scrub, 768
  procedure for, 766–767
Surgical specialties, 30
  and their descriptions, 31t
Surgical technician, 768
Surgical technologist, 768
Susceptible host, 563
Suture materials, 775–778
  and needles, 778
  size of, 777–778
  types of, 776–777, 779f
    use, size and, 778t
Suture needles, 778f
Sutures, 776, 789, 791
  procedure for assisting with repair using, 790
  procedure for removing, 792
Sweat, 362
Sweat glands, 364f
Swimmer's ear, 429
Symbols, in CPT manual, 308
Sympathetic nervous system, 414–415, 526
  summary of effects of, 414t
Sympathy, 71
Symptoms, 592
Synapses, 408
Synaptic cleft, 408
Synarthrotic joints, 380
Syncope, 616, 822–823
Synergist, 397
Syphilis, 20
Syringes, 1053–1056
  types of, 1054f
Systemic circulation, 442, 444f
Systemic lupus erythematosus, 469
Systems, 347
  organ, with major functions, 349f
Systolic blood pressure, 442, 526
  estimated, 623
  procedure for measuring, using palpatory
    method, 624

T

Tachycardia, 452, 606, 669
  caused by allergic reactions, 661
Tachypnea, 613
Talipes (clubfoot), 358
Tape measures, 635
Taste buds, 431, 431f
  types of, 491
Taste, sense of, 430–431

Tax table, 264f
Tax withholding, 260–261
Tay-Sachs disease (TSD), 358
T cells, 462, 464, 583
Teaching hospitals, 31
Teaching methods
  developing teaching plan, 1089
  guidelines for effective health instruction, 1084
  handling noncompliance, 1091
  for older adults, 1087–1088
  patient, 1085t–1087t
  and patients with disabilities, 1089
  and strategy, 1083–1084, 1087
Team. *See also* Employees
  accountability, 324
  atmosphere, creating, 323–324
  personality and skills, 323–324
  purpose and goals, 324
  roles, 324
  size, 323
Technology
  advancements in, 194
  Internet, 201
  patient education regarding computer, 198
Teeth, 491–493
  deciduous and permanent, 492f
  main portions of, 492–493
Telangiectasias, 365
Telephone triage, 121–122, 732
Telnet, 201
Temperatures, common laboratory, 844t
Temporal lobe, 409, 410
Tendinitis. *See* Tendonitis
Tendonitis, 401
Tendons, 401
Tension headaches, 417
TENS unit, 1007–1008
Terminal digit filing system, 215
  procedure for filing record numerically
    using, 217
Terminal illness, assisting patient with, 1135–1136
  religious, cultural, and personal experiences, 82
  stages of grief, 82
Testes, 527, 542, 543–544
  structure and function of, 527f
Testicular examination, 696
Testimony, court, 52
  pointers for, 52
Testosterone, 526, 540, 544
  declining levels of, 540
Tests
  comprehending importance of results of, 847
  confidentiality regarding patient, 863
  pregnancy, 894
  proficiency, 841
  pulmonary function, 957, 970–975
  qualitative, 836
  quantitative, 836
  results of, 211
  serology, 875
  strep, 876
Tetanus, 401–402, 1073, 1075
Thalamus, 410–411
Thalassemia, 747

Thermometers
  disposable, 606
  electronic or digital, 601, 605–606
  non-mercury glass, 600
  tympanic, 606
  types of, 600
Thesaurus, 183
Third-party
  checks, 252
  payers, billing, 231
Thoracic cavity, 351
Thready pulse, 610
Throat
  culture, 867, 870–871
    procedure for obtaining, 870
  examination of, 722
Thrombocytes, 444
Thrombophlebitis, 453–454
  example of, 453f
Thrombus, 679
Thymosin, 450
Thymus gland, 449, 450, 450f, 462, 528f
  hormones of, 527
Thyroid gland, 524
Thyroid-stimulating hormone, 523
Thyrotoxicosis, 524
Thyrotropin-releasing hormone (TRH), 522
Thyroxine, 524
Tickler files, 151, 219, 255
Tidal volume, 810, 970
Time, consideration for patient's, 136
Time management, 330–331, 1116–1117
  to do list, 1117t
Time patterns, 152–153
Time zones, 123
  map of, 124f
Tinnitus, 430
Tissue, 347
  cardiac muscle, 347
  in nervous system, 407
  radiolucent and radiopaque, 930
  types of, in human body, 348f
  types of muscle, 347, 395–396, 395f
T lymphocytes, 464
Tomography, 942
Tongue, 431f
  pain sensitivity in, 432
  taste buds on, 491
Tongue depressors, 635, 722
Tonsils, 449, 450f, 463–464, 475
  normal and enlarged, 464f
Topical medications, 1049
Tort law, 44–45
Torts
  definition of, 45
  intentional, 44t, 45
  unintentional, 45
Total lung capacity, 971
Touch, sense of, 421–432
Tourniquets, 829
Toxoplasmosis, 584
TPR (temperature, pulse, and respiration), 595
Trachea, 476, 493
Traction, 1007

Tracts, 408
Transcribers, 164
  procedure for operating, 165
Transcutaneous electric nerve stimulation (TENS), 1007–1008
Transducer, 945
Trans fats, 1103–1104
Transient ischemic attack (TIA), 680–681, 817
Transmission-based Precautions, 566, 568
Transplants, organ, 22
Transverse fissure, 409
Transverse fracture, 388
Traveler's checks, 251
Treatment, payment, and operations (TPO), 88
Trendelenburg position, 643f, 644–645
Triage, 152, 802
Tricare, 270, 275, 286
Trichomoniasis, 699
Tricuspid valve, 437
Triiodothyronine, 524
True ribs, 383
Trust, establishing, 84–85
Truth in Lending Act (1969), 47t
  Regulation Z, 232
Tuberculin skin test, 1067, 1070–1071
  procedure for performing, 1070
  questions to ask before administering, 1070
  results of, 1071
Tuberculosis (TB), 19, 20, 485, 584, 1067
Tubular secretion, 512
Tumors, 364, 662–663
  benign, 662, 663
  malignant, 662–663
  use of x-rays in diagnosis and treatment of, 930
Tuning forks, 635, 717, 720
Turgor, 646
Turner's syndrome, 358
Tympanic membrane, 428
Tympanic membrane thermometers, 606
  procedure for measuring temperature using, 608
Tympanometry, 720
Tympanum, 708
Type 1 diabetes, 531, 534
Type 2 diabetes, 531
Type AB blood, 447
Type A behavior, 1126
Type A blood, 446
Type B behavior, 1126
Type B blood, 447
Type O blood, 447
Typhoid fever, 857

U

Ulcer, 663f
Ulcerative colitis, 499
Ultrasound, 692, 944–945
  fetal, 945
  scanning, 945
  treatments using, 995–996
Ultrasound technologist, 36
Ultraviolet radiation, 993–994
Unethical behavior, accusations of, 57
Uniform Anatomical Gift Act, 44, 52

Unintentional torts, 45
Unit clerk, 38
United States Medical Licensing Examination (USMLE), 25
United States Pharmacopeia–National Formulary (USP–NF), 1024
Unit numbering filing system, 216
Universal donors, 447
Universal Precautions, 100, 101, 220, 565–566, 568–571, 574–580, 582, 838, 839. *See also* Standard Precautions
  guidelines, overseeing of, 837
Unmyelinated cells, 407–408
Upper GI series, 938
  guidelines for, 939
Upper respiratory system, 474
Ureters, 512
Urethra, 512
  male, 544
Urethritis, 555
Urge incontinence, 513, 515
Urgent surgery, 764
Urinalysis
  chemical characteristics, 886–890
  defined, 880
  importance of asepsis in, 880
  physical characteristics, 884–886
  reagent tablet testing, 890–891
  routine, 884–894
  testing, normal values for, 891
Urinary bladder, 512
Urinary meatus, 512
Urinary system, 509–518, 510f, 699–703
  common disorders associated with, 513–518.
    See also specific disorders
  disorders and diseases of, 514t
  effect of aging on, 680, 753
  functions of, 510–511, 699
  organs of, 511–512
  procedures and diagnostic tests relating to, 701t–702t
Urinary tract infections, 513–514
  proper hygiene and prevention of, 515
Urine, 512–513, 871. *See also* Urine samples
  automated chemical analyzers for, 891
  cells that may be found in, 892–894
  collection device, procedure for applying pediatric, 742
  culture, procedure for performing, 872
  formation of, 512, 513f
  pregnancy testing, 894
  procedure for evaluating physical characteristics of, 885
  procedure for testing for sugar in, using tablets, 890
  procedure for testing, with reagent strips, 888
  samples, 699–700
  sediment chart, 895f
Urine samples, 871
  catheterization specimen, 883
  clean-catch midstream specimen, 883–884
    procedure for collecting, 883
  collection of, 880–884
  cultural considerations regarding, 836
  microscopic examination, 892–894
  morning specimen (first void), 881
  pediatric specimen, 884
  routine, 880
    guidelines for collecting, 881

twenty-four hour specimen, 881
  guidelines for collecting, 882
two-hour postprandial specimen, 882
vital information provided by, 889–890
Urine specimen. *See* Urine samples
Urobilinogen, 889
Urticaria, 660
Usenet (Network News Transfer Protocol), 201
Usual, customary, and reasonable, 228, 276–277
Uterine cancer, 552–553
Uterine fibroids, 553
Uterine tubes, 538–539
Uterus, 538
Uvula, 491

V

Vaccinations, 18, 464, 565, 746
Vaccines, 18, 20–21, 465, 746, 1072–1073
  diphtheria, 1073
  DTaP, 1075
  Hepatitis A, 1075
  Hib, 1075
  measles, mumps, and rubella, 1075
  pertussis, 1073
  pneumococcal, 1075
  polio, 1076
  production of, 1073
  required by law, 53t
  tetanus, 1073, 1075
  varicella, 1075
Vagina, 541
Vaginitis, 553–554
Vagotomy, 505
Values, 66
Varicella, 1075
Varicose veins, 454
Vas deferens, 544
Vasectomy, 797
Vasoconstrictors, 524
Vasopressin, 524
Vastus lateralis muscle, 1058
Veins, 440
  circulation in, 443f
  in older individuals, 903
Vendors, 166
Venereal diseases, 20, 550–552
Venipuncture
  anatomy of arm for, 907f
  equipment, 905–907, 905f
  legal issues regarding, 904
  methods, 905
  patient preparation for, 907–908
  procedure for performing, using Vacutainer method, 910–913
  sites, 907
  unexpected events occurring when performing, 908
Venipuncture technicians, 37
Venom, 660
Ventilation, 478
Ventral cavity, 351
Ventricles, 436
  of brain, 409–410

Ventrogluteal muscle
  injecting, 1060f
  as injection site, 1061
Verbal communication, 70–71, 1128
  conveying positive attitude with, 71
  word selection and, 71
Vertebrae, 381–382
Vertebral cavity, 353
Vertebral column, 381–382
Vesicle, 663f
Vestibule, 541
Vials, 1055
  procedure for withdrawing medication from single-dose
    or multiple-dose, 1056–1057
Vibrios, 857
Videotapes, health care, 162
Virology, 563
Viruses, 563, 858
Vision insurance, 276
Vistech Consultant system, 713
Visual acuity, 708
  assessment of, 709
  measuring distance acuity, 709, 711
  near vision acuity, 711
  procedure for screening for color vision acuity, 712
  procedure for testing, using Snellen eye chart, 710
  and refractive errors, 708–709
Visual learners, 68
Visually impaired patients, 82
Vital capacity, 971
Vital signs, 595–596
  in children, 734, 738
  components of, 595. See also specific vital signs
  in infants, 598
  legal consequences of incorrect documentation of, 617
  procedure for measuring pediatric, 736–737
  taking, during emergencies, 805
  using Standard Precautions while measuring, 596
Vitamin deficiency anemias, 454
Vitamins, 754, 1105, 1106t–1108t
Vitreous humor, 424
Voice, active and passive, 174
Voice box. See Larynx
Voice over Internet Protocol (VoIP), 201
Voice recognition technology (VRT), 164–165
Void, 880
  first, morning specimen, 881
Voluntary muscles, 396
Voucher checks, 251
Vulva, 541

W

W-2 form, 265
  example of, 265f
W-4 form, 261
  example of, 263f
Walkers, 1002
  procedure for teaching patient to correctly use, 1005
Warranties, 165
Warrants, 249
Warts, 373
  changes in, 364
Waste, disposal of infectious, 570. See also Hazardous
  medical waste

Water, 1105
  in body, function of, 1105
  therapy, 1116
Wave scheduling, 145
Web MD, 1024
Weed, Lawrence, 651
Weight, 594
  conversion chart for pounds and kilograms, 594t
  indications provided by, 593–594
  measuring infants', 738
    procedure for, 739
  procedure for measuring, 595
Weights and measures, 1012
  apothecary system, 1012
  common abbreviations for, 1013t
  common household measure, 1014t
  liquid measurements, 1015t
  metric system, 1012–1013
Well-child visits, 733
Wellness, compliance and, 90
Western blot test, 584
West's nomogram, 1019
  chart, 1019f
Wet mount, 863
  preparation, 865–866
  slide, procedure for preparing, 867
Wheals, 663f
  formed as reaction to scratch testing of
    allergens, 662f
Wheelchairs, 1002
  transfer technique for, 1002–1003
    from bed or examining table to, 1004
    to chair or examination table from, 1006
Wheezes, 616
White blood cell count, 919
  differential, 919, 921
White blood cells, 442, 444, 464, 902
  types of, 921
"White coat" syndrome, 81, 619t
White matter, 408, 410, 411
Whooping cough, 1073
Windpipe, 476
Word processing, 164
  error correction in, 177–178
Word selection, 71
Workers' compensation, 275–276
  claim forms, 289
World Health Organization (WHO), 300, 302, 484
World Wide Web, 201, 281
Worms, 859
Wounds, 827
  bandaging of, 791
  classification of, 828f
  cleansing, 788–789
  complications, 788
  concepts relating to dressing, 827–829
  explaining care for, 784
  healing process, 788
  materials for closure of, 779
  specimens from, 875
  types of, 788
Write-it-once system, 250–252
Writing. See also Written communication
  tips for clear, 1084

Written communication, 1128–1129
 letter writing, 172–181
 using fax machine for, 188–189

X

X-ray film
 ownership of, 951
 processing, 950–951
 storage of records and, 951
X-rays, 678, 678f, 930
 characteristics of, 930–931
 helping children maintain correct position during
  taking of, 933
 positions and images produced, examples of, 934f
 principles of, 930

procedure for general, 935
 procedures requiring special preparations, 932t
X-ray technologist, 36
X-ray treatment. *See* Radiation therapy

Y

Yeast, 859
 in urine, 894
Yellow fever, 20
Young's rule, 1019

Z

ZIP codes, 185
Z-track injection method, 1067f